LEVER'S HISTOPATHOLOGY OF THE SKIN

LEVER'S HISTOPATHOLOGY OF THE SKIN

NINTH EDITION

Editor-in-Chief

DAVID E. ELDER, MB, CHB, FRCPA

Professor of Pathology and Laboratory Medicine,
Vice-Chair for Anatomic Pathology
Hospital of the University of Pennsylvania
Philadelphia, Pennsylvania

Associate Editors

ROSALIE ELENITSAS, MD

Associate Professor of Dermatology,
Director of Dermatopathology
Hospital of the University of Pennsylvania
Philadelphia, Pennsylvania

BERNETT L. JOHNSON, Jr., MD

Professor of Dermatology,
Professor of Pathology and Laboratory Medicine,
Senior Medical Director
Hospital of the University of Pennsylvania
Philadelphia, Pennsylvania

GEORGE F. MURPHY, MD

Professor of Pathology
Harvard Medical School;
Director of Dermatopathology
Brigham and Women's Hospital
Boston, Massachusetts

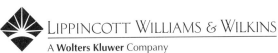

LIPPINCOTT WILLIAMS & WILKINS
A **Wolters Kluwer** Company
Philadelphia · Baltimore · New York · London
Buenos Aires · Hong Kong · Sydney · Tokyo

Acquisitions Editor: Jim Merritt
Developmental Editor: Michelle LaPlante
Project Manager: Nicole Walz
Production Editor: Print Matters, Inc.
Senior Manufacturing Manager: Benjamin Rivera
Compositor: Compset, Inc.
Printer: Quebecor World-Kingsport

© 2005 by LIPPINCOTT WILLIAMS & WILKINS
530 Walnut Street
Philadelphia, PA 19106 USA
LWW.com

Printed in the USA

Library of Congress Cataloging-in-Publication Data

Lever's histopathology of the skin.—9th ed. / editor-in-chief, David E. Elder ;
   associate editors, Rosalie Elenitsas, Bernett L. Johnson Jr., George F. Murphy.
      p. ; cm.
   Includes bibliographical references and index.
   ISBN 0-7817-3742-7 (alk. paper)
   1. Skin—Histopathology. I. Title: Histopathology of the skin. II. Lever,
Walter F. (Walter Frederick), 1909–1992. III. Elder, David E.
   [DNLM: 1. Skin Diseases—pathology. WR 105 L661 2004]
  RL95.L48 2004
  616.5'07—dc22

                         2004048810

10 9 8 7 6 5 4 3 2 1

This book is dedicated to our families: Peggy, Kate, and Ken; John, Mary Rose and Nicole; Mary-Martha, Susanne, Logan, Keith, and Brian; and Sharon, Erin and Emily, whose support and love enabled this work to be accomplished.

CONTRIBUTORS

Zsolt Argenyi, MD Professor of Pathology and Dermatology, Department of Pathology and Division of Dermatology, University of Washington, Director of Dermatopathology, University of Washington Medical Center, Seattle, WA

Sarah K. Barksdale, MD Quest Diagnostics, Teterboro, NJ

Raymond L. Barnhill, MD, MSc Professor of Pathology, University of Miami Medical Center Global Pathology Laboratory, Miami FL

Walter H.C. Burgdorf, MD Clinical Lecturer, Department of Dermatology, Ludwig Maximilian University, Munich, Germany

Klaus J. Busam, MD Department of Pathology, Sloan-Kettering Cancer Center, New York, NY

Eduardo Calonje, MD Head, Dermatopathology, Honorary Senior Lecturer, Dermatology, St. John's Institute of Dermatology, London, United Kingdom

Edward Chan, MD Clinical Assistant Professor, Department of Dermatology, University of Pennsylvania, Philadelphia, PA

Félix Contreras, MD Professor, Department of Pathology, Universidad Autonoma, Chairman, Pathology, La Paz Hospital, Madrid, Spain

A. Neil Crowson, MD Clinical Associate Professor, Departments of Dermatology and Pathology, University of Oklahoma and Regional Medical Laboratory, St. John Medical Center, Tulsa, OK

David E. Elder, MB, ChB, FRCPA Professor of Pathology and Laboratory Medicine, Vice-Chair, Department of Anatomic Pathology, University of Pennsylvania, Philadelphia, PA

Rosalie Elenitsas, MD Associate Professor, Department of Dermatology, Director, Dermatopathology, University of Pennsylvania, Philadelphia, PA

Lori A. Erickson, MD Assistant Professor, Department of Pathology, Mayo Clinic, Rochester, MN

Robert J. Friedman, MD Clinical Assistant Professor, Department of Dermatology, New York University Medical Center, New York, NY

Earl J. Glusac, MD Associate Professor, Departments of Pathology and Dermatology, Yale University School of Medicine, New Haven, CT

Thomas D. Griffin, MD Associate Clinical Professor, Department of Dermatalogy, Drexel University College of Medicine, Philadelphia, PA

Eckart Haneke, MD Professor, Institute of Dermatology, Inst. Derm. Klinikk, Sandvika, Norway

Terence J. Harrist, MD Medical Director of Pathology Services, Pathology Services, Inc, Cambridge, MA

John L.M. Hawk, MD Professor of Dermatology, Skin Sciences, St. John's Institute of Dermatology, Guys, Kings & St. Thomas School of Medicine, London, United Kingdom

Peter J. Heenan, MBBS, FRCPath, FRCPA Clinical Associate Professor, Department of Pathology, The University of Western Australia, Queen Elizabeth II Medical Centre, Nedlands, Western Australia

Kim M. Hiatt, MD Assistant Professor, Department of Pathology, University of Arkansas for Medical Sciences, Little Rock, AR

Molly Hinshaw, MD Assistant Professor of Dermatology, Department of Dermatology, University of Wisconsin – Madison, Madison, WI

Paul Honig, MD Professor of Pediatrics and Dermatology, University of Pennsylvania, Director, Pediatric Dermatology, The Children's Hospital of Philadelphia, Philadelphia, PA

Thomas D. Horn, MD, MBA Professor of Dermatology, University of Arkansas for Medical Sciences, Chief of Dermatology, Central Arkansas Veterans Healthcare System, Little Rock, AR

Michael D. Ioffreda, MD Assistant Professor, Department of Dermatology, Penn State Milton S. Hershey Medical Center, Hershey, PA

Christine Jaworsky, MD Associate Professor, Department of Dermatology, Case Western Reserve University, Staff Physician, MetroHealth Medical Center, Cleveland, OH

Bernett L. Johnson, Jr., MD   Professor, Departments of Dermatology and Pathology and Laboratory Medicine, Senior Medical Director, University of Pennsylvania, Philadelphia, PA

Waine C. Johnson, MD   Clinical Professor, Department of Dermatology, Drexel University College of Medicine, Philadelphia, PA

Edward R. Heilman, MD   Associate Professor of Dermatopathology, SUNY Downstate, New York, NY, Dermpath Diagnostics New York, Port Chester, NY

Jacqueline M. Junkins-Hopkins, MD   Assistant Professor, Director of CEQI, Department of Dermatology, University of Pennsylvania, Philadelphia, PA

Hideko Kamino, MD   Director, Dermatopathology Section, New York University Medical Center, New York, NY

Gary R. Kantor, MD   Clinical Professor, Department of Dermatology and Department of Pathology and Laboratory Medicine, Drexel University College of Medicine, Philadelphia, PA

Nigel Kirkham, MD   Director, Department of Pathology, Royal Sussex County Hospital, Brighton, United Kingdom

Walter Klein, MD   Department of Pathology, Johns Hopkins University, Baltimore, MD

B. Jack Longley, MD   Professor and Vice Chairman, Department of Dermatology, University of Wisconsin Medical School, Attending Physician, Department of Dermatology, University of Wisconsin Health, Madison, WI

Sebastian Lucas, FRCPath   Professor of Clinical Histopathology, Department of Histopathology, Guy's, King's and St. Thomas' School of Medicine at St. Thomas' Hospital, Consultant Histopathologist, Department of Histopathology, St. Thomas' Hospital, London, United Kingdom

Cynthia Magro, MD   Professor of Pathology, Division of Dermatopathology, Department of Pathology, Ohio State University, Columbus, OH

John Maize, MD   Clinical Professor, Department of Dermatology, Medical University of South Carolina, Charleston, SC, Medical Director, Dermpath Diagnostics, Maize Center for Dermatopathology, Mt. Pleasant, SC

John Maize, Jr., MD   Clinical Instructor, Department of Dermatology, Medical University of South Carolina, Charleston, SC, Dermatopathologist, Dermpath Diagnostics, Maize Center for Dermatopathology, Mt. Pleasant, SC

N. Scott McNutt, MD   Professor of Pathology, Department of Pathology, Weill Medical College of Cornell University, Director, Dermatopathology, New York Presbyterian Hospital, Cornell Campus, New York, NY

John Metcalf, MD   Director of Dermatopathology, Professor, Departments of Pathology and Dermatology Medical University of South Carolina, Charleston, SC

Martin Mihm, Jr., MD   Clinical Professor, Departments of Dermatology and Pathology, Harvard Medical School, Boston, MA

Michael E. Ming, MD, MSCE   Assistant Professor, Director, Pigmented Lesion Clinic, Department of Dermatology, University of Pennsylvania, Philadelphia, PA

Narciss Mobini, MD   Assistant Professor, Dermatopathology Section, New York University Medical Center, New York, NY

Abelardo Moreno, MD   Pathologist, Department of Pathology Hospital University de Bellott, Barcelona, Spain

George F. Murphy, MD   Professor of Pathology, Harvard Medical School; Director of Dermatopathology, Brigham and Women's Hospital, Boston, MA

Narayan S. Naik, MD   Department of Dermatology, New York University Medical Center, New York, NY

Carlos H. Nousari, MD   Former Chairman, Department of Dermatology, Cleveland Clinic Florida, Weston, FL

Bruce D. Ragsdale, MD   Adjunct Professor, Arizona State University, Tempe, AZ, Director, Western Dermatopathology Services, San Luis Obispo, CA

Richard J. Reed, MD   Emeritus Clinical Professor, Department of Pathology, Tulane School of Medicine, New Orleans, LA

Brian Schapiro, MB, ChB   Dermatopathologist, Skin Pathology Services, Department of Pathology, St. Joseph Mercy Hospital, Ann Arbor, MI

Roland Schwarting, MD   Professor, Department of Pathology, Anatomy, and Cell Biology, Jefferson Medical College, Thomas Jefferson University, Philadelphia, PA

Klaus Sellheyer, MD   The Cleveland Clinic Foundation Section of Dermatopathology, Cleveland, OH

John T. Seykora, MD, PhD   Assistant Professor, Department of Dermatology, University of Pennsylvania, Philadelphia, PA

Philip E. Shapiro, MD   Associate Clinical Professor of Dermatology, Yale University School of Medicine,

New Haven, CT, Director, Dermatopathology Laboratory of New England, Meridan, CT

Richard L. Spielvogel, MD   Clinical Professor, Department of Dermatology and Department of Pathology and Laboratory Medicine, Drexel University College of Medicine, Philadelphia, PA

Sonia Toussaint, MD   Assistant Director, Department of Dermatology, Hospital Dr. Manuel Gea Gonzalez, Mexico City, Mexico

Edward Wilson-Jones, FRCP, FRCPath   Emeritus Professor of Dermatology, St. John's Institute of Dermatology, St. Thomas' Hospital, London, United Kingdom

Hong Wu, MD, PhD   Howard Hughes Medical Institute, Chevy Chase, MD

Xiaowei Xu, MD, PhD   Assistant Professor, Department of Pathology and Laboratory Medicine, University of Pennsylvania, Philadelphia, PA

Albert C. Yan, MD   Assistant Professor, Department of Pediatrics and Dermatology, University of Pennsylvania, School of Medicine, Director, Children's Hospital of Philadelphia, Philadelphia, PA

Bernhard Zelger, MD   Associate Professor, Clinical Department of Dermatology and Venerology, Innsbruck Medical University, Innsbruck, Austria

PREFACE TO THE NINTH EDITION

This work represents, in many ways, an incremental revision and update of the previous edition, which itself was a somewhat more extensive revision of the series of editions produced over more than 40 years by Walter Lever, M.D. In this second generation of the revised editions, the principles that made "Lever" such a success for so long continue to be applied. These include, first and foremost, a continued organization of the book along the lines of a traditional clinicopathologic classification of cutaneous disease. This enables us to discuss lesions according to their clinical and etiological relationships, paralleling the organization of the major clinical texts. In some other dermatopathology works, a greater emphasis has been placed on histological patterns of disease as the underpinning of the chapter organization. This has advantages in enabling beginners to develop an appropriate differential diagnosis for a given pattern of disease, but can be confusing in that etiologically and clinically disparate conditions tend to be discussed in juxtaposition to each other, and also in that polymorphous conditions need to be discussed in multiple different places.

We have taken into account the modern emphasis on pattern recognition in several ways. First, within each chapter, the conditions considered are, when appropriate, organized and discussed along pattern lines. Second, we have, as in the past, included a chapter that presents an algorithmic classification of skin diseases according to histologic pattern features. It is intended that this chapter may serve as a means of developing a differential diagnosis from an unknown slide, following which references are provided to discussion of the disorders in other areas of the book. In addition, we have prepared a companion volume "Synopsis and Atlas of Lever's Histopathology of the Skin", which greatly extends the number of illustrations including a larger number of clinical images, and is organized completely on the basis of histologic patterns. Unlike some other pattern based works, this chapter includes neoplastic disorders among the inflammatory conditions. This, it becomes clear to the reader that a lichenoid actinic keratosis or in situ melanoma may share features with (and potentially be misdiagnosed as) a plaque of lichen planus or a patch of lupus. This Atlas, which was produced as a companion to the last edition of the "Big Lever", will be updated and extended to incorporate the new information in this present edition of "Lever".

The histological descriptions continue to be liberally illustrated with photomicrographs. In keeping with current practice and taking advantage of modern technology, the figures in this edition are mostly presented in color. Most of the figures in the previous edition have been replaced with new color photomicrographs or clinical images. The number of figures has also been substantially increased compared to previous editions, for a total of more than 1000 figures in this edition.

In another area of emphasis, we have continued the practice of providing clinical review prior to exposition of the histologic features for each group of disorders. This in our opinion greatly enhances the value of the work, not only for pathologists and others whose primary training is not in clinical dermatology, but also for dermatologists in training, and, no doubt, for some who are more advanced in the field as well.

At the other end of the spectrum of clinical science, we have continued and updated the classic work's emphasis on "histogenesis" by emphasizing underlying mechanisms of disease. The term "histogenesis", to us, includes mechanisms of development of histological patterns of disease and might equally well be (and sometime is) labeled "pathogenesis". In this edition, more than in any other because of the explosion of knowledge, molecular mechanisms of pathogenesis are presented for perhaps almost a majority of the diseases. However, it is interesting that, in most cases, these molecular mechanisms, while of explanatory interest, have not yet supplanted traditional histopathology and immunohistology as the "gold standard" for diagnosis of most of the conditions discussed in the book.

As in the past, the book does not attempt to be a compendium of all known skin diseases. However, we have tried to make it a reference work for those skin diseases in which histopathology plays an important role in diagnosis. We are grateful for this opportunity and are excited to present another edition of this revered work to a new generation of readers. At the same time, we hope that members of earlier generations, who have used "Lever" as their primary skin pathology training and reference source, will continue to find this new edition useful in their continuing development and in their daily practices.

David E. Elder
2004

PREFACE TO THE FIRST EDITION

This book is based on the courses of dermatopathology that I have been giving in recent years to graduate students of dermatology enrolled at Harvard Medical School and Massachusetts General Hospital. The book is written primarily for dermatologists; I hope, however, that it may be useful also to pathologists, since dermatopathology is given little consideration in most textbooks of pathology.

I have attempted to keep this book short. Emphasis has been placed on the essential histologic features. Minor details and rare aberrations from the typical histologic picture have been omitted. I have allotted more space to the cutaneous diseases in which histologic examination is of diagnostic value than to those in which the histologic picture is not characteristic. In spite of my striving for brevity I have discussed the histogenesis of several dermatoses, because knowledge of the histogenesis often is of great value for the understanding of the pathologic process.

Primarily for the benefit of pathologists who usually are not too familiar with dermatologic diseases, I have preceded the histologic discussion of each disease with a short description of the clinical features.

A fairly extensive bibliography has been supplied for readers who are interested in obtaining additional information. In the selection of articles for the bibliography preference has been given, whenever possible, to those written in English.

I wish to express my deep gratitude to Dr. Tracy B. Mallory and Dr. Benjamin Castleman of the Pathology Laboratory at the Massachusetts General Hospital for the training in pathology they have given me. It has been invaluable to me. Their teaching is reflected in this book. Furthermore, I wish to thank Mr. Richard W. St. Clair, who with great skill and patience produced all the photomicrographs in this book.

Walter F. Lever

CONTENTS

LEVER'S HISTOPATHOLOGY OF THE SKIN

INTRODUCTION TO DERMATOPATHOLOGIC DIAGNOSIS

DAVID E. ELDER
GEORGE F. MURPHY
ROSALIE ELENITSAS
BERNETT L. JOHNSON JR.

Readers of this book in its eight previous editions have relied on it to aid them in making accurate histologic diagnoses of cutaneous disease. A diagnosis is a clinical tool that assists in the process of codifying patients into disease groups that tend to share a common outcome, and a common set of responses to therapy. The histologic diagnosis in turn is used by clinicians to aid in the management of patients. The most accurate diagnosis is the one that most closely correlates with clinical outcome and helps direct the most appropriate clinical intervention. Thus, there is a close relationship between diagnosis and prognostication. By emphasizing certain key observations that have value in identifying particular diseases, this book aids observers to make appropriate histologic diagnoses, and to provide an estimate of prognosis, in most skin biopsies. Where applicable, ultrastructural, immunohistochemical, and molecular aids to diagnosis are discussed. These advances have resulted in increased specificity for many diagnoses. For example, immunofluorescence has long been used to differentiate among vesiculobullous disorders (Chapter 9). In another example, an amelanotic dermal tumor composed of large mitotically active cells that are positive in an immunohistochemical reaction for the HMB-45 or Melan-A antigens is almost certainly a malignant melanoma. In the absence of the immunologic criteria, these specific diagnoses could not have been made as reliably (Chapter 28). In the next several years, it can be expected that molecular criteria will increasingly be utilized for diagnosis and prognosis. For example, a fusion transcript for EWS-ATF1 detected by reverse transcriptase–polymerase chain reaction (RT-PCR) or potentially by fluorescence *in situ* hybridization (FISH) might currently be utilized to distinguish between a primary clear cell sarcoma, and a malignant melanoma involving the soft tissue, a distinction that is not always possible to make with certainty by traditional means (1). Despite the incremental advances of molecular techniques in diagnosis and prognosis, it may seem surprising that morphology is still the basis of diagnosis for most neoplasms and many inflammatory dermatoses. Yet, a histologic image represents a true synthesis of all molecular events acting in a given microscopic "scene," which encompasses not only the concerted expression of genes including oncogenes and suppressor genes, but also the sum total of all epigenetic effects such as gene methylation, posttranslational modification, and the spatially and temporally segregated interactions of proteins and other gene products. This level of complexity of information cannot be captured by any high-throughput molecular testing that has yet been conceived.

Although histopathology remains the gold standard for most dermatologic diagnoses, it must be recognized that not all lesions are amenable to definitive "specific" histologic diagnosis. Specificity, or the "true negativity rate," is the frequency of a negative test result in individuals who actually do not have the disease of interest. Specificity studies are hard to do because they require large-scale studies of normal populations, and because of the need for a "gold standard" for the disease, independent of the test under consideration. Most studies in the literature begin with data demonstrating the "sensitivity" or "true positive rate," which is a measure of the frequency of a positive test result in individuals with the disease (2). These data do not, however, indicate that a diagnostic test is reliable. As Foucar has stated, "Specificity rules. High or low sensitivity is a feature that makes a highly specific test more or less valuable" (2). For example, most melanomas are positive for the immunohistochemical marker S-100. However, almost all benign melanocytic neoplasms are also positive for the same marker. Mitoses in the dermal component of the neoplasm, on the other hand, are common in melanomas but rare in most benign neoplasms, and are therefore a useful, relatively specific but not pathognomonic marker for melanoma (Chapter 28).

The histologic features of many inflammatory dermatoses in particular are nonspecific or, at best, only suggestive of a specific diagnosis. Even among the more readily characterized papulosquamous dermatoses, such as psoriasis or lichen planus (Chapter 7), the histologic picture is more typically "compatible with" rather than "diagnostic of" the clinical process. Sometimes, however, the histopathology can contribute by ruling out an important diagnosis, even though an exact diagnosis cannot be made. For example, review of a biopsy of a psoriasiform plaque may rule out mycosis fungoides (Chapter 31), but may not be able to establish the specific diagnosis of psoriasis (Chapter 7). The obvious diagnostic limitations of histology extend to infectious and neoplastic processes as well. For example, infectious granulomas of different etiologies are not readily distinguishable, unless the causative organism can be demonstrated. This may not be possible without additional testing such as bacterial or fungal cultures (Chapters 21 to 23). The same applies to noninfectious inflammatory disorders such as pyoderma gangrenosum where infection needs to be ruled out as an etiologic possibility (Chapter 16). Similarly, in the neoplastic realm, histology may not suffice to distinguish between keratoacanthoma and squamous cell carcinoma (3) (Chapter 29), or between Spitz nevus and melanoma (4) (Chapter 28).

Some of these "difficult" diagnoses result from the existence of important data that are undetectable by routine histologic methods, such as sparse organisms in a granulomatous process. In other instances, the data might be detectable if sought, but are obscure. For example, many granulomatous processes can be more specifically characterized if more sensitive staining for organisms is done, as in a Grocott or acid-fast stain. If the observer does not think of infection, and orders the stain, the diagnosis is never made. In many other situations, however, such as the diagnosis of keratoacanthoma versus squamous cell carcinoma or of Spitz nevus versus melanoma, the available data may have been assiduously collected by the observer using complex algorithms published for these purposes, yet the diagnosis remains obscure, and agreement among observers is difficult or impossible to obtain. In such cases, there is typically a continuum of the traits that underlie diagnosis, and individuals in the vicinity of the diagnostic cut-point are more likely to be misclassified than others (5).

In a recently published "Tutorial on Melanocytic Lesions," a panel of six experts in pigmented lesion pathology reviewed 71 "difficult" cases (6). While agreement was substantial for many of the different categories of lesions, the categories of Spitz nevi and other variants of nevi and of nevoid melanoma were more difficult. Unanimity in diagnosis was reached in only 11 of 38 cases, and in 6 cases the opinions of the experts were equally divided between benign and malignant. In another category, that of six examples of "pseudomelanomas" in children, agreement on a benign diagnosis was almost unanimous, yet one of these patients had died of metastatic disease. In another study of 30 lesions selected for their difficulty, evaluation of 17 "Spitzean" lesions yielded no clear consensus as to diagnosis; "in only one case did six or more pathologists agree on

a single category, regardless of clinical outcome." In addition, some lesions that proved fatal were categorized by most observers as either Spitz nevi or atypical Spitz tumors (7). Thus, agreement on a diagnosis does not necessarily mean that the diagnosis is correct. Therefore, the best opinion that can be rendered about these lesions is that the true diagnosis is unknown, and the likely behavior of the lesion is uncertain.

Following practice in other areas of pathology where similar problems exist (8–18), such lesions in our opinion are best categorized as "tumors of uncertain malignant potential" (TUMP). In these cases, we always provide a differential diagnosis, and therapy is usually tailored with the "worst-case scenario" taken into consideration. Even this latter assumption is not without potential for controversy, however; it is not at all clear, for example, that therapy devised for routine cases of melanoma should be uncritically applied to melanocytic tumors of uncertain potential ("MELTUMP") (Chapter 29). In these "borderline" or "difficult" lesions, the clinical utility of histology may be aided by effective communication between clinician and pathologist with appropriate attention to the clinical and epidemiologic context of the lesion under study, and also by ancillary testing such as comparative genomic hybridization (CGH) or FISH for assessment of gene amplification profiles that have recently been shown to differ between Spitz nevi and melanomas (19). Even when all clinical, histologic, and molecular information is at hand, however, a consensus diagnosis may be impossible, and there is no prospective assurance that any diagnosis is biologically "correct."

Foucar (20) has elegantly discussed the difficulties inherent in making a histologic diagnosis (and these considerations apply to other forms of diagnosis as well), and the issues have also been well covered by Sackett et al. (21). A major source of difficulty in making an exact diagnosis in pathology, as in clinical medicine, is that the information required to make the diagnosis is frequently incomplete at some level, or at multiple levels. At the most fundamental level, there may simply be no extant standard for a particular diagnosis. For example, histopathology is often taken to be a gold standard for diagnosis of a particular disease. However, if the histopathologic parameters that are considered to define this disease have been determined in a clinically defined series of cases, their independence and specificity should be called into question. A histologic study of nummular dermatitis, however complete and accurate it may be, will not glean any information that reliably distinguishes between this diagnosis and that of another spongiotic dermatitis (Chapter 7). Patches of early mycosis fungoides biopsied from patients with established plaque stage lesions may well represent examples of "early" mycosis fungoides, yet similar histologic changes in a patient with only a solitary lesion may or may not progress to established disease (Chapter 31).

Another serious problem in histopathologic diagnosis results from the fact that specificity studies to determine the prevalence of criteria in diagnostically challenging cases are frequently not available. For example, early studies of the HMB-45 antibody determined that it had 100% specificity for melanoma cells in the dermis or deeper tissues (22). After the specificity studies were extended, however, it was recognized that this antigen is expressed not only in melanoma, but also in blue nevi (23) and in other benign lesions (Chapter 28).

Foucar has pointed out that the diagnostic process is an example of complex decision-making that has intrinsic uncertainty, usually resulting from one or more of the following: (a) the large number of variables that can be evaluated in an attempt to solve the problem results in novel combinations of variables that cannot be managed consistently by problem solvers; (b) one or more key variables lack clear definition; or (c) one or more key variables is hidden from the problem solver (20). To the uncertainty inherent in these complex problems can be added (d) the uncertainty (discussed above) of the specificity of the individual findings, and (e) the uncertainty that results from deficiencies in the observer's ability to evaluate and categorize histologic findings. Even the most expert observers have inherent and often unrecognized deficiencies that result in less than perfect reproducibility of histopathologic observations, and thus of diagnoses (24). Furthermore, there are limitations in the ability of even the most expert observers to communicate their diagnostic acumen to others (20).

The diagnostic difficulties that result from uncertainty are compounded when there is also failure to agree upon the criteria for diagnosis. In a study of inter- and intra-observer reproducibility for the diagnosis of dysplastic nevi, intraobserver reproducibility was substantial, and interobserver concordance was fair, despite differences in criteria. It was concluded that, although experienced dermatopathologists in this study used different diagnostic criteria for histologic dysplasia, their usage was consistent (25). In another study where observers agreed to abide by predetermined criteria, and were provided reference photomicrographs illustrative of the criteria, agreement was substantial to excellent for the histopathologic diagnosis of 112 melanocytic tumors, including typical and dysplastic nevi and melanomas. It was concluded that, using predetermined criteria, melanocytic dysplasia can be reproducibly graded among diverse general dermatopathologists (26).

In another example, the criteria for diagnosis of vertical growth phase in thin melanomas have been rigorously evaluated in two large studies. In one of the studies, 94 slides of malignant melanoma were circulated to six pathologists in two university departments. For each slide, the growth phase of the lesion, Breslow thickness, and Clark level were determined by each observer. The aims of the study were "to evaluate agreement among nonspecialist pathologists in identifying the vertical growth phase in malignant melanoma and to compare agreement for the growth phase with agreement for Breslow thickness and the Clark level." It was found that, although overall agreement for the growth phase was moderate, agreement among experienced observers was good. (27).

Although this was outside of the scope of the study, is it is likely that, with increased experience, the nonspecialist pathologists would attain the same level of agreement. In another similar study, 148 pathologists participated in two circulations of melanoma slides, and the results were compared with those of a national Melanoma Pathology Panel, which had developed and evaluated diagnostic criteria. After a first circulation of slides in which only fair agreement was achieved, a second circulation of slides was accompanied by diagnostic criteria and diagrams. In this second circulation, there was a higher level of agreement for overall diagnosis, using the categories benign, melanocytic intraepidermal neoplasia, and melanoma with vertical growth phase ($\kappa = 0.68$). In their conclusions, these authors emphasized the importance of standardized diagnostic criteria to ensure accurate reporting of incidence and correct management of patients (28).

As discussed by Foucar (20), differences in criteria may result from the use of different assumptions for the development of criteria. At the simplest level of diagnosis, an individual pathologist might establish a set of criteria that establish a diagnosis "by definition." Such a definitional diagnosis reduces uncertainty for that individual to a minimum. At a somewhat more advanced level, criteria are used that are considered likely to be acceptable to other pathologists, constituting a "consensus gold standard." At this level of diagnosis, difficulties in communicating a clear definition of the criteria among pathologists introduce uncertainty due to lack of reproducibility, and this uncertainty increases with the number of variables under consideration, and the resultant increasing subjectivity of the diagnostic exercise.

The most advanced measure of the level of diagnostic problem solving, according to Foucar, is represented by the attempt to assign a biologically correct label, one that precisely predicts a disease's course (20). Attempts to fully resolve this more difficult level of prediction are likely in most cases, if not all, to be frustrated by the uncertainties enumerated above, especially the existence of hidden variables—"host resistance," "virulence," "environmental effects," and so on—that are not evident to the observer of a histologic slide, however expert and diligent he or she may be. Efforts to improve on diagnostic efficacy at this level might, for example, pursue information at the ultrastructural or molecular level. However, the accurate and complete prediction of a particular disease outcome will always prove to be an elusive goal.

Prognostication—the prediction of disease outcome—is an important biological indicator of diagnostic efficacy. In some instances, many of them neoplasms, a histologic diagnosis is predictive of biologic behavior, such as the capacity for distant metastasis. Then, follow-up studies of outcome can serve as an appropriate gold standard for validation of diagnostic utility. Indeed, a 100% statistical probability of survival for a given neoplasm could be regarded as equivalent to a diagnosis of benignancy, illustrating a strong relationship between diagnosis and prognosis.

Even when such studies are available, however, the prediction of outcome is usually in terms of statistical probabilities, which are not absolute. The information needed to accurately predict outcome in any given individual case is frequently not available to the histologic observer. For example, the outcome of a viral infection may depend on the presence or absence of antibodies in the patient's serum, which cannot be determined from observation of histologic sections. Similarly, even the most advanced and seemingly lethal primary malignant melanoma has a certain probability of survival, even after utilizing the most sophisticated prognostic models (29).

Another advanced measure of the biological relevance of a diagnostic system is through the correlation of traditional diagnostic labels with molecular findings. In the studies of Bastian et al. (30), nevi have been distinguished from melanomas, a subset of atypical Spitz nevi has been distinguished from among the usual forms of this condition, and the acral-lentiginous subset of melanoma has been distinguished from other types, all through the use of comparative genomic hybridization to identify molecular lesions that appear to have specificity for these traditionally defined variants of melanocytic neoplasia (Chapter 29). In a patient with a suspected infection, a PCR test for "foreign" DNA can be diagnostic of the presence of an infectious agent (Chapters 20–25). These types of correlations can be expected to increase in the future, strengthening the relationship between our present empirically based classification schemas and the underlying biology.

It is likely that the best approximation to the goal of improving diagnostic specificity will be achieved by a detailed correlation of findings at the molecular, histologic, and gross anatomic levels with the physical findings and clinical history, interpreted in the context of the whole patient and his or her environment, with long-term follow-up serving as the "gold standard." In the "real world" of clinical medicine, a histologic description and differential diagnosis for a difficult case is often more likely to be useful than a single "specific" diagnosis that may be correct in its own frame of reference, but wrong or misleading in the total clinicopathologic context of a particular patient. The former is the traditional method of clinical practice, which should be aided but not supplanted by the tools of histopathology. The information in this book has been designed to assist in this clinical diagnostic process.

REFERENCES

1. Antonescu CR, Tschernyavsky SJ, Woodruff JM, et al. Molecular diagnosis of clear cell sarcoma: detection of EWS-ATF1 and MITF-M transcripts and histopathological and ultrastructural analysis of 12 cases. *J Mol Diagn* 2002;4:44–52.
2. Foucar E. Diagnostic decision-making in anatomic pathology. *Am J Clin Pathol* 2001;116[Suppl]:S21–S33.
3. Rank BK, Dixon PL. Another look at keratoacanthoma. *Aust N Z J Surg* 1979;49:654–658.
4. Piepkorn M. On the nature of histologic observations: the case of the Spitz nevus. *J Am Acad Dermatol* 1995;32:248–254.
5. Brenner H. How independent are multiple "independent" diagnostic classifications? *Stat Med* 2004;15:1377–1386.
6. Cerroni L, Kerl H. Tutorial on melanocytic lesions. *Am J Dermatopathol* 2001;23:237–241.
7. Barnhill RL, Argenyi ZB, From L, et al. Atypical Spitz nevi/tumors: lack of consensus for diagnosis, discrimination from melanoma, and prediction of outcome. *Hum Pathol* 1999;30:513–520.
8. Lasota J, Dansonka-Mieszkowska A, Stachura T, et al. Gastrointestinal stromal tumors with internal tandem duplications in 3' end of KIT juxtamembrane domain occur predominantly in stomach and generally seem to have a favorable course. *Mod Pathol* 2003;16:1257–1264.
9. Lee AH, Denley HE, Pinder SE, et al. Excision biopsy findings of patients with breast needle core biopsies reported as suspicious of malignancy (B4) or lesion of uncertain malignant potential (B3). *Histopathology* 2003;42:331–336.
10. Marion-Audibert AM, Barel C, Gouysse G, et al. Low microvessel density is an unfavorable histoprognostic factor in pancreatic endocrine tumors. *Gastroenterology* 2003;125:1094–1104.
11. Moore SW, Satge D, Sasco AJ, et al. The epidemiology of neonatal tumours. Report of an international working group. *Pediatr Surg Int* 2003;19:509–519.
12. Folpe AL, Fanburg-Smith JC, Miettinen M, et al. Atypical and malignant glomus tumors: analysis of 52 cases, with a proposal for the reclassification of glomus tumors. *Am J Surg Pathol* 2001;25:1–12.
13. Medina PM, Valero Puerta JA, Perez MD. Atypical stromal hyperplasia of the prostate (stromal proliferation of uncertain malignant potential). *Arch Esp Urol* 2000;53:722–723 (in Spanish).
14. Nucci MR, Prasad CJ, Crum CP, et al. Mucinous endometrial epithelial proliferations: a morphologic spectrum of changes with diverse clinical significance. *Mod Pathol* 1999;12:1137–1142.
15. Lin BT, Bonsib SM, Mierau GW, et al. Oncocytic adrenocortical neoplasms: a report of seven cases and review of the literature. *Am J Surg Pathol* 1998;22:603–614.
16. Menaker GM, Sanger JR. Granular cell tumor of uncertain malignant potential. *Ann Plast Surg* 1997;38:658–660.
17. Soumakis S, Panayiotides J, Protopapa E, et al. Quantitative pathology in uterine smooth muscle tumours: the case for the standard histologic classification criteria. *Eur J Gynaecol Oncol* 1997;18:203–207.
18. Carr NJ, Sobin LH. Unusual tumors of the appendix and pseudomyxoma peritonei. *Semin Diagn Pathol* 1996;13:314–325.
19. Bastian BC, LeBoit PE, Pinkel D. Mutations and copy number increase of HRAS in Spitz nevi with distinctive histopathological features. *Am J Pathol* 2000;157:967–972.
20. Foucar E. Debating melanocytic tumors of the skin: does an "uncertain" diagnosis signify borderline diagnostic skill? [Letter]. *Am J Dermatopathol* 1995;17:626–634.
21. Sackett DL, Haynes RB, Tugwell P. Early diagnosis. In: Sackett DL, Haynes RB, Tugwell P, eds. *Clinical epidemiology. A basic science for clinical medicine.* Boston/Toronto: Little, Brown and Company, 1985:139–155.
22. Gown AM, Vogel AM, Hoak D, et al. Monoclonal antibodies specific for melanocytic tumors distinguish subpopulations of melanocytes. *Am J Pathol* 1986;123:195.
23. Sun J, Morton TH, Gown AM. Antibody HMB-45 identifies the cells of blue nevi. *Am J Surg Pathol* 1990;14:748–751.
24. Farmer ER, Gonin R, Hanna MP. Discordance in the histopathologic diagnosis of melanoma and melanocytic nevi between expert pathologists. *Hum Pathol* 1996;27:528–531.

25. Piepkorn MW, Barnhill RL, Cannon-Albright LA, et al. A multiobserver, population-based analysis of histologic dysplasia in melanocytic nevi. *J Am Acad Dermatol* 1994;30:707–714.

26. Weinstock MA, Barnhill RL, Rhodes AR, et al. Reliability of the histopathologic diagnosis of melanocytic dysplasia. The Dysplastic Nevus Panel. *Arch Dermatol* 1997;133:953–958.

27. McDermott NC, Hayes DP, al-Sader MH, et al. Identification of vertical growth phase in malignant melanoma. A study of interobserver agreement. *Am J Clin Pathol* 1998;110:753–757.

28. Cook MG, Clarke TJ, Humphreys S, et al. A nationwide survey of observer variation in the diagnosis of thin cutaneous malignant melanoma including the MIN terminology. *J Clin Pathol* 1997;50:202–205.

29. Rivers JK, McCarthy SW, Shaw HM, et al. Patients with thick melanomas surviving at least 10 years: histological, cytometric and HLA analyses. *Histopathology* 1991;18:339–346.

30. Bastian BC. Understanding the progression of melanocytic neoplasia using genomic analysis: from fields to cancer. *Oncogene* 2003;22:3081–3086.

BIOPSY TECHNIQUES

ROSALIE ELENITSAS
MICHAEL E. MING

The technique used to obtain a specimen for microscopic evaluation may have a significant impact on the ability of the dermatopathologist to arrive at the correct diagnosis. Commonly used skin biopsy techniques are punch biopsy, superficial and deep shave biopsy, deep incisional biopsy, complete excision, and curettage. The choice of technique depends on multiple factors, including the clinical differential diagnosis and a mental review of the pathology of each disorder, anatomic site, morphology of the lesion, particularly its size and shape, overall physical health of the patient, and cosmetic concerns (1).

Selection of the appropriate lesion to biopsy when evaluating an inflammatory disorder is crucial. In most instances, histologic examination of a fully developed lesion will give more information than examination of an early or involuting lesion. However, vesicobullous lesions, ulcers, and pustular lesions are exceptions to this rule. For their histologic examination, a very early lesion is required; otherwise, secondary changes such as regeneration, degeneration, scarring, or secondary infection may obscure essential features and make recognition of the primary pathologic process impossible. The ideal candidate lesion for biopsy has not been scratched or traumatized, and is untouched by topical or systemic therapy, especially anti-inflammatory agents. If there are lesions in different stages of evolution, multiple biopsy specimens may be helpful. If one is considering diagnoses such as connective tissue nevus, anetoderma, atrophoderma, and some pigmentation disorders, the dermatopathologist may wish to compare involved and uninvolved skin. In those cases, one can perform a scalpel biopsy incorporating a portion of the lesion and adjacent normal skin.

When performing scalp biopsies for alopecia, many laboratories prefer two specimens: one for transverse (horizontal) sectioning and one for standard "vertical" sections. The punch instrument should be inserted into the skin parallel to the direction of hair growth, and the biopsy should extend well into the subcutis to be certain that the bulbs of terminal follicles are included (2). In scarring alopecia, it is important that a biopsy be performed in an area of erythema with visible hair shafts; a biopsy of a completely scarred area of alopecia will show only end-stage nonspecific changes.

Punch biopsy is the standard procedure for obtaining samples of inflammatory dermatoses but is often used for neoplasms as well. In most instances, a specimen obtained with a 4-mm biopsy punch is adequate for histologic study. A 3-mm punch may be preferable for small lesions or biopsies from the face or other areas where cosmesis is a concern. Either a 6-mm punch biopsy or a deep incisional biopsy using a scalpel should be performed if panniculitis is suspected to ensure that adequate amounts of subcutaneous fat are obtained. After the skin specimen has been loosened with the biopsy punch, it should be handled very gently and, above all, should not be grasped with forceps except at the very edge. Crush artifact from forceps makes a specimen of an inflammatory process essentially useless, with lymphoma and leukemic infiltrates being particularly susceptible to crush. Often, a punch biopsy specimen can be squeezed gently out of its socket or carefully speared with the syringe needle that was used for injection of the local anesthetic. Sharp scissors can be used to cut through the subcutaneous fat at the base of the specimen. All punch biopsy specimens for inflammatory disease should extend to the subcutaneous fat, because in many dermatoses, characteristic histologic features are found in the lower dermis or in the subcutaneous fat.

Shave biopsies may be either superficial or extend more deeply into the skin, but in general should extend at least into the papillary dermis. Superficial shave biopsies should be employed only for lesions in which characteristic histologic changes are expected to be present in the epidermis or the superficial dermis, such as seborrheic keratoses, solar keratoses, verrucae, benign nevi, and basal cell carcinomas. This method has the advantage of leaving the lower portion of the dermis intact so that, immediately afterward, lesions such as basal cell carcinomas can be fully removed by curettage with or without electrodesiccation. In addition, cosmesis is often improved by using the superficial shave biopsy technique. A variant of the deep shave biopsy is the saucerization technique, in which the blade is introduced at roughly a 45-degree angle. To aid in the control of the size of the tissue to be removed, some physicians score the skin before performing a shave biopsy. Shave biopsies are inadequate for differentiating between squamous cell carcinoma and keratoacanthoma, and a superficial shave biopsy is contraindicated if melanoma is included in the differential diagnosis due to concerns that a melanoma might be transected at the base. A transected melanoma specimen may be more difficult to diagnose, and accurate assessment of tumor thickness may be more difficult. Because of the thick stratum corneum, a shave biopsy of acral skin may produce a superficial specimen extending only to the mid-epidermis or papillary dermis. This is especially important when considering a biopsy of an acral pigmented lesion; in this situation, a punch biopsy or small excision is often the best method.

To carry out a shave biopsy, either the skin is raised as a fold and cut with the blade parallel to the skin surface, or a curved razor blade is used. Aluminum chloride is recommended for hemostasis; Monsel's solution (ferric subsulfate) and electrocautery are alternatives, but they may affect the interpretation of subsequent biopsies or reexcisions (3).

Deep incisional biopsies using a scalpel may be helpful when evaluating panniculitis as described above, or when assessing deep dermal or subcutaneous nodules. Complete excision is often used to obtain an initial specimen for diagnosis when examining atypical pigmented lesions or when evaluation of margins is necessary. Curettage is the least satisfactory of the above methods of obtaining material for histologic examination, because the submitted material usually is scanty and superficial, and has lost its architecture and may show crush artifact. Even if curettage is performed well, fragmentation and distortion cannot be avoided. Curettage of a melanoma that clinically resembles a seborrheic keratosis or pigmented basal cell carcinoma may prevent accurate diagnosis and may make assessment of microscopic features such as ulceration or regression more difficult.

The biopsy specimen should be placed in fixative immediately on removal from the patient to prevent autolysis. It should not be allowed to dry, and the dermatologist should check the specimen bottle to ensure that the tissue has not adhered to the side of the bottle or remained inside the punch. Patient information should be placed on the bottle itself, not on the lid, which could be accidentally placed on a different bottle. As fixative, 10% buffered formalin can be used in nearly all instances (see Chapter 4). However, if the specimen is mailed in winter, 10% aqueous formalin, which freezes at 11°C, may allow formation of ice crystals in the specimen. This causes damage and distortion in the specimen, particularly in epithelial cells, and makes adequate histologic evaluation impossible. Freezing can be prevented by the addition to the formalin of 95% ethyl alcohol, 10% by volume. An alternative is to let the specimen stand in the formalin solution at room temperature for at least 6 hours before mailing.

Every specimen submitted for histologic diagnosis should be accompanied by detailed clinical information, including a differential diagnosis. The histopathologist's ability to render an accurate diagnosis often depends on the available clinical information, and clinicopathologic correlation is the key to providing optimal patient care. Previous biopsies at the same site, specific requests (e.g., special stains for infectious organisms), and special handling should also be indicated on the requisition sheet sent to the laboratory with the specimen. If, for instance, a stain for lipids is to be carried out, the specimen must not be processed in the automatic processor (see Chapter 4). Handling of biopsies for immunofluorescence is discussed in Chapter 4.

REFERENCES

1. Bart RS, Kopf AW. Techniques of biopsy of cutaneous neoplasms. *J Dermatol Surg Oncol* 1979;5:979.
2. Headington JT. Transverse microscopic anatomy of the human scalp. *Arch Dermatol* 1984;120:449.
3. Olmstead PM, Lund HZ, Leonard DD. Monsel's solution: a histologic nuisance. *J Am Acad Dermatol* 1980;3:492.

HISTOLOGY OF THE SKIN

GEORGE F. MURPHY

OVERVIEW

Understanding of the normal histology of skin is central to definition of all that is termed cutaneous pathology. The journey to define the normal histology of human skin is a relatively short one in terms of spatial dimensions. From an *en face* view of the skin surface, characterized by desquamating scale, furrows, and evidence of adnexal growth, to the normal ultrastructure of key organelles within underlying cellular constituents, we span a magnification range of no more than 10^5 (a range of greater than 35 powers of 10 separate the distance from the first celestial impression of the Milky Way galaxy to the realm of subatomic particles here on planet Earth) (1). And yet, the histology of the skin is amazingly complex. Divided into two seemingly separate but functionally interdependent layers (epidermis and dermis), skin is composed of cells with myriad functions ranging from mechanical and photoprotection, immunosurveillance, nutrient metabolism, and repair.

The epidermal layer is composed primarily of keratinocytes (>90%), with minority populations of Langerhans cells, melanocytes, neuroendocrine (Merkel) cells, and unmyelinated axons. Architecturally, the epidermal layer has an undulant undersurface in two-dimensional sections, with downward invaginations termed *rete*, and interdigitating mesenchymal cones termed *dermal papillae* (not to be confused with follicular papillae of the hair bulb). In reality, three-dimensional reconstruction reveals epidermal rete to form a honeycomb of interconnected ridges, with dermal papillae representing rounded conical invaginations not dissimilar to the undersurface of an egg carton. Separated from the epidermis by a structurally and chemically complex basement membrane zone, the dermis consists of endothelial and neural cells and supporting elements, fibroblasts, dendritic and nondendritic monocyte/macrophages, factor XIIIa–expressing dermal dendrocytes, and mast cells enveloped within a matrix of collagen and glycosaminoglycan. Adnexae extend from the epidermis into the dermis and consist of specialized cells for hair growth, epithelial renewal (stem cells), and temperature regulation. Adnexal epithelium also appears to provide a safe haven for certain precursor cells (e.g., for melanocytes and dendritic cells) in an environment sequestered from deleterious environmental influences at the skin surface. The subcutis is an underlying cushion formed by cells engorged with lipid and nourished by vessels that grow within thin intervening septae. The developmental anatomy of skin is important not only in understanding the basis for mature structural-functional relationships, but also in terms of certain skin tumors that recapitulate embryologic cutaneous structure.

KERATINOCYTES OF THE EPIDERMIS

Embryology

The development of in utero skin biopsy techniques gives practical importance to understanding of the normal evolutionary histology of fetal skin. The epidermis begins as a single layer of ectodermal cells (2,3). By 5 weeks of gestational age, this has differentiated at least focally into two layers, the basal layer or stratum germinativum and the overlying periderm, and by 10 weeks, an intervening layer, the stratum intermedium, develops (Fig. 3-1). Cells forming the periderm are large, bulge from the epidermal surface, and are bathed in amniotic fluid. By 19 weeks, there are several layers of intermediate cells, and the periderm has begun to flatten (Figs. 3-1 and 3-2). Keratinization is well developed by 23 weeks within the stratum intermedium in association with small keratohyaline granules. At this juncture, most of the periderm cells have shed, and the keratinizing cells that remain beneath represent the newly formed stratum corneum (3).

By ultrastructure, the histogenesis of the epidermis involves early formation of immature desmosomes and early hemidesmosomes, and distinct basement membrane (6 to 7 weeks of gestational age) (4,5). Anchoring filaments are observed several weeks later, and the basement membrane appears structurally mature by the end of the first trimester (6). The surface cells of the periderm display numerous microvilli and cytoplasmic microvesicles, increasing the area in contact with amniotic fluid and suggesting active inter-

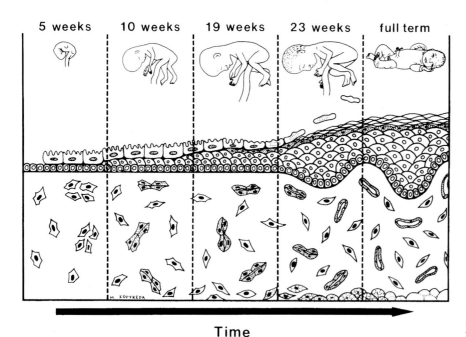

| 5 weeks | 10 weeks | 19 weeks | 23 weeks | full term |

Time

FIGURE 3-1. Schematic overview of embryonic development of human skin. (Courtesy of Michael Ioffreda, M.D.)

change between the periderm cells and the amniotic fluid (2). Tonofilaments are sparse until 16 weeks, when dense accumulations are observed in cells of the intermediate layer as evidence of beginning keratinization (3).

Normal Microanatomy

Two types of cells constitute the epidermis: keratinocytes and dendritic cells. The keratinocytes differ from the dendritic cells, or clear cells, by possessing intercellular bridges and ample amounts of stainable cytoplasm. As they differentiate into horny cells, the keratinocytes are arranged in four layers: basal cell layer (stratum basalis), squamous cell layer (stratum spinosum), granular layer (stratum granulosum), and horny layer (stratum corneum) (Fig. 3-3). The terms *stratum malpighii* and *rete malpighii* are often applied

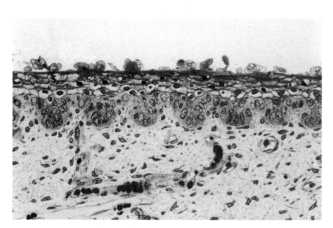

FIGURE 3-2. Histology of epidermis and dermis of 18-week normal human fetal skin (1-micron-thick plastic-embedded section).

to the three lower layers, which contain the basal, squamous, and granular cells, and comprise the nucleated, viable epidermis. An additional layer, the stratum lucidum, can be recognized in areas having a thick stratum granulosum and corneum forming the lowest portion of the horny layer, especially on the palms and soles.

Stratum Basalis

The basal cells form a single layer, are columnar, and lie with their long axis perpendicular to the dividing line between the epidermis and the dermis. They have a more basophilic cytoplasm than cells of the stratum spinosum, often contain melanin pigment transferred from adjacent melanocytes which parallels skin color, and contain a dark-staining oval or elongated nucleus (Fig. 3-4). They are connected with each other and with the overlying squamous cells by intercellular bridges or desmosomes (discussed in detail later). At their base, the basal cells are attached to the subepidermal basement membrane zone by modified desmosomes, termed hemidesmosomes. Basal cells and overlying squamous cells contain keratin intermediate filaments termed tonofilaments that form the developing cytoskeleton; these cells and related cytoskeletal proteins ultimately give rise to the anucleate stratum corneum at the epidermal surface (Figs. 3-5 and 3-6).

Most of the mitotic activity in normal human epidermis occurs in the basal cell layer. Even mitoses that appear to be located at a level above the basal cell layer often are found on serial sectioning to be in juxtaposition with a dermal papilla and thus to represent basal cells (6). A more efficient method of determining the location of proliferating cells in the human epidermis consists of either the intrader-

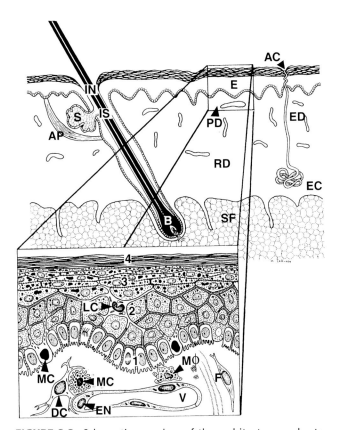

FIGURE 3-3. Schematic overview of the architecture and cytologic constituents of normal human skin. Projection demonstrates cellular components of epidermis and superficial dermis in greater detail, with epidermal strata denoted numerically (*1*, stratum basalis; *2*, stratum spinosum; *3*, stratum granulosum; *4*, stratum corneum). *E*, epidermis; *PD*, papillary dermis; *RD*, reticular dermis; *SF*, subcutaneous fat; *SC*, stratum cornuem; *SG*, stratum granulosum; *SS*, stratum spinosum; *SB*, stratum basalis; *LC*, Langerhans cell; *M*, melanocyte; *IN*, follicular infundibulum; *IS*, follicular isthmus; *B*, follicular bulb; *AP*, arrector pili muscle; *S*, sebaceous gland; *AC*, eccrine acrosyringium; *ED*, dermal eccrine duct; *EC*, coil of eccrine gland; *V*, vessel; *EN*, endothelial cell; *MC*, mast cell; *M*ϕ, macrophage; *DC*, perivascular dendritic cell; *F*, fibroblast; *ECM*, extracellular matrix. (Courtesy of Michael Ioffreda, M.D.)

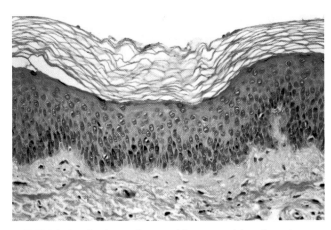

FIGURE 3-4. Histology of normal human epidermis and upper dermis (arm skin).

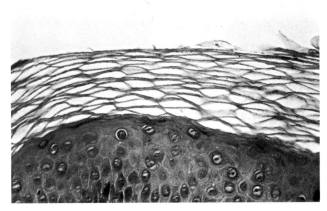

FIGURE 3-5. Histology of normally anucleate stratum corneum, the terminal differentiation product of underlying basal and suprabasal cells. Note the characteristic "basket-weave" architecture typical of nonacral sites.

mal injection of tritiated thymidine *in vivo* or the incubation of skin sections with antibodies to the cell cycle proliferation marker, Ki-67, *in vitro*. The tritiated thymidine method labels all cells in the S phase of DNA synthesis, which is approximately seven times longer than the mitotic or M phase. Thus, many more tritiated-thymidine-labeled cells can be visualized than mitoses. With the labeling method, 45% of the labeled cells in normal human epidermis were found in one study to be suprabasal in location; however, after the examination of tracings of serial sections, the corrected value was 32% (7). Ki-67 labeling is a useful way of determining cycling cells in paraffin sections, and as with tritiated thymidine, the vast majority of labeled cells in normal skin are within the basal cell layer of the epidermis (Fig. 3-7). In palm skin of nonhuman primates, populations of mitotically quiescent basal cells have been described that retain pulsed thymidine labels in contrast to actively dividing cells, where dilution of label occurs. These cells reside at tips of epidermal rete ridges, and have characteristics of stem cells (8). Recent studies have defined similar populations in the bulge region of the hair follicle (9). Moreover, unlike other basal cells that express cytokeratin 14, basal cells in the general region where stem cells reside

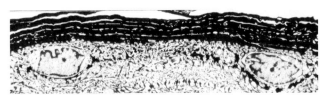

FIGURE 3-6. Ultrastructure of stratum corneum showing transition of intracellular tonofilaments within viable cells to anucleate stratum corneum at the epidermal surface. The darker granules directly beneath the stratum corneum represent keratohyaline granules.

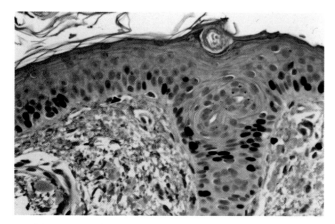

FIGURE 3-7. Evidence of basal cell layer replicative potential by Ki-67 immunostaining. Note the predominance of labeled cells in the basal cell layer of the epidermis and the included portion of a follicular infundibulum.

also express cytokeratin 15, indicating that biosynthetic heterogeneity exists within the basal layer with regard to expression of cytoskeletal elements.

Stratum Spinosum

The polyhedral cells of the stratum spinosum overlying the basal cell layer form a mosaic usually five to ten layers thick. They become flattened toward the surface, with their long axis arranged parallel to the skin surface (Figs. 3-5 and 3-6). The cells are separated by spaces that are traversed by intercellular bridges. These intercellular spaces stain slightly with the PAS stain and with Alcian blue and colloidal iron, suggesting that they contain neutral mucopolysaccharides and acid mucopolysaccharides (glycosaminoglycans). Pretreatment with hyaluronidase largely prevents staining with colloidal iron, indicating that hyaluronic acid is an important component of the glycosaminoglycans (10).

The tonofilaments within the cytoplasm of the keratinocytes of the stratum spinosum are loose bundles of electron-dense filaments (Fig. 3-5), each filament measuring 7 to 8 nm in diameter. These structures correlate with keratin proteins, as may be demonstrated by immunohistochemistry (Fig. 3-8). The tonofilaments at one end are attached to the attachment plaque of a desmosome, and the other end lies free in the cytoplasm near the nucleus. The desmosomes correlate with the intercellular bridges. Each desmosome possesses two electron-dense attachment plaques, one at either end, that are located in the cytoplasm of the two keratinocytes which the desmosome connects. Next to each attachment plaque lies the trilaminar plasma membrane of the two keratinocytes. Each trilaminar plasma membrane is 8 nm thick and consists of two electron-dense lines, called the inner and the outer leaflets, enclosing an electron-lucent line. In the center of the desmosome lies the intercellular cement substance, which shows greatest electron density

in the portion directly adjoining the outer leaflet of the trilaminar plasma membrane representing the cell surface coat (11). The cell surface coat often cannot be separated visually from the outer leaflet, and the two components have been referred to also as the intermediate dense layer (12). The remaining central portion of the intercellular cement appears electron lucent, except for a thin electron-dense line exactly in the center of the intercellular cement and the desmosome called the *intercellular contact layer* (11). The irregular location of the desmosomes shows that the plasma membrane of keratinocytes is remarkably convoluted.

The intercellular cement substance between two adjacent keratinocytes, referred to also as glycocalyx, contains glycoproteins, which are stainable *in vivo* and *in vitro* with ruthenium red and with lanthanum. Staining with either of these agents often results in greater electron density along the cell surface than in the center of the intercellular space because of a higher concentration of cement substance there as cell surface coat (13). The fact that the intercellular cement substance has a gel-like consistency explains why it on the one hand provides cohesion between the epidermal cells and on the other hand allows the rapid passage of water-soluble substances such as ruthenium red through the intercellular spaces and, furthermore, allows the opening up of desmosomes and individual cell movement (14).

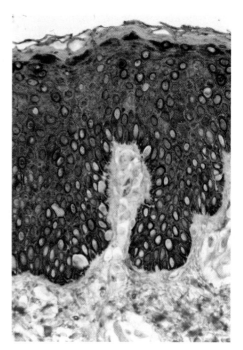

FIGURE 3-8. Immunohistochemistry for keratin proteins within the normal epidermis. This antiserum, which detects cytokeratins of various molecular weights, demonstrates diffuse staining within epidermal cells that contain keratin intermediate filaments.

Recent studies have begun to establish the molecular basis for keratinocyte-keratinocyte adhesion within the stratum spinosum and other epidermal layers. A key family of molecules is the cadherins, derived from multiple genes and representing Ca (++)-dependent cell adhesion molecules with a characteristic single-spanning transmembrane structure (15). Desmosomal cadherins are desmogleins and desmocollins (16) that localize to desmosomes and are linked to intracytoplasmic intermediate filaments by plakoglobin and desmoplakin. Within the desmosome complex, desmogleins within the cell membrane bind to plakoglobin through their cytoplasmic domain. Intermediate keratin filaments anchor at the desmosomal plaque, possibly by way of the carboxy-terminal domain of plakoglobin. The structural importance of these molecules in uniting keratinocytes cytoskeletons within the epidermis is indicated by the disorders pemphigus vulgaris and pemphigus foliaceus, where autoantibodies to members of the desmoglein subfamily of the cadherin supergene family result in clinical blisters due to loss of cell–cell adherence (acantholysis) (17,18). Desmoglein 3 is normally concentrated between immediately suprabasal keratinocytes, while desmoglein 1 is distributed principally among keratinocytes directly beneath the stratum corneum. Indeed, a remarkable correlation has been established between desmoglein expression in normal skin and pathologic lesions where specific desmogleins are disrupted with regard to the plane of blister formation due to loss of cell–cell adhesion.

Stratum Granulosum

The cells of the granular cell layer are flattened and their cytoplasm is filled with keratohyaline granules that are deeply basophilic and irregular in size and shape (Fig. 3-6). The thickness of the granular layer in normal skin is generally proportional to the thickness of the horny layer: it is only one to three cell layers thick in areas in which the horny layer is thin but measures up to ten layers in areas with a thick horny layer, such as the palms and soles (Fig. 3-9A and B). There often is an inverse relationship between the presence and thickness of the granular cell layer and parakeratosis (e.g., psoriasis, where extensive parakeratosis is associated with a markedly attenuated to absent stratum granulosum).

In the process of keratinization, the keratohyaline granules form two structures: the interfibrillary matrix or filaggrin, which cements the keratin filaments together, and the inner lining of the horny cells, the so-called marginal band. Whereas the tonofibrils contain only small amounts of sulfur as sulfhydryl groups, the interfibrillary matrix and the marginal band contain about ten times the amount of sulfur that is present in the tonofibrils, predominantly as disulfide bonds of cystine (19,20). Consequently, the tonofibrils are soft and flexible, while the matrix and marginal band provide necessary strength and stability (20). Thus, the keratin of the epidermis represents "soft" keratin, in contrast to the "hard" keratin of the hair and nails, in which keratohyaline granules are lacking and the tonofibrils themselves harden through the incorporation of disulfide bonds (21). "Soft" keratin desquamates as the result of enzymatic action, but the "hard" keratin of the hair and nails does not, thus requiring periodic cutting.

The granular cell layer represents the keratogenous zone of the epidermis, in which the dissolution of the nucleus and other cell organelles is prepared. In contrast to the stratum basalis and stratum spinosum, in which lysosomal enzymes, such as acid phosphatase and aryl sulfatase, are present as only a few granular aggregates, there is diffuse staining for lysosomal enzymes in the granular cell layer. These diffusely staining lysosomal enzymes probably play an important role in the autolytic changes occurring in the granular layer (22).

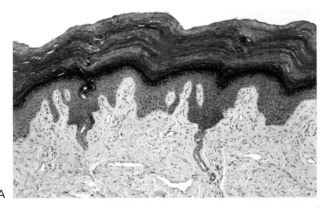 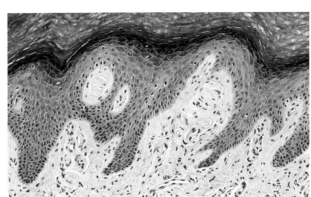

A   B

FIGURE 3-9. Histology of acral skin. Note the normally compacted and thickened stratum corneum **(A)** and the markedly thickened stratum granulosum **(B)**, as compared to non acral sites. (See Figs. 3-3, 3-4, and 3-5 for comparison.)

Stratum Corneum

Unlike the nucleated cells of the other epidermal layers that have been discussed, the cells of the normal stratum corneum are anucleate, and thus are technically dead. Thus the horny layer stains eosinophilic as a result of omission of basophilic nuclei. The thickness of the horny layer is often difficult to ascertain in formalin-fixed specimens, because some of the outer cell layers frequently detach themselves. Most of the horny layer is apt to show a basket-weave pattern in formalin-fixed specimens because of the presence of large intracellular spaces. These spaces are the result of inadequate fixation of soluble constituents within the horny cells by the formalin and the subsequent removal of these constituents by water, ethanol, and xylene during histologic processing. Thus, the portion of the cytoplasm that contains disulfide bonds of cystine has shrunk to form a shell along the cell membrane (23). In contrast, glutaraldehyde fixation used for electron microscopy causes precipitation of the formalin-soluble substances within the horny cells and allows staining of the contents of the horny cells with stains such as uranyl acetate and lead citrate. With a fluorescent stain it can be shown that the cells of the horny layer are arranged in orderly vertical stacks (24).

In certain formalin-fixed sections the lowest portion of the stratum corneum appears after processing and staining as a thin homogeneous eosinophilic zone, referred to as the stratum lucidum. This zone is most pronounced in areas in which the horny layer is thick, especially on the palms and soles. The stratum lucidum differs histochemically from the rest of the horny layer by being rich in protein-bound lipids contained in the Odland bodies (see below). It also has been called the stratum conjunctus, in contrast to the overlying stratum disjunctus with its basket-weave pattern (23).

Regional Variation

The epidermal layer may vary considerably from one body site to the next. Whereas the epidermis of the eyelid, axilla and knee/elbow all show a slightly verrucous architecture, eyelid epidermis gives rise to numerous vellus hair follicles, axilla to apocrine glands, and knee/elbow epidermis is thicker with a more prominent stratum corneum. Acral skin demonstrates progressive thickening and compaction of stratum corneum with progression from dorsal to ventral surfaces; nose skin displayed prominent, closely packed sebaceous lobules; and scalp skin gives rise to anagen follicles with bulbs that descend deeply into subcutaneous fat. Recognition of these regional variations is essential to avoiding misdiagnosis of pathology in otherwise normal skin.

Mucosal Epithelium

Skin shows considerable variation among different body sites, and appreciation of such normal differences is critical to accurate diagnostic assessment. Perhaps the most profound differences exist at mucosal and paramucosal sites. For example, with the exception of the dorsum of the tongue and the hard palate, the mucous membrane of the mouth possesses neither a granular nor a horny layer. Where these layers are absent, the epithelial cells in their migration from the basal layer to the surface first appear vacuolated, largely as a result of their glycogen content, then shrink, and finally desquamate. Electron microscopic examination reveals poor development of tonofilaments. The number of tonofilaments diminishes in the upper layers and they become dispersed. Large aggregates of glycogen are present in the cells. The epithelial cells of the oral mucosa show only few well-developed desmosomes. Instead, they show numerous microvilli at their borders. They are held together by an amorphous, moderately electron-dense intercellular cement substance, the resolution of which causes the detachment of the uppermost cells (25).

Specialized Structure and Function

Superficial Cellular Cohesion

The number of tonofilaments increases in the upper portion of the squamous layer. The earliest formation of keratohyaline granules consists of the aggregation of electron-dense ribonucleoprotein particles largely along tonofilaments. The keratohyaline granules increase in size through peripheral aggregation of ribonucleoprotein particles, and they surround more and more tonofilaments (26). By extending along numerous tonofilaments, the keratohyaline granules assume an irregular, often star-shaped outline and may reach a size of 1 to 2 μm. After ultimately ensheathing all tonofilaments, they form in the horny cells the electron-dense interfilamentous protein matrix of mature epidermal keratin. Keratohyaline granules are biochemically complex. One component is a histidine-rich protein called filaggrin precursor (27). When granular cells are converted to cornified cells, filaggrin precursor is broken down into many units of filaggrin. Filaggrin then aggregates with keratin filaments and acts as a "glue" for keratin filaments.

Terminal Differentiation

The transformation of granular cells into horny cells usually is abrupt. Fixation with glutaraldehyde and osmium tetroxide as used for electron microscopy preserves the internal structure of horny cells (Fig. 3-6), in contrast to formalin fixation for light microscopy. By electron microscopy, the cytoplasm of the cells in the lower portion of the horny layer shows relatively electron-lucent tonofilaments, about 8 nm thick, embedded in an interfilamentous substance having the same high degree of electron density as the keratohyaline granules (28). In the upper portions of the horny layer, however, the cells lose their filamentous structure. Together with the sudden keratinization of the horny cells, an electron-dense, homogeneous marginal band forms in their peripheral cytoplasm in close approximation to the trilaminar plasma membrane. Fully developed, the marginal band measures 16 nm thick, compared with 8 nm for the trilaminar plasma membrane. In the lowermost horny layer the trilaminar plasma membrane is preserved outside the marginal band; in the midportion of the horny layer it becomes discontinuous and then desquamates so that the marginal band serves as the real cell membrane (25). In the uppermost portion of the horny layer, even the marginal band often disappears concomitant with the degeneration and desquamation of the horny cells. Immunohistochemistry reveals that involucrin, a structural component of mature squamous epithelium, is incorporated into the marginal band as part of the formation of the protein envelope that characterizes squamous cells immediately prior to terminal differentiation (29). Desmosomal contacts are at first still present in the horny layer but disappear before desquamation of the horny cells.

Barrier Function

Odland bodies, also called membrane-coating lamellar granules, and keratinosomes, are small organelles that are discharged from the granular cells into the intercellular space and have two important functions: they establish a barrier to water loss, and they mediate stratum corneum cell cohesion. Lamellar granules appear first in the perinuclear cytoplasm in the stratum spinosum. Higher up in the epidermis, they rapidly increase in number and size (30). Both within and outside the granular cells, lamellar granules are round or oval, measure approximately 300 nm to 500 nm in diameter, and possess a trilaminar membrane and a laminated interior. The lamellar granules fuse with the plasma membrane of a granular cell, secreting its contents into the intercellular spaces (31). They contain neutral sugars linked to lipids and/or proteins; hydrolytic enzymes, possibly charged with degrading intercellular materials; and free sterols. The stratum granulosum interstices contain free sterols and sugars; the stratum corneum intercellular spaces stain as a pure neutral lipid mixture with abundant free sterols but no sugars (31). Sugars are cleaved at the granular-cornified layer interface by sugar-specific glycosidases.

An indication that the lamellar granules contribute to the physiologic water barrier was observed by Schreiner and Wolff in 1969 (32). When these investigators injected intradermally *in vivo* a solution of horseradish peroxidase as an electron microscopic tracer protein, they found that it penetrated the basement membrane and the intercellular spaces of the epidermis up to the upper portion of the granular layer, where lamellar granules block the intercellular spaces. Conclusive evidence was provided by Elias et al. (33), who showed by freeze-fracture techniques that the lamellar gran-

ules fuse and completely fill the intercellular spaces at the level of the granular layer. They concluded that the lipids formed in these organelles act as hydrophobic material, which is important to the barrier function. A similar permeability barrier exists in the oral mucosa. Lamellar granules may also contribute to cohesion between the cells of the lower stratum corneum as a result of the lipids that they contain. The action of enzymes, such as steroid sulfatase, removes the lipids from the upper stratum corneum and brings about desquamation of the cells there (34).

Enzyme Activity

Primary lysosomes that are membrane bound and contain a variety of hydrolytic enzymes, such as acid phosphatase, aryl sulfatase, and β-galactosidase, are seen in small numbers within keratinocytes, largely but not exclusively in the basal cell layer and lower squamous cell layer (13). These primary lysosomes are seen in the Golgi area, where they arise, and elsewhere in the cytoplasm. A great number of lysosomal enzymes are demonstrable in the granular layer and in the lowermost horny layer. However, on electron microscopic examination, only a very small proportion of these lysosomal enzymes is seen inside of primary lysosomes; most of the lysosomal enzymes are found free in the cytoplasm as irregularly shaped aggregates that are not membrane bound (35). Lysosomal enzymes are found also in the lamellar granules, while located within granular cells and after their discharge into the intercellular space (36). In addition to primary lysosomes, some secondary lysosomes, also called phagolysosomes, are present in the lower epidermis, especially in the basal cells. They digest phagocytized melanosomes, usually as melanosome complexes (see below). In cases of epidermal injury, such as sunburn or contact dermatitis, numerous phagosomes containing cellular organelles are present in the keratinocytes, which, as the result of the influx of lysosomal enzymes from primary lysosomes, become phagolysosomes (36).

Immune Functions of Keratinocytes

In recent years, the epidermal keratinocyte has been recognized as a potent source of immunogenic molecules. Although the list is ever increasing, keratinocytes are capable of producing interleukins (Il-1α, Il-1β, Il-6, Il-8); colony stimulating factors (Il-3, GM-CSF, G-CSF, M-CSF); interferons (IFN-α, IFN-β); tumor necrosis factors (TNF-α); transforming growth factors (TGF-α, TGFβ); and growth factors (platelet-derived growth factor, fibroblast growth factor) (37). Some of these substances are expressed constitutively, while others are synthesized only after signal transduction initiated by external or systemic cues (38). Accordingly, keratinocytes may play an active role in elaboration if molecular signals that facilitate lymphocyte homing and local activation, enabling certain dermal cells to mature, and regulating synthesis of extracellular matrix molecules. Because basal keratinocytes may be more potent producers and secretors of certain immunogenic molecules than more superficial epidermal cells, one must rethink the concept of keratinocyte maturation generally derived from efficiency of keratin synthesis.

MELANOCYTES

Embryology

The appearance of melanocytes in the epidermis takes place in a craniocaudal direction, in accordance with the development of the neural crest, from which the melanocytes are derived. By use of light microscopy on sections that have been treated with impregnation by Masson's ammoniated silver nitrate technic or exposed to the dopa reaction, melanocytes can be identified in the epidermis of the head region during the latter part of the third fetal month; in the more caudal body regions, the earliest formed melanin can be observed only in the latter part of the fourth month. Because melanocytes are functionally immature during their migration through the fetal dermis, they cannot be identified by histochemical methods until they have reached the epidermis (39). Electron microscopy allows an earlier recognition of melanocytes in the epidermis than is possible by light microscopy. Melanocytes with recognizable melanosomes may be seen in the fetal epidermis at a gestational age of 8 to 10 weeks (40), and using immunohistochemistry for HMB-45 protein, by 50 days estimated gestational age (41). Synthesis of melanin within the melanosomes occurs on the head in the latter part of the third month and elsewhere in the fourth month.

Normal Microanatomy

In sections stained with hematoxylin-eosin, melanocytes appear as randomly dispersed cells within the basal cell layer having a small, dark-staining nucleus and, largely as the result of shrinkage, a clear cytoplasm. They are found wedged between the basal cells of the epidermis, and because they are difficult to appreciate, are best demonstrated by special stains (Fig. 3-10). Although the number of melanocytes in relation to basal cells varies with the body region and increases with repeated exposure to ultraviolet light, the average number of clear cells in hematoxylin-eosin-stained vertical sections is one of ten cells in the basal layer (42). However, not all clear cells seen in routine sections necessarily are melanocytes; occasionally, basal keratinocytes show the same shrinkage artifact and are indistinguishable from melanocytes (43). Melanin is transferred by means of the dendritic processes (Fig. 3-10B) from the melanocytes to the basal keratinocytes, where it is first stored and later degraded. As a rule, a greater amount of melanin is present in the basal keratinocytes than in the melanocytes, and often basal cells at the tips of rete ridges are preferentially more melanized. Because only about 10% of the cells in the basal layer are melanocytes, each melanocyte supplies several keratinocytes with melanin, forming with them an epidermal melanin unit (44).

In persons with a light skin color, staining with hematoxylin-eosin may reveal few or no melanin granules in the basal cell layer. In persons with a dark skin color, especially individuals of African heritage, melanin granules are present in the basal cell layer as well as throughout the epidermis, including the horny layer, and in some instances in the upper dermis within macrophages, called melanophages. Accordingly, ethnic background as well as body site are critical in separating normal variations from true pathology.

Special Stains

Several special stains facilitate the light microscopic visualization of melanocytes and their products. Silver stains indicate the presence of melanin, which is both argyrophilic and argentaffin. Argyrophilia is based on the ability of melanin to be impregnated with silver nitrate solutions,

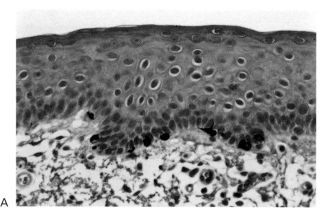
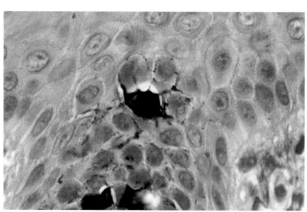

A · B

FIGURE 3-10. Immunohistochemical demonstration of normal melanocytes within the epidermal basal cell layer **(A)**. Note the dendritic extensions at higher magnification **(B)**. This cell appears to be suprabasal as a result of a tangential plane of section.

which, upon reduction with hydroquinone to silver, stains black. Because melanin is argentaffin, ammoniated silver nitrate may be reduced by phenolic groups in the melanin, forming black silver precipitate (Fontana–Masson method). Neither of these methods is entirely specific for melanin, however. Melanin may be bleached by strong oxidizing agents, such as hydrogen peroxide or potassium permanganate, a method that permits more specific identification (45), and is of use in heavily melanized tumors where pigment may obscure nuclear detail. The dopa reaction (46) is not of practical importance in routine diagnostic dermatopathology, but is instructive with regard to the biochemistry of melanization. Briefly, fresh, unfixed tissue sections or enzymatically separated epidermal sheets are incubated in a 0.01% solution of 3,4-dihydroxyphenylalanine (dopa) (47), staining melanocytes dark brown to black. The reaction imitates physiologic melanin formation, which begins by tyrosinase-dependent hydroxylation of tyrosine to dopa and the oxidation of dopa to dopaquinone, which is subsequently polymerized into melanin. Thus, the dopa reaction is in essence an assay for tyrosinase activity in melanosomes. Immunohistochemical detection of melanocytes is most commonly accomplished by antibodies to S-100 protein. This protein, originally isolated from bovine brain extract, is present in the cytoplasm of a variety of cells, including those of neural melanocytic lineage. Specialized macrophages, some epithelial cells, and a variety of nonmelanocytic cell types contain S-100 protein. In human epidermis, only melanocytes, which tend to reside within the basal layer, and Langerhans cells, with cell bodies mostly within the mid-epidermis, are reactive.

HMB-45 antibody reacts with a cytoplasmic epitope in cells of most but not all melanoma and in a minority of nevi. Melan-A is a melanosome-associated marker that has a high degree of specificity for melanocytes (Figs. 3-10). Activated and fetal melanocytes may be positive, but normal "resting" melanocytes are most often negative.

Ultrastructure

Melanocytes differ from keratinocytes by possessing no tonofilaments or desmosomes (Fig. 3-11A). Typically they "hang" down into the superficial dermis, but like basal keratinocytes, they are separated from the extracellular matrix by the basement membrane zone. At their base, where they lie in close apposition to the lamina densa, melanocytes show structures resembling the half-desmosomes of basal keratinocytes (48). Each of these structures consists of a cytoplasmic dense plate attached to the inner leaflet of the trilaminar plasma membrane and, except for being slightly smaller, has the same appearance as the attachment plaque of a half-desmosome. Anchoring filaments extend from the outer leaflet of the plasma membrane to the lamina densa. However, there is no subbasal cell dense plaque as in basal keratinocytes. Melanosomes are the most characteristic organelles of the melanocyte, and although they are commonly transferred to adjacent keratinocytes, identification of various stages of their formation within a cell assists in its ultrastructural identification as a melanocyte (Fig. 3-11B). Melanosomes in their development from stage I to stage IV gradually move from the cytoplasm of the melanocyte into the dendritic processes. However, even in

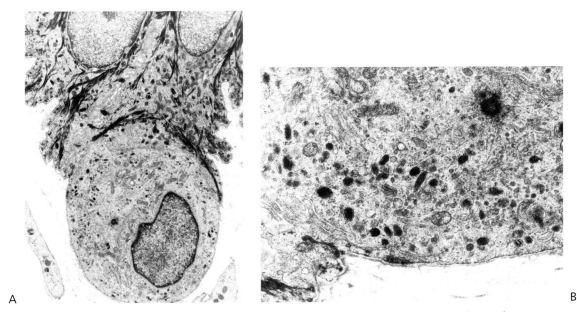

A   B

FIGURE 3-11. Ultrastructure of melanocytes. These cells characteristically "hang down" from basal cell layer and are devoid of tonofilaments of desmosomes **(A)**. They contain characteristic melanosomes in varying stages of melanization **(B)**.

the dendritic processes, stage II melanosomes may be seen. As melanosomes mature, their content of melanin increases, and their concentration of melanogenic enzyme decreases (49).

Stage I melanosomes are round, measure about 0.3 μm in diameter, and possess very intense enzyme activity concentrated along filaments. They contain no melanin (50). Stage II melanosomes are ellipsoid and measure approximately 0.5 μm in length, as do the melanosomes of stages III and IV. They contain longitudinal filaments that are cross-linked with one another. Enzyme activity is present both on the enveloping membrane and on the filaments. Melanin deposition on the cross-linked filaments begins at this stage. Stage III melanosomes have only little tyrosinase activity but show continued melanin deposition, partially through nonenzymatic polymerization. Stage IV melanosomes no longer possess tyrosinase activity. Melanin, which is formed entirely by nonenzymatic polymerization, fills the entire organelle and obscures its internal structure.

Regional Variation

The density of melanocytes has been most precisely determined on biopsy specimens 4 mm in diameter where the epidermis is separated from the dermis by incubation of the specimen in a 2N solution of sodium bromide. The resultant epidermal sheet is treated with a 1:1,000 solution of dopa for 2 hours to 4 hours and then is fixed in formalin, cleared, and mounted (47,51). It has thus been determined that the concentration of melanocytes in such epidermal sheets varies in different areas but is quite constant for any particular region. The highest concentration of melanocytes has been found on the face and the male genitals, about 2,000/mm^2, and the lowest on the trunk, about 800/mm^2 (51,52). No significant difference in the density of distribution of melanocytes for any given area of the skin exists between African American and Caucasoid skin. In the former, the melanocytes are uniformly highly reactive, whereas the melanocytes of Caucasoids, when not exposed to sunlight, are highly variable in dopa reactivity (53). In addition, African American skin contains larger and more highly dendritic melanocytes than Caucasoid skin (51,52).

Regional variation of melanocyte number and morphology may also be influenced by environmental factors, such as sun exposure. After a single exposure to ultraviolet light *in vivo*, the skin of Caucasoids, when examined with the dopa reaction, shows no increase in the density of the melanocyte population but does show an increase in the size and functional activity of the existing melanocytes (54). Repeated exposure to ultraviolet light, however, causes an increase in the concentration of dopa-positive melanocytes, as well as an increase in their size and functional activity (53,55). Thus, examination of habitually exposed and of unexposed skin from adjacent anatomic sites, such as the lateral and medial aspects of the upper arm, has shown a twofold higher concentration of melanocytes in habitually exposed skin (47). These studies are potentially relevant to utilization of S-100 immunohistochemistry in determining subtle increases or decreases in melanocyte populations as compared to age- and site-matched normal skin.

Specialized Structure and Function

Melanogenesis

Enzymatic melanogenesis (52,56,57) involves tyrosinase as the melanogenic enzyme. Tyrosinase is a copper-containing enzyme that catalyzes the hydroxylation of tyrosine to dihydroxyphenylalanine (dopa) and the oxidation of dopa to dopa-quinone. However, before tyrosinase can act on tyrosine, two cupric atoms present in tyrosinase must be reduced to cuprous atoms. It is believed that, in addition to being a substrate, dopa activates this reduction, thereby acting as a co-factor in the reaction. The conversion of tyrosine to melanin by tyrosinase is characterized by a variable lag period. When tyrosinase is present in low concentrations, as in epidermal melanocytes of nonirradiated skin, this lag period is markedly prolonged, and no use of tyrosine by tyrosinase is detectable. In contrast, in skin exposed *in vivo* to ultraviolet light (44), as well as in epidermal sheets (58) and in hair bulbs (52), tyrosinase activity is detectable with tyrosine as substrate. Because there is no lag period with dopa as substrate, tyrosinase in epidermal melanocytes can be readily demonstrated even in nonirradiated skin when skin sections are incubated in dopa rather than in tyrosine. The enzyme acting on dopa is therefore thought to be tyrosinase, rather than dopa-oxidase.

The melanogenic enzyme tyrosinase is synthesized in the Golgi-associated endoplasmic reticulum, in which tyrosinase condenses in membrane-limited vesicles. This process has been observed by electron microscopy in epidermal melanocytes after *in vivo* ultraviolet irradiation with either dopa or tyrosine as substrate (59). Subsequently, these tyrosinase units are transferred to dilated tubules of the smooth endoplasmic reticulum. There, tyrosinase is incorporated into a structural protein matrix containing filaments that have a distinctive periodicity. This then represents a stage I melanosome (60). Few stage I and II melanosomes have acid phosphatase activity, but the proportion of acid phosphatase-positive melanosomes increases in stage III, reaching a maximum in stage IV (61). This enzyme may play a role in the degradation or transfer of melanosomes. Detailed analysis of nonmelanosomal regulatory factors in melanogenesis has revealed coated vesicles to be richest in tyrosinase and catalase, whereas premelanosomes have the highest concentrations of peroxidase (62). Among relevant metal ions, premelanosomes contain higher amounts of copper, zinc, and iron than coated vesicles.

Melanin Transfer

The transfer of melanosomes from melanocytes to epidermal keratinocytes and to hair cortex cells is the result of active phagocytosis of the tips of melanocytic dendrites by keratinocytes and hair cortex cells, as demonstrated in tissue cultures (63) and in epidermal reconstructs seeded with melanocytes (64). With electron microscopy, one can observe that pseudopod-like cytoplasmic projections of keratinocytes or hair cortex cells are wrapped around the tips of dendrites. After such a projection has completely enveloped the tip of a dendrite, it is pinched off. At first, the melanosomes in the pinched-off dendrite are separated from the cytoplasm of the keratinocyte by the plasma membranes of the dendrite and of the keratinocyte (65). After the breakdown of these two plasma membranes, the melanosomes are dispersed throughout the cytoplasm of the keratinocyte, tending to be most concentrated above the nucleus. In the nonexposed skin of Caucasoids, especially those with light skin, such transferred melanosomes are found almost exclusively in the basal cell layer and, to a slight degree, in the layer of keratinocytes above the basal cell layer. However, in African Americans, in whom melanosomes are also principally seen in the basal cell layer, moderate quantities of melanosomes are found throughout the epidermis, including the stratum corneum (66).

The melanosomes present in keratinocytes of Caucasoid skin lie largely aggregated within membrane-bound melanosome complexes containing two or three melanosomes, and only a small proportion of melanosomes are singly dispersed. The melanosomes present within complexes often show signs of degeneration (66,67). In contrast, in skin of African and Australian aborigine heritage, the great majority of melanosomes lie singly dispersed, and relatively few melanosome complexes are found (66–68). The reason for the lack of aggregation of melanosomes in the latter racial groups seems to be their larger size. In Caucasoids, melanosomes range in length from 0.3 µm to 0.5 µm; in African Americans, they range in length from 0.5 µm to 0.8 µm (69). Because the membrane-bound melanosome complexes show considerable acid phosphatase activity, it is clear that they represent phagolysosomes in which the

melanosomes are being degraded (70). Thus, melanosomes appear to be removed more rapidly in Caucasoids than in individuals of African descent. It may be concluded that the difference in skin color is due to the following five factors: in African American skin, (a) there is greater production of melanosomes in melanocytes, (b) individual melanosomes show a higher degree of melanization, (c) melanosomes are larger, as a consequence of which, (d) there is a higher degree of dispersion in the keratinocytes, and (e) there is a slower rate of degradation (69). However, the predominant size of the melanosomes does not depend only on racial factors. Thus, topical treatment of the skin with trimethylpsoralen followed by irradiation with ultraviolet A light leads to an increase in the size of melanosomes in Caucasoids (71).

MERKEL CELLS

Embryology

Merkel cells arise, between weeks 8 and 12 of gestational age, from precursor stages of epithelial cells of early fetal epidermis that still express simple epithelial cytokeratins. *In situ* differentiation from epidermal ectoderm versus immigration of cells from the neural crest is supported by studies of fetal skin without Merkel cells transplanted to nude mice and subsequently found to contain mature Merkel cells within the engrafted tissue (72). Some Merkel cells detach from the epidermis and migrate temporarily into the upper dermis, where some of them associate with small nerves. The numerous dense-cored neurosecretory granules that they contain are formed within them.

Normal Microanatomy

Merkel cells are present within the basal cell layer of the epidermis (Fig. 3-12), oral mucosa, and in the bulge region of hair follicles (73). They are quite scarce, are irregularly distributed, and are occasionally arranged in groups (74). It is

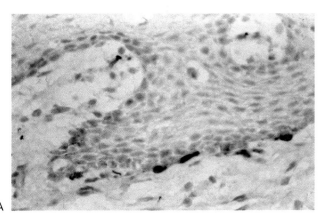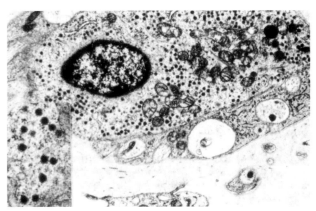

A B

FIGURE 3-12. Merkel cells in normal human skin. Immunohistochemistry reveals scattered positive cells within the basal cell layer **(A)**. By electron microscopy, Merkel cells contain characteristic neurosecretory granules **(B)**, *inset.*

assumed that the Merkel cell is a touch receptor (75). The Merkel cell cannot be recognized in light microscopic sections; however, in silver-impregnated sections, the meniscoid neural terminal that covers the basal portion of each Merkel cell can be seen as a Merkel disk (76). A sensory nerve fiber terminates at the disk. Immunohistochemistry for cytokeratin species (CK20) more typical of simple epithelial cells than keratinocytes permits differential identification of Merkel cells in tissue sections (Fig. 3-12A) (77).

On electron microscopic examination, Merkel cells usually are located directly above the basement membrane (Fig. 3-12B). They are quite easily recognized by electron microscopy, since they possess electron-dense granules, strands of intermediate filaments, and occasional desmosomes on their cell membranes connecting them with neighboring keratinocytes (75). The electron-dense granules vary in size between 80 nm and 200 nm and are membrane bound (Fig. 3-12B, inset). The filaments resemble tonofilaments and, like tonofilaments, are seen in some areas to converge upon desmosomes. In some sections, the Merkel disk can be seen above the basement membrane as a cushion on which the Merkel cell rests. It consists of a mitochondria-rich, nonmyelinated axon terminal (74).

Regional Variation

Merkel cells are most heavily concentrated in skin with high hair density and in glabrous epithelium of the digits, lips, regions of the oral cavity, and the outer root sheath of the hair follicle. These cells are present in mammals as so-called "touch-domes," also known as "Haarscheibe," a form of type I mechanoreceptor that surrounds tylotic hairs and the rete ridge collars about external root sheaths of hair follicles.

Specialized Structure and Function

Merkel cells are specialized epithelial cells that react with the intermediate filament cytokeratin and with desmosomal proteins (78,79). They also express a synaptophysin-like immunoreactivity similar to neuroendocrine carcinoma of the skin referred to also as Merkel cell carcinoma. The presence of synaptophysin-like immunoreactivity in Merkel cells supports the view that they are epithelial neuroendocrine cells and that they may possess a neurosecretory function (80). Merkel cells also contain neuron-specific enolase in their cytoplasm (81), but no neurofilaments (78).

LANGERHANS CELLS
Embryology

Langerhans cells are bone-marrow–derived cells that begin to appear in the epidermis by 7 weeks of gestation, recognizable as such by their positive staining for adenosine

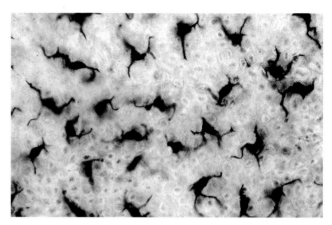

FIGURE 3-13. An epidermal sheet, removed and viewed en face, after ATPase enzyme histochemical staining. Note numerous evenly distributed, dendritic Langerhans cells.

triphosphatase (ATPase) (Fig. 3-13). At this stage, they are fewer, smaller, and less dendritic than at a later fetal stage. Although all Langerhans cells at this stage are ATPase positive, they are negative for their characteristic cell surface glycoprotein, CD1a (Fig. 3-14A). At a gestational stage of 60 days, Langerhans cells begin to express CD1a reactivity. By 80 to 90 days, the number of CD1a-positive cells increases abruptly, and after 90 days, the expression of CD1a is approximately equivalent to the number of ATPase-positive Langerhans cells (82). S-100 protein is not found in the Langerhans cells of fetal epidermis, but it can be demonstrated within 1 day after delivery (83). By electron microscopy, Langerhans cells can be identified by 10 to 11 weeks of gestation on the basis of the presence of Langerhans granules (Fig. 3-14B).

Normal Microanatomy

Langerhans cells are seen in histologic sections stained with hematoxylin-eosin as clear cells in the suprabasal epidermis. However, they cannot be reliably distinguished from occasional intraepidermal T-lymphocytes and macrophages, and their dendritic cytoplasmic processes cannot be resolved. Occasionally, focal hyperplasia of Langerhans cells results in an aggregate of these specialized histiocytes. The nuclei within such cellular clusters exhibit pallor and characteristic infoldings typical of Langerhans cells. In 1-micron, plastic-embedded sections, Langerhans cells are visualized as cells with (a) bodies generally situated in the midportion of the stratum spinosum, (b) nuclei with reniform to cleaved contours, and (c) delicate dendrites often extending to the level of the stratum corneum.

Because Langerhans cell detection is difficult in conventional sections, special stains are generally required for their detection and enumeration. Several enzyme histochemical stains may be used for identifying Langerhans cells and differentiating them from melanocytes. Among them are

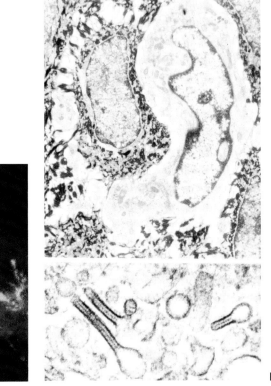

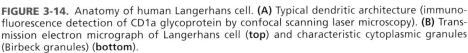

FIGURE 3-14. Anatomy of human Langerhans cell. **(A)** Typical dendritic architecture (immuno-fluorescence detection of CD1a glycoprotein by confocal scanning laser microscopy). **(B)** Transmission electron micrograph of Langerhans cell **(top)** and characteristic cytoplasmic granules (Birbeck granules) **(bottom)**.

adenosine triphosphatase (Fig. 3-13) and aminopeptidase (84). Langerhans are also positive for HLA-DR antigen and S-100 protein, although the former also reacts with cells forming the acrosyringium (85), and the latter is found in melanocytes. Langerhans cells can be demonstrated more specifically with monoclonal antibody to the prothymocyte differentiation cell surface glycoprotein, CD1a, when the antibody is labeled with either peroxidase or fluorescein (Fig. 3-14A) (86–88).

By electron microscopic examination, Langerhans cells show a markedly folded nucleus and no tonofilaments or desmosomes. Melanosomes are only rarely found in them and, if they are, they always are located within lysosomes, indicating that they have been phagocytized (89). Of great interest is the regular presence of an organelle, called the *Langerhans* or *Birbeck granule*, in the cytoplasm of Langerhans cells (Fig. 3-14B). The size of these granules varies considerably, from 100 nm to 1 μm (90). The granule has the three-dimensional shape of a disk and often shows a vesicle at one end and occasionally at both ends. A cross-section of the central portion has the appearance of a rod, and, if a vesicle is attached to the rod at one end, the Langerhans granule has the highly characteristic appearance of a tennis racquet. Viewed in rod-shaped cross-sections, the central portion has a central lamella showing

cross-striation with a periodicity of 6 nm (90). Langerhans granules form as a consequence of endocytotic, clathrin-associated invaginations of the cell membrane of Langerhans cells. This was first recognized on the basis of the presence of intradermally injected peroxidase within the granules of Langerhans cells even though the peroxidase molecule cannot cross the cell membrane (91). Also, on incubating Langerhans cells with a gold-labeled antibody directed against the CD1a glycoprotein of the cell membrane of the Langerhans cell it was found that the labeled CD1a was internalized and appeared within Langerhans granules (92). Cells that have the ultrastructural features of Langerhans cells but lack the Langerhans granule have been called indeterminate cells. They react specifically with the monoclonal antibody to CD1a (93,94).

Regional Variation

Langerhans cells are present in the epidermis in a concentration similar to that of melanocytes, between 460/mm² and 1,000/mm². In contrast to melanocytes, their number does not increase, but rather may decrease with repeated exposure to ultraviolet light (84). CD1a-positive Langerhans cells have been found to be less plentiful in trunk skin as compared to extremity skin (95). However, there appears to be considerable site variation among individuals, and the best comparison for determination of site-matched normal Langerhans cell numbers may be uninvolved skin directly adjacent to the lesion under study (95). The number of Langerhans cells may vary in contact allergic reactions. This is due to the fact that they are involved in the processing of antigen and its conveyance to lymphocytes subsequent to migration from skin to draining lymph nodes. Their number in the epidermis is increased in mycosis fungoides, where they are seen in contact with T-helper lymphocytes (96). Langerhans cells are present not only in the skin but also in the oral mucosa, vagina, lymph nodes, and thymus; occasionally, they are seen in the dermis (97).

Specialized Structure and Function

Langerhans cells originate in the bone marrow and are functionally and immunologically related to the monocyte-macrophage-histiocyte series (98). Langerhans cells constitute 2% to 4% of the total epidermal cell population (99). A few Langerhans cells are present in the dermis of normal skin. The histiocytes present in the cutaneous and visceral lesions of histiocytosis X contain Langerhans granules. These granules are indistinguishable in their electron microscopic appearance from those seen in epidermal Langerhans cells (100,101). Langerhans cells express immune response-associated antigens class II (HLA-DR in humans, Ia in mice) (102,103); Fc and C3 receptors; CD1a antigen (86–88); CD1c (M241) antigen (104); leukocyte common antigen (105); a membrane-bound ATPase (99); S-100 protein; and actin-like and vimentin filaments. These markers are compatible with an active role in cutaneous immunity.

Langerhans cells have antigen-presenting capacity. The recognition of a soluble protein and haptenated antigens by T-lymphocytes requires the initial uptake and processing by an HLA-DR–positive cell like the Langerhans cell, which then presents immunologically relevant moieties to the T-lymphocyte. Because of their antigen-presenting capacity, Langerhans cells play a crucial role in contact sensitization and in immunosurveillance against viral infections and neoplasms of the skin.

Ultraviolet (UV) radiation interferes with the antigen-presenting capacity of Langerhans cells. After UV irradiation fewer Langerhans cells could be demonstrated in the skin (106). It is likely that this initial decrease of Langerhans cells is due to a temporary loss of membrane markers, rather than to a destruction of the cells. Chronic repeated exposure to UV light may result in actual depletion of cells, contributing to potential for carcinogenesis. Similar depletion of Langerhans cells may result from application of potent topical corticosteroids (107) and in the setting of acquired immunodeficiency syndrome (108). With respect to the latter, viral particles have been identified in Langer-

hans cells (109), which interestingly express one of the HIV receptors, CD4 (110).

BASEMENT MEMBRANE ZONE
Normal Microanatomy and Ultrastructure

A subepidermal basement membrane zone not visible in sections stained with hematoxylin-eosin is seen on staining with the PAS stain (Fig. 3-15). It appears as a homogeneous band, 0.5 μ to 1 μ thick, at the epidermal–dermal junction (111). Its positive PAS reaction indicates a relatively large number of neutral mucopolysaccharides in this zone (112). Furthermore, impregnation with silver nitrate reveals in the uppermost dermis a meshwork of reticulum fibers. Staining with Alcian blue, which stains the band of polysaccharides and the reticulum meshwork, reveals that the band of polysaccharides is located above the reticulum layer (113). Direct immunofluorescence for basement membrane-associated proteins, such as bullous pemphigoid antigen, shows a light microscopic pattern similar to that observed with the PAS stain.

The light microscopic PAS-positive subepidermal basement membrane zone appears heterogeneous on electron microscopy (Fig. 3-16). It must be differentiated from the electron microscopic basement membrane, or lamina densa, which is a true membrane and, being only 35 nm to 45 nm thick, is submicroscopic. Thus, the light microscopic PAS-positive basement membrane zone is on the average 20 times thicker than the electron microscopic basement membrane, or lamina densa (111). A basement membrane zone similar to that seen at the epidermal–dermal border is present also around the cutaneous appendages.

The plasma membrane at the undersurface of basal cells shows half-desmosomes possessing only one intracytoplasmic attachment plaque to which tonofilaments from the interior of the basal cell are attached (Fig. 3-16). Beneath the plasma membrane of the basal cells, a rather electron-lucent zone called the lamina lucida, separates the trilaminar plasma membrane, about 8 nm wide, from the medium electron-dense basement membrane, or lamina densa (111). Within the electron-lucent zone, beneath each half-desmosome attachment plaque and extending parallel to it a plaque 7 nm to 9 nm thick, the sub-basal cell dense plate, lies about 10 nm from the outer leaflet of the basal cell plasma membrane (114,115). Filaments, 5 nm to 7 nm thick, called anchoring filaments, extend from the basal cell plasma membrane to the lamina densa, traversing the lamina lucida (Fig. 3-16). Filaments arising from the plasma membrane beneath the attachment plaque of a half-desmosome extend vertically to the underlying sub-basal cell dense plaque and from there to the lamina densa, whereas filaments not attached to sub-basal cell dense plaques show an irregular "criss-crossing" course from the basal cell plasma membrane to the lamina densa.

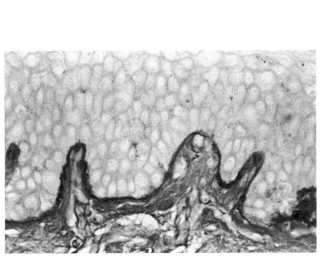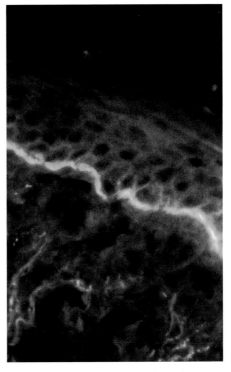

FIGURE 3-15. Demonstration of normal basement membrane zone separating epidermal and dermal layers by PAS stain **(A)**. By direct immunofluorescence staining for the basement membrane-associated structural protein, bullous pemphigoid antigen, a linear band is observed along the dermal–epidermal junction **(B)**.

Anchoring fibrils are short, curved structures with an irregularly spaced cross-banding of their central portions (116). They fan out at either end, the distal part inserting into the lamina densa and the proximal part terminating in the papillary dermis or looping around and merging in the lamina densa. They insert into amorphous patches con-

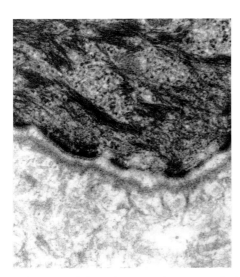

FIGURE 3-16. Transmission electron microscopy of the basement membrane separating the epidermis and dermis. Hemidesmosomes, lamina lucida, lamina densa, and anchoring fibrils may all be seen in this image.

taining type IV collagen, which is the main component of the lamina densa (116,117). Anchoring fibrils derive, at least in part, from the dermis and contain type VII collagen, as shown by immunoelectron microscopic localization of type VII collagen antibodies to anchoring fibrils (118). Besides anchoring fibrils, elastic fibers consisting of microfibril bundles and individual microfibrils approximately 10 nm in diameter are attached to the undersurface of the lamina densa. Three varieties of elastic tissue exist: oxytalan, elaunin, and elastic fibers (119). The oxytalan fibers consisting of microfibrils form a thin, superficial network perpendicular to the dermoepidermal junction. They originate from a plexus of elaunin fibers located parallel to the dermoepidermal junction in the upper dermis. The elaunin fibers are connected with the thicker elastic fibers of the middle and deep dermis. Effective anchoring of the epidermis to the dermis is a function largely of the anchoring fibrils; anchoring of the basement membrane by oxytalan fibers is quite sparse (120). Also, the diminution and ultimate disappearance of oxytalan fibers in aging skin indicates that they are of minor importance in the coherence between epidermis and dermis (119).

Molecular Anatomy

Immunoelectron microscopy has greatly assisted in correlating molecular composition and basement membrane

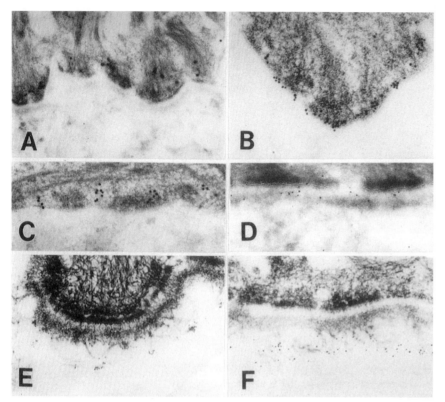

FIGURE 3-17. Immunoultrastructural mapping of molecular components of normal human basement membrane zone. **(A)** 230-kDa Bullous pemphigoid antigen in the intracellular portion of hemidesmosomes, where keratin filaments insert. **(B)** 180-kDa Bullous pemphigoid antigen, a transmembranous molecule along the plasma membrane of hemidesmosomes. **(C)** Desmoyokin, a nonhemidesmosomal and nondesmosomal plasma membrane protein here localizing to the basal cell membrane region adjacent to the basement membrane. **(D)** Laminin 5 (kalinin/nicein/epiligrin) within the lamina lucida. **(E)** Epidermolysis bullosa acquisita antigen showing localization to both ends of anchoring fibrils corresponding to the NC1 domain of type VII collagen. **(F)** Type VII collagen, collagenous domain, with typical central reactivity pattern within anchoring fibrils. (Courtesy of Hiroshi Shimizu, M.D., Ph.D.)

zone ultrastructure (Fig. 3-17). The cytoskeletal intermediate filaments within basal keratinocytes that insert into hemidesmosomes are composed predominantly of keratins 14 and 5 (see Yancey [121] for review). Hemidesmosomes contain bullous pemphigoid antigen 1 (BPAG1; 230 kD), bullous pemphigoid antigen 2 (BPAG2; 180 kD), integrin α6β4 (Fig. 3-13), and other molecules not as yet fully characterized. Bullous pemphigoid antigens are easily demonstrated by immunofluorescence as a smooth linear band that separates the epidermal and dermal layers (Fig. 3-15). Both BPAG2 and α6β4 integrin extend from the basal cell membrane into the lamina lucida, where anchoring filaments are observed by electron microscopy. Proteins associated with these anchoring filaments include laminin 5 (also called kalinin, nicein, epiligrin), and the surrounding lamina lucida is composed of laminin 1 and nidogen (entactin). The lamina densa is comprised primarily of type IV collagen. Although the molecular binding interactions are undoubtedly complex, it is known that α6β4 integrin is a receptor for laminin 1 and 5, and that laminin 5 (epiligrin) is a ligand for α3β1 integrin also expressed by basal keratinocytes. Such adhesive interactions are likely to contribute to the anchoring of basal cells to underlying lamina lucida. Nidogen within the lamina lucida is a 150-kD protein that facilitates adhesion between specific domains of laminin and type IV collagen within the adjacent lamina densa. The lamina densa itself is anchored to the underlying dermis in part by anchoring fibrils composed of type

VII collagen. Defects in basement membrane zone adhesive molecules due to autoantibodies or gene defects may result in disorders characterized by dermal–epidermal separation, as in bullous pemphigoid (BPAG1 and 2 are targets), cicatricial pemphigoid and Herlitz-type junctional epidermolysis bullosa (laminin 5 is the target), and epidermolysis bullosa acquisita and dystrophic epidermolysis bullosa (type VII collagen is the target).

HAIR FOLLICLES

Embryology

Hair germs, or primary epithelial germs, are first observed in embryos in the eyebrow region and the scalp during the third month of gestation (122). The general development of hair begins in the fourth fetal month in the face and scalp and gradually extends in a cephalo-caudal direction. Thus, during the fourth month, while some hair follicles on the head are already well matured and are producing hair, most of those on the trunk are barely differentiated (123). In addition, new primary epithelial germs keep developing between earlier ones so that, in any section obtained from the beginning of the fifth month up to birth, hair structures in different stages of development are found (124).

Hair germs, or primary epithelial germs, in their earliest stage of development consist of an area of crowding of deeply basophilic cells in the basal cell layer of the epider-

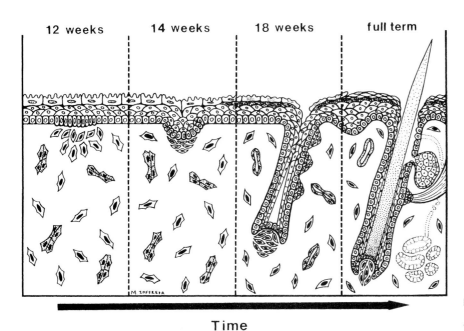

Time

FIGURE 3-18. Schematic overview of embryonic trichogenesis in human skin. (Courtesy of Michael Ioffreda, M.D.)

mis. Subsequently, the areas of crowding develop into buds that protrude into the dermis (Figs. 3-18 and 3-19). Beneath each bud lies a group of mesenchymal cells from which the dermal hair papilla is later formed. As the primary epithelial germ grows deeper into the dermis under induction by the underlying mesenchymal cells, it forms first the hair peg and then, as the hair matrix cells and the dermal hair papilla develop, the bulbous hair peg (125). Electron microscopic examination of hair germ buds and hair pegs of the embryo has revealed that relatively large cytoplasmic processes extend like pseudopodia from their basal cells through breaks in the basement membrane into the dermal mesenchyme. The mesenchymal cells that are concentrated beneath the hair germs are in contact with the basement membrane of the hair germs either directly or indirectly through various types of fibrils. Also, the mesenchymal cells are connected to each other through desmosome-like cell-to-cell contacts (122). These morphologic findings suggest that the "hair germ mesenchymal cells" pull down the hair germ as they move deeper in the dermal mesenchyme.

As the bulbous peg stage is reached, differentiation occurs in the lower and upper portions of the hair follicle and in the overlying epidermis. Differentiation in the lower portion of the follicle leads to the formation of the hair cone and subsequently to the formation of the hair, the cuticle, and the two inner root sheaths. The hair canal in the upper portion of the hair follicle, located at the level of the upper dermis, is formed by the premature death of the central core cells before they have become keratinized. In contrast, the intraepidermal portion of the hair canal is produced by means of premature keratinization and subsequent dissolution of the matrix cells of the cordlike hair canal extending obliquely through the epidermis. By the time the hair cone has reached the upper portion of the hair follicle, the hair canal is already open within the dermis and epidermis (126).

The hair follicles grow at a slant and, in the late hair peg or early bulbous stage, develop two or three bulges on their undersurface The lowest of the three bulges develops into the attachment for the arrector pili muscle; the middle bulge differentiates into the sebaceous gland. The uppermost bulge, if present, either involutes or develops into an apocrine gland. Apocrine glands develop only in certain regions (127). Formation of the intraepidermal portion of the hair canal through cellular destruction is found on electron microscopy to be associated with the presence of lyso-

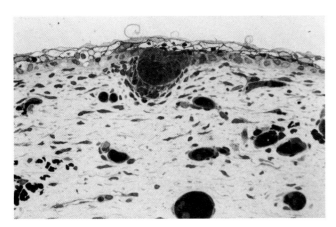

FIGURE 3-19. Histology of early trichogenesis, showing formation of primary epithelial germ with associated underlying mesenchymal condensation (1-micron-thick, plastic-embedded section).

some-like dense bodies. Thus, the intraepidermal portion of the hair canal seems to form by lysosomal digestion of cellular cytoplasm analogous to the formation of the intraepidermal eccrine duct and of the intrafollicular apocrine duct (126).

In sections treated with the dopa reaction or stained with ammoniated silver nitrate, melanocytes are distributed at random in primary epithelial germs and in hair pegs. During the bulbous peg stage, the melanocytes concentrate in the so-called pigment matrix region (the basal cell layer lying on top of the dermal hair papilla) and to a lesser degree in the lower hair bulb located lateral to the dermal hair papilla (124).

Normal Microanatomy

General Anatomical Features

The hair follicle, with its hair in longitudinal sections, consists of three parts: the lower portion, extending from the base of the follicle to the insertion of the arrector pili muscle; the middle portion, or isthmus, a rather short section, extending from the insertion of the arrector pili to the entrance of the sebaceous duct; and the upper portion, or infundibulum, extending from the entrance of the sebaceous duct to the follicular orifice. The lower portion of the hair follicle is composed of five major portions: the dermal hair papilla; the hair matrix; the hair, consisting inward to outward of medulla, cortex, and hair cuticle; the inner root

sheath, consisting inward to outward of inner root sheath cuticle, Huxley layer, and Henle layer; and the outer root sheath (Figs. 3-20 and 3-21). This bulb region gives rise to the formation of the hair shaft that occupies the overlying follicular canal (Fig. 3-22).

Cycles of Hair Growth

The histologic appearance of the hair follicle changes considerably during the hair cycle, which causes the hair to turn from an anagen hair into a catagen hair, then into a telogen hair, and finally into a new anagen hair. In the adult scalp, the anagen stage, the phase of active growth, lasts at least 3 years; catagen, the phase of regression, lasts about 3 weeks; and telogen, the resting period, lasts about 3 months. At any one time, approximately 84% of scalp hairs are in anagen stage, 2% in catagen, and 14% in telogen (128). These ratios are important in evaluating abnormalities in the hair cycle in biopsies of partially alopecic scalp. The daily hair growth rate averages about 0.4 mm on the scalp.

During its active growth, or anagen stage, the hair follicle shows at its lower pole a knob-like expansion, the hair bulb, composed of matrix cells and melanocytes. A small, egg-shaped dermal structure, the dermal hair papilla, protrudes into the hair bulb. The papilla induces and maintains the growth of the hair follicle (129). Because of the presence of large amounts of acid mucopolysaccharides in its ground substance, the dermal hair papilla stains posi-

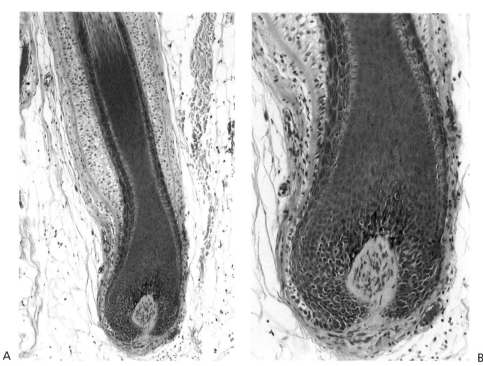

FIGURE 3-20. Histology of the lower portion of the human hair follicle. **(A)** and **(B)** Conventional histology. *(continued)*

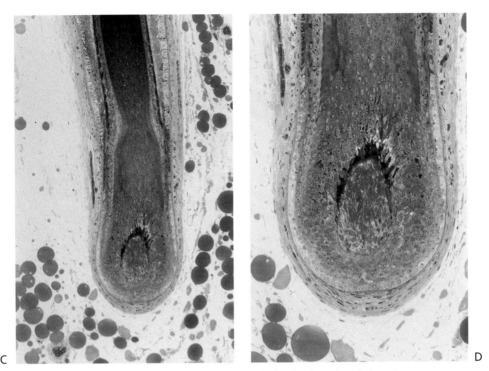

FIGURE 3-20. *(continued)* **(C)** and **(D)** One-micron-thick, plastic-embedded section.

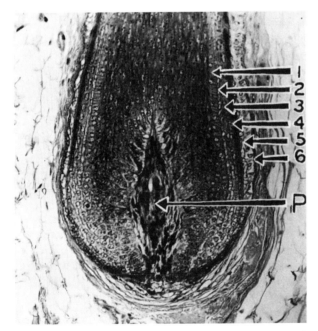

FIGURE 3-21. Lower portion of an anagen hair follicle. The follicular papilla (*P*), composed of connective tissue, protrudes into the hair bulb. The various linings of the hair can be recognized. From the outside to the inside, they are (*1*) the hair cuticle; (*2*) the inner root sheath cuticle; (*3*) the Huxley layer; (*4*) the Henle layer; (*5*) the outer root sheath; and (*6*) the glassy or vitreous layer.

tively with Alcian blue and metachromatically with toluidine blue. Because positive staining with Alcian blue takes place at pH 2.5 and at pH 0.5, it can be concluded that the ground substance of the hair papilla contains nonsulfated acid mucopolysaccharides, such as hyaluronic acid, and sulfated acid mucopolysaccharides, such as chondroitin sulfate (130). In addition, there is considerable alkaline phosphatase activity in the hair papilla during the anagen stage as a result of the presence of large numbers of capillary loops (131,132). In persons with dark hair, large amounts of melanin can be seen in the dermal hair papilla situated within melanophages.

Bulb and Lowermost Portion of Hair Follicle

The pluripotential cells of the hair matrix present in the hair bulb give rise to the hair and to the inner root sheath. In contrast, the outer root sheath represents a downward extension of the epidermis. The cells of the hair matrix have large vesicular nuclei and a deeply basophilic cytoplasm. Dopa-positive melanocytes are interspersed mainly between the basal cells of the hair matrix lying on top of the dermal hair papilla and, to a lesser degree, between the basal cells of the hair matrix located lateral to the hair papilla (124). Melanin, varying in quantity in accordance with the color of the hair, is produced in these melanocytes and is incorporated into the future cells of the hair through phagocytosis of the distal portion of dendritic processes by future hair

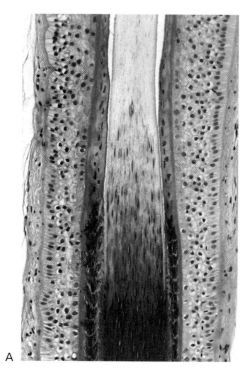
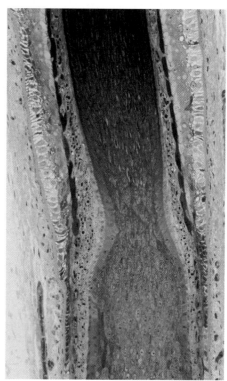

FIGURE 3-22. The mid to lower segment of the hair follicle showing transition zone demarcating the formation of the hair shaft within the follicular canal. Also note the highly glycogenated clear cells forming the outer root sheath of the follicle. **(A)** Conventional section. **(B)** One-micron-thick, plastic-embedded section.

cells. This transfer of melanin is analogous to that observed from epidermal melanocytes to keratinocytes.

As they move upward, the cells arising from the hair matrix differentiate into six different types of cells, each of which keratinizes at a different level. The outermost layer of the inner root sheath, the Henle layer, keratinizes first, thus establishing a firm coat around the soft central parts. The two apposed cuticles covering the inside of the inner root sheath and the outside of the hair keratinize next, followed by Huxley's layer. The hair cortex then follows, and the medulla is last (133).

The hair medulla of human hair is often difficult to find by routine light microscopy, because it may be discontinuous or even absent (134). It is more readily recognizable by polariscopic examination, because, unlike the cortex, the only partially keratinized medulla contains hardly any doubly refractile structures (135). If the medulla is seen by light microscopy in human hairs, it appears amorphous because of only partial keratinization.

The hair cortex consists of cells that, during their upward growth from the hair matrix, keratinize gradually by losing their nuclei and becoming filled with keratin fibrils. The process of keratinization takes place without the formation of keratohyaline granules, as seen in the keratinizing epidermis, or of trichohyalin granules, as seen in the inner root sheath. Thus, the keratin of the hair cortex represents hard keratin, in contrast to the keratin of the inner

root sheath, which, like that of the epidermis, represents soft keratin (136).

The hair cuticle (Fig. 3-21), located peripheral to the hair cortex, consists of overlapping cells arranged like shingles and pointing upward with their peripheral portion. The cells of the hair cuticle are tightly interlocked with the cells of the inner root sheath cuticle, resulting in the firm attachment of the hair to its inner root sheath. The hair and the inner root sheath move upward in unison (137).

The inner root sheath is composed of three concentric layers; from the inside to the outside, these are the inner root sheath cuticle (2 in Fig. 3-21), the Huxley layer (3 in Fig. 3-21), and the Henle layer (4 in Fig. 3-21). None of these three layers contains melanin. All three layers keratinize, unlike the cells of the hair cortex and of the hair cuticle, by means of trichohyalin granules. These granules resemble the keratohyaline granules of the epidermis, although they stain eosinophilic, in contrast to the basophilic-staining keratohyaline granules of the epidermis. Closest to the hair is the single-layered, inner root sheath cuticle, consisting of flattened overlapping cells that point downward in the direction of the hair bulb. Because the cells of the hair cuticle point upward, these two types of cells interlock tightly. Trichohyalin granules are few in the inner root sheath cuticle cells. The Huxley layer, which usually consists of two rows of cells, develops numerous trichohyalin granules at the level of the keratogenous zone of the hair. The Henle layer, only one cell layer thick and the first layer to undergo keratinization, already has many trichohyalin granules at its emergence from the hair matrix (138). After having become fully keratinized, the cells of all three layers composing the inner root sheath disintegrate when they reach the isthmus of the hair follicle, which extends from the area of attachment of the arrector pili muscle to the entrance of the sebaceous duct. The cells of the inner root sheath thus do not contribute to the emerging hair (139).

The outer root sheath (Figs. 3-21 and 3-22) extends upward from the matrix cells at the lower end of the hair bulb to the entrance of the sebaceous duct, where it changes into surface epidermis, which lines the upper portion, or infundibulum, of the hair follicle. The outer root sheath is thinnest at the level of the hair bulb, gradually increases in thickness, and is thickest in the middle portion of the hair follicle, the isthmus. In its lower portion, below the isthmus, the outer root sheath is covered by the inner root sheath and does not undergo keratinization. The outer root sheath cells have a clear, vacuolated cytoplasm because of the presence of considerable amounts of glycogen. In contrast to the surface epidermis lining the infundibulum, which contains active, melanin-producing melanocytes in its basal layer, the basal layer of the outer root sheath contains only inactive, amelanotic melanocytes demonstrable with toluidine blue. However, these inactive melanocytes can become melanin-producing cells after skin injuries, such as dermabrasion, when they increase in number and migrate upward into the regenerating upper portion of the outer root sheath and into the regenerating epidermis (140).

Follicular Isthmus

In the middle portion of the hair follicle, the so-called isthmus, which extends upward from the attachment of the arrector pili muscle (so-called bulge region) to the entrance of the sebaceous duct, the outer root sheath is no longer covered by the inner root sheath, which by then has keratinized and disintegrated. The outer root sheath therefore undergoes keratinization. This type of keratinization, referred to

as trichilemmal keratinization (141), produces large, homogeneous keratinized cells without the formation of keratohyaline granules. Trichilemmal keratinization is found also in catagen and telogen hairs and in trichilemmal cysts and trichilemmal tumors. The bulge region at the site of the arrector pili muscle insertion is poorly defined in human follicles and difficult to detect in routine sections. When it is visualized, it consists of several knobby protuberances and ridges composed of relatively undifferentiated follicular keratinocytes with putative stem cell capability (9).

The upper portion of the hair follicle above the entrance of the sebaceous duct, the infundibulum, is lined by surface epidermis, which, like the sebaceous duct, undergoes keratinization with the formation of keratohyaline granules. The infundibulum contains a number of dendritic nonkeratinocytes upon ultrastructural examination, and immunohistochemistry reveals numerous CD1a-positive Langerhans cells within the infundibula of normal adult anagen hairs.

The glassy or vitreous layer (6 in Fig. 3-21) forms a homogeneous, eosinophilic zone peripheral to the outer root sheath. Like the subepidermal basement membrane zone, it is PAS positive and diastase resistant, but it differs from the subepidermal basement membrane zone by being thicker and visible with routine stains. It is thickest around the lower third of the hair follicle. Peripheral to the vitreous layer lies the fibrous root sheath, which is composed of thick collagen bundles.

Sebaceous Glands

The sebaceous glands are well developed at the time of birth, most likely because of maternal hormones. After a few months, they undergo considerable atrophy. At puberty, as a result of increased androgen output, the sebaceous glands become greatly enlarged (142).

A sebaceous gland may consist of only one lobule, but often has several lobules leading into a common excretory duct composed of stratified squamous epithelium (Fig. 3-23A). Sebaceous glands, being holocrine glands, form their secretion by decomposition of their cells. In sebaceous

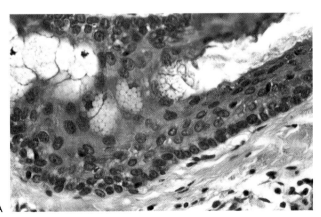
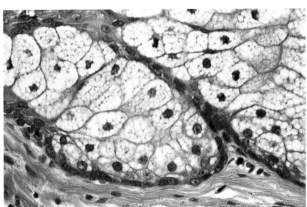

A   B

FIGURE 3-23. Sebaceous duct **(A)** and gland **(B)** budding from human anagen hair follicle.

glands of the skin, the pilosebaceous follicle into which the sebaceous duct leads may possess a large hair or a vellus hair that may be too small to reach the skin surface. There is no relationship between the size of the sebaceous gland and the size of the associated hair. For example, in the center of the face and on the forehead, where the sebaceous glands are very large, the associated hairs are of the vellus type.

Each sebaceous lobule possesses a peripheral layer of cuboidal, deeply basophilic cells that usually contain no lipid droplets (Fig. 3-23B). The more centrally located cells contain lipid droplets, which can be detected if lipid stains are used on formalin-fixed frozen sections, but in routinely processed sections in which the lipid has been extracted, the cytoplasm of these cells appears as a delicate network. The nucleus is centrally located. In the portion of the lobule located closest to the duct, the cells disintegrate. One sees coalesced lipid droplets in the excretory duct in lipid stains and amorphous material in routine stains.

The composition of lipids in the sebaceous glands is not uniform. Thus, under polarized light, doubly refractile lipids may be present in small to moderate amounts or may be absent (143). Histochemical examination reveals the presence of triglycerides and small amounts of phospholipids. Esterified cholesterol is present, but there is no free cholesterol. Waxes are also present, but they are not identifiable by histochemical means (143).

Electron microscopic studies have confirmed that the cells of the peripheral layer usually contain no lipid vacuoles. Analogous to the basal cells of the epidermis, they are attached to a basement membrane by half-desmosomes (144). In the cells located further inside, one can observe a marked increase in the volume of cytoplasm, the appearance of smooth endoplasmic reticulum, and the formation of fine lipid material within its cisterns. This indicates that the smooth endoplasmic reticulum synthesizes the lipid (144,145). In the Golgi region, the synthesized lipid material aggregates as lipid droplets. Toward the center of the sebaceous lobules, the cells, as a result of continued lipid synthesis, are almost completely filled with lipid droplets (Fig. 3-24). Although a true limiting membrane is clearly present around the lipid droplets in the incipient stages, none is detectable in mature droplets (146).

Lysosomal enzymes bring about the physiologic autolysis that occurs in the holocrine secretion. Histochemical staining of electron microscopic sections for lysosomal enzymes, such as acid phosphatase and aryl sulfatase, reveals an increasing number of lysosomes as the sebaceous cells become more lipidized. In the disintegrating cells located in the preductal region, the acid phosphatase and aryl sulfatase activity is most pronounced, but this activity is largely outside of lysosomes, because the lysosomes have released their contents in their function as "suicide bags" (147,148). Prior to the sudden disintegration of the sebaceous cells an abrupt conversion of −SH to S–S linkages of

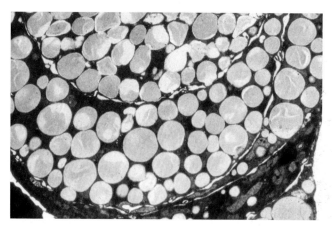

FIGURE 3-24. Transmission electron microscopy of sebaceous lobule. Lipid is visible as rounded homogeneous bodies filling the cytoplasm of mature sebocytes.

proteins occurs in sebaceous glands just as in epidermis and hair (149).

Regional Variation

Hair follicles vary considerably in different anatomic regions and according to age and sex. In adults, deep anagen hairs (extending into subcutaneous fat) are typically found on the scalp and male beard area, whereas vellus hairs typify the female face and nonbeard area facial regions of men. Hair of extremities and trunk generally can be differentiated from scalp hair by the more superficial location of the bulbs and diminished density. Sebaceous glands are present everywhere on the skin except on the palms and soles. On the skin, they are found in association with hair structures. In addition, free sebaceous glands that are not associated with hair structures occur in some areas of modified skin, such as the nipple and areola of both the male and female breasts. There, they occur over the entire surface of the nipple and in Montgomery's areolar tubercles, each of which contains several sebaceous lobules in association with a lactiferous duct. Free sebaceous glands are found also on the labia minora and the inner aspect of the prepuce. However, sebaceous glands occur only very rarely on the glans of the penis (150). The not-infrequent presence of free sebaceous glands on the vermilion border of the lips and on the buccal mucosa is known as Fordyce's condition. The meibomian glands of the eyelids are modified sebaceous glands.

Specialized Structure and Function

Hair Cycle

The hair cycle ensures that periodically, entirely new hair shafts are produced, as well as serves as an intrinsic regulator of maximum hair length. The hair cycle consists of the involutionary stage (catagen) and the end stage (telogen) of

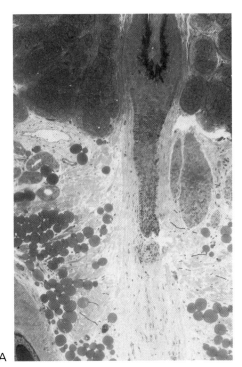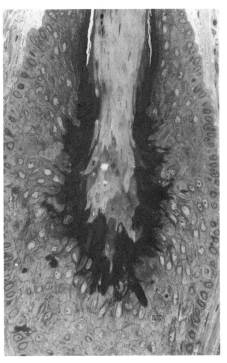

A   B

FIGURE 3-25. Follicular involution. Note the thin epithelial cord retracting within a fibrous sheath that demarcates the course of the preexisting anagen follicle **(A)**, and the formation of a club hair bordered by dense keratin **(B)**.

the old hair and its replacement by a young, new hair (early anagen). At the onset of the catagen stage, mitotic activity and melanin production in the hair bulb cease. Next, the bulb shrinks, setting the dermal hair papilla free (138). As the hair moves upward, the lower portion of the follicle involutes. The reduction in follicle size results from cell deletion by apoptosis, or programmed cell death (151). The lower follicle thus becomes a thin cord of epithelial cells (Fig. 3-25A) surrounded by the fibrous root sheath, which is wrinkled in thick folds. Also, as the hair moves upward, growth of the inner root sheath ceases, so that the lower end of the hair shaft becomes surrounded by dense keratin, referred to as trichilemmal keratin, that is formed by the outer root sheath without the interposition of keratohyaline granules (141) (Fig. 3-25B). This then represents the club hair of the catagen stage.

Next, the thin cord of epithelial cells retracts upward, faithfully followed by the underlying dermal hair papilla, which thus also moves upward. The cord of epithelial cells shortens until it forms only a small nipple-like downward protrusion from the club hair, called the secondary hair germ. Under it lies the dermal hair papilla. With the hair follicle decreased to about one third of its former length, the lowest portion of the hair follicle lies at the level of the attachment of the arrector pili. The lower portion of the hair is encased in trichilemmal keratin and completely surrounded by the outer root sheath. Folds of the fibrous root

sheath extend downward from the hair follicle. At this point, the hair has reached the telogen stage (152).

When regrowth of the hair begins, the secondary hair germ begins to elongate by cell division and grows down as an epithelial column together with the dermal hair papilla inside of the old, collapsed fibrous root sheath of the previous hair. As it is growing down, the lower end of the epithelial column becomes invaginated by the dermal hair papilla. A new hair bulb is formed, representing the early anagen stage. By subsequent differentiation, a new hair arises. Thus, the formation of an active hair follicle from the secondary germ recapitulates the embryonic pattern of development of the hair from the primary hair germ (152). Recent experimental data in rodents suggests that the primary site that gives rise to new hair germ during follicular regrowth is the bulge region of the follicle where a population of normally slow-cycling, relatively undifferentiated cells with features of stem cells reside (9). Stimulation of the bulge region, which persists throughout telogen, then gives rise to new hair germ and the developing anagen follicle (bulge activation hypothesis).

Hair Color

Three types of melanosomes are present in hair. Erythromelanin granules, seen in red hair, are polymorphous and have an irregular internal structure. The other two types of granules, homogeneous eumelanin granules and lamellated pheomelanin granules, are found in varying proportions in blond and dark hair and are round to oval. Dark hair contains more melanosomes than light hair, and the melanosomes are largely of the homogeneous eumelanin type; in light hair, lamellated pheomelanin melanosomes predominate (153).

In grey and white hair, the melanocytes in the basal layer of the hair matrix are greatly reduced in number or are absent. The melanocytes that are present show degenerative changes, especially of their melanosomes (154). The hair shafts contain only detritus of melanin or none at all (153).

Follicular Immunity

The number of CD1a-positive Langerhans cells in normal follicular infundibula raises questions concerning their role in follicular immunity. Such populations could be appropriately sequestered from harmful environmental agents, such as ultraviolet light, and thus serve as a reservoir of antigen presenting cells as well as an evolutionary rationale for preservation of hair follicles in *Homo sapiens* no longer in need of the thermal or protective benefits of hair shafts. Such follicle-associated immune tissue has been evidenced in clinical settings of primarily follicular pathology in contact dermatitis, as well as in sequential studies of human experimentally induced contact allergy where the first sentinel lymphocytes selectively home to follicular infundibula (155).

ECCRINE AND APOCRINE GLANDS

The apocrine glands differ from eccrine glands in origin, distribution, size, and mode of secretion. The eccrine glands primarily serve in the regulation of heat, and the apocrine glands represent scent glands.

Embryology

Eccrine glands are present in mammals, with the exception of anthropoid apes, only on the soles. Their presence in other parts of the skin in humans is a late development from the phylogenetic point of view. Accordingly, the eccrine glands develop in humans earlier on the palms and soles than elsewhere. On the palms and soles, eccrine gland germs are first seen early in the fourth gestational month (156). In the early part of the fifth fetal month, they develop in the axillae, and near the end of the fifth month, they begin to appear over the remainder of the body (123). The eccrine gland germs begin as areas of crowding of deeply basophilic cells in the basal layer of the epidermis. They differ from primary epithelial germs only slightly by

being narrower and by showing fewer mesenchymal cells at their base. Like hair follicles, eccrine glands may be seen at one time in different stages of development. In embryos 16 weeks old, some eccrine glands are already beginning to form coils on the palms and soles, while new eccrine gland germs are still forming in the epidermis (157).

At the time of lumen formation, the intradermal duct and the secretory segment show a wall composed of two layers of cells, an inner layer of luminal cells and an outer layer of basal cells. Although the dermal duct continues to consist of these two layers of cells throughout life, the two layers in the secretory segment undergo differentiation: the luminal cells differentiate into tall, columnar secretory cells extending from the basement membrane to the luminal border, and the basal cells differentiate into secretory cells or into myoepithelial cells, which appear as pyramidal, relatively small cells wedged at the base between secretory cells (156). The differentiation into secretory and myoepithelial cells in the secretory segment is well advanced on the palms and soles of embryos 22 weeks old. At the time of birth, the appearance of the eccrine glands resembles that of adult eccrine glands.

On electron microscopic examination, the embryonic lumen formation occurring in the eccrine dermal duct and in the secretory segment differs from the lumen formation occurring in the intraepidermal portion of the eccrine duct. (This difference exists also in the apocrine gland.) In the eccrine dermal duct, lumen formation results from a separation of desmosomes between apposing luminal cells and the subsequent formation of microvilli at the luminal surfaces. In the secretory portion, lumen formation also begins with the separation of luminal cells from one another and is followed by the appearance of numerous small secretory vesicles and dense secretory granules in the secretory cells (156).

In the intraepidermal portion of the eccrine duct, intracytoplasmic vacuoles form through lysosomal action within the inner cells of the intraepidermal eccrine duct units. These vacuoles enlarge, coalesce, and break through the plasma membrane. Through coalescence with similarly produced vacuoles from adjoining inner cells, a patent extracellular lumen is formed. After formation of the lumen, the intraepidermal eccrine duct unit undergoes keratinization—the outer cells at the level of the midsquamous layer and the inner cells at the level of the stratum granulosum (156).

In contrast to eccrine glands, apocrine glands develop only in certain areas. Wherever they form, they develop from the upper bulge of hair follicles that are in the early bulbous peg stage and show a hair cone. The formation of apocrine glands begins late in the fourth month and continues until late in embryonic life, as long as new hair follicles develop. In the earliest stage, a solid epithelial cord projects into the perifollicular mesenchyme at a right angle to the long axis of the hair follicle and then grows downward past the developing sebaceous gland and arrector pili bulge. By the time the tip of the epithelial cord has reached the level of the sebaceous gland, the intradermal ductal lumen begins to form, as does the intrafollicular lumen (127). At the time of birth, there is as yet no recognizable myoepithelial layer of cells around the secretory portion of the apocrine glands (123).

Electron microscopic examination shows that the apocrine dermal duct, like the eccrine duct, forms through separation of apposing luminal cells. In contrast, the intrafollicular lumen forms through lysosomal formation of intracytoplasmic vacuoles in neighboring cells and subsequent extracytoplasmic coalescence of these vacuoles (127). The formation of the intrafollicular portion of the apocrine duct is analogous to the formation of the intraepidermal portion of the eccrine duct.

Normal Microanatomy

Eccrine glands are composed of three segments: intraepidermal duct, intradermal duct, and secretory portion. The secretory portion makes up about one half of the basal coil, the other half being composed of duct. The basal coil lies either at the border between the dermis and the subcutaneous fat or in the lower third of the dermis. When located in the lower dermis, it is surrounded by fatty tissue that connects with the subcutaneous fat. Eccrine glands are highlighted by immunohistochemical stains for S-100 protein and carcinoembryonic antigen.

The intraepidermal eccrine duct extends from the base of a rete ridge to the surface and follows a spiral course (Fig. 3-26A). The cells composing the duct are different from the cells of the surrounding epidermis in that they are derived from dermal duct cells through mitosis and upward migration (158). For this reason, the intraepidermal eccrine duct has been referred to as acrosyringium or the epidermal sweat duct unit. The intraepidermal eccrine duct consists of a single layer of inner or luminal cells and two or three rows of outer cells. The ductal cells begin to keratinize, as evidenced by the presence of keratohyaline granules, at a lower level than the cells of the surrounding epidermis, in the middle squamous layer, and are fully keratinized at the level of the stratum granulosum of the surrounding epidermis (159). Before keratinization, the intraepidermal lumen is lined by an eosinophilic cuticle.

The intradermal eccrine duct is composed of two layers of small, cuboidal, deeply basophilic epithelial cells (Fig. 3-26B). Unlike the secretory portion of the eccrine gland, the eccrine duct has no peripheral hyaline basement membrane zone, but the lumen of the duct is lined with a deeply eosinophilic, homogeneous cuticle that is PAS-positive and diastase-resistant.

The secretory portion of the eccrine gland shows only one distinct layer composed of secretory cells (Fig. 3-26C).

The presence of only one distinct layer is due to the fact that the cells of the outer layer have become differentiated into either secretory or myoepithelial cells during the sixth to eighth months of embryonic life. The secretory cells lining the lumen consist equally of two types, clear cells and dark cells. The clear cells generally are broader at the base than they are near the lumen, appear somewhat larger than the dark cells, and contain very faint, small granules. The dark cells are broadest near the lumen and contain numerous basophilic granules (160). The clear cells contain PAS-positive, diastase-labile glycogen, and the dark cells contain PAS-positive, diastase-resistant mucopolysaccharides. The clear cells secrete abundant amounts of aqueous material together with glycogen; the dark cells secrete sialomucin (161). This substance contains both neutral and nonsulfated acid mucopolysaccharides, is positive for PAS and for Alcian blue at pH 2.4, and is resistant to diastase and hyaluronidase. Prolonged sweating leads to a depletion of glycogen in the clear cells (162). The myoepithelial cells possess a small spindle-shaped nucleus and long contractile fibrils. The fibrils run in a spiral, their long axes aligned obliquely to the direction of the secretory tubule. Delivery of sweat to the skin surface is greatly aided by myoepithelial contraction (163). Peripheral to the myoepithelial cells lies a hyaline basement membrane zone containing collagen fibers. The transition from the secretory to the ductal epithelium is abrupt (Fig. 3-26B). The lumen of the secretory portion of the eccrine gland, measuring approximately 20 μm in diameter, is small in comparison with that of the apocrine gland (compare Figs. 3-26C and 3-27). The lumen of the eccrine duct measures about 15 μm across.

The ultrastructure of the secretory portion of the eccrine gland reveals an admixture of clear cells containing glycogen granules, and dark cells containing large electron-dense granules situated within the luminal cytoplasm. The luminal membranes display short microvilli. Adjacent clear cells show prominent villous membrane folds that interdigitate, as well as intercellular canaliculi lined by microvilli.

Apocrine glands are tubular glands, the secretory cells of which pass through various stages. Schiefferdecker, who in 1917 first described these glands, observed that, during secretion, part of the cell was pinched off and released into the lumen (164). He referred to this process as decapitation secretion. He chose the name *apocrine* for these glands to indicate that part of the cytoplasm of the secretory cells was pinched off ("apo" means "off").

Apocrine glands, like eccrine glands, are composed of three segments: the intraepidermal duct, the intradermal duct, and the secretory portion. Because apocrine glands originate from the hair germ, or primary epithelial germ, the duct of an apocrine gland usually leads to a pilosebaceous follicle, entering it in the infundibulum, above the entrance of the sebaceous duct. An occasional apocrine duct, however, opens directly on the skin surface close to a

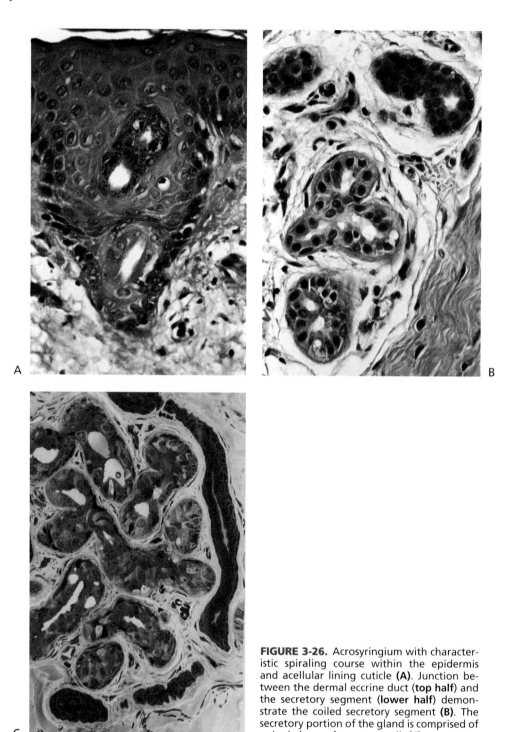

FIGURE 3-26. Acrosyringium with character-istic spiraling course within the epidermis and acellular lining cuticle **(A)**. Junction be-tween the dermal eccrine duct (**top half**) and the secretory segment (**lower half**) demon-strate the coiled secretory segment **(B)**. The secretory portion of the gland is comprised of a single layer of secretory cells **(C)**.

pilosebaceous follicle. In contrast to eccrine glands, the basal coil of apocrine glands, which is located in the subcu-taneous fat, is composed entirely of secretory cells and con-tains no ductal cells.

The ductal portion of the apocrine glands has the same histologic appearance as the eccrine duct, showing a double layer of basophilic cells and a periluminal eosinophilic cuti-cle. The intrafollicular or intraepidermal portion of the

apocrine duct is straight and not spiral in appearance, as is the intraepidermal eccrine duct.

The secretory portion of the apocrine gland shows a sin-gle layer of secretory cells, because the outer layer of cells consists of myoepithelial cells, just as in the eccrine gland. The secretory cells vary greatly in height, depending on the stage of secretion. Variation in height may be seen even in the cross-section of the same secretory tubule (165). The

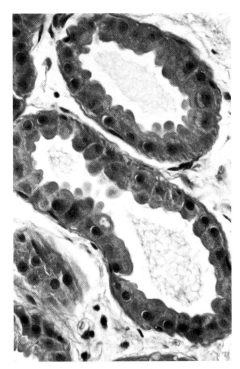

FIGURE 3-27. High magnification of apocrine gland segment showing typical decapitation-type secretion and characteristically dilated lumens.

secretory cells possess an eosinophilic cytoplasm. Except in the apical portion, they contain in their cytoplasm fairly large, PAS-positive, diastase-resistant granules, which appear much larger than similar granules seen in the dark secretory cells of eccrine glands. In addition, the apocrine granules frequently contain iron. Maturation of the secretory cells is indicated by the formation of a dome-shaped apical cap (Fig. 3-27). Most of the apical cap is nearly free of large granules, but it contains numerous small, smooth vesicles about 50 nm in diameter. Beneath the apical cap, numerous large granules, both of the dark and of the light type, are seen by electron microscopy. The luminal plasma membrane shows a moderate number of microvilli. The lumen of the secretory portion of apocrine glands is large, measuring up to 200 μm in diameter, ten times the average diameter of the lumen of eccrine glands (Fig. 3-27). The myoepithelial cells contain numerous contractile fibers extending in a spiral fashion around the secretory tubules. A hyaline basement membrane zone containing collagen is seen peripheral to the myoepithelium.

The type of secretion occurring in apocrine glands consists of the release of portions of cytoplasm into the lumen (Fig. 3-27). Because of the cytoplasm in the secretion, apocrine secretion, in contrast to eccrine secretion, is visible in histologic sections stained with hematoxylin-eosin. The apocrine secretion contains amorphous, PAS-positive, diastase-resistant material originating from the granules that have dissolved in the apical portion of the secretory cells

(166). This PAS-positive material, like the secretion of the dark cells in eccrine glands, consists of sialomucin (161).

Regional Variation

Eccrine glands are present everywhere in the human skin; however, they are absent in areas of modified skin that lack all cutaneous appendages, that is, the vermilion border of the lips, the nail beds, the labia minora, the glans penis, and the inner aspect of the prepuce. They are found in greatest abundance on the palms and soles and in the axillae.

Apocrine glands are encountered in only a few areas: in the axillae, in the anogenital region, and as modified glands in the external ear canal (ceruminous glands), in the eyelid (Moll's glands), and in the breast (mammary glands). Occasionally, a few apocrine glands are found on the face, in the scalp, and on the abdomen; they usually are small and nonfunctional (167). Apocrine glands develop their secretory portion and become functional only at puberty. The multiple protuberances present in the areola of the female breast and referred to as Montgomery's areolar tubercles each contain a lactiferous duct and several superficially located sebaceous lobules whose ducts lead into the lactiferous duct (168,169).

Specialized Structure and Function

The eccrine sweat gland is engineered for temperature regulation (170). With approximately 3 million glands in the human integument weighing 35μg/gland, the average human boasts about 100 g of eccrine glands capable of producing a maximum of approximately 1.8 l of sweat/hour! The eccrine secretory coil is richly invested in a stroma rich in unmyelinated nerve fibers that are believed to play an important role in regulation of sweat production. Cholinergic stimulation of eccrine clear cells has been shown to increase cytosolic Ca (++) in a biphasic manner. This results in stimulation of both K (+) and Cl (−) membrane channels, resulting in a net efflux of KCl along with Na (+) from the cell. Such electrolyte shifts, associated with eater loss, underscore major metabolic implications of excessive eccrine sweating. Aside from potentially critical temperature regulation, the eccrine gland may contribute to general cutaneous homeostasis. For example, patients with congenital anhidrotic ectodermal dysplasia suffer from heat intolerance that cannot be alleviated by simply adding moisture to the skin surface, suggesting that vasodilatation associated with sweating may in some way be linked to eccrine function (170). There is abundant biologically active Il-1 in sweat (171), as well as numerous proteolytic enzymes, raising the possibility that eccrine sweat may possess pro-inflammatory or protective functions.

The mechanisms and rationale for apocrine-type secretion remain elusive. Decapitation secretion in apocrine glands comparable to that seen by light microscopy has been found on electron microscopic examination by Kurosumi (172) and associates and by Schaumburg–Lever and Lever (164). Although Kurosumi and co-workers did not actually observe decapitation, they found detached apical caps. Schaumburg–Lever and Lever found three types of secretion: merocrine, apocrine, and holocrine. In the apocrine type of secretion, three stages were observed: formation of an apical cap, formation of a dividing membrane at the base of the apical cap, and formation of tubules above and parallel to the dividing membrane, supplying a new plasma membrane for both the undersurface of the apical cap and the top of the residual cell, bringing about detachment of the apical cap. Convincing proof of the detachment of entire apical caps in apocrine glands has been provided through scanning microscopy by Inoue (173), who observed on each secretory cell a cytoplasmic luminal protuberance about 2 μm in diameter. In the early stage of secretion, the protuberance was hemispheric, but later increased in height to form a linguiform process.

The raison d'être for apocrine secretion in humans remains an enigma, although it may simply be an evolutionary vestige (musk glands of the deer and scent glands of the skunk are modified apocrine-type structures). The characteristic odor in human axillary sweat has recently been shown to reside in volatile C_6-C_{11} acids, with the most abundant being 3-methyl-2-hexenoic acid (174). This initially odorless apocrine secretion is formed at the skin surface from protein precursors via saponification or bacteriolysis. Such chemical interactions are similar to those in lower mammals, where secreted proteins act as carriers of one or more pheromone signals.

SPECIALIZED KERATINIZATION: NAILS

The nail unit is a region of specialized keratinization of practical importance, since dermatosis, infections, and neoplasms may affect this region, prompting histologic sampling (175). The nail unit has six main components (see Fig. 3-28): (a) the nail matrix which gives rise to the nail plate; (b) the nail plate; (c) the cuticular system, consisting of the dorsal component, or cuticle, and the distal component, or hyponychium; (d) the nail bed, which includes the dermis and underlying bone and soft tissue beneath the nail plate; (e) an anchoring system of ligaments between bone and matrix proximally and between distal grooves distally; and (f) the nail folds proximally, laterally, and distally.

The dorsal surface proximal nail fold contains eccrine but not pilosebaceous units and undergoes epidermal-type keratinization with an intervening granular cell layer, resulting in the production of soft keratin. Its ventral surface forms the dorsal cuticle or eponychium of the nail. The epidermal layer of the ventral surface is devoid of rete ridges and undergoes onycholemmal keratinization. Keratohyalin granules

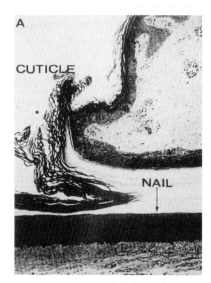
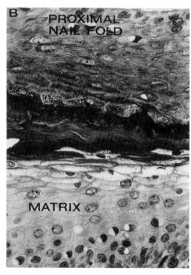
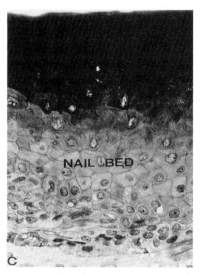

FIGURE 3-28. Photomicrograph of a saggital section 5 through the nail unit. **(A)** Distal tip of the proximal nail fold. Note the cuticle growing out of the nail plate. **(B)** Proximal margin of the proximal nail groove. Note the transition of the roof (the vertical surface) of the proximal nail fold with the matrix. Note the loss of keratohyalin granules. **(C)** Junction of matrix with the nail bed. Note the thin epithelium of the nail bed compared with that of the matrix. Neither epithelium contains keratohyalin granules. (Courtesy of Philip Fleckman, M.D., Karen A. Holbrook, Ph.D., and W.B. Saunders.)

are present in the epidermis of the ventral proximal nail fold, which produces the semihard keratin of the cuticle.

The nail matrix is responsible for the production of the "hard keratin" of the nail plate. This occurs via a process termed onychokeratinization, and as in trichilemmal keratinization, occurs by accretion of tonofilaments without the formation of intervening keratohyalin granules (176). This process involves thickening of the cellular envelope of the keratinizing cells to form a marginal band, analogous to similar changes in the surface epidermis (177). The nail matrix may be divided into two regions, one distal, responsible for the formation of the ventral portion of the nail plate, and clinically visible (the lunula); and the other proximal and responsible for the formation of the dorsal surface of the nail plate. The nail thickness is determined predominantly by the matrix, although the nail bed may contribute up to 20% as the nail grows (178). Melanocytes are present in the distal portion of the nail matrix (179), and Langerhans cells and Merkel cells have also been identified in this region (180).

The nail bed begins at the distal lunula and ends distally at the hyponychium, and also exhibits onycholemmal type of keratinization. The surface of the bed typically shows parallel longitudinal grooves that correlate with interdigitation of underlying rete ridges and dermal papillae. Clinically, the onychodermal band signifies the separation of the nail plate from the hyponychium where the normal volar epidermis and epidermal-type keratinization resumes.

DERMAL MICROVASCULAR UNIT

Not long ago, the dermis was considered to be a leathery cutaneous layer primarily responsible for housing and protection of vessels that served to nourish the keratinizing epidermis. Today we realize that the dermis is a dynamic microenvironment containing a repertoire of cells and matrix molecules arguably more complex and sophisticated than the epidermis and its appendages. The dermal microvascular unit is the heart of this new concept of the dermis, for it represents an intricate assemblage of cells responsible not only for cutaneous nutrition, but also for immune cell trafficking, regulation of vessel tone, and local hemostasis.

Endothelial Cells

General Microanatomy

The dermal microvasculature is divided into two important strata. The first, the superficial vascular plexus, defines the boundary between the papillary and the reticular dermis and extends within an adventitial mantle to envelop adnexal structures. This plexus forms a layer of anastomos-

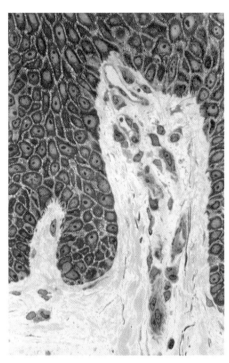

FIGURE 3-29. Histology of capillary loop originating from underlying superficial vascular plexus and extending into each dermal papilla.

ing arterioles and venules in close approximation to the overlying epidermis and is normally surrounded by other cellular components of the dermal microvascular unit (see below). Small capillary loops emanate from the superficial vascular plexus and extend into each dermal papilla (Fig. 3-29). The second plexus, the deep vascular plexus, is connected to the first by vertically oriented reticular dermal vessels and separates the reticular dermis from the subcutaneous fat. Many of these vessels are of larger caliber and communicate with branches that extend within fibrous septae that separate lobules of underlying subcutaneous fat.

The small arteries of the deep vascular plexus and the arterioles of the dermis possess three layers: an intima, composed of endothelial cells and an internal elastic lamina which stains for elastic tissue; a media, which contains two or more layers of muscle cells in the small arteries, but only a single layer of muscle cells in the arterioles of the lower dermis, and a discontinuous layer of muscle cells in the arterioles of the upper dermis; and an adventitia of connective tissue (181). The capillaries that are present throughout the dermis but especially in the papillary dermis are composed of a layer of endothelial cells surrounded by an incomplete layer of pericytes. A basement membrane, which stains positive with PAS, is present peripheral to the endothelial cells and surrounds the pericytes. There is alkaline phosphatase activity in the endothelial cells of all capillaries (131,182). Staining for alkaline phosphatase thus demonstrates well the capillary loop in each subepidermal dermal papilla, with the ascending, arterial limb of the loop staining more heavily than the descending, venous limb (131). The abundant capillaries present in the hair papilla of anagen hairs also stain heavily (131).

The walls of veins generally are thinner than those of arteries and less clearly divided into the three classic layers. The postcapillary venules resemble capillaries, because they consist of endothelial cells, pericytes, and a basement membrane (Fig. 3-30). The arteriolar and venous segments can be distinguished from each other on the basis of the basement membrane, which has a homogeneous appearance in the former and is multilaminated in the latter. Furthermore, terminal arterioles have elastin and smooth muscle cells in their walls, whereas postcapillary venules have only pericytes in their walls (184). The capillary loops leading from the subpapillary plexus to the dermal papillae and back can be divided into an intrapapillary portion and an extrapapillary portion. The extrapapillary ascending limb and the intrapapillary portion have the characteristics of an arterial capillary, that is, a homogeneous basement membrane, whereas the extrapapillary descending limb has venous characteristics, that is, a multilayered basement membrane (185). Although some investigators have observed areas of fenestration at the tips of the capillary loops between the endothelial cells (186), others have failed to find them (185). Endothelial cells characteristically show a well-developed endoplasmic reticulum, bundles of fairly thick cytoplasmic filaments with a diameter of 5 nm to 10 nm, and many pinocytotic vesicles at their luminal surface. Frequently, one can observe in endothelial cells a unique structure, the Weibel–Palade body. It is an electron-dense,

rod-shaped cytoplasmic organelle, measuring approximately 0.1 μm in diameter and up to 3 μm in length. It is composed of a number of small tubules, approximately 15 nm thick and arranged in the long axis of the rod (187). Peripheral to the endothelium lies a basement membrane. The peripheral row of cells, the pericytes, has long cytoplasmic processes and forms a discontinuous layer. They are completely surrounded by the capillary basement membrane. In larger capillaries, more than one layer of pericytes may be present, and transitional forms between pericytes and smooth muscle cells may be seen (188).

Endothelial cells of blood capillaries contain α-L-fucose, which can be demonstrated with Ulex europaeus (189), and they contain factor VIII–related antigen. Ulex and an antibody against factor VIII–related antigen are used as endothelial markers for the identification of neoplastic endothelial cells. Endothelial cells also express CD31 (190,191), a marker that may be the most sensitive for normal and neoplastic endothelial cells. In addition, endothelial cells of blood capillaries contain class I antigens (HLA-A,B,C) and class II antigen (HLA-DR) (192). HLA-DR is considered to play a role in antigen presentation and elicitation of an immune response (193), and endothelial cells as well as perivascular dermal dendritic cells are capable of dermal antigen presentation (see below). Laminin and type IV collagen are present within the vascular basement membranes. Blood capillaries contain vimentin intermediate filaments.

Specialized Structure and Function

Recent evidence indicates that endothelial cells are active participants in transmural shuttling of macromolecules as well as facilitators of normal and pathologic trafficking

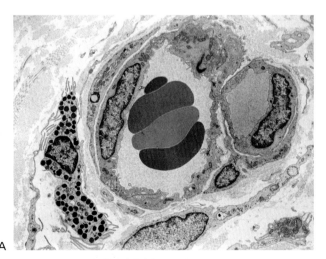
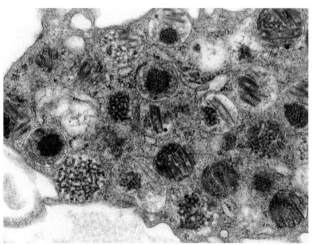

A   B

FIGURE 3-30. Transmission electron micrograph of dermal microvascular unit consisting of a plexus of central vessels and surrounding cells that form the junction between the papillary and reticular dermis **(A)**. Note endothelial cells lining the central postcapillary venule surrounded by pericytes and dermal immune cells, including granulated mast cells (granules depicted at higher magnification) **(B)**.

of immune cells. The luminal surface of the endothelial cell that lines the superficial postcapillary venule is the primary site of adhesive interactions that initiate subsequent diapedesis of leukocytes. The outer membrane of the Weibel–Palade body contains a glycoprotein termed CD62, which is rapidly transported to the luminal endothelial membrane upon exposure to histamine or thrombin (194, 195). This molecule mediates the initial loose rolling adhesion between circulating leukocytes and the endothelial surface. Subsequently, other cytokine-inducible glycoproteins are expressed in a cascade (E-selectin, vascular cell adhesion molecule-1 [VCAM-1], intercellular adhesion molecule-1 [ICAM-1]) on the endothelial surface, resulting in orchestrated and progressively stable leukocyte-endothelial adhesion (196–200). Some luminal molecules that are constitutively and diffusely expressed (e.g., CD31) redistribute to cell–cell junctions upon endothelial stimulation, thus creating a situation potentially conducive to concentrating adherent leukocytes at sites where transmural diapedesis may occur (200). Provocative signals for such events may come from inflammatory cells themselves, or from native cells in the perivascular space (see mast cells, below).

Glomus Cells

A special vascular structure, the glomus, is located within the reticular dermis in certain areas. Glomus formations occur most abundantly in the pads and nail beds of the fingers and toes, but also elsewhere on the volar aspect of the hands and feet, in the skin of the ears, and in the center of the face. The glomus is concerned with temperature regulation and represents a special arteriovenous shunt that, without the interposition of capillaries, connects an arteriole with a venule. When open, these shunts cause a great increase in blood flow in the area. Each glomus consists of an arterial and a venous segment. The arterial segment, called the Sucquet–Hoyer canal, branches from an arteriole and has a narrow lumen and a thick wall measuring 20 to 40 μm in diameter. The wall shows a single layer of endothelium, surrounded by a PAS-positive, diastase-resistant basement membrane zone, and a media that is densely packed with four to six layers of glomus cells (Fig. 3-31). These are large cells with a clear cytoplasm resembling epithelioid cells. Although myofibrils cannot be recognized within glomus cells with light microscopic staining methods, these cells have generally been regarded as smooth muscle cells (201). Peripheral to the glomus cells is a zone of loose connective tissue. Staining with silver salts shows many nerve fibers extending to the glomus cells within this zone. The venous segment of the glomus is thin-walled and has a wide lumen. This wide collecting venule functions as a reservoir and drains into a dermal venule. As many as four Sucquet–Hoyer canals may be found in a single glomus body, which is encapsulated (202).

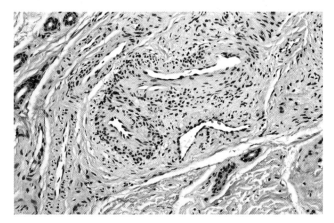

FIGURE 3-31. Glomus cells surrounding vessel from acral skin.

Electron microscopic study of the Hoyer–Hoyer canal reveals the glomus cells to be vascular smooth muscle cells. As such, each glomus cell is surrounded by a basement membrane. The cytoplasm of the glomus cells is filled with filaments with a diameter of about 5 nm. Cytoplasmic and peripheral dense bodies, 300 nm to 400 nm in diameter, are present in the glomus cells as a result of condensations of the myofilaments. Numerous nonmyelinated nerves ensheathed by Schwann cells are present peripheral to the glomus cells (203).

Mast Cells

Mast cells are bone marrow-derived cells that occur in the normal dermis in small numbers as oval to spindle-shaped cells with a centrally located round to oval nucleus. They are generally concentrated about blood vessels, specifically postcapillary venules (one to three cells/cross-sectional vessel profile). They contain in their cytoplasm numerous granules that do not stain with routine stains like hematoxylin-eosin. Therefore, mast cells in normal skin usually are indistinguishable from other perivascular cells, although one can occasionally recognize in mast cells a small amount of cytoplasm and the cell membrane. The granules stain with methylene blue, which is present in the Giemsa stain, with toluidine blue, and with Alcian blue. They also stain metachromatically with methylene blue and toluidine blue, that is, they stain in a color different from that possessed by the dye and appear purplish red rather than blue.

Electron microscopic examination of mast cells reveals numerous large and long villi at their periphery (Fig. 3-30). The mast cell granules appear as round, oval, or angular-shaped, membrane-bound structures. Mature granules measure up to 0.8 μm in diameter (204). They contain two components: lamellae and electron-dense, finely granular material (205). The lamellae appear in cross-sections as thick, curved, parallel filaments forming whorls or scrolls that may resemble fingerprints in their configuration. Each lamella is 7 to 12 nm wide, and their spacing is about 12 nm apart. At high magnification, the lamellae show transverse banding with a periodicity of approximately 6 nm. Tangential sectioning of the lamellae reveals paracrystalline lattices as a result of transverse banding. In some granules, distinct lamellae are not identifiable, and the internal appearance instead is finely granular. Other granules contain both lamellae and finely granular material. Recent immuno-ultrastructural observations indicate that the various granule subcompartments correlate with distribution of serine proteinases tryptase and chymase within granules (206). In addition, mast cells that populate connective tissue environments like dermis tend to contain granules with poorly formed scrolls and express both chymase and tryptase, whereas mast cells found primarily in mucosae and associated lamina propria have granules with well-formed scrolls and express tryptase but not chymase (207,208). Interestingly, one of these two granule types may be preferentially expressed in some cases of mastocytosis (209).

Degranulation of mast cells occurs after cross-linking of IgE on the cell surface, exposure to neuropeptides such as substance P, after nonspecific mechanical or thermal stimuli, or after exposure to a variety of exogenous secretagogues (compound 48/80, calcium ionophore, morphine sulfate). Degranulation generally occurs within minutes of exposure of the cell membrane to the secretagogue, and usually consists of the extrusion of entire granules, but some granules may undergo intracellular disintegration (204,210,211). Initial stages of degranulation consist of granule swelling with loss of internal substructure and electron density. Extrusion of granules takes place through extensive membrane fusion between the plasma membrane and perigranular membranes and is associated with formation of conduits resulting from fusion of the membranes of multiple granules. This results in extensive labyrinthine channels in the cell through which swollen, less electron-dense granules, all of which have lost their individual surrounding membranes, are released into the extracellular space (205,212). Concomitant with their release into the extracellular space, the granules release their preformed and stored mediators histamine, heparin, serine proteinases, and certain cytokines.

Immediate hypersensitivity reactions can be triggered by mast cells and basophils in "anaphylactically" sensitized persons through the presence on their cell surfaces of specific antibodies of the IgE type. When the specific antigen combines with these antibodies, an anaphylactic reaction is elicited through the degranulation of mast cells and the release of histamine from the granules (213). Histamine increases the permeability of postcapillary venules and, if released in sufficient amounts, may produce an anaphylactic shock. In delayed hypersensitivity reactions and in experimental allogeneic cytotoxic reactions, mast cells degranulate early, often preceding the initial influx of pioneer lymphocytes (214,215). Part of the reason for this lies in the recent discovery that human mast cells contain tumor necrosis factor α (TNF) (216), and local release of TNF as a consequence of mast cell degranulation induces expression of adhesion molecules such as E-selectin in adjacent postcapillary venules (217), with resultant leukocyte binding to the endothelial luminal membrane (218). Cooperation between the mast cell and the endothelial cell is also underscored by the observations that mast cells appear to situate in the laminin-rich perivascular space in association with expression of specific laminin receptors on their membranes (219), and that endothelial cells express mast cell growth factor (c-kit ligand) (220).

Neural Network

In sections stained with routine methods, one can recognize only the larger myelinated nerve bundles and the Meissner and Vater–Pacini end organs. The finer nerves require special staining, and accordingly the enormous importance of these structures to cutaneous homeostasis and pathology has been overlooked. Among the staining methods used are impregnation with silver salts (221), vital staining with methylene blue (222), and *in vitro* staining of thick sections with methylene blue (223). More recently, nerves have been identified by the S-100 technique (Fig. 3-32) and by using antibodies to specific neurofilaments, neuropeptides, and adhesion molecules (neural cell adhesion molecule-1). Nerves are composed of neuraxons, a cytoplasmic process that conducts neural impulses from cell bodies in the central nervous system, and Schwann cells (sheath cells or neurilemmal cells) enveloping the neuraxons (Fig. 3-32B). This primary functioning unit may or may not be myelinated and is surrounded by an endoneurium, a mucinous or fibrous matrix containing fibroblasts, which supports the primary functioning unit. A perineurium composed of elongated, flattened cells surrounds several primary functioning units and their endoneurial matrix (224).

The skin is supplied with sensory nerves and autonomic nerves, which permeate the entire dermis with nerve fibers showing frequent branching. Sensory and autonomic nerves differ in that sensory nerves possess a myelin sheath up to their terminal ramifications, but autonomic nerves do not. The autonomic nerves, derived from the sympathetic nervous system, supply the blood vessels, the arrectores pilorum, and the eccrine and apocrine glands. The sebaceous glands possess no autonomic innervation, and their functioning depends on endocrine stimuli. All autonomic nerves end in fine arborizations. So do the sensory nerves, except in a few areas in which there are, in addition to fine arborizations, special nerve end organs. Hair follicles, especially large hair follicles, are also surrounded below the entry of the sebaceous duct by a network of sensory nerves that lose their myelin sheaths a short distance

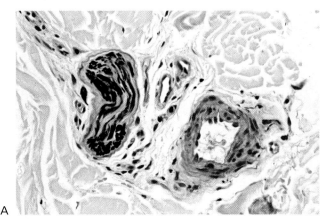
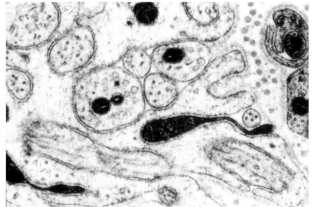

FIGURE 3-32. Dermal nerve fibers. S-100 immunohistochemical staining **(A)**. Transmission electron microscopy as individual axons enveloped by Schwann cells **(B)**.

from the outer root sheath and end in numerous arborizations of fine nonmyelinated fibers.

The papillary dermis is richly invested in unmyelinated nerve fibers, particularly about the dermal microvascular unit where axons often terminate in close proximity to mast cells (225). This relationship is of interest inasmuch as small neurosecretory granules within axons contain a variety of mediators, including neuropeptides that may serve as mast cell secretagogues, such as substance P. The development of confocal scanning laser microscopy has permitted assessment of complicated spatial relationships between axons and skin cells. Recently, superficial dermal axons containing another neuropeptide, calcitonin gene-related peptide (CGRP), were documented to enter the epidermis and to associate selectively with the cell bodies of Langerhans cells (226). Substance P-induced mast cell degranulation may elicit expression of endothelial-leukocyte adhesion molecules and thus be proinflammatory (227), and CGRP has been shown to diminish antigen presentation by Langerhans cells (228). Thus, the superficial dermal plexus of unmyelinated axons may represent a heretofore unappreciated influence of normal and perturbed cutaneous immunity.

Special Nerve End Organs

In the areas of hairless skin on the palms and the soles and in the areas of modified hairless skin at the mucocutaneous junctions, some of the sensory nerves end in special nerve end organs. They are of three types: mucocutaneous end organs, Meissner corpuscles (Fig. 3-33A), and Vater–Pacini corpuscles (Fig. 3-33B). Although it is customary to speak of them as end organs, they actually represent starting organs in a functional sense, because nerve impulses start there and are transmitted to the sensory cells of the spinal cord (229).

The mucocutaneous end organs, on the average 50 μm in diameter, are found in the modified hairless skin at the mucocutaneous junctions, namely, the glans, prepuce, clitoris, labia minora, perianal region, and vermilion border

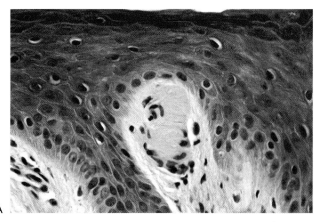
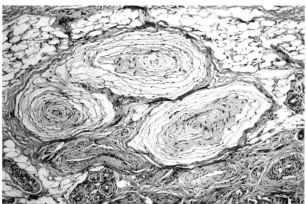

FIGURE 3-33. Meissner corpuscle within dermal papilla of human palm skin **(A)**. Vater–Pacini corpuscle within deep dermis of human sole skin **(B)**.

of the lip. They are in the papillary dermis. They cannot be recognized in routinely stained sections, in contrast to the Meissner corpuscles in the dermal papillae. Impregnation with silver nitrate reveals that from two to six myelinated nerve fibers enter each mucocutaneous end organ and, after losing their myelin sheaths, form many loops of nerve fibers resembling an irregularly wound ball of yarn. The electron microscopic features of mucocutaneous end organs are similar to those of Meissner corpuscles (230), despite minor differences in their light microscopic appearance. They show a subdivision into lobules, each containing a complex arrangement of axon terminals. These axon terminals are surrounded by concentric lamellar processes derived from so-called laminar cells, the nuclei of which are situated toward the periphery of the lobules. It is assumed that the laminar cells represent modified Schwann cells. The mucocutaneous end organs are always separated from the basal layer of the epidermis by a band of papillary dermal collagen.

Meissner corpuscles are located in dermal papillae (Fig. 3-33A) and mediate a sense of touch. They occur exclusively on the ventral aspects of the hands and feet, their number increasing distally. There are more Meissner corpuscles on the hands than on the feet. At the site of their greatest concentration, the fingertips, approximately every fourth papilla contains a Meissner corpuscle. The size of the Meissner corpuscles averages 30 μm by 80 μm in diameter. Owing to their size and their elongated shape, resembling that of a pinecone, they occupy the greater part of the papilla in which they are located. They possess a capsule composed of several layers of flattened Schwann cells that are arranged transverse to the long axis of the corpuscle. Impregnation with silver salts reveals that several myelinated nerves, as they approach the base or the side of the corpuscle, lose their myelin sheaths and then enter it. Within the corpuscle, the nerves take a meandering course upward. Electron microscopic studies reveal that the principal part of the Meissner corpuscle is made up of irregular layers of flattened, greatly elongated laminar cells. The nuclei of the laminar cells are located largely at the periphery of the corpuscle. The axons terminating within the Meissner corpuscle are surrounded by slender processes of the laminar cells. This enveloping of axons by laminar cells or their lamellar processes is analogous to the enveloping of axons by infolding of the plasma membrane of Schwann cells and indicates that the laminar cells are modified Schwann cells (231). The axon terminals and laminar cells are in direct contact with the epidermal basal cells at the upper end of the Meissner corpuscle without interposition of a basement membrane (232).

Vater–Pacini corpuscles are large, nerve end organs that are located in the subcutis and mediate a sense of pressure. They measure up to 1 mm in diameter and thus are detected easily by light microscopy (Fig. 3-33B). They are found most commonly below the skin of the volar aspects of the palms and soles, showing their greatest concentration at the tips of the fingers and toes. In addition, a few Vater–Pacini corpuscles occur in the subcutis of the nipple and of the anogenital region (230). Vater–Pacini corpuscles vary in shape. Some are ovoid, others have the appearance of a flattened sphere, and still others have an irregular shape. They consist of a stalk and of the body proper, the latter having a small core and a thick capsule. In the stalk, the single thick nerve supplying the Vater–Pacini corpuscle makes several turns and, just after entering the stalk, loses its myelin sheath. The core shows a granular substance surrounding the ascending meandering nerve. The thick capsule consists of 30 or more concentric, loosely arranged lamellae. On electron microscopic examination, the single nerve fiber present in the inner portion of the core retains its Schwann cell cytoplasmic covering for a short distance. The outer portion of the core shows closely packed, greatly elongated laminar cells. The thick capsule consists of at least 30 layers of flattened laminar cells separated from one another by fluid-filled spaces (233). The laminar cells of the Vater–Pacini corpuscle, analogous to those of the Meissner corpuscle, are modified Schwann cells.

Perivascular Dendritic Cells

In 1986, Headington introduced the term "dermal dendrocyte" to denote newly recognized dendritic cells in the human dermis (234). These cells were primarily but exclusively perivascular in location and differed from conventional bipolar fibroblasts by their stellate contours. Some of these cells appeared to represent "veil cells" that enshrouded venular walls with thin membrane flaps, as originally described by Braverman (235). Many of these cells were subsequently shown to express the membrane glycoprotein CD1c (236), HLA-DR, and certain macrophage markers as well as the cytoplasmic transglutaminase, Factor XIIIa (237) (Fig. 3-34). Heterogeneity of dermal dendro-

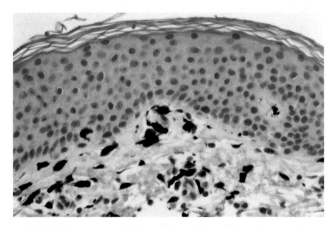

FIGURE 3-34. Factor XIIIa-positive "dermal dendrocytes" concentrated beneath the epidermal layer and about the dermal microvascular unit.

cytes within different dermal strata exists with regard to their expression of the hematopoietic progenitor antigen, CD34, and FXIIIa has been described (238).

Whereas dermal dendrocytes are dendritic only in cross-section, with three-dimensional reconstructions showing elaborate membranous flaps (238), truly dendritic cells also do exist in the perivascular space. These cells are Langerhans cell-like, although they generally do not contain Birbeck granules, strongly express HLA-DR, and are believed to be involved in dermal antigen presentation (239). Considerable plasticity among the various subpopulations of dermal perivascular dendritic cells may exist, and alterations in local microenvironment may induce phenotypic transformation from one subtype to another (240).

In general, perivascular dendritic cells are not identifiable as such in routinely prepared and stained sections, although immunohistochemistry for the relevant markers permits the ready identification and classification of these cell types. Dermal dendrocytes may be observed in certain situations where they acquire avid phagocytic potential, taking up hemosiderin, for example. Such phagocytic perivascular dendritic cells have been termed "dendrophages" (241).

Phagocytic Macrophages

Macrophages, also called histiocytes, are of bone marrow origin, circulate in the blood as precursors, and enter the tissue as monocytes (242). Upon proper stimulation, monocytes can develop into macrophages in the skin, which involves a considerable increase in cell size and changes in cellular composition and architecture, including increases in lysosomal enzymes, such as β-glucuronidase, acid phosphatase, lysozyme, and aryl sulfatase (242). Macrophages may develop further into epithelioid histiocytes and foreign body giant cells. Aggregates of activated macrophages are referred to as granulomas. Macrophages are most often concentrated in the perivascular space of normal skin, although depending on the nature and location of the stimulus for their activation, may be found anywhere in the dermis (or epidermis).

Macrophages constitute the "mononuclear phagocytic system," a concept that has replaced that of the reticuloendothelial system. The macrophages of the mononuclear phagocytic system, including the alveolar phagocytes in the lungs and the Kupffer cells in the liver, are the "professional" phagocytes, whereas the reticuloendothelial cells, including the dendritic reticulum cells in lymph nodes and the endothelial cells of blood vessels, are merely "facultative" phagocytes and are comparatively inadequate (243). As "professional" phagocytes, macrophages are capable of ingesting large particles and developing a high concentration of lysosomal enzymes that combine with the particles to for phagolysosomes. In contrast, the facultative phagocytosis carried out by endothelial cells consists merely of

pinocytosis of small particles without immune stimulation (243). Macrophages can also be stimulated by immunologic factors, having surface receptors for the Fc portion of IgG, for C3, and for immune-associated HLA-DR antigen (human leukocyte antigen-D subregion of the major histocompatibility complex) (244).

Monocytes are indistinguishable from lymphocytes, because both cells have a small, dark, rounded nucleus and very scanty cytoplasm that cannot be recognized in routine sections. Only slightly larger than lymphocytes, monocytes measure 12 to 15 μm in diameter (244). Monocytes can be differentiated from lymphocytes in histologic sections through staining for lysosomal enzymes, such as acid phosphatase, which are present in monocytes and absent in lymphocytes. In addition, monocytes but not lymphocytes express intracytoplasmic molecules that are probably associated with lysosomes, such as CD68, which may be detected immunohistochemically in paraffin sections (245).

Macrophages, because they are activated monocytes, are larger cells than monocytes and measure from 20 to 80 μm in diameter (244). They possess a vesicular, lightly staining, elongated nucleus with a clearly visible nuclear membrane. It is often impossible in routinely stained sections to distinguish macrophages from fibroblasts or from endothelial cells except through their respective locations or phagocytic activities. Macrophages that have ingested melanin are referred to as melanophages, and may be observed normally within the papillary dermis of darkly pigmented individuals. Macrophages that have ingested hemosiderin are termed siderophages, and may be suspected due to the characteristic yellow-green color and refractile nature of particulate hemosiderin. Iron stains (e.g., Prussian blue) will be confirmatory.

The origin of the tissue monocytes in human skin from blood monocytes has been established in healthy probands through transfusion of tritiated thymidine-labeled monocytes and their observation 3 hours later in skin window exudates (246). On the other hand, the dermal infiltrate of monocytes and macrophages in patients with chronic dermatitis is largely self-renewing, because the monocyte recruitment rate from the blood is low in these patients following the autotransfusion of labeled monocytes (246). Electron microscopic examination reveals in monocytes many primary lysosomes scattered through their cytoplasm as small dense bodies (247). Macrophages, which represent stimulated monocytes, differ from monocytes in that they are larger, show longer processes, and contain a larger number of lysosomes (248) (Fig. 3-35). Many macrophages contain phagocytized material within phagosomes, which, through the influx of the contents of primary lysosomes, have become phagolysosomes.

Emigrant Inflammatory Cells

Various types of cells, largely derived from the bone marrow, infiltrate the dermis and occasionally also the epidermis in the inflammatory dermatoses. Infiltration is initiated at the

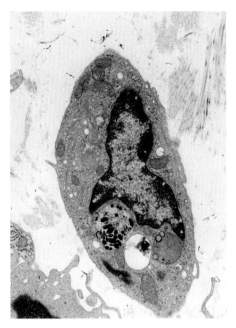

FIGURE 3-35. Ultrastructure of phagocytic macrophage within the dermis. Note intracytoplasmic lysosomes associated with engulfed cell breakdown products, including a large vacuole containing internalized melanosomes.

level of the dermal microvascular unit, accounting for the observation that upon detection, such cells are often partially or exclusively perivascular in location (Fig. 3-36). Such cells may also be present in normal skin in low numbers as part of the skin immune system. It is important for diagnostic purposes to identify the cell types, since many diagnostic algorithms for dermatitis classification and identification depend upon initial categorization by architecture followed by recognition of inflammatory cell type(s) (249). Three groups of cells are derived from the bone marrow: the granulocytic

group; the lymphocytic group, including plasma cells; and the monocytic or macrophagic group (discussed above).

Neutrophilic Granulocytes

The neutrophilic granulocyte, also called a neutrophil or polymorphonuclear leukocyte, is 10 to 15 μm in diameter and has a lobated nucleus consisting of several segments that are connected only by narrow bridges of nucleoplasm (Fig. 3-37). The cytoplasm contains numerous neutrophilic to slightly eosinophilic granules. On histochemical examination, the granules are seen to contain lysosomal enzymes and thus represent primary lysosomes. Two types of membrane-bound cytoplasmic granules or lysosomes are found to be present in neutrophils on electron microscopic examination: azurophilic and specific granules (250). The azurophilic granules, constituting about 20% of all granules, are relatively dense and large, measuring up to 1 μm in diameter. The more numerous specific granules average 300 nm in diameter. Among other substances, azurophilic granules contain (a) myeloperoxidase, which mediates the formation of hydrogen peroxide, essential for the killing of many microorganisms; (b) acid hydrolases, such as β-glucuronidase and acid phosphatase, capable of degrading dead bacteria and other necrotic material; (c) neutral proteases, such as collagenase and elastase, that may break down collagen and elastin; (d) cationic proteins, which cause an increase in vascular permeability; and (e) lysozyme, an enzyme that degrades and lyses bacterial cell walls. The specific granules also contain lysozyme and, in addition, collagenase, alkaline phosphatase, and lactoferrin, an iron-binding protein with bacteriostatic properties.

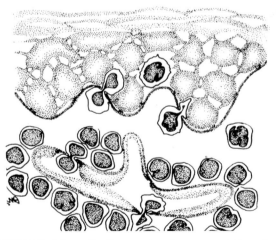

FIGURE 3-36. Schematic diagram showing accumulation of emigrant mononuclear cells characteristically about a postcapillary venule within the superficial microvascular plexus.

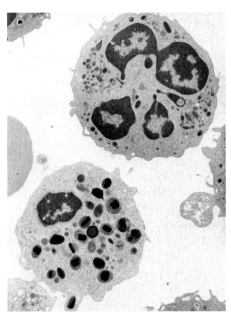

FIGURE 3-37. Ultrastructural comparison between neutrophilic (uppermost cell) and eosinophilic (lowermost cell) granulocytes.

Neutrophils are unusual in normal skin, but occur typically in a relatively small subset of dermatitides, including urticaria, immune complex–mediated necrotizing vasculitis, the spectrum of neutrophilic dermatosis (e.g., Sweet syndrome, pyoderma gangrenosum), and in various cutaneous infections. Neutrophils may participate, along with other cell types, in other inflammatory processes, such as psoriasis, seborrheic dermatitis, and pityriasis lichenoides et varioliformis acuta. In tissue sections, neutrophils are often recognized by virtue of their "popcorn" shaped nuclei within pale pink, faintly granular cytoplasm. Nuclear breakdown due to local necrosis or autodigestion results in fragmentation of the multiple nuclear lobes, resulting in the characteristic "nuclear dust" of vasculitis.

Functionally, neutrophilic granulocytes play an important role (a) in certain inflammatory responses (examples provided above); (b) in the phagocytosis and killing of microorganisms; and (c) in the immobilization and phagocytosis of antigen–antibody complexes in the presence of complement (251). Neutrophils fail to kill bacteria in chronic granulomatous disease where they are incapable of oxygen uptake from the surrounding media (252). Phagocytosis of organisms and antigen–antibody complexes by neutrophils is accompanied by their partial or complete degranulation, with associated discharge of lysosomal enzymes (253). Endocytotic uptake of microorganisms by neutrophils results in the formation of intracytoplasmic phagolysosomes where high enzyme concentrations result in microbial killing. Immune complexes, after activation of complement, may induce the local accumulation of neutrophils via chemotaxis. Phagocytosis of immune complexes by neutrophils and/or neutrophil degranulation may then occur (254). Exocytosis of neutrophil granules containing collagenase and elastase may result in local tissue damage, including necrosis of vessels containing immune complexes in their basement membranes (255).

Eosinophilic Granulocytes

The eosinophil, 12 to 17 μm in diameter, is characterized by strong eosinophilic granules in the cytoplasm and a characteristically bilobed nucleus (256). Eosinophil granules are larger than the granules of neutrophils. Although visible with routine stains, these granules stand out more clearly in brilliant red when a Giemsa stain is used. On electron microscopic examination, the granules of eosinophils are seen to be round to oval (Fig. 3-37). They consist of two components, a central, angular-shaped core, often referred to as the crystalloid, and a surrounding matrix. In electron microscopic sections stained with lead compounds, the crystalloid is more darkly stained than the matrix (257). The longer diameter of the granules measures 0.5 to 1.5 μm, and the shorter diameter 0.3 to 1 μm (257). The granules contain a variety of hydrolytic enzymes, particularly peroxidase and arylsulfatase, and therefore can be classified as lysosomes. The phagocytic potential of eosinophils seems to be limited to immune complexes and mast cell granules. During phagocytosis, which is analogous to that seen in neutrophils, the content of the eosinophilic granules is discharged into phagosomes (258).

Because eosinophils can phagocytize mast cell granules and certain antigen–antibody complexes, tissue eosinophilia in the skin can occur (a) as a result of anaphylactic or atopic hypersensitivity, (b) subsequent to the degranulation of mast cells, and (c) in certain diseases associated with deposits of antigen–antibody complexes in the skin. The tissue eosinophilia appearing in anaphylactic reactions and other forms of "immediate" allergy such as atopy is based on antibodies of the IgE type on the surface of mast cells. The anaphylactic reaction, classified as type I hypersensitivity reaction (259), occurs following the binding of a specific antigen to a specific antibody on the surface of the mast cells. This leads to degranulation of mast cells and to the release of vasoactive substances, especially histamine. Wherever degranulation of mast cells occurs, eosinophils may appear and phagocytize the released mast cell granules (253). Eosinophils thus may modify an anaphylactic reaction (260). Eosinophils are attracted in an anaphylactic reaction by sensitized mast cells, which release an eosinophil chemotactic factor of anaphylaxis (ECF-A). Eosinophils thus attracted to the site of an anaphylactic reaction accumulate around degranulating mast cells and phagocytize the free mast cell granules (261).

Diseases in which deposition of antigen–antibody complexes is the cause of eosinophilia include pemphigus vulgaris, particularly pemphigus vegetans, pemphigus foliaceus, bullous pemphigoid, and granuloma faciale. The reasons for the occasional presence of tissue eosinophilia in histiocytosis X and in Hodgkin's disease are not fully apparent. Parasitic infestations often are associated with eosinophilia both in the peripheral blood and in the tissue. It is likely that eosinophils function as effector cells in parasite destruction (258). Destruction of parasites, such as those causing schistosomiasis, is accomplished by means of the major basic protein (MBP) of the eosinophils. The MBP is localized in the crystalloid core of the eosinophil granules and accounts for more than 50% of the protein in the granules and for almost 25% of the total protein in the cell. Its toxicity provides a mechanism by which the eosinophil damages parasites. Release of MBP from degranulating eosinophils is, however, not always beneficial to the host. Release of MBP may partly account for the tissue damage seen in chronic hypersensitivity reactions (262).

Basophilic Granulocytes

Although basophils and mast cells have similar or identical functions and supplement each other, they are different cells both in origin and in anatomy (263). Both cells have their origin in the bone marrow, although basophils circulate in the peripheral blood, and mature mast cells are confined to connective tissue and mucosal tissue compartments. Basophils are relatively rare in human dermatitis, although they are active participants in certain forms of dermatitis in rodents (263). The demonstration of basophils in light microscopic sections requires the use of electron microscopic fixation and processing techniques; biopsy specimens must be embedded in plastic resin and sectioned at 1 μm. The sections then are stained with the Giemsa stain. Basophils possess a multilobed nucleus and large, diffusely arranged metachromatic granules, whereas mast cells have a unilobed nucleus and smaller, peripherally located metachromatic granules (264).

Lymphocytes

There are two types of peripheral lymphocytes: T- and B-lymphocytes, both of which arise in the bone marrow. One type migrates to the thymus, where it differentiates to a lymphocyte, and then proceeds to the peripheral lymphoid tissues as a thymus-derived or T-lymphocyte. In lymph nodes, T-lymphocytes are located predominantly in the interfollicular cortex, also called the paracortical areas. The other type of lymphocyte, the B-lymphocyte, matures in the bone marrow (265). The term B-lymphocyte, meaning bursa-derived lymphocyte, originally was given because, in birds, the bursa of Fabricius is held responsible for B-cell maturation (265). In humans, the term B-lymphocyte is used to mean bone-marrow–derived lymphocyte. In lymph nodes, B-lymphocytes largely occupy the lymph follicles, including their germinal centers. Whereas the T-lymphocyte is the effector cell for cellular immunity, the B-lymphocyte mediates humoral immunity. The lymph nodes and other lymphoid organs share three principal functions: (a) to concentrate within them antigens from all parts of the body, (b) to circulate the lymphocyte population through the lymphoid organs so that every antigen is exposed to antigen-specific lymphocytes, and (c) to carry the products of the immune response, the humoral antibodies and cells mediating cellular immunity, to the blood and tissue (265). T cells can exert important regulating functions on both T cells and B cells in the form of specific functional subsets termed helper T cells and suppressor T cells (266).

Lymphocytes measure on the average 8 μm in diameter and possess a relatively small, round nucleus that appears deeply basophilic because of the presence of numerous chromatin particles (Fig. 3-38). They have only a very narrow rim of cytoplasm that is hardly recognizable. It is usually impossible by light microscopy to distinguish lymphocytes from monocytes in routinely stained histologic sections; and, in several instances in which it was once assumed that lymphocytes were an important constituent of the dermal infiltrate, such as in contact dermatitis and sarcoidosis, it has been shown through demonstration of the presence of lysosomal enzymes within the cells and

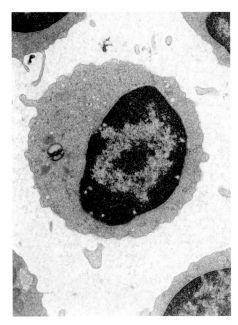

FIGURE 3-38. Transmission electron micrograph of mature lymphocyte; note chromatin-rich nucleus and organelle-poor cytoplasm.

through electron microscopy that many of the cells are monocytes rather than lymphocytes. It is therefore preferable to refer to cells with a histologic appearance of lymphocytes as lymphoid cells. Ultrastructurally, resting lymphocytes contain relatively few organelles within a thin cytoplasmic rim that surrounds a nucleus with coarsely aggregated heterochromatin (Fig. 3-38).

Although T and B cells are indistinguishable by light microscopy, they can be differentiated by *in vitro* tests. Human T-lymphocytes have receptors for sheep erythrocytes, so that, in the historically important E rosette assay, sheep erythrocytes (E) form rosettes around T-lymphocytes. Furthermore, T-lymphocytes undergo blastic transformation when exposed to mitogens such as phytohemagglutinin or concanavalin A, and anti–T-lymphocyte antisera have a specific cytotoxic effect on them (267,268). Antibodies are now available for the identification of T cells and B cells in routine paraffin sections (e.g., UCHL and L26, respectively). Specific detection of cell surface glycoproteins that correlate with T-cell functional subsets (CD4 for helper, CD8 for suppressor) or with T-cell maturation or activation (CD2, CD3, CD5, and Il-2 receptor, respectively) is most sensitively accomplished in fresh frozen-tissue sections. The same is true for classification of B-cell light chain expression (kappa vs. lambda). It is important to realize that normal skin will contain small numbers of perivascular T cells with the helper subtype predominating as part of the skin immune system.

T cells play an important role in normal cutaneous immunosurveillance and in delayed hypersensitivity reactions. Initial antigen uptake by Langerhans cells occurs during sensitization. After their migration to draining lymph nodes via dermal lymphatics (see below), Langerhans cells present antigen to naive T cells that undergo initial clonal expansion to become memory cells. Experimental data suggests that antigen-specific molecules capable of degranulating mast cells upon antigen reexposure may also occur at this step (269). In the challenge reaction, the dermal microvascular unit is activated (possibly in part due to mast cell degranulation), resulting in display of leukocyte adhesion molecules on the endothelial luminal surface that facilitate the recruitment of memory T cells. Upon local antigen presentation at the challenge site, these pioneer memory cells now capable of antigen recognition respond by elaboration of a cascade of cytokines that result in recruitment of secondary inflammatory cells.

The B-lymphocyte is the effector cell of humoral immunity. On antigenic stimulation, the primary follicles in lymph nodes, composed of small B-lymphocytes, develop into secondary follicles, consisting of a germinal center surrounded by a rim of small B-lymphocytes (265). In the germinal centers, small B-lymphocytes enlarge through an intermediate stage of centrocytes with cleaved nuclei into centroblasts, which are large cells with noncleaved nuclei (270). The centroblasts become immunoblasts as a result of antigenic stimulation and produce a clone of daughter cells that mature into immunoglobulin-secreting plasma cells (271,272). The differentiation of B-lymphocytes into plasma cells is helped by helper T cells and is suppressed by suppressor T cells (273). The plasma cells collect in the medullary cords of lymph nodes without circulating in the bloodstream but secrete immunoglobulins that circulate as "humoral" antibodies. Although these events most commonly occur in lymph nodes, identical alterations may take place in the dermis in response to locally introduced antigen, as is the case in cutaneous lymphoid hyperplasia with prominent germinal center formation (274,275).

Plasma Cells

Plasma cells have an abundant cytoplasm that is deeply basophilic, homogeneous, and sharply defined. The round nucleus is eccentrically placed and shows along its membrane coarse, deeply basophilic, regularly distributed chromatin particles, which give the nucleus a cartwheel appearance. The fact that patients with agammaglobulinemia lack plasma cells was responsible for early recognition of the fact that the plasma cell is the site of formation of all immunoglobulins that circulate as humoral antibodies. The synthesis of immunoglobulins takes place in plasma cells located mainly in the lymph nodes, the spleen, and the bone marrow. Because plasma cells are tissue cells and are not seen in the peripheral circulation, it can be assumed that, if they are present in the dermis, they have developed there from B-lymphocytes. Intracytoplasmic immunoglob-

ulins may be demonstrated immunohistochemically in paraffin-embedded tissue. Subclassification of cells according to kappa (approximately two-thirds of reactive plasma cells) and lambda (approximately one-third of reactive plasma cells) is also possible, and may facilitate in some instances detection of a neoplastic clone, where only one of the light chains is produced exclusively. On electron microscopy, plasma cells are characterized by the presence in their cytoplasm of an extensive system of cisternae lined by a rough endoplasmic reticulum. The cisternae usually are flat but may be irregularly dilated. Numerous ribosomes not only line the membranes of the endoplasmic reticulum, but also are present in the cytoplasm. The abundant ribosomes and the highly developed endoplasmic reticulum are involved in the synthesis of immunoglobulins. Thus, the cisternae are often filled with a homogeneous to granular substance that is released into the extracellular space.

Plasma cells are apt to be present in conspicuous numbers in several infectious diseases, such as early syphilis, rhinoscleroma, and granuloma inguinale. In the presence of many plasma cells, but especially in rhinoscleroma, round, hyaline, eosinophilic bodies called Russell bodies may be found inside and outside of plasma cells. They form within plasma cells as the result of a very active synthesis of immunoglobulins and may ultimately completely replace the plasma cells in which they have formed (276). They may possess a size twice that of normal plasma cells, measuring up to 20 μm in diameter. They contain varying amounts of glycoproteins and are as a rule Gram positive as well as PAS positive and diastase resistant (277). Russell bodies are initiated by intracisternal secretion, analogous to the secretion of immunoglobulins. When the plasma cell is overloaded with this material, first the nucleus and ultimately the entire cell lyse (276). Immunofluorescence staining shows the presence of immunoglobulins within the Russell bodies. Intense staining of Russell bodies is observed when anti–light-chain conjugates are used, but not when antiheavy chain conjugates are used (278).

DERMAL LYMPHATICS

Dermal lymphatics are often inconspicuous in normal skin because they do not have well-developed walls, as is the case with blood vessels. They are easily detected, however, when they become slightly ectatic as a result of increase lymphatic drainage, as in urticaria. Lymph vessels typically are not rounded in contour, but rather show angulations dictated by the fact that their lining lymphatics are buttressed by adjacent collagen bundles. In normal skin, the perilymphatic space is relatively devoid of other cells, and the lumen is lined by relatively flattened endothelial cells. Occasional valves may be observed emanating from the endothelial lining. By electron microscopy, the thin layer of endothelium does not contain Weibel–Palade bodies and is devoid of a basement membrane or surrounding pericytes. Lymphatic vessels show a negative or weakly positive reaction when incubated with *Ulex europaeus* and no reaction with an antibody against factor VIII–related antigen in most instances. They do not contain class I (HLA-A,B,C) or class II (HLA-DR) antigens (192). Endothelial cells of lymphatic vessels contain cytoplasmic filaments (279), which probably represent vimentin filaments.

DERMAL FIBROBLASTS

The dermis of a 2-month-old embryo consists of loosely arranged mesenchymal cells that are embedded in ground substance. During the third month, argyrophilic reticulum fibers appear. As these fibers increase in number and in thickness, they arrange themselves in bundles that no longer can be impregnated with silver and, instead, stain with the methods for collagen. Simultaneously, the mesenchymal cells develop into fibroblasts. Electron microscopic examination of the fetal dermis from week 6 to week 14 reveals, apart from Schwann cells identified by their association with neuraxons, three main types of cells: (a) stellate mesenchymal cells with long processes; (b) phagocytic macrophages of probable yolk-sac origin; and (c) cells containing granules, which could be either melanoblasts or mast precursors. From week 14 on, fibroblasts become numerous. In the normal adult dermis, fibroblasts appear as inconspicuous bipolar spindle cells with elongated ovoid nuclei. They cannot be reliably distinguished from other dermal spindle-shaped and dendritic cells. By electron microscopy, fibroblasts that actively synthesize collagen have a prominent rough endoplasmic reticulum composed of many membrane-lined cisternae with large numbers of attached ribo-

somes (Fig. 3-39). The dilated cisternae are filled with an amorphous material produced by the ribosomes lining the cisternae (280). This apparently amorphous material consists of triple helical procollagen molecules, each molecule being composed of three pro-α polypeptide chains. The procollagen molecules pass from the cisternae of the rough endoplasmic reticulum to the Golgi area, whence they are excreted into the extracellular space by means of secretory vesicles (281,282). Conversion of procollagen molecules into collagen molecules composed of three α chains then occurs outside the cell (283).

DERMAL MUSCLE CELLS
Smooth Muscle

Smooth or involuntary muscle of the skin occurs as arrectores pilorum as tunica dartos of the external genitals, and in the areola of the nipples. The muscle fibers of the arrectores pilorum arise in the connective tissue of the upper dermis and are attached to the hair follicle below the sebaceous glands. They are situated in the obtuse angle of the hair follicle. Thus, when contracted, they pull the hair follicle into a vertical position and produce the perifollicular elevations of "gooseflesh."

Smooth muscle is characterized by the absence of striation and by the location of the nucleus in the center of the muscle cell. Typically, the nuclei are "cigar-shaped," with rounded ends, a feature that may be diagnostically helpful in assessing dermal spindle cell proliferations and neoplasms. Argyrophilic reticulum fibers surround each muscle cell. Electron microscopic examination reveals that smooth muscle cells possess a basement membrane peripheral to the plasma membrane. The cytoplasm of the cells is filled with myofilaments, 5 nm in diameter, that form cytoplasmic and peripheral dense bodies as a result of condensations, just as the myofilaments do in myoepithelial cells, in vascular smooth muscle cells, and in glomus cells. The rather narrow spaces between the muscle cells are occupied by collagen fibrils and by Schwann cells with associated nonmyelinated axons.

Smooth muscle cells contain vimentin and desmin as intermediate filaments. In addition, they show a positive reaction when incubated with an antibody against S-100 protein.

Striated Muscle

Striated or voluntary muscle is found in the skin of the neck as platysma and in the skin of the face as muscles of expression. The striated muscle bundles take their origin either from a fascia or from the periosteum, or they form a closed ring, as in the musculus sphincter oris. They extend through the subcutaneous tissue into the lower dermis. The muscle fibers, like skeletal muscle, show characteristic cytoplasmic cross-striations. Their nuclei are located at the

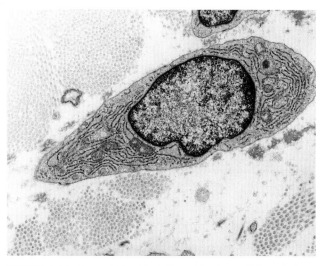

FIGURE 3-39. Dermal fibroblast viewed by transmission electron microscopy and showing dilated cisternae of rough endoplasmic reticulum and surrounding collagen fibers in cross-section.

periphery of the fibers immediately beneath the sar-colemma, the limiting membrane of the fibers.

EXTRACELLULAR MATRIX

The extracellular matrix of the dermis consists of collagenous and elastic fibers embedded into ground substance. All three components are formed by fibroblasts.

Collagen Fibers

Collagen represents by far the most abundant constituent of the connective tissue of the dermis. On light microscopy, collagen consists of fibers (Fig. 3-40). The diameter of collagen fibers is quite variable, ranging from 2 μm to 15 μm. The collagen fibers are present either as a finely woven network or as thick bundles. Collagen as a finely woven meshwork of collagen fibers is found in the papillary layer of the dermis, which includes not only the subepidermal papillae situated between the rete ridges but also the subpapillary layer forming a narrow ribbon between the rete ridges and the subpapillary blood vessels (Fig. 3-40). This is referred to as the papillary dermis. In addition, the pilosebaceous units and the eccrine and apocrine glands are encircled by a thin meshwork of collagen fibers similar to that present in the papillary dermis. Therefore, the papillary and the periadnexal dermis are regarded as an anatomical unit, the adventitial dermis. The blood

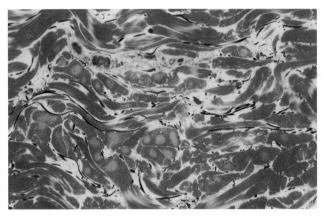

FIGURE 3-41. One micron-thick, plastic-embedded section of reticular dermis. By this technique, the pale thicker collagen fibers are separable from the more darkly stained thinner elastin fibers.

vessels of the dermis are also surrounded by a thin layer of fine collagen fibers. Biochemically, the papillary dermis is composed primarily of type III collagen.

The rest of the dermis, constituting by far the largest portion of the dermis and referred to as the reticular dermis, shows the collagen fibers united into thick bundles (Figs. 3-40 and 3-41). These collagen bundles extend in various directions horizontally, and thus some are cut lengthwise and others across in histologic sections. As a rule, collagen bundles that are cut lengthwise appear

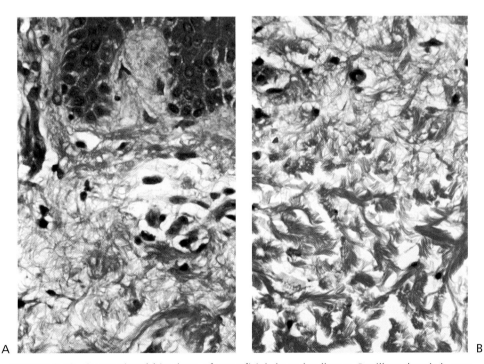

FIGURE 3-40. Conventional histology of superficial dermal collagen. Papillary dermis is composed of relatively delicate fibers **(A)** and **(B, upper half)** that interface with the thicker fibers of the underlying reticular dermis in **(B, lower half)**.

slightly wavy. Biochemically, reticular dermal collagen is composed primarily of type I collagen.

Reticulum fibers are not recognizable with routine stains, but, being argyrophilic, they can be impregnated with silver nitrate, which, by being subsequently reduced to silver, stains black. Reticulum fibers represent a special type of thin collagen fiber that measures from 0.2 to 1 µm in diameter. The argyrophilia shown by reticulum fibers, in contrast to collagen fibers, probably is related to the fact that reticulum fibers correspond to the distribution of type III collagen rather than type I collagen.

Argyrophilic reticulum fibers are the first-formed fibers during embryonic life and in various pathologic conditions associated with increased fibroblastic activity. In normal skin, even though collagen is being continuously replaced, the formation of new collagen is not preceded by an argyrophilic phase. Rather, all newly formed collagen consists of large fibers. However, there are a few areas in which normally small collagen fibers are present as reticulum fibers without transforming into larger, nonargyrophilic collagen fibers. This occurs above all in the basement membrane zone, the region of the adventitial dermis that lies closest to the epidermis and its appendages. In addition, reticulum fibers are present normally around blood vessels and as a basket-like capsule around each fat cell.

The biosynthesis of collagen begins within the fibroblast by the assembly of three pro-α polypeptide chains into a triple helical procollagen molecule (283). After excretion into the extracellular space, the three pro-α chains of each procollagen molecule are shortened by 30% to 40% through removal of the carboxy-terminal and amino-terminal peptide extensions brought about by the action of two enzymes produced by the fibroblast: carboxy-terminal peptidase and amino-terminal peptidase (282). This results in conversion of the procollagen molecule into the collagen molecule. Although the additional peptides present in procollagen keep it soluble and prevent its intracellular polymerization, collagen molecules polymerize readily. The collagen molecule is a rigid rod in which each of the three coiled α chains consists of about 1,000 amino acids (283). The collagen molecule is about 300 nm long and 1.5 nm wide (284,285). Collagen fibrils form by both lateral and longitudinal association of collagen molecules. However, the collagen fibrils vary in diameter as a result of varying degrees of polymerization of collagen molecules, with younger collagen fibrils being thinner than older fibrils. In the normal dermis, the thickness of collagen fibrils ranges from 70 nm to 140 nm; most of the fibrils are approximately 100 nm thick (286).

Collagen fibrils possess characteristic cross-striations with a periodicity of 68 nm. The periodicity of the cross-striations in the collagen fibrils can be explained as follows. Each collagen molecule possesses along its length of 300 nm five charged regions 68 nm apart, and although neighboring collagen molecules overlap each other, they always have their charged regions lying side by side. This parallel alignment of the charged regions produces the cross-striations (285). Reticulum fibrils possess the same 68-nm periodicity of their cross-striations as collagen fibrils but have a smaller diameter than collagen fibrils, varying between 40 nm and 65 nm rather than between 70 nm and 140 nm (287). Furthermore, reticulum and collagen differ in the number of fibrils present in the cross-section of each fiber and in the amount of ground substance present within and around each fiber. The amount of ground substance around the fibrils and on the surface of the fiber may explain the presence of argyrophilia in reticulum fibers and its absence in collagen fibers (287).

Seven different types of collagen have been recognized that differ in composition and antigenicity. Type I collagen, the predominant collagen in postfetal skin, is found in the large fiber bundles of the reticular dermis. Reticulum fibers are composed of type III collagen. Although type III collagen is the prevalent type of collagen in early fetal life, in postfetal life it is limited to the subepidermal and periappendageal regions, that is, the basement membrane zones and the perivascular region (288). Basement membrane collagen (basal lamina collagen) is type IV, and the collagen of cartilage is type II. Type V collagen has been recognized in fetal membranes and vascular tissue (289). Type VII collagen occurs in different basement membranes including those of the skin and forms a major structural component of anchoring fibrils (290). The skin of the human fetus contains a large percentage of type III collagen, in contrast to the skin of the adult, which contains a large proportion of type I collagen (291).

Among the differences in composition are the following. In type I collagen, the three α chains in the collagen molecule consist of two different kinds: two identical α chains designated as α-1(I), and a third chain called α-2. In type II collagen, the collagen molecules are composed of three identical, genetically distinct α chains, α-1(II). Type III collagen is also composed of three identical, distinct α chains (282). Type IV collagen consists of procollagen composed of three identical pro-α chains that have retained their nonhelical extensions. Types V and VI collagen have not yet been adequately characterized. Type VII collagen consists of three α chains, with the terminal regions being noncollagenous (290).

Elastic Fibers

Elastic fibers appear in the dermis at 22 weeks, much later than the collagenous fibers. At this time, acid orcein stains show elastic tissue in the reticular dermis either as granular material interspersed with occasional short fibers or as a delicate network of branching fibers. As gestation progresses, elastic fibers increase in quantity. At 32 weeks, a well-developed network of elastic fibers indistinguishable from that seen in term infants is present in both the papillary and the

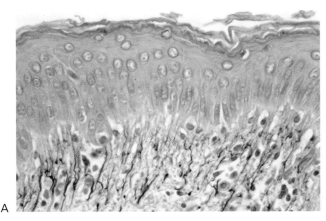
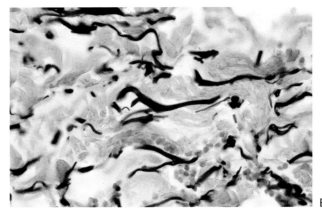

A   B

FIGURE 3-42. Histochemical demonstration of elastin fibers, within papillary dermis **(A)** and reticular dermis **(B)** (silver stain).

reticular dermis (292). Young elastic fibers, as seen in a 22-week-old fetal dermis, show masses of peripheral microfibrils surrounding a small amorphous electron-lucent core representing elastin, with only a few internal microfibrils. As the embryo matures, the amount of elastin and the number of microfibrils within the elastin increase while the number of peripheral microfibrils decreases (293).

In light microscopic sections that are routinely stained, elastic fibers are inconspicuous. With special elastic tissue stains, such as orcein or resorcin-fuchsin or in plastic-embedded sections, they are found entwined among the collagen bundles (Figs. 3-41 and 3-42). Because elastic fibers are thin in comparison with collagen bundles, measuring from 1 μm to 3 μm in diameter, and are wavy, only a small portion of any fiber is seen in histologic sections, giving even normal elastic fibers a fragmented appearance. The elastic fibers are thickest in the lower portion of the dermis, where they are arranged, like collagen bundles, chiefly parallel to the surface of the skin. Elastic fibers become thinner as they approach the epidermis. In the papillary dermis, they form an intermediate plexus of thinner elaunin fibers running parallel to the dermal–epidermal junction (Fig. 3-42A). From this plexus, thin fibers termed oxytalan fibers run upward in the papillary dermis perpendicular to the dermal–epidermal junction and terminate at the PAS-positive basement membrane zone.

The elastic fiber of the dermis consists of two components: the microfibrils and the matrix elastin. The microfibrils are electron-dense and measure 10 nm to 12 nm in diameter. They are aggregated at the periphery of the elastic fiber, giving the fiber its characteristic frayed appearance by ultrastructure. In addition, microfibrils are present within the elastin as strands 15 nm to 80 nm in diameter, extending in a longitudinal direction (294). The microfibril component amounts to only 15% of the elastic fiber, whereas the amorphous electron-lucid elastin makes up 85% of the fiber (295). It is the elastin that stains with elas-

tic tissue stains, is removable by elastase, and is markedly extensible, whereas the microfibrils are the elastic resilient component of the elastic fiber (294).

Elastic fibers undergo significant changes during life. One change, representing aging, is best studied in nonexposed skin. The other change, elastotic degeneration, is the result of chronic sun exposure and will be described elsewhere. In young children up to the age of 10 years, the elastic fibers may not be fully matured, so that microfibrils predominate (296). Physiologic aging is a gradual process and usually becomes quite apparent by ages 30 to 50. There is a gradual decrease in the number of peripheral microfibrils, so that ultimately there may be none and, instead, the surface of the elastic fiber appears irregular and granular (296). The microfibrils within the elastin matrix become thicker and show electron-lucent holes of varying sizes (297). In very old persons, fragmentation and disintegration of some of the elastic fibers may be observed. Oxytalan fibers that consist of microfibrils diminish and ultimately disappear in aging skin.

Ground Substance

The ground substance, an amorphous substance that fills the spaces between collagen fibers and collagen bundles, contains glycosaminoglycans, or acid mucopolysaccharides (Fig. 3-43). These glycosaminoglycans are covalently linked to peptide chains to form high-molecular-weight complexes called proteoglycans (298). Glycosaminoglycans are present in normal skin in such small amounts that they cannot be demonstrated with either routine or special histologic staining methods except in the hair papilla of anagen hair, which contains both nonsulfated and sulfated acid mucopolysaccharides. However, through the study of tissues with an active growth of fibroblasts, as seen in the papillary dermis in dermatofibroma and in the connective tissue around the tumor islands of basal cell epithelioma, it

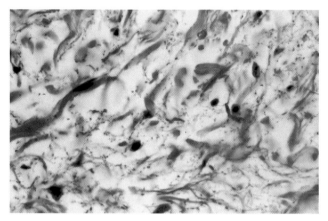

FIGURE 3-43. Ground substance. Although these mucopolysaccharides are normally inconspicuous by conventional light microscopy, in this case they are pathologically increased, and thus visible as thin pale blue-grey strands within widened spaces separating reticular dermal collagen.

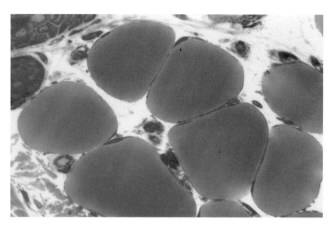

FIGURE 3-44. Mature adipose tissue forming the subcutaneous layer.

is known that the dermal ground substance consists largely of nonsulfated acid mucopolysaccharides such as hyaluronic acid (130). In healing wounds, however, in which new collagen is laid down, the ground substance contains sulfated and nonsulfated acid mucopolysaccharides (299).

The nonsulfated acid mucopolysaccharides consist largely of hyaluronic acid, are stainable with Alcian blue at pH 3.0 but not at pH 0.5, and show metachromasia with toluidine blue at pH 3.0 but not at pH 1.5. The sulfated acid mucopolysaccharides consist largely of chondroitin sulfate, are stainable with Alcian blue at pH 0.5 as well as at pH 3.0, and show metachromasia with toluidine blue at pH 1.5 as well as at pH 3.0. Both nonsulfated and sulfated acid mucopolysaccharides stain with colloidal iron. Testicular hyaluronidase hydrolyzes hyaluronic acid but not the sulfated acid mucopolysaccharides (130).

SUBCUTANEOUS FAT

Fat cells begin to develop in the subcutaneous tissue toward the end of the fifth month. Histologic examination at that time shows (a) spindle-shaped, lipid-free mesenchymal cells as precursor cells; (b) young-type fat cells containing two or more small lipid droplets; and (c) mature fat cells possessing one large central lipid droplet and a peripherally located nucleus, so-called signet-ring cells. Although some of the cells containing multiple, small lipid droplets resemble the multivacuolated mulberry cells present in brown fat and in hibernoma, only a few such cells occur in embryonic white fat. Brown and white fat are two separate entities incapable of interconversion (300).

Mature subcutaneous fat consists of lobules composed of adipocytes with cytoplasm markedly expanded by non-

vacuolated or membrane-bound lipid, which displaces the cell nucleus eccentrically to produce a thin, fusiform contour compressed along the inner plasma membrane (Fig. 3-44). The lipid dissolves in routinely processed specimens, although it is visible in glutaraldehyde-fixed, plastic-embedded specimens. It may be stained histochemically in frozen section obtained from fresh or "wet" tissue retrieved while still in formalin. The lobules that form the subcutis are separated by thin fibrous septae through which small vessels course. The septae provide structural stability to the subcutaneous layer by compartmentalizing it and by connecting the lowermost reticular dermis to the fascial planes that underlie the subcutis.

REFERENCES

1. Morrison P, Morrison P. *Powers of ten.* Redding, CT: Scientific American Library, 1982.
2. Breathnach AS. Embryology of human skin. *J Invest Dermatol* 1971;57:133–143.
3. Holbrook KA, Odland GF. The fine structure of developing human epidermis: light, scanning, and transmission electron microscopy of the periderm. *J Invest Dermatol* 1975;65:16–38.
4. Hashimoto K, Gross BG, Dibella RJ, et al. The ultrastructure of the skin of human embryos. IV. The epidermis. *J Invest Dermatol* 1966;47:317–335.
5. Matsunaka M, Mishima Y. Electron microscopy of embryonic human epidermis at seven and ten weeks. *Acta Derm Venereol (Stockh)* 1969;49:241–250.
6. Van Scott EJ, Ekel TM. Kinetics of hyperplasia in psoriasis. *Arch Dermatol* 1963;88:373–381.
7. Penneys NS, Fulton JE Jr, Weinstein GD, et al. Location of proliferating cells in human epidermis. *Arch Dermatol* 1970;101:323–327.
8. Lavker RM, Sun T-T. Heterogeneity in epidermal basal keratinocytes: morphological and functional correlations. *Science* 19;215:1239–1241.
9. Cotsarelis G, Sun T-T, Lavker RM. Label-retaining cells reside in the bulge area of the pilosebaceous unit: implications for follicu-

lar stem cells, hair cycle and skin carcinogenesis. *Cell* 1990;61: 1329–1337.

10. Cerimele D, Del Forno C, Serri F. Histochemistry of the intercellular substance of the normal and psoriatic human epidermis. *Arch Dermatol Res* 1978;262:27–36.

11. Hashimoto K, Lever WF. The cell surface coat of normal keratinocytes and of acantholytic keratinocytes in pemphigus. *Br J Dermatol* 1970;83:282–290.

12. Odland GF. The fine structure of the interrelationship of cells in the human epidermis. *J Biophys Biochem Cytol* 1958;4:529–538.

13. Wolff K, Schreiner E. An electron microscopic study on the extraneous coat of keratinocytes and the intercellular space of the epidermis. *J Invest Dermatol* 1968;51:418–430.

14. Wolff K, Wolff-Schreiner EC. Trends in electron microscopy of skin. *J Invest Dermatol* 1976;67:39–57.

15. Amagi M. Adhesion molecules. I. Keratinocyte-keratinocyte interactions, cadherins and pemphigus. *Prog Dermatol* 1995;104: 146–151.

16. Buxton RS, Magee AI. Structure and interactions of desmosomal and other cadherins. *Semin Cell Biol* 1992;3:157–167.

17. Amagai M, Klaus KV, Stanley JR. Autoantibodies against a novel epithelial cadherin in pemphigus vulgaris. a disease of cell adhesion. *Cell* 1991;67. 869–877.

18. Shimuzu H, Masunaga T, Ishiko A, et al. Demonstration of desmosomal antigens by electron microscopy using cryofixed and cryosubstituted skin with silver-enhanced gold probe. *J Histochem Cytochem* 1994;42:687–692.

19. Matoltsy AG. Desmosomes, filaments, and keratohyaline granules: their role in stabilization and keratinization of the epidermis. *J Invest Dermatol* 1975;65:127–142.

20. Matoltsy AG. Keratinization. *J Invest Dermatol* 1976;67:20–25.

21. Schwarz E. Biochemie der epidermalen Keratinisation. In: Marchionini A, ed. *Handbuch der Haut- und Geschlechtskrankheiten*, vol. 1, part 4A. Berlin: Springer-Verlag, 1979:1–115.

22. Lazarus GS, Hatcher VB, Levine N. Lysosomes and the skin. *J Invest Dermatol* 1975;65:259–271.

23. Spearman RIC. Some light microscopical observations on the stratum corneum of the guinea pig, man and common seal. *Br J Dermatol* 1970;83:582–590.

24. Christophers E. Cellular architecture of the stratum corneum. *J Invest Dermatol* 1971;56:165–169.

25. Hashimoto K. Cellular envelopes of keratinized cells of the human epidermis. *Arch Klin Exp Dermatol* 1969;235:374–385.

26. Bell RF, Kellum RE. Early formation of keratohyalin granules in rat epidermis. *Acta Derm Venereol (Stockh)* 1967;47:350–353.

27. Dale BA. Filaggrin, the matrix protein of keratin. *Am J Dermatopathol* 1985;7:65–68.

28. Brody I. An electron microscopic study of the fibrillar density in the normal human stratum corneum. *J Ultrastruct Res* 1970;30: 209–217.

29. Murphy GF, Flynn TC, Rice RH, et al. Involucrin expression in normal and neoplastic human skin. a marker for keratinocyte differentiation. *J Invest Dermatol* 1884;82:453–457.

30. Wolff-Schreiner EC. Ultrastructural cytochemistry of the epidermis [review]. *Int J Dermatol* 1977;16:77–102.

31. Elias PM. Epidermal lipids, barrier function, and desquamation. *J Invest Dermatol* 1983;80[Suppl]:44–49.

32. Schreiner E, Wolff K. Die Permeabilität des epidermalen Intercellularraums für kleinmolekulares Protein. *Arch Klin Exp Dermatol* 1969;235:78–88.

33. Elias PM, Goerke J, Friend DS. Mammalian epidermal barrier layer lipids: composition and influence on structure. *J Invest Dermatol* 1977;69:535–546.

34. Epstein EH Jr, Williams ML, Elias PM. Editorial. Steroid sulfatase, X-linked ichthyosis, and stratum corneum cell cohesion. *Arch Dermatol* 1981;117:761–763.

35. Braun-Falco O, Rupec M. Die Verteilung der sauren Phosphatase bei normaler und psoriatischer Verhornung. *Dermatologica* 1967;134:225–242.

36. Wolff K, Schreiner E. Epidermal lysosomes: electron microscopic cytochemical studies. *Arch Dermatol* 1970;101:276–286.

37. Bos JD, Kapsenberg ML. The skin immune system:progress in cutaneous biology. *Immunol Today* 1993;14:75–78.

38. Katz SI. The skin as an immunologic organ: allergic contact dermatitis as a paradigm. *J Dermatol* 1993;20:593–603.

39. Becker SW Jr, Zimmermann AA. Further studies on melanocytes and melanogenesis in the human fetus and newborn. *J Invest Dermatol* 1955;25:103–112.

40. Sagebiel RW, Odland GF. Ultrastructural identification of melanocytes in early human embryos. *J Invest Dermatol* 1970;54: 96(abst).

41. Holbrook KA, Underwood RA, Vogel AM, et al. The appearance, density and distribution of melanocytes in human embryonic and fetal skin revealed by the anti-melanoma monoclonal antibody HMB-45. *Anat Embryol* 1989;180:443.

42. Cochran AJ. The incidence of melanocytes in normal skin. *J Invest Dermatol* 1970;55:65–70.

43. Clark WH Jr, Watson MC, Watson BEM. Two kinds of "clear" cells in the human epidermis. *Am J Pathol* 1961;39:333–344.

44. Fitzpatrick TB. Human melanogenesis. *Arch Dermatol Syph* 1952;65:379–391.

45. Pearse AGE. *Histochemistry: theoretical and applied*, 3rd ed. Edinburgh: Churchill Livingstone, 1972.

46. Bloch B. Das Problem der Pigmentbildung in der Haut. *Arch Dermatol Syph Berlin* 1917;124:129–143.

47. Gilchrest BA, Blog FB, Szabo G. Effects of aging and chronic sun exposure on melanocytes in human skin. *J Invest Dermatol* 1979;73:141–143.

48. Tarnowski WM. Ultrastructure of the epidermal melanocyte dense plate. *J Invest Dermatol* 1970;55:265–268.

49. Fitzpatrick TB, Miyomato M, Ishikawa K. The evolution of concepts of melanin biology. *Arch Dermatol* 1967;96:305–323.

50. Toshima S, Moore GE, Sandberg AA. Ultrastructure of human melanoma in cell culture. Electron microscopic studies. *Cancer* 1968;21:202–216.

51. Staricco RJ, Pinkus H. Quantitative and qualitative data on the pigment cells of adult human epidermis. *J Invest Dermatol* 1957; 28:33–45.

52. Fitzpatrick TB, Szabo G. The melanocytes: cytology and cytochemistry. *J Invest Dermatol* 1959;32:197–209.

53. Quevedo WC Jr, Szabo G, Virks J, et al. Melanocyte populations in UV-radiated human skin. *J Invest Dermatol* 1965;45:295–298.

54. Pathak MA, Sinesi SJ, Szabo G. The effect of a single dose of ultraviolet radiation on epidermal melanocytes. *J Invest Dermatol* 1965;45:520–528.

55. Mishima Y, Tanay A. The effect of alpha-methyldopa and ultraviolet irradiation on melanogencis. *Dermatologica* 1968;136: 105–114.

56. Lerner AB, Fitzpatrick TB. Biochemistry of melanin formation. *Physiol Rev* 1950;30:91–126.

57. Lerner AB. On the etiology of vitiligo and gray hair. *Am J Med* 1971;51:141–147.

58. Szabo G. Tyrosinase in the epidermal melanocytes of white human skin. *Arch Dermatol* 1967;76:324–329.

59. Hunter JAA, Mottaz JH, Zelickson AS. Melanogenesis: ultrastructural histochemical observations on ultraviolet irradiated human melanocytes. *J Invest Dermatol* 1970;54:213–221.

60. Jimbow K, Quevedo WC Jr, Fitzpatrick TB, et al. Some aspects of melanin biology [review]. *J Invest Dermatol* 1976;67:72–89.

61. Nakagawa H, Rhodes A, Fitzpatrick TB, et al. Acid phosphatase in melanosome formation: a cytochemical study in normal human melanocytes. *J Invest Dermatol* 1984;83:140–144.

62. Shibata T, Prota G, Mishima Y. Non-melanosomal regulatory factors in melanogenesis. *J Invest Dermatol* 1993;100:274–280.

63. Cruickshank CND, Harcourt SA. Pigment donation in vitro. *J Invest Dermatol* 1964;42:183–184.

64. Valyi-Nagy IT, Murphy GF, Mancianti M-L, et al. Phenotypes and interactions of human melanocytes and keratinocytes in an epidermal reconstruction model. *Lab Invest* 1990;62:314–324.

65. Mottaz JH, Zelickson AS. Melanin transfer: a possible phagocytic process. *J Invest Dermatol* 1967;49:605–610.

66. Olson RL, Nordquist J, Everett MA. The role of epidermal lysosomes in melanin physiology. *Br J Dermatol* 1970;83:189–199.

67. Szabo G, Gerald AB, Pathak MA, et al. The ultrastructure of racial color differences in man. *J Invest Dermatol* 1970;54: 98(abst).

68. Minwalla L, Zhao Y, LePoole IC, et al. Keratinocytes play a role in regulating distribution patterns of recipient melanosomes in vitro. *J Invest Dermatol* 2001;117:341–347.

69. Flaxman BA, Sosio AC, Van Scott EJ. Changes in melanosome distribution in Caucasoid skin following topical application of N mustard. *J Invest Dermatol* 1973;60:321–326.

70. Wolff K, Schreiner E. Melanosomal acid phosphatase. *Arch Dermatol Forsch* 1971;241:255–272.

71. Toda K, Kathak MA, Parrish JA, et al. Alteration of racial differences in melanosome distribution in human epidermis after exposure to ultraviolet light. *Nature* 1972;236:143–145.

72. Moll I, Lane AT, Franke WW, et al. Intraepidermal formation of Merkel cells in xenografts of human skin. *J Invest Dermatol* 1990;94:359.

73. Moll I. Merkel cell distribution in human hair follicles of the fetal and adult scalp. *Cell Tiss Res* 1994;277:131–138.

74. Hashimoto K. Fine structure of Merkel cell in human oral mucosa. *J Invest Dermatol* 1972;58:381–387.

75. Kidd RL, Krawczyk WS, Wilgram GF. The Merkel cell in human epidermis. Its differentiation from other dendritic cells. *Arch Dermatol Forsch* 1971;241:374–384.

76. Smith KR Jr. The ultrastructure of the human Haarsheibe and Merkel cells. *J Invest Dermatol* 1970;54:150–159.

77. Moll R, Moll I, Franke WW. Identification of Merkel cells in human skin by specific cytokeratin antibodies: changes in cell density and distribution in fetal and adult plantar epidermis. *Differentiation* 1984; 28:136.

78. Saurat JH, Merot Y, Didierjean L, et al. Normal rabbit Merkel cells do not express neurofilament proteins. *J Invest Dermatol* 1984;82:641–642.

79. Ortonne JP, Darmon M. Merkel cells express desmosomal proteins and cytokeratins. *Acta Derm Venereol (Stockh)* 1985;65: 161–164.

80. Ortonne JP, Petchot-Bacque JP, Verrando P, et al. Normal Merkel cells express a synaptophysin-like immunoreactivity. *Dermatologica* 1988;177:1–10.

81. Masuda T, Ikida S, Tajima K, et al. Neuron-specific enolase (NSE). A specific marker for Merkel cells in human epidermis. *J Dermatol* 1986;13:67–69.

82. Foster A, Holbrook KA, Farr AG. Ontogeny of Langerhans' cells in human embryonic and fetal skin. *J Invest Dermatol* 1986;86: 240–243.

83. Penneys NS, Stoer C, Buck B, et al. Langerhans' cells in fetal and newborn skin and newborn thymus. *Arch Dermatol* 1984;120: 1082(abst).

84. Wolff K, Winkelmann RK. The influence of ultraviolet light on the Langerhans cell population and its hydrolytic enzymes in guinea pigs. *J Invest Dermatol* 1967;48:531–539.

85. Murphy GF, Shepard RS, Harrist TJ, et al. Ultrastructural documentation of HLA-DR antigen reactivity in normal human acrosyringeal epithelium. *J Invest Dermatol* 1983;81:181–183.

86. Murphy GF, Bhan AK, Sato S, et al. A new immunologic marker for human Langerhans cells. *N Engl J Med* 1981;304:791–792.

87. Fithian E, Kung P, Goldstein G, et al. Reactivity of Langerhans cells with hybridoma antibody. *Proc Natl Acad Sci U S A* 1981; 78:2541.

88. Murphy GF, Bhan AK, Sato S, et al. Characterization of Langerhans cells by the use of monoclonal antibodies. *Lab Invest* 1981; 45:465–468.

89. Breathnach AS, Wyllie LMA. Melanin in Langerhans cells. *J Invest Dermatol* 1965;45:401–403.

90. Niebauer G, Krawczyk WS, Wilgram GF. Ber Die Langerhans-Zell organelle bei Morbus Letterer-Siwe. *Arch Klin Exp Dermatol* 1970;239:125–137.

91. Hashimoto K. Langerhans' cell granule. An endocytic organelle. *Arch Dermatol* 1971;104:148–160.

92. Hanau D, Fabre M, Schmitt DA, et al. Human epidermal Langerhans cells internalize by receptor-mediated endocytosis T6 surface antigen. Birbeck granules are involved in the intracellular traffic of the T6 antigen. *J Invest Dermatol* 1987;89:172–177.

93. Murphy GF, Bhan AK, Harrist TJ, et al. In situ identification of T6-positive cells in normal human dermis by immunoelectron microscopy. *Br J Dermatol* 1983;108:423–431.

94. Chu A, Eisinger M, Lee JS, et al. Immunoelectron microscopic identification of Langerhans cells using a new antigenic marker. *J Invest Dermatol* 1982;78:177–180.

95. Horton JJ, Allen MH, Macdonald DM. An assessment of Langerhans cell quantification in tissue sections. *J Am Acad Dermatol* 1984;11:591–593.

96. Mackie RM, Turbitt ML. The use of a double-label immunoperoxidase monoclonal antibody technique in the investigation of patients with mycosis fungoides. *Br J Dermatol* 1982;106:379–384.

97. Kiistala U, Mustakallio KK. The presence of Langerhans cells in human dermis with special reference to their potential mesenchymal origin. *Acta Derm Venereol (Stockh)* 1968;48:115–122.

98. Tamaki K, Stingl G, Katz SI. The origin of Langerhans cells. *J Invest Dermatol* 1980;74:309–311.

99. Wolff K, Stingl G. The Langerhans cell. *J Invest Dermatol* 1983; 80[Suppl]:17–21.

100. Wolff, K. The Langerhans cell. *Curr Probl Dermatol* 1972; 4: 79–145.

101. Nezelof C, Basset F, Rousseau MF. Histiocytosis X: arguments for a Langerhans cell origin. *Biomedicine* 1973;18:365–371.

102. Shimada S, Katz SI. The skin as an immunologic organ. *Arch Pathol Lab Med* 1988;112:231–234.

103. Breathnach S, Katz SI. Cell-mediated immunity in cutaneous disease. *Hum Pathol* 1986;17:161–167.

104. Murphy GF, Bronstein BR, Knowles RW, et al. Ultrastructural documentation of M241 glycoprotein on dendritic cells in normal human skin. *Lab Invest* 1985;52:264–269.

105. Flotte TJ, Murphy GF, Bhan AK. Demonstration of T200 on human Langerhans cell surface membranes. *J Invest Dermatol* 1984;82:535–537.

106. Krueger GG, Emam M. Biology of Langerhans cells: analysis by experiments to deplete Langerhans cells from human skin. *J Invest Dermatol* 1984;82:613–617.

107. Belsito DV, Flotte TJ, Lim HW, et al. Effect of glucocorticosteroids on epidermal Langerhans cells. *J Exp Med* 1982;155: 291.

108. Belsito DV, Sanchez MR, Baer RL, et al. Reduced Langerhans cell Ia antigen and ATPase activity in patients with acquired immunodeficiency syndrome. *N Engl J Med* 1984;310:1279.

109. Tschachler E, Groh V, Popovic M, et al. Epidermal Langerhans cells-a target for HTLV-III/LAV infection. *J Invest Dermatol* 1987;88:233,1987.

110. Wood GS, Warner NL, Warnke RA. Leu3/4 antibodies react with cells of monocyte/macrophage and Langerhans cell lineage. *J Immunol* 1983;131:212.

111. Bourlond A, Vandooren-Deflorenne R. La membrane basale sous-épidermique. Sa structure et son ultrastructure. *Arch Belg Derm Syph* 1968;24:119–135.

112. Stoughton R, Wells G. A histochemical study on polysaccharides in normal and diseased skin. *J Invest Dermatol* 1950;14: 37–51.

113. Cooper JH. Microanatomical and histochemical observations on the dermal–epidermal junction. *Arch Dermatol* 1958;77:18–22.

114. Hashimoto K, Lever WF. An ultrastructural study of cell junctions in pemphigus vulgaris. *Arch Dermatol* 1970;101:287–298.

115. Tarnowski WM. Ultrastructure of the epidermal melanocyte-dense plate. *J Invest Dermatol* 1970;55:265–268.

116. Eady RAJ. The basement membrane. *Arch Dermatol* 1988;124: 709–712.

117. Eady RAJ. Babes, blisters and basement membranes: from sticky molecules to epidermolysis bullosa. *Clin Exp Dermatol* 1986;12:161–170.

118. Bruckner-Tuderman L, Ruegger S, Odermatt B, et al. Lack of type VII collagen in unaffected skin of patients with severe recessive dystrophic epidermolysis bullosa. *Dermatologica* 1988; 176:57–64.

119. Frances C, Robert L. Elastin and elastic fibers in normal and pathologic skin. *Int J Dermatol* 1984;23:166–179.

120. Kobayasi T. Dermoepidermal junction of normal skin. *J Dermatol (Tokyo)* 1978;5:157–165.

121. Yancey KB. Adhesion molecules. II. Interactions of keratinocytes with epidermal basement membrane. *Prog Dermatol* 1995;104:1008–1014.

122. Hashimoto K. The ultrastructure of the skin of human embryos. V. The hair germs and perifollicular mesenchymal cells. *Br J Dermatol* 1970;83:167–176.

123. Serri F, Montagna W, Mescon H. Studies of the skin of the fetus and the child. *J Invest Dermatol* 1962;39:199–217.

124. Mishima Y, Widlan S. Embryonic development of melanocytes in human hair and epidermis. *J Invest Dermatol* 1966;46:263–277.

125. Pinkus H. Embryology of hair. In: Montagna W, Ellis RA, eds. *The biology of hair growth*. New York: Academic Press, 1958: 1–23.

126. Hashimoto K. The ultrastructure of the skin of human embryos. IX. Formation of the hair cone and intraepidermal hair canal. *Arch Klin Exp Dermatol* 1970;238:333–345.

127. Hashimoto K. The ultrastructure of the skin of human embryos. VII. Formation of the apocrine gland. *Acta Derm Venereol (Stockh)* 1970;50:241–251.

128. Thiers BH, Galbraith GMP. Alopecia areata. In: Thiers BH, Dobson RL, eds. *Pathogenesis of skin diseases*. New York: Churchill Livingstone, 1986:57–64.

129. Kollar EJ. The induction of hair follicles by embryonic dermal papillae. *J Invest Dermatol* 1970;55:374–378.

130. Johnson WC, Helwig EB. Histochemistry of the acid mucopolysaccharides of skin in normal and in certain pathologic conditions. *Am J Clin Pathol* 1963;40:123–131.

131. Kopf AW, Orentreich N. Alkaline phosphatase in alopecia areata. *Arch Dermatol* 1957;76:288–295.

132. Cormia F. Vasculature of the normal scalp. *Arch Dermatol* 1963;88:692–701.

133. Pinkus H. Anatomy and histology of skin. In: Graham JH, Johnson WC, Helwig EB, eds. *Dermal pathology*. Hagerstown, MD: Harper & Row, 1972:1–24.

134. Zaun H. Histologie, Histochemie und Wachstumsdynamik des Haarfollikels. In: Marchionini A, ed. *Handbuch der Haut- und Geschlechtskrankheiten. Ergänzungswerk*, vol. 1, part 1. Berlin: Springer-Verlag, 1968:143–183.

135. Garn SM. The examination of hair under the polarizing microscope. *Ann N Y Acad Sci* 1951;53:649–652.

136. Leppard BJ, Sanderson KV, Wells RS. Hereditary trichilemmal cysts. *Clin Exp Dermatol* 1976;2:23–32.

137. Bandmann HJ, Bosse K. Histologie und Anatomie des Haarfollikels im Verlauf des Haarcyclus. *Arch Klin Exp Dermatol* 1966;227:390–409.

138. Montagna W. *The structure and function of skin*, 2nd ed. New York: Academic Press, 1962.

139. Parakkal PF, Matoltsy AG. A study of the differentiation products of the hair follicle cells with the electron microscope. *J Invest Dermatol* 1964;43:23–34.

140. Staricco RG. The melanocytes and the hair follicle. *J Invest Dermatol* 1960;35:185–194.

141. Pinkus H. "Sebaceous cysts" are trichilemmal cysts. *Arch Dermatol* 1969;99:544–555.

142. Strauss JS, Pochi PE. Histology, histochemistry, and electron microscopy of sebaceous glands in man. In: Marchionini A, ed. *Handbuch der Haut- und Geschlechtskrankheiten, Ergänzungswerk*, vol. 1, part 1. Berlin: Springer-Verlag, 1968:184–223.

143. Suskind RK. The chemistry of the human sebaceous gland. I. Histochemical observations. *J Invest Dermatol* 1951;17:37–54.

144. Cashion PD, Skobe Z, Nalbandian J. Ultrastructural observations on sebaceous glands of the human oral mucosa (Fordyce's disease). *J Invest Dermatol* 1969;53:208–216.

145. Rupec M. Zur Ultrastruktur der Talgdrüsenzelle. *Arch Klin Exp Dermatol* 1969;234:273–292.

146. Niizuma K. Lipid droplets of the sebaceous glands: some observations from tannic acid fixation. *Acta Derm Venerol (Stockh)* 1979;59:401–405.

147. Rupec M, Braun-Falco O. Zur Frage lysosomaler Aktivität in normalen menschlichen Talgdrüsen. *Arch Klin Exp Dermatol* 1968;232:312–324.

148. Rowden G. Aryl sulfatase in the sebaceous glands of mouse skin. *J Invest Dermatol* 1968;51:41–50.

149. Ito M, Suzuki M, Motoyoshi K, et al. New findings on the proteins of sebaceous glands. *J Invest Dermatol* 1984;82:381–385.

150. Hyman AB, Brownstein MH. Tyson's glands. *Arch Dermatol* 1969;99:31–36.

151. Weedon D, Strutton G. Apoptosis As the mechanism of the involution of hair follicles in catagen formation. *Acta Derm Venereol (Stockh)* 1981;61:335–339.

152. Kligman AM. The human hair cycle. *J Invest Dermatol* 1959; 33:307–316.

153. Mahrle G, Orfanos CE. Haarfarbe und Haarpigment. *Arch Dermatol Forsch* 1973;248:109–122.

154. Herzberg J, Gusek W. Das Ergrauen des Kopfhaares. *Arch Klin Exp Dermatol* 1970;236:368–384.

155. Waldorf HA, Walsh LJ, Schechter NM, et al. Early cellular events in evolving cutaneous delayed hypersensitivity in humans. *Am J Pathol* 1991;138:477–486.

156. Hashimoto K, Gross BG, Lever WF. The ultrastructure of the skin of human embryos. I. The intraepidermal eccrine sweat duct. *J Invest Dermatol* 1965;45:139–151.

157. Hashimoto K, Gross BG, Lever WF. The ultrastructure of human embryo skin. II. The formation of intradermal portion of the eccrine sweat duct and of the secretory segment during the first half of embryonic life. *J Invest Dermatol* 1966;46: 513–529.

158. Christophers E, Plewig G. Formation of the acrosyringium. *Arch Dermatol* 1973;107:378–382.

159. Hashimoto K, Gross BG, Lever WF. Electron microscopic study of the human adult eccrine gland. I. The duct. *J Invest Dermatol* 1966;46:172–185.

160. Montagna W, Chase HB, Lobitz WC Jr. Histology and cytochemistry of human skin. IV. The eccrine sweat glands. *J Invest Dermatol* 1963;20:415–423.

161. Headington JT. Primary mucinous carcinoma of skin. Histochemistry and electron microscopy. *Cancer* 1977;39:1055–1063.

162. Dobson RL, Sato K. The secretion of salt and water by the eccrine sweat gland. *Arch Dermatol* 1972;105:366–370.

163. Hurley HJ, Witkowski JA. The dynamics of eccrine sweating in man. *J Invest Dermatol* 1962;39:329–338.

164. Schiefferdecker P. Die Hautdrüsen des Menschen und der Säugetiere, ihre biologische und rassenanatomische Bedeutung, sowie die Muscularis sexualis. *Biol Ztrbl* 1917;37:534–562.

165. Schaumburg-Lever G, Lever WF. Secretion from human apocrine glands. *J Invest Dermatol* 1975;64:38–41.

166. Montes LF, Baker BL, Curtis AC. The cytology of the large axillary sweat glands in man. *J Invest Dermatol* 1960;35:273–291.

167. Hurley HJ, Shelley WB. *The human apocrine sweat gland in health and disease*. Springfield, IL: Charles C. Thomas, 1960.

168. Montagna W, Yun JS. The glands of Montgomery. *Br J Dermatol* 1972;86:126–133.

169. Smith DM JR, Peter TG, Donegan WL. Montgomery's areolar tubercle. *Arch Pathol Lab Med* 1982;106:60–63.

170. Sato K, Kane N, Soos G, et al. The eccrine sweat gland. basic science and disorders of eccrine sweating. *Prog Dermatol* 1995;29:1–11.

171. Sato K, Sato F. Interleukin-1 in human sweat is functionally active and derived from the eccrine sweat gland. *Am J Physiol* 1994;266:950–959.

172. Kuroisumi K, Yamagishi M, Sekine M. Mitochondrial deformation and apocrine secretory mechanism in the rabbit submandibular organ as revealed by electron microscopy. *Z Zellforsch* 1961;55:297–312.

173. Inoue T. Scanning electron microscope study of the human axillary apocrine glands. *J Dermatol (Tokyo)* 1979;6:299–308.

174. Spielman AI, Zeng X-N, Leyden JJ, et al. Proteinaceous precursors of human axillary odor. isolation of two novel odor-binding proteins. *Experentia* 1995;51:40–47.

175. Scher R, Daniel CR. *Nails: therapy, diagnosis, surgery*. Philadelphia: WB Saunders, 1990.

176. Hashimoto K. Ultrastructure of the human toenail. II. Keratinization and formation of the marginal band. *J Ultrastruct Res* 1971;36:391.

177. Hashimoto K. The marginal band: a demonstration of thickened cellular envelope of the human nail cell with the aid of lanthanum staining. *Arch Dermatol* 1971;103:387–393.

178. Johnson M, Shuster S. Continuous formation of a nail along the bed. *Br J Dermatol* 1993;128:277–280.

179. Higashi N. Melanocytes of the nail matrix and nail pigmentation. *Arch Dermatol* 1971;97:570.

180. Hashimoto K. Ultrastructure of the human toenail. I. Proximal nail matrix. *J Invest Dermatol* 1971;56:235.

181. Moretti G. The blood vessels of the skin. In: Marchionini A, ed. *Handbuch der Haut- und Geschlechtskrankheiten, Ergänzungswerk*, vol. 1, part 1. Berlin: Springer-Verlag, 1968:491–623.

182. Kopf AW. The distribution of alkaline phosphatase in normal and pathologic human skin. *Arch Dermatol* 1957;75:1–37.

183. Klingmuller G. Die Darstellung alkalischer Phosphatase in Capillaren. *Hautarzt* 1958;9:84–88.

184. Yen A, Braverman IM. Ultrastructure of the human dermal microcirculation: the horizontal plexus of the papillary dermis. *J Invest Dermatol* 1976;66:131–142.

185. Braverman IM, Yen A. Ultrastructure of human dermal microcirculation. II. The capillary loop of the dermal papillae. *J Invest Dermatol* 1977;68:44–52.

186. Seifert HW, Klingmuller G. Elektronenmikroskopische Struktur normaler Kapillaren und das Verhalten alkalischer Phosphatase. *Arch Dermatol Forsch* 1972;242:97–110.

187. Thorgeirsson G, Robertson AL Jr. The vascular endothelium—pathobiologic significance. *Am J Pathol* 1978;93:803–848.

188. Weber K, Braun-Falco O. Ultrastructure of blood vessels in human granulation tissue. *Arch Dermatol Forsch* 1973;248:29–44.

189. Holthofer H, Virtanen I, Kariniemi A-L, et al. Ulex europaeus I lectin as a marker for vascular endothelium in human tissues. *Lab Invest* 1982;47:60–66.

190. Albelda SM, Oliver P, Romer L, et al. EndoCAM: a novel endothelial cell–cell adhesion molecule. *J Cell Biol* 1990;110:1227–1237.

191. Berger R, Albelda S, Berd D, et al. Expression of platelet-endothelial cell adhesion molecule-1 (PECAM-1) during melanoma-induced angiogenesis in vivo. *J Invest Dermatol* 1992;98:584–589.

192. Suzuki Y, Hashimoto K, Crissman J, et al. The value of blood group-specific lectin and endothelial associated antibodies in the diagnosis of vascular proliferations. *J Cutan Pathol* 1986;13:408–419.

193. Smolle J. HLA-DR antigen-bearing keratinocytes in various dermatologic diseases. *Acta Derm Venereol* 1985;65:9–13.

194. Jones DA, Abbasi O, McIntire LV, et al. P-selectin mediates neutrophil rolling on histamine-stimulated endothelial cells. *Biophys J* 1991;65:1560–1569.

195. Thorlacius H, Raud J, Rosengren-Beezley S, et al. Mast cell activation induces P-selectin-dependent leukocyte rolling and adhesion in postcapillary venules in vivo. *Biochem Biophys Res Commun* 1994;203:1043–1049.

196. Albelda SM, Smith CW, Ward PA. Adhesion molecules and inflammatory injury. *FASEB* 1994;8:504–512.

197. Butcher EC. Leukocyte-endothelial cell recognition. three (or more) steps to specificity and diversity. *Cell* 1991;67:1033–1036.

198. Walsh LJ, Murphy GF. Role of adhesion molecules in cutaneous inflammation and neoplasia. *J Cutan Pathol* 1992;19:161–171.

199. Mcever RP. Selectins: novel receptors that mediate leukocyte adhesion during inflammation. *Thrombosis and Haemostasis* 1991;65:22–28.

200. Ioffreda M, Elder DE, Albelda SM, et al. TNFa induces E-selectin expression and PECAM–1 (CD31) redistribution in extracutaneous tissues. *Endothelium* 1993;1:47–54.

201. Mescon H, Hurley HJ, Moretti G. The anatomy and histochemistry of the arteriovenous anastomosis in human digital skin. *J Invest Dermatol* 1956;27:133–145.

202. Pepper M, Laubenheimer R, Cripps DJ. Multiple glomus tumors. *J Cutan Pathol* 1977;4:244–257.

203. Goodman TF. Fine structure of the cells of the Suquet–Hoyer canal. *J Invest Dermatol* 1972;59:363–369.

204. Hashimoto K, Tarnowski WM, Lever WF. Reifung und Degran-ulierung der Mastzellen in der menschlichen Haut. *Hautarzt* 1967;18:318–324.

205. Lagunoff D. Contributions of electron microscopy to the study of mast cells. *J Invest Dermatol* 1972;58:296–211.

206. Whitaker-Menezes D, Schechter NM, Murphy GF. Serine proteinases are regionally segregated within mast cell granules. *Lab Invest* 1995;72:34–41.

207. Irani AA, Bradford TR, Kepley CL, et al. Detection of MCT and MCTC types of human mast cells by immunohistochemistry using new monoclonal anti-tryptase and anti-chymase antibodies. *J Histochem Cytochem* 1989;37:1509–1515.

208. Craig SS, Schechter NM, Schwartz LB. Ultrastructural analysis of maturing human T and TC mast cells identified by immunoelectron microscopy. *Lab Invest* 1988;58:682–691.

209. Mirowski G, Austen KF, Horan RF, et al. Characterization of the cellular dermal infiltrates in human cutaneous mastocytosis. *Lab Invest* 1990;63:52–62.

210. Kobayasi T, Asboe-Hansen G. Degranulation and regranulation of human mast cells. *Acta Derm Venereol (Stockh)* 1969;49: 369–372.

211. Kaminer MS, Lavker RM, Walsh D, et al. Extracellular localization of human connective tissue mast cell granule contents. *J Invest Dermatol* 1991;96:1–8.

212. Uvnas B. Chemistry and storage function of mast cell granules. *J Invest Dermatol* 1978;71:76–80.

213. Kaliner MA. Editorial. The mast cell, a fascinating riddle. *N Engl J Med* 1979;301:498–499.

214. Lewis RE, Buchsbaum M, Whitaker D, et al. Intercellular adhesion molecule expression in the evolving cutaneous delayed hypersensitivity reaction. *J Invest Dermatol* 1989;93:672–677.

215. Murphy GF, Sueki H, Teuschler C, et al. Role of mast cells in early epithelial target cell injury in experimental acute graft-versus-host disease. *J Invest Dermatol* 1994;102:451–461.

216. Walsh LJ, Trinchieri G, Waldorf HA, et al. Human dermal mast cells contain and release tumor necrosis factor-α which induces endothelial leukocyte adhesion molecule-1. *Proc Natl Acad Sci U S A* 1991;88:4220–4224.

217. Klein LM, Lavker RM, Matis WL, et al. Degranulation of human mast cells induces an endothelial antigen central to leukocyte adhesion. *Proc Natl Acad Sci U S A* 1989;86:8972–8976.

218. Christofidou-Solomidou M, Murphy GF, Albelda SM. Induction of E-selectin-dependent leukocyte recruitment by mast cell degranulation in human skin grafts transplanted on SCID mice. *Am J Pathol* 1996;148:177–188.

219. Walsh LJ, Kaminer MS, Lazarus GS, et al. Role of laminin in localization of human dermal mast cells. *Lab Invest* 1991;65: 433–440.

220. Weiss RR, Whitaker-Menezes, Longley J, et al. Human dermal endothelial cells express membrane-associated mast cell growth factor. *J Invest Dermatol* 1995;104:101–106.

221. Winkelmann RK. Silver impregnation method for peripheral nerve endings. *J Invest Dermatol* 1955;24:57–64.

222. Woollard HH, Weddell G, Harpman JA. Observations on neurohistological basis of cutaneous pain. *J Anat* 1940;74:413–440.

223. Arthur RP, Shelley WB. The innervation of human epidermis. *J Invest Dermatol* 1959;32:397–413.

224. Reed RJ. Cutaneous manifestations of neural crest disorders. *Int J Dermatol* 1977;16:807–826.

225. Wiesner-Menzel L, Schultz B, Vakilzadeh F, et al. Electron microscopical evidence for a direct contact between nerve fibers and mast cells. *Acta Derm Venereol* 1981;61:465–475.

226. Hosoi J, Murphy GF, Egan CL, et al. Regulation of Langerhans cell function by nerves containing calcitonin gene-related peptide. *Nature* 1993;363:159–163.

227. Matis WL, Lavker RM, Murphy GF. Substance P induces the expression of an endothelial-leukocyte adhesion molecule by microvascular endothelium. *J Invest Dermatol* 1990;94:492–495.

228. Ashina A, Hosoi I, Bruvers S, et al. Regulation of Langerhans cell protein antigen presentation by calcitonin gene-related peptide, granulocyte-macrophage colony stimulating factor, and tumor necrosis factor α. *J Invest Dermatol* 1993;100: 489(abst).

229. Orfanos CE, Mahrle G. Ultrastructure and cytochemistry of human cutaneous nerves. *J Invest Dermatol* 1973;61:108–120.

230. Macdonald DM, Schmitt D. Ultrastructure of the human mucocutaneous end organ. *J Invest Dermatol* 1979;72:181–186.

231. Cauna N, Ross LL. The fine structure of Meissner's touch corpuscles of human fingers. *J Biophys Biochem Cytol* 1960;8:467–482.

232. Hashimoto K. Fine structure of the Meissner corpuscle of human palmar skin. *J Invest Dermatol* 1973;60:20–28.

233. Pease DC, Quilliam TA. Electron microscopy of the Pacinian corpuscle. *J Biophys Biochem Cytol* 1957;3:331–344.

234. Headington JT. The dermal dendrocyte. In: Callen JP, et al., eds. *Advances in dermatology*, vol. 1. Chicago: Year Book Medical, 1986:159.

235. Braverman IM, Sibley J, Keh-Yen A. A study of veil cells around normal, diabetic, and aged cutaneous microvessels. *J Invest Dermatol* 1986;86:57–67.

236. Nestle FO, Zheng XG, Thompson CB, et al. Characterization of dermal dendritic cells obtained from normal human skin reveals phenotypic and functionally distinctive subsets. *J Immunol* 1993;151:6535.

237. Cerio R, Griffiths CEM, Cooper KD, et al. Characterization of factor XIIIa positive dermal dendritic cells in normal and inflamed skin. *Br J Dermatol* 1989;121:421.

238. Sueki H, Whitaker D, Buchsbaum M, et al. Novel interactions between dermal dendrocytes and mast cells in human skin: implications for hemostasis and matrix repair. *Lab Invest* 1993;69: 160–172.

239. Meunier L, Gonzalez-Ramos A, Cooper KD. Heterogeneous populations of class II MHC+ cells in human dermal cell suspensions. *J Immunol* 1993;151:4067–4074.

240. Murphy GF, Messadi D, Fonferko E, et al. Phenotypic transformation of macrophages to Langerhans cells in the skin. *Am J Pathol* 1986;123:401–406.

241. Nickoloff BJ, Griffiths CEM. Not all spindle-shaped cells embedded in a collagenous stroma are fibroblasts: recognition of the "collagen-associated dendrophage." *J Cutan Pathol* 1990; 17:252–259.

242. Hirsh BC, Johnson WC. Concepts of granulomatous inflammation. *Int J Dermatol* 1984;23:90–100.

243. Wells GS. The pathology of adult-type Letterer–Siwe disease. *Clin Exp Dermatol* 1979;4:407–417.

244. Lasser A. The mononuclear phagocytic system. a review. *Hum Pathol* 1983;14:108–126.

245. Pulford KAF, Rigney EM, Jones M, et al.:KP1. a new monoclonal antibody that detects a monocyte/macrophage associated antigen in routinely processed tissue sections. *J Clin Pathol* 1989;42:414–421.

246. Meuret G, Marwendel A, Brand ET. Makrophagenrekrutierung aus Blutmonocyten bei Entzündungsreaktionen der Haut. *Arch Dermatol Forsch* 1972;245:254–266.

247. Papadimitriou JM, Spector WG. The origin, properties and fate of epithelioid cells. *J Pathol* 1971;105:187–203.

248. Spector WG. Epithelioid cells, giant cells, and sarcoidosis. *Ann N Y Acad Sci* 1976;278:3–6.

249. Murphy GF. *Dermatopathology*. Philadelphia: WB Saunders, 1995.

250. Weissmann G, Smolen JE, Hoffstein S. Polymorphonuclear leukocytes as secretory organs of inflammation. *J Invest Dermatol* 1978;71:95–99.

251. Wilkinson DS. Pustular dermatoses. *Br J Dermatol* 1969;81 [Suppl 3]:38–45.

252. Wade BH, Mandell GL. Polymorphonuclear leukocytes: dedicated professional phagocytes. *Am J Med* 1983;74:686–693.

253. Parish WE. Investigations on eosinophils. *Br J Dermatol* 1970; 82:42–64.

254. Henson PM. Pathological mechanisms in neutrophil-mediated injury. *Am J Pathol* 1972;68:593–612.

255. Lazarus GS, Daniels JR, Lian J, et al. Role of granulocyte collagenase in collagen degradation. *Am J Pathol* 1972;68: 565–578.

256. Berretty PJM, Cormane RH. The eosinophilic granulocyte. *Int J Dermatol* 1978;17:776–784.

257. Poole JCF. Electron microscopy of polymorphonuclear leukocytes. *Br J Dermatol* 1969;81[Suppl 3]:11–18.

258. Zucker-Franklin D. Eosinophilic function related to cutaneous disorders. *J Invest Dermatol* 1978;71:100–105.

259. Gell PGH, Coombs RRA. Classification of hypersensitivity reactions. In: Gell PGH, Coombs RRA, eds. *Clinical aspects of immunology*, 2nd ed. Oxford: Blackwell Scientific Publications, 1968.

260. Berretty PJM, Cormane RH. Eosinophilic granulocytes and skin disorders. *Int J Dermatol* 1981;20:531–540.

261. Goetzl EJ, Wasserman SI, Austen KF. Eosinophil polymorphonuclear leukocyte function in immediate hypersensitivity. *Arch Pathol* 1975;99:1–4.

262. Butterworth AE, David JR. Eosinophil function. *N Engl J Med* 1981;304:154–156.

263. Dvorak HF, Dvorak AM. Basophils, mast cells, and cellular immunity in animal and man. *Hum Pathol* 1972;3:454–456.

264. Katz SI. Recruitment of basophils in delayed hypersensitivity reactions. *J Invest Dermatol* 1978;71:70–75.

265. Weissman IL, Warnke R, Butcher EC, et al. The lymphoid system. Its normal architecture and the potential for understanding the system through the study of lymphoproliferative diseases. *Hum Pathol* 1978;9:25–45.

266. Stingl G, Knapp W. Immunological markers for characterization of subpopulations of mononuclear cells. *Am J Dermatopathol* 1981;3:215–223.

267. Claudy AL. The immunological identification of the Sézary cell. *Br J Dermatol* 1974;91:597–600.

268. Luckasen JR, Sabad A, Goltz RW, et al. T and B lymphocytes in atopic eczema. *Arch Dermatol* 1974;110:375–377.

269. Askenase PW. Delayed-type hypersensitivity (DTH) recruitment of T cell subsets via antigen-specific non-IgE antibodies. relevance to asthma, autoimmunity and immune responses to tumors and parasites. In: Coffman R, ed. *The regulation and functional significance of T cell subsets: progress in chemical immunology.* Basel: S. Karger, 1993.

270. Gerard-Marchant R, Hamlin I, Lennert K, et al. Classification of non-Hodgkin's lymphoma. *Lancet* 1974;2:406–408.

271. Wilson Jones E. Prospectives in mycosis fungicides in relation to other lymphomas. *Trans St John's Hosp Dermatol Soc* 1975;61:16–30.

272. Rywlin AM. Non-Hodgkin's malignant lymphomas: brief historical review and simple unifying classification. *Am J Dermatopathol* 1980;2:17–25.

273. Aisenberg AC. Cell lineage in lymphoproliferative disease. *Am J Med* 1983;74:679–685.

274. Murphy GF, Mihm MC. Benign, dysplastic, and malignant lymphoid infiltrates of the skin. An approach based on pattern analysis. In: Murphy GF, Mihm MC Jr, eds. *Lymphoproliferative Disorders of the Skin.* Boston: Butterworths, 1986:123–141.

275. Murphy GF, Elder D. *Non-melanocytic tumors of the skin.* Washington, DC: Armed Forces Institute of Pathology, 1991.

276. Erlach E, Gebhart W, Niebauer G. Ultrastructural investigations on the morphogenesis of Russell bodies. *J Cutan Pathol* 1976;3:145(abst).

277. Tappeiner J, Pfleger L, Wolff K. Das Vorkommen und histochemische Verhalten von Russellschen Körperchen bei plasma-cellulären Hautinfiltraten. *Arch Klin Exp Dermatol* 1965;222:71–90.

278. Blom J, Wiik A. Russell bodies—immunoglobulins? *Am J Clin Pathol* 1983;79:262–263.

279. Doroczy J. Die Struktur der dermalen Lymphkapillaren und ihre funktionelle Interpretation. *Hautarzt* 1984;35:630–638.

280. Scarpelli DG, Goodman RM. Observations on the fine structure of the fibroblast from a case of Ehlers–Danlos syndrome with the Marfan syndrome. *J Invest Dermatol* 1968;50:214–219.

281. Ross R, Benditt EP. Wound healing and collagen formation. V. Quantitative electron microscopic radioautographic observations of proline-H3 utilization by fibroblasts. *J Cell Biol* 1965;27:83–89.

282. Uitto J, Lichtenstein JR. Defects in the biochemistry of collagen in diseases of connective tissue. *J Invest Dermatol* 1976;66:59–79.

283. Nigra TP, Friedland M, Martin GR. Controls of connective tissue synthesis: collagen metabolism. *J Invest Dermatol* 1972;59:44–49.

284. Lazarus GS. Collagen, collagenase and clinicians. *Br J Dermatol* 1972;26:193–199.

285. Grant ME, Prockop DJ. The biosynthesis of collagen. *N Engl J Med* 1972;286:194–199.

286. Hayes RL, Rodnan GP. The ultrastructure of skin in progressive sclerosis (scleroderma). *Am J Pathol* 1971;63:433–442.

287. Schmidt W. Die normale Histologie von Corium und Subcutis. In: Marchionini A, ed. *Handbuch der Haut- und Geschlechtskrankheiten, Ergänzungswerk*, vol. 1, part 1. Berlin: Springer-Verlag, 1968:430–490.

288. Meigel WN, Gay S, Weber L. Dermal architecture and collagen type distribution. *Arch Dermatol Res* 1977;259:1–10.

289. Byers PH, Barsh GS, Holbrook KA. Molecular pathology in inherited disorders of collagen metabolism. *Hum Pathol* 1982;13:89–95.

290. Leigh IM, Eady RAJ, Heagerty AHM. Type VII collagen is a normal component of epidermal basement membrane. *J Invest Dermatol* 1988;90:639–642.

291. Stenn KS. Collagen heterogeneity of skin. *Am J Dermatopathol* 1979;1:87–88.

292. Deutsch TA, Esterly NB. Elastic fibers in fetal dermis. *J Invest Dermatol* 1975;65:320–323.

293. Varadi DP. Study on the chemistry and fine structure of elastic fibers from normal adult skin. *J Invest Dermatol* 1972;59:238–246.

294. Hashimoto K, Dibella RJ. Electron microscopic studies of normal and abnormal elastic fibers of the skin. *J Invest Dermatol* 1967;48:405–423.

295. Varadi DP. Studies on the chemistry and fine structure of elastic fibers from normal adult skin. *J Invest Dermatol* 1972;59:238–246.

296. Stadler R, Orfanos CE. Reifung und Alterung der elastischen Fasern. *Arch Dermatol Forsch* 1978;262:97–111.

297. Marsch WC, Schober E, Nurnberger F. Zur Ultrastruktur und Morphogenese der elastischen Faser und der aktinischen Elastose. *Z Hautkr* 1979;54:43–46.

298. Winand R. Biosynthesis, organization and degradation of mucopolysaccharides. *Arch Belg Derm Syph* 1972;28:35–40.

299. Jacques J, Cameron HCS. Changes in the ground-substance of healing wounds. *J Pathol* 1969;99:337–340.

300. Seemayer TA, Knaack J, Wang NS, et al. On the ultrastructure of hibernoma. *Cancer* 1975;36:1785–1793.

LABORATORY METHODS

ROSALIE ELENITSAS
CARLOS H. NOUSARI
JOHN T. SEYKORA

There are a number of important steps in preparing histologic sections prior to their interpretation by the dermatopathologist. Failure to handle the tissue properly may make it difficult to provide an accurate diagnosis or appropriate margins.

PREPARATION OF SPECIMENS

Fixation

It is important to properly fix a skin biopsy to stabilize proteins and prevent tissue decay. The specimen should be placed in fixative immediately after it is removed from the patient; artifacts may result if it is allowed to dry. The fixative of choice is a 10% neutral-buffered formalin solution. The volume of formalin should be 10 to 20 times the volume of the specimen. During winter, either 95% ethyl alcohol, 10% by volume, should be added to the formalin solution or the specimen should be allowed to stand in the formalin solution at room temperature for at least 6 hours before mailing.

Adequate time should be allowed for fixation. Fixation time is 1 to 2 hours per millimeter thickness. Large specimens, such as excised tumors, should be cut in the laboratory into slices 4 to 5 mm thick for further fixation, generally overnight. These specimens will also require greater volumes of formalin.

Grossing

After fixation, ink should be applied to the deep and lateral margins of an excisional specimen for which examination of margins has been requested. The specimen should be appropriately cut for the examination of margins. Some examples are demonstrated in Fig. 4-1. It is important to remember that these cuts are only representative of the margins, since it is almost impossible to evaluate every marginal cell. If the surgeon has placed a localizing suture, a different color of ink should be applied to that margin or some other method of labeling should be used to identify the margins. Four-mm and 6-mm punch biopsies are generally bisected, and specimens less than 3 mm in size should be submitted *en toto*. If a laboratory does not handle many skin specimens, discussion with the embedding technician may be appropriate to facilitate optimal orientation of the blocks.

Demonstration of Enzyme Activities

With few exceptions, specimens should not be placed in formalin for the demonstration of enzyme activities. Instead, they should be delivered to the laboratory wrapped in water-moistened gauze and placed in a clean container, because frozen sections cut on a cryostat are typically used for enzyme staining. Staining for enzyme activities is not routinely done, and therefore should not be requested without first checking with the laboratory.

Although immunohistochemistry has largely replaced histochemistry for routine diagnostic use, demonstration of dopa-oxidase activity in melanocytes could potentially aid in distinguishing a malignant melanoma from tumors not composed of melanocytes. Also, certain enzymes, such as succinic dehydrogenase and phosphorylase (eccrine), and acid phosphatase and beta-glucuronidase (apocrine) can be detected in glandular tumors. However, these differentials are not usually significant clinically.

Several enzyme reactions can be carried out on formalin-fixed, paraffin-embedded tissue: (1) demonstration of naphthol AS-D chloroacetate esterase activity, with naphthol AS-D chloroacetate as substrate (present in mature and immature granulocytes, except in myeloblasts and mast cells); and (2) demonstration of lysozyme with the antilysozyme immunohistochemical technique (lysozyme being present in mature and immature granulocytes, even in myeloblasts, and in histiocytes) (see Chapter 31) (1).

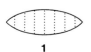 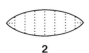 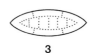

1   2   3

FIGURE 4-1. Preparation of blocks from a skin ellipse. After the margins have been painted with ink, the specimen is sectioned for processing and later embedding. In example 1, the tissue is cut as if one is slicing a loaf of bread; this is one of the most common methods used in dermatopathology laboratories. Example 2 allows for better evaluation of the "tips" of the ellipse; however, embedding of these small pieces is more difficult. Often only the center section of the "tips" is embedded, or the tips may be cut in half and embedded flat, especially for smaller specimens (example 3). In example 3, the entire margin is theoretically visualized; however, this method requires the technician to meticulously embed and orient small pieces of tissue and is not recommended for most specimens in most routine laboratories. (From Rapini R. Comparison of methods for checking surgical margins. *J Am Acad Dermatol* 1990;23:288, with permission.)

In two diseases, scleredema of Buschke and amyloidosis, unfixed frozen sections may show a more conclusive reaction to specific staining methods than is obtainable with formalin-fixed material. It is therefore recommended that, in these two diseases, only part of the tissue be fixed in formalin and the remainder be used for frozen sections. In scleredema, demonstration of hyaluronic acid with toluidine blue at pH 7.0 may be more intense in unfixed, frozen sections than in formalin-fixed sections. In amyloidosis, the reactions of the amyloid with crystal violet or Congo red may be conclusive only in unfixed, frozen sections (see Chapter 17).

Processing

The purpose of processing is to remove the extractable water from the skin and to provide a supporting matrix (paraffin) so that the tissue can be cut with minimal distortion. After fixation, routine specimens are processed in an automatic processor. An exception is specimens that are to be stained for lipids. Because lipids are extracted by the xylene used for the processing of specimens, frozen sections are cut and postfixed in 10% neutral-buffered formalin for lipid staining.

In the automated histology processor, the specimens pass first through increasing concentrations of ethanol for dehydration, then through xylene for lipid extraction and clearing of alcohol. Finally, the tissues are infiltrated with several changes of hot, melted paraffin (or Paraplast), to provide a matrix so that the tissue can be stabilized and cut easily. This processing takes between 4 and 12 hours; in most laboratories, processing is run overnight. The next morning, the specimens are embedded with the cut surface face down into the cassette base mold, in the liquid paraffin, which is allowed to harden. To prevent tangentially oriented sections, it is important that this cut surface be firmly embedded in the base of this mold. The specimens

are then cut on a rotary microtome into sections 5 to 7 μm thick.

Staining

Routine sections are usually stained with hematoxylin-eosin, the most widely used routine stain. With this staining method, nuclei stain blue or "basophilic," and collagen, muscles, and nerves stain red or "eosinophilic." Special stains are employed when particular structures need to be demonstrated. For details, see below and the *Manual of Histologic Staining Methods of the Armed Forces Institute of Pathology* (2).

HISTOCHEMICAL STAINING

Histochemistry, especially immunohistochemistry, at both the light microscopic and electron microscopic level, has gained increasing importance in recent years and has been largely responsible for the expansion of histopathology from a purely descriptive science to one that is dynamic and functional. Many enzyme histochemical methods are used only for research and have the limitation of usually requiring fresh tissue in the place of formalin-fixed tissue.

Most histochemical "special" stains can be carried out on formalin-fixed, paraffin-embedded material. Their primary uses in dermatopathology are listed in Table 4-1.

The periodic acid-Schiff (PAS) stain demonstrates the presence of certain polysaccharides, particularly glycogen and mucoproteins containing neutral mucopolysaccharides, by staining them red. The PAS reaction consists of the oxidation of adjacent hydroxyl groups in 1,2-glycols to aldehydes and the staining of the aldehydes with fuchsin-sulfuric acid. The PAS reaction is of value also in the study of basement membrane thickening, such as in lupus erythematosus or porphyria cutanea tarda. Furthermore, because the cell walls of fungi are composed of a mixture of cellulose and chitin and thus contain polysaccharides, fungi stain bright pink-red with the PAS reaction.

For the distinction of neutral mucopolysaccharides and fungi from glycogen deposits, it is necessary to compare two serial sections, one exposed to diastase before staining and the other not. Because glycogen is digested by the diastase, and thus no longer colored red by the PAS reaction, it can be easily distinguished from neutral mucopolysaccharides and fungi that are diastase-resistant. Because glycogen is present in outer root sheath cells and eccrine gland cells, demonstration of glycogen may be of diagnostic value in adnexal tumors with outer root sheath or eccrine differentiation. Demonstration of neutral mucopolysaccharides is of value in Paget's disease of the breast and in extramammary Paget's disease.

The Alcian blue reaction demonstrates the presence of acid mucopolysaccharides by staining them blue. Acid mu-

TABLE 4-1. HISTOCHEMICAL STAINS USED IN DERMATOPATHOLOGY

Stain	Purpose of stain	Results
Hematoxylin-eosin	Routine	Nuclei: blue Collagen, muscles, nerves: red
Masson trichrome	Collagen	Collagen: blue or green Nuclei, muscles, nerves: dark red
Verhoeff-van Gieson	Elastic fibers	Elastic fibers: black Collagen: red Nuclei, muscles, nerves: yellow
Pinkus acid orcein	Elastic fibers	Elastic fibers: dark brown
Silver nitrate	Melanin, reticulum fibers (argyrophilic)	Melanin, reticulum fibers: black
Fontana-Masson	Melanin (argentaffin)	Melanin: black
Methenamine silver	Fungi, Donovan bodies, Frisch bacilli (rhinoscleroma), basement membranes	Black
Grocott	Fungi	Fungus cell walls: black
Periodic acid-Schiff/diastase (PAS)	Glycogen, neutral MPS*, fungi	Glycogen: red; diastase labile Neutral MPS*, fungi: red; diastase resistant
Alcian blue, pH 2.5	Acid MPS*	Blue
Alcian blue, pH 0.5	Sulfated MPS*	Blue
Toluidine blue	Acid MPS*	Blue
Colloidal iron	Acid MPS*	Blue
Hyaluronidase	Hyaluronic acid	Hyaluronidase labile
Mucicarmine	"Epithelial" mucin	Red
Giemsa	Mast cell granules, acid MPS*, myeloid granules, Leishmania	MCG,† acid MPS*: metachromatically purple Myeloid granules, Leishmania: red
Fite	Acid-fast bacilli	Red
Pert potassium ferrocyanide	Hemosiderin (iron)	Blue
Alkaline Congo red	Amyloid	Pink-red, green birefringence in polarized light
Von Kossa	Calcium	Black
Scarlet red	Lipids	Red
Oil red O	Lipids	Red
Dopa (in unfixed tissue)	Tyrosinase in melanocytes	Black dopa-melanin
Naphthol-AS-D-chloroacetate esterase	Mast cells, neutrophils, myelocytes	Granules stain red
Warthin-Starry	Spirochetes	Black
Dietere and Steiner	Spirochetes, bacillary angiomatosis	Black

*MPS = mucopolysaccharides.
†MCG = mast cell granules.
Note: All stains except those for lipids, can be carried out on formalin-fixed paraffin-embedded specimens. The stains for lipids require formalin-fixed frozen sections.

copolysaccharides are present in the dermal ground substance, but in amounts too small to be demonstrable in normal skin. However, in the dermal mucinoses, there is a great increase in nonsulfated acid mucopolysaccharides, mainly hyaluronic acid, so that the mucin stains with Alcian blue (see Chapter 17). In extramammary Paget's disease of the anus with rectal carcinoma (see Chapter 30) and in cutaneous metastases of carcinoma of the gastrointestinal tract containing goblet cells (see Chapter 36), tumor cells in the skin, like their parent cells, secrete sialomucin. Sialomucin contains nonsulfated acid mucopolysaccharides staining with Alcian blue, as well as PAS-positive neutral mucopolysaccharides. Whereas nonsulfated acid mucopolysaccharides stain with Alcian blue at pH 2.5 but not

at pH 0.5, strongly acidic sulfated-acid mucopolysaccharides, such as heparin in mast cell granules and chondroitin sulfate in cartilage, stain with alcian blue both at pH 2.5 and at pH 0.5.

Several special stains for elastic tissue are available. The most commonly used stains are the Verhoeff–van Gieson (Fig. 4-2) or Weigert resorcin-fuchsin. Additional techniques, such as the Luna stain and Miller stain, may allow better visualization of elastic fibers than traditional methods (3). These stains are beneficial in the diagnosis of anetoderma, connective tissue nevi, mid-dermal elastolysis, and other alterations of elastic tissue.

The Geimsa stain is frequently utilized to highlight mast cells. Geimsa contains methylene blue, a metachro-

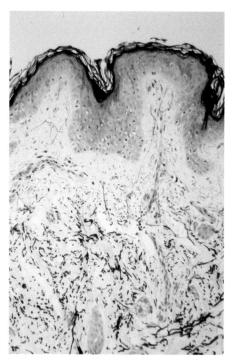

FIGURE 4-2. Elastic fibers. This Verhoeff–van Gieson stain demonstrates the darkly staining normal elastic fibers of the skin.

matic stain. The granules of a mast cell will stain metachromatically purple (Fig. 4-3).

POLARISCOPIC EXAMINATION

Polariscopic examination is the examination of histologic sections under the microscope with polarized light, with light from which all rays except those vibrating in one plane are excluded. For polariscopic examination, two

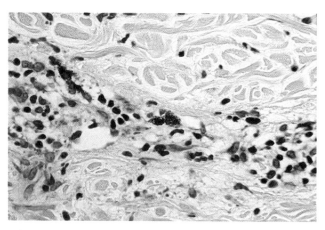

FIGURE 4-3. Geimsa stain. Mast cell cytoplasmic granules are purple.

disks made of polarizing plastics are placed on the microscope. One disk is placed below the condenser of the microscope and acts as the polarizer. The second disk is placed in the eyepiece of the microscope or on top of the glass slide and acts as the analyzer. When one of the two disks is rotated so that the path of the light through the two disks is broken at a right angle, the field is dark. However, when doubly refractile substances are introduced between the two disks, they break the polarization and are visible as bright white bodies in the dark field.

Polariscopic examination is useful in evaluating lipid deposits, certain foreign bodies, gout, and amyloid. With regard to lipids, it is not fully known why certain lipids are doubly refractile and others are not. In general, cholesterol esters are doubly refractile, but free cholesterol, phospholipids, and neutral fat are not. Only formalin-fixed, frozen sections can be used for a polariscopic examination for lipids.

Doubly refractile lipids are regularly present in the tuberous and plane xanthomas and xanthelasmata (but not always in the eruptive xanthomas) of hyperlipoproteinemia, in the cutaneous lesions of diffuse normolipemic plane xanthoma (see Chapter 26), and in the vascular walls of angiokeratoma corporis diffusum (Fabry disease) (see Chapter 26). Doubly refractile lipids are present, as long as the cutaneous lesions contain a sufficient amount of lipid, in histiocytosis X (Hand–Schüller–Christian type) (see Chapter 27), in juvenile xanthogranuloma (see Chapter 27), in erythema elevatum diutinum (extracellular cholesterosis) (see Chapter 8), and in dermatofibroma (lipidized "histiocytoma") (see Chapter 33).

Doubly refractile lipids are absent in lipid-containing lesions, as a rule, in necrobiosis lipoidica (see Chapter 14), in hyalinosis cutis et mucosae or lipoid proteinosis (see Chapter 17), and in multicentric reticulohistiocytosis and solitary reticulohistiocytic granuloma (see Chapter 26).

Among foreign bodies, silica causes granulomas showing doubly refractile spicules. These granulomas are caused either by particles of soil or glass (silicon dioxide) or by talcum powder (magnesium silicate) (see Chapter 14). Wooden splinters, suture material, and starch granules are also doubly refractile. An example of polariscopic examination is seen in Fig. 4-4.

Gout tophi show double refraction of the urate crystals if the crystals are sufficiently preserved. They are preserved by the use of alcohol rather than formalin for fixation (see Chapter 17). Amyloid shows a characteristic green birefringence in polarized light after staining with alkaline Congo red (see Chapter 17).

IMMUNOFLOURESCENCE TESTING

Two immunofluorescence methods are commonly used in dermatology: direct immunofluorescence testing, which

FIGURE 4-4. Polariscopic examination. In this talc granuloma, polaroscopy reveals hundreds of refractile foreign bodies within the dermis.

probes for immunoreactants localized in patients' own skin or mucous membranes, and indirect immunofluorescence testing, which is utilized to identify and titer circulating autoantibodies in the patient's serum. A modified indirect immunofluorescence technique using the patient's own skin as a substrate known as immunomapping, is used to determine the site of cleavage or abnormalities in the distribution of mutated proteins in various forms of hereditary epidermolysis bullosa.

DIRECT IMMUNOFLUORESCENCE

Direct immunofluorescence testing has a valuable diagnostic role in several autoimmune and inflammatory mucocutaneous diseases including autoimmune-mediated blistering diseases, dermatitis herpetiformis, Henoch–Schoenlein purpura (IgA vasculitis), and cutaneous lupus erythematosus. The role of direct immunofluorescence as a diagnostic procedure is important but not critical in other dermatoses such as dermatomyositis, cutaneous porphyrias, pseudoporphyria, lichen planus, and vasculitides other than Henoch–Schoenlein purpura (4).

Biopsy Techniques

A 3- to 4-mm punch biopsy is generally adequate. In the autoimmune blistering disease group, an inflamed but unblistered perilesional area is the ideal specimen. Blis-

tered lesional sampling is the most common cause of false negative results. On the other hand, sampling too distant from the blistering can cause false negative results. In a few cases of pemphigus, pemphigoid and epidermolysis bullosa acquisita even false negative results can occur in lesional blistered lesions. Of note, due to the often focal and skipping nature of the immunoreactants in dermatitis herpetiformis, a shave biopsy often provides of a broader surface to evaluate dermal papillae than a punch biopsy.

The performance of an adequate perilesional biopsy in mucosal lesions is often not feasible, thus a high incidence of false negative and even false positive may occur in these specimens. In patients with desquamative gingivitis secondary to mucous membrane pemphigoid, an easy way to obtain sampling is the so-called "peeling technique" where, rubbing the perilesional affected gingivae with a cotton swab induces a "fresh peeling of the mucosa." In most cases of the mucous membrane pemphigoid, the hemidesmosomal antigen 180 and 230 kD are the autoantigens; therefore, the hemidesmosomes will be available for interpretation in the peeled gingivae specimens and a linear immunostaining with "capping" phenomenon is observed (5a).

It has been reported that there is a theoretically higher incidence of false negative results in bullous pemphigoid lesions from lower extremities; however, this finding has not been confirmed by others.[5a]

In asymptomatic dermatitis[5a] herpetiformis patients who have strictly adhered to a gluten-free diet for less than 6 months, or even in patients that have not done so but remain lesion-free due to dapsone therapy, wide-shaved specimens from the elbows or any other classically affected area will still show the typical IgA deposits at the tips of dermal papillae (6).

Autoimmune and inflammatory disorders other than autoimmune blistering diseases in which direct immunofluorescence plays an important role, the specimens should be taken from lesional areas including cutaneous lupus erythematosus, dermatomyositis, vasculitides, lichen planus, cutaneous porphyria, and pseudoporphyria.

Transport and Processing of Biopsy Specimens

Tissue for immunofluorescence studies should be obtained fresh and kept moist until it is quickly frozen. Skin specimens can be kept on saline-moistened gauze in a small Petri dish for 24 hours but not longer before processing. For longer delay times, the specimens should be put into Michel's transport medium. This medium is composed of 5% ammonium sulfate, the potassium inhibitor N-ethylmaleimide, and magnesium sulfate in citrate buffer (pH 7.25). This solution is stable at room temperature but must be kept in tightly capped container to prevent absorption of CO_2 and acidification. Specimens stored in Michel's medium are stable for at least 2 weeks at room temperature. However, specimens stored in Michel's and kept in the refrigerator can be preserved for several weeks or even months. This method of transportation has made the direct immunofluorescence technique much more readily applicable. When the specimen is received in a laboratory, the ammonium sulfate is washed out and the specimen is oriented and embedded in OCT (optimal cutting temperature) compound and then the specimen is snap frozen. The tissue is then sectioned at 6 μm. The frozen sections are incubated with antihuman antibodies to IgG, IgA, IgM, C3, and fibrinogen. These antibodies are linked to a fluorescent label such as fluorescein isothiocyanate to allow visualization using a fluorescence microscope (4).

Direct Immunofluorescence Interpretation

Autoimmune Blistering Diseases

Sensitivity of direct immunofluorescence with active autoimmune blistering disease should be close to 100%. If not, it is likely due to technical reasons (7). In pemphigus vulgaris and pemphigus foliaceus, the IgG immunostaining on the epithelial cell surfaces can be granular and/or linear, resulting in a characteristic "chicken wire" pattern. Nonspecific patchy granular staining along the basement membrane is not uncommon, especially in mucosal lesions. In paraneoplastic pemphigus, the IgG "chicken wire" immunostaining tends to be linear, thick, and homogenous throughout the epidermis and mucosal specimens including those from bronchi with or without a concomitant linear basement membrane (8). Lichenoid mucosal and even cutaneous lesions in paraneoplastic pemphigus tend to show focal granular IgG and other immunoreactants along the basement membrane without the typical "chicken wire" pattern. The presence of low titers of circulating autoantibodies may preclude differentiation among the subepithelial autoimmune blistering disorders using indirect immunofluorescence or any other serologic test. In these cases, a technique called salt-split direct immunofluorescence often circumvents this problem. This technique consists of thawing the frozen specimen formerly used for routine direct immunofluorescence and incubating it in 1 molar (M) NaCl for 48 to 72 hours, allowing for separation of the epidermis from the dermis. This salt will cleave the basement membrane zone through the lamina lucida, leaving the hemidesmosomes on the epidermal side and deeper-seated proteins such as type VII collagen and epiligrin on the dermal side of the artificially induced blister. Therefore, in virtually all cases of bullous pemphigoid, the linear IgG immunostaining will be localized on the epidermal side (occasionally epidermal and dermal) and in epidermolysis bullosa acquisita on the dermal side.

Cutaneous Lupus Erythematosus

Direct immunofluorescence has a significant value in the evaluation of patients with active cutaneous connective tissue disease. The intensity of the deposits of immunoreactants along the basement membrane in these patients correlates with the degree of interface/lichenoid dermatitis/mucositis.

In discoid lupus erythematosus, the most common immunoreactant visualized with direct immunofluorescence is IgM, and in systemic lupus erythematosus and in subacute cutaneous lupus erythematosus, IgG. Of note, most patients with anti-Ro positive, subacute cutaneous-lupus erythematosus may have a characteristic granular IgG speckling pattern along the basement membrane and throughout the epidermis. The lupus band test, described as positive when granular IgG is present along the basement membrane zone in specimens from sun-protected nonlesional areas, has been rapidly abandoned due to its unreliability and current availability of more reliable methods to early diagnosis and prediction of systemic disease in lupus erythematosus (9).

Cutaneous Vasculitides

Direct immunofluorescence evaluation is a very important diagnostic tool in the work-up of cutaneous small vessel vasculitis, especially Henoch–Schöenlein purpura. The best immunofluorescence diagnostic yield in Henoch–Schöenlein purpura is obtained from 1- to 2-day old lesions. As lesions get older, the IgA deposits get degraded and cleared. Since most patients have older lesions at the time of evaluation, a high index of suspicion is required and exhaustive search for scant granular IgA deposits in very superficial papillary dermis is mandatory before ruling out Henoch–Schöenlein purpura.

Hypocomplementemic urticarial vasculitis is another small-vessel vasculitis in which direct immunofluorescence plays a critical diagnostic role. In this type of cutaneous vasculitis, granular IgG and C3 deposits are seen in and around small dermal vessels and along the basement membrane zone. The presence of basement membrane granular immunostaining among other clinical and serologic findings in patients with hypocomplementemic urticarial vasculitis have led some authors to believe that this vasculitis is no more than a subset of systemic lupus erythematosus (10).

Other Autoimmune and Inflammatory Skin Diseases

Lichen planus lesions, mainly the mucosal variant, are characterized by typical, yet not pathognomonic, linear and shaggy fibrin deposits, and patchy granular IgM and C3 along the basement membrane. The direct immunofluorescence findings in cutaneous porphyrias are indistinguishable from those seen in pseudoporphyria. These findings are characterized by thick and glassy linear IgG and IgA deposits in superficial dermal vessels in a "doughnut pattern" and along the basement membrane. It is thought that immunoglobulins get trapped and bound to glycoproteins in a thickened basement membrane zone and degenerated blood vessels in this disorder.

INDIRECT IMMUNOFLUORESCENCE

Indirect immunofluorescence is a semiquantitative procedure in which a double immunolabeling is carried out to evaluate the presence and titer of circulating antibodies, or to specifically localize antigen in the skin.

Indirect Immunofluorescence in the Evaluation of Circulating Antiepithelial Antibodies

Blood is drawn into a tube without anticoagulant, and the serum is serially diluted. Substrates most commonly used are 6-μm frozen sections of monkey esophagus, human salt-split skin, and murine bladder. The substrate is incubated with serum dilutions for 30 minutes at room temperature and then washed; antibodies bound to the substrates are detected by incubation with FITC-labeled, goat anti-human IgG and or IgA.

Monkey esophagus is probably the best single substrate for the evaluation of antiepithelial surface antibodies specifically for pemphigus vulgaris and paraneoplastic pemphigus. Pemphigus foliaceus has a high incidence of false negative results with this substrate. Low titers of antiepithelial surface antibodies up to 1:80 or even higher can also be seen in control sera (11). In pemphigus vulgaris and foliaceus, antidesmoglein antibodies give a "chicken wire staining," which is more predominant on superficial epithelial cells, whereas in paraneoplastic pemphigus, the antiplakin antibodies give a pattern that is consistently homogeneous throughout the epithelium and even sometimes associated with immunostaining along the basement membrane zone.

Transitional epithelium is a plakin-rich substrate, and thus murine bladder is a common substrate for the screening of circulating antiplakin antibodies in paraneoplastic pemphigus (12). Exceptional cases of pemphigus vulgaris, foliaceus, and pemphigoid would have concomitant low-titer antidesmoplakin antibodies (Fig. 4-5).

Monkey esophagus is also a useful substrate in the indirect immunofluorescence screening for subepidermal autoimmune blistering disease. However, human salt-split skin renders better definition of the subtypes of subepidermal blistering disorders. Disorders characterized by antibodies to

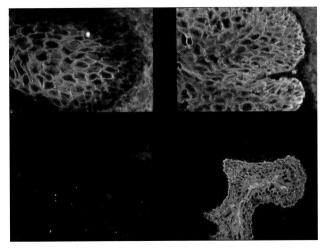

FIGURE 4-5. Differentiation between pemphigus vulgaris and paraneoplastic pemphigus using indirect immunofluorescence. *Left upper quadrant:* Pemphigus vulgaris. Indirect immunofluorescence showing IgG bound to epithelial cell surface of the stratified squamous epithelium of monkey esophagus. Of note, the "chicken wire" pattern is more prominent in the most superficial aspects of the epithelium. *Left lower quadrant:* Pemphigus vulgaris. Indirect immunofluorescence showing no IgG bound to epithelial cell surface of transitional epithelium of murine bladder. Transitional epithelium does not have desmogleins, the autoantigens of pemphigus vulgaris and foliaceus. *Right upper quadrant:* Paraneoplastic pemphigus. Indirect immunofluorescence showing IgG bound to epithelial cell surface of the stratified squamous epithelium of monkey esophagus. Of note, the "chicken wire" pattern is consistent throughout the epithelium and also along the basement membrane zone. Plakins, the autoantigens in paraneoplastic pemphigus are ubiquitous desmosomal and hemidesmosomal proteins present in squamous and non squamous epithelia. *Right lower quadrant:* Paraneoplastic pemphigus. Indirect immunofluorescence showing IgG bound to epithelial cell surface of transitional epithelium of the bladder. Transitional epithelium is rich in plakins.

hemidesmosomal proteins BP180 and BP230, including those seen in bullous and gestational pemphigoid, some cases of mucous membrane pemphigoid, and linear IgA bullous disease, are associated with a linear immunostaining on the epidermal side (roof) of the salt-split human skin.

On the other hand, patients with circulating antibodies reacting against type VII collagen and antiepiligrin (laminin 5) as is seen in epidermolysis bullosa acquisita and antiepiligrin mucous membrane pemphigoid respectively, have circulating IgG autoantibodies that bind the dermal side of the salt-split human skin.

More sensitive and specific assays for the evaluation of circulating autoantibodies including ELISA for antidesmoglein and anti–BP180 antibodies, immunoblotting, and immunoprecipitation for pemphigoid, epidermolysis bullosa acquisita, antiepiligrin, and immunoprecipitation for paraneoplastic pemphigus have been lately incorporated in the diagnostic armamentarium of autoimmune blistering diseases.

Indirect Immunofluorescence for Evaluating Cleavage Site in Hereditary Epidermolysis Bullosa

This technique offers a practical yet useful diagnostic tool in hereditary epidermolysis bullosa by revealing the site of the defect in these mechanobullous disorders. Thus, this technique classifies these disorders into epidermolytic, functional, and dermolytic categories (Table 4-2).

In brief, this technique is performed as follows: a fresh induced blister is obtained by twisting a rubber-ended pencil, and then this artificially induced blister skin specimen is incubated with anti–type IV collagen and anti–BP 180 antigen. Next, according to localization of the immunolabeling of these antibodies, the site of cleavage can de deducted.

In some cases of generalized, atrophic, benign epidermolysis bullosa, where the mutated protein is the BP 180 Ag, the immunostaining in the floor of the induced blister given by the anti–BP 180 may be focal or absent. Specific antibodies to the mutated protein are also used for complementary diagnostic purposes. These antibodies include anti-plectin antibodies EB simplex with muscular dystrophy, anti-$\alpha 6\beta 4$ in junctional epidermolysis bullosa with pyloric atresia, anti–laminin 5 antibodies for most cases of junctional epidermolysis bullosa, anti–type VII collagen for most cases of dystrophic form of hereditary epidermolysis bullosa. These specific antibodies are intended to identify a disrupted linear staining due to an even distribution of the probed mutated protein (13). The definite diagnosis of hereditary epidermolysis bullosa is made with electron microscopy and genetic analysis.

IMMUNOHISTOCHEMISTRY

Introduction to Techniques

Immunohistochemistry techniques have been available since the early 1970s, but they have been used widely for diagnostic pathology only since the early 1980s. They are mainly used to diagnose poorly differentiated malignant tumors and lymphoma. They can also be beneficial in the diagnosis of bullous diseases (14). With the refinement of techniques, immunohistochemistry methods have achieved the same sensitivity for many antigens in paraffin-embedded tissues as the direct immunofluorescence method in frozen sections. Compared to frozen sections, paraffin-embedded tissues offer the advantage of better preservation of cellular details and permanency of the reaction, so that the specimens can be preserved and stored. Most monoclonal antibodies, especially those necessary for the diagnosis of lymphoma, have required frozen section studies, but monoclonal antibodies are presently being produced that can be applied to formalin-fixed, paraffin-embedded tissue, such as antibodies for the identification of B cells, T cells, and macrophages.

Sections that will be incubated with polyclonal or monoclonal antibodies should be mounted on glass slides specially coated or charged to ensure better adherence (15). Many laboratories currently employ the Microprobe Slide Staining System (Fisher Scientific, Pittsburgh, PA), using slides with a positively charged surface.

Certain antibodies, including antibodies against keratins, lysozyme, or chymotrypsin require protease digestion if formalin-fixed, paraffin-embedded sections are used. Other "antigen retrieval" methods include the use of heat, either by microwaving or steaming the sections, and pretreatment of the sections with acid (HCl).

Immunohistologic Techniques

In most laboratories, immunopathology techniques are well established. Historically, several techniques have been used; the peroxidase-antiperoxidase (PAP) technique has been replaced by more sensitive techniques, namely, the avidin-biotin-peroxidase complex (ABC), the alkaline phosphatase–anti-alkaline phosphatase (APAAP), and the streptavidin peroxidase or alkaline phosphatase techniques. In all of these methods, the antibody is used to localize an enzyme (peroxidase or phosphatase) to sites of antigen expression in tissue sections. An appropriate "chromogen" is then added. A chromogen is a reagent that has the property of developing a color that can be visualized at sites of localization of the enzyme-antibody-antigen complex.

TABLE 4-2. INDIRECT IMMUNOFLUORESCENCE FOR THE EVALUATION OF SITE OF CLEAVAGE IN HEB

Type of HEB	Anti-BP180 Immunostaining	Anti-Type IV Collagen Immunostaining
Epidermolytic (simplex)	Floor	Floor
Junctional	Roof	Floor
Dermolytic	Roof	Roof

HEB, hereditary epidermolysis bullosa.

Alkaline Phosphatase–Anti-Alkaline Phosphatase Technique

This is an unlabeled antibody bridge technique that utilizes three antibodies; the first and third antibodies are from the same species and are monoclonal. The second antibody is polyclonal from the rabbit, and forms a bridge between the first and third antibody (16). The third antibody is linked to the enzyme alkaline phosphatase. After applying these antibodies with the linked enzyme, an alkaline phosphatase substrate is added containing a compatible indole chromogen such as INT/BCIP (which yields a red color after the phosphatase-catalyzed reaction), naphthol fast red (red color), or NBT/BCIP (blue). This method may be useful for pigmented tumors since the blue or red reagents can be distinguished easily from melanin (15).

Avidin-Biotin-Peroxidase Complex and Streptavidin Peroxidase or Alkaline Phosphatase Techniques

The avidin-biotin technique takes advantage of the strong interaction of avidin with biotin (17,18). Avidin is a glycoprotein found in egg white that has a strong affinity to biotin, a vitamin of low molecular weight. The streptavidin technique is exactly analogous, but achieves one to two orders of magnitude greater sensitivity by using streptavidin in place of avidin. This method is now becoming standard. In these techniques, the primary antibody (which may be monoclonal or polyclonal) binds directly with the specific antigen in or on the cells to form a stable antigen–antibody complex within the tissue section. A secondary antibody that has been labeled with biotin (biotinylated), and is directed against the same species and immunoglobulin type, binds to the primary antibody, leaving the biotinylated end available. A peroxidase or alkaline phosphatase detection system can be used. In a peroxidase method, the biotinylated complex is detected by avidin or streptavidin that has been conjugated to the peroxidase enzyme. A peroxidase-oriented chromogen is then added, such as diaminobenzidine (yielding a brown color) or aminoethylcarbazole (red color, and therefore useful for pigmented lesions). The alkaline phosphatase-streptavidin method is analogous to the streptavidin-peroxidase method, but in this case the biotinylated complex is detected with an alkaline phosphatase–linked streptavidin, and requires a compatible chromogen such as the indole reagents INT/BCIP (red color), naphthol fast red (red), or NBT/BCIP (blue). This technique in our experience achieves the greatest sensitivity of all immunohistochemical methods.

The origin of an undifferentiated cell can usually be determined with the application of monoclonal or polyclonal antibodies. A "panel approach" using multiple markers is the best method for evaluating problem neoplasms. Positive and negative controls should be used. If tumor cells unexpectedly do not show a positive reaction with a certain antibody, several possibilities exist, including technical difficulties with the assay. One may encounter nonspecific staining as well as aberrant immunoreactivity (observed staining with a particular antibody where it is theoretically unexpected). Caution should be taken not to make a diagnosis based on immunohistochemistry alone. Unfortunately, there is no antibody that distinguishes between benign and malignant cells.

APPLICATIONS OF IMMUNOHISTOPATHOLOGY

Diagnosis of Tumors (Excluding Lymphomas)

The most important antibodies for routine dermatopathology and their occurrence in certain cells and tissues are listed in Table 4-3. The most frequently used antibodies in dermatopathology are discussed below. The list of currently available antibodies is extensive; detailed information is available in literature reviews (19–23).

Antibodies Against Cytoskeletal Antigens

The cytoskeleton of a cell consists of intermediate filaments measuring 7 to 11 nm in diameter, actin-containing microfilaments, and tubulin-containing microtubules (24–26). Intermediate filaments are smaller than microtubules (25 nm) but larger than microfilaments (6 nm); hence, the designation intermediate.

Antibodies against intermediate filaments (IFs) help to identify the origin of an anaplastic cell. Malignant tumors usually retain the intermediate filament-type characteristic of the tissue of origin, and metastases generally continue to express these intermediate filaments (27). There are six groups of intermediate filaments. Types 1 and 2 IFs include cytokeratins, which are present in epithelia. Type 3 IFs include vimentin, found in mesenchymal cells; melanocytes, desmin found in most muscle cells; and GFAP (glial fibrillary acidic protein) found in glial cells and astrocytes. Type IV IFs include neurofilaments that are components of neurons. Nuclear lamins constitute type V IFs, while nestin comprises the type 6, and is found in some stem cells. In dermatopathology, keratin antibodies are used to differentiate epithelial from nonepithelial (melanocytic, hematopoietic, and mesenchymal) tumors. A mixture of antibodies against low and intermediate keratins such as AE1 and AE3 (AE1/3) is commonly used (28). An additional antibody to low molecular–weight keratins such as CAM 5.2 may be beneficial in poorly differentiated carcinomas (29). The keratin marker CK20 has useful specificity for Merkel–cell carcinoma (30).

Atypical spindle cell tumors, for example, are often difficult to diagnose with routine stains. The differential diag-

TABLE 4-3. COMMON ANTIGENS THAT CAN BE DETECTED IN FORMALIN-FIXED, PARAFFIN-EMBEDDED SECTIONS

Antigen	Location
Cytokeratins, including AE1, AE3, CAM 5.2, CK20	Epidermis and its appendages and their tumors
Vimentin	Mesenchymal cells, melanocytes, lymphomas, sarcomas, melanomas
Desmin	Smooth and skeletal muscle, muscle tumors
Leukocyte common antigen (LCA)	Benign leukocytes, lymphoma, leukemia
UCHL-1	T lymphocytes
L-26	B lymphocytes
Epithelial membrane antigen (EMA)	Sweat and sebaceous glands, carcinoma, epithelioid sarcoma
Carcinoembryonic antigen (CEA)	Eccrine and apocrine glands and their tumors, Paget cells
S-100 protein	Melanocytes, Langerhans cells, eccrine and apocrine glands and their tumors, Schwann cells, nerves, interdigitating reticulum cells, chondrocytes, melanomas, adipose tissue, liposarcomas, histiocytosis X
HMB-45	Melanoma cells, some nevus cells
Chromogranin	Neuroendocrine cells, Merkel cell carcinoma, eccrine gland cells
Synaptophysin	Neuroendocrine cells, Merkel cell carcinoma
Lysozyme	Macrophages, granulocytes, myeloid cells
Alpha$_1$-antitrypsin, alpha$_1$-antichymotrypsin	Macrophages, "fibrohistiocytic" neoplasms including MFH, but nonspecific in most routine practice
Factor VIII–related antigen	Endothelial cells, angiosarcomas, Kaposi's sarcoma
Ulex europasus agglutinin I	Endothelial cells, keratinocytes, angiosarcomas, Kaposi's sarcoma
CD31	Endothelial cells
CD34	Endothelial cells, bone marrow progenitor cells, cells of dermatofibrosarcoma protuberans
Smooth muscle actin	Smooth muscle cells and tumors, myofibroblastic cells
MART-1/MelanA	Melanocytes, nevi, melanoma
Factor XIIIa	Dermatofibromas, certain fibrohistiocytic cells (see text)

Note: Few if any of these reagents are perfectly specific for their target antigens. Every test must be interpreted in the context of all the available histologic and clinical information.

nosis for such lesions includes spindle-cell, squamous-cell carcinoma, atypical fibroxanthoma, leiomyosarcoma, and spindle-cell malignant melanoma. The most important antibodies are listed in Table 4-4 (31).

Vimentin

Vimentin is an intermediate filament originally isolated from chick embryo fibroblasts. It is found in fibroblasts, endothelial cells, macrophages, melanocytes, lymphocytes, and smooth muscle cells. Antibodies to vimentin are found in both benign and malignant counterparts of these cells (32). There have also been reports of positivity in epithelial tumors (33); however, normal epidermis is negative for this

antibody. Because of the nonspecific nature of the antibody, it is useful only as a panel approach to support mesenchymal or melanocytic differentiation.

Carcinoembryonic Antigen and Epithelial Membrane Antigen

Carcinoembryonic antigen (CEA) has been found in normal eccrine and apocrine cells, in benign sweat gland tumors, and in mammary and extramammary Paget's disease of the skin. Incubation with anti-CEA can be helpful in distinguishing Paget cells from atypical melanocytes in melanoma *in situ*. However, reactivity of melanomas with CEA has been reported (see Chapter 28) (34). Carcinoem-

TABLE 4-4. DIFFERENTIAL DIAGNOSIS OF MALIGNANT SPINDLE CELL TUMORS

Diagnosis	Keratin	Vimentin	Desmin	S-100	HMB-45	Factor VIII
Squamous cell carcinoma	+	−	−	−	−	−
Atypical fibroxanthoma	−	+	−	−	−	−
Melanoma	−	+	−	+	+	−
Leiomyosarcoma	−	+	+	−	−	−
Angiosarcoma	−	−	−	−	−	+

Note: Few if any of these reagents are perfectly specific for their target antigens. Every test must be interpreted in the context of all the available histologic and clinical information.

bryonic antigen typically stains adenocarcinomas from most organ systems. Most epithelial tumors react with antibodies against epithelial membrane antigen (EMA), including squamous cell carcinoma, breast carcinoma, and large-cell lung carcinoma. EMA will also stain normal sweat and sebaceous glands, although epidermis is unreactive with this antibody. Epithelioid sarcoma is also stained by EMA (see Chapter 33).

Neuron-Specific Enolase

Neuron-specific enolase (NSE) is an acidic enzyme found in neuroendocrine cells, neurons, and tumors derived from them. Merkel-cell carcinoma contains NSE; however, NSE can be detected in a variety of other tumors, including malignant melanoma, and therefore has low specificity. The keratin marker CK20 has better specificity for Merkel-cell tumors than for melanoma and other neuroendocrine tumors (35).

Chromogranin

The soluble proteins of chromaffin granules are called chromogranin (36). Chromogranins consist of three families of acidic proteins: chromogranin A, B, and C. They are normally found in most endocrine cells (e.g., thyroid, parathyroid, anterior pituitary). In the skin, chromogranin A has been found in Merkel-cell carcinoma (37). In contrast, nevi and melanoma do not contain chromogranin.

Synaptophysin

Synaptophysin is a 38–kD glycoprotein that participates in calcium-dependent release of neurotransmitters (38). It is a neuroendocrine antigen with a distribution similar to chromogranin. Positive staining with antibodies to synaptophysin is useful in the diagnosis of neuroendocrine tumors such as Merkel–cell carcinoma. Interestingly, normal Merkel cells are negative for this antibody. Similar to chromogranin, melanocytic tumors do not stain with synaptophysin.

S-100 Protein

S-100 protein is an acidic protein that binds Ca2+ and Zn2+. It was called S-100 because of its solubility in 100% ammonium sulfate at neutral pH. It is found in the cytoplasm and in the nucleus. S-100 protein can be detected in a large variety of cells: melanocytes, Langerhans cells, eccrine and apocrine gland cells, nerves, muscles, Schwann cells, myoepithelial cells, chondrocytes, and their malignant counterparts. Histiocytes may also stain positively with S-100 protein. The polyclonal antibody against S-100 works well on paraffin sections. Its high sensitivity contrasts with a low specificity, a feature that supports the concept of a panel approach to immunohistochemistry.

Useful applications of the antibody against S-100 protein include (a) diagnosing of spindle-cell melanoma and desmoplastic melanoma; (b) distinguishing between melanocytes and lymphocytes in halo nevi; (c) differentiating between pigmented actinic keratoses and lentigo maligna; and (d) diagnosing poorly differentiated cutaneous metastases.

HMB-45

HMB-45 is a monoclonal antibody that was initially generated from an extract of metastatic melanoma. Both primary and metastatic melanomas reveal cytoplasmic staining with HMB-45; spindle-cell melanomas and desmoplastic melanomas are frequently negative. This antibody reacts with a melanosomal protein, GP-100, which tends to be expressed in immature or proliferating cells. Unfortunately, HMB-45 may react with melanocytes in nevi, including dysplastic nevi and Spitz nevi (39). Therefore, it should not be used for the differential diagnosis between a malignant melanoma and a benign nevus. Most desmosplastic melanomas as well as some metastatic melanomas may show negative staining with HMB-45 (39).

MART-1/Melan A

Melanoma antigen recognized by T cells (MART-1) is a relative new melanocytic differentiation marker. The antigen is expressed in normal melanocytes, common nevi, Spitz nevi and malignant melanoma (Fig. 4-6). Monoclonal antibodies to MART-1/Melan A are commercially available and are suitable for both frozen tissue and formalin-fixed paraffin-embedded tissue. Negative staining is frequently seen in neurotized nevi and desmoplastic melanomas (40). In the skin, Melan A mRNA has only been found in melanocytic lesions and angiomyolipomas (41). Immunoreactivity can also be seen in the adrenal cortex, Leydig cell of the testes and granulosa cells of the

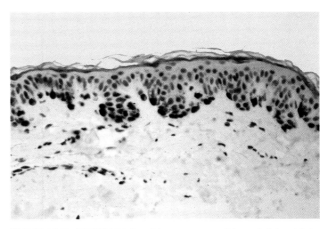

FIGURE 4-6. MART-1/Melan A immunoperoxidase staining highlights normal melanocytes in the basal layer of the epidermis.

ovary, and tumors derived from these cells. This antibody is a useful addition when evaluating intraepidermal melanocytes (vitiligo, early melanoma *in situ*), as well as amelanotic melanomas.

CD34

CD34 is a heavy glycosylated molecule that is expressed on virtually all human hematopoietic progenitor cells. Expression is normally lost during maturation in the skin. Both benign and malignant vascular tumors express this antigen. In dermatopathology, CD34 positivity in dermatofibrosarcoma protuberans is useful in differentiating these lesions from dermatofibromas, which are CD34 negative and factor XIIIa positive (42). Other cutaneous neoplasms that express CD34 include solitary fibrous tumor, giant-cell fibroblastoma, neurofibroma, epithelioid sarcoma, spindle cell lipoma, sclerotic fibroma, and fibrous papule of the nose.

Factor VIII–Related Antigen and Ulex Europaeus Agglutinin I

Factor VIII–related antigen (von Willebrand factor; vWF) is a large glycoprotein produced by endothelial cells and therefore useful in benign and malignant vascular neoplasms. However, some studies have demonstrated factor VIII positivity in only 50% of hemangiomas and 5% to 25% of malignant endothelial tumors (43,44).

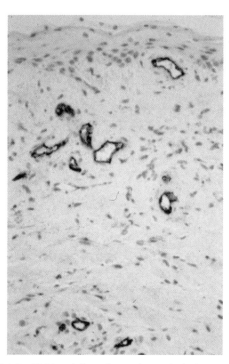

FIGURE 4-7. CD31 staining of vascular endothelium.

Ulex europaeus agglutinin I (UEA) is a lectin that reacts specifically with α-L-fucose present in endothelial cells, keratinocytes, and most eccrine glands. Ulex is a reliable marker for endothelial cells of blood vessels and lymphatics, although it is less specific than factor VIII–related antigen (45).

CD31

CD31 is a marker of endothelial differentiation that is normally expressed in endothelial cells and selected hematopoietic elements (46) (Fig. 4-7). This 130-kD glycoprotein, whose major function is to mediate platelet adhesion in vascular endothelial cells, is also known as "platelet endothelial cell adhesion molecule" (PECAM). CD31 is a sensitive marker for vascular tumors except Kaposi's sarcoma (47). It is a more sensitive marker for cutaneous angiosarcoma than factor VIII–related antigen.

Factor XIIIa

Factor XIIIa, a blood coagulation factor, is responsible for stabilizing newly formed clots by cross-linking fibrin. It is present in fibroblast-like mesenchymal cells, dermal dendrocytes, platelets, megakaryocytes, peritoneal and alveolar macrophages, normal adipose tissue, monocytes, placenta, and uterine and prostate tissue. As noted above, using factor XIIIa in combination with CD34 can be helpful in differentiating dermatofibroma from dermatofibrosarcoma protuberans. Factor XIIIa has also been reported to be positive in a multitude of other lesions, including fibrous papule, atypical fibroxanthoma, xanthogranuloma, multinucleate cell angiohistiocytoma, epithelioid cell histiocytoma, and atypical cells in radiation dermatitis (48,49,50).

Antibodies Against Lysozyme, α1-Antitrypsin, α1-Antichymotrypsin

These antibodies have been regarded as markers of mononuclear phagocytic cells. Although once felt to be markers for "fibrohistiocytic" neoplasms, they have also been identified in carcinomas and melanomas, making them less specific.

Antibodies Against Leukocyte Common Antigen

Antibodies against leukocyte common antigen (LCA) help to distinguish between undifferentiated lymphomas and carcinomas. LCA is found on all leukocytes, including granulocytes, lymphocytes, monocytes, macrophages, mast cells, and Langerhans cells. The lymphomas and leukemias

TABLE 4-5. IMMUNOHISTOCHEMISTRY OF BASOPHILIC SMALL CELLS IN THE DERMIS

Diagnosis	S-100	Synaptophysin	LCA*	Keratin
Lymphoma	−	−	+	−
Merkel cell carcinoma	−	+	−	+†
Carcinoma	+/−	−	−	+
Melanoma	+	−	−	−

*LCA = Leukocyte common antigen.
†Perinuclear staining.
Note: Few if any of these reagents are perfectly specific for their target antigens. Every test must be interpreted in the context of all the available histologic and clinical information. Poorly differentiated carcinoma may be keratin negative, or only positive with low-molecular-weight keratin antibodies.

react with the antibody against leukocyte common antigen; carcinomas and melanomas are negative. In addition to LCA, lysozyme and chloroacetate esterase aid in the diagnosis of leukemia cutis (51). LCA is particularly useful in the evaluation of tumors composed of small atypical basophilic cells in the dermis (Table 4-5). Other antigens useful in the analysis of suspected lymphomas include B- and T-cell markers: L-26 (CD-20, B cells) or MB2 (B cells) and UCHL-1 (CD-45RO, T cells) (see Chapter 31).

Diagnosis of Lymphomas

The application of monoclonal antibodies for the diagnosis of lymphomas is expanding. However, there is no antibody that distinguishes between benign and malignant lymphocytes. Hence, the difficult distinction between lymphoma and pseudolymphoma remains.

Although many antibodies are best used on frozen sections, an increasing number of commonly available antibodies can be used on formalin-fixed paraffin-embedded tissue. The quality of certain markers such as kappa and lambda light chains has been variable in paraffin sections, and is more reliable on frozen sections. Monoclonal antibodies can determine the cell types in a lymphoma or pseudolymphoma: helper or suppressor T cells, B cells, plasma cells, or macrophages. A confusing issue is that B-cell lymphomas may contain reactive T-cell infiltrates, which can outnumber B cells. The predominance of a T-helper lymphocytic infiltrate with epidermotropism of the T-helper subtype is highly suggestive of cutaneous T-cell lymphoma. In contrast, a mixture of T-helper and T-suppressor phenotypes is most consistent with a reactive profile (e.g., spongiotic dermatitis). In dense nodular infiltrates, the presence of germinal center formation with B-lymphocyte aggregates surrounded by a mantle of T cells favors lymphocytoma cutis over lymphoma. A detailed discussion of antibodies helpful in the diagnosis of lymphoma is found in Chapter 31.

Molecular studies can provide additional information in the evaluation of atypical lymphoid infiltrates. Detection of a characteristic gene rearrangement coding for B- and T-cell antigen receptors will identify the presence or absence of a clonal population of lymphocytes (52). These applications are an important supplement to routinely available technology; however, they must always be interpreted in the context of the clinical presentation and findings on routine histology. Although clonality studies can assist in early detection of cutaneous T-cell lymphoma, non-neoplastic processes such as pityriasis lichenoides, pseudolymphoma, and lichen planus occasionally show T-cell clonality (53–55).

Electron Microscopy

Transmission electron microscopy may be beneficial in the diagnosis of poorly differentiated skin neoplasms for which immunohistochemistry is negative (56). Using electron microscopy, the identification of intercellular junctions (epithelial tumors), melanosomes (melanocytic tumors), or Weibel-Palade bodies (endothelial cells) can provide an important diagnostic aid. Other uses of diagnostic electron microscopy include the subtype determination of epidermolysis bullosa and the diagnosis of metabolic storage diseases (e.g., Fabry disease) or amyloidosis. For optimum results, fresh tissue should be fixed in Karnovsky medium (paraformaldehyde-glutaraldehyde) and stored in the refrigerator until processing; although electron microscopy rarely can be performed from paraffin-embedded tissue, there may be extensive distortion precluding valuable interpretation.

REFERENCES

1. Neiman RS, Barcos M, Berard C, et al. Granulocytic sarcoma. *Cancer* 1981;48:1426.
2. Luna LG, ed. *Manual of Histologic Staining Methods of the Armed Forces Institute of Pathology*, 3rd ed. New York: McGraw-Hill, 1968.
3. Roten SV, Bhat S, Bhawan J. Elastic fibers in scar tissue. *J Cutan Pathol* 1996;23:37.
4. Nousari HC, Anhalt GJ. Skin diseases. In: Rose NR, Hamilton RG, Detrick B, eds. *Manual of Clinical Laboratory Immunology*. Washington, DC: ASM Press, 2002:1032.
5. Siegel MA, Anhalt GJ. Direct immunofluorescence of detached gingival epithelium for diagnosis of cicatricial pemphigoid. Report of five cases. *Oral Surg Oral Med Oral Pathol* 1993;75:296–302.
5a. Weigand DA. Effect of anatomic region on immunofluorescence diagnosis of bullous pemphigoid. *J Am Acad Dermatol* 1985;12:274.
6. Zone JJ, Meyer LJ, Petersen MJ. Deposition of granular IgA relative to clinical lesions in dermatitis herpetiformis. *Arch Dermatol* 1996;132:912–918.
7. Nousari HC, Anhalt GJ. Pemphigus and pemphigoid. *Lancet* 1999;325:667–672.

8. Nousari HC, Deterding R, Wojtczack H, et al. The mechanism of respiratory failure in paraneoplastic pemphigus. *N Engl J Med* 1999;340:1406–1410.

9. Mimouni D, Nousari CH. Systemic lupus erythematosus and the skin. In: Lahita R., ed. *Systemic Lupus Eythematosus*, 4th ed. San Diego: Elsevier Science, 2003:chapter 29.

10. Davis MD, Daoud MS, Kirby B, et al. Clinicopathologic correlation of hypocomplementemic and normocomplementemic urticarial vasculitis. *J Am Acad Dermatol* 1998;38:899–905.

11. Collins BA, Colvin RB, Nousari HC, et al. Immunofluorescence methods for diagnosis of renal and skin diseases. In: Rose NR, Hamilton RG, Detrick B, eds. *Manual of Clinical Laboratory Immunology*. Washington, DC: ASM Press, 2002: 393–401.

12. Nousari HC, Anhalt GJ. Pemphigus vulgaris, paraneoplastic pemphigus and pemphigus foliaceus. In: Kanitakis J, Vassileva S, Woodley D, eds., *Diagnostic Immunohistochemistry of the Skin*. London: Chapman & Hall Medical, 1998:74–83.

13. Zambruno G, Ortonne J-P, Meneguzzi G. Inherited epidermolysis bullosa. In: Kanitakis J, Vassileva S, Woodley D, eds. *Diagnostic Immunohistochemistry of the Skin*. London: Chapman & Hall Medical, 1998:126–142.

14. Pardo RJ, Penneys NS. Location of basement membrane type IV collagen beneath subepidermal bullous diseases. *J Cutan Pathol* 1990;17:336.

15. Schaumburg-Lever G. The alkaline phosphatase anti-alkaline phosphatase technique in dermatopathology. *J Cutan Pathol* 1987; 14:6.

16. Cordell JL, Falini B, Erber WN, et al. Immunoenzymatic labeling of monoclonal antibodies using immune complexes of alkaline phosphatase and monoclonal anti-alkaline phosphatase (APAAP complexes). *J Histochem Cytochem* 1984;33:219.

17. Hsu SM, Raine L. Protein A, avidin and biotin in immunohistochemistry. *J Histochem Cytochem* 1981;29:1349.

18. Elias JM. Immunohistochemical methods. In: Elias JM, ed. *Immunohistology: A Practical Approach to Diagnosis*. Chicago: American Society for Clinical Pathology Press, 1990:1.

19. Wallace ML, Smoller BR. Immunohistochemistry in diagnostic dermatopathology. *J Am Acad Dermatol* 1996;34:163.

20. Wick MR, Swanson PE, Ritter JH, Fitzgibbon JF. The immunohistology of cutaneous neoplasia: a practical perspective. *J Cutan Pathol* 1993;20:481.

21. Hudson AR, Smoller BR. Immunohistochemistry in diagnostic dermatopathology. *Derm Clin* 1999;17:667–689.

22. Hibshoosh H, Lattes R. Immunohistochemical and molecular genetic approaches to soft tissue tumor diagnosis: a primer. *Semin Oncol* 1997;24:515–525.

23. Mangini J, Li N, Bhawan J. Immunohistochemical markers of melanocytic lesions. *Am J Dermatopathol* 2002;24:270–281.

24. Murphy GF. Cytokeratin typing of cutaneous tumors: a new immunochemical probe for cellular differentiation and malignant transformation. *J Invest Dermatol* 1985;84:1.

25. Ho CL, Liem RK. Intermediate filaments in the nervous system: implications in cancer. *Cancer Metastasis Rev* 1996;15: 483–947.

26. Fuchs E. The cytoskeleton and disease: genetic disorders of intermediate filaments. *Ann Rev Genet* 1996;30:197–231.

27. Osborn M. Component of the cellular cytoskeleton: a new generation of markers of histogenetic origin. *J Invest Dermatol* 1984; 83:443.

28. Nelson WG, Sun TT. The 50- and 58-kdalton keratin classes as molecular markers for stratified squamous epithelia: cell culture studies. *J Cell Biol* 1983;97:244–251.

29. Inaloz HS, Ayyalaraju RS, Holt PJ, et al. A case of sarcomatoid carcinoma of the skin. *J Eur Acad Dermatol Venereol* 2003;17: 59–61.

30. Chan JK, Suster S, Wenig BM, et al. Cytokeratin 20 immunoreactivity distinguishes Merkel cell (primary cutaneous neuroendocrine) carcinomas and salivary gland small cell carcinomas from small cell carcinomas of various sites. *Am J Surg Pathol* 1997;21:226–234.

31. Argenyi ZB. Spindle cell neoplasms of the skin: a comprehensive diagnostic approach. *Semin Dermatol* 1989;8:283.

32. Leader M, Collins M, Patel J, et al. Vimentin: an evaluation of its role as a tumour marker. *Histopathology* 1987;11:63.

33. Iver PV, Leong AS. Poorly differentiated squamous cell carcinomas of the skin can express vimentin. *J Cutan Pathol* 1992; 19:34–39.

34. Sanders DSA, Evans AT, Allen CA, et al. Classification of CEA-related positivity in primary and metastatic malignant melanoma. *J Pathol* 1994;173:343.

35. Moll R, Lowe A, Laufer J, et al. Cytokeratin 20 in human carcinomas. *Am J Pathol* 1992;140:427.

36. Schober M, Fischer-Colbrie R, Schmid KW, et al. Comparison of chromogranin A, B, and secretogranin II in human adrenal medulla and phaeochromocytoma. *Lab Invest* 1987;57:385.

37. Lloyd RV, Cano M, Rosa P, et al. Distribution of chromogranin A and chromogranin I (chromogranin B) in neuroendocrine cells and tumors. *Am J Pathol* 1988;130:296.

38. Weidenmann B, Franke WW. Identification and localization of synaptophysin: an integral membrane glycoprotein of MW 38,000 characteristic of presynaptic vesicles. *Cell* 1985;45: 1017.

39. Wick MR, Swanson PE, Rocamora A. Recognition of malignant melanoma by monoclonal antibody HMB-45: an immunohistochemical study of 200 paraffin-embedded cutaneous tumors. *J Cutan Pathol* 1988;15:201.

40. Busam KJ, Chen YT, Old LJ, et al. Expression of Melan-A (MART-1) in benign melanocytic nevi and primary cutaneous malignant melanoma. *Am J Surg Pathol* 1998;22:976–982.

41. Jungbluth AA, Busam KJ, Gerald WL, et al. A103, an anti-Melan-A monoclonal antibody for the detection of malignant melanoma in paraffin-embedded tissues. *Am J Surg Pathol* 1998:22:595–602.

42. Goldblum JR, Tuthill RJ. CD34 and factor XIIIa immunoreactivity in dermatofibrosarcoma protuberans and dermatofibroma. *Am J Dermatopathol* 1997;19:147–153.

43. Swanson PE, Wick MR. Immunohistochemical evaluation of vascular neoplasms. *Clin Dermatol* 1991;9:243.

44. Wick MR, Manivel JC. Vascular neoplasms of the skin: a current perspective. *Adv Dermatol* 1989;4:185.

45. Meittinen M, Lindenmayer AE, Chaubal A. Endothelial cell markers CD31, CD34 & BNH9 antibody to H- and Y- antigens: evaluation of their specificity and sensitivity in the diagnosis of vascular tumors and comparison with von Willebrand factor. *Mod Pathol* 1994:7:82.

46. Albelda SM, Muller WA, Buck CA, et al. Molecular and cellular properties of PECAM-1 (ends CAM/CD31): a novel vascular cell–cell adhesion molecule. *J Cell Biol* 1991:115:1059.

47. DeYoung BR, Swanson PE, Argenyi ZB, et al. CD31 immunoreactivity in mesenchymal neoplasms of the skin. *J Cutan Pathol* 1995;22:215–222.

48. Wilson Jones E, Cerio R, Smith NP. Epithelioid cell histiocytoma: a new entity. *Br J Dermatol* 1989;120:185–195.

49. Nemeth AJ, Penneys NS. Factor XIIIa is expressed by fibroblasts in fibrovascular tumors. *J Cutan Pathol* 1989;16:266–271.

50. Moretto JC, Soslow RA, Smoller BR. Atypical cells in radiation dermatitis express factor XIIIa. *Am J Dermatopathol* 1998;20: 370–372.

51. Ratnam KV, Su WPD, Ziesmer SC, et al. Value of immunohistochemistry in the diagnosis of leukemia cutis: study of 54 cases using paraffin-section markers. *J Cutan Pathol* 1992;19:193.

52. Weinberg JM, Rook AH, Lessin SR. Molecular diagnosis of lymphocytic infiltrates of the skin. *Arch Dermatol* 1993;129: 1491.

53. Weiss LM, Wood GS, Ellisen LW, et al. Clonal T-cell populations in pityriasis lichenoides et varioliformis acuta (Mucha–Haberman disease). *Am J Pathol* 1987;126:417–421.

54. Schiller PI, Flaig MJ, Puchta U, et al. Detection of clonal T-cells in lichen planus. *Arch Dermatol Res* 2000;292:568–569.

55. Wood GS, Tung RM, Haeffner AC, et al. Detection of clonal T-cell receptor gene rearrangements in early mycosis fungoides/Sezary syndrome by polymerase chain reaction and denaturing gradient gel electrophoresis. *J Invest Dermatol* 1994;103:34–41.

56. Murphy GF, Dickersin GR, Harrist TJ, et al. The role of diagnostic electron microscopy in dermatology. In: Moschella S, ed. *Dermatology Update*. New York: Elsevier Press, 1981;355.

ALGORITHMIC CLASSIFICATION OF SKIN DISEASE FOR DIFFERENTIAL DIAGNOSIS

DAVID E. ELDER
ROSALIE ELENITSAS
BERNETT L. JOHNSON JR.
GEORGE F. MURPHY

INTRODUCTION

The diagnosis of disease concerns the ability to classify disorders into categories that predict clinically important attributes such as prognosis, or response to therapy. This permits appropriate interventions to be planned for particular patients. Understanding this process involves mastery of the stages of disease, the mechanisms of changes in morphology over time, and the molecular, cellular, gross clinical and epidemiological reasons for the differences among diseases.

The process of cutaneous diagnosis at its simplest level might involve the matching of a large number of attributes contained in classical descriptions of skin diseases with the presence or absence of the same attributes in a particular case under consideration. As there are hundreds of potential diagnostic categories, each having potentially scores of attributes, it is evident that an efficient strategy must be employed to enable diagnoses to be considered, dismissed, or retained for further consideration. Observation of an experienced dermatopathologist reveals a rapidity of accurate diagnosis that precludes the simultaneous consideration of more than a few variables. Indeed, the process of diagnosis by an experienced observer is quite different from that employed by the novice, and is based on the rapid recognition of combinations or patterns of criteria (1,2). Just as the recognition of an old friend occurs by a process that does not require the serial enumeration of particular facial features, this process of pattern recognition occurs almost instantly, and is based on broad parameters that do not at least initially require detailed evaluation.

In clinical medicine, patterns may present as combinations of symptoms and signs, or even of laboratory values, but in dermatopathology, the most predictive diagnostic patterns are recognized through the scanning lens of the microscope, or even before microscopy, as the micro-scopist holds the slide up to the light, to evaluate its profile and distribution of colors. Occasionally, a specific diagnosis can be made during this initial stage of pattern recognition, by a process of "gestalt" or instant recognition, but this should be tempered with a subsequent moment of healthy analytical scrutiny. More often, the scanning magnification pattern suggests a small list of possible diagnoses, a "differential diagnosis." Then, features that are more readily recognized at higher magnification may be employed to differentiate among the possibilities. Put in the language of science, the scanning magnification pattern suggests a series of hypotheses, which are then tested by additional observations (1). The tests may be observations made at higher magnification, the results of special studies such as immunohistochemistry, or external findings such as the clinical appearance of the patient, or the results of laboratory investigations. For example, a broad plaque-like configuration of small blue dots near the dermal–epidermal junction could represent a lichenoid dermatitis, or a lichenoid actinic keratosis. At higher magnification, the blue dots are confirmed to be lymphocytes, and one might seek evidence of parakeratosis, atypical keratinocytes, and plasma cells in the lesion, a combination which would rule out lichen planus and establish a diagnosis of actinic keratosis.

Most diagnoses in dermatopathology are established either by the "gestalt" method, or by the process of hypothesis generation and testing (differential diagnosis and investigation) just described, but in either case the basis of the methods is the identification of simple patterns recognizable with the scanning lens that suggest a manageably short list of differential diagnostic considerations. This *pattern recognition method* was first developed in a series of lectures given in Boston by Wallace Clark (3), and has been refined since for inflammatory skin disease by Ackerman (4), for inflammatory and neoplastic skin disease by Hood et al. (5), and most recently by Murphy (6), Barnhill (7), Maize et al. (8), Weedon (9), and McKee (10). The latter authors have published texts based more or less extensively on pattern classification. The present work, however, has been organized upon more traditional lines, in which diseases are discussed on the basis of pathogenesis (mechanisms) or etiology as well as upon reaction patterns. Such a classification has the advantage of placing disorders such as infections in a common relationship to one another, facilitating the description of their many common attributes. From a histopathologic point of view, however, the novice must learn that some infections, such as syphilis, can resemble disorders as disparate as psoriasis, lichen planus, cutaneous lymphoma, or granulomatous dermatitis.

Because there is a limited number of reaction patterns in the skin, morphologic simulants of disparate disease processes are common in the skin, as elsewhere. For this reason, classification methods based on patterns and those based on pathogenesis are incompatible with each other. To partially circumvent this problem, the present section of this book presents a pattern-based classification of cutaneous pathology based on *location in the skin*, on *reaction patterns*, and where applicable on *cell type*, indexed to the more detailed descriptions of the disease entities discussed in other sections of the book. The section has been based (with permission) on the original lecture notes prepared by Wallace H. Clark Jr., M.D., in 1965, and on the published works cited above, especially that of Hood et al. (5).

The classification is presented here in tabular form and is redundant, in that a particular disease entity may appear in several positions in the table, because of the morphological heterogeneity of disease processes, which are often based on evolutionary or involutional morphologic changes as a disease waxes and wanes. The order of presentation of particular entities in any given position in the table reflects the authors' rough opinion of the relative frequency of the entities in the list, as encountered in a typical dermatopathology practice. For example, lichenoid drug eruption may be more common than lichen planus in most hospital-based practices. However, lichen planus is the "prototypic" lichenoid dermatitis, while drug eruptions may adopt any of a number of morphologies as reflected by their appearance in the psoriasiform, lichenoid, perivascular, and bullous categories as well as elsewhere. The "prototypic" member of each category is underlined for easy reference to the detailed descriptions, because such entities constitute the descriptive standard in a given category, and they are also the standard against which other entities are evaluated. For example, a "naked" epithelioid cell granuloma may suggest sarcoidosis, while the presence of lymphocytes and necrosis in addition to granulomas might suggest tuberculosis, plasma cells might suggest syphilis, and neuritis might suggest leprosy.

The classification tables may be used as the basis of an algorithmic approach to differential diagnosis, or as a guide to the descriptions in the other sections of this book. For example, a psoriasiform dermatitis with plasma cells may represent syphilis or mycosis fungoides, whose descriptions are to be found in Chapters 21 and 31, respectively. Terms such as "psoriasiform" and "lichenoid" are defined briefly, and appropriate page references are provided in this section so that the reader may review more specific criteria for the distinctions among morphologic simulants. This system of hypothesis generating and testing should lead not only to more efficient use of this book in the evaluation and diagnosis of an unknown case, but should also facilitate the development of pattern recognition skills as more subtle diagnostic clues are absorbed into the diagnostic repertoire to allow for "tempered gestalt" diagnosis in an increasing percentage of cases.

This chapter is intended as a guide to differential diagnosis but should not be construed as an infallible diagnostic tool. Diagnosis should be based not only on the diagnostic considerations presented here, but also on those discussed elsewhere in this book and in the literature, all considered in a clinical and epidemiologic context appropriate to the individual patient.

REFERENCES

1. Sackett DL, Haynes RB, Guyatt GH, et al. *Clinical epidemiology. A basic science for clinical medicine.* 2nd ed. Boston: Little Brown, 1991.
2. Foucar E. Diagnostic decision-making in surgical pathology. In: Weidner N, ed. *Difficult diagnosis in surgical pathology.* Philadelphia: WB Saunders, 1995.
3. Reed RJ, Clark WH Jr. Pathophysiologic reactions of the skin. In: Fitzpatrick TB, ed. *Dermatology in general medicine.* New York: McGraw-Hill, 1971:192–216.
4. Ackerman AB. *Histologic diagnosis of inflammatory skin diseases: a method by pattern analysis.* Philadelphia: Lea and Febiger, 1978.
5. Hood AF, Kwan TH, Mihm MC, et al. *Primer of dermatopathology.* Boston: Little, Brown and Company, 1993.
6. Murphy GF. *Dermatopathology.* Philadelphia: WB Saunders, 1995.
7. Barnhill RL, ed. *Textbook of dermatopathology.* New York: McGraw-Hill, 1998.
8. Maize JC, ed. *Cutaneous pathology.* Philadelphia: Churchill Livingstone, 1998.
9. Weedon D. *Skin pathology.* London: Churchill Livingstone, 2002.
10. McKee P. *Pathology of the skin, with clinical correlations.* Philadelphia: Lippincott, 1989.

Part 1. Site Categories of Cutaneous Pathology

In this part, the major categories of cutaneous disease based on their location in the skin and subcutis are briefly discussed, with page references to later, more expanded, discussion.

I. Disorders Mostly Limited to the Epidermis and Stratum Corneum (77,98,105)

The stratum corneum is usually arranged in a delicate mesh-like or "basket-weave" pattern. It may be shed (exfoliated), or thickened (hyperkeratosis) with or without retention of nuclei (parakeratosis or orthokeratosis, respectively). Usually, alterations in the stratum corneum result from inflammatory or neoplastic changes that affect the whole epidermis and, more often than not, the superficial dermis. Only a few conditions, mentioned in this section, show pathology mostly or entirely limited to the stratum corneum.

II. Neoplastic Localized Epithelial or Melanocytic Proliferations (79,98,106)

Localized proliferations may be reactive but are often neoplastic. The epidermis (keratinocytes) may proliferate without extension into the dermis, extend into the dermis and may be squamous or basaloid. Melanocytes within the epidermis may proliferate with or without cytologic atypia (nevi, dysplastic nevi, melanoma *in situ*), in a proliferative epidermis (superficial spreading melanoma *in situ*, Spitz nevi) or an atrophic epidermis (lentigo maligna); they can also extend into the dermis as proliferative infiltrates (invasive melanoma with or without vertical growth phase). There may be an associated variably cellular often mixed inflammatory infiltrate, or inflammation may be essentially absent.

III. Inflammation of the Superficial Cutaneous Reactive Unit (82,98,109)

The epidermis, papillary dermis, and superficial capillary–venular plexus in the superficial reticular dermis react together in many dermatological conditions, and have been termed the "superficial cutaneous reactive unit" by Clark. Many dermatoses are associated with infiltrates of lymphocytes with or without other cell types, around the superficial vessels. The epidermis in pathologic conditions can be thinned (atrophic), thickened (acanthosis), edematous (spongiosis) and/or infiltrated by inflammatory cells (exocytosis). The epidermis may proliferate in response to chronic irritation or infection (bacterial, yeast, deep fungal, or viral). The epidermis may proliferate in response to dermatologic conditions (psoriasis, atopic dermatitis, prurigo). The papillary dermis and superficial vascular plexus

may have a variety of inflammatory cells, can be edematous, may have increased ground substance (hyaluronic acid), and may be sclerotic or homogenized.

IV. Acantholytic, Vesicular, and Pustular Disorders (85,99,115)

Keratinocytes may separate from each other resulting in separation and rounding up of keratinocyte cell bodies (acantholysis). This may occur on the basis of immunologic antigen–antibody mediated damage, on the basis of edema and inflammation (spongiosis), infections (impetigo or herpes viral infection), or on the basis of structural deficiencies of cell adhesion (Darier's disease). These processes produce spaces within the epidermis (vesicles, bullae, pustules).

V. Inflammation of the Reticular Dermis (87,94,119)

The dermis serves as a reaction site for a variety of inflammatory, infiltrative and desmoplastic (fibrogenic) processes. These include infiltrations of a variety of cells (lymphocytes, histiocytes, eosinophils, plasma cells, melanocytes, etc.); perivascular and vascular reactions; infiltration with organisms and foreign bodies; and proliferations of dermal fibers and precursors of dermal fibers as reactions to a variety of stimuli. The infiltrates may be characterized as perivascular, diffuse, or granulomatous.

VI. Neoplastic Nodules and Cysts of the Reticular Dermis (90,100,126)

Neoplasms of the reticular dermis may arise from any of the tissues included in the dermis—lymphoreticular tissue, connective tissue, and epithelial tissue of the skin appendages. In addition, metastases commonly present in the dermis.

VII. Inflammatory Disorders of Skin Appendages (93,100,133)

The hair, sebaceous glands, eccrine glands, apocrine glands, and nails may be involved in inflammatory processes (hidradenitis, folliculitis). Some neoplasms may masquerade as inflammatory processes.

VIII. Disorders of the Subcutis (94,100,135)

Reactions in the subcutis are mostly inflammatory, although neoplastic proliferations of the subcutis do occur (lipoma). Pathological conditions centered in the dermis may infiltrate the subcutis.

Part 2. Site, Pattern, and Cytologic Categories of Cutaneous Pathology

In the following listings, the categories of cutaneous disease based on location in the skin (categories I, II, III, etc.), architectural pattern (categories A, B, C, etc.), and cytology (categories 1, 2, 3, etc.) are presented. A single prototypic example of each disease category is listed, and a prototypic example of each major pattern category is illustrated and italicized in the text.

I. DISORDERS MOSTLY LIMITED TO THE EPIDERMIS AND STRATUM CORNEUM

A. Hyperkeratosis With Hypogranulosis

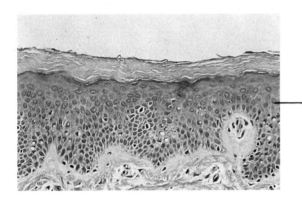

1. No Inflammation
   ichthyosis vulgaris

B. Hyperkeratosis With Normal or Hyper Granulosis

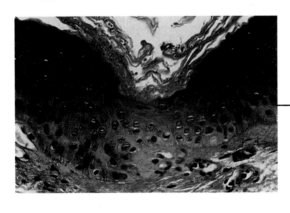

1. No Inflammation
   lamellar ichthyosis

2. Scant Inflammation
   dermatophytosis

C. Hyperkeratosis With Parakeratosis

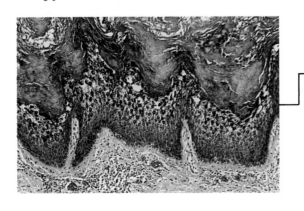

1. No Inflammation
   epidermolytic hyperkeratosis

2. Scant Inflammation
   scurvy

D. Localized or Diffuse Hyperpigmentations

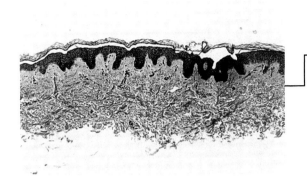

1. No Inflammation
   actinic lentigo

2. Scant Inflammation
   postinflammatory hyperpigmentation

E. Localized or Diffuse Hypopigmentation/Depigmentation

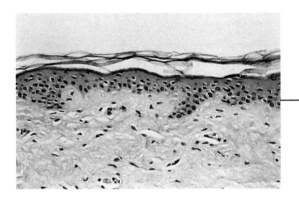

1. With or Without Slight Inflammation
   vitiligo

II. LOCALIZED SUPERFICIAL EPIDERMAL OR MELANOCYTIC PROLIFERATIONS

A. Localized Irregular Thickening of the Epidermis

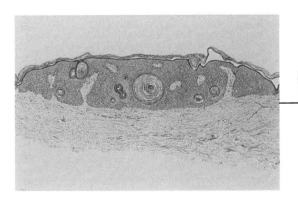

1. Epidermal Proliferation
   seborrheic keratosis

2. Melanocytic Proliferation
   melanoma in situ (superficial spreading type)

B. Localized Lesions With Thinning of the Epidermis

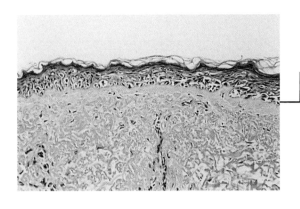

1. With Melanocytic Proliferation
   melanoma in situ (lentigo maligna type)

2. Without Melanocytic Proliferation
   actinic keratosis

C. Localized Lesions With Elongated Rete Ridges

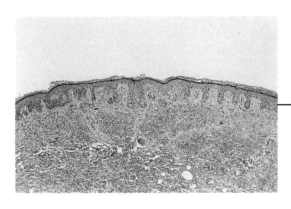

1. With Melanocytic Proliferation
   lentiginous junctional nevus

2. Without Melanocytic Proliferation
   epidermal nevus

D. Localized Lesions With Pagetoid Epithelial Proliferation

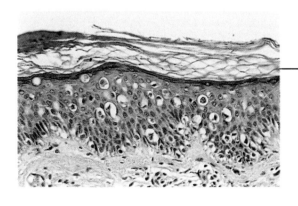

1. Keratinocytic Proliferation
   pagetoid squamous cell carcinoma in situ

2. With Melanocytic Proliferation
   melanoma in situ (superficial spreading type)

3. Glandular Epithelial Proliferation
   Paget's disease (mammary or extramammary)

4. Lymphoid Proliferation
   Pagetoid reticulosis, localized (Woringer-Kolopp)

E. Localized Papillomatous Epithelial Lesions

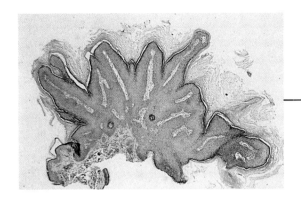

1. With Viral Cytopathic Effect
   verruca vulgaris

2. No Viral Cytopathic Effect
   verruciform xanthoma

F. Irregular Proliferations Extending into the Dermis

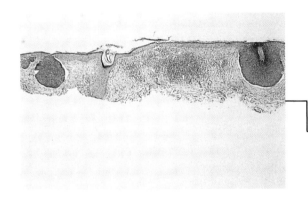

1. Squamous Differentiation
   squamous cell carcinoma, superficial

2. Basaloid Differentiation
   basal cell carcinoma, superficial type

G. Superficial Polypoid Lesions

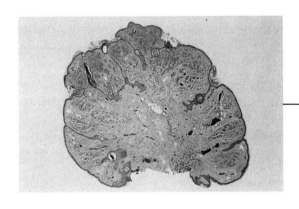

1. Melanocytic Lesions
   polypoid dermal and compound nevi

2. Stromal Lesions
   soft fibroma

III. DISORDERS OF THE SUPERFICIAL CUTANEOUS REACTIVE UNIT

A. Superficial Perivascular Dermatitis

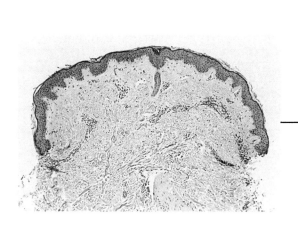

1. Lymphocytes Predominant
   morbilliform viral exanthem
   a. With Eosinophils
      arthropod bite reaction
   b. With Neutrophils
      erysipelas
   c. With Plasma Cells
      secondary syphilis
   d. With Extravasated Red Cells
      pityriasis rosea
   e. Melanophages Prominent
      postinflammatory hyperpigmentation

2. Mast Cells Predominant
   urticaria pigmentosa, nodular type

B. Superficial Perivascular Dermatitis With Spongiosis (Spongiotic Dermatitis)

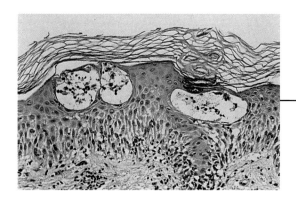

1. Lymphocytes Predominant
   nummular eczema
   a. With Eosinophils
      allergic contact dermatitis
   b. With Plasma Cells
      syphilis, primary or secondary lesions
   c. With Neutrophils
      seborrheic dermatitis

C. Superficial Perivascular Dermatitis With Epidermal Atrophy (Atrophic Dermatitis)

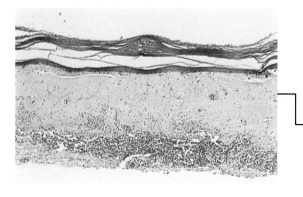

1. Scant Inflammatory Cells
   radiation dermatitis

2. Lymphocytes Predominant
   parapsoriasis/early mycosis fungoides
   a. With Papillary Dermal Sclerosis/Matrix Changes
      lichen sclerosus et atrophicus

D. Superficial Perivascular Dermatitis With Psoriasiform Proliferation (Psoriasiform Dermatitis)

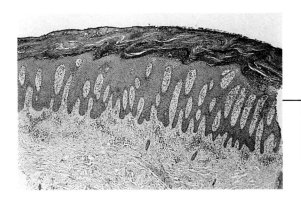

1. Lymphocytes Predominant
   chronic atopic dermatitis
   a. With Plasma Cells
      secondary syphilis
   b. With Eosinophils
      chronic allergic contact dermatitis

2. Neutrophils Prominent
   psoriasis vulgaris

E. Superficial Perivascular Dermatitis With Irregular Epidermal Proliferation (Hypertrophic Dermatitis)

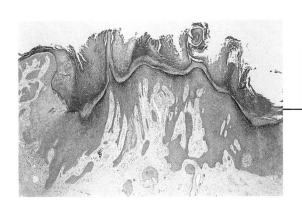

1. Lymphocytes Predominant
   prurigo nodularis
   a. Plasma Cells Present
      rupial secondary syphilis, condyloma lata

2. Neutrophils Prominent
   deep fungal infection

3. Neoplastic
   squamous cell carcinoma

F. Superficial Dermatitis With Lichenoid Infiltrates (Lichenoid Dermatitis)

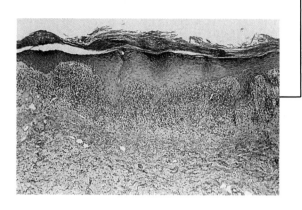

1. Lymphocytes Exclusively
   lichen planus

2. Lymphocytes Predominant
   lichen planus–like keratosis (benign lichenoid keratosis)
   a. Eosinophils Present
      lichenoid drug eruption
   b. Plasma Cells Present
      secondary syphilis
   c. With Melanophages
      postinflammatory hyperpigmentation

3. Histiocytes Predominant
   lichen nitidus

4. Mast Cells Predominant
   urticaria pigmentosa, papulonodular

G. Superficial Vasculitis and Vasculopathies

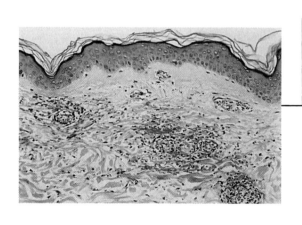

1. Neutrophilic Vasculitis
   cutaneous necrotizing (leukocytoclastic) vasculitis

2. Mixed Cell and Granulomatous Vasculitis
   Churg-Strauss vasculitis

3. Vasculopathies With Scant Inflammation
   malignant atrophic papulosis (Degos)

4. Thrombotic, Embolic, and Other Microangiopathies
   disseminated intravascular coagulation

H. Superficial Perivascular Dermatitis With Interface Vacuoles (Interface Dermatitis)

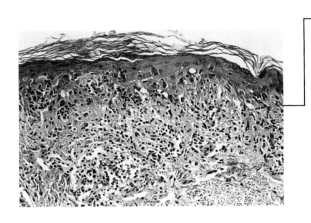

1. Apoptotic Cells Prominent (Cytotoxic Dermatitis)
   erythema multiforme

2. Apoptotic Cells Usually Absent
   dermatomyositis

3. Variable Apoptosis
   cytotoxic drug eruption

4. Basement Membranes Thickened
   lupus erythematosus

IV. ACANTHOLYTIC, VESICULAR, AND PUSTULAR DISORDERS

A. Subcorneal or Intracorneal Separation

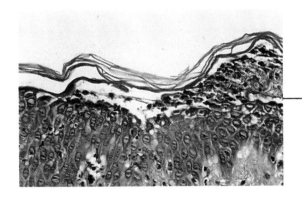

1. Scant Inflammatory Cells
   staphylococcal scalded skin

2. Neutrophils Prominent
   impetigo contagiosa

3. Eosinophils Predominant
   erythema toxicum neonatorum

B. Intraspinous Keratinocyte Separation, Spongiotic

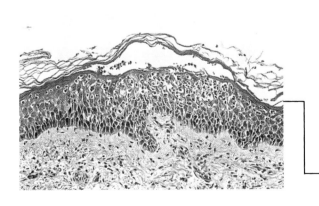

1. Scant Inflammatory Cells
   miliaria rubra

2. Lymphocytes Predominant
   nummular eczema
   a. Eosinophils Present
      allergic contact dermatitis

3. Neutrophils Predominant
   pustular psoriasis

C. Intraspinous Keratinocyte Separation, Acantholytic

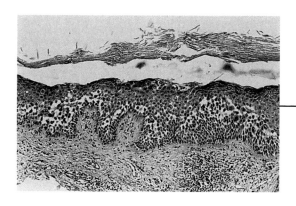

1. Scant Inflammatory Cells *Hailey-Hailey disease*

2. Lymphocytes Predominant herpes simplex, varicella-zoster a. Eosinophils Present   pemphigus vegetans

3. Mixed Cell Types acantholytic solar keratosis

D. Suprabasal Keratinocyte Separation

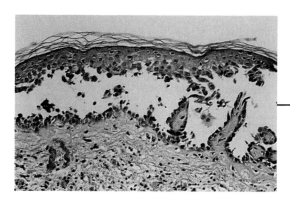

1. Scant Inflammatory Cells transient acantholytic dermatosis (Grover)

2. Lymphocytes and Plasma Cells acantholytic solar keratosis

3. Lymphocytes and Eosinophils *pemphigus vulgaris*

E. Subepidermal Vesicular Dermatitis

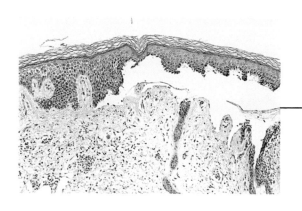

1. Scant/No Inflammation porphyria cutanea tarda

2. Lymphocytes Predominant bullous lichen planus

3. Eosinophils Prominent *bullous pemphigoid*

4. Neutrophils Prominent dermatitis herpetiformis

5. Mast Cells Prominent bullous mastocytosis

V. PERIVASCULAR, DIFFUSE, AND GRANULOMATOUS INFILTRATES OF THE RETICULAR DERMIS

A. Superficial and Deep Perivascular Infiltrates without Vascular Damage or Vasculitis

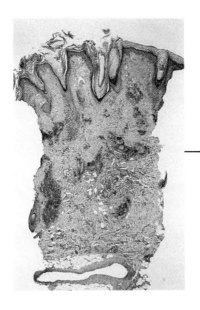

1. Lymphocytes Predominant
   discoid lupus erythematosus (DLE)

2. Neutrophils Predominant
   acute febrile neutrophilic dermatosis (Sweet's)

3. Lymphocytes and Eosinophils
   papular urticaria

4. Plasma Cells Present
   scleroderma/morphea

5. Mixed Cell Types
   erythema chronicum migrans

B. Vasculitis and Vasculopathies

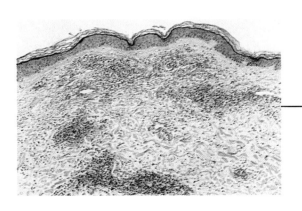

1. Scant Inflammatory Cells
   Degos disease (malignant atrophic papulosis)

2. Lymphocytes Predominant
   "lymphocytic vasculitis"

3. Neutrophils Prominent
   leukocytoclastic vasculitis

4. Mixed Cell Types and/or Granulomas
   allergic granulomatosis (Churg-Strauss)

5. Thrombotic and Other Microangiopathies
   disseminated intravascular coagulation

C. Diffuse Infiltrates of the Reticular Dermis

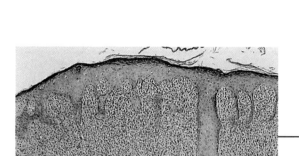

1. Lymphocytes Predominant cutaneous lymphoid hyperplasia/lymphocytoma cutis

2. Neutrophils Predominant acute febrile neutrophilic dermatosis (Sweet's)

3. "Histiocytoid" Cells Predominant lepromatous leprosy

4. Plasma Cells Prominent plasmacytoma, myeloma

5. Mast Cells Predominant *urticaria pigmentosa*

6. Eosinophils Predominant eosinophilic cellulitis (Well's syndrome)

7. Mixed Cell Types syphilis (primary, secondary, or tertiary)

8. Melanocytic Cells nevus of Ota, nevus of Ito

9. Extensive Necrosis calciphylaxis

D. Diffuse or Nodular Infiltrates of Reticular Dermis With Epidermal Proliferation

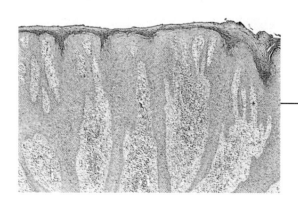

1. With Mixed Cellular Infiltrates *verruciform xanthoma*

E. Nodular Inflammatory Infiltrates of the Reticular Dermis: Granulomas, Abscesses, and Ulcers

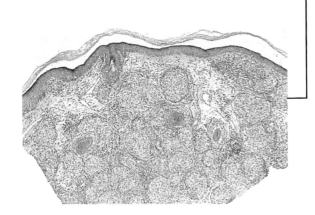

1. Epithelioid Cell Granulomas Without Necrosis
   sarcoidosis (lupus pernio and other types)

2. Epithelioid Cell Granulomas With Necrosis
   tuberculosis (lupus vulgaris and other types)

3. Palisading Granulomas
   granuloma annulare

4. Mixed Cell Granulomas
   keratin granuloma (ruptured cyst)

5. Inflammatory Nodules With Prominent Eosinophils
   angiolymphoid hyperplasia with eosinophils

6. Inflammatory Nodules With Mixed Cell Types
   sporotrichosis

7. Abscesses
   acute or chronic bacterial abscesses

8. Inflammatory Nodules With Prominent Necrosis
   aspergillosis

9. Chronic Ulcers and Sinuses
   pyoderma gangrenosum

F. Dermal Matrix Fiber Disorders

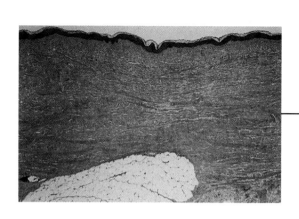

1. Collagen Increased
   scleroderma/morphea

2. Collagen Reduced
   atrophoderma

3. Elastin Altered
   pseudoxanthoma elasticum

4. Elastin Reduced
   cutis laxa

5. Perforating
   elastosis perforans serpiginosa

G. Deposition of Material in the Dermis

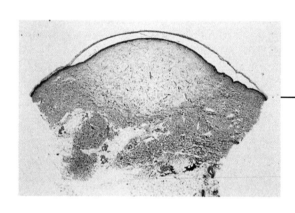

1. Increased Normal Matrix Constituents
   focal dermal mucinosis

2. Material Not Normally Present in the Dermis
   gout

3. Parasitic Infestations of the Dermis and/or Subcutis
   larva migrans (*Ancylostoma*)

VI. TUMORS AND CYSTS OF DERMIS AND SUBCUTIS

A. Small Cell Tumors

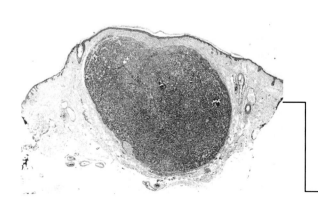

1. Tumors of Lymphocytes or Hemopoietic Cells
   tumor-stage mycosis fungoides

2. Tumors of Lymphocytes and Mixed Cell Types
   cutaneous lymphoid hyperplasia/lymphocytoma cutis

3. Tumors of Plasma Cells
   cutaneous plasmacytoma and myeloma

4. Small Round Cell Tumors
   eccrine spiradenoma

B. Large Polygonal and Round Cell Tumors

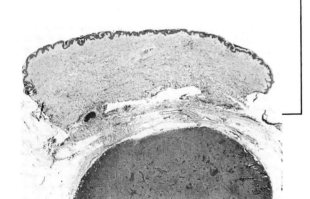

1. Squamous Cell Carcinomas primary squamous cell carcinoma

2. Adenocarcinomas metastatic adenocarcinoma

3. Melanocytic Tumors *metastatic melanoma*

4. Eccrine Tumors nodular hidradenoma

5. Apocrine Tumors hidradenoma papilliferum

6. Pilar Tumors trichoepithelioma

7. Sebaceous Tumors sebaceous adenoma and epithelioma

8. "Histiocytoid" Tumors xanthomas (eruptive, plane, tuberous, tendon)

9. Tumors of Large Lymphoid Cells cutaneous anaplastic large cell lymphoma (Ki-1)

10. Mast Cell Tumors mastocytosis

11. Tumors With Prominent Necrosis epithelioid sarcoma

12. Miscellaneous and Undifferentiated Epithelial Tumors undifferentiated carcinoma (large cell, small cell)

C. Spindle Cell, Pleomorphic, and Connective Tissue Tumors

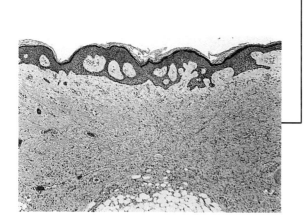

1. Fibrohistiocytic Spindle Cell Tumors *benign fibrous histiocytoma (dermatofibroma)*
2. Schwannian/Neural Spindle Cell Tumors neurofibromas
3. Spindle Cell Tumors of Muscle leiomyoma
4. Melanocytic Spindle Cell Tumors desmoplastic melanoma, including amelanotic
5. Tumors and Proliferations of Angiogenic Cells pyogenic granuloma
6. Tumors of Adipose Tissue nevus lipomatosus superficialis
7. Tumors of Cartilaginous Tissue soft tissue chondroma
8. Tumors of Osseous Tissue osteoma cutis

D. Cysts of the Dermis and Subcutis

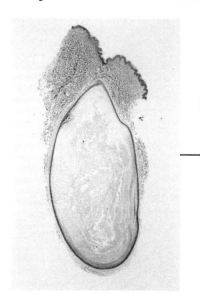

1. Pilar Differentiation *epidermal cyst*
2. Eccrine and Similar Differentiation eccrine hidrocystoma
3. Apocrine Differentiation apocrine hidrocystoma

VII. INFLAMMATORY DISORDERS OF SKIN APPENDAGES

A. Pathology Involving Hair Follicles

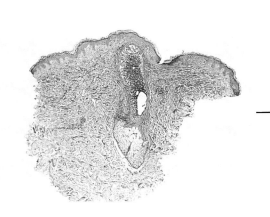

1. Scant Inflammation
   androgenic alopecia

2. Lymphocytes Predominant
   alopecia areata
   a. With Eosinophils Present
      eosinophilic pustular folliculitis

3. Neutrophils Prominent
   acute bacterial folliculitis

4. Plasma Cells Prominent
   acne keloidalis nuchae

5. Fibrosing and Suppurative Follicular Disorders
   hidradenitis suppurativa

B. Pathology Involving Sweat Glands

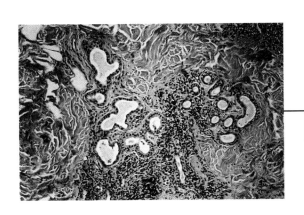

1. Scant Inflammation
   eccrine nevus

2. Lymphocytes Predominant
   lupus erythematosus
   a. With Plasma Cells
      cheilitis glandularis
   b. With Eosinophils
      insect bite reactions
   c. With Neutrophils
      neutrophilic eccrine hidradenitis

C. Pathology Involving Nerves

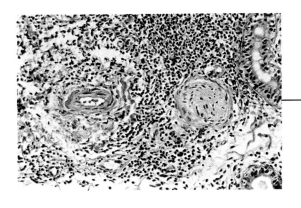

1. Lymphocytic Infiltrates
   herpes zoster

2. Mixed Inflammatory Infiltrates
   leprosy

3. Neoplastic Infiltrates
   neurotropic melanoma

D. Pathology of Nails

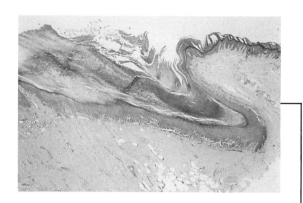

1. Lymphocytic Infiltrates lichen planus

2. Lymphocytes With Neutrophils tinea unguium, onychomycosis

3. Bullous Diseases Darier's disease

4. Parasitic Infestations scabies

5. Melanocytic Proliferation *malignant melanoma, acral-lentigmone type*

VIII. DISORDERS OF SUBCUTIS

A. Subcutaneous Vasculitis and Vasculopathy (Septal or Lobular)

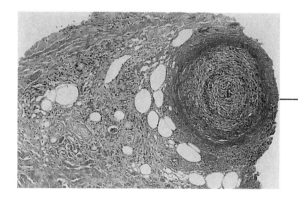

1. Neutrophilic *subcutaneous polyarteritis nodosa*

2. Lymphocytic nodular vasculitis

3. Granulomatous Churg-Strauss vasculitis

B. Septal Panniculitis without Vasculitis

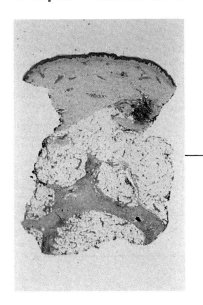

1. Lymphocytes and Mixed Infiltrates
   erythema nodosum and variants

2. Granulomatous
   subcutaneous granuloma annulare

3. Sclerotic
   scleroderma, morphea

C. Lobular Panniculitis without Vasculitis

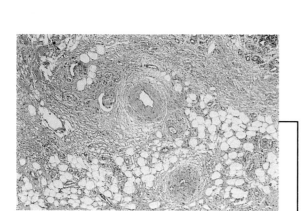

1. Lymphocytes Predominant
   lupus panniculitis

2. Lymphocytes and Plasma Cells
   scleroderma

3. Neutrophilic
   infection (cellulitis)

4. Eosinophils Prominent
   eosinophilic fasciitis

5. Histiocytes Prominent
   cytophagic histiocytic panniculitis

6. Mixed With Foam Cells
   Weber-Christian disease

7. Granulomatous
   subcutaneous sarcoidosis

8. Crystal Deposits, Calcifications
   sclerema neonatorum

9. Necrosis Prominent
   pancreatic panniculitis

10. Embryonic Fat Pattern
    lipoatrophy

11. Miscellaneous
    lipomembranous panniculitis

D. Mixed Lobular and Septal Panniculitis

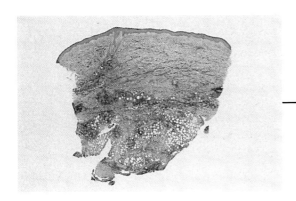

1. With Hemorrhage or Sclerosis
   traumatic panniculitis

2. Prominent Neutrophils
   necrotizing fasciitis (bacterial infection)

3. Prominent Lymphocytes
   nonspecific panniculitis

4. With Cytophagic Histiocytes
   histiocytic cytophagic panniculitis (late lesion)

5. With Granulomas
   mycobacterial panniculitis

E. Subcutaneous Abscesses

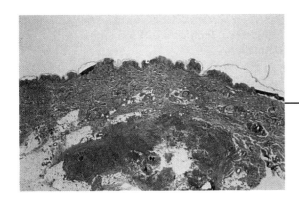

1. With Neutrophils
   deep fungus infection

Part 3. Site, Pattern, and Cytologic Categories of Cutaneous Pathology

In the following listings, the categories of cutaneous disease based on location in the skin (categories I, II, III, etc.), architectural pattern (categories A, B, C, etc.), and cytology (categories 1, 2, 3, etc.) are presented with page references for convenient access to the detailed disease listings that follow in Part 4.

Part 4. Disease Listings Categorized by Site, Pattern, and Cytology

In this section, the cutaneous diseases are listed in categories based on their location in the skin, architectural patterns, and cytology. The listings may be used as a basis for differential diagnosis generation, and for review of material covered elsewhere in this text.

In the lists that follow, the term "predominant" is used to describe an infiltrate in which the majority of the cells are of a certain type, usually lymphocytes or neutrophils. Many dermatoses are composed of infiltrates that are predominantly lymphocytic, with only an occasional other cell type, which are listed as, for example, "1. lymphocytes predominant." Many other dermatoses contain a diagnostically significant admixture of other cell type(s) as a minority population; these are listed in subsequent sections as "1a. with eosinophils," "1b. with plasma cells," and so on, with the understanding that lymphocytes predominate in these dermatoses also. Infiltrates in which there is an approximately equal admixture of multiple cell types are listed as "mixed" infiltrates. As in earlier sections, a prototypic condition for each section is italicized.

I. DISORDERS MOSTLY LIMITED TO THE EPIDERMIS AND STRATUM CORNEUM

The stratum corneum is usually arranged in a delicate mesh-like or "basket-weave" pattern. It may be shed (exfoliated), or thickened (hyperkeratosis) with or without retention of nuclei (parakeratosis or orthokeratosis respectively). The granular layer may be normal, increased (hypergranulosis), or reduced (hypogranulosis). Usually, alterations in the stratum corneum result from inflammatory or neoplastic changes that affect the whole epidermis and, more often than not, the superficial dermis. Only a few conditions, mentioned in this section, show pathology mostly or entirely limited to the stratum corneum.

A. Hyperkeratosis With Hypogranulosis

1. No Inflammation

B. Hyperkeratosis With Normal or Hypergranulosis

The stratum corneum is thickened, the granular cell layer is normal or thickened, and the dermis shows only sparse perivascular lymphocytes. There is no epidermal spongiosis or exocytosis.

1. No Inflammation

The upper dermis contains only sparse perivascular lymphocytes.

2. Scant Inflammation

Lymphocytes are minimally increased about the superficial plexus. There may be a few neutrophils in the stratum corneum.

C. Hyperkeratosis With Parakeratosis

The stratum corneum is thickened, the granular cell layer is reduced, there is parakeratosis. The dermis may show only sparse perivascular lymphocytes, although some of these conditions in other instances may show more substantial inflammation. There is no epidermal spongiosis or exocytosis.

1. No Inflammation

The upper dermis contains only sparse perivascular lymphocytes.

2. Scant Inflammation

Lymphocytes are minimally increased about the superficial plexus. There may be a few lymphocytes and/or neutrophils in the stratum corneum.

D. Localized or Diffuse Hyperpigmentations

Increased melanin pigment is present in basal keratinocytes, without melanocytic proliferation.

1. No Inflammation

The upper dermis contains only sparse perivascular lymphocytes.

2. Scant Inflammation

Lymphocytes are minimally increased about the superficial plexus. There may be a few lymphocytes and/or neutrophils in the stratum corneum. Melanophages may be present in the papillary dermis.

E. Localized or Diffuse Hypopigmentations

Melanin pigment is reduced in basal keratinocytes, with (vitiligo) or without (early stages of chemical depigmentation) a reduction in the number of melanocytes.

1. With or Without Slight Inflammation

Lymphocytes may minimally increase about the dermal–epidermal junction, as in the active phase of vitiligo, or may be absent, as in albinism.

II. LOCALIZED SUPERFICIAL EPIDERMAL OR MELANOCYTIC PROLIFERATIONS

Localized proliferations may be reactive but are often neoplastic. The epidermis (keratinocytes) may proliferate without extension into the dermis, may extend into the dermis, and may be squamous or basaloid. Melanocytes within the epidermis may proliferate with or without cytologic atypia (nevi, dysplastic nevi, melanoma *in situ*), in a proliferative epidermis (superficial spreading melanoma *in situ*, Spitz nevi) or an atrophic epidermis (lentigo maligna); they can also extend into the dermis as proliferative infiltrates (invasive melanoma with or without vertical growth phase). There may be an associated variably cellular often mixed inflammatory infiltrate, or inflammation may be essentially absent.

A. Localized Irregular Thickening of Epidermis

Localized irregular epidermal proliferations are usually neoplastic.

1. Localized Epidermal Proliferations

The epidermis is thickened secondary to a localized proliferation of keratinocytes (acanthosis). The proliferation can be cytologically atypical, as in squamous cell carcinoma *in situ*, or bland, as in eccrine poroma.

2. Superficial Melanocytic Proliferations

The epidermis may be thickened (acanthosis) and is associated with a proliferation of single or nested melanocytic cells. The proliferation can be malignant as in superficial spreading melanoma or benign as in nevi.

B. Localized Lesions With Thinning of Epidermis

A thinned epidermis is characteristic of aged or chronically sun-damaged skin. The epidermis is thinned secondary to diminished number and to decreased size of keratinocytes.

1. With Melanocytic Proliferation

The epidermis is thinned (atrophic) and there is proliferation of single or small groups of atypical melanocytes, resulting in the localization of melanocytes in contiguity with one another, in the basal layer of the epidermis.

2. Without Melanocytic Proliferation

The epidermis is thinned without proliferation of keratinocytes or melanocytes. Each melanocyte is separated from the next by several keratinocytes.

C. Localized Lesions With Elongated Rete Ridges

Elongation of the rete ridges without melanocytic proliferation is termed "psoriasiform hyperplasia" because this pattern is seen in psoriasis. Elongated rete with melanocytic proliferation and predominance of single cells over nests is termed a "lentiginous" pattern. The prototype of this pattern, also seen in a more exaggerated form in dysplastic nevi and in the "lentiginous" melanomas, is the lentigo simplex.

1. With Melanocytic Proliferation

The epidermal rete ridges are elongated and within these rete there is melanocytic proliferation.

2. Without Melanocytic Proliferation

The epidermis is thickened (acanthotic). Melanocytes are normal as are keratinocytes. The only change is acanthosis.

D. Localized Lesions With Pagetoid Epithelial Proliferation

A neoplastic proliferation of one cell type distributed as single cells or nests within a benign epithelium is termed "Pagetoid" after Paget's disease of the breast (mammary carcinoma cells proliferating in the skin of the nipple).

1. Keratinocytic Proliferation

The epidermis has atypical keratinocytes scattered within mature epithelium at all or multiple levels; there is loss of normal maturation. Mitoses are increased and there may be individual cell necrosis.

2. Melanocytic Proliferation

Atypical melanocytes are seen at all levels within the otherwise mature but often hyperplastic epidermis.

3. Glandular Epithelial Proliferations

Atypical large clear cells with glandular differentiation (mucin production, occasionally lumen formation) proliferate in a normally maturing epidermis.

4. Lymphoid Proliferations

Atypical, large clear lymphoid cells proliferate in a normally maturing epidermis.

E. Localized Papillomatous Epithelial Lesions

A "papilla" may be likened to a "finger" of stroma with a few blood vessels, collagen fibers, and fibroblasts, covered by a "glove" of epithelium, which may be reactive or neoplastic, benign or malignant.

1. With Viral Cytopathic Effects

The epidermis is acanthotic with vacuolated cells often having enlarged and somewhat irregular nuclei (koilocytes), the granular cell layer is usually thickened with enlarged keratohyaline granules, and there is parakeratosis in tall columns overlying the thickened epidermis at the tops of the papillae. Large inclusions are seen in molluscum contagiosum.

2. No Viral Cytopathic Effect

The epidermis proliferates. The cells may be basophilic or "basaloid" in type (seborrheic keratoses). There may be increased stratum corneum and elongation of the dermal papillae (squamous papilloma), or there may be basilar keratinocyte atypia (actinic keratosis).

F. Irregular Proliferations Extending into the Dermis

Irregular or asymmetrical proliferations of keratinocytes extending into the dermis are usually neoplastic. The differential diagnosis includes reactive pseudoepitheliomatous hyperplasia, which may be seen around chronic ulcers or in association with other inflammatory conditions.

1. Squamous Differentiation

The epidermis is irregularly thickened, the maturation is abnormal, and there may be keratinocyte atypia (squamous cell carcinoma). The proliferation is often associated with a thick parakeratotic scale.

2. Basaloid Differentiation

The proliferation is of basal cells from the epidermis, extending into the dermis. The epidermis can be thickened, normal, or atrophic.

G. Superficial Polypoid Lesions

A polyp is any lesion that protrudes from a surface. While a papilloma consists of elongated papillae representing a "finger" of stroma covered by a "glove" of epithelium, a polyp is more like a hand within which the papillae ("fingers") may be elongated or, more usually, normal or attenuated. Thus, polypoid lesions may also be papillomatous, or not. Many of the neoplasms listed in Section VI may also present as polypoid neoplasms.

1. Melanocyti Lesions

2. Stromal Lesions

3. Other Neoplasms

See Section VI (Tumor and Cysts of Dermis and Subcutis).

III. DISORDERS OF SUPERFICIAL CUTANEOUS REACTIVE UNIT

The epidermis, papillary dermis, and superficial capillary-venular plexus react together in many dermatologic conditions, and were termed the *superficial cutaneous reactive unit* by Clark. Many dermatoses are associated with infiltrates of lymphocytes with or without other cell types, around the superficial vessels. The epidermis in pathologic conditions can be thinned (atrophic), thickened (acanthosis), edematous (spongiosis), and/or infiltrated (exocytosis). The epidermis may proliferate in response to chronic irritation, infection (bacterial, yeast, deep fungal, or viral). The epidermis may proliferate in response to dermatologic conditions (psoriasis, atopic dermatitis, prurigo). The papillary dermis and superficial vascular plexus may have a variety of inflammatory cells, can be edematous, may have increased ground substance (hyaluronic acid), may be sclerotic or homogenized.

A. Superficial Perivascular Dermatitis

Many dermatoses are associated with infiltrates of lymphocytes with or without other cell types, around the vessels of the superficial capillary-venular plexus. The vessel walls may be quite unremarkable, or there may be slight to moderate endothelial swelling. Eosinophilic change ("fibrinoid necrosis"), a hallmark of true vasculitis, is not seen. The term "lymphocytic vasculitis" may encompass some of the conditions mentioned here, but is of doubtful validity in the absence of vessel wall damage. The epidermis is variable in its thickness, amount and type of exocytotic cells, and in the integrity of the basal cell zone (liquefaction degeneration). In some of the entities listed here, the perivascular infiltrate may in some examples also involve vessels of the mid and deep vessels. These conditions are also listed in Section V (Perivascular, Diffuse and Granulomatous Infiltrates of the Reticular Dermis, p. 119).

1. Superficial Perivascular Dermatitis, Lymphocytes Predominant

Lymphocytes are seen about the superficial vascular plexus. Other cell types are rare or absent.

1a. Superficial Perivascular Dermatitis With Eosinophils

In addition to lymphocytes, eosinophils are present in varying numbers, with both a perivascular and interstitial distribution.

1b. Superficial Perivascular Dermatitis With Neutrophils

In addition to lymphocytes, neutrophils are present in varying numbers, with both a perivascular and interstitial distribution.

If vasculitis is present, refer to Section III.G.

1c. Superficial Perivascular Dermatitis With Plasma Cells

Plasma cells are seen about the dermal vessels as well as in the interstitium. They are most often admixed with lymphocytes.

1d. Superficial Perivascular Dermatitis With Extravasated Red Cells

A perivascular lymphocytic infiltrate is associated with extravasation of erythrocytes, without fibrinoid necrosis of vessels.

1e. Superficial Perivascular Dermatitis, Melanophages Prominent

There is a perivascular infiltrate of lymphocytes, with an admixture of pigment-laden melanophages, indicative of prior damage to the basal layer, and "pigmentary inconti-

nence." Some degree of residual interface damage may also be evident.

2. Superficial Perivascular Dermatitis, Mast Cells Predominant

Mast cells are the main infiltrating cells seen in the dermis. Lymphocytes are also present, and there may be a few eosinophils.

B. Superficial Dermatitis With Spongiosis (Spongiotic Dermatitis)

Spongiotic dermatitis is characterized by intercellular edema in the epidermis. In mild or early lesions, the intercellular space is increased with stretching of desmosomes but the integrity of the epithelium is intact. In more severe spongiotic conditions, there is separation of keratinocytes to form spaces (vesicles). For this reason, the spongiotic dermatoses are also discussed later in Section IV (Acantholytic, Vesicular, and Pustular Disorders).

1. Spongiotic Dermatitis, Lymphocytes Predominant

There is marked intercellular edema (spongiosis) within the epidermis. In the dermis, perivascular lymphocytes are predominant.

1a. Spongiotic Dermatitis With Eosinophils

There is marked intercellular edema (spongiosis) within the epidermis. In the dermis, lymphocytes are predominant. Eosinophils can be found in most examples of atopy and allergic contact dermatitis, and are numerous in incontinentia pigmenti.

1b. Spongiotic Dermatitis With Plasma Cells

There is marked intercellular edema (spongiosis) within the epidermis. In the dermis, perivascular lymphocytes are predominant, and plasma cells are present.

1c. Spongiotic Dermatitis With Neutrophils

There is marked intercellular edema (spongiosis) within the epidermis. Lymphocytes are present in the dermis. There is focal and shoulder parakeratosis, with a few neutrophils in the stratum corneum.

C. Superficial Dermatitis With Epidermal Atrophy (Atrophic Dermatitis)

Most inflammatory dermatoses are associated with epithelial hyperplasia. Only a few chronic conditions exhibit epidermal atrophy.

1. Epidermal Atrophy, Scant Inflammatory Infiltrates

The epidermis is thinned, only a few cell layers thick. There is a scanty lymphocytic infiltrate about the superficial capillary-venular plexus.

2. Epidermal Atrophy, Lymphocytes Predominant

The epidermis is thinned, but not as marked as in aged or irradiated skin. In the dermis there are many lymphocytes about the superficial capillary-venular plexus.

2a. Epidermal Atrophy With Papillary Dermal Sclerosis/Matrix Changes

The epidermis is thinned, there can be hyperkeratosis. The dermis is homogenized and edematous, inflammation is minimal.

D. Superficial Dermatitis With Psoriasiform Proliferation (Psoriasiform Dermatitis)

Psoriasiform proliferation is a form of epithelial hyperplasia characterized by uniform elongation of rete ridges. Although the surface may be slightly raised to form a plaque, the epidermal proliferation tends to extend downward into the dermis, in contrast to a papillomatous pattern in which the rete ridges are elongated upwards above the plane of the epidermal surface and a papilloma (such as a wart) is formed. The prototype is psoriasis, in which the suprapapillary plates are thinned. In most other psoriasiform conditions, the suprapapillary plates are thickened, but not as much as the elongated rete. Because of the increased epithelial turnover, there is often associated hypogranulosis and parakeratosis.

1. Psoriasiform Epidermal Proliferation, Lymphocytes Predominant

The epidermis is evenly and regularly thickened in a psoriasiform pattern, spongiosis is variable (rare to absent in psoriasis, common in seborrheic and inflammatory dermatoses). There is an infiltrate of lymphocytes about dermal vessels.

1a. Psoriasiform Epidermal Proliferation With Plasma Cells

The epidermis is evenly thickened and may be spongiotic. There may be exocytosis of lymphocytes. The stratum corneum is variable, often parakeratotic. Plasma cells are found about the superficial vessels in varying numbers, admixed with lymphocytes.

1b. Psoriasiform Epidermal Proliferation With Eosinophils

The epidermis is evenly thickened and may be spongiotic, and there may be exocytosis of inflammatory cells, including eosinophils. Eosinophils are easily identified in the dermis and may be numerous in some conditions (e.g., incontinentia pigmenti).

2. Psoriasiform Epidermal Proliferation, Neutrophils Prominent (Neutrophilic/Pustular Psoriasiform Dermatitis)

The epidermis is evenly thickened, and there is exocytosis (migration of inflammatory cells through the epidermis) of neutrophils. These may collect into abscesses in the epidermis at the level of the stratum corneum (Munro microabscess). The stratum corneum is thickened and parakeratotic, and contains neutrophils.

E. Superficial Dermatitis With Irregular Epidermal Proliferation (Hypertrophic Dermatitis)

Irregular thickening and thinning of the epidermis is seen in some reactive conditions, but the possibility of squamous cell carcinoma should also be considered. As in other conditions associated with increased epithelial turnover, there may be hypogranulosis and parakeratosis.

1. Irregular Epidermal Proliferation, Lymphocytes Predominant

The epidermis is irregularly thickened, with areas of normal thickness, of acanthosis and of thinning. Lymphocytes are the predominant inflammatory cell about the dermal vessels.

1a. Irregular Epidermal Proliferation, Plasma Cells Present

The epidermis is irregularly acanthotic. Plasma cells are found about the dermal vessels admixed with lymphocytes.

2. Irregular Epidermal Proliferation, Neutrophils Prominent

The epidermis has focal areas of acanthosis, neutrophils can be seen as exocytotic cells, and are found in the dermis in abscesses and about dermal vessels without there being a primary vasculitis.

3. Irregular Epidermal Proliferation, Neoplastic

The epidermis is irregularly acanthotic. There is an associated neoplastic infiltrate in the epidermis or dermis, or in both.

F. Superficial Dermatitis With Lichenoid Infiltrates (Lichenoid Dermatitis)

Lichenoid inflammation is a dense "band-like" infiltrate of small lymphocytes clustered about the dermal–epidermal junction and obscuring the interface. The epidermis is variable in its thickness, amount of exocytotic lymphocytes, and the integrity of the basal cell zone (liquefaction degeneration). Hypergranulosis due to delayed epidermal maturation is a commonly associated feature. For the same reason, there may be orthokeratotic hyperkeratosis. Apoptotic or necrotic keratinocytes are often present. In lichen planus, these are called Civatte bodies. Pigmentary incontinence (melanin-laden macrophages in the papillary dermis) is common, as in any condition in which there is destruction of basal keratinocytes.

1. Lichenoid Dermatitis, Lymphocytes Exclusively

The band-like infiltrate is composed almost exclusively of lymphocytes. Eosinophils and plasma cells are essentially absent.

2. Lichenoid Dermatitis, Lymphocytes Predominant

The band-like lichenoid infiltrate is composed almost exclusively of lymphocytes. A few plasma cells and eosinophils may also be present.

2a. Lichenoid Dermatitis, Eosinophils Present

Eosinophils are found in the lichenoid dermal infiltrate, about the dermal vessels and in some instances around the adnexal structures.

2b. Lichenoid Dermatitis, Plasma Cells Present

Plasma cells are found in the lichenoid infiltrate; their number is variable, but they do not as a rule comprise the major portion of the dermal infiltrate.

2c. Lichenoid Dermatitis With Melanophages

Most of the conditions listed as lichenoid dermatoses may be associated with release of pigment from damaged basal keratinocytes into the papillary dermis "pigmentary incontinence." If a specific dermatosis cannot be identified, the appearances may be classified as postinflammatory hyperpigmentation.

3. Lichenoid Dermatitis, Histiocytes Predominant

Histiocytes are the predominant cell type in the dermal infiltrate.

G. Superficial Vasculitis and Vasculopathies

Endothelial swelling, eosinophilic degeneration of the vessel wall ("fibrinoid necrosis"), and infiltration of the vessel wall by neutrophils, with nuclear fragmentation or leukocytoclasia resulting in "nuclear dust," define true vasculitis. There are extravasated red cells in the vessel walls and adjacent dermis. If the vasculitis is severe, ulceration or subepidermal separation ("bullous vasculitis") can occur. "Lymphocytic vasculitis" in which there is no vessel wall damage is a controversial term and is discussed under lymphocytic infiltrates. A "vasculopathy" includes any abnormality of the vessel wall that does not meet the criteria above for vasculitis, such as fibrosis or hyalinization of the vessel wall without inflammation or necrosis.

1. Neutrophilic Vasculitis

In the dermis, vessels are necrotic, fibrinoid is present and there are perivascular and intravascular neutrophils with leukocytoclasia and nuclear dust.

2. Mixed Cell and Granulomatous Vasculitis

There is vessel wall damage, and a mixed infiltrate in the dermis that includes eosinophils, plasma cells, histiocytes, and giant cells.

3. Vasculopathies With Scant Inflammation

There is fibrosis or hyalinization of the vessel walls, with few inflammatory cells.

4. Thrombotic, Embolic, and Other Microangiopathies

There are thrombi or emboli within the lumens of small vessels. In other microangiopathies, the vessel walls may be thickened with compromise of the lumen (amyloidosis, calciphylaxis).

H. Superficial Dermatitis With Interface Vacuoles (Interface Dermatitis)

1. Vacuolar Dermatitis, Apoptotic/Necrotic Cells Prominent

Lymphocytes approximate the dermal–epidermal junction. Vacuolar degeneration is present in the basal cell zone. Apoptotic keratinocytes are found in the epidermis in variable numbers, visualized as round eosinophilic anuclear structures. The dermis usually has perivascular lymphocytes and may show pigment incontinence.

2. Vacuolar Dermatitis, Apoptotic Cells Usually Absent

There is basilar keratinocyte vacuolar destruction, apoptotic cells are rare or absent. The dermis has perivascular lymphocytes and may show pigment incontinence.

3. Vacuolar Dermatitis, Variable Apoptosis

Vacuolar degeneration is associated with variable numbers of apoptotic cells in the epidermis. The dermis may have increased ground substance and there may be pigmentary incontinence.

4. Vacuolar Dermatitis, Basement Membranes Thickened

Vacuolar degeneration is associated with variable numbers of apoptotic cells in the epidermis. The basement membrane zone is thickened by deposition of eosinophilic hyaline material.

IV. ACANTHOLYTIC, VESICULAR, AND PUSTULAR DISORDERS

Keratinocytes may separate from each other on the basis of immunologic antigen-antibody mediated damage resulting in separation and rounding up of keratinocyte cell bodies (acantholysis), on the basis of edema and inflammation (spongiosis), or perhaps on the basis of structural deficiencies of cell adhesion (Darier's disease). These processes produce intraepidermal spaces (vesicles, bullae, pustules).

A. Subcorneal or Intracorneal Separation

There is separation within or just below the stratum corneum. Inflammatory cells may be sparse, or may consist predominantly of neutrophils.

1. Sub/Intracorneal Separation, Scant Inflammatory Cells

There is separation within or just below the stratum corneum, associated with scant inflammation, usually lymphocytic.

2. Sub/Intracorneal Separation, Neutrophils Prominent

There is separation in or just below the stratum corneum. Neutrophils are prominent in the stratum corneum and in the superficial epidermis, and can often be found in the dermis.

3. Sub/Intracorneal Separation, Eosinophils Predominant

There is separation in or just below the stratum corneum, with (pemphigus) or without acantholytic keratinocytes. Eosinophils are present in the epidermis, and occasionally there is eosinophilic spongiosis. The separation is associated with a dermal infiltrate that contains eosinophils.

B. Intraspinous Keratinocyte Separation, Spongiotic

There are spaces within the epidermis (vesicles, bullae). There may be dyskeratosis or acantholysis, and a few eosinophils may be present in the epidermis.

1. Intraspinous Spongiosis, Scant Inflammatory Cells

The infiltrate in the dermis is scant, and lymphocytic or eosinophilic.

2. Intraspinous Spongiosis, Lymphocytes Predominant

In the dermis, lymphocytes predominate. Eosinophils can be found in most examples of atopy, and allergic contact dermatitis.

2a. Intraspinous Spongiosis, Eosinophils Present

The number of eosinophils seen is variable from many in incontinentia pigmenti and pemphigus vegetans to few in atopic dermatitis.

3. Intraspinous Spongiosis, Neutrophils Predominant

Neutrophils are seen in the epidermis, stratum corneum and in the dermis. Aggregations of neutrophils in the superficial spinous layer constitute the spongiform pustules of Kogoj characteristic of psoriasis.

If vasculitis is present, refer to Section III.G or V.B.

C. Intraspinous Keratinocyte Separation, Acantholytic

There are spaces within the epidermis (vesicles, bullae). The process of separation is acantholysis. Keratinocytes within the spinous layer detach or separate from each other or from basal keratinocytes. There may be dyskeratosis, and a few eosinophils may be present in the epidermis. The infiltrate in the dermis is variable, composed of lymphocytes with or without eosinophils.

1. Intraspinous Acantholysis, Scant Inflammatory Cells

The infiltrate in the dermis is scant, and lymphocytic or eosinophilic.

2. Intraspinous Acantholysis, Predominant Lymphocytes

In the dermis, lymphocytes are predominant. In erythema multiforme and related lesions there is necrosis of individual cells (apoptosis) that may become confluent.

2a. Intraspinous Acantholysis, Eosinophils Present

The number of eosinophils seen is variable from many in incontinentia pigmenti and pemphigus vegetans to few in atopic dermatitis.

3. Intraspinous Separation, Neutrophils or Mixed Cell Types

Inflammatory cells in the dermis include lymphocytes and plasma cells, with or without eosinophils, neutrophils, mast cells, and histiocytes.

D. Suprabasal Keratinocyte Separation

There is separation between the keratinocytes of the basal layer and those of the spinous layer.

1. Suprabasal Vesicles, Scant Inflammatory Cells

The suprabasal separation may be associated with scant inflammation, and frequently with dyskeratotic or atypical keratinocytes.

2. Suprabasal Separation With Keratinocytes Atypia, Lymphocytes, and Often Plasma Cells

Suprabasal separation is associated with keratinocyte atypia.

3. Suprabasal Vesicles, Lymphocytes, and Eosinophils

There is suprabasal separation with eosinophils in the epidermis (eosinophilic spongiosis), and in the dermis.

E. Subepidermal Vesicular Dermatitis

A subepidermal blister refers to separation of the epidermis from the dermis. The roof of the blister is composed of an intact or (partially) necrotic epithelium.

1. Subepidermal Vesicles, Scant/No Inflammation

The infiltrate in the dermis in most of these conditions is scant (few lymphocytes, eosinophils, neutrophils).

2. Subepidermal Vesicles, Lymphocytes Predominant

The epidermis is separated from the dermis, predominantly due to liquefaction of the basal cell layer. In PMLE massive papillary dermal edema is the cause. The infiltrate in the dermis is primarily lymphocytic.

3. Subepidermal Vesicles, Eosinophils Prominent

The subepidermal blister is associated with a dermal infiltrate rich in eosinophils. Eosinophils may extend into the overlying epidermis.

4. Subepidermal Vesicles, Neutrophils Prominent

A neutrophilic infiltrate is seen often in dermal papillae at the dermal–epidermal junction adjacent to the subepidermal blister, or in the blister.

5. Subepidermal Vesicles, Mast Cells Prominent

The epidermis is separated from the dermis. There is an infiltrate in the superficial dermis composed almost entirely of mast cells, with or without a few eosinophils. This may be associated with separation of the epidermis from the dermis.

V. PERIVASCULAR, DIFFUSE, AND GRANULOMATOUS INFILTRATES OF RETICULAR DERMIS

The dermis serves as a reaction site for a variety of inflammatory, infiltrative and desmoplastic processes. These include infiltrations of a variety of cells (lymphocytes, histiocytes, eosinophils, plasma cells, melanocytes, etc.); perivascular and vascular reactions; infiltration with organisms and foreign bodies; proliferations of dermal fibers and precursors of dermal fibers as reactions to a variety of stimuli.

A. Superficial and Deep Perivascular Infiltrates without Vascular Damage or Vasculitis

In some of the diseases considered here, the infiltrates are predominantly in the upper reticular dermis (urticarial eruptions), while others are both superficial and deep (gyrate erythemas). Most of these also involve the superficial plexus. A few diseases are mainly deep (some examples of lupus erythematosus, scleroderma)

1. Perivascular Infiltrates, Lymphocytes Predominant

In the dermis there is no vasculitis, only a perivascular surround of lymphocytes as the predominant cell.

2. Perivascular infiltrates, Neutrophils Predominant

Neutrophils are seen in perivascular or perivascular and diffuse patterns in the dermis. Edema is prominent in some instances (Sweets).

If vasculitis is present, refer to Section V.B.

3. Perivascular Infiltrates, Lymphocytes, and Eosinophils

Lymphocytes and eosinophils are mixed in the infiltrate. Lymphocytes are always seen; eosinophil numbers may vary being greatest in bite reactions and often (although variable and sometimes very few) in eosinophilic fasciitis.

If vasculitis is present, refer to Section V.B.

4. Perivascular Infiltrates With Plasma Cells

In addition to lymphocytes, plasma cells are found in the dermal infiltrate.

B. Vasculitis and Vasculopathies

True vasculitis is defined by eosinophilic degeneration of the vessel wall ("fibrinoid necrosis"), infiltration of the vessel wall by neutrophils, with neutrophils, nuclear dust and extravasated red cells in the vessel walls and adjacent dermis. Some of the conditions mentioned here lack these prototypic findings, and may be termed "vasculopathies" (e.g., Degos disease).

1. Vascular Damage, Scant Inflammatory Cells

Although there is significant vascular damage, there is little early inflammatory response.

2. Vasculitis, Lymphocytes Predominant

The term "lymphocytic vasculitis" is controversial, but there are some conditions in which perivascular and intramural lymphocytes may be associated with some degree of vasculopathy, not usually including frank fibrinoid necrosis. Most of these conditions are discussed elsewhere as "perivascular lymphocytic infiltrates." In angiocentric lymphomas, the cells infiltrating the vessel walls are neoplastic, but the process may be mistaken for an inflammatory reaction.

3. Vasculitis, Neutrophils Prominent

Neutrophils are prominent in the infiltrate, with fibrinoid necrosis and nuclear dust; eosinophils and lymphocytes are also found.

4. Vasculitis, Mixed Cell Types, and/or Granulomas

Histiocytes and giant cells are a part of the infiltrate. Lymphocytes and eosinophils can also be found depending on the diagnosis. Giant cell arteritis is a true inflammation of the artery wall (true arteritis), although there is no fibrinoid necrosis.

5. Thrombotic and Other Microangiopathies

The dermal vessels contain fibrin, red cells and platelet thrombi, and/or eosinophilic protein precipitates.

C. Diffuse Infiltrates of Reticular Dermis

Diffuse infiltrates of the reticular dermis may show some relation to vessels or to skin appendages, or may be randomly distributed in the reticular dermis.

1. Diffuse Infiltrates, Lymphocytes Predominant

Lymphocytes are seen almost to the exclusion of other cell types.

2. Diffuse Infiltrates, Neutrophils Predominant

Neutrophils are the main infiltrating cell although lymphocytes can be found.

3. Diffuse Infiltrates, "Histiocytoid" Cells Predominant

Histiocytes or histiocytoid cells are found in great numbers in the dermal infiltrate. Some may be foamy, and others may contain organisms. The leukemic cells of myeloid leukemia may be easily mistaken for histiocytes and may have histiocytic differentiation (myelomonocytic leukemia).

4. Diffuse Infiltrates, Plasma Cells Prominent

Plasma cells are found in the diffuse dermal infiltrate, though they may not be the predominant cell.

5. Diffuse Infiltrates, Mast Cells Predominant

Mast cells compose almost the entire dermal infiltrate. There may be an admixture of eosinophils.

6. Diffuse Infiltrates, Eosinophils Predominant

Eosinophils are prominent although not the only infiltrating cell. Lymphocytes are also found, and plasma cells may also be present.

7. Diffuse Infiltrates, Mixed Cell Types

The diffuse infiltrate contains plasma cells, lymphocytes, histiocytes and a variety of acute inflammatory cells.

8. Diffuse Infiltrates, Pigment Cells

The diffuse infiltrate contains bipolar, cuboidal or dendritic cells with brown cytoplasmic pigment.

9. Diffuse Infiltrates, Extensive Necrosis

Vascular and dermal necrosis are found secondary to vascular occlusion, or to destruction by organisms.

D. Diffuse or Nodular Infiltrates of Reticular Dermis With Epidermal Proliferation

Ill-defined nodules or diffuse infiltrates of inflammatory cells, usually including lymphocytes, plasma cells, and neutrophils, are present in the dermis, and the epidermis is irregularly thickened.

1. Epidermal Proliferation With Mixed Cellular Infiltrates

E. Nodular Inflammatory Infiltrates of Reticular Dermis: Granulomas, Abscesses, and Ulcers

A granuloma is defined as a collection of histiocytes, which may have abundant cytoplasm and confluent borders ("epithelioid histiocytes"), often with Langhans-type giant cells. Granulomas may be associated with necrosis or may palisade around areas of necrobiosis, may be mixed with other inflammatory cells, may include foreign-body giant cells, and may contain ingested foreign material or pathogens (acid-fast bacilli, fungi). An abscess is a localized area of suppurative necrosis, containing abundant neutrophils mixed with necrotic debris, and usually surrounded by a reaction of granulation tissue and fibrosis.

1. Epithelioid Cell Granulomas Without Necrosis

Large epithelioid histiocytes are common in the infiltrate as well as giant cells. The infiltrate may also contain a few plasma cells as well as lymphocytes.

2. Epithelioid Cell Granulomas With Necrosis

The presence of necrosis in an epithelioid cell granuloma of the skin strongly suggests tuberculosis except in lesions of the face. Epithelioid sarcoma may simulate a necrotizing granuloma.

3. Palisading Granulomas

There are foci of altered collagen ("necrobiosis") surrounded by histiocytes, and lymphocytes. Histiocytic giant cells may also be seen in the infiltrate. The lesions of epithelioid sarcoma are associated with true tumor necrosis, but may superficially resemble rheumatoid nodules.

4. Mixed Cell Granulomas

Lymphocytes and plasma cells are present in addition to epithelioid histiocytes, which may form loose clusters, and giant cells, which may be quite inconspicuous. In many of these granulomatous infiltrates, organisms are found. Keratin granuloma is the most common mixed granuloma. Flakes of keratin may be appreciated as fibers, often gray rather than pink, in the cytoplasm of giant cells.

5. Inflammatory Nodules With Prominent Eosinophils

The nodular dermal infiltrates contain many eosinophils often admixed with lymphocytes.

6. Inflammatory Nodules With Mixed Cell Types

A variety of cells in the infiltrate, including neutrophils, histiocytes, plasma cells, giant cells, and lymphocytes.

7. Inflammatory Nodules With Necrosis and Neutrophils (Abscesses)

Inflammatory nodules characterized by central suppurative necrosis, with neutrophils adjacent to the necrosis, and often with granulation tissue, mixed inflammatory cells including epithelioid histiocytes and giant cells, and fibrosis at the periphery.

8. Inflammatory Nodules With Prominent Necrosis

Necrosis is a striking feature along with variable but sometimes sparse infiltrates of inflammatory cells, which may include plasma cells, epithelioid histiocytes, neutrophils, lymphocytes, and hemorrhage. Organisms may be demonstrable. Epithelioid sarcoma may simulate an inflammatory lesion.

9. Chronic Ulcers and Sinuses Involving the Reticular Dermis

A chronic ulcer is characterized by central suppurative necrosis, with neutrophils adjacent to the necrosis, and often with granulation tissue, fibrosis, and reactive epithelium at the periphery. A sinus extends deeper into the dermis than most ulcers, in a serpentine fashion. A fistula is an abnormal communication between two epithelial-lined surfaces. The histological architecture of fistulas and sinuses is similar to that of chronic ulcers.

F. Dermal Matrix Fiber Disorders

The dermis serves as a reaction site for a variety of inflammatory, infiltrative and desmoplastic processes. These may include accumulations or deficiencies of dermal fibrous and nonfibrous matrix constituents as reactions to a variety of stimuli.

1. Fiber Disorders, Collagen Increased

Dermal collagen is increased with production at the dermal subcutaneous interface. Inflammation is seen at this site. The inflammatory cells are lymphocytes, plasma cells, and eosinophils. Fibroblasts in some instances are increased.

2. Fiber Disorders, Collagen Reduced

Collagen may be reduced focally or diffusely as part of an inborn error of collagen fiber metabolism, or as an acquired phenomenon.

3. Fiber Disorders, Elastin Increased or Prominent

Abnormal elastic fibers are increased focally in the dermis and may become calcified (PXE), or there is diffuse elastosis in the superficial reticular dermis of sun-exposed skin.

4. Fiber Disorders, Elastin Reduced

Elastin may be reduced focally or diffusely as part of an inborn error of its metabolism, or as an acquired phenomenon.

5. Fiber Disorders, Perforating

Abnormal elastin or collagen fibers may be extruded through the epidermis, which may form channels that extend down into the dermis.

G. Deposition of Material in Dermis

The dermis serves as a reaction site for a variety of inflammatory, infiltrative, and desmoplastic processes, which may include accumulations of matrix molecules that may either be indigenous to the normal dermis, or foreign to it.

1. Increased Normal Nonfibrous Matrix Constituents

Ground substance (hyaluronic acid) is increased, associated with a varying inflammatory infiltrate that can include lymphocytes, plasma cells, and eosinophils.

2. Deposition of Material Not Normally Present in the Dermis

Materials not present in substantial amounts in the normal dermis are deposited, as crystals (gout), amorphous deposits (calcinosis), hyaline material (colloid milium, amyloidosis, porphyria), or as pigments.

3. Parasitic Infestations of Dermis and/or Subcutis

Macroscopically visible parasitic agents may infest the dermis and subcutis.

VI. TUMORS AND CYSTS OF DERMIS AND SUBCUTIS

Neoplasms in the reticular dermis may arise from any of the tissues included in the dermis—lymphoreticular tissue, connective tissue, and epithelial tissue of the skin appendages. In addition, metastases commonly present in the dermis and subcutis.

A. Small Cell Tumors

A neoplastic nodule is a circumscribed collection of neoplastic cells in the dermis. Abscesses, granulomas, and cysts may also present as nodules. Cysts are considered separately. In general, neoplastic nodules can be differentiated from reactive and inflammatory nodules by the presence of a monotonous population of cells consistent with a clonal proliferation, while inflammatory nodules are composed of inflammatory cell types (lymphocytes, neutrophils, histiocytes, etc.), generally in a heterogeneous mixture.

1. Tumors of Lymphocytes or Hemopoietic Cells

Nodular infiltrates or extensive diffuse infiltrates of normal and/or atypical lymphocytes are found in the dermis.

2. Tumors of Lymphocytes and Mixed Cell Types

Nodular infiltrates or extensive diffuse infiltrates of normal lymphocytes are found in the dermis. Other reactive cell types (plasma cells, histiocytes) are admixed.

3. Tumors of Plasma Cells

Nodular plasma cell infiltrates, with scattered lymphocytes.

4. Small Round Cell Tumors

Tumors of small cells with scant cytoplasm, and with small dark nuclei, constitute a group of tumors that can usually be distinguished from one another with appropriate immunohistochemical investigations, in conjunction with light microscopic and clinical information. Some of these tumors arise in the deep soft tissue, but they may rarely present in a deep skin biopsy.

B. Large Polygonal and Round Cell Tumors

1. Squamous Cell Carcinomas

Proliferations of atypical cells with more or less abundant cytoplasm, contiguous cell borders, evidence of keratinization, and/or desmosomes occupy the dermis as nodular masses. Most primary squamous cell carcinomas show evidence of epidermal origin, often with associated squamous cell carcinoma *in situ.*

2. Adenocarcinomas

Proliferations of atypical cells with more or less abundant cytoplasm, and with evidence of gland formation and/or mucin production occupy the dermis as nodular masses. The possibility of metastatic adenocarcinoma must be considered and differentiated from the possibility of a primary cutaneous adenocarcinoma of skin appendages (refer to eccrine, apocrine, pilar, sebaceous tumor sections below).

3. Melanocytic Tumors

The proliferations in the dermis are melanocyte derived, pigmented or amelanotic, benign, atypical, or malignant. Superficial lesions may involve the epidermis (junctional component). There may be a fibrous and inflammatory host response. S100 and HMB45 stains may be of value in recognizing melanocytic differentiation in amelanotic tumors.

4. Eccrine Tumors

Proliferations of eccrine ductal (small dark cells usually forming tubules at least focally) or glandular tissue or both in a hyalinized or sclerotic dermis. The inflammatory infiltrate is mainly lymphocytic.

5. Apocrine Tumors

Tumors in the dermis are composed of proliferations of apocrine ductal and glandular epithelium (large pink cells with decapitation secretion). The stroma is sclerotic and well vascularized, and the inflammatory cells are mainly lymphocytes.

6. Pilar Tumors

The dermal infiltrating tumor is composed of epithelium that differentiates toward hair, or is a proliferation of portions of the follicular structure and its stroma. The inflammatory cell infiltrate is mainly lymphocytic, and the dermis is fibrocellular.

7. Sebaceous Tumors

The dermal masses are proliferations of the germinative epithelium and of mature sebocytes. The admixture of these cells varies from one tumor to the other. The dermis is fibrocellular.

8. "Histiocytoid" Tumors

"Histiocytes" may have foamy cytoplasm reflecting the accumulation of lipids, or may have eosinophilic or amphophilic cytoplasm surrounding an ovoid nucleus with open chromatin. Some nonhistiocytic lesions whose cells may simulate histiocytes are also included here.

9. Tumors of Large Lymphoid Cells

Large lymphoid cells may be mistaken for carcinoma or melanoma cells, but may be distinguished morphologically by their tendency to less cohesive growth in large sheets, by the absence of epithelial or melanocytic differentiation, and by immunopathology.

10. Mast Cell Tumors

Mast cells predominate in a nodular dermal infiltrate, with scattered eosinophils.

11. Tumors With Prominent Necrosis

Necrosis is a striking feature in epithelioid sarcoma, which may be in consequence be mistaken for a granulomatous process. In addition, many advanced malignancies, often metastatic, have prominent necrosis.

12. Miscellaneous and Undifferentiated Epithelial Tumors

Proliferations of atypical cells with more or less abundant cytoplasm and contiguous cell borders occupy the dermis as nodular masses.

C. Spindle Cell, Pleomorphic, and Connective Tissue Proliferations

A proliferation of elongated tapered "spindle cells" are found in the dermis; these may be of fibrohistiocytic, muscle, neural (Schwannian), melanocytic, or unknown origin. Immunohistochemistry may be essential in making these distinctions.

1. Fibrohistiocytic Spindle Cell Proliferations

There is a proliferation of spindle to pleomorphic cells that may synthesize collagen, or be essentially undifferentiated. In the absence of specific markers for fibroblasts, immunohistochemistry is of little diagnostic utility except to rule out nonfibrous spindle cell tumors. Morphology is critical for accurate diagnosis.

2. Schwannian/Neural Spindle Cell Tumors

These tumors are composed of elongated, narrow spindle cells that tend to have serpentine S-shaped nuclei, and to be arranged in "wavy" fiber bundles. Immunohistochemistry for S100 is useful, but not specific.

3. Spindle Cell Tumors of Muscle

Smooth muscle cells have more abundant cytoplasm than fibroblasts or Schwann cells. The cytoplasm is trichrome positive, and reacts with muscle markers desmin and muscle-specific actin. The nuclei tend to have blunt ends. In neoplasms, the cells tend to be arranged in whorled bundles.

4. Melanocytic Spindle Cell Tumors

Melanocytic spindle cell tumors may have many attributes of schwannian tumors described above. S100 is positive, and HMB45 is often negative in the spindle cell melanomas. Diagnosis of melanoma then depends on recognizing melanocytic differentiation—pigment synthesis, or a characteristic intraepidermal *in situ* or microinvasive component.

5. Tumors and Proliferations of Angiogenic Cells

There is a dermal proliferation of vascular endothelium. Factor VIII staining may be helpful in demonstrating endothelial differentiation. The many variants of benign hemangiomas should be carefully considered in the differential diagnosis of Kaposi's sarcoma and angiosarcoma.

6. Tumors of Adipose Tissue

7. Tumors of Cartilaginous Tissue

8. Tumors of Osseous Tissue

D. Cysts of Dermis and Subcutis

A cyst is a space lined by epithelium; its contents are usually a product of its lining. Some cysts are inclusion or retention cysts of normal structures (hair follicle–related cysts). Others are benign neoplasms. Some malignant neoplasms may be cystic. These tend to be larger and asymmetric, with a poorly circumscribed and infiltrative border. Their epithelial lining is proliferative, with cytologic atypia.

1. Pilar Differentiation

Cystic proliferations are present in the dermis; these show spaces surrounded by epithelium of follicular origin and differentiation. Keratin is usually seen in the cystic cavity. Associated cells may be sparse or may include lymphocytes and plasma cells.

2. Eccrine and Similar Differentiation

Cystic proliferations are present in the dermis, these show spaces surrounded by eccrine epithelium (small dark epithelial cells). The epithelium of ciliated and bronchogenic cysts is not eccrine but may resemble that of an eccrine cyst.

3. Apocrine Differentiation

Cystic proliferations are present in the dermis; these show spaces surrounded by apocrine epithelium (large pink cells with decapitation secretion). There may be lymphocytes and plasma cells (syringocystadenoma).

VII. INFLAMMATORY AND OTHER BENIGN DISORDERS OF SKIN APPENDAGES

The hair, sebaceous glands, eccrine glands, apocrine glands, and nails may be involved in inflammatory processes (hidradenitis, folliculitis). Some neoplasms may masquerade as inflammatory processes.

A. Pathology Involving Hair Follicles

Inflammatory processes may present as alopecia, or as follicular localization of inflammatory rashes. Acne and related conditions present as dilatation of follicles that are filled with keratin.

1. Scant Inflammation

There is follicular alteration with a sparse infiltrate of cells, mainly lymphocytes.

2. Lymphocytes Predominant

There is follicular alteration with an inflammatory infiltrate mainly of lymphocytes.

2a. With Eosinophils Present

Eosinophils are prominent in the infiltrate and may infiltrate the follicular structures.

3. Neutrophils Prominent

There is a follicular alteration with an inflammatory infiltrate containing neutrophils, which may result in disruption of the follicle.

4. Plasma Cells Prominent

Plasma cells are seen in abundance in the infiltrate. In most instances they are admixed with lymphocytes.

5. Fibrosing and Suppurative Follicular Disorders

There is extensive fibrosis of the dermis, often with keratin tunnels of follicular origin, and with embedded hairs with associated foreign-body inflammation. Neutrophils and plasma cells are seen in abundance in the infiltrate, in addition to lymphocytes.

B. Pathology Involving Sweat Glands

The sebaceous glands, eccrine glands, and apocrine glands may be involved in inflammatory processes (hidradenitis).

1. Scant Inflammation

Sweat glands are abnormal in color or size and number, but there is little or no inflammation.

2. Lymphocytes Predominant

There is a predominantly lymphocytic infiltrate in and around the sweat glands.

2a. With Plasma Cells

There is a predominantly lymphocytic infiltrate in and around the sweat glands. Plasma cells are also present as a minority population.

2b. With Eosinophils

There is an inflammatory infiltrate with eosinophils in and around the sweat glands.

2c. With Neutrophils

There is an inflammatory infiltrate with neutrophils in and around the sweat glands.

C. Pathology Involving Nerves

Specific inflammatory involvement of nerves is uncommon in dermatopathology.

1. Lymphocytic Infiltrates

Neurotropic spread of neoplasms, especially neurotropic melanoma, may be associated with a dense lymphocytic infiltrate that may tend to obscure a subtle infiltrate of neoplastic spindle cells. Certain infections may also be associated with inflammation of nerves.

2. Mixed Inflammatory Infiltrates

There is a mixed inflammatory infiltrate involving nerves.

3. Neoplastic Infiltrates

Many neoplasms may occasionally involve nerves. The involvement by carcinomas (basal cell, squamous cell, metastatic) is commonly in the perineural space, while involvement by neurotropic melanoma tends to occupy the endoneurium and to be associated with a dense lymphocytic infiltrate that may tend to obscure a subtle infiltrate of neoplastic spindle cells.

D. Pathology of Nails

Several inflammatory dermatoses more often seen elsewhere in the skin may present incidentally or exclusively in the nails. The reaction patterns may vary from those seen elsewhere, because of the unique responses of the nail unit to injury.

1. Lymphocytic Infiltrates

2. Lymphocytes With Neutrophils

3. Bullous Diseases

4. Parasitic Infestations

VIII. DISORDERS OF SUBCUTIS

The reactions in the subcutis are mostly inflammatory, although tumors (proliferations) of the subcutis do occur (lipoma). Pathologic conditions arising in the dermis may infiltrate the subcutis.

A. Subcutaneous Vasculitis and Vasculopathy (Septal or Lobular)

True vasculitis is defined by the presence of necrosis and inflammation in vessel walls. Other forms of vasculopathy include thrombosis and thrombophlebitis, fibrointimal hyperplasia, and neoplastic infiltration of vessel walls.

1. Neutrophilic

Neutrophils and disrupted nuclei are present in the wall of the vessel, with associated eosinophilic "fibrinoid" necrosis.

2. Lymphocytic

The concept of "lymphocytic vasculitis" is a controversial one. Many disorders characterized by lymphocytes within the walls of vessels are best classified as lymphocytic infiltrates. The term "vasculitis" may be appropriate when there is vessel wall damage, as in nodular vasculitis, even in the absence of neutrophils and "fibrinoid."

3. Granulomatous

The inflammatory infiltrate in the vessel walls is composed of mixed cells including more or less epithelioid histiocytes, and giant cells. Other cell types including lymphocytes and plasma cells, and sometimes neutrophils and eosinophils, are commonly present also.

B. Septal Panniculitis Without Vasculitis

1. Septal Panniculitis, Lymphocytes, and Mixed Infiltrates

The inflammation predominantly involves the subcutaneous septa, although there may be "spillover" into the fat lobules. The infiltrate is mainly lymphocytic although other cells can be found including plasma cells and acute inflammatory cells.

2. Septal Panniculitis, Granulomatous

Subcutaneous granulomas may present as ill-defined collections of epithelioid histiocytes, as well-formed epithelioid-cell granulomas, and as palisading granulomas in which histiocytes are radially arranges around areas of necrosis or necrobiosis.

3. Septal Panniculitis, Sclerotic

Sclerosis of the panniculitis may begin as a septal process and extend into the lobules.

C. Lobular Panniculitis Without Vasculitis

The inflammation is mainly confined to the lobules, although there may be some septal involvement.

1. Lobular Panniculitis, Lymphocytes Predominant

Lymphocytes are the primary infiltrating cells.

2. Lobular Panniculitis, Lymphocytes, and Plasma Cells

Lymphocytes and plasma cells are the primary infiltrating cells.

3. Lobular Panniculitis, Neutrophilic

Lymphocytes and neutrophils are the primary infiltrating cells.

4. Lobular Panniculitis, Eosinophils Prominent

Lymphocytes and eosinophils are the primary infiltrating cells.

5. Lobular Panniculitis, Histiocytes Prominent

Lymphocytes and histiocytes are the primary infiltrating cells.

6. Lobular Panniculitis, Mixed With Foam Cells

Lymphocytes, plasma cells, and a variety of infiltrating cells can be seen including giant cells and foamy histiocytes.

7. Lobular Panniculitis, Granulomatous

Lymphocytes and histiocytes are the primary infiltrating cells.

8. Lobular Panniculitis, Crystal Deposits, Calcifications

Crystalline deposits derived from free fatty acids or other precipitated salts are present in the fat lobules.

9. Lobular Panniculitis, Necrosis Prominent

There is fat necrosis with a resulting mixed infiltrate.

10. Lobular Panniculitis, Embryonic Fat Pattern

Due to atrophy or failure of normal morphogenesis, immature small fat cells are present in the lobules.

11. Lobular Panniculitis, Miscellaneous

Lymphocytes, plasma cells, and a variety of infiltrating cells can be seen including giant cells and histiocytes.

D. Mixed Lobular and Septal Panniculitis

Neoplastic infiltrates and inflammation due to trauma or infection do not respect anatomic compartments of the subcutis.

1. With Hemorrhage or Sclerosis

Inflammation due to trauma is likely to be associated with hemorrhage, neutrophilic inflammation, and sclerosis in late lesions.

2. With Many Neutrophils

Neutrophilic inflammation diffusely involves the subcutis.

3. With Many Lymphocytes

Lymphocytic infiltrates diffusely involve the subcutis.

4. With Cytophagic Histiocytes

Histiocytes with phagocytized erythrocytes diffusely infiltrate the subcutis.

5. With Granulomas

There is granulomatous inflammation diffusely involving the subcutis.

E. Subcutaneous Abscesses

A collection of neutrophils in the subcutis, usually surrounded by granulation tissue and fibrosis.

1. With Neutrophils

The center of the abscess contains pus, which is viscous because of the presence of DNA fragments derived from neutrophils and dead organisms.

CONGENITAL DISEASES (GENODERMATOSES)

BERNETT L. JOHNSON JR.
PAUL HONIG

ICHTHYOSIS

A classification of ichthyosis includes four major and three minor forms. In addition, there are a number of syndromes that are associated with ichthyosis.

Ichthyosis Vulgaris

Ichthyosis vulgaris, which is inherited in an autosomal dominant fashion, is a common disorder. It develops a few months after birth. The skin shows scales that are large and adherent on the extensor surfaces of the extremities, resembling fish scales, and are small elsewhere. The flexural creases are spared. Keratosis pilaris is often present, and the palms and soles may show hyperkeratosis.

A noninherited form of the disease may appear in patients with lymphoma, particularly Hodgkin's disease (1), but this form has been reported also in association with carcinoma (2) and sarcoidosis. The expression of profilaggrin is reduced in this disorder. Profilaggrin mRNA in keratinocytes cultured from subjects with ichthyosis vulgaris is unstable and has a shorter half-life compared with that in normal cells. Therefore, a stabilizing factor may be absent or functionally inactive (6).

Histopathology. The characteristic finding is the association of a moderate degree of hyperkeratosis with a thin or absent granular layer (Fig. 6-1). The hyperkeratosis often extends into the hair follicles, resulting in large keratotic follicular plugs. The dermis is normal.

Histogenesis. Labeling with tritiated thymidine shows a normal rate of epidermal proliferation (3). The hyperkeratosis is regarded as a retention keratosis resulting from increased adhesiveness of the stratum corneum (3). The reason for this, as seen by electron microscopy, is a delay in the dissolution of the desmosomal disks in the horny layer. Keratohyaline granules are regularly seen on electron microscopy, in contrast to light microscopy. The stratum granulosum, however, consists of only a single layer, and

the keratohyaline granules appear small and crumbly or spongy, evidence of defective synthesis. The reason for the inadequate formation of keratohyaline granules lies in a defect in the synthesis of filaggrin, a histidine-rich protein (4). Defective profilaggrin expression in ichthyosis vulgaris may be a result of selectively impaired post-transcriptional control (5). In noninherited ichthyosis vulgaris associated with neoplasia, the keratohyaline granules have been described as being small but showing a normal structure, indicating a reduced but not an abnormal synthesis (10).

Differential Diagnosis. Although the noninflamed but dry skin of patients with atopic dermatitis clinically resembles ichthyosis vulgaris, on histologic examination it does not show the features of ichthyosis vulgaris but rather increased epidermal thickness, patchy parakeratosis, and slight hypergranulosis in places, as seen in chronic dermatitis (10).

X-Linked Ichthyosis

X-linked ichthyosis is recessively inherited, about 90% caused by gene deletion. It is only rarely present at birth. Although female heterozygotes are frequently affected, males have a more severe form of the disorder. The thickness of the adherent scales increases during childhood (8). In contrast to ichthyosis vulgaris, the flexural creases may be involved.

Histopathology. There is hyperkeratosis. The granular layer is normal or slightly thickened but not thinned as in dominant ichthyosis vulgaris. The epidermis may be slightly thickened (10).

Histogenesis. X-linked ichthyosis, like ichthyosis vulgaris, shows a normal rate of epidermal proliferation. The disorder is a retention hyperkeratosis characterized by delayed dissolution of the desmosomal disks in the horny layer. In contrast to that of ichthyosis vulgaris, the synthesis of keratohyaline granules in X-linked ichthyosis is not defective, and the rate of synthesis is slightly increased (11). The cause of the retention hyperkeratosis in X-linked ichthyosis is the virtual absence of steroid sulfatase activity.

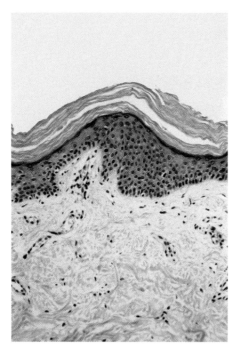

FIGURE 6-1. Ichthyosis vulgaris. Hyperkeratosis with a diminished and focally absent granular cell layer (original magnification × 100).

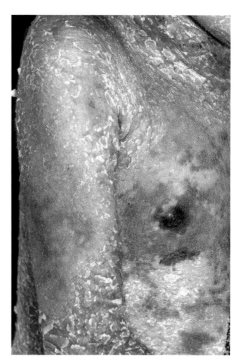

FIGURE 6-2. Epidermolytic hyperkeratosis. Generalized erythema, scaling, and a reepithelialized right axilla (previously denued).

This was first recognized in skin fibroblasts (12), but was found subsequently also in the entire epidermis and in leukocytes (13). X-linked ichthyosis is caused by an extensive deletion of the steroid sulfatase gene (9). Steroid sulfatase normally acts on cholesteryl sulfate, a product of the Odland bodies that is discharged with them from the granular cells into the intercellular space and provides cell cohesion in the lower stratum corneum. Failure of steroid sulfatase to remove cholesteryl sulfate results in persistent cell cohesion even in the upper stratum corneum, and interferes with the normal process of desquamation (14).

Epidermolytic Hyperkeratosis

Epidermolytic hyperkeratosis, an autosomal dominantly inherited disease also known as *bullous congenital ichthyosiform erythroderma*, shows from the time of birth generalized erythema (Fig. 6-2). Within a few days after birth, there is thick, brown, verrucous scaling (Fig. 6-3). The flexural surfaces of the extremities show marked involvement, often consisting of furrowed hyperkeratosis. Vesicles and bullae are usually encountered only during the first few years.

Histopathology. A characteristic histologic picture is seen in the epidermis (Fig. 6-4) and is referred to either as epidermolytic hyperkeratosis (3) or as granular degeneration (15). It is present in bullous as well as in nonbullous areas. There are variously sized clear spaces around the nuclei in the upper stratum spinosum and in the stratum granulo-

sum. Peripheral to the clear spaces the cells show indistinct boundaries formed by lightly staining material or by keratohyaline granules. One observes a markedly thickened granular layer containing an increased number of irregularly shaped keratohyaline granules and compact hyperkeratosis (16). When bullae form, they arise intraepidermally through separation of edematous cells from one another (17). The upper dermis shows a moderately severe, chronic inflammatory infiltrate. Mitotic figures are five times more numerous than in normal epidermis (3).

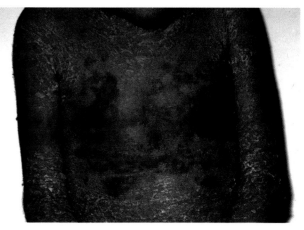

FIGURE 6-3. Epidermolytic hyperkeratosis. Erythema and thick "scales" in older child.

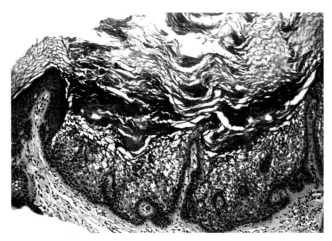

FIGURE 6-4. Epidermolytic hyperkeratosis. There is vacuolization of the upper and midspinus layer. There is hyperkeratosis with large keratohyaline granules in the vacuolated expanded granular cell layer (original magnification × 100).

Pathogenesis. Defects in keratin genes (KRT1 and KRT10) (20) are now known to be associated with this disorder. Mutations were found in the carboxy terminal of the rod domain of keratin 1 and the aminoterminal of the rod domain of keratin 10 (18). The essential electron microscopic features are excessive production of tonofilaments and excessive and premature formation of keratohyaline granules, so that at the periphery of the cells numerous keratohyaline granules are embedded in thick shells of irregularly clumped tonofilaments (15,189). The desmosomes appear normal, but the association of tonofilaments and desmosomes is disturbed, so that many desmosomes are attached to only one keratinocyte instead of connecting two neighboring keratinocytes. Because of this disturbance in desmosomal attachment, blister formation takes place and real acantholysis occurs (21). Labeling with tritiated thymidine reveals greatly increased proliferative activity in the epidermis (3). It can be concluded that keratinization is both excessive and abnormal.

Differential Diagnosis. Although the histologic picture of epidermolytic hyperkeratosis is diagnostic for the type of ichthyosis called epidermolytic hyperkeratosis, it is not specific for it. Hyperkeratosis is found also in several other seemingly unrelated conditions (22,23): epidermolytic keratosis palmaris et plantaris, solitary epidermolytic acanthoma, disseminated epidermolytic acanthoma, and linear epidermal nevus, usually of the systematized type. This latter entity was thought to be an entirely different condition than epidermolytic hyperkeratosis but with similar histologic findings. However, it is now known that epidermal nevi of the epidermolytic hyperkeratotic type are a mosaic genetic disorder of suprabasal keratin (i.e., point mutations of 10k alleles of epidermal cells in keratinocytes from lesional skin) that can be transmitted to offspring producing generalized epidermolytic hyperkeratosis (23). Epidermo-

lytic hyperkeratosis can be an incidental finding in a variety of conditions (25,26).

Autosomal Recessive Ichthyosis

In many instances, it is possible to subdivide recessive ichthyosis into two types. A less severe type, *congenital ichthyosiform erythroderma*, shows fine white scales with fairly pronounced erythroderma and has a tendency to improve at the time of puberty. The more severe type, *lamellar ichthyosis*, shows large, plate-like scales and severe ectropion but only slight erythroderma. In both forms the flexural surfaces and the palms and soles are involved (13,27). Several hypotheses have been proposed for this condition, including a transglutaminase acylation defect (28), or a defect in lamellar body secretion (29) and LOX genes (30). The condition results from deleterious mutations in the transglutaminase 1(TGM1) gene. However, the disease is genetically heterogeneous; some families were found to be unlinked to TGM1 and 2q33–3J (32).

In rare instances, autosomal recessive ichthyosis is associated with storage of neutral lipid in multiple tissues, the Chanarin–Dorfman syndrome (31). It is easily recognized by the presence of lipid vacuoles in leukocytes.

Histopathology. The histologic findings in both congenital ichthyosiform erythroderma and lamellar ichthyosis are nonspecific. As a rule, however, congenital ichthyosiform erythroderma shows only mild thickening of the stratum corneum with foci of parakeratosis, whereas lamellar ichthyosis has a markedly thickened stratum corneum without areas of parakeratosis (33).

In the Chanarin–Dorfman syndrome, lipid stains reveal prominent neutral lipid droplets in some of the epidermal cells (31).

CHILD Syndrome

This rare but clinically striking dermatosis shows from birth unilateral ichthyosiform erythroderma and ipsilateral underdevelopment of the limbs (Fig. 6-5). It is known under the acronym for congenital hemidysplasia with ichthyosiform erythroderma and limb defects, or CHILD syndrome (34). Since nearly all published cases have been female, it is likely that the disease is the result of an X-linked dominant gene defect that is lethal in the hemizygote male fetus. Peroxisomal abnormalities have been found in fibroblasts from involved skin in these children (35). More recently, this disorder has been shown to result from mutations in genes encoding enzymes involved in sequential steps in the conversion of lanosterol to cholesterol (36).

Histopathology. On a thickened epidermis, one observes pronounced hyperkeratosis with prominent parakeratotic foci (37).

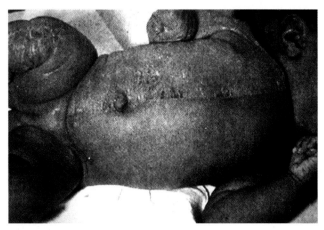

FIGURE 6-5. CHILD syndrome. Note unilateral erythema, scaling, and underdevelopment of limbs.

Harlequin Ichthyosis

Harlequin ichthyosis is a rare condition that is frequently but not invariably fatal (31). It is probably of autosomal recessive inheritance since in one family five siblings had the disease. At birth, the child is encased in a thick, horny cuirass with deep fissures. Marked ectropion and eclabium are present. Fetal skin biopsy is the only available method for prenatal diagnosis.

Histopathology. There is usually a massive hyperkeratosis, the stratum corneum being 20 to 30 times thicker than the stratum malpighii (39). The appearance of the stratum granulosum is variable; it may be normal or it may be flattened to absent. A stain for fat has shown small droplets of neutral fat distributed uniformly throughout the cornified cells. Some cases have shown papillomatosis in addition to the massive hyperkeratosis or areas of parakeratosis.

Pathogenesis. An abnormality in lamellar body formation and secretion (40) may exist, which results in inadequate delivery of desmosomal proteases to the stratum corneum (29) leading to failure to degrade corneodesmosomes and, therefore, massive hyperkeratosis (41).

Erythrokeratodermia Variabilis

A rare, dominantly inherited disorder, erythrokeratodermia variabilis starts in infancy rather than at birth. It has two morphologic components. First, areas of erythema expand centrifugally and coalesce into circinate figures. These lesions fluctuate, sometimes rapidly, in their configuration and extent, and thus are "variable." Second, persistent hyperkeratotic plaques develop both within the areas of erythema and in areas of apparently normal skin (42). In rare cases, referred to as *progressive symmetric erythrokeratodermia*, only persistent erythematous hyperkeratotic plaques are present, and they are limited to the extremities (43).

Histopathology. The changes are nonspecific. In the hyperkeratotic plaques, they consist of hyperkeratosis with moderate papillomatosis and acanthosis. The granular layer appears normal, being two to three cell layers thick (42).

Histogenesis. Labeling with tritiated thymidine shows a normal rate of proliferation. It is likely that the hyperkeratosis is due to decreased shedding of horny cells and is of the retention type (42). A mutation in the genes gjb3 and gjb4, which affect connexins 31 and 30.3, has been described (44).

Ichthyosis Linearis Circumflexa

A recessive disorder that is present at birth or starts shortly thereafter, ichthyosis linearis circumflexa shows extensive migratory polycyclic lesions of erythema and scaling (45). Some of the areas show at their periphery a distinctive "double-edged" scale. The presence of extensive erythema causes a resemblance to psoriasis. The dermatosis persists through life. In more than half of the reported cases, hair anomalies have been present in the scalp, usually trichorrhexis invaginata, the so-called Netherton's syndrome (46).

Histopathology. The areas of erythema and scaling show nonspecific changes with some resemblance to psoriasis, such as elongation of the rete ridges and hyperkeratosis, as well as parakeratosis (47).

The double-edged scale frequently shows in the upper stratum malpighii intracellular edema and irregular spongiosis resulting in multilocular vesicles or vesiculopustules within the horny layer (48). In other cases, focal accumulations of PAS-positive, diastase-resistant, and homogeneous material representing exuded serum protein are seen within a parakeratotic stratum corneum (49). The presence of such exudative changes, however, is not specific or characteristic for ichthyosis linearis circumscripta, as has been claimed (50).

Histogenesis. Electron microscopic examination has shown the presence of multilocular vesicles that are filled with an amorphous substance compatible with serum protein (51).

Syndromes Associated with Ichthyosis

There is an expanding list of syndromes that combine ichthyosis with neuroectodermal and mesodermal defects (52). Some of the syndromes described in the literature may be chance associations (53). Among the well-established syndromes are the *Sjögren–Larsson syndrome*, which is characterized by lamellar ichthyosis in association with mental retardation and spastic paresis (54); skin fibroblasts and leukocytes from these patients are deficient in activity of the enzyme fatty alcohol, NAD oxidoreductase (55); and due to a gene defect in FALDH (56). *Rud's syndrome*, showing generalized ichthyosis with hypogonadism, mental deficiency, and epilepsy (57); *Conradi's syndrome*, in which ichthyosis with a whorled pattern is associated with skeletal and ocular abnormalities (58) with a gene defect in EBP affecting Delta 8, Delta 7 sterol isomerase (empopamil-binding protein) (60). Some forms are associated with peroxisome abnormalities (59). *Netherton's syndrome*, which consists of a combination of either ichthyosis linearis circumflexa or, less commonly, lamellar ichthyosis with trichorrhexis invaginata; IBIDS syndrome, ichthyosis associated with brittle hair, impaired intelligence, decreased fertility, and short stature (52); and PIBIDS syndrome, showing photosensitivity and IBIDS. Patients with these syndromes have sulfur-deficient, sparse hair, including KID syndrome, keratitis associated with ichthyosis and deafness (61); neutral lipid-storage disease, ichthyosis with cataracts, deafness, ataxia, and lipid droplets in many circulating cells (62); and multiple sulfatase deficiencies, a combination of ichthyosis, neurodegeneration, organomegaly, and skeletal dysplasia (includes steroid sulfatase deficiency). The only syndrome showing specific histologic changes in the skin is *Refsum's syndrome*.

Refsum's Syndrome

An autosomal recessive disorder, Refsum's syndrome is characterized by generalized ichthyosis, cerebellar ataxia, progressive paresis of the extremities, and retinitis pigmentosa.

Histopathology. The skin shows hyperkeratosis, hypergranulosis, and acanthosis. In the basal and suprabasal cells of the epidermis are variably sized vacuoles that, on staining for lipids, are seen to contain lipid accumulations (63).

Pathogenesis. The primary metabolic defect in Refsum's syndrome is an accumulation of phytanic acid, which results from a deficiency of alpha-phytanic acid alpha-hydroxylase (64). Refsum's disease is caused by mutations in the phytanoyl-CoA hydroxylase gene (65).

KERATOSIS PALMARIS ET PLANTARIS

Three major autosomal dominant forms and two autosomal recessive forms of keratosis palmaris et plantaris exist. Evidence is accruing that indicates abnormalities in intracellular structural proteins (e.g., loricrin, keratins), desmosomal proteins, gap junction components (e.g., connexins), and enzymes (e.g., catheptins) lead to the varying palmoplantar keratodermas. Gene defects causing many types of hereditary palmoplantar keratodermas have been discovered (68). The three dominantly inherited forms follow:

Keratosis palmaris et plantaris of Unna–Thost, showing either diffuse or localized, occasionally linear hyperkerato-

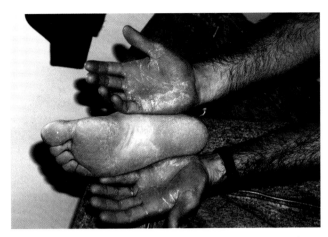

FIGURE 6-6. Keratosis palmeris et plantaris of Unna–Thost. Thickened palms and soles of the father, whose child has similar findings.

sis of the palms and soles (Fig. 6-6). A division into two types, a circumscribed type with limitation to the palms and soles and an extending type with gradual progression to the dorsa of the hands and feet, ankles and wrists, and elbows and knees, is not tenable because both types may occur in the same family (66).

Epidermolytic keratosis palmaris et plantaris, although clinically indistinguishable from the Unna–Thost type, histologically shows epidermolytic hyperkeratosis. Apparently this form is quite common (67). This variant has been associated with mutations in keratin type 9 localized within the keratin gene cluster on chromosome 17q 12-q21 and keratin type 1 on chromosome 12q13 (68).

Keratosis palmo-plantaris punctata (or *papulosa*) has multiple keratotic plugs.

The two recessively inherited forms follow:

Keratosis palmaris et plantaris of the Meleda type, showing diffuse involvement of the palms and soles and a marked tendency toward progression to the dorsa of the hands and feet, ankles and wrists, and elbows and knees (69).

The *Papillon–Lefèvre syndrome* shows the clinical characteristics of the Meleda type in association with periodontosis resulting in the loss first of the deciduous teeth and later of the permanent teeth (70). An abnormality in cathepsin C localized to chromosome 11q14.1 has been found (68).

In addition, keratosis palmaris et plantaris occurs in three syndromes: (a) pachyonychia congenita, keratins 6b,9,16,17 on 12q13 (17q12-q21) (68); (b) hidrotic ectodermal dysplasia, (connexin 30 on 13q12) (68); and (c) the Richner–Hanhart syndrome associated with tyrosinemia (tyrosine tyrosinase on 16q22 (1-q22.3) (68).

Histopathology. In keratosis palmaris et plantaris of the Unna–Thost and Meleda types, as well as in the Papillon–Lefèvre syndrome, the histologic picture is nonspecific, consisting of considerable hyperkeratosis, hypergranulosis, acanthosis, and a sparse inflammatory infiltrate of lymphocytes in the upper dermis (69,70).

In epidermolytic keratosis palmaris et plantaris, the histologic picture is identical to that seen in epidermolytic hyperkeratosis. Many cells in the middle and upper stratum malpighii appear vacuolated, and scattered cavities are present as a result of ruptured cell walls. Keratohyaline granules are numerous and large (71–73).

In keratosis palmo-plantaris punctata, there is massive hyperkeratosis over a sharply limited area, with depression of the underlying Malpighian layer below the general level of the epidermis. There is an increase in the thickness of the granular layer. The dermis is free of inflammation (74). In two cases reported as punctate keratoderma, a cornoid lamella was seen in the center of the hyperkeratotic plug; these cases represent punctate porokeratosis with the lesions limited to the palms and soles, rather than keratosis palmo-plantaris punctata (75,76).

ACROKERATOELASTOIDOSIS

Acrokeratoelastoidosis is a rare, autosomal dominantly inherited condition in which firm, shiny papules are seen at the periphery of the palms and soles with extension to the dorsa of the fingers and the sides of the feet (77,78) (Fig. 6-7).

Histopathology. The essential histologic feature in the papules consists of diminution and fragmentation of the elastic fibers, especially in the deeper portions of the dermis (77,78). Some of the fragmented elastic fibers appear thickened and tortuous (79).

Histogenesis. On electron microscopic examination, the elastic fibers in the reticular dermis appear disaggregated, with fragmentation of the microfibrils (78,80).

Differential Diagnosis. In *focal acral hyperkeratosis*, the lesions have the same clinical appearance as in acrokeratoelastoidosis. There may or may not be a familial predisposition, but the elastic tissue stains fail to reveal any abnormalities (81,82). In *degenerative collagenous plaques of the hands*, the lesions develop late in life; there is no involvement of the feet and no familial predisposition. These histologic changes consist of basophilic degeneration of the elastic tissue (83,84).

PACHYONYCHIA CONGENITA

A disorder with autosomal dominant inheritance, pachyonychia congenita is characterized by the following triad: (a) subungual hyperkeratosis with accumulation of hard, keratinous material beneath the distal portion of the nails (Fig. 6-8), lifting the nails from the nail bed; (b) keratosis palmaris et plantaris with thick callosities, especially on the soles, that are tender and are often associated with blister formation; and (c) thick white areas on the oral mucosa (Fig. 6-9) that resemble those seen in white sponge nevus and possess no tendency toward malignant degeneration (85). Follicular hyperkeratosis may occur, mainly on the elbows and knees. Several clinical variants have been described. Type I shows prominent palmoplantar hyperkeratosis and extensive follicular hyperkeratosis that also involves the trunk. Type II (most common) manifests scalloped tongue and oral leukokeratosis. Type III develops corneal thickenings and cataracts. Type IV (Jackson–Lawler variant) develops cysts of the head, neck, and chest at puberty. They may also manifest hidradenitis suppurativa and milia. A late onset type may also exist.

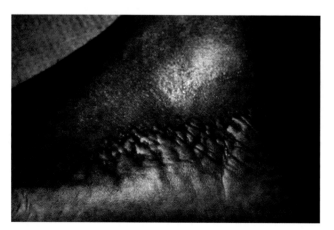

FIGURE 6-7. Acrokeratoelastoidosis. Firm papules at side of foot.

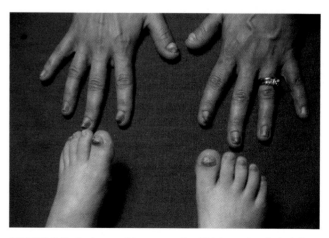

FIGURE 6-8. Pachyonychia congenita. Thickened nails in infant with this syndrome.

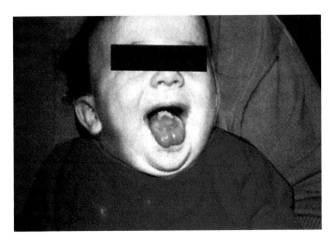

FIGURE 6-9. Pachyonychia congenita. Note whitened mucosa at back of tongue.

Histopathology. The nail bed shows marked hyperkeratosis. As in a normal nail bed, there is no granular layer (85). The blisters that may be seen beneath and around the plantar callosities arise in the upper layers of the stratum malpighii through increasing intracellular edema and vacuolization. Unlike friction blisters, they show no areas of necrosis (86). The oral lesions show thickening of the oral epithelium with extensive intracellular vacuolization, exactly as seen in white sponge nevus, and without evidence of dyskeratosis (87).

Pathogenesis. A defect in keratin synthesis in types I and II is suggested by mutations of K6b, K9, K16, and K17 mapped to chromosome 12q13 or 17q12-q21 (88,89).

DYSKERATOSIS CONGENITA

Dyskeratosis congenita usually is inherited as an X-linked recessive disorder, most likely location Xq28, occurring only in males, but in some instances it is transmitted in an autosomal dominant fashion, in which case females also may be affected (90). It is characterized by the following triad: (a) dystrophy of the nails, with failure of the nails to form a nail plate; (b) white thickening (leukokeratosis) of the oral and occasionally also of the anal mucosa; and (b) extensive areas of netlike pigmentation of the skin suggestive of poikiloderma atrophicans vasculare but with less atrophy and telangiectasia. Carcinoma may develop in areas of buccal and anal leukokeratosis. In many cases, a Fanconi type of anemia develops that may begin with leukopenia and thrombocytopenia but ends in severe pancytopenia (91).

Histopathology. In dyskeratosis congenita, the areas of netlike pigmentation show as their only constant feature melanophages in the upper dermis (92). In contrast to poi-

kiloderma atrophicans vasculare, atrophy of the epidermis, vacuolization of basal cells, and inflammatory infiltration of the upper dermis are either absent (93) or are mild and thus not diagnostic (92). Oral biopsies may show squamous cell carcinoma *in situ* or invasive squamous cell carcinoma.

Pathogenesis. The gene responsible for X-linked dyskeratosis congenita (9DKC1) encodes a protein called Dyskeratin essential for ribosome biogenesis and telomerase RNP assembly. X-linked and autosomal dyskeratosis congenita have reduced telomere lengths but normal telomerase activity (94,96).

POROKERATOSIS

Porokeratosis has a wide variety of manifestations, but with the exception of the punctate type, it is characterized by a distinct peripheral keratotic ridge that corresponds histologically to the cornoid lamella (Fig. 6-10). Porokeratosis is inherited in an autosomal dominant pattern. Five different forms can be distinguished (95).

The *plaque type*, as originally described by Mibelli, shows a single or a few lesions several centimeters in diameter. Rarely, there are numerous lesions (97). The border often consists of a raised wall, having on its top a furrow filled with keratotic material. The lesions have a tendency toward peripheral extension.

Disseminated superficial actinic porokeratosis, the most common type, shows lesions that often are most pronounced in sun-exposed areas and may be exacerbated by exposure to the sun (98). However, the term "actinic" cannot be applied to all cases. In some instances, the lesions

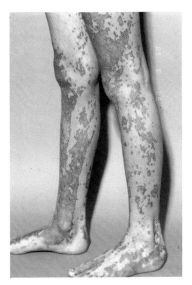

FIGURE 6-10. Porokeratosis. Linear hyperkeratosis along the feet and legs.

are distributed mainly in areas not exposed to the sun (99), and in some cases immunosuppression has been the eliciting factor (100). The extensor surfaces of the extremities are the most common site of involvement. The lesions in disseminated superficial porokeratosis are small and are surrounded only by a narrow, slightly raised, hyperkeratotic ridge without a distinct furrow (98).

Linear porokeratosis may involve only a segment of the body or may have a generalized distribution. The lesions clinically resemble those of linear verrucous epidermal nevus (101,102).

Porokeratosis plantaris, palmaris, et disseminata is characterized by the appearance in adolescence or early adult life of many lesions on the palms and soles and, subsequently, by the involvement of other areas of the body with large numbers of small superficial lesions (103–105).

Punctate porokeratosis, limited to the palms and soles, shows numerous punctate, 1- to 2-mm seed-like keratotic plugs without tendency to centrifugal enlargement. They may be moderately tender to pressure (106).

Development of squamous cell carcinoma or of Bowen's disease within lesions of porokeratosis has been repeatedly reported in patients with solitary lesions (107) and in persons with disseminated lesions (103) or linear lesions (108). In one reported instance with many lesions and multiple squamous cell carcinomas, visceral metastases resulted in death (97).

Histopathology. It is essential that the specimen for biopsy be taken from the peripheral, raised, hyperkeratotic

ridge. On histologic examination, the ridge then shows a keratin-filled invagination of the epidermis. In the plaque type of porokeratosis, the invagination extends deeply downward at an angle, the apex of which points away from the central portion of the lesion. In the center of this keratin-filled invagination rises a parakeratotic column, the so-called cornoid lamella, representing the most characteristic feature of porokeratosis of Mibelli (109) (Fig. 6-11). Within the parakeratotic column, the horny cells appear homogeneous and possess pyknotic nuclei. In the epidermis beneath the parakeratotic column, the keratinocytes are irregularly arranged and have pyknotic nuclei with perinuclear edema. In the upper stratum malpighii, some cells possess an eosinophilic cytoplasm as a result of premature keratinization (110). Usually no granular layer is found at the site at which the parakeratotic column arises, but elsewhere the keratin-filled invagination of the epidermis has a well-developed granular layer.

The histologic changes in the other forms of porokeratosis are similar to those seen in the plaque type but less pronounced, the central invagination being rather shallow, especially in disseminated superficial actinic porokeratosis (Fig. 6-12A). The shallow parakeratotic invagination then stands out by showing homogeneous cells rather than the basket-weave pattern seen in the surrounding orthokeratotic stratum corneum (Fig. 6-12B).

Because the peripheral raised ridge in porokeratosis slowly moves centrifugally, it stands to reason that the invagination is not bound to a definite structure, such as the sweat pore, as originally assumed by Mibelli. Although the invagination occasionally may be seen within a sweat pore or a pilosebaceous follicle, it is found most commonly in the epidermis independent of these cutaneous appendages (111). Overexpression of the P53 tumor-suppressor protein has been found in porokeratosis (112). The epidermis overlying the central portion of a lesion of porokeratosis may be either flattened or normal in thickness or, rarely, acanthotic. A nonspecific perivascular infiltrate of chronic inflammatory cells is present in the dermis.

Pathogenesis. The presence of a clone of abnormal epidermal cells located at the base of the parakeratotic column explains the lesions of porokeratosis. As a result of a gradual centrifugal movement of this clone, the furrow is slanted, its apex pointing away from the center of the lesion (111).

Electron microscopic examination reveals that, in the epidermis beneath the parakeratotic column, many keratinocytes show signs of degeneration. They show a pyknotic nucleus, large perinuclear vacuoles that are separated from one another by cytoplasmic strands, and condensation of tonofilaments at their periphery (113). At the base of the parakeratotic column, dyskeratotic cells composed of nuclear remnants and aggregated tonofilaments are seen (114). The parakeratotic column is composed chiefly of cells with a pyknotic nucleus and a cytoplasm possessing high electron density because of the presence of many par-

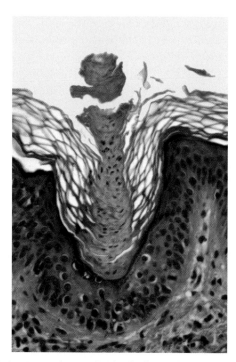

FIGURE 6-11. Porokeratosis of Mibelli. Stacked parakeratosis in an area of delled epidermis. The underlying granular cell layer is diminished to absent (original magnification × 200).

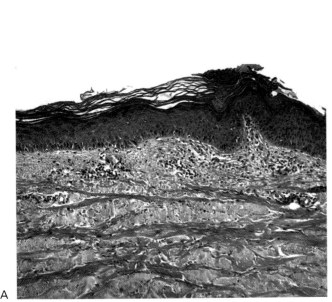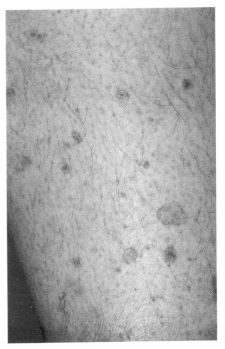

A   B

FIGURE 6-12. Disseminated actinic porokeratosis. **A:** Numerous pink-brown thin plaques on the leg, with a characteristic raised peripheral rim. (Photograph by William K. Witmer.) **B:** A parakeratotic column arises that is quite superficially located. Overlying an effaced epidermis, a lymphocytic infiltrate is seen in the dermis; × 45.

tially degraded organelles. In addition, a few dyskeratotic cells are present (114).

Differential Diagnosis. Even though cornoid lamellation is a typical finding for porokeratosis, it is found in a variety of other conditions (115), especially in verruca vulgaris and solar keratosis. A histologic distinction of punctate porokeratosis from plantar or palmar warts may be impossible, and clinical data, such as age of onset, inheritance, and number and size of lesions may be needed. For discussion of porokeratotic eccrine duct nevus, see section on nevus comedonicus.

XERODERMA PIGMENTOSUM

In xeroderma pigmentosum, an autosomal recessive disorder, excessive solar damage to the skin develops at an early age. Consequently, the lesions occur chiefly in areas of the skin habitually exposed to sunlight. Three stages are recognized. In the first stage, which usually starts when the child is 1 or 2 years old, slight diffuse erythema is associated with scaling and small areas of hyperpigmentation resembling freckles. In the second stage, atrophy of the skin, mottled pigmentation, and telangiectases give the skin an appearance similar to that of a chronic radiodermatitis. Solar keratoses arise in areas of scaling. In the third stage, which usually starts in adolescence but sometimes much earlier in the patient's life, various types of malignant tumors of the

skin appear, often causing death. They include squamous cell carcinoma, basal cell epithelioma, and, rarely, fibrosarcoma. In about 3% of patients with xeroderma pigmentosum, malignant melanomas arise. In some patients, they show no tendency to metastasize but in others they metastasize rapidly (116). Multiple malignant melanomas have been observed (117). The eyes also are affected, showing conjunctivitis and often keratitis with corneal opacities.

A very rare form of xeroderma pigmentosum is the *De Sanctis–Cacchione syndrome,* which in addition to severe skin lesions shows neurologic manifestations, especially microcephaly, retarded growth, and cerebellar ataxia (118).

Histopathology. In the first stage, the histopathologic appearance is not specific, but the diagnosis is suggested by a combination of changes that normally are not seen in the skin of young persons. They are hyperkeratosis, thinning of the stratum malpighii with atrophy of some of the rete ridges and elongation of others, a chronic inflammatory infiltrate in the upper dermis, and irregular accumulations of melanin in the basal cell layer, with or without an increase in the number of melanocytes.

In the second stage, the hyperkeratosis and irregular hyperpigmentation already present in the first stage are more pronounced. The epidermis shows atrophy in some areas and acanthosis in others. There may be disorder in the arrangement of the epidermal nuclei, and in some areas the epidermis may show atypical downward growth, so that the histologic picture in such areas is identical with that of solar keratosis. The upper dermis shows basophilic degeneration of the collagen and solar elastosis, as also is seen in solar degeneration.

In the third, or tumor, stage, histologic evidence of the various malignant tumors mentioned earlier is found.

Pathogenesis. In patients with xeroderma pigmentosum (with the exception of those who have the so-called XP variant; see below), skin cells in tissue culture show a decrease in their ability to repair the damage induced by sunlight to their DNA. This repair is brought about by *excision repair*, a system whereby damaged single-strand regions of DNA are excised and replaced with new sequences of bases (119). The reason for the inadequate excision repair is that the DNA-endonuclease that initiates the excision process is deficient. *In vitro* testing of skin fibroblasts from different patients with xeroderma pigmentosum shows considerable variation in the excision defect, the extent of repair replication varying between 0% and 90% of normal. Affected siblings are usually similar to each other in degree of repair replication. However, no correlation exists between the level of repair replication and the severity of clinical symptoms (120).

There are at least five patients known in whom excision repair is normal but the cells are defective in a DNA repair mode referred to as postreplication repair. This represents the so-called XP variant form. In cells of this variant form, the rate of conversion from low- to high-molecular-weight DNA is defective (121). Mutated genes in this condition include XP(A-G) and h RAD 30 with affected protein function complementation group A-G and DAN polymerase (122).

Electron microscopic examination of the epidermis has revealed in pigmented areas marked pleomorphism and a definite increase in the number of melanosomes. In some cases, very large melanosomes, referred to as giant melanosomes, are present in both melanocytes and keratinocytes (123). Even epidermis that is protected from light and shows no clinical abnormalities exhibits significant cellular alterations.

ECTODERMAL DYSPLASIA

The ectodermal dysplasias share abnormalities of the hair, nails, teeth, and sweat glands. Additionally other abnormalities including mental retardation are described. Over 170 different clinical conditions have been reported as ectodermal dysplasias, many of which have clinical overlap. For the purpose of simplification, we will discuss *hidrotic* and *anhidrotic* (now called hypohidrotic) forms (124).

The *hidrotic* form, which has an autosomal dominant inheritance, is primarily a disorder of keratinization and is characterized by hypotrichosis, dystrophic nails, and palmoplantar hyperkeratosis. It is sometimes associated with dental hypoplasia (125). The degree of alopecia varies from

slight to total (128). A mutated gene gap junction protein beta-b (GJB6) on chromosome 13q12, which encodes connexin 30, has been described (126).

The *anhidrotic* (hypohidrotic) form is an X-linked recessive disorder (the mutated gene LEDA affects ectodysplasia (127) and is localized to Xq12-q13.1), occurring in its full expression only in males. Females, as heterozygotes, may be mildly affected, with reduced sweating and faulty dentition. Males affected with anhidrotic ectodermal dysplasia show the tetrad of anhidrosis or hypohidrosis, hypotrichosis, dental hypoplasia, and a characteristic facies (129) (Fig. 6-13). Frequently, there is also dystrophy of the nails (129). The greatly reduced or absent function of the eccrine glands results in intolerance to heat. The face shows prominent frontal bosses and a depressed nasal bridge (Fig. 6-14). In addition, the mucous glands of the mouth and respiratory tract may be absent (131). The lack of mammary glands and nipples has been noted (130).

Histopathology. Both the hidrotic and the anhidrotic forms show hypoplasia of the hair and the sebaceous glands, with a decrease in their number, size, and degree of maturation (125,130).

In the anhidrotic form, there is, in addition, either a total absence or severe hypoplasia of the eccrine glands. In the case of hypoplasia, eccrine glands are present in only a few areas, especially the axillae and palms, but even in these areas, they are sparse and poorly developed. The secretory cells may be small and flat, so that they resemble endothelial rather than epithelial cells, and the excretory ducts may be composed of a single instead of a double layer of epithelial cells (132). The apocrine glands of the axillae are present in some patients with the anhidrotic form; in others, these glands are hypoplastic and cannot be distinguished

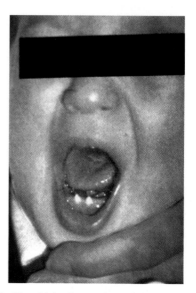

FIGURE 6-13. Hypohidrotic ectodermal dysplasia. Characteristic pegged teeth.

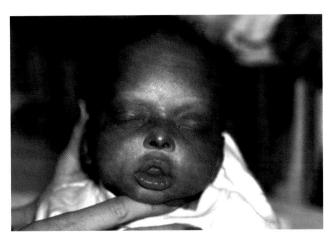

FIGURE 6-14. Hypohidrotic ectodermal dysplasia. In addition to frontal bossing and a flat nasal bridge, this infant demonstrates hyperpigmentation of the eyelids and surrounding skin, as well as patulous lips.

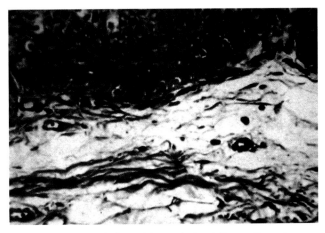

FIGURE 6-15. Focal dermal hypoplasia. Adipose tissue is present very near the epidermis, separated from it by only a few collagen fibers (original magnification × 200).

from hypoplastic eccrine glands; in others, both eccrine and apocrine glands are absent.

Focal Dermal Hypoplasia Syndrome

The focal dermal hypoplasia syndrome, or Goltz's syndrome, is probably due to an X-linked dominant gene lethal in homozygous males. Therefore, the syndrome occurs largely in females. Its occasional occurrence in males may be the result of a new mutation (133). The mode of inheritance thus is similar to that of incontinentia pigmenti.

The cutaneous manifestations of the focal dermal hyperplasia syndrome include widely distributed linear areas of hypoplasia of the skin resembling striae distensae; soft, yellow nodules, often in linear arrangement; and large ulcers due to congenital absence of skin that gradually heal with atrophy. One must remember that there are varied presentations of this syndrome (134). Frequent additional abnormalities include lack of a digit, which may be associated with syndactyly and which results in the very characteristic "lobster-claw deformity"; colobomata of the eyes, microphthalmia, or agenesis of an eye (135); and hypoplasia of hair, nails, or teeth (136). The presence of fine, parallel, vertical striations in the metaphysis of the long bones on radiography, referred to as osteopathia striata, is a reliable diagnostic marker of Goltz's syndrome (137).

Histopathology. The linear areas of hypoplasia of the skin show a marked diminution in the thickness of the dermis, the collagen being present as thin fibers not united into bundles (137). The soft, yellow nodules represent accumulations of fat that largely replace the dermis, so that the subcutaneous fat extends upward to the epidermis in some areas (136–138) (Fig. 6-15). Thin fibers of collagen and even some bundles of collagen resembling

those of normal dermis may be located between the subepidermal adipose tissue and the subcutaneous fat (137).

Pathogenesis. Electron microscopic examination shows, in addition to collagen fibrils 70 nm or more in diameter, many fine filamentous structures measuring 5 to 70 nm in diameter. There are two types of fat cells, one unilocular and the other multilocular, the latter representing young lipocytes (139).

Differential Diagnosis. Fat cells are seen in the dermis in the nevus lipomatosus of Hoffmann and Zurhelle as well, but the extreme attenuation of the collagen that occurs in some areas of the skin in patients with focal dermal hypoplasia syndrome is not seen in nevus lipomatosus. Several females with deletions of the distal short arm of X(Xp22.3–p22.2) have recently been described who have overlapping features of this syndrome.

APLASIA CUTIS CONGENITA

Aplasia cutis congenita consists of a localized absence of skin at the time of birth (Fig. 6-16). Most commonly, one observes a single ulcer or several ulcers on the scalp that measure only 1 to 3 cm in diameter and heal uneventfully. In some instances, intrauterine healing has occurred. Occasionally, large defects of the skin are present, but even then, as a rule, healing takes place within several months (140,141). The condition includes a diverse group of disorders in which localized absence of skin occurs alone or in association with a wide variety of abnormalities (142).

Histopathology. Ulcers extend through the entire thickness of the dermis, exposing the subcutaneous fat (143). Healed areas show, besides a flattened epidermis, fibrosis in the dermis and complete absence of adnexal structures (140).

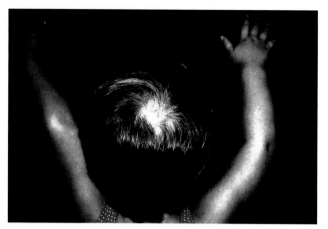

FIGURE 6-16. Aplasia cutis congenita. Two areas of congenitally absent skin (scarred and hairless).

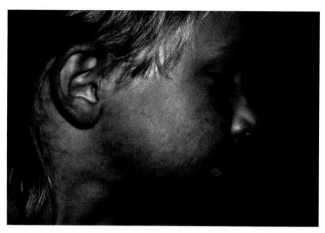

FIGURE 6-18. Poikiloderma congenitale. Older child with poikilodermatous changes of the cheek and ear.

Differential Diagnosis. Aplasia cutis should not be confused with congenital absence of the skin, where only epidermis is absent. This is a variant of epidermolysis bullosa (Bart's syndrome) (144).

POIKILODERMA CONGENITALE (ROTHMUND–THOMSON SYNDROME)

Poikiloderma congenitale is inherited in an autosomal recessive pattern due to mutations in the DNA helicase gene RECQLA on gene map locus 8q24.3 (145). It begins a few months after birth with erythema on the face (Fig. 6-17), and subsequently extends to the dorsa of the hands and feet and occasionally also to the arms, legs, and buttocks. Later

on, slight atrophy develops with telangiectases and mottled hyper- and hypo-pigmentation, so that the appearance is that of poikiloderma atrophicans vasculare (Fig. 6-18). Exposure to light aggravates the lesions. Most patients show dwarfism and hypogonadism. In about 40% of the patients, cataracts develop between ages 4 and 7 (146). Recent evidence suggests that children with this syndrome have a reduced DNA repair capacity (147).

Histopathology. During the early phase occurring in infancy and early childhood, there is hydropic degeneration of the basal layer leading to "pigment incontinence" with presence of melanophages in the upper dermis (130). A mild chronic inflammatory infiltrate is intermingled with the melanophages and may show a bandlike arrangement close to the flattened epidermis (146) (Fig. 6-19). The histologic changes thus may be identical with those seen in the early stage of poikiloderma atrophicans vasculare. In

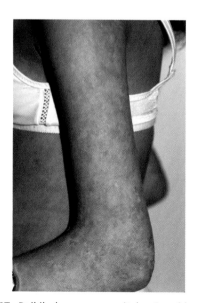

FIGURE 6-17. Poikiloderma congenitale. An older child with poikiloderma, atrophy, and hyperpigmentation.

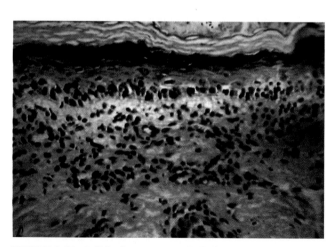

FIGURE 6-19. Poikiloderma congenitale (Rothman–Thompson), early. This section from a young child shows flattening of the epidermis, hydropic degeneration of the basal layer, and a bandlike inflammatory infiltrate in the upper dermis (original magnification × 200).

later childhood and adult life, the epidermis is flattened, and dilated capillaries as well as melanophages are present in the upper dermis, but there is no longer any inflammatory infiltrate.

Bloom's Syndrome (Congenital Telangiectatic Erythema)

Bloom's syndrome, with autosomal recessive inheritance due to mutations in the gene encoding DNA helicase RecQ protein like-2 on gene map locus 15q26.1 (149) resembles poikiloderma congenitale by showing (a) telangiectatic erythema of the face starting in infancy and often extending to the forearms and hands, (b) sensitivity to sunlight, (c) café au lait macules in over 50% of patients (150), and (d) growth retardation (Fig. 6-20). It differs from poikiloderma congenitale by (a) the lack of netlike hyper- and hypo-pigmentation (151); (b) the absence of hypogonadism (testicular atrophy and sterility are common in male patients) and cataracts; (c) the occasional presence of immunoglobulin deficiencies, especially of IgA and IgM (152,153); (d) a high incidence of nonspecific chromosomal breakage (152) and a great increase in the frequency of another type of chromosome instability, sister chromatid exchanges (154); and (e) an increased risk for malignant disease, especially leukemia, lymphoma, and carcinoma of the alimentary tract (155).

Histopathology. The epidermis is flattened and may show hydropic degeneration of the basal cell layer (154). There is dilatation of the capillaries in the upper dermis, which may be associated with a perivascular mononuclear infiltrate (150–154); however, there may be absence of any infiltrate (151).

Pathogenesis. Bloom's syndrome shows impairment of both cellular and humoral immunity, although this is not as pronounced as in ataxia-telangiectasia (see below). Evidence of impaired cellular immunity is the occasional absence of delayed hypersensitivity reactions (153) and the tendency toward development of malignant disease. Evidence of impaired humoral immunity is the occasional presence of immunoglobulin deficiencies. However, in contrast to ataxia-telangiectasia, susceptibility to infections is not pronounced.

Differential Diagnosis. Pigmentary incontinence is not pronounced in Bloom's syndrome, as it is in poikiloderma congenitale. The presence of hydropic degeneration of the basal cell layer and of a perivascular infiltrate may cause difficulties in differentiation from lupus erythematosus. However, no linear deposits of immunoglobulin are seen at the dermal-epidermal junction in Bloom's syndrome (154).

ATAXIA-TELANGIECTASIA

Ataxia-telangiectasia is transmitted in an autosomal recessive mode. The ataxia is evident already in infancy, whereas the telangiectases do not appear until childhood. They usually appear first on the bulbar conjunctivae, with subsequent extension to the cheeks, ears, and neck, and often also to other areas, such as the buttocks and extremities. A marked susceptibility to infections, particularly sinopulmonary infections, exists. Death from chronic respiratory infection or lymphoma-leukemia is common in the second or third decade of life (156).

Histopathology. The upper dermis shows numerous markedly dilated vessels that belong to the subpapillary venous plexus (157).

Pathogenesis. All patients have severe defects in both humoral and cellular immunity. In approximately 75% of the patients there is an absence or extreme deficiency of the serum IgA, and in about 80% a great IgE deficiency (158). Autopsies have established maldevelopment of the thymus as an integral part of ataxia-telangiectasia (159). Increased number of T cells with gamma/delta chains in the T-cell receptors rather than alpha/beta chains may produce defects in immunity (160). Chromosomal breakage is common, but there is no increased rate of sister chromatid exchanges (157). Mutations at the ATM gene that affect protein kinase have been mapped to gene locus 11q22.3 (161).

PROGERIA OF THE ADULT (WERNER'S SYNDROME)

Werner's syndrome, which has an autosomal recessive mode of inheritance, does not manifest itself until the second or third decade of life. The subcutaneous fat and the musculature of the extremities undergo atrophy, so that the

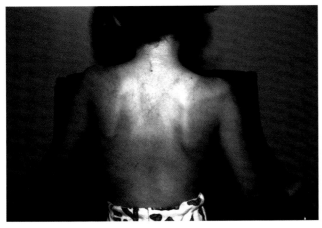

FIGURE 6-20. Bloom's syndrome. Erythema of the shoulders with photodistributed skin changes on the back.

patient exhibits thin arms and legs. The skin of the extremities gradually becomes taut, and ulcers may develop on the legs. As signs of premature senility, patients show graying of the hair, cataracts, and atherosclerosis in early adult life. Diabetes of the late-onset type (162) and hypogonadism due to interstitial fibrosis of the testes (163) are common. Death usually occurs in the fifth decade of life because of atherosclerosis.

Histopathology. On the arms and legs, where the skin is taut, the epidermis is thin and devoid of rete ridges, and the dermis shows fibrosis with or without hyalinization of the collagen. The pilosebaceous structures degenerate. The subcutaneous fatty tissue is largely replaced by newly synthesized, hyalinized collagen that merges with the collagen of the overlying dermis (164).

Pathogenesis. Poor growth and decreased life span of cultured skin fibroblasts have been found (165). The cause is due to mutation in the RECQL2 gene, which encodes a homolog of the E coli RecQDNA helicase on gene map locus 8p12–11.2 (149).

Differential Diagnosis. Differentiation from a late lesion of scleroderma may be difficult, because fibrosis and hyalinization of the collagen are seen also in scleroderma (162). In its late stage, scleroderma may also show no inflammatory infiltrate, so that differentiation has to be made on the basis of the patient's history and clinical manifestations.

EPIDERMOLYSIS BULLOSA

On the basis of clinical, histologic, and electron microscopic findings, three groups of epidermolysis bullosa (EB) are recognized: epidermal, junctional, and dermal (Table 6-1).

In all types of EB, the blisters form as a result of minor trauma. Because of great differences in prognoses, identification of the type of EB is often very important. In families with the potential of having an infant born with one of the frequently or potentially fatal forms of EB, such as *EB letalis* (Fig. 6-21) or generalized *EB dystrophica-recessive* (Fig. 6-

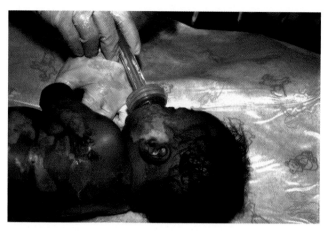

FIGURE 6-21. Junctional epidermolysis bullosa. Erosions of the face, arm, and trunk.

22), a prenatal biopsy at 18 to 20 weeks of gestation is recommended. On electron microscopy, EB letalis shows abnormalities of the hemidesmosomes while generalized EB dystrophica-recessive shows absence of anchoring fibrils.

There is more variability in the clinical course in some forms of EB than was previously appreciated (166). For example, within the epidermal type of EB, which usually has a good prognosis, some cases of *EB herpetiformis*, which is known also as the Dowling–Meara variant, may show generalized blistering that at times is associated with mortality during early infancy (167) (Fig. 6-23). Also, the junctional form of EB can result in scarring as *cicatricial junctional EB* (168). Occasionally dermal EB may be transient and heal within a few months (169,170). It is likely that the majority of cases published as Bart's syndrome, which was originally described as congenital absence of the skin (171), belong in this group 172,173).

Histopathology. If a fresh blister is available, a specimen for biopsy may be taken from its edge. However, it is advisable to carry out a biopsy also on an induced blister because it will show a blister free of secondary changes. In an

TABLE 6-1. COMPARISON OF THE CLINICAL FEATURES AND PROGNOSIS IN EPIDERMOLYSIS BULLOSA

Type	Epidermolysis bullosa	Distribution	Inheritance	Oral	Scarring	Prognosis
Epidermal	EB simplex	Generalized	Dominant	+	−	Good
	EB Cockayne	Feet, hands	Dominant	−	−	Good
	EB Dowling–Meara (Herpetiform)	Generalized	Dominant	+	Atrophy	Improves by school age
Junctional	EB letalis	Generalized	Recessive	+	−	Usually fatal
	EB benign	Generalized	Recessive	+/−	Atrophy	Good
Dermal	EB dystr-dom	Extremities	Dominant	+/−	+	Good
	EB dystr-rec	Generalized	Recessive	++	+++	Poor
	EB dystr-rec	Localized	Recessive	+	+	Good
	EB dystr-inversa	Mainly trunk	Recessive	+	+, late	Good
	EB acquisita	Generalized	—	+	+	Good

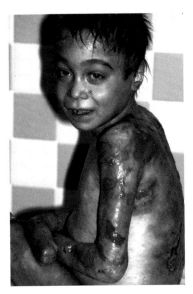

FIGURE 6-22. Recessive dystrophic epidermolysis bullosa. Child with mitten deformity of hands, as well as generalized blisters and scarring.

existing blister the location of the blister may have changed as the result of regeneration of keratinocytes at the base of the blister or degeneration of the keratinocytes over the blister. The mode of artificially producing a blister depends on the degree of vulnerability of the skin, but in most instances gentle friction with a cotton swab or a pencil eraser is used. The preferred type of biopsy is either a shave or an ellipse. The use of a punch is not recommended because the applied torsion will frequently cause total separation and even loss of the epidermis (174).

Even though electron microscopic examination (discussed below) is informative, the light microscopic features seen in the various forms of EB are of diagnostic value.

In *epidermal EB*, which includes EB simplex, EB of feet and hands of Weber and Cockayne (175), and EB herpeti-

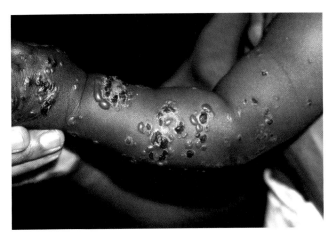

FIGURE 6-23. Epidermal epidermolysis bullosa. Herpetiform blistering on the leg.

formis (Dowling–Meara) (176,177), the primary separation in experimentally induced blisters always occurs within the basal cell layer. Spontaneously arising blisters may be found subepidermally as the result of complete disintegration of the basal cell layer; in bullae of more than one day's duration the cleavage may be found intraepidermally or subcorneally as a result of epidermal regeneration (175). In sections stained with the PAS technique, the PAS–positive basement membrane zone is located on the dermal side of the blister (178).

In *junctional EB,* the trauma of having a specimen taken for biopsy generally is sufficient to induce separation. This separation is located between the epidermis and the dermis, with the PAS–positive basement membrane zone usually remaining with the dermis (179). Autopsy has revealed, in some cases of EB letalis, extensive subepithelial separation also in the gastrointestinal, respiratory, and urinary tracts (179,180). There are no morphologic or enzymatic abnormalities to distinguish the atrophic benign form of junctional EB from EB letalis (182).

In *EB dystrophica-dominant* and *EB dystrophica-recessive,* light microscopy shows dermal–epidermal separation. A PAS stain is of little help in ascertaining the exact level of cleavage because the PAS–positive basement membrane zone often appears hazy (179). If recognizable, it is seen in contact with the detached epidermis or it appears split. In EB dystrophica-dominant, scarring is mild, but in generalized EB dystrophica-recessive, extensive erosions may occur, resulting in ulcerations and severe scarring. Severe oral involvement can lead to esophageal stenoses (183). In especially severe cases, death may occur. The ulcers and scars of the skin, mouth, and esophagus may give rise to squamous cell carcinomas, which tend to metastasize (184).

EB acquisita is not a genodermatosis but an autoimmune disorder.

Pathogenesis. If possible, all specimens of artificially induced blisters should be subjected to electron microscopic examination and immunofluorescence mapping (179). The latter procedure consists of exposing cryostat sections to specific antisera against type IV collagen (localized in the lamina densa or basal lamina), against laminin (localized in the lower portion of the lamina lucida), and against bullous pemphigoid antigen (localized in the upper portion of the lamina lucida in the vicinity of the hemidesmosomes). For the latter test, bullous pemphigoid antibodies contained in many bullous pemphigoid sera are used.

In the epidermal types of EB, electron microscopic examination shows that cleavage is the result of degenerative cytolytic changes occurring in the lower portion of the basal cells between the dermal–epidermal junction and the nucleus (EM 4). Immunofluorescence mapping shows all three antigens (type IV collagen, laminin, bullous pemphigoid antigen) to be located beneath the cleavage. Studies in several families with the Dowling–Meara form of epidermolysis bullosa revealed point mutations of keratin genes for KRT5 and KRT14 on chromosome 12 and 17, respectively (185). Various mutations in the KRT5 gene can lead to Koebner type of EBS or the Weber–Cockayne type.

In the junctional types of EB electron microscopic examination often shows the hemidesmosomes to be abnormal, especially in EB letalis. They may be reduced in size or number, and may lack their sub-basal cell-dense plaque (186). There are, however, exceptions. In one fatal case of EB letalis, the hemidesmosomes were structurally and numerically normal. Also, one patient with nonlethal junctional EB showed similar abnormalities of the hemidesmosomes as seen in the majority of patients in the lethal group (187). It is possible that the abnormalities of the hemidesmosomes are a secondary phenomenon, and that the basic cause of the junctional types of EB is a biochemical disorder of a lamina lucida constituent. In favor of this theory is the fact that normal skin shows separation at the dermal–epidermal junction when cultured with blister fluid of patients with EB letalis (188). Immunofluorescence mapping shows type IV collagen and laminin on the floor of the blister; bullous pemphigoid antigen is present mainly on the blister roof, but also in a more spotty distribution and to a much lesser extent on the blister floor (179). Mutations have been found in any of three polypeptides of laminin-5: alpha-3(LAMA 3); beta 3 (LAMB 3); and gamma-2 (LAMC2). The gene is responsible for encoding a portion of Laminin 5. This mutation may have significance in reducing adhesion between the epidermis and dermis (189). A newly found mutation of the gene encoding beta$_4$ integrin has been found in the subset of EB letalis with pyloric atresia (190).

The dermal types of EB, on electron microscopy, show abnormalities in regard to their anchoring fibrils. Generalized recessive dystrophic EB shows absence of the anchoring fibrils even in nonlesional unscarred skin. On the other hand, in both dominant dystrophic EB and localized recessive dystrophic EB, structurally normal anchoring fibrils are present but in significantly reduced number (191). The complete absence of anchoring fibrils in generalized recessive dystrophic EB could be established through the lack of a reaction with monoclonal antibodies to anchoring fibrils (192). Because type VII collagen is a major structural component of the anchoring fibrils, immunofluorescence staining with polyclonal antibodies to type VII collagen reveals complete absence of staining, even in the unaffected skin of patients with severe dystrophic recessive EB (193). Similarly, there was no reaction with periodic acid-thiosemicarbazide-silver proteinate, which stains anchoring fibrils selectively (194). Mutations in the gene encoding type VII collagen (COL 7A1) located at chromosome band 3p21 has been reported to cause these abnormal findings in the dystrophic forms of epidermolysis bullosa (195,196). Immunofluorescence mapping shows all three basement membrane zone constituents—bullous pemphigoid anti-

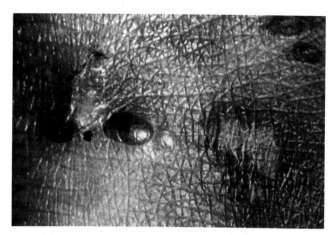

FIGURE 6-24. Epidermolysis bullosa acquisita. A blister surrounded by two scars.

gen, laminin, and type IV collagen—on top of the cleavage (179).

Epidermolysis Bullosa Acquisita

EB acquisita starts in childhood or adult life (196) with blisters at sites of trauma resulting in atrophic scars which in some cases are not pronounced (Figs. 6-24 and 6-25). Milia may not appear until the disorder has been present for many years. Oral lesions are seen occasionally. A significant proportion of patients with EB acquisita have circulating IgG antibodies (198).

Histopathology. The bullae are located beneath the epidermis and thus are indistinguishable in their location from those seen in bullous pemphigoid. The prevalence of eosinophils in the infiltrate of bullous pemphigoid often helps in distinguishing the two diseases. However, because the findings by light microscopic immunofluorescence are identical in the two diseases, patients with EB acquisita

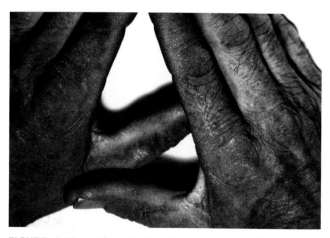

FIGURE 6-25. Epidermolysis bullosa acquisita. Blistering and scarring on backs of hands.

have been misdiagnosed frequently as having bullous pemphigoid before the recognition of the different location of the respective antibodies on immunoelectron microscopy. "Salt-split" skin combined with immunofluorescence has proven to be an aid in distinguishing EBA from BP. The early studies demonstrated EB acquisita antibodies on the dermal side (floor) of the salt split skin and BP antibodies on the epidermal side (roof) (199,200). Later studies have found BP as well as EB acquisita antibodies on the floor of the salt split (201). In spite of these latter studies, this technique still has value in differentiating these two conditions.

Histogenesis. Since EB acquisita on direct immunofluorescence shows subepidermal deposits of IgG and C3, and on indirect immunofluorescence often shows circulating antibodies against IgG, a misdiagnosis of bullous pemphigoid has been made in some cases (202), or in the case of pronounced scarring, a misdiagnosis of cicatricial pemphigoid (203). Immunoelectron microscopy, however, has shown a different location of the IgG deposits in these two disease groups: in bullous pemphigoid and cicatricial pemphigoid they are located in the lamina lucida (204); in EB acquisita they are found in the upper dermis just beneath or contiguous to the lamina densa (198). Similarly, whereas type IV collagen and laminin are located at the floor of the blister in bullous pemphigoid, they are seen on the roof of the blister in EB acquisita. Because antibody to human type IV collagen functions also in formalin fixed, paraffin embedded tissue sections, standard immunoperoxidase methods have revealed type IV collagen to be associated with the blister roof in EB acquisita and with the blister base in bullous pemphigoid and cicatricial pemphigoid (205).

FAMILIAL BENIGN PEMPHIGUS (HAILEY–HAILEY DISEASE)

Familial benign pemphigus is inherited as an autosomal dominant trait, with a family history obtainable in about two-thirds of the patients. Genetic studies have localized the gene on chromosome 3q (206), specifically 3q21-q24, the area responsible for ATP dependent calcium transport (207). It is characterized by a localized, recurrent eruption of small vesicles on an erythematous base. By peripheral extension, the lesions may assume a circinate configuration. The sites of predilection are the intertriginous areas, especially the axillae and the groin. Only very few instances of mucosal lesions have been reported, of the mouth (208,209), the labia majora (209), and the esophagus (210).

Histopathology. Although, as in *Darier's disease*, early lesions may show small suprabasal separations, so called lacunae, fully developed lesions show large separations, that is, vesicles and even bullae, in a predominantly suprabasal position (Fig. 6-26). Villi, which are elongated papillae lined

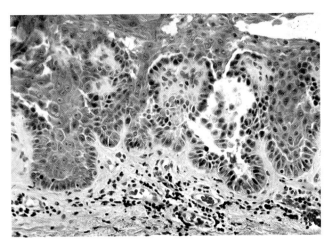

FIGURE 6-26. Familial benign pemphigus (Hailey–Hailey). The bulla is largely in a suprabasal position. The extensive loss of intercellular bridges with partial coherence of cells gives the detached epidermis the appearance of a dilapidated brick wall. On the right side within the granular layer, a corps rond can be seen (original magnification × 40).

by a single layer of basal cells, protrude upward into the bulla, and, in some cases, narrow strands of epidermal cells proliferate downward into the dermis. Many cells of the detached stratum malpighii show loss of their intercellular bridges, so that acantholysis affects large portions of the epidermis. Individual cells and groups of cells usually are seen in large numbers in the bulla cavity. In spite of the extensive loss of intercellular bridges, the cells of the detached epidermis in many places show only slight separation from one another because a few intact intercellular bridges still hold them loosely together. This quite typical feature gives the detached epidermis the appearance of a dilapidated brick wall.

Many of the cells of the stratum malpighii that have lost all or most of their intercellular bridges show a fairly normal cytoplasm and a normal nucleus in which mitotic activity has even been observed (211,212). Some of the acantholytic cells, however, have a homogenized cytoplasm, suggesting premature partial keratinization. In some instances, such acantholytic cells with premature keratinization resemble the grains of Darier's disease. Occasionally, a few corps ronds are present in the granular layer (Fig. 6-26) (211–213).

Differential Diagnosis. Histologically, familial benign pemphigus shares certain features with both Darier's disease and pemphigus vulgaris. In all three diseases, one finds predominantly suprabasal separation of the epidermis caused by acantholysis and resulting in lacunae or bullae and villi formation.

Differentiation of familial benign pemphigus from Darier's disease as a rule is not very difficult, because in Darier's disease, (a) the suprabasal separations usually are smaller, thus appearing as lacunae rather than as bullae; (b) acantholysis is less pronounced, being limited to the lower epidermis, especially the suprabasal region; and (c) dyskeratosis consisting of the formation of corps ronds and grains is much more evident.

Pemphigus vulgaris often resembles familial benign pemphigus to a striking degree, and, in some specimens, histologic differentiation of these two diseases may be impossible. As a rule, however, in pemphigus vulgaris there is less extensive acantholysis, limited largely to the suprabasal region, so that the detached epidermis appears normal and lacks the appearance of a dilapidated brick wall, and more severe degeneration of the acantholytic cells within and near the bulla cavity. The presence of eosinophils in the bulla points toward a diagnosis of pemphigus vulgaris, but their absence does not rule it out. In case of doubt, immunofluorescence will decide the issue.

There used to be much discussion as to whether familial benign pemphigus represents a vesicular variant of Darier's disease. Two points in favor of the basic unity of the two diseases were stressed: the alleged simultaneous presence of both diseases in the same patient, and the occurrence of corps ronds in both diseases. However, it has become apparent that patients described as having both diseases were either cases of Darier's disease with vesicular lesions (214) or cases of familial benign pemphigus with the presence of corps ronds (214,215). Evidence against a relationship is also the fact that, in affected families, always only one of the two diseases occurs.

KERATOSIS FOLLICULARIS (DARIER'S DISEASE)

Darier's disease is usually transmitted in an autosomal dominant pattern. It has been found to be due to mutations in the ATP2A2 gene on chromosome T2, which encodes the sarcoplasmic/endoplasmic reticulum calcium pump ATPase SERCA2. The gene is 12q23–24.1 (207). In typical cases, there is a more or less extensive, persistent, slowly progressive eruption consisting of hyperkeratotic or crusted papules often showing a follicular distribution. By coalescence, verrucous crusted areas may form. The so-called seborrheic areas are sites of predilection (Fig. 6–27A and B). The oral mucosa is involved occasionally (216). In some cases of Darier's disease, one finds on the dorsa of the hands and feet keratotic papules that resemble those seen in *acrokeratosis verruciformis of Hopf* (217).

Special clinical variants of keratosis follicularis are a hypertrophic type, a vesiculobullous type, and a linear or zosteriform type. In the hypertrophic type, widespread, markedly thickened, and hyperkeratotic lesions are seen, especially in the intertriginous areas (218). In the vesiculobullous type, vesicles and small bullae are seen in addition to papules (219,220). In the linear or zosteriform

type, usually limited to one side, there are either localized or widespread lesions that may be present at birth (221), but in most cases have arisen in infancy, childhood, or adult life (222). The question has been raised as to whether this type of lesion represents a linear epidermal nevus with acantholytic dyskeratosis rather than Darier's disease (221) and the designation *acantholytic dyskeratotic epidermal nevus* has been suggested (222). It is quite likely that some of the cases with scattered papular lesions of limited extent arising in adult life and diagnosed as acute, eruptive Darier's disease (223) or acute adult-onset Darier-like dermatosis in reality represented transient acantholytic dermatosis. A recent review on the clinical aspects of this condition has been written (224).

Histopathology. The characteristic changes in Darier's disease follow: (a) a peculiar form of dyskeratosis resulting in the formation of corps ronds and grains, (b) suprabasal acantholysis leading to the formation of suprabasal clefts or lacunae, and (c) irregular upward proliferation into the lacunae of papillae lined with a single layer of basal cells, or so-called villi (Fig. 6-27C). There are also papillomatosis, acanthosis, and hyperkeratosis. The dermis shows a chronic inflammatory infiltrate. In some cases, there is downward proliferation of epidermal cells into the dermis.

The corps ronds occur in the upper stratum malpighii, particularly in the granular and horny layers; grains are found in the horny layer and as acantholytic cells within the lacunae. Corps ronds possess a central homogeneous, basophilic, pyknotic nucleus that is surrounded by a clear halo. By virtue of size and the conspicuous halo, corps ronds stand out clearly (Fig. 6-28). Peripheral to the halo lies basophilic dyskeratotic material as a shell (225). The nonstaining halo in some instances is partially replaced by homogeneous, eosinophilic dyskeratotic material (226). Compared with the corps ronds, the grains are much less conspicuous. They resemble parakeratotic cells but are somewhat larger. The nuclei of grains are elongated and often grain-shaped, and are surrounded by homogeneous dyskeratotic material that usually stains basophilic but may stain eosinophilic. The lacunae represent small, slitlike intraepidermal vesicles most commonly located directly above the basal layer. They contain acantholytic cells and show premature partial keratinization. Because of shrinkage, some of them are elongated, and these then appear identical with the grains in the horny layer. The villi projecting into the lacunae may be quite tortuous, so that, on histologic examination, some of them appear in cross section as rounded dermal structures lined by a solitary row of basal cells (Fig. 6-27C).

Hyperkeratosis and papillomatosis may cause the formation of keratotic plugs, which often fill the pilosebaceous follicles but are found also outside of follicles. That Darier's disease is not exclusively a follicular disorder is also proved by the fact that areas devoid of follicles, such as palms, soles, and the oral mucosa, may be affected.

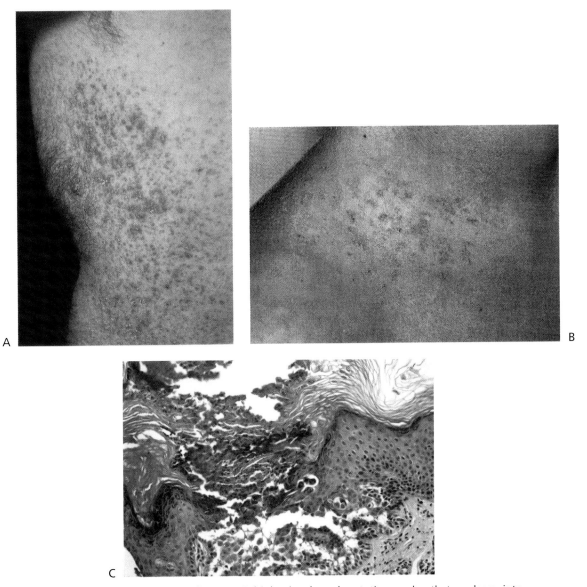

FIGURE 6-27. A: Darier's disease. Multiple tiny hyperkeratotic papules that coalesce into plaques present on the trunk. **B:** Crusted papules in a follicular distribution at the base of the neck and upper chest. **C:** Low magnification. Hyperkeratosis and papillomatosis are evident. Numerous lacunae (*L.*) are present. On the left are elongated papillae lined by a single layer of cells, so-called villi (*V.*). Corps ronds (*C.R.*) are present in the granular layer, and grains are seen in the horny layer. The lacunae contain desquamated cells (*C.*) (original magnification × 100).

In hypertrophic lesions of Darier's disease, one can occasionally observe considerable acanthosis, either as proliferations of basal cells or as pseudocarcinomatous hyperplasia. Proliferations of basal cells consist of long, narrow cords composed of two rows of basal cells separated by a narrow lacunar space (227).

The vesiculobullous lesions, which occur in rare instances, differ from lacunae merely in size; they contain numerous shrunken cells with the appearance of grains (219,220).

The keratotic papules that may occur on the dorsa of the hands and feet and that clinically resemble those seen in acrokeratosis verruciformis of Hopf in most instances, on serial sectioning show mild dyskeratotic changes and often suprabasal clefts as well (217). They are a manifestation of Darier's disease and not of acrokeratosis verruciformis.

The lesions on the oral mucosa are analogous in appearance to those observed on the skin and thus show lacunae and dyskeratosis, although definite well-formed corps ronds generally are absent (228).

The occasional reports of patients having both Darier's disease and familial benign pemphigus or a transition from one of these two diseases to the other are discussed in the differential diagnosis of familial benign pemphigus.

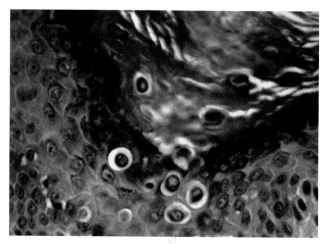

FIGURE 6-28. Darier's disease. Hyperkeratosis is present and corps ronds are in the thickened stratum corneum and epidermis. Suprabasalar acantholysis is present; × 400.

Pathogenesis. Whereas histologically a distinction between Darier's disease and familial benign pemphigus is generally possible, with dyskeratosis being the predominating factor in Darier's disease and acantholysis in familial benign pemphigus, this distinction is not as clearly evident in electron microscopic examination. The reason for this is that for electron microscopy only a small specimen can be processed, which in either of the two diseases shows predominantly acantholysis in some instances and dyskeratosis in others and only rarely shows both. In both diseases, however, acantholysis precedes dyskeratosis.

Acantholysis has been thought by some authors to be due to the loss of the intercellular contact layer within desmosomes, both in Darier's disease (229,230) and in familial benign pemphigus (231). The two halves of the desmosomes then pull apart, after which the tonofilaments become detached from them. Another group of authors believes that there is some basic defect in the tonofilament—desmosome complex in Darier's disease (226–232) and in familial benign pemphigus (233)—resulting in separating of tonofilaments from the attachment plaques of desmosomes and subsequently leading to the disappearance of desmosomes and thus to acantholysis. It is likely that both processes take place simultaneously in both Darier's disease (225) and familial benign pemphigus (234).

The cause for the acantholysis in Darier's disease and familial benign pemphigus is not yet definitely known. The faulty synthesis of the intercellular substance has long been suspected (235,236). It seems likely that mutations underlying Darier's disease and Hailey–Hailey disease would affect structural components but both disorders mapped to chromosome regions devoid of any known candidate gene. Further studies suggested that intercellular communication is crucial for epidermal differentiation. This was corroborated when mutations found in ATP2A2 caused Darier's

disease and disclosed a role for the SERCA2 pump in the calcium signaling pathway that regulates cell-to-cell adhesion and differentiation of the epidermis (237).

In association with the loss of desmosomes, excessive amounts of tonofilaments form within the keratinocytes around the nucleus as thick, electron-dense bundles. A defect of the tonofilaments would best explain the dyskeratotic features of both Darier's disease and familial benign pemphigus. In Darier's disease, in which the dyskeratosis is much more pronounced than in familial benign pemphigus, thick bundles of tonofilaments, often in association with large keratohyaline granules, form large aggregates of homogenized dyskeratotic material. The corps ronds, on electron microscopic examination, are characterized by extensive cytoplasmic vacuolization (238). They show in their center an irregularly shaped nucleus surrounded by a halo of autolyzed electron-lucid cytoplasm and at their periphery a shell of tonofilaments (EM 16) (225–229). The grains are seen on electron microscopic examination to consist of nuclear remnants surrounded by dyskeratotic bundles of tonofilaments.

In familial benign pemphigus, after loss of the desmosomes, excessive amounts of tonofilaments form within the keratinocytes and aggregate around the nucleus as thick, electron-dense bundles, often in a whorling configuration; however, even though dyskeratosis is present, it is less pronounced than in Darier's disease, and most of the keratinocytes keratinize normally, only very few becoming grains or corps ronds as the result of dyskeratotic degeneration.

On intralesional injection of tritiated thymidine, one group (239) observed labeling of many acantholytic keratinocytes in familial benign pemphigus but not in Darier's disease, suggesting to them that in familial benign pemphigus the epidermal cells participated in the renewal of the epidermis but did not do so in Darier's disease, probably because these cells were undergoing keratinization. However, another group (240) could not confirm this observation.

Differential Diagnosis. Although acantholytic dyskeratosis in association with corps ronds is highly characteristic of Darier's disease, it occurs also in several other conditions (241–243): in warty dyskeratoma, a solitary lesion with a deep central invagination; in transient or persistent acantholytic dermatosis, in which the lesions consist of discrete papules; in focal acantholytic dyskeratoma, manifesting itself as a solitary papule; and as an incidental small focus in a variety of unrelated lesions. Occasionally, a few corps ronds are seen also in familial benign pemphigus (see preceding text).

ACROKERATOSIS VERRUCIFORMIS OF HOPF

In acrokeratosis verruciformis, an autosomal dominant disorder, numerous flat, hyperkeratotic, occasionally verrucous papules are present on the distal part of the extremi-

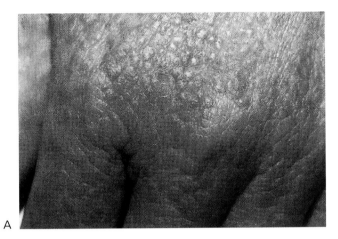

A

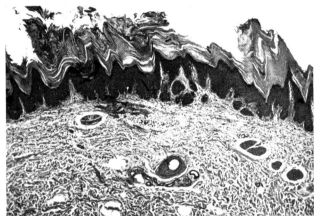

B

FIGURE 6-29. A: Acrokeratosis verruciformis of Hopf. Flat papules on back of hands. **B:** A well-circumscribed lesion shows hyperkeratosis and papillomatosis. The latter is associated with elevations of the epidermis resembling church spires (original magnification × 100).

ties, predominantly on the dorsa of the hands (Fig. 6-29A) and feet (244).

Histopathology. The papules show considerable hyperkeratosis, an increase in thickness of the granular layer, and acanthosis. In addition, there is slight papillomatosis, which is frequently but not always associated with circumscribed elevations of the epidermis resembling church spires (Fig. 6-29B) (245,246). The rete ridges are slightly elongated and extend to a uniform level.

Histogenesis. A possible relationship between acrokeratosis verruciformis and Darier's disease has been repeatedly discussed. On the one hand, there is no question that acrokeratosis verruciformis usually occurs as an independent entity, often in several family members (241) and occasionally even in many family members (247) but also as a solitary incidence (246). On the other hand, a relationship to Darier's disease is suggested by several observations:

- Patients with Darier's disease not infrequently show lesions that are indistinguishable from acrokeratosis

verruciformis both clinically and histologically (245–248).

- Some of the lesions of presumed acrokeratosis verruciformis occurring in patients with Darier's disease show dyskeratosis and lacunae as seen in Darier's disease, whereas others do not.
- Patients with apparent histologic lesions of acrokeratosis verruciformis may later develop histologic lesions of Darier's disease.

Admittedly, there can be considerable clinical resemblance between the acral lesions of both diseases, but, if multiple specimens for biopsy are taken and serial sections carried out, clear histologic evidence of Darier's disease is obtained only in those patients who have Darier's disease (249). It seems that there is only one instance in which both diseases were seen in different members of the same family (250), and this may well have been coincidence. Rather than taking the view that the two diseases result from a single dominant defect with variable expressivity (250), it is best to regard acrokeratosis verruciformis as an independent entity.

Differential Diagnosis. Although elevations of the epidermis with the configuration of church spires are quite typical of acrokeratosis verruciformis, they may be absent and are not specific for that disease. Particularly, they are present in the hyperkeratotic type of seborrheic keratosis. Even though seborrheic keratoses usually are larger than the lesions of acrokeratosis verruciformis, clinical data may be necessary for the differentiation of these two conditions. Also, acrokeratosis verruciformis may resemble verrucae clinically, but it differs from verruca plana by the absence of vacuolization in the cells of the upper epidermis and from verruca vulgaris by the absence of parakeratosis.

PSEUDOXANTHOMA ELASTICUM

In this disorder, genetically abnormal elastic fibers with a tendency toward calcification occur in the skin and frequently also in the retina and within the walls of arteries, particularly the gastric mucosal arteries, coronary arteries, and large peripheral arteries. The inheritance is usually autosomal recessive but is occasionally autosomal dominant. It seems that two recessive and two dominant forms exist (251). Struk predicts that allelic heterogeneity with different variants of a single disease gene residing on 16p13.1 accounts for both recessive and dominant forms of pseudoxanthoma elasticum (252). The classic disorder in this classification is recessive type 1. In the dominant type 1, the cutaneous and internal manifestations are more severe than in recessive type 1, whereas in dominant type 2 they are less severe. The very rare recessive type 2 shows only cutaneous involvement, which, however, is extensive (253).

The accuracy of the Pope classification has been disputed, leading to a new classification (254).

The cutaneous lesions usually appear first in the second or third decade of life and are generally progressive in extent and severity. They consist of soft, yellowish, coalescing papules, and the affected skin appears loose and wrinkled. The sides of the neck, the axillae, and the groin are the most common sites of lesions (Fig. 6-30). In the eyes, so-called angioid streaks of the fundi may cause progressive impairment of vision. Involvement of the arteries of the gastric mucosa may lead to gastric hemorrhage; involvement of coronary arteries may result in attacks of angina pectoris, although myocardial infarction is rare; involvement of the large peripheral arteries may cause intermittent claudication (255). Radiologic examination in such cases reveals extensive calcification of the affected peripheral arteries (256).

In rare instances, the coexistence of pseudoxanthoma elasticum with elastosis perforans serpiginosa has been reported, with perforation and transepidermal elimination present only in the lesions of elastosis perforans serpiginosa (257). Calcific elastosis, which has been referred to also as perforating pseudoxanthoma elasticum or localized acquired pseudoxanthoma elasticum, is not related to pseudoxanthoma elasticum. The absence of skin lesions should not be used to exclude pseudoxanthoma elasticum in patients with an inherited predisposition and suspicious manifestations, such as angioid streaks or gastric bleeding. In these patients, biopsies of scars or of flexural skin may show the characteristic changes of pseudoxanthoma elasticum in the deep dermis (254).

Histopathology. Histologic examination of the involved skin reveals in the middle and lower thirds of the dermis considerable accumulations of swollen and irregularly

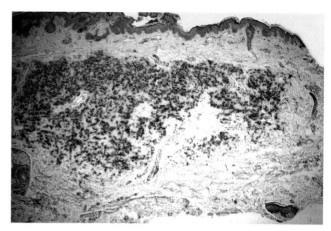

FIGURE 6-31. Pseudoxanthoma elasticum. Low magnification, H&E stained tissue showing calcified altered elastic fibers in the midreticular dermis (original magnification × 100).

clumped fibers staining like elastic fibers; that is, they stain deeply black with orcein or Verhoeff's stain (Figs. 6-31 and 6-32). Although normally elastic fibers do not stain with routine stains such as hematoxylin-eosin, the altered elastic fibers in pseudoxanthoma elasticum stain faintly basophilic because of their calcium imbibition. Staining for calcium with the von Kossa method also shows these fibers well. In the vicinity of the altered elastic fibers, there may be accumulations of a slightly basophilic mucoid material, which stains strongly positive with the colloidal iron reaction or with Alcian blue (258). The number of collagen bundles is reduced in such areas, and numerous reticulum fibers are seen on impregnation with silver (259). In some cases with pronounced elastic tissue calcification a macrophage and giant cell reaction may be present (260).

The angioid streaks occur in Bruch's membrane, which is located between the retina and the choroid and possesses numerous elastic fibers in its outer portion, the lamina

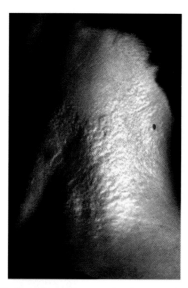

FIGURE 6-30. Pseudoxanthoma elasticum. Yellow coalescing papules at the side of neck.

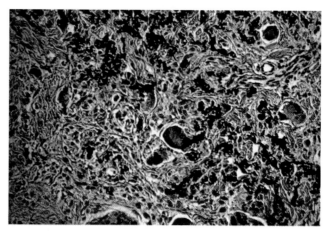

FIGURE 6-32. Pseudoxanthoma elasticum, high magnification, elastic tissue stain. The elastic fibers show marked degeneration (original magnification × 100).

elastica. Calcification of these fibers causes fissures to form in the lamina elastica. These fissures result in repeated hemorrhages and exudates, which in turn cause degenerative changes in the retina consisting of scar formation and pigment shifting (260,261).

Gastric bleeding is the result of calcification of elastic fibers in the thin-walled arteries located immediately beneath the gastric mucosa. The internal elastic lamina is particularly affected. In muscular arteries, such as the coronary arteries and the large peripheral arteries, calcification begins in the internal and external elastic laminae, leading to their fragmentation, and subsequently extends to the media and intima (255). Calcification of the elastic fibers in the endocardium is a common occurrence but is clinically silent (262).

Histogenesis. Electron microscopic examination shows that the calcification occurs in normal-appearing elastic fibers (259,262–265). In some patients, especially in young persons, only some of the elastic fibers in the lower dermis are calcified, and the calcification is variable in degree. In adult patients, however, most elastic fibers show considerable calcification and, as a result, degeneration. Early calcification of elastic fibers consists either of diffuse granular deposits throughout the elastic fiber or of dense aggregates that may be located in the center or near the margin of the fiber (EM 5). With progression of the calcification, the elastic fibers ultimately become fully calcified, showing marked swelling and bizarre distortions. In addition, heavy calcium deposits may be seen in the ground substance adjacent to elastic fibers and free in the ground substance. The presence of calcified material outside of elastic fibers can be explained by the disintegration of completely calcified elastic fibers (265).

Besides varying numbers of normal collagen fibrils, irregularly twisted collagen fibrils and granulofilamentous aggregates are present. It appears unlikely that the process of calcification begins in the granulofilamentous material, as maintained by some authors who regard this material as an abnormal precursor of elastic fibers (264–266). It is probable that this misinterpretation has resulted from the examination of advanced lesions containing disintegrated calcified elastic fibers within the granulofilamentous material (262). In favor of a primary location of the calcification within elastic fibers is the important observation that, in decalcified sections of endocardial lesions, the internal structure of the calcified segments of elastic fibers is very similar to that of the adjacent noncalcified segments.

Differential Diagnosis. Solar elastosis, like pseudoxanthoma elasticum, shows abnormal elastic tissue. However, in solar elastosis this material is located in the upper third of the dermis and is present as dense masses rather than as individual altered fibers. Furthermore, these dense masses always show negative staining for calcium. If associated with a perforation, calcific elastosis is easily distinguished from pseudoxanthoma elasticum. In the absence of a perforation the two are indistinguishable, and clinical data are necessary for differentiation.

CONNECTIVE TISSUE NEVUS

The connective tissue nevus represents a hamartoma in which the amount of collagen is increased, but the amount of elastic tissue may be increased, normal, or decreased. The lesions consist of slightly elevated, slightly indurated nodules that may be grouped together in one or several plaques or may be widely disseminated (Fig. 6-33). A connective tissue nevus can occur without alterations in other organs and without being genetically determined (267); without alterations in other organs, being inherited as an autosomal dominant trait (268); or with osteopoikilosis, being inherited in an autosomal dominant pattern (269). The shagreen patches of tuberous sclerosis do not strictly belong in the category of connective tissue nevi, since they always consist only of excessive amounts of collagen and thus are "collagen nevi" rather than connective tissue nevi (270).

Connective tissue nevi associated with osteopoikilosis are also referred to as *Buschke–Ollendorff syndrome*, because these authors first recognized the frequent simultaneous occurrence of these two types of lesions. The skin lesions in this syndrome consist of firm, pale papules and plaques in asymmetric distribution with a tendency to grouping (269–272). Individual members of affected families may have skin lesions without bone lesions, and vice versa. The bone lesions of osteopoikilosis are asymptomatic and, on x-ray examination, consist of round or oval densities 2 to 10 mm in diameter in the long bones and in the bones of the hands, feet, and pelvis.

Histopathology. A clear separation of collagenoma and elastoma is not always possible, because in many instances

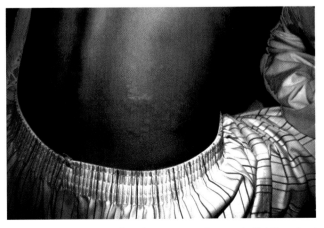

FIGURE 6-33. Connective tissue nevus. Grouped slightly raised nodules producing an irregular surface on the lower posterior chest.

both collagenous and elastic fibers are increased, as indicated by the fact that most lesions of connective tissue nevus feel firm to the touch. The increase in the amount of collagen may be difficult to ascertain if the collagen bundles are normal in appearance. In some lesions of collagenoma (268) and lesions of the connective tissue nevus–osteopoikilosis syndrome (279–272), the collagen bundles are thickened and homogenized.

Most cases of the connective tissue nevus–osteopoikilosis syndrome clearly show a marked increase in the amount of elastic fibers, which are present as broad, interfacing bands, without showing signs of degeneration (273,274) (Fig. 6-34).

Pathogenesis. On electron microscopic examination, connective tissue nevi show a variable picture. In some cases, the elastic fibers appear thick and are surrounded by a thready material (267). In the Buschke–Ollendorff syndrome (275), the elastic fibers lack their microfibrillar component so that only electron-lucent elastin is present (276).

Differential Diagnosis. Pseudoxanthoma elasticum is the major differential disease. The connective tissue nevus does not show elastic tissue fragmentation and calcification, as does pseudoxanthoma elasticum.

LINEAR MELORHEOSTOTIC SCLERODERMA

Melorheostosis is characterized by linear hyperostosis of an extremity. It may be associated with thickening and hypertrichosis of the overlying skin. Although not familial, its start in infancy suggests a congenital disorder (277).

Histopathology. The skin shows thickening of the dermis caused by the extension of normal-appearing collagen and elastic tissue in strands and lobules into the subcutaneous fat (278).

Pathogenesis. Hyperplasia of the skin is related to the underlying cortical hyperostosis. The normal appearance of the thickened dermis indicates that the process does not represent localized scleroderma (278).

WINCHESTER SYNDROME

A rare autosomal recessive disorder described only in the offspring of consanguineous parents, Winchester syndrome is characterized by dwarfism, small-joint destruction, corneal opacities, thickening and hypertrichosis of the skin, and hypertrophic lips and gingivae (279).

Histopathology. In the early stage, the skin shows proliferation of fibroblasts in the lower portions of the dermis with extension into the subcutaneous tissue. At a later stage, the collagen appears homogenized and contains only few fibroblasts (280). Some areas may show an increase in both the number of fibroblasts and the density of the collagen bundles (281).

Pathogenesis. An abnormal function of the fibroblasts is the likely cause for all manifestations. Electron microscopic examination has shown dilated and vacuolated mitochondria in the fibroblasts (280).

EHLERS–DANLOS SYNDROME

The Ehlers–Danlos syndrome (EDS) has been divided into more than ten types on the basis of clinical, genetic, and biochemical information (282). The common clinical features are hyperextensibility of the skin; fragility of the skin with impaired wound healing, resulting in the formation of atrophic scars; and hypermobility of the joints, which may lead to dislocations (Fig. 6-35). Occasionally, one observes at sites of traumatic hematomas raisin-like pseudotumors that are raised and soft and have a wrinkled surface. In

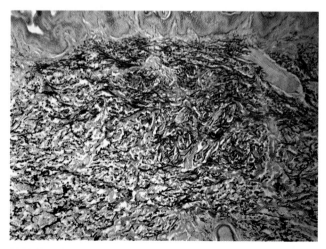

FIGURE 6-34. Connective tissue nevus. The elastic fibers are markedly increased in number and size without showing signs of degeneration (original magnification × 100).

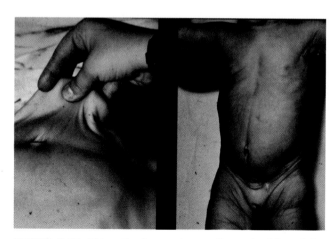

FIGURE 6-35. Ehlers–Danlos syndrome. Hyperelasticity of the skin.

some cases, firm, spheroid subcutaneous nodules form at sites of traumatic fat necrosis. Patients rarely live beyond the second decade of life because of ruptures of large arteries or of the gastrointestinal tract (283).

EDS types I, II, and III, the most common forms of this syndrome, are inherited in an autosomal dominant pattern and are distinguished by the extent and severity of the symptoms; type I is the gravis type, type II the mitis form, and type III the benign hypermobile type. No biochemical defect has been detected. Absence of the inferior labial frenulum and the lingual frenulum has recently been described in EDS II and EDS III (284). EDS I and II are allelic with mutations in pro-alpha-1 (V) collagen chains (COL5A1) causing both types (285). Type II EDS can also be caused by a missense mutation in the COL5A2 gene (286). Mutations in more than one gene can lead to the type III phenotype (287).

EDS type IV, the arterial form, is inherited as an autosomal dominant or recessive trait. The skin of persons with this disorder is thin and fragile. Ecchymoses are very common. This tendency toward rupture is explained by the fact that there is a deficiency of type III collagen (COL3A1 gene) in the skin and in other tissues. Even though cultured fibroblasts are capable of normal synthesis of collagen type III, they show poor secretion of it into the medium (288).

EDS type V has an X-linked recessive inheritance pattern and clinical features similar to those of type I. The fibroblasts produce only 15% to 30% of the normal amount of lysyl oxidase. This deficiency results in deficient intramolecular cross-linking in the collagen molecule (282). An abnormality in the expression of COL5A1 may be the issue here (291).

EDS type VI, the ocular type, with autosomal recessive inheritance, is characterized by severe scoliosis and intraocular bleeding (289). There is a deficiency in lysyl hydroxylase in this form of the disorder. The gene for this enzyme maps to 1p36.3. p36.2 (287).

EDS type VII, the arthrochalasis type, also with autosomal dominant or recessive inheritance, shows marked looseness of joints resulting in multiple joint dislocations. The skin and tendons of patients with this form of EDS contain collagen polypeptides with a length intermediate between pro-alpha (procollagen) chains and alpha (collagen) chains. This is due to a structural mutation in the pro-alpha 2 chain that prevents the normal enzymatic removal of the aminopropeptide from it (290). A mutation at one of at least two loci COL1A1 and COL1A2 can produce this autosomal dominant phenotype (291). The autosomal recessive subtype may be due to mutations in the ADMTS2 gene (292).

EDS type VIII, the periodontal type, inherited as an autosomal dominant trait, is characterized by severe periodontitis and moderate skin fragility. Its biochemical defect is thought to be due to decreased production of type III collagen.

EDS type IX, the occipital horn syndrome (X-linked cutis laxa), with X-linked recessive inheritance, shows moderate skin extensibility, joint hypermobility, bladder diverticula, herniae, and rhizomelic limb shortening. The defect is due to abnormal copper metabolism caused by a mutation in the Cu^{++} transporting ATPase alpha peptide and a decrease in lysyl oxidase. This disorder may be allelic with Menkes syndrome (293).

EDS type X, the fibronectin type, with autosomal recessive inheritance, shows stria, moderate skin extensibility, joint hypermobility, and a platelet aggregation defect caused by dysfunction of the plasma fibronectin (291) gene map locus 2q34.

Histopathology. Except for areas of the skin that have been altered secondarily by trauma, most patients with types I to III show no abnormalities either in the thickness of the skin or in the appearance of the collagen or of the elastic fibers. Only an exceptional patient shows thin collagen fibers that are not united to collagen bundles. In these cases, the skin may also be reduced in thickness and show a relative increase in amount of elastic fibers (294). These changes are more pronounced in the type I (gravis) than in the types II and III, and are more evident when a large excision biopsy is carried out, rather than a punch biopsy. They are often seen best in the collagen bundles of the connective tissue septae of the hypodermis, with the collagen bundles appearing thin and rare (295).

E-D type IV shows the most pronounced degree of dermal thinning of all types, usually to half or three quarters of normal thickness. There is a relative abundance of elastic fibers that appear shortened and fragmented. This probably is secondary to changes in collagen fiber morphology (296).

The raisin-like pseudotumors that arise at the site of hematomas show fibrosis and numerous capillaries; they may also show accumulations of foreign body giant cells (297). The spheroid subcutaneous nodules consist of partially necrotic adipose tissue that may contain areas of dystrophic calcification and that is surrounded by a thick layer of dense collagen (298).

Histogenesis. The enzyme deficiencies observed in the various types of the EDS suggest a disturbance in collagen biosynthesis. In several electron microscopic studies, no abnormalities were observed in the normal skin of patients with EDS (299,300); however, other studies have reported abnormalities. In a study comparing healing experimental wounds in a patient with EDS with those in normal persons, the fibroblasts of the patient with EDS showed a paucity of rough-surfaced endoplasmic reticulum, and the bundles of collagen appeared small and sparse (302). Similar abnormalities were observed also in the normal-appearing skin of five patients with various types of EDS. The fibroblasts were smaller than in the skin of normal control persons, the endoplasmic reticulum was underdeveloped, and ribosome content was diminished. In addition, some collagen fibrils possessed an irregular outline, and lateral aggregation of the fibrils into bundles was reduced (301,

302). Scanning electron microscopic examination in various types of EDS has revealed thinner collagen bundles than normal and, within the bundles, gross disorganization of the collagen fibers (300). Scanning electron microscopy has shown that the hyperextensibility in the EDS is due to defective "wicker work" of the collagen fiber bundles.

CUTIS LAXA (ELASTOLYSIS)

Cutis laxa, also called dermatochalasis and generalized elastolysis, is characterized by loose, pendulous skin resulting in a prematurely aged appearance (Fig. 6-36). There are congenital and acquired types of occipital horn syndrome (see type IX in section on Ehlers–Danlos syndrome) and acquired. In the congenital type, the usual mode of inheritance is autosomal recessive (303), although autosomal dominant transmission due to a mutation in the elastin gene has been described in a few relatively mild cases (304). The occipital horn syndrome is X-linked (293). The acquired type has no genetic background (304).

In both the congenital and the acquired types, internal organs are frequently involved. There may be pulmonary emphysema causing death in infancy in some of the congenital cases (303–306) or later in life in some of the acquired cases (305). The congenital form may show wormian bones of the lambdoidal suture and osteoporosis. The deficiency in lysyl oxidase is due to a mutation on the encoding gene located on chromosome 5q (308). In addition, there may be diverticula in the gastrointestinal tract or in the bladder. Also, rectal prolapse and inguinal, umbilical, and hiatal hernias have been observed (303). About half of the cases of acquired cutis laxa are preceded or accompanied by a cutaneous eruption showing urticaria (307), erythematous plaques (309), or a vesicular eruption (310). The occipital horn syndrome is discussed in the section on Ehlers–Danlos syndrome and should be categorized as a disorder of copper metabolism.

Histopathology. In cases without an inflammatory infiltrate, changes are limited to the elastic fibers and depend on the stage and the severity of the disease. In the early stage, the elastic fibers are diminished either throughout the dermis or largely in the upper dermis or the lower dermis (311). Those elastic fibers that are present may be considerably thickened in their midportion and may taper to a point at either end. Their borders may be indistinct and they may stain unevenly, showing a granular appearance (Fig. 6-37). Ultimately, no intact elastic fibers may be identifiable. Instead, fine, dust-like orceinophilic granules may be scattered in the dermis.

In cases in which an inflammatory infiltrate is present, it may consist of a nonspecific chronic inflammatory infiltrate of lymphocytes and histiocytes. However, it may also contain neutrophils. If vesicles are present, they are subepidermal in location and may show papillary microabscesses composed of neutrophils and eosinophils suggestive of dermatitis herpetiformis.

In patients with involvement of internal organs, the lungs and gastrointestinal tract show the same granular changes in the elastic fibers as seen in the skin.

Histogenesis. Electron microscopic examination shows degenerative changes in the elastic fibers that vary somewhat from case to case. In some instances, the elastic fibers show normal microfibrils but a deficiency of the amorphous, electron-lucent elastin (306–312); in other instances, the elastin is preserved and the microfibrils are absent. In most electron microscopic examinations, the most

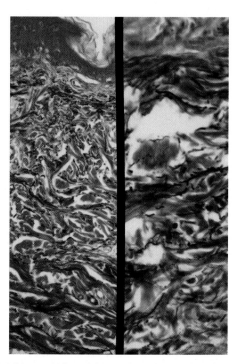

FIGURE 6-37. Cutis laxa, elastic tissue stain. The degenerated elastic fibers stain unevenly, resulting in a granular appearance and indistinct border. Split views 100×/4,000×.

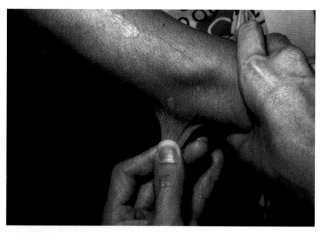

FIGURE 6-36. Cutis laxa. Child with pendulous skin.

significant finding is the presence of electron-dense amorphous or granular aggregates in the vicinity of the elastic fibers (313). The presence of this electron-dense material outside of elastic fibers suggests that, instead of a primary elastolysis, as generally assumed, a defect in the synthesis of elastic fibers causes the disease (306–309).

Another controversy concerns the role of the cutaneous eruption that precedes or accompanies many of the reported cases of acquired cutis laxa. The traditional view has been that the inflammatory infiltrate is in some way responsible for the damage to the elastic fibers (314). However, in one reported case, sequential biopsies seemed to indicate that the changes in the elastic fibers induced the inflammatory infiltrate, and the possibility therefore exists that the inflammatory infiltrate is a consequence of changes in the fibers.

PACHYDERMOPERIOSTOSIS

An idiopathic and an acquired form of pachydermoperiostosis exist, the latter being secondary to carcinoma of the lung. The idiopathic form is transmitted as an autosomal dominant trait, males being more severely affected than females (315). The manifestations include (a) clubbing of the digits, with periosteal proliferation of the bones of the hands and feet; (b) hyperplasia of the soft parts of the forearms and legs, with periosteal proliferation of the corresponding bones; and (c) thickening and furrowing of the skin of the face and scalp (cutis verticis gyrata). In abortive forms, there may be only clubbing of the fingers with periosteal proliferation of the bones of the hands and forearms (316).

Histopathology. The skin of the face shows thickening of the dermis, with thick fibrous bands extending into the subcutaneous tissue (317). In addition to an increase in the amount and size of the collagen bundles in the dermis, there is an increase in the number of fibroblasts and in the amount of ground substance. The latter stains with colloidal iron, and because it is composed largely of hyaluronic acid, it stains with Alcian blue at pH 2.5 but not at pH 0.45.

URTICARIA PIGMENTOSA

Urticaria pigmentosa, although occasionally showing an autosomal dominant mode of transmission (318,319), with a possible relationship to mutations in the KIT gene (320) in most instances occurs without a family history. It can be divided into four forms: (a) urticaria pigmentosa arising in infancy or early childhood without significant systemic lesions (321); (b) urticaria pigmentosa arising in adolescence or adult life without significant systemic lesions (322); (c) systemic mast cell disease; and (d) mast cell leukemia.

In the first form, the cutaneous lesions often improve or even clear at puberty (323). Systemic lesions are absent as a rule and, if present, usually are few in number. Progression into systemic mast cell disease is very rare (see later). In the second form, urticaria pigmentosa arising in adolescence or adult life, systemic lesions are often present but as a rule are rather static in their course (324,325). However, spontaneous regression has never been documented in adults, in contrast to children (326). In only a few patients is there progression to the third form, systemic mast cell disease, which shows extensive and progressive involvement of internal organs (see section on systemic lesions). The fourth form, mast cell leukemia, is very rare. It is characterized by the presence of cytologically malignant mast cells in many organs of the body, especially in the bone marrow and the peripheral blood, and is a rapidly fatal disease (327). Usually there are no skin lesions (328).

Patients with extensive mast cell infiltration of the skin or the internal organs commonly have attacks of flushing, palpitation, or diarrhea as a result of degranulation of mast cells and the release of histamine.

Five types of cutaneous lesions are seen in urticaria pigmentosa (323). Two types can occur in both the infantile and the adult forms. One is the maculopapular type, the most common type, consisting usually of dozens or even hundreds of brown lesions that urticate on stroking (Fig. 6-38A); the other type exhibits multiple brown nodules or plaques, and, on stroking, shows urtication and occasionally blister formation (Fig. 6-38B). The third type, seen almost exclusively in infants, is characterized by a usually solitary, large cutaneous nodule, which on stroking often shows not only urtication but also large bullae. In rare instances, solitary nodules have been described as arising in adults without giving rise to bullae (329). The fourth type, the diffuse erythrodermic type, always starts in early infancy and shows generalized brownish red, soft infiltration of the skin, with urtication on stroking. Multiple blisters may form during the first 2 years of life on stroking and also spontaneously. When bullae are a predominant clinical feature, the term *bullous mastocytosis* has been applied (330,331). Although visceral lesions are common in the diffuse erythrodermic type, they usually improve and only very rarely progress to fatal systemic mast cell disease. On rare occasions, death occurs in early infancy, apparently as a result of histamine shock with no or insignificant mast cell infiltration of visceral organs (332). The fifth type of lesion, telangiectasia macularis eruptiva perstans, which usually occurs in adults, consists of an extensive eruption of brownish red macules showing fine telangiectasias, with little or no urtication on stroking (333).

Histopathology. In all five types of lesions, the histologic picture shows an infiltrate composed chiefly of mast cells, which are characterized by the presence of metachromatic granules in their cytoplasm. These granules are not visible

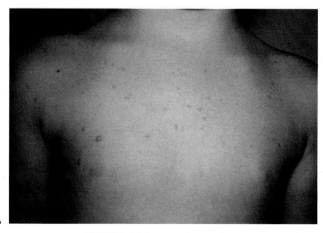

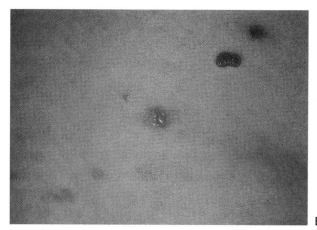

FIGURE 6-38. A: Urticaria pigmentosa. Multiple papular lesions of Urticaria Pigmentosa. **B:** Blister formation.

with routine stains but can be seen well after staining with a Giemsa stain or with toluidine blue. Also, the method using naphthol AS-D chloroacetate esterase, often called Leder's method, makes mast cell granules appear red and thus quite conspicuous (334).

In the maculopapular type and in telangiectasia macularis eruptiva perstans, the mast cells are limited to the upper third of the dermis and are generally located around capillaries. In some mast cells, the nuclei may be round or oval, but in most mast cells, they are spindle shaped (Fig. 6-39). Because the mast cells may be present only in small numbers, and because in sections stained with hematoxylin-eosin, their nuclei resemble those of fibroblasts or pericytes, the diagnosis may be missed unless special staining is employed (335).

In cases with multiple nodules or plaques or with a solitary large nodule, the mast cells lie closely packed in tumor-like aggregates (Figs. 6-40 and 6-41). The infiltrate may extend through the entire dermis and even into the subcutaneous fat (336). Whenever the mast cells lie in dense aggregates, their nuclei are cuboidal rather than spindle shaped, and they show ample eosinophilic cytoplasm and a well-defined cell border. Because of the shape of their

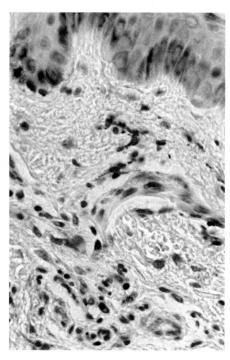

FIGURE 6-39. Urticaria pigmentosa, maculopapular (adult type). Scattered mast cells are seen, some cuboidal in shape. The greatest numbers are about dermal vessels. The epidermis is hyperpigmented (original magnification × 100).

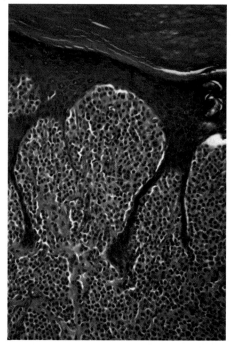

FIGURE 6-40. Urticaria pigmentosa, nodular type. Mast cells fill the expanded papillary dermis (H&E stain, original magnification × 100).

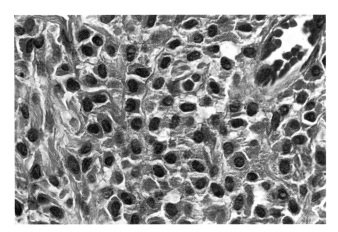

FIGURE 6-41. Urticaria pigmentosa, nodular type. Cuboidal mast cells that fill and expand the papillary dermis. These cells closely resemble nevus cells. Special stains will differentiate (original magnification × 400).

nuclei and ample cytoplasm, they have a rather distinctive appearance, so that the diagnosis usually can be made even before special staining has been carried out.

In the diffuse, erythrodermic type, one observes in the upper dermis a dense, band-like infiltrate of mast cells with a rather uniform appearance showing round to oval nuclei and a distinctly outlined cytoplasm (337).

Eosinophils may be present in small numbers in all types of urticaria pigmentosa with the exception of telangiectasia macularis eruptiva perstans, in which eosinophils are generally absent because of the small numbers of mast cells within the lesions. If a biopsy is taken shortly after the lesion has been stroked, one observes an increased number of eosinophils and extracellular mast cell granules as an indication that granules have been released by the cells (338).

The bullae that may occur in infants with multiple or solitary nodules or with the diffuse erythrodermic type arise subepidermally (339). Because of regeneration of the epidermis at the base of the bulla, older bullae may be located intraepidermally. The bullous cavity often contains mast cells as well as eosinophils (340). The pigmentation of lesions of urticaria pigmentosa is due to the presence of increased amounts of melanin in the basal cell layer and occasionally also of melanophages in the upper dermis.

Systemic Lesions

It is important to distinguish between asymptomatic systemic involvement of limited degree and true systemic mast cell disease, in which the lesions are symptomatic, widespread, and progressive.

Asymptomatic systemic involvement of a limited degree may occur in urticaria pigmentosa of children, but it is not common. It occurs most commonly in the erythrodermic and nodular types and consists of bone and bone marrow involvement or of hepatosplenomegaly. In urticaria pig-

mentosa of adults, systemic lesions are more common. For instance, in routine bone marrow biopsies, as many as 75% of adult patients show mast cell infiltration of bone marrow, in contrast to only 18% of children; radiologic survey of the skeleton has revealed bone changes in 44% of adult patients with urticaria pigmentosa, but in only 5% of children (341). On radiologic examination, bones with mast cell infiltration may show areas of increased lucency intermingled with areas of increased density owing to the fact that mast cell aggregates in the bone marrow can cause focal bone resorption as well as reactive bone formation (342).

In true systemic mast cell disease, massive infiltration of the bones may cause collapse of several vertebrae or a fracture of long bones (343). Myelofibrosis may occur, resulting in anemia, leukopenia, and thrombocytopenia (313). Pancytopenia may cause death. Systemic mastocytosis, besides involving the bone marrow and bones, generally involves various groups of lymph nodes and the liver and spleen, resulting in hepatosplenomegaly. In some cases, the gastrointestinal tract, lungs, and meninges are also infiltrated with mast cells (326). Mature mast cells may be found in the peripheral blood.

Histogenesis. As seen by both light microscopy and electron microscopy, the mast cells of urticaria pigmentosa do not differ from normal mast cells either in structure or in mode of degranulation (EM 18) (345,346). Because mast cells contain histamine and release it during degranulation, chemical analysis of cutaneous lesions of urticaria pigmentosa reveals a considerably higher level of histamine than is found in normal skin (347).

The increased melanin pigmentation in lesions of urticaria pigmentosa is the result of stimulation of epidermal melanocytes by mast cells. It is not caused by any substance present within the mast cells. In one case of nodular urticaria pigmentosa, however, some mast cells showed dual granulation containing mast cell granules and melanosomes, as well as granules representing intergrades between mast cell granules and melanosomes (348).

Differential Diagnosis. Even if numerous mast cells are present, an absolutely reliable diagnosis of urticaria pigmentosa requires the demonstration of mast cell granules with the Giemsa stain, Leder's method, or toluidine blue stain. On routine staining, the mast cells in macular lesions may resemble fibroblasts or pericytes, but those in nodular or erythrodermic lesions may resemble the histiocytes that are seen in Letterer–Siwe disease or in eosinophilic granuloma. Differentiation of urticaria pigmentosa from these two diseases on routine staining can be particularly difficult because, in all three diseases, the infiltrate may contain eosinophils. In contrast with Letterer–Siwe disease, the cells of urticaria pigmentosa have no tendency to invade the epidermis. Occasionally, the cuboidal mast cells in nodular urticaria pigmentosa resemble nevus cells, but they show no tendency to lie in nests and show no junction activity.

The macular type of urticaria pigmentosa, especially telangiectasia maculosa eruptiva perstans, occasionally may be difficult to diagnose even with the Giemsa stain because the number of mast cells may be so small that it does not differ significantly from the number normally present (341). Some inflammatory dermatoses, such as atopic dermatitis, lichen simplex chronicus, and lichen planus, may contain a high percentage of mast cells in their inflammatory cell infiltrates (349). In urticaria pigmentosa, however, the infiltrate consists exclusively of mast cells, except for a slight admixture of eosinophils as a result of the degranulation of some of the mast cells.

INCONTINENTIA PIGMENTI

Incontinentia pigmenti is an X-linked dominantly inherited disorder. Females with the abnormal gene on only one of their two X chromosomes are heterozygous for this condition and are not severely affected, but males with the abnormal gene on their single X chromosome are hemizygous for this condition and hence are so severely affected that they die in utero. This explains the predominance of female patients with this disorder (350). Of 609 reported cases, only 16 have been in boys. The fact that these boys were no more severely affected than their female counterparts suggests that the disease in all living male patients is the result of spontaneous mutation (351). The familial form of this disorder IP2 (or classical incontinentia pigmentosa) is localized to the Xq28 region (352). It is due to a mutation in the IKK-gamma gene, which is also called NEMO.

The disorder has four stages. The first stage, consisting of erythema and bullae arranged in lines, either is present at birth or starts shortly thereafter. The extremities are predominantly affected. There is also marked blood eosinophilia. In the second stage, which occurs after about 2 months, the vesicular lesions gradually are superseded by linear, verrucous lesions that persist for several months. As the verrucous lesions subside, widely disseminated areas of irregular, spattered, or whorled pigmentation develop. This pigmentation, representing the third stage, is most pronounced on the trunk (Fig. 6-42A). It diminishes gradually after several years and may even clear completely. The fourth stage is seen in adult females. Subtle, faint, hypochromic or atrophic lesions in a linear pattern are most apparent on the lower extremities (354).

In about 80% of the cases, incontinentia pigmenti is associated with various congenital abnormalities, particularly of the central nervous system, eyes, and teeth. Partial alopecia at the vertex is also often seen (351).

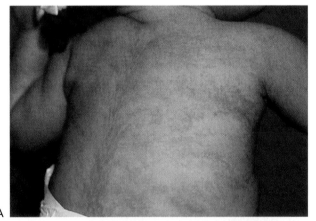

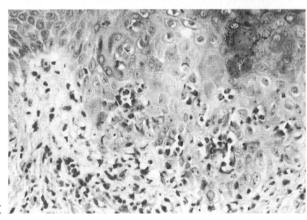

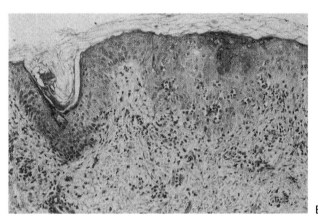

FIGURE 6-42. A: Incontinentia pigmenti. Streaking and whorled pigmentation on the trunk. **B:** The transition stage between vesicular and acanthotic. Many eosinophils are seen in the dermis and in the focally a acanthotic and spongiotic epidermis. **C:** High magnification of Fig. 6-42B, showing eosinophilic spongiosis and acanthosis.

Histopathology. The vesicles seen during the first stage arise within the epidermis and are associated with spongiosis. They are of the type seen in dermatitis (355). However, they differ from the vesicles of dermatitis by the numerous eosinophils within them and around them in the epidermis (eosinophilic spongiosis) (Fig. 6-42B and C). The epidermis between the vesicles often shows single dyskeratotic cells and whorls of squamous cells with central keratinization. Like the epidermis, the dermis shows an infiltrate containing many eosinophils and some mononuclear cells.

The alterations in the second stage consist of acanthosis, irregular papillomatosis, and hyperkeratosis. Intraepidermal keratinization, consisting of whorls of keratinocytes and of scattered dyskeratotic cells, is often more pronounced than in the first stage. The basal cells show vacuolization and a decrease in their melanin content. The dermis shows a mild, chronic inflammatory infiltrate intermingled with melanophages. This infiltrate extends into the epidermis in many places.

The areas of pigmentation seen in the third stage show extensive deposits of melanin within melanophages located in the upper dermis. Usually, this dermal hyperpigmentation is found in association with a diminution of pigment in the basal layer, the cells of which show vacuolization and degeneration (356). In some cases, however, the cells of the basal layer contain abundant amounts of melanin (357,358).

A different pattern has recently been described on the skin of the legs of an infant in whom the vesiculation had produced superficial scarring and depigmentation. The light-colored skin lacked melanocytes and appendages as the result of scarring, and the darker skin showed a normal degree of pigmentation without incontinence of pigment (359).

Pathogenesis. The fact that the first two stages of incontinentia pigmenti are seen predominantly on the extremities and the third stage mainly on the trunk has led to the assumption by some authors that the pigmentary changes of the third stage occur independently of the bullous and verrucous lesions of the first two stages and represent some sort of nevoid anomaly. Electron microscopic studies, however, have revealed common features, albeit to varying extents, in all three stages of incontinentia pigmenti, and thus suggest that the three stages are related to each other (360–362). Even in the first stage, many keratinocytes and melanocytes show degenerative changes resulting in the migration of macrophages to the epidermis, where they phagocytize dyskeratotic keratinocytes and melanosomes. Subsequently, the macrophages return to the dermis (EM 6). The macrophages seen in the dermis in the second and third stages contain many melanosome complexes and thus are easily recognizable as melanophages even by light microscopy, whereas the macrophages in the first stage contain only few melanosome complexes and therefore can be identified as melanophages only in the electron microscope (360). The phagocytosis of melanin by dermal macrophages in the first stage of the disease (361) and the pres-

ence of dyskeratotic keratinocytes in the epidermis during all three stages of the disease have been confirmed.

The presence of eosinophils in epidermal and dermal infiltrates can be explained by the presence in the early vesicular stage of basophils, which release eosinophil chemotactic factor of anaphylaxis (363). Eosinophil chemotactic activity has been demonstrated in patients with incontinentia pigmenti in the blister fluid (364), and in eluates of crusted scales overlying the lesions (365).

HYPOMELANOSIS OF ITO

Hypomelanosis of Ito was originally called incontinentia pigmenti achromians, but because the disorder shows no pigmentary incontinence, this term has been largely abandoned. However, it is now felt that hypomelanosis of Ito is not an entity, but rather a symptom of many different states of mosaicism and is due to an X autosome translocation involving Xp11 (366).

The hypomelanosis seen in this disorder may be present at birth. However, it usually develops during the first year of life. In some instances, the loss of pigment does not begin until childhood. There is a tendency for the pigmentary loss to become more pronounced at first but to be followed by partial repigmentation in adult life. The pattern and distribution of the hypopigmentation in hypomelanosis of Ito is similar to the pattern of hyperpigmentation seen in incontinentia pigmenti (Fig. 6-43). Although first

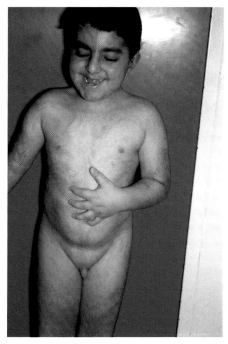

FIGURE 6-43. Hypomelanosis of Ito. Streaking hypopigmentation on trunk.

reported in Japanese patients, hypomelanosis of Ito has since been observed in many ethnicities/races.

Congenital abnormalities are found in 50% of the cases (367). Most common are mental retardation and seizure disorders, but there also may be abnormalities of the eyes, hair, teeth, or the musculoskeletal system (368). Abnormal chromosomal constitutions are common (369).

Histopathology. In the hypopigmented areas, a Fontana–Masson stain shows a decrease in the amount of melanin granules in the basal cell layer, with a complete absence of melanin in some areas (370). With the dopa reaction, the hypopigmented areas are seen to contain fewer and smaller melanocytes than normal, with sparse, short dendrites (371).

Pathogenesis. The electron microscopic findings show a significant decrease in the number of melanosomes within melanocytes and keratinocytes (368–371). In addition, some melanocytes show degenerative changes and an absence of melanosomes (372).

REFERENCES

1. Stevanovic DV. Hodgkin's disease of the skin. *Arch Dermatol* 1960;82:96.
2. Flint GL, Flam M, Soter NA. Acquired ichthyosis: a sign of non-lymphoproliferative malignant disorder. *Arch Dermatol* 1975; 111:1446.
3. Frost P, Van Scott EJ. Ichthyosiform dermatoses. *Arch Dermatol* 1966;94:113.
4. Sybert VP, Dale BA, Molbrook KA. Ichthyosis vulgaris: identification of a defect in synthesis of fillagrin correlated with an absence of keratohyaline granules. *J Invest Dermatol* 1985;84: 191.
5. Nirunsukiri W, Presland RB, Brumbaugh SG, et al. Decreased profillagrin expression in ichthyosis vulgaris is a result of selectively impaired posttranscriptional control. *J Biol Chem* 1995; 270:871.
6. Nirunsukiri W, Zhang SH, Heckman P. Reduced stability and bi-allelic, coequal expression of profilaggren mRNA in keratinocytes cultured from subjects with ichthyosis vulgaris. *J Invest Dermatol* 1998;110:854.
7. Finley AY, Nicholls S, King CS, et al. The dry non-eczematous skin associated with atopic eczema. *Br J Dermatol* 1980;103: 249.
8. Frost P. Ichthyosiform dermatoses. *J Invest Dermatol* 1973;60: 541.
9. Sugawara T, Fujimoto Y, Fugimoto S. Molecular analysis of X-linked ichthyosis in Japan. *Horm Res* 2001:56:82.
10. Feinstein A, Ackerman AB, Ziprkowski L. Histology of autosomal dominant ichthyosis vulgaris and X-linked ichthyosis. *Arch Dermatol* 1970;101:524.
11. Anton-Lamprecht L. Zur ultrastruktur hereditarer verhornungsstorungen: IV. X-chromosomal-recessive ichthyosis. *Arch Dermatol Forsch* 1974;248:361.
12. Shapiro LJ, Weiss R, Webster D, et al. X-linked ichthyosis due to steroid-sulphatase deficiency. *Lancet* 1978;1:70.
13. Williams ML, Elias P. X-linked ichthyosis: elevated cholesterol sulfate in pathological stratum corneum. *J Invest Dermatol* 1981; 76:312(abst).
14. Epstein EH Jr, Williams ML, Elias PM. Editorial: steroid sulfatase, X-linked ichthyosis, and stratum corneum cohesion. *Arch Dermatol* 1981;117:761.
15. Ishibashi Y, Klingmuller G. Erythrodermia ichthyosiformis congenita bullosa Brocq. *Arch Klin Exp Dermatol* 1968;232: 205.
16. Ackerman AB. Histopathologic concept of epidermolytic hyperkeratosis. *Arch Dermatol* 1970;102:253.
17. McCurdy J, Beare JM. Congenital bullous ichthyosiform erythroderma. *Br J Dermatol* 1976;79:294.
18. Rothnagel JA, Dominey AM, Dempsy LD, et al. Mutations in the rod domains of keratins 1 and 10 in epidermolytic hyperkeratosis. *Science* 1992;257:1128.
19. Schnyder UW. Inherited ichthyosis. *Arch Dermatol* 1970;102:240.
20. Irvine AD, Mc Lean WH. Human keratin diseases: the increasing spectrum of disease and subtlety of the phenotype–genotype correlation. *Br J Dermatol* 1999;140:815.
21. Anton-Lamprecht I, Schnyder UW. Ultrastructure in inborn errors of keratinization. *Arch Dermatol Forsch* 1974;250:207.
22. Mehregan AH. Epidermolytic hyperkeratosis. *J Cutan Pathol* 1978;5:76.
23. Niizuma K. Isolated epidermolytic acanthoma. *Dermatologica* 1979;159:30.
24. Paller AS, Synder AJ, Chan YM, et al. Genetic and clinical mosaicism in a type of epidermal nevus. *N Engl J Med* 1994;331: 1408.
25. Mitchel EJ, Schneiderman P, Grossman ME, et al. Epidermolytic hyperkeratosis with polycyclic psoriasiform plaques resulting from a mutation in the keratin 1 gene. *Exp Dermatol* 1999;8:501.
26. Arin MJ, Longley MA, Epstein EH, et al. Identification of a novel mutation in keratin 1 in a family with epidermolytic hyperkeratosis. *Exp Dermatol* 2000;9;9:16.
27. Hazell M, Marks R. Clinical histology and cell kinetic discriminants between lamellar ichthyosis and nonbullous congenital ichthyosiform erythroderma. *Arch Dermatol* 1985;121:489.
28. Hohl D, Huber M, Frenk E. Analysis of the cornified cell envelope in lamellar ichthyosis. *Arch Dermatol* 1993;129:618.
29. Menon GK, Williams ML, Ghadally R, et al. Lamellar bodies as delivery systems of hydrolytic enzymes: implications for normal cohesion and abnormal desquamation. *Br J Dermatol* 1992;126: 337.
30. Jobard F, Lefevre C, Karaduman A, et al. Lipoxygenase-3 (ALOXE3) and 12(R)–lipoxygenase(ALOX12B) are mutated in non-bullous congenital ichthyosiform erythroderma (NCIE) linked to chrosome 17p13.1. *Hum Mol Genet* 2002;11:107.
31. Elias PM, Williams ML. Neutral lipid storage disease with ichthyosis. *Arch Dermatol* 1985;121:1000.
32. Parmentier ML, Lakdar H, Blanchet–Bardon C, et al. Mapping of a second locus for lamella ichthyosis to chromosome 2q33–35 1996. *Hum Mol Genet* 1996;5:862.
33. Williams ML, Elias PM. Heterogeneity in autosomal recessive ichthyosis. *Arch Dermatol* 1985;121:477.
34. Happle R. X-chromosomal vererbte dermatosen. *Hautarzt* 1982; 33:73.
35. Emami S, Rizzo WB, Hanley KP, et al. Peroxisomal abnormality in fibroblast from involved skin of CHILD syndrome. *Arch Dermatol* 1992;128:1213.
36. Kelley RI, Herman GE. Inborn errors of sterol bioysnthesis. *Annu Rev Genomics Hum Genet* 2001;2:299.
37. Christiansen JV, Petersen HO, Søgaard H. The CHILD syndrome: congenital hemodysplasia with ichthyosiform and limb defects. *Acta Derm Venereol Suppl (Stockh)* 1984;64:165.
38. Roberts LJ. Long-term survival of a harlequin fetus. *J Am Acad Dermatol* 1989;21:335.
39. Luderschmidt C, Dorn M, Bassermann R, et al. Kollodiumbaby und harlekinfetus. *Hautarzt* 1980;31:154.

40. Milner ME, O'Guin WM, Holbrook KA, et al. Abnormal lamellar granules in harlequin ichthyosis. *J Invest Dermatol* 1992;99: 824.

41. Williams ML. Ichthyosis: mechanisms of disease. *Pediatr Dermatol* 1992;9:365.

42. Vandersteen PR, Muller SA. Erythrokeratodermia variabilis. *Arch Dermatol* 1971;103:362.

43. Nir M, Tanzer F. Progressive symmetric erythrokeratodermia. *Dermatologica* 1978;156:268.

44. Richard G. Conexin disorders of the skin. *Adv Dermatol* 2001; 17:243.

45. Judge MR, Morgan G, Harper JI. A clinical and immunological study of Netherton's syndrome. *Br J Dermatol* 1994;131:615.

46. Mehvorah B, Frenk E, Brooke EM. Ichthyosis linearis circumflexa Comèl. *Dermatologica* 1974;149:201.

47. Altman J, Stroud J. Netherton's syndrome and ichthyosis linearis circumflexa: psoriasiform ichthyosis. *Arch Dermatol* 1969;100: 550.

48. Hersle K. Netherton's disease and ichthyosis linearis circumflexa. *Acta Derm Venereol Suppl (Stockh)* 1972;52:298.

49. Thorne EG, Zelickson AS, Mottaz JH, et al. Netherton's syndrome: an electron microscopic study. *Arch Dermatol Res* 1975; 253:177.

50. Mehvorah B, Frenk E. Ichthyosis linearis circumflexa Comèl with trichorrhexis invaginata (Netherton's syndrome). *Dermatologica* 1974;149:193.

51. Zina AM, Bundino S. Ichthyosis linearis circumflexa Comèl and Netherton's syndrome: an ultrastructural study. *Dermatologica* 1979;158:404.

52. Jorizzo JL, Crounse RG, Wheeler CE Jr. Lamellar ichthyosis, dwarfism, mental retardation, and hair shaft anomalies. *J Am Acad Dermatol* 1980;2:309.

53. Wells RS. Some genetic aspects of dermatology: a review. *Clin Exp Dermatol* 1980;5:1.

54. Heijer A, Reed WB. Sjögren–Larsson syndrome. *Arch Dermatol* 1965;92:545.

55. Rizzo WB, Dammann AL, Craft DA, et al. Sjögren–Larsson syndrome: inherited defect in the fatty alcohol cycle. *J Pediatr* 1989; 115:228.

56. Rixxo WB. Inhereted disorders of fatty alcohol metabolism. *Mol Genet Metab* 1998;65:63.

57. Maldonado RR, Tamayo L, Carnevale A. Neuroichthyosis with hypogonadism (Rud's syndrome). *Int J Dermatol* 1975; 14:347.

58. Edidin DV, Esterly NB, Bamzai AK, et al. Chondrodysplasia punctata: Conradi–Hunermann syndrome. *Arch Dermatol* 1977; 113:1431.

59. Emami S, Hanley KP, Esterly NB, et al. X-Linked dominant ichthyosis with peroxisomal deficiency: an ultrastructural and ultracytochemical study of the Conradi–Hunermann syndrome and its murine homolog, the Bare Patches Mouse. *Arch Dermatol* 1994;130:325.

60. Derry JM, Gormally E, Means GD, et al. Mutations in a delta8 delta7 sterol isosomerase in the tattered mouse and X-linked dominant chondrodysplasia punctata. *Nat Genet* 1999; 22:286.

61. Skinner BA, Greist MC, Norins AL. The keratins, ichthyosis and deafness (KID) syndrome. *Arch Dermatol* 1981;177:285.

62. Williams ML, Coleman RA, Placzek D, et al. Neutral lipid storage disease with ichthyosis: evidence for a function defect in phospholipid linked triacylglycerol metabolism in cultured fibroblasts. *Biochem Biophys Acta* 1991;1096:162.

63. Davies MG, Marks R, Dykes PJ, et al. Epidermal abnormalities in Refsum's disease. *Br J Dermatol* 1977;97:401.

64. Rand RE, Baden HP. The ichthyoses: a review. *J Am Acad Dermatol* 1983;8:285.

65. Jansen GA, Otman R, Ferdmandusse S, et al. Refsum disease si caused by mutations in the gene phytanol-CoA hydroxylase gene. *Nat Genet* 1997;17:190.

66. Kansky A, Arzensek J. Is palmoplantar keratoderma of Greither's type a separate nosologic entity? *Dermatologica* 1979;158:244.

67. Hamm H, Happlf R, Butterfass T, et al. Epidermolytic keratoderma of Vorner: is it the most common type of hereditary palmoplantar keratoderma? *Dermatologica* 1988;177:138.

68. Kimyai-Asadi A, Kotcher LB, Jih MH. The mohecular basis of hereditary palmoplantar keratodermas. *J Am Acad Dermatol* 2002;47:327–43.

69. Salamon T, Bogdanovic B, Lazovic-Tepava CO. Die krankheit von Mljet. *Dermatologica* 1969;138:433.

70. Bach JN, Levan NE. Papillon–Lefevre syndrome. *Arch Dermatol* 1968;97:154.

71. Klaus S, Weinstein GD, Frost P. Localized epidermolytic hyperkeratosis: a form of keratoderma of the palms and soles. *Arch Dermatol* 1970;101:272.

72. Moulin G, Bouchet B. La keratodermie palmo-plantaire familiale avec hyperkeratose epidermolytique. *Ann Dermatol Venereol* 1977;104:38.

73. Fritsch P, Honigsmann H, Jaschke E. Epidermolytic hereditary palmoplantar keratoderma. *Br J Dermatol* 1978;99:561.

74. Buchanan RN Jr. Keratosis punctata palmaris et plantaris. *Arch Dermatol* 1963;88:644.

75. Brown FC. Punctate keratoderma. *Arch Dermatol* 1971;104:682.

76. Herman PS. Punctate porokeratotic keratoderma. *Dermatologica* 1973;147:206.

77. Bogle MA, Hwang LY, Tschen JA. Acrokeratoelastoidosis. *J Am Acad Dermatol* 2002;47:448.

78. Jung EG, Beil FU, Anton-Lamprecht I, et al. Akrokeratoelastoidosis. *Hautarzt* 1974;25:7.

79. Highet I, Rook A, Anderson JR. Acrokeratoelastoidosis. *Br J Dermatol* 1982;106:337.

80. Johansson EA, Kariniemi AL, Niemi KM. Palmoplantar keratoderma of punctate type: acrokeratoelastoidosis costa. *Acta Derm Venereol Suppl (Stockh)* 1980;60:149.

81. Dowd PM, Hartman RRM, Black MM. Focal acral hyperkeratosis. *Br J Dermatol* 1989;109:97.

82. Blum SL, Cruz PD Jr, Siegel DM. Focal acral hyperkeratosis. *Arch Dermatol* 1987;123:1225.

83. Burks JW, Wise LJ, Clark WH Jr. Degenerative collagenous plaques of the hands. *Arch Dermatol* 1960;82:362.

84. Ritchie EB, Williams HM Jr. Degenerative collagenous plaques of the hands. *Arch Dermatol* 1966;93:202.

85. Kelly EW Jr, Pinkus H. Report of a case of pachyonychia congenita. *Arch Dermatol* 1958;77:724.

86. Schonfeld PHIR. The pachyonychia congenita syndrome. *Acta Derm Venereol Suppl (Stockh)* 1980;60:45.

87. Witkop CJ, Gorlin RJ. Four hereditary mucosal syndromes. *Arch Dermatol* 1961;84:762.

88. Mc Lean WHI, Rugg EL, Lunny DP, et al. Keratin-16 and keratin-17 mutations cause pachyonychia congenita. *Nat Genet* 1995;9:273.

89. Terrinoni A, Smith FJ, Diama B, et al. Novel and recurrent mutations in the genes encoding keratins K616 and K17 in 13 cases of pachyonychia congenital. *J Invest Dermatol* 2001;117: 1391.

90. Tchou PK, Kohn T. Dyskeratosis congenita: an autosomal dominant disorder. *J Am Acad Dermatol* 1982;6:1034.

91. Gutman A, Frumkin A, Adam A, et al. X-linked dyskeratosis congenita with pancytopenia. *Arch Dermatol* 1978;114:1667.

92. Bryan HG, Nixon RK. Dyskeratosis congenita and familial pancytopenia. *JAMA* 1965;192:203.

93. Costello MJ, Buncke CM. Dyskeratosis congenita. *Arch Dermatol* 1956;73:123.

94. Vulliamy TJ, Knight SW, Mason PJ, et al. Very short telomeres in the peripheral blood of patients with X-linked and autosomal dyskeratosis congenital. *Blood Cells Mol Dis* 2001, 27:353.

95. Chernosky ME. Editorial: porokeratosis. *Arch Dermatol* 1986; 122:869.

96. Knight SW, Vulliamy TJ, Morgan B, et al. Identification of novel DKCL mutations in patients with dyskeratosis congenital. Implications for pathophysiology and diagnosis. *Hum Genet* 2001;108:299.

97. Brodkin RH, Rickert RR, Fuller FW, et al. Malignant disseminated porokeratosis. *Arch Dermatol* 1987;123:1521.

98. Chernosky ME, Freeman RG. Disseminated superficial actinic porokeratosis (DSAP). *Arch Dermatol* 1967;96:611.

99. Schwarz T, Seiser A, Gschnait F. Disseminated superficial actinic porokeratosis. *J Am Acad Dermatol* 1984;11:724.

100. Neumann RA, Knobler RM, Metze D, et al. Disseminated superficial porokeratosis and immunosuppression. *Br J Dermatol* 1988;119:375.

101. Rahbari H, Cordero AA, Mehregan AH. Linear porokeratosis. *Arch Dermatol* 1974;109:526.

102. Nabai H, Mehregan AH. Porokeratosis of Mibelli: a report of two unusual cases. *Dermatologica* 1979;159:325.

103. Guss SB, Osbourn RA, Lutzner MA. Porokeratosis plantaris, palmaris et disseminata. *Arch Dermatol* 1971;104:366.

104. Shaw JC, White CR Jr. Porokeratosis plantaris, palmaris et disseminata. *J Am Acad Dermatol* 1984;11:454.

105. Brasch J, Scheuer B, Christophers E. Porokeratosis plantaris, palmaris et disseminata. *Hautarzt* 1985;36:459.

106. Himmelstein R, Lynnfield YL. Punctate porokeratosis. *Arch Dermatol* 1984;120:263.

107. Oberste-Lehn H, Moll B. Porokeratosis Mibelli und stachelzellcarcinom. *Hautarzt* 1968;19:399.

108. Coskey RJ, Mehregan A. Bowen disease associated with porokeratosis of Mibelli. *Arch Dermatol* 1975;111:1480.

109. Mibelli V. Contributo allo studio della ipercheratosi dei canali sudoriferi. *G Ital Mal Ven* 1983;28:313.

110. Braun-Falco O, Balsa RE. Zur histochemie der cornoiden lamelle. *Hautarzt* 1969;28:543.

111. Reed RJ, Leone P. Porokeratosis: a mutant clonal keratosis of the epidermis. *Arch Dermatol* 1970;101:340.

112. Magee JW, McCalmont TH, LeBoit PE. Over expression of P53 tumor supressor protein in porokeratosis. *Arch Dermatol* 1994;130:187.

113. Mann PR, Cort DF, Fairburn EA, et al. Ultrastructural studies on two cases of porokeratosis of Mibelli. *Br J Dermatol* 1974; 90:607.

114. Sato A, Anton-Lamprecht I, Schnyder UW. Ultrastructure of inborn errors of keratinization: VII. Porokeratosis mibelli and disseminated superficial actinic porokeratosis. *Arch Dermatol Res* 1976;255:271.

115. Wade TR, Ackerman AB. Cornoid lamellation: a histologic reaction pattern. *Am J Dermatopathol* 1980;2:5.

116. McGovern VJ. Melanoblastoma, with particular reference to its incidence in childhood. *Australas J Dermatol* 1962;6:190.

117. Tullis GD, Lynde CW, McLean DI. Multiple melanomas occurring in a patient with xeroderma pigmentosum. *J Am Acad Dermatol* 1984;11:364.

118. Reed WB, Sugarman Gl, Mathis RA. DeSanctis–Cacchione syndrome. *Arch Dermatol* 1977;113:1561.

119. Cleaver JE. Xeroderma pigmentosum. Genetic and environmental influences in skin carcinogenesis. *Int J Dermatol* 1978; 17:435.

120. Akiba H, Kato T, Seiji M. Enzyme defects in xeroderma pigmentosum. *J Dermatol* 1976;3:163.

121. Friedberg EC. Recent studies on the DNA repair defects. *Arch Pathol* 1978;102:3.

122. Berneburg M, Lehmann AR. Xeroderma pigmentosum and related disorders: defects in DNA repair and transcription. *Adv Genet* 2001;43:71.

123. Guerrier CJ, Lutzner MA, Devico V, et al. An electron microscopical study of the skin in 18 cases of xeroderma pigmentosum. *Dermatologica* 1973;146:211.

124. Priolo M, Lagana C. Ectodermal dysplasias: a new clinical-genetic classification. *J Med Genet* 2001;38:579.

125. Pierard GE, Van Neste D, Letot B. Hidrotic ectodermal dysplasia. *Dermatologica* 1979;158:168.

126. Lamartine J, Munhoz EG, Kibar Z, et al. Mutations in GJB6 cause hidrotic ectodermal dysplasia. *Nat Genet* 2000;26:142.

127. Kere J, Srivastava AK, Montonen O, et al. X-linked anhidrotic (hypohidrotic ectodermal dysplasia is caused by mutations in a novel transmembrane protein. *Nat Genet* 1996;73:409.

128. McNaughton PZ, Pierson DL, Rodman RG. Hidrotic ectodermal dysplasia in a black mother and daughter. *Arch Dermatol* 1976;112:1448.

129. Clarke A, Phillips DIM, Brown R, et al. Clinical aspects of X-linked hypohidrotic ectodermal dysplasia. *Arch Dis Child* 1987; 62:989.

130. Martin-Pascual A, De Unamuno P, Aparicio M, et al. Anhidrotic (or hypohidrotic) ectodermal dysplasia. *Dermatologica* 1977;154:235.

131. Reed WB, Lopex DA, Landing B. Clinical spectrum of anhidrotic ectodermal dysplasia. *Arch Dermatol* 1970;102:134.

132. Malagon V, Taveras JE. Congenital anhidrotic ectodermal and mesodermal dysplasia. *Arch Dermatol* 1956;74:253.

133. Happle R, Lenz W. Striation of bone in focal dermal hypoplasia: manifestation of functional mosaicism. *Br J Dermatol* 1977;96:133.

134. Kilmer SL, Grix AW, Isseroff RR. Focal dermal hypoplasia. Four cases with varying presentations. *J Am Acad Dermatol* 1993;28:1839.

135. Gottlieb SK, Fisher BK, Violin GA. Focal dermal hypoplasia. *Arch Dermatol* 1973;108:551.

136. Goltz RW, Henderson RR, Hitch JM, et al. Focal dermal hypoplasia syndrome. *Arch Dermatol* 1970;101:1.

137. Howell JB, Reynolds J. Osteopathia striata. *Trans St Johns Hosp Dermatol Soc* 1974;60:178.

138. Lever WF. Hypoplasia cutis congenita (case presentation). *Arch Dermatol* 1964;90:340.

139. Tsuji T. Focal dermal hypoplasia syndrome: an electron microscopical study of the skin lesions. *J Cutan Pathol* 1982;9:271.

140. Harari Z, Pusmanik A, Dvoretsky I, et al. Aplasia cutis congenita with dystrophic nail changes. *Dermatologica* 1976;153:363.

141. Levin DL, Nolan KS, Esterly NB. Congenital absence of skin. *J Am Acad Dermatol* 1980;2:203.

142. Frieden IJ. Aplasia cutis congenita: a clinical review and proposal for classification. *J Am Acad Dermatol* 1986;14:646.

143. Deeken JH, Caplan RM. Aplasia cutis congenita. *Arch Dermatol* 1970;102:386.

144. Bart BJ. Epidermolysis bullosa and congenital localized absence of skin. *Arch Dermatol* 1970;101:78.

145. Lindor NM, Furuichi Y, Kiato S, et al. Rothman–Thomson syndrome due to RECQ4 helicase mutations: report andclinical and molecular comparisons with Bloom's and Werner's syndromes. *Am J Med Genet* 2000;90:223.

146. Rook A, Davis R, Stevanovic D. Poikiloderma congenitale: Rothmund–Thomson syndrome (review). *Acta Derm Venereol Suppl (Stockh)* 1959;39:392.

147. Venos EM, Collins M, Jane WD. Rothmund–Thomson syndrome: review of the world literature. *J Am Acad Dermatol* 1992;27:750.

148. Dick DC, Morley WN, Watson JT. Rothmund–Thomson syndrome and osteogenic sarcoma. *Clin Exp Dermatol* 1982;7:119.

149. Nakura J, Ye L, Morishima A, et al. Helicases and aging. *Cell Mol Life Sci* 2000;57:716.
150. Gretzula JL, Hevia O, Weber PJ. Bloom's syndrome. *J Am Acad Dermatol* 1987;17:479.
151. Braun-Falco O, Marghescu S. Kongenitales telangiektatisches erythem (Bloom syndrom) mit diabetes insipidus. *Hautarzt* 1966;17:155.
152. Landau IW, Sasaki MS, Newcomer VD, et al. Bloom's syndrome. *Arch Dermatol* 1966;94:687.
153. Bloom D, German J. The syndrome of congenital telangiectatic erythema and stunted growth. *Arch Dermatol* 1971;103:545.
154. Dicken CH, Dewald G, Gordon H. Sister chromatid exchanges in Bloom's syndrome. *Arch Dermatol* 1978;114:755.
155. Sawitsky A, Bloom D, German J. Chromosomal breakage and acute leukemia in congenital telangiectatic erythema and stunted growth. *Ann Intern Med* 1966;65:487.
156. Swift M, Morrell D, Massey RB, et al. Incidence of cancer in 161 families affected by ataxia-telangiectasia. *N Engl J Med* 1991;325:1831.
157. Gschnait F, Grabner G, Brenner W, et al. Ataxia telangiectatica (Louis–Bar syndrom). *Hautarzt* 1979;30:527.
158. Smith LL, Conerly SL. Ataxia telangiectasia or Louis–Bar syndrome. *J Am Acad Dermatol* 1985;12:681.
159. McFarlin DE, Strober W, Waldmann TA. Ataxia-telangiectasia (review). *Medicine (Baltimore)* 1972;51:281.
160. Carbonari M, Cherc M, Paganelli R, et al. Relative increase of T cells expressing the gamma/delta rather than the alpha/beta receptor in ataxia-telangiectasia. *N Engl J Med* 1990;322:73.
161. Spacey SD, Gatti RA, Bebb G. The molecular basis and clinical management of ataxia telangiectasia. *Can J Neurol Sci* 2000;27:184.
162. Epstein CJ, Martin GM, Schultz AL, et al. Werner's syndrome (review). *Medicine (Baltimore)* 1966;45:177.
163. Tritsch H, Lischka G. Werner's Syndrom, kombiniert mit Pseudo-Klinefelter syndrom. *Hautarzt* 1968;19:547.
164. Fleischmajer R, Nedwich A. Werner's syndrome. *Am J Med* 1973;54:111.
165. Bauer EA, Silverman N, Busiek D, et al. Diminished response of Werner's syndrome fibroblasts to growth factors PDFG and FGF. *Science* 1986;234:1240.
166. Fine JD. Editorial: changing clinical and laboratory concepts in inherited epidermolysis bullosa. *Arch Dermatol* 1988;124:523.
167. Buchbinder LH, Lucky AW, Dallard E, et al. Severe infantile epidermolysis bullosa simplex: Dowling–Meara type. *Arch Dermatol* 1986;122:190.
168. Haber RM, Hanna W, Ramsay CA, et al. Cicatricial junctional epidermolysis bullosa. *J Am Acad Dermatol* 1985;12:836.
169. Hashimoto K, Matsumoto M, Iacobelli D. Transient bullous dermolysis of the newborn. *Arch Dermatol* 1985;121:1429.
170. Fisher GB Jr, Greer KE, Cooper PH. Congenital self-healing (transient) mechanobullous dermatosis. *Arch Dermatol* 1988;124:240.
171. Bart BJ, Gorlin RJ, Anderson VE, et al. Congenital localized absence of skin and associated abnormalities resembling epidermolysis bullosa. *Arch Dermatol* 1966;93:296.
172. Voss M. Epidermolysis bullosa dystrophica Bart (Bart-Syndrom). *Hautarzt* 1985;36:351.
173. Smith SZ, Cram DL. A mechanobullous disease of the newborn: Bart's syndrome. *Arch Dermatol* 1978;114:81.
174. Eady RAJ, Tidman MJ. Diagnosing epidermolysis bullosa [Comment]. *Br J Dermatol* 1983;108:621.
175. Haneke E, Anton-Lamprecht I. Ultrastructure of blister formation in epidermolysis bullosa hereditaria: V. Epidermolysis bullosa simplex localisata type Weber–Cockayne. *J Invest Dermatol* 1982;78:219.
176. Anton-Lamprecht I, Schnyder UW. Epidermolysis bullosa Dowling–Meara. *Dermatologica* 1982;164:221.
177. Medenic A, Mojsilovic L, Fenske NA, et al. Epidermolysis bullosa herpetiformis with mottled pigmentation and an unusual punctate keratoderma. *Arch Dermatol* 1986;122:900.
178. Hintner H, Stingl G, Schuler G, et al. Immunofluorescence mapping of antigen determinants within the dermal-epidermal junction in mechanobullous diseases. *J Invest Dermatol* 1981;76:113.
179. Pearson RW. The mechanobullous diseases. In: Fitzpatrick TB, Amdt KA, Clark WH Jr, et al., eds. *Dermatology in General Medicine*. New York: McGraw-Hill, 1971:621.
180. Schachner L, Lazarus GS, Dembitzer H. Epidermolysis bullosa hereditaria letalis. *Br J Dermatol* 1977;96:51.
181. Lowe LB. Hereditary epidermolysis bullosa. *Arch Dermatol* 1967;95:587.
182. Paller AS, Fine JD, Kaplan S, et al. The generalized atrophic benign form of junctional epidermolysis bullosa. *Arch Dermatol* 1986;122:704.
183. Bergenholtz A, Olsson O. Die epidermolysis bullosa hereditaria dystrophica mit oesophagusveranderungen. *Arch Klin Exp Dermatol* 1963;271:518.
184. Reed WB, College J Jr, Prancis MJO, et al. Epidermolysis bullosa dystrophica with epidermal neoplasms. *Arch Dermatol* 1974;110:894.
185. Epstein EH. Molecular basis of epidermolysis bullosa. *Science* 1992;256:799.
186. Oakley CA, Wilson N, Ross JA, et al. Junctional epidermolysis bullosa in two siblings: clinical observations, collagen studies, and electron microscopy. *Br J Dermatol* 1984;111:533.
187. Tidman MJ, Eady RAJ. Hemidesmosome heterogeneity in junctional epidermolysis bullosa revealed by morphometric analysis. *J Invest Dermatol* 1986;86:51.
188. Matsumoto M, Hashimoto K. Blister fluid from epidermolysis bullosa letalis induces dermal-epidermal separation *in vitro*. *J Invest Dermatol* 1986;87:117.
189. McGrath JA, Pulkkinen L, Christiano AM, et al. Altered lamin-5 expression due to mutations in the gene encoding the beta-3 chain (LAMB 3) in generalized atrophic benign epidermolysis bullosa. *J Invest Dermatol* 1995;104:467.
190. Pulkkinen L, Uitto J. Mutation analysis and molecular genetics of epidermolysis bullosa. *Matrix Biol* 1999;18:29.
191. Tidman MJ, Eady RAJ. Evaluation of anchoring fibrils and other components of the dermal-epidermal junction in dystrophic epidermolysis bullosa by a quantitative ultrastructural technique. *J Invest Dermatol* 1985;84:374.
192. Goldsmith LA, Briggaman RA. Monoclonal antibodies to anchoring fibrils for the diagnosis of epidermolysis bullosa. *J Invest Dermatol* 1983;81:464.
193. Bruckner-Tuderman L, Ruegger S, Odermatt B, et al. Lack of type VII collagen in unaffected skin of patients with severe recessive dystrophic epidermolysis bullosa. *Dermatologica* 1988;176:57.
194. Nanchahal J, Tidman MJ. A study of the dermo-epidermal junction in dystrophic epidermolysis bullosa using the periodic add-thiosemicarbazide-silver proteinate technique. *Br J Dermatol* 1985;113:397.
195. Uitto J, Christiano AM. Molecular basis for the dystrophic forms of epidermolysis bullosa: mutations in the type VII collagen gene. *Arch Dermatol Res* 1994;287:16.
196. Dunhill MGS, Richards AJ, Milana G, et al. Genetic linkage to the type VII collagen gene (COL7A1) in 26 families with generalized recessive dystrophic epidermolysis bullosa and anchoring fibril abnormalities. *J Med Genet* 1994;31:745.
197. Lacour JP, Bernard P, Rostain G, et al. Childhood acquired epidermolysis bullosa. *Pediatr Dermatol* 1995;12:16.

198. Gammon WR, Briggaman RA, Woodley DT, et al. Epidermolysis acquisita: a pemphigoid-like disease. *J Am Acad Dermatol* 1984;11:820.

199. Woodley DT. Immunofluoresence on salt-split skin for the diagnosis of epidermolysis bullosa acquisita. *Arch Dermatol* 1990; 126:229.

200. Valeski JE, Kumar V, Beutner EH, et al. Differentation of bullous pemphigoid from epidermolysis bullosa acquisita on frozen skin biopsies. *Int J Dermatol* 1992;31:37.

201. Pang BK, Lee YS, Ratnam VK. Floor pattern salt-split skin cannot distinguish bullous pemphigoid from epidermolysis bullosa acquisita: use of toad skin. *Arch Dermatol* 1993;129:744.

202. Gammon WR, Briggaman RA. The incidence of epidermolysis bullosa acquisita among patients diagnosed as bullous pemphigoid. *J Invest Dermatol* 1984;2:407(abst).

203. Dahl MGC. Epidermolysis bullosa acquisita: a sign of cicatricial pemphigoid. *Br J Dermatol* 1979;101:475.

204. Fine JD, Neiser GR, Katz SI. Immunofluorescence and immunoelectron microscopic studies in cicatricial pemphigoid. *J Invest Dermatol* 1984;82:39.

205. Pardo R, Penneys N. The location of basement membrane type IV collagen in subepidermal bullous diseases. *J Cutan Pathol* 1988;15:334(abst).

206. Peluso AM, Bonifast J, Ikeda S, et al. Hailey–Hailey disease sublocalization of the gene on chromosome 3Q and identification of a kindred with an apparent deletion. *J Invest Dermatol* 1995;104:598.

207. Hu Z, Bonifas JM, Beech J, et al. Mutations in ATP2Cl, encoding a calcium pump, cause Hailey–Hailey Disease. *Nat Genet* 2000;24:61.

208. Botvinick I. Familial benign pemphigus with oral mucous membrane lesions. *Cutis* 1973;12:371.

209. Heinze R. Pemphigus chronicus benignus familiaris (Gougerot/Hailey–Hailey) mit schleimhautbeteiligung bei einer diabehkerin. *Dermatol Monatsschr* 1979;165:862.

210. Kahn D, Hutchinson E. Esophageal involvement in familial benign chronic pemphigus. *Arch Dermatol* 1974;109:718.

211. Winer LH, Leeb AJ. Benign familial pemphigus. *Arch Dermatol* 1953;67:77.

212. Herzberg JJ. Pemphigus Gougerot/Hailey–Hailey *Arch Klin Exp Dermatol* 1955;202:21.

213. Ellis FA. Vesicular Darier's disease (so-called benign familial pemphigus). *Arch Dermatol Syph* 1950;61:715.

214. Niordson AM, Sylvest B. Bullous dyskeratosis follicularis and acrokeratosis verruciformis. *Arch Dermatol* 1965;92:166.

215. Nicolis G, Tosca A, Marouli O, et al. Keratosis follicularis and familial benign chronic pemphigus in the same patient. *Dermatologica* 1979;159:346.

216. Ferris T, Lamey PJ, Rennies JS. Darier's disease: oral features and genetic aspects. *Br Dent J* 1990;168:71.

217. Panja RK. Acrokeratosis verruciformis (Hopf): a clinical entity? *Br J Dermatol* 1977;96:643.

218. Wheeland RG, Gilmore WA. The surgical treatment of hypertrophic Darier's disease. *J Dermatol Surg Oncol* 1985;11:420.

219. Piérard J, Geerts ML, Vandeputte H, et al. A propos de quelques cas de dyskeratose folliculaire. *Arch Belg Dermatol* 1968;24:381.

220. Hori Y, Tsuru N, Niimura M. Bullous Darier's disease. *Arch Dermatol* 1982;118:278.

221. Demetree JW, Lang PG, St Clair JT. Unilateral, linear, zosteriform epidermal nevus with acantholytic dyskeratosis. *Arch Dermatol* 1979;115:875.

222. Starink TM, Woerdeman MJ. Unilateral systematized keratosis follicularis: a variant of Darier's disease or an epidermal nevus (acantholytic dyskeratotic epidermal nevus)? *Br J Dermatol* 1981;105:207.

223. Fishman HC. Acute, eruptive Darier's disease (keratosis follicularis). *Arch Dermatol* 1975;111:221.

224. Burge SM, Wilkerson JD. Darier–White disease: a review of the clinical features in 163 patients. *J Am Acad Dermatol* 1992; 27:40.

225. Sato A, Anton-Lamprecht I, Schnyder UW. Ultrastructure of dyskeratosis in Morbus Darier. *J Cutan Pathol* 1977;4:173.

226. Piérard J, Kint A. Die Dariersche krankheit. *Arch Klin Exp Dermatol* 1968;231:382.

227. Krinitz K. Tumorose veranderungen bei Morbus Darier. *Hautarzt* 1966;7:445.

228. Weathers DR, Olansky S, Sharpe LO. Darier's disease with mucous membrane involvement. *Arch Dermatol* 1969;100:50.

229. Mann PR, Haye KR. An electron microscope study on the acantholytic and dyskeratotic processes in Darier's disease. *Br J Dermatol* 1970;82:561.

230. Biagini G, Costa AM, Laschi R. An electron microscope study of Darier's disease. *J Cutan Pathol* 1975;2:47.

231. De Dobbeleer G, Achten G. Disrupted desmosomes in induced lesions of familial benign chronic pemphigus. *J Cutan Pathol* 1979;6:418.

232. Caulfield JB, Wilgram GF. An electron-microscope study of dyskeratosis and acantholysis in Darier's disease. *J Invest Dermatol* 1963;41:57.

233. Wilgram GF, Caulfield JB, Lever WF. An electron microscopic study of acantholysis and dyskeratosis in Hailey and Hailey's disease. *J Invest Dermatol* 1962;39:373.

234. Gottlieb SK, Lutzner MA. Hailey–Hailey disease: an electron microscopic study. *J Invest Dermatol* 1970;54:368.

235. Abell E. Immunopathological investigation of glycocalyx material in Darier's and Hailey–Hailey disease. *J Invest Dermatol* 1983;80:355(abst).

236. Ishibashi Y, Kajiwara Y, Andoh I, et al. The nature and pathogenesis of dyskeratosis in Hailey–Hailey's disease and Darier's disease. *J Dermatol* 1984;11:335.

237. Sakuntabhai A, Ruiz-Perez V, Carter S, et al. Mutations in ATP2A2, encoding a Ca 2+ pupm, cause Darier's disease. *Nat Genet* 1999;21:271.

238. Gottlieb SK, Lutzner MA. Darier's disease. *Arch Dermatol* 1973;107:225.

239. Lachapelle JM, De La Brassinne M, Geerts MI. Maladies de Darier et de Hailey–Hailey: etude comparative de l'incorporation dethymidine tritiee dans les cellules epidermiques. *Arch Belg Dermatol* 1973;29:241.

240. Pierard-Franchimont C, Pierard GE. Suprabasal acantholysis. *Am J Dermatopathol* 1983;5:421.

241. Ackerman AB. Focal acantholytic dyskeratosis. *Arch Dermatol* 1972;106:702.

242. Palmer DD, Perry HO. Benign familial chronic pemphigus. *Arch Dermatol* 1962;86:493.

243. Schanne R, Burg G, Braun-Falco O. Zur nosologischen beziehung der dyskeratosis follicularis (Darier) und des pemphigus benignus chronicus familiaris (Hailey–Hailey). *Hautarzt* 1985;36:504.

244. Panja RK. Acrokeratosis verruciformis (Hopf): a clinical entity? *Br J Dermatol* 1977;96:643.

245. Waisman M. Verruciform manifestations of keratosis follicularis. *Arch Dermatol* 1960;81:1.

246. Schueller WA. Acrokeratosis verruciformis of Hopf. *Arch Dermatol* 1972;106:81.

247. Niedelman ML, McKusick VA. Acrokeratosis verruciformis (Hopf). *Arch Dermatol* 1962;86:779.

248. Penrod JN, Everett MA, McCreight WG. Observations on keratosis follicularis. *Arch Dermatol* 1960;82:367.

249. Beerman H. In discussion of Waisman M: verruciform manifestations of keratosis follicularis. *Arch Dermatol* 1960;81:1.

250. Herndon JH Jr, Wilson JD. Acrokeratosis verruciformis (Hopf) and Darier's disease. *Arch Dermatol* 1966;93:305.

251. Pope FM. Historical evidence for the genetic heterogeneity of pseudoxanthoma elasticum. *Br J Dermatol* 1975;92:493.

252. Struk B, Neldner KH, Rao VS, et al. Mapping of both autosomal recessive and dominant variants of Pseudoxanthoma elasticum to chromosome 16p13.1. *Hum Mol Genet* 1997;6:1823.

253. Pope FM. Two types of autosomal recessive pseudoxanthoma elasticum. *Arch Dermatol* 1974;110:209.

254. Lebwohl M, Nelder K, Pope M, et al. Classification of pseudoxanthoma elasticum: report of a consensus conference. *J Am Acad Dermatol* 1994;30:103.

255. Mendelsohn G, Bulkley BH, Hutchins GM. Cardiovascular manifestations of pseudoxanthoma elasticum. *Arch Pathol* 1978; 102:298.

256. Eddy DD, Farber EM. Pseudoxanthoma elasticum. *Arch Dermatol* 1962;86:729.

257. Caro J, Sher A, Rippey JJ. Pseudoxanthoma elasticum and elastosis perforans serpiginosum. *Dermatologica* 1975;150:36.

258. Huang SN, Steele HD, Iqumar G, et al. Ultrastructural changes of elastic fibers in pseudoxanthoma elasticum. *Arch Pathol* 1967;83:108.

259. Danielsen L, Kohayasi T, Larsen HW, et al. Pseudoxanthoma elasticum. *Acta Derm Venereol Suppl (Stockh)* 1970;50:355.

260. Goodman RM, Smith EW, Paton D, et al. Pseudoxanthoma elasticum: a clinical and histopathological study (review). *Medicine (Baltimore)* 1963;42:297.

261. Kreysel HW, Lerche W, Janner M. Beobachtungen zum Gronblad-Strandberg-Syndrom (angioid streaks, pseudoxanthoma elasticum). *Hautarzt* 1967;8:24.

262. Akhtar M, Brody H. Elastic tissue in pseudoxanthoma elasticum: ultrastructural study of endocardial lesions. *Arch Pathol* 1975;99:667.

263. Hashimoto K, Dibella RJ. Electron microscopic studies of normal and abnormal elastic fibers of the skin. *J Invest Dermatol* 1967;48:405.

264. Martinez-Hernandez A, Huffer WE. Pseudoxanthoma elasticum: dermal polyanions and the mineralization of elastic fibers. *Lab Invest* 1974;31:181.

265. McKee PH, Cameron CHS, Archer DB, et al. A study of four cases of pseudoxanthoma elasticum. *J Cutan Pathol* 1977;4:146.

266. Saito Y, Klingmuller G. Elektronmikroskopische untersuchungen zur morphogenese elastischer fasern bei der senilen elastose und dem pseudoxanthoma elasticum. *Arch Dermatol Res* 1977;260:179.

267. Danielsen L, Kobayasi T, Jacobsen GK. Ultrastructural changes in disseminated connective tissue nevi. *Acta Derm Venereol Suppl (Stockh)* 1977;57:93.

268. Uitto J, Santa-Cruz J, Eisen AZ. Familial cutaneous collagenoma: genetic studies on a family. *Br J Dermatol* 1979;101: 185.

269. Morrison JGL, Wilson Jones E, Macdonald DM. Juvenile elastoma: the Buschke–Ollendorff syndrome. *Br J Dermatol* 1977; 97:417.

270. Kobayasi T, Wolf-Jurgensen P, Danielsen L. Ultrastructure of shagreen patch. *Acta Derm Venereol Suppl (Stockh)* 1973;53:275.

271. Schorr WF, Opitz JM, Reyes CN. The connective tissue nevus: osteopoikilosis syndrome. *Arch Dermatol* 1972;106:208.

272. Nevin NC, Thomas PS, Davis RI, et al. Melorheostosis in a family with autosomal dominant osteopoikilosis. *Am J Med Genet* 1999;82:409.

273. Cole GW, Barr RJ. An elastic tissue defect in dermatofibrosis lenticularis disseminata. *Arch Dermatol* 1982;118:44.

274. Verbov J, Graham R. Buschke–Ollendorff syndrome: disseminated dermatofibrosis with osteopoikilosis. *Clin Exp Dermatol* 1986;11:17.

275. Buschke A, Ollendorff H. Ein fall von dermatofibrosis lenticularis disseminata und osteopathia condensans disseminata. *Dermatol Wochenschr* 1928;86:257.

276. Reymond JL, Stoebner P, Beani JC, et al. Buschke–Ollendorf syndrome: an electron microscopic study. *Dermatologica* 1983; 166:64.

277. Miyachi Y, Hori OT, Yamada A, et al. Linear melorheostotic scleroderma with hypertrichosis. *Arch Dermatol* 1979;115:1233.

278. Wagers LT, Young AW Jr, Ryan SF. Linear melorheostotic scleroderma. *Br J Dermatol* 1972;86:297.

279. Winter RM. Winchester syndrome. *J Med Genet* 1989;26:772.

280. Cohen AH, Hollister DW, Reed WB. The skin in the Winchester syndrome. *Arch Dermatol* 1975;111:230.

281. Nabai H, Mehregan AH, Mortezai A, et al. Winchester syndrome: report of a case from Iran. *J Cutan Pathol* 1977;4:281.

282. Wenstrup RJ, Florer JB, Willing MC, et al. Haplo-insufficiency for COL5A1 expression is a common molecular mechanism underlying the classical form Ehlers Danlos syndrome. *Am J Hum Genet* 2000;66:1766.

283. McFarland W, Fuller DE. Mortality in Ehlers Danlos syndrome due to spontaneous rupture of large arteries. *N Engl J Med* 1964;271:1309.

284. DeFelice C, Toto P, DiMaggio G, et al. Absence of the inferior labial and lingual frenula in Ehlers Danlos syndrome. *Lancet* 2001;357:1500.

285. Burrows NP, Nichols AC, Yates JRW, et al. The gene encoding collagen alpha IV COL5A1 is linked to mixed Ehlers–Danlos syndrome type I/II. *Invest Dermatol* 1996;106:1273.

286. Richards AJ, Martin S, Nichols AC, et al. A single base mutation in COL5A2 causes Ehlers–Danlos syndrome type II. *J Med Genet* 1998;35:846.

287. Narcisi P, Richards AJ, Ferguson SD, et al. A family with Ehlers–Danlos syndrome type II/articular hypermobility syndrome has a glycine 637 to serene substitution in type III collagen. *Hum Genet* 1994;3:1617.

288. Temple AS, Hinton P, Narcisi P, et al. Detection of type III collagen in skin fibroblasts from patients with Ehlers–Danlos syndrome type IV by immunofluorescence. *Br J Dermatol* 1988; 118:17.

289. Pinnell SR, Crane SM, Kenzora JE, et al. A heritable disorder of connective tissue. *N Engl J Med* 1972;286:1013.

290. Prockop DJ, Kivirikko KL, Tuderman L, et al. The biosynthesis of collagen and its disorders. *N Engl J Med* 1979;301:77.

291. Byers PH, Davic M, Atkinson M, et al. Ehlers–Danlos syndrome type VIIA and VIIB result from splice-junction mutations or genomic deletions that involve exon6 in the COL1A1 and COL1A2 genes of type I collagen. *Am J Med Genet* 1997; 72:94.

292. Colige A, Sieron Al, Li SW, et al. Human Ehlers–Danlos syndrome type IIIC and bovine dermatosparaxis are caused by mutations in the procollagen 1N-proteinase gene. *Am J Hum Genet* 1999;65:308.

293. Das S, Levinson B, Vulpe C, et al. Similar splicing mutations of Menkes/mottled copper transporting ATPase gene in occipitap horn syndrome and the blotchy mouse. *Am J Hum Genet* 1995; 56:570.

294. Sulica VL, Cooper PH, Pope FM, et al. Cutaneous histologic features in Ehlers–Danlos syndrome. *Arch Dermatol* 1979;115: 40.

295. Pierard GE, Pierard-Franchimont C, Lapiere CM. Histopathological aid at the diagnosis of the Ehlers–Danlos syndrome, gravis and mitis types. *Int J Dermatol* 1983;22:300.

296. Pope FM, Nicholls AC, Narcisi P, et al. Type III collagen mutations in Ehlers–Danlos syndrome type IV and other related disorders. *Clin Exp Dermatol* 1988;13:285.

297. Ronchese F. Dermatorrhexis. *Am J Dis Child* 1936;51:1403.

298. Cullin SI. Localized Ehlers–Danlos syndrome. *Arch Dermatol* 1979;115:332.

299. Wechsler HL, Fisher ER. Ehlers–Danlos syndrome. *Arch Pathol* 1964;77:613.

300. Black CM, Gathercole LJ, Bailey AJ, et al. The Ehlers–Danlos syndrome: an analysis of the structure of the collagen fibres of the skin. *Br J Dermatol* 1980;102:85.

301. Scarpelli DG, Goodman RM. Observations on the fine structure of the fibroblast from a case of Ehlers–Danlos syndrome with the Marfan syndrome. *J Invest Dermatol* 1968;50:214.

302. Sevenich M, Schultz-Ehrenburg U, Orfanos CE. Ehlers–Danlos syndrome eine fibroblasten-und kollagenkrankheit. *Arch Dermatol Res* 1980;267:237.

303. Goltz RW, Hult AM, Goldfarb M, et al. Cutis laxa. *Arch Dermatol* 1965;92:373.

304. Zhang MC, He L, Yong SL, et al. Cutis laxa arising from a frame shift mutation in the elastic gene. *Am J Genet* 1997; 61[Suppl]:A353.

305. Reed WB, Horowitz RE, Beighton P. Acquired cutis laxa. *Arch Dermatol* 1971;103:661.

306. Hashimoto K, Kanzaki T. Cutis laxa. *Arch Dermatol* 1975;111: 861.

307. Scott MA, Kauh YC, Luscome HA. Acquired cutis laxa associated with multiple myeloma. *Arch Dermatol* 1976;112:853.

308. Khakoo A, Thomas R, Trompeter R. Congenital cutis laxa and lysyl oxidase deficiency. *Clin Genet* 1997;51:109.

309. Nanko H, Jepsen LV, Zachariae H, et al. Acquired cutis laxa (generalized elastolysis). *Acta Derm Venereol Suppl (Stockh)* 1979;59:315.

310. Kerl H, Burg G, Hashimoto K. Fatal, penicillin-induced, generalized, postinflammatory elastolysis (cutis laxa). *Am J Dermatopathol* 1983;5:267.

311. Reed WB, Horowitz RE, Beighton P. Acquired cutis laxa. *Arch Dermatol* 1971;103:661.

312. Ledoux-Corbusier M. Cutis laxa, congenital form with pulmonary emphysema: an ultrastructural study. *J Cutan Pathol* 1983; 10:340.

313. Sayers CP, Goltz RW, Mottaz J. Pulmonary elastic tissue in generalized elastolysis (cutis laxa) and Marfan's syndrome. *J Invest Dermatol* 1975;65:451.

314. Harris RB, Heapy MR, Perry HO. Generalized elastolysis (cutis laxa). *Am J Med* 1979;65:815.

315. Rimoin DL. Pachydermoperiostosis (idiopathic cubbing and periostosis). *N Engl J Med* 1965;272:923.

316. Curth HO, Firschein IL, Alpert M. Familial clubbed fingers. *Arch Dermatol* 1961;83:828.

317. Hambrick GW, Carter DM. Pachydermoperiostosis. *Arch Dermatol* 1966;94:594.

318. Shaw JM. Genetic aspects of urticaria pigmentosa. *Arch Dermatol* 1968;97:137.

319. Bazex A, Dupre A, Christol B, et al. Les mastocytoses familiales. *Ann Dermatol Syphiligra* 1971;98:241.

320. Rosbotham JL, Malik NM, Syrris P, et al. Lack of a c-Kit mutation in familial urticaria pigmentosa. *Br J Dermatol* 1999;140: 849.

321. Kettelhut BV, Metcalfe DD. Pediatric mastocytosis. *Ann Allergy* 1994;73:197.

322. Longley J, Duffy TP, Kohn S. The mast cell and mast cell disease. *J Am Acad Dermatol* 1995;32:545.

323. Klaus SN, Winkelmann RK. Course of urticaria pigmentosa in children. *Arch Dermatol* 1962;86:68.

324. Iwatsuki K, Tadahiro A, Tagami H, et al. Immunofluorescent study in purpura pigmentosa chronica. *Acta Derm Venereol Suppl (Stockh)* 1980;60:341.

325. Caplan RM. The natural course of urticaria pigmentosa. *Arch Dermatol* 1963;6.

326. Roberts PL, McDonald HB, Wells RF. Systemic mast cell disease in a patient with unusual gastrointestinal and pulmonary abnormalities. *Am J Med* 1968;45:638.

327. Friedman BL, Will JJ, Freidman DG, et al. Tissue mast cell leukemia. *Blood* 1958;13:70.

328. Horny HP, Parwaresch MR, Lennert K. Bone marrow findings in systemic mastocytosis. *Hum Pathol* 1985;16:808.

329. Baraf CS, Shapiro L. Solitary mastocytoma. *Arch Dermatol* 1969;99:589.

330. Orkin M, Good RA, Clawson CC, et al. Bullous mastocytosis. *Arch Dermatol* 1970;101:547.

331. Welch EA, Alper JC, Bogaars H, et al. Treatment of bullous mastocytosis with disodium cromoglycate. *J Am Acad Dermatol* 1983;9:349.

332. Allison J. Skin mastocytosis presenting as a neonatal bullous eruption. *Australas J Dermatol* 1967;9:83.

333. Cramer JH. Telangiectasia macularis eruptiva perstans, eine sonderform der urticaria pigmentosa. *Hautarzt* 1964;15:370.

334. Wong E, Morgan EW, MacDonald DM. The chloroacetate esterase reaction for mast cells in dermatopathology. *Acta Derm Venereol Suppl (Stockh)* 1982;62:431.

335. Mihm MC, Clark WH, Reed RJ, et al. Mast cell infiltrates of the skin and the mastocytosis syndrome. *Hum Pathol* 1973;4: 231.

336. Johnson WC, Helwig EB. Solitary mastocytosis (urtcaria pigmentosa). *Arch Dermatol* 1961;84:806.

337. Braun-Falco O, Jung J. Uber klinische und experimentelle beobachtungen bei einem fall von diffuser haut-mastocytose. *Arch Klin Exp Dermatol* 1961;39.

338. Drennan JM. The mast cells in urticaria pigmentosa. *J Pathol Bacteriol* 1951;63:513.

339. Miller RO, Shapiro L. Bullous urticaria pigmentosa in infancy. *Arch Dermatol* 1965;91:595.

340. Dewar WA, Milene JA. Bullous urticaria pigmentosa. *Arch Dermatol* 1955;71:717.

341. Rodermund OR, Klingmuller G, Rohner HG. Interne befunde bei mastozytose. *Hautarzt* 1980;31:175.

342. Sostre S, Handler HL. Bony lesions in systemic mastocytosis. *Arch Dermatol* 1977;113:1245.

343. Naveh Y, Ludatscher R, Gellei B, et al. Ultrastructural features of mast cells in systemic mastocytosis. *Acta Derm Venereol Suppl (Stockh)* 1970;55:443.

344. Monheit GD, Murad T, Conrad M. Systemic mastocytosis and the mastocytosis syndrome. *J Cutan Pathol* 1979;6:42.

345. Freeman RG. Diffuse urticaria pigmentosa. *Am J Clin Pathol* 1967;48:187.

346. Hashomoto K, Gross BG, Lever WF. An electron microscopic study of the degranulation of mast cell granules in urticaria pigmentosa. *J Invest Dermatol* 1966;46:139.

347. Davis MJ, Lawler JC, Higdon RS. Studies on an adult with urticaria pigmentosa. *Arch Dermatol* 1958;77:224.

348. Okun MR, Bhawan J. Combined melanocytoma-mastocytoma in a case of nodular mastocytosis. *J Am Acad Dermatol* 1979; 1:338.

349. Mixhail GR, Miller-Milinska A. Mast cell population in human skin. *J Invest Dermatol* 1964;43:249.

350. Gordon H, Gordon W. Incontinentia pigmenti: clinical and genetical studies of two familial cases. *Dermatologica* 1961;140: 150.

351. Carney RG Jr. Incontinentia pigmenti: a world statistical analysis. *Arch Dermatol* 1976;112:535.

352. Wijker M, Ligtenberg MJL, Schoute F, et al. The gene for hereditary bullous dystrophy: X-linked macular type maps to the XQ27.3 region. *Am J Hum Genet* 1995;56:1096.

353. International Incontinentia Pigmenti Consortium. Genomic rearrangement in NEMO impairs NF-kappaB activation and is a cause of incontinentia pigmenti. *Nature* 2000;405:466.

354. Dutheil P, Valpres P, Hors Cayla MC, et al. Incontinentia pigmenti late sequelae and genotypic diagnosis: a three generation study of four patients. *Pediatr Dermatol* 1995;12:107.
355. Epstein S, Vedder IS, Pinkus H. Bullous variety of incontinentia pigmenti (Bloch–Sulzberger). *Arch Dermatol Syph* 1952;65:557.
356. Sultzberger MB. Incontinentia pigmenti (Bloch–Sulzberger). *Arch Dermatol Syph* 1938;38:57.
357. Vilanova X, Aguade JP. Incontinentia pigmenti. *Ann Dermatol Syphiligra* 1959;86:247.
358. Rubin L, Becker SW Jr. Pigmentation in the Bloch–Sulzberger syndrome (incontinentia pigmenti). *Arch Dermatol* 1956;74:263.
359. Ashley JR, Burgdorf WHC. Incontinentia pigmenti: pigmentary changes independent of incontinence. *J Cutan Pathol* 1987;14:248.
360. Schaumburg-Lever G, Lever WF. Electron microscopy of incontinentia pigmenti. *J Invest Dermatol* 1973;61:151.
361. Gurrier LJW, Wong CK. Ultrastructural evolution of the skin in incontinentia pigmenti (Bloch–Sulzberger). *Dermatologica* 1974;149:10.
362. Caputo R, Gianotti F, Innocenti M. Ultrastructural findings in incontinentia pigmenti. *Int J Dermatol* 1975;14:46.
363. Schmalstieg FC, Jorizzo JL, Tschen J, et al. Basophils in incontinentia pigmenti. *J Am Acad Dermatol* 1984;10:362.
364. Tsuda S, Higushi M, Ichiki M, et al. Demonstration of eosinophil chemotactic factor in the blister fluid of patients with incontinentia pigmenti. *J Dermatol* 1985;12:363.
365. Takematsu H, Terui T, Torinuki W, et al. Incontinentia pigmenti: eosinophil chemotactic activity of the crusted scales in the vesiculobullous stage. *Br J Dermatol* 1986;115:61.
366. Kaster W, Ehrig T, Happle R. Hyopmelanosis of Ito no entity but a cutaneous sign of mosacism. In: Nordlund JJ, BoisseyR, Hearings Y, et al., eds. *The Pigmenteary System and Its Disorders.* New York: Oxford University Press, 1988.
367. Sultzberger MB. Incontinentia pigmenti (Bloch–Sulzberger). *Arch Dermatol Syph* 1938;38:57.
368. Cambazard F, Hermier C, Thivol ET Jr, et al. Hypomelanose de Ito: revue de littérature à propos de 3 cas. *Ann Dermatol Venereol* 1986;113:15.
369. Sybert VP. Hypomelanosis of Ito: a description not a diagnosis. *Acta Dermatol Venerol Suppl (Stockh)* 1977;57:216.
370. Grosshans EM, Stoebner P, Bergoend H, et al. Incontinentia pigmenti achromians (Ito). *Dermatologica* 1971;142:65.
371. Nordlund JJ, Klaus SN, Gino J. Hypomelanosis of Ito. *Acta Derm Venereol Suppl (Stockh)* 1977;57:261.
372. Morohashi M, Hashimoto K, Goodman TF Jr, et al. Ultrastructural studies of vitiligo, Vogt–Koyanagi syndrome and incontinentia pigmenti achromians. *Arch Dermatol* 1977;113:755.

7

NONINFECTIOUS ERYTHEMATOUS, PAPULAR, AND SQUAMOUS DISEASES

NARCISS MOBINI
SONIA TOUSSAINT
HIDEKO KAMINO

URTICARIA

Urticaria is characterized by the presence of abrupt onset, transient and recurrent wheals, which are raised erythematous and edematous areas of skin that are often pruritic. When large wheals occur and the edema extends to the subcutaneous or submucosal tissues, the process is referred to as angioedema (1). Acute episodes of urticaria generally last only several hours. When episodes of urticaria last up to 24 hours and recur over a period of at least 6 to 8 weeks, the condition is considered chronic urticaria. When urticaria and angioedema occur simultaneously, the condition tends to have a chronic course.

In approximately 15% to 25% of patients with chronic urticaria, an eliciting stimulus or underlying predisposing condition can be identified (2). The various causes of urticaria include soluble antigens in foods, drugs, and insect venom; contact allergens; physical stimuli such as pressure, vibration, solar radiation, and cold temperature; occult infections and malignancies; and some hereditary syndromes such as familial cold urticaria and Muckle–Wells syndrome (amyloidosis, nerve deafness, and urticaria), both inherited as an autosomal dominant trait and linked to chromosome 1q44. Schnitzler syndrome is characterized by a chronic urticaria and a monoclonal gammopathy with evolution in 15% of patients to lymphoplasmacytic neoplasms (3).

Recent evidence suggests that at least 30% of chronic idiopathic urticarias may have an autoimmune basis for their condition (4,5). (See pathogenesis discussion.)

In *hereditary angioedema*, a rare form of dominantly inherited angioedema, recurrent attacks of edema involve not only the skin but also the oral, upper respiratory, and gastrointestinal tracts. Itching is absent and there is no associated urticaria. However, lesions may be painful. Attacks are commonly precipitated by trauma, such as dental extraction or by emotional stress. Patients may later manifest autoimmune disorders such as systemic or discoid lupus erythematosus.

Urticarial vasculitis is a syndrome consisting of recurrent episodes of urticarial lesions often associated with arthralgia and abdominal pain and rarely with glomerulonephritis and obstructive pulmonary disease (6). The individual skin lesions tend to persist for 1 to 3 days and may resolve with purpura or hyperpigmentation (7). Lesions in urticarial vasculitis are not necessarily acral in distribution. Urticarial vasculitis should be suspected when individual lesions persist for more than 24 hours and produce burning or stinging sensations (8). Urticarial vasculitis may be normo- or hypo-complementemic. The latter is less frequent and can occur in up to 30% of cases (9). Organ involvement is more common in hypocomplementemic urticarial vasculitis than in the normocomplementemic form (7). Urticarial vasculitis is usually idiopathic but may be associated with infectious mononucleosis, infectious hepatitis, serum sickness, systemic lupus erythematosus, Sjögren's syndrome, mixed cryoglobulinemia, polycythemia rubra vera (10), and B-cell lymphoma (11). Urticarial vasculitis may antedate other manifestations of collagen vascular disease by months or years (12). Accordingly, the appropriate serologic studies should be performed and periodically monitored.

Histopathology. In *acute urticaria* one observes interstitial dermal edema, dilated venules with endothelial swelling, and a paucity of inflammatory cells. In *chronic urticaria*, interstitial dermal edema and a perivascular and interstitial mixed-cell infiltrate with variable numbers of lymphocytes, eosinophils, and neutrophils are present (13) (Figs. 7-1 and 7-2).

In *angioedema*, the edema and infiltrate extend into the subcutaneous tissue. In *hereditary angioedema*, there is subcutaneous and submucosal edema without infiltrating inflammatory cells (14).

In *urticarial vasculitis*, the dermis shows an early leukocytoclastic vasculitis characterized by (a) an infiltrate predominantly within and around the walls of small blood vessels composed largely of neutrophils, some of which show fragmentation of their nuclei (leukocytoclasis); (b)

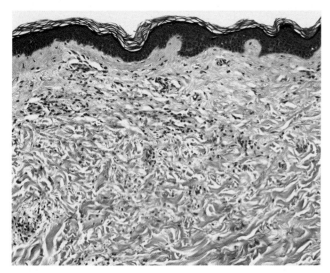

FIGURE 7-1. Urticaria. Sparse superficial perivascular and interstitial inflammatory infiltrate.

minimal to absent deposits of fibrin in the vessel walls; and (c) slight to moderate extravasation of erythrocytes (15).

Pathogenesis. On electron microscopic examination, common urticaria reveals mast cell and eosinophil degranulation. In chronic urticaria, IgG autoantibodies cross-link the alpha chain of the high-affinity receptor for IgE on mast cells (Fc epsilon RI), which results in histamine release. It appears that complement, especially C5a, augments histamine release (16,17). In addition, other chemotactic mediators are also released from mast cells, which induce a sequential up-regulation of endothelial adhesion molecules (P-selectin, E-selectin, ICAM-1, and VCAM-1) and of beta 2 integrins on leukocytes (18). The presence of these autoantibodies against Fc epsilon RI of the IgE receptor or IgE itself is detected in at least 30% of the patients with chronic urticaria.

Most patients with hereditary angioedema have a low serum level of the esterase inhibitor of the first component of complement (C1INH). Exhaustion of this inhibitor allows activation of C1. This leads to activation of C4 and C2, with the generation of a C2 fragment possessing kinin-like activity and causing increased vascular permeability (2). A smaller proportion of patients with hereditary angioedema have a deficit in functional C1-esterase inhibitor.

In urticarial vasculitis, circulating immune complexes are found in about one-half of the patients. By direct immunofluorescence testing, strong granular deposits of immunoreactants were seen along the dermoepidermal junction and perivascular areas (12,19). Positive immunofluorescence findings are more common in patients with the hypocomplementemic form of urticarial vasculitis (8). Renal biopsy in patients with hypocomplementemia frequently shows glomerulonephritis (6).

PRURITIC URTICARIAL PAPULES AND PLAQUES OF PREGNANCY

Pruritic urticarial papules and plaques of pregnancy (PUPPP) is a fairly common entity, first described in 1979 by Lawley et al. (20). The condition has a predilection for primigravidas in the third trimester of pregnancy. The rash usually starts on the abdomen and is composed of intensely pruritic erythematous urticarial papules, which may be surmounted by vesicles. The proximal parts of the extremities are also affected. There is no increased incidence of the rash in subsequent pregnancies (21). The rash usually involutes spontaneously after delivery. Fetal outcome appears to be unaffected.

Histopathology. Microscopic findings most commonly show a superficial and mid-dermal perivascular lymphohistiocytic infiltrate with variable numbers of eosinophils and neutrophils, together with edema of the superficial dermis. Epidermal involvement is variable and consists of focal spongiosis, parakeratosis, and mild acanthosis (20–22).

Pathogenesis. A possible correlation has been proposed between susceptibility to develop PUPPP and increased maternal weight gain, and twin/triplet pregnancies (23, 24). In cultures of human keratinocytes, lesional epidermis of PUPPP has shown positive progesterone receptor (PR) expression detected by immunohistochemistry and reverse transcriptase polymerase chain reaction (RT-PCR). Nonlesional epidermis however, has not revealed any PR positivity (25). In addition, a paternal factor hypothetically generated or expressed by the fetal portion of the placenta has been invoked as the cause of PUPPP in two families with unusual conjugal patterns (26). Direct immunofluo-

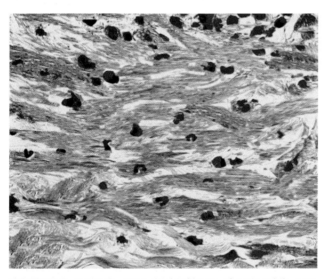

FIGURE 7-2. Urticaria. Interstitial infiltrate of eosinophils, neutrophils, and lymphocytes.

rescence studies may be negative or show nonspecific immunoreactants in the dermal blood vessels or at the dermoepidermal junction (27).

ERYTHEMA ANNULARE CENTRIFUGUM

Erythema annulare centrifugum is also known as gyrate erythema and represents a hypersensitivity reaction manifesting as arcuate and polycyclic areas of erythema. The condition has been categorized into superficial and deep variants. The deep form was originally described by Darier and is characterized by annular areas of palpable erythema with central clearing and absence of surface changes (28). The superficial variant differs only by the presence of a characteristic trailing scale, a delicate annular rim of scale that trails behind the advancing edge of erythema (29,30). Small vesicles may occur.

The lesions may attain considerable size (up to 10 cm across) over a period of several weeks, may be mildly pruritic, and have a predilection for the trunk and proximal extremities. Most cases resolve spontaneously within 6 weeks; however, the condition may persist or recur for years. In a recent study of 66 patients with erythema annulare centrifugum, the lower extremities were the most frequently involved area and the superficial variant was more common than the deep form, 78% versus 22%, respectively (31).

Histopathology. In the superficial variant of gyrate erythema, there is a superficial, perivascular, tightly cuffed

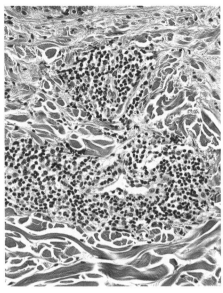

FIGURE 7-4. Gyrate erythema, deep form. Dense perivascular lymphocytic infiltrate.

lymphohistiocytic infiltrate with endothelial cell swelling and focal extravasation of erythrocytes in the papillary dermis. In addition, there are focal epidermal spongiosis and focal parakeratosis (29,30).

In the classic deep form or indurated type, a superficial and deep perivascular lymphocytic infiltrate characterized by a tightly cuffed "coat-sleeve–like" pattern is present in the mid and deep dermis (32) (Figs. 7-3 and 7-4).

Pathogenesis. The exact pathogenesis of erythema annulare centrifugum is not clear. Erythema annulare centrifugum has been associated with occult infections, dermatophytosis, candidiasis, medications, and, rarely, underlying malignancy such as lymphoma (33). The rash responds poorly to topical steroids. Treatment of any underlying disorder, if identifiable, is indicated.

Differential Diagnosis. The rather striking coat-sleeve–like perivascular arrangement of the infiltrate seen in the deep form of gyrate erythema is encountered also in secondary syphilis. However, in secondary syphilis numerous plasma cells and histiocytes are usually present, and the intima and endothelial cells are swollen. The presence of increased deposits of connective tissue mucin distinguishes tumid lupus erythematosus from deep gyrate erythema.

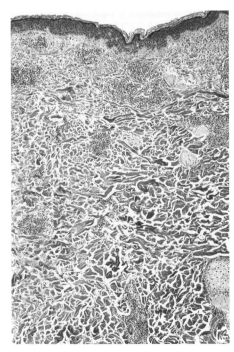

FIGURE 7-3. Gyrate erythema, deep form. Superficial and deep, dense perivascular lymphocytic infiltrate.

ERYTHEMA GYRATUM REPENS

Erythema gyratum repens is a very rare, but clinically highly characteristic, dermatosis first reported in 1952 by Gammel (34). It represents a paraneoplastic syndrome that is associated with internal malignancy in 82% of patients (35). The most common malignancies reported are lung/bronchial, esophageal, and breast carcinomas. The eruption typically is very pruritic and is composed of concentric and parallel bands of erythema and scale producing a "wood-grain" pattern on the skin. The trunk and extremities are preferentially involved; however, the entire integument may be affected. The rash of erythema gyratum repens constantly migrates at a fairly rapid rate (up to 1 cm per day). Ichthyosis and palmar/plantar hyperkeratosis have been observed concomitantly in 16% and 10% of patients, respectively (36). The condition is known to remit with treatment and eradication of the associated malignancy.

Histopathology. The histologic picture usually shows mild acanthosis, spongiosis, focal parakeratosis, and a superficial perivascular lymphohistiocytic infiltrate that may also include eosinophils, neutrophils, and melanophages (36,37).

Pathogenesis. Several authors have described granular deposition of C3, C4, or IgG at the basement membrane zone on direct immunofluorescence suggesting that erythema gyratum repens may have an immunologic basis (38–40). In particular, Caux et al. (40) noted that the deposits are located in the sublamina densa region using immunoelectron microscopy.

ERYTHEMA DYSCHROMICUM PERSTANS

Erythema dyschromicum perstans, also called ashy dermatosis, is an extensive asymptomatic eruption. It begins with disseminated macules showing an elevated, red active border, which, by peripheral extension and coalescence, form large patches with a polycyclic outline. Although the macules may at first be erythematous before assuming their characteristic bluish gray color, they often appear blue-gray from the very beginning. The disease progresses slowly, and the discoloration persists. The most common areas of involvement are the trunk, arms, and face. Most patients with this disorder are Latin American (41).

Histopathology. In the early active stage or in the erythematous active border, there is vacuolar alteration of the basal layer. The papillary dermis shows a mild to moderate perivascular infiltrate of lymphocytes and histiocytes intermingled with melanophages (42,43). There may also be exocytosis of lymphocytes into the basal layer and occasional necrotic keratinocytes or colloid bodies resembling those seen in lichen planus may be present (44). Late lesions show aggregates of melanophages in the papillary dermis (42).

Pathogenesis. Electron microscopic examination reveals many vacuoles delimited by a membrane within the affected keratinocytes as the ultrastructural counterpart of the vacuolar alteration. This is associated with widening of the intercellular spaces and retraction of desmosomes to either one cell or the other. Additional findings include discontinuities in the subepidermal basement membrane and the presence in the dermis of melanophages containing aggregates of melanosomes enclosed by a lysosomal membrane (45). It can be assumed that the vacuolar alteration of basal keratinocytes is the cause of the pigmentary incontinence and of the formation of the colloid bodies.

Direct immunofluorescence studies have shown IgG deposition on necrotic keratinocytes at the dermal–epidermal junction, and immunohistochemical stains have revealed that in early lesions the dermal inflammatory infiltrate is composed primarily of T-lymphocytes, including both CD4+ (helper-inducer) and CD8+ (cytotoxic-suppressor) subtypes (46).

It has been shown that the expression of intercellular adhesion molecule 1 (ICAM-1) and HLA-DR molecule on basal layer keratinocytes is increased. The dermal cell infiltrate expressed the activation molecule AIM/CD69 and the cytotoxic cell marker CD94 (47). Damage and necrosis of the basal keratinocytes resulting in formation of colloid bodies and pigmentary incontinence suggests a possible relationship of erythema dyschromicum perstans to lichen planus pigmentosus, also called lichen planus actinicus or subtropicus (44,48,49). However, lichen planus pigmentosus shows a different clinical presentation characterized by dark brown macules located predominantly on exposed areas and flexural folds; histologically it sometimes has a more pronounced lichenoid distribution of the infiltrate (43,50). Lichen planopilaris coexisting with erythema dyschromicum perstans has been reported (51).

Differential Diagnosis. Erythema dyschromicum perstans may show similarities with the inflammatory infiltrate and pigmentary incontinence seen in interface drug reactions, especially in the late stage of fixed-drug eruption (42).

PRURIGO SIMPLEX

Prurigo simplex is characterized by intensely pruritic, erythematous urticarial papules that are seen in symmetric distribution, especially on the trunk and extensor surfaces of the extremities of middle-aged patients. Some patients may have an atopic background or may exhibit dermographism (52). In contrast to dermatitis herpetiformis, which prurigo simplex may resemble in clinical appearance, there is no grouping of lesions (53). In other cases, prurigo simplex greatly resembles arthropod bites (papular urticaria).

Histopathology. The histologic picture of the early papules shows mild acanthosis, spongiosis with an occasional small spongiotic vesicle, and parakeratosis. The upper dermis contains a mild lymphocytic inflammatory infiltrate in a largely perivascular arrangement (54). An admixture of eosinophils is present in some cases (53,55). Excoriated papules show partial absence of the epidermis, and they are covered with a crust containing degenerated nuclei of inflammatory cells (53). On serial sectioning, most of the histologic changes may be found to be located around hair follicles, which then show spongiosis and exocytosis of lymphocytes in the follicular infundibulum, and a perifollicular infiltrate (56). In other instances, there is distinct sparing of the follicular structures (55).

Differential Diagnosis. The diagnosis of dermatitis herpetiformis is easily excluded by the absence in prurigo simplex of neutrophilic microabscesses at the tips of dermal papillae and of neutrophils, eosinophils, and nuclear dust in the dermal infiltrate. A negative direct immunofluorescence study of perilesional skin excludes dermatitis herpetiformis or urticarial bullous pemphigoid (52). The histologic picture of prurigo simplex resembles that of a subacute eczematous dermatitis, except that the extent of its papular lesions is much more limited. Histologic differentiation from papular urticaria is not possible (53).

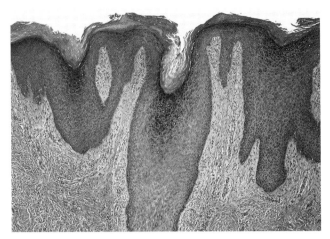

FIGURE 7-5. Prurigo nodularis. Marked irregular acanthosis, focal hypergranulosis, and compact orthokeratosis with parakeratosis.

PRURIGO NODULARIS

Prurigo nodularis is a chronic dermatitis characterized by discrete, raised, firm hyperkeratotic papulonodules, usually from 5 to 12 mm in diameter but occasionally larger. They occur chiefly on the extensor surfaces of the extremities and are intensely pruritic. The disease usually begins in middle age and women are more frequently affected than men (57). Prurigo nodularis may coexist with lesions of lichen simplex chronicus and there may be transitional lesions (58).

The cause remains unknown but local trauma, insect bites, atopic background, and metabolic or systemic diseases have been implicated as predisposing factors in some cases (58–61).

Histopathology. Pronounced hyperkeratosis and irregular acanthosis are observed. In addition, there may be papillomatosis and irregular downward proliferation of the epidermis and adnexal epithelium (62) approaching pseudoepitheliomatous hyperplasia (63) (Fig. 7-5). The papillary dermis shows a predominantly lymphocytic inflammatory infiltrate and vertically oriented collagen bundles. Occasionally, prominent neural hyperplasia may be observed (63); however, this is an uncommon finding and is not considered to be an essential feature for the diagnosis of prurigo nodularis (64). In some cases, silver stains or cholinesterase stains demonstrate the increased number of cutaneous nerves (57).

Eosinophils and marked eosinophil degranulation may be seen more frequently in patients with an atopic background (59). Dermal Langerhans cells are shown to be increased in prurigo nodularis compared to normal controls (65). The identification of enlarged dendritic mast cells, containing fewer cytoplasmic granules within the lesional dermis has recently been described (66).

Pathogenesis. It is generally assumed that the neural proliferation in prurigo nodularis is a secondary phenomenon due to chronic trauma by scratching. Still, it may be that the extreme pruritus is related to the increased number of dermal nerves (63). A recent study has shown that nerve growth factor (NGF) and its receptors are overexpressed in lesional skin of prurigo nodularis, compared to normal controls, with the inflammatory cell infiltrate being the source of NGF with resulting neural hyperplasia (67).

On electron microscopic examination, it is evident that the neural proliferation involves both axons and Schwann cells (63). Many nerve fibers are demonstrable also with immunostains for S-100 protein (68), neurofilament, and myelin basic protein (69). Immunohistochemical analysis has confirmed that they are mostly sensory nerves by demonstrating the presence of sensory neuropeptides (70). In addition, Merkel cells are reported to be increased in number in the basal cell layer of the affected interfollicular epidermis, suggesting that these specialized sensory receptors interacting with the neural fibers may participate in the pathogenesis of the disease (71).

Differential Diagnosis. Lichen simplex chronicus may have a similar histologic picture, although less exuberant and less circumscribed (64). Multiple keratoacanthomas, which often show less of a central crater than solitary keratoacanthomas, may be difficult to distinguish from prurigo nodularis because both show marked epidermal and epithelial hyperplasia (72).

PSORIASIS

Psoriasis may be divided into *psoriasis vulgaris, generalized pustular psoriasis,* and *localized pustular psoriasis.*

Psoriasis Vulgaris

Clinical Features. Psoriasis vulgaris is a common chronic inflammatory skin disorder that affects approximately 1.5% to 2% of the population in Western countries. It is characterized by pink to red scaly papules and plaques. The lesions are of variable size, sharply demarcated, dry, and usually covered with layers of fine, silvery scales. As the scales are removed by gentle scraping, fine bleeding points are usually seen, the so-called Auspitz sign. The scalp, sacral region, and extensor surfaces of the extremities are commonly involved, although in some patients the flexural and intertriginous areas are mainly affected (inverse psoriasis). An acute variant, guttate or eruptive psoriasis, is often seen in younger patients and is characterized by an abrupt eruption of small lesions associated with acute group A β-hemolytic streptococcal infections (73). Involvement of the nails is common; the most frequent alteration of the nail plate surface is the presence of pits (74). In severe cases, the disease may affect the entire skin and present as generalized erythrodermic psoriasis. Pustules are generally absent in psoriasis vulgaris, although pustules on palms and soles occasionally occur. Rarely, one or a few areas show pustules, and this is referred to as "psoriasis with pustules." Also rarely, severe psoriasis vulgaris develops into generalized pustular psoriasis. Oral lesions such as stomatitis areata migrans (geographic stomatitis) and benign migratory glossitis (geographic tongue) may be seen in psoriasis vulgaris as well as in generalized pustular psoriasis (75,76).

Psoriatic arthritis characteristically involves the terminal interphalangeal joints, but frequently the large joints are also affected so that a clinical differentiation from rheumatoid arthritis is often difficult. However, the rheumatoid factor is generally absent.

Generalized Pustular Psoriasis

Clinical Features. Generalized pustular psoriasis includes (a) acute generalized pustular psoriasis (von Zumbusch type and acute exanthematous type); (b) generalized pustular psoriasis of pregnancy (impetigo herpetiformis); (c) infantile and juvenile pustular psoriasis; and (d) subacute annular or circinate pustular psoriasis (77).

This cutaneous eruption is characterized by the presence of variable numbers of sterile pustules appearing in erythematous and scaly lesions associated with moderate to severe constitutional symptoms (78). Several exacerbations may occur, and in the intervals between them, lesions of ordinary psoriasis may be seen.

The four variants of generalized pustular psoriasis show considerable resemblance and overlapping in their clinical picture and also have a similar histologic appearance. They differ mainly in the mode of onset and the distribution of the lesions. Frequently, all four diseases show oral pustules, particularly on the tongue (79).

Acute generalized pustular psoriasis of von Zumbusch, is generally diagnosed when the pustular eruption occurs in patients with preexisting psoriasis, either of the plaque type (80) or of the erythrodermic type (81). Frequently, the

eruption occurs after systemic steroid therapy withdrawal (77,82). The *exanthematous type of generalized pustular psoriasis* refers to a group of patients with later onset of psoriasis, atypical distribution of the lesions, and a rapid and apparently spontaneous pustular eruption (83).

Generalized pustular psoriasis of pregnancy is a rare pustular eruption that appears during the last trimester of pregnancy. It starts with flexural lesions of psoriasis followed by a generalized pustular eruption. It may occur repeatedly during successive pregnancies (84). Some authors have considered it to be the same disease as *impetigo herpetiformis* (77), but others claim that they stand as separate entities (85,86).

In some instances of *subacute annular pustular psoriasis*, the annular or gyrate lesions show a clinical resemblance to subcorneal pustular dermatosis (87,88). Figurate lesions are more frequently seen in subacute or chronic forms of generalized pustular psoriasis (77). Annular pustular psoriasis, though usually generalized, in some instances may be localized (89).

Very rarely, children develop generalized pustular psoriasis also known as *infantile and juvenile pustular psoriasis*. In these patients, the disease has a benign course with frequent spontaneous remissions (90).

Localized Pustular Psoriasis

Clinical Features. There are three types of localized pustular psoriasis: (a) "psoriasis with pustules" (82,83), in which only one or a few areas of psoriasis show pustules and the tendency to change into a generalized pustular psoriasis is low; (b) localized acrodermatitis continua of Hallopeau, which occasionally evolves into generalized acrodermatitis continua; and (c) pustular psoriasis of the palms and soles, with two variants—the chronic palmoplantar pustulosis, also called pustulosis palmaris et plantaris, and the acute palmoplantar pustulosis or "pustular bacterid." Both variants of the third type are occasionally seen in association with psoriasis vulgaris (77). The relationship of Reiter's disease to psoriasis will be discussed in the description of Reiter's disease.

Acrodermatitis continua of Hallopeau is the term used when the pustular eruption involves the distal portions of the hands and feet. In the localized type of acrodermatitis continua, these are the only areas affected, while in the generalized type of acrodermatitis continua, extensive areas of the skin in addition to the acral portions of extremities are involved (83). Atrophy of the skin and permanent nail loss may occur on the fingers and toes.

Pustulosis palmaris et plantaris is a chronic, relapsing disorder occurring on the palms, soles, or both. Crops of small, deep-seated pustules are seen within areas of erythema and scaling. In the earliest stage, the lesions may appear as vesicles or vesiculopustules. During the subsiding stage, the pustules appear as brown macules. The sites of predilection are the mid-palms and thenar eminences of the hands, and the heels and insteps of the feet (91). In pustulosis palmaris et plantaris, in contrast to acrodermatitis continua of Hallopeau, the acral portions of the fingers and toes are spared. An acute variant called "pustular bacterid" (92) describes a rare eruption of large and sterile pustules on hands and feet.

Psoriasis and Acquired Immunodeficiency Syndrome

Clinical Features. The association between psoriasis and HIV infection is commonly seen. The prevalence of psoriasis is reported to be 1.3% to 2.5% in the HIV-positive population (93,94). Clinically, psoriasis may have a more severe course with sudden exacerbations and may be refractile to treatment (93,95). Extensive erythrodermic psoriasis may occur (96). Palmoplantar involvement, flexural (inverse) psoriasis, and psoriatic arthritis were found to be more frequent in patients who developed psoriasis after the HIV infection (94). Although a direct relation between the stage of HIV infection and the severity of psoriasis has not been found, a trend of low, peripheral T-cell CD4+ (helper-inducer) counts and a more severe clinical course has been noted (94).

Psoriasis Vulgaris

Histopathology. The histologic picture of psoriasis vulgaris varies considerably with the stage of the lesion and usually is diagnostic only in early scaling papules and near the margin of advancing plaques.

The earliest pinhead-sized macules or smooth-surfaced papules show subtle histologic changes with a preponderance of dermal changes (97,98). At first, there is capillary dilatation and edema in the papillary dermis, with a lymphocytic infiltrate surrounding the capillaries. The lymphocytes extend into the lower portion of the epidermis, where slight spongiosis develops. Then focal changes occur in the upper portion of the epidermis, where granular cells become vacuolated and disappear, and mounds of parakeratosis are formed. The neutrophils usually are seen only at the summits of some of the mounds of parakeratosis and appear scattered through an otherwise orthokeratotic cornified layer (Fig. 7-6). These mounds of parakeratosis with neutrophils represent the earliest manifestation of Munro microabscesses (98). At this stage, which is characterized clinically by an early scaling papule, a histologic diagnosis of psoriasis can often be made. In some cases, when there is marked exocytosis of neutrophils, they may aggregate in the uppermost portion of the spinous layer to form small spongiform pustules of Kogoj. Lymphocytes remain

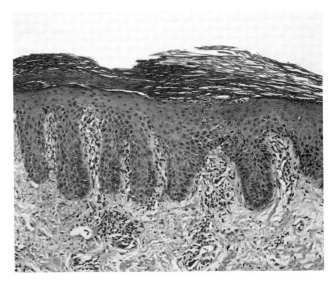

FIGURE 7-6. Early psoriasis. Mounds of parakeratosis with neutrophils, thin granular layer, moderate acanthosis, focal spongiosis, increased mitotic figures, dilated blood vessels at the tip of the dermal papillae, and perivascular infiltrate of lymphocytes and a few neutrophils.

confined to the lower epidermis, which, as more and more mitoses occur, becomes increasingly hyperplastic. The epidermal changes are at first focal, but later on become confluent, leading clinically to plaques.

In the fully developed lesions of psoriasis, as best seen at the margin of enlarging plaques, the histologic picture is characterized by (a) acanthosis with regular elongation of the rete ridges with thickening in their lower portion; (b) thinning of the suprapapillary epidermis with the occasional presence of small spongiform pustules; (c) pallor of the upper layers of the epidermis; (d) diminished to absent granular layer; (e) confluent parakeratosis; (f) presence of Munro microabscesses; (g) elongation and edema of the dermal papillae; and (h) dilated and tortuous capillaries (Fig. 7-7).

Of all the listed features, only the spongiform pustules of Kogoj and Munro microabscesses are truly diagnostic of psoriasis and, in their absence, the diagnosis can rarely be made with certainty on a histologic basis. The changes in active psoriasis are discussed in detail below.

The rete ridges show considerable elongation and extend downward to a uniform level, resulting in regular acanthosis (Fig. 7-8). They are often slender in their upper portion but show thickening ("clubbing") in their lower portion. Not infrequently, adjacent rete ridges seem to coalesce at their bases due to tangential sectioning. Usually, intercellular and intracellular edema is absent in the rete ridges and keratinocytes located well above the basal layer show deep basophilia. In addition, mitoses are not limited to the basal layer as in normal skin, but are also seen above the basal layer. This, together with a considerable lengthening of the basal cell layer due to elongation of the rete ridges, results in a marked increase in the number of mi-

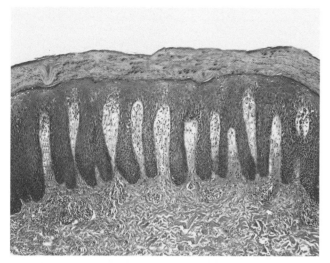

FIGURE 7-7. Psoriasis, well-developed plaque. Markedly elongated rete ridges, absent granular layer, parakeratosis with neutrophils, and dilated tortuous vessels in the dermal papillae.

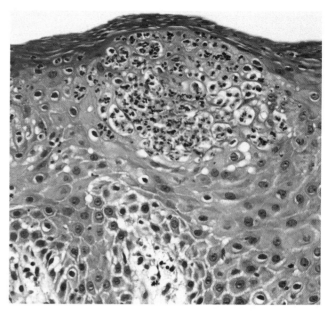

FIGURE 7-9. Psoriasis. Closer view of a spongiform pustule of Kogoj formed by collections of neutrophils in the spinous and granular layers.

toses. This increase has been calculated to be 27 times the number of mitoses in uninvolved skin (99).

The suprapapillary epidermis appears relatively thin in comparison with the markedly elongated rete ridges, and the cells in the upper layers of the epidermis may appear enlarged and pale stained as a result of intracellular edema and hypogranulosis. Keratinocytes beneath the parakeratotic cornified layer may be intermingled with neutrophils (100). The histologic picture is then that of a small spongiform pustule of Kogoj (Fig. 7-9). Although it is only a mi-

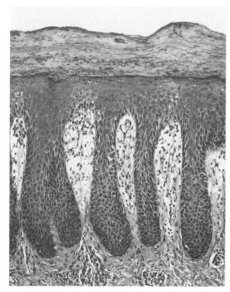

FIGURE 7-8. Psoriasis, well-developed plaque. Acanthosis with club-shaped rete ridges of even length, suprabasal mitoses, thin suprapapillary epidermal plates, absent granular layer, pallor of the upper epidermis, and confluent parakeratosis with collections of neutrophils.

cropustule, it is nevertheless of the same type as the much larger macropustules seen in pustular psoriasis. Such a spongiform pustule, highly diagnostic for psoriasis and its variants, shows aggregates of neutrophils within the interstices of a sponge-like network formed by degenerated and thinned epidermal cells (101).

In some instances, the cornified layer consists entirely of confluent parakeratosis forming a plate-like scale with a concomitant absence or diminution of the granular layer. However, occasional focal orthokeratosis with preservation of the underlying granular cells is present.

Munro microabscesses are located within the parakeratotic areas of the cornified layer (Fig. 7-10). They consist of accumulations of neutrophils and pyknotic nuclei of neutrophils that have migrated there from capillaries in the papillae through the suprapapillary epidermis. As a rule, Munro microabscesses are easily found in early lesions but are few in number or absent in long-standing lesions (102).

The dermal papillae, in accordance with the elongation and basal thickening of the rete ridges, are elongated and club shaped. They show edema, and the capillaries within them appear dilated and tortuous. A relatively mild inflammatory infiltrate is present in the upper dermis and the papillae. It consists of lymphocytes, except in early lesions, in which neutrophils are also present in the upper portion of the papillae (103).

An entirely typical histologic picture as described above is not always found, even if the biopsy specimens are taken from clinically typical lesions of psoriasis (104). Orthokeratosis often appears intermingled with parakeratosis. In such cases, one may see vertically adjoining areas of orthokeratosis and parakeratosis, focal parakeratosis, or occa-

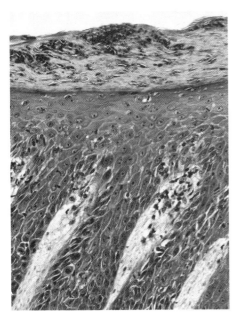

FIGURE 7-10. Psoriasis, plaque lesion. Closer view of the neutrophilic collections within the parakeratotic cornified layer (Munro microabscess). Note thin suprapapillary epidermal plates and dilated blood vessels in the dermal papillae.

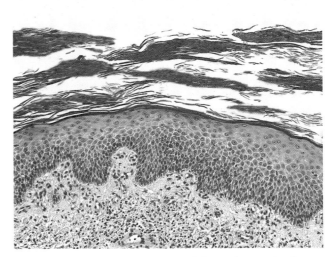

FIGURE 7-11. Eruptive psoriasis. Multilayered mounds of parakeratosis admixed with basketweave orthokeratosis, slight acanthosis, and dilated blood vessels in the dermal papillae.

sionally, alternating layers of orthokeratosis and parakeratosis. The latter pattern indicates a fluctuation in the activity of the psoriasis.

The bleeding points that may be produced by gentle scraping of the skin (Auspitz sign) correspond to the tips of dermal papillae. They are attributable to the following histologic changes: parakeratosis, intracellular edema of keratinocytes in the suprapapillary epidermis, thinning of the suprapapillary plates, and dilatation of the capillaries in the upper portion of the papillae.

Guttate or *eruptive psoriasis* shows the histologic features of an early or active lesion of psoriasis, where there is more pronounced inflammatory infiltrate and less acanthosis as compared with a well-developed chronic plaque of psoriasis. Because of its acute onset, one may observe the remaining normal basket-weave orthokeratotic cornified layer overlying the mounds of parakeratosis with neutrophils, which, in turn, may appear loosely arranged (Fig. 7-11).

The histologic picture of *erythrodermic psoriasis* in some instances shows enough of the characteristics of psoriasis to allow this diagnosis. Frequently, however, the histologic appearance is indistinguishable from that of a chronic eczematous dermatitis (105).

Generalized Pustular Psoriasis

Histopathology. Whereas in ordinary psoriasis, the spongiform pustule of Kogoj is a very small micropustule and is seen only in early, active lesions, it occurs as a macropustule in all variants of generalized pustular psoriasis and repre-

sents their characteristic histologic lesion. The spongiform pustule forms through the migration of neutrophils from the papillary dermal capillaries to the upper layer of epidermis, where they aggregate within the interstices of a sponge-like network formed by degenerated and thinned epidermal cells (101). As the size of the pustule increases, the epidermal cells in the center of the pustule undergo complete cytolysis so that a large single cavity forms (Fig. 7-12). At the periphery of the pustule, however, the network of thinned epidermal cells persists for a much longer time. As the neutrophils of the spongiform pustule move

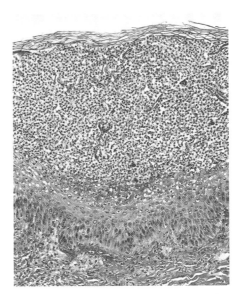

FIGURE 7-12. Pustular psoriasis. Large collections of neutrophils with spongiosis in the upper spinous layer and granular layer.

up into the cornified layer, they become pyknotic and assume the appearance of a large Munro abscess (80,106).

In addition to the large spongiform pustules, the epidermal changes in generalized pustular psoriasis are very much like those seen in psoriasis vulgaris, consisting of parakeratosis and elongation of the rete ridges. The upper dermis contains an infiltrate of lymphocytes, and neutrophils can often be seen migrating from the capillaries in the papillae into the epidermis (107). The oral lesions show the same spongiform pustule formation as those seen on the skin (79).

In the healing stage, the lesions of all types of generalized pustular psoriasis may present the same histologic appearance as ordinary psoriasis (80).

Localized Pustular Psoriasis

Histopathology. In the variants of localized pustular psoriasis, "psoriasis with pustules" (82,83) and localized annular pustular psoriasis, the histologic picture is the same as that described for generalized pustular psoriasis.

In localized acrodermatitis continua of Hallopeau, the nail bed is mainly affected, showing marked epithelial hyperplasia with variable numbers of spongiform pustules, and orthokeratosis with mounds of parakeratosis with neutrophils. The nail matrix is only occasionally involved (108).

In pustulosis palmaris et plantaris, there is a fully developed large intraepidermal unilocular pustule. It is elevated only slightly above the surface but presses onto the underlying dermis. Many neutrophils are present within the cavity of the pustule. The epidermis surrounding the pustule shows slight acanthosis, and an inflammatory infiltrate can be seen beneath the pustule (109). In many instances, one can observe typical, though small, spongiform pustules in the epidermal wall of the pustule, most commonly at the junction of the lateral walls and the overlying epidermis (109–113). These spongiform pustules are identical to those seen in the walls of the pustules of generalized pustular psoriasis.

Very early lesions may show spongiosis and exocytosis of lymphocytes in the lower epidermis overlying the tips of dermal papillae (112). This may be followed by the formation of a small intraepidermal vesicle containing mostly lymphocytes (109,112). Subsequently, there is a massive exocytosis of neutrophils, which penetrate the intercellular spaces of the vesicle wall, where the histologic picture of spongiform pustules is then seen (109). In the acute form, pustular bacterid, leukocytoclastic vasculitis has been described (114).

Psoriasis and AIDS

Histopathology. The histological picture in most cases is similar to that of psoriasis. In others, the histologic sections may show acanthosis without thinning of the suprapapillary

epidermis, slight spongiosis, rare necrotic keratinocytes, and a superficial perivascular infiltrate of lymphocytes and histiocytes that occasionally contains some plasma cells (115). As in other dermatitides related to AIDS, eosinophils may be present in the inflammatory infiltrate.

Pathogenesis of Psoriasis Vulgaris

Although the cause of psoriasis is still unknown, there is increasing evidence of a complex interaction between altered keratinocytic proliferation and differentiation, inflammation, and immune dysregulation.

Electron Microscopy. The earliest recognizable morphologic events in psoriasis have been investigated in lesions that cleared with corticosteroid under occlusion and were then allowed to relapse. The earliest indications of relapse, as seen by electron microscopy, are swelling and intercellular widening of endothelial cells. This is followed by the appearance around postcapillary venules of mast cells showing degranulation. Hours later, activated macrophages migrate into the lower epidermis, where there is loss of desmosome-tonofilament complexes. Only then lymphocytes and neutrophils are seen (116).

Ultrastructurally, in well-developed lesions, psoriatic keratinocytes from the suprabasal layers of the epidermis show significant abnormalities. The tonofilaments are decreased in number and in diameter and lack their normal aggregation. The size and number of keratohyaline granules are greatly reduced, and occasionally these are absent (117,118). The cornified cells possess thin tonofilaments and often retain organelles and a nucleus as parakeratotic cells. They often fail to form a marginal band and to lose their outer plasma membrane (119). Basal keratinocytes may show cytoplasmic processes protruding into the dermis through gaps in the basal lamina. The presence of these herniations correlates with psoriatic activity. They are more numerous in active and untreated lesions and are absent in completely resolved and uninvolved psoriatic skin (120). The intercellular spaces between all epidermal cells are widened because of a deficiency in the glycoprotein-rich cell surface coat, so that intercellular adhesion is limited to the desmosomes (119,121). Electron microscopic studies have confirmed the view that the keratinocytes in psoriasis are defective and not just immature owing to accelerated epidermal proliferation. Although a correlation exists in psoriasis between an increased rate of mitosis and parakeratosis, rapid proliferation of the epidermis does not cause parakeratosis (122).

Ultrastructural studies of the spongiform pustule of Kogoj, one of the most characteristic histologic structures encountered in psoriasis, reveal that it is located in the uppermost portion of the spinous and granular layers, where neutrophils lie intercellularly in a multilocular pustule in which the sponge-like network is composed of degenerated and flattened keratinocytes (101).

The ultrastructure of the capillary loops in the dermal papillae shows them to be different from normal capillary loops. Normal skin microvasculature has a homogeneous-appearing basement membrane and no bridged fenestrations between endothelial cells. In psoriasis, however, the capillaries show a wider lumen, bridged fenestrations and gaps between endothelial cells, edematous areas in the cytoplasm of endothelial cells, pericytes and myocytes, extravasation of red blood cells and inflammatory cells and a thickened multilayered basement membrane (123). This finding may be a result of the deposition of amorphous substances and accumulation of collagen fibrils in the basement membrane zone (124).

Epidermal Cell-Cycle Kinetics

The rate of epidermal cell replication is markedly accelerated in active lesions of psoriasis, as shown by the higher than normal number of basal and suprabasal mitotic figures and the greater number of premitotic cells labeled by tritiated thymidine (125). The mitotic activity within different lesions of psoriasis and even within the same lesion can vary considerably and seems to correlate with the degree of parakeratosis. Thus, psoriatic epidermis with 91% to 100% parakeratosis shows on the average five times as many mitotic figures as psoriatic epidermis with only 0% to 20% parakeratosis (104). The frequent finding in psoriasis of alternating layers of orthokeratosis and parakeratosis suggests that epidermal growth activity fluctuates in the lesions (104). Step sections of early "punctate" papules show a mitotically very active parakeratotic center surrounded by a zone with a thickened granular layer and a relatively low mitotic rate (126).

Early calculations made it appear likely that, in psoriatic lesions, there was a great acceleration of the transit time of cells from the basal cell layer to the uppermost row of the squamous cell layer, from approximately 53 days in normal epidermis to only 7 days in the epidermis of active psoriatic lesions (125).

Further investigations (127) have found that (a) the germinative cell cycle is shortened from 311 to 36 hours, indicating that psoriatic keratinocytes proliferate approximately eight-fold faster than do normal keratinocytes; (b) there is a doubling of the proliferative cell population in psoriasis from 27,000 to 52,000 cells/mm^2 of epidermal surface area; and (c) 100% of the germinative cells of the epidermis enter the growth fraction instead of only 60% for normal subjects. However, in another study (128), it was shown that the germinative cell-cycle time in normal epidermis is around 200 hours and in psoriatic epidermis about 100 hours, a twofold rather than an eight-fold acceleration.

The source of the cycling cells in the suprabasal layers of the epidermis is not yet well defined. They could be an expanded population of basal keratinocytes or could be recruited from the transient-amplifying cells (TAC), which refer to suprabasal keratinocytes committed to terminal differentiation, that might undergo rounds of amplifying divisions above the basal layer (129). Based on keratin studies, it is believed that proliferating keratinocytes may result from recruitment of TAC (129) because they express K1/K10 and predominantly K6/K16 keratins and not K5/K14 as basal keratinocytes do (130).

Recent studies have suggested that psoriatic epidermis shows aberrant expression of apoptosis-related molecules representing suppressed apoptotic process, which might be related to proliferative characteristic of the epidermis in this disease (131).

Keratinocyte Differentiation

Keratinocytes undergo the process of differentiation as they migrate upward through the epidermis from the basal layer to the cornified layer. During this process, different structural proteins are synthesized. One such protein family is the keratins, which are intermediate filaments found in the cytoplasm of all the epithelial cells. Studies have revealed that the keratin pair K5/K14 is expressed in basal keratinocytes (132) and keratins K1/K10 are found in the suprabasal layers. Involucrin, one of the major precursor proteins of the cornified cell envelope, is detected higher in the granular and cornified layers (133). In psoriatic skin, basal keratinocytes continue to express K5/K14; however, keratins K1/K10 are replaced by the so-called hyperproliferation-associated keratins K6 and K16. In addition, involucrin is expressed prematurely in the lower suprabasal layers (130,134). Keratin 17, normally expressed in the deep, outer root sheath of the hair follicle, has been found also in the upper suprabasal keratinocytes within the interfollicular psoriatic epidermis (130).

Immunopathology

Immunologic factors play a very important role in the pathogenesis of psoriasis. Psoriasis is now regarded as a T cell mediated disorder. It has been shown that both CD4+ T-lymphocytes and CD8+ T-lymphocytes are found in the papillary dermis and the epidermis of the psoriatic lesions. CD8+ T-lymphocytes seem to be dominant in the epidermis, whereas the CD4+ T-lymphocytes are the predominant subset in the dermis. Presence of CD8+ T cells within the epidermis is thought to be a key event in the pathogenesis of psoriasis (135), with up to one-third of them expressing the activation markers (136). Recent data suggest that lesions of psoriasis exhibit clonal expansion of epidermal T-lymphocytes detected by quantitative competitive polymerase chain reaction that examined the T-cell receptor, beta-chain variable-region genes. Recurrent lesions also show the recruitment of the identical expanded T-cell clones. Nonlesional skin did not show the presence of the same T-cell receptor rearrangements. These findings suggest that a stable antigen-specific pathogenic T-cell response may play a role in disease perpetuation in psoriasis (137–139). The activation of T-lymphocytes may be due to bacterial superantigens such as group A beta-hemolytic streptococci. It is suggested that amino acid sequences from streptococcal M-protein share the sequences with keratin 17, therefore an epitope on keratin 17 or keratin 6 may be a target for autoreactive lymphocytes in psoriasis (140,141). Group A streptococcal-reactive CD8+ and to a lesser extent CD4+ T cells in psoriatic epidermis may play a role in the pathogenesis of both poststreptococcal guttate psoriasis (142) and chronic plaque psoriasis (143). Activated CD4+ T-lymphocytes produce a variety of cytokines including interleukin-2 (IL-2), tumor necrosis factor-alpha (TNF-α) and gamma-interferon (γ-IFN), which is also produced by CD8+ T-lymphocytes (144).

Keratinocytes stimulated by TNF-α may produce interleukin-8 (IL-8), which is a potent T-lymphocyte and neutrophil chemoattractant present in increased amounts in psoriatic epidermis. This cytokine may be involved in the formation of Munro microabscesses (145).

γ-IFN is thought to play an important role in the initiation of psoriatic lesions as demonstrated by the induction of pinpoint lesions of psoriasis at sites of γ-IFN injection in previously uninvolved skin (146).

γ-IFN induces the expression of the intercellular adhesion molecule-1 (ICAM-1) in keratinocytes and endothelial cells. This molecule mediates the adhesion and trafficking of lymphocytes into the epidermis by binding to its ligand LFA-1 (lymphocyte function-associated antigen-1) expressed on lymphocyte membranes (145). In addition, γ-IFN inducible protein (IP-10) is overexpressed by keratinocytes in psoriatic lesional skin (147). IP-10 is detected in epidermis during cellular immune responses and may have chemotactic as well as mitogenic properties. However, it has been shown that keratinocytes from lesional psoriatic skin have altered responses to γ-IFN (148). Psoriatic keratinocytes are shown not to be responsive to the growth inhibition effects of γ-IFN (149), suggesting that decreased responsiveness of keratinocytes to γ-IFN may contribute to the hyperproliferation and altered differentiation of epidermal cells in psoriasis (150).

Pathogenesis of Localized Pustular Psoriasis

A relationship of pustulosis palmaris et plantaris with psoriasis is not generally accepted, although two facts favor a close relationship: the relatively common occurrence of psoriasis in patients with pustulosis palmaris et plantaris, reported in 19% to 48% of the patients (151–153), and the common presence of spongiform pustules in the walls of the pustules of pustulosis palmaris et plantaris. The argument that the primary occurrence of a mononuclear reaction in pustulosis palmaris et plantaris speaks against a relationship with psoriasis (109) can be countered by the fact that a mononuclear infiltrate precedes the appearance of neutrophils in psoriasis as well. Also, a leukotactic factor

identical to that noted in psoriasis has been found in pustulosis palmaris et plantaris (154).

Pathogenesis of Psoriasis and AIDS

There is evidence of the role of both CD8+ and CD4+ T-lymphocytes and γ-IFN in the pathogenesis of psoriasis in AIDS (115,155). Paradoxically, as T-helper lymphocyte counts decline, it appears that psoriatic lesions exacerbate until a preterminal stage when the dermatitis improves. The latter event is probably a consequence of a decreased local production of γ-IFN due to the increasing number of infected T-helper lymphocytes or a diminished number of dermal lymphocytes available to produce this cytokine (115). However, in a recent study, it has been shown that γ-IFN serum levels were much higher in HIV+ psoriatic patients than HIV− subjects (156).

The immunodysregulation resulting from HIV infection may trigger psoriasis in those genetically predisposed by carrying HLA-Cw*0602 allele. HLA-Cw*0602 could act as a cross-reactive target for cytotoxic T-lymphocytes responding to peptides from microorganisms. Human retrovirus-5 has been implicated in the pathogenesis of psoriatic arthropathy but not psoriasis (155). Immunohistochemical studies have shown similar proportions of T-lymphocyte subtypes in psoriasis of HIV+ patients and in psoriasis of immunocompetent hosts (157). Furthermore, there is evidence of identical keratinocyte expression of γ-IFN–induced protein 10 in both groups (115). These two findings suggest that the cellular immune reactions involved in the pathogenesis of psoriasis may be similar in AIDS and non-AIDS patients (157).

Differential Diagnosis of Psoriasis

Two histologic features are of great value in the diagnosis of psoriasis vulgaris: (a) mounds of parakeratosis with neutrophils at their summits (Munro microabscesses); and (b) spongiform micropustules of Kogoj in the uppermost layers of the spinous layer. Dilatation and tortuosity of capillaries in the papillae may also be of help in the diagnosis. All other features, such as acanthosis with elongation of the rete ridges and parakeratosis, can be found also in chronic eczematous dermatitis, such as *atopic dermatitis, nummular dermatitis,* or *allergic contact dermatitis,* which then may appear to be "psoriasiform." However, the elongation of rete ridges is uneven. Although mild spongiosis may be seen in psoriasis, the presence of marked spongiosis and especially of coagulated serum as evidence of crusting in the cornified layer are features speaking against psoriasis, except in psoriasis on volar skin in which spongiosis may be prominent. In addition, eosinophils, which are commonly found in allergic contact dermatitis and mainly in HIV+ patients, are rarely seen in the psoriatic infiltrate. Difficulties may arise in treated lesions of psoriasis and in those with superimposed allergic contact dermatitis secondary to topical treatments. *Lichen simplex chronicus* is considered in the differential diagnosis of fully developed psoriatic plaques. In contrast to psoriasis, it shows a prominent granular layer, more irregular acanthosis, and fibrosis of the papillary dermis with collagen bundles aligned perpendicularly to the skin surface (158). *Seborrheic dermatitis* may be very difficult to distinguish from psoriasis vulgaris, especially if overlap occurs. Accentuated spongiosis, mounds of parakeratosis with neutrophils predominantly at the follicular ostia, and more irregular acanthosis are histologic features suggestive of seborrheic dermatitis. *Pityriasis rubra pilaris* shares some histologic features with psoriasis, namely, acanthosis and parakeratosis. However, it could be differentiated from well-developed lesions of psoriasis by the presence of thick suprapapillary plates, broader and shorter ridges, preserved granular layer and alternating ortho and parakeratosis. It also lacks Munro microabscesses and neutrophils in the infiltrate (159). Although the Kogoj spongiform pustule is highly diagnostic of the psoriasis group of diseases, including Reiter's disease, histologically typical spongiform pustules may occur also in *pustular dermatophytosis*, *bacterial impetigo*, *pustular drug eruptions*, and *candidiasis*, particularly if pustules are clinically present (160). PAS and Gram stains are useful to identify the infectious microorganisms. Aggregates of neutrophils with pyknotic nuclei within areas of parakeratosis may occur in conditions other than psoriasis, but they generally differ from Munro microabscesses by being larger and less well circumscribed and by often showing crusting.

Because of the clinical and, particularly, the histologic resemblance of the tongue lesions in pustular psoriasis with those seen in geographic tongue, it has been suggested that geographic tongue represents an abortive form of pustular psoriasis (161).

REITER'S DISEASE

Reiter's disease is a sterile arthritis associated in most cases with a distant infection causing enteritis or urethritis. Reiter's disease predominantly affects young men and consists of the triad of urethritis, arthritis, and conjunctivitis. Although as a rule the arthritis occurs in attacks and is followed by recovery, it progresses in some cases to cause permanent damage to the affected joints (162,163). Cutaneous lesions occur in about half of affected patients. Lesions have a predilection for the glans penis (balanitis circinata), the palms and soles (keratoderma blennorrhagicum), and the subungual areas.

In uncircumcised men, balanitis circinata presents as superficial crusted erosions forming a serpiginous pattern. In circumcised men, the condition presents as erythematous hyperkeratotic and coalescent papules on the glans (164). Lesions on the palms and soles are erythematous, mollusk-like plaques with central keratotic excrescences. Pustular le-

sions may also develop. The subungual lesions consist of hyperkeratosis with opacification of the nail plate and eventual shedding of the nail plate may occur. The prevalence of Reiter's disease in HIV-infected individuals is less than 1%; however, the disease appears to be more severe in immunocompromised patients (164).

Histopathology. Early pustular lesions on the palms or soles show a spongiform macropustule in the upper epidermis (162,165). In addition, one observes parakeratosis and elongation of the rete ridges.

As the lesions age, the parakeratotic cornified layer thickens considerably, which correlates with the keratotic excrescences seen clinically. The parakeratotic cornified layer is intermingled with the pyknotic nuclei of neutrophils. In old lesions, spongiform pustules are no longer seen and the histologic picture shows acanthosis and orthokeratosis with only a few areas of parakeratosis, but occasionally the histologic picture resembles psoriasis (162).

Pathogenesis. Most cases of Reiter's disease are probably caused by microorganisms that infect the urogenital or gastrointestinal systems such as *Chlamydia trachomatis*, *Ureaplasma urealyticum*, Shigella, Salmonella, Campylobacter, Cyclospora, and Yersinia species. *Chlamydia trachomatis* has been cultured from urethral samples in nearly half of the patients and is thought to be capable of triggering Reiter's syndrome in susceptible men (166). Although joint cultures are negative for bacteria in Reiter's disease, hybridization studies have detected chlamydial RNA in synovial specimens (167). The occurrence of Reiter's syndrome following BCG immunotherapy for bladder cancer has been reported (168). Eighty percent of Reiter's disease patients are HLA-B27 positive (164); however, the precise role of this MHC class I antigen in the development of this disease remains unclear.

A close relationship to psoriasis has been assumed for the cutaneous lesions because of their clinical resemblance to psoriasis and the presence of spongiform pustules (162). Similarly, the arthritis of Reiter's disease resembles that of psoriasis not only clinically but also by the absence of rheumatoid factor (163).

Differential Diagnosis. The early spongiform pustule seen in Reiter's disease is indistinguishable from the spongiform pustule seen in pustular psoriasis. Slightly older lesions often can be identified as representing Reiter's disease in contradistinction to psoriasis by the presence of a markedly thickened cornified layer.

PARAPSORIASIS

There are still three entities described as parapsoriasis: *small plaque parapsoriasis*, *large plaque parapsoriasis*, and *parapsoriasis variegata*.

Large plaque parapsoriasis and *parapsoriasis variegata* are best considered as early stages of cutaneous T-cell lymphoma (169). These are discussed in Chapter 31.

The *small plaque parapsoriasis* is known also as xantho-erythrodermia perstans of Crocker (170) and as digitate dermatosis (171). Pink to yellow, slightly scaly, oval or elongated, often finger print–like patches 1 to 5 cm in diameter, the plaques are symmetrically distributed over the trunk and the proximal portions of the extremities following the tension lines of the skin (172). The eruption is usually asymptomatic, has a chronic course, and tends to persist. In some instances, cases diagnosed originally as small plaque type, later on showed reticulate pigmentation and atrophy, requiring reclassification as the large plaque type (173).

Histopathology. The *small plaque parapsoriasis* shows focal epidermal involvement consisting of slight spongiosis, exocytosis of lymphocytes, mild acanthosis, and parakeratosis (171,174). Elongated mounds of parakeratosis with collections of plasma above a basket-weave cornified layer is a characteristic finding (Fig. 7-13). In the papillary dermis, there is a mild superficial perivascular lymphocytic infiltrate that in some instances is more pronounced and resembles that seen in the large plaque type; such cases require inclusion in the large plaque category (173,175). It must be conceded that, in some instances, a clinical or histologic distinction of small plaque parapsoriasis from large plaque parapsoriasis is difficult, so that only the subsequent course decides the issue (173).

Pathogenesis. The inflammatory infiltrate in small plaque parapsoriasis is dominated by CD4+ (helper-inducer) T-lymphocytes with a small proportion of the CD8+ (cyto-toxic-suppressor) T-lymphocytes subset. Langerhans cells are increased in the epidermis and dermis (176).

Relationship to Lymphoma. Because of the division of parapsoriasis en plaque into a small plaque type and a large

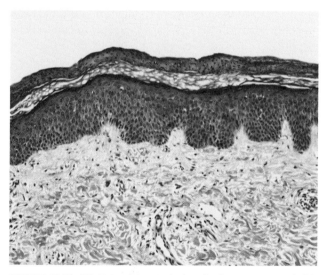

FIGURE 7-13. Digitate dermatosis (small plaque parapsoriasis). Characteristic elongated mound of parakeratosis with collections of plasma above a basketweave cornified layer, preserved granular layer, and minimal acanthosis. There is a sparse superficial perivascular lymphocytic infiltrate.

plaque type and the gradual acceptance of the term *digitate dermatosis* for the small plaque type, the relationship of parapsoriasis to mycosis fungoides has been clarified. It is generally accepted that small plaque parapsoriasis, or digitate dermatosis, is a benign disorder without the potential of transformation into mycosis fungoides (169,171,173, 177,178). However, it has been shown that in some cases there is a dominant clonal rearrangement of the infiltrating T-lymphocytes (176). This finding has led to the hypothesis that small plaque parapsoriasis could be placed into the category of "abortive lymphomas," which includes conditions where clonality can be demonstrated, but conversion into a systemic lymphoma does not occur (179). Another study detected a clonal T-cell proliferation in the peripheral blood but not in the skin of patients with small plaque parapsoriasis, suggesting that this disorder is not related to mycosis fungoides where there is clonal T-cell proliferation in both peripheral blood and skin (180).

PITYRIASIS ROSEA

Pityriasis rosea is a self-limited dermatitis lasting from 4 to 7 weeks. It frequently starts with a herald patch followed by a disseminated eruption. The lesions, found chiefly on the trunk, neck, and proximal extremities, consist of round to oval salmon-colored patches following the lines of cleavage and showing peripherally attached, thin, cigarette paper–like scales. Several typical and atypical clinical variants have been described including papular, vesicular, urticarial, purpuric, and recurrent forms (181).

Histopathology. The patches of the disseminated eruption show a superficial perivascular dermal infiltrate that consists predominantly of lymphocytes, with occasional eosinophils and histiocytes. Lymphocytes extend into the epidermis (exocytosis), where there is spongiosis, intracellular edema, mild to moderate acanthosis, areas of decreased to absent granular layer, and focal parakeratosis with plasma (182–184). Intraepidermal spongiotic vesicles (182,183) and a few necrotic keratinocytes (185) are found in some cases. A common feature is the presence of extravasated erythrocytes in the papillary dermis, which sometimes extend into the overlying epidermis (185,186) (Fig. 7-14). Occasionally, multinucleated keratinocytes in the affected epidermis can be seen (186). Late lesions from the disseminated eruption are more likely to have a psoriasiform pattern (182) and a slight increased number of eosinophils in the inflammatory infiltrate (184). The herald patch may have, in addition to the histopathologic changes described above, more pronounced acanthosis, deeper and denser perivascular inflammatory infiltrate, and papillary dermal edema (186).

Pathogenesis. The cause of pityriasis rosea is still unknown, although a viral etiology such as human herpesvirus 7 (HHV-7) is suspected (187). Cell-mediated im-

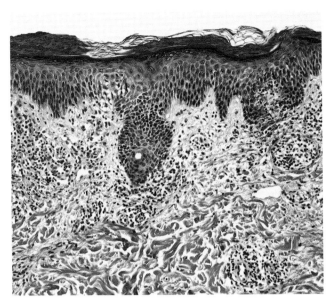

FIGURE 7-14. Pityriasis rosea. Superficial perivascular infiltrate of lymphocytes and extravasated erythrocytes that extend to the epidermis, where there is moderate acanthosis, spongiosis, decreased granular layer, and mounds of parakeratosis.

munity may be involved in the pathogenesis of pityriasis rosea due to the presence of activated helper-inducer T-lymphocytes (CD4+/HLA-DR+) in the epidermal and dermal infiltrate (188) in association with a highly increased number of Langerhans cells (CD1a+) (189,190) and the expression of HLA-DR+ antigen on the surface of keratinocytes located around the area of lymphocytic exocytosis (191).

Differential Diagnosis. The differential diagnosis includes superficial gyrate erythema and small plaque parapsoriasis (digitate dermatosis). The histopathologic picture in superficial gyrate erythema could be identical to that seen in milder forms of pityriasis rosea. Elongated mounds of parakeratosis with plasma, sparse superficial perivascular lymphocytic infiltrate, minimal exocytosis and spongiosis are features of small plaque parapsoriasis (174).

GIANOTTI–CROSTI SYNDROME (PAPULAR ACRODERMATITIS OF CHILDHOOD AND PAPULOVESICULAR ACROLOCATED SYNDROME)

Papular acrodermatitis of childhood was first described by Gianotti in 1955 (192). It is clinically characterized by a nonpruritic, symmetrical eruption of monomorphic erythematous papules on the face, extremities, and buttocks lasting about 3 weeks. It was originally described in association with lymphadenopathy and hepatitis B viral infection (193). However, in recent years, it has become

apparent that similar acral papular eruptions may occur with several other viruses, such as Epstein–Barr virus, coxsackie virus, parainfluenza virus, vaccine-related virus, and cytomegalovirus, among others (194–197). In such cases, there is often no hepatitis or lymphadenopathy. These eruptions were classified by Gianotti (193) in a separate category as "papular or papulovesicular acrolocated syndrome." However, further studies (197,198) have failed to identify repeatable clinical differences between papular acrodermatitis of childhood and papulovesicular acrolocated syndrome. The term Gianotti–Crosti syndrome now applies to all self-limited, acrolocated, papular eruptions that occur in association with an underlying viral infection (199).

Histopathology. There is a superficial and mid-dermal perivascular infiltrate of lymphocytes and histiocytes with some lymphocytes extending to the overlying epidermis where there is focal spongiosis and parakeratosis. In some cases, there is associated papillary dermal edema and extravasation of erythrocytes. In some instances true lymphocytic vasculitis has been described with lymphocytes in the vessel walls and extravasated erythrocytes into the upper dermis (194). Gianotti–Crosti syndrome associated with Epstein–Barr virus is reported to have marked papillary dermal edema with minimal spongiosis and rare eosinophils in the dermal infiltrate (200). The inflammatory pattern may also present as a lichenoid interface dermatitis (201).

Pathogenesis. Immunohistochemical stains have shown that the inflammatory infiltrate is composed predominantly of CD4+ (helper-inducer) T-lymphocytes and about 20% of CD8+ (suppressor-cytotoxic) T-lymphocytes. There is also an increased number of Langerhans cells in the epidermis. A virus-induced type IV hypersensitivity reaction has been proposed (202). The surface antigen of the hepatitis B virus is detectable in the sera of all cases of papular acrodermatitis of childhood due to hepatitis B virus by radioimmunoassay. Cases in which serologic studies for hepatitis B virus are negative require studies for other viruses by means of throat swabs and stool samples and by testing for antibodies (195).

MUCOCUTANEOUS LYMPH NODE SYNDROME (KAWASAKI DISEASE)

The mucocutaneous lymph node syndrome, first reported in 1967 (203), is most common in Japanese or Korean children under 5 years of age, although it can occur in all races (204) either sporadically or epidemically. A definitive diagnosis is established by the presence of unexplained fever lasting 5 or more days and of at least four out of five clinical criteria: (a) bilateral conjunctivitis; (b) erythematous oral mucosa, injected or dry fissured lips, and "strawberry tongue"; (c) erythema and indurated edema of hands and feet often followed by periungual desquamation; (d) polymorphous skin rash; and (e) cervical nonsuppurative lymphadenopathy (205). Measles and group A β-hemolytic streptococcal infections may closely resemble Kawasaki disease and must be excluded (206).

The course of the disease could be divided in three clinical phases: acute, subacute, and convalescent. The first phase is the febrile period in which all the diagnostic signs may be seen (207). The rash appears around the third to fifth day of illness and may have different morphologic patterns such as maculopapular, morbilliform, scarlatiniform, or urticarial (208). It involves the trunk and extremities and in some cases has a peculiar perineal distribution (209).

Recently a psoriasiform skin eruption that occurs during either the acute or convalescent phase has been described, with some lesions being pustular (210). There are many other associated systemic manifestations, but cardiovascular complications account for the death of 2% of the children with the disease (203). Twenty percent of untreated patients may develop coronary artery aneurysms (211), and myocardial infarction secondary to aneurysmal thrombosis is the principal cause of death (212). A rare and serious complication is the development of peripheral ischemia and gangrene (213).

Histopathology. The histologic changes in the skin consist of a sparse perivascular infiltrate of lymphocytes and histiocytes (203), marked papillary dermal edema, and dilatation of blood vessels (214). Mild exocytosis of lymphocytes can be seen (215). An uncommon pustular variant of Kawasaki disease shows sterile intraepidermal spongiform pustules with neutrophils (216).

Pathogenesis. Electron microscopic studies have revealed swelling and focal degenerative changes of endothelial cells from the superficial and deep vascular plexuses of the skin (214). Immunohistochemical stains have shown that the inflammatory infiltrate has predominantly CD4+ (helper-inducer) T-lymphocytes and CD14+ macrophages, with only a few CD8+ (suppressor-cytotoxic) T-lymphocytes and no CD20+ B-lymphocytes (215). There is also expression of HLA-DR by keratinocytes and endothelial cells (215). In the acute stage of the disease, interleukin-1 alpha (IL-1α) and tumor necrosis factor-alpha (TNF-α) can be detected in the epidermis. TNF-α is also found on blood vessel walls (215). All these findings support the hypothesis of a cell-mediated immune reaction in the pathogenesis of the disease, possibly triggered by a virus (217), conventional antigen (218), or superantigen (219). It has been suggested that vascular endothelial growth factor (VEGF), also known as vascular permeability factor, together with hepatocyte growth factor (HGF) might play an important role in the pathophysiology of Kawasaki disease; and their serum levels could be a powerful predictor for the development of coronary artery lesions (220,221). The detection of autoantibodies against a 70-kD protein from vascular

smooth muscle cells may also contribute to the coronary and systemic vasculitis in Kawasaki disease (222).

LICHEN PLANUS

Lichen planus is a subacute or chronic dermatosis that may involve skin, mucous membranes, hair follicles, and nails (223).

In glabrous skin, the eruption is characterized by small, flat-topped, shiny, polygonal, violaceous papules that may coalesce into plaques. The papules often show a network of white lines known as Wickham's striae. Pruritus is usually pronounced. The disease has a predilection for the flexor surfaces of the forearms, legs, and the glans penis. The eruption may be localized or extensive, and Koebner's phenomenon is commonly seen (224).

The oral lesions of lichen planus are frequently found, either as sole manifestation of the disease or associated with cutaneous involvement (225). They usually involve the buccal and glossal mucosa and most often consist of a lacy, reticular network of white coalescent papules (226). Besides the reticular type, other lesional patterns have been described, such as plaque-like, atrophic, papular, erosive, and bullous (223,227).

The nails are involved in about 10% of cases and show roughening, longitudinal ridging, and, rarely, thinning and destruction (228). Pterygium formation is a frequent finding.

A common variant is *hypertrophic lichen planus*, which is usually found on the shins and consists of thickened and often verrucous plaques. In contrast, *vesicular lichen planus* is rare. It shows vesicles situated only on some of the preexisting lesions (229,230). It is different from so-called *lichen planus pemphigoides* in which the eruption is more disseminated and the bullae are more extensive (231), arising from papules of lichen planus and from normal-appearing skin (230,232–234). Although lichen planus pemphigoides and bullous pemphigoid manifest in different ways clinically, the same antigen may be involved in the immunopathogenesis of these two diseases. (See pathogenesis discussion.)

Lichen planopilaris designates the folliculotropic variant of lichen planus, which predominantly involves the scalp. Initially, there may be only follicular papules or perifollicular erythema; however, with progressive hair loss, irregularly shaped atrophic patches of scarring alopecia develop on the scalp. The axillae and the pubic region may also be affected and the alopecia in these areas may be cicatricial (235). Hyperkeratotic follicular papules may also be seen on glabrous skin (236). The association of scarring alopecia of hair-bearing areas and hyperkeratotic follicular papules on glabrous skin is known as Graham–Little syndrome. Lichen planopilaris may also coexist with typical lesions of lichen planus on skin, mucous membranes, or nails. Linear lichen planopilaris of the face resolving with scarring has also been described (237).

Ulcerative lichen planus, a rare but quite characteristic variant of lichen planus, shows bullae, erosions, and painful ulcerations on the feet and toes resulting in atrophic scarring and permanent loss of the toenails. It is usually associated with patches of atrophic alopecia of the scalp and with cutaneous and oral lesions of lichen planus (238–240).

Lichen planus actinicus, or *pigmentosus*, occurs mainly in Middle Eastern countries, where between 20% and 30% of lichen planus cases are of this type (241,242). It tends to be more common in children or young adults. The lesions develop in spring and summer on sun-exposed areas, especially the face. Three different forms have been described: annular (the most common type), pigmented (resembling melasma) (243), and dyschromic (244). The lesions are typically annular plaques with central slate blue to light brown pigmentation and well-defined, slightly raised, hypopigmented borders. Pruritus is minimal or absent.

The *overlap syndrome*, *lichen planus/lupus erythematosus*, refers to a heterogeneous group of patients bearing at the same time, skin lesions with clinical, histological, and/or immunological features typical of both diseases (245). The cutaneous findings in these unusual cases consist of erythematous to purplish scaly patches and plaques, some of them with central atrophy, with a predilection for photodistributed areas (246) or acral portions of extremities (245).

Twenty-nail dystrophy may be encountered in adults as well as children. The nails have longitudinal ridging and distal notching and splitting. With time they become thin and roughened. Clinically, the nail changes resemble those seen in lichen planus (247,248). Other manifestations of lichen planus are usually absent. In children, the nail changes tend to involute spontaneously after a few years. In familial cases, it tends to have an unremitting course. Congenital cases have been described (249). Twenty-nail dystrophy may be idiopathic or may be associated with alopecia areata, atopic dermatitis, lichen planus, or psoriasis.

The coexistence of *lichen nitidus* with lichen planus is frequent enough to have suggested to some authors that they are variants of the same disease (250).

Malignant transformation of cutaneous lichen planus occurs in less than 1% of cases (251). In hypertrophic lichen planus of the leg, development of squamous cell carcinoma or keratoacanthoma is an exceptional occurrence (252,253). There have been reports of squamous cell carcinoma arising occasionally on long-standing lesions of lichen planus situated on mucous membranes or the vermillion border (254–257). The incidence of carcinoma evolving in oral lichen planus is about 0.5% (258–260), with a range of 0. 3% to 3% (257,261). Development of carcinoma in ulcers of the feet in ulcerative lichen planus has been reported to occur rarely in lesions that had not been previously grafted (262,263).

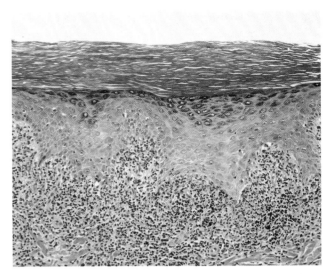

FIGURE 7-15. Lichen planus. Dense band-like infiltrate predominantly of lymphocytes in the papillary dermis that extends to the epidermis, where there is vacuolar alteration of the basal layer, necrotic keratinocytes, irregular acanthosis, wedge-shaped hypergranulosis, and compact orthokeratosis.

Histopathology. Typical papules of lichen planus show (a) compact orthokeratosis, (b) wedge-shaped hypergranulosis, (c) irregular acanthosis, (d) vacuolar alteration of the basal layer, and (e) a band-like dermal lymphocytic infiltrate in close approximation to the epidermis (Figs. 7-15 and 7-16). This constellation of findings is sufficiently diagnostic that a histologic diagnosis can be rendered in more than 90% of cases (264).

The cornified layer shows compact orthokeratosis and contains very few, if any, parakeratotic cells, a fact that is important for the diagnosis. The thickening of the granular layer is uneven and wedge shaped. The granular cells appear increased in size and contain coarse and more abundant keratohyaline granules. On step sectioning, the areas of wedge-shaped hypergranulosis are found to be contigu-

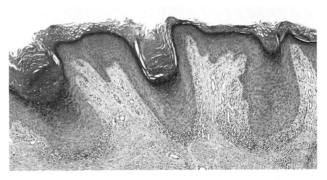

FIGURE 7-16. Hypertrophic lichen planus. Marked irregular acanthosis, hypergranulosis, and compact orthokeratosis. The vacuolar alteration and the lymphocytic inflammatory infiltrate is accentuated at the base of the rete ridges.

ous to intraepidermal adnexal structures, namely acrosy-ringia and acrotrichia (265). Wickham's striae are believed to be caused by a focal increase in the thickness of the granular layer and of the total epidermis (266).

The acanthosis in lichen planus is irregular and affects the spinous layer of the rete ridges as well as the suprapapillary plates. The keratinocytes of the spinous layer often appear larger and eosinophilic, possibly because of advanced keratinization. The rete ridges show irregular lengthening, and some of them are pointed at their lower end, giving them a saw-toothed appearance. The dermal papillae between elongated rete ridges are often dome shaped (267).

The cells of the basal layer are not clearly visible in early lesions because the dense dermal infiltrate obscures the dermal–epidermal junction with vacuolar alteration and necrosis of the basal keratinocytes. In fully developed lesions, the basal layer has the appearance of flattened squamous cells.

The infiltrate in the upper dermis is band-like and sharply demarcated at its lower border and is composed almost entirely of lymphocytes intermingled with macrophages. A few eosinophils and/or plasma cells may be seen. Melanophages are seen in the upper dermis, often in considerable number, as a result of damage to the basal cells with subsequent pigment incontinence. In some instances, the dermal lymphocytic infiltrate is seen in juxtaposition to the acrosyringium and vacuolar alteration of the acrosyringeal basal cell layer is a prominent finding (*acrosyringeal lichen planus*) (268).

In old lesions, the cellular infiltrate decreases in density, but the number of melanophages increases. In areas in which a basal cell layer has regenerated, the dermal infiltrate no longer lies in close approximation to the epidermis. *Hypertrophic lichen planus* shows considerable acan-

thosis, papillomatosis, hypergranulosis, and hyperkeratosis. The interface vacuolar changes are discrete and often limited to the base of the rete ridges (Fig. 7-16).

Necrotic keratinocytes are present in most of cases in the lower epidermis and especially in the papillary dermis. They are also referred to as colloid, hyaline, cytoid, or Civatte bodies. They average 20 μm in diameter and have a homogeneous, eosinophilic appearance (see Fig. 7-17). They are PAS positive and diastase resistant. Even though necrotic keratinocytes are found most commonly in lichen planus, they may occur in any interface dermatitis in which damage to the basal cells occurs, including graft-versus-host disease (GVHD), lichen nitidus, lupus erythematosus, drug reactions, and in inflamed keratoses such as lichenoid actinic keratosis and lichen planus-like keratosis. They may even be seen in normal skin (269). In lichen planus, the number of necrotic keratinocytes may be so large that they are seen lying in clusters in the uppermost dermis (245). Their aggregation may result in perforation of the epidermis with subsequent transepidermal elimination (270).

Occasionally, small areas of artifactual separation between the epidermis and the dermis, known as Max–Joseph spaces, are seen (264) (Fig. 7-18). In some instances, the separation occurs *in vivo* and subepidermal blisters form (*vesicular lichen planus*). These vesicles form as a result of extensive damage to the basal cells (229,231).

Oral lichen planus. The oral lesions of lichen planus differ in their histologic appearance from those of the skin, as one would expect, since the oral mucosa normally shows parakeratosis without the presence of a granular layer. Thus, the lesions of the mouth often show parakeratosis rather than orthokeratosis, although alternating areas of both types of keratinization with the presence of a granular layer may be observed (227) (Fig. 7-19). Also, rather than showing acan-

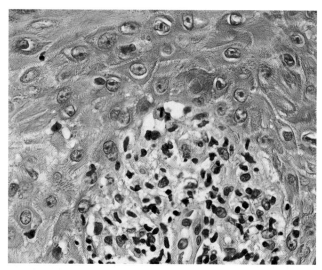

FIGURE 7-17. Lichen planus. Closer view shows lymphocytes and melanophages in the papillary dermis, vacuolar alteration of the basal layer, pink-staining necrotic keratinocytes (Civatte bodies), and enlarged keratinocytes with eosinophilic cytoplasm.

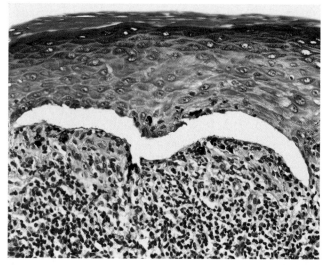

FIGURE 7-18. Lichen planus. Artifactual cleft between the epidermis and the lichenoid infiltrate known as a Max–Joseph space.

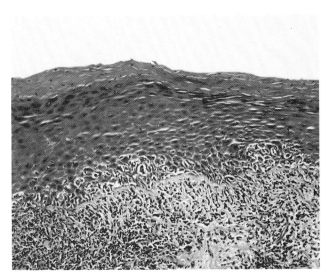

FIGURE 7-19. Oral lichen planus. Similar lichenoid inflammatory pattern as seen in the skin except for less hypergranulosis and confluent parakeratosis.

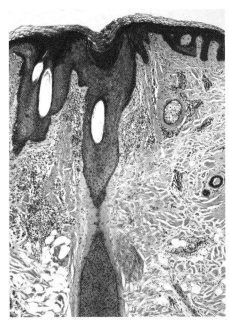

FIGURE 7-21. Lichen planopilaris, developed lesion. Perifollicular fibrosis and inflammation with epithelial atrophy at the infundibuloisthmic portion, give rise to an hourglass configuration.

thosis, the epithelium often is atrophic. Ulcerations may develop either through the rupture of vesicles or as a result of necrosis of the atrophic epithelium.

Lichen planopilaris. Most early lesions of lichen planopilaris show a focally dense, band-like perifollicular lymphocytic infiltrate at the level of the infundibulum and the isthmus where the hair "bulge" is located. Initially, the inferior segment of the hair follicle is spared. Vacuolar changes of the basal layer of the outer root sheath and necrotic keratinocytes are often seen. In addition, orthokeratosis, follicular plugging, and wedge–shaped hypergranulosis of the infundibulum are observed (Fig. 7-20).

Interfollicular epidermis is often spared but it can occasionally be involved (271). In more developed lesions perifollicular fibrosis and epithelial atrophy at the level of the infundibulum and isthmus are characteristic findings giving rise to an hourglass configuration (Fig. 7-21). It is hypothesized that damage to the hair bulge, where the stem cells of the hair follicle supposedly reside, results in permanent scarring alopecia. Advanced cases show alopecia with vertically oriented fibrotic tracts containing clumps of degenerated elastic fibers that replaced the destroyed hair follicles. This end-stage scarring alopecia in which no visible hair follicles remain is called pseudopelade of Brocq (272).

The hyperkeratotic follicular papules that are occasionally seen on glabrous skin in association with lichen planopilaris of the scalp exhibit similar changes; however, perifollicular fibrosis is usually slight and the process does not eventuate in scarring (273).

Ulcerative lichen planus. In ulcerative lichen planus, specimens taken from skin adjacent to the ulcer generally show active lichen planus (238,240,262).

Lichen planus actinicus. In some instances, the histologic picture of lichen planus actinicus is similar to the typical lichen planus but with a tendency toward thinning of the epidermis at the center of the lesion and more evident pigmentary incontinence in the upper dermis (43,242). Because of the histologic resemblance in some cases, a relationship between lichen planus actinicus and erythema dyschromicum perstans has been postulated (274); however, they have significant clinical differences (43).

Overlap syndrome—lichen planus/lupus erythematosus. In some cases of the overlap syndrome, the histologic features

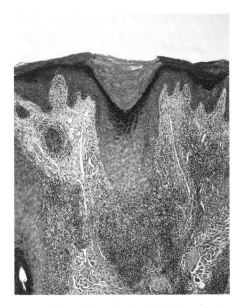

FIGURE 7-20. Lichen planopilaris. Follicular plugging, hypergranulosis, and dense band-like perifollicular lymphocytic infiltrate that obscures the infundibular epithelium.

and direct immunofluorescence findings are more consistent with lichen planus. In others, the immunofluorescence testing favors lupus erythematosus (246), and still in another subset of patients there are lesions of lichen planus that coexist, rather than overlap, with those of lupus erythematosus (275,276).

Twenty-nail dystrophy. Histologic data on twenty-nail dystrophy are available in only a few cases. Twenty-nail dystrophy is a manifestation of diverse underlying processes; therefore, its histology will vary (248,249). Biopsies may show typical lichen planus involving the nail matrix (247,277). However, spongiosis may be prominent as in cases associated with atopic dermatitis.

Lichen planus pemphigoides. In lichen planus pemphigoides, biopsies taken from bullae arising from uninvolved skin show subepidermal bullae with an infiltrate that is not band-like and that contains eosinophils (230).

Pathogenesis. The eosinophilia of the keratinocytes and the increase in thickness of the granular and cornified layers suggest a decreased epidermal turnover. However, in spite of severely damaged basal cells, measurements of cell proliferation in lichen planus with tritiated thymidine have shown an increase in cell proliferation (278).

Electron microscopy. On electron microscopy, the basal keratinocytes in lichen planus, together with their desmosomes and hemidesmosomes, show degenerative changes (279). Whereas the tonofilaments in the basal cells are decreased in early lesions, they are increased in later lesions (280). Because of the presence of degenerated and necrotic keratinocytes in the basal layer, it is assumed that the basal cells in later lesions are largely regenerated cells. The dermal infiltrate, extending to the epidermis, causes damage to the lamina densa such as fragmentation (EM 12). This may be followed by duplication and irregular folding of the lamina densa (281). The dermal infiltrate contains mainly lymphocytes but also macrophages. Some of the lymphocytes have hyperconvoluted nuclei and appear indistinguishable from Sézary cells.

Necrotic keratinocytes or colloid bodies are located largely in the papillary dermis but also in the lower most epidermis (EM 12). They can be seen to develop from damaged keratinocytes through filamentous degeneration. This is followed by their discharge into the dermis (282). Necrotic keratinocytes consist of aggregates of filament bundles, with each filament measuring approximately 10 nm in diameter. The use of antikeratin immune sera has resulted in their intense staining (283). Necrotic keratinocytes often still contain cell organelles, such as melanosomes and mitochondria, but only rarely contain nuclear material (284). Fibrin deposits in the upper dermis are a common finding in electron microscopy studies.

In the vesicular lesions of lichen planus, electron microscopic examination shows cytolysis of basal keratinocytes; the blister cavity is, therefore, situated below the spinous layer (285).

Immunofluorescence. In lichen planus, fibrinogen deposition can be demonstrated by direct immunofluorescence as shaggy deposits at the dermal–epidermal junction (286). Only occasionally are there granular deposits of IgM (287), or linear deposits of C3 (288), or both IgG and C3 (289) in the basement membrane zone. Necrotic keratinocytes are demonstrable in lichen planus by direct immunofluorescence staining in about 87% of cases (286). They stain mainly for IgM but often also for IgG, IgA, C3 and fibrin. Although necrotic keratinocytes are found occasionally in many other conditions with damage to the basal cell layer, such as lupus erythematosus, they are highly suggestive of lichen planus if they are present in large numbers or arranged in clusters. Their staining for IgM facilitates their recognition (269).

In lichen planopilaris, direct immunofluorescence in many specimens shows deposition of IgM and/or IgA, IgG, and, rarely, C3 at the level of the infundibulum and isthmus (290). The necrotic keratinocytes may react with anti-IgM antibody. There is often deposition of fibrinogen in a shaggy pattern surrounding the affected follicles. The dermal–epidermal junction is virtually always negative for deposition of immunoreactants (271).

In lichen planus pemphigoides, direct immunofluorescence of perilesional skin shows the presence of IgG and C3 in a linear arrangement along the basement membrane zone (230,291), and on immunoelectron microscopy, C3 is seen to be localized within the lamina lucida, analogous to its location in bullous pemphigoid (232). It has been shown that circulating IgG autoantibodies are directed against the bullous pemphigoid antigen 180 (BP180, type XVII collagen), a transmembrane hemidesmosomal glycoprotein of the basal keratinocytes that spans the lamina lucida (292,293). Immunoelectron microscopic studies have also confirmed the location of the antigen being at the same site as the bullous pemphigoid antigen; the basal cell hemidesmosomes on the epidermal side of salt-split skin (294). However, it is suggested that the immunoglobulin subclass of the autoantibody and/or the epitope that is recognized may be different in these two diseases (292). One study has shown that in addition to BP180 antigen, the autoantibodies were also directed against a 200-kD antigen (295).

In the overlap syndrome lichen planus/lupus erythematosus, some patients show immunofluorescence testing consistent with lichen planus; in another group direct immunofluorescence shows deposition of immunoglobulins and C3 at the dermal–epidermal junction in a linear granular pattern as in cutaneous lupus erythematosus (246).

Immunohistochemistry. The infiltrating cells in lichen planus are predominantly T-lymphocytes with very few B-lymphocytes. More than 90% are activated T-lymphocytes expressing HLA-DR antigen and some interleukin-2 receptor (296). The identification of various subtypes of T-lymphocytes has given contradictory results with regards to the predominance of CD4+ helper-inducer T-lymphocytes and CD8+ suppressor-cytotoxic T-lymphocytes in the infiltrate (297–299). It is likely that both subsets participate in the immunologic reaction. It has been shown that in older lesions of oral lichen planus the suppressor T-lymphocytes predominate. The epitheliotropic lymphocytes have also been shown to be of the same subtype, supporting a cell-mediated cytotoxic mechanism against epithelial cells (298,300). In the epidermis adjacent to the infiltrate, basal keratinocytes express HLA-DR surface antigen and intercellular adhesion molecule-1 (ICAM-1) (301); both of which are implicated to enhance the interaction between lymphocytes and their epidermal targets resulting in keratinocyte destruction (299). It is probable that these surface antigens are induced by cytokines (γ-IFN and TNF-α) released by lymphocytes from the infiltrate (302,303). Immunophenotyping studies on T-lymphocytes extracted from specimens of lichen planus have shown that the majority of clones were CD8+ T-lymphocytes, displayed suppressor activity, and expressed αβT-cell receptor (304) or a distinctive γδT-cell receptor (305). Clonal expansion of α2β3T-cell receptor of the V-gene family has been reported, suggesting that a superantigen could be involved in the pathogenesis of the disease (306).

The number of Langerhans cells in the epidermis is increased very early in the disease (265), especially near keratinocytes expressing HLA-DR+ antigen (307). Immuno-electron studies have shown close contacts of lymphocytes with Langerhans cells and macrophages. Specific conjugations between CD4+ (helper-inducer) T-lymphocytes and dendritic (HLA-DR+) cells and between CD8+ (cytotoxic-suppressor) T-lymphocytes and degenerated basal keratinocytes have been observed in lesional epithelium of oral mucosa. These cell-to-cell interactions suggest that a cell-mediated immune mechanism is operative (308).

Differential Diagnosis. It should be borne in mind that parakeratosis is not a feature of lichen planus of the skin and that, if more than focal parakeratosis is present, a diagnosis of lichen planus should not be made on histologic grounds.

Focal parakeratosis and adjacent solar lentigines in an otherwise typical histologic picture of lichen planus should be regarded as lichen planus–like keratosis, even more so if it is a solitary and nonpruritic lesion (309). Lichenoid drug eruptions may be differentiated from lichen planus by the presence of focal parakeratosis with concomitant absence of the granular layer, necrotic keratinocytes in the basal and spinous layers, exocytosis of lymphocytes to the upper layers of the epidermis, and a deeper inflammatory infiltrate with numerous eosinophils (310).

Differentiation from lichenoid lupus erythematosus is based on (a) atrophy of the epidermis in addition to acanthosis, (b) absence of eosinophilia of the keratinocytes in the spinous layer, (c) a superficial band-like infiltrate with a superficial and deep perivascular and periadnexal infiltrate, (d) the presence of a thickened PAS-positive basement membrane, and (e) dermal mucin deposits. Direct immunofluorescence findings may also be helpful; in lupus erythematosus, linear or granular deposits of immunoglobulins and C3 predominate in lesional skin, while in lichen planus, clusters of necrotic keratinocytes with absorbed immunoglobulins and complement are found. Langerhans cells (CD1a+/S-100+) are decreased in number in discoid and systemic lupus erythematosus; in contrast, they are increased in early lichen planus (299). The epidermal changes in chronic GVHD may be similar to lichen planus; however, the inflammatory infiltrate tends to be perivascular instead of band-like. In addition, the number of Langerhans cells in GVHD is decreased and nearly all intraepidermal lymphocytes are cytotoxic-suppressor T cells (311). In long-standing hypertrophic lichen planus, the basal layer may show hardly any residual damage and the infiltrate may no longer be band-like, rendering differentiation from lichen simplex chronicus at times difficult (312). However, in hypertrophic lichen planus, deeper sections still may show areas of damage to the basal layer at the base of the rete ridges.

On the lips and in the mouth, the differentiation of lichen planus from early squamous cell carcinoma *in situ* ("dysplastic leukoplakia") may cause difficulties clinically as well as histologically. Both diseases may show hyperkeratosis and an inflammatory infiltrate close to the epidermis/epithelium. Yet a thorough microscopic study reveals more atypical keratinocytes in squamous cell carcinoma *in situ*. Furthermore, squamous cell carcinoma *in situ* is more apt than lichen planus to show irregular downward proliferation of the rete ridges and numerous plasma cells.

Lichen planopilaris of the scalp must be differentiated in its early phase from discoid lupus erythematosus, which affects the hair follicles as well as the interfollicular epidermis. Lupus erythematosus shows vacuolar degeneration of the basal cells both in the epidermis and in the hair follicles without disappearance of basal cells. In addition, it also shows a thickened epidermal basement membrane and an interfollicular superficial and deep perivascular infiltrate. In their late stages, both lichen planopilaris and lupus erythematosus may result in permanent scarring alopecia, which is known as pseudopelade of Brocq (272).

LICHEN PLANUS–LIKE KERATOSIS

Lichen planus–like keratosis (LPLK), also known as "benign lichenoid keratosis," was originally described in 1966 as "solitary lichen planus" (313) and as "solitary lichen planus–like keratosis" (314). It is a common lesion that occurs predominantly on the trunk and upper extremities of adults between the fifth and seventh decades, but occurrence on the face and lower extremities have also been reported (315–318). LPLK consists of a nonpruritic papule or slightly indurated plaque that is nearly always solitary, although cases with more than one skin lesion have been reported. It usually measures 5 to 20 mm in diameter and its color varies from bright red to violaceous to brown. Its surface may be smooth or slightly verrucous (319). Lichen planus–like keratosis probably represents the inflammatory stage of involuting solar lentigines (320).

Histopathology. Histologic examination shows, at least in a part of the lesion, a lichenoid pattern that may be indistinguishable from lichen planus (309,313,314). As in lichen planus, there is vacuolar alteration of the basal cell layer and a band-like lymphocytic infiltrate that obscures the dermal–epidermal junction. Necrotic keratinocytes are commonly seen and may be numerous (319). As in lichen planus, the epidermis often shows increased eosinophilia, hypergranulosis, and hyperkeratosis (321). In contrast to lichen planus, however, parakeratosis is fairly common (316) (Fig. 7-22). Although usually focal (309), at times parakeratosis is prominent (319). In addition, eosinophils and plasma cells in the infiltrate are more frequently found in some cases of LPLK as opposed to lichen planus, in which they are rarely seen (309,322). A residual solar lentigo at the edge of the lesion supports the diagnosis of LPLK (323). Immunohistochemical studies have shown that LPLK has significantly fewer Langerhans cells in the epidermis compared to lichen planus (324). The epidermal and dermal lymphocytes were shown to mainly consist of CD8+ T cells and partly CD20+ B cells. CD4+ T cells were scarce. However, epidermal lymphocytes in lichen planus were mainly CD8+ T cells and dermal lymphocytes were CD4+ or CD8+ T cells. In lichen planus, CD20+ B cells were fewer than in LPLK. Memory T cells express a skin-homing receptor called cutaneous lymphocyte-associated antigen (CLA). This antigen is strongly expressed in lichen planus but not in LPLK, suggesting that in lichen planus, disease-related lymphocytes infiltrate the epidermis, whereas in LPLK the lymphocytes may be nonspecific infiltrating cells (318).

Direct immunofluorescence studies have revealed the linear deposition of IgM at the basement membrane zone (325). Even though some keratinocytes may show pyknotic hyperchromatic nuclei, no definite nuclear atypia is seen. If marked keratinocytic atypia is found in association with a lichenoid inflammatory pattern, a lichenoid actinic keratosis should be considered in the differential diagnosis (326).

Pathogenesis. LPLK has been noted to involute spontaneously (327). LPLK may be the inflammatory stage of regressing solar lentigines and reticulated seborrheic keratoses (320,322,323). These precursor lesions could be the targets of an immune cell–mediated reaction (309).

KERATOSIS LICHENOIDES CHRONICA

A rare asymptomatic dermatosis, keratosis lichenoides chronica was first described by Kaposi in 1895 as "lichen ruber acuminatus verrucosus et reticularis" (328), and received its present name in 1972 (329). It usually begins in adulthood between 20 and 50 years of age, being extremely rare in children (330,331). It shows an extensive eruption, symmetrically distributed, predominantly on dorsal aspects of extremities and trunk consisting of red to violaceous papulonodules covered with a thick, adherent scale and arranged often in a characteristic linear and occasionally reticular pattern. These lesions may coalesce to form erythematous scaly or hyperkeratotic plaques (332,333). Very frequently there is associated seborrheic dermatitis-like eruption of the face, palmoplantar hyperkeratosis (332), and in some cases, nail changes with warty hypertrophy of the periungual tissues, which has been described as a distinctive feature of the disease (334). Mucosal membrane involvement is common and includes oral ulcers, nodular infiltration of the epiglottis and larynx, blepharitis, and keratoconjunctivitis among others (329,332,333,335). Although the disease is characterized by a chronic and progressive course, spontaneous resolution has been reported (336).

The disease has been reported in association with lymphoma (337), following trauma (338), and after a drug-induced erythroderma (339).

Histopathology. In most cases, there is a lichenoid inflammatory pattern with areas of vacuolar alteration of the basal cell layer, necrotic keratinocytes, and a band-like inflammatory infiltrate of lymphocytes, histiocytes, and numerous plasma cells that obscures the dermal–epidermal junction (332,340). The epidermis shows areas of acanthosis as well as atrophy covered by a hyperkeratotic cornified layer showing focal parakeratosis and follicular plugging

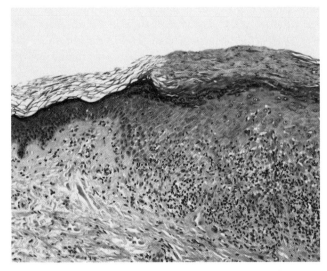

FIGURE 7-22. Lichen planus–like keratosis. Lichenoid inflammatory pattern with numerous necrotic keratinocytes, granular layer of uneven thickness, orthokeratosis, and parakeratosis with a residual solar lentigo.

(341). Prominent, dilated dermal capillaries are seen in cases with associated telangiectasias (342).

Differential Diagnosis. Although the histologic picture may closely resemble that of lichen planus, the presence of parakeratosis, alternating areas of atrophy and acanthosis, numerous plasma cells, and a heavier infiltrate than is usually seen in lichen planus may help in the differentiation. In addition, the clinical appearance of keratosis lichenoides chronica is quite different from that of lichen planus.

LICHEN NITIDUS

Lichen nitidus is a chronic and usually asymptomatic dermatitis that begins commonly in childhood or early adulthood (343). It is characterized by round, flat-topped, flesh-colored papules 2 to 3 mm in diameter that may occur in groups but do not coalesce. The lesions appear frequently as a localized eruption affecting predominantly the arms, trunk, or penis. In some patients, the eruption may become generalized (344), and Koebner's phenomenon may be observed (345). There are a few cases reported to occur on palms, soles, nails, and mucous membranes (346). The clinical course is unpredictable and spontaneous resolution may be seen (343).

Histopathology. Each papule of lichen nitidus consists of a well-circumscribed mixed-cell granulomatous infiltrate that is closely attached to the lower surface of the epidermis and confined to a widened dermal papilla. The infiltrate is composed of lymphocytes, mono- and a few multi-nucleated epithelioid histiocytes. The dermal infiltrate often extends slightly into the overlying epidermis, which is flattened and shows vacuolar alteration of the basal cell layer, focal subepidermal clefting, diminished granular layer, and focal parakeratosis (343). Transepidermal perforation of the infiltrate through the thinned epidermis may occur (347). At each lateral margin of the infiltrate, rete ridges tend to extend downward and seem to clutch the infiltrate in the manner of a "claw clutching a ball" (Fig. 7-23). The palmar lesions have shown to have the infiltrate mostly disposed around the bases of the rete ridges, similar to that found in hypertrophic lichen planus (348). Follicular involvement in lichen nitidus has been described (349).

Relationship Between Lichen Planus and Lichen Nitidus. There are controversial facts regarding the relationship that might exist between lichen planus and lichen nitidus. The view that lichen nitidus represents a variant of lichen planus has been supported by several authors because both diseases are occasionally present simultaneously (344), ultrastructural findings are similar (350), and, in some cases of lichen planus, small miliary papules may have a histologic appearance consistent with lichen nitidus (351). However, the subsequent evolution is different; in lichen nitidus the papule remains small and develops parakeratosis and epidermal flattening, whereas in lichen planus

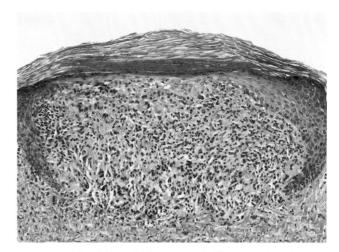

FIGURE 7-23. Lichen nitidus. Dense infiltrate of lymphocytes and histiocytes in an expanded dermal papilla, thin suprapapillary epidermis with vacuolar alteration of the basal layer, and focal parakeratosis.

the papule develops acanthosis and hyperkeratosis (344). Occasional deposits of fibrinogen can be observed by direct immunofluorescence in lichen nitidus, in contrast to lichen planus, where most of the lesions have globular deposits of immunoglobulins at the dermal–epidermal junction (352). Furthermore, immunohistochemical studies have revealed diverse cell populations in the inflammatory infiltrate of each disease (353). Lichen nitidus has a significantly smaller proportion of CD4+ (helper-inducer) and HECA-452+ (skin-homing receptor) T-lymphocytes, compared to lichen planus, suggesting different immunologic pathways (353).

LICHEN STRIATUS

Lichen striatus is a fairly uncommon dermatitis that, as a rule, occurs in children from 5 to 15 years of age, but may be seen in adults (354). It usually manifests itself as a unilateral eruption along Blaschko's lines (355) on the extremities, trunk, or neck as either a continuous or an interrupted band composed of minute, slightly raised, erythematous papules, which may have a scaly surface. The lesions appear abruptly and usually involute within a year. They are occasionally pruritic (356). Hypopigmented lesions may be seen in dark-skinned patients (357). A few cases with associated onychodystrophy (358,359), rare cases of multiple or bilateral presentations (360,361), and simultaneous occurrence of lichen striatus in siblings (362) have been reported.

Histopathology. Although lichen striatus has been recognized by its variable histologic picture (354,357,363), some constant microscopic findings may be present (364). There is usually a superficial perivascular inflammatory infiltrate of lymphocytes admixed with a variable number of

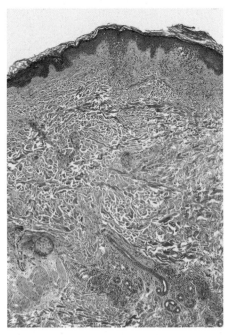

FIGURE 7-24. Lichen striatus. Superficial and deep perivascular, perieccrine and perifollicular infiltrate of lymphocytes and histiocytes that extends to the epidermis, which shows acanthosis and spongiosis.

histiocytes. Plasma cells and eosinophils are rarely seen (354) (Fig. 7-24). Focally, in the papillary dermis the infiltrate may have a band-like distribution with extension into the lower portion of the epidermis, where there is vacuolar alteration of the basal layer and necrotic keratinocytes. In these areas, the papillary dermis occasionally contains melanophages (354,363). Additional epidermal changes consist of spongiosis and intracellular edema often associ-

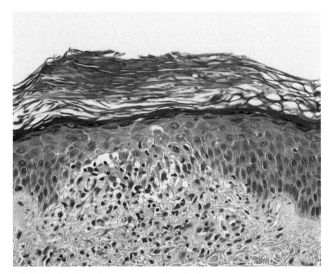

FIGURE 7-25. Lichen striatus. Closer view shows an infiltrate of lymphocytes and histiocytes, exocytosis of lymphocytes, acanthosis, spongiosis, and focal parakeratosis.

ated with exocytosis of lymphocytes and focal parakeratosis (Fig. 7-25). Less frequently, there are scattered necrotic keratinocytes in the spinous layer as well as subcorneal spongiotic vesicles filled with Langerhans cells (364). A very distinctive feature is the presence of inflammatory infiltrate in the reticular dermis around hair follicles and eccrine glands (354,364) (Fig. 7-24). An unusual perforating variant of lichen striatus has been described, which shows transepidermal elimination of clusters of necrotic keratinocytes (365).

Pathogenesis. In lichen striatus it has been found that the inflammatory cells reaching the epidermis are CD8+ (suppressor-cytotoxic) T-lymphocytes (364,366) with the Langerhans cells population in the epidermis either decreased or increased. These findings suggest a cell-mediated immunologic mechanism where cytotoxic events against keratinocytes could be taking place during the evolution of the disease (364).

Differential Diagnosis. Lichen striatus may show histologic features similar to other interface dermatitides such as lichen planus, lichen nitidus, or graft-versus-host disease. In contrast to lichen striatus, the inflammatory infiltrate of lichen nitidus is only focally present in widened dermal papillae and contains more histiocytes. The presence of epidermal spongiosis and a deeper dermal inflammatory infiltrate around adnexal structures are features rarely seen in lichen planus.

INFLAMMATORY LINEAR VERRUCOUS EPIDERMAL NEVUS

Inflammatory linear verrucous epidermal nevus (ILVEN) presents as a persistent, linear, intensely pruritic lesion. It is composed of erythematous, slightly verrucous, scaly papules arranged in one or several lines. Although the usual time of onset is early childhood, the disease may arise in adults (367). The most common location is on a lower extremity. On rare occasions the lesions are bilateral (368).

ILVEN in association with arthritis (369) and lichen amyloidosus (370) has been reported. ILVEN is considered to be a variant of epidermal nevi; however, it is described in the papulosquamous disorders due to its clinical and histologic similarities to psoriasis and lichen striatus.

Histopathology. One observes hyperkeratosis with foci of parakeratosis, moderate acanthosis, elongation and thickening of the rete ridges with a "psoriasiform" appearance, papillomatosis, and, occasionally, slight spongiosis with exocytosis of lymphocytes (371).

Frequently, a rather characteristic histologic feature is a sharply demarcated alternation of orthokeratosis and parakeratosis in the cornified layer (Fig. 7-26). The parakeratotic areas are slightly raised, lack a granular layer, and show a compact eosinophilic cornified layer with nuclear preservation. The orthokeratotic areas instead are slightly

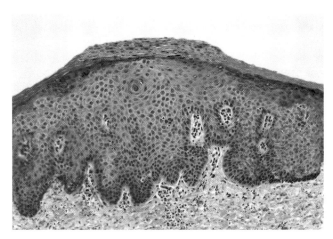

FIGURE 7-26. Inflammatory linear verrucous epidermal nevus (ILVEN). Moderate acanthosis with elongated rete ridges and alternating elevated foci of parakeratosis with absent granular layer and depressed foci of orthokeratosis with preserved granular layer.

depressed with underlying hypergranulosis (368,372,373). Underneath the parakeratotic areas, there is mild exocytosis of lymphocytes and slight spongiosis (374). The papillary dermis shows a mild to moderate perivascular inflammatory infiltrate of lymphocytes and histiocytes.

Pathogenesis. Electron microscopy and immunohistochemical studies have shown that keratinocyte differentiation is altered in the parakeratotic areas.

Ultrastructurally, keratinocytes have prominent Golgi apparatus and vesicles in their cytoplasm. The intercellular spaces in upper layers of the epidermis are widened by deposits of an electron-dense homogeneous substance. The cytoplasm of parakeratotic corneocytes contains remnants of nucleus and membrane structures and a few lipid droplets. The marginal band formation inside the plasma membrane is incomplete, suggesting a deficient keratinization process (374).

Involucrin expression has a very characteristic pattern in ILVEN. The orthokeratotic epidermis shows increased involucrin expression, whereas the parakeratotic areas are almost negative for involucrin staining (374). This pattern differs from that of psoriasis, in which involucrin is expressed prematurely in most of the suprabasal keratinocytes (375).

More than 90% of the mononuclear cells in the dermal infiltrate are CD4+ (helper-inducer) T-lymphocytes; in contrast, the majority of the epidermal infiltrating T-lymphocytes are CD4 negative (376).

Differential Diagnosis. The clinical appearance of lichen striatus and ILVEN may be indistinguishable. However, ILVEN, in contrast to lichen striatus, is pruritic and persistent. Histologically, lichen striatus tends to have a lichenoid pattern, and ILVEN a psoriasiform pattern. Furthermore, careful search of step sections will usually reveal in

ILVEN alternate areas of orthokeratosis with a thickened granular layer and of parakeratosis without a granular layer. The view that they are one and the same diseases (377) does not appear warranted.

While alternating orthokeratosis and parakeratosis can be seen in psoriasis and occasionally Munro microabscesses can be found in ILVEN, the differential diagnosis of these two entities could be sometimes difficult to assess and clinicopathologic correlation is necessary (378).

PITYRIASIS RUBRA PILARIS

Pityriasis rubra pilaris is an erythematous squamous disorder characterized by follicular keratotic papules and perifollicular erythema that coalesce to form orange-red scaly plaques that frequently contain islands of normal-appearing skin (379). As the erythema extends, the follicular component is often lost, but it persists longest on the dorsa of the proximal phalanges. The lesions spread caudally and may progress to a generalized erythroderma (380). Other clinical findings are palmoplantar keratoderma and scaling of the face and scalp. Five types can be recognized (380). However, only three types are common enough to deserve mention. *Type I classical adult type* and *type III classical juvenile type* are seen in 55% and 10% of patients, respectively. They are considered to be the same disease in different age groups (381). In both groups, the majority of the patients clear on average within 3 years (381,382). *Type IV*, the *circumscribed juvenile type*, accounts for approximately one-quarter of the patients. It affects children and is characterized by sharply demarcated areas of follicular hyperkeratosis and erythema on the knees and elbows. It may improve in the late teens (381). There is a familial form of pityriasis rubra pilaris inherited as an autosomal dominant trait (383).

Pityriasis rubra pilaris has been reported to occur in association with malignancies (384,385) and arthritis/arthropathy (386,387).

Histopathology. The histologic picture of a fully developed erythematous lesion shows acanthosis with broad and short rete ridges, slight spongiosis, thick suprapapillary plates, focal or confluent hypergranulosis, and alternating orthokeratosis and parakeratosis oriented in both vertical and horizontal directions (159) (Fig. 7-27). In the dermis, there is a mild superficial perivascular lymphocytic infiltrate and moderately dilated blood vessels (159,388).

Areas corresponding to follicular papules show dilated infundibula filled out with an orthokeratotic plug, and often display perifollicular shoulders of parakeratosis and a mild perifollicular lymphocytic infiltrate (389) (Fig. 7-28). Erythrodermic lesions have a thinned or absent cornified layer, plasma exudates, and a diminished granular zone (159).

Differential Diagnosis. Even though pityriasis rubra pilaris and psoriasis bear a similar clinical appearance, they

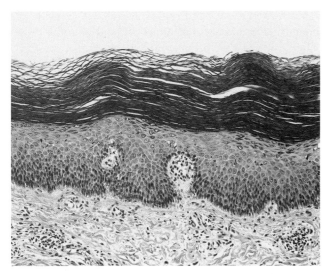

FIGURE 7-27. Pityriasis rubra pilaris. Moderate acanthosis with short and broad rete ridges, focally thin granular layer, and alternating vertical and horizontal foci of orthokeratosis and parakeratosis.

are not alike histologically. Psoriasis differs from pityriasis rubra pilaris by the presence of neutrophils and Munro microabscesses, more pronounced parakeratosis in mounds, thin suprapapillary plates, elongated rete ridges, and tortuous blood vessels (388). Pityriasis rubra pilaris has a more prominent granular layer with less epidermal spongiosis and inflammatory infiltrate (159). Moreover, it has been demonstrated that pityriasis rubra pilaris has a lower keratinocyte proliferation rate compared to psoriasis, suggesting differences in cell kinetic characteristics (388,390,391).

Pathogenesis. The cause of pityriasis rubra pilaris is unknown. There is evidence that suggests an abnormal epidermal differentiation based on the presence of suprabasal

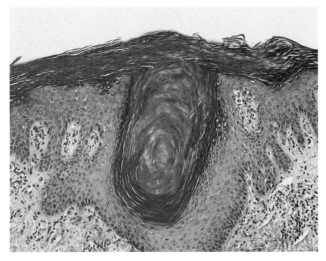

FIGURE 7-28. Pityriasis rubra pilaris, follicular lesion. Dilated follicular infundibulum with hyperkeratotic plug.

staining with monoclonal antibody against AE1 and the detection of cytokeratins K6 and K16, which are not expressed in normal skin (383).

PITYRIASIS LICHENOIDES

Pityriasis lichenoides is an uncommon cutaneous eruption usually classified in two forms that differ in severity. Simultaneous appearance of the two types (392) and transitions between them often occur, suggesting that they are variants of the same disease (393,394). Both are rarely pruritic or painful, with crops of self-healing lesions affecting young adults (393) and occasionally children (392,395).

The milder form, called *pityriasis lichenoides chronica*, is characterized by recurrent crops of brown-red papules 4 to 10 mm in size, mainly on the trunk and extremities, that are covered with a scale and generally involute within 3 to 6 weeks with postinflammatory pigmentary changes (174).

The more severe form, called *pityriasis lichenoides et varioliformis acuta* (PLEVA), also referred to as Mucha–Habermann disease, consists of a fairly extensive eruption, present mainly on the trunk and proximal extremities. It is characterized by erythematous papules that develop into papulonecrotic, occasionally hemorrhagic or vesiculo-pustular lesions that resolve within a few weeks, usually with little or no scarring. In occasional patients, some lesions increase in size to necrotic ulcers of 1 to 2 cm in diameter healing with an atrophic or varioliform scar. Although the individual lesions follow an acute course, the disorder is chronic, extending over several months or even years because of the development of crops of new lesions. Cases of PLEVA occurring during pregnancy and affecting the vagina/cervical mucosa with resultant premature rupture of the membranes and/or premature labor have been reported (396,397). Very rarely, patients with PLEVA have a sudden, severe flare-up of their disease, characterized by innumerable coalescent necrotic ulcerations associated with high fever and systemic manifestations (398–400).

Histopathology. In pityriasis lichenoides chronica, the mild form, one observes a superficial perivascular infiltrate composed of lymphocytes that extends into the epidermis, where there is vacuolar alteration of the basal layer, mild spongiosis, a few necrotic keratinocytes, and confluent parakeratosis. Melanophages and small numbers of extravasated erythrocytes are commonly seen in the papillary dermis (174,393).

In PLEVA, the more severe form, there is a perivascular and dense band-like, predominantly lymphocytic infiltrate in the papillary dermis that extends into the reticular dermis in a wedge-shaped pattern (Fig. 7-29). The infiltrate obscures the dermal–epidermal junction with pronounced

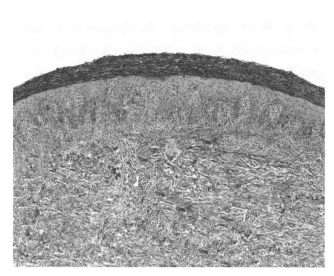

FIGURE 7-29. Pityriasis lichenoides et varioliformis acuta. Lichenoid inflammatory pattern with a superficial and deep perivascular lymphocytic infiltrate.

vacuolar alteration of the basal layer, marked exocytosis of lymphocytes and erythrocytes, and intercellular and intracellular edema leading to variable degrees of epidermal necrosis (Fig. 7-30). Ultimately, erosion or even ulceration may occur. The overlying cornified layer shows parakeratosis and a scaly crust with neutrophils in the more severe cases (393,401).

Variable degrees of papillary dermal edema, endothelial swelling, and extravasated erythrocytes are seen in the

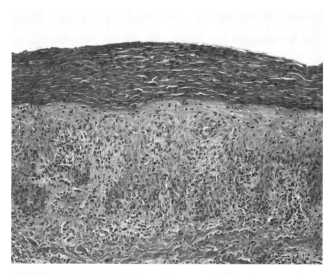

FIGURE 7-30. Pityriasis lichenoides et varioliformis acuta. Closer view reveals lichenoid inflammatory pattern with an infiltrate of lymphocytes, extravasated erythrocytes, irregular acanthosis, pallor of the upper layers of the epidermis, spongiosis, necrotic keratinocytes, and confluent mounds of parakeratosis with plasma, neutrophils, and lymphocytes.

majority of cases. Although occasionally small deposits of fibrin are present within the vessel walls, severe vascular damage is rarely found (393) except in the severe febrile ulceronecrotic variant of PLEVA, where lymphocytic vasculitis with leukocytoclasis is a fairly common feature (398,400).

Differential Diagnosis. Occasionally, the histologic picture of PLEVA can be mimicked by other diseases such as pityriasis rosea, vesicular insect bites, and subacute eczematous dermatitis. The presence of a deeper inflammatory infiltrate, extensive epidermal necrosis, and absence of intraepidermal spongiotic microvesicles may help distinguish PLEVA from pityriasis rosea and subacute eczematous dermatitis. Numerous eosinophils in a vertically oriented dermal infiltrate are more commonly seen in insect bites (402). The differential diagnosis with lymphomatoid papulosis is discussed in Chapter 31.

Pathogenesis. Most of the cells in the inflammatory infiltrate are activated T-lymphocytes (HLA-DR+/CD3+) (394,401,403) that uniformly express CD7 and rarely lack other T-cell antigens (CD2, CD5) (394,404). Two constant findings in PLEVA are the predominance of CD8+ (cytotoxic-suppressor) over CD4+ (helper-inducer) T-lymphocytes in the infiltrate, and the expression of HLA-DR on the surrounding keratinocytes (394,401, 403,404), suggesting a direct cytotoxic immune reaction in the pathogenesis of epidermal necrosis. Recent studies have suggested that PLEVA is a clonal T-cell disorder (405–407). Some cases of pityriasis lichenoides chronica, although less frequent than PLEVA, also exhibited a clonal T-cell receptor gene rearrangement (405,408). It does not appear that cases of clonal PLEVA have a higher risk of developing malignant lymphoma (405,409). However, there are rare reports of few patients with pityriasis lichenoides who have been associated with cutaneous lymphoma (410,411). It is suggested that monoclonal expansion of T cells most likely results from a host immune response to an as yet unidentified antigen, perhaps a viral one (405,412).

REFERENCES

1. Aoki T, Kojima M, Horiko T. Acute urticaria: history and natural course of 50 patients. *J Dermatol* 1994;21:73.
2. Cooper KD. Urticaria and angioedema: diagnosis and evaluation. *J Am Acad Dermatol* 1991;25:166.
3. Lipsker D, Veran Y, Grunenberger F, et al. The Schnitzler syndrome. Four new cases and review of the literature. *Medicine (Baltimore)* 2001;80:37.
4. Hide M, Francis DM, Grattan CE, et al. Autoantibodies against the high-affinity IgE receptor as a cause of histamine release in chronic urticaria. *N Engl J Med* 1993;328:1599.
5. Greaves MW. Chronic urticaria. *N Engl J Med* 1995;332:1767.
6. Soter NA. Chronic urticaria as a manifestation of necrotizing venulitis. *N Engl J Med* 1977;296:1440.

7. Sanchez NP, Winkelmann RK, Schroeter AL. The clinical and histopathologic spectrums of urticarial vasculitis. *J Am Acad Dermatol* 1982;7:599.

8. Gammon WR. Urticarial vasculitis. *Dermatol Clin* 1985;3:97.

9. Mehregan DR, Hall MJ, Gibson LE. Urticarial vasculitis: a histopathologic and clinical review of 72 cases. *J Am Acad Dermatol* 1992;26:441.

10. Farell AM, Sabroe RA, Bunker CB. Urticarial vasculitis associated with polycythemia rubra vera. *Clin Exp Dermatol* 1996;21:302.

11. Wilson D, McCluggage WG, Wright GD. Urticarial vasculitis: a paraneoplastic presentation of B-cell non Hodgkin's lymphoma. *Rheumatology (Oxford)* 2002;41:476.

12. Bisaccia E, Adamo V, Rozan SW. Urticarial vasculitis progressing to systemic lupus erythematosus. *Arch Dermatol* 1988;124:1088.

13. Huston DP, Bressler RB. Urticaria and angioedema. *Med Clin North Am* 1992;76:805.

14. Soter NA, Wasserman SI. Urticaria, angioedema [Review]. *Int J Dermatol* 1979;18:517.

15. Soter NA, Austen KF, Gigli I. Urticaria and arthralgias as manifestations of necrotizing angiitis (vasculitis). *J Invest Dermatol* 1974;63:485.

16. Monroe EW, Schulz CI, Maize JC, et al. Vasculitis in chronic urticaria. *J Invest Dermatol* 1981;76:103.

17. Kikuchi Y, Kaplan AP. A role for C5a in augmenting IgG-dependent histamine release from basophils in chronic urticaria. *J Allergy Clin Immunol* 2002;109:114.

18. Haas N, Hermes B, Henz BM. Adhesion molecules and cellular infiltrate: histology of urticaria. *J Invest Dermatol Symp Proc* 2001;6:137.

19. Davis MD, Daoud MS, Kirby B, et al. Clinicopathologic correlation of hypocomplementemic and normocomplementemic urticarial vasculitis. *J Am Acad Dermatol* 1998;38:899.

20. Lawley TJ, Hertz HC, Wade TR, et al. Pruritic urticarial papules and plaques of pregnancy. *JAMA* 1979;241:1696.

21. Callen JP, Hanno R. Pruritic urticarial papules and plaques of pregnancy (PUPPP). *J Am Acad Dermatol* 1981;5:401.

22. Yancey KB, Russel RP, Lawley TJ. Pruritic urticarial papules and plaques of pregnancy. *J Am Acad Dermatol* 1984;10:473.

23. Cohen LM, Capeless EL, Krusinski PA, et al. Pruritic urticarial papules and plaques of pregnancy and its relationship to maternal-fetal weight gain and twin pregnancy. *Arch Dermatol* 1989;125:1534.

24. Elling SV, McKenna P, Powell FC. Pruritic urticarial papules and plaques of pregnancy in twin and triplet pregnancies. *J Eur Dermatol Venereol* 2000;14:378.

25. Im S, Lee ES, Kim W, et al. Expression of progesterone receptor in human keratinocytes. *J Korean Med Sci* 2000;15:647.

26. Weiss R, Hull P. Familial occurrence of pruritic urticarial papules and plaques of pregnancy. *J Am Acad Dermatol* 1992;26:715.

27. Aronson IK, Bond S, Fiedler VC, et al. Pruritic urticarial papules and plaques of pregnancy: clinical and immunopathologic observations in 57 patients. *J Am Acad Dermatol* 1998;39:933. Erratum in *J Am Acad Dermatol* 1999;40:611.

28. Darier J. De l'erytheme annulaire centrifuge. *Ann Dermatol Syphilol* 1916;6:57.

29. Ackerman AB. *Histologic Diagnosis of Inflammatory Skin Diseases*, Second Edition. Baltimore, Williams & Wilkins. 1997;623.

30. Bressler GS, Jones RE Jr. Erythema annulare centrifugum. *J Am Acad Dermatol* 1981;4:597.

31. Kim KJ, Chang SE, Choi JH, et al. Clinicopathologic analysis of 66 cases of erythema annulare centrifugum. *J Dermatol* 2002;29:61.

32. Tyring SK. Reactive erythemas: erythema annulare centrifugum and erythema gyratum repens. *Clin Dermatol* 1993;11:135.

33. Ural AU, Ozcan A, Avcu F, et al. Erythema annulare centrifugum as the presenting sign of CD30 positive anaplastic large cell lymphoma: association with disease activity. *Hematologica (Budap)* 2001;31:81.

34. Gammel JA. Erythema gyratum repens. *Arch Dermatol* 1952;66:494.

35. Eubanks LE, McBurney E, Reed R. Erythema gyratum repens. *Am J Med Sci* 2001;321:302.

36. Boyd AS, Neldner KH, Menter A. Erythema gyratum repens: a paraneoplastic eruption. *J Am Acad Dermatol* 1992;26:757.

37. Leavell US, Winternitz WW, Black JH. Erythema gyratum repens and undifferentiated carcinoma. *Arch Dermatol* 1977;95:343.

38. Holt PJA, Davies MG. Erythema gyratum repens: an immunologically mediated dermatosis. *Br J Dermatol* 1977;96:343.

39. Albers SE, Fenske NA, Glass LF. Erythema gyratum repens: direct immunofluorescence microscopic findings. *J Am Acad Dermatol* 1993;29:493.

40. Caux F, Lebbe C, Thomine E, et al. Erythema gyratum repens. A case studied with immunofluorescence, immunoelectron microscopy and immunohistochemistry. *Br J Dermatol* 1994;131:102.

41. Dominguez-Soto L, Hojyo-Tomoka T, Vega-Memije E, et al. Pigmentary problems in the tropics. *Dermatol Clin* 1994;12:777.

42. Knox JM, Dodge BG, Freeman RG. Erythema dyschromicum perstans. *Arch Dermatol* 1968;97:262.

43. Vega ME, Waxtein L, Arenas R, et al. Ashy dermatosis and lichen planus pigmentosus: a clinicopathologic study of 31 cases. *Int J Dermatol* 1992;31:90.

44. Tschen JA, Tschen EA, McGavran MH. Erythema dyschromicum perstans. *J Am Acad Dermatol* 1980;2:295.

45. Soter NA, Wand C, Freeman RG. Ultrastructural pathology of erythema dyschromicum perstans. *J Invest Dermatol* 1969;52:155.

46. Miyagawa S, Komatsu M, Okuchi T, et al. Erythema dyschromicum perstans: immunopathologic studies. *J Am Acad Dermatol* 1989;20:882.

47. Baranda L, Torres-Alvarez B, Cortes-Franco R, et al. Involvement of cell adhesion and activation molecules in the pathogenesis of erythema dyschromicum perstans (ashy dermatitis). The effect of clofazimine therapy. *Arch Dermatol* 1997;133:325.

48. Bhutani LK, Bedi TR, Pandhi RK, et al. Lichen planus pigmentosus. *Dermatologica* 1974;149:43.

49. Naidorf KF, Cohen SR. Erythema dyschromicum perstans and lichen planus. *Arch Dermatol* 1982;118:683.

50. Sanchez NP, Pathak MA, Sato SS, et al. Circumscribed dermal melaninoses: classification, light, histochemical, and electron microscopic studies on three patients with the erythema dyschromicum perstans type. *Int J Dermatol* 1982;21:25.

51. Metin A, Calka O, Ugras S. Lichen planopilaris coexisting with erythema dyschromicum perstans. *Br J Dermatol* 2001;145:522.

52. Sheretz EF, Jorizzo JL, White WL, et al. Papular dermatitis in adults: subacute prurigo, American style? *J Am Acad Dermatol* 1991;24:697.

53. Braun-Falco O, von Eickstedt UM. Beitrag zur urticaria papulosa chronica. *Hautarzt* 1957;8:534.

54. Kocsard E. The problem of prurigo. *Australas J Dermatol* 1962;6:156.

55. Rosen T, Algra RJ. Papular eruption in black men. *Arch Dermatol* 1980;116:416.

56. Uehara M, Ofuji S. Primary eruption of prurigo simplex subacuta. *Dermatologica* 1976;153:49.

57. Doyle JA, Connolly SM, Hunziker N, et al. Prurigo nodulans: a reappraisal of the clinical and histologic features. *J Cutan Pathol* 1979;16:392.

58. Rowland Payne CME, Wilkinson JD, McKee PH, et al. Nodular prurigo: a clinicopathological study of 46 patients. *Br J Dermatol* 1985;113:431.

59. Tanaka M, Aiba S, Matsumura N, et al. Prurigo nodularis consists of two distinct forms: early-onset atopic and late-onset nonatopic. *Dermatology* 1995;190;269.

60. Rien BE, Lemont H, Cohen RS. Prurigo nodularis in association with uremia. *J Am Podiatry Assoc* 1982;72:321.

61. Fina L, Grimalt R, Berti E, et al. Nodular prurigo associated with Hodgkin's disease. *Dermatologica* 1991;182:243.

62. Miyauchi H, Uehara M. Follicular occurrence of prurigo nodularis. *J Cutan Pathol* 1988;15:208.

63. Runne U, Orfanos CE. Cutaneous neural proliferation in highly pruritic lesions of chronic prurigo. *Arch Dermatol* 1977;113:787.

64. Lindley RP, Rowland P. Neural hyperplasia is not a diagnostic prerequisite in nodular prurigo. *J Cutan Pathol* 1989;16:14.

65. Johansson O, Liang Y, Heilborn JD, et al. Langerhans cells in prurigo nodularis investigated by HLA-DR and S-100 immunofluorescence double staining. *J Dermatol Sci* 1998;17:24.

66. Liang, Jacobi HH, Marcusson JA, et al. Dendritic mast cells in prurigo nodularis skin. *Eur J Dermatol* 1999;9:297.

67. Johansson O, Liang Y, Emtestam L. Increased nerve growth factor- and tyrosine kinase A–like immunoreactivities in prurigo nodularis skin: an exploration of the cause of neurohyperplasia. *Arch Dermatol Res* 2002;293:614.

68. Harris B, Harris K, Penneys NS. Demonstration by S-100 protein staining of increased numbers of nerves in the papillary dermis of patients with prurigo nodularis. *J Am Acad Dermatol* 1992;26:56.

69. Aso M, Hashimoto K, Hamzavi A. Immunohistochemical studies of selected skin diseases and tumors using monoclonal antibodies to neurofilament and myelin proteins. *J Am Acad Dermatol* 1985;13:37.

70. Molina FA, Burrows NP, Jones RR, et al. Increased sensory neuropeptides in nodular prurigo: a quantitative immunohistochemical analysis. *Br J Dermatol* 1992;127:344.

71. Nahass GT, Penneys NS. Merkel cells and prurigo nodularis. *J Am Acad Dermatol* 1994;31:86.

72. Ereaux LP, Schopflocher P. Familial primary self-healing squamous epithelioma of skin. *Arch Dermatol* 1965;91:589.

73. Telfer NR, Chalmers RJG, Whale K, et al. The role of streptococcal infection in the initiation of guttate psoriasis. *Arch Dermatol* 1992;128:39.

74. Faber EM, Nall ML. Natural history of psoriasis in 5,600 patients. *Dermatologica* 1974;148:1.

75. Morris LF, Phillips CM, Binnie WH, et al. Oral lesions in patients with psoriasis: a controlled study. *Cutis* 1992;49:339.

76. Pogrel MA, Cram D. Intraoral findings in patients with psoriasis with a special reference to ectopic geographic tonge (erythema circinata). *Oral Surg Oral Med Oral Pathol* 1988;66:184.

77. Baker H. Pustular psoriasis. *Dermatol Clin* 1984;2:455.

78. Zelickson BD, Muller SA. Generalized pustular psoriasis. *Arch Dermatol* 1991;127:1339.

79. Wagner G, Luckasen JR, Goltz RW. Mucous membrane involvement in generalized psoriasis. *Arch Dermatol* 1976;112:1010.

80. Shelley WB, Kirschbaum JO. Generalized pustular psoriasis. *Arch Dermatol* 1961;84:73.

81. Braverman IM, Cohen I, O'Keefe EO. Metabolic and ultrastructural studies in a patient with pustular psoriasis (Von Zumbusch). *Arch Dermatol* 1972;105:189.

82. Schuppener JH. Ausdrucksformen pustulöser psoriasis. *Dermatol Wochenschr* 1958;138:841.

83. Baker H, Ryan TJ. Generalized pustular psoriasis. *Br J Dermatol* 1968;80:771.

84. Katzenellenbogen I, Feuerman EI. Psoriasis pustulosa and impetigo herpetiformis: single or dual entity? *Acta Derm Venereol (Stockh)* 1966;46:86.

85. Pierard GE, Pierard-Franchimont C, de la Brassine M. Impetigo herpetiformis and pustular psoriasis during pregnancy. *Am J Dermatopathol* 1983;5:215.

86. Lotem M, Katzenelson V, Rotem A, et al. Impetigo herpetiformis: a variant of pustular psoriasis or a separate entity? *J Am Acad Dermatol* 1989;20:338.

87. Resneck JS, Cram DL. Erythema annulare-like pustular psoriasis. *Arch Dermatol* 1973;108:687.

88. Adler DJ, Rower JM, Hashimoto K. Annular pustular psoriasis. *Arch Dermatol* 1981;117:313.

89. Zala L, Hunziker T. Lokalisierte form der psoriasis von typ des erythema annulare centrifugum mit pustulation. *Hautarzt* 1984;35:53.

90. Zelickson BD, Muller SA. Generalized pustular psoriasis in childhood: report of thirteen cases. *J Am Acad Dermatol* 1991;24:186.

91. Ashhurst PJC. Relapsing pustular eruptions of the hands and feet. *Br J Dermatol* 1964;776:169.

92. Andrews GC, Machacek GF. Pustular bacterids of the hands and feet. *Arch Dermatol Syphilol* 1935;32:837.

93. Duvic M, Johnson TM, Rapini RP, et al. Acquired immunodeficiency syndrome–associated psoriasis and Reiter's syndrome. *Arch Dermatol* 1987;123:1622.

94. Obuch ML, Maurer TA, Becker B, Berger TG. Psoriasis and human immunodeficiency virus infection. *J Am Acad Dermatol* 1992;27:667.

95. Lazar AP, Roenigk HH. AIDS and psoriasis. *Cutis* 1987;39:347.

96. Johnson TM, Duvic M, Rapini RP, et al. AIDS exacerbates psoriasis. *N Engl J Med* 1985;313:22,1415.

97. Braun-Falco O, Christophers E. Structural aspects of initial psoriatic lesions. *Arch Dermatol Forsch* 1974;251:95.

98. Ragaz A, Ackerman AB. Evolution, maturation, and regression of lesions of psoriasis. *Am J Dermatopathol* 1979;1:199.

99. Van Scott EJ, Ekel TW. Kinetics of hyperplasia in psoriasis. *Arch Dermatol* 1963;88:373.

100. Gordon M, Johnson WC. Histopathology and histochemistry of psoriasis. *Arch Dermatol* 1967;95:402.

101. Rupec M. Zur ultrastruktur der spongiformen pustel. *Arch Klin Exp Dermatol* 1970;239:30.

102. Burks JW, Montgomery H. Histopathologic study of psoriasis. *Arch Dermatol Syphilol* 1943;48:479.

103. Pinkus H, Mehregan AH. The primary histologic lesion of seborrheic dermatitis and psoriasis. *J Invest Dermatol* 1966;46:109.

104. Cox AH, Watson W. Histologic variations in lesions of psoriasis. *Arch Dermatol* 1972;106:503.

105. Abrahams J, McCarthy JT, Sanders ST. 101 cases of exfoliative dermatitis. *Arch Dermatol* 1963;87:96.

106. Muller SA, Kitzmiller KW. Generalized pustular psoriasis. *Acta Derm Venereol (Stockh)* 1962;42:504.

107. Kingery FAJ, Chinn HD, Saunders TS. Generalized pustular psoriasis. *Arch Dermatol* 1961;84:912.

108. Piraccini BM, Fanti PA, Morelli R, et al. Hallopeau's acrodermatitis continua of the nail apparatus: a clinical and pathological study of 20 patients. *Acta Derm Venereol (Stockh)* 1994;74:65.

109. Pierard J, Kint A. La pustulose palmo-plantaire chronique et recidivante. *Ann Dermatol Venereol* 1978;105:681.

110. Pierard J, Kint A. Les "bacterides pustuleuses" d'Andrews. *Arch Belg Dermatol Syphiligr* 1966;22:83.

111. Lever WF. In discussion with Pay D: pustular psoriasis. *Arch Dermatol* 1969;99:641.

112. Uehara M, Ofuji S. The morphogenesis of pustulosis palmaris et plantaris. *Arch Dermatol* 1974;109:518.
113. Thorman J, Heilesen B. Recalcitrant pustular eruptions of the extremities. *J Cutan Pathol* 1975;2:19.
114. Tan RS. Acute generalized pustular bacterid. *Br J Dermatol* 1974;91:209.
115. Smoller BR, McNutt S, Gray MH, et al. Detection of the interferon-gamma–induced protein 10 in psoriasiform dermatitis of acquired immunodeficiency syndrome. *Arch Dermatol* 1990;126:1457.
116. Schubert C, Christophers E. Mast cells and macrophages in early relapsing psoriasis. *Arch Dermatol Res* 1985;277:352.
117. Brody I. The ultrastructure of the epidermis in psoriasis vulgaris as revealed by electron microscopy. *J Ultrastruct Res* 1962;6:304.
118. Hashimoto K, Lever WF. Elektronenmikroskopische untersuchungen der hautveränderungen bei psoriasis. *Dermatol Wochenschr* 1966;152:713.
119. Orfanos CE, Schaumburg-Lever G, Mahrle G, et al. Alterations of cell surfaces as a pathogenetic factor in psoriasis. *Arch Dermatol* 1973;107:38.
120. Heng MCYL, Kloss SG, Kuehn CD, et al. The significance and pathogenesis of basal keratinocyte herniations in psoriasis. *J Invest Dermatol* 1986;87:362.
121. Mercer EH, Maibach HI. Intercellular adhesion and surface coats of epidermal cells in psoriasis. *J Invest Dermatol* 1968;51:215.
122. Christophers C, Braun-Falco O. Mechanisms of parakeratosis. *J Dermatol* 1970;82:268.
123. Braverman IM, Yen A. Ultrastructure of the human dermal microcirculation: II. The capillary loops of the dermal papillae. *J Invest Dermatol* 1977;68:44.
124. Mordovtsev VN, Albanova VI. Morphology of skin microvasculature in psoriasis. *Am J Dermatopathol* 1989;11:33.
125. Weinstein GD, Van Scott EJ. Autoradiographic analysis of turnover times of normal and psoriatic epidermis. *J Invest Dermatol* 1965;45:257.
126. Soltani K, Van Scott EJ. Patterns and sequence of tissue changes in incipient and evolving lesions of psoriasis. *Arch Dermatol* 1972;106:484.
127. Weinstein GD, McCullough JL, Ross PA. Cell kinetic basis for pathophysiology of psoriasis. *J Invest Dermatol* 1985;85:579.
128. Gelfant S. The cell cycle in psoriasis: a reappraisal. *Br J Dermatol* 1976;95:577.
129. McKay IA, Leigh IM. Altered keratinocyte growth and differentiation in psoriasis. *Clin Dermatol* 1995;13:105.
130. Leigh IM, Navsaria H, Purkis PE, et al. Keratins (K16 and K17) as markers of keratinocyte hyperproliferation in psoriasis in vivo and in vitro. *Br J Dermatol* 1995;133:501.
131. Takahashi H, Manabe A, Ishida-Yamamoto A, et al. Aberrant expression of apoptosis-related molecules in psoriatic epidermis. *J Dermatol Sci* 2002;28:187.
132. Nelson W, Sun TT. The 50- and 58-kdalton keratin classes as molecular markers for stratified squamous epithelia: cell culture studies. *J Cell Biol* 1983;97:244.
133. Hohl D. The cornified cell envelope. *Dermatologica* 1990;180:201.
134. Stoler A, Kopan R, Duvic M, et al. Use of monospecific antisera and cRNA probes to localize the major changes in keratin expression during normal and abnormal epidermal differentiation. *J Cell Biol* 1988;107:427.
135. Koga T, Duan H, Urabe K, et al. In situ localization of IFN-gamma-positive cells in psoriatic lesional epidermis. *Eur J Dermatol* 2002;12:20.
136. Bos JD, Zonneveld I, Das PK, et al. The skin immune system (SIS): distribution and immunophenotype of lymphocyte subpopulations in normal human skin. *J Invest Dermatol* 1987;88;569.
137. Vollmer S, Menssen A, Prinz JC. Dominant lesional T cell receptor rearrangements persist in relapsing psoriasis but are absent from nonlesional skin: evidence for a stable antigen-specific pathogenic T cell response in psoriasis vulgaris. *J Invest Dermatol* 2001;117:1296.
138. Lin WJ, Norris DA, Achziger M, et al. Oligoclonal expansion of intraepidermal T cells in psoriasis skin lesions. *J Invest Dermatol* 2001;117:1546.
139. Chang JC, Smith LR, Froning KJ, et al. CD8+ T-cells in psoriatic lesions preferentially use T-cell receptors V beta 3 and/or V beta 13. 1 genes. *Ann N Y Acad Sci* 1995;756:370.
140. Gudmundsdottir AS, Sigundsdottir H, Sigurgeirsson B, et al. Is an epitope on keratin 17 a major target for autoreactive T lymphocytes in psoriasis? *Clin Exp Immunol* 1999;117:580.
141. Valdimarsson H, Sigmundsdottir H, Jonsdottir I. Is Psoriasis induced by streptococcal superantigens and maintained by M-protein–specific T cells that cross-react with keratin? *Clin Exp Immunol* 1997;107[Suppl 1]: 21.
142. Leung DYM, Walsh P, Giorno R, et al. A potential role for superantigens in the pathogenesis of psoriais. *J Invest Dermatol* 1993;100:225.
143. Ovigne JM, Baker BS, Davison S, et al. Epidermal CD8+ T cells reactive with group A streptococcal antigens in chronic plaque psoriasis. *Exp Dermatol* 2002;11:357.
144. Baker BS, Fry L. The immunology of psoriasis. *Br J Dermatol* 1992;126:1.
145. Griffiths CEM, Voorhees JJ. Immunological mechanisms involved in psoriasis. *Springer Semin Immunopathol* 1992;13:441.
146. Fierlbeck G, Rassner G, Muller C. Psoriasis induced at the injection site or recombinant interferon gamma. *Arch Dermatol* 1990;126:351.
147. Gottlieb AB, Luster AD, Posnett DN, et al. Detection of gamma interferon-induced protein IP-10 in psoriatic plaques. *J Exp Med* 1988;168:941.
148. Nickoloff BJ, Griffiths CEM, Barker JNWN. The role of adhesion molecules, chemotactic factors and cytokines in inflammatory and neoplastic skin diseases: 1990 update. *J Invest Dermatol* 1990;94:151S.
149. Baker BS, Powles AV, Valdimarsson H, et al. An altered response by psoriatic keratinocytes to gamma interferon. *Scand J Immunol* 1988;28:735.
150. Nickoloff BJ, Mitra RS, Elder JT, et al. Decreased growth inhibition by recombinant gamma interferon is associated with increased transforming growth factor-alpha production in keratinocytes cultured from psoratic lesions. *Br J Dermatol* 1989;121:161.
151. Everall J. Intractable pustular eruption of the hands and feet. *Br J Dermatol* 1957;69:269.
152. Enfors W, Molin L. Pustulosis palmaris et plantaris. *Acta Derm Venereol (Stockh)* 1971;51:289.
153. Thomsen K. Pustulosis palmaris et plantaris treated with methotrexate. *Acta Derm Venereol (Stockh)* 1971;51:397.
154. Tagami H, Ofuji S. A leukotactic factor in the stratum corneum of pustulosis palmaris et plantaris. *Acta Derm Venereol (Stockh)* 1978;58:401.
155. Mallon E. Retroviruses and psoriasis. *Curr Opin Infect Dis* 2000;13:103.
156. Bruer-McHam JN, Marshall GD, Lewis DE, et al. Distinct serum cytokines in AIDS-related skin diseases. *Viral Immunol* 1998;11:215.
157. Ichihashi N, Seishima M, Takahashi T, et al. A case of AIDS manifesting pruritic papular eruptions and psoriasiform lesions: an immunohistochemical study of the lesional dermal infiltrates. *J Dermatol* 1995;22:428.

158. Barr RJ, Young EM. Psoriasiform and related papulosquamous disorders. *J Cutan Pathol* 1985;12:412.

159. Soeprono FF. Histologic criteria for the diagnosis of pityriasis rubra pilaris. *Am J Dermatopathol* 1986;8:277.

160. Degos R, Garnier G, Civatte J. Pustulose par *Candida albicans* avec lésions psoriasiformes rappelant le psoriasis pustuleux. *Bull Soc Fr Dermatol Syphiligr* 1962;69:231.

161. Dawson TAJ. Tongue lesions in generalized pustular psoriasis. *Br J Dermatol* 1974;91:419.

162. Perry HO, Mayne JG. Psoriasis and Reiter's syndrome. *Arch Dermatol* 1965;92:129.

163. Khan MY, Hall WH. Progression of Reiter's syndrome to psoriatic arthritis. *Arch Intern Med* 1965;116:911.

164. Altman EM, Centeno LV, Mahal M, et al. AIDS-associated Reiter's syndrome. *Ann Allergy* 1994;72:307.

165. Weinberger HW, Ropes MW, Kulka JP, et al. Reiter's syndrome: clinical and pathologic observations [Review]. *Medicine (Baltimore)* 1962;41:35.

166. Martin DH, Pollock S, Kuo CC, et al. *Chlamydia trachomatis* infections in men with Reiter's syndrome. *Ann Intern Med* 1984;100:207.

167. Rahman MU, Cheema MA, Schumacher HR, Hudson AP. Molecular evidence for the presence of chlamydia in the synovium of patients with Reiter's syndrome. *Arthritis Rheum* 1992;35:521.

168. Hogarth MB, Thomas S, Seifert MH, Tariq SM. Reiter's Syndrome following intravesical BCG immunotherapy. *Postgrad Med J* 2000;76:791.

169. Burg B, Dummer R, Nestle FO, et al. Cutaneous lymphomas consist of a spectrum of nosologically different entities including mycosis fungoides and small plaque parapsoriasis. *Arch Dermatol* 1996;132:567.

170. Radcliffe-Crocker H. Xanthoerythrodermia perstans. *Br J Dermatol* 1905;17:119.

171. Hu CH, Winkelmann RK. Digitate dermatosis: a new look at symmetrical small plaque parapsoriasis. *Arch Dermatol* 1973;107:65.

172. Yeager JK, Posnak EJ, Cobb MW. Digitate dermatosis. *Cutis* 1991;48:457.

173. Samman PD. The natural history of parapsoriasis en plaques (chronic superficial dermatitis) and prereticulotic poikiloderma. *Br J Dermatol* 1972;87:405.

174. Benmaman O, Sanchez JL. Comparative clinicopathological study on pityriasis lichenoides chronica and small plaque parapsoriasis. *Am J Dermatopathol* 1988;10:189.

175. Binazzi M. Some research on parapsoriasis and lymphoma. *Arch Dermatol Res* 1977;258:17.

176. Haeffner AC, Smoller BR, Zepter K, et al. Differentiation and clonality of lesional lymphocytes in small plaque parapsoriasis. *Arch Dermatol* 1995;131:321.

177. Bonvalet D, Colau-Gohm K, Belaich S, et al. Les differentes formes du parapsoriasis en plaques. *Ann Dermatol Venereol* 1977;104:18.

178. Heid E, Desvaux J, Brändle J, et al. Der verlauf der parapsoriasis en plaques (Brocq'sche Krankheit). *Z Hautkr* 1977;52:658.

179. Burg B, Dummer R. Small plaque (digitate) parapsoriasis is an "abortive cutaneous T-cell lymphoma" and is not mycosis fungoides. *Arch Dermatol* 1995;131:336.

180. Muche JM, Lukowsky A, Heim J, et al. Demonstration of frequent occurrence of clonal T cells in the peripheral blood but not in the skin of patients with small plaque parapsoriasis. *Blood* 1999;94:1409.

181. Parsons JM. Pityriasis rosea update. *J Am Acad Dermatol* 1986;15:159.

182. Bunch LW, Tilley JC. Pityriasis rosea. *Arch Dermatol* 1961;84:79.

183. Aiba S, Tagami H. Immunohistologic studies in pityriasis rosea. *Arch Dermatol* 1985;121:761.

184. Panizzon R, Bloch PH. Histopathology of pityriasis rosea Gibert: qualitative and quantitative light- microscopic study of 62 biopsies of 40 patients. *Dermatologica* 1982;165:551.

185. Okamoto H, Imamura S, Aoshima T, et al. Dyskeratotic degeneration of epidermal cells in pityriasis rosea: Light and electron microscopic studies. *Br J Dermatol* 1982;107:189.

186. Bonafe JL, Icart J, Perpere M, et al. Etude histopathologique, ultrastructurale, immunologique et virologique du pityriasis rose de Gibert. *Ann Dermatol Venereol* 1982;109:855.

187. Blauvett A. Skin diseases associated with human herpesvirus 6,7, and 8 infection. *J Invest Dermatol Symp Proc* 2001;6:197.

188. Yoshiike T, Aikawa Y, Wongwaisayawan H, et al. HLA-DR antigen expression on peripheral T cell subsets in pityriasis rosea and herpes zoster. *Dermatologica* 1991;82:160.

189. Baker BS, Lamber S, Powles AV, et al. Epidermal DR+T6–dendritic cells in inflammatory skin diseases. *Acta Derm Venereol (Stockh)* 1988;68:209.

190. Bos JD, Huisman PM, Kreg SR, et al. Pityriasis rosea (Gibert): abnormal distribution pattern of antigen presenting cells *in situ*. *Acta Derm Venereol (Stockh)* 1985;65:132.

191. Aiba S, Tabami H. HLA-DR antigen expression on the keratinocyte surface in dermatosis characterized by lymphocytic exocytosis (e.g., pityriasis rosea). *Br J Dermatol* 1984;3:285.

192. Gianotti F. Rilievi di una particolare casistica tossinfettiva caratterizzata da eruzione eritemato-infiltrativa desquamativa a focolai lenticolari, a sede elettiva acroesposata. *G Ital Dermatol* 1955;96:678.

193. Gianotti F. Papular acrodermatitis of childhood and other papulo-vesicular acro-located syndromes. *Br J Dermatol* 1979;100:49.

194. Spear KL, Winkelmann RK. Gianotti–Crosti syndrome: a review of ten cases not associated with hepatitis B. *Arch Dermatol* 1984;120:891.

195. Taieb A, Plantin P, Du Pasquier P, et al. Gianotti–Crosti syndrome: a study of 26 cases. *Br J Dermatol* 1986;115:49.

196. Baldari U, Monti A, Righini MG. An epidemic of infantile papular acrodermatitis (Gianotti–Crosti syndrome) due to Epstein–Barr virus. *Dermatology* 1994;188:203.

197. Draelos ZK, Hansen RC, James WD. Gianotti–Crosti syndrome associated with infections other than hepatitis B. *JAMA* 1986;256:2386.

198. Caputo R, Gelmetti C, Ermacora E, et al. Gianotti–Crosti syndrome: a retrospective analysis of 308 cases. *J Am Acad Dermatol* 1992;26:207.

199. Blauvelt A, Turner ML. Gianotti–Crosti syndrome and human immunodeficiency virus infection. *Arch Dermatol* 1994;130:481.

200. Smith KJ, Skelton H. Histopathologic features seen in Gianotti–Crosti syndrome secondary to Epstein–Barr virus. *J Am Acad Dermatol* 2000;43:1076.

201. Stefanato CM, Goldberg LJ, Andersen WK, et al. Gianotti–Crosti syndrome presenting as lichenoid dermatitis. *Am J Dermatopathol* 2000;22:162.

202. Margyarlaki M, Drobnitsch I, Schneider I. Papular acrodermatitis of childhood: Gianotti–Crosti disease. *Pediatr Dermatol* 1991;8:224.

203. Kawasaki T, Kosaki F, Owaka S, et al. A new infantile acute febrile mucocutaneous lymph node syndrome (MLNS) prevailing in Japan. *Pediatrics* 1974;54:271.

204. Melish ME, Hicks RV. Kawasaki syndrome: clinical features, pathophysiology, etiology and therapy. *J Rheumatol* 1990;17:2.

205. Dajani AS, Bisno AL, Chung KJ, et al. Diagnostic guidelines for Kawasaki disease. American Heart Association Committee

on Rheumatic Fever, Endocarditis, and Kawasaki Disease. *Am J Dis Child* 1990;144:1218.

206. Burns JC, Mason WH, Glode MP, et al. Clinical and epidemiologic characteristics of patients referred for evaluation of possible Kawasaki disease. *J Pediatr* 1991;118:680.

207. Wortmann DW. Kawasaki syndrome. *Semin Dermatol* 1992; 11:37.

208. Ducos MH, Taieb A, Sarlangue J, et al. Manifestations cutanees de la maladie de Kawasaki: a propos de 30 observations. *Ann Dermatol Venereol* 1993;120:589.

209. Friter BS, Lucky AW. The perineal eruption of Kawasaki syndrome. *Arch Dermatol* 1988;124:1805.

210. Eberhard BA, Sundel RP, Newuger JW, et al. Psoriatic eruption in Kawasaki disease. *J Pediatr* 2000;137:578.

211. Suzuki A, Kamiya T, Kuwahara N, et al. Coronary arterial lesions of Kawasaki disease: cardiac catheterization findings of 1100 cases. *Pediatr Cardiol* 1986;7:3.

212. Kato H, Ichinose E, Kawasaki T. Myocardial infarction in Kawasaki disease: clinical analyses in 195 cases. *J Pediatr* 1986; 108:923.

213. Tomita S, Chung K, Mas M, et al. Peripheral gangrene associated with Kawasaki disease. *Clin Infect Dis* 1992;14:121.

214. Hirose S, Hamashima Y. Morphological observations on the vasculitis in the mucocutaneous lymph node syndrome: a skin biopsy study of 27 patients. *Eur J Pediatr* 1978;129:17.

215. Sato N, Sagawa K, Sasaguri Y, et al. Immunopathology and cytokine detection in the skin lesions of patients with Kawasaki disease. *J Pediatr* 1993;122:198.

216. Kimura T, Miyazawa H, Watanabe K, et al. Small pustules in Kawasaki disease: a clinicopathological study of four patients. *Am J Dermatopathol* 1988;10;218.

217. Shingadia D, Bose A, Booy R. Could a herpes virus be the cause of Kawasaki disease? *Lancet Infect Dis* 2002;2:310.

218. Shulman ST, De Inocencio J, Hirsch R. Kawasaki disease. *Pediatr Clin North Am* 1995;42:1205.

219. Leung DY, Meissner HC, Fulton DR, et al. Superantigens in Kawasaki syndrome. *Clin Immunol Immunopathol* 1995;77: 119.

220. Ohno T, Yuge T, Kariyazono H, et al. Serum hepatocyte growth factor combined with vascular endothelial growth factor as a predictive indicator for the occurrence of coronary artery lesions in Kawasaki disease. *Eur J Pediatr* 2002;161: 105.

221. Terai M, Yasukawa K, Narumoto S, et al. Vascular endothelial growth factor in acute Kawasaki disease. *Am J Cardiol* 1999;83: 337.

222. Suzuki H, Muragaki Y, Uemura S, et al. Detection of autoantibodies against a 70 KDa protein derived from vascular smooth muscle cells in patients with Kawasaki disease. *Eur J Pediatr* 2002;161:324.

223. Boyd AS, Neldner KH. Lichen planus. *J Am Acad Dermatol* 1991;2593.

224. Boyd AS, Neldner KH. The isomorphic response to Koebner. *Int J Dermatol* 1990;29:401.

225. Conklin RJ, Blasberg B. Oral lichen planus. *Dermatol Clin* 1987;5:663.

226. Bricker SL. Oral lichen planus: a review. *Semin Dermatol* 1994; 13:87.

227. Shklar G. Erosive and bullous oral lesions of lichen planus. *Arch Dermatol* 1968;97:411.

228. Samman PD. The nails in lichen planus. *Br J Dermatol* 1961; 73:288.

229. Sarkany I, Caron GA, Jones HH. Lichen planus pemphigoides. *Trans St Johns Hosp Dermatol Soc* 1964;50:50.

230. Saurat JH, Guinepain MT, Didierjean L, et al. Coexistence d'un lichen plan et d'un pemphigoide bulleuse. *Ann Dermatol Venereol* 1977;104:368.

231. Gawkrodger DJ, Stavropoulos PG, McLaren KM, et al. Bullous lichen planus and lichen planus pemphigoides: clinicopathological comparisons. *Clin Exp Dermatol* 1989;14:150.

232. Hintner H, Tappeiner G, Honigsmann H, et al. Lichen planus and bullous pemphigoid. *Acta Derm Venereol Suppl (Stockh)* 1979;85:71.

233. Mora RG, Nesbitt LT Jr, Brantley JB. Lichen planus pemphigoides: clinical and immunofluorescence findings in four cases. *J Am Acad Dermatol* 1983;8:331.

234. Allen CM, Camisa C, Grimwood R. Lichen planus pemphigoides: report of a case with oral lesions. *Oral Surg Oral Med Oral Pathol* 1987;63:184.

235. Silvers DN, Katz BE, Young AW. Pseudopelade of Brocq is lichen planopilaris: report of four cases that support this nosology. *Cutis* 1993;51:99.

236. Waldorf DS. Lichen planopilaris. *Arch Dermatol* 1966;93:684.

237. Kuster W, Kind P, Holzle E, et al. Linear lichen planopilaris of the face. *J Am Acad Dermatol* 1989;21:1331.

238. Cram DL, Kierland RR, Winkelmann RK. Ulcerative lichen planus of the feet. *Arch Dermatol* 1966;93:692.

239. Thormann J. Ulcerative lichen planus of the feet. *Arch Dermatol* 1974;110:753.

240. Weidner F, Ummenhofer B. Lichen ruber ulcerosus (dystrophicans). *Z Hautkr* 1979;54:1008.

241. Katzenellenbogen I. Lichen planus actinicus: lichen planus in subtropical countries. *Dermatologica* 1962;124:10.

242. Dilaimy M. Lichen planus subtropicus. *Arch Dermatol* 1976; 112:125.

243. Salman SM, Kibbi AG, Zaynoun S. Actinic lichen planus: a clinicopathologic study of 16 patients. *J Am Acad Dermatol* 1989;20:226.

244. Bouassida S, Boudaya S, Turki H, et al. Actinic lichen planus: 32 cases. *Am J Dermatol Venereol* 1998;125:408.

245. Camisa C, Neff JC, Olsen RG. Use of indirect immunofluorescence in the lupus erythematosus/lichen planus overlap syndrome: an additional diagnostic clue. *J Am Acad Dermatol* 1984;11:1050.

246. Davies MG, Gorkiewicz A, Knight A, et al. Is there a relationship between lupus erythematosus and lichen planus? *Br J Dermatol* 1977;96:145.

247. Scher RK, Fischbein R, Ackerman AB. Twenty-nail dystrophy: a variant of lichen planus. *Arch Dermatol* 1978;114:612.

248. Wilkinson JD, Dawber RPR, Bowers RP, et al. Twenty-nail dystrophy of childhood. *Br J Dermatol* 1979;100:217.

249. Kechijian P. Twenty nail dystrophy of childhood. *Cutis* 1985; 35:38.

250. Kawakami T, Soma Y. Generalized lichen nitidus appearing subsequent to lichen planus. *J Dermatol* 1995;22:434.

251. Sigurgeirsson B, Lindelof B. Lichen planus and malignancy: an epidemiologic study of 2071 patients and a review of the literature. *Arch Dermatol* 1991;127:1684.

252. Kronenberg K, Fretzin D, Potter B. Malignant degeneration of lichen planus. *Arch Dermatol* 1971;104:304.

253. Allen JV, Callen JP. Keratoacanthomas arising in hypertropic lichen planus. *Arch Dermatol* 1981;117:519.

254. Fowler CB, Rees TD, Smith BR. Squamous cell carcinoma on the dorsum of the tongue arising in a long-standing lesion of erosive lichen planus. *J Am Dent Assoc* 1987;115:707.

255. Katz RW, Brahim JS, Travis WD. Oral squamous cell carcinoma arising in a patient with long-standing lichen planus: a case report. *Oral Surg Oral Med Oral Pathol* 1990;70:282.

256. Marder MZ, Deesen KC. Transformation of oral lichen planus to squamous cell carcinoma: a literature review and report of case. *J Am Dent Assoc* 1982;105:55.

257. Kaplan B, Barnes L. Oral lichen planus and squamous carcinoma: case report and update of the literature. *Arch Otolaryngol* 1985;111:543.

258. Fulling HJ. Cancer development in oral lichen planus. *Arch Dermatol* 1973;108:667.

259. Holmstrup P, Pindborg JJ. Erythroplakic lesions in relation to oral lichen planus. *Acta Derm Venereol Suppl (Stockh)* 1979; 85:77.

260. Murti PR, Daftary DK, Bhonsle RB, et al. Malignant potential of oral lichen planus: observation in 722 patients from India. *J Oral Pathol* 1986;15:71.

261. Castano E, Lopez-Rios F, Alvarez-Fernandez JG, et al. Verrucous carcinoma in association with hypertrophic lichen planus. *Clin Exp Dermatol* 1997;22:23.

262. Male O, Azambuja R. Diagnostische und therapeutische probleme beim lichen ruber ulcerosus. *Z Hautkr* 1975;50:403.

263. Crotty CP, Su WP, Winkelmann RK. Ulcerative lichen planus: follow-up of surgical excision and grafting. *Arch Dermatol* 1980;116:1252.

264. Ellis FA. Histopathology of lichen planus based on analysis of one hundred biopsies. *J Invest Dermatol* 1967;48:143.

265. Ragaz A, Ackerman AB. Evolution, maturation, and regression of lesions of lichen planus. *Am J Dermatopathol* 1981;3:5.

266. Rivers JK, Jackson R, Orizaga M. Who was Wickham and what are his striae? *Int J Dermatol* 1986;25:611.

267. Gougerot H, Civatte A. Criteres cliniques et histologiques des lichens planus cutanes et muqueux: delimitation. *Ann Dermatol Syphilol* 1953;80:5.

268. Enhamre A, Lagerholm B. Acrosyringeal lichen planus. *Acta Derm Venereol (Stockh)* 1987;67:346.

269. Grubauer G, Romani N, Kofler H, et al. Apoptosic keratin bodies as autoantigen causing the production of IgM-anti-keratin intermediate filament autoantibodies. *J Invest Dermatol* 1986;87:466.

270. Hanau D, Sengel D. Perforating lichen planus. *J Cutan Pathol* 1984;11:176.

271. Mehregan DA, Van Hale HM, Muller SA. Lichen planopilaris: clinical and pathologic study of forty-five patients. *J Am Acad Dermatol* 1992;27:935.

272. Dawber PRP. What is pseudopelade? *Clin Exp Dermatol* 1992; 17:305.

273. Matta M, Kibbi AG, Khattar J, et al. Lichen planopilaris: a clinicopathologic study. *J Am Acad Dermatol* 1990;22:594.

274. Tschen JA, Tschen EA, McGavran MH. Erythema dyschromicum perstans. *J Am Acad Dermatol* 1980;2:295.

275. Van der Horst JC, Cirkel PKS, Nieboer C. Mixed lichen planus-lupus erythematosus disease: a distinct entity? *Clin Exp Dermatol* 1983;8:631.

276. Grabbe S, Kolde G. Coexisting lichen planus and subacute cutaneous lupus erythematosus. *Clin Exp Dermatol* 1995;20:249.

277. Colver GB, Dawber RPR. Is childhood idiopathic atrophy of the nails due to lichen planus? *Br J Dermatol* 1987;116:702.

278. Ebner H, Gebhart W, Lassmann H, et al. The epidermal cell proliferation in lichen planus. *Acta Derm Venereol (Stockh)* 1977;57:133.

279. Medenica M, Lorincz A. Lichen planus: an ultrastructural study. *Acta Derm Venereol (Stockh)* 1977;57:55.

280. Clausen J, Kjaergaard J, Bierring F. The ultrastructure of the dermo-epidermal junction in lichen planus. *Acta Derm Venereol (Stockh)* 1981;61:101.

281. Ebner H, Gebhart W. Epidermal changes in lichen planus. *J Cutan Pathol* 1976;3:167.

282. Hashimoto K. Apoptosis in lichen planus and several other dermatoses. *Acta Derm Venereol (Stockh)* 1976;56:187.

283. Gomes MA, Staquet MJ, Thivolet J. Staining of colloid bodies by keratin antisera in lichen planus. *Am J Dermatopathol* 1981; 3:341.

284. Ebner H, Gebhart W. Light and electron microscopic studies on colloid and other cytoid bodies. *Clin Exp Dermatol* 1977;2: 311.

285. Ebner H, Erlach E, Gebhart W. Untersuchungen über die blasenbildung beim lichen ruber planus. *Arch Dermatol Forsch* 1973;247:193.

286. Abell E, Presbury DG, Marks R, et al. The diagnostic significance of immunoglobulin and fibrin deposition in lichen planus. *Br J Dermatol* 1975;93:17.

287. Baart de la Faille-Kuyper EH, Baart de la Faille H. An immunofluorescence study of lichen planus. *Br J Dermatol* 1974; 90:365.

288. Varelzidis A, Tosca A, Perissios A, et al. Immunohistochemistry in lichen planus. *Dermatologica* 1979;159:137.

289. Morel P, Perron J, Crickx B, et al. Lichen plan avec depots lineaires d'IgG et de C3 a la junction dermo-epidermique. *Dermatologica* 1981;163:117.

290. Ioannades D, Bystryn JC. Immunofluorescence abnormalities in lichen planopilaris. *Arch Dermatol* 1992;128:214.

291. Sobel S, Miller R, Shatin H. Lichen planus pemphigoides. *Arch Dermatol* 1976;112:1280.

292. Zillikens D. BP 180 as the common autoantigen in blistering diseases with different clinical phenotypes. *Keio J Med* 2002; 51:21.

293. Hsu S, Ghohestani RF, Uitto J. Lichen planus pemphigoides with IgG autoantibodies to the 180 kd bullous pemphigoid antigen (type XVII collagen). *J Am Acad Dermatol* 2000;42:136.

294. Song Y, Naito K, Yaguchi H, et al. Lichen planus pemphigoides: report of a case and binding sites of circulating anti-basement membrane zone antibodies. *Nippon Hifuka Gakkai Zasshi* 1989;99:1111.

295. Yoon KH, Kim SC, Kang DS, et al. Lichen planus pemphigoides with circulating autoantibodies against 200 and 180 KDa epidermal antigens. *Eur J Dermatol* 2000;10:212.

296. Sundquist KG, Wanger L. Expression of lymphocyte activation markers in benign cutaneous T cell infiltrates: discoid lupus erythematosus versus lichen ruber planus. *Acta Derm Venereol (Stockh)* 1989;69:292.

297. Buechner SA. T-cell subsets and macrophages in lichen planus. *Dermatologica* 1984;169:325.

298. Ishii T. Immunohistochemical demonstration of T cell subsets and accessory cells in oral lichen planus. *J Oral Pathol* 1987;16: 356.

299. Shiohara T, Moriya N, Tanaka K, et al. Immunopathologic study of lichenoid skin diseases: correlation between HLA-DR positive keratinocytes or Langerhans' cells and epidermotropic T cells. *J Am Acad Dermatol* 1988;18:67.

300. Matthews JB, Scully CM, Potts AJ. Oral lichen planus: an immunoperoxidase study using monoclonal antibodies to lymphocyte subsets. *Br J Dermatol* 1984;3:587.

301. Bennion SD, Middleton MH, David-Bajar KM, et al. In three types of interface dermatitis, different patterns of expression of intercellular adhesion molecule-1 (ICAM-1) indicate different triggers of disease. *J Invest Dermatol* 1995;105:71S.

302. Griffiths CE, Voorhees JJ, Nickoloff BJ. Characterization of intercellular adhesion molecule-1 and HLA-DR expression in normal and inflamed skin: modulation by recombinant gamma interferon and tumor necrosis factor. *J Am Acad Dermatol* 1989;20:617.

303. Dustin ML, Singer KH, Tuck DT, et al. Adhesion of T lymphoblasts to epidermal keratinocytes is regulated by interferon gamma and is mediated by intercellular adhesion molecule-1 (ICAM-1). *J Exp Med* 1988;167:1323.

304. Surgeman PB, Savage NW, Seymour GJ. Phenotype and suppressor activity of T-lymphocyte clones extracted from lesions of oral lichen planus. *Br J Dermatol* 1994;131:319.

305. Gadenne AS, Struke R, Dunn D, et al. T-cell lines derived from lesional skin of lichen planus patients contain a distinctive population of T-cell receptor gamma delta-bearing cells. *J Invest Dermatol* 1994;103:347.

306. Simark-Mattsson C, Bergenholtz G, Jontell M, et al. T cell receptor V-gene usage in oral lichen planus: increased frequency of T cell receptors expressing V alfa2 and V beta3. *Clin Exp Immunol* 1994;98:503.

307. Farthing PM, Matear P, Cruchley AT. Langerhans' cell distribution and keratinocyte expression of HLA-DR in oral lichen planus. *J Oral Pathol* Med 1992;21:451.

308. Hirota J, Osaki T. Electron microscopy study on cell-to-cell interactions in oral lichen planus. *Pathol Res Pract* 1992;188: 1033.

309. Prieto VG, Casal M, McNutt NS. Lichen planus-like keratosis: a clinical and histological reexamination. *Am J Surg Pathol* 1993;17:259.

310. Van den Haute V, Antoine JL, Lachapelle JM. Histopathological discriminant criteria between lichenoid drug eruption and idiopathic lichen planus: retrospective study on selected samples. *Dermatologica* 1989;179:10.

311. Rocken M: Zur pathogenese des lichen ruber planus, ein modernes konzept. *Z Hautkr* 1988;63:911.

312. Haber H, Sarkany I. Hypertrophic lichen planus and lichen simplex. *Trans St Johns Hosp Dermatol Soc* 1958;41:61.

313. Lumpkin LR, Helwig EB. Solitary lichen planus. *Arch Dermatol* 1966;93:54.

314. Shapiro L, Ackerman AB. Solitary lichen planus-like keratosis. *Dermatologica* 1966;132:386.

315. Laur WE, Posey RE, Waller JD. Lichen planus-like keratosis: a clinicopathologic correlation. *J Am Acad Dermatol* 1981;4:329.

316. Scott MA, Johnson WC. Lichenoid benign keratosis. *J Cutan Pathol* 1976;3:217.

317. Le Coz CJ. Lichen planus-like keratosis or (solitary) benign lichenoid keratosis. *Ann Dermatol Venereol* 2000;127:219.

318. Jang KA, Kim SH, Choi JH. Lichenoid keratosis: a clinicopathologic study of 17 patients. *J Am Acad Dermatol* 2000;43: 511.

319. Goette DK. Benign lichenoid keratosis. *Arch Dermatol* 1980; 116:780.

320. Goldenhersh MA, Barnhill RL, Rosenbaum HM, et al. Documented evolution of a solar lentigo into a solitary lichen planus-like keratosis. *J Cutan Pathol* 1986;13:308.

321. Frigg AF, Cooper PH. Benign lichenoid keratosis. *Am J Clin Pathol* 1985;83:439.

322. Berger TG, Graham JH, Goette DK. Lichenoid benign keratosis. *J Am Acad Dermatol* 1984;11;635.

323. Mehregan AH. Lentigo senilis and its evolution. *J Invest Dermatol* 1975;65:429.

324. Prieto VG, Casal M, McNutt NS. Immunohistochemistry detects differences between lichen planus-like keratosis, lichen planus, and lichenoid actinic keratosis. *J Cutan Pathol* 1993;20: 143.

325. Inui S, Itami S, Kobayashi T, et al. A case of lichen planus-like keratosis:deposition of IgM in the basement membrane zone. *J Dermatol* 2000;27:615.

326. Tan CY, Marks R. Lichenoid solar keratosis: prevalence and immunologic findings. *J Invest Dermatol* 1982;79:365.

327. Berman A, Herszenson S, Winkelmann RK. The involuting lichenoid plaque. *Arch Dermatol* 1982;118:93.

328. Kaposi M. Lichen ruber acuminatus and lichen ruber planus. *Arch Dermatol Syphilol* 1895;31:1.

329. Margolis MG, Cooper GA, Johnson SAM. Keratosis lichenoides chronica. *Arch Dermatol* 1972;105:739.

330. Torrelo A, Mediero IG, Zasmbrano A. Keratosis lichenoides chronica in a child. *Pediatr Dermatol* 1994:11:46.

331. Patrizi A, Neri I, Passasrini B, et al. Keratosis lichenoides chronica: a pediatric case. *Dermatology* 1995;191:264.

332. Masouye I, Saurat JH. Keratosis lichenoides chronica: the century of another Kaposi's disease. *Dermatology* 1995;191:188.

333. Braun-Falco O, Bieber T, Heider L. Chronic lichenoid keratosis: disease variant or disease entity? *Hautarzt* 1989;40:614.

334. Baran R, Panizzon R, Goldberg L. The nails in keratosis lichenoides chronica: characteristics and response to treatment. *Arch Dermatol* 1984;120:1471.

335. Duperrat B, Carton FX, Denoeux JP, et al. Keratose lichenoide striae. *Ann Dermatol Venereol* 1977;104:564.

336. van der Kerkhof PCM. Spontaneous resolution of keratosis lichenoides chronica. *Dermatology* 1993;187:200.

337. Lombardo GA, Annessi G, Baliva G, et al. Keratosis lichenoides chronica. Report of a case associated with B-cell lymphoma and leg panniculitis. *Dermatology* 2000;201:261.

338. Haas N, Czaika V, Sterry W. Keratosis lichenoides chronica following trauma. A case report and update of the last literature review. *Hautarzt* 2001;52:629.

339. Criado PR, Valente NY, Sittart JA, et al. Keratosis lichenoides chronica: report of a case developing after erythroderma. *Australas J Dermatol* 2000;41:247.

340. Nabai H, Mehregan AH. Keratosis lichenoides chronica. *J Am Acad Dermatol* 1980;2:217.

341. Petrozzi JW. Keratosis lichenoides chronica. *Arch Dermatol* 1976;112:709.

342. David M, Filhaber A, Rotem A, et al. Keratosis lichenoides chronica with prominent telangiectasia: response to etretinate. *J Am Acad Dermatol* 1989;21:1112.

343. Lapins JA, Willoughby C, Helwig EB. Lichen nitidus: a study of forty-three cases. *Cutis* 1978:21:634.

344. Kawakami T, Soma Y. Generalized lichen nitidus appearing subsequent to lichen planus. *J Dermatol* 1995;22:434.

345. Maeda M. A case of generalized lichen nitidus with Koebner's phenomenon. *J Dermatol* 1994;21:273.

346. Munro CS, Cox NH, Marks JM, et al. Lichen nitidus presenting as palmoplantar hyperkeratosis and nail dystrophy. *Clin Exp Dermatol* 1993;18:381.

347. Itami A, Ando I, Kukita A. Perforating lichen nitidus. *Int J Dermatol* 1994;33:382.

348. De Eusebio Murillo E, Sanchez Yus E, Novo Lens R. Lichen nitidus of the palms: a case with peculiar histopathologic features. *Am J Dermatopathol* 1999;21:161.

349. Madhok R, Winkelmann RK. Spinous, follicular lichen nitidus associated with perifollicular granulomas. *J Cutan Pathol* 1988; 15:248.

350. Fimiani M, Alessandrini C, Castelli A, et al. Ultrastructural observations in lichen nitidus. *Arch Dermatol Res* 1986;279:77.

351. Wilson HTH, Bett DCG. Miliary lesions in lichen planus. *Arch Dermatol* 1961;83:74.

352. Waisman M, Dundon BC, Michel B. Immunofluorescent studies in lichen nitidus. *Arch Dermatol* 1973;107:200.

353. Smoller BR, Flynn TC. Immunohistochemical examination of lichen nitidus suggests that it is not a localized papular variant of lichen planus. *J Am Acad Dermatol* 1992;27:232.

354. Reed RJ, Meek T, Ichinose H. Lichen striatus: a model for the histologic spectrum of lichenoid reactions. *J Cutan Pathol* 1975;2:1.

355. Taieb A, el Youbi A, Grosshans E, et al. Lichen striatus: a Blaschko linear acquired inflammatory skin eruption. *J Am Acad Dermatol* 1991;25:637.

356. Vasily D, Bhatia SG. Lichen striatus. *Cutis* 1981;28:442.

357. Patrone P, Patrizi A, Bonci A, et al. Lichen striatus: studio clinico ed istologico di 8 casi. *G Ital Dermatol Venereol* 1990;125: 267.

358. Karp DL, Cohen BA. Onychodystrophy in lichen striatus. *Pediatr Dermatol* 1993;10:359.

359. Tosti A, Peluso AM, Misciali C, et al. Nail lichen striatus: clinical features and long-term follow-up of five patients. *J Am Acad Dermatol* 1997;36:908.

360. Mopper C, Horwitz DC. Bilateral lichen striatus. *Cutis* 1971;8: 140.

361. Aloi F, Solaroli C, Pippione M. Diffuse and bilateral lichen striatus. *Pediatr Dermatol* 1997;14:36.

362. Patrizi A, Neri I, Fiorentini C, et al. Simultaneous occurrence of lichen striatus in siblings. *Pediatr Dermatol* 1997;14:293.

363. Stewart WM, Pietrini LP, Thomine E. Lichen striatus: criteres histologiques. *Ann Derm Venereol* 1977;104:132.

364. Gianotti R, Restano L, Grimalt R, et al. Lichen striatus—a chameleon: an histopathological and immunohistological study of forty-one cases. *J Cutan Pathol* 1995;22:18.

365. Pujol RM, Toneu A, Moreno A, et al. Perforating lichen striatus. *Acta Derm Venereol (Stockh)* 1988;68:171.

366. Zhang Y, Mc Nutt NS. Lichen striatus. Histological, immunohistochemical and ultrastructural study of 37 cases. *J Cutan Pathol* 2001;28:65.

367. Goldman K, Don PC. Adult onset of inflammatory linear verrucous epidermal nevus in a mother and her daughter. *Dermatology* 1994;189:170.

368. Landwehr AJ, Starink TM. Inflammatory linear verrucous epidermal naevus. *Dermatologica* 1983;166:107.

369. Al-Enezi S, Huber AM, Krafchick BR, et al. Inflammatory linear verrucous epidermal nevus and arthritis: a new association. *J Pediatr* 2001;138:602.

370. Zhuang L, Zhu W. Inflammatory linear verrucous epidermal nevus coexisting with lichen amyloidosus. *J Dermatol* 1996;23: 415.

371. Altman J, Mehregan AH. Inflammatory linear verrucous epidermal nevus. *Arch Dermatol* 1971;104:385.

372. Dupre A, Christol B. Inflammatory linear verrucose epidermal nevus. *Arch Dermatol* 1977;113:767.

373. Toribio J, Quinones PA. Inflammatory linear verrucose epidermal nevus. *Dermatologica* 1975;150:65.

374. Ito M, Shimizu N, Fujiwara H, et al. Histopathogenesis of inflammatory linear verrucose epidermal naevus: histochemistry, immunohistochemistry and ultrastructure. *Arch Dermatol Res* 1991;283:491.

375. Bernard BA, Reano A, Darmon YM, et al. Precocious appearance of involucrin and epidermal transglutaminase during differentiation of psoriatic skin. *Br J Dermatol* 1986;114: 279.

376. Welch ML, Smith KJ, Skelton HG, et al. Immunohistochemical features in inflammatory linear verrucous epidermal nevi suggest a distinctive pattern of clonal dysregulation of growth. *J Am Acad Dermatol* 1993;29:242.

377. Laugier P, Olmos L. Naevus lineaire inflammatoire (NEVIL) et lichen striatus: deux aspects d'une meme affection. *Bull Soc Fr Dermatol Syphiligr* 1976;83:48.

378. De Jong EMGJ, Rulo HFC, Van de Kerkhof PCM. Inflammatory linear verrucous epidermal naevus (ILVEN) versus linear psoriasis: a clinical, histological and immunohistochemical study. *Acta Derm Venereol (Stockh)* 1991;71:343.

379. Fox BJ, Odom RB. Papulosquamous diseases: a review. *J Am Acad Dermatol* 1985;12:597.

380. Griffiths WAD. Pityriasis rubra pilaris. *Clin Exp Dermatol* 1980;5:105.

381. Griffiths WAD. Pityriasis rubra pilaris: the problem of its classification [Letter]. *J Am Acad Dermatol* 1992;26:140.

382. Gelmetti C, Schiuma AA, Cerri D, Gianotti F. Pityriasis rubra pilaris in childhood: a long-term study of 29 cases. *Pediatr Dermatol* 1986;2:446.

383. Vanderhooft SL, Francis JS, Holbrook KA, et al. Familial pityriasis rubra pilaris. *Arch Dermatol* 1995;131:448.

384. Kloos C, Muller UA, Hoffken , et al. Paraneoplastic pityriasis rubra pilaris in metastatic adenocarcinoma without diagnosable primary. *Dtsch Med Wochenschr* 2002;127:437.

385. Huynh NT, Hunt MJ, Cachia AR, et al. Merkel cell carcinoma and multiple cutaneous squamous cell carcinomas in a patient with pityriasis rubra pilaris. *Australas J Dermatol* 2002;43:48.

386. Conaghan PG, Sommer S, Mc Gonagle D, et al. The relationship between pityriasis rubra pilaris and inflammatory arthritis: case report and response of the arthritis to anti-tumor necrosis factor immunotherapy. *Arthritis Rheum* 1999; 9:1998.

387. Behr FD, Bangert JL, Hansen RC. Atypical pityriasis rubra pilaris associated with arthropathy and osteoporosis: a case report with 15 year follow-up. *Pediatr Dermatol* 2002; 19:46.

388. Braun-Falco O, Ryckmanns F, Schmoeckel C, et al. Pityriasis rubra pilaris: a clinico-pathological and therapeutic study with special reference to histochemistry, autoradiography, and electron microscopy. *Arch Dermatol Res* 1983;275:287.

389. Niemi KM, Kousa M, Storgards K, et al. Pityriasis rubra pilaris. *Dermatologica* 1976;152:109.

390. Kanitakis J, Hoyo E, Chouvet B, et al. Keratinocyte proliferation in epidermal keratinocyte disorders evaluated through PCNA/cyclin immunolabelling and AgNOR counting. *Acta Derm Venereol (Stockh)* 1993;73:370.

391. Griffiths WAD, Pieris S. Pityriasis rubra pilaris: an autoradiographic study. *Br J Dermatol* 1982;107:665.

392. Gelmetti C, Rigoni C, Alessi E, et al. Pityriasis lichenoides in children: a long-term follow-up of eighty-nine cases. *J Am Acad Dermatol* 1990;23:473.

393. Willemze R, Scheffer E. Clinical and histologic differentiation between lymphomatoid papulosis and pityriasis lichenoides. *J Am Acad Dermatol* 1985;13:418.

394. Wood GS, Strickler JG, Abel EA, et al. Immunohistology of pityriasis lichenoides et varioliformis acuta and pityriasis lichenoides chronica. *J Am Acad Dermatol* 1987;16:559.

395. Longley J, Demar L, Feinstein RP, et al. Clinical and histologic features of pityriasis lichenoides et varioliformis acuta in children. *Arch Dermatol* 1987;123:1335.

396. Brazzini B, Gheresetich I, Urso C, et al. Pityriasis lichenoides et varioliformis acuta during pregnancy. *J Eur Acad Dermatol Venereol* 2001;15:458.

397. Eskandar MA. Pityriasis lichenoides at varioliformis acuta in pregnancy. *Saudi Med J* 2001;22:1127.

398. Maekawa Y, Nakamura T, Nogami R. Febrile ulceronecrotic Mucha-Habermann's disease. *J Dermatol* 1994;21:46.

399. De Cuyper C, Hindryckx P, Deroo N. Febrile ulceronecrotic pityriasis lichenoides et varioliformis acuta. *Dermatology* 1994; 189:50.

400. Lopez-Estebaranz JL, Vanaclocha F, Gil R, et al. Febrile ulceronecrotic Mucha-Habermann disease. *J Am Acad Dermatol* 1993;29:903.

401. Muhlbauer JE, Bhan AK, Harrist TJ, et al. Immunopathology of pityriasis lichenoides acuta. *J Am Acad Dermatol* 1984;10: 783.

402. Hood AF, Mark EJ. Histopathologic diagnosis of pityriasis lichenoides et varioliformis acuta and its clinical correlation. *Arch Dermatol* 1982;118:478.

403. Giannetti A, Girolomoni G, Pincelli C, et al. Immunopathologic studies in pityriasis lichenoides. *Arch Dermatol Res* 1988; 280:S61.

404. Varga FJ, Vonderheid EC, Olbricht SM, et al. Immunohistochemical distinction of lymphomatoid papulosis and pityriasis lichenoides et varioliformis acuta. *Am J Pathol* 1990;136; 979.

405. Weinberg JM, Kristal L, Chooback L, et al. The clonal nature of pityriasis lichenoides. *Arch Dermatol* 2002;138: 1063.

406. Dereure O, Levi E, Kadin ME. T cell clonality in pityriasis lichenoides et varioliformis acuta: a heteroduplex analysis of 20 cases. *Arch Dermatol* 2000;136:1483.

407. Weiss LM, Wood GS, Ellisen LW, et al. Clonal T-cell populations in pityriasis lichenoides et varioliformis acuta (Mucha-Habermann disease). *Am J Pathol* 1987;126:417.

408. Shieh S, Mikkola DL, Wood GS. Differentiation and clonality of lesional lymphocytes in pityriasis lichenoides chronica. *Arch Dermatol* 2001;137:305.

409. Kadin M. T-cell clonality in pityriasis lichenoides. Evidence for a premalignant or reactive immune disorder? *Arch Dermatol* 2002;138:1089.

410. Fortson JS, Schoroeter AL, Esterly NB. Cutaneous T-cell lymphoma (parapsoriasis en plaque): an association with pityriasis lichenoides et varioliformis acuta in young children. *Arch Dermatol* 1990;126:1449.

411. Panizzon RC, Speich R, Dassi H. Atypical manifestations of pityriasis lichenoides chronica: development into paraneoplasia and non-Hodgkin lymphomas of the skin. *Dermatology* 1992; 184:65.

412. McKee PH. Pityriasis lichenoides in vascular diseases. In: McKee PH, ed. *Pathology of the Skin with Clinical Correlations*, 2nd ed. London: Mosby-Wolfe, 1996:5.8.

8

VASCULAR DISEASES

RAYMOND L. BARNHILL
KLAUS J. BUSAM
CARLOS H. NOUSARI
XIAOWEI XU
SARAH K. BARKSDALE

This chapter discusses vasculitides, vasculopathies, and several other disease processes with vascular injury that can affect the skin. The spectrum of clinical manifestations of such diseases is broad and depends on several factors including the number, size, and type of vessels involved (arterial vs. venous); the extent of vascular damage; the presence or absence of inflammation; the type of inflammatory infiltrate (neutrophilic vs. lymphocytic); the infiltrate's distribution (superficial dermis vs. deep dermis or subcutis); and other parameters.

In general, severe vascular damage with vascular occlusion leads to ischemic damage, and may result in necrosis, blister formation, and/or ulceration. Nonocclusive vascular disease may be associated with damage to the structural integrity of the vessel wall and may lead to leakage of blood, resulting in dermal hemorrhage and edema. Dermal hemorrhage is clinically seen as purpura. Hemorrhages less than 3 mm in diameter are called petechiae while larger lesions are called ecchymoses. If an inflammatory infiltrate is present, purpura may become palpable.

CRITERIA FOR VASCULITIS

Considerable controversy surrounds the criteria for vasculitis. The essential difficulty is the dynamic nature of vascular injury. The appearance of the injured vessels and the inflammatory cells present change as lesions evolve over time. Furthermore, the degree of vascular injury varies depending on the severity of the insult. The spectrum of vascular reaction to injury ranges from endothelial cell swelling and leakiness to frank fibrinoid necrosis and fibrin deposition. Thus, criteria for recognizing microvascular injury are somewhat arbitrary.

While the minimum criteria for vasculitis have remained controversial, in general, vasculitis must have two components: (a) an inflammatory cell infiltrate, and (b) evidence of vascular injury (Table 8-1). Vasculitis is an in-

flammatory process, and thus the absence of inflammation precludes the diagnosis even though vascular alterations may be present. However, in the late healing state, the inflammatory cell infiltrate may be minimal. The inflammatory cells involved may include neutrophils, lymphocytes, or monocytes/macrophages. The type of infiltrating cell may correlate to some extent with the chronology of the process, but not always.

Evidence of vascular injury is the second major component of vasculitis. Criteria for vascular injury have included (a) evidence of vessel leakiness such as edema and extravasation of erythrocytes, (b) evidence of vessel destruction such as necrosis of endothelium and deposition of fibrinoid material within the vascular lumina or vessel walls, and (c) evidence of inflammatory compromise of the vascular walls including infiltration by inflammatory cells and leukocytoclasis of the surrounding inflammatory cell infiltrate (Fig. 8-1). As mentioned above, there is a continuum of injury. However, for several years pathologists have required a certain degree of injury, as manifested by deposition of fibrinoid material and/or necrosis of the vessel itself, as a primary indicator of a true vasculitis. Certain changes, including edema, extravasation of erythrocytes, infiltration of vessel walls, leukocytoclasis, and thrombosis may occur with minimal evidence of vascular injury. Pathologists should strive not to overinterpret such changes as vasculitis when definitive evidence of vessel injury is lacking. For instance, leukocytoclasis also may result from necrosis of a neutrophilic infiltrate itself without fibrinoid necrosis of vessels. Similarly, fibrin thrombi may be present in non-inflamed vessels in the setting of hypercoagulable states.

Determining whether the vascular injury is primary or secondary is another major problem in interpreting vasculitis. Primary vascular injury implies that the vascular insult is the predominant disease process. Secondary vascular injury indicates that another disease process outside the vessels is the primary pathologic process. An example of the latter is vascular alteration noted near cutaneous ulcera-

TABLE 8-1. DEFINITIONS OF VASCULAR INJURY

Primary vascular injury
Vasculopathy
  Fibrinoid deposition, thrombosis with limited to no
    inflammation
  Infiltration of vessel wall by inflammatory cells with other-
    wise minimal alteration
  Leukocytoclasis of tissue infiltrate with minimal alteration of
    vessel—that is, swelling only, absence of fibrinoid necrosis
Vasculitis
  Perivascular inflammatory cell infiltrate* (neutrophilic,
    eosinophilic, lymphocytic, histiocytic, or mixed)
  Fibrinoid necrosis*—necrosis of vessel wall with deposition of
    fibrinoid material
  Other changes often present but not essential: edema,
    extravasation of erythrocytes, leukocytoclasis, infiltration
    of vessel wall by inflammatory cells, swelling of endothelial
    cells, luminal thrombosis
Secondary vascular injury†
Vasculopathy or vasculitis
Secondary to another insult such as external trauma or
  ulceration
Variable vascular alterations with sparing of some vessels
Peripheral perivascular fibrinoid deposition

*Essential for diagnosis.
†Distinguishing between primary and secondary vasculitis is often
not possible.

tion. In many instances, distinguishing clearly between a primary and a secondary vascular insult is not possible. However, secondary vascular injury is often variable with sparing of some vessels within the zone of tissue injury. Other indications of secondary vascular injury include deposition of fibrinoid material at the periphery of the vessel wall and focal thrombosis without significant infiltration by inflammatory cells.

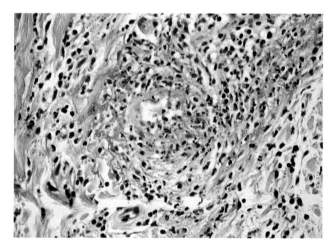

FIGURE 8-1. Hypersensitivity vasculitis showing an upper dermal small blood vessel with full-blown features of neutrophil-rich vasculitis. The specimen was obtained from a 2-day-old purpuric papule.

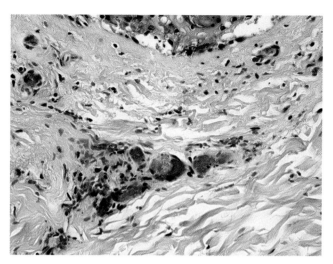

FIGURE 8-2. Vasculopathic reaction, disseminated intravascular coagulation. Pink fibrin thrombi are present within vessels that do not show evidence of damage or inflammation in their walls.

The term *vasculopathy* may be used to describe certain degrees of vascular alteration and injury that fail to satisfy the criteria for vasculitis. Such vascular alterations might include vascular thrombosis with little other evidence of injury (Fig. 8-2), deposition of fibrinoid material with little or no inflammation, and minimal infiltration of vessel walls with little or no leukocytoclasis.

EVALUATION OF VASCULITIS

The classification of inflammatory vascular reactions—specifically that of vasculitides—is difficult for a variety of reasons (1–4). Clinically different entities lack histologic specificity, and the same disease process may show a spectrum of histologic changes depending on the stage of the disease, level of activity, and type of treatment that might have modified its course. In an attempt to standardize nomenclature for vasculitides, an international conference has proposed a system primarily based on vessel size (3–6). Classification based on vessel size is helpful because there is some correlation with the clinical presentation. Purpura typically reflects small-vessel injury. Cutaneous nodules suggest the involvement of medium-size arteries. However, classification based on vessel size alone is of limited value in dermatopathology, because most cutaneous vasculitides affect primarily small dermal vessels.

A practical approach (Table 8-2) for the histopathologist in evaluating small-vessel inflammatory reactions is first to decide whether or not clear-cut vascular damage is present and sufficient for a designation as vasculitis, and then to assess the composition of the inflammatory infiltrate (neutrophilic/leukocytoclastic vs. eosinophilic vs. lymphocytic vs. granulomatous); its distribution (superfi-

TABLE 8-2. APPROACH TO VASCULITIS

1. Determine if vasculitis or vasculopathy is present or absent.
2. Primary or secondary
3. Size of vessel and type
   a. Large
   b. Medium
   c. Small
4. Composition of infiltrate
   a. Neutrophilic/leukocytoclastic
   b. Eosinophilic
   c. Lymphocytic
   d. Histiocytic/granulomatous
5. Evaluation for infection
6. Serologic and immunopathologic evaluation
   a. Evaluation for ANCA, ANA, rheumatoid factor, cryoglobulins
   b. Immunofluorescence and other studies for the detection of immune complexes—for example, IgA fibronectin aggregates
7. Clinical context
   a. Cutaneous involvement only
   b. Extent of systemic involvement

cial, superficial and deep, or deep only); and to look for associated findings, such as microorganisms, that might narrow the differential diagnosis. The context of the histologic findings is important—for example, vasculitic changes may merely be secondary events in the setting of an ulcer resulting from nonvasculitic causes, such as herpes virus infection or trauma. Lesions also have life spans and a leukocytoclastic vasculitis may evolve into a predominantly lymphocytic or even granulomatous process.

Histopathology alone is inadequate to classify a vasculitic disease process. Integration of data from other laboratory tests, clinical findings, and even arteriography may be critical to arrive at a diagnosis. In particular, clinical and radiographic findings are needed to assess the degree of systemic involvement and range in size of arteries involved. Infection must be excluded via special stains, cultures, and other laboratory studies. Specific systemic diseases that may be associated with vasculitis such as collagen vascular diseases must be excluded.

Antineutrophil cytoplasmic antibodies (ANCAs) are serologic markers that have allowed a new classification of certain vasculitides. These markers may reflect biologic re-

lationships between disease processes (5–7). ANCAs are best demonstrated by a combination of indirect immunofluorescence of normal peripheral blood neutrophils followed by enzyme-linked immuno-absorbant assay (ELISA) to detect specific autoantibodies. Indirect immunofluorescence assays reveal two staining patterns: cytoplasmic (c-ANCA) and perinuclear (p-ANCA). ELISAs show that the majority of c-ANCAs are autoantibodies to proteinase 3, and most p-ANCAs are specific for myeloperoxidase (MPO). These antibodies are especially helpful, in combination with clinical features, in the differential diagnosis of three small-vessel vasculitides: Wegener's granulomatosis syndrome (WG), Churg–Strauss syndrome (CSS), and microscopic polyarteritis (MPA). WG is usually associated with c-ANCA, MPA with either p- or c-ANCA, and CSS with p-ANCA (Table 8-3). These three syndromes are termed "pauci-immune vasculitides," as vascular injury is not associated with immunoglobulin deposition in vessel walls, in contrast to the immune complex mediated small-vessel injury seen in entities such as Henoch–Schönlein purpura. The pathogenesis of the vascular injury and the role of ANCAs in these disease processes are still unclear. ANCAs may play a role in inducing vasculitis by activating circulating neutrophils and monocytes, causing them to adhere to vessels, degranulate, and release toxic metabolites, thereby causing vascular injury. On the other hand, ANCA may be an epiphenomenon unrelated to the pathogenesis of these diseases.

The following subsections discuss the histologic features and clinical differential diagnoses of inflammatory vascular reactions affecting the skin. Vasculitides are categorized first by vessel size. The only large-vessel vasculitis with cutaneous or subcutaneous findings mentioned here is temporal (giant cell) arteritis. Vasculitis affecting medium- and small-size arteries, and, in particular, small-vessel vasculitides, are discussed in more detail. Small-vessel vasculitides are classified according to the composition of the inflammatory infiltrate: neutrophilic/leukocytoclastic versus lymphocytic versus granulomatous vasculitis.

Vasculitis of Large- and Medium-Size Vessels: Temporal (Giant Cell) Arteritis

Giant cell arteritis of the elderly primarily affects large- or medium-size arteries in the temporal region. Although the

TABLE 8-3. ANCA-POSITIVE VASCULITIDES

Disease process	Antimyeloperoxidase (p-ANCA)	Antiserine proteinase (c-ANCA)
Wegener's syndrome	Rare (5%)	Common (80%)
Microscopic polyangitis (polyarteritis)	Common (50–60%)	Common (45%)
Churg-Strauss syndrome	Common (70%)	Rare (7%)

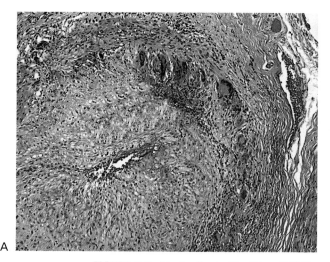
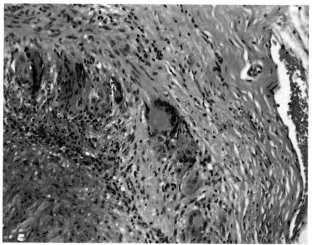

FIGURE 8-3. Giant cell arteritis. **(A)** and **(B)** Biopsy of the temporal artery shows a predominantly mononuclear cell infiltrate with a few giant cells in the region of the internal elastic lamina.

etiology of temporal arteritis is unknown, in some cases, actinic degeneration of the internal elastic lamina may provoke granulomatous inflammation in a reaction similar to actinic granuloma.

The arteritis may be unilateral or bilateral and associated with involvement of other cranial arteries—in particular, retinal arteries. The clinical presentation may include pain and tenderness of the forehead and possible sudden visual impairment. Erythema and edema of the skin overlying the involved arteries are commonly seen, although occasionally the scalp may ulcerate (8). The involved artery may be palpable. Clinical laboratory data include a significantly elevated erythrocyte sedimentation rate (ESR).

Although the clinical presentation is strongly suggestive of the diagnosis, a biopsy is often performed for confirmation prior to the initiation of systemic steroid therapy. However, results of diagnostic tests are not always positive.

Histopathology. Involved arteries show an inflammatory process of mainly lymphocytes and macrophages that may extend throughout the entire arterial wall (Fig. 8-3). Classically, fragmentation of the lamina elastica and elastophagocytosis by multinucleated giant cells are seen. However, depending on the stage of the disease process, giant cells may not be present, and the inflammatory infiltrate is often unevenly distributed. Step sections may be needed for identification. In some instances, neutrophils may be present, but this finding should not impede the diagnosis. An Elastica–van Gieson stain greatly facilitates the evaluation of elastic fibers. Disruption of the internal elastic lamina is not sufficient for diagnosis, because this is nonspecific. In late stages, thickening of the intima by deposits of fibrin-like material and myofibroblastic proliferation with subsequent luminal narrowing may be the only findings.

Differential Diagnosis. Not all cases of arteritis involving the temporal artery represent examples of temporal arteritis. Infection-related vasculitis, connective tissue disease,

and polyarteritis nodosa might enter into the differential diagnosis. The latter processes often show necrotizing neutrophilic vasculitides (depending on the stage), and diagnosis is dependent on serologic studies, the absence of infection, and clinical findings.

Vasculitis Affecting Medium- and Small-Size Vessels

Vasculitides affecting medium-size vessels include Kawasaki syndrome, Takayasu arteritis, infections, Buerger's disease, polyarteritis nodosa, MPA, WG, CSS, rheumatoid vasculitis, and giant cell (temporal) arteritis. As noted above, there are several methods of classifying vasculitides available. WG, MPA, and CSS can be categorized as ANCA-associated vasculitides. Temporal arteritis, WP, and CSS can also be classified as vasculitides associated with granulomatous inflammation.

Kawasaki Disease

Kawasaki disease is a necrotizing arteritis that usually affects young children, with a peak age incidence at age 1 year (9). Mucocutaneous findings are common and include a polymorphous exanthematous macular rash, conjunctival congestion, dry reddened lips, "strawberry tongue," oropharyngeal reddening, and swelling of the hands and feet—especially the palms and soles. Typically a nonpurulent cervical lymphadenopathy is associated. Desquamation of the skin of the fingers typically occurs after 1 to 2 weeks, often followed by thrombocytosis. The most serious clinical complications are related to arteritis and thrombosis of coronary arteries.

Histology. Cutaneous vasculitis is rare. The macular rash is usually accompanied by nonspecific histologic changes. Characteristic arteritis is typically found in visceral sites, such as the coronary arteries.

Mondor's Disease and Other Superficial Thrombophlebitides

Mondor's disease is a thrombophlebitis of the subcutaneous veins of the chest region and is often manifested clinically by a cord-like induration (26). Generalized symptoms are usually not a feature, and resolution within weeks is the norm.

Histopathology. In early lesions, a polymorphonuclear infiltrate may be present. However, most biopsied lesions show subcutaneous veins with organizing thrombi and fibrous thickened walls that give them a cord-like appearance at scanning magnification.

Pathogenesis. In the majority of cases, the etiology remains unknown; however, local interference with venous flow may be a factor. Trauma, connective tissue disease, breast carcinoma (in rare cases), and a variety of other conditions have been associated.

Superficial thrombophlebitis of small- to medium-size veins may be encountered at other anatomic sites, most commonly in the lower extremities. Tenderness and erythema of the overlying skin is the common presentation. Histologic changes are nonspecific and typically show or-ganizing thrombi and a variably dense mononuclear cell infiltrate.

Thromboangiitis Obliterans (Buerger's Disease)

Buerger's disease is a distinctive condition characterized by a segmental, thrombosing inflammatory process affecting intermediate and small arteries and sometimes veins. The vessels of the upper and lower extremities are most commonly involved. The condition almost exclusively affects smokers. Cutaneous findings are manifestations of ischemic injury.

Histopathology. Active lesions are characterized by luminal thrombotic occlusion and a mixed inflammatory cell infiltrate of the vessel wall, characteristically with microabscesses. Later, the thrombus is organized and its lumen may be recanalized (Fig. 8-4). A granulomatous reaction may be present as well.

Differential Diagnosis. The histologic findings in Buerger's disease have been thought to be characteristic. The

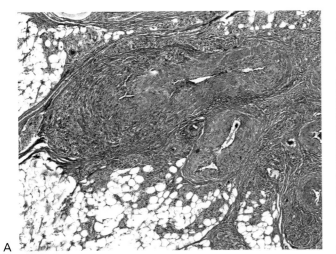

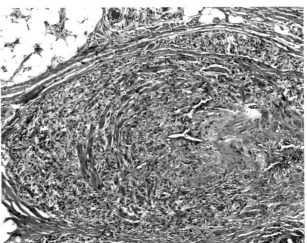

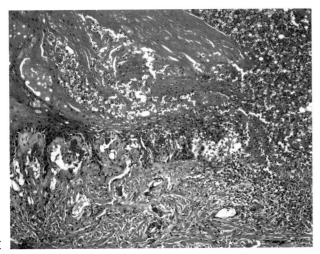

FIGURE 8-4. Thromboangiitis obliterans (Buerger's disease). A mixed inflammatory infiltrate is present in the wall of a large vein and its lumen is recanalized in a 35-year-old man **(A)** and **(B)** with associated ischemic ulceration n in the distal extremity **(C)**.

prevalent current opinion is that these findings are nonspecific and probably occur in other processes, including nonspecific thrombosis and inflammation of intermediate-size arteries and veins.

Polyarteritis Nodosa

Kussmaul and Maier reported in 1866 the case of a 27-year-old man with fever, abdominal pain, muscle weakness, peripheral neuropathy, and renal disease (11). They termed the fatal illness *periarteritis nodosa* (PAN), referring to nodular protuberances along the course of medium-size muscular arteries, which histologically were characterized by inflammation predominantly at the periphery of the vessel walls, with vessel wall destruction. Ferrari noted in 1903 the more characteristic presence of inflammatory cells within all levels of the affected vessels, and suggested the term *polyarteritis* instead of *periarteritis* (12).

Clinical Features. PAN is more common in men than women, usually occurring between ages 20 and 60 years. Clinical manifestations may be dramatic and protean. Fever, malaise, weight loss, weakness, myalgias, arthralgias, and anorexia are common symptoms reflecting the systemic nature of the disease. Other findings may reflect infarction of specific organs. Renal involvement, present in about 75% of patients, is the most common cause of death. Hematuria, proteinuria, hypertension, and azotemia may result from both infarction owing to disease of renal arteries or sometimes focal, segmental necrotizing glomerular lesions, suggesting involvement of small vessels. Acute abdominal crises, strokes, myocardial infarction, and mononeuritis multiplex result from involvement of relevant arteries. Arteriography of visceral arteries often shows multiple aneurysms that are highly suggestive of PAN. ANCAs are generally absent in patients with predominately medium-size vessel involvement. Symptoms such as asthma, Löffler's syndrome, and rashes may be related to the hypereosinophilia sometimes seen in these patients. Cutaneous manifestations include subcutaneous nodules that may pulsate or ulcerate, ecchymoses, and gangrene of fingers and toes. Livedo reticularis, bullae, papules, scarlatiniform lesions, and urticaria occur in some patients. A limited form of PAN without visceral involvement may exist but this concept is controversial (13). The so-called cutaneous polyarteritis nodosum may not be limited to the skin, but may also affect muscle, peripheral nerves, and joints. The course of disease is described as benign, but protracted with steroid dependence.

Histopathology. The characteristic lesion of classic PAN is a panarteritis involving medium- and small-size arteries (Fig. 8-5). Even though in classic PAN the arteries show the characteristic changes in many visceral sites, affected skin often shows only small-vessel disease, and arterial involvement is typically focal. The changes affecting cutaneous small vessels are usually those of a necrotizing leuko-

cytoclastic vasculitis. If there is a clinical presentation of cutaneous nodules, panarteritis similar to visceral lesions is usually detected. In classic PAN, the lesions typically are in different stages of development (i.e., fresh and old). Early lesions show degeneration of the arterial wall with deposition of fibrinoid material. There is partial to complete destruction of the external and internal elastic laminae. An infiltrate present within and around the arterial wall is composed largely of neutrophils showing evidence of leukocytoclasis, although it often contains eosinophils. At a later stage, intimal proliferation and thrombosis lead to complete occlusion of the lumen with subsequent ischemia and possibly ulceration. The infiltrate also may contain a significant number of lymphocytes, histiocytes, and some plasma cells, which may extend far into the surrounding perivascular tissue and may be predominant at a certain stage. In the healing stage, there is fibroblastic proliferation extending into the perivascular area. The small vessels of the middle and upper dermis often exhibit a nonspecific lymphocytic perivascular infiltrate.

Differential Diagnosis. Vasculitis indistinguishable from PAN may be observed in infections (bacterial, e.g., pseudomonas; viral, e.g., hepatitis B or HIV); in connective tissue diseases (lupus erythematosus, rheumatoid arthritis); in WG; in CSS; and in other settings—for example, acute myelogenous leukemia—without explanation. MPA can overlap considerably with PAN as discussed below.

Pathogenesis. The pathogenesis of classic PAN is poorly understood. Direct immunofluorescence testing of skin lesions of PAN shows some immune deposits in dermal vessels. However, they may reflect a secondary event after vascular injury from another cause. ANCAs are generally absent in patients with predominately medium-size vessel involvement, and thus are not involved in the pathogenesis of these cases of PAN.

Microscopic Polyangiitis

Davson, Ball, and Platt distinguished *classic* and *MPA nodosa* (14). Classic polyarteritis nodosa is to a greater degree a disease of medium-size vessels so that ischemic glomerular lesions are common but glomerulonephritis is rare. Microscopic polyarteritis nodosa, also termed *microscopic polyangiitis* (MPA), on the other hand, refers to a systemic small-vessel vasculitis primarily affecting arterioles and capillaries that is typically related to focal necrotizing glomerulonephritis with crescents. Involvement of the small vessels of the kidneys, lungs, and skin gives MPA a particular clinical picture, and separates MPA from classic polyarteritis nodosum.

Clinical Features. The majority of patients with MPA are male and over 50 years of age. Prodromal symptoms include fever, myalgias, arthralgias, and sore throat. The most common clinical feature is renal disease, manifesting as microhematuria, proteinuria, or acute oliguric renal failure.

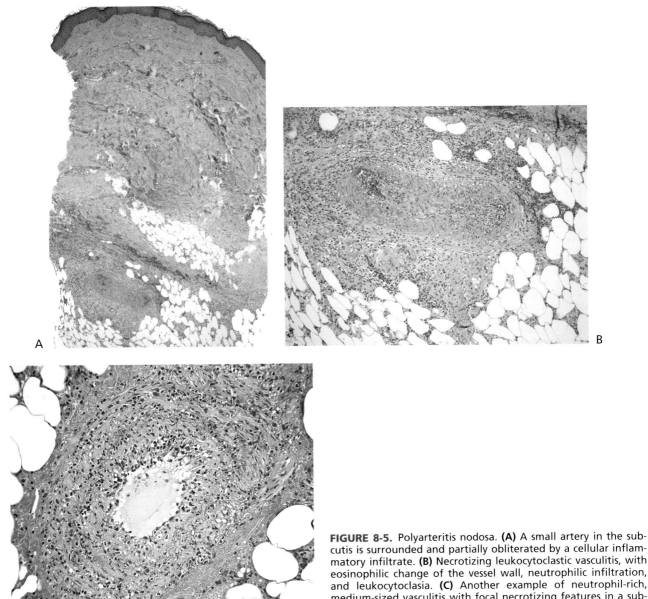

FIGURE 8-5. Polyarteritis nodosa. **(A)** A small artery in the subcutis is surrounded and partially obliterated by a cellular inflammatory infiltrate. **(B)** Necrotizing leukocytoclastic vasculitis, with eosinophilic change of the vessel wall, neutrophilic infiltration, and leukocytoclasia. **(C)** Another example of neutrophil-rich, medium-sized vasculitis with focal necrotizing features in a subcutaneous vessel in a patient with polyarteritis nodosa.

Although cutaneous involvement is rare in classic PAN, 30% to 40% of patients with MPA have skin changes. These include palpable purpura, splinter hemorrhages, and ulcerations. Tender erythematous nodules and livedo reticularis typical of classic PAN are exceedingly rare in MPA. Pulmonary involvement without granulomatous tissue reaction occurs in approximately one-third of patients. Other organ systems (e.g., gastrointestinal tract, central nervous system, serosal and articular surfaces) also may be affected, but this is less common. Serious clinical complications usually arise from renal and pulmonary disease.

Histopathological Features. A leukocytoclastic vasculitis primarily affecting arterioles, venules, and capillaries is observed. Necrotizing vasculitis of medium-size arteries typi-

cal of classic PAN is present on occasion. Cutaneous granulomatous inflammation is not a feature of MPA.

Differential Diagnosis. MPA and classic PAN may not be distinguishable in every case, practically speaking. Glomerulonephritis, typical skin signs, ANCA positivity, and lack of arteriography findings (aneurysms and stenoses reflecting medium-size vessel involvement) favor MPA over classic PAN (15). MPA also tends not to be associated with viral hepatitis in contradistinction to some cases of classic PAN. Biopsy findings are less useful in distinguishing between these two syndromes, as the size of diseased vessels detected is highly dependent on biopsy site, size of specimens, and number of tissue samples. Thus, lack of medium-size vessel involvement in a biopsy by no means excludes classical PAN. Conversely, detection of small-vessel involvement also does not exclude classical PAN, which may show small-vessel disease. A number of cases of vasculitis show overlapping features leading to the introduction of the term "overlapping syndrome of vasculitis" to encompass vasculitis affecting both small- and medium-size arteries (16). The differential diagnosis also includes Wegener's vasculitis and other small-vessel vasculitides that are occasionally ANCA positive, such as certain drug reactions. The granulomatous inflammation of WG should be lacking in MPA; however, these two entities share many features, and some are of the opinion that the distinction of MPA from WG is largely artificial (17).

Granulomatous Vasculitis and Granulomatous Vascular Reactions

Over the lifespans of many inflammatory reactions involving blood vessels, histiocytes may predominate at a certain stage and form granulomas (1,4) (Fig. 8-6). Granuloma formation may occur with no or minimal vascular wall damage, or may be associated with fibrinoid degeneration of the vessel wall. In the latter situation, a granulomatous vasculitis is present. The main disease processes that need to be considered in the differential diagnosis of a granulomatous vascular reaction are listed in Table 8-4.

TABLE 8-4. DIFFERENTIAL DIAGNOSIS OF GRANULOMATOUS VASCULAR REACTIONS

Infection
Wegener's granulomatosis
Churg-Strauss syndrome
Polyarteritis nodosa
Cutaneous Crohn's disease
Drug reaction
Connective tissue disease
Granuloma annulare
Necrobiosis lipoidica
Paraneoplastic phenomena
Angiocentric T-cell lymphoma (lymphomatoid granulomatosis)
Erythema nodosum and erythema nodosum-like reactions

The two main disease processes in which granulomatous vasculitis has been described as prominent and fairly characteristic, although nonspecific, are WG and CSS, which are discussed in more detail here. However, the most common cutaneous histologic finding in both diseases is leukocytoclastic vasculitis. The granulomatous inflammation seen in the skin usually is not angiodestructive. Other disease processes that enter the differential diagnosis are also mentioned.

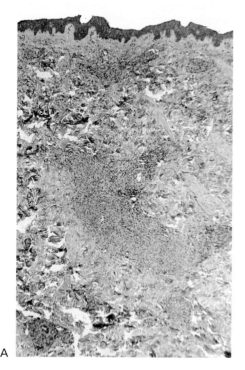
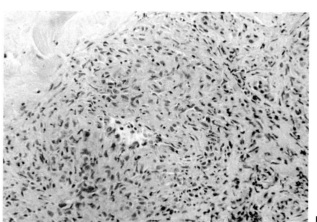

FIGURE 8-6. Granulomatous vasculitis. Note perivascular histiocytic/granulomatous infiltrate **(A)**, and focal vascular damage **(B)**.

Churg–Strauss Syndrome

The classic clinicopathologic syndrome of Churg–Strauss is characterized by asthma, fever, hypereosinophilia, eosinophilic tissue infiltrates, necrotizing vasculitis, and extravascular granuloma formation. Short of an autopsy, the classic pathologic triad of necrotizing vasculitis, eosinophilic tissue infiltration, and extravascular granulomas is extremely difficult to demonstrate because of the focality of the process (18). A broader definition of CSS requiring asthma, hypereosinophilia >1.5 × 10⁹/L, and systemic vasculitis involving two or more extrapulmonary organs has been suggested. Considerable overlap with other systemic vasculitides, and with other inflammatory disorders associated with eosinophils, such as eosinophilic pneumonitis, has brought the legitimacy of CSS into question.

Clinical Features. Despite multiple reports, CSS appears to be rare. Between 1950 and 1995, only 120 cases were identified at the Mayo clinic (19). The incidence of CSS is similar in males and females. It typically presents in the third or fourth decade of life. Patients tend to display several phases of disease development, from nonspecific symptoms of asthma and allergic rhinitis (prodromal phase), to a phase of hypereosinophilia with eosinophilic pneumonitis or gastroenteritis (second phase) and, finally, to systemic vasculitis (third phase). The internal organs most commonly involved are the lungs, the gastrointestinal tract, and, less commonly, the peripheral nerves and the heart. In contrast to PAN, renal failure is rare. The three disease phases do not always occur sequentially but may on occasion present simultaneously. There is also a limited form of allergic granulomatosis, in which, in addition to preexisting asthma, the lesions are confined to the conjunctiva, skin, and subcutaneous tissue.

Two types of cutaneous lesions occur in about two-thirds of all patients: (a) hemorrhagic lesions varying from petechiae to extensive ecchymoses, sometimes accompanied by necrotic ulcers and often associated with areas of erythema (similar to Henoch-Schönlein purpura); and (b) cutaneous–subcutaneous nodules. The most common sites of skin lesions are the extremities, but the trunk may also show involvement. In some instances, the petechiae and ecchymoses are generalized.

Diagnostically helpful laboratory findings include an elevated peripheral eosinophil count. CSS is also associated with ANCA. Serum samples from patients with CSS obtained during an active phase of the disease contain anti-MPO (p-ANCA) in the majority of cases (approximately 70%). The levels of anti-MPO have been found to correlate with disease activity. Anti-MPO is found less often in patients with limited forms of the disease. Antiserine proteinase antibodies (c-ANCA) may infrequently be found in patients with CSS (approximately 7%).

Histopathology. The areas of cutaneous hemorrhage typically show leukocytoclastic vasculitis (LCV). However, eosinophils may be conspicuous. In some instances, the dermis shows a granulomatous reaction called palisading necrotizing granuloma composed predominantly of radially arranged histiocytes and, frequently, multinucleated giant cells centered around degenerated collagen fibers (Fig. 8-7). The central portions of the granulomas contain degenerated collagen fibers and disintegrated cells, particularly eosinophils, in great numbers. These palisading granulomas can be embedded in a diffuse inflammatory exudate rich in eosinophils. In the subcutaneous tissue, the granulomas may attain considerable size through expansion and confluence, giving rise to the clinically apparent cutaneous–subcutaneous nodules. Initially thought to be characteristic histologic features, these granulomas were referred to as Churg–Strauss granulomas. However, they are not always present and are not a prerequisite for the diagnosis. Moreover, more recent studies have shown that similar findings can also be observed in other disease processes, such as connective tissue diseases (rheumatoid arthritis and lupus erythematosus), WG, PAN, lymphoproliferative disorders, subacute bacterial endocarditis, chronic active hepatitis, and inflammatory bowel disease (Crohn's disease and ulcerative colitis) (20).

Differential Diagnosis. CSS is a clinicopathologic entity. As such, a diagnosis of CSS depends on the clinical picture of respiratory disease, particularly a history of asthma, p-ANCA positivity, and histology compatible and supportive of this diagnosis, especially granulomatous inflammation, necrotizing angiitis, and eosinophilia. The principal differential diagnosis is from PAN, MPA, WG, and the conditions mentioned above that may show extravascular necrotizing granulomas. There appears to be significant overlap with WG and PAN. Particular patients may shift from one disease category to another over time.

Wegener's Granulomatosis

WG was first recognized as a distinct clinicopathologic disease process in 1936, when Wegener reported three patients with a "peculiar rhinogenic granulomatosis." Goodman and Churg summarized postmortem studies in 1954, from which evolved the classic triad of this clinicopathologic complex characterized by (a) necrotizing and granulomatous inflammation of the upper and lower respiratory tracts; (b) glomerulonephritis; and (c) systemic vasculitis (21). Liebow and Carrington (18), and later Deremee et al. (22), described limited variants of the disease involving the respiratory tract only.

With the recognition of an association between ANCAs and WG, the concept of WG has been modified and the necessity of demonstrating granulomatous inflammation as a prerequisite for the diagnosis of WG has been challenged. A less restrictive definition has been proposed (3) as *Wegener's vasculitis.* Subsumed under this less restrictive cate-

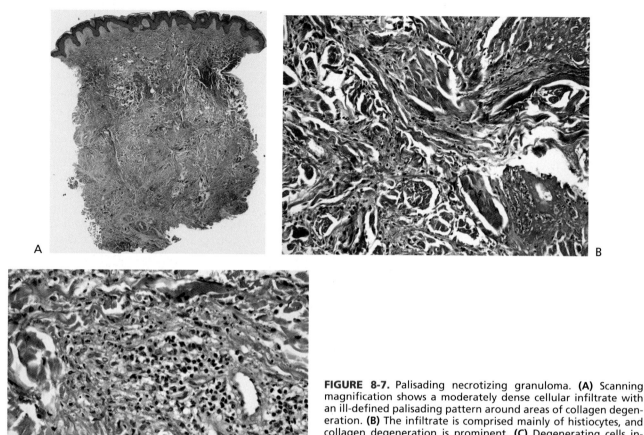

A

B

C

FIGURE 8-7. Palisading necrotizing granuloma. **(A)** Scanning magnification shows a moderately dense cellular infiltrate with an ill-defined palisading pattern around areas of collagen degeneration. **(B)** The infiltrate is comprised mainly of histiocytes, and collagen degeneration is prominent. **(C)** Degenerating cells including eosinophils are present in some foci. This lesion, formerly called "Churg–Strauss granuloma," is not diagnostic of any particular entity, and in addition to Wegener's syndrome, may also be seen in connective tissue diseases, periarteritis nodosa, lymphoproliferative disorders, subacute bacterial endocarditis, chronic active hepatitis, and inflammatory bowel disease (see text).

gory are ANCA-positive patients with clinical presentations of WG, such as sinusitis, pulmonary infiltrates, and nephritis, and documented necrotizing vasculitis, but without biopsy-proven granulomatous inflammation. Both classic WG and Wegener's vasculitis are considered different manifestations of *Wegener's syndrome*, a more generic term proposed by the Working Classification of ANCA-Associated Vasculitides (3).

Two-thirds of patients with WG are male, and the mean age range for diagnosis is 35 to 54 years. The vast majority of patients are Caucasians. Clinical presentation is extremely variable, ranging from an insidious course with a prolonged period of nonspecific constitutional symptoms and upper respiratory tract findings to abrupt onset of severe pulmonary and renal disease. The most commonly involved anatomic sites include upper respiratory tract, lower respiratory tract, and kidneys. Other organ systems that are commonly affected include joints and skin. Migratory, polyarticular arthralgia of large and small joints is found in up to 85% of patients with WG. Cutaneous involvement is

extremely variable in different series, ranging from less than 20% to more than 50% of patients. Skin involvement may manifest as in macular erythematous rash, purpura, papules, papulonecrotic lesions, and nodules with and without ulceration. Occasionally cutaneous lesions are the first manifestation of WG. However, because of their nonspecific appearance, they are infrequently recognized as presentations of WG.

The development of assays for ANCA has greatly facilitated the diagnosis of WG and the monitoring of disease activity. In a series of 182 patients with WG, sera from 15 of 16 of the patients with active disease and 3 of 9 of the patients in remission were positive for antiserine proteinase (c-ANCA) (23).

Histopathology. The majority of skin biopsies in patients with WG show nonspecific histopathology, and not all of them are directly related to the pathophysiology of WG (24). Such nonspecific reaction patterns include perivascular lymphocytic infiltrates. However, in about 25% to 50% of patients, cutaneous lesions have fairly characteristic histopathologic findings. The more frequent distinct reaction patterns include necrotizing/leukocytoclastic small-vessel vasculitis and granulomatous inflammation (24,25). Minute foci of tissue necrosis are surrounded by histiocytes and are similar to lesions described in open lung biopsies from WG patients. The palisading granulomas resembling those of CSS may occur, except that the center of the WG granuloma contains necrobiotic collagen and basophilic fibrillar necrotic debris admixed with neutrophils (Fig. 8-7). True granulomatous vasculitis appears to be rare.

Differential Diagnosis. Other conditions causing LCV and granulomatous reactions include CSS, metastatic Crohn's disease, rheumatoid arthritis, and sarcoidosis. Granulomatous vascular reactions may also be a manifestation of T-cell lymphomas, such as angiocentric T-cell lymphoma or panniculitic T-cell lymphoma. The distinction between CSS and WG relies primarily on clinical findings. In contrast to WG, CSS is associated with asthma, lacks lesions in the upper respiratory tract, rarely shows severe renal involvement, and typically is accompanied by eosinophilia or eosinophilic infiltrates and p-ANCA positivity. The distinction between MPA and WG may be difficult clinically; however, MPA should lack granulomatous inflammation.

Small-Vessel Neutrophilic/ Leukocytoclastic Vasculitis

A large number of different disease processes can be accompanied by small-vessel vasculitis with predominantly neutrophilic infiltrates. The main diseases to be considered (4,5) are listed in Table 8-5.

Histopathology of Neutrophilic Small-Vessel Vasculitis

Neutrophilic small-vessel vasculitis is a reaction pattern of small dermal vessels, almost exclusively postcapillary venules, characterized by a combination of vascular damage and an infiltrate composed largely of neutrophils (Fig. 8-8). Because there is often fragmentation of nuclei (karyorrhexis or leukocytoclasis), the term *leukocytoclastic vasculitis* (LCV) is frequently used. Depending on its severity, this process may be subtle and limited to the superficial dermis, or be pandermal and florid and associated with necrosis and ulceration. If edema is prominent, a subepidermal blister may form. If the neutrophilic infiltrate is dense and there is pustule formation, the term *pustular vasculitis* may be applied (Fig. 8-9). In a typical case of LCV, the dermal vessels show swelling of the endothelial cells and deposits of strongly eosinophilic strands of fibrin within and around their walls. The deposits of fibrin and the marked edema together give the vessel walls a "smudgy" appearance referred to as fibrinoid degeneration. Actual necrosis of the perivascular collagen, however, is seen only rarely in conjunction with ulcerative lesions. If the vascular

TABLE 8-5. DIFFERENTIAL DIAGNOSIS OF CUTANEOUS NEUTROPHILIC SMALL-VESSEL VASCULITIS, CATEGORIZED ON THE BASIS OF PROPOSED PATHOGENIC MECHANISMS

Infection
   Bacterial (gram-positive/-negative organisms, mycobacteria, spirochetes)
   Rickettsial
   Fungal
   Viral
Immunologic injury
   Immune-complex mediated
      Henoch-Schönlein purpura
      Urticarial vasculitis
      Cryoglobulinemia
      Serum sickness
      Connective tissue diseases
     Autoimmune-diseases
     Infection-induced immunologic injury (e.g., hepatitis B or C, streptococcal)
   Drug-induced
   Paraneoplastic processes
   Behçet's disease
      Erythema elevatum diutinum
   Antineutrophil antibody associated
      Wegener's granulomatosis
      Microscopic polyangiitis
      Churg-Strauss syndrome
      Some drug-induced vasculitis
   Unknown
      Polyarteritis nodosa

changes are severe, luminal occlusion of vessels may be observed. The cellular infiltrate is present predominantly around the dermal blood vessels or within the vascular walls, so that the outline of the blood vessels may appear

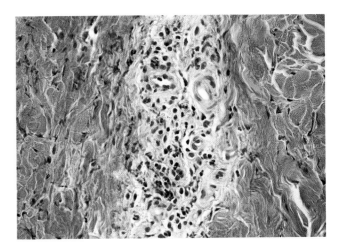

FIGURE 8-8. Hypersensitivity vasculitis showing a upper dermal small blood vessel with neutrophil-rich vasculitis and other adjacent postcapillary venules with a perivascular mononuclear cell infiltrate without features of vasculitis. The specimen was obtained from a 6-day-old purpuric macule.

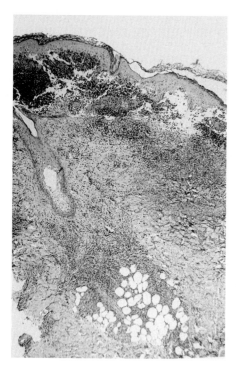

FIGURE 8-9. Pustular vasculitis. Subepidermal blister formation with many polymorphonuclear cells and vascular damage are present.

indistinct. The infiltrate consists mainly of neutrophils and of varying numbers of eosinophils and mononuclear cells. The infiltrate also is scattered throughout the upper dermis in association with fibrin deposits between and within collagen bundles. Extravasation of erythrocytes is commonly present.

As with any inflammatory process, the appearance of the reaction pattern depends on the stage at which the biopsy is taken. In older lesions, the number of neutrophils may be decreased and the number of mononuclear cells increased so that mononuclear cells may predominate and a designation of a lymphocytic or even granulomatous vasculitis or vascular reaction might be made.

Pathogenesis. Many disease processes may exhibit LCV. The major causes of vasculitis are infection and immune-mediated inflammation. Table 8-5 categorizes vasculitides on the basis of suggested pathogenetic mechanisms. Although T-cell–mediated inflammation has been implicated in large-vessel vasculitides, antibody-mediated inflammation seems to play a prominent role in small-vessel vasculitis. Its final common pathway typically involves neutrophils and monocyte activation with adherence to endothelial cells, infiltration of the vessel wall, and release of lytic enzymes and toxic radicals. This final pathway of vascular injury may be initiated by (a) the deposition of immune complexes, (b) direct binding of antibodies to antigens in vessel walls, and (c) activation of leukocytes by antibodies with specificity for leukocyte antigens

(ANCAs). It must be stressed that an immune-complex etiology has been invoked much too often to explain all forms of vasculitis and particularly small-vessel vasculitis. In many instances, immune complexes are not the primary events in vascular injury but simply epiphenomena.

Diagnostic Approach to Neutrophilic Small-Vessel Vasculitis

As already mentioned, the clinical and histologic manifestations are fairly nonspecific for a particular category of vasculitis. For example, palpable purpura may be the clinical appearance of dermal leukocytoclastic small-vessel vasculitis secondary to infection (e.g., gonococcal sepsis); immune-complex–mediated vasculitis (e.g., cryoglobulinemia or Henoch-Schönlein purpura); ANCA-associated vasculitis (e.g., WG); allergic vasculitis (e.g., reaction to a drug); vasculitis associated with connective tissue; or a paraneoplastic phenomenon. It is important therefore, to interpret the histologic findings only in the context of clinical information to reach an appropriate diagnosis. Often, additional laboratory data, such as from microbiologic cultures, special stains for organisms, or immunofluorescence or serologic studies, are needed. Because the treatment for infectious vasculitides is so radically different from the treatment for immune-mediated diseases, the most important diagnostic step in the evaluation of a vasculitis is to rule out an infectious process. If noninfectious vasculitis is suspected, evidence for systemic vasculitis must be sought. Clinical findings—such as hematuria, arthritis, myalgia, enzymatic assays for muscle or liver enzymes, and serologic analysis for ANCAs, antinuclear antibodies, cryoglobulins, hepatitis B and C antibodies, IgA-fibronectin aggregates, and complement levels—are important to further delineate the disease process. Exposure to a potential allergen, such as a drug, that might have elicited a hypersensitivity reaction should be sought. Evidence of an allergic pathogenesis is reassuring because it suggests that the vasculitic process may be self-limited and not associated with systemic vasculitis. As mentioned previously, it is also important to address the possibility that the histologic findings of vasculitis may be a secondary phenomenon, as, for example, in ulceration from localized trauma.

The following subsections discuss the main clinical settings in which LCV occurs.

Infectious Vasculitis

An infectious process needs to be ruled out early in the evaluation of an LCV (1,4). Microorganisms may invade vessels directly or damage them by an immune-mediated mechanism. *Neisseria meningitides* is a common cause of infectious cutaneous leukocytoclastic vasculitis. Meningococci may be found within endothelial cells and neutrophils at sites of vascular inflammation. However, other Gram-positive or Gram-negative bacteria and fungi also

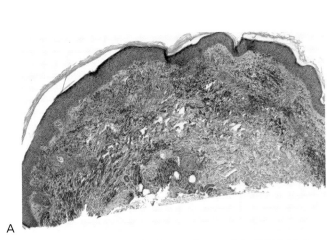
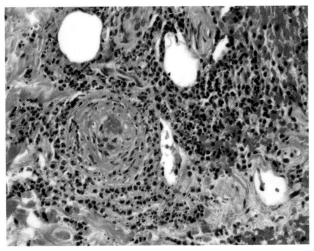

A   B

FIGURE 8-10. Septic vasculitis. **(A)** Multiple vessels are surrounded by a dense inflammatory infiltrate and/or contain eosinophilic thrombotic material. There is marked associated purpuric hemorrhage. **(B)** A small vessel contains fibrin in its lumen and shows fibrinoid change of its wall, with a prominent neutrophilic infiltrate in the wall and in the adjacent tissue. Culture was positive for Pseudomonas. Organisms are difficult to appreciate in the figure.

may cause cutaneous small-vessel vasculitis (Fig. 8-10). Staphylococcal sepsis can lead to neutrophilic vasculitis with purpura or nodular lesions, which may contain microabscesses. Rickettsial infections, such as Rocky Mountain spotted fever (RMSF), are characterized by invasion of endothelial cells by organisms causing vascular damage. Inflammation, however, is often minimal in RMSF. Direct immunofluorescence microscopy may demonstrate the organism. Clinically, the spectrum of changes ranges from small macules to papules and purpura. Acid-fast organisms can also cause vasculitis. Lucio's phenomenon (erythema necroticans) and erythema nodosum leprosum (ENL) are syndromes that may arise during the course of lepromatous leprosy. In both cases, biopsies show vascular damage, including LCV. Histologically, Lucio's phenomenon shows necrotizing small-vessel vasculitis, and Fite–Faraco staining reveals large aggregates of acid-fast bacilli within the vascular walls and endothelium and throughout the dermis. Ischemia and necrosis of the epidermis, dermis, and adnexal structures often with ulceration are seen. Some researchers have suggested that the massive endothelial mycobacterial burden in Lucio's phenomenon may directly lead to vascular damage (26).

Henoch-Schönlein Purpura

Henoch-Schönlein purpura (H-SP) is clinically characterized by palpable purpura of the buttocks and lower extremities, abdominal pain, and hematuria (27). It typically affects children following streptococcal upper respiratory tract infections, and is usually self-limited with a resolution expected 6 to 16 weeks after the onset of symptomatology.

Complications generally arise from renal involvement that may even necessitate kidney transplantation. IgA myeloma has also resulted in HSP-like manifestations (28).

Histology. Henoch-Schönlein purpura cannot be distinguished histologically from other forms of LCV, although the degree of vascular damage is often not as great as that usually observed in typical LCV. Immunofluorescence studies typically demonstrate the deposition of IgA in capillaries (Fig. 8-11). Such a limited extent of vascular damage is also commonly observed in urticarial vasculitis (see text below), and clinical findings may be necessary for distinction of H-SP from urticarial vasculitis. IgA-associated vasculitis may occur outside of the symptom complex of HSP (29). However, serologic detection of IgA-fibronectin aggregates may be associated with greater likelihood of renal or systemic disease in patients with cutaneous LCV (30).

Urticarial Vasculitis

Persistent wheals (lasting >24 hours by convention) with faint purpura are a typical clinical finding of urticarial vasculitis. Often residual purpura are seen after resolution of the urticarial lesions (31). Urticarial vasculitis is not a specific disease but rather a manifestation of a vasculitis that is associated with increased vascular permeability. The course of urticarial vasculitis is generally benign and episodic, lasting several months. However, urticarial vasculitis sometimes occurs in lupus erythematosus and may be the initial clinical manifestation of that disease. Approximately one-third of all patients with vasculitic urticaria have decreased complement levels (hypocomplementemic vasculitis) (Fig. 8-12). They may have systemic findings, such as arthralgias

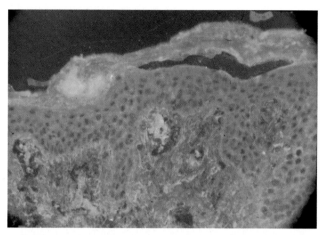

FIGURE 8-11. Direct immunofluorescence showing granular IgA deposits in very superficial dermal vessels. This immunofluorescence finding is diagnostic for IgA vasculitis (Henoch Schönlein purpura). Other immunoreactants were negative or significantly weaker.

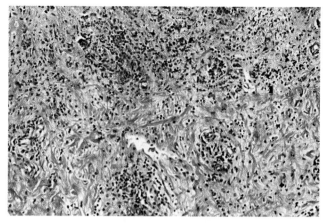

FIGURE 8-13. Neutrophil-rich small vessel vasculitis of upper and mid-dermal vessels associated with interstitial spillage of neutrophils from a patient with hypocomplementemic urticarial vasculitis.

and adenopathy and may be more likely to have underlying systemic lupus erythematosus (32).

Histopathology. The histology of urticarial vasculitis ranges from mild to fully developed LCV (Fig. 8-13).

Cryoglobulinemias and Other Small-Vessel Vasculitides Associated with Paraproteins

Small-vessel vasculitis may be associated with paraproteins—that is, abnormal serum proteins (1,33). Such paraproteins include cryoglobulins, cryofibrinogens, macroglobulins, and gamma-heavy chains. Cryoglobulins are serum immunoglobulins that precipitate when the serum is cooled and redissolve upon rewarming. There are three major types of cryoglobulinemia. In type I cryoglobulinemia, monoclonal IgG or IgM cryoglobulins are found, often associated with lymphoma, leukemia, Waldenström's macroglobulinemia, or multiple myeloma, or without known underlying disease. In type II cryoglobulinemia, the cryoprecipitate consists of both monoclonal and polyclonal cryoglobulins, with one cryoglobulin acting as an antibody against the other. These cryoglobulins are circulating immune complexes. The most common combination is IgG-IgM (Fig. 8-14). In type III cryoglobulinemia, the immunoglobulins are polyclonal. Type II and III or mixed cryoglobulinemias are frequently associated with connective tissue disorders, such as lupus erythematosus, rheumatoid arthritis, and Sjögren's syndrome, or may be related to

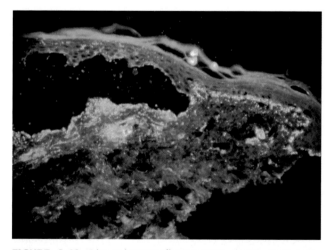

FIGURE 8-12. Direct immunofluorescence showing granular IgG deposits in superficial dermal vessels and along the basement membrane zone. This combined vasculitic and with lupus type immunofluorescence finding is characteristic of hypocomplementemic urticarial vasculitis.

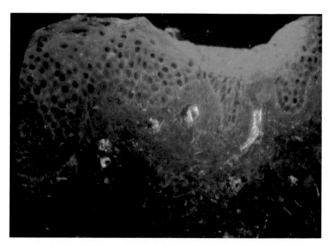

FIGURE 8-14. Direct immunofluorescence showing dense granular IgM deposits in superficial small vessels in a patient with cryoglobulinemia type 2. This specimen also showed concomitant dense granular C3 in same blood vessels.

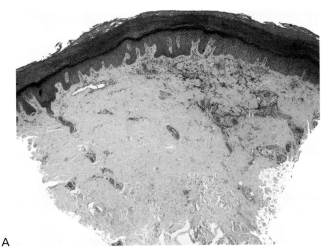
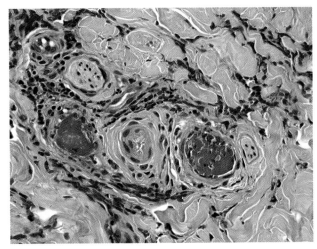

FIGURE 8-15. (A) Cryoglobulinemia. Vessels in the reticular dermis contain brightly eosinophilic material. **(B)** The deposition is associated with little or no damage to the vessel walls in this case.

infection—in particular, hepatitis C infection. Idiopathic forms of type II and III cryoglobulinemias are also termed essential mixed cryoglobulinemia.

Clinically, cutaneous lesions in patients with cryoglobulinemia may manifest as chronic palpable purpura, urticaria-like lesions, livedo reticularis, acrocyanosis, digital gangrene, and leg ulcers. Raynaud's phenomenon is common. Systemic manifestations may include arthralgia, hepatosplenomegaly, lymphadenopathy, and glomerulonephritis.

Histopathology. In type I cryoglobulinemia, amorphous material (precipitated cryoglobulins) is deposited subjacent to endothelium and throughout the vessel wall as well as within the vessel lumen, resulting in a thrombus-like appearance (Fig. 8-15). These precipitates stain pink with hematoxylin and eosin and bright red with PAS stain, as opposed to less intense staining of fibrinoid material. Some capillaries are filled with red blood cells, and extensive extravasation of erythrocytes may be present. An inflammatory infiltrate is usually lacking in contrast to mixed cryoglobulinemia, which typically shows an LCV (Fig. 8-16). PAS-positive intramural and intravascular cryoprecipitates may be found also in mixed cryoglobulinemia, although less frequently than in type I cryoglobulinemia.

Other small-vessel vasculitides with the histologic pattern of an LCV may be found in association with Waldenström's hyperglobulinemia (hyperglobulinemic purpura), and in Schnitzler's syndrome, which manifests as chronic urticaria with macroglobulinemia (usually monoclonal IgM) and other paraproteinemias.

Serum Sickness

This syndrome of a morbilliform urticarial eruption, fever, and lymphadenopathy occurs 7 to 10 days after a primary antigen exposure, or 2 to 4 days after a repeat exposure. The antigen may be a drug, from an arthropod sting or from a previous infection, or therapeutic serum globulins (34). Serum sickness is usually a self-limited condition. The LCV of serum sickness has no distinctive histologic features.

Connective Tissue Disease

Rheumatoid arthritis, lupus erythematosus, and other diseases in the spectrum of connective tissue disease may develop LCV (35). Clinical and serologic information is critical to the correct interpretation of the cutaneous findings in these clinical settings.

Autoimmune Diseases

Primary Sjögren's syndrome is not associated with connective tissue disease, but may present with purpura in addi-

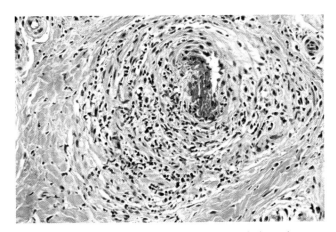

FIGURE 8-16. Cryoglobulinemia. A small mid dermal artery showing neutrophil rich vasculitis secondary to hepatitis C associated cryoglobulinemia type 2.

tion to ocular and glandular involvement (1). The histologic reaction pattern is often an LCV.

ANCA-Associated Vasculitis

The pauci-immune vasculitides associated with ANCA are discussed in more detail above. MPA, WG, and CSS may all be associated with cutaneous LCV.

Drug-Induced Vasculitis

A hypersensitivity reaction to a drug may result in an LCV (1,4). Penicillin, thiazides, and sulfonamides are the most common drugs used to induce LCV. Drugs also may induce the pattern of pustular vasculitis.

Paraneoplastic Vasculitis

A wide spectrum of vasculitic processes has been associated with neoplastic disorders (36). The most common associations include polyarteritis nodosa with hairy cell leukemia and cutaneous small-vessel vasculitis with lymphoproliferative disorders and some carcinomas.

Behçet's Disease

Behçet's disease is a multisystem disease characterized by oral aphthous lesions and at least two of the following criteria: genital aphthae, synovitis, posterior uveitis, cutaneous pustular vasculitis, and meningoencephalitis (37). This HLA-B51 associated disease is common in the Middle East and Japan, but rare in Northern Europe and the United States. The clinical presentation is extremely variable, and so is the vascular involvement, which can range from active inflammatory lesions to aneurysms, arterial or venous occlusions or varices.

Histopathology. The histopathologic spectrum of mucocutaneous inflammatory vascular lesions includes, depending on the stage and activity of the lesion, neutrophilic, lymphocytic, and granulomatous vascular reactions. Biopsy specimens of early lesions typically show a neutrophilic vascular reaction and Behçet's disease is sometimes classified as a neutrophilic dermatosis/neutrophilic vascular reaction. However, fully developed necrotizing leukocytoclastic vasculitis may develop. If the neutrophilic infiltrate is very dense, the pattern of pustular vasculitis may be found (Fig. 8-9).

Pathogenesis. The etiology of Behçet's disease remains unknown. The vascular injury is presumably immune mediated, because immune-complex deposition has been demonstrated in vessel walls (37). Disorders of neutrophils are also being discussed with regard to the etiology of this disease (37). However, the occurrence of cutaneous vasculitis as well as the vascular injury seen in other organ systems suggest that Behçet's disease is best classified as a systemic vasculitis (38).

Localized Fibrosing Small-Vessel Vasculitis

Erythema elevatum diutinum (EED) and granuloma faciale (GF) are very similar chronic fibrosing conditions that show evidence of vascular damage. Sometimes, one or both may be classified with the neutrophilic dermatoses. Both entities are hypothesized to be reactions to localized persistent immune complex deposition or hypersensitivities to a persistent antigen. EED- and GF-like reactions may occasionally be seen in clinical settings atypical for either entity (39).

Erythema Elevatum Diutinum

This rare condition is characterized by persistent, initially red to violaceous and later brown to yellow papules, nodules, and plaques (40). The lesions, typically distributed symmetrically on the extensor surfaces of the extremities, are initially soft and then evolve into fibrous nodules.

Histopathologic Features. In the early stage of erythema elevatum diutinum (EED), nonspecific LCV is observed. In later stages, granulation tissue and fibrosis form with a diffuse mixed-cell infiltrate showing a predominance of neutrophils. The capillaries may still show deposits of fibrinoid material or merely fibrous thickening. Fully developed lesions of EED may be indistinguishable from neutrophilic dermatoses discussed below, Behçet's disease or neutrophilic drug reaction. Granuloma faciale may also resemble EED but is distinguished by clinical localization to the face, sparing of the superficial papillary dermis (a "grenz zone"), and prominence of eosinophils and plasma cells in addition to neutrophils. Occasional cases show neutrophilic microabscesses in the tips of dermal papillae that might suggest dermatitis herpetiformis (41). In old, fibrotic lesions of EED, an orderly array of spindle cells and collagen bundles are often parallel to the skin surface with vertically arranged capillaries similar to a scar (Fig. 8-12). Lipid material also may be present as cholesterol clefts. Serial sections may be required to demonstrate vascular damage in late lesions. These older lesions of EED must be differentiated from Kaposi's sarcoma, dermatofibroma, or granuloma annulare. Neutrophils, nuclear dust, and fibrin owing to persistent vascular damage may be present, helping to distinguish these lesions from dermatofibromas or scars. The irregularly arranged, jagged vascular spaces of Kaposi's sarcoma are absent and many of the spindle cells have the immunohistochemical and electron microscopic features of macrophages. Focal areas of basophilic collagen caused by nuclear dust in EED can resemble the mucin seen in granuloma annulare, but do not stain with Alcian blue.

Pathogenesis. EED probably is not a distinct disease entity, but rather a clinicopathologic reaction pattern, most often developing in with either a monoclonal or polyclonal gammopathy, in particular IgA hyperglobulinemia. Inflammatory bowel disease, rheumatoid arthritis, and systemic lupus erythematosus may also be associated with EED. HIV-infected patients also develop EED, which can clinically mimic Kaposi's sarcoma (42).

Granuloma Faciale

Clinically granuloma faciale (GF) presents as one or several asymptomatic, soft, brown-red, slowly enlarging papules or plaques, almost always on the face of older individuals. Rare upper respiratory tract forms have been described (43).

Histopathologic Features. A dense polymorphous infiltrate is present mainly in the upper half of the dermis, but may extend into the lower dermis and occasionally even into the subcutaneous tissue. Quite characteristically, the infiltrate does not invade the epidermis or the pilosebaceous appendages, *but* is separated from them by a narrow "grenz" zone of normal collagen (Fig. 8-17). The pilosebaceous structures tend to remain intact. The polymorphous infiltrate consists primarily of neutrophils and eosinophils, but mononuclear cells, plasma cells, and mast cells also are present. Vascular damage in GF is seen but often is limited, and thus perhaps GF is best termed a neutrophilic vascular reaction (44). Frequently, the nuclei of some of the neutrophils are fragmented, especially in the vicinity of the capillaries, thus forming nuclear dust. Often, there is some evidence of vasculitis with deposition of fibrinoid material within and around vessel walls. Occasionally, some hemorrhage is noted. Foam cells and fibrosis frequently are observed in older lesions.

Differential Diagnosis. Granuloma faciale can appear similar to erythema elevatum diutinum, although a grenz zone and prevalence of eosinophils and plasma cells favors granuloma faciale. Other neutrophilic dermatoses can be distinguished from granuloma faciale by the lack of a grenz zone and clinical features. Frank leukocytoclastic vasculitis should not be seen in granuloma faciale. In acneiform lesions and folliculitises, pilosebaceous units are invaded by inflammatory cells and may be destroyed or disrupted.

Pathogenesis. Vascular damage may be important to the pathogenesis of this lesion as direct immunofluorescence data suggest an immune complex–mediated event with deposition of mainly IgG in and around vessels.

Neutrophilic Dermatoses

The histopathologist occasionally encounters lesions consisting of a neutrophilic infiltrate, sometimes even with leukocytoclasis, and some degree of vascular damage (37). However, the extent of vascular damage is insufficient for necrotizing vasculitis—that is, fibrinoid necrosis is lacking. Occasionally such a histologic picture may be seen in an early lesion of vasculitis. However, several clinical conditions characterized by neutrophilic infiltrates rarely develop necrotizing vasculitis and need to be distinguished from vasculitis. These entities are categorized as neutrophilic dermatoses, and are characterized by (a) a neutrophilic infiltrate histologically, (b) a lack of microorganisms on special stains and cultures, and (c) clinical improvement on systemic steroid treatment (45). Vascular damage has been observed in these conditions, but it remains unclear whether the vascular injury plays an etiologic role or is merely an epiphenomenon. A relationship between these entities may be indicated by their

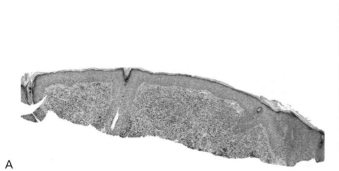
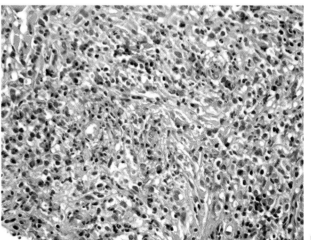

A   B

FIGURE 8-17. Granuloma faciale. **(A)** Cellular infiltrate in the dermis, separated from the epidermis by an uninvolved or "grenz" zone. **(B)** The infiltrate is contains numerous neutrophils and eosinophils. Vascular damage is minimal.

occasion co-occurrence in patients with predisposing conditions.

Acute Febrile Neutrophilic Dermatosis (Classic Sweet's Syndrome and Sweet's-Like Neutrophilic Dermatosis)

R.D. Sweet in 1964 described a disease process that he termed "acute febrile neutrophilic dermatosis," which was characterized by abrupt onset of fever, leukocytosis, and erythematous plaques infiltrated by neutrophils (45,46). This condition typically occurs in middle-aged women after nonspecific infections of the respiratory or gastrointestinal tract. The lesions tend to be found on the face or extremities and only rarely involve the trunk and respond to steroid treatment. Despite the numerous neutrophils, the lesions are sterile. Vesicles and pustules may also arise. Involvement of noncutaneous sites, such as eyes, joints, oral mucosa, and visceral sites (lungs, liver, kidneys) has been reported (46). Various disorders have been associated with neutrophilic dermatoses similar to those seen in Sweet's syndrome (Sweet's-like neutrophilic dermatosis). About 20% of cases are associated with malignancy. Cutaneous eruptions with inflammatory vascular reactions, which on occasion simulate the lesions of Sweet's syndrome, may also occur in association with hereditary periodic fever, which comprises several syndromes including familial Mediterranean fever, hyper-IgD syndrome, and tumor-necrosis-factor (TNF), receptor-associated periodic syndrome (47).

Histopathology. Typically, a dense perivascular infiltrate composed largely of neutrophils is seen assuming a band-like distribution throughout the papillary dermis (Fig. 8-18). Some of the neutrophils may show nuclear fragmentation (leukocytoclasis). In addition, the infiltrate may contain scattered lymphocytes and histiocytes and occasional eosinophils. The density of the infiltrate varies and may be limited in a small proportion of cases. Vasodilation and swelling of endothelium with moderate erythrocyte extravasation, as well as prominent edema of the upper dermis, are characteristic. In some instances, subepidermal blister formation may result. Extensive vascular damage is not a feature of Sweet's syndrome. The histologic appearance varies depending on the stage of the process. In later stages, lymphocytes and histiocytes may predominate. Sweet's-like neutrophilic dermatoses often show a similar histologic picture. However, the reaction pattern may on occasion be quite different for instance manifesting as deep subcutaneous localized suppurative panniculitis. The infiltrate of Sweet's syndrome is not characteristic enough to exclude infection on histologic findings alone. As always, to arrive at the correct interpretation of a neutrophilic infiltrate, cultures need to be obtained and special stains need to be performed to exclude an infectious etiology.

Pathogenesis. The etiology of Sweet's syndrome is unknown but is thought to be a hypersensitivity reaction. The three major concepts that have been discussed are immune-complex vasculitis, altered T-cell activation, and altered function of neutrophils. All lack, however, sufficient experimental support. The vascular alterations seen in Sweet's may be secondary to the massive extravasation of activated neutrophils. Direct immunofluorescence studies are generally negative in Sweet's syndrome (45).

Bowel-Associated Dermatosis-Arthritis Syndrome

This syndrome was initially described in patients after jejunoileal bypass surgery. Subsequently, however, the spectrum of the syndrome has expanded to include other dis-

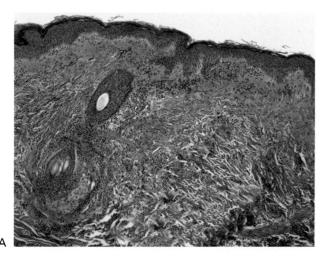
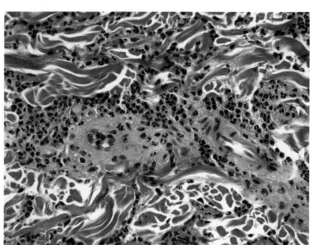

A   B

FIGURE 8-18. Sweet's syndrome. **(A)** There is a dense infiltrate in the upper dermis, consisting mainly of neutrophils, without leukocytoclasia. **(B)** Vascular damage is slight.

ease processes with typical cutaneous findings and associated bowel disease (1). Patients may have inflammatory bowel disease or a blind loop after peptic ulcer surgery. The cutaneous lesions are characterized by initial small macules that develop through a papular phase into pustules on a purpuric base. The evolution usually occurs within a 2-day period. The lesions typically reach a size of 0.5 to 1.5 cm. They are typically distributed on the upper part of the body, especially the arms, rather than on the dependent sites of the legs. Cutaneous lesions often occur in crops and are episodical (1 to 2 weeks), with a tendency to recur within months. Fever, myalgias, and arthralgias may accompany the disease process.

Histopathology. The histopathologic changes are usually those of neutrophilic vascular reactions with little or none of the vascular damage observed in Sweet's syndrome and other neutrophilic dermatoses. However, frank necrotizing small-vessel vasculitis may occasionally be noted. In fully developed lesions, the neutrophilic infiltrate and papillary dermal edema may be florid, and subepidermal pustule formation is seen. If vascular damage is observed in such a context, the term "pustular vasculitis" is applied.

Pathogenesis. One suggested etiology involves antigens derived from intestinal bacteria triggering an immune-complex–mediated reaction with vascular insults (48).

Pyoderma Gangrenosum

Pyoderma gangrenosum (PG) is included in this chapter as well as in Chapter 16, because in these and other authors' opinions, it represents a clinicopathologic manifestation that falls within the spectrum of neutrophilic dermatoses (1). As with other neutrophilic dermatoses, infection must be excluded in order to arrive at the correct diagnosis.

Several clinical types have been described: ulcerative PG, with an undermined border; pustular PG with discrete, painful pustules; painful bullae with progression to a superficial ulceration; vegetative PG with a painless ulcer, a nonundermined exophytic border (49). Classically, lesions begin as tender papulopustules or folliculitis that eventually may ulcerate. In the fully developed stage, the lesions have a distinctive raised, undermined border with a dusky purple hue. Again, as with neutrophilic dermatoses in general, pyoderma gangrenosum may occur as an isolated cutaneous phenomenon or may be a cutaneous manifestation associated with various systemic disease processes, such as inflammatory bowel disease, connective tissue diseases, and lymphoproliferative lesions.

Histopathology. The histologic findings are nonspecific and the diagnosis is primarily clinical. Most authors studying early lesions have reported a primarily neutrophilic infiltrate, which frequently involves follicular structures (50). Others, however, have stated that the lesions begin with a lymphocytic reaction (51). Degrees of vessel involvement range from none to fibrinoid necrosis. In the majority of biopsied lesions,

a neutrophilic infiltrate is present with some, but limited, vascular damage. Outright vasculitis has been reported and has led to speculations about its possible role in the etiology of PG. Focal vasculitis is often observed in fully developed lesions, but appears secondary to the inflammatory process. The infiltrate tends to be deeper and more extensive than that in classic Sweet's syndrome. The pattern of pustular vasculitis may be present. Fully developed lesions exhibit ulceration, necrosis, and a mixed inflammatory cell infiltrate (Fig. 8-19). Involvement of the deep reticular dermis and subcutis may exhibit primarily mononuclear cell and granulomatous inflammatory reactions.

Lymphocytic Small-Vessel Vasculitis

A histologic diagnosis of a lymphocytic vasculitis may be made if there is sufficient evidence of vascular damage and the inflammatory infiltrate is predominantly lymphocytic (Fig. 8-20). Often, the vascular damage is subtle and in many cases there may be disagreement among dermatopathologists on whether or not the term "vasculitis" is warranted (52). Clear-cut evidence of vasculitis is indisputable if an inflammatory infiltrate is present together with fibrinoid necrosis of the vascular wall. However, these findings are rarely or only focally present in the majority of conditions that have been said to manifest lymphocytic vasculitis.

The disease processes in which lymphocytic vasculitis is commonly observed are listed in Table 8-6. Lymphocytic vasculitis may also be seen in a stage of an otherwise leukocytoclastic or granulomatous vasculitis or in a process that at other times may even be noninflammatory and manifested perhaps as a vasculopathy (e.g., atrophie blanche).

Lymphomatoid Vasculitis and Vascular Reactions

The terms "lymphomatoid vasculitis" and "lymphomatoid vascular reaction" may be used if there is a lymphocytic vasculitis or lymphocytic vascular reaction with significant cytologic atypia of the lymphoid cells (Table 8-7). Although lymphoid nuclear irregularities of some degree may be present in many lymphocytic vascular reactions, probably as a reflection of an activated state of the lymphocytes, lymphoid atypia tends to be particularly well developed in lymphomatoid and some viral processes. The differential diagnosis includes, then, vascular damage in the context of cutaneous lymphoma, such as angiocentric T-cell lymphoma and other lymphomas (53).

Pigmented Purpuric Dermatitis

Historically, four variants of purpura pigmentosa chronica have been described: purpura annularis telangiectodes of Majocchi, progressive pigmentary dermatosis of Schamberg, pigmented purpuric dermatitis of Gougerot and

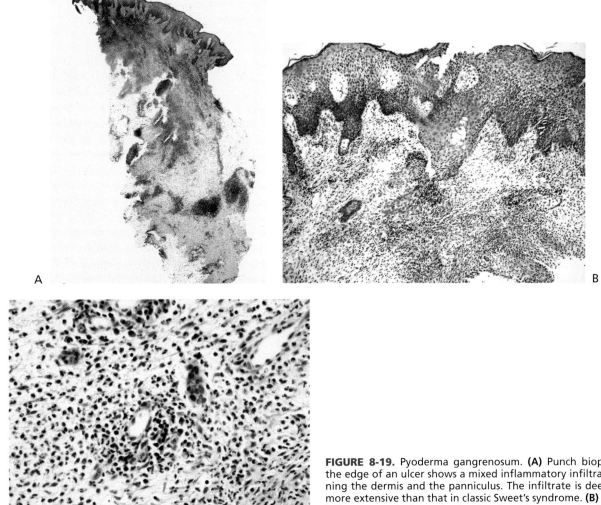

A

B

C

FIGURE 8-19. Pyoderma gangrenosum. **(A)** Punch biopsy from the edge of an ulcer shows a mixed inflammatory infiltrate spanning the dermis and the panniculus. The infiltrate is deeper and more extensive than that in classic Sweet's syndrome. **(B)** A mixed inflammatory infiltrate in the dermis with spongiosis of the epidermis at the edge of the ulcer. **(C)** Neutrophils and lymphocytes surround a vessel, but there is no frank vasculitis.

Blum, and eczematoid-like purpura of Doucas and Kapentanakis. These entities are all closely related and often cannot be reliably distinguished on clinical and histologic grounds (54). In practice, subclassification may not be necessary. Lichen aureus is a closely related localized variant. The general terms *pigmented purpuric dermatitis*, *chronic purpuric dermatitis*, and *purpura pigmentosa chronica* appear suitable for this disease spectrum.

Clinically, the primary lesion consists of discrete puncta. Gradually, telangiectatic puncta may appear as a result of capillary dilatation, with pigmentation as a result of hemosiderin deposits. In some cases, telangiectasia (Majocchi's disease) predominates; in others, pigmentation (Schamberg's disease) predominates. In Majocchi's disease, the lesions are usually irregular in shape and occur predominantly on the lower legs. In some cases, the findings may mimic those of stasis. Not infrequently, clinical signs of in-

flammation are present, such as erythema, papules, and scaling (Gougerot–Blum disease), or papules, scaling, and lichenification (eczematoid-like purpura). The disorder is often limited to the lower extremities, but it may be extensive. Mild pruritus may be present. These are no systemic symptoms related to this disease process. A localized variant of PPD is lichen aureus, in which one or a few patches are present, most commonly on the legs (55). The patches are composed of closely set, flat papules of a rust, copper, or orange color. In some cases, petechiae are present within the patches. Lichen aureus shows a male predilection and a peak incidence in the fourth decade. The lesions of lichen aureus tend to persist. They typically occur on the lower legs, but may affect many other sites.

Histopathology. The basic process is a lymphocytic perivascular infiltrate limited to the papillary dermis (Fig. 8-21). Epidermal alterations may include slight acanthosis

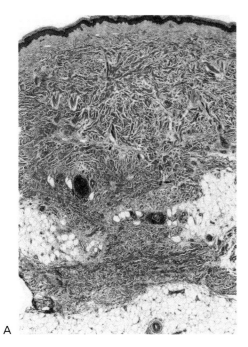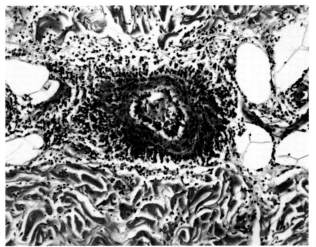

A   B

FIGURE 8-20. Lymphocytic vasculitis. **(A)** A small vessel in the reticular dermis is surrounded by an inflammatory infiltrate. **(B)** The infiltrate is comprised of lymphocytes. There is damage to the vessel wall.

and basal layer vacuolopathy. There is also some variability in the pattern of the dermal infiltrate. In some instances, the infiltrate may assume a band-like or lichenoid pattern, particularly in the lichenoid variant of Gougerot–Blum disease, and may involve the reticular dermis in a perivascular distribution. Evidence of vascular damage may be present, and the reaction pattern may then be termed lymphocytic vasculopathy, vasculitis, or capillaritis. However, the extent of vascular injury is usually mild and often insufficient to justify the term "vasculitis." Vascular damage commonly consists only of endothelial cell swelling and dermal hemorrhage. Extravasated red blood cells and sub-

tle deposits of hemosiderin are usually found in the vicinity of the capillaries. However, less commonly fibrinoid material is deposited in vessel walls. In some instances, the infiltrate involves the epidermis and may be associated with mild spongiosis and patchy parakeratosis, particularly in some cases of pigmented purpuric lichenoid dermatitis of Gougerot and Blum and eczematoid-like purpura of Doucas and Kapetanakis. The pattern of the infiltrate often is both perivascular and interstitial, infiltrating the papillary dermis between vessels.

In old lesions, the capillaries often show dilatation of their lumen and proliferation of their endothelium. Ex-

---

TABLE 8-6. DIFFERENTIAL DIAGNOSIS OF LYMPHOCYTIC VASCULITIS AND LYMPHOCYTIC VASCULAR REACTIONS

Arthropod bites
Drug-induced and other hypersensitivity reactions
Infection-associated reactions (e.g., viral)
Connective tissue diseases
Behçet's disease
Purpuric dermatitides
PLEVA/PLC/LYP
Cutaneous lymphoma
Autoimmune diseases
Pernio
Polymorphous light eruption
Atrophie blanche
Infestations (e.g., scabies)

TABLE 8-7. DIFFERENTIAL DIAGNOSIS OF LYMPHOMATOID VASCULITIS AND VASCULAR REACTION

T-cell lymphoproliferative disorders
Peripheral T-cell lymphoma
Angiocentric T-cell lymphoma
Lymphomatoid papulosis
Lymphomatoid granulomatosis
Angioimmunoblastic lymphadenopathy
Pigmented purpuric dermatitis-like eruptions
Lymphomatoid drug eruptions
Lymphomatoid contact dermatitis
Connective tissue disease
Viral processes
Florid hypersensitivity reactions
   Arthropod bites
   Scabies infestations

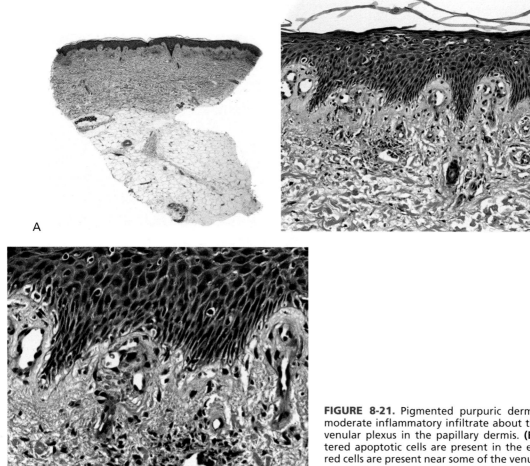

A

B

C

FIGURE 8-21. Pigmented purpuric dermatosis. **(A)** There is a moderate inflammatory infiltrate about the superficial capillary-venular plexus in the papillary dermis. **(B)** Spongiosis and scattered apoptotic cells are present in the epidermis. Extravasated red cells are present near some of the venules. **(C)** The vessel walls are thickened, without vasculitis. Hemosiderin pigment is not prominent in this example.

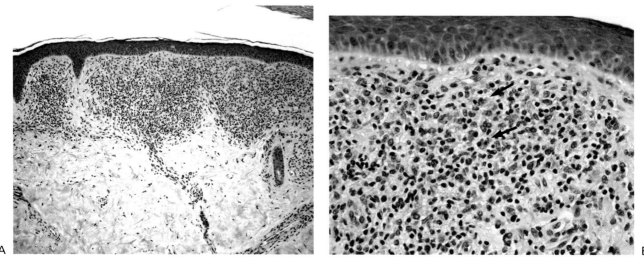

A

B

FIGURE 8-22. Lichen aureus. A dense lichenoid infiltrate in the papillary dermis **(A)**, with hemo-siderin-laden macrophages **(B)** (*arrows*), accounting for the golden clinical color of these lesions.

travasated red blood cells may no longer be present, but one frequently finds hemosiderin, although in varying amounts. The inflammatory infiltrate is less pronounced than in the early stage.

In lichen aureus, a dense lymphohistiocytic infiltrate is present in the superficial dermis, typically distributed in a band-like fashion and often associated with an increase in dermal capillaries. Exocytosis of mononuclear cells into the epidermis may be seen. Scattered within the infiltrate are hemosiderin-laden macrophages (Fig. 8-22). The absence or near absence of Civatte bodies or basal layer vasculopathy facilitates the differential diagnosis from lichenoid dermatitides, such as lichen planus or lichen striatus.

Differential Diagnosis. PPD may resemble stasis dermatitis because inflammation, dilatation of capillaries, extravasation of erythrocytes, and deposits of hemosiderin occur in both. However, in stasis dermatitis, the process extends much deeper into the dermis, and more pronounced epidermal changes and fibrosis of the dermis are usually present. Changes of intravascular red blood cell sludge and some fibrin deposits also may be seen in stasis, indicating a low flow state. As mentioned earlier, the histologic pattern of PPD may resemble or possibly be an abnormal T-cell process. Careful evaluation of the lesion for epidermotropism and lymphoid atypia, and (of particular importance) good clinicopathologic correlation, are needed to arrive at the correct diagnosis. However, suspicious or equivocal lesions require monitoring and possibly further evaluation for possible progression to cutaneous T-cell lymphoma.

Pathogenesis. The etiology of PPD is essentially unknown, and there are probably several different factors involved. Some cases of chronic purpuric dermatitis may be related to a hypersensitivity reaction to drugs. However, in the majority of cases, the etiology of this process is unclear. Stasis changes are seen in some individuals with PPD, suggesting venous insufficiency may be a contributing factor (51). Eruptions with the clinical and histologic appearance of a pigmented purpuric dermatitis have also been associated with subsequent development of a T-cell lymphoproliferative disorder in some patients. Thus, it is possible that some PPD may be the initial manifestation of T-cell lymphoproliferative disease (55,56).

VASCULOPATHIC REACTIONS

A vasculopathic reaction as defined in Table 8-1 refers to the histologic finding of vascular damage in the absence of vasculitis. Vasculopathic reactions may be associated with (a) coagulopathies, (b) metabolic disorders leading to alterations of the vessel wall, (c) structural deficiencies of the perivascular connective tissue, or (d) miscellaneous other disease processes.

Coagulopathies

Any coagulopathy may be accompanied by vasculopathic changes. The extent of vascular damage is variable. Vascular damage may occur in the setting of altered platelet counts, such as in idiopathic thrombocytopenic purpura, in coagulation factor deficiencies (e.g., inherited or acquired protein C and S deficiencies), coagulopathies associated with connective tissue disease (e.g., lupus anticoagulant, antiphospholipid antibody syndrome) (Fig. 8-23),

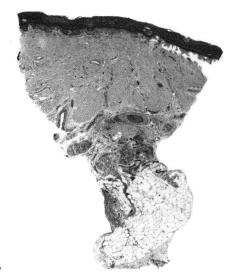

A

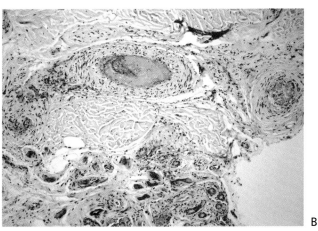

B

FIGURE 8-23. Antiphospholipid syndrome. **(A)** A vessel in the deep dermis contains an eosinophilic fibrin thrombus. The affected vessels are commonly more superficial in this condition. **(B)** The thrombus is not associated with inflammation of the vessel wall. Other small vessels in the vicinity are also affected.

and platelet thrombosis in heparin necrosis. Extensive vascular damage with luminal occlusion by thrombotic material may develop in coumarin necrosis, in thrombotic thrombocytopenic purpura, and in disseminated intravascular coagulation—specifically in the setting of purpura fulminans (57).

In mild forms, clinical manifestations may be subtle and limited to petechiae. In severe forms of coagulopathies, large areas of ecchymosis may be present, typically located on the extremities. Large hemorrhagic bullae may overlie the ecchymoses, and some of the ecchymotic areas may undergo necrosis.

Histopathology. The histologic features are nonspecific for any particular disorder. In mild forms of coagulopathies, the only histologic manifestation may be dermal hemorrhage—that is, extravasation of red blood cells into perivascular connective tissue. With increasing severity of the disease process, intravascular fibrin thrombi may be found (Fig. 8-2). In severe forms (e.g., thrombotic thrombocytopenic purpura, coumarin necrosis, and purpura fulminans), thrombotic vascular occlusion may lead to hemorrhagic infarcts, epidermal and dermal necrosis, or subepidermal bulla formation. In severe systemic intravascular coagulation, internal organs may also show widespread thrombosis of small vessels and hemorrhagic necrosis.

Calciphylaxis

Calciphylaxis is an uncommon complication of renal failure usually in combination with secondary or tertiary hyperparathyroidism. Obesity, female gender, and poor nutritional status are some putative risk factors. Painful violaceous lesions that may be indurated often develop in areas of livedo reticularis on the trunk and extremities, and can rapidly progress to form bullae, ulcers, eschars, and gangrene. The prognosis is extremely poor, especially for proximal disease, even with aggressive treatment by parathyroidectomy (58). Fulminant sepsis may develop from infection of necrotic or gangrenous tissue.

Histopathologic Features. The principal histologic findings include (a) calcification of soft tissue and small vessels; (b) nonspecific intimal proliferation of small vessels, often resulting in luminal narrowing; (c) variable fibrin thrombi; and (d) frequent ischemic necrosis of skin and subcutis (Fig. 8-24). The small vessels involved by this process cannot be identified as either arterial or venous. Foreign body–giant cell reaction to calcium and mixed inflammatory cell infiltrates that are neutrophil rich may be seen.

Cutaneous calcium deposits may be seen in a number of other conditions, especially cutaneous calcinosis and metastatic calcifications. Calcinosis usually lacks prominent vascular involvement. Other crystal-induced inflammatory diseases such as gout, pseudogout, or oxalosis that are associated with a giant cell reaction to crystal deposits

and surrounding fibrosis may resemble calciphylaxis (58). Histopathologically, pancreatic panniculitis may suggest calciphylaxis. However, the polymorphous infiltrate and ghost-like cells seen in panniculitis are absent in calciphylaxis (59). If a biopsy of calciphylaxis lacks significant calcium deposits due to sampling error, the findings may be limited to ischemic damage or mimic a coagulopathy.

Pathogenesis. The relationships between the calcification, thrombosis, and ischemic necrosis in calciphylaxis are unclear. Although vascular calcification is common in uremic patients, calciphylaxis is rare. Elevation of the calcium and phosphorous product along with a poorly defined precipitating or challenging event or agent are hypothesized to be necessary for calcium deposition in cutaneous tissues. However, the list of putative sensitizing agents is long and the calcium and phosphorus product may be within normal limits. The development of a hypercoagulable state may be an additional important element in the pathogenesis of this entity but is not present in all cases (60).

Metabolic Vasculopathies

Vasculopathies may arise also from metabolic disorders. Deposition of endogenously produced material, as in diabetes mellitus, amyloidosis, or porphyria, may lead to vessel fragility. Hemorrhage and ischemic damage to the area of skin supplied by the affected vessels are seen. The basic histologic vascular alteration in the above-mentioned disorders is the deposition of amorphous material in the walls of dermal capillaries. The details of the histopathology of these disorders are discussed in more detail in other chapters of this book.

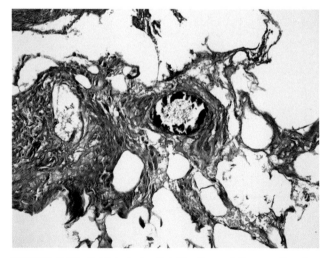

FIGURE 8-24. Calciphylaxis. Calcification of the media of a small vessel in the panniculus, with delicate fibroplasia of the intima. There may be interstitial deposition of calcium as well.

Atherosclerosis is by far the most common form of vasculopathy. However, atherosclerosis is primarily a disease of large vessels supplying visceral organs, and thus not discussed here in detail. Cutaneous changes are usually rare and are secondary manifestations of peripheral ischemia. Luminal occlusion may result from intimal thickening and lipid deposition, superimposed thrombosis, or, less frequently, cholesterol emboli. Because cholesterol microemboli can cause cutaneous findings mimicking vasculitis, this phenomenon is discussed in more detail below.

Cutaneous Cholesterol Embolism

Cholesterol crystal embolization is usually a disease of the elderly with significant atherosclerosis (61). Atheromatous plaque material may detach spontaneously. However, more commonly, plaque material is dislodged by an invasive procedure, such as arterial catheterization. Microemboli or cholesterol crystals typically lead to ischemic changes. Cutaneous manifestations are common, often affect the lower extremities, and include livedo reticularis, purple discoloration, gangrene of toes, and small, painful ulcerations on the legs. Occasionally, a few nodules or indurated plaques may occur. A typical clinical sign is adequate distal pulsation, indicating that the ischemia is arteriolar rather than arterial.

Histopathology. Cholesterol emboli may be found as needle-shaped clefts within the lumina of small vessels. The intravascular clefts, which are in effect dissolved cholesterol crystals, may be single or multiple and are commonly associated with amorphous eosinophilic material, macrophages, or foreign-body giant-cell reactions. Vascular walls exhibit intimal fibrosis and often obliteration of lumina in older lesions. In many instances, only fibrin thrombi are observed. Often a deep biopsy and multiple sections of biopsy material are needed to reveal such emboli, which are distributed focally and therefore are difficult to find.

Vasculopathies Resulting from Deficiencies in Connective Tissue

Lastly, structural deficiencies in the perivascular connective tissue may cause vascular fragility and lead to dermal hemorrhage. Such alterations underlie the hemorrhages that accompany senile purpura and scurvy.

Histopathology. In senile purpura, extravasation of red blood cells is encountered in atrophic skin with solar elastosis and normal-appearing capillaries. In scurvy, dermal hemorrhage is found predominantly in the vicinity of hair follicles without evidence of capillary changes. Hemosiderin-laden macrophages are usually noted (62). Other findings associated with scurvy include intrafollicular keratotic plugs and coiled hair.

Other Clinical Presentations Associated with Vasculopathic Reactions

Livedo Reticularis

Livedo reticularis is persistent red-blue mottling of the skin in a net-like pattern and differs from cutis marmorata by not subsiding with warming of the skin. This condition is a nonspecific sign of sluggish blood flow from any cause. Associations include vasculitis or vasculopathy in the context of several different systemic or localized disease processes, such as infection, atrophie blanche, cholesterol emboli, and connective tissue disease. Frequently, however, the condition is idiopathic and limited to the lower extremities. Generalized livedo reticularis has also been described as part of a potentially severe arterio-occlusive syndrome (Sneddon's syndrome) that is often complicated by cerebrovascular disease (63).

Histopathology. A biopsy specimen taken from an erythematous area may be normal, whereas a biopsy specimen from a white area may show a vessel with a thickened wall and the lumen occluded by a thrombus. In other cases, deeply situated dermal arterioles have shown obliterative changes. Other changes observed in livedo reticularis are intravascular aggregates of red blood cells, suggesting a low flow state.

Atrophie Blanche

Atrophie blanche is a common condition that usually affects middle-aged or elderly females (64). Synonymous terms are livedoid vasculitis, livedo reticularis with seasonal ulceration, and segmental hyalinizing vasculitis. Typically located on the lower portions of the legs, particularly on the ankles and the dorsa of the feet, this condition begins as purpuric macules and papules, which develop into small, painful ulcers with a tendency to recur. Healing of the ulcers results in the white atrophic areas that have given the disease its name. A fully developed case of atrophie blanch shows irregularly outlined, whitish atrophic areas with peripheral hyperpigmentation and telangiectasia. Many of the patients have associated livedo reticularis. The condition also may be seasonal, with the greatest disease activity in the summer and winter months.

Histopathology. The histologic findings are nonspecific and vary with the stage of the lesion. However, in all stages, vascular changes are present. In early lesions, fibrinoid material may be noted in the vessel wall or vessel lumen (Fig. 8-25). Infarction with hemorrhage and an inflammatory infiltrate may be present as well. In late atrophic lesions, the epithelium is thinned and the dermis is sclerotic, with little if any cellular infiltrate. The walls of the dermal vessels may show thickening and hyalinization of the intima. Luminal occlusion by intimal proliferation and/or fibrinoid material and sometimes recanal-

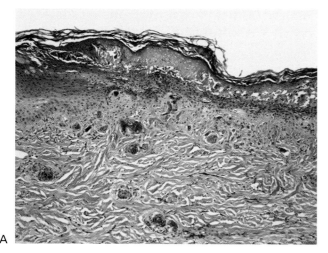
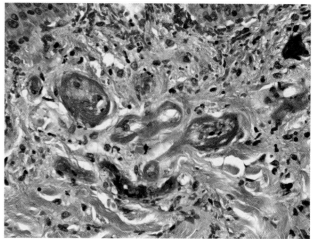

FIGURE 8-25. Atrophie blanche. **(A)** An early lesion characterized by an area of epidermal necrosis with underlying vasculopathy. **(B)** The superficial portion of the epidermis is necrotic. Vessel walls are thickened and contain fibrinoid/thrombotic material.

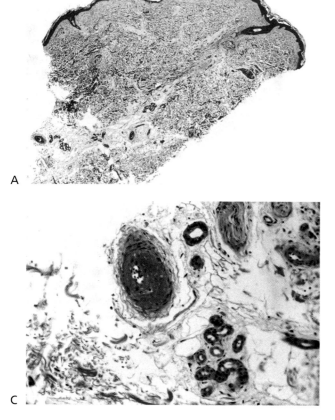

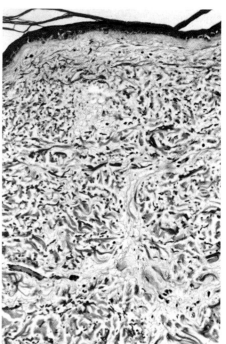

FIGURE 8-26. Degos lesion. Atrophic epidermis overlies a wedge-shaped area of dermis **(A)**, with mucin deposition **(B)**, and a thrombosed vessel at the base **(C)**. This Degos lesion was observed in a patient with dermatomyositis.

ized thrombotic vessels may be seen. In some cases, the vessels in the superficial dermis are predominantly affected; in others, the vessels in the middle and even deep dermis are mostly affected.

Pathogenesis. The etiology of atrophie blanche is unknown. Immune-complex deposits that have been observed in late lesions are likely secondary changes (65). A primary disturbance of fibrinolysis in the endothelium of affected microvessels has been postulated (66).

Degos' Syndrome

Degos had initially described a cutaneointestinal syndrome, in which distinct skin findings ("drops of porcelain") were associated with recurrent attacks of abdominal pain that often ended in death from intestinal perforations (67). The skin lesions of this syndrome arise in crops of asymptomatic, slightly raised, yellowish red papules that gradually develop an atrophic porcelain-white center. These papules tend to affect the trunk and proximal extremities. Degos chose the name *malignant atrophic papulosis* (MAP) for these lesions to emphasize the serious clinical course of the cutaneointestinal disease that he was describing. At that time, the cutaneous lesions were then thought to be specific and pathognomonic for this unique disease entity (Degos' disease). Currently, such skin lesions are considered to be a clinicopathologic reaction pattern that can be associated with a number of conditions (68). Lesions similar if not identical to MAP have been noted in connective tissue diseases such as lupus erythematosus, dermatomyositis, and progressive systemic sclerosis, in atrophie blanche, and in Creutzfeldt–Jakob disease (69).

Histopathology. The classic lesion shows a wedge-shaped area of altered dermis covered by atrophic epidermis with slight hyperkeratosis. Dermal alterations may include frank necrosis. More common, however, are edema, extensive mucin deposition, and slight sclerosis (Fig. 8-26). A sparse perivascular lymphocytic infiltrate may be seen although the dermis is largely acellular. Typically, vascular damage is noted in the vessels at the base of the "cone of necrobiosis." Vascular alterations may be subtle and manifest as endothelial swelling. However, more characteristically, intravascular fibrin thrombi may be noted suggesting that the dermal and epidermal changes result from ischemia. Altered vessels usually lack an inflammatory infiltrate. The histopathology observed may vary with the evolution of the lesions. Early lesions may be more mucinous and mimic tumid lupus while more evolved lesions are more sclerotic (70).

Pathogenesis. The etiology of Degos' syndrome is unclear. The findings have been ascribed to a coagulopathy, vasculitis, or mucinosis. However, convincing evidence to support any single causal factor is lacking.

REFERENCES

1. Callen JP. Cutaneous vasculitis: relationship to systemic disease and therapy. *Curr Probl Dermatol* 1993;5:45.
2. Fauci AS. The spectrum of vasculitis. *Ann Intern Med* 1978; 89:660.
3. Jennette JC, Falk RJ, Andrassy K, et al. Nomenclature of systemic vasculitides: proposal of an international consensus conference. *Arthritis Rheum* 1994;37:187.
4. Jennette JC. Vasculitis affecting the skin. *Arch Dermatol* 1994; 130:899.
5. Jennette JC, Falk RJ. Diagnostic classification of antineutrophil cytoplasmic autoantibody-associated vasculitides. *Am J Kidney Dis* 1991;16:184.
6. Jennette JC, Falk RJ. Anti-neutrophil cytoplasmic antibodies and associated diseases: a review. *Am J Kidney Dis* 1990;15:517.
7. Goeken J. Antineutrophil cytoplasmic and anti-endothelial cell antibodies: new mechanisms for vasculitis. *Curr Opin Dermatol* 1995;19:75.
8. Baum EW, Sams WM Jr, Payne RR. Giant cell arteritis: a systemic disease with rare cutaneous manifestations. *J Am Acad Dermatol* 1982;6:1081.
9. Landing BH, Larson EJ. Pathologic features of Kawasaki disease (mucocutaneous lymph node syndrome). *Am J Cardiovasc Pathol* 1987;4:75.
10. Johnson WC, Wallrich R, Helwig EB. Superficial thrombophlebitis of the chest wall. *JAMA* 1962;180:103.
11. Kussmaul A, Maier K. Ueber eine bisher nicht beschriebene eigenthümliche Arterienerkrankung (Periarteriitis nodosa), die mit Morbus Brightii und rapid fortschreitender allgemeiner Muskellähmung einhergeht. *Dtsch Arch Klin Med* 1866;1:484.
12. Ferrari E. Veber polyarteritis acuta nodosa (sogerannte periarteritis nodosa) undihre Beziehurgen zur polymyositis and polyneuritis acuta. *Beitr Pathol Anat* 1903;34:350.
13. Diaz-Perez JL, Winkelman RK. Cutaneous periarteritis nodosa. *Arch Dermatol* 1974;110:407–414.
14. Davson J, Ball J, Platt R. The kidney in periarteritis nodosa. *Q J Med* 1948;17:175.
15. Guillevin L, Lhote F, Amouroux J, et al. Antineutrophil cytoplasmic antibodies, abnormal angiograms and pathological findings in polyarteritis nodosa and Churg–Strauss syndrome: indications for the classification of vasculitides of the polyarteritis nodosa group. *Br J Rheum* 1996;35:958–964.
16. deShazo RD, Levinson AI, Lawless OJ, et al. Systemic vasculitis with co-existent large and small-vessel involvement: a classification dilemma. *JAMA* 1977;238:1940–1942.
17. Modesto A, Keriven O, Dupre-Goudable C, et al. There is no real difference between Wegener's granulomatosis and micropolyarteritis. *Contrib Nephrol* 1991;191–194.
18. Liebow AA, Carrington CB. Hypersensitivity reactions involving the lung. *Trans Stud Coll Physicians (Philadelphia)* 1966; 34:47.
19. Davis MD, Daoud MS, McEvoy MT, et al. Cutaneous manifestations of Churg–Strauss syndrome: a clinicopathologic correlation. *J Am Acad Dermatol* 1997;37:199–203.
20. Finan MC, Winkelman RK. The cutaneous extravascular necrotizing granuloma (Churg–Strauss granuloma) and systemic disease: a review of 27 cases. *Medicine (Baltimore)* 1983;62:142.
21. Goodman GC, Churg J. Wegener's granulomatosis. *Arch Pathol* 1954;58:533.
22. Deremee RA, McDonald TJ, Harrison EG Jr, et al. Wegener's granulomatosis. *Mayo Clin Proc* 1976;51:777.
23. Arana RM, Hubscher O, Eimon A, Casanova MB, Fonseca R, Turin M. Anticytoplasm antibodies of polymorphonuclear neutrophils in Wegener's granulomatosis and other autoimmune

diseases, and in patients undergoing hemodialysis. *Medecina* (B. Aires) 1993;53:113–116.

24. Barksdale SK, Hallahan CW, Kerr GS, et al. Cutaneous pathology in Wegener's granulomatosis. *Am J Surg Pathol* 1995;19:161.

25. Fauci AS, Wolff SM. Wegener's granulomatosis: studies in 18 patients and a review of the literature. *Medicine (Baltimore)* 1973; 52:535.

26. Pursley TV, Jacobson RR, Apisarnthanarax P. Lucio's phenomenon. *Arch Dermatol* 1980;116:201–204.

27. Mills JA, Michael BA, Bloch DA, et al. The American College of Rheumatology 1990 criteria for the classification of Henoch–Schönlein purpura. *Arthritis Rheum* 1990;33:1114.

28. Birchmore D, Sweeney C, Choudhury D, et al. IaA multiple myeloma presenting as Henoch–Schoenlein purpura/polyarteritis nodosa overlap syndrome. *Arthritis Rheum* 1996;39:698–703.

29. Magro CM, Crowson AN. A clinical and histologic study of 37 cases of immunoglobulin A-associated vasculitis. *Am J Dermatopathol* 1999;21:234–240.

30. Jennette JC, Wieslander J, Tuttle R, et al. Serum IgA-fibronectin aggregates in patients with IgA nephropathy and Henoch-Schönlein purpura: diagnostic valve and pathogenic implications. The glomerulor disease collaborative network. *Am J Kidney Dis* 1991;18:466.

31. Mehregan DR, Hall MJ, Gibson LE. Urticarial vasculitis: a histopathologic and clinical review of 72 cases. *J Am Acad Dermatol* 1992;26:441–448.

32. Davis MDP, Daoud MS, Kirby B, et al. Clinicopathologic correlation of hypocomplementemic and normocomplementemic urticarial vasculitits *J Am Acad Dermatol* 1998;38:899–905.

33. Cohen SJ, Pittelkow MR, Su WP. Cutaneous manifestations of cryoglobulinemia: clinical and histopathologic study of 72 patients. *J Am Acad Dermatol* 1992;26:38.

34. Patel A, Prussick R, Buchanan WW, et al. Serum sickness-like illness and leukocytoclastic vasculitis after intravenous streptokinase. *J Am Acad Dermatol* 1991;24:652.

35. Lakhanpal S, Conn DL, Lie JT. Clinical and prognostic significance of vasculitis as early manifestation of connective tissue disease syndromes. *Ann Intern Med* 1984;101:743.

36. Sanchez-Guerro J, Gutierrez-Urena S, Vidaller A, et al. Vasculitis as a paraneoplastic syndrome: report of 11 cases and review of the literature. *J Rheumatol* 1990;17:1458.

37. Jorizzo JL, Solomon AR, Zanolli MD, et al. Neutrophilic vascular reactions. *Arch Dermatol* 1988;19:983.

38. Chen KR, Kawahara Y, Miyakawa S, et al. Cutaneous vasculitis in Behçet's disease: a clinical and histopathologic study of 20 patients. *J Am Acad Dermatol* 1997;36:689–696.

39. Carlson JA, LeBoit PE. Localized chronic fibrosing vasculitis of the skin: an inflammatory reaction that occurs in settings other than erythema elevatum diutinium and granuloma faciale. *Am J Surg Pathol* 1997;21:698–705.

40. LeBoit PE, Yen TSB, Wintroub B. The evolution of lesions in erythema elevatum diutinum. *Am J Dermatopathol* 1986;8:392.

41. Sangüeza OP, Pilcher B, Sangüeza MD. Erythema elevatum diutinum: a clinicopathological study of eight cases. *Am J Dermatopathol* 1997;19:214–222.

42. Requena L, Yus ES, Martin L, et al. Erythema elevatum diutinum in a patient with acquired immunodeficiency syndrome. *Arch Dermatol* 1991;127:1819–1822.

43. Burns BV, Roberts PF, De Carpentier J, et al. Eosinophilic angiocentric fibrosis affecting the nasal cavity. A mucosal variant of the skin lesion granuloma faciale. *J Laryngol Otol* 2001;115: 223–226.

44. Pinkus H. Granuloma faciale. *Dermatologica* 1952;105:85–99.

45. Von Den Driesch P. Sweet's syndrome: acute febrile neutrophilic dermatosis. *J Am Acad Dermatol* 1994;31:535.

46. Sweet RD. Acute febrile neutrophilic dermatosis. *Br J Dermatol* 1964;74:349.

47. Drenth JPH, van der Meer JWM. Hereditary periodic fever. *N Engl J Med* 2001;345:1748–1757.

48. Ely PH. The bowel bypass syndrome: a response to bacterial peptidoglycans. *J Am Acad Dermatol* 1980;2:473.

49. Powell FC, Su WPD, Perry HO. Pyoderma gangrenosum: classification and management. *J Am Acad Dermatol* 1996;34:395–409.

50. Holt PJA, Davis MG, Saunders KC, et al. Pyoderma gangrenosum. *Medicine (Baltimore)* 1980;59:114.

51. Su WP, Schroeter AL, Perry HO, et al. Histopathologic and immunopathologic study of pyoderma gangrenosum. *J Cutan Pathol* 1986;13:323.

52. Massa MC, Su WPD. Lymphocytic vasculitis: is it a specific clinicopathologic entity? *J Cutan Pathol* 1984;11:132.

53. Thomas R, Vuitch F, Lakhanpl S. Angiocentric T-cell lymphoma masquerading as cutaneous vasculitis. *J Rheumatol* 1994;21:760.

54. Randall SJ, Kierland RR, Montgomery H. Pigmented purpuric eruptions. *Arch Dermatol Syphiligr* 1951;64:177.

55. Waisman M, Waisman M. Lichen aureus. *Arch Dermatol* 1976; 112:696.

56. Barnhill RL, Braverman IM. Progression of pigmented purpura-like eruptions to mycosis fungoides: report of three cases. *J Am Acad Dermatol* 1988;19:25.

57. Robboy SJ, Mihm MC, Colman RC, et al. The skin in disseminated intravascular coagulation. *Br J Dermatol* 1973;88:221.

58. Fischer AH, Morris DJ. Pathogenesis of calciphylaxis: study of 3 cases with literature review. *Hum Pathol* 1995;26:1055–1064.

59. Lugo-Somolinos A, Sanchez JL, Menedez-Coll J, et al. Calcifying panniculitis associated with polycystic kidney disease and chronic renal failure. *J Am Acad Dermatol* 1990;22:743–747.

60. Mehta RL, Scott G, Sloand JA, et al. Skin necrosis associated with acquired protein C deficiency in patients with renal failure and calciphylaxis. *Am J Med* 1990;88:252–257.

61. Falanga V, Fine MJ, Kapoor WN. The cutaneous manifestations of cholesterol crystal embolization. *Arch Dermatol* 1986;122: 1194.

62. Walker A. Chronic scurvy. *Br J Dermatol* 1968;80:625.

63. Sneddon IB. Cerebro-vascular lesions and livedos reticularis. *Br J Dermatol* 1975;77:180.

64. Stiefler RE, Bergfeld WF. Atrophie blanche [review]. *Int J Dermatol* 1982;21:1.

65. Shornick JK, Nichoces BK, Bergstresser PR, et al. Idiopathic atrophie blanche. *J Am Acad Dermatol* 1983;8:792.

66. McCalmont CS, McCalmont TH, Jorizzo JC, et al. Livedo vasculitis: vasculitis or thrombotic vasculopathy? *Clin Exp Dermatol* 1992;17:4.

67. Degos R, Delort J, Tricot R. Dermatite papulo-squameuse atrophiante. *Bull Soc Fr Dermatol Syphiligr* 1942;49:148,281.

68. Doutre MS, Beylot C, Bioulac P, et al. Skin lesion resembling malignant atrophic papulosis in lupus erythematosus. *Dermatologica* 1987;175:45.

69. Magrinat G, Kerwin KS, Gabriel DA. The clinical manifestations of Degos' syndrome. *Arch Pathol Lab Med* 1989;113:354.

70. Harvell JD, Williford PL, White WL. Benign cutaneous Degos' disease: a case report with emphasis on histopathology as papules chronologically evolve. *Am J Dermatopathol* 2001;23:116–123.

NONINFECTIOUS VESICULOBULLOUS AND VESICULOPUSTULAR DISEASES

HONG WU
BRIAN SCHAPIRO
TERENCE J. HARRIST

CLASSIFICATION OF BLISTERS

Definition

A blister is a fluid-filled cavity formed within or beneath the epidermis. The fluid consists of tissue fluid and plasma. A variable component of inflammatory cells may also be present. Blisters may occur in many dermatoses. At first glance, this observation seems to imply that blistering is too general or nonspecific for use in clinical gross evaluation. However, the character of blisters in a given disorder tends to be uniform and to have reproducible characteristics. One useful distinction is the categorization of blisters into *vesicles* (blisters <0.5 cm in diameter) and *bullae* (blisters >0.5 cm in diameter). For example, vesicles characteristically occur in dermatitis herpetiformis as opposed to pemphigoid, in which bullae are most commonly observed.

Mechanisms of Blister Formation

The mechanisms observable in routine sections for some diseases are shown in Table 9-1. *Spongiosis* is the accumulation of extracellular fluid within the epidermis with resultant separation of the keratinocytes. Pronounced spongiosis leads to disruption of desmosomes and subsequent blister formation. Thus, the epidermis has a "spongy" appearance microscopically and the increasing accumulation of fluid leads to a vesicle and, in some instances, to a bulla. Marked spongiosis may terminate in reticular degeneration (below). Spongiosis is almost always associated with an infiltrate of lymphocytes within the epidermis and around superficial vessels. However, spongiosis is a passive event associated with increased permeability of the superficial vascular plexus, particularly the postcapillary venules.

Acantholysis results from the loss of appropriate keratinocyte cell–cell contact. Histologic evidence of acantholysis includes the presence of rounded keratinocytes with condensed cytoplasm and large nuclei with peripheral condensation of chromatin and prominent nucleoli.

Reticular degeneration results from ballooning degeneration (intracellular edema) with secondary rupture of the keratinocytes. The remaining desmosomal attachments often connect strands of ruptured keratinocytic membranes and cytoplasm to intact keratinocytes, giving the epidermis an irregular meshwork appearance.

Cytolysis is the disruption of keratinocytes. It occurs in the normal epidermis when the structural (keratin) matrix and desmosomal plaques of the keratinocyte are overwhelmed by high levels of physical agents such as friction and heat. Friction (mechanical energy applied parallel to the epidermis) leads to the shearing of keratinocytes one from another and of the keratinocytes themselves, giving the characteristic clear fluid-filled blisters. Minimal friction may lead to cytolysis in subjects whose keratinocytes do not have normal structural matrix and desmosomes, such as in epidermolysis bullosa simplex and epidermolysis bullosa of the Cockayne–Weber type.

Basement membrane zone disruption or destruction results from primary structural deficiencies as well as from both humoral and cellular immunologically mediated damage. When blisters arise at the epidermal basement membrane zone, any of the specific subanatomic compartments can be affected: (a) the basal keratinocytes, and particularly their lower portions; (b) the lamina lucida, an electron-lucid area immediately subjacent to the plasma membrane; (c) the lamina densa, composed principally of type IV collagen; and (d) the sublamina densa zone.

Pathologic Evaluation

When blisters are encountered microscopically, systematic analysis can lead to diagnosis in most cases. The critical interpretive assessments to be approached in sequence are as follows: (a) the blister separation plane (Table 9-2); (b) the mechanism(s) of blister formation (Table 9-1); and (c) the character of the inflammatory infiltrate, including its pres-

TABLE 9-1. DISEASES AND MECHANISMS OF BLISTER FORMATION

Disease	Blister Formation Mechanisms
Spongiosis	Eczematous dermatitis
	Miliaria
	Pemphigus (early)
	Transient acantholytic dermatosis (one pattern)
Acantholysis	Pemphigus
	Transient acantholytic dermatosis (some patterns)
	Hailey–Hailey disease
	Darier's disease
	Irritant dermatitis (some)
Reticular degeneration	Viral infections
	Eczematous dermatitis (late stage)
Cytolysis	Epidermolysis bullosa simplex
	Epidermolytic hyperkeratosis
	Friction blister
	Erythema multiforme (in part)
	Irritant dermatitis (some)
Basement membrane zone destruction	Bullous pemphigoid
	Cicatricial pemphigoid
	Linear IgA dermatosis
	Dermatitis herpetiformis
	Epidermolysis bullosa acquisita
	Epidermolysis bullosa letalis
	Epidermolysis bullosa dystrophica

TABLE 9-2. SELECTED DISEASES WITH SPECIFIC SEPARATION PLANES

1. Intraepidermal
1.1. Subcorneal/granular
    Miliaria crystallina
    Staphylococcal scalded skin syndrome
    Pemphigus foliaceus and variants
    Bullous impetigo
    IgA pemphigus
    Subcorneal pustular dermatosis
    Erythema toxicum neonatorum
    Transient neonatal pustular melanosis
    Acropustulosis of infancy
    Spinous
1.2. Spongiotic dermatitis
    Friction blister (may extend into dermis)
    Miliaria rubra
    Incontinentia pigmenti
    IgA pemphigus
    Epidermolytic hyperkeratosis
    Hailey–Hailey disease
    Suprabasal
1.3. Pemphigus vulgaris and variants
    Paraneoplastic pemphigus
    Darier's disease
2. Subepidermal
2.1. *Basal keratinocyte necrosis, cytolysis, or damage*
    Epidermolysis bullosa simplex
    Thermal injury (some)
    Erythema multiforme
    Herpes gestationis
2.2. *Epidermal basement membrane zone destruction or disruption*
2.2.1. *Lamina lucida*
    Bullous pemphigoid
    Cicatricial pemphigoid
    Herpes gestationis
    Dermatitis herpetiformis
    Linear IgA dermatosis
    Porphyria cutanea tarda
    Epidermolysis bullosa letalis (junctional)
    Suction blister
    Thermal injury (some)
    Sublamina densa
    Bullous systemic lupus erythematosus
    Epidermolysis bullosa acquisita
    Linear IgA dermatosis (IgA-mediated epidermolysis bullosa acquisita)
    Epidermolysis bullosa dystrophica
3. Dermal
    Penicillamine-induced blisters (iatrogenic)

ence or absence, its pattern, and the specific cell types involved (Table 9-3).

Six principal problems are encountered using this algorithm. The first is that the separation plane may change as blisters age. Spongiotic microvesicles may move into the stratum corneum as crust. The epidermal blister roofs may become necrotic not allowing assessment of the original blister plane. However, the basal keratinocytes may retain their columnar appearance in the blister roof (or base). Allowing for separation into either suprabasal or sub-basal blister formation. Also, basal keratinocytes are the most melanized cells in the epidermis. Searching for the melanized basal keratinocytes (i.e., the basal unit), even if they are necrotic, may allow assessment of the original blister plane. Some blister roofs may be viable for a week or so; in this case the viable keratinocytes may become elongated and line the base of the blister. Similarly, the re-epithelialized subepidermal or suprabasal blisters are initially lined by flat squamous keratinocytes rather than columnar or cuboidal keratinocytes. When re-epithelialization first occurs, there are no normal retia, and the flat squamous keratinocytes migrate on a matrix of fibrinogen not normal papillary dermis. Second, microscopic slit-like spaces occur within the epidermis in the group of clefting diseases—Darier's disease, Hailey–Hailey disease, and Grover's disease—mimicking true blisters. However, these clefts are

small and do not contain fibrin and tissue fluid. This group of disorders, furthermore, only rarely presents clinically with blisters. Third, evaluation of routine histologic preparations may not allow one to accurately assess the specific mechanism of blister formation. This is particularly true in the subepidermal vesiculobullous disorders. Fourth, the cell types infiltrating the lesions in the vesiculobullous diseases change as the lesions age. Fifth, the histologic descriptions of many of the subepidermal blistering disorders are

TABLE 9-3. PRINCIPAL INFILTRATING INFLAMMATORY CELLS IN SELECTED VESICULOBULLOUS DERMATOSES

Dermatosis	Principal Cell Type	Infiltrate
Porphyria Variegated Cutanea tarda		Absent
Epidermolysis bullosa acquisita (classic)		Absent
Bullous pemphigoid (cell-poor)	Eosinophils	Minimal
Spongiotic dermatitis	Lymphocytes	Present
Erythema multiforme	Lymphocytes	Present
Bullous pemphigoid (cell-rich)	Eosinophils	Present
Herpes gestationis	Eosinophils	Present
Dermatitis herpetiformis	Neutrophils	Present
Linear IgA dermatosis	Neutrophils	Present
Epidermolysis bullosa acquisita (inflammatory)	Neutrophils or mixed neutrophils and eosinophils	Present
Bullous systemic lupus erythematosus	Neutrophils Interface dermatitis	Present
Cicatricial pemphigoid	Mixed neutrophils and eosinophils Lymphocytic, bandlike (mucosa only) Eosinophils	Present
Paraneoplastic pemphigus	Lymphocytes-interface dermatitis (lichen planus or erythema multiforme-like)	Present

Note: These descriptions are accurate in the vast majority of cases in each dermatosis; however, occasionally the cell types may differ, rendering immunofluorescence testing mandatory. Other inflammatory cells may be present as a minor component, but on occasion are of significant numbers.

not accompanied by the rigorous immunologic evaluation required today. For example, many cases originally reported as bullous pemphigoid and cicatricial pemphigoid are now known to be better classified as epidermolysis bullosa acquisita and linear IgA bullous dermatosis. Many of the subepidermal blistering disorders may strikingly mimic each other clinically, leading to inappropriate diagnosis and making the histologic descriptions in the literature suspect. Lastly, in order to rapidly improve the rash and symptomology of the patient, clinicians often embark on therapeutic regimens for the presumed clinical diagnosis. The therapy often consists of topical or systemic steroids and inhibitors of inflammation. Histopathologic examination of a biopsy is only pursued when the therapeutic response is nil or partial, calling into question the clinical diagnosis. Many submit biopsies without notifying the dermatopathologist of the therapy. Such therapy often suppresses the inflammatory infiltrate, the epidermal response, the "triple response of Lewis" and other histopathologic changes. The evolution and temporal relationship of histologic changes of dermatitides under various therapies are *not* sufficiently documented to allow optimal, or perhaps, even accurate diagnostic study. Biopsies should be taken of virgin disease not of therapeutically altered skin if at all possible. If therapy has been instituted, it should be stopped, if possible, at least a week before biopsy.

With these points in mind, the specific disorders and groups of disorders will be discussed.

SPONGIOTIC DERMATITIS

Definition and Evaluation

Spongiotic dermatitis may be acute, subacute, or chronic. The process is dynamic, and each specific type of dermatitis may progress from the acute to the chronic phase. Although the term *spongiotic dermatitis* is occasionally used interchangeably with *eczema*, the word "eczema" lacks specific meaning (1). *Spongiosis* refers to the accumulation of edema fluid between keratinocytes, in some cases progressing to vesicle or even bulla formation.

In *acute spongiotic dermatitis*, the stratum corneum is normal and the epidermis is of normal thickness. The degree of spongiosis is variable, extending from slight to marked, with intraepidermal vesiculation in the latter instance. The surrounding keratinocytes may be stellate, surrounded by clear spaces representing the site of fluid collection (Fig. 9-1). Papillary dermal edema is present, correlating with the degree of spongiosis. A lymphohistiocytic infiltrate is present around the superficial plexus, with exocytosis of lymphocytes into spongiotic foci.

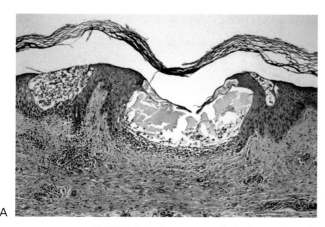
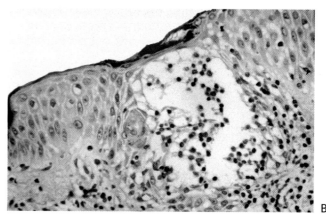

FIGURE 9-1. Acute spongiotic dermatitis: allergic contact dermatitis. **(A)** Spongiosis with vesicles containing fluid and inflammatory cells. **(B)** Exocytosis of lymphocytes and eosinophils into the spongiotic epidermis.

In *subacute spongiotic dermatitis*, there is usually mild to moderate spongiosis, occasionally with microvesiculation. The epidermis is moderately acanthotic. The parakeratotic stratum corneum may contain aggregates of coagulated plasma and scattered lymphocytes and neutrophils, forming a crust (Fig. 9-2). There is a superficial perivascular lymphohistiocytic infiltrate, which is less prominent than in the acute phase. Impetiginization by Gram-positive cocci (staphylococci and streptococci) may lead to neutrophilic crust.

In *chronic dermatitis*, there is hyperkeratosis with areas of parakeratosis, often hypergranulosis, and moderate to marked acanthosis (Fig. 9-3). Spongiosis may be present focally, often minimal in degree. The inflammatory infiltrate is often sparse, and papillary dermal fibrosis may be a prominent feature. The degree of spongiosis and quantity of the infiltrate reflect the present activity of the underlying dermatitis. The other changes reflect lichen simplex chronicus.

Specific Types of Spongiotic Dermatitis

Allergic Contact Dermatitis

The prototype of acute spongiotic dermatitis is allergic contact dermatitis, secondary to exposure to poison ivy. Usually between 24 and 72 hours after exposure to the antigen, the patient develops pruritic, edematous, erythematous papules and plaques, and, in some cases, vesicles. Linear papules and vesicles are common in allergic contact dermatitis to poison ivy, reflecting the points of contact between the plant and the skin. Other common causes of allergic contact dermatitis include nickel, paraphenylenediamine, rubber compounds, fragrances, and preservatives in cosmetics. The degree of histologic alterations to these antigens may be less striking than that secondary to poison ivy.

Histopathology. Early lesions are acute spongiotic dermatitis. If vesicles develop, they may contain clusters of

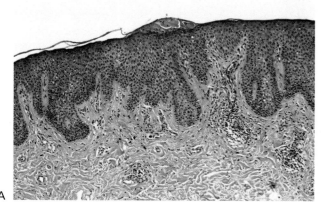
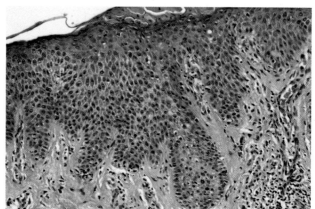

FIGURE 9-2. Subacute spongiotic dermatitis: nummular dermatitis. **(A)** There is irregular acanthosis, spongiosis and superficial perivascular inflammatory infiltrate. Parakeratosis containing plasma is also present. **(B)** Spongiosis is accompanied by exocytosis of inflammatory cells.

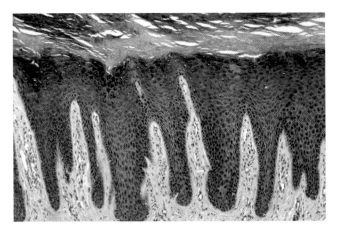

FIGURE 9-3. Lichen simplex chronicus. There is hyperkeratosis, hypergranulosis and irregular psoriasiform acanthosis with minimal spongiosis. Vertically oriented collagen in the papillary dermis is characteristic.

Langerhans cells. There is superficial dermal infiltrate of lymphocytes, macrophages and Langerhans cells with accentuation around the small vessels. Eosinophils may be present in the dermal infiltrate as well as within areas of spongiosis (Fig. 9-1). In patients with continued exposure to the antigen, the biopsy may show a subacute or, later, a chronic spongiotic dermatitis, often with lichen simplex chronicus due to rubbing.

Pathogenesis. Allergic contact dermatitis represents a type IV, cell-mediated, delayed hypersensitivity reaction. The immunologic reaction consists of an afferent limb, the sensitization or induction phase, and an efferent limb, the elicitation phase. The allergen is usually of low molecular weight (a hapten), and lipid soluble. After penetrating the skin, the hapten binds to a carrier protein to form a complete antigen (2), which is processed by antigen-presenting cells, principally the epidermal Langerhans cells, and possibly other cutaneous dendritic cells. These cells then migrate to the draining lymph nodes, where they present the antigen to T-lymphocytes. The process triggers antigen-specific commitment and production of memory and effector T cells. Following subsequent exposure of the sensitized subject to the same allergen, an accelerated and more aggressive secondary immune response will be elicited. Both CD4+ and CD8+ subtypes of T-lymphocytes participate in contact hypersensitivity reactions (3). The homing of lymphocytes to the antigen in exposed skin requires various cell adhesion molecules, such as lymphocyte function–associated antigen-1 (LFA-1) (4). Lymphocytes liberate various cytokines in the affected area of skin, including interleukins IFN-γ and TNF-α, leading to a further influx of inflammatory cells, particularly nonsensitized lymphocytes and eosinophils. Chemokines appear to be crucial regulators of both induction and expression of allergic contact dermatitis.

Irritant Contact Dermatitis

This inflammatory reaction occurs after exposure to an irritant, a toxic compound that causes a reaction in most individuals who come into contact with it. Common irritants include alkalis, such as soaps, detergents, lye, and ammonia-containing compounds. The irritant response is determined by the type of chemical, its concentration, the mode of exposure, the body site, the barrier function locally, and the age of the patient. Atopy is a predisposing factor. The clinical morphology varies; sometimes it is indistinguishable from allergic contact dermatitis.

Chemical burns, usually caused by strong alkalis and acids, lead to immediate painful erythema progressing to vesiculation, necrosis, and, if severe, ulceration. Acute irritant reactions produce a monomorphic picture with scaling, redness, vesicles, pustules, or erosions, and are caused by such mild irritants as detergents and water with additives. Agents producing this pattern include tretinoin, benzalkonium chloride, dithranol, adhesive tapes, and cosmetics. Chronic irritant contact dermatitis is characterized by dryness, chapping, and absence of vesicles. This reaction pattern is produced by repetitive contact to water, detergent, and solvents.

Histopathology. The histologic picture varies from extensive ulceration, to simply diffuse hyperkeratosis or parakeratosis with congestion and ectasia, to a spongiotic pattern essentially identical to allergic contact dermatitis. The variable features reflect the protean factors discussed above. Some correlations are worthy of note. In some instances, there is significant necrosis with nuclear karyorrhexis and cytoplasmic pallor (Bandmann's achromia) (5). In severe reactions, the necrosis may extend into the dermis. Some irritants such as cantharidin and trichloroethylene produce acantholysis and neutrophilic infiltration in the epidermis (6) (Fig. 9-4). Other contactants may specifically target vascular endothelium. Some reactions, however, may be

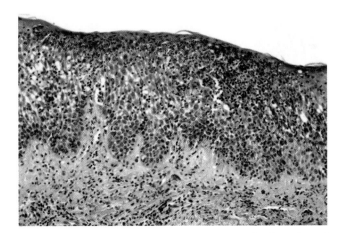

FIGURE 9-4. Irritant dermatitis. There is superficial epidermal necrosis together with spongiosis and infiltrate of neutrophils.

entirely spongiotic, such as those due to weak irritants, strong irritants in low concentration, and those in the "irritable skin syndrome." Because of these observations and those made in positive patch test sites, routine histopathological changes do not reliably separate irritant from allergic contact reactions, although necrosis, neutrophilic infiltration, and acantholysis are more frequent in the former. In the recovery phase of irritant dermatitis, mild epidermal hyperplasia, sometimes psoriasiform, is often present. Psoriasiform hyperplasia may develop in chronic irritant reactions. In other words, most common irritants lead to subacute and chronic spongiotic dermatitis histologic features identical to those of allergic contact reactions.

Pathogenesis. The pathogenesis of irritant contact dermatitis is not completely understood. Contrary to popular belief, recent studies indicate that very complex reaction patterns occur involving immunologic components in the irritant response. There are surprisingly more similarities than differences between irritant contact dermatitis and allergic contact dermatitis in morphology, clinical manifestation, chemokine expression, and involvement of T cells (7–9).

Dyshidrotic Dermatitis

This entity is characterized by recurrent, severely pruritic, deep-seated vesicles that classically involve the lateral aspects of the fingers and, in some cases, the toes. Episodes may be precipitated by infections, "id" reactions, contact reactions, and emotional stress. In chronic cases, there may be more extensive involvement of the palms and soles. Although the eruption develops acutely, it may become chronic with erythema, lichenification, and fissuring. Secondary impetiginization is common.

Histopathology. Spongiosis and intraepidermal vesiculation occur in acute lesions (Fig. 9-5). There is a superficial perivascular lymphohistiocytic infiltrate with exocytosis of lymphocytes into spongiotic zones. The infiltration is usu-

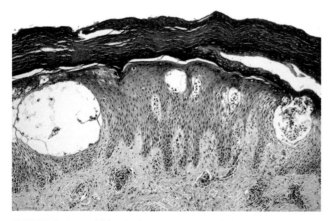

FIGURE 9-5. Dyshidrotic dermatitis. In acral skin, large intraepidermal vesicles are held intact by the thick stratum corneum.

ally mild. In acute lesions, the compact, thickened stratum corneum of acral skin remains intact, and the epidermal thickness is normal. With chronicity, spongiosis diminishes, acanthosis and parakeratosis predominate, and serum may be identified within the stratum corneum. Difficulty in diagnosis may occur because of the formation of vesiculopustules in older lesions. A periodic acid–Schiff (PAS) stain should always be performed on vesicular lesions of the palms and soles, because tinea manus/pedis may mimic dyshidrotic dermatitis histologically.

Autoeczematization or Id Reaction

A sudden generalized or localized vesicular dermatitis developing in association with a defined local dermatitis or infection is known as an "id" reaction. The lesions are pinhead-sized, acuminate or flat-topped, papules. The patient most often has bullous tinea pedis or kerion, thus the name, "dermatophytid." In some cases, patients have a severe localized dermatitis, such as stasis dermatitis, with subsequent development of widespread papulovesicular lesions (10). Other forms of id reactions exist.

Histopathology. The features are those of acute spongiotic dermatitis, often with micro- or macro-vesiculation. Eosinophils may be present (11). There is often some edema of the superficial papillary dermis with some large lymphocytes (presumably activated) in the upper dermis (12). The infiltrating cells are T cells—those within the epidermis are principally CD8+, and those within the dermis are principally CD4+ (13).

Pathogenesis. An id reaction is a secondary vesicular dermatitis of sudden onset that cannot be identified as a common dermatosis, and that is not due to a direct external contactant, infective agent, direct spread of local infection, or associated common dermatosis (14). It has been postulated to be a hypersensitivity dermatitis to an autoantigen; however, this has never been proven. Several other possibilities exist. First, the reaction may represent a conditioned hyperirritability or responsiveness precipitated by the local infection or dermatitis (15). Acute local chemical irritation may lower the threshold for an irritant reaction to the same chemical at remote sites. Second, localized dermatitis leads to local production of cytokines by keratinocytes. If the cytokines are hematogenously disseminated, they may lead to distant skin hyperirritability. Lastly, dissemination of antigen (but not of whole infectious agents) from the local site may occur with then a secondary response developing at a site of distant deposition. Microbial antigens have been identified in an id reaction in a patient with tuberculoid leprosy (16).

Photoallergic Dermatitis

Photoallergy is increased reactivity of skin to ultraviolet and visible light and is brought about by a chemical agent on an immunologic basis (17). The eruption of photoallergic dermatitis may be due to topical application of, or oral ingestion of, a photosensitizing agent, resulting in a photocontact dermatitis or photodrug eruption, respectively. Agents that may elicit a photocontact dermatitis include soaps and cleansers (containing halogenated salicylanilide), perfumes (such as musk ambrette), topical sulfonamides, sunscreens, benzocaine, and diphenhydramine (18). Common causes of photodrug eruption include thiazide diuretics, oral hypoglycemics, and phenothiazines. The eruption is pruritic and composed of erythematous papules and confluent plaques on sun-exposed skin, usually the face, dorsal aspect of the arms, and the "V" of the neck.

Histopathology. The features are similar to that of an acute allergic contact dermatitis, showing moderate to severe spongiosis, in some cases with vesiculation, and a superficial perivascular lymphohistiocytic infiltrate with exocytosis. A deeper perivascular infiltrate and eosinophils are more common in photoallergic dermatitis induced by systemic ingestion of medications. With chronic exposure to the antigen, there is progression to chronic dermatitis, with diminished spongiosis, less intense inflammation, and more acanthosis. Phototoxic reactions are "sunburn" reactions with epidermal apoptosis and necrosis with intraepidermal to subepidermal blisters—the changes paralleling the degree of damage. Neutrophils are prominent.

Nummular Dermatitis

The eruption is characterized by pruritic, coin-shaped (nummular), erythematous, scaly, crusted plaques. The lesions tend to develop on the extensor surfaces of the extremities.

Histopathology. Nummular dermatitis is the prototype of subacute spongiotic dermatitis (Fig. 9-2). There is mild to moderate spongiosis, usually without vesiculation. Irregular acanthosis with some exocytosis of inflammatory cells is usually present. The parakeratotic stratum corneum contains aggregates of coagulated plasma, forming a crust. Mild papillary dermal edema and vascular dilatation may be present. There is superficial perivascular infiltrate of lymphocytes, some eosinophils, and occasional neutrophils and plasma cells.

Pathogenesis. The etiology of this entity is unknown. The routines and ultrastructural changes in nummular dermatitis resemble those of contact dermatitis. Intercellular edema is the most conspicuous finding (19). There is shearing and loss of desmosomes as spongiosis becomes marked.

Atopic Dermatitis

The eruption is characterized by areas of severe pruritus, erythema, scaling, and excoriation, and with chronicity, lichenification, and lichen simplex chronicus. Many of the cutaneous changes are due to chronic rubbing and scratching. Most patients are diagnosed in childhood, and approximately one-third of cases are diagnosed before 1 year of age (20). There is a female predominance, and many patients have other atopic disorders such as allergic rhinitis or asthma. In infants, the lesions predominate on the face and extensor surfaces of the extremities, but later affect the flexural surfaces. The classically involved sites in older children and adults are the popliteal, antecubital fossae, and the sides of the neck. Secondary bacterial infection is common.

Histopathology. In early phases, there is mild spongiosis, exocytosis of lymphocytes, and parakeratosis. Lymphocytes and scattered histiocytes are present around the superficial vascular plexus. In long-standing lesions, the rete ridges are regularly elongated, with less prominent spongiosis and cellular infiltrate. Hyperkeratosis and wedge-shaped hypergranulosis with areas of parakeratosis develop. There appear to be increased numbers of small vessels with a thickening of their walls that involves both endothelial cells and the basement membrane (21). Eosinophils are less conspicuous than in allergic contact or nummular dermatitis. With time, the changes may be those of lichen simplex chronicus.

Pathogenesis. Understanding of the disease remains incomplete. Atopic dermatitis develops as a result of complex interactions of genetic, environmental, and immunologic factors. Allergic reactions appear to play a role in some patients, but in other patients, factors such as disturbance of skin function, infection, and stress may be more important. Factors identified as being involved in the pathogenesis of atopic dermatitis include the differentiation of helper T cells, increased life span of eosinophils, multiple roles of IgE, the pattern of local cytokine expression, infectious agents, and superantigens (22). The initiation of atopic dermatitis appears to be driven by allergen-induced activation of type 2 T-helper cells (Th-2 cells), leading to increased levels of interleukin-4, -10 and -13, and elevated IgE ensues. IgE contributes to the inflammatory cell infiltrate by several mechanisms, including immediate/late phase reaction, allergen presentation by IgE-bearing Langerhans cells, and allergen-induced activation of IgE-bearing macrophages.

The mononuclear cell infiltrate in the lesions probably reflects a combination of both IgE dependent mast cell/basophil degranulation and Th-2 cell-mediated responses elicited during acute exposure to allergens, including ingestants, inhalants, or contact aeroallergens such as human dander, grass pollens, and house dust mites (23).

The pattern of local cytokine expression plays an important role in modulating tissue inflammation and depends on the activity or duration of the skin lesion. Acute skin inflammation is associated with a predominance of IL-4 and IL-13 expression, and little INF-γ. But in chronic lesions, there are increased INF-γ–producing cells (24,25). In addition, atopic dermatitis can be exacerbated by fungal, bacterial and viral skin infections. In particular, *Staphylococcus aureus* may exacerbate or maintain skin inflammation in atopic dermatitis by secreting a group of toxins known to act as superantigens (26).

No specific single gene is a unique marker for atopic dermatitis. There is some allelic association with chromosomes 5q31, 11q13, 14q11, and 3q21. Chromosome 5q31 contains the IL-4 gene cluster family. Because IL-4 is central to the induction of IgE synthesis by B cells, it has been suggested that polymorphisms in the chromosome 5q31 region are linked to the gene controlling total serum IgE in atopic individuals. Another possible candidate gene found on chromosome 11q13 is the high-affinity IgE receptor (27,28).

Lichen Simplex Chronicus

The vast majority of patients with pruritus who chronically rub the skin may develop lichen simplex chronicus. It often develops in the setting of atopic dermatitis or allergic contact dermatitis. The lesions are pruritic, thick plaques often with excoriation, in which the normal skin markings are accentuated, the latter finding known as lichenification. Uncommonly, some patients develop macular or lichen amyloidosis. Some patients, due to the character of their underlying disease such as dermatitis herpetiformis, only rarely develop lichen simplex chronicus. Lastly, skin with severe chronic dermatoheliosis does not develop typical lichen simplex chronicus.

Histopathology. Lichen simplex chronicus is the prototype for chronic dermatitis (Fig. 9-3). There is hyperkeratosis interspersed with areas of parakeratosis, acanthosis with irregular elongation of the rete ridges, hypergranulosis, and broadening of the dermal papillae. Slight spongiosis may be observed, but vesiculation is absent. Minimal papillomatosis is sometimes present. Excoriations, which are punctate ulcerations lined by necrotic superficial papillary dermis, fibrin, and neutrophils, are often present; however, they are often present in many pruritic dermatoses. There may be a sparse superficial perivascular infiltrate without exocytosis. In the papillary dermis, there are an increased number of fibroblasts and vertically oriented collagen bundles. As rubbing increases in intensity and chronicity, epidermal hyperplasia becomes more florid, and the fibrosis more marked. Search for features of dermatitis associated with chronic rubbing and scratching may give a hint as to the initial underlying dermatitis.

Seborrheic Dermatitis

Clinically, patients develop erythema and greasy scale on the scalp, ears, eyebrows, nasolabial areas, and central chest. Rarely, patients with seborrheic dermatitis develop generalized lesions. In infants, the scalp ("cradle cap"), face,

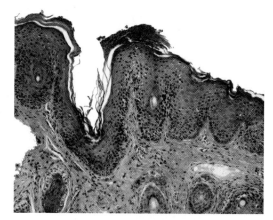

FIGURE 9-6. Seborrheic dermatitis. There is neutrophilic parakeratosis on the follicular ostial shoulder. The epidermis is hyperplastic. Spongiosis is minimal in this biopsy.

and diaper areas are often involved. It is a rare cause of erythroderma. Seborrheic dermatitis is seen with increased frequency in patients with Parkinson's disease (29), epilepsy, congestive heart failure, chronic alcoholism, zinc deficiency, and HIV infection. Patients with HIV infection often have severe refractory disease and atypical distribution (30,31).

Histopathology. The histopathologic features are a combination of those observed in psoriasis and spongiotic dermatitis. Mild cases may exhibit only slight subacute spongiotic dermatitis. The stratum corneum contains focal parakeratosis, with a predilection for the follicular ostia, a finding known as "shoulder parakeratosis" (Fig. 9-6). Occasional pyknotic neutrophils are present within parakeratotic foci (neutrophilic parakeratosis), sometimes with fluid (neutrophilic crust). There is moderate acanthosis with regular elongation of the rete ridges, mild spongiosis, and focal exocytosis of lymphocytes. The dermis contains a sparse mononuclear cell infiltrate. In HIV-infected patients, the epidermis contains apoptotic keratinocytes, and the dermal infiltrate usually contains plasma cells (31).

Pathogenesis. The pathogenesis is unknown, the role of *Malassezia sp.* (*Pityrosporum*) in the etiology is controversial, even though many patients have a good response to oral or topical ketoconazole (32,33).

Stasis Dermatitis

Patients with long-standing venous insufficiency and lower extremity edema may develop pruritic, erythematous, scaly papules, and plaques on the lower legs, often in association with brown pigmentation and hair loss. Ulceration is a frequent complication of long-standing statis dermatitis.

Histopathology. The variable epidermis is hyperkeratotic with focal parakeratosis, acanthosis, atrophy and focal spongiosis. There is proliferation of small blood vessels in the papillary dermis, forming lobular aggregates (glomeruloid proliferation). The proliferation may be florid, mimicking Kaposi's sarcoma (acroangiodermatitis) (34). There is a superficial perivascular lymphocytic infiltrate that surrounds thickened capillaries and venules. The reticular dermis is often fibrotic. Extravasated erythrocytes and hemosiderin are usually present superficially, but they may be identified about the deep vascular plexus as well.

Differential Diagnosis of Spongiotic Dermatitis

Acute spongiotic dermatitis may be seen histologically in pityriasis rosea, guttate parapsoriasis, spongiotic drug eruptions, arthropod bite reactions, and dermatophyte infections. Lesions of pityriasis rosea contain discontiguous suprapapillary, as opposed to diffuse, areas of spongiosis, exocytosis of lymphocytes, and overlying mounds of (lenticular) parakeratosis. The spongiosis varies from micro- to macro-vesicular. In addition, extravasated erythrocytes may be present within these foci in the epidermis. Guttate parapsoriasis is similar to pityriasis rosea, but it lacks the intraepidermal erythrocytes and has less lymphohistiocytic infiltrate. Spongiotic drug eruptions tend to have a deeper infiltrate with eosinophils than other forms of acute spongiotic dermatitis. In arthropod bite reactions, the epidermal changes are focal, corresponding to the site of attack, and the infiltrate is wedge-shaped. Bite or sting parts are often not found. A periodic acid–Schiff (PAS) stain is necessary to exclude dermatophyte infection.

Pityriasis lichenoides, dermatophyte infection, spongiotic drug eruption, or an arthropod bite reaction may show histopathologic features similar to subacute *spongiotic dermatitis*. In pityriasis lichenoides et varioliformis acuta, the lesions are circumscribed, and apoptotic keratinocytes, dry neutrophil-rich scale, bandlike interface dermatitis, areas of epidermal necrosis, and a deeper perivascular infiltrate are present. Dermatophyte infections characteristically have neutrophils within the stratum corneum, along with fungal hyphae; however, PAS stain is often necessary to identify the fungal hyphae.

Conditions that reveal *chronic dermatitis* include pellagra and other nutritional deficiencies, mycosis fungoides, and psoriasis, particularly if altered by therapy. In the nutritional deficiencies, upper epidermal pallor, necrosis, and neutrophilic infiltrate are characteristic. In mycosis fungoides, psoriasiform epidermal hyperplasia may be present, but the lymphocytes have nuclear atypia and cerebriform morphology with epidermotropism, in the absence of spongiosis. Lesions of psoriasis may resemble lichen simplex chronicus, but thinning of the suprapapillary plates, confluent parakeratosis, neutrophils within the stratum corneum and upper epidermis, and dilated tortuous capillaries are distinctive.

Other Disorders with Spongiotic Dermatitis

Erythroderma and Generalized Exfoliative Dermatitis

Erythroderma is characterized by generalized erythema and scale, often in association with fever. The eruption is nonspecific and may be caused by a variety of underlying conditions. In one study, 74.4% were associated with a pre-existing dermatosis, 14.6% were idiopathic, and 5.5% were related to drugs and malignancy (35). Psoriasis is the most common pre-existing dermatosis; others include spongiotic dermatitis, pityriasis rubra pilaris, photosensitivity syndromes, and, rarely, statis dermatitis, dermatophytosis, pemphigus foliaceus, and even bullous pemphigoid. Many drugs have been incriminated, such as phenytoin, thiazides, nonsteroidal anti-inflammatory drugs (NSAIDs), and recombinant cytokines. A small percentage of erythroderma is associated with lymphoma, most frequently cutaneous T-cell lymphoma, in the form of Sézary syndrome or erythrodermic mycosis fungoides. The "red man syndrome" is erythroderma without knowing underlying causes. Some cases may progress to mycosis fungoides after many years.

Histopathology. A careful search for histologic features of any of the above listed etiologies must be undertaken; however, the nature of underlying dermatosis is not always discernible in the erythrodermic phase, and the changes are often those of either a nonspecific subacute or chronic dermatitis. Erythrodermic lesions associated with underlying psoriasis resemble early lesions of psoriasis with only mild epidermal hyperplasia, mild spongiosis, mounds of parakeratosis with a few neutrophils, and red cell extravasation in the papillary dermis (36). Blood vessels in the upper dermis are usually dilated. In cases of erythroderma related to mycosis fungoides, atypical cells with cerebriform nuclei are present in the infiltrate. Eosinophils may be present. Drug-related cases may simulate mycosis fungoides with exocytosis, lymphocytic atypia, and presence of eosinophils. The presence of rare apoptotic keratinocytes may be a clue to drug etiology.

The histopathologic findings are helpful in establishing the etiologic diagnosis in only about 40% of cases (37). Repeat biopsies and hematologic studies at regular intervals are recommended in patients without definitive diagnosis.

Miliaria

Miliaria develops when sweating is associated with obstruction of the intraepidermal sweat duct. There are three types: miliaria crystallina, miliaria rubra, and miliaria profunda.

Miliaria crystallina develops when the sweat duct is obstructed within the stratum corneum. Asymptomatic, small, superficial, noninflammatory vesicles resembling dewdrops develop, mainly on the trunk, after severe sunburn or with profuse sweating during a febrile illness. The vesicles rapidly subside when sweating ceases or the horny layer overlying the vesicles exfoliates. In some cases, the eruption may be present at birth (38).

Miliaria rubra (prickly heat) ensues when the sweat duct is obstructed within the deeper layers of the epidermis. It generally develops during and after excessive sweating in skin covered by clothing. It may also occur after prolonged covering of the skin by occlusive polyethylene wraps. Anhidrosis and heat intolerance result, particularly when the trunk is occluded (39,40). The lesions consist of pruritic small papulovesicles surrounded by erythema. Pustules may develop.

Miliaria profunda usually develops after recurrent episodes of miliaria rubra, particularly in tropical climates. The sweat duct is occluded at the dermal–epidermal junction. Lesions are nonpruritic, flesh-colored papules and can result in widespread anhidrosis.

Histopathology. In miliaria crystallina, one observes intracorneal or subcorneal vesicles that are in continuity with the underlying sweat duct. A sparse to moderate infiltrate of neutrophils is seen at the periphery of the vesicle. The surrounding epidermis is spongiotic, and there is papillary dermal edema as well as sparse superficial perivascular inflammation.

In miliaria rubra, spongiotic vesicles are found in the stratum malpighii. Serial sectioning shows these vesicles to be in continuity with a sweat duct. Periductal lymphocyte infiltration and spongiosis are seen, as is an infiltrate in the underlying dermis (41) (Fig. 9-7). In many instances, the distal, intraepidermal sweat duct is filled with amorphous "casts" that are PAS-positive and diastase resistant.

In miliaria profunda, the features are similar to those of miliaria rubra but the inflammatory changes involve the lower epidermis and superficial dermis.

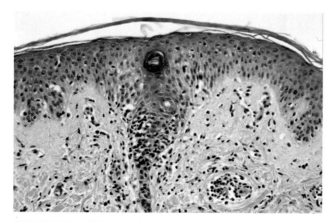

FIGURE 9-7. Miliaria rubra. There is spongiosis about and within the epidermal eccrine duct. Lymphocytes are present in the areas of spongiosis.

Pathogenesis. In miliaria crystallina, the obstruction of the sweat duct within the stratum corneum is caused either by mild damage to the epidermis from a preceding sunburn or by excessive hydration of the stratum corneum. In neonates, excess hydration of the stratum corneum in utero in combination with immature eccrine ducts may cause swelling of the ductal epithelial cells and occlusion of the duct (38).

In miliaria rubra, increased environmental temperature plays an important role (42). Aerobic bacteria are thought to contribute to the obstruction of the acrosyringium. In favor of this view are the frequent presence of *S. aureus* within the sweat ducts (43), and the fact that the development of miliaria rubra under an occlusive polyethylene film can be prevented by application of antibacterial solutions (44).

The PAS-positive, diastase-resistant, amorphous plug within the acrosyringium may occur as a result of injury to the luminal cells, inflammation, and ductal and periductal spongiosis. These changes occur after 48 hours of occlusion and resolve after 14 days, when old damaged stratum corneum is desquamated. Tape stripping can restore sweating, which supports a reversible high-level blockage (40).

Immunologic Deficiency Diseases Associated with Spongiotic Dermatitis

Familial Leiner's Disease

In this syndrome, infants develop generalized seborrheic dermatitis, severe diarrhea, recurrent local and systemic infections, and marked wasting. Death is usually due to septicemia. A dysfunction of the fifth component of complement (C5) exists, in addition to other cellular and humoral immune defects (45).

Hyperimmunoglobulin E Syndrome (Job's syndrome)

In this disease, patients have recurrent pyogenic infections, atopic dermatitis, extreme elevation of serum IgE, and defective neutrophil chemotaxis (46). The infectious complications include recurrent cold staphylococcal abscesses, furunculosis, otitis, sinusitis, and staphylococcal pneumonia (47).

Wiskott–Aldrich Syndrome

This X-linked recessive disorder affects males and is characterized by recurrent, systemic bacterial and viral infections, purpura due to thrombocytopenia, and an atopic dermatitis-like eruption. Because of progressive deterioration of cellular immunity, death due to infection or lymphoma ensues in the first decade of life (48).

Chronic Granulomatous Disease

This X-linked recessive disorder affects males, beginning in infancy with perioral dermatitis. The dermatitis often progresses to granulomatous lesions accompanied by cervical adenitis (49). Suppurative and granulomatous infections develop in the skin, lungs, bone, and liver, most commonly due to *S. aureus*. Death occurs in most cases in childhood or adolescence. The defect lies in decreased capacity of neutrophils to generate hydrogen peroxide and kill catalase-positive bacteria and fungi (50). *In vitro*, neutrophils are unable to reduce nitroblue tetrazolium dye after phagocytosis, a useful screening test for the disease.

PEMPHIGUS GROUP

As first demonstrated in 1943, acantholysis is the characteristic feature of the bullae of pemphigus (51). The acantholysis results from *in vivo* bound antibodies first discovered in 1964 (52). Pemphigus is now characterized as autoimmune blistering disease presenting clinically with flaccid intraepithelial blisters, erosions, and ulcerations of the skin and mucous membranes, histologically with acantholysis, and immunologically with *in vivo* bound and circulating autoantibodies against the cell-membrane components of keratinocytes important in cell–cell adhesion. These antibodies are demonstrable by direct immunofluorescence (DIF) testing of skin, and indirect immunofluorescence (IIF) testing of serum. The use of these techniques is now the accepted practice in the diagnosis of all anti-body-mediated primary vesiculobullous disorders (Table 9-4). Pemphigus can be divided into five types: (a) pemphigus vulgaris, with its reactive state, pemphigus vegetans; (b) pemphigus foliaceus, with its lupus-like variant, pemphigus erythematosus, and its endemic variant, fogo selvagem; (c) drug-induced pemphigus; (d) IgA pemphigus; and (e) paraneoplastic pemphigus.

Pathophysiology of Pemphigus

The target antigens of pemphigus (Table 9-5) are located in the desmosomes, the most prominent adhesion junctions in stratified squamous epithelium. The desmosome complex contains desmogleins and desmocollins as transmembrane constituents, and plakoglobin, plakophilin, and desmoplakin as cytoplasmic constituents (Fig. 9-8). Desmogleins and desmocollins are members of the cadherin supergene family (53,54), a group of calcium-dependent proteins that play an important role in the formation and maintenance of tissue integrity. The cadherin molecules form dimers as their functional unit, with the extracellular domain from one cell binding to an opposing cell. The cytoplasmic domain of the cadherin associates with plakoglobin, which links intermediate filaments (i.e., keratins) to the desmosome through desmoplakin. Three desmoglein and three democollin genes have been identified. Of the three desmogleins, desmoglein 1 is a 160-kD molecule that expressed primarily in the upper layers of the epidermis. It is the target antigen in pemphigus foliaceus. Desmoglein 2 is found in simple epithelia and basal epidermis. Des-

TABLE 9-4. DIRECT INFILTRATING INFLAMMATORY TESTING IN VESICULOBULLOUS DERMATOSES

Dermatosis	Principal Immunoreactant	Site	Pattern
Pemphigus, all variants except:	IgG	ICS	Lace-like
IgA pemphigus	IgA	ICS	Lace-like
Paraneoplastic pemphigus	IgG	ICS	Lace-like
	C3, IgG	BMZ	Linear
	C3, IgG	BMZ	Granular
Bullous pemphigoid	C3, IgG	BMZ	Linear
Cicatricial pemphigoid	C3, IgG	BMZ	Linear
Herpes gestationis	C3	BMZ	Linear
Epidermolysis bullosa acquisita	C3, IgG	BMZ	Linear
Bullous systemic lupus erythematosus	C3, IgG	BMZ	Linear
	C3, IgG	BMZ	Granular
Dermatitis herpetiformis	IgA	BMZ	Granular
Linear IgA dermatosis	IgA	BMZ	Linear
Erythema multiforme	C3, IgM	BMZ	Granular
	C3, IgM	Vessels	Granular
Porphyria/pseudoporphyria	IgG	BMZ	Glassy broad
Bullous dermatosis of hemodialysis	IgG	Vessels	Glassy broad

Note: Other immunoglobulins may be present, but they are less intense when present and less frequently observed.
ICS, squamous intercellular substance; BMZ, epidermal basement membrane zone.

TABLE 9-5. TARGET ANTIGENS IN PEMPHIGUS

Diseases	Auto-antibodies	Antigens	Location of Antigens
Pemphigus vulgaris			
Mucosal mainly	IgG	Desmoglein 3 (130 kD)	Desmosomes
Mucocutaneous	IgG	Desmoglein 3 (130 kD)	
		Desmoglein 1 (160 kD)	
Pemphigus foliaceus	IgG	Desmoglein 1 (160 kD)	Desmosomes
Paraneoplastic pemphigus	IgG	Desmoglein 1 (160 kD)	Desmosomes or hemidesmosomes
		Desmoglein 3 (130 kD)	
		Desmoplakin I (250 kD)	
		Envoplakin (210 kD)	
		Periplakin (190 kD)	
		Plectin (500 kD)	
		BPAG1 (230 kD)[a]	
		γ-Catenin (plakoglobin- 82 kD)	
Drug-induced pemphigus	IgG	Desmoglein 3 (130 kD)	Desmosomes
		Desmoglein 1 (160 kD)	
IgA pemphigus			
SPD type	IgA	Desmocollin 1 (110/100 kD)	Desmosomes
IEN type	IgA	Desmoglein 1 (160 kD)	
		Desmoglein 3 (130 kD)	

[a]BPAG1, bullous pemphigoid antigen.

moglein 3 is a 130-kD molecule that localizes primarily in the spinous layer and mucous membrane. It is the target antigen in pemphigus vulgaris (55). Since mucosal epithelium express mainly desmoglein 3 but skin expresses both desmoglein 1 and 3, damage by antibodies to desmoglein 3 results in oral lesions at an early stage of pemphigus vulgaris. If desmoglein 1 antibodies are present, cutaneous lesions appear to result and the disease tends to be more se-

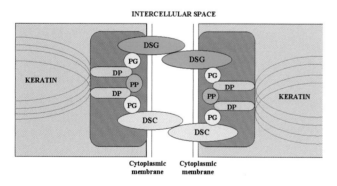

Dsg - Desmoglein   Dsc - Desmocollin   PG - Plakoglobin   DP - Desmoplakin   PP - Plakophilin

FIGURE 9-8. The desmosome. The desmosome complex includes desmogleins and desmocollins as transmembrane components, and plakoglobin, plakophilin, and desmoplakin as cytoplasmic components. The cytoplasmic domains of desmoglein and desmocollin associate with plakoglobin, which links intermediate filaments (keratin) to the desmosome through desmoplakin.

vere (55a). Less is known about the desmocollins. Some cases of IgA pemphigus have had autoantibodies to the desmocollins.

Pemphigus Vulgaris

This condition develops primarily in older individuals, presenting with large and flaccid bullae. They break easily and leave denuded areas that tend to increase in size by progressive peripheral detachment of the epidermis, leading in some cases to widespread cutaneous involvement. The lesions characteristically involve the oral mucosa, scalp, midface, sternum, groin, and pressure points. Oral lesions are almost invariably present and may be the first manifestation of the disease (10% of cases) (56). Before corticosteroids became available, mortality of this disease was high because of fluid loss and superinfection.

Histopathology. It is important that early blisters, preferably small ones, are selected for biopsy. Care should be given to keeping the epidermis attached to the dermis, since the torque applied in punch biopsies may separate the blister roof from the blister base. Therefore, one may use a refrigerant spray before excising the blister with a punch biopsy, or excise it with a scalpel. If no recent blister is available, an old one may be moved into the neighboring skin by gentle vertical pressure with a finger (positive Nikolsky sign) (57). The newly created cleavage will reveal early and specific histologic changes.

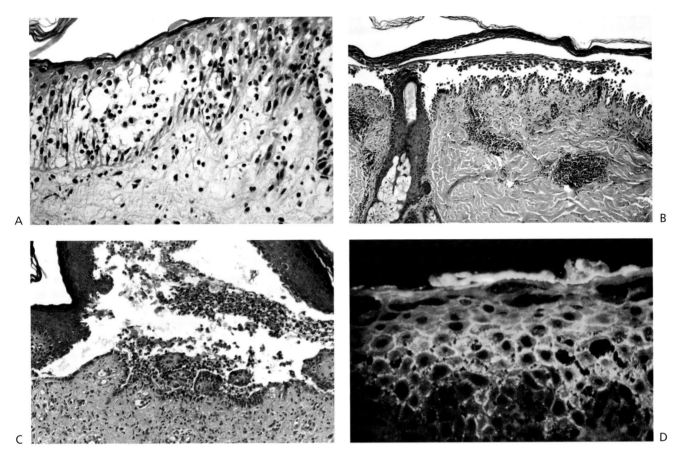

FIGURE 9-9. Pemphigus vulgaris. **(A)** The earliest changes consist of intercellular edema with eosinophilic spongiosis leading to loss of intercellular bridges in the lower epidermis. **(B)** An intraepidermal acantholytic blister has a suprabasal cleavage plane. Acantholysis may extend into adnexal structures and stratum spinosum. **(C)** The suprabasal blister contains acantholytic cells, neutrophils and eosinophils. Note the dermal papillae lined by a single layer of basal keratinocytes, so-called villi. **(D)** There is lace-like squamous intercellular space deposition of IgG in the lower epidermis (direct immunofluorescence).

The earliest recognized change may be either rare eosinophilic spongiosis, or more commonly, "spongiosis" in the lower epidermis (Fig. 9-9A). This "spongiosis" may actually represent the earliest manifestation of acantholysis rather than true spongiosis as defined earlier. Acantholysis leads first to the formation of clefts, and then to blisters in a predominantly suprabasal location (58,59) (Fig. 9-9B and C). The intraepithelial acantholysis may extend into adnexal structures, or occasionally be higher in the stratum spinosum. The basal keratinocytes, although separated from one another through the loss of attachment, remain firmly attached to the dermis like a "row of tombstones" (58). Within the blister cavity, the acantholytic keratinocytes, singularly or in clusters, have rounded, condensed cytoplasm about an enlarged nucleus with peripherally palisaded chromatin and enlarged nucleoli. There is little inflammation in the early phase of blister formation. If present, it is usually a sparse, lymphocytic perivascular infiltrate accompanied by dermal edema. If, however, eosinophilic spongiosis is apparent, numerous eosinophils may infiltrate the dermis. The phenomenon of eosinophilic spongiosis occurs occasionally in other blistering diseases, particularly in their early phases, including acute contact dermatitis, pemphigus foliaceus, bullous pemphigoid, herpes gestationis, drug eruptions, spongiotic arthropod bite reactions (60), and transient acantholytic dermatosis. Several important changes ensue as the lesions age. First, a mixed inflammatory cell reaction consisting of neutrophils, lymphocytes, macrophages, and eosinophils may develop (58). Because of the instability of the blister roof, erosion and ulceration may occur. Older blisters may also have several layers of keratinocytes at the blister base because of keratinocyte migration and proliferation. Lastly, there may be considerable downward growth of epidermal strands, giving rise to so-called villi (Fig. 9-9C). The evaluation of patients with only oral lesions is difficult, because intact blisters are rarely encountered due to the trauma of mastication, and biopsies may show only erosion and ulceration. Indeed, it is best to sample the edge of a denuded area with intact mucosa in an attempt to demonstrate the typical pathologic changes. Clinicians frequently cannot distinguish between an ulcer and the intact mucosa, as both are often white and shaggy. In patients with only oral lesions, biopsies of intact oral mucosa for DIF testing are more sensitive than biopsies of lesions for routine light microscopic evaluation (61). However, biopsy from the maxillary and upper buccal mucosa is necessary when there is extensive ulceration. Serum constituents may invade into the squamous intercellular substance. Cytologic examination using a Tzanck preparation is useful for the rapid demonstration of acantholytic epidermal keratinocytes in the blisters of pemphigus vulgaris. For this purpose, a smear is taken from the underside of the roof and from the base of an early, freshly opened bulla. Giemsa stain is applied with subsequent rinsing and air-drying (62). Because acantholytic keratinocytes are occasionally seen in various nonacantholytic vesiculobullous or pustular diseases as a result of secondary acantholysis, cytologic examination represents merely a preliminary test and should not supplant histologic examination (63).

Immunofluorescence Testing. The edge of a blister with intact surrounding normal skin, uninvolved skin adjacent to a blister or adjacent erythematous skin should be supplied for study. The tissue may be snap-frozen or transported in Michel's medium. DIF testing is a very reliable and sensitive diagnostic test for pemphigus vulgaris, in that it demonstrates IgG in the squamous intercellular/cell surface areas in up to 95% of cases, including early cases and those with very few lesions, and in up to 100% of cases with active disease (64) (Fig. 9-9D). It remains positive, often for many years after clinical disease has subsided (65). Negative DIF findings when the patient is in remission may be a good prognostic indicator (66). At this time, DIF testing is incorrectly thought by most to be free of false positives; however, false positives may occur. On occasion, it may be difficult to distinguish intercellular staining of pemphigus from nonspecific staining that may occur, for example, in spongiotic dermatitis, psoriasis, bullous impetigo, and epidermis adjacent to ulcers secondary to a number of disorders may have squamous intercellular substance IgG due to insulation of serum into the intercellular substance. Often IgM, IgA, fibrinogen, and albumin are present as well indicating nonspecific insulation and trapping in the false-positive tests.

In recent years, immunoperoxidase methods have achieved roughly the same sensitivity as the IF method, but they have not replaced IF testing as the prime diagnostic tool (67,68).

Unfixed frozen sections of guinea pig esophagus, monkey esophagus (65), or normal human skin (69) are used as substrate for indirect IF testing. In general, monkey esoph-

agus is the best substrate for IIF studies. IgG is demonstrated in the squamous intercellular substance in 80% to 90% of cases (70), and the titer correlates with disease activity (71). False-positive indirect tests occur. In a series of 1500 patients with circulating pemphigus antibodies, approximately 1% had no evidence of clinical disease (72). Antibodies that mimic or that may give *in vitro* deposition in stratified squamous epithelium in the absence of pemphigus have been reported in burns, penicillin allergy, toxic epidermal necrolysis, systemic lupus erythematosus, myasthenia gravis, bullous pemphigoid, cicatricial pemphigoid, lichen planus, and in patients with antibodies directed against blood groups A and B (72–74). Such antibodies are present in low titer and are thought to be nonpathogenic. Antidesmoglein autoantibodies are sometimes found in patients with no bullous disease. For example, they have been found in patients with silicosis (75), and in relatives of patients with pemphigus vulgaris (76).

Pathogenesis. Compelling evidence has accumulated that IgG autoantibodies against desmoglein 3 and desmoglein 1 are pathogenic and play a primary role in inducing the blister formation in pemphigus. Affinity-purified IgG from pemphigus vulgaris sera recognized the extracellular domain of desmoglein 3 and cause suprabasal acantholysis when injected into neonatal mice (77). Furthermore, when antidesmoglein 3 IgG from pemphigus vulgaris is immunoabsorbed with the extracellular domains of desmoglein 3, those sera no longer have the ability to cause blisters in neonatal mice (78). Although the pathogenic role of antidesmoglein 3 autoantibodies in blister formation is assured, the exact sequence of events that occur after antibody binding is not totally understood. Conformational epitope mapping of desmoglein 3 in pemphigus vulgaris suggest that the amino terminal residue 1–161 is the target of autoantibodies (79). This segment is in the extracellular domain that is essential for cell–cell adhesion. One possibility is that these antibodies interfere directly with the adhesive interaction of desmogleins between cells by steric hindrance. Another possibility is that the disruption of cell–cell adhesion is mediated by signal transduction. Proteinases, likely induced by pemphigus antigen–antibody union, are thought to play an important role in acantholysis (80). Although complement fixation by pemphigus antibody may promote acantholysis (81), acantholysis occurs in experimental systems in the absence of complement (80). What stimulates the formation of autoantibodies is unknown, although drugs, viral infection, trauma, ionizing radiation, and PUVA therapy have been implicated because they preceded the onset of pemphigus. Pemphigus vulgaris is rarely associated with internal cancer, Castleman's disease, thymoma, myasthenia gravis, localized scleroderma, Grave's disease, and systemic lupus erythematosus.

Ultrastructural Study. The intercellular cement substance, or glycocalyx, is partially or entirely resolved in lesions with early acantholysis (82). There is widening of the intercellular spaces with intact desmosomes. As the intercellular space is widened, there is separation of the two opposing attachment plaques of the desmosomes, so that single attachment plaques, with adherent tonofilaments, are seen at the periphery of keratinocytes (83). As acantholysis progresses, the desmosomes gradually disappear and the keratinocytes develop numerous cytoplasmic processes that often interdigitate with one another. All of the early ultrastructural changes in pemphigus vulgaris are extracellular. Only subsequent to the dissolution of the desmosomes does retraction of the tonofilaments to the perinuclear area develop with ultimate degeneration of the acantholytic cells. The cohesion of the basal keratinocytes with the basement membrane zone is not affected in pemphigus vulgaris because of the preservation of structures connecting the basal keratinocytes with the dermis. Immunoelectron microscopy shows that the immunoglobulins are deposited on the surface of the keratinocytes in a discontinuous globular pattern in the extracellular domains of desmosomes (84).

Differential Diagnosis. In early blisters that are free of secondary changes, such as the degeneration or regeneration of epidermal cells, the histopathology of pemphigus vulgaris is characteristic. Important differential diagnoses include Hailey–Hailey disease and transient acantholytic dermatosis. Hailey–Hailey disease has full-thickness ("dilapidated brick wall") acantholysis, epidermal hyperplasia, and an impetiginized scale crust. The acantholysis does not extend down follicles as it does in pemphigus. Transient acantholytic dermatosis may exhibit small foci of intraepidermal acantholysis, but these are only a few retia wide in contrast to the uniform widespread acantholysis observed in biopsies of pemphigus vulgaris. Disorders that are characterized by focal acantholytic dyskeratosis are readily separated from pemphigus vulgaris by the presence of abnormal granular keratinocytes and parakeratotic cells, so-called corps ronds and corps grains. Although light microscopic examination of pemphigus lesions is important, positive DIF is the gold standard in diagnosis at this time, and must be pursued in all cases in which pemphigus vulgaris is considered.

Pemphigus Vegetans

This is an uncommon variant of pemphigus vulgaris, comprising only 1% to 2% of cases (64,70). Historically, pemphigus vegetans has been divided into the Neumann type and Hallopeau type. In the Neumann type, the disease begins and ends as pemphigus vulgaris, but many of the denuded areas heal with verrucous vegetations that may contain small pustules in early stages. The Hallopeau type is relatively benign, having pustules as the primary lesions instead of bullae. Their development is followed by the formation of gradually enlarging verrucous vegetations, especially in intertriginous areas (58).

Histopathology. In the Neumann type, the early lesions consist of bullae and denuded areas that have the same histologic picture as that of pemphigus vulgaris. As the lesions age, however, there is formation of villi and verrucous epidermal hyperplasia. Numerous eosinophils are present within the epidermis and dermis, producing both eosinophilic spongiosis and eosinophilic pustules (Fig. 9-10A). Acantholysis may not be present in older lesions. In the Hallopeau type, the early lesions consist of pustules arising on normal skin with acantholysis and formation of small clefts, many in a suprabasal location. The clefts are filled with numerous eosinophils and degenerated acantholytic epidermal cells (Fig. 9-10B). Early lesions may reveal more eosinophilic abscesses than in the Neumann type (85). The subsequent verrucous lesions are histologically identical to the Neumann type.

Immunofluorescence Testing. DIF examination reveals squamous intercellular IgG in all reported cases (86,87).

Pathogenesis. Pemphigus vegetans is a variant of pemphigus vulgaris in which verrucous vegetations develop. It is unclear why such vegetations develop in some cases of

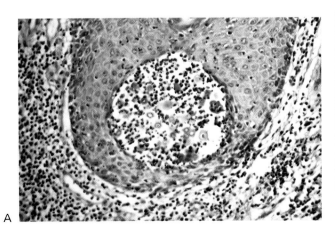
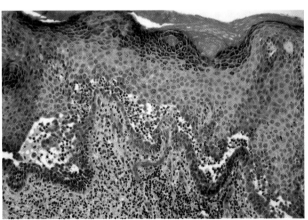

A   B

FIGURE 9-10. Pemphigus vegetans. **(A)** Intraepidermal abscesses are composed of eosinophils and a few acantholytic keratinocytes. **(B)** There is marked acanthosis and suprabasal clefts containing eosinophils.

pemphigus vulgaris and not in others. However, they tend to develop in areas of relative occlusion and maceration with subsequent bacterial infection suggesting a response to superinfection.

Differential Diagnosis. The principal differential diagnosis is pyoderma vegetans, a condition often associated with inflammatory bowel disease, particularly ulcerative colitis. It can mimic pemphigus vegetans clinically and histologically (88). In pyoderma vegetans, neutrophils are more commonly found, and intraepidermal eosinophilic abscesses and acantholysis are rare. Direct immunofluorescence is negative in pyoderma vegetans (88). Halogenoderma and blastomycosis-like pyoderma must be excluded as well (Chapters 11 and 21).

Pemphigus Foliaceus

Usually developing in middle-aged individuals, pemphigus foliaceus may have a chronic generalized course or may rarely present as an exfoliative dermatitis. Patients may present with flaccid bullae that usually arise on an erythematous base or as scaling patches without evident blisters. Erythema, oozing, and crusting are present. Because of their superficial location, the blisters break easily, leaving shallow erosions rather than the denuded areas seen in pemphigus vulgaris. Oral lesions do not occur. The Nikolsky sign is positive, and Tzanck preparation reveals acantholytic granular keratinocytes. Fogo selvagem (endemic pemphigus foliaceus) is clinically, histologically, and immunologically indistinguishable from pemphigus foliaceus (89,90). It develops in those who live or visit areas close to rivers and streams in Brazil, the peak incidence being at the end of the rainy season. The cause of fogo selvagem is unknown, but substantial epidemiologic evidence suggests that it is precipitated by an environmental factor. A case control study found that farmers exposed to black fly (*Simulium pruinosum*) bites were much more likely to develop fogo selvagem than farmers who were not bitten (91). Sunlight may exacerbate the condition (92).

Histopathology. The earliest change consists of acantholysis in the upper epidermis, within or adjacent to the granular layer, leading to a subcorneal bulla in some instances (Fig. 9-11A and B). More commonly, enlargement of the cleft leads to detachment of the stratum corneum without bulla being seen. The number of acantholytic keratinocytes is usually small, often requiring a careful search to identify them. Secondary clefts may develop, leading to detachment of the epidermis in its mid level. These clefts may extend to above the basal layer, rarely giving rise to limited areas of suprabasal separation (93). In the setting of a subcorneal blister, dyskeratotic granular keratinocytes are diagnostic for this disorder. Eosinophilic spongiosis may be prominent with intraepidermal eosinophilic pustules (94–96). Thus, the histologic features of pemphigus foliaceus may have three patterns: (a) eosinophilic spongiosis;

(b) a subcorneal blister, often with few acantholytic keratinocytes; and (c) a subcorneal blister with dyskeratotic granular keratinocytes (Fig. 9-11B), diagnostic for this disorder. The character of the inflammatory infiltrate is variable and depends on the age of the lesion, whether a blister is present, whether the superficial portion of the epidermis has been detached, and whether there is impetiginization or necrosis of the blister roof.

Immunofluorescence Testing. DIF testing of perilesional skin is positive in the vast majority of cases. Two patterns of pemphigus antibody deposition have been described. In most cases, there is full-thickness squamous intercellular substance deposition of IgG. Rarely, IgG may be localized only to the superficial portion of the epidermis (97) (Fig. 9-11C). IIF testing of serum reveals squamous intercellular substance deposition of IgG in 80% to 90% of cases (73).

Pathogenesis. As in pemphigus vulgaris, the autoantibodies of pemphigus foliaceus are pathogenic. During the course of the disease, the antibody levels fluctuate, and have some correlation with disease activity. The pemphigus foliaceus antigen, desmoglein 1 is expressed more intensely in the upper layers of the epidermis (55), which explains the superficial cleavage plane of pemphigus foliaceus. Interestingly, in staphylococcal scald skin syndrome (SSSS), the exfoliative exotoxin produced by *S. aureus* specifically binds and cleaves desmoglein 1, resulting in blister formation at identical levels of pemphigus foliaceus (98). In addition, desmoglein 1 is concentrated in the upper torso, and is less prominent in the buccal mucosa, scalp, and lower torso, correlating with lesion distribution (99). Recently, there is a report of a subset of pemphigus foliaceus patients exhibiting pathogenic autoantibodies against both desmoglein 1 and desmoglein 3 (100). Similarly, patients with pemphigus vulgaris similar to this subset of patients may have antibodies to desmoglein 1 and desmoglein 3 in various quantities, possibly explaining the variable (high to mid to superficial) cleavage plane in the epidermis in some patients.

Ultrastructural Study. There is early loss of intercellular cement substance within the lower epidermis associated with a decrease in the number of desmosomes and formation of tortuous microvilli from the keratinocyte surface. However, acantholysis is most pronounced in the upper layers of the epidermis (82,83). In the mid-epidermis, many keratinocytes have perinuclear arrangement of the tonofilaments and homogenization of the perinuclear tonofilament bundles as evidence of dyskeratosis. Marked dyskeratosis distinguishes pemphigus foliaceus from pemphigus vulgaris (101).

Differential Diagnosis. The differential diagnosis includes SSSS, impetigo, and subcorneal pustular dermatosis (Sneddon–Wilkinson). IF testing may be required to separate SSSS from pemphigus foliaceus, since a small number of acantholytic cells may be observed in SSSS. The lesions of pemphigus foliaceus may become impetiginized and sec-

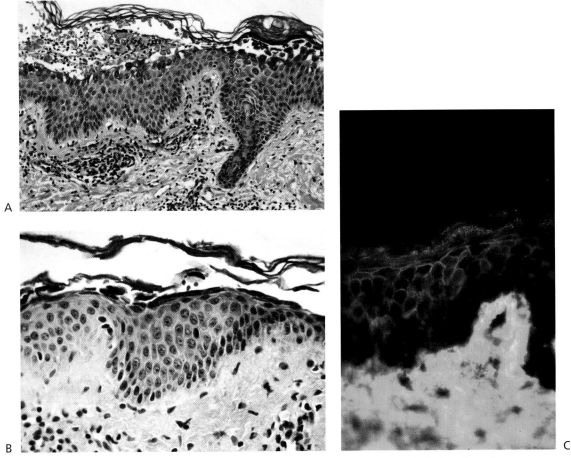

FIGURE 9-11. Pemphigus foliaceus. **(A)** A subcorneal blister with acantholytic cells and neutrophils in the cavity. **(B)** In the setting of a subcorneal blister, these dyskeratotic acantholytic granular cells are diagnostic of pemphigus foliaceus. **(C)** The intercellular IgG is deposited in the intercellular spaces throughout the epidermis. Rarely, as in this case, the IgG is present in greater quantity in the superficial layers.

ondarily altered, producing pustules as in impetigo and subcorneal pustular dermatosis. Pemphigus foliaceus contains more acantholytic keratinocytes than do the other two disorders, and pustules are the primary lesions in subcorneal pustular dermatosis. Because the lesions of pemphigus foliaceus may become superinfected, the finding of bacteria does not confirm a diagnosis of bullous impetigo; therefore, IF testing is critical. Subcorneal pustular dermatosis usually produces large dome-shaped subcorneal pustules rather than the flaccid flat pustules of pemphigus foliaceus.

Pemphigus Erythematosus

Also known as Senear–Usher syndrome, pemphigus erythematosus is a variant of pemphigus foliaceus that gets its name from its lupus erythematosus–like clinical appearance, in which the erythematous plaques and patches are in a butterfly distribution. They may remain localized to this area or may become generalized. No oral lesions are observed (102).

Histopathology. The light microscopic features are identical to those of pemphigus foliaceus (58,103) (Fig. 9-12). Interface dermatitis may also be apparent in rare cases, making distinction from lupus erythematosus difficult.

Immunofluorescence Testing. DIF testing of perilesional skin reveals squamous intercellular substance deposition of IgG in greater than 75% of cases, and granular deposition of IgM and IgG (i.e., a positive lupus band test) at the dermo–epidermal junction. IIF studies using monkey esophagus as substrate reveal squamous intercellular substance deposition of IgG in 80% of cases. Antinuclear antibodies are observed in 30% to 80% of cases (102).

Ultrastructural Study. Pemphigus erythematosus is identical to pemphigus foliaceus in its ultrastructural alterations.

Differential Diagnosis. The differential diagnosis is the same as in pemphigus foliaceus. The presence of interface dermatitis in some cases leads to confusion with lupus ery-

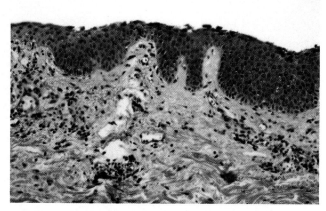

FIGURE 9-12. Pemphigus erythematosus. The histologic appearances are identical to those of pemphigus foliaceus. In this biopsy, the roof of the blister is eroded, a frequent event, leaving a diminished but acantholytic granular layer.

thematosus and paraneoplastic pemphigus. Subcorneal acantholysis is not a feature of lupus erythematosus.

Pemphigus Herpetiformis

Pemphigus herpetiformis combines the clinical features of dermatitis herpetiformis with the immunologic and histologic features of pemphigus, usually the foliaceus type (104). This variant deserves recognition only because of its clinical presentation. Patients present with pruritic, erythematous, vesicular, or papular lesions, often in herpetiform pattern. Mucous membranes are uncommonly involved.

Histopathology. There is eosinophilic spongiosis with or without acantholysis. Variable numbers of neutrophils may be present, leading to neutrophilic spongiosis or subcorneal pustules with both eosinophils and neutrophils.

Immunofluorescence Testing. Because the clinical presentation and histologic findings are often atypical, the most reliable basis for diagnosis of pemphigus herpetiformis is immunopathology. Direct immunofluorescence on perilesional skin shows the deposition of IgG on the surface of keratinocytes primarily in the upper epidermis (104). Indirect immunofluorescence has demonstrated circulating IgG antiepithelial cell surface autoantibodies in most patients with pemphigus herpetiformis. Most cases have circulating antibodies to desmoglein I, the pemphigus foliaceus antigen. A few cases with antibodies to the pemphigus vulgaris antigen, desmoglein 3, have been reported (105).

Drug-Induced Pemphigus

Although immunologic features identical to those of idiopathic pemphigus are reported in most cases of drug-induced pemphigus (106), evidence indicates that some drugs may induce acantholysis without production of anti-

bodies (107). The offending drugs, most frequently penicillamine, captopril, and penicillin derivatives, often contain sulfhydryl groups (108). The earliest clinical manifestation is that of a nonspecific morbilliform or urticarial eruption. In penicillamine-induced pemphigus, the eruption is characteristic and has been labeled "toxic prepemphigus rash" (107,109). Subsequently, the characteristic lesions of pemphigus develop. Upon cessation of drug therapy, the rash regresses in those patients who do *not* have pemphigus antibodies in contrast to those patients with pemphigus antibodies, in whom the rash frequently persists. This latter subset has the clinical waxing and waning course of pemphigus.

Histopathology. The findings in the early eruption are nonspecific, consisting of spongiosis, parakeratosis, and a variable dermal infiltrate. Well-developed lesions are essentially identical to those of pemphigus foliaceus or pemphigus vulgaris. Eosinophilic spongiosis may be prominent.

Immunofluorescence Testing. DIF testing is positive in approximately 90% of patients with drug-induced pemphigus (107,110). IIF study of serum reveals circulating squamous intercellular substance IgG antibodies in 70% of cases (110). The antibody titers are usually low and do not appear to correlate with the severity of disease (109).

Pathogenesis. In those cases in which there is antibody production with subsequent acantholysis, the pathogenesis appears to be identical to that of idiopathic pemphigus. Because the pemphigus antigens have disulfide bonds, sulfhydryl-containing drugs may bind to them (111,112). These drugs have been shown to localize in high concentration in the epidermis. Therefore, the drug appears to directly affect the keratinocyte adhesion molecules, interferes with their function, and causes subsequent acantholysis, explaining those cases of drug-induced pemphigus that do not have pemphigus antibodies.

IgA Pemphigus

IgA pemphigus is a pruritic pustular eruption characterized by squamous intercellular IgA deposits and intraepidermal neutrophils. It occurs primarily in middle-aged and elderly individuals, but several cases have been described in children (113,114). The clinical findings are similar to those in pemphigus foliaceus or subcorneal pustular dermatosis. There are flaccid pustules that arise on an erythematous base. They often appear in an annular arrangement (115). The most common sites of involvement are the axilla and groin, but the trunk, proximal extremities, and lower abdomen can also be involved. Mucous membrane involvement is rare. Mild leukocytosis, eosinophilia, and IgA kappa paraproteinemia may be present (116).

IgA pemphigus is a clinically heterogeneous group reflecting differences in the autoantigens involved (117). In general, patients may develop one of two types: a subcorneal pustular dermatosis (SPD) type, or an intraepider-

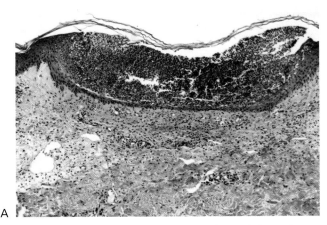
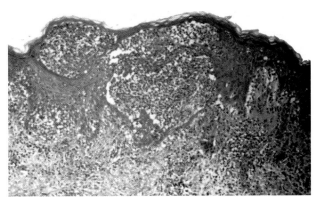

A

B

FIGURE 9-13. IgA pemphigus. **(A)** In subcorneal pustular dermatosis type, intraepidermal pustule with numerous neutrophils is seen subcorneally. **(B)** In intraepidermal neutrophilic type, the neutrophils are in the suprabasal and stratum spinosum.

mal neutrophilic dermatosis (IEN) type (113,118,119). The presence of cases with overlap features supports the notion that this is one disease with variable expression.

Histopathology. Two patterns are observed that parallel the two clinical presentations (Fig. 9-13A and B). In the SPD type, there are subcorneal vesicopustules or pustules with minimal acantholysis. In the IEN type, there are intraepidermal vesicopustules or pustules contain small to moderate numbers of neutrophils. One case of IgA pemphigus, which resembled pemphigus foliaceus without neutrophil infiltration, has been described (120).

Immunofluorescence Testing. DIF testing reveals IgA deposition in the squamous intercellular substance throughout the epidermis with increased intensity in the upper layers in some cases of the subcorneal pustular type. Complement and other immunoglobulins are usually not present (113). However, some cases may have both IgG and IgA present and thus may make a specific diagnosis difficult (i.e., pemphigus vulgaris vs. IgA pemphigus) unless evaluation for antigen specificity is available (121). IIF results are positive in fewer than 50% of reported cases (122–125). In the SPD type, IgA autoantibodies were shown to recognize desmocollin 1 (126). In the IEN type, the autoantigens remain to be identified; the antibodies have been variously characterized as reacting to desmoglein 1 or desmoglein 3 in a subset of patients (117,127,128).

Differential Diagnosis. The subcorneal pustular dermatosis variant is identical to Sneddon–Wilkinson disease. Indeed, many cases reported as Sneddon–Wilkinson disease, in which IF testing was not performed, likely represent the subcorneal pustular dermatosis variant of IgA pemphigus. Pustular psoriasis, bullous impetigo, and pemphigus vulgaris are the principal differential diagnoses. Pustular psoriasis may not be distinguishable on routine light microscopic study, and therefore IF testing may be required.

Paraneoplastic Autoimmune Multiorgan Syndrome: Paraneoplastic Pemphigus

Paraneoplastic pemphigus (PNP), originally described by Anhalt (129), was shown to be associated with underlying neoplasms. The most commonly associated neoplasms included non-Hodgkin's lymphoma (42%), chronic lymphocytic leukemia (29%), Castleman's disease (10%), thymoma (6%), spindle cell sarcoma (6%), and Waldenström's macroglobulinemia (6%). The age of onset is variable, although the majority of patients are between the ages of 45 and 70 years.

Cutaneous lesions are quite polymorphic. The most consistent clinical feature of PNP is the presence of intractable stomatitis, which present as erosion and ulceration that affect all surfaces of the oropharynx and characteristically extend onto the lips mimicking Stevens–Johnson syndrome. Small airway occlusion, secondary to pulmonary epithelial injury can be fatal. Autoantibodies are deposited in the kidneys, bladder, and muscle. The extent and diversity of the clinical presentations and immunopathologic mechanisms led to the suggestion that PNP, a disease of epithelial adhesion, represents one manifestation of a heterogeneous autoimmune syndrome, paraneoplastic autoimmune multiorgan syndrome (PAMS) (129a). At least six different clinical variants are recognized: bullous pemphigoid-like, cicatricial pemphigoid-like, pemphigus-like, erythema multiforme-like, graft-versus-host disease–like, and lichen planus-like (129a,130–132,132a,132b).

Histopathology. The histologic features are variable, depending on the various clinical presentations. The lesions show a unique combination of erythema multiforme-like, lichen planus-like, pemphigus vulgaris-like and pemphigoid-like features. The principal findings are suprabasal

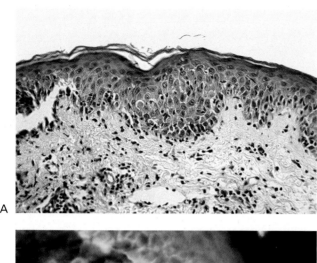

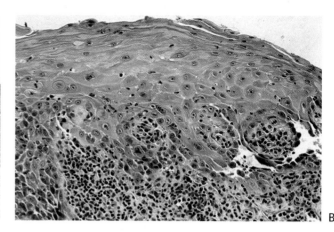

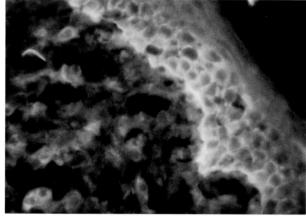

FIGURE 9-14. Paraneoplastic pemphigus. **(A)** Erythema multiforme-like pattern. There is a cell-poor interface dermatitis with apoptosis of keratinocytes. There are also pemphigus vulgaris-like changes with a suprabasal blister. **(B)** Lichen planus-like pattern. There is a cell-rich lichenoid dermatitis associated with a suprabasal blister. **(C)** There are both intercellular and basement membrane staining with IgG by direct immunofluorescence.

acantholysis as seen in pemphigus vulgaris with, in addition, basal apoptosis, in association with a vacuolar interface dermatitis (erythema multiforme-like) with or without lichenoid inflammation (lichen planus-like) (133) (Fig. 9-14A and B). Paraneoplastic pemphigus may present exclusively with lichenoid interface dermatitis in the absence of acantholysis (134). In pemphigoid-like lesions, a subepidermal blister is present (132b).

Immunofluorescence Testing. DIF testing of perilesional skin and mucosa reveals IgG in the squamous intercellular substance in concert with immune reactant deposition at the dermo–epidermal junction (Fig. 9-14C). At the dermo–epidermal junction, granular deposition of complement is noted most frequently (131). Linear deposition of complement, IgG, and IgM, and granular deposition of complement and IgG have been identified in one case each (130). When present, basement membrane zone staining helps to distinguish PNP from other forms of pemphigus in which basement membrane zone immunoglobulin and complement deposition are generally not present (135). Whereas circulating PNP antibodies bind to squamous keratinocytes in routine substrates in the majority of cases, the antibodies bind to rat bladder epithelium in all cases.

Pathogenesis. Patients with PNP (PNP) develop IgG autoantibodies against multiple antigens (Table 9-5). It ap-

pears that all the members of the plakin family, as well as desmogleins, are targeted by IgG autoantibodies in PNP. While antidesmoglein antibodies play a role in inducing the loss of cellular adhesion of keratinocytes and blister formation, the pathophysiologic relevance of the antiplakin autoantibodies is unclear. The intracellular location of plakin proteins makes them unlikely initial targets. One could speculate that damage to cell membranes induced by antidesmoglein IgG provides access into the cell for antiplakin autoantibodies; the latter then bind to their target antigens, inhibit their functions, and perhaps precipitate some of the unique features of PNP, such as dyskeratosis. In addition to the humoral autoimmunity, autoreactive cellular responses mediated by CD8+ cytotoxic T-lymphocytes, natural killer cells, and monocytes/macrophages appear to be important in the pathogenesis of PAMS (129a).

SUBEPIDERMAL BULLOUS DISEASE

Subepidermal bullous diseases are disorders in which a blister forms along the dermo–epidermal junction. This group of diseases includes conditions with different clinical presentations, histologic findings, and pathogenesis. Both inherited and acquired alterations in key adhesion proteins at

TABLE 9-6. TARGETS COMMON TO AUTOIMMUNE AND INHERITED BLISTERING DISEASES

Protein Target	Structural Target	Autoimmune Disease	Genetic Disease
BPAG1 (BP230)	HD	BP	None identified
BPAG2 (BP180, type XVII collagen)	HD-anchoring filament complexes	BP, PG, CP, LABD	GABEB
A6β4 integrin subunit β4	HD-anchoring filament complexes	Ocular CP	Junctional EB with pyloric atresia
Laminin 5	Lamina lucida-lamina densa interface	Antiepiligrin CP	Junctional EB–Herlitz
Type VII collagen	Anchoring fibrils	EB acquisita, bullous systemic lupus erythematosus	Dystrophic EB

BP, bullous pemphigoid; CP, cicatricial pemphigoid; EB, epidermolysis bullosa; HD, hemidesmosome; PG, pemphigoid gestationis; LABD, linear IgA bullous dermatosis.

or in dermo–epidermal junction result in blister formation. In the subgroup of autoimmune subepidermal bullous diseases, major target antigens bound by autoantibodies from patients have been characterized (Table 9-6). Importantly, some of the genes encoding these autoantigens harbor mutations responsible for various mechanobullous diseases, that is, epidermolysis bullosa (EB). To understand subepidermal bullous disease, it is essential to have some knowledge of the epidermal basement membrane zone and the various target proteins associated with it (Fig. 9-15).

Proceeding from the epidermis to the dermis, there are four distinct structural components of the epidermal basement membrane:

- Intermediate filament, hemidesmosomal plaques, and plasma membranes of the basal keratinocytes
- Lamina lucida that contains delicate anchoring filaments connecting hemidesmosomes in basal keratinocytes to the underlying lamina densa
- Lamina densa that provides the basement membrane with much of its strength. The main component is type IV collagen
- Sublaminar densa region containing anchoring fibrils (type VII collagen), anchoring plaques, and filamentous proteins of the papillary dermis

Along the basal surface of the keratinocytes of dermo–epidermal junction, keratin intermediate filaments (keratin 5 and 14) attach to hemidesmosomes (HD) on the basal plasma membrane. Major intracellular components of HD include the 230-kD bullous pemphigoid antigen (BPAg1) and plectin. The transmembrane components of the HD include α6β4 integrin and the 180-kD bullous pemphigoid antigen (BPAg2). Both extend to the lamina lucida at the site where anchoring filaments are located. The anchoring filaments straddle the lamina lucida between HD and the lamina densa. Antibodies to the BPAg1 are of the most common autoimmune subepidermal bullous disease, bullous pemphigoid (136). BPAg2 is targeted by autoantibodies from patients with bullous pemphigoid, pemphigoid gestationis (PG), cicatricial pemphigoid (CP), and a subgroup of linear IgA bullous dermatosis (LABD) (137–139). Some patients with generalized atrophic benign epidermolysis bullosa (GABEB) have a congenital deficiency of BPAg2. Mutation of the β4 subunit of α6β4 integrin leads to junctional EB associated with pyloric atresia (140).

The lamina lucida is the weakest link in the dermo–epidermal junction and it is the cleavage plane in salt-split skin. Multiple antigens are associated with the lamina lucida, particularly the anchoring filaments. The antigens include laminin 5, laminin 6, uncein, nidogen, and epiligrin. Autoantibodies to epiligrin, the α3 subunit of laminin 5, result in one form of cicatricial pemphigoid. Nonsense mutations of the laminin 5 gene are associated

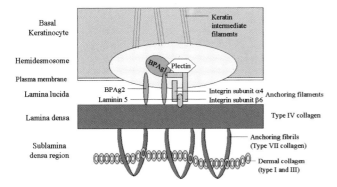

FIGURE 9-15. Schematic model of dermoepidermal junction. Along the basal surface of the keratinocytes, keratin intermediate filaments attach to hemidesmosomes (HD) on the basal plasma membrane. Major intracellular components of HD include the bullous pemphigoid antigen (BPAg1) and plectin. The transmembrane components of the HD include α6β4 integrin and the bullous pemphigoid antigen (BPAg2). Both extend to the lamina lucida at the site where anchoring filaments are located. The anchoring filaments straddle the lamina lucida between HD and the lamina densa. Multiple antigens are associated with the lamina lucida, including laminin 5 and epiligrin. The lamina densa is an electron-dense layer that lies parallel and contiguous to the lamina lucida. The main component is type IV collagen. In the sublamina densa region, the lamina densa and the overlying epidermis are tethered to the papillary dermis by anchoring fibrils. Type VII collagen is the major component of anchoring fibrils.

with the Herlitz subtype of junctional epidermolysis bullosa (141).

The lamina densa is an electron-dense layer that lies parallel to and contiguous to the lamina lucida. The main component is type IV collagen, which is thought to provide the basement membrane with much of its strength. Other antigenic components are laminin 1, nidogen, and heparan sulfate proteoglycans.

In the sublamina densa region, the lamina densa and the overlying epidermis are tethered to the papillary dermis by anchoring fibrils, a series of looping elements along the underside of the lamina densa that serve as attachment sites for collagens in the papillary dermis. Type VII collagen is the major component of anchoring fibrils. Autoantibodies against type VII collagen have been identified in epidermolysis bullosa acquisita (EBA), bullous systemic lupus erythematosus and some variants of linear IgA disease (IgA-mediated EBA) (143–145). Nonsense mutations of type VII collagen gene (COL7A1) are associated with dystrophic EB.

Bullous Pemphigoid

First described in 1953, bullous pemphigoid affects primarily elderly patients with large tense bullae arising on urticarial erythematous bases or on nonerythematous skin (146). The course is chronic and benign. In contrast to pemphigus, the Nikolsky sign is negative. The lesions involve the trunk, extremities, and intertriginous areas, with the oral mucosa involved in about one third of the cases. Bullous pemphigoid may start as a nonspecific eruption suggestive of urticaria or dermatitis, and can persist for weeks or months (147,148). Rarely, bullous pemphigoid may present as an erythroderma.

Histopathology. In early lesions, papillary dermal edema in combination with a cell-poor or cell-rich perivascular lymphocytic and eosinophilic infiltrate is present (Fig. 9-16A). The blister arises at the dermo–epidermal junction (146,149). In the cell-rich pattern, the blisters arise on erythematous skin (Fig. 9-16B). Eosinophilic papillary abscesses may develop with numerous perivascular and inter-

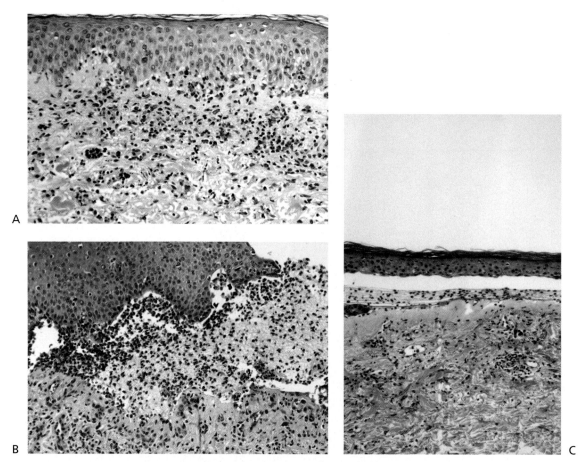

FIGURE 9-16. Bullous pemphigoid. **(A)** Prebullous phase, eosinophils are present at the dermoepidermal junction and in the dermis. **(B)** Cell-rich variant, subepidermal blister formation and an inflammatory infiltrate composed predominantly of eosinophils and a few neutrophils in the dermis and bullous cavity. **(C)** Cell-poor variant, subepidermal blister with few inflammatory cells.

stitial eosinophils intermingled with lymphocytes and neutrophils in the superficial and deep dermis. Early lesions may have the histologic features of eosinophilic cellulitis (Well's syndrome). Eosinophilic spongiosis may occur. The cell-poor pattern is observed when blisters develop on relatively normal skin (Fig. 9-16C), in which there is usually a scant perivascular lymphocytic infiltrate with few eosinophils, some scattered throughout the dermis and others near the epidermis (149,150). The blister lumen contains few inflammatory cells. Epithelial migration and regeneration may result in an intraepidermal location in older blisters. Similar to pemphigus vegetans, a pseudocarcinomatous hyperplasia of the epidermis, subepidermal bullae, and accumulations of eosinophils and lymphocytes may be seen (151,152).

Immunofluorescence Testing. DIF testing of perilesional skin has shown linear C3 deposition (Fig. 9-17A) (Table 9-4). At the dermo–epidermal junction in virtually 100% of cases and IgG in 65% to 95% (73). IIF studies reveal circulating anti–basement membrane zone IgG antibodies in 70% to 80%. Similarly deposited IgA and IgM are observed in about 25% of cases. No correlation exists between the antibody titer and the clinical severity of the disease (153,154). The IgG is located within the lamina lucida (155,156), where it appears bound specifically to the hemidesmosomes (157).

Salt-split skin IF studies (incubation of normal or patient skin in 1 mol/L NaCl results in a split in the lamina lucida) are an important diagnostic tool. The technique was first developed in 1984, in which normal human skin was used as a substrate and patient serum as test (indirect salt-split skin technique) (158). The epidermis is reliably split from the underlying dermis through the lamina lucida. Pemphigoid antibodies bind solely to the lower aspect of the basal keratinocytes (the blister roof). In 80% of cases; in about 20% of cases, the antibodies bind to both the lower basal keratinocytes (the roof), and the superior aspect of the base (the blister floor) (Table 9-7). Rarely, it has been reported that pemphigoid antibodies may bind solely to the floor (159,160); however, these reports have not been substantiated.

Perilesional skin submitted for DIF examination may also be salt-split (direct salt-split skin technique) (161,162). When this technique is used in pemphigoid, IgG is present on the roof or on the roof and the floor (Fig. 9-17B and C). Localization to only the dermal base has not been reported in bullous pemphigoid using this technique (Table 9-7). This pattern is characteristic for EBA (Fig. 9-20C).

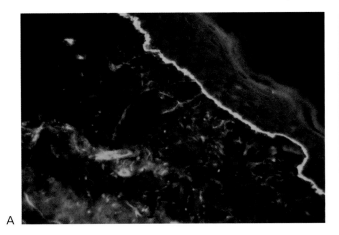
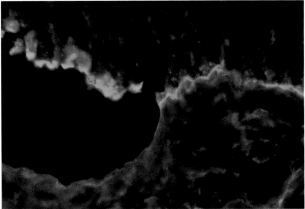
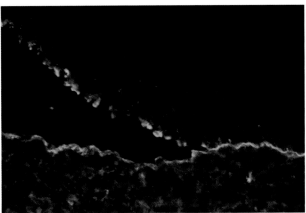

FIGURE 9-17. Bullous pemphigoid, direct immunofluorescent. **(A)** There is linear deposition of IgG in the basement membrane zone (direct immunofluorescence). **(B,C)** Salt split direct immunofluorescence studies reveal IgG deposition on epidermal side **(B)** or at both epidermal and dermal side **(C)** of the blister. When present on the roof, note the semilunar pattern, corresponding to the curvature of the basal keratinocytes.

TABLE 9-7. SPLIT-SKIN IMMUNOFLUORESCENCE RESULTS (INDIRECT METHOD)

Roof Only	Roof and Base	Base Only
Bullous pemphigoid (80%), Herpes gestationis	Bullous pemphigoid (~15%), Herpes gestationis	According to some, bullous pemphigoid IgG may localize to the base in the indirect method in 5% of cases. This is not our experience (i.e., that of TJH), and the status of these cases is uncertain.
Cicatricial pemphigoid	Cicatricial pemphigoid	Antiepiligrin cicatricial pemphigoid Epidermolysis bullosa acquisita Bullous systemic lupus erythematosus Porphyria cutanea tarda
Linear IgA dermatosis	Linear IgA dermatosis	IgA epidermolysis bullosa acquisita

[a]In the direct methods (see Amato et al. [148] and Bushkell et al. [149]), this finding (bullous pemphigoid antibodies localizing to the base) has not been reported, and has not occurred in the experience of TJH.

Pathogenesis. Pemphigoid antibodies bind to two antigens, a 230-kD protein (BPAg1), and a second, 180-kD protein (BPAg2) (163,164). The principal antigen, BPAg1, is associated with the cytoplasmic attachment site of hemidesmosomes and is largely within the basal keratinocyte. BPAg2 is a hemidesmosomal antigen that extends to the lamina lucida. The distribution of these antigens within the skin correlates with lesion location (165). A blistering disorder clinically similar to pemphigoid has antibodies that recognize a 105-kD protein synthesized by both keratinocytes and fibroblasts (166,167).

Given the known data, a sequence of pathogenetic events may be proposed. Pemphigoid antibodies bind with BPAg1 and BPAg2, activating the complement cascade. The anaphylatoxins, C3a and C4a, are elaborated, activating mast cells. Mast cell activation may be augmented by pemphigoid IgG4, which has homocytotropic properties for mast cells (168). The mast cells degranulate, releasing a variety of inflammatory mediators, including eosinophil chemotactic factor, neutrophil chemotactic factor, leukotriene B4, proteolytic enzymes, and eosinophil stimulating factor (169,170). Eosinophil infiltration ensues with subsequent degranulation and release of major basic protein and other proteolytic enzymes. The vessels are hyperpermeable, probably because of the release of vascular permeability factor (VPF) by keratinocytes (171). Lamina lucida separation develops from injury of basal keratinocytes, disruption of hemidesmosomes, and proteolysis (172). The role of infiltrating lymphocytes that are predominantly CD4+ is unclear. IL-1 and IL-2, as well as INF-γ, have been identified in blister fluids (173).

Ultrastructural Study. Pemphigoid antibodies bind within the lamina lucida, in particular, to the hemidesmosomes (155,156). The blister arises within the lamina lucida in both the cell-poor and cell-rich lesions. In cell-poor lesions (174), there is disruption of the anchoring filaments without lamina densa fragmentation (175,176). In contrast, inflammatory lesions of bullous pemphigoid with numerous eosinophils and mononuclear cells in the dermis result in greater local destruction or blister formation in the lamina lucida with fragmentation of the lamina densa (155,177).

Clinical Variants

Drug-Associated Bullous Pemphigoid

Furosemide, phenacetin, and various penicillins have been associated with bullous pemphigoid (178–180). It is possible that drug hypersensitivity may not be a cause of pemphigoid, but that the patients had subclinical pemphigoid with a superimposed drug eruption that produces damage to the dermo–epidermal junction. The combination hits the threshold of basal damage necessary to produce subepidermal blister formation.

Pemphigoid Localized to Lower Extremities

Some patients, usually women, present with tense bullae localized to the lower extremities (181). Histologically, these reveal a cell-poor pattern and have positive IF findings less frequently (50%) than routine bullous pemphigoid. At least in one instance, it has been shown that the IgG is directed against BPAg1 (182). The exact nosology of the DIF cases is unclear. In our estimation, they likely represent subepidermal blisters in ischemic lower extremities secondary to chronic stasis dermatitis or other causes of chronic ischemic dermatitis such as diabetic microangiopathy, due to the high metabolic activity of basal keratinocytes and inhibition of hemidesmosome formation and maintenance. The hemidesmosome turnover rate is quite rapid, at 4 to 6 hours.

Vesicular Pemphigoid

This variant is worthy of designation only because of its clinical similarity to dermatitis herpetiformis, which may lead to misdiagnosis.

Differential Diagnosis. Histologic differentiation of bullous pemphigoid from pemphigus vulgaris is not difficult because of the difference in cleavage planes and the mechanism of blister formation. Bullous pemphigoid is frequently indistinguishable from herpes gestationis; however, herpes gestationis may have greater quantities of infiltrating neutrophils and more basal keratinocyte damage. Epidermolysis bullosa acquisita (inflammatory variant) may have greater numbers of infiltrating neutrophils, but differentiation may be impossible. Dermatitis herpetiformis is characterized by a subepidermal infiltrate of neutrophils with papillary microabscesses. Similarly, linear IgA dermatosis is characterized, in the vast majority of cases, by a neutrophil-rich infiltrate. Erythema multiforme is an interface dermatitis characterized by basal vasculopathy, basal apoptosis, and a tagging lymphohistiocytic infiltrate along the dermo–epidermal junction. Diabetic blisters are noninflammatory, subepithelial in location, and often associated with fibrosis. Some patients with pemphigoid may present only with a superficial perivascular lymphoeosinophilic infiltrate without migration of eosinophils to the dermo–epidermal junction. This histologic reaction pattern is most commonly associated with morbilliform drug eruptions. Rarely, the changes of eosinophilic cellulitis (Well's syndrome) may also herald the presence of pemphigoid. Bullous drug eruptions may present with subepidermal vesicles and eosinophils, and later lesions of dermatitis herpetiformis may contain eosinophils. An IF study is necessary to make a specific diagnosis.

Cicatricial Pemphigoid

Historically, a bullous disorder characterized by a chronic course, scarring, and predilection for mucosal surfaces is known as cicatricial pemphigoid. Most patients are elderly, and there is a male predilection. Oral blisters are present in virtually all cases, and ocular involvement is observed in 75% and cutaneous involvement in 33%. The oral lesions are usually small blisters that subsequently erode and ulcerate. Other mucosal surfaces, including the larynx, esophagus, nose, vulva, and anus, may also be involved. Scarring is less evident in these locations than in the conjunctiva, where erythema, without blisters and ulceration, and subsequent scarring are the rule. Unilateral blindness occurs in up to 20% of cases. The cutaneous lesions are of two types: (a) an extensive eruption of bullae that heals without scarring (146,183,184); and (b) areas of erythema mainly on the face and scalp in which bullae erupt intermittently followed by atrophy and scarring (185,186). Both types of lesions may be present in the same patient (187,188). In the Brunsting–Perry variant, there are no mucosal lesions, but rather one to several circumscribed erythematous patches on which recurrent crops of blisters appear with atrophic scarring. The patches are usually confined to the head and neck area (189,190). Other clinical variants include a

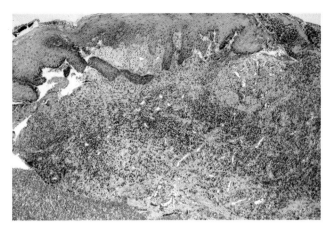

FIGURE 9-18. Cicatricial pemphigoid. There is fibrosis beneath the subepidermal blister containing fibrin. There is often a cell-rich lichenoid infiltrate.

widespread nonscarring bullous eruption in which scarring lesions develop only on the head (191), and widespread bullae that heal with atrophic scars (192,193).

Histopathology. In cutaneous lesions, a subepidermal blister develops that may extend down adnexa (Fig. 9-18). Neutrophils, histiocytes, and lymphocytes predominate in the inflammatory infiltrate. Eosinophils may or may not be numerous. Lamellar fibrosis beneath the epidermis is a hallmark but may not be present in the initial lesions. Mucosal lesions generally have a lichenoid lymphocytic infiltrate in which neutrophils or eosinophils or both may be present (194). The changes are often nonspecific in both mucosal and cutaneous lesions, but the above features should lead to consideration of cicatricial pemphigoid.

Immunofluorescence Testing. DIF studies reveal linear IgG and C3 in lesional and perilesional skin in approximately 80% of cases. In three series, a total of 35 of 46 patients had linear deposits (195–197). In most, both IgG and C3 were present, occasionally in association with IgA or IgM. Rarely, only C3 was present (196). In other cases labeled cicatricial pemphigoid, linear IgA was the only immunoglobulin found (197,198). Therefore, these cases are now best considered linear IgA bullous dermatosis. Patients with cicatricial conjunctivitis that display only linear IgA deposits and are best considered a scarring variant of linear IgA dermatosis (199–201). With respect to the Brunsting–Perry type, nine of ten patients had linear IgG at the dermo–epidermal junction, three of whom had concomitant linear C3 (190,202,203).

IIF testing of serum yields variable results depending on the substrate used (monkey esophagus, guinea pig esophagus, normal human skin, salt-split skin). It appears that circulating antibodies in this disorder may be more readily demonstrated when salt-split human skin is used as substrate, in which IgG may be localized only to the roof or, as in the antiepiligrin subgroup, to the base of the induced separation (204,205) (Table 9-7).

The difference in clinical presentation, as well as the localization of the immunoreactants may be explained by differing antigenic specificity of the antibodies. The known autoantigens include (a) epiligrin (206) or laminin 5 (the antigen associated with previously termed antiepiligrin CP); (b) β4 subunit of the α6β4 integrin (the antigen is predominantly associated with ocular CP) (207); and (c) BPAg2 (208) and BPAg1 (164). It is noteworthy that autoantibodies from patients with CP tend to target the C-terminus of BPAg2, whereas those from patients with BP, pemphigoid gestationis, and lamina-lucida type linear IgA bullous dermatosis typically target the NC16A domain of BPAg2. All of these antigens occur within the lamina lucida, with epiligrin present in the lower lamina lucida. This may explain the localization of the antibody to the artifactually created blister base in salt-split skin preparations (Table 9-5). At this point in time, cicatricial pemphigoid is best considered not one disease but several diseases with a similar clinical phenotype of scarring, predilection for mucosal and conjunctival surfaces, and subepidermal bullae. Many cases in the literature labeled cicatricial pemphigoid without adequate immunologic study may be labeled linear IgA disease or EBA involving principally mucosal surfaces.

Ultrastructural Study. Electron microscopic examination revealed in two studies that the oral and cutaneous lesions possess an intact basement membrane zone at the base of the blister (184,209). In another study of both the oral and cutaneous lesions, the basement membrane zone was destroyed (210).

Paraneoplastic Autoimmune Multiorgan Syndrome: Paraneoplastic Pemphigus

As mentioned earlier, patients with PNP may present clinical, histologic, and immunohistologic features reminiscent of bullous pemphigoid or cicatricial pemphigoid.

Herpes Gestationis

This is a blistering disorder that usually develops during the second to third trimester in pregnant women. It is estimated to occur in 1 in 50,000 pregnancies (211). Intensely pruritic, urticarial lesions usually develop on the abdomen with subsequent involvement of the extremities, hands, and feet. They usually progress to tense vesicles and bullae, some herpetiform. The disorder may recur with subsequent pregnancies, menstrual periods, or the use of birth control pills. The course for the mother is benign. There was a debate concerning the possibility of an increased incidence and risk of fetal morbidity and mortality. However,

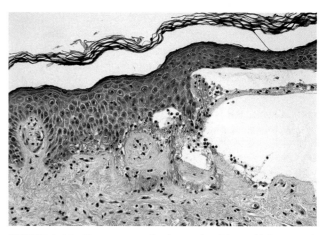

FIGURE 9-19. Herpes gestationis. A subepidermal blister with eosinophils and neutrophils. The epidermis shows focal spongiosis.

data obtained in the 1990s indicates that no such risk can be confirmed (212). There is an association with prematurity and small-for-gestational-age weights (213). The infant, however, may be born with a mild, transient, vesiculobullous eruption secondary to transplacental transfer of the mediating antibody (214,215).

Histopathology. In zones of erythema and edema, there is a perivascular infiltrate composed of lymphocytes and eosinophils. There is marked papillary dermal edema. There may be spongiosis (216), which may be eosinophilic in type. Focal necrosis of the basal keratinocytes, which has been emphasized by some authors, leads to a subepidermal blister (217) (Fig. 9-19).

Immunofluorescence Testing. DIF testing reveals linear deposition of C3 in perilesional skin in virtually all patients (214). IgG is similarly deposited in 30% to 40% (215, 218). Immunoelectron microscopic study has revealed IgG and C3 to reside within the lamina lucida. Using routine IIF studies of serum, it is uncommon to demonstrate circulating anti–squamous basement membrane zone antibody. Using *in vitro* complement fixation, a circulating anti–basement membrane zone IgG is demonstrable in most cases. At this point in time, the use of the label, *HG factor*, for these IgG antibodies is of historical interest only. The BPAg2 is the principal antigen, but the BPAg1 is recognized in some patients as well (219,220); BPAg2 is a component of type XVII collagen (221).

Ultrastructural Study. The epidermis at the periphery of bullae shows significant damage, most pronounced in basal keratinocytes, with resultant complete or partial necrosis of epidermal cells (222). Despite the fact that basal keratinocytes show severe damage, the basal cell plasma membrane and the lamina densa are well preserved and are present at the floor of the blister. The hemidesmosomes may be intact in some areas (223).

VESICULOBULLOUS DERMATOSES WITH AUTOIMMUNITY TO TYPE VII COLLAGEN

Epidermolysis Bullosa Acquisita

Classically, EBA is a noninherited disorder of acquired skin fragility (224,225). This presentation of EBA was the only one recognized until recently. Blisters develop on non-inflammatory bases with a predilection for acral areas. Scarring and milia formation ensue. A characteristic nail dystrophy and alopecia are noted. This presentation is associated with malignant lymphoma, amyloidosis, and colitis or enteritis. Some patients with EBA may have significant involvement of oral and conjunctival mucosa and therefore may be *cicatricial pemphigoid-like* (226). However, acral lesions are prominent and nail dystrophy is noted. In this type, biopsy from mucosal lesions reveals inflammatory, subepidermal bullae with scarring and milia similar to cicatricial pemphigoid.

In 1984, five patients with EBA had clinical, histologic, and immunohistologic features characteristic of bullous pemphigoid (225). They had generalized, pruritic, erythematous macules and papules on which bullae arose. There was less tendency for the lesions to develop acrally and greater involvement of flexural surfaces than in the previously described forms of EBA. At presentation, neither scarring nor milia were discerned; however, delicate scars developed later at the sites of blister formation.

Histopathology. The *bullous pemphigoid-like* presentation described above is the most common form of EBA. The subepidermal blisters are inflammatory. The predominant infiltrating cells are lymphocytes and neutrophils in perivascular and focal interstitial array. Eosinophils are present in variable numbers (Fig. 9-20A). In the classic form, the subepidermal blisters are noninflammatory (Fig. 9-20B), and fibrosis and milia formation are often present.

Immunofluorescence Testing. Examination of perilesional skin using DIF reveals linear deposition of complement at the basement membrane zone in the vast majority of cases. IgG is by far the most common immunoglobulin found, but IgM and IgA may be present as well. Increasing numbers of immunoglobulin subclasses noted at the dermo–epidermal junction favor a diagnosis of EBA over bullous pemphigoid. The presence of linear C3 at the dermo–epidermal junction alone favors bullous pemphigoid over EBA. However, use of routine DIF cannot reliably distinguish between bullous pemphigoid and EBA. IIF reveals circulating anti–basement membrane zone antibodies in up to 50% (224,227,228).

Use of the salt-split skin technique leads to the appropriate diagnosis in most cases (229) (Fig. 9-20C). The anti-

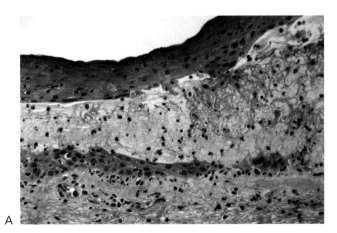

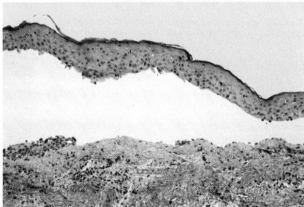

FIGURE 9-20. Epidermolysis bullosa acquisita. **(A)** Inflammatory type. Some neutrophils and eosinophils are in the blister cavity and the superficial dermis. The blister is partially re-epithelialized. **(B)** Noninflammatory type with a subepidermal blister. **(C)** Salt-split direct immunofluorescence reveals linear deposition of IgG in the blister base.

bodies in EBA have specificity for the globular carboxyl terminus of type VII collagen and are deposited beneath the lamina densa (230,231). Therefore, on salt-split skin studies, IgG is on the floor and not on the roof of the split (229) (Table 9-7).

Bullous Systemic Lupus Erythematosus

Vesicles and bullae may develop in patients with systemic lupus erythematosus. In contrast to dermatitis herpetiformis, they are nonpruritic and may be widespread. In contrast to dermatitis herpetiformis, the lesions are neither symmetrical nor do they have a predilection for extensor surfaces of arms, elbows, or scalp. The lesions may be photodistributed. These patients rarely have classic lesions of discoid, systemic, or subacute cutaneous lupus erythematosus when they develop blisters. In cases from the literature, the vast majority have had a previous history of lupus erythematosus, and most authors have required definitive American Rheumatologic Association (ARA) criteria before making the diagnosis in those patients with bullous lesions. However, at least three patients (who later developed other stigmata of lupus) have presented with a blistering eruption but without previous signs or symptoms of connective tissue disease (232–235). Bullous lupus erythematosus is most common in women, particularly black women (236–240). Most of these cases were exquisitely sensitive to dapsone therapy, with rapid involution of the lesions. No correlation with clinical activity of lupus erythematosus was apparent (239). Some patients with EBA will progress to systemic lupus erythematosus (SLE). (See also Chapter 10.)

Histopathology. Three histologic patterns have been identified in such lesions. The first is striking basal layer vacuolization with subsequent blister formation. The second is vasculitis with subepidermal blister and pustule formation (Fig. 9-21A and B). The third and most common is a dermatitis herpetiformis-like histologic pattern. Approximately 25% of cases are said to have a small-vessel, neutrophil-rich leukocytoclastic vasculitis beneath the blister (239). Histologic features more routinely identified with lupus erythematosus are not present. Another histologic finding that is not emphasized in most case reports is the presence of dermal mucin and hyaluronic acid as defined by Alcian blue stain at pH 2.5 (241). The frequency of mucin deposition is unknown.

Immunofluorescence Testing. In all reported cases, IgG and C3 are deposited at the epidermal basement membrane zone. The pattern was linear in more than 50% and was referred to as "granular bandlike" in approximately 25%. IgM and IgA were present in approximately 50% and 60% of cases, respectively. The conflicting pattern of immune reactant deposition is difficult to explain. In these reports, the pattern varies from a "thick band" to a "fine

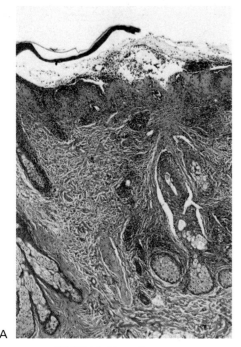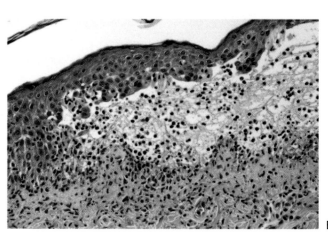

FIGURE 9-21. Bullous systemic lupus erythematosus. **(A)** There is a subepidermal blister and perifollicular inflammatory cell infiltrate. **(B)** The neutrophils are predominant in the blister and superficial dermis.

ribbonlike" or "tubular" pattern. The ribbonlike or linear pattern represents antibodies that are bound to rigid, anatomically compartmentalized antigens such as in bullous pemphigoid or epidermolysis bullosa acquisita. In general, granular patterns represent deposition of circulating immune complexes *in situ* or *in situ* binding of antigen and antibody in noncompartmentalized zones. Therefore, perhaps some of the cases represent tubular or linear deposition obscured by confluent granular bands (positive lupus band test). IIF study of serum rarely reveals circulating anti–squamous basement membrane zone antibodies that are detected against type VII collagen (234). It should be noted, however, that salt-split skin preparations may be a more sensitive substrate than whole-skin mounts.

A salt-split skin preparation using patient serum reveals localization to the split floor as in EBA (Table 9-7). Lastly, Western immunoblots reveal binding to either 290-kD or 145-kD dermal proteins, components of type VII collagen (242). However, antibodies to type VII collagen are not present in all cases.

Ultrastructural Study. Immunoelectron microscopic examination reveals electron-dense deposits of IgG at the lower edge of the basal lamina and immediately subjacent dermis in an identical location to the antibody in EBA (242).

SUBEPIDERMAL IGA-MEDIATED VESICULOBULLOUS DERMATOSES

Dermatitis Herpetiformis

This is an intensely pruritic, chronic recurrent dermatitis that has a slight male predilection. The lesions usually develop in young to middle-aged adults as symmetrical grouped papulovesicles, vesicles, or crusts on erythematous bases. Oral lesions are absent (243). The elbows, knees, buttocks, scapula, and scalp are commonly involved. There is a high incidence (about 90%) of gluten-sensitive enteropathy, and an increased but rare risk of lymphoma (244). Dermatitis herpetiformis in association with SLE has also been reported (245).

Histopathology. The typical histologic features are best observed in erythematous skin adjacent to early blisters. In these zones, neutrophils accumulate at the tips of dermal papillae (246). With an increase in size to microabscesses, a significant admixture of eosinophils may be noted. As microabscesses form, a separation develops between the tips of the dermal papillae and the overlying epidermis, so that early blisters are multiloculated (Fig. 9-22A). The presence of fibrin in the papillae may give them a bluish appearance (247). Within 1 to 2 days, the rete ridges lose their attachment to the dermis, and the blisters then become unilocular (Fig. 9-22B), and clinically apparent (248). At this time, the characteristic papillary microabscesses may be observed at

the blister periphery. For this reason, the inclusion of perivesicular skin in the biopsy specimen is of utmost value. The papillary dermis beneath the papillae may have a relatively intense inflammatory infiltrate of neutrophils and some eosinophils. Many neutrophils may exhibit leukocytoclasis. Subjacent to this, a perivascular infiltrate composed of lymphocytes, neutrophils, and eosinophils may be apparent (249). In one study, the diagnostic finding of papillary microabscesses was present in all patients (250). In another study of 105 biopsy specimens, they were present in only 52% (251). Apoptotic keratinocytes may be noted above the papillary microabscesses.

Immunofluorescence Testing. In 1967, Cormane described the presence of granular deposits of IgA within the dermal papillae in both lesional and nonlesional skin (252). IgA is found alone or in combination with other immune reactants in over 95% of cases when uninvolved skin of the forearm or buttock is tested (Fig. 9-22C). Fibrillary IgA deposits may also be present. Early in the course of the disease, IgA deposits may be absent, and repeat DIF is necessary (253). Some recommend that biopsies be taken from clinically normal skin immediately adjacent to erythema, because false-negative results may occur when blistered or inflamed skin is evaluated (254,255). The presence of IgA within the skin is not altered by dapsone therapy. After as long as 2 years, a gluten-free diet results in the disappearance of IgA from the skin. Negative results of DIF testing of two appropriately selected biopsy sites are a strong indication that the patient does not have dermatitis herpetiformis.

Circulating IgA antibodies that react against reticulin, smooth muscle endomysium, the dietary antigen gluten, bovine serum albumin, and β-lactoglobin may be present. Only the presence of IgA endomysial antibodies is of diagnostic importance but their presence is not specific nor very sensitive (256). Using monkey or pig gut as substrate, IIF has been used to detect antiendomysial antibodies, which are present in 52% to 100% of patients (257,258).

Pathogenesis. Three important findings must be considered in the pathogenesis of dermatitis herpetiformis. First, the disease is associated with a gluten-sensitive enteropathy; second, granular IgA is deposited in the skin; and third, patients have a high frequency of certain HLA antigens. HLA-B8, DR3, and Dqw2 have been identified in high frequency in patients with dermatitis herpetiformis and celiac disease (259–261). The majority of patients show focal celiac sprue–like changes on jejunal biopsy (262). Patients with celiac disease develop IgA autoantibodies to tissue transglutaminase, which degrades gliadin. Antitissue transglutaminase antibodies and antiendomysial antibodies are detected in patients with dermatitis herpetiformis (262a). Recently, papillary dermal-bound IgA-immune precipitates in dermatitis herpetiformis have been shown to contain epidermal transglutaminase (262b).

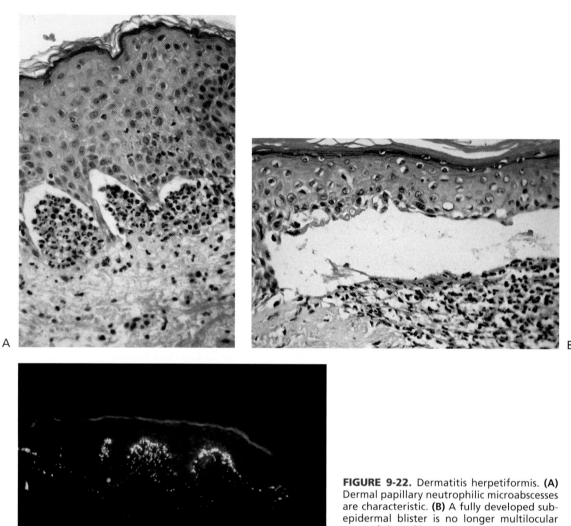

FIGURE 9-22. Dermatitis herpetiformis. **(A)** Dermal papillary neutrophilic microabscesses are characteristic. **(B)** A fully developed sub-epidermal blister is no longer multilocular most of the infiltrating cells are neutrophils. **(C)** There is granular and thready IgA predominantly at the tips of dermal papillae (direct immunofluorescence).

The IgA deposition results in activation of the complement system followed by chemotaxis of neutrophils into the papillary dermis (263). Enzymes released from these neutrophils degrade laminin and type IV collagen, contributing to blister formation (264).

Ultrastructural Study. The changes in dermatitis herpetiformis resemble those observed in the inflammatory bullae of bullous pemphigoid (177). Neutrophils are the major inflammatory cell in the former, whereas eosinophils predominate in the latter. Fibrin appears earlier and in greater amount in dermatitis herpetiformis, particularly in dermal papillae. While it has been shown immunohistochemically that the early blister forms above the apparently intact lamina lucida (265). In more advanced lesions the lamina densa has been destroyed, as is noted in the "inflammatory bullae" of bullous pemphigoid (246,250).

Linear IgA Dermatosis

A group of bullous disorders mediated by IgA antibodies with differing specificities for epidermal basement membrane zone antigens has been labeled *linear IgA dermatosis* (LAD). There are two relatively definitive clinical phenotypes that are based on patient age and clinical features—adult linear IgA dermatosis and childhood linear IgA dermatosis (chronic benign bullous dermatosis of childhood). They differ slightly in their clinical presentations but have identical immunopathological features. Third, a clinical phenotype similar to cicatricial pemphigoid has been described. Fourth, a subset of patients has been described with drug-induced linear IgA dermatosis. On the basis of immunoelectromicroscopic localization of the IgA deposition, there are at least two distinct types of LAD: a lamina lucida type and a sublamina densa type. Some of the sub-lamina densa type LAD are best classified as IgA epidermolysis bullosa acquisita.

Adult Type

Vesicles and bullae develop in patients usually over 40 years of age, with a slight female predilection. The lesions are less symmetrical and less pruritic than those in dermatitis herpetiformis but are distributed in similar locations. Ocular and oral lesions may be present in up to 50% of cases. Plantar and palmar bullae may develop in contrast to dermatitis herpetiformis. Cutaneous lesions in LAD are heterogeneous and may mimic other bullous diseases. Linear IgA dermatosis has been associated with an increased risk of lymphoma (266). Ulcerative colitis has been correlated with LAD in various studies, one of which found ulcerative colitis in 7.1% of LAD patients (267). A rare association with SLE has been reported (268).

Histopathology. The features are similar, if not identical, to dermatitis herpetiformis (Fig. 9-23A and B). According to some, there is less tendency for papillary microabscess formation and greater tendency for uniform neutrophil infiltration along the entire dermo–epidermal junction and rete in inflamed skin (269). Rarely, one may observe a principally lymphocytic infiltrate, sometimes with numerous neutrophils (268).

Immunofluorescence Testing. As this test defines the disease, DIF reveals linear IgA along the basement membrane zone in perilesional skin in 100% of cases (Fig. 9-23C). In the lamina lucida type of LAD, IgA antibodies bind to the epidermal side of salt-split skin, whereas in the sublamina densa type, such as IgA-mediated epidermolysis bullosa acquisita, IgA antibodies bind to the dermal side of salt-split skin (Table 9-7).

In the vast majority of cases, IgA1 is present, but rarely is IgA2 present. When IgG and IgA are present, some detailed immunologic study may be needed to allow differential diagnosis with bullous pemphigoid (270). It has been suggested that if the IgA deposits are more intense than the IgG deposits, and C3 deposition is strong, then linear IgA dermatosis is the best diagnosis (271). However, it is best considered a distinct disorder labeled *linear IgA/IgG dermatosis* until more data are available. One patient presented with linearly deposited IgG initially and only subsequently developed linear IgA deposits (272). Low titers of circulating anti–squamous basement membrane zone IgA have been identified in only 20% to 30% of cases (272–275). A recent study, however, has noted such antibodies in up to 75% of patients (276,277).

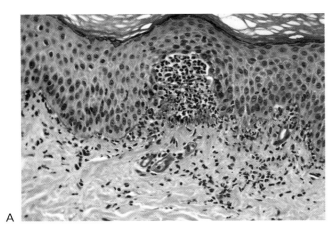

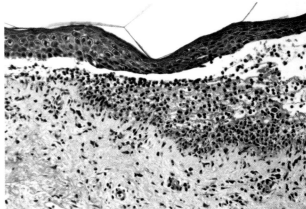

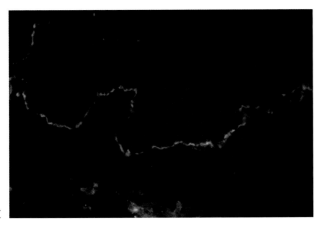

FIGURE 9-23. Linear IgA bullous dermatosis. **(A)** An earlier lesion, the neutrophils are along the dermoepidermal junction and concentrated in the dermal papillae. **(B)** There is a subepidermal blister with inflammatory cells and fibrin in the lumen and in the base. Most of the inflammatory cells are neutrophils. A few eosinophils are also present. **(C)** Direct immunofluorescence study reveals deposition of IgA in a linear pattern along the basement membrane zone.

Pathogenesis. In the lamina lucida type LAD, the antigens against which the IgA is directed include a 97-kD and a 120-kD protein that may be found in epidermal and dermal extracts (278). Both of them are part of the shed ectodomain of the 180-kD bullous pemphigoid antigen (BPAg 2) (279,280). In the sublamina densa type, the antigen in many instances is unknown. In some cases, the antigen is type VII collagen, specifically the NC-1 domain, the immunodominant epitope for the epidermolysis bullosa acquisita (282). The events of the inflammatory cascade in IgA-mediated diseases are not well understood.

Ultrastructural Study. The antibodies are deposited principally within the lamina lucida and less commonly beneath the lamina densa (IgA-mediated EBA) (282).

Drug-Associated Linear IgA Dermatosis

It is important to note that drug therapy has frequently been associated with adult-type linear IgA dermatosis. Vancomycin, lithium, diclofenac, captopril, cefamandole, and somatostatin have been associated with such presentations (283–286). Histologically, the changes are identical to idiopathic linear IgA dermatosis in most cases. In some cases, there is an associated lymphoeosinophilic infiltrate in combination with the interface neutrophilic infiltration.

Childhood Type

Originally known as chronic bullous dermatosis of childhood (287). This disorder presents in prepubertal, often preschool children, and rarely in infancy. Vesicles or bullae develop on an erythematous or normal base, occasionally giving rise to a so-called "string of pearls," a characteristic lesion in which peripheral vesicles develop on a polycyclic plaque (288). They involve the buttocks, lower abdomen, and genitalia, and characteristically have a perioral distribution on the face. Oral lesions may occur (289). The disorder usually remits by age 6 to 8, but 12% in one series experienced persistent disease (277,290).

Histopathology. The features are similar to those of the adult-type disease. Some cases, however, resemble bullous pemphigoid because of the presence of eosinophils (289, 291).

Immunofluorescence Testing. DIF testing reveals linearly deposited IgA in virtually 100% of cases (292). At this time, the targeted antigens are thought to be identical to those noted in the adult-type disease.

NONINFECTIOUS VESICULOPUSTULAR DERMATOSES
Erythema Toxicum Neonatorum

A benign, asymptomatic eruption affecting about 40% of term infants usually within 12 to 48 hours after birth, erythema toxicum neonatorum lasts 2 to 3 days and consists of blotchy macular erythema, papules, and pustules that tend to develop at sites of pressure. The eruption is associated with blood eosinophilia.

Histopathology. The macular erythema is characterized by sparse eosinophils in the upper dermis, largely in a perivascular location, and mild papillary dermal edema.

The papules show an accumulation of numerous eosinophils and some neutrophils in the area of the follicle and overlying epidermis. Papillary dermal edema is more intense and eosinophils more numerous.

Mature pustules are subcorneal and are filled with eosinophils and occasional neutrophils. The pustules form as a result of the upward migration of eosinophils to the surface epidermis from within and around the hair follicles (293).

Pathogenesis. The etiology is unknown. However, two hypotheses have been offered. The first is high-viscosity ground substance in the newborn, which because of osmotic changes at birth, causes tissue dilution and inflammation with minor trauma (294). Second, the eruption has been suggested to be a minor acute graft-versus-host reaction caused by maternal–fetal transfer of lymphocytes during delivery (295). The cell types have been evaluated and include Langerhans cells, eosinophils, neutrophils, and macrophages along E-selectum–expressing cells, and the cytokines, IL-1 alpha and IL-1 beta, and chemokines IL-8 and eotaxin negative (295a).

Differential Diagnosis. Eosinophilic pustular folliculitis is similar to erythema toxicum neonatorum histologically, but has completely different clinical features and has a predilection for the scalp (296). The subcorneal pustules of impetigo and transient neonatal pustular melanosis are not follicular in origin and contain primarily neutrophils rather than eosinophils. A smear of a pustule is helpful to characterize the predominant inflammatory cell. Although many eosinophils are present in the vesicles of incontinentia pigmenti, the vesicle is intraepidermal rather than subcorneal, and spongiosis is present. In addition, necrotic keratinocytes may be prominent in incontinentia pigmenti but are absent in erythema toxicum neonatorum.

Transient Neonatal Pustular Melanosis

Affecting 4.4% of black newborns and 0.6% of white newborns, flaccid vesicopustules with a predilection for the face, trunk, and diaper area develop at birth (297). These rupture after 1 to 2 days, leaving hyperpigmented macules with collarettes of scale. The development of typical lesions of erythema toxicum neonatorum has been observed days later (298). Perhaps the two eruptions represent the same disease in different phases, or their coexistence may be on the basis of the frequent occurrence of erythema toxicum neonatorum.

Histopathology. The vesicopustules consist of intracorneal or subcorneal aggregates of neutrophils with an admixture of eosinophils. Fragmented hair shafts may reside within the blister cavity (298). Within the dermis is an inflammatory infiltrate with some neutrophils and eosinophils. The macules show focal basal hypermelaninosis (297). There is no melanin in the dermis.

Acropustulosis of Infancy

Recurrent crops of intensely pruritic vesicles or pustules, 1 to 3 mm in diameter, are often mistaken for scabies. They develop primarily in black infants at birth or during the first year of life (299,300). The lesions occur predominantly on the distal extremities, heal with hyperpigmentation, and resolve in most cases by age 2. Rare cases have been reported in older children (301).

Histopathology. The intraepidermal or subcorneal vesicopustules contain neutrophils and sparse eosinophils. There is mild papillary dermal edema and a sparse, mixed, superficial perivascular infiltrate (302,303).

Pathogenesis. The etiology of infantile acropustulosis is unknown. The disease may be associated with atopic dermatitis and elevated serum IgE levels (303). Direct and IIF studies have been negative.

Differential Diagnosis. Impetigo, subcorneal pustular dermatosis, candidiasis, and transient neonatal pustular melanosis may be identical to acropustulosis of infancy, so that clinical data are necessary for differentiation. Special stains are necessary to rule out an infectious etiology.

Subcorneal Pustular Dermatosis

Subcorneal pustular dermatosis (Sneddon–Wilkinson disease) is a chronic disorder first described in 1956, and is characterized by sterile pustules that have a predilection for flexural surfaces and the axillary and inguinal folds (304). Many cases have been shown to be a variant of IgA pemphigus (305a,305b). It usually spares the face and mucous membranes. The pustules develop in an annular or serpiginous arrangement. Pus characteristically accumulates in the lower half of large pustules (305).

Subcorneal pustular dermatosis may be associated with a monoclonal gammopathy, most commonly an IgA paraproteinemia. Some of these cases eventuate in an IgA myeloma (306), and may have IgA squamous intercellular substance deposits.

Histopathology. The pustules are subcorneal and contain neutrophils, with only an occasional eosinophil (Fig. 9-24). The underlying slightly edematous stratum malpighii contains a small number of neutrophils. Only a few spongiform pustules are formed. In some instances, a few acantholytic cells are in the base of the pustule, most likely because of proteolytic enzymes present in the pustular contents. They may be partially attached to the epidermis or may lie free in the pustule among the neutrophils (307). The dermal papillae contain dilated capillaries and a perivascular infiltrate composed of neutrophils and a few eosinophils and mononuclear cells (308).

Immunofluorescence Testing. While most original DIF studies were reported as negative, as more cases accumulate, many cases have squamous intercellular IgA, indicating that they are best considered IgA pemphigus (intraepidermal IgA pustulosis) (305b).

Pathogenesis. The squamous intercellular substance IgA leads to neutrophilic infiltration. In some patients, elevated levels of TNF-α in the serum and pustules may be responsible for neutrophil activation (309).

Ultrastructural Study. The edge of the pustules shows cytolytic changes in the upper epidermis, especially in the granular layer. Dissolution of the plasma membrane and of the cytoplasm of granular cells causes the formation of a subcorneal split. The transepidermal migration of neutrophils and their subcorneal accumulation are regarded as events secondary to the cellular destruction in the stratum granulosum seen in one study (310).

Differential Diagnosis. The differential diagnosis includes other entities that show subcorneal pustules. Histologic differentiation from impetigo may be impossible unless bacteria can be demonstrated with a Gram stain. Cultures may be necessary for diagnosis. Histologic differentiation from pemphigus foliaceus or pemphigus erythematosus may also be difficult, since both diseases show subcorneal blisters with acantholysis. Although the acantholysis tends to be more pronounced in pemphigus than in subcorneal pustular dermatosis. Clinical information, immunofluorescence testing, and a therapeutic trial of sulfones may be necessary for definitive diagnosis.

Although subcorneal pustules occur in both pustular psoriasis and subcorneal pustular dermatosis, spongiform pustules occur only in pustular psoriasis (305). Some authors regard subcorneal pustular dermatosis as a variant of pustular psoriasis (311,312); but with the association to IgA gammopathies and squamous intercellular substance deposits of IgA, this view is discredited.

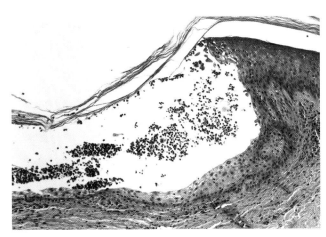

FIGURE 9-24. Subcorneal pustular dermatosis. There is a subcorneal vesicle filled with neutrophils. A few acanthotic keratinocytes are mixed with numerous neutrophils. Only a few spongiform pustules are formed.

Erythema Multiforme

Erythema multiforme is an acute, self-limited dermatosis that may be divided into a minor and major form, the latter also known as Stevens–Johnson syndrome, which is characterized by a severe and sometimes fatal disease with fever and systemic symptoms. Oral lesions are usually present. As the name implies, the lesions may be multiform, including macules, papules, vesicles, and bullae. Patients with erythema multiforme minor have recurrent lesions affecting primarily the extremities, with red papules; some evolve into typical target or iris lesions. Approximately 50% of individuals will give a history of preceding herpetic infection (312a, 312b).

Toxic epidermal necrolysis is widely, but not universally, regarded as the severe end of the spectrum of erythema multiforme major or Stevens–Johnson syndrome (313, 314). Some clinicians have arbitrarily diagnosed toxic epidermal necrolysis when blisters and peeling involved more than 30% of the total body surface area and Steven–Johnson syndrome when mucosal lesions were present and blistering involved less than 30% of the body surface (315).

Patients with Stevens–Johnson syndrome (a) often present with fever, have truncal involvement, and a more purpuric macular eruption, which progress to central blister formation and epidermal necrosis. Atypical target lesions may be present (316). Involvement of the oral, conjunctival, nasal, and genital mucosa is common. In toxic epidermal necrolysis, a widespread blotchy erythema develops. This is soon followed by the development of large, flaccid bullae and detachment of the epidermis in large sheets, leaving the dermis exposed and giving a moist, eroded appearance (317). The disease has a high mortality rate because of fluid loss and sepsis. Nearly 90% of Steven–Johnson syndrome or toxic epidermal necrolysis cases are caused by medications, most commonly NSAIDs, sulfonamides, α-lactam antibiotics, and nonsteroidal anti-inflammatory drugs (318). Although the presence or absence of mucosal lesions has been used to differentiate the various forms of bullous erythema multiforme, in a recent study no correlation was found, and overall 90% of patients had mucosal lesions (319).

Histopathology. Erythema multiforme is considered the prototype of the vacuolar form of interface dermatitis (320). Because of its acute nature, there is an orthokeratotic stratum corneum. The earliest changes include vacuolization of the basal cell layer, tagging of lymphocytes along the dermo–epidermal junction, and a sparse, superficial, perivascular lymphoid infiltrate (Fig. 9-25). Mild spongiosis and exocytosis are seen. Necrosis of individual keratinocytes in the basal unit occurs, the hallmark of erythema multiforme. Satellite cell necrosis, characterized by intraepidermal lymphocytes in close association with necrotic keratinocytes, is frequently present.

In more papular, edematous lesions, there is papillary dermal edema and more significant spongiosis and inflam-

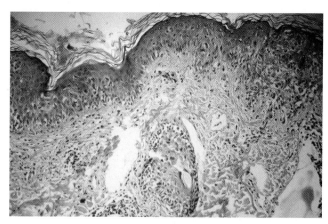

FIGURE 9-25. Erythema multiforme. There is a superficial perivascular and interface dermatitis with apoptotic keratinocytes. Lymphocytes are "tagging" along the dermoepidermal junction with apoptotic keratinocytes, which have eosinophilic cytoplasm and pyknotic nucleus. The stratum corneum is normal.

mation. Intraepidermal vesicles associated with exocytosis may be noted rarely (321).

In toxic epidermal necrolysis, there are numerous necrotic keratinocytes, even full-thickness epidermal necrosis, and a subepidermal bulla. The dermal inflammatory infiltrate is sparser in toxic epidermal necrolysis than in erythema multiforme (Fig. 9-26). Extravasated erythrocytes are commonly found within the blister cavity. Melanophages within the papillary dermis occur in late lesions.

In addition to the clinical differences, some histologic differences have been noted between drug-induced and herpes simplex–associated erythema multiforme (322). In the former, there is more widespread keratinocyte necrosis, microscopic blister formation, and more pigmentary incontinence. In cases associated with herpes simplex virus

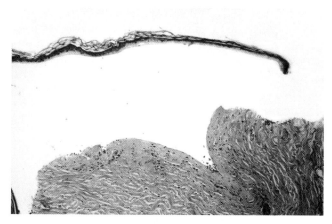

FIGURE 9-26. Toxic epidermal necrolysis. There is a cell-poor subepidermal blister and epidermal necrosis. The dermal inflammatory infiltrate is sparse.

infection, there is more exocytosis, liquefaction degeneration of the basal layer, and papillary dermal edema. Nuclear dust may be identified in the papillary dermis in the latter (322). Although one study has noted a significant number of eosinophils in drug-induced erythema multiforme (323), this has not been noted by others (324). In our estimation, a generous number of eosinophils excludes erythema multiforme. One study has found that an acrosyringeal concentration of apoptotic keratinocytes in erythema multiforme is a clue to a drug etiology (325). Erythema multiforme-like changes and eosinophils can be seen in biopsies taken from the hypersensitivity reactions to phenytoin, carbamazepine and related drugs, which we label erythema multiforme-like drug eruptions. Interestingly, the clinical picture does not resemble erythema multiforme.

Some authors have previously classified erythema multiforme into a dermal type, epidermal type, and mixed dermal-epidermal type (326); however, this classification is no longer widely accepted (322,324). The predominance of epidermal or dermal changes reflects the site of biopsy within an individual lesion and when, in the temporal evolution of the disease, the biopsy is taken. In addition, many cases of primarily "dermal erythema multiforme" may represent hypersensitivity reactions in which interface dermatitis is not the characteristic reaction pattern.

Immunofluorescence Testing. In many patients with erythema multiforme, deposits of IgM and C3 are found in the walls of the superficial dermal vessels (327,328). Granular deposits of C3, IgM, and fibrinogen may also be present along the dermo–epidermal junction (322,329). In postherpetic erythema multiforme, herpetic antigen may be observed in association with the deposits on immunofluorescence testing. In toxic epidermal necrolysis, diffuse epidermal deposition of immunoglobulin and complement in necrotic keratinocytes may be observed (330). Nonspecific deposition of immune reactants in apoptotic or necrotic keratinocytes may be observed in other forms of erythema multiforme and other disorders with apoptosis, lymphocyte satellite necrosis and epidermal necrosis.

Pathogenesis. Although many precipitating factors (infections, vaccinations, drugs and neoplasms) have been implicated in erythema multiforme, the most frequent etiology for the minor form is herpes simplex virus infection, while drugs are often incriminated in the major. Other infections associated with erythema multiforme include Epstein-Barr virus (331), cytomegalovirus (332), and Lyme disease (333). Mycoplasma pneumoniae is uncommonly associated with Steven–Johnson syndrome (334). Numerous drugs have been implicated. NSAIDS are most commonly involved, followed by sulfonamides, anticonvulsants, penicillins, tetracycline, and doxycycline (335,336).

Erythema multiforme appears to result from a cell-mediated immune reaction. In the case of herpes simplex, Polymerase chain reaction and *in situ* hybridization have detected herpes simplex virus DNA within lesions of erythema multiforme (337,338). The virus remains in the skin for up to 3 months after the lesions have healed (339). Some authors hypothesize that disease development begins with deposition and expression of HSV genes, leading to recruitment of HSV-specific CD4$^+$ T cells with production of interferon-gamma (IFN-γ). This step initiates an inflammatory cascade that includes increased infiltration of leukocytes, monocytes, natural killer (NK) cells, and T cells (340). The infiltrate consists largely of CD4$^+$ (helper) lymphocytes in the dermis, and CD8$^+$ (cytotoxic) cells in the epidermis. The mononuclear cells that are associated with necrotic keratinocytes in the process referred to as "satellite cell necrosis" are largely CD8$^+$ cytotoxic lymphocytes similar to those occurring in graft-versus-host disease (341). In drug-induced, erythema multiforme major/Stevens–Johnson syndrome/toxic epidermal necrolysis, TNF-α produces the epidermal destruction (342).

Ultrastructural Study. The basal lamina is located on the floor or the roof of the blister (326). The basal cells show marked intracytoplasmic damage with a loss of organelles. Neutrophils and macrophages, rich in lysosomes, are present in the lower epidermis phagocytizing the damaged keratinocytes. In the midepidermis, large, electron-dense, dyskeratotic bodies correspond to the cells with eosinophilic necrosis seen by light microscopy (326,343). The damaged epidermal cells often contain few or no organelles (326). Large granular lymphocytes have been identified within the epidermis in close contact with keratinocytes, a finding that supports cell-mediated cytotoxic injury to keratinocytes (344).

Differential Diagnosis. Necrotic keratinocytes are also a characteristic feature in fixed drug eruptions, pityriasis lichenoides, connective tissue disease, subacute radiation dermatitis, phototoxic dermatitis, acute graft-versus-host disease, viral exanthems, and some drug eruptions. In patients with widespread desquamation or detachment, the differential diagnosis includes toxic epidermal necrolysis and SSSS. Whereas the former involves subepidermal separation, the latter results from separation of the epidermis subcorneally or within the granular layer. Frozen section evaluation of the blister roof is a rapid diagnostic tool to determine the level of the split.

Graft-Versus-Host Disease

Graft-versus-host disease (GVHD) occurs in situations in which donor immunocompetent T cells transferred into allogenic hosts incapable of rejecting them. The sources of the T cells include primarily peripheral blood stem cell and bone marrow transplants (345), and, infrequently, unirradiated blood products (346), solid organ transplants (347), and maternofetal lymphocyte engraftment (348). Graft-versus-host-like reaction has been reported in patients with a thymoma or lymphoma (349,350).

The disease can be divided into an acute and a chronic phase. Acute GVHD typically occurs between 7 and 21 days after transplantation but may be seen as late as 3 months; chronic GVHD arises after a mean of 4 months, but may occur as soon as 40 days post-transplantation. The two phases were originally defined on the basis of time of presentation (351,352). However, the use of donor lymphocytes and the withdrawal of immunosuppression in relapsed patients have obscured these time-based divisions. In addition, many patients have both phases, either merging with one another or separated by an asymptomatic period (353). The frequency of acute GVHD depends on the disparity of HLA antigens (354). The risk of chronic GVHD is 11 times greater if the patients had prior acute GVHD.

In the *acute phase*, the classic triad includes skin lesions, hepatic dysfunction, and diarrhea. The clinical severity is judged on the extent of the cutaneous eruption, total bilirubin, and stool volume. The eruption is characterized by extensive macular erythema, a morbilliform eruption, purpuric lesions, violaceous scaly papules and plaques, bullae, or in some cases a toxic epidermal necrolysis-like epidermal detachment. There is a predilection for the cheeks, ears, neck, upper chest, and palms and soles. Occasionally, follicular papules are seen simulating a folliculitis (355). Oral lesions may be present. About 30% of patients die from complications of acute GVHD. The overall clinical stage, during the first 40 days after transplantation, is useful in identifying patients with progressive and fatal disease

(351). Cutaneous GVHD may be due to a synergistic effect from local irradiation (356).

In the *chronic phase*, an early lichenoid stage and a late sclerodermoid stage can be distinguished. Each stage can occur without the other (357). Although usually generalized, the involvement is in rare instances localized to a few areas (353). In the lichenoid stage, both the cutaneous and oral lesions may be clinically similar to those in lichen planus (358). In addition, the skin may show extensive erythema and irregular hyperpigmentation. A poikilodermatous phase may precede the eventual sclerodermoid stage. Other late manifestations include a lupus erythematosus-like eruption, cicatricial alopecia, chronic ulcerations (353), pyogenic granuloma and angiomatous lesions (359).

Histopathology. The early changes in acute phase consist of focal basal vacuolation and sparse superficial perivascular lymphocytic infiltrate with exocytosis of individual cells into the epidermis and follicular epithelium. The number of lymphocytes correlate positively with the probability of developing more severe acute GVHD (360,361). In association with the perivascular infiltrate, there is marked endothelial cell swelling and narrowing of the vascular lumen. Established lesions show more pronounced vacuolation, focal spongiosis, lymphocytic infiltration and dyskeratosis at all levels of epidermis (362,363). The *acute phase* has been divided into four histopathologic grades (364,365). In grade 1 disease, there is focal or diffuse vacuolization of the basal cell layer. In grade 2 lesions, spongiosis and dyskeratotic keratinocytes are identified (Fig. 9-27A), some

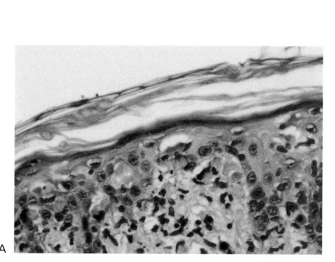
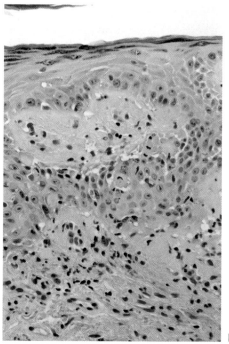

FIGURE 9-27. Graft versus host disease. **(A)** An acute lesion with interface changes and apoptosis of keratinocytes. **(B)** There is lichenoid dermatitis with basal vacuolopathy and apoptosis. There is fibrosis of the papillary dermis.

accompanied by two or more epidermal lymphocytes, a phenomenon known as "satellite cell necrosis." The necrotic keratinocytes contain a pyknotic nucleus and eosinophilic cytoplasm. Grade 3 lesions are characterized by subepidermal cleft formation, and in grade 4 there is complete loss of the epidermis. In cases with follicular papules, the involved follicles show degenerate changes in the cells of the follicular epithelium similar to those in the epidermis (355). In rare cases, basal vacuolization and dyskeratosis of the follicular epithelium may be the only changes (366).

In the *chronic phase*, the early lichenoid stage may still show evidence of satellite cell necrosis within the epidermis (366) (Fig. 27B). The overall histologic picture greatly resembles that of lichen planus with hyperkeratosis, hypergranulosis, acanthosis, apoptotic keratinocytes, and a mononuclear cell infiltrate immediately below the epidermis with pigmentary incontinence (358). As in lichen planus, apoptotic keratinocytes may "drop" into the upper dermis (367). There may be areas of separation of the basal cell layer from the dermal papillae resembling the clefts seen in severe lichen planus (353). A rare manifestation is so called "columnar epidermal necrosis," characterized by small foci of total epidermal necrosis accompanied by a lichenoid tissue reaction (368).

In the late sclerodermoid phase, the epidermis is atrophic, with the keratinocytes being small, flattened, and hyperpigmented. Basal layer vacuolization, inflammation, and colloid body formation are rare or absent (353). The dermis is thickened, with sclerosis extending into the subcutaneous tissue resulting in septal hyalinization. The adnexal structures are destroyed (369,370). Subepidermal bullae were present in one reported case (370).

Immunofluorescence Testing. Epithelial basement membrane zone granular IgM and complement deposition is present in 39% of patients with the acute form and in 86% of patients with the chronic form of GVHD (372). In addition, IgM and C3 have been found in the walls of dermal vessels (368,372).

Pathogenesis. Acute and chronic forms of the disease have a different pathogenesis (373). In acute GVHD, it is believed that preparative regimen before the infusion of the graft cause extensive tissue damage, which releases inflammatory cytokines and expose recipient major histocompatibility complex (MHC) antigens. Recognition of the host antigen by donor T cells, and activation and proliferation of them is crucial in the initial phase. The greater the disparity between donor and recipient MHC, the greater the T-cell response. In identical pairs, the donor T cells recognize minor antigen difference. Infiltration of both CD4+ and CD8+ T cells or with either one of them predominating has been reported (375–378). γδ T cells represent a minority of infiltrates (379–380). B cells are not found.

The inflammatory cytokines (ILs, GM-CSF, TNF-α, IFN-γ) produced by activated T cells and by tissue damage during the preparative regimen also activate mononuclear

phagocytes and natural killer (NK) cells (381). Both Fas/FasL-dependent apoptosis and perforin/granzyme-dependent killing are important in GVHD-induced damage (382). In skin, young rete ridge keratinocytes (383), follicular stem cells (375), and Langerhans cells (357,358,375) are preferred targets. However, the exact mechanisms by which the skin, liver, and gastrointestinal tract are targeted are not clear.

Less is understood about the pathophysiology of chronic GVHD. The role of donor T cells against the recipient's tissue has been demonstrated. In addition, autoreactivity has also been suggested. Most immunohistochemical studies have shown that CD8+ T cells predominate. TNF-α and IL-1α are constantly produced by keratinocytes in the lesional skin (387).

Ultrastructural Study. The necrotic keratinocytic cytoplasm is filled with numerous aggregated tonofilaments (388). Granule-producing cytotoxic lymphocytes, natural killer–like cells, have been identified in direct cytolytic attack on epithelial cells undergoing apoptosis (389,390).

Differential Diagnosis. The acute phase of GVHD is similar to erythema multiforme, with scattered necrotic keratinocytes and the formation of subepidermal clefts through hydropic degeneration of basal cells. In severe cases, the fulminant lesions resemble toxic epidermal necrolysis. These patients are also at increased risk for drug eruptions, chemotherapy-induced eruptions and radiation dermatitis, all of which may be indistinguishable from acute GVHD (391,392). If there is follicular dyskeratosis, the diagnosis is much more likely to be acute GVHD. The presence of eosinophils is not necessarily in favor of drug reaction, as eosinophils are occasionally observed in GVHD. Epidermal changes identical to acute GVHD may be seen in bone marrow transplant patients without cutaneous lesions (394).

The *eruption of lymphocyte recovery* occurs predominantly in patients after receiving cytoreductive therapy (without bone marrow transplant) for acute myelogenous leukemia (394). The eruption is typically morbilliform and develops between 6 and 21 days of chemotherapy, correlating with the earliest recovery of lymphocytes to the circulation. In contrast to patients with GVHD, these patients do not develop diarrhea or liver abnormalities. Resolution occurs over several days. Histopathologically, a superficial perivascular mononuclear cell infiltrate, basal vacuolization, spongiosis, and rare dyskeratotic keratinocytes are present. The changes may be indistinguishable from those of early allogeneic or autologous GVHD, and clinical information is essential (395). The systemic administration of recombinant cytokines prior to marrow recovery leads to a relatively heavy lymphocytic infiltrate with nuclear pleomorphism and hyperchromasia (396).

Distinguishing between the lichenoid lesions of GVHD and lichen planus is often impossible. However, late sclerotic lesions can be differentiated from scleroderma by the marked atrophy of the epidermis. Active synthesis of collagen takes place largely in the upper third of the dermis; in scleroderma, collagen is synthesized mainly in the lower dermis and in the subcutaneous tissue (367).

Transient Acantholytic Dermatosis (Grover's Disease)

First described in 1970, transient acantholytic dermatosis is characterized by pruritic, discrete papules, and papulovesicles on the chest, back, and thighs (397). In rare instances, vesicles and even bullae are seen (398).

Most patients are middle-aged or elderly men. Although the disorder is transient in the majority of patients, lasting from 2 weeks to 3 months, it can persist for several years (399,400). The condition has been reported coexisting with other dermatosis, such as asteatotic eczema, allergic contact dermatitis, atopic eczema, psoriasis, and pemphigus foliaceus (404–406). There have been reports of patients with transient acantholytic dermatosis and malignancy, most commonly lymphoproliferative and genitourinary neoplasms (405–407).

Histopathology. Focal acantholysis and dyskeratosis ("focal acantholytic dyskeratosis") are present. Because these foci are small, they are sometimes found only when step sections are obtained. The acantholysis may occur in four histologic patterns, resembling Darier's disease (Fig. 9-28), Hailey–Hailey disease, pemphigus vulgaris, or spongiotic dermatitis. Two or more of these patterns may be found in the same specimen (400). There is usually a superficial dermal infiltrate of lymphocytes and sometimes eosinophils.

Immunofluorescence Testing. In general, IF results are often said to be negative (407). However, in one study, 5 of 11 patients had C3 deposition in several locations in the epidermis and at the dermo–epidermal junction, but there was no consistent pattern (408). Two other patients were

reported to have granular basement membrane zone staining of C3 alone or in combination with IgM on direct IF (409). IgA and IgM were also noted in colloid bodies, and papillary dermal vascular staining was identified.

Pathogenesis. Despite the histologic similarity to Darier's disease, Grover's disease does not share an abnormality in ATP2A2 gene (410), which encodes a keratinocyte Ca (2+) pump. Mutation of ATP2A2 is responsible for Darier's disease. Although its pathogenesis remains unknown, there appears to be a relationship to excessive sweating, fever, and bed confinement. Some authors have hypothesized that heat or sweat urea that leaks from the intraepidermal portion of the sweat duct into the surrounding epidermis causes acantholysis (411). Others dispute this theory, and have found the sweat duct to be intact (412). Finally, interleukin-4 may be responsible for acantholysis, either by induction of plasminogen activator or by stimulation of antibody production (413). The expression of syndecan-1, a proteoglycan important for keratinocytes intercellular adhesion is markedly decreased in Grover's disease. The same phenomenon also occurs in other acantholytic conditions, such as pemphigus and herpes simplex infection, suggestive of decreased intercellular adhesion that is characteristic of these lesions (414).

Ultrastructural Study. In the pemphigus-like zones, there is intradesmosomal separation (415), fewer desmosomes, and perinuclear aggregation of tonofilament bundles (416). In the Darier type, features similar to those of Darier disease are present (417).

Differential Diagnosis. The features that help differentiate transient acantholytic dermatosis from the four diseases that it resembles are the focal nature of the histologic changes and the mixture of patterns. The presence of eosinophils in the superficial dermal infiltrate of Grover's disease serves as a distinguishing feature from Darier's disease, in which they are usually absent. It is important to have clinical information for a definitive diagnosis. IF studies are rarely necessary to exclude pemphigus.

DERMATOPATHIES PRODUCED BY EXTERNAL ENERGY

Friction Blisters

These blisters develop mainly on the soles as a result of prolonged walking, and on the palms and the palmar surfaces of the fingers as a result of repetitive actions required in certain occupations or sports. They may occur also as self-inflicted artifacts (418).

Histopathology. In both naturally occurring and experimentally produced friction blisters, intraepidermal cleavage develops as a result of cytolysis and necrosis of keratinocytes in the upper stratum malpighii (419) (Fig. 9-29). The roof of the blister is composed of the stratum corneum, stratum granulosum, and amorphous cellular de-

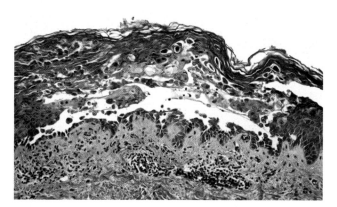

FIGURE 9-28. Transient acantholytic dermatosis. There is hypergranulosis with acantholytic dyskeratotic keratinocytes. The clefts extend to a suprabasal location.

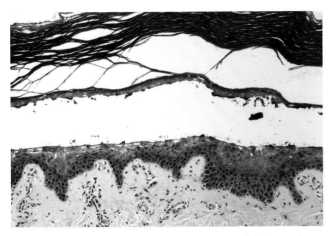

FIGURE 9-29. Friction blister. The intraepidermal blister splits at the level just beneath the stratum granulosum. A thin layer of amorphous cellular debris is present on both sides of the blister.

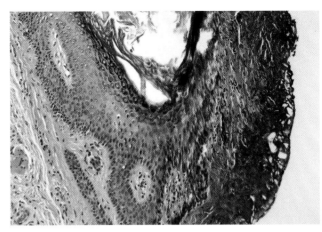

FIGURE 9-30. Electrodesiccation. The keratinocytes are elongated with nuclear pyknosis and cytoplasmic eosinophilia. The collagen is more basophilic compared to the unaffected tissue on the left.

bris (420). Most of the degenerated keratinocytes are pale and are located at the floor of the cleft. The deeper part of the epidermis consists of undamaged cells (418).

Pathogenesis. Friction blisters are caused by shearing forces within the epidermis. They form only where the epidermis is thick and firmly attached to the underlying tissue (418).

Ultrastructural Study. Electron microscopy reveals clumped tonofilaments, intracellular edema, small vacuoles at the cell periphery, and areas devoid of organelles (421).

Electric Burns

It is important that dermatopathologists be familiar with the cutaneous effects of electric current as they are used during electrodesiccation and electrocautery.

Histopathology. Electrodesiccation and electrocautery cause a separation of the epidermis from the dermis. A diagnostic histologic feature is the fringe of elongated, degenerated cytoplasmic processes that protrudes from the lower end of the detached basal cells into the subepidermal space (Fig. 9-30). The nuclei of the basal cells appear stretched vertically. In addition, the upper dermis is homogenized because of coagulation necrosis (422).

Thermal Burns

In the evaluation of thermal burns, the depth of penetration is of great importance because first- and second-degree burns heal readily, whereas third-degree burns require grafting.

Histopathology. First-degree burns are those in which the lower epidermis, particularly the basal cell layer, remains viable, and only the upper epidermis is affected by heat coagulation. In the affected areas, the nuclei may appear pyknotic and contain perinuclear halos. In a more advanced

stage, the nuclei stain faintly eosinophilic or not at all, like "architectural ghosts" (423).

Second-degree burns often show subepidermal blisters and are characterized by partial-thickness dermal necrosis. The lower portion of the cutaneous appendages remains intact, allowing re-epithelization to occur. Superficial second-degree burns are associated with necrosis of the surface epidermis and of only a small amount of superficial dermal collagen; in deep second-degree burns, much of the dermal collagen and the cutaneous appendages are injured (424). In partial-thickness dermal necrosis, the depth of epithelial damage in the cutaneous appendages is a good indicator of the depth of irreversible damage to the collagen. The border between heat coagulated and normal epithelium is sharp (425). At a later stage, an inflammatory reaction develops at the junction of the viable and nonviable tissue.

Third-degree burns show full-thickness dermal necrosis with destruction of all cutaneous appendages. The coagulation necrosis may extend to the subcutaneous tissue and to the underlying muscle (424).

Suction Blisters and Purpura

Negative pressure applied over a circumscribed area may form a subepidermal blister that arises in the lamina lucida. A second reaction, noninflammatory purpura, may also result. The changes may be secondary to overcoming the adhesive forces in the lamina lucida or in vessels (425).

REFERENCES

1. Ackerman AB, Ragaz A. A plea to expunge the word "eczema" from the lexicon of dermatology and dermatopathology. *Am J Dermatopathol* 1982;4:315.

2. Eisen HN, Orris L, Belman S. Elicitation of delayed allergic skin reactions with haptens: the dependence of elicitation on hapten combination with protein. *J Exp Med* 1952;95:473.

3. Kimber I, Dearman RJ. Allergic contact dermatitis: the cellular effectors. *Contact Dermatitis* 2002;46:1–5.

4. Kondo S, Kono T, Brown WR, et al. Lymphocyte function-associated antigen-1 is required for maximum elicitation of allergic contact dermatitis. *Br J Dermatol* 1994;131:354–359.

5. Lachapelle JM. Current concepts and new prospects. *Arch Belg Dermatol Syphiligr* 1973;20:83–92.

6. Willis CM, Stephens SJM, Wilkinson JD. Differential patterns of epidermal leukocyte infiltration in patch test reactions to structurally unrelated chemical irritants. *J Invest Dermatol* 1993; 101:364.

7. Brand CU, Hunziker T, Schaffner T, et al. Activated immuno-competent cells in human skin lymph derived from irritant contact dermatitis: an immunomorphological study. *Br J Dermatol* 1995;132:39–45.

8. Brasch J, Burgard J, Sterry W. Common pathogenetic pathways in allergic and irritant contact dermatitis. *J Invest Dermatol* 1992;98:166–170.

9. Levin CY, Maibach HI. Irritant contact dermatitis: is there an immunologic component? *Int Immunopharmacol* 2002;2:183–189.

10. Kasteler JS, Petersen MJ, Vance JE, et al. Circulating activated T lymphocytes in autoeczematization. *Arch Dermatol* 1992;128:795.

11. Ackerman AB. *Histologic diagnosis of inflammatory diseases.* Philadelphia: Lea and Febiger, 1976.

12. Weedon D. *Skin pathology,* 2nd ed. Edinburgh: Churchill-Livingstone, 2002.

13. Bruynzeel DP, Nieboer C, Boorsma DM, et al. Allergic reactions, "spillover" reactions and T cell subsets. *Arch Dermatol Res* 1983;275:80.

14. Shelley WB. Id reaction. In: *Consultations in dermatology.* Philadelphia: Saunders, 1972:262.

15. Roper SS, Jones HE. An animal model for altering the irritability threshold of normal skin. *Contact Dermatitis* 1985;13:91.

16. Choudri SH, Magro CM, Crowson AN, et al. An id reaction to *Mycobacterium leprae*: first documented case. *Cutis* 1995;54:282.

17. Epstein JH. Phototoxicity and photoallergy. *Semin Cutan Med Surg* 1999;18:274–284.

18. De Leo VA, Harber LC. Contact photodermatitis. In: Fisher AA, ed. *Contact dermatitis,* 3rd ed. Philadelphia: Lea and Febiger, 1986:454.

19. Braun-Falco O, Petry G. Feinstruktur der epidermis bei chronischem nummulärem ekzem. *Arch Klin Exp Dermatol* 1966;224: 63.

20. Diepgen TL, Fartasch M. Recent epidemiological and genetic studies in atopic dermatitis. *Acta Derm Venereol Suppl (Stockh)* 1992;176:13.

21. Soter NA, Mihm MC Jr. Morphology of atopic eczema. *Acta Dermatol Venereol Suppl (Stockh)* 1980;92:11–15.

22. Leung DY, Soter NA. Cellular and immunologic mechanisms in atopic dermatitis. *J Am Acad Dermatol* 2001;44:S1–12.

23. Ring J, Darsow U, Behrendt H. Role of aeroallergens in atopic eczema: proof of concept with the atopy patch test. *J Am Acad Dermatol* 2001;45:S49–S52.

24. Teraki Y, Hotta T, Shiohara T. Increased circulating skin-homing cutaneous lymphocyte-associated antigen (CLA)+ type 2 cytokine-producing cells, and decreased CLA+ type 1 cytokine-producing cells in atopic dermatitis. *Br J Dermatol* 2000;143: 373–378.

25. Cooper KD, Stevens SR. T cells in atopic dermatitis. *J Am Acad Dermatol* 2001;45:S10–S12.

26. Leung DY. Atopic dermatitis and the immune system: the role of superantigens and bacteria. *J Am Acad Dermatol* 2001;45: S13–S16.

27. Coleman R, Trembath RC, Harper JI. Genetic studies of atopy and atopic dermatitis. *Br J Dermatol* 1997;136:1–5.

28. Wollenberg A, Bieber T. Atopic dermatitis: from the genes to skin lesions. *Allergy* 2000;55:205–213.

29. Binder RL, Jonelis FJ. Seborrheic dermatitis in neuroleptic-induced parkinsonism. *Arch Dermatol* 1983;119:473–475.

30. Froschl M, Land HG, Landthaler M. Seborrheic dermatitis and atopic eczema in human immunodeficiency virus infection. *Semin Dermatol* 1990;9:230–232.

31. Soeprono FF, Schinella RA, Cockerell CJ, et al. Seborrheic-like dermatitis of acquired immunodeficiency syndrome. *J Am Acad Dermatol* 1986;14:242.

32. Ashbee HR, Ingham E, Holland KT, et al. The carriage of Malassezia furfur serovars A, B and C in patients with pityriasis versicolor, seborrheic dermatitis and controls. *Br J Dermatol* 1993;129:533–540.

33. Faergemann J, Bergbrant IM, Dohse M, et al. Seborrhoeic dermatitis and Pityrosporum (Malassezia) folliculitis: characterization of inflammatory cells and mediators in the skin by immunohistochemistry. *Br J Dermatol* 2001;144:549–556.

34. Rao B, Unis M, Poulos E. Acroangiodermatitis: a study of ten cases. *Int J Dermatol* 1994;33:179.

35. Pal S, Haroon TS. Erythroderma: a clinico-etiologic study of 90 cases. *Int J Dermatol* 1998;37:104–107.

36. Tomasini C, Aloi F, Solaroli C, et al. Psoriatic erythroderma: a histopathologic study of forty-five patients. *Dermatology* 1997; 194:102–106.

37. Botella-Estrada R, Sanmartin O, Oliver V, et al. Erythroderma: a clinicopathologic study of 56 cases. *Arch Dermatol* 1994;130: 1503.

38. Straka BF, Cooper PH, Greer KE. Congenital miliaria crystallina. *Cutis* 1991;47:103.

39. Pandolf KB, Griffin TB, Munro EH, et al. Heat intolerance as a function of percent of body surface involved with miliaria rubra. *Am J Physiol* 1980;239:R233.

40. Sulzberger MB, Harris DR. Miliaria and anhidrosis III: Multiple small patches and the effects of different periods of occlusion. *Arch Dermatol* 1972;105:845.

41. Loewenthal LJA. The pathogenesis of miliaria. *Arch Dermatol* 1961;84:2.

42. Lillywhite LP. Investigation into the environmental factors associated with the incidence of skin disease following an outbreak of miliaria rubra at a coal mine. *Occup Med* 1992;42:183.

43. Lyons RE, Levine R, Auld D. Miliaria rubra: a manifestation of staphylococcal disease. *Arch Dermatol* 1962;86:282.

44. Hölzle E, Kligman AM. The pathogenesis of miliaria rubra: role of the resident microflora. *Br J Dermatol* 1978;99:117.

45. Jacobs JC, Miller ME. Fatal familial Leiner's disease. *Pediatrics* 1972;49:225.

46. Stanley J, Perez D, Gigli I, et al. Hyperimmunoglobulin E syndrome. *Arch Dermatol* 1978;114:765.

47. Donabedian H, Gallin JI. The hyperimmunoglobulin E recurrent-infection (Job's) syndrome. *Medicine (Baltimore)* 1983;62: 195.

48. Rosen FS. The primary immunodeficiencies: dermatologic manifestations. *J Invest Dermatol* 1976;67:402.

49. Weston WL. Disorders of phagocytic function. *Arch Dermatol* 1976;112:1589.

50. Dilworth JA, Mandell GL. Adults with chronic granulomatous disease of "childhood." *Am J Med* 1977;63:233.

51. Civatte A. Diagnostic histopathologique de la dermatite polymorphe douloureuse ou maladie de Duhring-Brocq. *Ann Dermatol Syphiligr* 1943;3:1.

52. Beutner EH, Jordon RE. Demonstration of skin antibodies in sera of pemphigus vulgaris patients by indirect immunofluorescent staining. *Proc Soc Exp Biol Med* 1964;117:505.

53. Amagai M, Klaus-Kovtun V, Stanley JR. Autoantibodies against a novel epithelial cadherin in pemphigus vulgaris, a disease of cell adhesion. *Cell* 1991;67:869–877.

54. Koch PJ, Walsh MJ, Schmelz M, et al. Identification of desmoglein, a constitutive desmosomal glycoprotein, as a member of the cadherin family of cell adhesion molecules. *Eur J Cell Biol* 1990;53:1–12.

55. Kowalczyk AP, Anderson JE, Borgwardt JE, et al. Pemphigus sera recognize conformationally sensitive epitopes in the amino-terminal region of desmoglein-1. *J Invest Dermatol* 1995;105: 147–152.

55a. Harman KE, Gratian MJ, Bhogal BS, et al. A study of desmoglein 1 autoantibodies in pemphigus vulgaris: racial differences in frequency and the association with a more severe phenotype. *Br J Dermatol* 2000;143:343–348.

56. Younus J, Ahmed AR. The relationship of pemphigus to neoplasm. *J Am Acad Dermatol* 1990;23:482.

57. Asboe-Hansen G. Blister-spread induced by finger pressure, a diagnostic sign of pemphigus. *J Invest Dermatol* 1960;34:5.

58. Lever WF. *Pemphigus and pemphigoid*. Springfield, IL: Charles C. Thomas, 1965.

59. Tappeiner J, Pfleger L. Pemphigus vulgaris: dermatitis herpetiformis. *Arch Klin Exp Dermatol* 1962;214:415.

60. Crotty C, Pittelkow M, Muller SA. Eosinophilic spongiosis: a clinicopathologic review of seventy-one cases. *J Am Acad Dermatol* 1983;8:337.

61. Arndt K, Harrist TJ. Case records of the Massachusetts General Hospital: weekly clinicopathological exercises. Case 26–1980. *N Engl J Med* 1980;303:35.

62. Wheeland RG, Burgdorf WHC, Hoshow RA. A quick Tzanck test. *J Am Acad Dermatol* 1983;8:258.

63. Graham JH, Bingul O, Burgoon CB. Cytodiagnosis of inflammatory dermatoses. *Arch Dermatol* 1963;87:118.

64. Korman NJ. Pemphigus. *J Am Acad Dermatol* 1988;18:1219.

65. Judd KP, Lever WF. Correlation of antibodies in skin and serum with disease severity in pemphigus. *Arch Dermatol* 1979;115: 428.

66. Ratnam KV, Pang BK. Pemphigus in remission: value of negative direct immunofluorescence in management. *J Am Acad Dermatol* 1994;30:547.

67. Kuhn A, Mahrle G, Steigleder GK. Immunohistologische untersuchungen von immundermatosen am rekonstituiertem paraffinschnitt. *Hautarzt* 1988;39:351.

68. Cerio R, Macdonald DM. Routine diagnostic immunohistochemical labeling of extracellular antigens in formol saline solution-fixed, paraffin-embedded cutaneous tissue. *J Am Acad Dermatol* 1988;19:747.

69. Bhogal B, Wojnarowska F, Black MM, et al. The distribution of immunoglobulins and the C3 component of complement in multiple biopsies from the uninvolved and perilesional skin in pemphigus. *Clin Exp Dermatol* 1986;11:49.

70. Korman NJ. Pemphigus. *Immunodermatology* 1990;8:689.

71. Fitzpatrick RE, Newcomer VD. The correlation of disease activity and antibody titers in pemphigus. *Arch Dermatol* 1980;116: 285.

72. Ahmed AR, Workman S. Anti-intercellular substance antibodies: presence in serum samples of 14 patients without pemphigus. *Arch Dermatol* 1983;119:17.

73. Harrist TJ, Mihm MC. Cutaneous immunopathology: the diagnostic use of direct and indirect immunofluorescence techniques in dermatologic disease. *Hum Pathol* 1979;10:625.

74. Grop PJ, Inderbitzen TM. Pemphigus antigen and blood group substance A and B. *J Invest Dermatol* 1967;49:285.

75. Ueki H, Kohda M, Nobutoh T, et al. Antidesmoglein autoantibodies in silicosis patients with no bullous diseases. *Dermatology* 2001;202:16–21.

76. Brandsen R, Frusic-Zlotkin M, Lyubimov H, et al. Circulating pemphigus IgG in families of patients with pemphigus: comparison of indirect immunofluorescence, direct immunofluorescence, and immunoblotting. *J Am Acad Dermatol* 1997;36: 44–52.

77. Amagai M, Karpati S, Prussick R, et al. Autoantibodies against the amino-terminal cadherin-like binding domain of pemphigus vulgaris antigen are pathogenic. *J Clin Invest* 1992;90:919–926.

78. Amagai M, Hashimoto T, Shimizu N, et al. Absorption of pathogenic autoantibodies by the extracellular domain of pemphigus vulgaris antigen (Dsg3) produced by baculovirus. *J Clin Invest* 1994;94:59–67.

79. Futei Y, Amagai M, Sekiguchi M, et al. Use of domain-swapped molecules for co-informational epitope mapping of desmoglein 3 in pemphigus vulgaris. *J Invest Dermatol* 2000;115:829–834.

80. Schiltz JR. Pemphigus acantholysis: a unique immunologic injury. *J Invest Dermatol* 1980;74:359.

81. Hashimoto T, Sugiura M, Kurihara S, et al. *In vitro* complement activation by intercellular antibodies. *J Invest Dermatol* 1982;78: 316.

82. Hashimoto K, Lever WF. An electron microscopic study of pemphigus vulgaris of the mouth with special reference to the intercellular cement. *J Invest Dermatol* 1967;48:540.

83. Hashimoto K, Lever WF. The intercellular cement in pemphigus vulgaris: an electron microscopic study. *Dermatologica* 1967; 135:27.

84. Zhou S, Ferguson DJ, Allen J, et al. The location of binding sites of pemphigus vulgaris and pemphigus foliaceus autoantibodies: a post-embedding immunoelectron microscopic study. *Br J Dermatol* 1997;136:878–883.

85. Ahmed AR, Blose DA. Pemphigus vegetans, Neumann type and Hallopeau type. *Int J Dermatol* 1984;23:135.

86. Nelson CG, Apisarnthanarax P, Bean SF, et al. Pemphigus vegetans of Hallopeau: immunofluorescence studies. *Arch Dermatol* 1977;114:627.

87. Lever WF. Pemphigus and pemphigoid: a review of the advances made since 1964. *J Am Acad Dermatol* 1979;1:2.

88. Bianchi L, Carrozzo AM, Orlandi A, et al. Pyoderma vegetans and ulcerative colitis. *Br J Dermatol* 2001;144:1224–1227.

89. Beutner EH, Prigenzi LS, Hale LS, et al. Immunofluorescent studies of autoantibodies to intracellular areas of epithelia in Brazilian pemphigus foliaceus. *Proc Soc Exp Biol Med* 1968;127: 81.

90. Crosby DL, Diaz LA. Endemic pemphigus foliaceus. *Dermatol Clin* 1993;11:453.

91. Clovis, Borges, Chaul, et al. Environmental risk factors in endemic pemphigus foliaceus (fogo selvagem). *J Invest Dermatol* 1992;98:847.

92. Reis VM, Toledo RP, Lopez A, et al. UVB-induced acantholysis in endemic pemphigus foliaceus (fogo selvagem) and pemphigus vulgaris. *J Am Acad Dermatol* 2000;42:571–576.

93. Perry HO. Pemphigus foliaceus. *Arch Dermatol* 1961;83:57.

94. Emerson RW, Wilson Jones E. Eosinophilic spongiosis in pemphigus. *Arch Dermatol* 1968;97:252.

95. Jablonska S, Chorzelski TP, Beutner EH, et al. Herpetiform pemphigus: a variable pattern of pemphigus. *Int J Dermatol* 1975;14:353.

96. Lagerholm B, Frithz A, Borglund E. Light and electron microscopic aspects of pemphigus herpetiformis (eosinophilic spongiosis) in comparison with other acantholytic disorders. *Acta Derm Venereol (Stockh)* 1979;59:305.

97. Bystryn JC, Abel E, Defeo C. Pemphigus foliaceus: subcorneal intercellular antibodies of unique specificity. *Arch Dermatol* 1974;110:857.

98. Amagai M. Desmoglein as a target in autoimmunity and infection. *J Am Acad Dermatol* 2003;48:244–252.

99. Ioannides D, Hytiroglou P, Phelps RG, et al. Regional variation in the expression of pemphigus foliaceus, pemphigus erythematosus, and pemphigus vulgaris antigens in human skin. *J Invest Dermatol* 1991;96:159.

100. Arteaga LA, Prisayauh PS, Simon JP, et al. A subset of pemphigus foliaceus patients exhibits pathogenetic autoantibodies against both desmoglein 1 and desmoglein 3. *J Inv Dermatol* 2002;118:806–811.

101. Wilgram GF, Caulfield JB, Madgic EB. An electron microscopic study of acantholysis and dyskeratosis in pemphigus foliaceus. *J Invest Dermatol* 1964;43:287.

102. Amerian ML, Ahmed AR. Pemphigus erythematosus: presentation of four cases and review of the literature. *J Am Acad Dermatol* 1984;10:215.

103. Perry HO, Brunsting LA. Pemphigus foliaceus. *Arch Dermatol* 1965;91:10.

104. Robinson ND, Hashimoto T, Amagai M, et al. The new pemphigus variants. *J Am Acad Dermatol* 1999;40:649–671.

105. Ishii K, Amagai M, Komai A, et al. Desmoglein 1 and desmoglein 3 are the target autoantigens in herpetiform pemphigus. *Arch Dermatol* 1999;135:943–947.

106. Korman NJ, Eyre RW, Zone J, et al. Drug-induced pemphigus: autoantibodies directed against the pemphigus antigen complexes are present in penicillamine and captopril-induced pemphigus. *J Invest Dermatol* 1991;96:273.

107. Pisani M, Ruocco V. Drug induced pemphigus. *Clin Dermatol* 1986;4:118.

108. Ruocco V, Sacerdoti G. Pemphigus and bullous pemphigoid due to drugs. *Int J Dermatol* 1991;30:307.

109. Ruocco V, de Luca M, Pisani M, et al. Pemphigus provoked by D-penicillamine: an experimental approach using *in vitro* tissue cultures. *Dermatologica* 1982;164:236.

110. Yokel BK, Hood AF, Anhalt GJ. Induction of acantholysis in organ explant culture by penicillamine and captopril. *Arch Dermatol* 1989;125:1367.

111. Eyre RW, Stanley JR. Human autoantibodies against a desmosomal complex with a calcium-sensitive epitope are characteristic of pemphigus foliaceus patients. *J Exp Med* 1987;165:1719.

112. Eyre RW, Stanley JR. Identification of pemphigus vulgaris antigen extracted from normal human epidermis and comparison with pemphigus foliaceus antigen. *J Clin Invest* 1988;81:807.

113. Hodak E, David M, Ingber A, et al. The clinical and histopathological spectrum of IgA-pemphigus: a report of two cases. *Clin Exp Dermatol* 1990;15:433.

114. Saurat JH, Merot Y, Salomon D, et al. Pemphigus-like IgA deposits and vesiculopustular dermatosis in a 10-year-old girl. *Dermatologica* 1987;20:89.

115. Beutner EH, Chorzelski TP, Wilson RM, et al. IgA pemphigus foliaceus. *J Am Acad Dermatol* 1989;20:89.

116. Burrows D, Bingham EA. Subcorneal pustular dermatosis and IgA gammopathy. *Br J Dermatol* 1984;11:91.

117. Harman KE, Holmes G, Bhogal BS, et al. Intercellular IgA dermatosis (IgA pemphigus)—two cases illustrating the clinical heterogeneity of this disorder. *Clin Exp Dermatol* 1999;24:464–466.

118. Teraki Y, Amagai Z, Hashimoto T, et al. Intercellular IgA dermatosis of childhood. *Arch Dermatol* 1991;127:221.

119. Ebihara T, Hashimoto T, Iwatsuki K, et al. Autoantigens for IgA anti-intercellular antibodies of intercellular IgA vesiculopustular dermatosis. *J Invest Dermatol* 1991;97:742.

120. Neumann E, Dmochowski M, Bowszyc M, et al. The occurrence of IgA pemphigus foliaceus without neutrophilic infiltration. *Clin Exp Dermatol* 1994;19:56.

121. Ohno H, Miyagawa S, Hashimoto T, et al. Atypical pemphigus with concomitant IgG and IgA anti-intercellular autoantibodies associated with monoclonal IgA gammopathy. *Dermatology* 1994;189[Suppl]:115.

122. Hashimoto T, Inamoto N, Nakamura K, et al. Intercellular IgA dermatosis with clinical features of subcorneal pustular dermatosis. *Arch Dermatol* 1987;123:1062.

123. Piette W, Burken RP, Ray TL. Intraepidermal neutrophilic dermatosis: presence of circulating pemphigus-like IgA antibody specific for monkey epithelium. *J Invest Dermatol* 1987;88:512.

124. Tagami H, Iwatsuki K, Iwase Y, et al. Subcorneal pustular dermatosis with vesiculobullous eruption: demonstration of subcorneal IgA deposition and a leukocyte chemotactic factor. *Br J Dermatol* 1983;109:581.

125. Nishikawa T, Shimizu H, Hashimoto T. Role of IgA intercellular anti-bodies: report of clinically and immunologically atypical cases. In: Orfanos CE, Stadler R, Gollnick H, eds. *Proceedings of the 17th World Congress of Dermatology.* New York: Springer-Verlag, 1987:383.

126. Hashimoto T, Kiyokawa C, Mori O, et al. Human desmocollin 1 (Dsc 1) is an autoantigen for the subcorneal pustular dermatosis type of IgA pemphigus. *J Invest Dermatol* 1997;109:127–131.

127. Miyagawa S, Hashimoto T, Ohno H, et al. Atypical pemphigus associated with monoclonal IgA gammopathy. *J Am Acad Dermatol* 1995;32:352–357.

128. Hashimoto T, Komai A, Futei Y, et al. Detection of IgA autoantibodies to desmogleins by an enzyme-linked immunosorbent assay: the presence of new minor subtypes of IgA pemphigus. *Arch Dermatol* 2001.

129. Anhalt GJ. Paraneoplastic pemphigus. *Adv Dermatol* 1997;77–97.

129a. Nguyen VT, Ndoye A, Bassler KD, et al. Classification, clinical manifestations, and immunopathological mechanisms of the epithelial variant of paraneoplastic autoimmune multiorgan syndrome: a reappraisal of paraneoplastic pemphigus. *Arch Dermatol* 2001;137:193–206.

130. Mutasim DF, Pelc NJ, Anhalt GJ. Paraneoplastic pemphigus. *Dermatol Clin* 1993;11:473.

131. Anhalt GJ, Kim SC, Stanley JR, et al. Paraneoplastic pemphigus: an autoimmune mucocutaneous disease associated with neoplasia. *N Engl J Med* 1990;323:1729.

132. Bystryn JC, Hodak E, Gao SQ, et al. A paraneoplastic mixed bullous skin disease associated with anti-skin antibodies and a B-cell lymphoma. *Arch Dermatol* 1993;129:870.

132a. Musette P, Joly P, Gilbert D, et al. A paraneoplastic mixed bullous skin disease: breakdown in tolerance to multiple epidermal antigens. *Br J Dermatol* 2000;143:149–53.

132b. Setterfield J, Shirlaw PJ, Lazarova Z, et al. Paraneoplastic cicatricial pemphigoid. *Br J Dermatol* 1999;141:127–31.

133. Horn TD, Anhalt GJ. Histologic features of paraneoplastic pemphigus. *Arch Dermatol* 1992;128:1091.

134. Stevens SR, Griffiths EM, Anhalt GJ, et al. Paraneoplastic pemphigus presenting as a lichen planus pemphigoides-like eruption. *Arch Dermatol* 1993;129:866.

135. Mehregan DR, Oursler JR, Leiferman KM, et al. Paraneoplastic pemphigus: a subset of patients with pemphigus and neoplasia. *J Cutan Pathol* 1993;20:203–210.

136. Mueller S, Klaus-Kovtun VS, Stanley JR. A 230-kD basic protein is the major bullous pemphigoid antigen. *J Invest Dermatol* 1989;92:33–38.

137. Marinkovich MP, Taylor TB, Keene DR, et al. LAD-1, the linear IgA bullous dermatosis autoantigen, is a novel 120-kDa anchoring filament protein synthesized by epidermal cells. *J Invest Dermatol* 1996;106:734–738.

138. Zillikens D, Giudice GJ. BP180/type XVII collagen: its role in acquired and inherited disorders or the dermal-epidermal junction. *Arch Dermatol Res* 1999;291:187–194.

139. Schmidt E, Zillikens D. Autoimmune and inherited subepidermal blistering diseases: advances in the clinic and the laboratory. *Adv Dermatol* 2000;16:113–158.

140. Vidal F, Aberdam D, Miquel C, et al. Integrin beta 4 mutations associated with junctional epidermolysis bullosa with pyloric atresia. *Nat Genet* 1995;10:229–234.

141. Tyagi S, Bhol K, Natarajan K, et al. Ocular cicatricial pemphigoid antigen: partial sequence and biochemical characterization. *Proc Natl Acad Sci U S A* 1996;93:14714–14719.

142. Pulkkinen L, Christiano AM, Gerecke D, et al. A homozygous nonsense mutation in the beta 3 chain gene of laminin 5 (LAMB3) in Herlitz junctional epidermolysis bullosa. *Genomics* 1994;24:357–360.

143. Woodley DT, Burgeson RE, Lunstrum G, et al. Epidermolysis bullosa acquisita antigen is the globular carboxyl terminus of type VII procollagen. *J Clin Invest* 1988;81:683–687.

144. Gammon WR, Woodley DT, Dole KC, et al. Evidence that anti-basement membrane zone antibodies in bullous eruption of systemic lupus erythematosus recognize epidermolysis bullosa acquisita autoantigen. *J Invest Dermatol* 1985;84:472–476.

145. Chorzelski TP, Jablonska S, Maciejowska E. Linear IgA bullous dermatosis of adults. *Clin Dermatol* 1991;9:383–392.

146. Lever WF. Pemphigus. *Medicine (Baltimore)* 1953;32:1.

147. Asbrink E, Hovmark A. Clinical variations in bullous pemphigoid with respect to early symptoms. *Acta Derm Venereol (Stockh)* 1981;61:417.

148. Amato DA, Silverstein J, Zitelli J. The prodrome of bullous pemphigoid. *Int J Dermatol* 1988;27:560.

149. Bushkell LL, Jordon RE. Bullous pemphigoid: a cause of peripheral blood eosinophilia. *J Am Acad Dermatol* 1983;8:648.

150. Rook AJ, Waddington E. Pemphigus and pemphigoid. *Br J Dermatol* 1953;65:425.

151. Winkelmann RK, Su WPD. Pemphigoid vegetans. *Arch Dermatol* 1979;115:446.

152. Kuokkanen K, Helin H. Pemphigoid vegetans. *Arch Dermatol* 1981;117:56.

153. Sams WM, Jordon RD. Correlation of pemphigoid and pemphigus antibody with activity of disease. *Br J Dermatol* 1971;84:7.

154. Person JR, Rogers RS III. Bullous and cicatricial pemphigoid: clinical, histologic, pathogenic, and immunopathological correlations. *Mayo Clin Proc* 1977;52:54.

155. Schaumburg-Lever G, Rule A, Schmidt-Ullrich B, et al. Ultrastructural localization of in vivo bound immunoglobulins in bullous pemphigoid. *J Invest Dermatol* 1975;64:47.

156. Holubar K, Wolfe K, Konrad K, et al. Ultrastructural localization of immunoglobulins in bullous pemphigoid skin. *J Invest Dermatol* 1975;64:220.

157. Mutasim DF, Anhalt GJ, Diaz LA. Linear immunofluorescence staining of the basement membrane zone produced by pemphigoid antibodies: the result of hemidesmosome staining. *J Am Acad Dermatol* 1987;16:75.

158. Gammon WR, Briggaman RA, Inman AO, et al. Differentiating anti-lamina lucida and anti-sublamina densa anti-BMZ antibodies by indirect immunofluorescence on 1.0 M sodium chloride-separated skin. *J Invest Dermatol* 1984;82:139.

159. Pang BK, Lee YS, Ratnam KV. Floor-pattern salt-split skin cannot distinguish bullous pemphigoid from epidermolysis bullosa acquisita. *Arch Dermatol* 1993;129:744.

160. Logan RA, Bhogal B, Das AK, et al. Localization of bullous pemphigoid antibody: an indirect immunofluorescence study of 228 cases using a split-skin technique. *Br J Dermatol* 1987;117:471.

161. Wuepper KD. Repeat direct immunofluorescence to discriminate pemphigoid from epidermolysis bullosa acquisita. *Arch Dermatol* 1990;126:1365(correspondence).

162. Gammon WR, Kowalewski C, Chorzelski TP, et al. Direct immunofluorescence studies of sodium chloride-separated skin in the differential diagnosis of bullous pemphigoid and epidermolysis bullosa acquisita. *J Am Acad Dermatol* 1990;22:664.

163. Meuller S, Klaus-Kovtun V, Stanley JR. A 230kD basic protein is the major bullous pemphigoid antigen. *J Invest Dermatol* 1989;92:33.

164. Labib RS, Anhalt GJ, Patel HP, et al. Molecular heterogeneity of the bullous pemphigoid antigens as detected by immunoblotting. *J Immunol* 1986;136:1231.

165. Goldberg DJ, Sablonski M, Bystryn JC. Regional variation in the expression of bullous pemphigoid antigen and location of lesions in bullous pemphigoid. *J Invest Dermatol* 1984;82:326.

166. Cotell SL, Lapiere JC, Chen JD, et al. A novel 105-kDa lamina lucida autoantigen: association with bullous pemphigoid. *J Invest Dermatol* 1994;103:78.

167. Chan LS, Cooper KD. A novel immune-mediated subepidermal bullous dermatosis characterized by IgG autoantibodies to a lower lamina lucida component. *Arch Dermatol* 1994;130:343.

168. Nakagawa T, De Weck AL. Membrane receptors for the IgG4 subclass of human basophils and mast cells. *Clin Rev Allergy* 1983;1:197.

169. Varigos GA, Morstyn G, Vadas MA. Bullous pemphigoid blister fluid stimulates eosinophil colony formation and activates eosinophils. *Clin Exp Immunol* 1982;50:555.

170. Grando SA, Glukhensky BT, Drannik GN, et al. Mediators of inflammation in blister fluids from patients with bullous pemphigoid and pemphigus vulgaris. *Arch Dermatol* 1989;125:925.

171. Brown LF, Harrist TJ, Yeo KT, et al. Increased expression of vascular permeability factor (vascular endothelial growth factor) in bullous pemphigoid, dermatitis herpetiformis and erythema multiforme. *J Invest Dermatol* 1995;104:744.

172. Stahle-Backdahl M, Inoue M, Giudice GJ, et al. 92-kD gelatinase is produced by eosinophils at the site of blister formation in bullous pemphigoid and cleaves the extracellular domain of recombinant 180-kD bullous pemphigoid autoantigen. *J Clin Invest* 1994;93:2022.

173. Kaneko F, Minagawa T, Takiguchi Y, et al. Role of cell-mediated immune reaction in blister formation of bullous pemphigoid. *Dermatology* 1992;184:34.

174. Braun-Falco O, Rupec M. Elektronenmikroskopische untersuchungen zur dynamik der acantholyse bei pemphigus vulgaris. *Arch Klin Exp Dermatol* 1967;230:1.

175. Kobayashi T. The dermo-epidermal junction in bullous pemphigoid. *Dermatologica* 1967;134:157.

176. Lever WF, Hashimoto K. The etiology and treatment of pemphigus and pemphigoid. *J Invest Dermatol* 1969;53:373.

177. Schaumburg-Lever G, Orfanos CE, Lever WF. Electron microscopic study of bullous pemphigoid. *Arch Dermatol* 1972;106:662.

178. Fellner MJ, Katz JM. Occurrence of bullous pemphigoid after furosemide therapy. *Arch Dermatol* 1976;112:75.

179. Kashihara M, Danno K, Miyachi Y, et al. Bullous pemphigoid-like lesions induced by phenacetin. *Arch Dermatol* 1984;120:1196.

180. Hodak E, Ben-Shetrit A, Ingber A, et al. Bullous pemphigoid: an adverse effect of ampicillin. *Clin Exp Dermatol* 1990;15:50.

181. Person JR, Rogers RS III, Perry HO. Localized pemphigoid. *Br J Dermatol* 1976;95:531.

182. Soh H, Hosokawa H, Miyauchi H, et al. Localized pemphigoid shares the same target antigen as bullous pemphigoid. *Br J Dermatol* 1991;125:73.

183. Behlen CH, Mackay DM. Benign mucous membrane pemphigus with a generalized eruption. *Arch Dermatol* 1965;92:566.

184. Brauner GJ, Jimbow K. Benign mucous membrane pemphigoid. *Arch Dermatol* 1972;106:535.

185. Lever WF. Pemphigus conjunctivae with scarring of the skin. *Arch Dermatol Syphilol* 1942;46:875, and 1944;49:113.

186. Hardy KM, Perry HO, Pingree GC, et al. Benign mucous membrane pemphigoid. *Arch Dermatol* 1971;104:467.

187. Kleine-Natrop HE, Haustein UF. "Benignes Schleimhautpemphigoid" mit rascher Erblindung und generalisierten vernarbenden Hautveränderungen. *Hautarzt* 1968;19:6.

188. Tagami H, Imamura S. Benign mucous membrane pemphigoid. *Arch Dermatol* 1974;109:711.

189. Brunsting LA, Perry HO. Benign pemphigoid? A report of seven cases with chronic scarring, herpetiform plaques about the head and neck. *Arch Dermatol* 1957;75:489.

190. Michel B, Bean SF, Chorzelski T, et al. Cicatricial pemphigoid of Brunsting–Perry: immunofluorescent studies. *Arch Dermatol* 1977;113:1403.

191. Hanno R, Foster DR, Bean SF. Brunsting–Perry cicatricial pemphigoid associated with bullous pemphigoid. *J Am Acad Dermatol* 1980;3:470.

192. Provost TT, Maize JC, Ahmed AR, et al. Unusual subepidermal bullous diseases with immunologic features of bullous pemphigoid. *Arch Dermatol* 1979;115:156.

193. Braun-Falco O, Wolff HH, Ponce E. Disseminiertes vernarbendes pemphigoid. *Hautarzt* 1981;32:233.

194. Rogers RS III, Seehafer JR, Perry HO. Treatment of cicatricial (benign mucous membrane) pemphigoid with dapsone. *J Am Acad Dermatol* 1982;6:215.

195. Bean SF. Cicatricial pemphigoid: immunofluorescent studies. *Arch Dermatol* 1974;110:552.

196. Griffith MR, Fukuyama K, Tuffanelli D, et al. Immunofluorescent studies in mucous membrane pemphigoid. *Arch Dermatol* 1974;109:195.

197. Rogers RS III, Perry HO, Bean SF, et al. Immunopathology of cicatricial pemphigoid: studies of complement deposition. *J Invest Dermatol* 1977;68:39.

198. Reunala T, Rantala J, Histanen J, et al. Linear IgA deposition in benign mucous membrane pemphigoid. *J Cutan Pathol* 1984;11:232(abst).

199. Leonard JN, Wright P, Williams DM, et al. The relationship between linear IgA disease and benign mucous membrane pemphigoid. *Br J Dermatol* 1984;110:307.

200. Leonard JN, Hobday CM, Haffenden GP, et al. Immunofluorescent studies in ocular cicatricial pemphigoid. *Br J Dermatol* 1988;118:209.

201. Wojnarowska F, Marsden RA, Bhogal B, et al. Childhood cicatricial pemphigoid with linear IgA deposits. *Clin Exp Dermatol* 1984;9:407.

202. Jacoby WD Jr, Bartholome CW, Ramchand SC, et al. Cicatricial pemphigoid (Brunsting–Perry type): case report and immunofluorescence findings. *Arch Dermatol* 1978;114:779.

203. Ahmed AR, Salm M, Larson R, et al. Localized cicatricial pemphigoid (Brunsting–Perry). *Arch Dermatol* 1984;120:932.

204. Kelly SE, Wojnarowska F. The use of chemically split tissue in the detection of circulating anti-basement membrane antibodies in bullous pemphigoid and cicatricial pemphigoid. *Br J Dermatol* 1988;118:31.

205. Fine JD, Neises GR, Katz SI. Immunofluorescence and immunoelectron microscopic studies in cicatricial pemphigoid. *J Invest Dermatol* 1984;82:39.

206. Domloge-Hultsch N, Anhalt GJ, Gammon WR, et al. Anti-epiligrin cicatricial pemphigoid: a subepithelial bullous disorder. *Arch Dermatol* 1994;130:1521.

207. Bhol KC, Dans MJ, Simmons RK, et al. The autoantibodies to alpha 6 beta 4 integrin of patients affected by ocular cicatricial pemphigoid recognize predominately epitopes within the large cytoplasmic domain of human beta 4. *J Immunol* 2000;165:2824–2829.

208. Bernard P, Prost C, Lecerf V, et al. Studies of cicatricial pemphigoid autoantibodies using direct immunoelectron microscopy and immunoblot analysis. *J Invest Dermatol* 1990;94:630.

209. Susi FR, Shklar G. Histochemistry and fine structure of oral lesions of mucous membrane pemphigoid. *Arch Dermatol* 1971;104:244.

210. Caputo R, Bellone AG, Crosti C. Pathogenesis of the blister in cicatricial pemphigoid and in bullous pemphigoid. *Arch Dermatol Forsch* 1973;247:181.

211. Shornick JK, Bangert JL, Freeman RG, et al. Herpes gestationis: clinical and histologic features of twenty-eight cases. *J Am Acad Dermatol* 1983;8:214.

212. Shornick JK. Herpes gestationis. *Dermatol Clin* 1993;11:527.

213. Shornick JK, Black MM. Fetal risks in herpes gestationis. *J Am Acad Dermatol* 1992;26:63.

214. Chorzelski TP, Jablonska S, Beutner EH, et al. Herpes gestationis with identical lesions in the newborn. *Arch Dermatol* 1976;112:1129.

215. Katz A, Minta JO, Toole JWP, et al. Immunopathologic study of herpes gestationis in mother and infant. *Arch Dermatol* 1977;113:1069.

216. Piérard J, Thiery M, Kint A. Histologie et ultrastructure de l'herpes gestationis. *Arch Belg Dermatol Syphiligr* 1969;25:321.

217. Hertz KC, Katz SI, Maize J, et al. Herpes gestationis: a clinicopathological study. *Arch Dermatol* 1976;112:1543.

218. Provost TT, Tomasi TB. Evidence for complement activation via the alternate pathway in skin diseases. *J Clin Invest* 1973;52:1779.

219. Kelly SE, Bhogal BS, Wojnarowska F, et al. Western blot analysis of the antigen in pemphigoid gestationis. *Br J Dermatol* 1990;122:445.

220. Morrison LH, Labib RS, Zone JJ, et al. Herpes gestationis autoantibodies recognize a 180kD human epidermal antigen. *J Clin Invest* 1988;81:2023.

221. Li K, Tamai K, Tan EM, et al. Cloning of type XVII collagen. *J Biochem* 1993;268:8825.

222. Schaumburg-Lever G, Saffold OE, Orfanos CE, et al. Herpes gestationis: histology and ultrastructure. *Arch Dermatol* 1973;107:888.

223. Yaoita H, Gullino M, Katz SI. Herpes gestationis: ultrastructure and ultrastructural localization on in vivo-bound complement. *J Invest Dermatol* 1976;66:383.

224. Roenigk HH Jr, Ryan JG, Bergfeld WG. Epidermolysis bullosa acquisita: report of three cases and review of all published cases. *Arch Dermatol* 1971;103:1.

225. Gammon WR, Briggaman RA, Woodley DT, et al. Epidermolysis bullosa acquisita: a pemphigoid-like disease. *J Am Acad Dermatol* 1984;11:820.

226. Dahl MV. Epidermolysis bullosa acquisita: a sign of cicatricial pemphigoid? *Br J Dermatol* 1979;101:475.

227. Yaoita H, Briggaman RA, Lawly TJ, et al. Epidermolysis bullosa acquisita: ultrastructural and immunologic studies. *J Invest Dermatol* 1981;76:288.

228. Woodley DT, Gammon WR. Epidermolysis bullosa acquisita. *Immunol Ser* 1989;46:547.

229. Gammon WR, Fine JD, Briggaman RA. Autoimmunity to type VII collagen: features and roles in basement membrane zone injury. In: Fine JD, ed. *Bullous diseases*. New York: Igaku Shoin, 1993:75.

230. Nieboer C, Boorsma DM, Woerdeman MJ, et al. Epidermolysis bullosa acquisita: immunofluorescence, electron microscopic and immunoelectron microscopic studies in four patients. *Br J Dermatol* 1980;102:383.

231. Woodley DT, Burgeson RE, Lunstrum G, et al. The epidermolysis bullosa acquisita antigen is the globular carboxy terminus of type VII procollagen. *J Clin Invest* 1988;81:683.

232. Olansky AJ, Briggaman RA, Gammon WR, et al. Bullous systemic lupus erythematosus. *J Am Acad Dermatol* 1982;7:511.

233. Miller JA, Dowd DM, Dudeney C, et al. Vesiculobullous eruption in systemic lupus erythematosus: demonstration of common anti-DNA antibody idiotype at the dermoepidermal junction. *J R Soc Med* 1968;79:365.

234. Barton DD, Fine JD, Gammon WR, et al. Bullous systemic lupus erythematosus: an unusual clinical course and detectable circulating antibodies to the epidermolysis bullosa acquisita antigen. *J Am Acad Dermatol* 1986;15:369.

235. Kettler AH, Bean SF, Duffy JO, et al. Systemic lupus erythematosus presenting as a bullous eruption in a child. *Arch Dermatol* 1988;124:1083.

236. Pedro SD, Dahl MV. Direct immunofluorescence of bullous systemic lupus erythematosus. *Arch Dermatol* 1973;107:118.

237. Jacoby RA, Abraham AA. Bullous dermatosis and systemic lupus erythematosus in a 15-year-old boy. *Arch Dermatol* 1979; 115:1094.

238. Penneys NS, Wiley HS. Herpetiform blisters in lupus erythematosus. *Arch Dermatol* 1979;115:1427.

239. Hall RP, Lawley TJ, Smith HR, et al. Bullous eruption of systemic lupus erythematosus: dramatic response to dapsone therapy. *Ann Intern Med* 1979;97:165.

240. Camisa C, Sharma HM. Vesiculobullous systemic lupus erythematosus: a report of two cases and a review of the literature. *J Am Acad Dermatol* 1983;9:924.

241. Tsuchida T, Furue M, Kashiwado T, et al. Bullous systemic lupus erythematosus with cutaneous mucinosis and leukocytoclastic vasculitis. *J Am Acad Dermatol* 1994;31:387.

242. Gammon WR, Woodley DT, Dole KC, et al. Evidence that anti-basement membrane zone antibodies in bullous eruption of systemic lupus erythematosus recognized epidermolysis bullosa acquisita autoantigen. *J Invest Dermatol* 1985;84:472.

243. Tolman MM, Moschella SL, Schneiderman RN. Dermatitis herpetiformis: specific entity or clinical complex? *J Invest Dermatol* 1959;32:557.

244. Bose SK, Lacour JP, Bodokh I, et al. Malignant lymphoma and dermatitis herpetiformis. *Dermatology* 1994;188:177–181.

245. Aronson AJ, Soltani R, Aronson IK, et al. Systemic lupus erythematosus and dermatitis herpetiformis: concurrence with Marfan's syndrome. *Arch Dermatol* 1979;115:68.

246. Piérard J. De l'aspect histologique des plaques érythémateuses de la dermatite herpétiforme de Duhring. *Ann Dermatol Syphiligr (Paris)* 1963;90:121.

247. Clark WH, Yip SY, Tolman MB. The histiogenesis of dermoepidermal separation in dermatitis herpetiformis. *Clin Res* 1968;61:433(abst).

248. MacVicar DN, Graham JH, Burgoon CF Jr. Dermatitis herpetiformis, erythema multiforme and bullous pemphigoid: a comparative histopathological and histochemical study. *J Invest Dermatol* 1963;41:289.

249. Eng AM, Moncada B. Bullous pemphigoid and dermatitis herpetiformis: histologic differentiation. *Arch Dermatol* 1974;110: 51.

250. Kint A, Geerts ML, De Brauwere D. Diagnostic criteria in dermatitis herpetiformis. *Dermatologica* 1976;153:266.

251. Connor BL, Marks R, Wilson Jones E. Dermatitis herpetiformis. *Trans St Johns Hosp Dermatol Soc* 1972;58:191.

252. Cormane R. Immunofluorescent studies of the skin in lupus erythematosus and other diseases. *Pathol Eur* 1967;2:170.

253. Zone JJ, Carioto LA, LaSalle BA, et al. Granular IgA is decreased or absent in never involved skin in dermatitis herpetiformis. *Clin Res* 1985;33:159.

254. Van der Meer JB. Granular deposits of immunoglobulins in the skin of patients with dermatitis herpetiformis: an immunofluorescent study. *Br J Dermatol* 1969;81:493.

255. Chorzelski TP, Beutner EH, Jablonska S, et al. Immunofluorescence studies in the diagnosis of dermatitis herpetiformis and its differentiation from bullous pemphigoid. *J Invest Dermatol* 1971;56:373.

256. Beautner EH, Chorzelski TB, Kumar V, et al. Sensitivity and specificity of IgA-class antiendomysial antibodies for dermatitis herpetiformis and findings relevant to their pathogenic significance. *J Am Acad Dermatol* 1986;15:464–473.

257. Kadunce DP, Meyer LJ, Zone JJ. IgA class antibodies in dermatitis herpetiformis: reaction with tissue antigens. *J Invest Dermatol* 1989;93:253.

258. Kumar V, Hemedenger E, Chorzelski T, et al. Reticulin and endomysial antibodies in bullous diseases. Comparison of specificity and sensitivity. *Arch Dermatol* 1987;123:1179.

259. Katz SI, Hertz KC, Rogentine GN, et al. HLA-B8 and dermatitis herpetiformis in patients with IgA deposits in skin. *Arch Dermatol* 1977;113:155.

260. Strober W. Immunogenic factors. In: Katz SI, moderator. Dermatitis herpetiformis: the skin and the gut. *Ann Intern Med* 1980;93:857.

261. Hall RP, Sanders ME, Duquesnoy RJ, et al. Alterations in HLA-DP and HLA-DQ antigen frequency in patients with dermatitis herpetiformis. *J Invest Dermatol* 1989;93:501.

262. Marks J, Shuster S, Watson A. Small bowel changes in dermatitis herpetiformis. *Lancet* 1966;2:1280.

262a. Kumar V, Jarzabek-Chorzelska M, Sulej J, et al. Tissue transglutaminase and endomysial antibodies-diagnostic markers of gluten-sensitive enteropathy in dermatitis herpetiformis. *Clin Immunol* 2001;98:378–382.

262b. Sardy M, Karpati S, Merkl B, et al. Epidermal transglutaminase (TGase 3) is the autoantigen of dermatitis herpetiformis. *J Exp Med* 2002;195:747–757.

263. Graeber M, Baker BS, Garioch JJ, et al. The role of cytokines in the generation of skin lesions in dermatitis herpetiformis. *Br J Dermatol* 1993;129:530–532.

264. Karttunen T, Autio-Harmainen H, Rasanen O, et al. Immunohistochemical localization of epidermal basement membrane laminin and type IV collagen in bullous lesions of dermatitis herpetiformis. *Br J Dermatol* 1984;111:389–394.

265. Pardo RJ, Penneys NS. Location of basement membrane type IV collagen beneath subepidermal bullous diseases. *J Cutan Pathol* 1990;17:336.

266. Godfrey K, Wojnarowska F, Leonard J. Linear IgA disease of adult: association with lymphoproliferative malignancy and possible role of other triggering factors. *Br J Dermatol* 1990; 123:447–452.

267. Paige DG, Leonard JN, Wojnarowska F, et al. Linear IgA disease and ulcerative colitis. *Br J Dermatol* 1997;136:779–782.

268. Lau M, Kaufmann-Grunzinger I, Raghunath M. A case report of a patient with features of systemic lupus erythematosus and linear IgA disease. *Br J Dermatol* 1991;124:498.

269. Smith SB, Harrist TJ, Murphy GF, et al. Linear IgA bullous dermatosis v. dermatitis herpetiformis. *Arch Dermatol* 1984; 120:324.

270. Adachi A, Tani M, Matsubayashi S, et al. Immunoelectron microscopic differentiation of linear IgA bullous dermatosis of adults with coexistence of IgA and IgG deposition from bullous pemphigoid. *J Am Acad Dermatol* 1992;27:394.

271. Petersen MJ, Gammon WR, Briggaman RA. A case of linear IgA disease presenting as initially with IgG immune deposits. *J Am Acad Dermatol* 1986;14;1014.

272. Leonard JN, Haffenden GP, Ring NP, et al. Linear IgA disease in adults. *Br J Dermatol* 1982;107:301.

273. Mobacken H, Kastrup W, Ljunghall K, et al. Linear IgA dermatosis: a study of ten adult patients. *Acta Derm Venereol (Stockh)* 1983;63:123.

274. Wojnarowska F, Whitehead P, Leigh IM, et al. Identification of the target antigen in chronic bullous disease of childhood and linear IgA disease of adults. *Br J Dermatol* 1991;124:157.

275. Peters MS, Rogers RS. Clinical correlations of linear IgA deposition at the cutaneous basement membrane zone. *J Am Acad Dermatol* 1989;20:761.

276. Wojnarowska F, Marsden RA, Black MM. An updated review of the chronic acquired bullous diseases of childhood. *Br J Dermatol* 1983;109:40.

277. Wojnarowska F, Marsden RA, Bhogal B. Chronic bullous disease of childhood, childhood cicatricial pemphigoid, and linear IgA disease of adults. *J Am Acad Dermatol* 1988;19:792.

278. Zone JJ, Taylor TB, Meyer LJ. Identification of the cutaneous basement membrane zone antigen and isolation of antibody in linear immunoglobulin A bullous dermatosis. *J Clin Invest* 1990;85:812.

279. Zone JJ, Taylor TB, Meyer LJ, et al. The 97 kDa linear IgA bullous disease antigen is identical to a portion of the extracellular domain of the 180 kDa bullous pemphigoid antigen, BPAg2. *J Invest Dermatol* 1998;110:207–210.

280. Marinkovich MP, Taylor TB, Keene DR, et al. LAD-1, the linear IgA bullous dermatosis autoantigen, is a novel 120-kDa anchoring filament protein synthesized by epidermal cells. *J Invest Dermatol* 1996;106:734–738.

281. Zambruno G, Kanitakis J. Linear IgA dermatosis with IgA antibodies to type VII collagen. *Br J Dermatol* 1996;135:1004–1005.

282. Prost C, DeLuca C, Combemale P, et al. Diagnosis of adult linear IgA dermatosis by immunoelectron microscopy in 16 patients with linear IgA deposits. *J Invest Dermatol* 1989;92:39.

283. Carpenter S, Berg D, Sidhu-Malik N, et al. Vancomycin-associated linear IgA dermatosis. *J Am Acad Dermatol* 1992;26:45.

284. Baden LA, Apovian C, Imber MM, et al. Vancomycin-induced linear IgA bullous dermatosis. *Arch Dermatol* 1988;124:1186.

285. Gabrielsen TO, Staerfelt F, Thune PO. Drug-induced bullous derma-tosis with linear IgA deposits along the basement membrane. *Acta Derm Venereol (Stockh)* 1981;61:439.

286. McWhirter JD, Hashimoto K, Fayne S, et al. Linear IgA bullous dermatosis related to lithium carbonate. *Arch Dermatol* 1987;123:1120.

287. Jordon RE, Bean SF, Trifshauser CT, et al. Chronic bullous dermatitis herpetiformis: Negative immunofluorescent tests. *Arch Dermatol* 1970;101:629.

288. Van der Meer JB, Remme JJ, Nelkins MJJ, et al. IgA antibasement membrane antibodies in a boy with pemphigoid. *Arch Dermatol* 1977;113:1462.

289. Marsden RA, McKee PH, Bhogal B, et al. A study of benign chronic bullous dermatosis of childhood. *Clin Exp Dermatol* 1980;5:159.

290. Burge S, Wojnarowska F, Marsden A. Chronic bullous dermatosis of childhood persisting into adulthood. *Pediatr Dermatol* 1988;5:246.

291. Esterly NB, Furey NL, Kirschner BS, et al. Chronic bullous dermatosis of childhood. *Arch Dermatol* 1977;113:42.

292. McGuire J, Nordlund J. Bullous disease of childhood. *Arch Dermatol* 1973;108:284.

293. Freeman RG, Spiller R, Knox JM. Histopathology of erythema toxicum neonatorum. *Arch Dermatol* 1960;82:586.

294. Stone OJ. High viscosity of newborn extracellular matrix is the etiology of erythema toxicum neonatorum. Neonatal jaundice? Hyaline membrane disease? *Med Hypotheses* 1990;33:15.

295. Bassukas ID. Is erythema toxicum neonatorum a mild self-limited acute cutaneous graft-versus-host reaction from maternal-to-fetal lymphocyte transfer? *Med Hypotheses* 1992;38:334.

295a. Marchini G, Ulfgren AK, Lore K, et al. Erythema toxicum neonatorum: an immunohistochemical analysis. *Pediatr Dermatol* 2001;18:177–187.

296. Lucky AW, Esterly NB, Heskel N, et al. Eosinophilic pustular folliculitis in infancy. *Pediatr Dermatol* 1984;1:202–206.

297. Ramamurthy RS, Reveri M, Esterly NB, et al. Transient neonatal pustular melanosis. *J Pediatr* 1976;88:831.

298. Ferrandiz C, Coroleu W, Ribera M, et al. Sterile transient neonatal pustulosis is a precocious form of erythema toxicum neonatorum. *Dermatology* 1992;185:18.

299. Jarratt M, Ramsdell W. Infantile acropustulosis. *Arch Dermatol* 1979;115:834.

300. Newton JA, Salisbury J, Marsden A, et al. Acropustulosis of infancy. *Br J Dermatol* 1986;115:735.

301. Dromy R, Raz A, Metzker A. Infantile acropustulosis. *Pediatr Dermatol* 1991;8:284.

302. Bundino S, Zina AM, Ubertalli S. Infantile acropustulosis. *Dermatologica* 1982;165:615.

303. Palungwachira P. Infantile acropustulosis. *Australas J Dermatol* 1989;30:97.

304. Sneddon IB, Wilkinson DS. Subcorneal pustular dermatosis. *Br J Dermatol* 1956;68:385.

305. Sneddon IB, Wilkinson DS. Subcorneal pustular dermatosis. *Br J Dermatol* 1979;100:61.

305a. Gniadecki R, Bygum A, Clemmensen O, et al. IgA pemphigus: the first two Scandinavian cases. *Acta Derm Venereol* 2002;82:441–445.

305b. Wallach D. Intraepidermal IgA pustulosis. *J Am Acad Dermatol* 1992;27:993–1000.

306. Atukorala DN, Joshi RK, Abanmi A, et al. Subcorneal pustular dermatosis and IgA myeloma. *Dermatology* 1993;187:124.

307. Burns RE, Fine G. Subcorneal pustular dermatosis. *Arch Dermatol* 1959;80:72.

308. Wolff K. Ein beitrag zur nosologie der subcornealen pustulösen dermatose (Sneddon–Wilkinson). *Arch Klin Exp Dermatol* 1966;224:248.

309. Grob JJ, Mege JL, Capo C, et al. Role of tumor necrosis factor-α in Sneddon–Wilkinson subcorneal pustular dermatosis: a model of neutrophil priming in vivo. *J Am Acad Dermatol* 1991;25:944.

310. Metz J, Schröpl F. Elktronenmikroskopische untersuchungen bei subcornealer pustulöser dermatose. *Arch Klin Exp Dermatol* 1970;236:190.

311. Sanchez N, Ackerman AB. Subcorneal pustular dermatosis: a variant of pustular psoriasis. *Acta Derm Venereol Suppl (Stockh)* 1979;85:147.

311a. Weston WL, Brice SL, Jester JD, et al. Herpes simplex virus in childhood erythema multiforme. *Pediatrics* 1992;89:32–4.

311b. Schofield JK, Tatnall FM, Leigh IM. Recurrent erythema multiforme: clinical features and treatment in a large series of patients. *Br J Dermatol* 1993;128:542–545.

312. Chimenti S, Ackerman AB. Is subcorneal pustular dermatosis of Sneddon and Wilkinson an entity sui generis? *Am J Dermatopathol* 1981;3:363.

313. Lyell A. A review of toxic epidermal necrolysis in Britain. *Br J Dermatol* 1967;79:662.

314. Ruiz-Maldonado R. Acute disseminated epidermal necroses. *J Am Acad Dermatol* 1985;13:623.

315. Rasmussen JE. Erythema multiforme: should anyone care about the standards of care? *Arch Dermatol* 1995;131:726–729.

316. Assier H, Bastuji-Garin S, Revuz J, et al. Erythema multiforme with mucous membrane involvement and Stevens–Johnson

syndrome are clinically different disorders with distinct causes. *Arch Dermatol* 1995;131:539.

317. Lyell A. Toxic epidermal necrolysis: an eruption resembling scalding of the skin. *Br J Dermatol* 1956;68:355.

318. Schöpf E, Stühmer A, Rzany B, et al. Toxic epidermal necrolysis and Stevens–Johnson syndrome. *Arch Dermatol* 1991;127:839.

319. Bastuji-Garin S, Rzany B, Stern RS, et al. Clinical classification of cases of toxic epidermal necrolysis, Stevens–Johnson syndrome, and erythema multiforme. *Arch Dermatol* 1993;129:92.

320. Leboit PE. Interface dermatitis: how specific are its histopathologic features? *Arch Dermatol* 1993;129:1324.

321. Bedi TR, Pinkus H. Histopathological spectrum of erythema multiforme. *Br J Dermatol* 1976;95:243.

322. Howland WW, Golitz LE, Weston WL, et al. Erythema multiforme: clinical, histopathologic, and immunologic study. *J Am Acad Dermatol* 1984;10:438.

323. Patterson JW, Parsons JM, Blaylock WK, et al. Eosinophils in skin lesions of erythema multiforme. *Arch Pathol* 1989;113:36.

324. Ackerman AB, Ragaz A. Erythema multiforme. *Am J Dermatopathol* 1985;7:133.

325. Zohdi-Mofid M, Horn TD. Acrosyringeal concentration of necrotic keratinocytes in erythema multiforme: a clue to drug etiology. *J Cutan Pathol* 1997;24:235–240.

326. Orfanos CE, Schaumburg-Lever G, Lever WF. Dermal and epidermal types of erythema multiforme. *Arch Dermatol* 1974;109:682.

327. Imamura S, Yanase K, Taniguchi S, et al. Erythema multiforme: demonstration of immune complexes in the sera and skin lesions. *Br J Dermatol* 1980;102:161.

328. Bushkell LL, Mackel SE, Jordon RE. Erythema multiforme: direct immunofluorescence studies and detection of circulating immune complexes. *J Invest Dermatol* 1980;74:372.

329. Finan MC, Schroeter AL. Cutaneous immunofluorescence study of erythema multiforme: correlation with light microscopic patterns and etiologic agents. *J Am Acad Dermatol* 1984;10:497.

330. King T, Helm TN, Valenzuela R, et al. Diffuse intraepidermal deposition of immunoreactants on direct immunofluorescence: a clue to the early diagnosis of epidermal necrolysis. *Int J Dermatol* 1994;33:634.

331. Hughes J, Burrow NP. Infections mononucleosis presenting as erythema multiforme. *Clin Exp Dermatol* 1993;18:373–374.

332. Koga T, Kubota Y, Nakayawa J. Erythema multiforme-like eruptions induced by cytomegalovirus infection in an immunocompetent adult. *Acta Derm Venereol* 1999;79:166.

333. Schuttelaar M-LA, Lacijendecker R, Heinhnis RJ, et al. Erythema multiforme and persistent erythema as early cutaneous manifestations of Lyme disease. *J Am Acad Dermatol* 1997;37:873–875.

334. Tay Y-K, Huft JC, Weston WL. Mycoplasma pneumoniae infection is associated with Stevens–Johnson syndrome, not erythema multiforme (Von Hebra). *J Am Acad Dermatol* 1996;35:757–760.

335. Chan HL, Stern RS, Arndt KA, et al. The incidence of erythema multiforme, Stevens–Johnson syndrome and toxic epidermal necrolysis: a population-based study with particular reference to reactions caused by drugs among out patients. *Arch Dermatol* 1990;126:43–47.

336. Rzany B, Correia O, Kelly JP, et al. Risk of Stevens–Johnson syndrome and toxic epidermal necrosis during the first weeks of antiepileptic therapy: a case control study. *Lancet* 1999;353:2190–2194.

337. Aslanzadeh J, Helm KF, Espy MJ, et al. Detection of HSV-specific DNA in biopsy tissue of patients with erythema multi-

forme by polymerase chain reaction. *Br J Dermatol* 1992;126:19.

338. Brice SL, Krzemien D, Weston WL, et al. Detection of herpes simplex virus DNA in cutaneous lesions of erythema multiforme. *J Invest Dermatol* 1989;93:183.

339. Brice SL, Leahy MA, Ong L, et al. Examination of non-involved skin, previously involved skin, and peripheral blood for herpes simplex virus DNA in patients with recurrent herpes-associated erythema multiforme. *J Cutan Pathol* 1994;21:408.

340. Aurelian L, Ono F, Burnett J. Herpes simplex virus (HSV) associated erythema multiforme (HAEM): a viral disease with an autoimmune component. *Dermatol Online J* 2003;9:1.

341. Margolis R, Tonnesen MG, Harrist TJ, et al. Lymphocyte subsets and Langerhans cells/indeterminate cells in erythema multiforme. *J Invest Dermatol* 1983;81:403.

342. Paquet P, Paquet F, Al Saleh W, et al. Immunoregulatory effector cells in drug-induced toxic epidermal necrolysis. *Am J Dermatopathol* 2000;22:413–417.

343. Prutkin L, Fellner MJ. Erythema multiforme bullosum. *Acta Derm Venereol (Stockh)* 1971;51:429.

344. Ford MJ, Smith KL, Croker BP, et al. Large granular lymphocytes within the epidermis of erythema multiforme lesions. *J Am Acad Dermatol* 1992;27:460.

345. Glucksberg H, Strob R, Fefer A, et al. Clinical manifestations of graft-versus-host disease in human recipients of marrow from HLA-matched sibling donors. *Transplantation* 1975;18:295.

346. Anderson KC, Weinstein HJ. Transfusion-associated graft-versus-host disease. *N Engl J Med* 1990;323:315.

347. Schmuth M, Vogel W, Weinlich G, et al. Cutaneous lesions as the presenting sign of acute graft-versus-host disease following liver transplantation. *Br J Dermatol* 1999;141:901–904.

348. Morhenn VB, Maibach HI. Graft vs. host reaction in a newborn. *Acta Derm Venereol (Stockh)* 1974;54:133.

349. Holder J, North J, Bourke J, et al. Thymoma-associated cutaneous graft-versus-host- like reaction. *Clin Exp Dermatol* 1997;22:287–290.

350. Scarisbrick JJ, Wakelin SH, Russell-Jones R. Cutaneous graft-versus-host-like reaction in systemic T-cell lymphoma. *Clin Exp Dermatol* 1999;24:382–383.

351. Darmstadt GL, Donnenberg AD, Vogelsang GB, et al. Clinical, laboratory, and histopathologic indicators of progressive acute graft-versus-host disease. *J Invest Dermatol* 1992;99:397.

352. Fujii H, Hiketa T, Matsumoto Y, et al. Clinical characteristics of chronic cutaneous graft-versus-host disease in Japanese leukemia patients after bone marrow transplantation: low incidence and mild manifestations. *Bone Marrow Transplant* 1992;10:331.

353. Shulman HM, Sale GE, Lerner KG, et al. Chronic cutaneous graft-versus-host disease in man. *Am J Pathol* 1978;91:545.

354. Johnson ML, Farmer ER. Graft-versus-host reactions in dermatology. *J Am Acad Dermatol* 1998;38:369–392.

355. Friedman KJ, Leboit PE, Farmer ER. Acute follicular graft-vs-host reaction. *Arch Dermatol* 1988;124:688.

356. Desbarats J, Seemayer TA, Lapp WS. Irradiation of the skin and systemic graft-versus-host disease synergize to produce cutaneous lesions. *Am J Pathol* 1994;144:883.

357. James WD, Odom RB. Graft-v.-host disease. *Arch Dermatol* 1983;119:683.

358. Saurat JH, Gluckman E, Russel A, et al. The lichen planus-like eruption after bone marrow transplantation. *Br J Dermatol* 1975;93:675.

359. Barnadas MA, Brunet S, Sureda A, et al. Exuberant granulation tissue associated with chronic graft-versus-host disease after transplantation of peripheral blood progenitor cells. *J Am Acad Dermatol* 1999;41:876–879.

360. Hymes SR, Farmer ER, Lewis PG, et al. Cutaneous graft-versus-host reaction: prognostic features seen by light microscopy. *J Am Acad Dermatol* 1985;12:468.

361. Horn TD, Bauer DJ, Vogelsang GB, et al. Reappraisal of histologic features of the acute cutaneous graft-versus-host reaction based on an allogeneic rodent model. *J Invest Dermatol* 1994; 103:206.

362. Sale GE, Lerner KG, Berker EA, et al. The skin biopsy in the diagnosis of acute graft-versus-host disease in man. *Am J Pathol* 1977;89:621–636.

363. Farmer ER. The histopathology of graft-versus-host disease. *Adv Dermatol* 1986;1:173–188.

364. Lerner KG, Kao GF, Storb R, et al. Histopathology of graft-versus-host reaction (GvHR) in human recipients of marrow from HLA-matched sibling donors. *Transplant Proc* 1974;6:367.

365. Horn TD. Acute cutaneous eruptions after bone marrow ablation: roses by other names? *J Cutan Pathol* 1994;21:385–392.

366. Chaudhuri SPR, Smoller BR. Acute cutaneous graft versus host disease: a clinicopathologic and immunophenotypic study. *Int J Dermatol* 1992;31:270.

367. Janin-Mercier A, Saurat JH, Bourges M, et al. The lichen planuslike and sclerotic phases of the graft versus host disease in man. *Acta Derm Venereol (Stockh)* 1981;61:187.

368. Saijo S, Honda M. Sasahara E, et al. Columnar epidermal necrosis. A unique manifestation of transfusion-associated cutaneous graft-versus-host disease. *Arch Dermatol* 2000;136: 743–746.

369. Tanaka K, Sullivan KM, Shulman HM, et al. A clinical review: cutaneous manifestations of acute and chronic graft-versus-host disease following bone marrow transplantation. *J Dermatol* 1991;18:11.

370. Spielvogel RL, Goltz RW, Kersey JH. Scleroderma-like changes in chronic graft vs host disease. *Arch Dermatol* 1977;113:1424.

371. Hymes SR, Farmer ER, Burns WH, et al. Bullous scleroderma-like changes in chronic graft-versus-host disease. *Arch Dermatol* 1985;121:1189–1192.

372. Tsoi MS, Storb R, Jones E, et al. Deposition of IgM and C at the dermoepidermal junction in acute and chronic cutaneous graft-vs-host disease in man. *J Immunol* 1978;120:1485.

373. Ullman S. Immunoglobulins and complement in skin in graft-versus-host disease. *Ann Intern Med* 1976;85:205.

374. Parkman R, Rappeport J, Rosen F. Human graft versus host disease. *J Invest Dermatol* 1980;74:276.

375. Volc-Platzer B, Rappersberger K, Mosberger I, et al. Sequential immunohistologic analysis of the skin following allogeneic bone marrow transplantation. *J Invest Dermatol* 1988; 91:162.

376. Murphy GF, Whitaker D, Sprent J, et al. Characterization of target injury of murine acute graft-versus-host disease directed to multiple minor histocompatibility antigens elicited by either CD4+ or CD8+ effector cells. *Am J Pathol* 1991;138:983.

377. Kawai K, Matsumoto Y, Watanabe H, et al. Induction of cutaneous graft-versus-host disease by local injection of unprimed T cells. *Clin Exp Immunol* 1991;84:359.

378. Sakamoto H, Michaelson J, Jones WK, et al. Lymphocytes with a CD4+ CD8−CD3− phenotype are effectors of experimental cutaneous graft-versus-host disease. *Proc Natl Acad Sci U S A* 1991;88:10890.

379. Horn TD, Farmer ER. Distribution of lymphocytes bearing TCR in cutaneous lymphocytic infiltrates. *J Cutan Pathol* 1990;17:165.

380. Norton J, Al-Saffar N, Sloane JP. An immunohistological study of lymphocytes in human cutaneous graft-versus-host disease. *Bone Marrow Transplant* 1991;7:205.

381. Acevedo A, Aramburu J, Lopez J, et al. Identification of natural killer (NK) cells in lesions of human cutaneous graft-versus-host disease: Expression of a novel NK-associated surface antigen (Kp43) in mononuclear infiltrates. *J Invest Dermatol* 1991; 97:659.

382. Vogelsang GB, Lee L, Bensen-Kennedy D. Pathogenesis and treatment of graft-versus-host disease after bone marrow transplant. *Annu Rev Med* 2003;54:29–52.

383. Sale GE, Shulman HM, Gallucci BB, et al. Young rete ridge keratino-cytes are preferred targets in cutaneous graft-versus-host disease. *Am J Pathol* 1985;118:278.

384. Murphy GF, Lavker RM, Whitaker D, et al. Cytotoxic folliculitis in GvHD: evidence of follicular stem cell injury and recovery. *J Cutan Pathol* 1990;18:309.

385. Breathnach SM, Shimada S, Kovac Z, et al. Immunologic aspects of acute cutaneous graft-versus-host disease: decreased density and antigen-presenting function of Ia+ Langerhans cells and absent antigen-presenting capacity of Ia+ keratinocytes. *J Invest Dermatol* 1986;86:226.

386. Lever R, Turbitt M, Mackie R, et al. A prospective study of the histological changes in the skin in patients receiving bone marrow transplants. *Br J Dermatol* 1986;114:161.

387. Aractingi S, Chosidow O. Cutaneous graft-versus-host disease. *Arch Dermatol* 1998;134:602–612.

388. DeDobbeleer GD, Ledoux-Corbusier MH, Achtern GA. Graft versus host reaction: an ultrastructural study. *Arch Dermatol* 1975;111:1597.

389. Ferrara JLM, Guillen FJ, Van Dijken PJ, et al. Evidence that large granular lymphocytes of donor origin mediate acute graft-versus-host disease. *Transplantation* 1989;47:50.

390. Sale GE, Gallucci BB, Schubert MM, et al. Direct ultrastructural evidence of target-directed polarization by cytotoxic lymphocytes in lesions of human graft-versus-host disease. *Arch Pathol Lab Med* 1987;111:333.

391. Leboit PE. Subacute radiation dermatitis: a histologic imitator of acute cutaneous graft-versus-host disease. *J Am Acad Dermatol* 1989;20:236.

392. Drijkoningen M, De Wolf-Peeters C, Tricot G, et al. Drug-induced skin reactions and acute cutaneous graft-versus-host reaction: a comparative immunohistochemical study. *Blut* 1988; 56:69.

393. Elliott CJ, Sloane JP, Sanderson KV, et al. The histological diagnosis of cutaneous graft versus host disease: relationship of skin changes to marrow purging and other clinical variables. *Histopathology* 1987;11:145.

394. Horn TD, Redd JV, Karp JE, et al. Cutaneous eruptions of lymphocyte recovery. *Arch Dermatol* 1989;125:1512.

395. Bauer DJ, Hood AF, Horn TD. Histologic comparison of autologous graft-versus-host reaction and cutaneous eruption of lymphocyte recovery. *Arch Dermatol* 1993;129:855.

396. Horn T, Lehmkuhle MA, Gore A, et al. Systemic cytokine administration alters the histology of the eruption of lymphocyte recovery. *J Cutan Pathol* 1996;23:242–246.

397. Grover RW. Transient acantholytic dermatosis. *Arch Dermatol* 1970;101:426.

398. Lang I, Lindmaier A, Hönigsman H. Das spektrum der transienten akantholytischen dermatosen. *Hautarzt* 1986;37: 485.

399. Chalet M, Grover R, Ackerman AB. Transient acantholytic dermatosis. *Arch Dermatol* 1977;113:431.

400. Heenan PJ, Quirk CJ. Transient acantholytic dermatosis. *Br J Dermatol* 1980;102:515.

401. Grover RW, Rosenblaum R. The association of transient acantholytic dermatosis with other skin diseases. *J Am Acad Dermatol* 1989;11:253–256.

402. Chatet M, Grover R, Ackerman AB. Transient acantholytic dermatosis. A reevaluation. *Arch Dermatol* 1977;113:431–435.

403. Fleckman P, Stenn K. Transient acantholytic dermatosis associated with pemphigus foliaceus. Coexistence of two acantholytic disease. *Arch Dermatol* 1983;119:155–156.
404. Roger M, Valence C, Bressieux J, et al. Grover's disease associated with Waldenstrom's macroglobulineous and neutrophilic dermatosis. *Acta Derm Venereol* 2000;80:145–146.
405. Guana AL, Cohen PR. Transient acantholytic dermatosis in oncology patients. *J Clin Oncol* 1994;12:1703.
406. Manteaux AM, Rapini RP. Transient acantholytic dermatosis in patients with cancer. *Cutis* 1990;46:488.
407. Pehamberger H, Gschnait F, Konrad K, et al. Transient acantholytic dermatosis Grover. *Z Hautkr* 1977;52:841.
408. Bystryn JC. Immunofluorescence studies in transient acantholytic dermatosis (Grover's disease). *Am J Dermatopathol* 1979;1:325.
409. Millns JL, Doyle JA, Muller SA. Positive cutaneous immunofluorescence in Grover's disease. *Arch Dermatol* 1980;116:515.
410. Powell J, Sakuntabhai A, James M, et al. Grover's disease, despite histological similarity to Darier's disease, does not share an abnormality in the ATP2A2 gene. *Br J Dermatol* 2000 143:658.
411. Hu C-H, Michel B, Farber EM. Transient acantholytic dermatosis (Grover's disease): a skin disorder related to heat and sweating. *Arch Dermatol* 1985;121:1439.
412. Gretzula JC, Penneys NS. Transient acantholytic dermatosis: an immunohistochemical study. *Arch Dermatol* 1986;122:972.
413. Mahler SJ, De Villez RL, Pulitzer DR. Transient acantholytic dermatosis induced by recombinant human interleukin 4. *J Am Acad Dermatol* 1993;29:206.
414. Bayer-Garner I, Dilday B, Sanderson R, et al. Acantholysis and spongiosis are associated with loss of Syndecan-1 expression. *J Cutan Pathol* 2001;28:135–139.
415. Kanzaki T, Hashimoto K. Transient acantholytic dermatosis with involvement of oral mucosa. *J Cutan Pathol* 1978;5:23.
416. Wolff HH, Chalet MD, Ackerman AB. Transitorische akantholytische dermatose (Grover). *Hautarzt* 1977;28:78.
417. Grover RW, Duffy JL. Transient acantholytic dermatosis. *J Cutan Pathol* 1975;2:111.
418. Brehmer-Anderson E, Göransson K. Friction blisters as a manifestation of pathomimia. *Acta Derm Venereol (Stockh)* 1975;55:65.
419. Naylor PFD. Experimental friction blisters. *Br J Dermatol* 1955;67:327.
420. Sulzberger MB, Cortese TA Jr, Fishman L, et al. Studies on blisters produced by friction. *J Invest Dermatol* 1966;47:456.
421. Hunter JAA, McVittie E, Comaish JS. Light and electron microscopic studies of physical injury to the skin. II. Friction. *Br J Dermatol* 1974;90:491.
422. Winer LH, Levin GH. Changes in the skin as a result of electric current. *Arch Dermatol* 1958;78:386.
423. Sevitt S. Histological changes in burned skin. In: *Burns: pathology and therapeutic application*. London: Butterworth & Co., 1957:18.
424. Foley FD. Pathology of cutaneous burns. *Surg Clin North Am* 1970;50:1200.
425. Metzker A, Merlob P. Suction purpura. *Arch Dermatol* 1992;128:822.

CONNECTIVE TISSUE DISEASES

CHRISTINE JAWORSKY

LUPUS ERYTHEMATOSUS

Lupus erythematosus (LE) is a disease that affects multiple organ systems and has a broad range of clinical manifestations. It may take the form of an isolated cutaneous eruption or a fatal systemic illness.

A combination of clinical and laboratory data was used to devise the "Criteria for the Classification of Systemic Lupus Erythematosus" by the American Rheumatism Association in 1972, amended in 1982 (1), and later slightly modified (2). These criteria were developed for classification of patients with systemic lupus erythematosus as opposed to other rheumatic diseases. They are also widely used to diagnose patients with lupus erythematosus. This classification is based on 11 criteria:

- Malar rash
- Discoid rash
- Photosensitivity
- Oral ulcers, usually painless
- Arthritis, nonerosive, involving two or more peripheral joints, with tenderness, swelling, or effusion
- Serositis (pleurisy or pericarditis)
- Renal disorder (persistent proteinuria exceeding 0.5 g/day or cellular casts)
- Neurologic disorders (seizures or psychosis)
- Hematologic disorders (hemolytic anemia, leukopenia of less than 4,000/mm^3, lymphopenia of less than 1,500/mm^3, or thrombocytopenia of less than 100,000/mm^3)
- Immunologic disorder (positive LE-cell preparation, anti-DNA in abnormal titer, antibody to Sm nuclear antigen, or false-positive serologic test for syphilis)
- Antinuclear antibody

A person is judged to have systemic lupus erythematosus (SLE) if any four or more of the 11 criteria are present serially or simultaneously. Furthermore, a diagnosis of SLE is indicated in any patient who has at least three of the following four symptoms: (a) a cutaneous eruption consistent with lupus erythematosus; (b) renal involvement; (c) serositis; or (d) joint involvement (3). A diagnosis of SLE

requires confirmation by laboratory tests. Even though the prognosis of SLE has been greatly improved by early diagnosis and modern methods of treatment, the mortality rate of the disease is between 15% and 25% (4). Death usually results from infection or severe nephritis (5).

The importance of adequate laboratory data for evaluation of the seriousness of the illness and its prognosis has long been recognized. Histologic examination of affected tissues in conjunction with serologic and immunofluorescence studies is essential for proper evaluation of a patient with LE.

Cutaneous changes of lupus erythematosus may be subdivided according to the morphology of the clinical lesion and/or its duration (acute, subacute, or chronic). Differentiation between LE subtypes is based upon the constellation of clinical, histologic, and immunofluorescence findings (6). Histologic findings alone may not be sufficient to correctly classify the subtype of the eruption (7). Not every case of lupus erythematosus can be assigned with certainty to a category because intermediate forms and transitions from one type to another occur.

Chronic Cutaneous Lupus Erythematosus

Discoid Lupus Erythematosus

Characteristically, lesions of discoid lupus erythematosus (DLE) consist of well-demarcated, erythematous, slightly infiltrated, "discoid" plaques that often show adherent thick scales and follicular plugging. Early and active lesions usually display surrounding erythema (Fig. 10-1A). Old lesions often appear atrophic and have hypo- or hyper-pigmentation. Occasionally lesions may show verrucous hyperkeratosis, especially at their periphery (8). Hypopigmentation within previously affected areas is frequent. Rarely, neoplasms have been reported in lesions of lupus erythematosus and have included basal cell carcinoma, squamous cell carcinoma, and atypical fibroxanthoma (9).

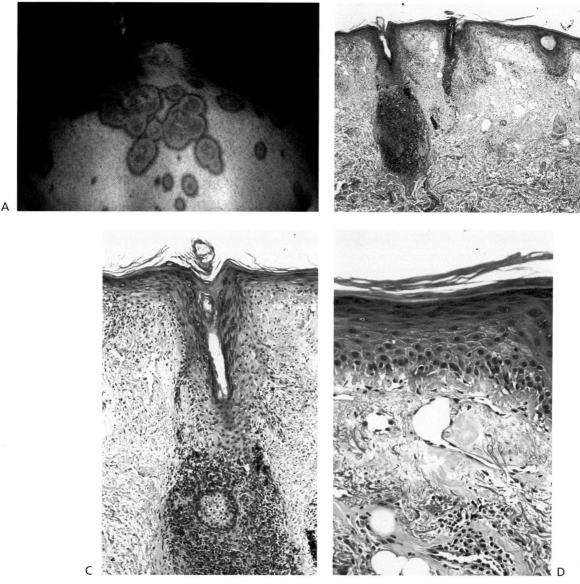

FIGURE 10-1. Discoid lupus erythematosus. **A:** An adult with discoid plaques of lupus erythematosus on the upper back: areas of erythema show stromal inflammation, while paler zones demonstrate scarring. **B:** The epidermis has lost its rete ridge pattern and shows follicular plugging. There is a brisk mononuclear inflammatory infiltrate near the dermal-epidermal junction, which obscures folliculo-dermal junctions. **C:** Vacuolization of basilar keratinocytes within a follicular ostium. Note the slightly basophilic stromal background indicative of mucin deposition. **D:** A thickened basement membrane may be noted in H&E stained sections. The infiltrate is composed of predominantly lymphocytes admixed with occasional plasma cells. *(continued)*

In many instances, the discoid cutaneous lesions are limited to the face, where the malar areas and the nose are predominantly affected. In addition, the scalp, ears, oral mucosa, and vermilion border of the lips may be involved. In patients with involvement of the head and neck unaccompanied initially by systemic lupus erythematosus (SLE), conversion of DLE to SLE is infrequent (10% risk).

In patients with *disseminated discoid lupus erythematosus*, discoid lesions are seen predominantly on the upper trunk and upper limbs, usually, but not always in association with lesions on the head (10). SLE may eventually develop in some of these patients (11). Although discoid cutaneous lesions are typical of DLE, they are also seen in as many as 14% of the patients with SLE (12).

Histopathology. In most instances of *discoid lesions*, a diagnosis of lupus erythematosus is possible on the basis of a combination of histologic findings. Changes may be apparent at all levels of the skin, but all need not be present in every case. The findings are summarized below:

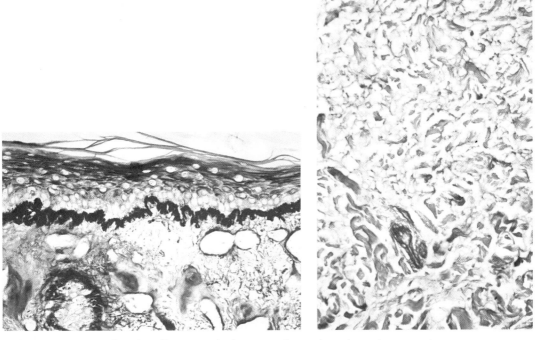

FIGURE 10-1. *(continued)* **E:** PAS stain demonstrating an irregular and tortuous basement membrane zone. **F:** Alcian blue stains highlight abundant mucin deposits among collagen bundles.

- Stratum corneum: hyperkeratosis with follicular plugging
- Epithelium: thinning and flattening of the stratum malpighii, hydropic degeneration of basal cells, dyskeratosis, and squamatization of basilar keratinocytes
- Basement membrane: thickening and tortuosity
- Stroma: a predominantly lymphocytic infiltrate arranged along the dermal–epidermal junction, around hair follicles and other appendages, and in an interstitial pattern; interstitial mucin deposition; edema, vasodilatation, and slight extravasation of erythrocytes
- Subcutaneous: slight extension of the inflammatory infiltrate may be present.

The stratum corneum is usually hyperkeratotic. Parakeratosis is not conspicuous, and it may be absent. Keratotic plugs are found mainly in dilated follicular openings (Fig. 10-1B and C), but they may occur in the openings of eccrine ducts as well. Follicular channels in the dermis may contain concentric layers of keratin instead of hairs.

The most significant histologic change in lupus erythematosus is hydropic degeneration of the basal layer, also referred to as liquefaction degeneration. This change is characterized by vacuolar spaces beneath and between basilar keratinocytes (Fig. 10-1C). In its absence, a histologic diagnosis of lupus erythematosus should be made with caution and only when other histologic findings greatly favor a diagnosis of LE. In addition to liquefaction degeneration,

basilar keratinocytes may show individual cell necrosis (apoptosis) and acquire elongated contours like their superficial counterparts, rather than retaining their normal columnar appearance (squamatization). Frequently, the undulating rete ridge pattern is lost, and replaced by a linear array of squamatized keratinocytes (Fig. 10-1D).

The epidermal changes vary with the clinical character of lesions; there may be thinning and flattening of the stratum malpighii. A clinically verrucous lesion shows a hyperplastic, papillomatous epidermis with hyperkeratotic scale that simulates a hypertrophic solar keratosis or even a superficially invading squamous cell carcinoma (13). In lesions of DLE that clinically do not show adherent scaling or keratotic plugging, the epidermis may show few or no changes and, in particular, no hydropic changes in the basal layer (14).

The basement membrane, normally delicate and inconspicuous, appears thickened and tortuous in long-standing lesions (Fig. 10-1E). This change becomes more apparent with periodic acid-Schiff (PAS) stains (PAS positive, diastase resistant), and may be found not only at the dermal–epidermal interface but along follicular–dermal junctions as well. These findings correlate with locations of immunoreactant deposits found on direct immunofluorescence testing of affected skin. By contrast, in areas of pronounced hydropic degeneration of the basal cells, the PAS-positive subepidermal basement zone may be fragmented and even absent (15). Capillary walls may also show thickening, homogenization, and an increase in the intensity of the PAS reaction.

The inflammatory infiltrate in the dermis is usually lymphocytic admixed with plasma cells (Fig. 10-1C and D). Its distribution is a clue to the diagnosis of LE. In active lesions, the infiltrate can be found approximating the dermal–epidermal junction associated with hydropic degeneration. In hair-bearing areas, the infiltrate is located around hair follicles and the sebaceous glands (Fig. 10-1C). Frequently, one can observe hydropic changes in the basal layer of the hair follicles, which may be of diagnostic value in the absence of dermal–epidermal changes. By impinging on pilosebaceous units, the infiltrate causes their gradual atrophy and disappearance. A patchy inflammatory infiltrate also may be present in the upper dermis in an interstitial pattern and around eccrine coils. Occasionally, the infiltrate extends into the subcutaneous fat.

The dermis shows edema and often small foci of extravasated erythrocytes. In dark-skinned persons, melanin is frequently seen within melanophages in the upper dermis because hydropic degeneration in the basal cells causes these cells to lose their melanin (pigmentary incontinence). Vascular channels may be dilated and surrounded by edema. Obliterative and proliferative changes are absent. An increase in the ground substance, hyaluronic acid, is common in the middle and lower dermis, and is best demonstrated with colloidal iron or Alcian blue stains (16) (Fig. 10-1F). Fibrinoid deposits in the dermis are encountered only rarely in discoid lesions, and then only in early discoid lesions.

Colloid bodies, referred to in lichen planus as Civatte bodies, are apoptotic keratinocytes that present as round to ovoid, homogeneous, eosinophilic structures (Fig. 10-2). They may be seen in lesions of DLE, but also in other

inflammatory processes where there is damage to basilar keratinocytes (poikiloderma, lichen planus, fixed drug eruptions, lichenoid keratoses). They measure approximately 10 μm in diameter, and are present in the lower epidermis or in the papillary dermis. When located in the dermis, colloid bodies are PAS positive and diastase resistant and, on direct immunofluorescence staining, often are found to contain immunoglobulins (IgG, IgM, IgA), complement, and fibrin. This staining does not represent an immunologic phenomenon but is the result of passive absorption.

Differential Diagnosis. The epidermal changes seen in DLE must be differentiated from lichen planus since both diseases may show hydropic degeneration of the basal cell layer. In lichen planus, there are wedge-shaped hypergranulosis and triangular elongation of rete ridges described as "saw-toothing," which are not observed in DLE; in DLE, the epidermis frequently appears flattened. In addition, in lichen planus the infiltrate is superficial (not superficial and deep) and stromal mucin deposition is not seen. (For a discussion of the overlap syndrome lichen planus and lupus erythematosus, see Chapter 7.)

Patchy dermal lymphocytic infiltrates may be seen in five disorders that begin with the letter "l" (called the *five L's*). They are lupus erythematosus, lymphocytic lymphoma, lymphocytoma cutis, polymorphous light eruption of the plaque type, and lymphocytic infiltration of the skin of Jessner.

In the absence of significant subepidermal vacuolization, LE must be differentiated from the other four diseases:

In *lymphocytic lymphoma* atypical lymphocytes are present, are tightly packed, have an interstitial distribution ("Indian filing"), and do not surround pilosebaceous units as in LE.

In *lymphocytoma cutis* (see Chapter 32), the infiltrate usually is heavier than in lupus erythematosus, may have an interstitial component, shows no tendency to arrange itself around pilosebaceous structures, and often contains an admixture of larger, paler lymphocytes arranged in lymphoid follicles, mimicking germinal center formation.

In the plaque type of *polymorphous light eruption* there is often a prominent band of papillary dermal edema. The infiltrate is more intense in the superficial than deep dermis and is occasionally admixed with neutrophils. It does not have a folliculocentric arrangement, and is not usually accompanied by stromal mucin deposition (Chapter 12).

In *Jessner's lymphocytic infiltration of the skin*, the dermal infiltrate may be indistinguishable from that seen in early, nonscarring or purely dermal lesions of lupus erythematosus. The presence of increased numbers of B-lymphocytes in the infiltrate may help distinguish this from LE (17) (see below).

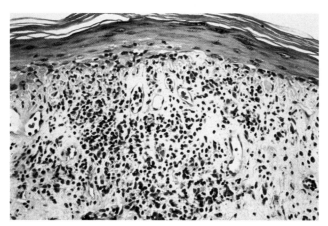

FIGURE 10-2. Discoid lupus erythematosus. Hyperkeratotic stratum corneum overlying an epidermis that has lost its rete ridge pattern. There is squamotization of basilar keratinocytes, formation of colloid bodies, and an interstitial lymphoplasmacytic inflammatory infiltrate.

Verrucous Lupus Erythematosus

An exaggerated proliferative epithelial response, which occurs in approximately 2% of patients with chronic cutaneous LE, manifests as verrucous-appearing lesions (Fig. 10-3A). Clinically, two types of lesions have been reported in this subset of LE. Lesions may simulate lichen planus or keratoacanthomas. They occur on the face (nose, chin, lips), arms, dorsal aspects of the hands, and occasionally the back. The presence of lesions typical of DLE elsewhere is a helpful clue to the diagnosis.

Histologically, the epidermis is papillomatous, hyperplastic, and surmounted by hyperkeratotic scale. Large numbers of dyskeratotic keratinocytes are usually noted in the lower portion of the epithelium, associated with a band-like mononuclear infiltrate along the dermal–epidermal junction (Fig. 10-3B). Older lesions display a thick-ened basement membrane zone (Fig. 10-3C). A second pattern consists of a cup-shaped keratin-filled crater surrounded by an acanthotic epidermis with elongated rete ridges and a sparse mononuclear infiltrate. These changes, in the presence of a deep dermal perivascular, periappendageal and interstitial infiltrate and mucin deposition, suggest a diagnosis of hypertrophic or verrucous LE (9).

Tumid Lupus Erythematosus

The dermal form of LE without surface/epithelial changes is known as tumid LE. Clinically, affected patients display indurated papules, plaques, and nodules without erythema, atrophy, or ulceration of the surface (Fig. 10-4A). Histologically, superficial and deep dermal perivascular, interstitial, and periappendageal lymphocytic infiltrates asso-

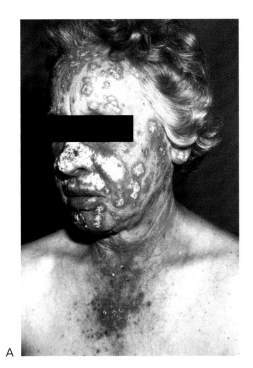

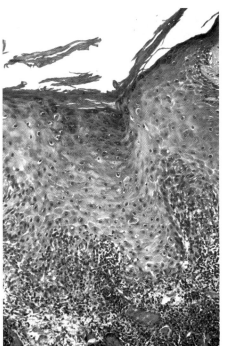

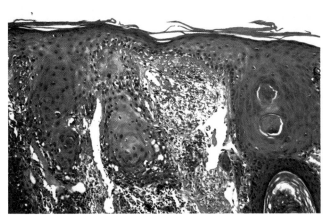

FIGURE 10-3. Hypertrophic or Verrucous lupus erythematosus. **A:** A woman with hyperkeratotic scaly plaques on an erythematous base in a photo distribution. **B:** A hyperplastic epidermis with hypergranulosis and a brisk lichenoid mononuclear infiltrate, histologically mimicking lichen planus. **C:** A hyperplastic epidermis with keratinocyte atypia. There is also a thickened basement membrane zone and interstitial mucin deposition.

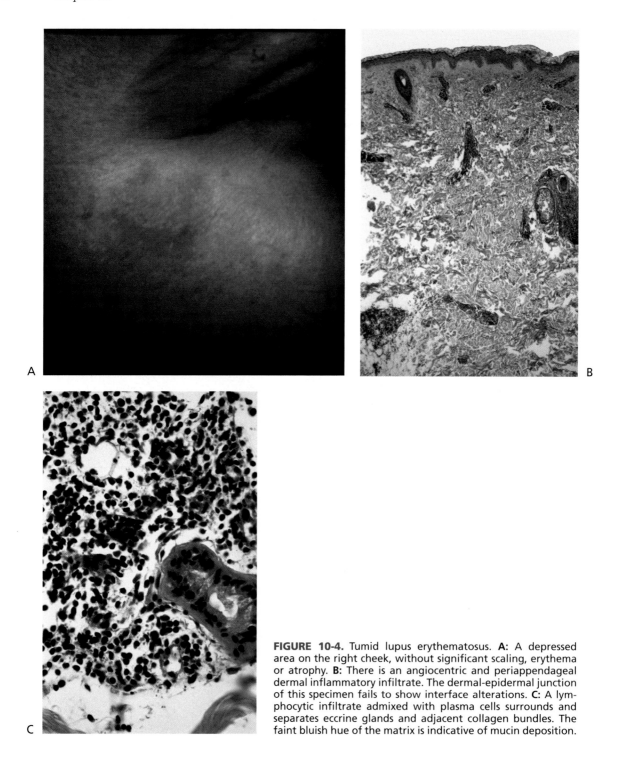

FIGURE 10-4. Tumid lupus erythematosus. **A:** A depressed area on the right cheek, without significant scaling, erythema or atrophy. **B:** There is an angiocentric and periappendageal dermal inflammatory infiltrate. The dermal-epidermal junction of this specimen fails to show interface alterations. **C:** A lymphocytic infiltrate admixed with plasma cells surrounds and separates eccrine glands and adjacent collagen bundles. The faint bluish hue of the matrix is indicative of mucin deposition.

ciated with stromal mucin deposits are observed (Fig. 10-4B and C) (18).

Lupus Erythematosus Profundus/Panniculitis

Lupus erythematosus may show changes in adipose tissue associated with the chronic cutaneous or systemic forms. Two-thirds of affected patients have discoid LE lesions.

Women are affected three to four times more often than men. Typically, multiple discrete, firm, deep nodules arise on the face, arms (particularly the deltoid area), chest, and/or buttocks. The legs and back may be affected as well. The overlying skin may be normal, erythematous, or atrophic. The panniculitis resolves, leaving depressed atrophic scars. Several observers believe that lupus erythematosus profundus may represent a lymphoproliferative disease related to connective tissue disease, which has an indolent biologic behavior (19).

Subcutaneous adipose tissue may be involved with or without inflammation in the dermis or dermal–epidermal junction. Salient histologic findings include a predominantly lobular lymphohistiocytic infiltrate often with plasma cells, occasionally forming germinal centers (Fig. 10-5A and B). Vascular changes include endothelial prominence, thrombosis, calcification, or perivascular fibrosis ("onion-skin" appearance). Fat necrosis with fibrin deposition often eventuates in hyalinization of adipose lobules (Fig. 10-5C and D). Stromal mucin deposition may be prominent in well-established lesions. The intensity of the infiltrates may lessen over time as the hyalinization progresses (Fig. 10-5D).

Subacute Cutaneous Lupus Erythematosus

Subacute cutaneous lupus erythematosus (SCLE) represents about 9% of all cases of lupus erythematosus. It is characterized by extensive erythematous, symmetric non-scarring and nonatrophic lesions that arise abruptly on the upper trunk, extensor surfaces of the arms, and dorsa of the

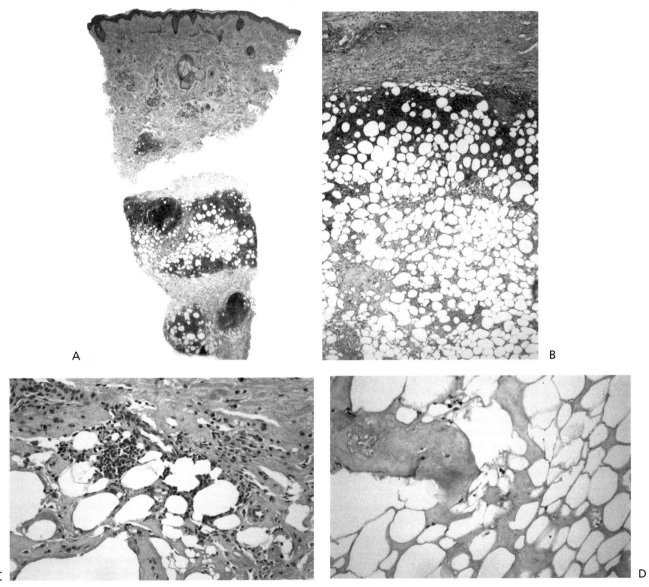

FIGURE 10-5. Lupus panniculitis. **A:** An intense inflammatory infiltrate is present at the dermal-subcutaneous interface and extends into adipose tissue in an interstitial pattern. **B:** The inflammatory infiltrate outlines individual adipocytes, giving it a lace-like pattern. **C:** With increased duration of lesions, the inflammation may become less intense. Damaged adipose tissue becomes hyalinized. **D:** An established noninflammatory lesion of lupus panniculitis, where adipose tissue is hyalinized and hypocellular. (Courtesy of Stephen C. Somach, MD.)

hands and fingers. This eruption has two clinical variants: (a) papulosquamous lesions, and (b) annular to polycyclic lesions. Frequently both types of lesions are seen. In some instances, vesicular and discoid lesions with scarring may coexist.

Patients with SCLE may have mild systemic involvement, particularly arthralgias. Approximately 50% fulfill criteria for SLE. Severe SLE, with renal or cerebrovascular disease, develops in only 10% of SCLE (20). Serologic studies show 70% of affected patients to have the anti-Ro (SS-A) antibody. Patients with SCLE often bear the HLA-DR2 and HLA-DR3 phenotype. SCLE may occur asynchronously with other connective tissue diseases such as Sjögren's syndrome and morphea.

Histopathology. See histopathology discussion of Neonatal Lupus Erythematosus section.

Neonatal Lupus Erythematosus

Neonatal lupus erythematosus has clinical and histologic skin changes and serologic findings similar to SCLE. Children of mothers with active SLE may develop LE-like symptoms in the neonatal period related to passage of maternal IgG antinuclear antibodies (particularly anti-Ro/SSA, anti-La/SSB, or anti-U1RNP autoantibodies) through the placenta. Anti-Ro/SSA are the predominant autoantibodies and are found in approximately 95% of cases. This may result in a transient syndrome characterized by widespread polycyclic, annular, and usually nonscarring lesions. There is associated photosensitivity, transient thrombocytopenia, mild hemolytic anemia, leukopenia, and congenital heart block. These changes have their onset at birth to 2 months and usually resolve in the first 6 months of life with decreasing levels of maternal antibodies. The heart block occurs in approximately 50% of affected infants, usually without associated skin lesions, and may be fatal. Of interest, individuals affected with transient neonatal LE may develop SLE as young adults (21).

Histopathology. Histologic changes in SCLE (and neonatal LE) differ in degree from those in the discoid lesions, and are most intense at the dermal–epidermal interface. They consist of the following:

- Hydropic degeneration of the basilar epithelial layer, sometimes severe enough to form clefts and subepidermal vesicles
- Colloid bodies in the lower epidermis and papillary dermis (common)
- Edema of the dermis that is more pronounced than in discoid lesions
- Focal extravasation of erythrocytes and dermal fibrinoid deposits (common)

Because of less prominent hyperkeratosis and inflammatory infiltrate than in discoid lesions (21) in comparison with chronic, and particularly discoid LE, it is not always possible to correctly categorize lesions based on histology alone since there is overlap. Pilosebaceous atrophy is helpful as a discriminating feature and correlates with DLE rather than SCLE.

Systemic Lupus Erythematosus

In SLE the cutaneous manifestations usually appear less suddenly than in SCLE and are less pronounced so that the signs and symptoms of systemic involvement usually overshadow the often subtle form of skin involvement. Usually systemic manifestations, especially joint manifestations, precede the cutaneous lesions. Only approximately 20% of SLE patients demonstrate prominent cutaneous features at the onset of their disease (22), but approximately 80% will exhibit cutaneous lesions in the course of their disease (23).

The cutaneous manifestations commonly consist of malar erythema, photosensitivity, palmar erythema, periungual telangiectases, diffuse hair loss as a result of telogen effluvium, and urticarial vasculitis and/or bullous lesions. The erythematous lesions of SLE consist of erythematous, slightly edematous patches without significant scaling and atrophy. As a rule, the patches are not sharply demarcated. The most common site of involvement is the malar region, but any area of the skin may be involved, particularly the palms and fingers. Occasionally, lesions show a petechial, vesicular, or ulcerative component. Rarely, in the late stage, some of the lesions may assume the appearance of poikiloderma atrophicans vasculare.

Well-defined "discoid" lesions with atrophic scarring, as seen typically in DLE, occur in about 15% of the patients with SLE. They may precede all other clinical manifestations of SLE. A relatively benign course characterizes SLE in most patients with preceding DLE (24); however, many patients typically have persistent multiple abnormal laboratory findings from the beginning. This is in contrast to cases of simple DLE, in which most abnormal laboratory findings, if present at all, are transient.

Two variants of SLE, *SLE with genetic deficiency of complement components* and *bullous LE*, bear mention. In the former, the onset of SLE occurs in early childhood and often affects several siblings because of the autosomal recessive mode of transmission (25). Deficiencies of C2 and C4 result in strikingly similar clinical pictures of extensive lesions similar to DLE with marked scaling, atrophy, and scarring associated with sensitivity to sunlight. In addition, there can be central nervous system involvement and glomerulonephritis, which may be fatal (26).

In *bullous SLE*, subepidermal blisters may arise in previously involved or uninvolved areas. They may form large hemorrhagic bullae to herpetiform vesicles, arise suddenly, and show clinical resemblance to lesions of bullous pemphigoid or dermatitis herpetiformis.

The coexistence of SLE and systemic scleroderma or dermatomyositis has been repeatedly described. It is

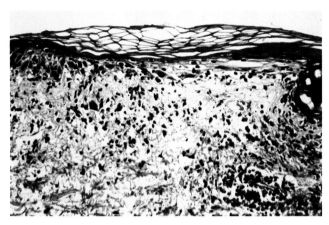

FIGURE 10-6. Subacute lupus erythematosus. A moderate mononuclear inflammatory infiltrate in the upper dermis associated with pronounced dermal edema. There is continuous subepidermal vacuolization, pigment incontinence, and focal hemorrhage.

known as overlap syndrome and refers to the coexistence of two related but separate diseases. This is in contrast to *mixed connective tissue disease*, which has become recognized as a disease entity.

For a discussion of the induction of SLE by various drugs, see Chapter 11.

Histopathology. Early lesions of SLE of the erythematous, edematous type may show only slight and nonspecific changes. In well-developed lesions, the histologic changes correspond to those described for subacute cutaneous LE (Fig. 10-6): hydropic degeneration of the basal cell layer occurs in association with edema of the upper dermis and extravasation of erythrocytes.

Fibrinoid deposits in the connective tissue of the skin are often seen in erythematous, edematous lesions, especially in patients with SLE. Such fibrinoid deposits consist of precipitation of fibrin in the ground substance. They appear as granular, strongly eosinophilic, PAS-positive, diastase-resistant deposits between collagen bundles, in the walls of dermal vessels, in the papillary dermis or beneath the epidermis in the basement membrane zone. Fibrinoid deposits are not specific for LE. They are seen in association with vascular injury, particularly in leukocytoclastic vasculitis.

The subcutaneous fat is often involved in SLE. Changes similar to those in lupus profundus may be seen, but are usually milder: there may be focal mucin deposition associated with a predominantly lymphocytic infiltrate. Adipocytes may be separated by edema and fibrinoid deposits. These histologic changes in the subcutaneous fat produce no clinically apparent lesions.

Occasionally, palpable purpuric lesions in SLE patients show a leukocytoclastic vasculitis histologically indistinguishable from leukocytoclastic vasculitis of other causes: there is endothelial cell swelling, a neutrophilic inflamma-

tory infiltrate, nuclear dust formation, perivenular fibrin deposition, and stromal hemorrhage. Urticaria-like lesions may occur, and show either a leukocytoclastic vasculitis or a perivascular mononuclear infiltrate not diagnostic of lupus erythematosus (27). Also, white atrophic lesions may occur in SLE that both clinically and histologically resemble those of malignant atrophic papulosis of Degos (28).

Bullous SLE shows two histologic inflammatory patterns: one is neutrophilic and the other mononuclear. The neutrophilic type simulates dermatitis herpetiformis or linear IgA bullous disease with the formation of papillary microabscesses (29) (Fig. 10-7A, B, and C). Nuclear dust is seen in the papillary microabscesses and in the upper dermis around and within the walls of blood vessels. Direct immunoelectron microscopic studies have localized immunoreactant deposits to beneath the lamina densa, and consist of IgG with or without IgM, and often IgA in a linear or granular pattern. Some patients may also have circulating antibasement-zone antibodies and antibodies directed against type VII collagen. The latter antibodies are similar but not identical to those in epidermolysis bullosa acquisita (30).

The subepidermal blister associated with a mononuclear inflammatory infiltrate arises in long-standing lesions of cutaneous lupus erythematosus (Fig. 10-8A and B). It likely corresponds to an altered dermal–epidermal interface resulting from inflammation and immunocomplex deposition. This type of change is a part of the spectrum of LE rather than a distinct entity.

Regarding *systemic lesions*, although the etiology of SLE is obscure, it is evident that much of the tissue damage results from deposition of antibody-antigen complexes in affected organ systems. These immune complexes are demonstrable in renal glomeruli, blood vessels, skin, and the choroid plexus of the brain.

Arthritis occurs most often; however, renal changes are the most important because they are the most common cause of death in SLE. Percutaneous renal biopsy allows determination of the type and degree of histologic changes in the kidneys, which are of prognostic significance regardless of the absence or severity of clinical renal disease (31). As in skin, immunoglobulin and complement (immunoreactant) deposits are detectable with immunofluorescence and electron microscopic studies.

Four subsets of renal disease have been categorized by the World Health Organization. *Mesangial* immunoglobulin and complement deposits are most frequently seen in SLE. If this process remains stable, there may be no clinical evidence of renal disease or mild proteinuria and/or hematuria. *Focal proliferative glomerulonephritis* (affecting less than 50% of glomerular tufts) shows mesangial changes and segmental deposits of immunoreactants in subendothelial and subepithelial areas and in the basement membranes. This process is associated with proteinuria and often hematuria. *Diffuse proliferative glomerulonephritis* (af-

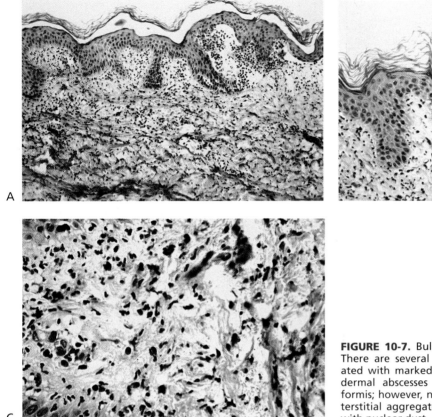

A

B

C

FIGURE 10-7. Bullous lupus erythematosus, neutrophilic. **A:** There are several broad-based subepidermal blisters associated with marked papillary dermal edema. **B:** The papillary dermal abscesses simulate findings of dermatitis herpetiformis; however, neutrophils also invade the epidermis. **C:** Interstitial aggregates of neutrophils in the dermis associated with nuclear dust.

fecting greater than 50% of glomeruli) shows changes similar to, but more extensive than, those in focal glomerulonephritis. Extensive immunoreactant endothelial and intramembranous deposits correspond to wire loops. Proteinuria and hematuria are common in affected patients; nephrotic syndrome eventually occurs in nearly all pa-

tients. If there is disease progression, death may occur within 2 years from uremia or active SLE. *Membranous glomerulonephritis* is present when there is fairly uniform thickening of the glomerular basement membrane associated with finely granular immunoreactant deposits along the basement membrane in subendothelial locations. This

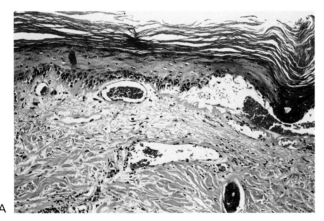

A

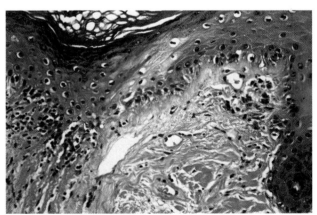

B

FIGURE 10-8. Bullous lupus erythematosus, mononuclear. **A:** A broad subepidermal cleft is present beneath an epidermis that has lost its rete ridge pattern and is surmounted by hyperkeratotic scale. The stroma contains perivascular and periappendageal inflammatory infiltrates. **B:** Adjacent to the zone of dermal-epidermal separation, there is a thickened eosinophilic basement membrane zone. Interface alterations are noted along intact dermal-epidermal junction: a mononuclear inflammatory infiltrate tags basilar keratinocytes, and is associated with subepidermal vacuolization.

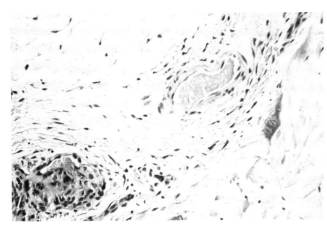

FIGURE 10-9. Lupus anticoagulant syndrome. High magnification of pale eosinophilic intravascular thrombi. There is a negligible inflammatory host response.

change is nearly always associated with proteinuria and often the nephrotic syndrome. In contrast with diffuse proliferative glomerulonephritis, renal insufficiency is often slowly progressive.

Serositis involving the pleura, epicardium, and peritoneum may show submucosal mononuclear inflammatory infiltrates associated with fibrinoid deposits. In the spleen, periarterial fibrosis around the follicular arteries is common and is highly characteristic of SLE. Thick, concentrically layered rings of sclerotic collagen fibers surround the arteries.

The *verrucous endocarditis of SLE*, the so-called Libman–Sacks endocarditis, occurs mainly on the mitral and tricuspid valves. In the subendothelial connective tissue there are collections of necrotic debris, fibrinoid material, and inflammatory cells forming small vegetations on the valve leaflets (32).

The *antiphospholipid syndrome* occurs in patients with SLE and other autoimmune diseases who develop immunoglobulins that can prolong phospholipid-dependent coagulation tests. These immunoglobulins occur in association with SLE and other autoimmune diseases, but are found unassociated with them as well. One of these is a lupus anticoagulant and occurs in about 10% of SLE patients. Affected patients are at greater risk for thromboembolic disease including deep venous thrombosis, pulmonary emboli, and other large vessel thrombosis. Other associated findings are recurrent fetal wastage, renal vascular thrombosis, thrombosis of dermal vessels (Fig. 10-9), and thrombocytopenia. Anticardiolipin antibody, a second type of antiphospholipid antibody, occurs five times more often than lupus anticoagulant antibody. It is associated with recurrent arterial and venous thrombosis, valvular abnormalities, cerebrovascular thromboses, and essential hypertension (Sneddon's syndrome) (33). Other cutaneous findings include livedo reticularis, necrotizing purpura, disseminated intravascular coagulation, and stasis ulcers of the ankles (34).

Pathogenesis and Laboratory Findings. The etiology of lupus erythematosus is considered to be multifactorial at this time and is summarized in Table 10-1. The serologic

TABLE 10-1. PATHOGENESIS OF LUPUS ERYTHEMATOSUS

Genetic	HLA-DR2	Mothers with newborns with neonatal LE
		Patients positive for anti–Ro/SSA
		Older patients with SLE
	HLA-DR3	Younger SLE patients with anti–native DNA antibodies
	HLA-B8	Increased frequency in:
	HLA-DR3	Mothers with newborns with neonatal LE
	HLA-DQ23	Females with primary Sjögren's syndrome
	HLA-DRw52	Female patients with Sjögren's syndrome/LE
Environmental precipitants	Drugs	Procainamide, hydralazine
	Ultraviolet light	
	Possibly diet	
Hormonal influences	Predisposition of females in childbearing years	
Autoimmunity	Every aspect of immune system affected:	
	B cells	Abnormal B lymphocyte maturation and activation
		Hypergammaglobulinemia
	T cells	Decreased peripheral T lymphocytes
		T-cell hyperactivity
		Increased % of CD29+ (memory helper) T cells
		Preferential loss of CD4, CD45R+ (suppressor inducer) cells in active LE
		Defective T suppressor function
	Natural killer cell	Normal number of NK cells but decreased NK-cell activity (deficient in active cytotoxicity)
	Antilymphocyte antibody	Lymphocytotoxic antibodies in sera of 80% of SLE patients
	Antinuclear antibodies	Nuclear membrane targets
		Chromatin targets
		Ribonucleoprotein targets

TABLE 10-2. ANTINUCLEAR ANTIBODIES

Appearance	Pattern	Target site	Associated antibodies	Associated disorder
	Homogenous	Chromatin	Anti-histone Anti-DNA	SLE False + SLE Drug-induced LE
	Rim	Chromatin Nuclear membrane	Anti-DNA Anti-laminin (rare)	SLE
	Fine speckled	Nuclear RNP Chromatin	Anti-Sm Anti-Ro/SSA Anti-La/SSB Anti-U1RNP Anti-Ku Anti-topoIsomerase 1 (SCL-70)	SLE, often with nephritis SLE, Sjögren's syndrome SLE, mixed CTD SLE, scleroderma, myositis Scleroderma
	Discrete speckled	Chromatin	Anti-centromere	CREST
	Nucleolar	Nucleolar RNP Nucleolar components	Anti-U3RNP Anti-RNA polymerase I Anti-Pm-Sci	Scleroderma

hallmark of lupus erythematosus is the production of autoantibodies. There is a wide variety of antibodies against different cellular targets. The initial screening test for antinuclear antibodies (ANAs) is indirect immunofluorescence, which provides limited but clinically useful information. Many other assays are available for more specific characterization of ANAs and include immuno-diffusion, enzyme-linked immunosorbent assays (ELISA), immunoprecipitation, and immunoblots.

Indirect immunofluorescence detects nuclear, homogenous, rim, speckled, and nucleolar patterns (Table 10-2). The fluorescence ANA test can be regarded as a specific marker for SLE in a rim pattern with a titer of 1:160 or higher and is often indicative of the presence of antinative or double-stranded DNA antibodies. At a titer of 1:20, about 20% of patients with DLE, most patients with systemic scleroderma, and as many as 5% of normal persons may have a positive reaction. The presence of anti-Sm is indicative of associated lupus nephritis. Antibodies against single-stranded DNA are nonspecific and are found in a variety of diseases. Anti-nRNP antibodies are of diagnostic significance only at high titers because they then indicate mixed connective tissue disease. ANA-negative sera should be examined for the presence of anti-Ro/SSA and La/SSB antibodies, characteristic of subacute and neonatal LE and SLE with genetic deficiency of complement components.

The LE cell test is of historical significance. It consisted of incubating patients' serum with normal white blood cells. In the presence of antibody to whole nucleoprotein (LE factor), damage to nuclei of leukocytes incited phago-cytosis of affected nuclei by unaffected white blood cells. If a smear of the incubated white blood cells is made and stained with Wright's stain, the phagocytized nuclear material may be observed within some of the neutrophils as a large, round, amorphous, smoky, basophilic body of such a large size that it presses the nucleus of the neutrophil against the cell membrane. This represents the LE cell.

Direct immunofluorescence studies detect immunoreactant deposits in affected tissues, particularly the skin and kidneys. A skin biopsy (3- to 4-mm punch) is submitted in saline-impregnated gauze or phosphate-buffered saline, snap frozen, sectioned, and incubated with fluorescein-conjugated antisera to IgA, IgM, IgG, and the third component of complement (C3). In a positive test, there is continuous granular deposition of usually two or more immunoreactants (in a band) along the dermal–epidermal junction. Variables that affect test results are the site of the biopsy (sun-exposed vs. sun-protected), duration of the lesion (acute, subacute, chronic), and preceding therapy. The frequency and implications of positive results in DLE and SLE are summarized in (35–37) Table 10-3.

Cautious sampling and interpretation of findings are necessary to avoid false-positive and false-negative results. The presence of only one type of immunoreactant, particularly in an intermittent distribution, may be seen in chronically sun-exposed skin or with underlying disorders such as rosacea. False-negative results are often found in acute or subacute lesions and treated lesions. Optimally, an established lesion (present for 3 months or longer) that has not been treated is submitted for study (38).

TABLE 10-3.   DIRECT IMMUNOFLUORESCENCE IN LUPUS ERYTHEMATOSUS

Site		Result	
		Discoid LE	Systemic LE
Sun exposed (e.g., dorsal forearm)	Involved	Positive in >90% of untreated lesions	Positive in 80%–90% of untreated lesions
Sun exposed (e.g., volar forearm)	Uninvolved	Almost always negative	Positive in >80% of untreated SLE
Non sun exposed (e.g., buttock)	Uninvolved	Negative	With active LE: positive in >91%
			With inactive SLE: positive in 33%
			Positive result may be indicative of renal involvement

Electron microscopic examination of the cutaneous lesions of both DLE and SLE shows marked changes in the basal cells and the lamina densa. The basal cells show vacuolization of their cytoplasm, which may progress to necrosis and disintegration of the cytoplasm. The colloid or Civatte bodies that may be seen in the epidermis and in the dermis are similar in appearance on electron microscopy to those observed in lichen planus. They are finely filamentous to amorphous granular in appearance and do not possess a delimiting membrane.

The antigen–antibody complexes have been localized with immunoelectron microscopy to beneath the lamina densa. They are seen as irregular aggregates in the uppermost portion of the dermis in the ground substance and occasionally on collagen fibrils. In some instances, small amounts of reaction product are seen also within the lamina densa and the lamina lucida. Localization of immune complexes in lupus erythematosus thus differs from their localization in bullous pemphigoid, in which they are situated entirely within the lamina lucida near the basal cells (see Chapter 9). In bullous SLE, direct immunoelectron microscopy of perilesional skin also shows the reaction product in a continuous band-like distribution below the lamina densa and a separation plane in the dermis below this band, indicating early bulla formation (39).

The presence of intracytoplasmic tubuloreticular structures has been reported in the cutaneous and renal lesions of SLE and in lesions of DLE. They bear a superficial resemblance to tubuloreticular structures and internal nucleoproteins of paramyxovirus. They are a nonspecific result of cell injury related to increased interferon alpha levels in lupus patients and are not specific for lupus erythematosus (39,40).

Jessner's Lymphocytic Infiltration of the Skin

Jessner's lymphocytic infiltration of the skin, first described in 1953 (41), is not a well-understood entity. It is characterized by asymptomatic papules or well-demarcated, slightly infiltrated red plaques, which may develop central clearing. In contrast to lesions of chronic lupus erythematosus, the surface shows no follicular plugging or atrophy. Lesions arise most often on the face, but may also involve the neck and upper trunk (42). Although this disorder has been reported to occur in childhood (43), affected patients are usually middle-aged men and women.

Variable numbers of lesions (one to many) often persist for several months or several years. They may disappear without sequelae, or recur at previously involved sites or elsewhere. The eruption may be precipitated or aggravated by sunlight. Antimalarial drugs and/or corticosteroids are useful in controlling this disorder.

Histopathology. The epidermis may be normal but often appears slightly flattened. In the dermis, there are moderately dense perivascular and diffuse infiltrates composed of small, mature lymphocytes admixed with occasional histiocytes and plasma cells (Fig. 10-10A and B). The infiltrate may extend around folliculo-sebaceous units and into subcutaneous adipose tissue.

The histologic differential diagnosis of lymphocytic infiltration of the skin includes the other four of the five "L's": lupus erythematosus, polymorphous light eruption, lymphocytoma cutis, and lymphoma. Lupus erythematosus is compared with lymphocytic infiltrate of the skin in Table 10-4. The latter entity is limited to sun-exposed skin and lacks the hyperkeratosis, atrophy, interface changes, and direct immunofluorescence findings noted in lupus. Therefore, lupus should be excluded with serologic and direct immunofluorescence studies.

Approximately 10% of cases of lupus that lack interface alterations and that show negative direct immunofluorescence studies may initially be placed into the holding category of "lymphocytic infiltrates of the skin". Polymorphous light eruptions usually show prominent papillary dermal edema (Chapter 12); however, plaque-type polymorphous light eruption may histologically overlap with lymphocytic infiltration of the skin. Clinical features may sometimes separate these two entities.

Immunohistochemical cell marker studies indicate that the predominant component of lymphocytic infiltration of the skin is a mature T lymphocyte. The relative sparsity of B-

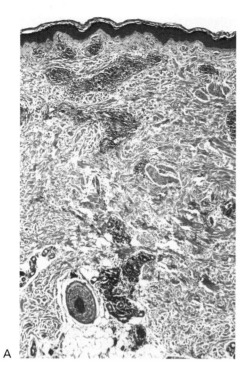
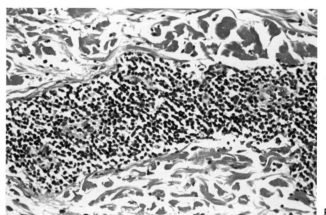

FIGURE 10-10. Jessner's lymphocytic infiltrate. **A:** The epidermis is normal. The dermis contains tightly cuffed lymphocytic infiltrates following blood vessels and focally surrounding appendages. **B:** Higher magnification shows a purely lymphocytic infiltrate around vascular channels.

lymphocytes may assist in separation of this entity from lymphocytoma cutis, which usually displays larger B-cell components with or without associated germinal center formation. Lymphoma cutis may be distinguished with cell-marker analysis, which may show a high proportion of B-lymphocytes with a less mature phenotype than expected in skin or cells with aberrant expression of cell-surface antigens.

TABLE 10-4.   DIFFERENCES BETWEEN LYMPHOCYTIC INFILTRATES OF THE SKIN AND DISCOID LUPUS ERYTHEMATOSUS

	Lymphocytic infiltrate of the skin	Discoid lupus erythematosus
Distribution	Sun-exposed areas	Sun-exposed areas with or without involvement of non sun-exposed areas
Clinical appearance		
Hyperkeratosis	Absent	Present
Healing with atrophy	Absent	Present
Histopathology		
Interface changes	Absent	Present
Immunofluorescence		
Involved skin	Negative	Positive in 90% of cases

Pathogenesis. Opinion varies as to whether Jessner's lymphocytic infiltrate of the skin is a distinct entity. The following four views have been expressed: (a) clinical, histologic, and immunohistochemical findings warrant its distinction as a separate entity (44); (b) although some cases represent an entity, others are DLE; (c) all cases are DLE; and (d) it represents an abortive or initial phase of any of the four other diseases with a patchy dermal infiltrate—that is, discoid lupus erythematosus, the plaque type of polymorphous light eruption, lymphocytoma cutis, and lymphocytic lymphoma. The last view appears to be the most likely (45).

The diagnosis of lymphocytic infiltration of the skin depends upon clinico-pathologic correlation and on longitudinal follow-up. It may be used as a preliminary diagnostic term until a more definitive diagnosis is possible.

MIXED CONNECTIVE TISSUE DISEASE

Overlapping findings of SLE, scleroderma, and polymyositis associated with the presence of high titers of anti-U1 RNP antibodies have been recognized since 1972 as the syndrome of *mixed connective tissue disease* (MCTD) (46). The clinical presentation includes, but is not limited to, edema of the hands, acrosclerosis, Raynaud's phenomenon, synovitis of one or more joints, and myositis that is documented with biopsy or serum elevations of muscle enzymes. Esophageal hypomotility and pulmonary disease may be seen as well. The diagnosis of MCTD may not be made at the outset since symptoms may present in an asynchronous fashion. The first clue to the diagnosis is usually a positive, high-titer speckled ANA.

Cutaneous lupus erythematosus lesions are found in approximately half of the patients, about as often as "sausage fingers" or sclerodactyly. They cover the entire spectrum of cutaneous lupus erythematosus. Most commonly there are diffuse, nonscarring, poorly demarcated subacute lesions, but some patients show acute malar eruptions as seen in SLE or persistent scarring lesions as seen in DLE.

Patients with high-titer anti-U1 RNP antibodies have a low prevalence of serious renal disease and life-threatening neurologic complications. Although the prognosis of MCTD compares favorably to that of SLE, death may occur from progressive pulmonary hypertension and cardiac complications (47).

Histopathology. If cutaneous lesions of lupus erythematosus are present, the histologic findings correspond to the type of lesion described in the section on DLE and SLE.

Histogenesis. MCTD, in contrast with most cases of SLE, has no antibodies to DNA. The absence of such antibodies accounts for the rarity of renal disease.

Indirect immunofluorescence studies show the presence of very high titers of serum antibodies directed against extractable ribonuclease-sensitive antigens known as small nuclear ribonucleoproteins (snRNP). They characterize MCTD but are not specific for it. They produce a fine, speckled ANA pattern at high dilutions. This speckled pattern corresponds to the widespread distribution of snRNP in the nucleus at sites of active gene transcription, where messenger RNA is being processed.

Direct immunofluorescence staining of normal skin shows deposition of IgG in a speckled (particulate) pattern in epidermal nuclei. Although this finding is typical of MCTD, it is found occasionally also in patients with SLE and other connective-tissue diseases (48). In addition, patients with MCTD may show a subepidermal lupus band in normal skin. Such a band has been observed in normal sun-exposed skin in about 20% of cases.

DERMATOMYOSITIS

Dermatomyositis manifests as an inflammatory myopathy with characteristic cutaneous findings. In the absence of cutaneous findings, the diagnosis of polymyositis is applied. Cutaneous findings alone, without muscular involvement, has been termed *amyopathic dermatomyositis* or *dermatomyositis sine myositis* (49).

Both dermatomyositis and polymyositis are uncommon diseases that have a similar incidence. Both have two peaks of occurrence: one in childhood and one between the ages of 45 and 65 (50). In some instances, the cutaneous eruption precedes the development of muscular weakness by many months or even by several years.

Diagnostic criteria for dermatomyositis include proximal symmetric muscle weakness, elevated muscle enzymes, lack of neuropathy on electromyelography, consistent muscle biopsy changes, and cutaneous findings. Involvement of the skeletal muscles causes progressive weakness, vague muscular pain, and later, muscle atrophy. The proximal muscles of the extremities and the anterior neck muscles often are the first to be involved. Involvement of the pharynx may result in dysphagia and aspiration of food, and involvement of the diaphragm and of the intercostal muscles may lead to respiratory failure.

Two distinctive cutaneous lesions are found in dermatomyositis. One is violaceous, slightly edematous periorbital patches that primarily involve the eyelids, known as the *heliotrope rash*. The other is discrete red-purple papules over the bony prominences, particularly the knuckles, knees, and elbows, known as *Gottron's papules*. These may evolve into atrophic plaques with pigmentary alterations and telangiectasia and are then known as *Gottron's sign*.

Other cutaneous findings include periungual telangiectasia, hypertrophy of cuticular tissues associated with splinter hemorrhages, photosensitivity, and poikiloderma. Often lesions resembling the erythematous–edematous lesions seen in subacute cutaneous or systemic lupus erythematosus may be found. Subcutaneous and periarticular calcification may be found, particularly in affected children. Calcinosis is usually seen centered in the proximal muscles of the shoulders and pelvic girdle.

Controversy exists over the association of dermatomyositis with malignancy (51). Interpretation of reports with incidences of 6% to 50% is hampered by the asynchronous development of malignancy in relation to the dermatomyositis. Some series fail to show a significant difference between affected patients and the control population. If malignancy arises with dermatomyositis, it usually occurs in the adult form. Some sources indicate this association is also present in the childhood form, while others view such reports with skepticism. Various tumors have been reported, with ovarian carcinoma perhaps being most frequent (52).

As with lupus erythematosus, the pathogenesis of the disease is uncertain. Associated antibodies include PM1, Jo1 (correlates with pulmonary fibrosis), Ku (associated with sclerodermatomyositis), and M2. On the whole, the prognosis of dermatomyositis is favorable, especially when treatment with corticosteroids is used. Mortality has been reported to be approximately 14% in some series, with metastatic malignancy a frequent cause of death (53).

Histopathology. The erythematous–edematous lesions of the skin in dermatomyositis may show only nonspecific inflammation. However, quite frequently the histologic changes are indistinguishable from those seen in SLE.

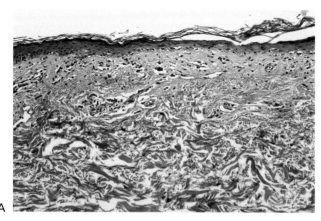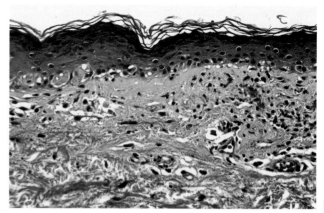

A   B

FIGURE 10-11. Dermatomyositis. **A:** An atrophic epidermis shows marked vacuolar alteration of basilar keratinocytes associated with a sparse lymphocytic inflammatory infiltrate around superficial dermal vessels. **B:** Marked vacuolar alteration of basilar keratinocytes associated with sparse lymphocytic infiltrates and papillary dermal melanophages.

There is epidermal atrophy, basement membrane degeneration, vacuolar alteration of basilar keratinocytes, a sparse lymphocytic inflammatory infiltrate around blood vessels, and interstitial mucin deposition (54) (Fig. 10-11A and B). With severe inflammatory changes, there may be associated subepidermal fibrin deposition. Immune complexes are not detected at the dermal–epidermal junction, as in lupus erythematosus.

Old cutaneous lesions with the clinical appearance of poikiloderma atrophicans vasculare usually show a band-like infiltrate under an atrophic epidermis with hydropic degeneration of the basal cell layer (see also the section on poikiloderma atrophicans vasculare). The Gottron's papules overlying the knuckles also show vacuolization of the basal cell layer, but acanthosis rather than epidermal atrophy (55). Subcutaneous tissue may show focal areas of panniculitis associated with mucoid degeneration of fat cells in early lesions. Extensive areas of calcification may be present in the subcutis at a later stage (see calcinosis cutis, Chapter 17).

Magnetic resonance imaging permits noninvasive assessment of muscle inflammation and may serve as a guide in locating a site for muscle biopsy. Tender proximal muscles of an extremity yield more useful information than atrophic, weak muscles, which show end-stage changes. Three types of changes may be observed in active disease: (a) interstitial inflammatory infiltrates composed of lymphocytes and macrophages; (b) segmental muscle fiber necrosis (loss of skeletal muscle transverse striation, hyalinization of the sarcoplasm, fragmentation and/or phagocytosis of degenerated muscle fragments); or (c) vasculopathy (56). The latter entity may be seen in the childhood form and shows immunocomplex deposition in vessel walls (57). Old lesions usually show a rather nonspecific picture of atrophy of the muscle fibers and diffuse interstitial fibrosis with relatively little inflammation.

Systemic Lesions

Changes in organs other than the skin and the striated muscles occur only rarely in dermatomyositis, in contrast to SLE and systemic scleroderma. The myocardium may show changes identical to those in the skeletal muscle but less severe. Ulcerative lesions in the gastrointestinal tract, caused by vascular occlusions, have also been described (58).

Histogenesis. On electron microscopic examination the degenerative changes include focal disintegration of myofilaments and myofibrils, vacuolization, and accumulation of lipid and lysosomes within muscle fibers. As in lupus erythematosus, nonspecific intracytoplasmic tubuloreticular structures may be found in skin and muscles.

Differential Diagnosis. Differentiation of the cutaneous lesions of dermatomyositis from those of subacute cutaneous or systemic lupus erythematosus may be impossible on a histologic basis. It may also be impossible on clinical grounds in cases in which muscular weakness is mild or absent, as it may be in the early stage of dermatomyositis. In such cases, laboratory tests are of great value. The most important is the lupus band test, which is always negative in lesions of dermatomyositis (59), whereas in lesions of lupus erythematosus it is positive in 90% of cases. Other tests that are usually negative in dermatomyositis and often positive in lupus erythematosus include urinalysis and renal function tests, as well as tests for antinuclear antibodies, anti-native DNA antibodies, and antibodies to ribonucleoprotein. However, patients with active myositis show an elevation of serum creatine kinase and aldolase.

Poikiloderma Atrophicans Vasculare

Poikiloderma atrophicans vasculare may be seen in three different settings: (a) in association with three genodermatoses; (b) as an early stage of mycosis fungoides; and (c) in association with dermatomyositis and, less commonly, lupus erythematosus.

The three genodermatoses in which the cutaneous lesions have the appearance of poikiloderma atrophicans vasculare follow: (a) poikiloderma congenitale of Rothmund–Thomson (Chapter 6), with the lesions of poikiloderma present largely on the face, hands, and feet, and occasionally also on the arms, legs, and buttocks; (b) Bloom's syndrome (Chapter 6), with poikiloderma-like lesions on the face, hands, and forearms; and (c) dyskeratosis congenita (Chapter 6), in which there may be extensive netlike pigmentation of the skin suggestive of poikiloderma atrophicans vasculare.

Poikiloderma-like lesions as features of early mycosis fungoides may be seen in one of two clinical forms: either as the large plaque type of parapsoriasis en plaques, also known as poikilodermatous parapsoriasis (Chapter 7), or as parapsoriasis variegata, also called parakeratosis variegata, which, in its early state, shows papules arranged in a netlike pattern (Chapter 7). Although these two types of parapsoriasis represent an early stage of mycosis fungoides, not all cases progress clinically into fully developed mycosis fungoides (60). Cases in which no progression toward mycosis fungoides is observed have been described also as *idiopathic poikiloderma atrophicans vasculare* (61).

The third group of diseases in which lesions of poikiloderma atrophicans vasculare occur is represented by dermatomyositis and SLE. Dermatomyositis is much more commonly seen as the primary disease than lupus erythematosus, and the association with dermatomyositis often is referred to as poikilodermatomyositis. In contrast to mycosis fungoides, in which poikilodermatous lesions are seen in the early stage, the lesions found in dermatomyositis and SLE generally represent a late stage.

Clinically, the term poikiloderma atrophicans vasculare is applied to lesions that, in the early stage, show erythema with slight, superficial scaling, a mottled pigmentation, and telangiectases. In the late stage the skin appears atrophic and the erythema is less pronounced than in the early stage, but the mottled pigmentation and the telangiectases are more pronounced. The clinical picture then resembles chronic radiodermatitis.

Histopathology. In its early stage poikiloderma atrophicans vasculare, without respect to its cause, shows moderate thinning of the stratum malpighii, effacement of the rete ridges, and hydropic degeneration of the basal cells. In the upper dermis there is a band-like infiltrate, which in places invades the epidermis. The infiltrate consists mainly of lymphoid cells but also contains a few histiocytes. Melanophages filled with melanin as a result of pigmentary incontinence are found in varying numbers within the infiltrate. In addition, there is edema in the upper dermis and the superficial capillaries are often dilated. In the late stage the epidermis is apt to be markedly thinned and flattened, but the basal cells still show hydropic degeneration. Melanophages and edema of the upper dermis are still present, and telangiectasia may be pronounced.

The amount and type of dermal infiltrate vary with the underlying cause. In poikiloderma atrophicans vasculare associated with one of the genodermatoses the mononuclear infiltrate is mild and may be absent in the late stage (62). Similarly, in the late stage of poikiloderma seen in association with dermatomyositis or SLE there is only slight dermal inflammation (54) (Fig. 10-12). In contrast, the amount of inflammatory infiltrate seen in poikiloderma associated with early mycosis fungoides increases rather than decreases with time. In addition, cells with large, hyperchromatic nuclei, so-called mycosis cells, are likely to be present and there is often marked epidermotropism of the

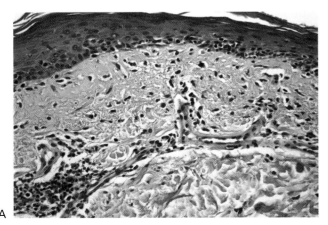
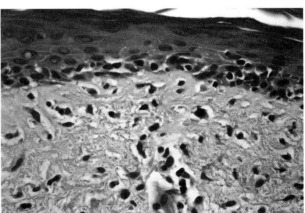

FIGURE 10-12. Poikiloderma. **A:** The epidermis appears flattened. The upper dermis contains a patchy lymphocytic infiltrate. **B:** The epidermis shows hydropic degeneration of the basal cells. There are scattered lymphocytes in the dermis and the basal epidermis.

infiltrate, which may result in Pautrier microabscesses. Cell-marker analysis of such cases has shown most cells to be T helper/inducer (CD4+) lymphocytes that lack Leu-8 and/or Leu-9 expression, as seen in cutaneous T-cell lymphoma (63).

SCLERODERMA

Scleroderma (Gr. *skleros*, hard, and *derma*, skin) is a connective tissue disorder characterized by thickening and fibrosis of the skin. Two types of scleroderma exist: circumscribed scleroderma (*morphea*), and systemic scleroderma (*progressive systemic sclerosis*). They are somewhat analogous to the purely cutaneous form of lupus erythematosus (DLE) and the cutaneous plus visceral involvement in systemic lupus erythematosus. Rarely, morphea and systemic scleroderma may coexist. In such instances, the manifestations of morphea arise first and are extensive, whereas those of systemic scleroderma are mild and nonprogressive (64). Rarely, the manifestations of systemic scleroderma precede those of morphea (65).

There are also two variants of morphea: atrophoderma of Pasini and Pierini, and eosinophilic fasciitis of Shulman. The latter disease differs sufficiently from morphea so that it will be discussed separately.

Hardening of the skin (sclerodermoid changes) may also arise in association with genetic, metabolic, neurologic, and immunologic disorders, with occupational or chemical exposures, in association with malignancy or as a sequela of infection (66). Genetic disorders that may show sclerodermatous cutaneous changes include phenylketonuria, progeria, Rothmund–Thomson syndrome, and Werner's syndrome. Occupations at risk are jackhammer and chain-saw operators, and those exposed to polyvinyl chloride, silica, and epoxy resins. Patients with metabolic disorders such as porphyria cutanea tarda, primary systemic amyloidosis, Hashimoto's disease, carcinoid syndrome, and childhood diabetes mellitus may show similar cutaneous changes. Chronic graft-versus-host disease frequently shows sclerodermatous changes, while scattered reports in the literature indicate such changes may arise subsequent to silicone and paraffin injections for cosmetic procedures (67). Chemical agents have been known to induce thickening and hardening of the skin. Specific compounds include polyvinyl chloride, bleomycin, pentazocine, L-5 hydroxytryptophan and carbidopa (68), Spanish rapeseed oil (69), and L-tryptophan (eosinophilia-myalgia syndrome) (70).

Morphea

In morphea, or circumscribed scleroderma, the lesions usually are limited to the skin and to the subcutaneous tissue beneath the cutaneous lesions. Occasionally, however, the underlying muscles and rarely the underlying bones are also affected.

Morphea may be divided according to morphology and distribution of lesions into six types: guttate, plaque, linear, segmental, subcutaneous, and generalized. Eosinophilic fasciitis, even though it is the fascial component of subcutaneous morphea, is discussed separately because of its somewhat different clinical and histologic appearance.

Guttate lesions occur almost always in association with lesions of the plaque type. Guttate lesions are small and superficial; they resemble the lesions of lichen sclerosus et atrophicus but do not show hyperkeratosis or follicular plugging.

Lesions of the plaque type, the most common manifestation of morphea, are round or oval but through coalescence may assume an irregular configuration. They are indurated, have a smooth surface, and show an ivory color. As long as they are enlarging, they may show a violaceous border, the so-called lilac ring.

Lesions of the linear type occur predominantly on the extremities and on the anterior scalp. When one or several extremities are involved, there is often, in addition to induration of the skin, marked atrophy of the subcutaneous fat and of the muscles, resulting in contractures of muscles and tendons and ankyloses of joints. In children it may result in impaired growth of the affected limb (71). On the anterior portion of the scalp and on the forehead, linear morphea often has the configuration of the stroke of a saber (*coup de sabre*) (71).

Segmental morphea occurs on one side of the face, resulting in hemiatrophy. Occasionally, morphea en *coup de sabre* and facial hemiatrophy occur together (72). It is uncertain if Parry–Romberg facial hemiatrophy represents a part of the spectrum of linear scleroderma involving the face.

In subcutaneous morphea (morphea profunda) the involved skin feels thickened and bound to the underlying fascia and muscle. The involved plaques are ill defined, and the skin of these plaques is smooth and shiny (73).

Generalized morphea comprises very extensive cases showing a combination of several of the five types just described. It is seen mainly in children, in whom it has been described as disabling pansclerotic morphea (64), but it can also occur in adults. Rarely, bullous lesions are seen in patients with generalized morphea (74).

There are several reported cases of morphea, which involves the superficial reticular dermis, as contrasted with its usual involvement of the deep reticular dermis (75). The clinical impact of the depth of involvement is unclear at this point. The coexistence of lesions of morphea and lichen sclerosus et atrophicus is worthy of note.

There are conflicting data regarding *Borrelia burgdorferi* infection in cases of morphea. Studies indicating that such a relationship exists are primarily from Europe (76). Studies in North America, and some from Europe, have resulted in negative findings (77).

Histopathology. The different types of morphea cannot be differentiated histologically. Rather, they differ in regard to severity and to their depth of involvement of the skin. Therefore, it is of great importance that the specimen for biopsy includes adequate amounts of subcutaneous tissue, since most of the diagnostic alterations are seen in the lower dermis and in the subcutis.

Early inflammatory, intermediate, and late sclerotic stages exist. In the early inflammatory stage, found particularly at the violaceous border of enlarging lesions, the reticular dermis shows interstitial lymphoplasmacytic infiltrates among slightly thickened collagen bundles (Fig. 10-13A). As lesions become established, the inflammatory infiltrates surround eccrine coils and are associated with hypocellular collagen bundles and reduced numbers of surrounding adipocytes (Fig. 10-13B). A much more pronounced inflammatory infiltrate than that seen in the dermis often involves the subcutaneous fat and extends upward toward the eccrine glands. Trabeculae subdividing the subcutaneous fat are thickened because of the presence of an inflammatory infiltrate and deposition of new collagen. Large areas of subcutaneous fat are replaced by newly formed collagen, which is composed of fine, wavy fibers, rather than of bundles, and which stains only faintly with hematoxylin-eosin (78). Vascular changes in the early inflammatory stage generally are mild both in the dermis and in the subcutaneous tissue. They may consist of endothelial swelling and edema of the walls of the vessels (79).

In the late sclerotic stage, as seen in the center of old lesions, the inflammatory infiltrate has disappeared almost completely, except in some areas of the subcutis. The epidermis is normal. The collagen bundles in the reticular dermis often appear thickened, closely packed, and hypocellular, and stain more deeply eosinophilic than in normal skin (Fig. 10-13C and D). In the papillary dermis, where the collagen normally consists of loosely arranged fibers, the collagen may appear homogeneous.

The eccrine glands appear markedly atrophic, have few or no adipocytes surrounding them, and appear surrounded by newly formed collagen (Fig. 10-13B). Also, instead of lying near the dermal–subcutaneous junction as in normal skin, they seem to lie higher in the dermis as a result of the replacement of most of the subcutaneous fat by newly formed collagen. This collagen consists of thick, pale, sclerotic, homogeneous, or hyalinized bundles with only few fibroblasts (hypocellular). Few blood vessels are seen within the sclerotic collagen; they often have a fibrotic wall and a narrowed lumen. Elastic stains show thick elastic fibers arranged in parallel to hypocellular collagen strands and in parallel to the epidermal surface (Fig. 10-13E) (80).

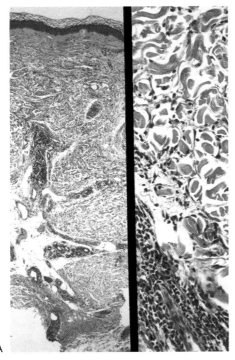 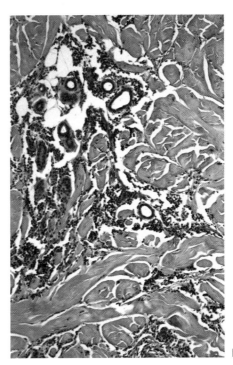

A   B

FIGURE 10-13. Morphea. **A:** The early inflammatory phase of morphea, where there is an interstitial lymphoplasmacytic infiltrate distributed among deep dermal collagen bundles. Collagen bundles are minimally swollen. **B:** Over time, collagen bundles become thickened, hypocellular and swollen. Lymphoplasmacytic inflammatory infiltrates separate such collagen strands, surround eccrine coils in the deep dermis, and are associated with loss of adipocytes around eccrine apparatus. *(continued)*

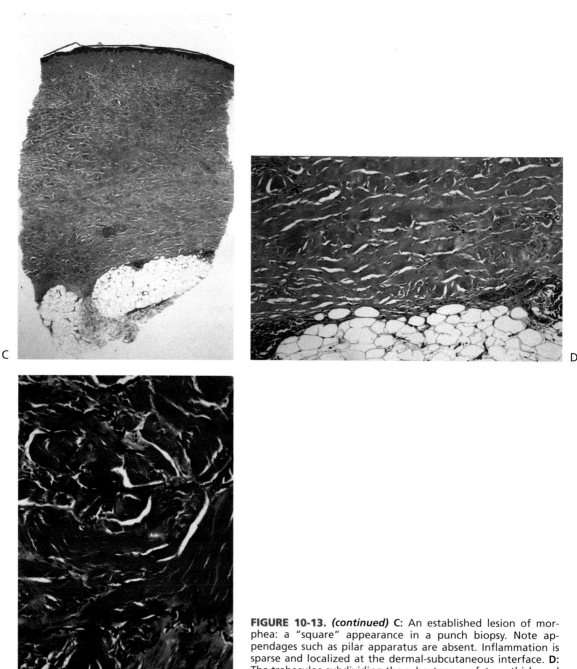

FIGURE 10-13. *(continued)* **C:** An established lesion of morphea: a "square" appearance in a punch biopsy. Note appendages such as pilar apparatus are absent. Inflammation is sparse and localized at the dermal-subcutaneous interface. **D:** The trabeculae subdividing the subcutaneous fat are thickened and there is a patchy lymphoplasmacytic infiltrate. Pale thickened collagen bundles appear arranged in parallel to each other. **E:** Elastic stains demonstrate thick, coarse elastic fibers separated by collagen. They have a somewhat parallel array.

The fascia and striated muscles underlying lesions of morphea may be affected in the linear, segmental, subcutaneous, and generalized types. The fascia shows fibrosis and sclerosis similar to that seen in subcutaneous tissue. The muscle fibers appear vacuolated and separated from one another by edema and focal collections of inflammatory cells (81).

Bullae, seen only on rare occasions in generalized and subcutaneous morphea, arise subepidermally, probably as a result of lymphatic obstruction, causing subepidermal edema.

Differential Diagnosis. Contrasting features of morphea and lichen sclerosus et atrophicus are summarized in Table 10-5. They include relatively little epidermal change in morphea, as compared with thinning of the rete ridges, follicular plugging, and interface alterations of lichen sclerosus. Reticular dermal changes of fibrosis and inflammation of morphea contrast with edema and loss of elastic tissue in

TABLE 10-5. CONTRASTING FEATURES OF MORPHEA AND LICHEN SCLEROSUS ET ATROPHICUS

	Morphea	Lichen sclerosus et atrophicus
Epidermis	Relatively normal	Thinning of rete
	No follicular plugging	Follicular plugging
Dermal-epidermal junction	No hydropic degeneration	Hydropic degeneration of basilar cells
	Subepidermal separation infrequent	Often subepidermal bullae
Dermis	Appears homogenized	Marked edema
	Papillary dermal collagen elastic fibers present	Elastic fibers absent
Subcutis	Inflammation	No inflammation or fibrosis
	Fibrosis	

lichen sclerosus. Histologic differentiation of the late stage of morphea from lichen sclerosus et atrophicus may cause difficulties, particularly in view of the fact that the two conditions may coexist.

Systemic Scleroderma

In systemic scleroderma, in addition to involvement of the skin and the subcutaneous tissue visceral lesions are present, leading to death in some patients. The indurated lesions of the skin are not sharply demarcated or "circumscribed," as in morphea, although a few well-demarcated morphea-like patches may occasionally be seen.

Cutaneous involvement usually starts peripherally on the face and hands, gradually extending to the forearms. Facial changes include a mask-like expressionless face, inability to wrinkle the forehead, a beak-like nose, and tightening of the skin around the mouth associated with radial folds. The hands show nonpitting edema involving the dorsa of the fingers, hands, and forearms. Gradually the fingers become tapered, the skin becomes hard, and flexion contractures form. These changes are referred to as acrosclerosis and are associated with Raynaud's phenomenon, which may precede other manifestations by months or even years. Microscopic examination of the nail-fold capillary beds shows tortuosity and redundancy of capillary loops with dilatation of the arterioles and venules. Such abnormalities may occasionally be seen in patients with localized scleroderma and herald coexisting or evolving systemic sclerosis (82).

Systemic sclerosis with limited scleroderma, known as CREST syndrome, is associated with Raynaud's phenomenon in virtually all affected patients. This variant of acrosclerosis, which frequently but not invariably has a favorable prognosis, consists of several or all of the following manifestations: Calcinosis cutis, Raynaud's phenomenon, involvement of the esophagus with dysphagia, sclerodactyly, and telangiectases. Death from visceral lesions is rather infrequent in the CREST syndrome (83).

In about 5% of cases, the cutaneous lesions first appear on the trunk as so-called *diffuse systemic scleroderma*, often sparing the peripheral portions of the extremities. Raynaud's phenomenon is absent in such patients. There are, however, transitional forms starting out as acrosclerosis with Raynaud's phenomenon but then extending to the proximal portions of the arms and to the trunk.

In both forms of systemic scleroderma, the skin in the involved areas is diffusely indurated and, as a result of diffuse fibrosis of the subcutaneous fat, becomes firmly bound to the underlying structures. The skeletal musculature is affected, resulting in weakness and atrophy. Contractures of the muscles and tendons and ankyloses of the joints may develop.

Occasional manifestations pertaining to the skin include diffuse hyperpigmentation, which is seen mainly in diffuse systemic scleroderma. Macular telangiectases on the face and hands, calcinosis cutis located on the extremities, and ulcerations, especially on the tips of the fingers and over the knuckles, occur predominantly in acrosclerosis. Also vascular ulcers on the lower extremities resembling those seen in atrophie blanche may occur in patients with acrosclerosis.

Histopathology. The histologic appearance of the skin lesions in systemic scleroderma is similar to that of morphea so that histologic differentiation of the two types is not possible. However, in early lesions of systemic scleroderma the inflammatory reaction is less pronounced than in morphea, so that only a mild inflammatory infiltrate is present around the dermal vessels, around the eccrine coils, and in the subcutaneous tissue. The vascular changes in early lesions are slight, as in morphea (84). In contrast, in the late stage, systemic scleroderma shows more pronounced vascular changes than morphea, particularly in the subcutis. These changes consist of a paucity of blood vessels, thickening and hyalinization of their walls, and narrowing of the lumen. Even in the late stage of systemic scleroderma, the epidermis appears normal, only occasionally showing disappearance of the rete ridges. Aggregates of calcium may also be seen in the late stage within areas of sclerotic, homogeneous collagen of the subcutaneous tissue (see also calcinosis cutis, Chapter 17).

Systemic Lesions

Internal organs are often affected in scleroderma, but their involvement varies greatly in extent and degree. Involvement does not necessarily imply functional compromise, and in many affected patients systemic scleroderma ultimately comes to a standstill. The clinical symptoms produced by reduced pliability, vascular compromise, and subsequent loss of function can be found in the gastrointestinal tract, lungs, heart, and kidneys as well as the skin. In the gastrointestinal tract submucosal fibrosis and replacement of the muscularis by fibrosis with intimal thickening of blood vessels give rise to difficulties in swallowing, regurgitation, malabsorption, and eventually ileus. In the lungs, interstitial fibrosis, degeneration of alveolar spaces, and intimal thickening of arteries result in dyspnea and cor pulmonale. Cases of pulmonary carcinoma (predominantly bronchioloalveolar) have been observed and are associated with the presence of pulmonary fibrosis (85). The most serious consequences arise in the kidneys. Adventitial fibrosis may affect interlobar, arcuate, and interlobular arteries, while mucoid degeneration affects arcuate and interlobular arteries. Uremia occurs more frequently than rapidly evolving renal failure and hypertension. The latter entity, termed scleroderma renal crisis, is associated with "onion-skin" hyperplasia of arterial walls and may be fatal (86).

Pathogenesis and Laboratory Findings. The pathogenesis of systemic scleroderma, as with lupus erythematosus, is uncertain and may be multifactorial. Histogenetic factors are essentially the same in morphea and systemic scleroderma; they differ only in degree and extent.

The triad of vascular compromise, collagen matrix aberrations, and presence of serologic autoimmune indicators contribute in variable degrees to symptoms and clinical findings in scleroderma and morphea (Table 10-6). Although a relationship to retroviral disease has been suggested, it is speculative and may reflect molecular mimicry of viral antigens (87).

Microvascular Changes

Involved vessels are primarily precapillary arterioles. Changes in the microvasculature have been noted in clinically normal skin. Perivascular edema and functional changes in endothelial cells can be detected early (88). Precapillary arterioles then show endothelial proliferation and mononuclear inflammatory infiltrates, followed by intimal proliferation and luminal narrowing (89). Corresponding electron microscopic findings include vacuolization and destruction of endothelial cells, reduplication of the basement membrane, enlargement of the rough endoplasmic reticulum in pericytes and fibroblasts, and perivascular fibrosis. Although widespread arteriolitis may be present in early stages, only rarely does it progress to a necrotizing arteriolitis and eventuate in periarteritis nodosa (90).

A role for adhesion molecules in the evolution of lesions of scleroderma has been suggested: they are thought to bind mononuclear cells to endothelial cells and facilitate transvascular migration of inflammatory cells into the con-

nective tissue. Interactions with connective-tissue components may lead to the release of cytokines and growth factors, resulting in up-regulation of matrix production by fibroblasts and changes in fibroblast phenotype, eventuating in fibrosis (91).

Collagen Matrix Aberrations

Analysis of collagen in affected skin has shown excess production of connective-tissue components normally present in the dermis, including types I, III, V, VI, and VII collagen, fibronectin, and proteoglycans (92,93). Other studies suggest that fibroblasts in localized and systemic scleroderma express some markers of smooth muscle differentiation (myofibroblasts), which may account for their different biologic behavior (94). Some observers have found loss of CD34+ dendritic cells in affected areas, a finding of uncertain significance (75,95).

Serologic/Immunologic Markers

Most patients with systemic sclerosis (greater than 90%) and approximately 50% with localized scleroderma (morphea) have a positive ANA. The pattern may be homogenous, speckled, or nucleolar. When using human laryngeal carcinoma cell lines, HEp2, more than 90% of patients with morphea or acrosclerosis have a detectable anticen-

TABLE 10-6. PATHOGENIC FACTORS IN SCLERODERMA

Vascular aberrations	Raynaud's phenomenon
	Intimal hyperplasia of blood vessels
	Adventitial fibrosis
	Vascular abnormalities in other visceral organs
	Microvascular abnormalities
	Enlargement and tortuosity of capillary loops
	Capillary loop dropout
	Thickened and reduplicated basement membrane
	Loss of endothelium
Immunologic factors	T helper cell (CD4+) infiltrates
	Reduction in T-suppressor (CD8+) cells
	Increased soluble interleukin 2 receptors correlate with disease progression and mortality
	Decreased interleukin 1 production by peripheral mononuclear cells
Serologic markers	ANA+ in more than 90% of patients
	Low/absent anti-native (double stranded) DNA, anti-Sm, rare anti-nRNP
	Speckled ANA pattern correlates with anti-centromere antibody on HEp-2 cells and CREST and a relatively favorable prognosis
	Anti-DNA-Topoisomerase 1 (Sci-70)

tromere antibody. In patients with systemic sclerosis this antibody is not usually detected. Instead, 20% to 40% of them have antibodies to Scl-70. This antigen has been identified as DNA–topoisomerase I, an intracellular enzyme involved in the uncoiling of DNA before it is transcribed. Antibodies to this enzyme hinder its function. The presence of antibodies to Scl-70 correlates with systemic sclerosis, while the presence of anticentromere antibodies correlates with morphea or CREST and suggests a more favorable prognosis (96).

In some cases of systemic scleroderma, epidermal nucleolar IgG deposition is seen even in clinically normal skin as a result of high serum concentrations of antibody to nucleolar antigen (97). Although subepidermal and vascular deposits are regularly absent in the skin in scleroderma, kidney biopsies in patients with renal involvement show diffuse vascular deposits of immunoglobulins, predominantly IgM, or of complement in the intima of the interlobular and arcuate arteries, which by light microscopy often exhibit fibromucinous alterations (98).

Atrophoderma of Pasini and Pierini

In atrophoderma of Pasini and Pierini there are areas on the trunk, particularly the back, in which the skin appears slightly depressed and has a slate-gray color but shows no other surface changes. The lesions are asymptomatic, bilateral, symmetrical, and sharply but often irregularly demarcated, measuring from 1 to 10 cm in diameter. They often show a "cliff-drop" border, which is largely an optical effect of the slate-gray discoloration. In old lesions, the center of the depressed area may feel slightly indurated.

Histopathology. The histologic changes in early lesions usually are slight and nonspecific, consisting of some thickening of the collagen bundles and a mild, scattered, chronic inflammatory infiltrate (99). Older lesions show no inflammatory infiltrate, but in the deeper layers of the dermis, they may show collagen bundles that not only are thickened but also appear tightly packed. In addition, indurated areas may show homogeneous, hyalinized collagen bundles (100).

Because the collagen bundles in the skin of the back normally are rather thick, it may be difficult to determine whether the collagen shows any changes. It is therefore desirable to take a biopsy specimen not only from the lesion but also from normal skin, either from an area nearby or from the opposite side with subcutaneous fat for comparison.

Pathogenesis. Some authors believe that atrophoderma of Pasini and Pierini is a disease entity, as suggested by the original describers. In favor of this view is that in atrophoderma, the atrophy comes first and the sclerosis possibly appears later, whereas in morphea, the sclerosis comes first and the atrophy appears later (101).

Most observers view the clinical presentation of atrophoderma to be distinct from morphea: atrophoderma

has an earlier onset (second to third decade) and protracted course of 10 to 20 years, and lesions lack a violaceous ring, which characteristically surrounds lesions of morphea. Microscopic findings show similarities to morphea, however, suggesting that atrophoderma of Pasini and Pierini may be a distinct, abortive variant of morphea (102). To support this view there are instances of coexistent morphea and atrophoderma, as well as reports of transformation of lesions of morphea into atrophoderma (101). A relationship of this disorder to *Borrelia burgdorferi* infection has been reported but needs more studies to be confirmed (103).

EOSINOPHILIC FASCIITIS (SHULMAN'S SYNDROME)

First described in 1974 (104), eosinophilic fasciitis is a scleroderma-like disorder characterized by inflammation and thickening of the deep fascia. It has a rapid onset associated with pain, swelling, and progressive induration of the skin leading to exaggerated deep grooving of the skin around superficial veins. This disorder is often accompanied by a peripheral eosinophilia and hypergammaglobulinemia, and has been associated with aplastic anemia. Eosinophilic fasciitis may have its onset with unusual physical exertion; however, more recently it has been reported in association with l-tryptophan ingestion (105). The latter association is known as eosinophilia-myalgia syndrome, which is clinically and histologically similar to eosinophilic fasciitis.

Eosinophilic fasciitis often involves one or more extremities. The induration may cause a decreased range of motion and, in severe cases, even joint contractures (106). In only a few cases are there lesions on the trunk, and the face is almost invariably spared. In nearly all reported cases, Raynaud's phenomenon and visceral lesions of scleroderma have been absent. Only very few instances of incontestable eosinophilic fasciitis have shown evidence of Raynaud's phenomenon (107) or mild pulmonary fibrosis (108). The disorder has a varied course: some patients improve spontaneously, others improve with corticosteroids, while still others may have relapses and remissions.

Histopathology. A deep-wedge biopsy to skeletal muscle including fascia is essential to making the diagnosis of eosinophilic fasciitis. The fascia is markedly thickened, appears homogeneous, and is permeated by a mononuclear inflammatory infiltrate (Fig. 10-14A, B, and C). In some instances, the infiltrate in the fascia contains an admixture of eosinophils (109). The underlying skeletal muscle in some cases shows myofiber degeneration, severe inflammation with a component of eosinophils, and focal scarring; in other cases, however, it is not involved.

In most cases the adipose tissue shows no significant changes, except that the fibrous septa separating deeply located fat lobules are thicker, paler staining, and more ho-

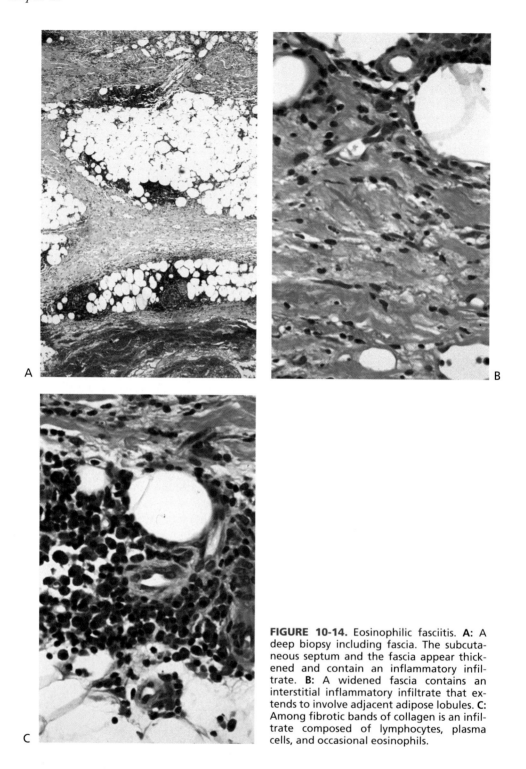

A

B

C

FIGURE 10-14. Eosinophilic fasciitis. **A:** A deep biopsy including fascia. The subcutaneous septum and the fascia appear thickened and contain an inflammatory infiltrate. **B:** A widened fascia contains an interstitial inflammatory infiltrate that extends to involve adjacent adipose lobules. **C:** Among fibrotic bands of collagen is an infiltrate composed of lymphocytes, plasma cells, and occasional eosinophils.

mogeneous and hyaline than normal dermal connective tissue. In other cases, however, the collagen in the lower reticular dermis appears pale and homogeneous, and the entire subcutaneous fat is replaced by horizontally oriented, thick, homogeneous collagen containing only few fibroblasts and merging with the fascia (110).

Pathogenesis. Whereas at first the impression prevailed that eosinophilic fasciitis was a new syndrome, it soon be-

came apparent that the disorder represents a variant of morphea (106). Eosinophilic fasciitis shares many features with generalized morphea: they both may show inflammation and fibrosis of the fascia, as well as blood eosinophilia and hypergammaglobulinemia. Also, antinuclear antibodies are present in a significant number of cases (111). The term morphea profunda, analogous to lupus erythematosus profundus, has been applied to this disorder (112). Nevertheless, because of its acute onset in most cases, its usual limitation to the structures underlying the skin, and its tendency to resolve, eosinophilic fasciitis deserves recognition as a distinct variant of morphea (113).

LICHEN SCLEROSUS ET ATROPHICUS

Lichen sclerosus (LS) encompasses the disorders known as *lichen sclerosus et atrophicus, balanitis xerotica obliterans* (LS of the male glans and prepuce), and *kraurosis vulvae* (LS of the female labia majora, labia minora, perineum, and perianal region) (114). Lichen sclerosus is an inflammatory disorder of unknown etiology that affects patients 6 months of age to late adulthood. In both males and females, genital involvement is the most frequent, and often the only, site of involvement. Extragenital lesions may occur with or without coexisting genital lesions.

Lesions of LS are characterized by white polygonal papules that coalesce to form plaques. Comedo-like plugs on the surface of the plaque correspond to dilated appendageal ostia. The plugs may disappear as the lesion ages, leaving a smooth, porcelain-white plaque. Solitary or generalized lesions may become bullous and hemorrhagic.

In males, involvement of the glans and prepuce often result in phimosis. Although the literature is dominated by reports of LS in incompletely or uncircumcised men (115), occurrences in circumcised men are reported as well (116). Neoplasms have been infrequently documented in association with LS; however, a cause-and-effect relationship has not been established (114).

In females, contiguous involvement of the labial, perineal, and anal areas has been described clinically as "figure 8" or "keyhole" lesions (117). Many cases of childhood LS in girls resolve by menarche (118). If lesions persist, atrophy of the labia and narrowing of the vaginal orifice may ensue. In contrast to lichen sclerosus et atrophicus of the skin, which rarely itches, there is often severe pruritus in the vulvar region. Although neoplasms have been reported in association with LS, the current consensus is that LS is not itself a premalignant condition (119). Since neoplasms have arisen in areas adjacent to lesions of LS, long-range follow-up of patients with lichen sclerosus et atrophicus of the vulva is advisable.

Of interest, lesions of LS may koebnerize (be provoked by trauma) (120) as well as coexist with morphea (120, 121). In extensive cases of morphea, lichen sclerosus et atrophicus may become superimposed on some of the lesions. It is then best recognized by recognizing pale superficial dermal collagen, as compared with hypocellular compacted deep dermal collagen, and the presence of follicular plugging (122,123).

Histopathology. Salient histologic findings in cutaneous lesions of lichen sclerosus et atrophicus follow: (a) hyperkeratosis with follicular plugging; (b) atrophy of the stratum malpighii with hydropic degeneration of basal cells; (c) pronounced edema and homogenization of the collagen in the upper dermis; and (d) an inflammatory infiltrate in the mid-dermis.

The hyperkeratosis is so marked that the horny layer is often thicker than the atrophic stratum malpighii, which may be reduced to a few layers of flattened cells (Fig. 10-15A and B). The cells of the basal layer show hydropic degeneration. The rete ridges often are completely absent, although they may persist in a few areas and show some irregular downward proliferation. In such prolifera-

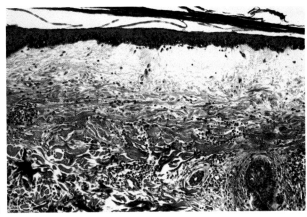
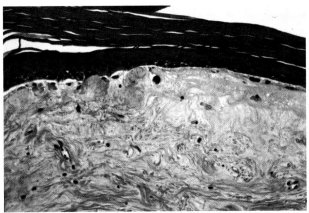

FIGURE 10-15. Lichen sclerosus. **A:** Lichen sclerosus showing a subepidermal zone of pallor. A "trilayered" or "striped" appearance: compact hyperortho-keratotic scale and atrophic epidermis (dark pink/red), a pale dermis (white), and subjacent, variably dense interstitial lymphocytic inflammatory infiltrate (blue) delineating the depth of this process. **B:** A well-established lesion, showing a thick hyperkeratotic scale, an atrophic epidermis, and pale superficial dermal stroma with melanophages. Intermittent cleft-like spaces separate an atrophic epidermis from a pale dermis.

tions, hydropic degeneration of the basal cells usually is pronounced.

Plugging of appendageal ostia by keratotic plugs is often associated with atrophy and disappearance of appendageal structures. Keratotic plugging is not apparent in mucosal lesions. In the latter areas, particularly the vulva, squamous hyperplasia adjacent to the atrophic epidermis can be found in about one-third of patients with LS. There may

be varying degrees of "dysplasia" consisting of disorderly arrangement of the cells and enlarged hyperchromatic nuclei. Transition into carcinoma, however, is said to be rare (124).

Beneath the epidermis is a broad zone of pronounced lymphedema (Fig. 10-15A and B). Within this zone, the collagenous fibers are swollen and homogeneous and contain only a few nuclei. They stain poorly with eosin and

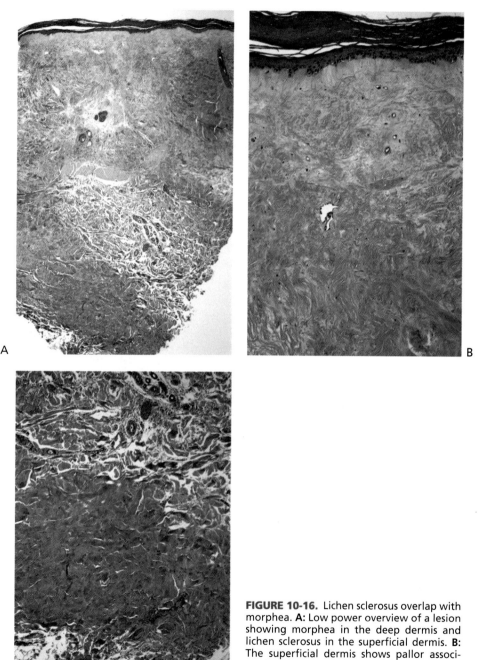

FIGURE 10-16. Lichen sclerosus overlap with morphea. **A:** Low power overview of a lesion showing morphea in the deep dermis and lichen sclerosus in the superficial dermis. **B:** The superficial dermis shows pallor associated with loss of the overlying epidermal rete ridge pattern and hyperkeratosis. **C:** The deep dermis shows compacted, hypocellular collagen bundles and loss of appendageal structures.

other connective tissue stains. The blood and lymph vessels are dilated, and there may be areas of hemorrhage. Elastic fibers are sparse and, in old lesions, are absent within the area of lymphedema (125). In areas of severe lymphedema, clinically visible bullae may form; they are found in subepidermal locations (126). Shrinkage within the area of lymphedema may occur during the process of dehydration of the specimen, resulting in the formation of pseudobullae, which often are located intradermally.

Except in lesions of long duration, an inflammatory infiltrate is present in the dermis. The younger the lesion, the more superficial is the location of the infiltrate. In very early lesions and at the periphery of somewhat older lesions, the infiltrate may be found in the uppermost dermis, in direct apposition to the basal layer. Soon, however, a narrow zone of edema and homogenization of the collagen displaces the inflammatory infiltrate farther down, so that in well-developed lesions, the infiltrate is found in the mid-dermis. The infiltrate can be patchy, but it is often band-like and composed of lymphoid cells admixed with plasma cells and histiocytes. In old lesions in which the infiltrate is slight or absent, the collagen bundles in the midportion and lower dermis may appear swollen, homogeneous, and hyperchromatic, thus appearing sclerotic (hence lichen *sclerosus*). Cases of overlap of morphea and LS may be seen and demonstrate the histologic changes of both disorders in their respective locations of the dermis (Fig. 10-16A, B, and C).

Pathogenesis. Changes in the dermal matrix have been detected in LS. By electron microscopy, collagen fibrils often lack cross-striation and in cross-sections sometimes have the appearance of empty tubes, suggesting degeneration of collagen fibrils (127). In some areas, new immature collagen of reduced and variable diameter (40 to 80 nm) is seen (128). Ultrastructural studies also have shown degeneration of subepidermal elastin and increases in ground substance (129).

In the epidermis, intercellular edema separates epidermal cells that show degenerative changes. There is nearly a complete absence of melanosomes within the keratinocytes. This is the result either of degeneration and disappearance of the melanocytes (128) or of inhibition of the transfer of melanosomes from the melanocytes to the keratinocytes (130).

Differential Diagnosis. Very early lesions may resemble lichen planus because of the apposition of the inflammatory infiltrate to the basal layer. However, the basal cells are not replaced by flattened squamous cells, as in lichen planus, but appear hydropic, and a subepidermal zone of edema usually has already begun to form in some areas in lichen sclerosus et atrophicus.

Old lesions of lichen sclerosus et atrophicus with thickening and hyperchromasia of the collagen bundles in the midportion and lower dermis and only a slight inflammatory infiltrate may resemble morphea. Nevertheless, the epidermis in morphea, although it may be thin, shows neither hydropic degeneration of the basal cells nor follicular plugging, and the upper dermis in morphea has elastic fibers and shows no zone of edema (125). Still, in lesions in which lichen sclerosus et atrophicus develops either secondarily to morphea or simultaneously with it, there are, in addition to the epidermal and subepidermal changes of lichen sclerosus et atrophicus, changes indicative of morphea in the lower dermis and subcutaneous fat. A definite diagnosis of both lichen sclerosus et atrophicus and morphea in the same lesion can be made only if the newly formed collagen extends into the subcutaneous fat and consists of faintly staining, homogeneous collagen (131).

REFERENCES

1. Tan EM, Cohen AS, Fries JF, et al. The 1982 revised criteria for the classification of systemic lupus erythematosus. *Arthritis Rheum* 1982;25:1271.
2. Wechsler HL. Lupus erythematosus. A clinician's coign of vantage [Editorial]. *Arch Dermatol* 1983;119:877.
3. Ropes M. Observations on the natural course of disseminated lupus erythematosus. *Medicine (Baltimore)* 1964;43:387.
4. Hahn BH. Management of systemic lupus erythematosus. In: Kelley WN, Harris ED Jr, Ruddy S, et al., eds. *Textbook of Rheumatology*, 4th ed. Philadelphia: Saunders, 1994;1043.
5. Ginzler EM, Schorn K. Outcome and prognosis in systemic lupus erythematosus. *Rheum Dis Clin North Am* 1988;14:67.
6. David-Bajar KM, Bennion SD, DeSpain JD, et al. Clinical, histologic, and immunofluorescent distinctions between subacute cutaneous lupus erythematosus and discoid lupus erythematosus. *J Invest Dermatol* 1992;99:251.
7. Jerdan MS, Hood AF, Moore GW, et al. Histopathologic comparison of the subsets of lupus erythematosus. *Arch Dermatol* 1990;126:52.
8. Uitto J, Santa-Cruz DJ, Eisen AZ, et al. Verrucous lesions in patients with discoid lupus erythematosus. *Br J Dermatol* 1978; 98:507.
9. de Berker D, Dissaneyeka M, Burge S. The sequelae of chronic cutaneous lupus erythematosus. Lupus 1992;1:181.
10. O'Loughlin S, Schroeter AL, Jordon RE. A study of lupus erythematosus with particular reference to generalized discoid lupus. *Br J Dermatol* 1978;99:1.
11. Millard LG, Rowell NR. Abnormal laboratory test results and their relationship to prognosis in discoid lupus erythematosus. *Arch Dermatol* 1979;115:1055.
12. Estes D, Christian CL. The natural history of systemic lupus erythematosus by prospective analysis. *Medicine (Baltimore)* 1971; 50:85.
13. Vinciullo C. Hypertrophic lupus erythematosus: differentiation from squamous cell carcinoma. *Australas J Dermatol* 1986;27:76.
14. Bielicky T, Trapl J. Nichtvernarbender chronischer erythematodes. *Arch Klin Exp Dermatol* 1963;217:438.
15. Ueki H, Wolff HH, Braun-Falco O. Cutaneous localization of human gamma globulins in lupus erythematosus. *Arch Dermatol Forsch* 1974;248:297.
16. Panet-Raymond G, Johnson WC. Lupus erythematosus and polymorphous light eruption. *Arch Dermatol* 1973;108:785.
17. Akasu R, Kahn HJ, From L. Lymphocyte markers on formalin-fixed tissue in Jessner's lymphocytic infiltrate and lupus erythematosus. *J Cutan Pathol* 1992;19:59.

18. Ruiz H, Sanchez JL. Tumid lupus erythematosus. *Am J Dermatopathol* 1999;12:356.

19. Magro CM, Crowson AN, Kovatich AJ, et al. Lupus profundus, indeterminate lymphocytic lobular panniculitis and subcutaneous T-cell lymphoma: a spectrum of subcuticular T-cell lymphoid dyscrasia. *J Cutan Pathol* 2001;28:235.

20. Sontheimer RD. Subacute cutaneous lupus erythematosus: a decade's perspective. *Med Clin North Am* 1989;73:1073.

21. Lee LA. Neonatal lupus erythematosus. *J Invest Dermatol* 1993; 100:9S.

22. Provost TT. Subsets in systemic lupus erythematosus. *J Invest Dermatol* 1979;72:110.

23. Gilliam JN. Systemic lupus erythematosus and the skin. In: Lahita RG, ed. *Systemic Lupus Erythematosus.* New York: John Wiley & Sons, 1987;615.

24. Callen JP. Chronic cutaneous lupus erythematosus. *Arch Dermatol* 1982;118:412.

25. Mascart-Lemone F, Hauptmann G, Goetz J, et al. Genetic deficiency of C4 presenting with recurrent infections and a systemic lupus erythematosus-like disease. *Am J Med* 1983;75:295.

26. Tappeiner G, Hintner H, Scholz S, et al. Systemic lupus erythematosus in hereditary deficiency of the fourth component of complement. *J Am Acad Dermatol* 1982;7:66.

27. Provost TT, Zone JJ, Synkowski D, et al. Unusual cutaneous manifestations of systemic lupus erythematosus. Urticaria-like lesions: correlation with clinical and serologic abnormalities. *J Invest Dermatol* 1980;75:495.

28. Callen JP. Mucocutaneous changes in patients with lupus erythematosus: The relationship of these lesions to systemic disease. *Rheum Dis Clin North Am* 1988;14:79.

29. Camisa C. Vesiculobullous systemic lupus erythematosus: a report of four cases. *J Am Acad Dermatol* 1988;18:93.

30. Gammon WR, Briggaman RA, Bullous SLE: a phenotypically distinctive but immunologically heterogeneous bullous disorder. *J Invest Dermatol* 1993;100:28S.

31. Schur PH. Clinical features of SLE. In: Kelley WN, Harris ED Jr, Ruddy S, et al, eds. *Textbook of Rheumatology,* 4th ed. Philadelphia: Saunders, 1994:1017.

32. Klemperer P, Pollack AD, Baehr G. Pathology of disseminated lupus erythematosus. *Arch Pathol* 1941;32:569.

33. Asherson RA, Baguley E, Pal C, et al. Antiphospholipid syndrome: five year follow-up. *Ann Rheum Dis* 1991;50:805.

34. Bick RL, Baker WF Jr. The antiphospholipid and thrombosis syndromes. *Med Clin North Am* 1994;78:667.

35. Tuffanelli DL. Cutaneous immunopathology: recent observations. *J Invest Dermatol* 1975;65:143.

36. Provost TT, Andres G, Maddison PJ, et al. Lupus band test in untreated SLE patients. *J Invest Dermatol* 1980;74:407.

37. Gately LE, Nesbitt LT. Update on immunofluorescent testing in bullous diseases and lupus erythematosus. *Dermatol Clin* 1994; 1:133.

38. Jaworsky C, Murphy GF. Special techniques in dermatology. *Arch Dermatol* 1989;125:963.

39. Olansky AJ, Briggaman RA, Gammon WR, et al. Bullous systemic lupus erythematosus. *J Am Acad Dermatol* 1982;7:511.

40. Woods VG Jr. Pathogenesis of systemic lupus erythematosus. In: Kelley WN, Harris ED, Ruddy S, et al., eds. *Textbook of Rheumatology,* 4th ed. Philadelphia: Saunders, 1994:999.

41. Jessner M, Kanof NB. Lymphocytic infiltration of the skin. *Arch Dermatol Syphiligr* 1953;68:447.

42. Toonstra J, Wildschut A, Boer J, et al. Jessner's lymphocytic infiltration of the skin. *Arch Dermatol* 1989;125:1525.

43. Higgins CR, Wakeel RA, Cerio R. Childhood Jessner's lymphocytic infiltrate of the skin. *Br J Dermatol* 1994;131:99.

44. Konttinen YT, Bergroth V, Johansson E, et al. A long-term clinicopathologic survey of patients with Jessner's lymphocytic infiltration of the skin. *J Invest Dermatol* 1987;89:205.

45. Cerio R, Oliver GF, Spaull J, et al. The heterogeneity of Jessner's lymphocytic infiltrate. *J Cutan Pathol* 1988;15:300(abst).

46. Sharp GC, Irvin WS, Tan EM, et al. Mixed connective tissue disease: an apparently distinct rheumatic disease syndrome associated with a specific antibody to an extractable nuclear antigen (ENA). *Am J Med* 1972;52:148.

47. Ueda N, Mimura K, Meada H, et al. Mixed connective tissue disease with fatal pulmonary hypertension and a review of the literature. *Virchows Arch A Pathol Anat Histopathol* 1984;404: 335.

48. Burrows NP, Bhogal BS, Russel Jones R, et al. Clinicopathological significance of cutaneous epidermal nuclear staining by direct immunofluorescence. *J Cutan Pathol* 1993;20:159.

49. Callen JP, Tuffanelli DL, Provost TT. Collagen vascular disease: an update. *J Am Acad Dermatol* 1994;28:477.

50. Cronin ME, Plotz PH. Idiopathic inflammatory myopathies. *Rheum Dis Clin North Am* 1990;16:655.

51. Callen JP. Malignancy in polymyositis/dermatomyositis. *Clin Dermatol* 1988;6:55.

52. Whittmore SE, Rosenshein NB, Provost TT. Ovarian cancer in patients with dermatomyositis. *Medicine (Baltimore)* 1994;73: 153.

53. Bohan A, Peter JB, Bowman RL, et al. A computer-assisted analysis of 153 patients with polymyositis and dermatomyositis. *Medicine (Baltimore)* 1977;56:255.

54. Janis JF, Winkelmann RK. Histopathology of the skin in dermatomyositis. *Arch Dermatol* 1968;97:640.

55. Hanno R, Callen JP. Histopathology of Gottron's papules. *J Cutan Pathol* 1985;12:389.

56. DeGirolami UU, Smith TW. Teaching monograph: pathology of skeletal muscle diseases. *Am J Pathol* 1982;107:231.

57. Kissel JT, Mendell JR, Rammohan KW. Microvascular deposition of complement membrane attack complex in dermatomyositis. *N Engl J Med* 1986;314:329.

58. Wainger CK, Lever WF. Dermatomyositis: a report of three cases with postmortem observations. *Arch Dermatol Syph* : 196.

59. Harrist TJ, Mihm MC Jr. Cutaneous immunopathology: the diagnostic use of direct and indirect immunofluorescence techniques in dermatologic diseases [Review]. *Hum Pathol* 1979; 10:625.

60. Samman PD. The natural history of parapsoriasis en plaques (chronic superficial dermatitis) and prereticulotic poikiloderma. *Br J Dermatol* 1972;87:405.

61. Steigleder GK. Die poikilodermien-genodermien und genodermatosen? *Arch Dermatol Syph (Berlin)* 1952;194:461.

62. Braun-Falco O, Marghescu S. Kongenitales teleangiektatisches erythem (Bloom-Syndrom) mit diabetes insipidus. *Hautarzt* 1966;17:155.

63. Lindae ML, Abel EA, Hoppe RT, et al. Poikilodermatous mycosis fungoides and large-plaque parapsoriasis exhibit similar abnormalities of T-cell antigen expression. *Arch Dermatol* 1988; 124:366.

64. Diaz-Perez JL, Connolly SM, Winkelmann RK. Disabling pansclerotic morphea of children. *Arch Dermatol* 1980;116:169.

65. Ikai K, Tagami H, Imamura S, et al. Morphea-like cutaneous changes in a patient with systemic scleroderma. *Dermatologica* 1979;158:438.

66. Callen JP, Tuffanelli DL, Provost TT. Collagen-vascular disease: an update. *J Am Acad Dermatol* 1993;28:477.

67. Sahn EE, Garen PD, Silver RM, et al. Scleroderma following augmentation mammoplasty. *Arch Dermatol* 1990;126:1198.

68. Joly P, Lampert A, Thomine E, et al. Development of pseudobullous morphea and scleroderma-like illness during therapy with L-5 hydroxytryptophan and carbidopa. *J Am Acad Dermatol* 1991;25:332.

69. Toxic Epidemic Syndrome Study Group. Toxic epidemic syndrome: Spain, 1981. *Lancet* 1982;2:697.

70. Oursler JR, Farmer ER, Roubenoff R, et al. Cutaneous manifestations of the eosinophilia-myalgia syndrome. *Br J Dermatol* 1992;127:138.
71. Falanga V, Medsger TA Jr, Reichlin M, et al. Linear scleroderma: clinical spectrum, prognosis, and laboratory abnormalities. *Ann Intern Med* 1986;104:849.
72. Dilley JJ, Perry HO. Bilateral linear scleroderma en coup de sabre. *Arch Dermatol* 1968;97:688.
73. Su WPD, Greene SL. Bullous morphea profunda. *Am J Dermatopathol* 1986;8:144.
74. Synkowski DR, Lobitz WC Jr, Provost TT. Bullous scleroderma. *Arch Dermatol* 1981;117:135.
75. McNiff JM, Glusac EJ, Lazova RZ, et al. Morphea limited to the superficial reticular dermis: an underrecognized histologic phenomenon. *Am J Dermatopathol* 1999;21:315.
76. Buechner SA, Winkelmann RK, Lautenschlager S, et al. Localized scleroderma associated with Borrelia burgdorferi infection: clinical, histologic, and immunohistochemical observations. *J Am Acad Dermatol* 1993;29:190.
77. Weinecke R, Schlupen EM, Zochling N, et al. No evidence for Borrelia burgdorferi-specific DNA in lesions of localized scleroderma. *J Invest Dermatol* 1995;104:23.
78. Fleischmajer R, Nedwich A. Generalized morphea: I. Histology of the dermis and subcutaneous tissue. *Arch Dermatol* 1972;106:509.
79. O'Leary PA, Montgomery H, Ragsdale WE. Dermatohistopathology of various types of scleroderma [Review]. *Arch Dermatol* 1957;75:78.
80. Taylor RM. Sclerosing disorders. In: Farmer ER, Hood AF, eds. *Pathology of the Skin.* Norwalk, CT: Appleton and Lange, 1990:275.
81. Hickman JW, Sheils WS. Progressive facial hemiatrophy. *Arch Intern Med* 1964;113:716.
82. Maricq HR. Capillary abnormalities, Raynaud's phenomenon, and systemic sclerosis in patients with localized scleroderma. *Arch Dermatol* 1992;128:630.
83. Medsger TA, Masi AT, Rodnan GP, et al. Survival with systemic sclerosis (scleroderma). *Ann Intern Med* 1971;75:369.
84. Fleischmajer R, Nedwich A. Generalized morphea: I. Histology of the dermis and subcutaneous tissue. *Arch Dermatol* 1972;106:509.
85. Abu-Shakra M, Guillemin F, Lee P. Cancer in systemic sclerosis. *Arthritis Rheum* 1993;36:460.
86. Tuffanelli DL. Systemic scleroderma. *Med Clin North Am* 1989;73:1167.
87. Jablonska S, Blaszczyk M, Chorzelski TP, et al. Clinical relevance of immunologic findings in scleroderma. *Clin Dermatol* 1993;10:407.
88. Prescott RJ, Freemont AJ, Jones CJ, et al. Sequential dermal microvascular and perivascular changes in the development of scleroderma. *J Pathol* 1992;166:255.
89. Haustein UF, Herrmann K, Böhme HJ. Pathogenesis of progressive systemic sclerosis [Review]. *Int J Dermatol* 1986;25:286.
90. Toth A, Alpert LI. Progressive systemic sclerosis terminating as periarteritis nodosa. *Arch Pathol* 1971;92:31.
91. Postlewaithe AE. Connective tissue metabolism including cytokines in scleroderma. *Curr Opin Rheumatol* 1993;5:766.
92. Rudnicka L, Varga J, Christiano AM, et al. Elevated expression of type VII collagen in the skin of patients with systemic sclerosis: regulation by transforming growth factor-beta. *J Clin Invest* 1994;93:1709.
93. Varga J, Rudnicka L, Uitto J. Connective tissue alterations in systemic sclerosis [Review]. *Clin Dermatol* 1994;12:387.
94. Sappino AP, Masouyé I, Saurat JH, et al. Smooth muscle differentiation in scleroderma fibroblastic cells. *Am J Pathol* 1990;137:585.
95. Aiba S, Tabata N, Ohtani H, et al. CD34+ spindle-shaped cells selectively disappear from the skin lesion of scleroderma. *Arch Dermatol* 1994;130:593.
96. Aeschlimann A, Meyer O, Bourgeois P, et al. Anti-Scl-70 antibodies detected by immunoblotting in progressive systemic sclerosis: specificity and clinical correlations. *Ann Rheum Dis* 1989;48:992.
97. Prystowsky SD, Gilliam JN, Tuffanelli D. Epidermal nucleolar IgG deposition in clinically normal skin. *Arch Dermatol* 1971;114:536.
98. Lapenas D, Rodnan GP, Cavallo T. Immunopathology of the renal vascular lesion of progressive systemic sclerosis (scleroderma). *Am J Pathol* 1978;91:243.
99. Quiroga ML, Woscoff A. L'atrophodermie idiopathique progressive (Pasini-Pierini) et la sclérodermie atypique lilacée non indurée (Gougerot). *Ann Dermatol Syphiligr* 1961;88:507.
100. Miller RF. Idiopathic atrophoderma [Review]. *Arch Dermatol* 1965;92:653.
101. Weiner M. In discussion to Eshelman OM: idiopathic atrophoderma of Pasini and Pierini. *Arch Dermatol* 1965;92:737.
102. Kencka D, Blaszczyk M, Jablonska S. Atrophoderma Pasini—Pierini is a primary atrophic abortive morphea. *Dermatology* 1995;190:203.
103. Buechner SA, Rufli T. Atrophoderma of Pasini and Pierini. Clinical and histopathologic findings and antibodies to Borrelia burgdorferi in thirty-four patients. *J Am Acad Dermatol* 1994;30:441.
104. Shulman L. Diffuse fasciitis with hypergammaglobulinemia and eosinophilia: a new syndrome? *J Rheumatol* 1974;1:46 (abst).
105. Freundlich B, Werth VP, Rook AH, et al. L-Tryptophan ingestion associated with eosinophilic fasciitis but not progressive systemic sclerosis. *Ann Int Med* 1990;112:758.
106. Golitz LE. Fasciitis with eosinophilia: the Shulman syndrome. *Int J Dermatol* 1980;19:552.
107. Barriere H, Stalder JF, Berger M, et al. Syndrome de Shulman. *Ann Dermatol Venereol* 1980;107:643.
108. Tamura T, Saito Y, Ishikawa H. Diffuse fasciitis with eosinophilia. *Acta Derm Venereol (Stockh)* 1979;59:325.
109. Weinstein D, Schwartz RA. Eosinophilic fasciitis. *Arch Dermatol* 1978;114:1047.
110. Lupton GP, Goette DK. Localized eosinophilic fasciitis. *Arch Dermatol* 1979;115:85.
111. Jablonska S, Hamm G, Kencka D, et al. Fasciitis eosinophilica, Übergang in eine eigenartige sklerodermie (sklerodermie-fasciitis). *Z Hautkr* 1984;59:711.
112. Su WPD, Person JR. Morphea profunda. *Am J Dermatopathol* 1981;3:251.
113. Helfman T, Falanga V. Eosinophilic fasciitis. *Clin Dermatol* 1994;12:449.
114. Meffert JJ, Davis BM, Grimwood RE. Lichen sclerosus. *J Am Acad Dermatol* 1995;32:393.
115. Ledwig PA, Weigand DA. Late circumcision and lichen sclerosus et atrophicus of the penis. *J Am Acad Dermatol* 1989;20:211.
116. Loening-Baucke V. Lichen sclerosus et atrophicus in children. *Am J Dis Child* 1991;145:1058.
117. Clark JA, Muller SA. Lichen sclerosus et atrophicus in children. *Arch Dermatol* 1967;95:476.
118. Helm KF, Gibson LE, Muller SA. Lichen sclerosus et atrophicus in children and young adults. *Pediatr Dermatol* 1991;8:97.
119. Woodruff JD, Baens JS. Interpretation of atrophic and hypertrophic alterations in the vulvar epithelium. *Am J Obstet Gynecol* 1963;86:713.
120. Pock L. Koebner phenomenon in lichen sclerosus et atrophicus [Letter]. *Dermatologica* 1990;181:76.
121. Shono S, Imura M, Osaku A, et al. Lichen sclerosus et atrophicus, morphea and coexistence of both diseases. Histologic studies using lectins. *Arch Dermatol* 1991;127:1352.

122. Tremaine R, Adam JE, Orizaga M. Morphea coexisting with lichen sclerosus et atrophicus. *Int J Dermatol* 1990;29:486.
123. Wallace HJ. Lichen sclerosus et atrophicus [Review]. *Trans St Johns Hosp Dermatol Soc* 1971;57:9.
124. Hart WR, Norris HJ, Helwig EB. Relation of lichen sclerosus et atrophicus of the vulva to development of carcinoma. *Obstet Gynecol* 1975;45:369.
125. Steigleder GK, Raab WP. Lichen sclerosus et atrophicus. *Arch Dermatol* 1961;84:219.
126. Gottschalk HR, Cooper ZK. Lichen sclerosus et atrophicus with bullous lesions and extensive involvement. *Arch Dermatol* 1947;55:433.
127. Mann PR, Cowan MA. Ultrastructural changes in four cases of lichen sclerosus et atrophicus. *Br J Dermatol* 1973;89:223.
128. Kint A, Geerts ML. Lichen sclerosus et atrophicus: an electron microscopic study. *J Cutan Pathol* 1975;2:30.
129. Frances C, Weschler J, Meimon G, et al. Investigation of intercellular matrix macromolecules involved in lichen sclerosus. *Acta Derm Venereol (Stockh)* 1983;63:483.
130. Klug H, Sönnichsen N. Elektronenoptische untersuchungen bei lichen sklerosus et atrophicus. *Dermatol Monatsschr* 1972; 158:641.
131. Uitto J, Santa Cruz DJ, Bauer EA, et al. Morphea and lichen sclerosus et atrophicus: clinical and histopathologic studies in patients with combined features. *J Am Acad Dermatol* 1980; 3:271.

11

CUTANEOUS TOXICITIES OF DRUGS

THOMAS D. HORN
KIM M. HIATT

Drug reactions, which reportedly occur at a rate of approximately 2.2% of in-patients (1), arise by immunologic as well as nonimmunologic mechanisms. The risk of developing an adverse drug reaction is higher in women, the elderly, patients with Sjögren's syndrome, and AIDS patients (2). Nonimmunologic mechanisms encompass pharmacokinetics of drugs such as absorption, plasma protein binding, distribution, metabolism, and elimination. Genetic factors influence metabolic pathways, specifically oxidation, hydrolysis, and acetylation, and are suggested to be the mechanisms of toxicity reactions, such as occur in sulphonamide and anticonvulsant toxicities (3). Theories regarding immunologic mechanisms of drug-induced disease include cell-mediated reactions to altered cell surface proteins that effect a lymphocytic response. Molecular mimicry of endogenous peptides modified by binding with ingested drugs has also been suggested (4). Drugs can also stimulate an anaphylactic-type reaction by IgE-mediated or immune complex-mediated mechanisms. Drug–protein complexes cross-link IgE molecules on sensitized mast cells or basophils releasing chemical mediators, which result in systemic effects including urticaria, angioedema, anaphylaxis, and anaphylactoid reactions. Immune complex mechanisms rely on persistence of drug antigen in the serum long enough to elicit an antibody response. And finally, antibody-mediated reactions occur as a result of cell-bound, drug hapten complexing with IgG antibody, which stimulates complement fixation and cytolysis as occurs in some cases of drug-associated thrombocytopenic purpura (3). New drug formulations, in particular liposomal and transdermal delivery systems, are responsible for increasing numbers of cutaneous reactions, primarily by the nature of their preferential accumulation in target tissues such as skin (5,6).

Several medication-related cutaneous eruptions are considered elsewhere in the text, including urticaria (Chapter 7), erythema multiforme (Chapter 9), toxic epidermal necrolysis (Chapter 9), erythema nodosum (Chapter 20), erythroderma (Chapter 9), vasculitis (Chapter 8), and corticosteroid-induced acne (Chapter 18).

EXANTHEMIC DRUG ERUPTIONS

Eruptive and efflorescent cutaneous drug reactions are perhaps the most common adverse effects of medications. Morbilliform and pustular eruptions are considered under this heading. Virtually any drug may be associated with a morbilliform eruption; the nonspecific clinical and histologic changes make definitive implication of a specific agent difficult. The most common class of medications causing morbilliform eruptions is antibacterial antibiotics (7). The morbilliform rash consists of fine blanching papules, which appear suddenly, are symmetric, and often are brightly erythematous in Caucasian patients.

Various drugs are implicated in acute generalized exanthemic pustulosis (AGEP) (8,9). Widespread nonfollicular, sterile pustules develop within a period of hours after administration of the offending agent. Although enteroviral infection and mercury exposure are cited as causes, antibacterial antibiotics are most often implicated with a broad range of other medications as well, including acetaminophen and terbinafine (10). Fever, leukocytosis, purpura, and clinical features suggesting erythema multiforme accompany the pustules. *In vitro* studies have shown this to be a drug-specific process effected by CD4$^+$ T-cell–mediated release of the neutrophil chemoattractant, IL-8 (11). Unlike drug-induced macular and papular eruptions, in AGEP there is no up-regulation of MHC class II expression on keratinocytes (12).

Histopathology. The typical morbilliform drug eruption displays a variable, often sparse, mainly perivascular infiltrate of lymphocytes and eosinophils. Eosinophils may be absent. Some vacuolization of the dermal–epidermal junction with few apoptotic epidermal cells may be observed, but not to the degree typical of erythema multiforme or toxic epidermal necrolysis. Biopsies of acute generalized exanthematous pustulosis have subcorneal or intraepidermal pustules, papillary dermal edema and a lymphohistiocytic perivascular infiltrate with some eosinophils and neutrophils (Fig. 11-1A and B). Vasculitis and/or single cell keratinocyte necrosis may be present (9).

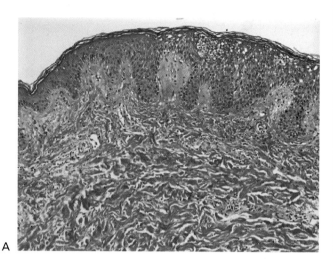

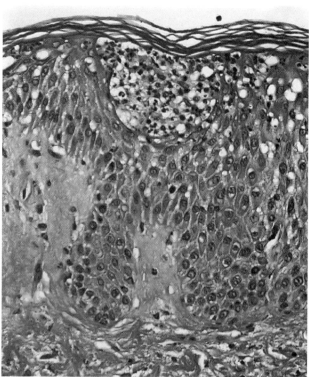

A

B

FIGURE 11-1. Acute generalized exanthematous pustulosis. **A:** Diffuse spongiosis is present with an upper dermal perivascular infiltrate and upper epidermal pustule. Ampicillin was the inciting drug. **B:** A subcorneal and intraspinous collection of neutrophils is present.

Differential Diagnosis. Distinction of morbilliform drug eruption from viral exanthem in the absence of eosinophils is generally not possible. More than occasional dyskeratotic epidermal cells should prompt consideration of erythema multiforme, toxic epidermal necrolysis, or fixed drug eruption. Based strictly on histologic descriptions, distinction of acute generalized exanthematous pustulosis from pustular psoriasis, subcorneal pustular dermatosis, and, in some instances, leukocytoclastic vasculitis cannot be made.

DRUG ERUPTIONS PRIMARILY CHARACTERIZED BY INTERFACE DERMATITIS

The histologic features comprising interface dermatitis (see Chapter 9) include vacuolar alteration of the basilar epidermis, necrotic keratinocytes, flattening of basilar keratinocytes, variable infiltration of the upper dermis by lymphocytes and histiocytes, variable exocytosis, and melanophages. These findings may be induced by drugs in several different but reproducible patterns including erythema multiforme, toxic epidermal necrolysis, lichenoid drug eruption, and fixed drug eruption.

ERYTHEMA MULTIFORME AND TOXIC EPIDERMAL NECROLYSIS

Erythema multiforme is characterized by target or "bull's-eye" erythematous edematous macules in varied distribution but with predilection for the palms and soles. In contrast, toxic epidermal necrolysis displays diffuse erythema with the patient complaining of tender skin. Blisters may develop in both disorders as well as mucosal and conjunctival involvement. Medications associated with increased risk for these entities include sulfonamides, trimethoprim-sulfamethoxazole, phenobarbital, carbamazepine, phenytoin, oxicam, nonsteroidal antiinflammatory agents, allopurinol, corticosteroids (13), cyclooxygenase inhibitors (14, 15), sustained release bupropion, nitroglycerine patch, and griseofulvin (16).

Histopathology. In the spectrum of interface dermatitides, erythema multiforme and toxic epidermal necrolysis display greater keratinocyte necrosis and less inflammation than other disorders (Fig. 11-2). Necrotic keratinocytes are found at all epidermal levels in the fully evolved lesion and may become confluent to form a thoroughly necrotic blister roof. Eventual subepidermal bullae may form (see Chapter 9). The etiology of the process can often not be determined by the histology, however, a dermal inflam-

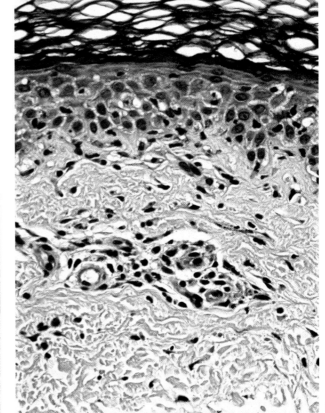

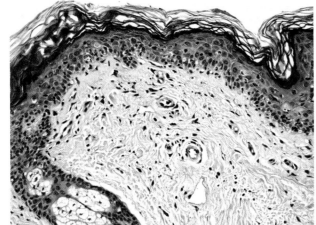

A   B

FIGURE 11-2. Drug-induced erythema multiforme. **A:** There is keratinocyte necrosis at all levels of the epidermis and a minimal inflammatory infiltrate. The dermal eosinophils suggest the drug-induced process. **B:** Keratinocyte necrosis and a mild dermal inflammatory infiltrate of lymphocytes and eosinophils are seen.

matory infiltrate containing eosinophils and acrosyringeal keratinocyte necrosis would suggest a drug-mediated process (17).

LICHENOID DRUG ERUPTION

Lichenoid drug eruption shares clinical similarity to lichen planus. Erythematous to violaceous papules and plaques develop on the trunk and extremities in association with drug ingestion. Implicated agents most commonly include quinacrine, quinidine and gold (18), but also include nonsteroidal anti-inflammatory drugs (19), antihypertensive medications (especially captopril), penicillamine, chloroquine, and hepatitis B vaccine (20).

Histopathology. Lichenoid drug eruption is also similar to lichen planus histologically (Fig. 11-3). In comparison with erythema multiforme and toxic epidermal necrolysis, lichenoid drug eruptions are more heavily inflamed with a more prominent interstitial pattern. Differentiation from lichen planus may not be possible. Numerous eosinophils, parakeratosis, and perivascular inflammation around the

mid and deep dermal plexuses are generally absent in lichen planus.

FIXED DRUG ERUPTION

Fixed drug eruptions show circumscribed erythematosus patches that recur persistently at the same site with each administration of the implicated drug. Increasing numbers of lesions may occur with each successive administration. The most common type of fixed drug eruption consists of one or several slightly edematous, erythematous patches that may develop dusky centers, become bullous and, on healing, leave pigmented macules. Fixed drug eruptions occur most commonly after the ingestion of trimethoprim-sulfamethoxazole, acetylsalicylic acid, phenolphthalein, tetracycline, barbiturates, and phenylbutazone, but also occur after ingestion of various other drugs (21).

Histopathology. The histologic changes observed in fixed drug eruption resemble erythema multiforme and toxic epidermal necrolysis (Fig. 11-4). The frequent presence of

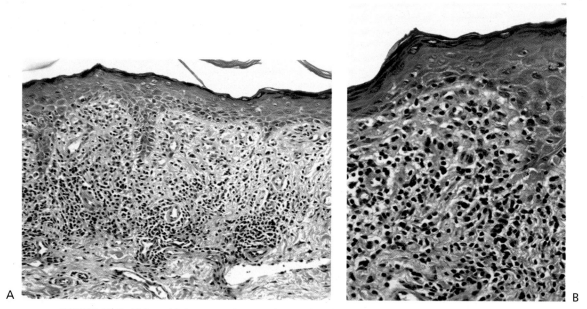

FIGURE 11-3. Lichenoid drug eruption. **A:** There is basal vacuolopathy, with Civatte bodies and a band-like inflammatory infiltrate. Eosinophils in the inflammatory infiltrate suggest the drug-induced nature of this eruption. **B:** The perivascular inflammatory infiltrate, eosinophils and increased pigment incontinence present in this lichenoid drug eruption are typically not seen in lichen planus.

hydropic degeneration of the basal cell layer leads to "pigmentary incontinence," which is characterized by the presence of melanin within macrophages in the upper dermis. Scattered necrotic keratinocytes with eosinophilic cytoplasm and pyknotic nuclei (often referred to as Civatte bodies, colloid bodies, or dyskeratotic cells) are frequently seen in the epidermis and represent apoptosis. Bullae form by detachment of the epidermis from the underlying dermis. Not infrequently, the epidermis shows extensive con-

fluent necrosis, even in areas in which it has not yet become detached. Confident distinction among fixed drug eruption, erythema multiforme, and toxic epidermal necrolysis, based on examination of a skin biopsy specimen alone, is not always possible. The inflammatory infiltrate may be composed purely of mononuclear cells or may be polymorphous.

Pathogenesis. On electron microscopic examination, the necrotic keratinocytes are filled with thick, homogenized

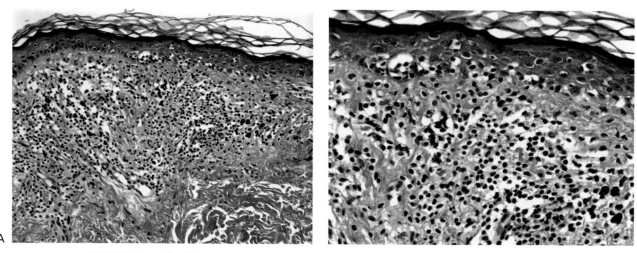

FIGURE 11-4. Fixed drug reaction. **A:** A lichenoid inflammatory infiltrate, scattered necrotic keratinocytes, basal vacuolopathy, and numerous melanin-laden macrophages are present. **B:** Higher power of the same lesion demonstrating the basal vacuolopathy, lymphocytic infiltrate, and pigmentary incontinence.

keratin tonofilaments and show only sparse remnants of organelles and nuclei. Keratinocytes located in the basal cell layer are often the most severely affected cells. The pigmentary incontinence develops when (a) lymphocytes migrate into the epidermis and cause damage to keratinocytes, which become necrotic; (b) macrophages invade the epidermis and phagocytize the necrotic keratinocytes together with their melanosomes; and (c) the macrophages return to the dermis, where they are able to digest all cellular remnants except for the melanosomes, which are resistant to digestion (22). The process of pigmentary incontinence in fixed drug eruptions is similar to that occurring in incontinentia pigmenti (see Chapter 6). Expression of keratinocyte intercellular adhesion molecule-1 (ICAM-1, CD54) is sharply limited to lesional epidermis in fixed drug eruption. Localized induction of this adhesion molecule by drugs may explain the sharply circumscribed clinical lesions (10).

TOXIC ACRAL ERYTHEMA

Hand-foot syndrome, palmar-plantar erythrodysesthesia syndrome, or toxic acral erythema refers to a transient painful erythema of the palms and soles, which becomes edematous and ultimately desquamates. Blisters may form leaving ulcerated epithelium. Numerous chemotherapeutic agents, including cytarabine, docetaxel, and 5-fluorouracil have been implicated. The cutaneous lesions attributable to docetaxel, an antineoplastic agent that interferes with normal microtubule function, are not limited to acral sites (24).

Histopathology. Histologically, the skin displays vacuolar degeneration of basilar keratinocytes with eventual cleft formation. Mild epidermal dysmaturation may be seen. Keratinocyte necrosis is also present in the lower third of the epidermis. In the dermis, there is a mild perivascular infiltrate of lymphocytes with few eosinophils.

DRUG-INDUCED SCLERODERMA-LIKE CONDITIONS

Numerous medications have been implicated in causing scleroderma-like conditions (25). Although the pathophysiology still remains unclear, disturbances in the vasculature and immune system leading to fibroblastic dysregulation and subsequent deposition of intercellular matrix proteins, has been proposed (26). Bleomycin, an antitumor agent, is known to cause similar changes in a reversible, dose-dependent fashion in both the skin and the lung due to drug accumulation in these organs deficient in specific metabolic enzymes (27,28). Multiple cycles of docetaxel are also associated with rapid development of transient scleroderma-like features in dependent areas (29,30). Scleroderma-like

changes have also been associated with other agents, including phytonadione (vitamin K_1) (31), L-tryptophan, pentazocine, ergot, bromocriptine, ketobemidone, morphine, cocaine, and appetite suppressants.

Histopathology. The features are those of idiopathic scleroderma (Chapter 10), including fibrosis of the dermis and subcutis, adnexal structure entrapment and atrophy and mild vascular dilatation with minimal to no inflammatory infiltrate.

BULLAE AND SWEAT GLAND NECROSIS IN DRUG-INDUCED COMA

A patient who is in a coma as a result of an accident, illness, or a large dose of a narcotic drug may show, within a few hours, areas of erythema at sites of pressure. Usually within 24 hours, vesicles and bullae develop in the erythematous patches. The incidence of bullae depends on the severity of the coma and is highest in patients who subsequently die. Coma caused by carbon monoxide poisoning can also produce the lesions (32). The bullae are located at sites subjected to pressure, such as the hands, wrists, scapulae, sacrum, knees, legs, ankles, and heels.

Histopathology. The epidermis shows varying degrees of necrosis (Fig. 11-5). In areas of complete necrosis of the epidermis, the bullae arise subepidermally, but, in areas of only diminished viability showing eosinophilia of the cytoplasm and decreased staining of the nuclei, small intraepidermal vesicles may be seen. Where the epidermis is necrotic in its upper layers but not in its lower layers, even large bullae can form intraepidermally. Blisters may also form in a suprabasal location and may contain some acantholytic cells (33).

The secretory cells of the sweat glands show necrosis characterized by eosinophilic homogenization of their cytoplasm and by pyknosis or absence of their nuclei (Fig. 11-5C and D). The sweat ducts usually appear less severely damaged but may also show pale staining or necrosis similar to that of the secretory cells (34). It is of interest that the sweat gland necrosis is limited to areas in which there are skin lesions. In patients who survive, the necrotic sweat gland epithelium is replaced by normal-appearing epithelial cells within about 2 weeks. In many instances, the pilosebaceous units are also affected with sebaceous gland necrosis and occasional necrosis of the outer and inner root sheaths.

The dermis beneath the bullae, and occasionally also the dermis around the sweat glands, contains a sparse polymorphous infiltrate composed of neutrophils, eosinophils, lymphocytes, and histiocytes. In addition, some extravasated erythrocytes are often present.

Pathogenesis. The necrosis of the epidermis and sweat glands is a result of both generalized and local hypoxia. The bullae, in turn, are the result of epidermal damage. Coma, whether the result of an accident, an illness, or a drug, causes generalized hypoxia by depressing blood circulation

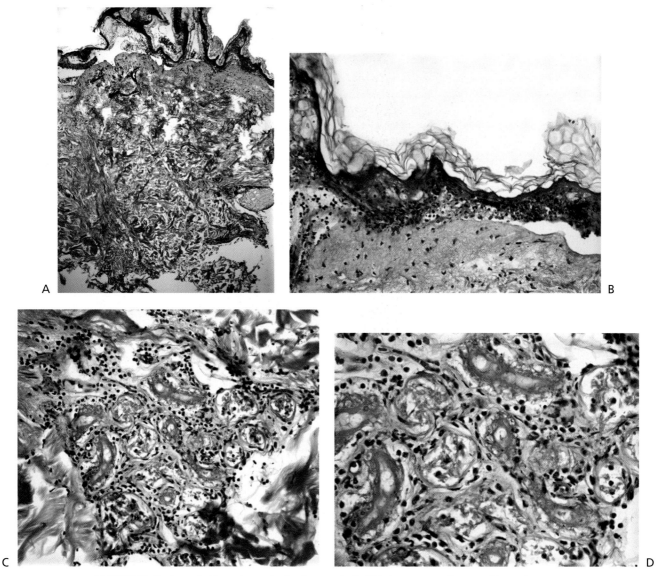

FIGURE 11-5. Coma bulla and sweat gland necrosis. **A:** This low power shows epidermal necrosis, subepidermal blister, and necrosis of the eccrine coil. **B:** There is full-thickness epidermal necrosis and subepidermal blister. **C:** Cytoplasmic eosinophilia along with absent and pyknotic nuclei characterize necrosis of this sweat gland. **D:** Higher power of *(C)* image.

and respiration. In the case of poisoning with carbon monoxide, its binding to hemoglobin acts as an additional factor (35). Pressure causes further local hypoxia by decreasing blood flow.

DRUG-INDUCED BULLOUS DISORDERS

Several medications are linked to the development of antibody-mediated pemphigus (Table 11-1). Among these, penicillamine is perhaps the most common; however, the growing list of implicated agents includes other thiol-, sulfur-, and amide-containing drugs (36). The majority of cases of penicillamine- and other thiol-induced

pemphigus present as pemphigus foliaceus, and have fewer immunofluorescence findings and a more favorable prognosis on drug withdrawal. Those cases attributed to non-thiol drugs, in particular those with an active amide group, may provoke disease indistinguishable from spontaneously occurring pemphigus vulgaris. Drug induction of subepidermal blisters is also recognized, with vancomycin-induced linear IgA dermatosis as a prime example (37). Oropharyngeal pemphigus secondary to interferon alpha-2a has also been reported (38).

Histopathology. Histologic examination reveals a picture identical with that seen in pemphigus vulgaris and/or pemphigus foliaceus not associated with drugs (39) (see Chapter 9). The autoantibody response to desmoglein 1 and

TABLE 11-1. DRUGS THAT CAUSE PEMPHIGUS

Penicillamine	Cephalexin
Captopril	Ceftazidime
Piroxicam	Pyrazolone derivatives
Bucillamine	Interleukin-2
Penicillin	Alpha-interferon
Ampicillin	Propanolol
Rifampin	Phenobarbital
Cefadroxil	Levodopa

desmoglein 3 is similar in both spontaneous and drug-induced disease (40).

Pathogenesis. Both biochemical and immunological mechanisms, not mutually exclusive, have been proposed. In the subset of patients in which tissue-bound antibodies cannot be found, a biochemical mechanism is suggested. These drugs directly bind to keratinocyte membranes forming bonds that interfere with cell-cell adhesion resulting in acantholysis (36). Predisposition to development of pemphigus vulgaris is linked to MHC II (41). It has been postulated that polymorphisms of the DR4 beta chain impart T-cell recognition of exogenous peptides that stimulate autoantibody production by B-lymphocytes (42). Additionally, immunologic acantholysis can be triggered by biochemical events that lead to formation of a neoantigen, with consequent autoantibody production (36). In most thiol drug–related cases, intercellular antibodies can be demonstrated, indicating that this class of drugs acts primarily through immunologically mediated acantholysis.

DRUG-INDUCED LUPUS ERYTHEMATOSUS

Drug-induced lupus erythematosus resembles mild systemic lupus erythematosus and is characterized by arthralgia or arthritis, and myalgia and may be accompanied by serositis, fever, hepatomegaly, splenomegaly, and skin manifestations. The cutaneous lesions are typical of systemic lupus erythematosus. Central nervous system and renal involvement are rare. The drugs most commonly implicated include procainamide, hydralazine, quinidine, chlorpromazine, isoniazid, methyldopa, and propylthiouracil (43). However, the number of medications associated with induction of lupus erythematosus is increasing. It is possible that the development of a systemic lupus erythematosus-like syndrome in a patient under medication with these drugs represents the uncovering of latent systemic lupus erythematosus.

Drug-induced systemic lupus erythematosus can be clinically, pathologically, and serologically indistinguishable from spontaneously arising systemic lupus erythematosus. However, cutaneous and renal manifestations are rare in drug-induced systemic lupus erythematosus, and pleuro-pulmonary manifestations are somewhat more common than in spontaneous disease. Clinical presentations resembling subacute cutaneous lupus erythematosus secondary to terbinafine have been reported (44,45). Usually, but not always, when the medication is discontinued, the clinical and laboratory manifestations subside.

Histopathology. The histologic picture of the cutaneous lesions is the same as in lupus erythematosus (see Chapter 10).

Pathogenesis. As in other autoimmune-related disorders, genetic predisposition, in particular, HLA-DR4, has a role in drug-induced lupus. Antinuclear antibodies are usually present and directed against single-stranded DNA or histones (46). Different drugs appear to be associated with different antihistone profiles (43). Anti–double-stranded DNA antibodies are usually absent. Hypocomplementemia is rare. The occurrence of a lupus band on direct immunofluorescence testing of normal-appearing skin is uncommon (47). The rate of drug acetylation has also been associated with disease onset. Rapid acetylators have a much lower incidence of hydralazine-induced lupus, whereas slow acetylators are at higher risk (48). Additionally, there is evidence that myeloperoxidase produced by neutrophils in conjunction with cells capable of generating superoxides, transforms lupus-inducing drugs to cytotoxic products. Elucidation of this process is still evolving (43).

DRUG-INDUCED PHOTOSENSITIVITY

Drug-induced photosensitivity can be subdivided into photoallergic and phototoxic drug eruptions. Photoallergic drug eruptions represent a T-cell–mediated reaction.

Photoallergic Drug Eruption

In photoallergy, ultraviolet light alters either the hapten or the avidity with which the hapten combines with the carrier protein to form a complete photoantigen (49). Among the photoallergenic drugs are the sulfonamides; the thiazides, such as chlorothiazide and tolbutamide, both of which are aromatic sulfonamides; griseofulvin; the phenothiazines, such as chlorpromazine; quinine; topical nonsteroidal anti-inflammatory medications, including piroxicam (50) and sunscreens (51). A photoallergic drug eruption causes photocontact dermatitis in all light-exposed areas. Like any allergic contact dermatitis, it causes itching.

Histopathology. The histologic appearance of photoallergic dermatitis is that of an allergic contact dermatitis and include spongiosis, mild acanthosis and a superficial perivascular lymphocytic infiltrate with eosinophils (52) (Fig. 11-6).

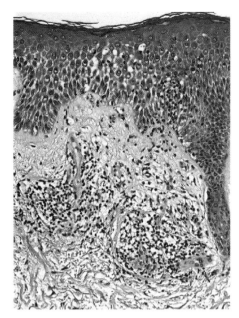

FIGURE 11-6. Photoallergic dermatitis. There is epidermal spongiosis with microvesicle formation, exocytosis of lymphocytes, and a perivascular lymphocytic infiltrate admixed with scattered eosinophils.

Phototoxic Drug Eruption

Certain internally administered drugs, in association with ultraviolet light, may produce a phototoxic dermatitis that resembles intensified sunburn. Among the drugs known to elicit a phototoxic response are all drugs capable of producing a photoallergic reaction, provided that they are given in sufficiently high concentrations (53). Other commonly prescribed phototoxic drugs are certain tetracyclines, such as demeclocycline hydrochloride and doxycycline (54), quinolones (55), and psoralens.

Histopathology. A phototoxic drug eruption, like a sunburn reaction, shows both vacuolated keratinocytes (sunburn cells) characterized by abundant, pale cytoplasm, and apoptotic keratinocytes characterized by reduced, eosinophilic cytoplasm (56). The dermis shows edema and enlargement of endothelial cells (Fig. 11-7).

PHOTODISTRIBUTED HYPERPIGMENTATION

Certain drugs, in particular, chlorpromazine, amiodarone, imipramine and desipramine, when given in sufficient doses for several years are known to produce reversible slate-gray discoloration on sun-exposed areas of the skin. Exposed parts of the bulbar conjunctivae may show brownish pigmentation (57). Similarly, photodistributed slate-gray, reticulated pigmentation has been described in patients on long-acting diltiazem hydrochloride (58).

Histopathology. In chlorpromazine, amiodarone, imipramine, and desipramine reactions, there is a variable amount of melanin in the basal layer of the epidermis (Fig. 11-8). Throughout the dermis, there is considerable accumulation of pigment-laden macrophages, predominantly in a perivascular pattern. The pigment has the staining properties of melanin in that it stains black with the Fontana–Masson silver stain and is decolorized by hydrogen peroxide. In patients on long-term chlorpromazine, this melanin-like material is found in many internal organs, throughout the entire mononuclear-phagocyte system and, to a lesser degree, in the parenchymal cells of the liver, kidneys, and endocrine glands, in myocardial fibers, and in cerebral neurons (59).

In contrast, the diltiazem reactions reveal lichenoid dermatitis with atrophic epidermis and basal vacuolar change. The papillary dermis is expanded with prominent and di-

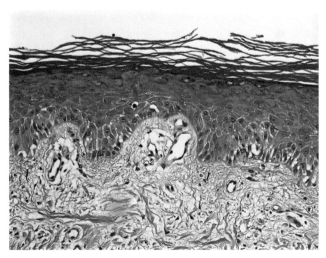

FIGURE 11-7. Phototoxic dermatitis. Vacuolated keratinocytes (sunburst cells) and apoptotic keratinocytes are present. The dermis shows edema and enlarged endothelial cells.

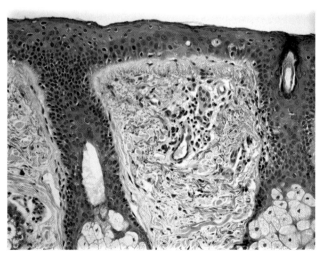

FIGURE 11-8. Chlorpromazine pigmentation. Pigment-laden macrophages, with a predominant perivascular pattern, are seen in this case of chlorpromazine pigmentation.

lated thin-walled vessels and a sparse inflammatory infiltrate as well as a perivascular and periadnexal lymphocytic infiltrate (58).

Histogenesis. Electron microscopic examination has confirmed the presence of many melanosome complexes within the lysosomes of dermal macrophages. In addition, 0.2 to 3 μm in diameter, round or bizarrely shaped electron dense bodies may be seen in macrophages, endothelial cells, pericytes, Schwann cells, and fibroblasts, usually within lysosomes (60). Both electron-dense bodies and melanosome complexes may be found within the same lysosome. While the dense bodies histochemically react like melanin, the striking sulfur peak on microprobe analysis strongly suggests the drug or its metabolite (60) are also present. As some drugs do bind to melanin (61), it seems likely that the electron-dense bodies represent complexes of melanin with drug. These complexes are subsequently carried from the dermis by way of the circulating blood leukocytes to the various internal organs (62). In diltiazem-related hyperpigmentation, only melanosomes, without drug or drug metabolite, are seen (58).

DRUG-INDUCED PSEUDOLYMPHOMA SYNDROME

Phenytoin, carbamazepine (63), sodium valproate (64), gemcitabine (65), gold (66), and the clonidine patch (67) are among the agents that have been associated with a pseudolymphoma syndrome characterized by generalized lymphadenopathy, hepatosplenomegaly, fever, arthralgia, and eosinophilia. Cutaneous findings range from a few erythematous plaques or nodules to a generalized macular and papular eruption and generalized exfoliative dermatitis

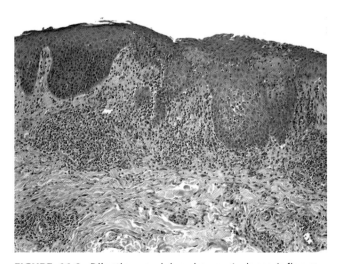

FIGURE 11-9. Dilantin pseudolymphoma. A dense inflammatory infiltrate with exocytosis of atypical-appearing lymphocytes and absence of spongiosis are seen in this phenytoin-induced pseudolymphoma.

(68–70). In all cases, there is improvement and ultimate clearing when the offending agent is discontinued.

Histopathology. On histologic examination of the skin, the infiltrate is often indistinguishable from that of mycosis fungoides (this syndrome is also known as "pseudo-mycosis fungoides") in that there are cerebriform nuclei in the dermal infiltrate and Pautrier microabscesses in the epidermis (68) (Fig. 11-9). In cutaneous nodules, the infiltrate may suggest a cutaneous lymphoma of the non-Hodgkin's type, because large masses of atypical lymphocytes are present in the dermis as well as in the subcutaneous tissue (71,72). T-cell receptor monoclonality has been demonstrated in some cases (64).

DRUG-INDUCED PSEUDOPORPHYRIA

Several medications are reported to cause cutaneous lesions resembling the blisters of porphyria cutanea tarda. Unlike porphyria cutanea tarda, other cutaneous manifestations are absent and no derangement in porphyrin metabolism has been identified. Healing occurs once the medication is discontinued. Implicated drugs include naproxen, furosemide, tetracycline, dapsone, and pyridoxine (73).

Histopathology. The blisters resemble the poorly or noninflamed subepidermal bullae of porphyria cutanea tarda (Chapter 17).

Histogenesis. The mechanism by which this reaction occurs is unknown. Unlike porphyria cutanea tarda, no deposits in the skin are revealed by direct immunofluorescence testing (Chapter 17) (73).

CUTANEOUS REACTIONS TO ANTINEOPLASTIC CHEMOTHERAPEUTIC DRUGS

In general, the cutaneous changes brought about by antineoplastic chemotherapeutic agents are the result of their antiproliferative effects disrupting cutaneous cellular metabolism. Clinical manifestations vary. Neutrophilic eccrine hidradenitis presents with erythematous, often acral, plaques several days after cytoreductive chemotherapy. Acral erythema unassociated with primary eccrine changes also occurs after chemotherapy (see above). Hyperpigmentation develops under occluded skin after thio-TEPA administration and in grouped linear streaks after bleomycin as well after long-term hydroxyurea therapy (74). Diffuse hyperpigmentation commonly occurs after antineoplastic chemotherapy. Erythema preceding the hyperpigmentation in these settings is minimal or absent. An acneiform follicular eruption has been reported secondary to administration of a monoclonal antibody to epidermal growth factor receptor (75). Anagen effluvium is a well-established effect of the antiproliferative nature of many chemotherapeutic agents.

Histopathology. Cytoreductive chemotherapy may cause a disruption of the normal pattern of keratinocyte maturation from small cuboidal cells in the basilar epidermis to flattened squamous cells in the stratum corneum. At intervening epidermal levels, keratinocytes are separated by widened intercellular spaces, lose polarity, and display irregular large nuclei, midepidermal mitotic figures, and apoptosis (Fig. 11-10). These changes, referred to as *epidermal dysmaturation*, may be observed in the epidermis after any significant cytoreductive therapy, and are not necessarily associated with clinical lesions. Upper dermal melanophages often accompany these changes. In this setting, "star-burst" mitotic figures are described after systemic etoposide administration (76). Numerous mid- and upper-level mitotic figures (so-called "mitotic arrest") are observed after podophyllotoxin application to condyloma. Etoposide and podophyllotoxin are vinca alkaloid derivatives, disrupting mitotic spindle formation by attaching to microtubule proteins.

Several entities in this section are unified by the theory of drug concentration in eccrine sweat. Specimens from patterned *postchemotherapy hyperpigmentation* show vacuolization of basilar epidermis, melanin incontinence, and apoptosis in occluded skin after administration of alkylating agents (77). Inflammation is sparse or absent. Squamous metaplasia of upper eccrine ducts, *syringosquamous metaplasia*, is described after cytoreductive therapies. The normally cuboidal cells lining the duct display irregularly increased amounts of eosinophilic cytoplasm with associated polymorphous inflammation, fibrosis, and necrosis (78) (Fig. 11-11). *Neutrophilic eccrine hidradenitis* consists of variable infiltration of the eccrine coil by neutrophils and lymphocytes with necrosis of secretory epithelium (Fig. 11-12). In-

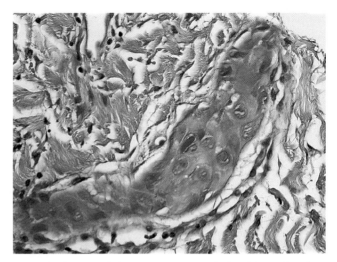

FIGURE 11-11. Syringosquamous metaplasia. This eccrine duct is lined by squamoid cells with ample eosinophilic cytoplasm and large nuclei rather than the normal cuboidal cells.

dividual cells or whole coils show increased cytoplasmic eosinophilia (Fig. 11-12B), degeneration of nuclei and loss of integrity of cell walls (79,80). Edema and mucinous change may be seen in the perieccrine adipose tissue.

Intradermal injection of bleomycin is cytotoxic to keratinocytes and eccrine epithelium resulting in epidermal and eccrine necrosis, infiltration of the skin by neutrophils, and expression of HLA-DR and ICAM-1 on keratinocytes (35).

The acneiform eruption secondary to anti-EGFR demonstrates a perifollicular infundibular T-cell lymphocytic infiltrate.

Histogenesis. The notion of concentration of antineoplastic chemotherapeutic agents in sweat serves to unify the

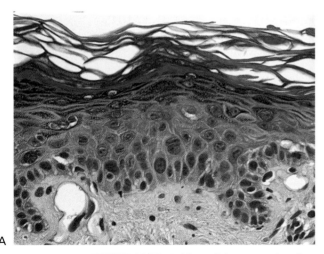
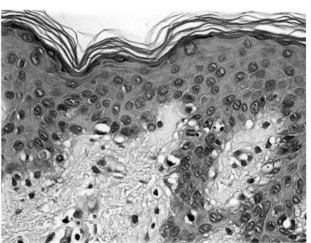

FIGURE 11-10. Epidermal dysmaturation due to antineoplastic chemotherapy. **A:** This relatively mild example illustrates loss of polarity and disorganization of keratinocytes, including binucleate cells. **B:** Dysmaturation is more advanced in this example, with loss of keratinocyte polarity, highly irregular nuclear contours, multinucleation, and apoptosis.

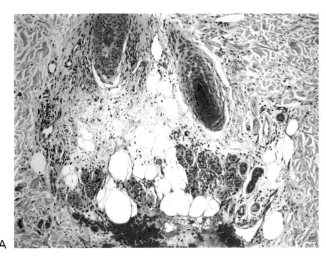
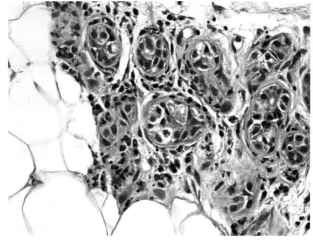

A   B

FIGURE 11-12. Neutrophilic eccrine hidradenitis. **A:** Neutrophils and occasional mononuclear cells are present in the perieccrine adventitia. There is infiltration of the eccrine coil by lymphocytes and neutrophils. Perieccrine edema is also present. Some epithelial cells display early necrosis with increased cytoplasmic eosinophilia. **B:** Neutrophilic and lymphocytic infiltrate of the eccrine coil and eccrine necrosis characterized by increased cytoplasmic eosinophilia, pyknotic nuclei, and dyscohesion. This eccrine coil displays more advanced necrosis.

clinical observation of patterned hyperpigmentation (beneath bandages and electrocardiogram pads in the case of thio-TEPA) and the histologic observations of neutrophilic eccrine hidradenitis and syringosquamous metaplasia. Changes after antineoplastic chemotherapy likely represent a mix of direct toxic effect on the various constituent cells of the skin with secondary inflammation incited by cell damage. Other chemotherapy-related cutaneous changes may also involve similar mechanisms—namely, intertriginous erosion/ulceration after isophosphamide (81) and flagellate hyperpigmentation after busulfan (82). Why specific agents affect specific cell populations in the skin in repeatable fashion is unclear. It is important to note that identification of epidermal dysmaturation assumes considerable importance in establishing the diagnosis of acute graft-versus-host reaction. When possible, the inflammation and apoptosis of a graft-versus-host reaction should be sought in areas unaffected or less affected by dysmaturation.

In the case of acneiform eruptions, it has been postulated that the inflammatory infiltrate is elicited by the presence of antibody on the surface of follicular epithelial cells (75).

CUTANEOUS ERUPTIONS RESULTING FROM ADMINISTRATION OF HUMAN RECOMBINANT PROTEINS

Technologic advances in recombinant DNA research have resulted in the availability of human recombinant cytokines (including colony-stimulating factors) for adminis-

tration to patients in order to effect immunologic manipulation for therapeutic benefit. Based on the actions of human cytokines, specific agents are administered, generally to immunocompromised patients, to enhance the number and/or activity of leukocytes, platelets, or erythrocytes. This action is aimed at hematopoietic cells in the marrow and/or mature leukocytes in the peripheral circulation or tissues.

Mucocutaneous effects of systemic administration of at least 13 cytokines are described (Table 11-2). The findings generally occur (a) at injection sites, (b) as variably distributed eruptions, or (c) as exacerbation or induction of other dermatologic disorders, such as psoriasis.

Etanecept, a recombinant tumor necrosis factor alpha receptor fused to the Fc fragment of IgG$_2$ and recombinant interferon-beta 1a and 1b have been associated with injection site reactions (83–85).

When asked to examine a skin biopsy specimen from an eruption suspected to be caused by a cytokine, the pathologist should know the temporal relation between administration of the cytokine and appearance of the eruption, white blood cell count, and actions of the cytokine. Ideally, the cutaneous eruption will have begun soon after initiation of cytokine therapy and the histopathology of the eruption will relate in some way to recognized effects of the cytokine.

Histopathology. The morbilliform eruption induced by pharmacologic doses of human recombinant, granulocyte-macrophage colony–stimulating factor (GM-CSF) illustrates these criteria (86,87). The upper dermis contains a perivascular and interstitial infiltrate of neutrophils, eosinophils, and lymphocytes (Fig. 11-13). The relative

TABLE 11-2. MUCOCUTANEOUS EFFECTS OF SYSTEMIC ADMINISTRATION OF CYTOKINES

Cytokine	Reported Association
Interleukin-1 alpha and beta	Phlebitis, mucositis
Interleukin-2	Diffuse erythema, exacerbation of psoriasis, and autoimmune diseases
Interleukin-3	Flushing
Interleukin-4	Edema
Interleukin-6	Erythematous eruption
GM-CSF	Diffuse eruption
G-CSF	Neutrophilic dermatoses, vasculitis
Tumor necrosis factor alpha	Erythroderma
Tumor necrosis factor alpha receptor/IgG$_2$ Fc	Injection site reaction
Interferon alpha	Alopecia, injection site reaction
Interferon beta	Mostly injection site reactions, including vasculitis
Interferon gamma	Exacerbated graft-versus-host reactions

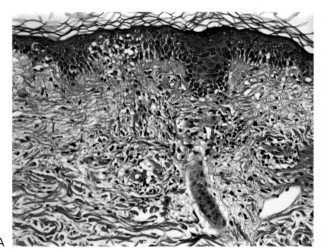

A

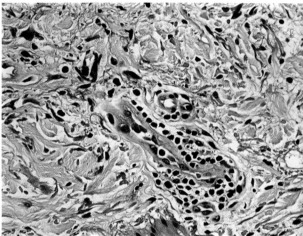

B

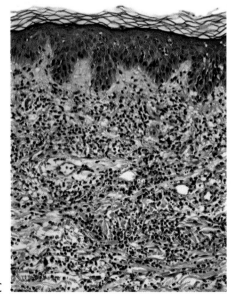

C

FIGURE 11-13. Granulocyte-macrophage colony stimulating factor (GM-CSF). **A:** A diffuse perivascular and interstitial inflammatory cell infiltrate is present with associated vascular dilatation and epidermal spongiosis. **B:** High power of a perivascular and interstitial inflammatory cell infiltrate. **C:** The density of the inflammatory infiltrate varies, and as seen in this case, may be extensive, simulating Sweet's syndrome.

proportion of cell types varies (Fig. 11-13C). Macrophages are increased in number and size and may contain melanin when situated in the upper dermis. The epidermis may display intercellular edema with exocytosis of inflammatory cells. Vasculitis is absent.

Granulocyte colony stimulating factor (G-CSF) is associated with the development of erythematous plaques that contain numerous neutrophils and upper dermal edema, thus resembling the skin lesions of Sweet's syndrome (88).

Findings at the site of etanercept injection include a superficial perivascular inflammatory infiltrate composed primarily of lymphocytes with eosinophils admixed with small numbers of neutrophils and macrophages. Mild dermal edema and vasodilation are also noted (83). Interferon injection sites have shown a mild perivascular lymphocytic infiltrate, and thrombosis of deep vessels without fibrinoid necrosis (84,85).

Pathogenesis. In the case of eruptions associated with GM-CSF and G-CSF, the histologic findings relate to the administration and known actions of the cytokine. In a period of peripheral neutropenia, one finds numerous granulocytes in tissue from these eruptions. Additionally, the effects of GM-CSF on macrophages are demonstrable in the skin by observing their expanded number and size. Immunostains to macrophage/monocyte markers may be useful to highlight this finding. Injection site reactions with etanercept are suggestive of a delayed-type hypersensitivity reaction while those of interferon-beta suggest enhancement of preexisting disease-related platelet activation (85).

CUTANEOUS MANIFESTATIONS OF ANTIRETROVIRAL THERAPY

Antiretroviral therapy options currently include protease inhibitors, non-nucleoside reverse transcriptase inhibitors and nucleoside reverse transcriptase inhibitors. While exanthematous eruptions and urticaria have been described with the use of these agents, they have also been associated with several unique findings. The lipodystrophy syndrome, identified originally with the use of protease inhibitors and subsequently with the use of nucleoside analogues (89,90), is characterized by peripheral lipoatrophy and central adiposity. Protease inhibitors and nucleoside analogues are associated with paronychia with pyogenic granulomas of the lateral nail fold. Unique patterns of hyperpigmentation involving nails, skin, and mucous membranes are seen secondary to melanocyte stimulation by zidovudine (91,92). The patterns of nail pigmentation include entire nail pigmentation, transverse banding, and multiple longitudinal bands of any or all nails of fingers and toes. Leukocytoclastic vasculitis and drug rash with eosinophilia and systemic symptoms (DRESS) are also associated with this group of agents (93).

Histopathology. Histologic features of the lipodystrophy syndrome secondary to protease inhibitors are the same as lipodystrophy from other causes (Chapter 20).

MINOCYCLINE PIGMENTATION

The prolonged administration of minocycline, a semisynthetic tetracycline, may result in three distinct types of cutaneous pigmentation: (1) a blue-black pigmentation occurring within areas of inflammation or scarring, usually on the face, especially in active or healed acne lesions; (2) a blue-gray pigmentation of previously normal skin, most commonly seen on the legs but also occurring on the forearms; and (3) a diffuse, muddy brown discoloration, sometimes accentuated in sun-exposed areas (94,95). A systemic minocycline-induced hypersensitivity syndrome presents 2 to 4 weeks after the start of therapy. Symptoms include fever, rash, peripheral eosinophilia and internal organ involvement. Internal organ involvement includes hepatitis or abnormal liver functions test results, pneumonitis, and renal abnormalities (96).

Histopathology. The histologic picture shows differences among the three types of pigmentation. The focal blue-black pigmentation of the face in the first type is associated with macrophages and reacts like hemosiderin (97) (Fig. 11-14). In contrast, the blue-gray pigmentation in the second type, most commonly observed on the legs, shows staining for iron and also reacts with the Fontana–Masson stain; and the muddy brown pigmentation in the third type reveals increased melanization of the basal cell layer and within macrophages in the upper dermis.

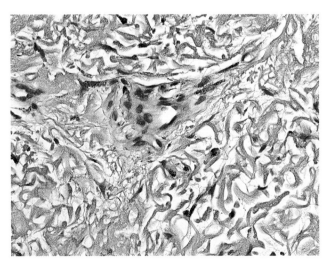

FIGURE 11-14. Minocycline hyperpigmentation. This is the localized variant of minocycline pigmentation. The pigment is present in macrophages and dermal dendrocytes with a predominant perivascular pattern.

Histogenesis. It appears likely that the iron-containing pigment in the first two types of pigmentation represents a drug metabolite–protein complex (94). The pigment in the second type that reacts with the Fontana–Masson stain does not contain melanin, because it does not bleach with hydrogen peroxide. The pigment in the third type reacts like melanin and may represent a phototoxic phenomenon. The pathogenesis of minocycline-induced hypersensitivity reaction has not been elucidated.

CLOFAZIMINE-INDUCED PIGMENTATION

Clofazimine is administered to patients with leprosy and may cause a pink to pink-brown dyspigmentation soon after initiation of therapy. The pigmentation resolves slowly after discontinuation of clofazimine. The most notably involved areas are the obvious leprosy lesions (98).

Histopathology. The upper dermis contains numerous foamy macrophages that possess cytoplasm with brown granular pigment. This pigment stains for lipofuscin, but not for melanin or iron.

Pathogenesis. Upon electron microscopy, the macrophages are found to contain phagolysosomes with either lipid or electron-dense granules with a lamellar substructure consistent with lipofuscin or ceroid pigment (98). The mechanism by which clofazimine causes these changes is unclear.

PENICILLAMINE-INDUCED DERMATOSES

The prolonged administration of penicillamine can cause alterations in collagen and elastic tissue that may result in areas of atrophy of the skin. Anetoderma and serpiginosa elastosis perforans are observed. Alteration of epidermal desmosomal elements may induce pemphigus (see above).

Penicillamine-Induced Atrophy of the Skin

Patients on prolonged penicillamine therapy may show atrophy of the skin of the face and neck; light blue, atrophic macules resembling anetoderma; easy bruising resulting in small hemorrhages into the skin followed by milia; or small, white papules at sites of venipuncture in the antecubital fossae (99).

Histopathology. The anetoderma shows diminution or absence of elastic tissue. The areas of easy bruising of the skin and the papules at sites of venipuncture show either diminution or degeneration and homogenization of collagen (100).

Histogenesis. The formation of elastic tissue and collagen involves the participation of aldehydes to produce stable cross-links. By reacting with aldehydes to form thiazolidine compounds, penicillamine impairs the formation of such stable cross-links (101).

Penicillamine-Induced Elastosis Perforans Serpiginosa

Elastosis perforans serpiginosa may occur in patients receiving prolonged treatment with penicillamine. Although the clinical picture does not differ from that of idiopathic elastosis perforans serpiginosa (see Chapter 15), the histologic and electron microscopic features of the altered elastic fibers are unique. Both penicillamine-induced atrophy of

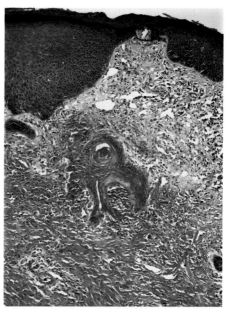

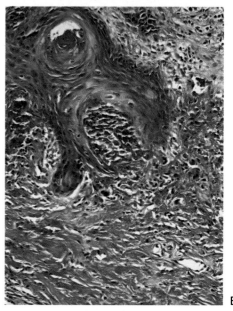

FIGURE 11-15. Penicillamine-induced elastosis serpiginosa. **A:** In this low-power image, thickened elastic fibers in a necrotic background are seen in the process of transepidermal elimination. Otherwise, the elastic fibers in the papillary dermis appear normal on routine stained sections. **B:** Higher power of image A. *(continued)*

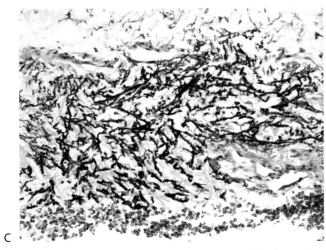
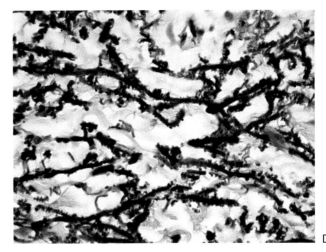

C

D

FIGURE 11-15. *(continued)* **C:** The elastic fibers in the mid-dermis show lateral budding, characteristic of penicillamine effect (Verhoeff–von Gieson elastic stain). **D:** Higher-power view of *(C)* image, showing the knobby appearance or lateral budding of the elastic fibers characteristic of penicillamine effect.

the skin and penicillamine-induced elastosis perforans serpiginosa may occur in the same patient (102).

Histopathology. In comparison with the idiopathic type of elastosis perforans serpiginosa, the penicillamine-induced type, on staining for elastic tissue, shows less hyperplasia of elastic fibers in the papillary dermis, except in areas of active transepidermal elimination (Fig. 11-15A and B). However, in the middle and deep layers of the dermis, a greater number of hyperplastic elastic fibers are present than in idiopathic elastosis perforans serpiginosa. These fibers have an appearance that is specific for penicillamine-induced elastosis perforans serpiginosa. Lateral budding is noted, with the buds arranged perpendicular to the principal fibers. The coarse elastic fibers thus show a serrated, sawtoothlike border, have been aptly compared to the twigs of a bramble bush and have been referred to as "lumpy-bumpy" (99) (Fig. 11-15C and D). Similar changes in individual elastic fibers are observed also in nonlesional skin and have been seen in a skeletal artery (100).

Pathogenesis. On electron microscopic examination, the affected elastic fibers show an inner core that closely resembles a normal elastic fiber with dark microfibrils embedded in electron-lucent elastin. Peripheral to this, a wide, homogeneous, electron-lucent coat is seen that has the appearance of elastin and shows numerous sac-like protuberances bulging outward between the adjacent collagen fibers (103).

HALOGEN ERUPTIONS

Ingestion of bromides may cause, besides a pustular eruption, the formation of vegetating, papillomatous plaques called *bromoderma.* The plaques, which usually occur on

the lower extremities, often show pustules at their peripheries. Although bromoderma often appears only after prolonged intake of bromides, it may arise soon after administration as well.

Iododerma, usually seen on the face, begins as a rule with multiple pustules that rapidly coalesce into vegetating plaques. Like bromoderma, the plaques of iododerma often show pustules at their peripheries, but they usually show less papillomatous proliferation and a softer consistency than bromoderma, and they often ulcerate. Iododerma is frequently associated with severe systemic signs and symptoms and may be fatal in rare instances (104). Although the eruption usually arises after prolonged ingestion of iodides, it may start within a few days, especially in patients with chronic renal disease. *Fluoroderma* has been described after the frequent application of a fluoride gel to the teeth for the purpose of preventing caries during ionizing radiation to the face (105). The lesions consist of scattered papules and nodules on the neck and in the preauricular regions.

Histopathology. The histologic picture in the halogen eruptions is suggestive rather than diagnostic. The difference between bromoderma and iododerma lies largely in the epidermal changes, which usually are much more pronounced in bromoderma, although there is some overlap. The dermal changes are essentially the same and vary with the age of the lesion.

In early lesions, the dermis in both bromoderma and iododerma shows a dense infiltrate of neutrophils, which, in areas of dermal necrosis, show nuclear dust. There may be intradermal abscesses. Eosinophils are present in most cases and may be numerous. Extensive extravasation of erythrocytes may also be seen. At a later stage, the proportion of mononuclear cells increases, and histiocytes may show abundant cytoplasm or large nuclei. The blood vessels are increased in number and dilated, and may show proliferation of endothelium.

The epidermal changes in bromoderma are often pronounced. In addition to papillomatosis, one may observe considerable downward epidermal proliferation, occasionally to such a degree as to produce the picture of pseudo-carcinomatous hyperplasia. The acanthosis may center on upper-level follicular epithelium. Frequently, intraepidermal abscesses are present (Fig. 11-16). The intraepidermal abscesses are filled with neutrophils, eosinophils, and some desquamated keratinocytes, most of which appear necrotic, although some resemble acantholytic cells. Some epithelial

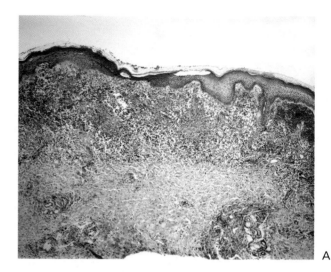

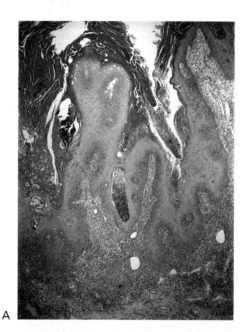

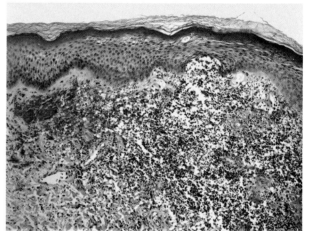

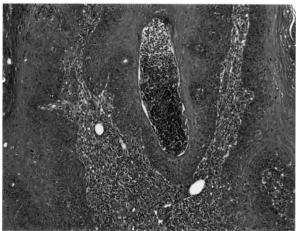

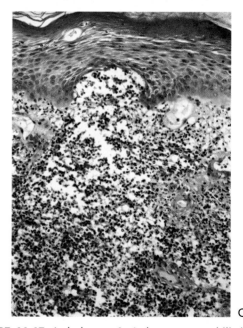

FIGURE 11-16. Bromoderma. **A:** This low-power image of bromoderma shows pseudoepitheliomatous hyperplasia with an intradermal abscess containing desquamated keratinocytes and neutrophils. Additionally, there is a dense superficial dermal inflammatory infiltrate composed of lymphocytes, plasma cells, scattered neutrophils, and rare eosinophils. **B:** There is downward proliferation of the epidermis, which encloses a large abscess. The dermis contains a dense inflammatory infiltrate.

FIGURE 11-17. Iododerma. **A:** A dense neutrophilic infiltrate with dermal necrosis is seen. There is less epidermal hyperplasia than would be seen in bromoderma. **B:** Dermal necrosis and a neutrophilic infiltrate. **C:** Higher power showing neutrophilic infiltrate.

islands in the upper dermis, instead of enclosing an abscess, are filled with keratin.

In iododerma, the epidermis may be eroded or ulcerated. At the margin of the ulcers, one may find intraepidermal abscesses. In old lesions, pseudoepitheliomatous hyperplasia may be encountered, although usually less than in bromoderma (105) (Fig. 11-17). Fluoroderma has been described only as a mild eruption, but it shares with iododerma and bromoderma the presence of eosinophils, neutrophils, and erythrocytes in the dermis and of microabscesses in the epidermis (105).

Pathogenesis. Even though there is often a very long interval between the first ingestion of iodides or bromides and the appearance of the cutaneous lesion, halogen eruptions appear to be an allergic phenomenon; once a person has become sensitized, the eruption recurs within a few days upon the readministration of iodides or bromides. Halogen eruptions probably arise on the basis of delayed hypersensitivity.

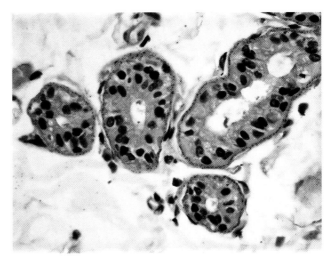

FIGURE 11-18. Argyria. Silver granules are present in the basement membrane surrounding the sweat glands. In some cases, the granules may be so dense that they form a solid black band.

ARGYRIA

Argyria is caused by prolonged ingestion or mucosal application of silver salts. When ingested, there is a slate-blue discoloration on the skin, especially in the sun-exposed areas. The oral mucosa, conjunctivae, fingernail beds (but not toenail) (106), intestines, liver, spleen, and peritoneum may also be involved (107,108). Argyria (and chrysiasis) has been reported after acupuncture (109) and in a silversmith following multiple cutaneous punctures by a silver filament (110).

Histopathology. In the dermis, there are extracellular fine, small, round, uniformly sized brown-black silver granules, both singly and clustered. The deposition is predominantly extracellular and found in both sun-exposed and unexposed skin. They are present in the greatest numbers in the basement membrane zone surrounding the sweat glands (Fig. 11-18) as well as in the connective tissue sheaths around the hair follicles and sebaceous glands, in the walls of capillaries, in the arrectores pilorum, and in the nerves (111). Silver granules are also found in the dermal papillae and scattered diffusely throughout the dermis. Elastic tissue stains reveal a predilection of the granules for elastic fibers, which explains the presence of fingerlike chains of granules projecting into the dermal papillae (110). In contrast, silver is not seen in the epidermis or its appendages. Although visible in routine stains, dark-field microscopy reveals brilliantly refractile, white particles against a dark background. In addition to silver, there is an increase in the amount of epidermal melanin, particularly in sun-exposed skin. Melanophages may also be scattered throughout the upper dermis. Deposits of silver are also found in internal organs. Incubation of sections in a solution consisting of 1% potassium ferricyanide

in 20% sodium thiosulfate will result in decolorization of silver.

Pathogenesis. Electron microscopy reveals extracellular aggregates of irregularly shaped granules varying in size from 200 to 400 nm in diameter, but ranging up to 1,000 nm (111).

The increase in the amount of melanin in the basal cell layer and occasionally also in the upper dermis suggests that the presence of silver in the skin may stimulate melanocyte activity. Increased epidermal melanin is observed also with deposits of other heavy metals, such as iron in hemochromatosis (see Chapter 17) and mercury in mercury pigmentation (see later). The pronounced slate-blue pigmentation in exposed skin is caused by increases in both melanin and silver (112).

CHRYSIASIS

Chrysiasis is slate-blue discoloration on sun-exposed skin caused by the prolonged parenteral administration of gold salts, generally for the treatment of rheumatoid arthritis.

Histopathology. Gold granules are found predominantly within cells, particularly within endothelial cells and macrophages (113). However, extracellular granules may also be observed. They are larger and more irregularly shaped than silver granules. While they are also light refractile with dark-field examination, the granules are orange-red birefringent on fluorescence microscopy (114).

Histogenesis. Electron microscopic examination shows the presence of electron-dense, angulated particles within phagolysosomes of endothelial cells and macrophages (113). X-ray spectroscopic analysis demonstrates a spectrum consistent with the presence of gold (113).

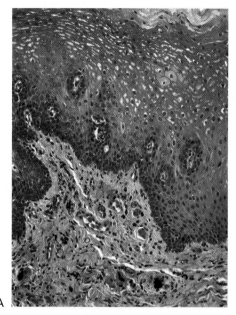
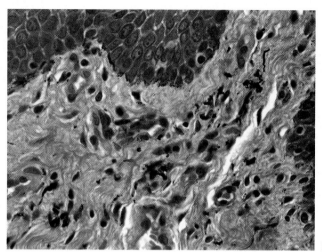

FIGURE 11-19. Mercury deposition. **A:** The large black-brown mercury deposits along with the multinucleate foreign body giant cell infiltrate seen in this case are characteristic of traumatic implantation. **B:** Extracellular and intracellular brown-black mercury granules are seen in the upper dermis. In this case, they are also seen in the basement membrane.

MERCURY PIGMENTATION

Regular application of a mercury-containing cream to the face and neck over many years may produce a slate-gray pigmentation of the skin in the areas to which the cream has been applied. Generally, the pigmentation is most pronounced on the eyelids, in the nasolabial folds, and in the folds of the neck (115). Most mercury-containing creams are no longer manufactured. Traumatic implantation of mercury may also occur.

Histopathology. Irregular, brown-black granules are found in the upper dermis, both extracellularly and within macrophages. In rare instances, granules are seen also in the basal cell layer of the epidermis. As in argyria and chrysiasis, dark-field microscopy reveals brilliantly refractile granules (116). Silver staining reveals normal or increased basalar melanin (116). Traumatic implantation of mercury results in variably sized, often large, amorphous deposits of mercury in the dermis and subcutis. Chronic changes include dermal fibrosis and granulomatous inflammation (Fig. 11-19).

Pathogenesis. Electron microscopic examination shows the mercury particles, which are approximately 14 nm in diameter, to be aggregated into irregular granules with diameters of up to 340 nm. The granules are associated with elastic fibers as well as along the collagen fibers. In macrophages, they are present within lysosomes or free in the cytoplasm (116). When seen in the epidermis, the mercury granules lie in the intercellular spaces of the basal cell layer (116).

Because the pigmentation is most pronounced in skin folds that are protected from the sun, and there may be no increase in the amount of melanin, it can be concluded that most of the pigmentation is caused by the mercury rather than the melanin.

REFERENCES

1. Bigby M, Jick S, Jick H, et al. Drug-induced cutaneous reactions. A report from the Boston Collaborative Drug Surveillance Program on 15438 consecutive inpatients 1975–1982. *JAMA* 1986;256:3358–3363.
2. Roujeau R-J, Stern RS. Serious adverse cutaneous reactions to drugs. *N Engl J Med* 1994;331:1272–1285.
3. Breathnach SM. Mechanisms of drug eruptions. Part I. *Australas J Dermatol* 1995;36:121–127.
4. Scharf SJ, Friedman A, Brautbar C, et al. HLA class II allelic variation and susceptibility to pemphigus vulgaris. *Proc Natl Acad Sci U S A* 1988;85:3504–3508.
5. Lotem M, Hubert A, Lyass O, et al. Skin toxic effect of polyethylene glycol-coated liposomal doxorubicin. *Arch Dermatol* 2000; 136:1475–1480.
6. Kreuter A, Gambichler T, Schlottmann, et al. Psoriasiform pustular eruptions from pegylated-liposomal doxorubicin in AIDS-related Kaposi's sarcoma [Letter]. *Acta Derm Venerol* 2001;81: 224.
7. Kuokkanen K. Drug eruptions: a series of 464 cases in the Department of Dermatology, University of Turku, Finland, during 1966–70. *Acta Allergologica* 1972;27:407–438.
8. Cropley TA, Fitzpatrick TBF. Dermatology diagnosis by recognition of clinical, morphologic patterns and syndromes. In: Fitzpatrick TB, Eisen AZ, Wolff K, et al., eds. *Dermatology in general medicine.* New York: McGraw-Hill, 1993:55.

9. Sideroff A, Halevy S, Bavinck J, et al. Acute generalized exanthematous pustuosis (AGEP)—a clinical reaction pattern. *J Cutan Pathol* 2001;28:113–119.
10. Dupin N, Gorin I. Acute generalized exanthematous pustulosis induced by terbinafine, *Arch Derm* 1996;132:1253–1254.
11. Britxchgi M, Steiner UC, Schmid S, et al. T cell involvement in drug-induced acute generalized exanthematous pustulosis. *J Clin Invest* 2001;107:1433–1441.
12. Yawalkar N, Egli F, Hari Y, et al. Infiltration of cytotoxic T cells in drug-induced cutaneous eruptions. *Clin Exp Allergy* 2000;30:847–855.
13. RoujeauAQ JC, Kelly JP, Naldi L, et al. Medication use and the risk of Stevens–Johnson syndrome or toxic epidermal necrolysis. *N Engl J Med* 1995;333:1600–1607.
14. Sarkat R, Kaur C, Kanwar AJ. Erythema multiforme due to refocoxib. *Dermatology* 2002;204:304–305.
15. Nikas SN, Kittas G, Karamaounas N, et al. Meloxicam-induced erythema multiforme. *Am J Med* 1999;107:532–534.
16. Thami GP, Kaur S, Kanwar AJ. Erythema multiforme due to griseofulvin with positive re-exposure test. *Dermatology* 2001;203:84–85.
17. Zohdi-Mofid M, Horn TD. Acrosyringeal concentration of necrotic keratinocytes in erythema multiforme: a clue to drug etiology. *J Cutan Pathol* 1997;24:235–240.
18. Oliver GF, Winkelmann RK, Muller SA. Lichenoid dermatitis: a clinicopathologic and immunopathologic review of sixty-two cases. *J Am Acad Dermatol* 1989;21:284–292.
19. Powell ML, Ehrlich A, Belsito DV. Lichenoid drug eruption to salsalate. *J Am Acad Dermatol* 2001;45:616–619.
20. Saywell CA, Wittal RA, Kossard S. Lichenoid reaction to hepatitis B vaccine. *Australas J Dermatol* 1997;38:152–154.
21. Kanwar AJ, Bharija SC, Singh M, et al. Ninety-eight fixed drug eruptions with provocation tests. *Dermatologica* 1988;177:274–279.
22. Van Hecke E, Kint A, Temmerman L. A lichenoid eruption induced by penicillamine. *Arch Dermatol* 1981;117:676–677.
23. Teraki Y, Moriya N, Shiohara T. Drug-induced expression of intercellular adhesion molecule-1 on lesional keratinocytes in fixed drug eruption. *Am J Pathol* 1994;145:550–560.
24. Zimmerman GC, Keeling JH, Burris HA, et al. Acute cutaneous reactions to docetaxel, a new chemotherapeutic agent. *Arch Dermatol* 1995;131:202–206.
25. Haustein UF, Haupt B. Drug-induced scleroderma and sclerodermiform conditions. *Clin Dermatol* 1998;16:353–366.
26. Clark JG, Starcher BC, Uitto J. Bleomycin-induced synthesis of type I procollagen by human lung and skin fibroblasts in culture. *Biochim Biophys Acta* 1980;631:359–357.
27. Cohen IS, Mosher MB, O'Keefe EJ, et al. Cutaneous toxicity of bleomycin therapy. *Arch Dermatol* 1973;107:553–555.
28. Finch WR, Rodnan GP, Buckingham RB, et al. Bleomycin-induced scleroderma. *J Rheumatol* 1980;7:651–659.
29. Cleveland MG, Ajaikumar BS, Reganti R. Cutaneous fibrosis induced by docetaxel, a case report. *Cancer* 2000;88:1078–1081.
30. Battafarano DF, Zimmerman GC, Older SA, et al. Docetaxel associated scleroderma-like changes of the lower extremities. *Cancer* 1995;76:110–115.
31. Wilkins K, DeKoven J, Assaad D. Cutaneous reactions associated with vitamin K1. *J Cutan Med Surg* 2000;4:164–168.
32. Leavell UW, Farley CH, McIntire JS. Cutaneous changes in a patient with carbon monoxide poisoning. *Arch Dermatol* 1969;99:429–433.
33. Herschthal D, Robinson MJ. Blisters of the skin in coma induced by amitriptyline and chloracepate dipotassium. *Arch Dermatol* 1979;115:499.
34. Brehmer-Andersson E, Pedersen NB. Sweat gland necrosis and bullous skin changes in acute drug intoxication. *Acta Dermatol Venereol* 1969;49:157–162.
35. Templeton SF, Solomon AR, Swerlick RA. Intradermal bleomycin infections into normal human skin: a histopathologic and immunopathologic study. *Arch Dermatol* 1994;130:577–583.
36. Brenner S, Bialy-Golan A, Ruocco V. Drug-induced pemphigus. *Clin Dermatol* 1998;16:393–397.
37. Carpenter S, Berg D, Sidhu-Malik N, et al. Vancomycin-associated linear IgA dermatoses. A report of three cases. *J Am Acad Dermatol* 1992;26:45–48.
38. Marinho RT, Johnson NW, Fatela NM, et al. Oropharyngeal pemphigus in a patient with chronic hepatitis C during interferon alpha-2a therapy. *Eur J Gastroenterol Hepatol* 2001;13:869–872.
39. Landau M, Brenner S. Histopathologic findings in drug-induced pemphigus. *Am J Dermatopathol* 1997;19:411–414.
40. Brenner S, Bialy-Golan A, Anhalt G. Recognition of pemphigus antigens in drug-induced pemphigus vulgaris and pemphigus foliaceus. *J Am Acad Dermatol* 1997;36:919–923.
41. Scharf SJ, Friedman A, Vrautvar C. HLA class II allelic variation and susceptibility to pemphigus vulgaris. *Proc Natl Acad Sci U S A* 1988;85:3504–3508.
42. Wucherpfenning KW, Srominger JL. Selective binding of self peptides to disease-associated major histocompatibility complex molecules: a mechanism of MHC-linked susceptibility to human autoimmune diseases. *J Exp Med* 1995;1818:1597–1601.
43. Pramatarov KD. Drug-induced lupus erythematosus. *Clin Dermatol* 1998;16:367–377.
44. Bonsmann G, Schiller M, Luger T, et al. Terbinafine-induced subacute cutaneous lupus erythematosus. *J Am Acad Dermatol* 2001;44:925–931.
45. Callen JP, Hughes AP, Kulp-Shorten C. Subacute cutaneous lupus erythematosus induced or exacerbated by terbinafine: a report of 5 cases. *Arch Dermatol* 2001;137:1196–1198.
46. Pauls JD, Gohill J, Fritzler MJ. Antibodies from patients with systemic lupus erythematosus and drug-induced lupus bind determinants on histone 5(H5). *Mol Immunol* 1990;27:701–711.
47. Grossman J, Callerame ML, Condemi JJ. Skin immunofluorescence studies on lupus erythematosus and other antinuclear antibody-positive disease. *Ann Intern Med* 1974;80:496–500.
48. Uetrecht JP, Woosley RL. Acetylator phenotype and lupus erythematosus. *Clin Pharmacokinet* 1981;6:118–134.
49. Harber LC, Baer RL. Pathogenic mechanisms of drug-induced photosensitivity. *J Invest Dermatol* 1972;58:327–342.
50. Ophaswongse S, Maibach H. Topical nonsteroidal antiinflammatory drugs: allergic and photoallergic contact dermatitis and phototoxicity. *Contact Dermatitis* 1993;29:57–64.
51. Cook N, Freeman S. Report of 19 cases of photoallergic contact dermatitis to sunscreens seen at the Skin and Cancer Foundation. *australas J Dermatol* 2001;42:257–259.
52. Willis I, Kligman AM. The mechanism of photoallergic contact dermatitis. *J Invest Dermatol* 1968;51:378–384.
53. Horio T, Miyauchi H, Asada Y, et al. Phototoxicity and photoallergy of quinolones in guinea pigs. *J Dermatol Sci* 1994;7:130–135.
54. Frost P, Weinstein GP, Gomez EC. Phototoxic potential of minocycline and doxycycline. *Arch Dermatol* 1972;105:681–683.
55. Lasarow RM, Isseroff RR, Gomez EC. Quantitative in vitro assessment of phototoxicity by a fibroblast-neutral assay. *J Invest Dermatol* 1992;98:725–729.
56. Gilchrest BA, Soter NA, Stoff JS, et al. The human sunburn reaction: histologic and biochemical studies. *J Am Acad Dermatol* 1981;5:411–422.
57. Hays GB, Lyle CB Jr, Wheeler CE Jr. Slate-grey color in patients receiving chlorpromazine. *Arch Dermatol* 1964;90:471.

58. Scherschun L, Lee M, Lim H. Diltiazem-associated photodistributed hyperpigmentation: a review of 4 cases. *Arch Dermatol* 2001;137:179–182.

59. Greiner AC, Nicolson GA. Pigmentary deposit in viscera associated with prolonged chlorpromazine therapy. *CMAJ* 1964;91:627.

60. Benning TL, McCormack KM, Ingram P, et al. Microprobe analysis of chlorpromazine pigmentation. *Arch Dermatol* 1988;124:1541–1544.

61. Blois MS Jr. On chlorpromazine binding in vivo. *J Invest Dermatol* 1965;45:475.

62. Sanatove A. Pigmentation due to phenothiazines in high and prolonged doses. *JAMA* 1965;191:263–268.

63. Welykyi S, Gradini R, Nakao J, et al. Carbamazepine-induced eruption histologically mimicking mycosis fungoides. *J Cutan Pathol* 1990;17:111–116.

64. Cogrel O, Beylot-Barry M, Vergier B, et al. Sodium valproate-induced cutaneous pseudolymphoma followed by recurrence with carbamazepine. *Br J Dermatol* 2001;144:1235–1238.

65. Marucci G, Sgarbanti E, Maestri A, et al. Gemcitabine-associated CD8+ CD30+ pseudolymphoma. *Br J Dermatol* 2001;145:650–652.

66. Kim KJ, Lee MW, Choi JH, et al. CD30-positive T-cell-rich pseudolymphoma induced by gold acupuncture. *Br J Dermatol* 2002;146:882–884.

67. Shelley WB, Shelley ED. Pseudolymphoma at site of clonidine patch. *Lancet* 1997;350:1223–1224.

68. Wolf R, Kahane E, Sandbank M. Mycosis fungoides-like lesions associated with phenytoin therapy. *Arch Dermatol* 1985;121:1181–1182.

69. Charlesworth EN. Phenytoin-induced pseudolymphoma syndrome. *Arch Dermatol* 1977;113:477–480.

70. Harris DW, Ostlere L, Buckley C, et al. Phenytoin-induced pseudolymphoma: a report of a case and review of the literature. *Br J Dermatol* 1992;127:403–406.

71. Adams JD. Localized cutaneous pseudolymphoma associated with phenytoin therapy: a case report. *Australas J Dermatol* 1981;22:28–29.

72. Braddock SW, Harrington D, Vose J. Generalized nodular cutaneous pseudolymphoma associated with phenytoin therapy: use of T-cell receptor gene rearrangement in diagnosis and clinical review of cutaneous reactions to phenytoin. *J Am Acad Dermatol* 1992;27:337–340.

73. Howard AM, Dowling J, Varigos G. Pseudoporphyria due to naproxen. *Lancet* 1985;1:819–820.

74. Radaelli F, Calori R, Faccini P, et al. Early cutaneous lesions secondary to hydroxyurea therapy. *Am J Hematol* 1998;58:82–83.

75. Busam KJ, Capodieci P, Motzer R, et al. Cutaneous side-effects in cancer patients treated with the antiepidermal growth factor receptor antibody C225. *Br J Dermatol* 2001;144:1169–1176.

76. Yokel BK, Friedman KJ, Farmer ER, et al. Cutaneous pathology following etoposide therapy. *J Cutan Pathol* 1987;14:326–330.

77. Horn TD, Beveridge RA, Egorin MJ, et al. Observations and proposed mechanism of N,N′,N″-triethylenethiophosphoramide (Thio-TEPA)-induced hyperpigmentation. *Arch Dermatol* 1989;125:524–527.

78. Hurt MA, Halvorson RD, Peter FC Jr, et al. Eccrine squamous syringometaplasia: a cutaneous sweat gland reaction in the histologic spectrum of "chemotherapy-associated eccrine hidradenitis." *Arch Dermatol* 1990;126:73–77.

79. Fitzpatrick JE, Bennion SD, Reed OM, et al. Neutrophilic eccrine hidradenitis associated with induction chemotherapy. *J Cutan Pathol* 1987;14:272–278.

80. Harrist TJ, Fine JD, Berman RS, et al. Neutrophilic hidradenitis: a distinctive type of neutrophilic dermatosis associated with myelogenous leukemia and chemotherapy. *Arch Dermatol* 1982;118:263–266.

81. Linassier C, Colombat P, Reisenleiter M, et al. Cutaneous toxicity of autologous bone marrow transplantation in nonseminomatous germ cell tumors. *Cancer* 1990;65:1143–1145.

82. Hymes SR, Simonton SC, Farmer ER, et al. Cutaneous busulfan effect in patients receiving bone marrow transplantation. *J Cutan Pathol* 1985;12:125–129.

83. Zeltser R, Valle L, Tanck C, et al. Clinical histological and immunophenotypic characteristics of injection site reactions associated with etanercept: a recombinant tumor necrosis factor [alpha] receptor: Fc fusion protein. *Arch Dermatol* 2001:137:893–899.

84. Garcia-F-Villalta M, Dauden E, Sanchez J, et al. Local reactions associated with subcutaneous injections of both beta-interferon 1a and 1b. *Acta Derm Venereol* 2001;81:152.

85. Elgart GW, Sheremata W, Ahn YS. Cutaneous reactions to recombinant human interferon beta-1b: the clinical and histologic spectrum. *J Am Acad Dermatol* 1997:37:553–558.

86. Horn TD, Burke PJ, Karp JE, et al. Intravenous administration of recombinant human granulocyte-macrophage colony-stimulating factor causes a cutaneous eruption. *Arch Dermatol* 1991;127:49–52.

87. Mehregan DR, Fransway AF, Edmonson JH, et al. Cutaneous reactions to granulocyte-monocyte colony-stimulating factor. *Arch Dermatol* 1992;128:1055–1059.

88. Park JW, Mehrotra B, Barnett BO, et al. The Sweet syndrome during therapy with granulocyte colony-stimulating factor. *Ann Int Med* 1992;116:996–998.

89. Williamson K, Rebolli AC, Manders SM. Protease inhibitor induced lipodystrophy. *J Am Acad Dermatol* 1999;40:635–636.

90. Saint-Marc T, Partisane M, Poizot-Martin I, et al. A syndrome of peripheral fat wasting (lipodystrophy) in patients receiving long-term nucleoside analogue therapy. *AIDS* 1999;13:1659–1667.

91. Greenberg RG, Berger TG. Nail and mucocutaneous hyperpigmentation with azidothymidine therapy. *J Am Acad Dermatol* 1990;22:327–330.

92. Obuch ML, Baker G, Roth RI, et al. Selective cutaneous hyperpigmentation in mice following zidovudine administration. *Arch Dermatol* 1992;28:508–513.

93. Ward HA, Russo GG, Shrum J. Cutaneous manifestations of antiretroviral therapy. *J Am Acad Dermatol* 2002;46:284–293.

94. Argenyi ZB, Finelli L, Bergfeld WF, et al. Minocycline-related cutaneous hyperpigmentation as demonstrated by light microscopy, electron microscopy and x-ray energy spectroscopy. *J Cutan Pathol* 1987;14:176–180.

95. Pepine M, Flowers DP, Ramos-Caro FA. Extensive cutaneous hyperpigmentation caused by minocycline. *J Am Acad Dermatol* 1993;28:292–295.

96. Knowles SR, Shapiro L, Shear NH. Serious adverse reactions induced by minocycline: report of 13 patients and review of the literature. *Arch Dermatol* 1996;132:934–939.

97. Altman DA, Fivenson DP, Lee MW. Minocycline hyperpigmentation: a model for in situ phagocytic activity of factor XIIIa positive dermal dendrocytes. *J Cutan Pathol* 1992;19:340–345.

98. Job CK, Yoder L, Jacobsen RR, et al. Skin pigmentation from clofazimine therapy in leprosy patients: a reappraisal. *J Am Acad Dermatol* 1990;23:236–241.

99. Poon E, Mason G, Oh C. Clinical and histological spectrum of elastotic changes induced by penicillamine. *Australas J Dermatol* 2002;43:147–151.

100. Fitzpatrick JE. New histopathologic findings in drug eruptions. *Dermatol Clin* 1992;10:19–36.

101. Siegel RC. Collagen cross-linking: effect of D-penicillamine on cross-linking in vitro. *J Biol Chem* 1977;252:254–259.

102. Meyrick Thomas RH, Kirby JDT. Elastosis perforans serpiginosa and pseudoxanthoma elasticum-like skin change due to D-penicillamine. *Clin Exp Dermatol* 1985;10:386–391.

103. Bolognia JL, Braverman I. Pseudoxanthoma-elasticum-like skin changes induced by penicillamine. *Dermatol* 1992;184:12–18.

104. O'Brien TJ. Iodic eruptions. *Australas J Dermatol* 1987;28:119–122.

105. Blasik LG, Spencer SK. Fluoroderma. *Arch Dermatol* 1979;115:1334–1335.

106. Plewig G, Lincke H, Wolff HH. Silver-blue nails. *Acta Derm Venereol (Stockh)* 1977;57:413–419.

107. Prescott RJ, Wells S. Systemic argyria. *J Clin Pathol* 1994;47:556–557.

108. Gherardi R, Brochard P, Chamek B, et al. Human generalized argyria. *Arch Pathol* 1984;108:181–182.

109. Suzuki H, Baba S, Uchigasaki S, et al. Localized argyria with chrysiasis caused by implanted acupuncture needles. *J Am Acad Dermatol* 1993;29:833–837.

110. Rongioletti F, Robert E, Buffa P, et al. Blue nevi-like dotted occupational argyria. *J Am Acad Dermatol* 1992;27:1015–1016.

111. Pezzarosa E, Alinovi A, Ferrari C. Generalized argyria. *J Cutan Pathol* 1983;10:361–363.

112. Johansson EA, Kanerva L, Niemi KM, et al. Generalized argyria with low ceruloplasmin and copper levels in the serum. A case report with clinical and microscopical findings and a trial of penicillamine treatment. *Clin Exp Dermatol* 1982;7:169–176.

113. Pelachyk JM, Bergfeld WF, McMahon JT. Chrysiasis following gold therapy for rheumatoid arthritis. *J Cutan Pathol* 1984;11:491–494.

114. Al-Talib RK, Wright DH, Theaker JM. Orange-red birefringence of gold particles in paraffin wax embedded sections: an aid to the diagnosis of chrysiasis. *Histopathology* 1994;24:176–178.

115. Lamar LM, Bliss BO. Localized pigmentation of the skin due to topical mercury. *Arch Dermatol* 1966;93:450–453.

116. Burge KM, Winkelmann RK. Mercury pigmentation: an electron microscopic study. *Arch Dermatol* 1970;102:51–61.

THE PHOTOSENSITIVITY DISORDERS

JOHN L. M. HAWK
EDUARDO CALONJE

Cutaneous disorders caused by ultraviolet radiation (UVR), or photodermatoses, comprise drug and chemical photosensitivity, the DNA repair-deficient disorders, the UVR-exacerbated dermatoses, and the largest and commonest group, the idiopathic, probably immunologically based photodermatoses. The latter are polymorphic (polymorphous) light eruption, actinic prurigo, hydroa vacciniforme, chronic actinic dermatitis (photosensitivity dermatitis and actinic reticuloid syndrome, persistent light reaction), and solar urticaria (1–3). Thus, recent investigation of this last group has yielded much evidence that the conditions included are all immunologically mediated. The first four are probably delayed-type hypersensitivity (DTH) reactions against UVR-induced skin antigen, with the exact clinical features perhaps determined by the cutaneous sites of antigen formation, and the last is probably an immediate-type of hypersensitivity response against similarly produced cutaneous or circulating substances. Confirmation of this hypothesis now requires definitive identification of the putative antigens for the conditions.

Drug and chemical photosensitivity, the DNA repair-deficient disorders, and the UVR-exacerbated dermatoses are considered elsewhere in this book; the idiopathic, probably immunologically based photodermatoses are now discussed here.

POLYMORPHIC (POLYMORPHOUS) LIGHT ERUPTION

Polymorphic (polymorphous) light eruption (PMLE) is a commonly occurring, transient, intermittent, UVR-induced eruption of nonscarring, erythematous, itchy papules, plaques, or vesicles of exposed skin. It is most severe in spring and summer and most common in young women (1–3). It is seen mostly at temperate latitudes, affecting up to one in five subjects of any skin coloring; attacks develop during sunny vacations and summer weather, often persisting or recurring, sometimes with gradual reduction in severity, from spring until fall. They follow around 15 minutes to a few hours of sun exposure, or occasionally a few days after a period with little exposure, and begin within hours of irradiation and last for hours, days, or rarely weeks. Some but not necessarily all exposed skin is affected, usually symmetrically; normally uncovered sites are most frequently spared. Diagnosis is made from the history and clinical findings in the presence of normal circulating antinuclear factor and extractable nuclear antibody titers, and of normal urinary, stool, and blood porphyrin concentrations. If there is diagnostic uncertainty, however, lesional histology generally provides good evidence for PMLE, while broad-spectrum or monochromatic irradiation skin tests may induce the typical eruption or else abnormal erythemal or papular responses. Treatment is for the most part prophylactic, and often effective. Often the limitation of UVR exposure, use of appropriate clothing, and regular application of high-protection, broad-spectrum sunscreens during exposure are satisfactory for mild disease, while short courses of low-dose psoralen ultraviolet A photochemotherapy (PUVA) or broad- or narrow-band (311 to 312 nm) ultraviolet B (UVB) phototherapy before summer begins are usually effective in more severe instances. If the eruption should develop despite these measures, however, a short course of systemic steroid therapy usually rapidly abolishes it, but the value of other previously advocated medications, such as antimalarials and beta-carotene, has not been confirmed in controlled trials.

Histopathology. The histologic findings vary according to age of the lesion sampled. Very early lesions show either a normal epidermis or mild spongiosis with focal lymphocyte exocytosis and an underlying mild or occasionally moderate, superficial and deep, perivascular and periadnexal, lymphohistiocytic inflammatory cell infiltrate (1–6) (Fig. 12-1); the lymphocytes have a T-helper phenotype (CD3/CD4 positive). Interestingly, in experimentally induced PMLE lesions, the infiltrate in the first 72 hours postinduction also has a predominant T-helper phenotype, but thereafter a mainly T-cytotoxic type (CD3/CD8 positive) (7). Occasional eosinophils and rare neutrophils may

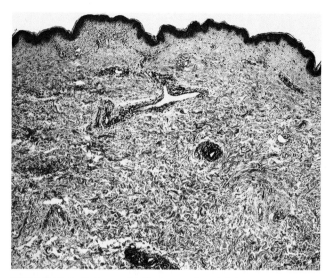

FIGURE 12-1. Polymorphic (polymorphous) light eruption. Early lesion showing superficial and deep, perivascular, and periappendageal, inflammatory infiltrate.

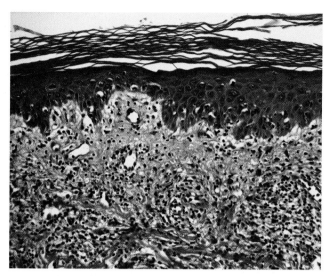

FIGURE 12-3. Polymorphous light eruption. Mild spongiosis and focal interface change with hydropic degeneration of basal cells; the latter may suggest lupus.

also be found. As lesions progress, there is marked edema of the papillary dermis and more prominent dermal inflammation (Fig. 12-2), along with occasional focal interface change and mild hydropic basal cell degeneration (6) (Fig. 12-3). In such cases, the histologic picture may resemble cutaneous lupus erythematosus (see below). Exceptionally, a fairly prominent dermal infiltrate may raise the possibility of lymphoma.

Pathogenesis. The eruption of PMLE is induced by exposure to UVR, particularly from strong summer sunlight. Artificial reproduction is less easy, and exact action spectra have not been conclusively determined. Nevertheless, the

responsible wavelengths appear to be UVB in around a quarter of patients, UVA in half, and both in the remainder; visible light may also rarely be responsible. The eruption itself very likely appears to be a DTH response in view of its pattern of dermal cellular infiltration, cytokine production, and adhesion molecule expression, arguably to UVR-induced, endogenous, cutaneous antigen (1–3). Further, it appears likely that a genetically determined impairment of normal UVR-induced cutaneous immunosuppressive activity may permit the reaction (8).

Differential Diagnosis. The diagnosis is generally apparent from the clinical history, in which sun exposure is nearly always clearly involved in causing the typical eruption, provided that circulating antinuclear and extractable nuclear antibody titers and urinary, stool, and blood porphyrin concentrations are normal. Histologically, PMLE must be differentiated from lupus erythematosus, the porphyrias, actinic prurigo, Jessner's lymphocytic infiltrate, cutaneous T-cell lymphoma, chilblains, and rosacea (1–3, 6). In cutaneous lupus erythematosus, the interface change is more prominent not only in the epidermis but also in adnexal structures; apoptotic keratinocytes are often seen and papillary dermal edema is not a feature. In addition, dermal mucin deposition may be seen in lupus and is absent in PMLE. Actinic prurigo usually displays changes secondary to excoriation, variable epidermal hyperplasia, and more prominent lymphocyte spongiosis and exocytosis; however, early lesions in both conditions may show very similar microscopic findings, except that dermal edema is usually absent in actinic prurigo. In Jessner's lymphocytic infiltrate, epidermal changes are absent, there is no papillary dermal edema, and the dermal mononuclear cell infiltrate tends to be more prominent. Cutaneous T-cell lymphoma is only rarely included in the differential

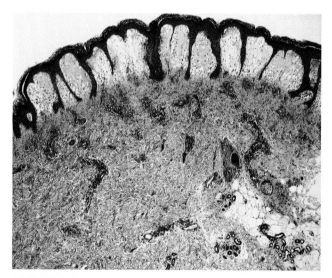

FIGURE 12-2. Polymorphic (polymorphous) light eruption. Established lesion showing prominent papillary dermal edema and moderately prominent, superficial and deep, perivascular and periadnexal, mononuclear inflammatory cell infiltrate.

diagnosis of PMLE, and mainly when the dermal infiltrate is prominent; however, the exocytosis of lymphocytes with irregular nuclear outlines is not a feature of the latter, which usually also shows variable spongiosis. The histology of chilblains, on the other hand, is almost identical to that of PMLE, particularly when there is prominent papillary dermal edema, but fortunately the clinical setting of each disease usually allows distinction. Rosacea shows no epidermal change, dermal edema is absent, the dermal infiltrate is mild and surrounds superficial small blood vessels and adnexal structures, and focal lymphocytic exocytosis into hair follicles is often seen.

ACTINIC PRURIGO

Actinic prurigo (AP) is a moderately rare, itchy, papular or nodular, excoriated, chronic summer eruption of the light-exposed and to a lesser extent covered skin of children, usually girls; it may resolve by early adulthood (1–3) and is more common in Native and mixed race Americans. The face and distal limbs are most often affected, while the proximal limbs and forehead beneath the hair fringe, less often exposed, are mostly spared; the buttocks, however, are often involved. Superficial, pitted, or linear scars may be present at the sites of previous lesions, and chronic cheilitis and conjunctivitis are possible. In addition, some patients may also describe acute attacks of rash following specific sunlight exposure episodes, similar to PMLE. Therapy is often helpful, consisting in mild cases of reduced sun exposure, the use of protective clothing, and the application of high-protection, broad-spectrum sunscreens, emollients, and topical steroids, while in more severe cases, low-dose PUVA or narrow-band UVB irradiation therapy, similar to that for PMLE, may sometimes be useful in appropriate patients. If not, oral thalidomide clears around three-quarters of affected subjects, although a marked risk of teratogenicity and the moderate possibility of peripheral neuropathy necessitate great care in its use (1–3).

Histopathology. The histology varies according to clinical evolution. Thus, early intact lesions show variable and often mild epidermal spongiosis, and a superficial and deep dermal, perivascular, mononuclear cell infiltration similar to that of PMLE, but in the absence of substantial papillary dermal edema (Fig. 12-4). This latter finding, however, may be seen in occasional biopsies, and histologic distinction from PMLE may then be impossible, requiring close clinicopathologic correlation (9). Occasional eosinophils are often seen. AP lesions are frequently excoriated; careful attention should be paid when a biopsy is performed to avoid lesions with such prominent secondary changes (6) (Fig. 12-5). Evolving lesions may also occasionally display focal interface change with hydropic degeneration of basal cells, such that distinction from cutaneous lupus may then be difficult (6) (Fig. 12-6). In rare cases, there may be a

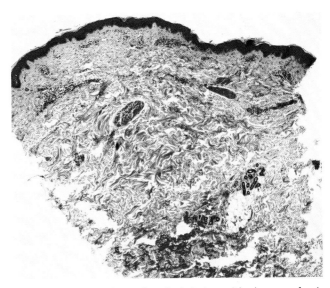

FIGURE 12-4. Actinic prurigo. Early lesion with absence of epidermal change, and mild to moderate superficial and deep, perivascular and periadnexal, mononuclear inflammatory cell infiltrate.

heavy, superficial, and deep dermal mononuclear cell infiltrate, with difficulty in distinction from lymphoma, especially if associated interface changes are present. In older lesions, there is usually variable lichenification (Fig. 12-7), focal papillary dermal fibrosis, a moderately heavy mononuclear cell infiltrate, and irregular epithelial hyperplasia similar to the features of chronic eczema, or even prurigo nodularis (1–3) (see Fig. 12-4). The AP inflammatory cell infiltrate has a T-helper phenotype (CD3/CD4 positive). AP must thus be differentiated from the same disorders as PMLE in its more unusual acute form, and from other

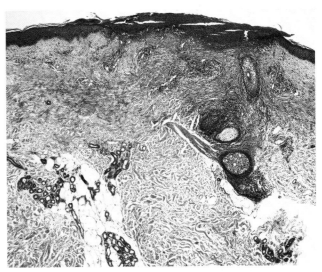

FIGURE 12-5. Actinic prurigo. Prominent superficial necrosis secondary to excoriation and fairly heavy perivascular and periadnexal inflammatory cell infiltrate.

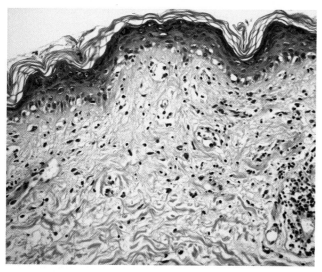

FIGURE 12-6. Actinic prurigo. Interface change may be more prominent than in polymorphic light eruption, and histologic distinction from lupus more difficult.

causes of chronic eczema or prurigo in its chronic forms. Finally, although AP histology may often be fairly non-specific, the lesions of AP cheilitis characteristically show a dense lymphocytic infiltrate with frequent well-formed lymphoid follicles (10,11), a finding regarded as potentially very helpful in cases of diagnostic doubt.

Pathogenesis. UVR exposure appears to be of prime importance in the causation of AP, given the greater severity of the disorder in summer and after sun exposure, and relatively frequent abnormal erythemal or papular skin responses to monochromatic irradiation. Such reactions occur in a half to two-thirds of patients, often to the UVB wavelengths alone but sometimes also the UVA (1–3); re-

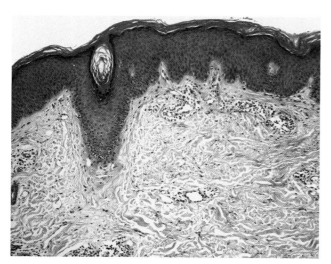

FIGURE 12-7. Actinic prurigo. Older lesion showing lichenification.

sponses to broad-spectrum irradiation have not been reported. The clinical behavior of acute AP, its histological appearances, and a familial association with PMLE give credence to suggestions that it may be a persistent form of PMLE, and thus also a DTH reaction against UVR-induced, endogenous, cutaneous antigen, but this remains speculative. However, the persistence of AP lesions compared with those of PMLE might well be determined by the patient's human leukocyte antigen (HLA) type. This is usually HLA-DR4, found in only 30% of normal subjects, or its subtype DRB1*0407, present in only 6% of normal European Caucasians but relatively common in Native Americans, in whom AP is also more prevalent (12).

Differential Diagnosis. AP must be differentiated from PMLE, lupus erythematosus, insect bites, scabies, lymphoma, nodular prurigo, and eczema. Its seasonal variation, affected sites, and sometimes positive light tests may assist in this differentiation, as well as its histology, particularly if a lesion is fresh. However, close clinicopathologic correlation is essential for reliable diagnosis. In biopsies with interface change, distinction from lupus erythematosus may be difficult, but in AP, such change is usually very patchy, focal, and limited to the epidermis, while apoptotic keratinocytes are usually absent. If a prominent dermal infiltrate is seen, the diagnosis of T-cell lymphoma may well come into consideration, but cytologic atypia and epidermotropism are lacking in AP. Finally, in its usual chronic forms, the distinction of AP from chronic eczema is impossible on histologic grounds alone.

HYDROA VACCINIFORME

Hydroa vacciniforme (HV) is a very rare, intermittent, UVR-induced, blistering, and scarring eruption of exposed skin, usually in children (1–3,13,14). The condition generally has onset by age 10 years with resolution by early adulthood. Usually sparse, occasionally coalescent, symmetrically scattered, and sometimes hemorrhagic vesicles and bullae are characteristic, particularly of the face, ears, and limbs; these then umbilicate and crust over days, healing thereafter in weeks to leave persistent, disfiguring pock scars. Treatment is very difficult. Avoidance of UVR exposure, clothing cover, and the application of high-protection, broad-spectrum sunscreens have limited efficacy; in resistant cases, courses of prophylactic low-dose UVB phototherapy or PUVA may sometimes help. All other therapies are at best marginally useful.

Histology. The main very characteristic histologic abnormality is that of progressive intra- and inter-cellular epidermal edema leading to prominent reticular degeneration, vesiculation, and finally confluent epidermal necrosis (Figs. 12-8 and 12-9). The vesicles contain fibrin and acute inflammatory cells, and overlie a dermal cellular infiltrate

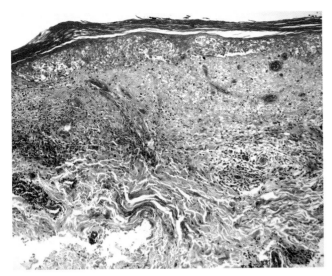

FIGURE 12-8. Hydroa vacciniforme. Prominent confluent epidermal necrosis associated with dermal perivascular inflammatory cell infiltrate.

of predominantly perivascular lymphocytes, histiocytes and neutrophils (1–3,13). A vasculitis is not seen. In some cases, there is focal necrosis of the superficial dermis. Prominent secondary changes in late lesions may obscure the characteristic findings.

Pathogenesis. The eruption of HV is induced by bright summer sunlight (1–3,13,14). Artificial induction is more difficult and requires repeated broad-spectrum or, less reliably, UVB skin exposure; exact action spectra have not been determined. Blood, urine, and stool porphyrin concentra-

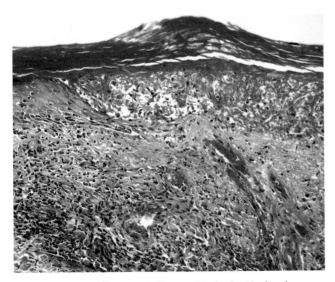

FIGURE 12-9. Hydroa vacciniforme. Marked reticular degeneration of the epidermis at the edge of the lesion and very superficial dermal necrosis with fibrin deposition.

tions, lesional viral studies, and circulating viral, antinuclear factor, and extractable nuclear antibody titers are generally normal, notwithstanding sporadic recent suggestions of occasional Epstein–Barr virus infection (15). Further, the dermal perivascular mononuclear cell infiltration of HV and its clinical resemblance to PMLE suggest possible similar pathogeneses for the two disorders. Arguably, both are DTH-type immunological responses to UVR-induced, endogenous, cutaneous antigen; in HV, the location of the putative antigen, a toxic photoproduct, or the intensity of the reaction, may conceivably lead to the scarring.

Differential Diagnosis. HV must be differentiated from cutaneous viral disorders, the porphyrias, lupus erythematosus, and the other idiopathic, probably immunologically based photodermatoses by its clinical features and largely diagnostic histopathology, provided always that appropriate viral studies, blood, urine, and stool porphyrin concentrations, and circulating antinuclear factor and extractable nuclear antibody titers are also normal. The pattern of necrosis is however remarkably similar to that seen in viral, including herpetic, infections, and hand, foot, and mouth disease. Nevertheless, distinction from herpetic infection is easy, as HV lesional biopsies lack viral inclusions, multinucleated keratinocytes and nuclei with ground glass appearance. In addition, in HV hair follicle necrosis is lacking. Distinction from hand, foot, and mouth disease, on the other hand, is more difficult, but the clinical settings of the two diseases are totally different. Finally, a T-cell lymphoma variant with facial necrotic lesions simulating HV has been described in Asian and Central American Indian children (15), but histologic distinction is not difficult as atypical lymphoid cells are readily apparent in the lymphomatous infiltrate.

CHRONIC ACTINIC DERMATITIS

Chronic actinic dermatitis (CAD) (photosensitivity dermatitis and actinic reticuloid syndrome, persistent light reaction) is a rare, persistent, often disabling, UVR- and occasionally visible light–induced eczema of exposed and sometimes also covered sites (1–3,16). The condition is most common in older men and at temperate latitudes, and most severe in summer. It may affect previously normal subjects, or patients with prior endogenous eczema, photoallergic or allergic contact dermatitis, perhaps oral drug photosensitivity, or even rarely PMLE; allergic contact sensitivity to ubiquitous airborne, sometimes photoactive, agents often coexists. There is an itchy, scattered, or confluent, subacute or chronic eczema of the exposed skin; this may be lichenified or excoriated or, in more severely affected patients, composed of erythematous, shiny, infiltrated, discrete or coalescent papules or plaques on a background of erythema, eczema, or normal skin. Erythroderma is also possible. Malignant transformation has occasionally been claimed but never convincingly demonstrated, although a CAD response from the onset of cutaneous T-cell lymphoma seems perhaps rarely possible. In the past, UVB- and UVA-induced (and occasionally also visible light-induced) pseudolymphomatous CAD has been known as actinic reticuloid; UVB-induced eczematous CAD, as photosensitive eczema or photosensitivity dermatitis; UVB-induced and UVA-induced eczematous CAD, as photosensitivity dermatitis; and CAD following photoallergic contact dermatitis, as persistent light reaction. CAD treatment is often difficult—the restriction of UVR exposure, wearing of appropriately protective clothing, application of high-protection broad-spectrum sunscreens, and avoidance of exacerbating contact allergens is only relatively rarely effective. If these measures fail, therefore, intermittent oral steroid therapy, low-dose PUVA under initial high-dose oral steroid cover, or immunosuppressive therapy with azathioprine or cyclosporine may be necessary; the disease does, however, sometimes slowly remit (17).

Histology. In early CAD, the histology (1–3,16,18) may resemble that of any other spongiotic process, including eczema and contact dermatitis, with epidermal spongiosis, lymphocytic exocytosis, and a superficial and deep, perivascular, lymphohistiocytic, inflammatory infiltrate. In older lesions, however, there is variable, often marked, acanthosis of the epidermis and infundibular portions of hair follicles (Fig. 12-10), while spongiosis and lymphocytic exocytosis may be focally prominent (Fig. 12-11). Secondary changes from excoriation are also frequent in both early and late disease, and consist of focal epidermal necrosis, scale-crust formation, dermoepidermal junction fibrin deposition, and neutrophils with nuclear dust. In

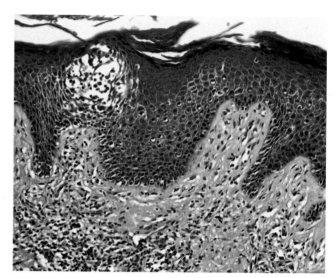

FIGURE 12-11. Chronic actinic dermatitis. Lichenification in association with prominent spongiotic changes and exocytosis of lymphocytes.

addition, there may be occasional Pautrier microabscess-like collections of cells, usually of the Langerhans type. In the papillary dermis, vertically streaked collagen, stellate fibroblasts, and small, multinucleated cells, often described as Montgomery giant cells (Fig. 12-12), are frequently present; these latter, however, may commonly occur in any chronic inflammatory process. Deep in the dermis, there is often a predominantly perivascular, usually dense, mononuclear cell infiltrate of mainly T-lymphocytes, histiocytes, eosinophils, and plasma cells; in severe CAD, this may be even more prominent, along

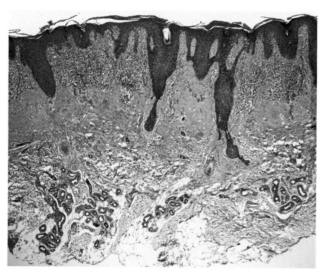

FIGURE 12-10. Chronic actinic dermatitis. Older lesion with prominent hyperplasia of epidermis and infundibular portion of hair follicles.

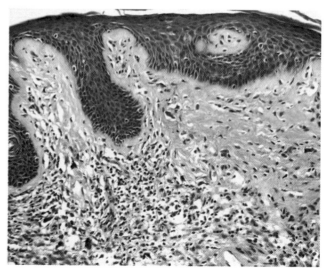

FIGURE 12-12. Chronic actinic dermatitis. Fibrosis of papillary dermis with mononuclear inflammatory cells and scattered small giant cells.

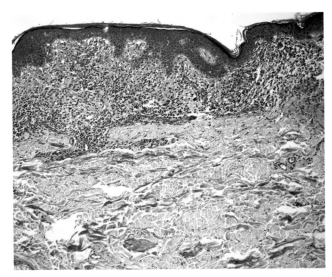

FIGURE 12-13. Chronic actinic dermatitis/actinic reticuloid. Prominent superficial dermal mononuclear cell infiltrate focally obscuring dermoepidermal junction.

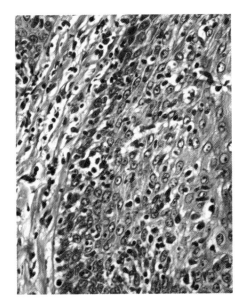

FIGURE 12-15. Chronic actinic dermatitis/actinic reticuloid. A Pautrier-like microabscess within infundibulum of hair follicle.

with marked focal epidermal lymphocyte exocytosis (Fig. 12-13), and a degree of irregularity of nuclear outline (Figs. 12-14 and 12-15). In such cases, formerly included within the term actinic reticuloid, distinction from cutaneous T-cell lymphoma may often be difficult, although it has been suggested that the T-lymphocytes in such cases have a diagnostically helpful, predominantly CD8 (cytotoxic) positive phenotype; most other reactive infiltrates and cutaneous T-cell lymphomas instead are mostly CD4 (helper) positive (19). Personal experience, however, suggests that this is not always so, as infiltrating helper T-lymphocytes are often prominent in CAD as well.

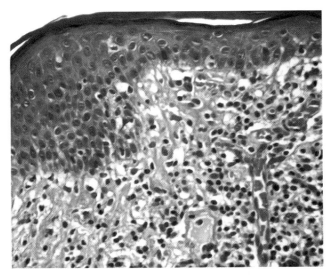

FIGURE 12-14. Chronic actinic dermatitis/actinic reticuloid. Focal epidermal exocytosis of lymphocytes, some displaying irregular nuclear outlines.

Pathogenesis. CAD is clinically and histologically reproducible at all skin sites in the absence of exogenous photosensitizer by UVB alone, UVB and UVA combined, or rarely UVB, UVA, and short visible radiation altogether. The clinical features and pattern of dermal cellular infiltration, cytokine production, and adhesion molecule activation are all essentially indistinguishable from those of allergic contact dermatitis. In that the latter is a known DTH response (1–3,16), therefore, it seems highly likely that the CAD reaction is also, presumably against photo-activated endogenous, cutaneous antigen. Further, action spectrum studies suggest that the UVR absorber initiating the process may conceivably be DNA or a similar or associated molecule (20). In addition, the concomitant airborne allergic contact dermatitis common in CAD may perhaps increase cutaneous immune responsiveness and thus putative antigen recognition. On the other hand, the frequently photoaged skin of CAD may conceivably lead instead or as well to diminished normal UVR-induced cutaneous immunosuppression, and again greater antigen recognition, as well as to easier antigen penetration and slower clearance, all further potentiating disease development.

Differential Diagnosis. CAD must be distinguished from other eczemas, in particular the seborrheic and atopic forms, from airborne and topical medicament contact dermatitis, and from cutaneous T-cell lymphoma. However, in that its histologic appearances are indistinguishable from those of other subacute or chronic spongiotic processes, or in its severe forms from cutaneous T-cell lymphoma, a clinical history is essential for firm diagnosis. Nevertheless, severe CAD is generally separable from lymphoma by its superficial dermal fibrosis, paucity of cytologically atypical lympho-cytes, and at least focal prominent spongiosis.

SOLAR URTICARIA

Solar urticaria (SU) is a rare UVR- or visible radiation–induced whealing of exposed skin; the more common primary SU occurs spontaneously, and the rare secondary form follows photosensitization to drugs or chemicals (1–3,21). Primary SU is slightly more common in women, with onset between the ages of 10 and 50 years. The eruption develops on exposed skin within 5 to 10 minutes, fading within an hour or two; regularly uncovered sites such as face and backs of hands are sometimes spared. A tingling sensation and patchy erythema generally precede separate or confluent whealing, the latter sometimes generalized and possibly associated with headache, nausea, bronchospasm, faintness, or systemic collapse. Secondary SU generally follows exposure to substances such as tar, pitch, dyes, drugs such as benoxaprofen, or rarely the endogenous metabolite protoporphyrin in erythropoietic protoporphyria. Avoidance of the inducing radiation, use of appropriate sunscreens, or medication with adequate doses of nonsedating antihistamines may help around half of patients. Resistant cases may instead respond to PUVA or plasmapheresis, but some SU patients do poorly with all therapies.

Histopathology. The epidermis appears unremarkable. In the dermis, there is edema as evidenced by mild collagen bundle separation, along with slight, rarely moderate, perivascular and interstitial inflammatory cell infiltration with

eosinophils, and occasionally also neutrophils and lymphocytes (1–3,21,22) (Fig. 12-16).

Pathogenesis. Any UVR or visible radiation waveband, specific for a given patient, may induce primary SU (1–3, 21). Whealing is probably mediated through allergic type I hypersensitivity to cutaneous or circulating, irradiation-induced allergen; presumed circulating antibodies have also been identified, very likely IgE in type. In secondary SU, the eruption apparently follows nonimmunological direct tissue injury. Histamine is probably the major chemical mediator in both forms.

Differential Diagnosis. Clinically, SU must be differentiated from other light-induced eruptions by its much shorter time course and characteristic whealing, and from other forms of urticaria, particularly heat induced; histological distinction, however, is not possible. The porphyrias, drug and chemical photosensitivity, and lupus erythematosus must also be excluded for final diagnosis.

REFERENCES

1. Hawk JLM. Cutaneous photobiology. In: Champion RH, Burton JL, Burns DA, et al., eds. *Rook/Wilkinson/Ebling Textbook of Dermatology*, 6th ed. Oxford: Blackwell Science, 1998: 973–993.
2. Hawk JLM, Norris PG. Abnormal responses to ultraviolet radiation: idiopathic. In: Freedberg IM, Eisen ZA, Wolff K, et al., eds. *Dermatology in General Medicine*, 5th ed. New York: McGraw-Hill, 1999:1573–1589.
3. Norris PG, Hawk JLM. The idiopathic photodermatoses: polymorphic light eruption, actinic prurigo and hydroa vacciniforme. In: JLM Hawk, ed. *Photodermatology*. London: Arnold, 1999:178–190.
4. Epstein JH. Polymorphous light eruption. *J Am Acad Dermatol* 1980;3:329–343.
5. Hölzle E, Plewig G, Hofmann C, et al. Polymorphous light eruption—experimental induction of lesions. *J Am Acad Dermatol* 1982;7:111–125.
6. Grabczynska, SA, McGregor JM, Hawk JLM, et al. The histologic spectrum of actinic prurigo and polymorphic light eruption. *Am J Dermatopathol* 2004 *(submitted for publication)*.
7. Norris PG, Morris J, McGibbon DM, et al. Polymorphic light eruption: an immunopathological study of evolving lesions. *Br J Dermatol* 1989;120:173–183.
8. van de Pas CB, Hawk JLM, Young AR, et al. Patients with polymorphic light eruption are resistant to UVR-induced suppression of the contact hypersensitivity response. *J Invest Dermatol* 2004;122:286–292.
9. Lane PR, Murphy F, Hogan DJ, et al. Histopathology of actinic prurigo. *Am J Dermatopathol* 1993;15:326–331.
10. Herrera-Geopfert R, Magaña M. Follicular cheilitis. A distinctive histopathologic finding in actinic prurigo. *Am J Dermatopathol* 1995;17:357–361.
11. Vega-Memije ME, Mosqueda-Taylor A, Irigoyen-Camacho ME, et al. Actinic prurigo cheilitis: clinicopathologic analysis and therapeutic results in 116 cases. *Oral Surg Oral Med Oral Pathol Oral Radiol Endod* 2002;94:83–91.
12. Menagé HduP, Vaughan RW, Baker CS, et al. HLA-DR4 may determine expression of actinic prurigo in British patients. *J Invest Dermatol* 1996;106:362–364.

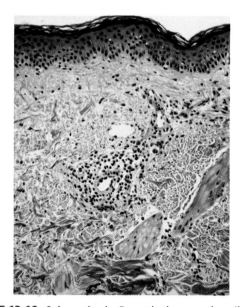

FIGURE 12-16. Solar urticaria. Dermal edema, and a mild interstitial and perivascular inflammatory cell infiltrate of lymphocytes and eosinophils.

13. Sonnex TS, Hawk JLM. Hydroa vacciniforme: a review of ten cases. *Br J Dermatol* 1988;118:101–108.
14. Gupta G, Man I, Kemmett D. Hydroa vacciniforme: a clinical and follow-up study of 17 cases. *J Am Acad Dermatol* 2000;42: 208–213.
15. Cho KH, Kim CW, Heo DS, et al. Epstein–Barr virus-associated peripheral T-cell lymphoma in adults with hydroa vacciniforme-like lesions. *Clin Exp Dermatol* 2001;26:242–247.
16. Menagé HduP, Hawk JLM. The idiopathic photodermatoses: chronic actinic dermatitis. In: JLM Hawk, ed. *Photodermatology*. London: Arnold, 1999;190–202.
17. Dawe RS, Crombie IK, Ferguson J. The natural history of chronic actinic dermatitis. *Arch Dermatol* 2000;136:1215–1220.
18. Toonstra J. Actinic reticuloid. *Semin Diagn Pathol* 1991;8:109–116.
19. Chu AC, Robinson D, Hawk JLM, et al. Immunologic differentiation of the Sézary syndrome due to cutaneous T-cell lymphoma and chronic actinic dermatitis. *J Invest Dermatol* 1986; 86:134–137.
20. Menagé HduP, Harrison GI, Potten CS, et al. The action spectrum for induction of chronic actinic dermatitis is similar to that for sunburn inflammation. *Photochem Photobiol* 1995;62:976.
21. Hölzle E. The idiopathic photodermatoses: solar urticaria. In: JLM Hawk, ed. *Photodermatology*. London: Arnold, 1999;203–210.
22. Leiferman K, Norris PG, Murphy GM, et al. Evidence for eosinophil degranulation with deposition of granule major basic protein in solar urticaria. *J Am Acad Dermatol*, 1989;21:75–80.

DISORDERS ASSOCIATED WITH PHYSICAL AGENTS: HEAT, COLD, RADIATION, AND TRAUMA

JACQUELINE M. JUNKINS-HOPKINS

Physical injury to the skin can result in a number of disorders of the epidermis, dermis, and/or subcutis, depending on the type of agent exposure. Direct injury to the skin by radiation and temperature-associated exposure results in distinct histopathologic skin alterations that are discussed in this chapter. Disorders due to direct physical injury and surgical-related injury also are discussed; however, cutaneous alterations associated with cosmetic-associated procedures such as reactions to injectable material (e.g., silicone) are discussed elsewhere. Conditions that have other pathogenesis, but may be related to temperature or physical exposure, such as Raynaud's phenomenon, physical urticaria, and cold panniculitis, are discussed in Chapters 10, 7, and 20, respectively.

HEAT-ASSOCIATED INJURIES

The effect of heat on the skin is determined by the skin thickness, and degree, extent, and duration of heat exposure. The source of the heat also influences the degree of tissue injury. For instance, dry heat results in charring and desiccation, while moist heat results in opaque coagulation. Immersion burns are more severe than flash and splatter burns, and electrical burns result in deep tissue necrosis (1). Exposure of the skin to extreme heat results in a first-, second- or third-degree burn, while prolonged or repetitive exposure to less intense heat results in changes of erythema ab igne. Surgery-related electrodesiccation-induced injury also has distinct histopathologic features, and is discussed at the end of the chapter.

BURNS

Tissue injury from direct exposure to heat is defined by the depth (partial or full thickness) or extent (first, second, or third degree) of tissue injury. The resultant tissue injury is a sequel of the release of inflammatory and vasoactive media-

tors released due to denaturation and coagulation of proteins, and edema from increased capillary permeability (2). Painful erythema and edema without vesiculation is seen in first-degree burns; vesiculation and blisters characterize superficial second-degree burns, which progress to pallor and anesthesia if both the epidermis and dermis are injured; and third-degree burns show massive necrosis with charring, denuded superficial tissue, granulation tissue, and scar formation (1). Deep second-degree burns and third-degree burns show overlapping features. Secondary bacterial infections may cause the injury of a superficial second-degree burn to extend deeper, with changes similar to a third-degree burn.

Histopathology. In first-degree burns, vasodilatation is the predominant feature. Epidermal and subepidermal edema may progress to partial thickness superficial epidermal necrosis. Full-thickness epidermal necrosis differentiates second from first-degree burns.

In superficial second-degree burns, partial to full-thickness necrosis and edema of the epidermis and subepidermal stroma result in blister formation. Typically, epidermal necrosis and separation from the dermis at the dermal–epidermal junction or within necrotic basilar keratinocytes are seen (Fig. 13-1). Although initially vasoconstriction occurs, biopsies show prominent vasodilatation and edema in the dermis. Necrotic changes may extend into the lower reticular dermis in deep second-degree burns, but the appendages tend to be spared, differentiating a second-degree from a third-degree burn.

In third-degree burns, full-thickness coagulation necrosis of the epidermis and dermis, including the appendages is seen (Fig. 13-1). The resultant scar is characterized by hyalinized collagen and absence of adnexal structures (Fig. 13-2).

Differential Diagnosis: Radiation dermatitis is differentiated from burn scars by the presence of atypical radiation fibroblasts in the former. Complete absence of the adnexal structures favors a burn scar, as the eccrine glands may be spared with radiation. In morphea/scleroderma, there is preservation of eccrine coils, and a lymphoplasmacellular infiltrate may be seen.

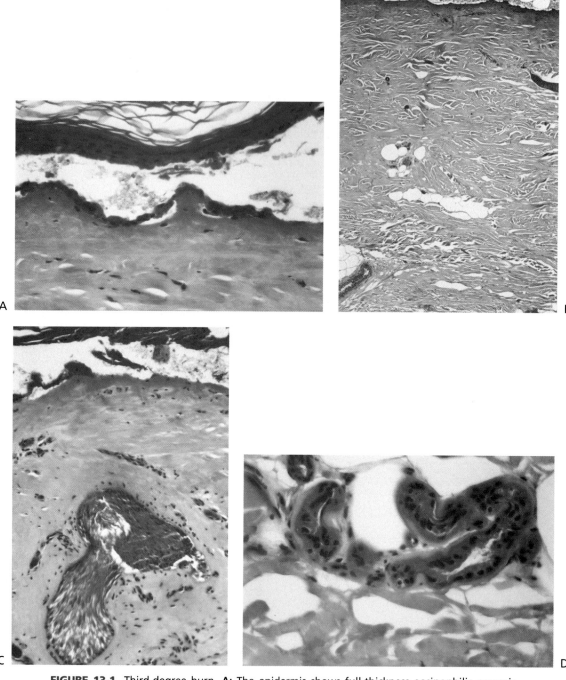

FIGURE 13-1. Third-degree burn. **A:** The epidermis shows full-thickness eosinophilic necrosis resulting in bullous disassociation from the dermis and incipient denution. This bulla formation can be seen in second- and third-degree burns. The collagen shows homogenized necrosis, with loss of distinction between collagen bundles. The fibroblasts are nonatypical, differentiating this from chronic radiation injury. **B:** There is pandermal eosinophilic homogenized alteration collagen, with necrosis of an eccrine gland. The epidermis shows bulla formation. **C:** Extension of the injury involving the pilosebaceous units differentiates a third-degree from a superficial second-degree burn. Burn injury to the pilosebaceous unit results in eosinophilic necrosis of the epithelium and elongation of the nuclei. The surrounding stroma shows coagulation of the collagen and vascular thrombosis. **D:** Eosinophilic alteration of an injured eccrine gland differentiates third- from second- and first-degree burns.

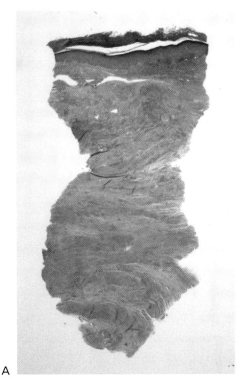

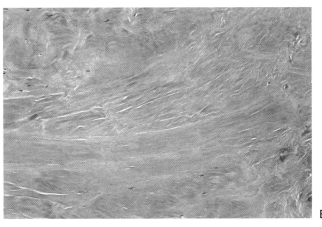

A
B

FIGURE 13-2. Chronic burn scar. **A:** The dermis and subcutis are diffusely sclerotic and homogenized, with compete absence of adnexal structures, including arrector pili muscles, differentiating this from radiation injury and scleroderma/morphea. The absence of vascular proliferation and presence of homogenized thickening of the collagen differentiates a chronic burn from a scar from other reparative causes. **B:** The sclerotic collagen is nearly devoid of fibroblasts, in particular atypical ones, differentiating this from chronic radiation injury.

Burn Scar–Associated Carcinoma

Carcinomas, especially basal cell carcinomas, may arise acutely, within 2 to 3 months after the injury (1). Delayed carcinomas arise after a latent period that ranges from 10 to 70 years, and include squamous more often than basal cell carcinomas. The occurrence of cancer developing in burn scars was noted in 1860 by Heurteux, and like trauma-induced carcinomas were described by Marjolin in 1828; these cancers are more aggressive than their sun-induced counterparts. Metastases may occur in approximately one-third of the cases. The carcinomas arise from the edges of wounds or from epithelial remnants entrapped in the scar, and thus may not occur as frequently if there has been grafting (1).

Acute Ultraviolet Burn

Mild ultraviolet-induced burns or sunburns resulting in erythema are characterized by the presence of scattered apoptotic keratinocytes, "sunburn cells," and variable subepidermal edema. Clinical blistering may result from severe burns due to full-thickness epidermal necrosis and/or dermal edema (Fig. 13-3). The preservation of appendages allows epidermal regeneration.

Ultraviolet Recall

This is also known as sunburn reactivation, and refers to the phenomenon in which a medication, typically methotrexate, induces an acute cutaneous eruption restricted to the area of previous sunburn (3). The recall phenomenon

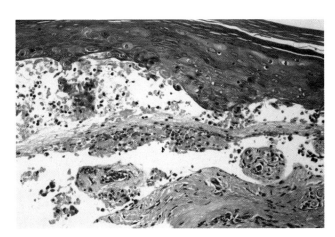

FIGURE 13-3. Acute ultraviolet radiation burn. This is an example of a UVA-induced burn showing full-thickness dyskeratotic keratinocytes throughout all layers of the epidermis, with subepidermal blister formation.

generally occurs if methotrexate was given 1 to 5 days after sunburn, not if the burn is concomitant or much earlier. With methotrexate, the reaction tends to show features of vesiculobullous sunburn, and in most cases is more severe than the initial sunburn. Some antibiotics have also been associated with a variety of ultraviolet recall reactions (3,4), which differ from the methotrexate reaction. Antibiotic-related reactions tend to occur at a later interval from the burn, with a less severe, more morbilliform-like drug reaction (3). Changes of toxic epidermal necrolysis have rarely been reported with trimethoprim sulfa (5).

ERYTHEMA AB IGNE

Clinically, erythema ab igne presents as reticulated brown to erythematous patches, typically on the shins, buttocks, or lower back (Fig. 13-4). This is associated with repetitive exposure to open hearths, stoves, or steam heaters. Prolonged repeated contact with heating pads or hot water bottles can also result in erythema ab igne.

Histopathology. Biopsies of erythema ab igne show variable histopathologic features, which are nonspecific in the absence of clinical-pathologic correlation. The bi-

opsy may appear normal on hematoxylin and eosin staining, with the exception of increased epidermal atrophy and/or rete effacement, and pigment incontinence. Interface dermatitis, characterized by mild basal vacuolization, necrotic keratinocytes, and subtle squamatization has been described in the early stages (6). The dermis shows dilation and congestion of postcapillary venules and a mild but variable perivascular infiltrate of lymphocytes, histiocytes, melanophages, and neutrophils (6–8) (Fig. 13-4). Elastic stains demonstrate an increased amount of elastic tissue in the upper and mid dermis, and Alcian blue stains may reveal an increase in hyaluronic acid. Deposition of iron has been described (7), but this may reflect the anatomic site of the lower legs (8). Basal keratinocytic atypia and frank squamous cell carcinoma *in situ* have been reported in erythema ab igne of the lower leg (9).

Differential Diagnosis. The elastic tissue alteration induced by ultraviolet radiation in solar elastosis is apparent on hematoxylin and eosin stains as solid and homogenized material, as opposed to erythema ab igne, which shows no perceptible elastic changes on routine staining. Erythema chronicum perstans may also show subtle interface dermatitis with pigment dropout, but is distinguished from erythema ab igne by the clinical presentation and the ab-

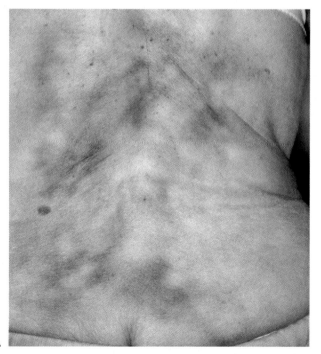

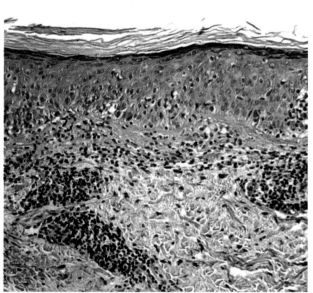

A B

FIGURE 13-4. Erythema ab igne. **A:** Clinically, reticulated brown patches are seen in erythema ab igne. This may present on the lower back where there has been frequent use of a heating pad. **B:** Erythema ab igne has variable histologic features. This hematoxylin and eosin stained biopsy shows a perivascular lymphocytic infiltrate in the superficial dermis that focally disrupts the dermal-epidermal interface. There is no discernible elastic fiber abnormality noted on routine staining. The absence of clumped basophilic elastic tissue differentiates erythema ab igne from solar elastosis. *(continued)*

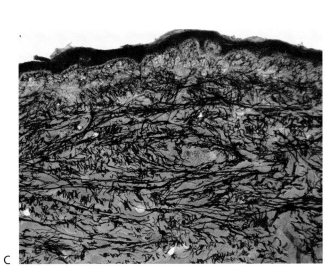

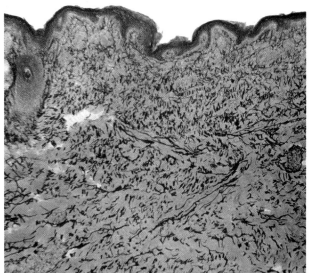

C

D

FIGURE 13-4. *(continued)* **C:** Staining for elastic tissue highlights the increased amount of elastic tissue, in comparison to uninvolved skin (see *D*), characteristic of erythema ab igne. **D:** Elastic staining of uninvolved skin, showing a normal distribution of elastic fibers, as compared with *(C)*. (Photographs courtesy of Waine Johnson, M.D.)

sence of increased elastic fibers. A hypersensitivity reaction with interface changes may show some overlapping features, but the clinical history should prompt elastic tissue staining, differentiating the two entities.

RADIATION-INDUCED SKIN ALTERATIONS

Cutaneous alterations due to irradiation include acute and chronic radiation dermatitis, radiation recall dermatitis, and secondary cutaneous neoplasms. The inflammatory changes that occur in the skin after irradiation, or radiation dermatitis, occur as a result of biochemical changes on x-ray penetrated cells, without a detectable rise in temperature. The resultant injury is determined by the threshold radiation dose. In addition to the dose of irradiation, host factors play a role in the development of radiation dermatitis, such as in ataxia telangiectasia homozygotes, which have up to three-fold normal radiation sensitivity (10). Patients with underlying conditions such as connective tissue disease, diabetes mellitus, and hyperthyroid disease have been reported to have an exaggerated reaction to radiotherapy (11). Concomitant use of radiation sensitizers, such as doxorubicin and taxane antineoplastic agents may predispose an individual to increased acute toxicity reactions to radiation (12). In contrast, radiation-induced cancer is a stochastic effect; thus, the risk of developing a neoplasm is independent of the dose. Fluoroscopically guided procedures may cause radiation dermatitis in areas of skin not directly in the radiation port, usually the back (11). Radiation recall dermatitis refers to precipitation of an inflammatory reaction limited to a site of a quiescent

radiation field, induced by administration of medication. Other cutaneous consequences of irradiation include vitiligo (13), lichen planus (14), and bullous pemphigoid (15).

Acute, Subacute, and Chronic Radiation Dermatitis

Changes of acute radiation dermatitis may become apparent between two weeks and three months post procedure. Phases of skin injury response have been outlined in detail (11). Erythema, desquamation, alopecia, xerosis, dyschromia, vascular compromise and proliferation with telangiectasia, blistering, epidermal and dermal atrophy and necrosis, and ulceration may be seen in the acute phases. Changes of chronic radiation dermatitis are noted at 1-year postradiation, but often represent progression of acute radiation dermatitis, and thus may be evident earlier. Epidermal atrophy, poikiloderma, hyperkeratosis, telangiectases, and fibrotic thickening of the dermis and subcutaneous tissue are seen. Late-onset dermal necrosis and changes of chronic radiation dermatitis with or without prior acute radiation may be seen years after the initial radiation. Nonhealing ulcers may be seen. Deep megavoltage radiation for noncutaneous malignancies may result in subcutaneous sclerosis that may extend into the underlying skeletal muscle (16).

Histopathology. Histopathologic changes of radiation dermatitis vary with the morphologic lesion biopsied (11).

Acute radiation dermatitis is characterized by scattered pyknotic keratinocytes and epidermal edema. Depending on the dose of radiation, epidermal necrosis with blister formation and sloughing of the epidermis (clinically referred to as "moist desquamation") may be seen. Hyperkeratosis is seen with dry desquamation. Dermal changes include collagen and endothelial cell edema, vasodilatation, erythrocyte extravasation, and fibrin thrombi of vessels. Variable inflammation is noted throughout the dermis, with involvement of the epidermis. Acute necrotic changes similar to that seen in the epidermis also may occur in the adnexal epithelium, eventuating in absence of pilosebaceous structures. Complete destruction of eccrine glands is not com-

mon. In severe radiation injury, necrosis of the epidermis and dermis results in chronic ulceration.

Late-stage or chronic radiation dermatitis is characterized by eosinophilic homogenized sclerosis of the dermal collagen, scattered large bizarre, atypical "radiation fibroblasts," absence of pilosebaceous units, and vascular changes (17) (Fig. 13-5). The deep vessels show fibrous thickening, sometimes with luminal obliteration and re-canalization, while superficially, telangiectases are prominent. The epi-

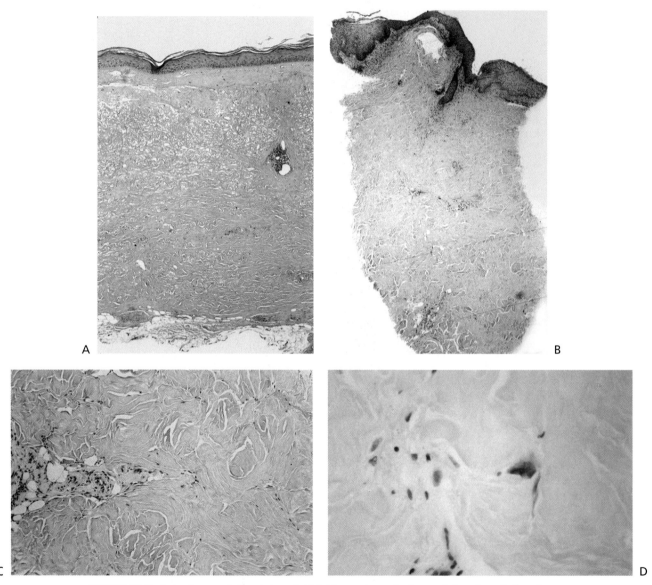

FIGURE 13-5. Late-stage radiation injury. **A:** This biopsy shows features of chronic radiation dermatitis, including epidermal atrophy, pandermal collagen sclerosis with mild lymphocytic inflammation and absence of hair follicles. **B:** A rectangular, "squared-off" silhouette is due to the sclerotic collagen alteration. This biopsy also demonstrates the variation of epidermal atrophy and hyperplasia that can be seen in radiation dermatitis. **C:** There is sclerotic collagen bundle thickening, with compression of eccrine glands. Preservation of eccrine glands differentiates this from a burn scar. **D:** Large bizarre and atypical radiation fibroblasts amid thickened collagen bundles differentiate radiation dermatitis from morphea and third-degree burn scars. These are sparsely scattered, in contrast to atypical cells of a sarcoma. *(continued)*

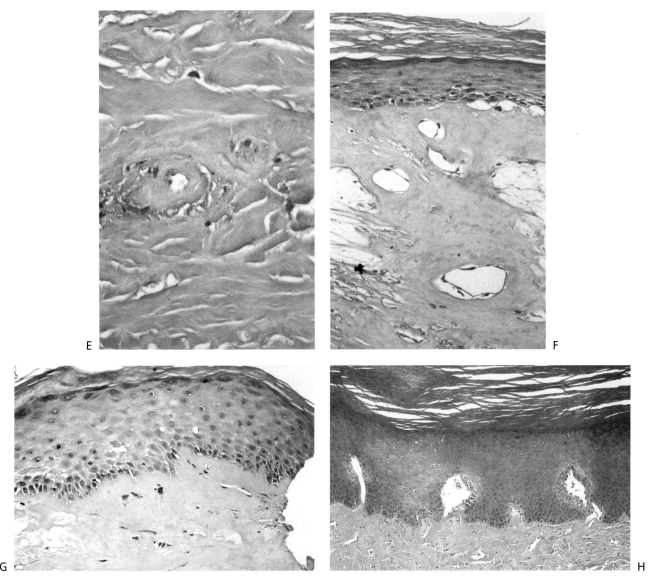

FIGURE 13-5. *(continued)* E: Sclerosis of endothelial cells is seen amidst thickened sclerotic collagen bundles. **F:** There is telangiectasia of the upper dermal vessels, with epidermal atrophy and sclerosis of papillary dermal collagen. **G:** The epidermis shows features of interface dermatitis, with liquefaction of the basal layer, rete effacement, and pigment dropout. **H:** The epidermis may show hyperplasia, incorporating the underlying telangiectatic vessels between the rete.

dermal changes include atrophy and hyperkeratosis, and features of an interface reaction (Fig. 13-5). A maturation disorder with nuclei atypia and individual cell keratinization may be seen. Juxtaposed to atrophic areas may be epidermal hyperplasia that may extend downward and encase the telangiectatic vessels.

The origin of the radiation fibroblast is not known. Immunohistochemical studies have shown diffuse positive cytoplasmic staining of the radiation fibroblasts with antibody to factor XIIIa, with only focal staining with antibody to CD34 in some cells (18). However, others have not demonstrated as consistent factor XIIIa staining.

The cells are negative for HHF-35 (muscle-specific actin), Ki-67, and P53 (19).

Subacute radiodermatitis applies to the phase of radiation injury in which there are overlapping features of acute and chronic radiation dermatitis. The histology is that of an interface dermatitis, with basal vacuolization and keratinocyte necrosis (20) (Fig. 13-6). The presence of satellite cell necrosis, characterized by close apposition of necrotic keratinocytes and CD8+, TIA-1+ T-lymphocytes, suggests cytotoxic lymphocyte mediated apoptosis is involved in the pathogenesis of subacute radiation dermatitis (21).

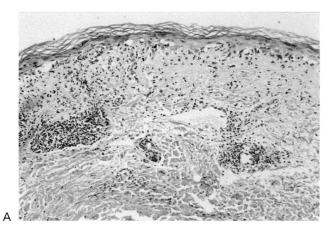

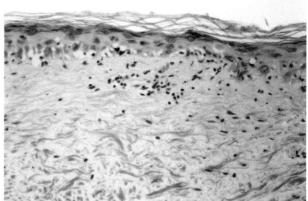

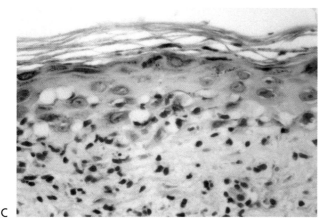

FIGURE 13-6. Subacute radiation dermatitis. **A:** In subacute radiation dermatitis, there is an inflammatory infiltrate involving the epidermis, papillary dermis, and vessels, without sclerotic collagen alteration. The epidermis is atrophic due to interface dermatitis. **B:** The interface dermatitis of subacute radiation dermatitis is indistinguishable from those of some other causes of interface dermatitis, such as fixed drug eruption and graft-versus-host disease, requiring clinical information to differentiate these entities. Lymphocytes disrupt the basal cell layer, and are associated with vacuolization of the basal keratinocytes, dyskeratotic keratinocytes, and pigment dropout. Note that the collagen is nonsclerotic, and the fibroblasts are nonatypical, in contrast to that in Figure 13-4B and C, which represent a later stage of this process. **C:** Satellite cell necrosis, or close approximation of lymphocytes with apoptotic keratinocytes is seen in subacute radiation dermatitis as well as in graft-versus-host disease and other cytotoxic dermatoses.

Radiation-induced malignancies include squamous cell carcinomas and basal cell carcinomas, predominantly (22), and these often occur in the background of chronic radiation dermatitis. The squamous cell carcinomas display aggressive, metastasizing behavior, and include spindled variants. True sarcoma-induced radiation malignancies are less common, and usually arise in heavily irradiated tissue with a latent period of 3 to 24 years. These include malignant fibrous histiocytoma, fibrosarcoma, osteosarcoma, liposarcoma, chondrosarcoma, and sarcomas of pluripotential mesenchymal cell derivation (23). Desmoplastic cutaneous leiomyosarcoma has also been reported (24). Mesenchymal sarcomas frequently occur on the chest wall after irradiation for breast carcinoma or Hodgkin's disease (25). Angiosarcomas, including spindled cell variants, may be seen at sites of prior irradiation, usually in conjunction with lymphedematous changes (26). Adjacent changes of chronic radiation dermatitis may be seen, but are not always present.

Differential Diagnosis. Subacute radiation dermatitis may be indistinguishable from graft-versus-host disease and fixed drug eruption (27,28). The latter is particularly difficult to differentiate from subacute radiation dermatitis in fluoroscopy-induced cases, since the changes often do not occur at the irradiation portal site; thus, the clinician may be unaware of the association with radiation injury. Morphea/scleroderma is favored over chronic radiation dermatitis by the absence of radiation fibroblasts. Lichen sclerosis may show similar telangiectasia and interface alteration, and there can be similarity in the papillary dermal pallor and homogenization, but the presence of deeper, thickened, eosinophilic collagen bundles with radiation fibroblasts favor radiation changes. Clinical correlation may be confirmatory. Deep burn scars show complete absence of all adnexal structures without abnormal fibroblasts, in contrast to radiation sclerosis, where the eccrine glands are often preserved. Radiation sarcomas should be differentiated from spindled squamous cell carcinoma by immunohistochemical staining (see Chapter 32).

Radiation Recall Dermatitis

The phenomenon of radiation recall has been extensively reviewed (29). Typical medications implicated include chemotherapeutic agents, especially the taxane family, methotrexate, and high-dose interferon alfa 2b (30). Ingestion or infusion of these medications results in an acute inflammatory reaction in a previously quiescent radiation field. It may occur from days to weeks, and sometimes years, after radiation therapy, and acute toxicity need not have occurred with the initial radiation. The exact pathophysiology of the reaction is currently unknown. Radiation recall reactions should be differentiated from radiosensitivity, which represents a reaction induced by drugs given less than 7 days after radiotherapy (29).

Histopathology. At sites of prior radiation therapy, a spectrum of epidermal changes similar to those in acute radiation dermatitis is seen, and includes bulla formation due to prominent interface dermatitis (31). Dermal changes may reflect an element of previous chronic radiation dermatitis, and include fibrosis and radiation fibroblasts.

COLD INJURY TO THE SKIN

Direct injury to the skin due to extremes in cold temperatures can be seen in frostbite and nonfreezing cold injury. In the latter, there is injury above the freezing point, associated with wet, immobile, venous stagnation conditions, such as trench foot. Both types of cold injury have a similar pathogenesis, which includes cyclic massive vasoconstriction and excessive vasodilation, endothelial cell leakage, erythestasis, arteriovenous shunting, segmental vascular necrosis, possibly due to decreased clearance of toxic substances, and massive thrombosis (32).

Frostbite

Frostbite is typically seen on acral sites, and results from tissue freezing. An increased susceptibility is seen in patients with alcohol consumption, constrictive clothing, peripheral vascular disease, smokers, and in windy conditions. Frostbite can be categorized based on the depth of injury. First degree is characterized by erythema and edema after thawing that does not blister and subsides within several days. In second degree, within the first 1 to 2 days following re-warming, there is blister formation. This is followed by necrotic eschar formation and eventual autoamputation of the affected area. In third degree, the entire dermis is edematous, and may remain so for a month or more (1).

Pernio (Chilblain)

Pernio (chilblain) is a distinct form of cold-induced injury in which humidity, in addition to cold, plays a role in inducing the condition (33). There are acute and chronic presentations. Chilblain classically presents in young to middle-aged women as painful, burning, and/or pruritic erythematous to violaceous or cyanotic macules, papules, deep nodules, and plaques on the fingers, toes, distal extremities, and rarely the face. Involvement of the thighs has been described in association with river crossings (34). The acute form is more common in young women. Lesions are noted within 12 to 14 hours of exposure in the acute form, and persist for 10 to 14 days. The lesions may become hemorrhagic, bullous, or ulcerated, but they tend to be self-limited. The chronic form has overlapping features with acute pernio, but occurs in middle-age women and, with repeated winter recurrences, may result in slow-to-heal ulcers and scarring. A genetic predisposition has been implied, as well as a history of peripheral vascular disease (33). A childhood variant has been described, and is associated with cryoproteins (35).

Pernio may arise in conjunction with histopathologic, clinical, and serologic features of lupus, and is referred to as chilblain lupus erythematosus or lupus pernio (36–39). Clinically, antibodies to SSA/Ro are seen, with associated Raynaud's phenomenon. Patients with chilblain lupus erythematosus may present without over lupus, but are at risk of progressing to systemic lupus erythematosus from 1 to 10 years later (39).

Histopathology. There is a superficial and deep T-lymphocytic infiltrate around the small venules and arterioles in the dermis and subcutis, with accentuation around the deep eccrine coils (Fig. 13-7). The interstitium may also be prominently involved in the superficial dermis. The infiltrate tends to be of moderate intensity, but may be dense. The most superficial vessels of the papillary dermis are less involved, but the infiltrate may show congestion. Papillary dermal edema is characteristic, and while it may be quite striking, its presence is variable. A superficial variant exists, lacking involvement of the deeper portions of the tissue, but showing papillary dermal edema. Lymphocytic vasculitis, characterized by endothelial cell swelling and edema and infiltration of the vessel walls by lymphocytes, without consistent presence of fibrinoid necrosis is seen (33) (Fig. 13-7). The epidermal changes range from scattered necrotic keratinocytes to epidermal pallor or necrosis. Effacing interface dermatitis is not typically seen in idiopathic pernio. In chilblain lupus erythematosus (lupus pernio), there are dermal changes of pernio with interface dermatitis of lupus and a positive lupus band test.

Differential Diagnosis. Pernio may be difficult to differentiate from lupus erythematosus. The presence of prominent dermal edema, eccrine coil accentuation of the infiltrate, and spongiosis favor pernio over lupus (38). Diagnostic criteria have been proposed to differentiate chilblain lupus erythematosus from idiopathic chilblains (40). The papular form of chilblains may be difficult to differentiate from erythema multiforme, and may require

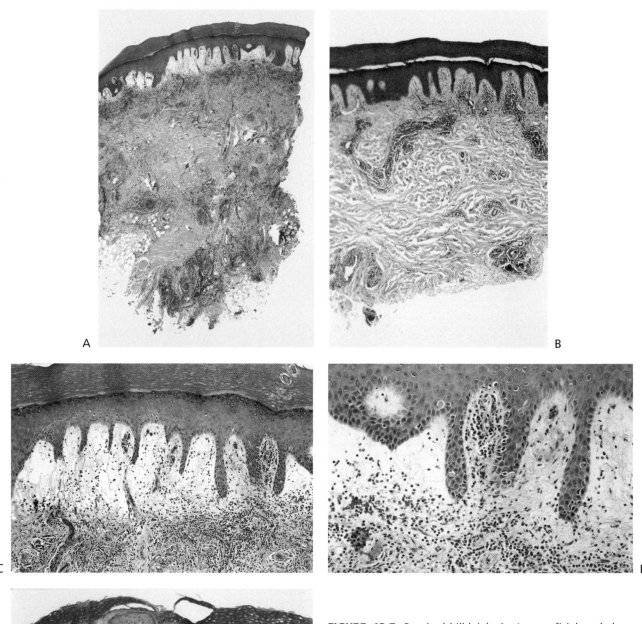

A

B

C

D

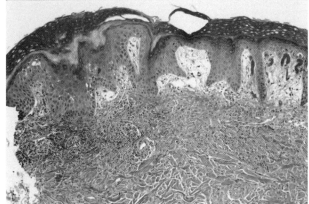

E

FIGURE 13-7. Pernio (chilblain). **A:** A superficial and deep perivascular and perieccrine lymphocytic infiltrate involving acral skin, with striking papillary dermal edema typifies perniosis. **B:** Although papillary dermal edema is characteristic, some cases of pernio may lack this feature. The deep perieccrine infiltrate helps to differentiate this from conditions such as erythema multiforme, which may show some similar features. **C:** Striking dermal edema may result in incipient dermolytic bulla formation. **D:** Involvement of the dermal papillary vessel may be minimal. Dyskeratosis may be present, but a frank interface reaction is not seen. If present, lupus or chilblain lupus should be considered. **E:** The degree of papillary dermal edema may vary. Lymphocytes may be interstitial to band-like, in addition to perivascular. Prominent vascular congestion is seen in the dermal papilla. *(continued)*

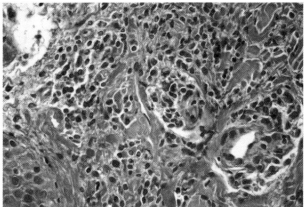

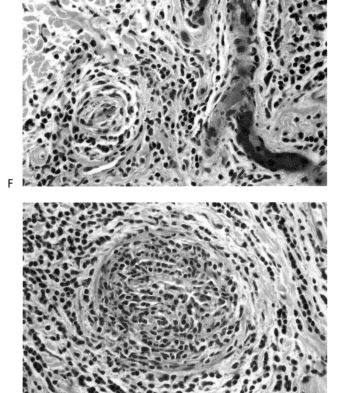

FIGURE 13-7. *(continued)* **F:** Various degrees of vascular damage may be seen. Here there are congestion and vaso-occlusion with early necrosis of one small venule. In a nearby vessel, there is infiltration of the vessel wall, consistent with the lymphocytic vasculitis of pernio. **G:** In pernio, the endothelial cells are often swollen and show infiltration by lymphocytes, without evidence of necrotizing vasculitis. **H:** Medium-sized vessels may occasionally be infiltrated by lymphocytes. A granulomatous, neutrophilic, and or eosinophilic component is not seen, differentiating pernio from other known causes of medium-sized vessel vasculitis.

clinical history to differentiate the two (41). The deep inflammatory component of pernio differentiates it from acral lesions of erythema multiforme. Polymorphous light eruption, dermal hypersensitivity, erythema annulare centrifugum, and Jessner's lymphocytic infiltrate can show a similar pattern of perivascular lymphocytic infiltrate. The presence of lymphocytic vasculitis and the clinical history of cold-induced acral lesions favor pernio. Other clinical and histologic mimickers of pernio include lesions of rheumatoid arthritis, cryofibrinogenemia, antiphospholipid syndrome, and others lack the papillary dermal edema of pernio (42). Occasionally, the lymphocytic infiltrate may be so intense as to simulate cutaneous lymphoma, but the absence of atypia and presence of superficial dermal edema favor pernio.

Cryotherapy-Induced Injury

Cryotherapy is a commonly used tool to destroy benign and premalignant or, on occasion, malignant cutaneous lesions. This procedure may also be employed prior to curettage of keratoses. The dermatopathologist may encounter freeze-related changes in this latter circumstance. Rapid freezing with liquid nitrogen results in the production of highly destructive intracellular ice crystals (2). The extent of injury is determined, in part, by the thickness of the stratum corneum, length of exposure to the liquid nitrogen and the degree of pressure applied (43). Cell types differ in their susceptibility to cold injury. The hypopigmentation seen with cryotherapy reflects the susceptibility of melanocytes to this form of injury.

Histopathology. Microscopic features may differ, depending on the interval between cryotherapy and biopsy. Typically in rapid freeze injury, the keratinocytes show a loss of cell outline, with ghost-like changes or homogenization of the epidermis (Fig. 13-8). This is associated with subepidermal–dermal bulla formation and subepidermal edema. The stratum corneum, being a devitalized structure, is not affected; thus, there will be preservation of parakeratosis (43). There may be loss of melanocytes or pigment at the site of a prior cryotherapy site, with melanocytic hyperplasia or pigment dropout in the adjacent skin (2). With more intense cryotherapy, coagulation rather than edema is seen in the dermis. This may result in coagulation necrosis of hair follicles and possibly eccrine glands, and scar formation of the surrounding collagen. A polymorphous infiltrate, which includes eosinophils, has been described (44). Hemorrhage and thrombosis may be seen in the dermal papilla.

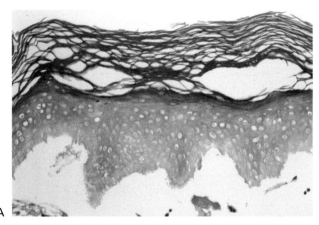
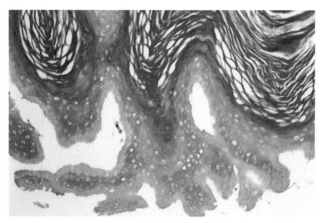

A   B

FIGURE 13-8. Cryotherapy-induced cold injury. **A:** There is pallor of the epidermal keratinocytes, with loss of the cellular outline. **B:** The cold injury has resulted in a subepidermal bulla. In cryotherapy of this seborrheic keratosis, there has been preservation of the stratum corneum architecture, probably due to the devitalized nature of this portion of the epidermis, while the remaining tissue shows homogenization of the epithelium, with disassociation of the epithelium from the dermis in a subepidermal fashion.

CUTANEOUS INJURY DUE TO PHYSICAL TRAUMA

Friction-Induced Blister

Prominent or repetitive shear-induced injury, especially on acral skin, such as the hands and feet results in bulla formation. This may or may not be accompanied by hemorrhage.

Histopathology. A friction blister has an intraepidermal plane of separation, often beneath the stratum granulosum, in the upper portions of the epidermis (Fig. 13-9). The surrounding keratinocytes show pallor and loss of the cell outline. The edge of the blister cavity shows a jagged

outline. The dermis does not show significant alteration or inflammation.

Differential Diagnosis. Other causes of paucicellular blister should be differentiated from friction blisters. Suction blisters and porphyria cutanea tarda have their plane of separation in a subepidermal location. Epidermolysis bullosa and epidermolysis bullosa acquisita may be acrally located, but show a subepidermal bulla and characteristic electron microscopic and immunofluorescence features, respectively (see Chapter 9). Although diabetic bullae are also acral-located noninflammatory blisters, and may have a partially intraepidermal plane, they tend to show a more prominently subepidermal split, without cytolytic keratinocytic changes.

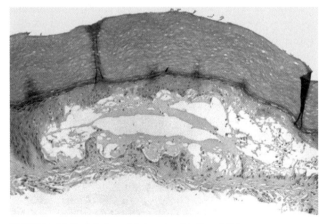

FIGURE 13-9. Friction blister. In friction blisters, one sees a noninflammatory intraepidermal blister, with pallor of the surrounding epidermis. The keratinocytes may show reticular degeneration or other sequelae of cytolysis or shearing.

Talon Noir (Black Heel, Calcaneal Petechiae)

Talon noir typically presents as an irregular black macule on thickly keratinized acral sites, such as the heels and toes. These are often biopsied to exclude acral melanoma. Talon noir often occur in association with athletic activity, and result from shearing forces that lead to stratum corneal hemorrhage (45).

Histopathology. Often, only the stratum corneum is sampled, and shows erythrocytes within layers of a thickened orthokeratotic stratum corneum (Fig. 13-10). Parakeratosis is common. There may be associated serosanguineous fluid, with superficial blister formation. When dermis is incorporated in the biopsy, erythrocytes may be seen in the dermal papillae and epidermis. Iron staining does not highlight this process.

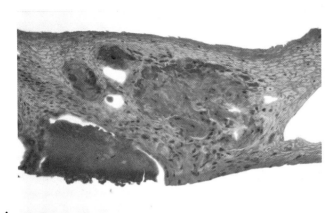

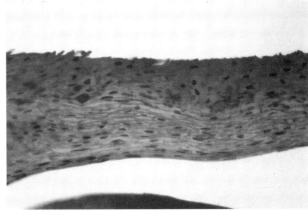

A

B

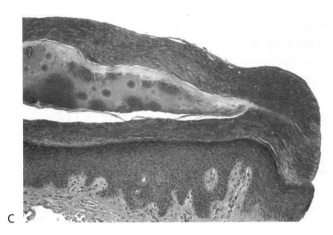

C

FIGURE 13-10. Talon noir (calcaneal petechiae). **A:** Talon noir occurs on acral skin, due to shearing or rubbing trauma; thus one sees a hyperkeratotic stratum corneum, often accompanied by parakeratosis. Often, only portions of the stratum corneum are sampled. The hemorrhage can be identified as loculated erythrocytes and serosanguinous fluid, or as small collections of intracorneal erythrocytes, some of which show degeneration. **B:** The hemorrhage may present as solitary intact or degenerating erythrocytes within the corneal layers. Hemosiderin will not be apparent on hematoxylin or iron staining. **C:** There may be features of a friction blister, with intracorneal hemorrhage accompanied by serosanguinous fluid, forming an intracorneal hemorrhagic bulla.

Acanthoma Fissuratum (Granuloma Fissuratum)

Acanthoma fissuratum occurs at the site of chronic low-grade pressure or rubbing trauma, at the site where eyeglasses sit in the nose or ear. Clinically, there is a pink to flesh-colored plaque or nodule with a central depression, located on the lateral bridge of the nose, near the medial canthus or near the cheek, or at the crease between the postauricular scalp and posterior ear, where the eye glass stem lies. This may be biopsied to exclude nonmelanoma skin cancer.

Histopathology. The epidermis shows prominent non-atypical acanthosis with mild orthohyperkeratosis and hypergranulosis. The rete are wide and blunt-ended, and centrally there is attenuation of the rete, which corresponds to the clinical depression (Fig. 13-11). Spongiosis and parakeratosis may be seen. The dermis shows a proliferation of small, slightly dilated vessels, with a fibrotic stroma and variable patchy chronic inflammation.

Differential Diagnosis. The epidermal and fibrovascular changes noted in acanthoma fissuratum are similar to those seen in chondrodermatitis nodularis helicis (Chapter 18). The latter is differentiated by the location

on the auricle and the presence of fibrinoid dermal necrosis and cartilaginous changes. Lichen simplex chronicus shows some similar features, but shows more dermal fibrosis and vertical orientation of the vessels in the dermal papillae.

Surgery-Associated Injury

Curettage surgery is frequently performed by dermatologists to biopsy, treat, or "define" a superficial basal or squamous cell carcinoma prior to excision. Curettage is frequently followed by electrodesiccation to further destroy remaining tumor and/or to assist in hemostasis.

Histopathology. Electrodesiccation-induced injury results in elongation and stretch distortion of the epithelial nuclei (Fig. 13-12). Basophilic collagen necrosis can be seen beneath a recent electrodesiccation-induced surgical ulcer or scar. This may present with lace-like coagulation necrosis of the collagen and epidermis. At a healing biopsy site, foci of this injured collagen may be seen engulfed by multinucleated giant cells. The dermis beneath a recent curettage ulcer base shows edema, vascular dilation, and congestion, without coagulation necrosis

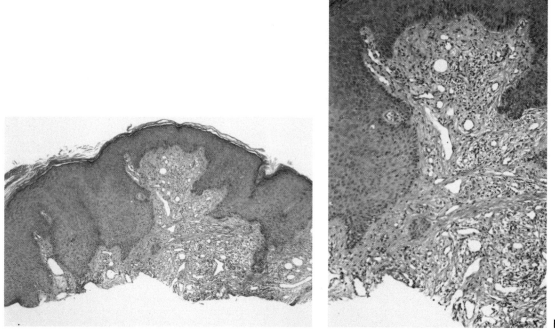

FIGURE 13-11. Acanthoma fissuratum (granuloma fissuratum). **A:** There is nonatypical acanthosis of the epidermis, with attenuation of the rete centrally. **B:** Within the dermis, there is a proliferation of slightly dilated small vessels, associated with fibrosis and a variable chronic inflammatory infiltrate. The term "granuloma" is a misnomer, as a granulomatous infiltrate is not seen.

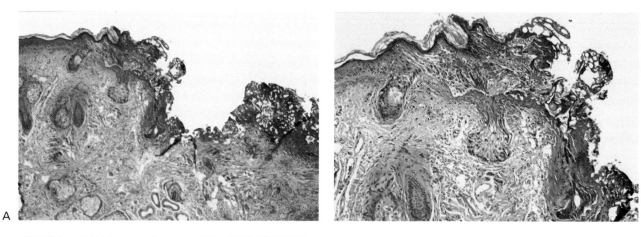

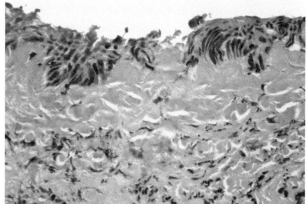

FIGURE 13-12. Electrodessication injury. **A:** There is ulceration of the epidermis and dermis with reticulated lace-like hemorrhagic and basophilic coagulation necrosis of the epidermis and superficial dermis. **B:** Near the edge of the ulcer, the epidermis and follicular epithelium show elongated alteration of the nuclei, with disassociation and blister formation. **C:** The epithelial cells typically show elongation of nuclei in electrodessication injury. Hyperchromasia of nuclei may be seen, simulating atypia, but the stretch artifact and absence of parakeratosis differentiates this from an actinic keratosis. *(continued)*

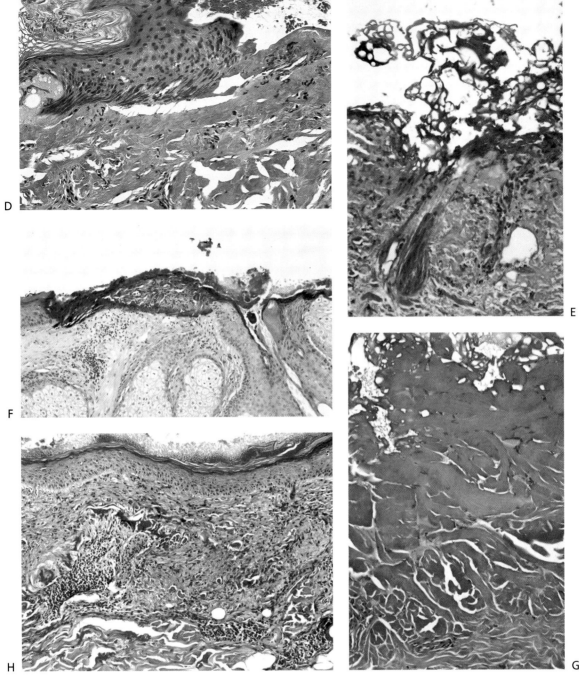

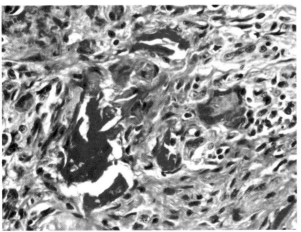

FIGURE 13-12. *(continued)* **D:** Incipient blister formation can be seen in association with elongation cytolysis of keratinocytes and/or coagulation necrosis of the dermis due to electrodessication heat injury. **E:** Electrodessication elongation effects on the follicular epithelium are similar to those seen in the epidermis. This higher-power view highlights the lace-like pattern of coagulation necrosis seen in some cases of electrodessication injury. **F:** This demonstrates another pattern of electrodessication injury, characterized by abrupt basophilic alteration of the collagen and epithelium. **G:** The dermal changes of electrodessication injury are characterized by homogenized basophilic coagulation necrosis and loss of the distinction between collagen bundles. In contrast, the deeper tissue shows minimally damaged collagen, with distinct separation of the collagen bundles. Superficially there is mild lace-like change. **H:** Within a healing surgical biopsy site, foci of basophilic desiccated collagen are noted beneath the reparative fibrosis. **I:** A foreign body reaction to altered collagen is noted, with engulfment of the basophilic injured collagen.

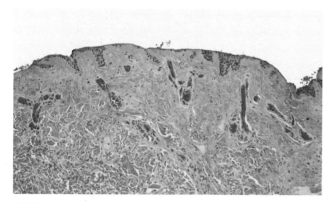

FIGURE 13-13. Curettage-induced ulceration. In contrast to desiccation-induced injury, there is no dermal collagen reaction. The ulcer base typically shows vascular congestion.

(Fig. 13-13). Dermal inflammation will be minimal, unless there are residual biopsy site changes. The epidermis is usually denuded, but there may be partial remnants of attached epidermis, without the stretch artifact typical of electrodesiccation.

Differential Diagnosis. The nuclei elongation of electrodesiccation injury should be differentiated from atypia of an actinic keratosis. Atypical melanocytic hyperplasia may show overlap features, but this can be differentiated with immunohistochemical stains for melanocytes (Chapter 28).

REFERENCES

1. Zalar GL, Harber LC. Reactions to physical agents. In: Moschella SL, Hurley HJ, eds., *Dermatology*. Philadelphia: WB Saunders, 1985:1672–1690.
2. Page EH, Shear NH. Temperature-dependent skin disorders. *J Am Acad Dermatol* 1988;18:1003.
3. Krishnan RS, Lewis AT, Kass JS, et al. Ultraviolet recall-like phenomenon occurring after piperacillin, tobramycin, and ciprofloxacin therapy. *J Am Acad Dermatol* 2001;44:1045.
4. Garza LA, Yoo EK, Junkins-Hopkins JM, et al. Photo recall effect in association with cefazolin. *Cutis* 2004;73:79.
5. Shelley WB, Shelley ED, Campbell AC, et al. Drug eruptions presenting at sites of prior radiation damage (sunlight and electron-beam). *J Am Acad Dermatol* 1984;11:53.
6. Hurwitz RM, Tisserand ME. Erythema ab igne. *Arch Dermatol* 1987;123:21.
7. Finlayson GR, Sams WM, Smith JG. Erythema ab igne: a histopathological study. *J Invest Dermatol* 1966;46:104.
8. Johnson WC Butterworth T. Erythema ab igne elastosis. *Arch Dermatol* 1971;104:128.
9. Arrington JH, Lockman DS. Thermal keratoses and squamous cell carcinoma in situ associated with erythema ab igne. *Arch Dermatol* 1979;115:1226.
10. Busch D. Genetic susceptibility to radiation and chemotherapy injury: diagnosis and management. *Int J Radiat Oncol Biol Phys* 1994;30:997.
11. Koenig TR, Wolff D, Metler FA, et al. Skin injuries from fluoroscopically guided procedures. Part I: characteristics of radiation injury. *AJR Am J Roentgenol* 2001;177:3.
12. Hanna YM, Baglan KL, Stromberg JS, et al. Acute and subacute toxicity associated with concurrent adjuvant radiation therapy and paclitaxel in primary breast cancer therapy. *Breast J* 2002;8:149.
13. Pajonk F, Weissenberger C, Witucki G, et al. Vitiligo at the site of irradiation in a patient with Hodgkin's disease. *Strahlenther Onkol* 2002;178:159.
14. Kim JH, Krivda SJ. Lichen planus confined to a radiation therapy site. *J Am Acad Dermatol* 2002;46:604.
15. Parikh SK, Ravi A, Kuo DY, et al. Bullous pemphigoid masquerading as acute radiation dermatitis: case report. *Eur J Gynaecol Oncol* 2001;22:322.
16. James WD, Odom RB. Late subcutaneous fibrosis following megavoltage radiotherapy. *J Am Acad Dermatol* 1980;3:616.
17. Young EM, Barr RJ. Sclerosing dermatoses. *J Cutan Pathol* 1985;12:426.
18. Moretto JC, Soslow RA, Smoller BR. Atypical cells in radiation dermatitis express factor XIIIa. *Am J Dermatopathol* 1998;20:370.
19. Meehan SA, LeBoit PE. An immunohistochemical analysis of radiation fibroblasts. *J Cutan Pathol* 1997;24:309.
20. LeBoit PE. Subacute radiation dermatitis: a histologic imitator of acute cutaneous graft-versus-host disease. *J Am Acad Dermatol* 1989;20:236.
21. Stone MS, Robson KJ, LeBoit PE. Subacute radiation dermatitis from fluoroscopy during coronary artery stenting: evidence for cytotoxic lymphocyte mediated apoptosis. *J Am Acad Dermatol* 1998;38:333.
22. Totten RS, Antypas PG, Dupertuis M, et al. Pre-existing roentgen-ray dermatitis in patients with skin cancer. *Cancer* 1957;10:1024.
23. Sook Seo I, Warner TFCS, Warren JS, et al. Cutaneous postirratiation sarcoma. *Cancer* 1985;56:761.
24. Diaz-Cascajo C, Borghi S, Weyers W. Desmoplastic leiomyosarcoma of the skin. *Am J Dermatopathol* 2000;22:251.
25. Souba WW, McKenna RJ, Meis J, et al. Radiation-induced sarcomas of the chest wall. *Cancer* 1986;57:610.
26. Kiyohara T, Kumakiri M, Kobayashi H, et al. Spindle cell angiosarcoma following irradiation therapy for cervical carcinoma. *J Cutan Pathol* 2002;29:96.
27. Hivnor CM, Kantor J, Seykora JT, et al. Subacute radiation dermatitis. *Am J Dermatopathol* 2004;6:210.
28. Schecter AK, Lewis MD, Robinson-Bostom L, et al. Cardiac catheterization-induced acute radiation dermatitis presenting as a fixed drug eruption. *J Drugs Dermatol* 2003;2:425–427.
29. Camidge R, Price A. Characterizing the phenomenon of radiation recall dermatitis. *Radiother Oncol* 2001;59:237.
30. Thomas R, Stea B. Radiation recall dermatitis from high-dose interferon alfa-2b. *J Clin Oncol* 2002;20:355–357.
31. Castellano D, Hitt R, Cortes-Funes H, et al. Side effects of chemotherapy. Case 2. Radiation recall reaction induced by gemcitabine. *J Clin Oncol* 2000;18:695.
32. Smith KJ, Germain M, Skalton H. Histopathologic features seen with radiation recall or enhancement eruptions. *J Cutan Med Surg* 2002;6:535.
33. Kukla JP. Cold injury to the skin. The pathogenic role of microcirculatory impairment. *Arch Environ Health* 1965;11:484.
34. Herman EW, Kezis JS, Silvers DN. A distinctive variant of pernio. Clinical and histopathologic study of nine cases. *Arch Dermatol* 1981;117:26.
35. Price RD, Murdoch DR. Perniosis (chilblains) of the thigh: report of five cases, including four following river crossings. *High Alt Med Biol* 2001;2:535.
36. Weston WL, Morelli JG. Childhood pernio and cryoproteins. *Pediatr Dermatol* 2000;17:97.

37. Doutre MS, Beylot C, Beylot J, et al. Chilblain lupus erythematosus: report of 15 cases. *Dermatology* 1992;184:26.

38. Pock L, Petrovska P, Becvar R, et al. Verrucous form of chilblain lupus erythematosus. *J Eur Acad Dermatol Venereol* 2001;15:448.

39. Cribier B, Djeridi N, Peltre B, et al. A histologic and immunohistochemical study of chilblains. *J Am Acad Dermatol* 2001;45:924.

40. Franceschini F, Calzavara-Pinton P, Qinsanini M, et al. Chilblains lupus erythematosus is associated with antibodies to SSA/Ro. *Lupus* 1999;8:215–9.

41. Su WP, Perniciaro C, Rogers RS 3rd, et al. Chilblains lupus erythematosus (lupus pernio): clinical review of the Mayo Clinic experience and proposal of diagnostic criteria. *Cutis* 1994;54:395.

42. Wessagowit P, Asawanonda P, Noppakun N. Papular perniosis mimicking erythema multiforme: the first case report in Thailand. *Int J Dermatol* 2000;39:527.

43. Crowson AN, Magro CM. Idiopathic perniosis and its mimics: a clinical and histological study of 38 cases. *Hum Pathol* 1997; 478–484.

44. Kee CE. Liquid nitrogen therapy. *Arch Dermatol* 1967;96:198.

45. Crissey JT, Peachy JC. Calcaneal petechiae. *Arch Dermatol* 1961; 83:501.

NONINFECTIOUS GRANULOMAS

EARL J. GLUSAC
PHILIP E. SHAPIRO

GRANULOMA ANNULARE

Granuloma annulare is an idiopathic palisaded granulomatous condition that is frequently encountered by dermatopathologists. It occurs most commonly in children and young adults but may affect all age groups. Females are affected somewhat more commonly than males. The lesions of granuloma annulare consist of small, firm, asymptomatic papules that are flesh-colored or pale red, and are often grouped in a ringlike or circinate fashion. There usually are several lesions, but there may be just one, or there may be many. The lesions are found most commonly on the arms, hands, legs, and feet. The trunk may also be involved, and rare sites of involvement include the palms, penis, and ear and periocular regions (1). Although chronic, the lesions usually subside after a number of years. Unusual variants of granuloma annulare include (a) a generalized form, consisting of hundreds of papules that are either discrete or confluent but only rarely show an annular arrangement (2,3); (b) perforating granuloma annulare, with umbilicated lesions occurring usually in a localized distribution (4–6), and rarely in a generalized distribution (7–9); (c) erythematous or patch granuloma annulare, showing large, slightly infiltrated erythematous patches, with a palpable border, on which scattered papules may subsequently arise (10,11); and (d) subcutaneous/deep granuloma annulare, in which subcutaneous nodules occur, especially in children, either alone or in association with intradermal lesions (12–19). The subcutaneous nodules have a clinical appearance similar to rheumatoid nodules, although there is no history of arthritis, and there is a greater tendency to occur on the legs, feet, and, occasionally, the head (15,20,21). A very rare, deep, destructive form of granuloma annulare has also been described (22,23).

A correlation between generalized papular granuloma annulare and diabetes mellitus has been observed by several authors (3,24,25). Granuloma annulare has been reported in at least 60 patients with HIV or AIDS, with a greater incidence of generalized disease in this population (26–30). Granuloma annulare-like lesions have also been reported

to develop at sites of resolved herpes zoster (31,32) and occasionally in association with tattoos (33), necrobiosis lipoidica (34), and sarcoidosis (35).

Histopathology. Histologically, granuloma annulare shows an infiltrate of histiocytes and a perivascular infiltrate of lymphocytes that is usually sparse. The histiocytes may be present in an interstitial pattern without apparent organization, or in palisades, surrounding areas with prominent mucin (Figs. 14-1, 14-2, and 14-3). Patterns between these two extremes occur, and typically a single biopsy will show histiocytes that are not palisaded, slightly palisaded, and well palisaded. Although degenerated collagen or small quantities of fibrin may be present (35), increased mucin is the hallmark of granuloma annulare. Increased mucin is almost always apparent on routinely stained sections as faint blue material with a stringy, finely granular appearance. Stains such as colloidal iron and alcian blue can be used to highlight mucin if it is not clearly apparent. Occasionally, sections will not reveal increased mucin, particularly those lacking a palisaded arrangement of histiocytes. In biopsies with well-developed palisades, the central mucinous area is commonly accompanied by a few nuclear fragments or neutrophils. Plasma cells are rarely present. A sparse infiltrate of eosinophils is seen in approximately half of cases, and occasional biopsies show abundant eosinophils (36,37). Multinucleated histiocytes are present more often than not, but they are usually few and often subtle. They can occasionally be seen to have engulfed short, thick, blue-gray elastic fibers (38). The histiocytic infiltrate is usually present throughout the full thickness of the dermis or the middle and upper dermis, but occasionally just the superficial or the deep dermis is involved (39). Mitotic figures are usually rare (<1/10 high-power fields [HPF]) but may be as frequent as 7/10 HPF in rare examples (40).

Rare examples of granuloma annulare show aggregates of epithelioid histiocytes, usually with some giant cells and a rim of lymphoid cells, which resemble the granulomas of sarcoidosis (35,39). These usually differ from sarcoidal granulomas, however, by showing poorer circumscription and lacking asteroid bodies. Vascular changes in granuloma annulare are variable but generally inconspicuous (41). In

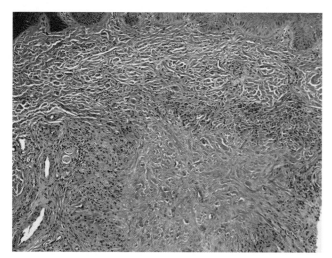

FIGURE 14-1. Granuloma annulare. A palisade of histiocytes surrounds mucin in the upper dermis.

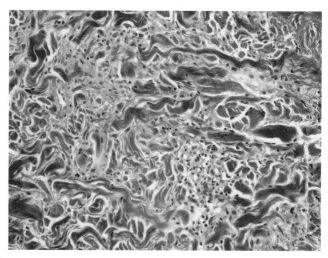

FIGURE 14-3. Granuloma annulare. Interstitial pattern granuloma annulare exhibits histiocytes between collagen bundles and perivascular lymphocytes.

some instances, however, there are fibrinoid deposits in vessel walls and occlusion of vascular lumina (42).

Among the variants of granuloma annulare mentioned, the usual histologic picture of palisaded and interstitial pattern is found in the generalized form (2). An interstitial pattern predominates in the erythematous and patch variants (10,11). In perforating granuloma annulare, at least part of the palisading granulomatous process is located superficially and is associated with disruption of the epidermis (4,5,7,8).

The subcutaneous nodules of deep granuloma annulare usually show large histiocytic palisades surrounding mucin and degenerated collagen (Fig. 14-4). These central, degenerated foci exhibit a pale appearance (43); however, examples in which mucin was not apparent or in which the central area appeared more fibrinoid have also been reported

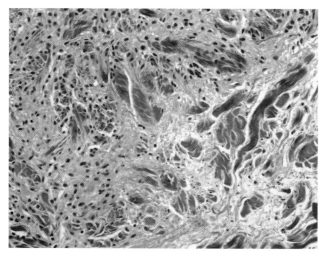

FIGURE 14-2. Granuloma annulare. Histiocytes surround mucin, which shows a feathery blue appearance, and a few fragments of neutrophils.

(20,21). As such, subcutaneous granuloma annulare may be histologically indistinguishable from rheumatoid nodule, an appearance that has led to the term *pseudorheumatoid nodule.*

Pathogenesis. The cause of granuloma annulare remains unknown. Possible precipitating events in small subsets of patients have included insect bites, warts, erythema multiforme, herpes zoster, exposure to sunlight, hepatitis B vaccine, and tuberculin skin tests (44–47). There is likely an increased incidence and increased disease severity in patients with diabetes mellitus. Thrombi or vasculitic changes have been noted in some examples, and it is possible that what we currently term *granuloma annulare* may represent a variety of disease processes.

Electron microscopic examination reveals degeneration of both collagen and elastic fibers in granuloma annulare (35). The macrophages (histiocytes) show a high content of primary lysosomes and considerable cytoplasmic activity with release of lysosomal enzymes into the extracellular space (48). Synthesis of types I and III collagen also occurs, probably as a reparative response (49). A cell-mediated immune response also appears to be involved, marked by prominent, activated helper T cells (50–52). One immunoperoxidase study of the histiocytic population showed staining for lysozyme, but not for other macrophage markers such as HAM 56 or CD68 (53). Another demonstrated positivity for these two markers (40).

Blood vessel deposits of IgM and the third component of complement (C3) have been observed by some investigators (51), but others have found them only rarely (54) or not at all (55). Thus, the existence of an immune complex vasculitis in granuloma annulare (51) appears unlikely.

Differential Diagnosis. Granuloma annulare and necrobiosis lipoidica may resemble one another histologically. Although much has been written about the difficulty of

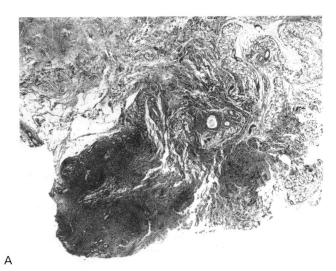
A

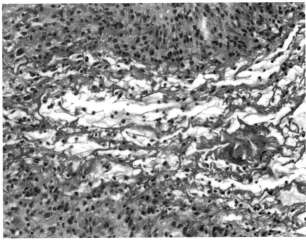
B

FIGURE 14-4. Deep granuloma annulare. **A:** A well-circumscribed subcutaneous nodule shows palisaded histiocytes surrounding mucin and fibrinoid material. **B:** Histiocytes in a palisade surround mucin and fibrinoid material.

separating these disorders histologically (41), it should be pointed out that the distinction can be easily accomplished clinically in most circumstances (56). Furthermore, although it is true that histologic distinction may be impossible, usually it can be accomplished by using the following criteria:

Although either disease may involve the dermis diffusely, necrobiosis lipoidica rarely involves just one focus of the dermis or predominantly the upper half of the dermis, whereas granuloma annulare often does.

Histiocytes in palisades that completely encircle altered connective tissue are more common in granuloma annulare, whereas histiocytes in linear array that are horizontally oriented in a somewhat tiered fashion are more typical of necrobiosis lipoidica.

Abundant mucin is typical of granuloma annulare and distinctly uncommon in necrobiosis lipoidica.

Necrobiosis lipoidica often shows dermal sclerosis and thickened subcutaneous septa, whereas granuloma annulare does not (the sclerosis often produces a straight edge to the sides of a punch biopsy, in contrast to the inward retraction and/or more irregular edge seen in biopsies without sclerosis).

Other features that are more characteristic of necrobiosis lipoidica include the presence of a larger number of giant cells, prominent deep dermal plasma cells, and more pronounced vascular changes, including thickened blood vessel walls. Furthermore, necrobiosis lipoidica is more likely to show extensive deposits of lipids or nodular lymphocytic infiltrates in the deep dermis or subcutis (57), although neither feature is commonly seen.

The interstitial type of granuloma annulare, in which palisades of histiocytes are not well developed, is less likely to be confused with necrobiosis lipoidica. This pattern is more likely to be mistaken for a process that can also show a superficial and deep lymphocytic infiltrate, such as the inflammatory stage of morphea, but the subtle presence of histiocytes in an interstitial pattern usually allows a definitive diagnosis of granuloma annulare. Mycosis fungoides can have a granulomatous infiltrate with a granuloma annulare–like pattern (58,59). Such examples of this cutaneous T-cell lymphoma can usually be recognized by the presence of at least some intraepidermal lymphocytes, a dermal lymphocytic infiltrate that is more dense around the superficial plexus than the deep one, and/or a lichenoid component to the infiltrate. The interstitial type of granuloma annulare may also resemble a xanthoma. Distinction is usually possible because in granuloma annulare a foamy appearance to the histiocytes is either completely lacking or very subtle; in xanthoma, at least some of the histiocytes are obviously foamy. Additionally, granuloma annulare tends to show an obvious perivascular lymphocytic infiltrate, whereas most xanthomas do not (60). Drug reactions may also mimic granuloma annulare, but these usually show interface changes that allow for their distinction (61). Rarely, infection with mycobacterium marinum may have few neutrophils and may produce a histologic picture resembling interstitial granuloma annulare (62).

Differentiation of subcutaneous granuloma annulare from a rheumatoid nodule is not always possible on histologic grounds, but subcutaneous granuloma annulare is more likely than rheumatoid nodule to show prominent mucin and less likely to show foreign-body giant cells or prominent stromal fibrosis (43).

Finally, it should be remembered that granuloma annulare and other palisading granulomas may be simulated by epithelioid sarcoma, a lesion that may also contain mucin. Clues to epithelioid sarcoma include ulceration, cytologic atypia, necrotic foci that include necrotic epithelioid cells, and history of recurrence. Although atypia tends not to be striking, the epithelioid cells in epithelioid sarcoma usually show more nuclear hyperchromasia and pleomorphism, more mitotic figures, larger size, and redder cytoplasm than do the histiocytes of granuloma annulare (63). Immunohistochemically, epithelioid sarcoma can be distinguished from granuloma annulare by positivity for epithelial membrane antigen and keratins. While a variety of keratins may be present in epithelioid sarcoma, the most common is cytokeratin 8/CAM 5.2, present in 94% of cases (64).

ANNULAR ELASTOLYTIC GIANT-CELL GRANULOMA

Annular elastolytic giant-cell granuloma is the name that is currently in vogue for a condition with unclear nosologic status, and it is uncertain whether or not it is truly distinct from granuloma annulare (65–67). It almost always occurs on sun-exposed skin, such as the face, neck, dorsum of hand, forearm, and arm; hence the previous name *actinic granuloma* (68,69). The appearance of lesions after prolonged tanning bed usage has been reported (70). However, there are a few reports of similar lesions involving sun-protected sites (71–74). The lesions clinically resemble granuloma annulare. They are typically large, somewhat annular plaques. The border may be serpiginous and is slightly raised, approximately 3 mm wide, and pearly or slightly red or brown. The central zone may show depigmentation and/or atrophy. Smaller papules may also occur, and lesions may be solitary, few, or numerous (68,75,76). Other names under which these lesions have been described include *atypical necrobiosis lipoidica of the face and scalp* (77), *Miescher's granuloma of the face* (76), and *granuloma multiforme* (75). A possibly related process occurs on the conjunctiva (78).

Histopathology. The histologic features are best appreciated in a radial biopsy that contains the central zone, elevated border, and skin peripheral to the ring (68,75, 76). The central zone shows the hallmark of the disease, that is, near or total absence of elastic fibers, best appreciated with an elastic tissue stain (e.g., Verhoeff–van Gieson) (Figs. 14-5, 14-6, and 14-7). The collagen in this zone may show horizontally oriented fibers producing a slight scar-like appearance (Fig. 14-5). By contrast, the zone peripheral to the annulus shows an increased amount of thick elastotic material with the staining properties of elastic tissue. The transitional zone at the raised border shows a granulomatous infiltrate with either of the patterns seen in granuloma annulare, that is, histiocytes arranged interstitially between collagen bundles or, less commonly, in a palisade. Occasionally, there are contiguous epithelioid histiocytes in small clusters. Multinucleated histiocytes are conspicuous, usually being large and containing as many as a dozen nuclei, mostly in haphazard arrangement, but sometimes in ringed array. Elastotic fibers are present adjacent to and within the giant cells (Fig. 14-6). Asteroid bodies that stain like elastic fibers may be found in the giant cells (76). The infiltrate also contains lymphocytes and often some plasma cells. Mucin is not present.

Differential Diagnosis. The principal differential diagnosis is granuloma annulare, which may in fact be an artificial distinction. Since engulfment of abnormal elastic fibers can also occur in granuloma annulare (38), as well as in other granulomatous processes, it has been argued that the elastophagocytosis of annular elastolytic giant-cell granuloma does not qualify it as a distinct entity different from granuloma annulare of sun-damaged skin (66). Although

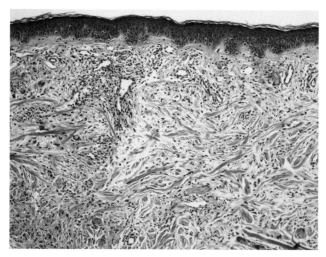

FIGURE 14-5. Annular elastolytic granuloma. Multinucleated histiocytes at left abut connective tissue at the center of the lesion that is slightly fibrotic; mucin is not apparent.

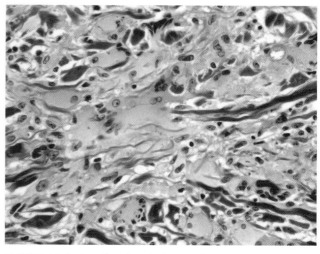

FIGURE 14-6. Annular elastolytic granuloma. Some multinucleated histiocytes have ingested blue-gray elastic fibers.

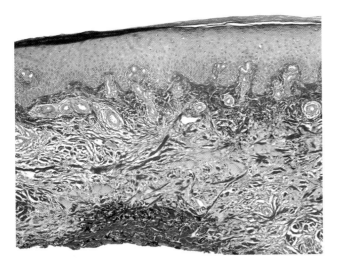

FIGURE 14-7. Annular elastolytic granuloma. Elastic tissue stain shows absence of elastic fibers in the center of the lesion.

some elastolysis has also been described in granuloma annulare (75), it is the complete loss of elastic tissue in the central zone that has been used as the primary basis for separating the diseases. Other features that have been evoked for distinguishing them is the presence of larger and more numerous giant cells, the absence of mucin in annular elastolytic giant-cell granuloma (68,79), and sparing of areas that lack elastic tissue, such as scars (74).

Necrobiosis lipoidica differs by the lack of a central zone of elastolysis and the presence of degenerated collagen, sclerosis, and, in some circumstances, lipids and vascular changes. Furthermore, annular elastolytic giant-cell granuloma involves mostly the upper and middle dermis, whereas necrobiosis lipoidica tends to affect the deep dermis and sometimes the subcutis at least as much as the upper dermis. Foreign body granulomas generally have more distinct collections of epithelioid histiocytes, lack zonation in density of elastic fibers, and often have identifiable foreign material.

NECROBIOSIS LIPOIDICA

Necrobiosis lipoidica is an idiopathic disorder typified by indurated plaques of the shins. In 1966, in a large series, Muller and Winkelman (80) reported that two-thirds of patients with necrobiosis lipoidica had overt diabetes at the time of diagnosis. Of the rest, all but 10% developed diabetes within 5 years, had abnormal glucose tolerance, or had a history of diabetes in at least one parent (25). In a more recent series, only 11% of patients had diabetes at presentation, with an additional 11% developing diabetes or impaired glucose tolerance over 15 years (81). Of all patients with diabetes, fewer than 1% develop necrobiosis lipoidica (25,81). Some reports have suggested that necro-

biosis lipoidica heralds more rapid progression of diabetes, in patients with that disorder (82).

In well-developed necrobiosis lipoidica, one observes one or several sharply but irregularly demarcated patches or plaques, usually on the shins (83). Usually they are bilateral and the condition is more often present in women (25). The lesions appear yellow-brown in the center and purplish at the periphery. Whereas the periphery of the lesions may show slight induration, the center of the lesions gradually becomes atrophic, shows telangiectases, and may ulcerate. When lesions first begin, red-brown papules can be observed. In addition to the shins, lesions may be present elsewhere on the lower extremities, including the ankles, calves, thighs, popliteal areas, and feet. In about 15% of the cases, lesions are present also in areas other than the legs, especially on the dorsa of the hands, fingers, and forearms. Rarely, the head and abdomen are affected. Necrobiosis lipoidica with lesions exclusively outside the legs is extremely rare; it is reported to occur in 1% of patients with necrobiosis lipoidica (80).

Lesions located in areas other than the legs may appear raised and firm and may have a papular, nodular, or plaque-like appearance without atrophy. Clinically they may resemble granuloma annulare (80). Involvement of the scalp by large, atrophic patches occurs occasionally. This is usually seen in association with lesions on the shins and elsewhere (84,85) but also, rarely, in isolation (86–88).

In rare instances, transfollicular elimination of necrotic material takes place in necrobiosis lipoidica, producing small hyperkeratotic plugs within a plaque (89,90). Necrobiosis lipoidica occasionally coexists with sarcoid (91) or granuloma annulare (34). Rare examples of squamous cell carcinoma arising in lesions of necrobiosis lipoidica have been reported (92,93).

Histopathology. On histologic examination, the epidermis may be normal, atrophic, or hyperkeratotic. In some instances, the surface of the biopsy shows ulceration. Usually the entire thickness of the dermis or its lower two-thirds is affected by a process that exhibits a variable degree of granulomatous inflammation, degeneration of collagen, and sclerosis (Figs. 14-8 and 14-9). Histologic changes of necrobiosis lipoidica may be seen in subcutaneous septae (94,95). Occasionally only the upper dermis is affected (39,41,56, 80,96). The granulomatous component is usually conspicuous, and the histiocytes may or may not be arranged in a palisade. Occasionally there are just a few scattered epithelioid histiocytes and giant cells. The latter picture is more likely to occur in sections in which sclerosis is extensive, and occasionally in such biopsies several sections must be examined before a granulomatous component becomes apparent. Giant cells are usually of the Langhans or foreign-body type; occasionally, Touton cells or asteroid bodies (97) are seen. If the histiocytes are arranged in a palisade, the palisades tend to be somewhat horizontally oriented and/or vaguely tiered. Occasionally, histiocytes may be seen to completely encircle

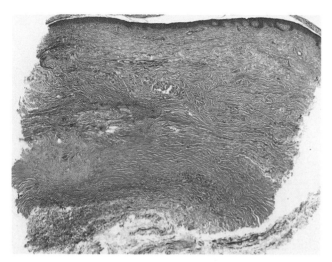

FIGURE 14-8. Necrobiosis lipoidica. The presence of sclerosis can be identified by the relatively straight edges of the punch biopsy. The infiltrate involves the full thickness of the dermis and is arranged in a tier-like fashion.

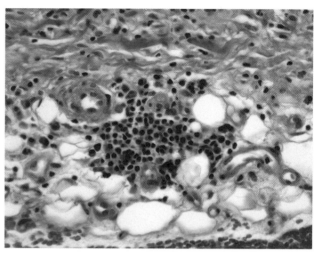

FIGURE 14-10. Necrobiosis lipoidica. Plasma cells at the dermal–subcutaneous junction are a typical finding.

altered connective tissue, particularly degenerated collagen, but, more commonly, altered connective tissue is incompletely surrounded by histiocytes. This alteration of connective tissue has also been referred to as "necrobiosis." The altered collagen appears different from normal collagen by having a paler, grayer hue and by appearing more fragmented and haphazardly arranged; it may also appear more compact or smudged (Fig. 14-9). Areas of sclerosis with a diminished number of fibroblasts can be seen. A clue to the presence of sclerosis can be found by looking at the edges of the biopsy specimen, which tend to be straight with less of the inward retraction of the dermis ordinarily associated with punch biopsies (Fig. 14-8). Increased mucin is usually inapparent or subtle in contrast to granuloma annulare. Other findings include a sparse to moderately dense, primarily perivascular lymphocytic infiltrate, plasma cells in the deep dermis in some biopsies (Fig. 14-10), involvement of the upper subcutis with thickened fibrous septa, and lipids (which may be present in foamy histiocytes [98], which may be inferred from the presence of cholesterol clefts, or which can be detected extracellularly with special stains on fresh tissue). Older lesions show telangiectases superficially. Blood vessels, particularly in the middle and lower dermis, often exhibit thickening of their walls with proliferation of their endothelial cells. The process may lead to partial and rarely to complete occlusion of the lumen. The thickened walls may be infiltrated with PAS-positive, diastase-resistant material (41). Vascular changes of this type are seen particularly near foci containing thickened, hyalinized collagen bundles. Whereas the vascular changes often are conspicuous in lesions of the lower legs, they usually are mild or absent elsewhere (87).

One cannot reliably determine if the patient has diabetes based on histologic findings; however, florid palisading and degeneration of collagen has been correlated with such (80).

Pathogenesis. The cause of necrobiosis lipoidica is unknown, and it is unclear whether the degeneration of collagen is a primary or a secondary event (83). Some authors have postulated that the degeneration of collagen is the result of vascular changes secondary to clinical or latent diabetes (99). However, evidence against a vascular cause includes the absence of vascular pathology in approximately one-third of biopsies examined (80), and the fact that affected vessels are often situated in the lower dermis and of a larger caliber than the vessels affected by diabetic microangiopathy. Abnormal glucose transport by fibroblasts has also been implicated (100).

Electron microscopic examination shows degenerative changes in collagen and elastin with loss of cross-striation in collagen fibrils. Collagen synthesis by fibroblasts is diminished (101).

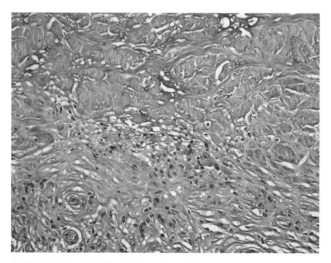

FIGURE 14-9. Necrobiosis lipoidica. Histiocytes, lymphocytes and degenerated collagen are present.

Direct immunofluorescence studies have shown that necrobiotic foci contain fibrinogen. Deposits of immunoglobulin and C3 have been found in the vessel walls (102, 103), but this is not a consistent finding (104).

Differential Diagnosis. Differentiation of necrobiosis lipoidica from granuloma annulare has been discussed in the section on granuloma annulare.

Occasionally, necrobiosis lipoidica shows discrete collections of epithelioid cells that may resemble those seen in sarcoidosis (84,105). However, significant alteration of the collagen is usually present in necrobiosis lipoidica and absent in sarcoidosis (84).

Necrobiotic xanthogranuloma with paraproteinemia can simulate necrobiosis lipoidica, but differs by showing a more dense, diffuse infiltrate with a greater number of foamy histiocytes, more extensive inflammation of the subcutis, and greater disruption of normal subcutaneous architecture.

A discussion of differentiation of necrobiosis lipoidica from annular elastolytic granuloma appears in the section on annular elastolytic granuloma earlier in this chapter.

RHEUMATOID NODULES

Rheumatoid nodules are deeply seated firm masses that occur in patients with rheumatoid arthritis, particularly over extensor prominences, such as the proximal ulna, olecranon process, and metacarpophalangeal and proximal interphalangeal joints (106). They may occur elsewhere, such as the back of the hands, over amputation stumps (107), and rarely in extracutaneous sites, such as the lung and heart (108,109). The nodules vary in size from a few millimeters to 5 cm and may be solitary or numerous (108). Rarely, rheumatoid nodules show a central draining perforation (110). Rheumatoid factor is almost always found in high titer. Rarely, nodules may precede apparent joint disease (106). The rapid appearance of many small rheuma-

toid nodules has been reported in some patients who have been treated with methotrexate. This presentation has been termed *accelerated rheumatoid nodulosis* (111,112). Rheumatoid nodules also occur in occasional patients with systemic lupus erythematosus who do not exhibit rheumatoid arthritis (113–115).

Pseudorheumatoid nodule is a term that has been applied to nodules in the subcutis that mimic rheumatoid nodules histologically but that develop in the absence of rheumatoid arthritis (or systemic lupus erythematosus) (13,14,21). These occur in children or adults. The subsequent development of rheumatoid arthritis occurs infrequently in adults and rarely, if ever, in children. Because some of these nodules occur in patients with other lesions that are typical of intradermal granuloma annulare (13, 14), the nodules are now generally considered to represent a subcutaneous variant of granuloma annulare.

Histopathology. Rheumatoid nodules occur in the subcutis and deep dermis. They exhibit one or several areas of fibrinoid degeneration of collagen that stain homogeneously red (Fig. 14-11). Nuclear fragments and basophilic material are often present, but mucin is almost always minimal or absent (43). These foci of degenerative change are surrounded by histiocytes in a palisade. Foreign-body giant cells are present in approximately 50% of biopsies (43). In the surrounding stroma, there is a proliferation of blood vessels associated with fibrosis. A sparse infiltrate of other inflammatory cells is associated with the histiocytes and surrounding stroma. Lymphocytes and neutrophils are most common, but mast cells, plasma cells, and eosinophils may be present. Occasionally, lipid is seen (13,43). Vasculitis has been described (116), but is not usually encountered (43). In perforating rheumatoid nodules, the central fibrinoid material connects to the overlying skin surface (110).

Pathogenesis. Factors that have been implicated in the formation of rheumatoid nodules include trauma, vasculitis, and a specific T-cell–mediated immune reaction (117,106).

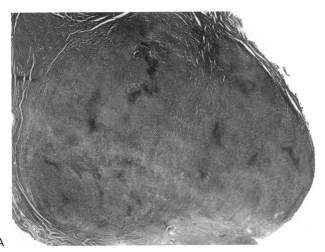
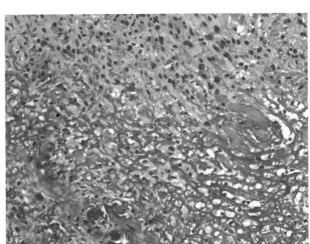

A

B

FIGURE 14-11. Rheumatoid nodule. **A:** A deeply seated, circumscribed nodule exhibits palisading around degenerated material. **B:** Fibrin is surrounded by histiocytes in palisaded arrangement.

Differential Diagnosis. The principal differential diagnosis is subcutaneous granuloma annulare, which was discussed in the section on granuloma annulare. A distinction should be made from epithelioid sarcoma, which was also covered in that section. Nonabsorbable sutures or other foreign material may produce periarticular palisaded granulomas like those of rheumatoid nodule (118,119); in such instances, there should be a history of previous surgery or trauma, and birefringent material may be visible under polarized light. Rheumatic fever produces nodules (rheumatic nodules), especially over the elbows, knees, scalp, knuckles, ankles, and spine (120), which were confused with rheumatoid nodules in the early part of the 20th century. Histologically, a rheumatic fever nodule is less likely to show central, homogeneous fibrinoid necrosis. A palisade of histiocytes is usually not as well developed, and fibrosis is minimal or absent (108,121). Rarely, an infectious process, such as cryptococcosis, can produce a deep palisaded granuloma. It can be differentiated from rheumatoid nodule because the palisade surrounds primarily necrotic debris and organisms, rather than fibrinoid material.

PALISADED NEUTROPHILIC AND GRANULOMATOUS DERMATITIS

In 1983, Finan and Winkelmann reported on 27 patients with a variety of systemic disorders who had cutaneous lesions comprised of a palisaded granulomatous infiltrate with prominent neutrophils. These patients often had umbilicated papules and nodules on the elbows and extensor surfaces of the digits (122). They termed this condition *Churg–Strauss granuloma* or *cutaneous extravascular necrotizing granuloma*. Of note, only a minority of these patients had Churg–Strauss disease, and many had a connective tissue disorder. Others observed similar lesions in patients with rheumatoid arthritis and described them under names such as *rheumatoid papules* (123,124) and *superficial ulcerating rheumatoid necrobiosis* (125,126). In 1994, Chu et al. (127) reported on nine patients with connective tissue disorders and cutaneous lesions similar to those described above. Biopsies from some of these patients showed histologic changes in early lesions that were judged to be a unique form of leukocytoclastic vasculitis. They proposed the terms *palisaded neutrophilic and granulomatous dermatitis* to cover the spectrum of lesions in this disorder: early vasculitic lesions, later palisaded granulomatous lesions, and late-stage lesions, which resembled necrobiosis lipoidica histologically (but not clinically). Interstitial granulomatous dermatitis with arthritis likely represents a variant of palisaded neutrophilic and granulomatous dermatitis in which patients present with long, linear, "rope-like" dermal lesions on the trunk, sometimes associated with more typical acral papules and nodules (128,129). Additional patients with similar histologic findings have been reported with other cutaneous manifestations such as annular indurated plaques (130–132).

Histopathology. There are three sometimes overlapping histologic patterns in this rare condition: (a) early lesions resembling leukocytoclastic vasculitis; (b) fully developed lesions with a granuloma annulare-like appearance, but which are associated with prominent neutrophils; and (c) a fibrosing, necrobiosis lipoidica-like final stage.

Early lesions show a superficial and deep, diffuse infiltrate of neutrophils with leukocytoclasis, amorphous stringy basophilic debris, and degenerated collagen (127,133). There is vasculitis with unusually broad cuffs of fibrin that separate the vessels from the surrounding basophilic material and altered collagen. Extravasated red cells are scant. Papillary dermal edema is typical, and the epidermis may be ulcerated or hyperplastic.

The fully developed lesions of this condition are more often encountered. They show a palisaded granulomatous infiltrate with some resemblance to granuloma annulare (127,133) (Figs. 14-12 and 13). While vasculitic changes are usually not conspicuous at this stage, neutrophilic dust and intact neutrophils are present in the centers of the palisades, accompanied by thickened, degenerated collagen bundles, fibrin, and mucin (Fig. 14-13).

The uncommonly encountered late or third stage findings include histiocytes in a palisade around degenerated collagen, fibrin, and scattered neutrophils (127), with fibrosis in the dermis between the granulomas. Wisps of mucin may be present at the periphery of granulomas, but not in their centers. There may also be a sparse, superficial and deep perivascular infiltrate of lymphocytes and eosinophils.

Pathogenesis. Palisaded neutrophilic and granulomatous dermatitis has been associated with a wide variety of conditions. While most are connective tissue disorders, such as rheumatoid arthritis or lupus erythematosus, others include lymphoproliferative disorders, bacterial endocarditis, inflammatory bowel disease, thyroid disease, diabetes melli-

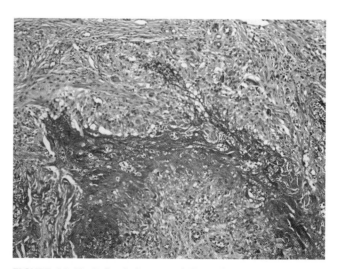

FIGURE 14-12. Palisaded neutrophilic and granulomatous dermatitis. This fully developed lesion exhibits palisades of histiocytes associated with neutrophils, basophilic debris, mucin, and degenerated collagen.

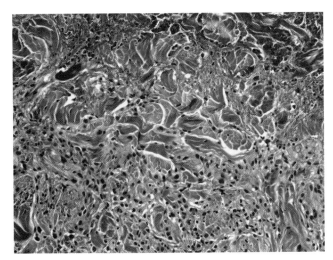

FIGURE 14-13. Palisaded neutrophilic and granulomatous dermatitis. Neutrophilic dust and intact neutrophils are present in the centers of the palisades, accompanied by degenerated collagen bundles, fibrin, and mucin.

tus and infections (127,134). This condition is thought to represent an unusual immune complex–mediated vasculitis. IgM and C3 have been identified in small vessel walls. The changes seen in fully developed lesions are thought to be a response to the vasculitic changes, accompanying ischemia and enzymatic degradation by neutrophils.

Differential Diagnosis. Early lesions of palisaded neutrophilic and granulomatous dermatitis may be distinguished from other forms of leukocytoclastic vasculitis by the presence of unusually broad cuffs of fibrin around vessel walls, which separate the vessels from abundant basophilic nuclear debris. Also, compared to most examples of leukocytoclastic vasculitis, early palisaded neutrophilic and granulomatous dermatitis shows fewer extravasated erythrocytes, a denser infiltrate of neutrophils and more nuclear debris diffusely throughout the dermis.

Fully developed lesions resemble granuloma annulare but differ from it by showing less prominent mucin, more fibrin, and thickening of collagen bundles. While granuloma annulare may occasionally show nuclear debris, it is not as prominent as in palisaded neutrophilic and granulomatous dermatitis. This disorder also shows intact neutrophils, while granuloma annulare only rarely does so. Churg–Strauss disease may show findings similar to palisaded neutrophilic and granulomatous dermatitis, but differs by showing a predominance of eosinophils rather than neutrophils. Lesions of Wegener's granulomatosis are more likely to show active vasculitic changes concurrent with the palisaded granulomatous component. Drug eruptions (135) and infections with a palisaded and neutrophilic response may also be seen.

SARCOIDOSIS

Sarcoidosis is a systemic granulomatous disease of undetermined etiology. A distinction is made between the rare sub-

acute, transient type of sarcoidosis and the usual chronic, persistent type.

In subacute, transient sarcoidosis, erythema nodosum is associated with hilar adenopathy, fever and, in some cases, migrating polyarthritis and acute iritis. The disease subsides in almost all patients within a few months without sequelae. Cutaneous manifestations other than erythema nodosum do not occur (136,137). Occasionally, there is enlargement of some of the subcutaneous lymph nodes, such as the submental or cervical nodes (138).

In chronic, persistent sarcoidosis, cutaneous lesions are encountered in approximately one-fourth of patients who are seen in medical departments (139). In contrast, cutaneous lesions are the only manifestation of sarcoidosis in about one-fourth of patients with sarcoidosis seen in dermatologic departments (140–142). In the United States, this disorder is much more common and is more severe in African Americans (143,144). It is rare in children (145–147). A rare genetic disorder, Blau syndrome, may present in childhood and mimic sarcoidosis. This autosomal dominant disorder is marked by granulomatous inflammation of the skin, uveal tract and joints, sparing the lungs (148,149).

The most common cutaneous lesions of sarcoidosis are brown-red or purple papules and plaques (150). Through central clearing, annular or circinate lesions may result. When papules or plaques of sarcoidosis are situated on the nose, cheeks, and ears, the term *lupus pernio* is applied (151). This presentation has been associated with upper respiratory involvement and greater disease severity (150,152).

A rare form of sarcoidosis is its lichenoid variant, in which small, papular lesions occur (153). Very rare manifestations of sarcoidosis include erythrodermic, ichthyosiform, atrophic, ulcerating, verrucous, angiolupoid, hypopigmented, alopecic and morpheaform variants. In erythrodermic sarcoidosis, the erythroderma may be generalized (154) or may consist of extensive, sharply demarcated, brown-red, slightly scaling patches with little or no palpable infiltration (155). In ichthyosiform sarcoidosis, ichthyotic changes favor the lower extremities (156) but at times they also may be present elsewhere on the skin (157, 158). Rarely, there are extensive atrophic lesions (159). They may undergo ulceration (160,161). Multiple ulcers have been described also in plaquelike lesions (162). Angiolupoid sarcoid is characterized by a prominent telangiectatic component (163). Lesions of hypopigmented sarcoid appear as macules with or without an associated papular or nodular component (164).

Subcutaneous nodules of sarcoidosis are also rare. Originally described by Darier and Roussy (165), they may occur in association with other cutaneous lesions (155,166) or alone (167). Sarcoidosis has been described in AIDS patients (168), and a transient form of chronic sarcoidosis has been reported in patients with hepatitis C undergoing treatment with interferon alfa and ribavirin (169).

382   *Chapter 14*

Systemic sarcoidosis occasionally coexists with granu-loma annulare (142). Cutaneous lesions of sarcoidosis may localize to areas of scarring, as in herpes zoster scars (170, 171). Tattoos (172,173), exogenous ochronosis (174), or other exogenous materials in the skin (175) may serve as a nidus for cutaneous lesions in patients with sarcoidosis. Two studies have demonstrated polarizable foreign mater-ial in approximately 20% of cutaneous sarcoidal lesions from patients with systemic sarcoidosis (176,177).

Histopathology. The lesions of erythema nodosum occur-ring in subacute, transient sarcoidosis have the same histo-logic appearance as "idiopathic" erythema nodosum (138).

Like lesions in other organs, the cutaneous lesions of chronic, persistent sarcoidosis are characterized by the pres-ence of circumscribed collections of epithelioid histiocytes, so-called epithelioid cell tubercles, which show little or no necrosis (Figs. 14-14 and 14-15).

The papules, plaques, and lupus pernio–type lesions show variously sized aggregates of epithelioid cells scattered irregularly through the dermis with occasional extension into the subcutis (178). In the erythrodermic form, the infiltrate shows small granulomas in the upper dermis in-termingled with numerous lymphocytes (155,179), and, rarely, also giant cells (180). Typical sarcoidal granulomas are found in the ichthyosiform lesions (157), in ulcerated areas (162), and in atrophic lesions (181,182). Verrucous sarcoid exhibits prominent associated acanthosis and hy-perkeratosis (183,184). Biopsies of hypopigmented sar-coid may reveal granulomas, which may have a perineural component, or fail to reveal granulomas (185). In subcu-

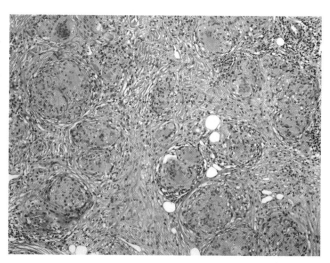

FIGURE 14-15. Sarcoid. Well-circumscribed, roundish collec-tions of epithelioid histiocytes, some multinucleated, with few lymphocytes.

taneous nodules, larger epithelioid cell tubercles lie in the subcutaneous fat (167).

In typical cutaneous lesions of sarcoidosis, the well-demarcated islands of epithelioid cells contain few, if any, giant cells. Those that are present are usually of the Langhans type. A moderate number of giant cells can be found in old lesions. These giant cells may be large and irregular in shape. Giant cells may contain asteroid bod-ies or Schaumann bodies. Asteroid bodies (Fig. 14-16), which are more common, are star-shaped eosinophilic structures that, when stained with phosphotungstic acid–hematoxylin, produce a center that is brown-red with radi-ating blue spikes (155). Schaumann bodies are round or oval, laminated, and calcified, especially at their periphery. They stain dark blue because of the presence of calcium.

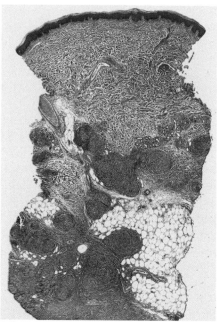

FIGURE 14-14. Sarcoid. There are well-circumscribed, nodular collections of epithelioid histiocytes in the dermis. This example also shows subcutaneous involvement, which is less common than purely dermal involvement.

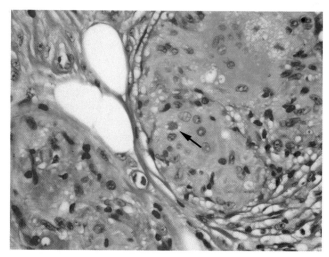

FIGURE 14-16. Sarcoid. Three star-shaped, eosinophilic aster-oid bodies are present, one at the arrow and two in the upper right.

Neither of these two bodies is specific for sarcoidosis, as they have been observed in a variety of other granulomas, including those of leprosy, tuberculosis, foreign body reactions, and necrobiotic xanthogranuloma (186).

Classically, sarcoid has been associated with only a sparse lymphocytic infiltrate, particularly at the margins of the epithelioid cell granulomas (see Fig. 14-15). Because of the scarcity of lymphocytes, the granulomas have been referred to as "naked" tubercles. However, lymphocytic infiltrates in sarcoid may occasionally be dense, as in tuberculosis (Fig. 14-17). Occasionally, small foci of fibrin or necrosis showing eosinophilic staining is found in the center of some of the granulomas (152,178) (Fig. 14-18). A reticulum stain of sarcoid reveals a network of reticulum fibers surrounding and permeating the epithelioid cell granulomas. If the granulomas of sarcoidosis involute, fibrosis extends from the periphery toward the center, with gradual disappearance of the epithelioid cells (178). Fibrosis, however, is minimal to absent in most examples of sarcoidosis, with the exception of the morpheaform variant, where it is prominent (187).

Systemic Lesions. The lungs are the most commonly involved organ in the chronic, persistent type of sarcoidosis, and respiratory symptoms are present in approximately 50% of patients (137). The lesions may be either nodular or diffuse with extensive parenchymal fibrosis.

In about 25% of the patients, ocular manifestations occur, most commonly chronic iridocyclitis. Splenomegaly is present in about 17%. In approximately 12%, osseous granulomas are present, most commonly in the phalanges of the fingers and toes. Involved phalanges appear swollen and deformed, often sausage-shaped (188). The skull may show circumscribed lytic lesions (189). About 8% of the patients have involvement of large salivary glands, usually the parotid. In about 5%, one encounters

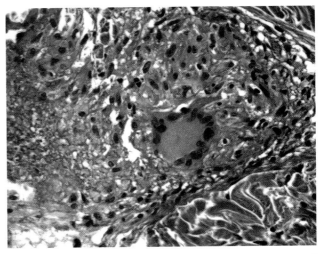

FIGURE 14-18. Sarcoid. On the left, there is fibrinoid material within the granulomatous component.

paresis of a cranial nerve, most commonly of the facial nerve (137). Oral mucosal involvement occurs very rarely (190). Asymptomatic enlargement of the hilar lymph nodes is present in 70%, of peripheral lymph nodes in 30%, and of the liver in 20% of patients (137,191).

Sarcoidosis, although usually a benign disease, is fatal in approximately 5% of patients (137,191). The most common cause of death from sarcoidosis is right ventricular failure resulting from massive pulmonary involvement. Pulmonary hemorrhage and superimposed tuberculosis are rare causes of death. Another potentially fatal complication is renal insufficiency resulting from hypercalcemia and hypercalciuria (192) or from sarcoidal glomerulonephritis (193). In very rare instances, death results from massive involvement of the myocardium (194) or liver (195). Hypopituitarism from involvement of either the pituitary gland or the hypothalamus is also a rare fatal complication (196).

The diagnosis of sarcoidosis in a patient with systemic disease is based upon clinical presentation, biopsy findings, and exclusion of other granulomatous processes. If skin lesions are present, they are an obvious choice for biopsy. In the absence of skin lesions, a Kveim test was frequently used in the past. The Kveim test involves intradermal injection of antigen derived from heat-sterilized suspension of sarcoidal tissue, particularly spleen or lymph node. The site is sampled 6 weeks later, with a positive result being the formation of a sarcoid-like granuloma (197,198). The test has a sensitivity of about 80%, with false-positive reactions occurring in less than 2% (199). However, Kveim antigen is neither widely available nor approved by the U.S. Food and Drug Administration. It is infrequently used at present (143). The most accepted alternative approach for confirming a presumptive diagnosis of systemic sarcoidosis is fiberoptic bronchoscopy with transbronchial lung biopsy (200). Endobronchial biopsy has also been shown to be

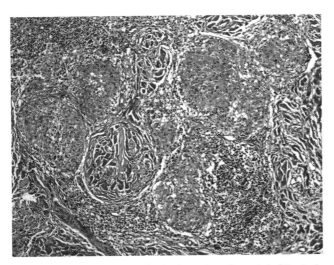

FIGURE 14-17. Sarcoid. A fairly dense lymphocytic infiltrate is associated with the epithelioid histiocytes, a less common finding than the usual "naked tubercles."

useful (201), as has asymptomatic gastrocnemius muscle biopsy (202). Less specific ancillary tests, such as serum angiotensin–converting enzyme levels, can provide supportive data (144).

Pathogenesis. The cause of sarcoidosis is unknown, and the disease may not have the same pathogenesis in all individuals. Alterations in immunologic status have long been recognized, including hypergammaglobulinemia, impaired delayed-type hypersensitivity reactions to cutaneous antigens (anergy), and a shift of helper T-lymphocytes from peripheral blood to sites of disease activity (203). However, these immunologic phenomena may represent a response to an as yet unidentified antigen (204). Mycobacteria, especially cell-wall deficient forms, have been postulated to represent the antigen source (204–207). *Mycobacterium tuberculosis* has been implicated by some studies, while others have suggested atypical mycobacteria (207,208). Other infectious causes such as *Rickettsia* (209) species have also been suggested.

Electron microscopic examination of epithelioid cells fails to show any evidence of bacterial fragments, unlike the macrophages seen in granulomas caused by mycobacteria, although the cells contain primary lysosomes, some autophagic vacuoles, and complex, laminated residual bodies (210). The giant cells form through the coalescence of epithelioid cells with partial fusion of their plasma membranes. Schaumann bodies likely arise from laminated residual bodies of lysosomes. Asteroid bodies consist of collagen showing the typical 64- to 70-nm periodicity. It seems likely that this collagen is trapped between epithelioid cells during the stage of giant-cell formation (210).

Differential Diagnosis. The histologic differentiation of sarcoidosis from lupus vulgaris may be very difficult, and it is occasionally impossible. There is no absolute histologic criterion by which the two diseases can be differentiated with certainty. However, as a rule, the infiltrate in sarcoidosis lies scattered throughout the dermis, whereas the infiltrate in lupus vulgaris is located close to the epidermis. Furthermore, sarcoidosis usually shows few lymphoid cells at the periphery of the granulomas, giving them the appearance of "naked" granulomas. By contrast, lupus vulgaris often shows a marked inflammatory reaction around and between the granulomas. The granulomas of sarcoidosis usually show much less central necrosis than the granulomas of lupus vulgaris (211); however, not all biopsies of tuberculosis show necrosis, and some biopsies of sarcoid do. The epidermis in sarcoidosis is usually normal or atrophic. In lupus vulgaris, in addition to atrophy, areas of ulceration, acanthosis, and pseudocarcinomatous hyperplasia are not uncommon. The absence of identifiable mycobacteria with acid-fast stain cannot be used to exclude tuberculosis, as the organisms in lupus vulgaris are scarce and may be difficult or impossible to find.

Foreign-body granulomas can also resemble sarcoidosis. Polariscopic examination in search of doubly refractile material, such as silica, should be performed on biopsies suspected of being sarcoidosis. The papular type of acne rosacea occasionally shows "naked" tubercles indistinguishable from those of sarcoidosis, but unlike sarcoid, they are usually perifollicular.

Tuberculoid leprosy, which may show granulomas in association with only a sparse lymphocytic infiltrate, can also be difficult to distinguish from sarcoidosis. Only 7% of cases of tuberculoid leprosy show acid-fast bacilli, and then only a few, so that they may easily be overlooked (212). The most likely place to find bacilli is within degenerated dermal nerves (the granulomas of tuberculoid leprosy form around dermal nerves that are undergoing necrosis). The granulomas of tuberculoid leprosy show small areas of central necrosis more often than those of sarcoidosis. Also, the granulomas of tuberculoid leprosy, in contrast with those of sarcoidosis, follow nerves and therefore often appear elongated (213). Clinical correlation may be required to distinguish between these two diseases. For example, in the United States, leprosy virtually can be excluded if a patient has not been in an endemic area (either in a foreign country or where it is carried in armadillos domestically, e.g., Texas and Louisiana) or has not had prolonged close contact with another individual with the disease.

FOREIGN-BODY REACTIONS

Foreign substances, when injected or implanted accidentally into the skin, can produce a nonallergic foreign-body reaction, or, in persons specifically sensitized to them, an allergic response (214). In addition, certain substances formed within the body may produce a nonallergic foreign-body reaction when deposited in the dermis or subcutis. Such endogenous foreign-body reactions are produced, for instance, by urates in gout and by keratinous material in pilomatricoma, as well as in ruptured epidermoid and trichilemmal cysts.

Histopathology. A nonallergic foreign-body reaction typically shows a granulomatous response marked by histiocytes and giant cells surrounding foreign material. Often, some of the giant cells are of the foreign-body type, in which the nuclei are in haphazard array. In addition, lymphocytes are usually present, as may be plasma cells and neutrophils. Frequently, some of the foreign material is seen within macrophages and giant cells, a finding that of course is of great diagnostic value. The most common cause of a foreign-body granuloma is rupture of a hair follicle or follicular cyst, and sometimes only the cyst contents, rather than residual cyst wall, is identifiable (Fig. 14-19). Exogenous substances producing nonallergic foreign-body reactions include silk and nylon sutures (Fig. 14-20), wood or other plant material (Fig. 14-21), paraffin and other oily substances, silicone gel, talc, surgical glove starch powder, and cactus spines. Some

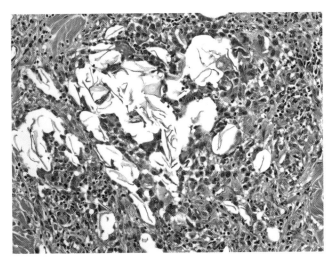

FIGURE 14-19. Ruptured epidermoid cyst. There are neutrophils and histiocytes surrounding grayish-pink cornified cells from the center of the cyst.

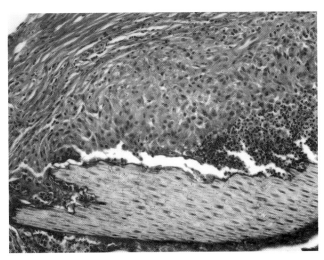

FIGURE 14-21. Foreign body reaction to a wood splinter. The wood splinter shows an orderly arrangement of rectangular cells, typical of plant material, surrounded by a nodular infiltrate with histiocytes, including multinucleated histiocytes and neutrophils.

of these substances—nylon sutures, wood, talc, surgical glove starch powder, and sea-urchin spines—are doubly refractile on polarizing examination. Double refraction often is very helpful in localizing foreign substances. Knife marks in the section may be an additional clue to the presence of particulate foreign matter (Fig. 14-22).

An allergic granulomatous reaction to a foreign body typically shows a sarcoidal or tuberculoid pattern consisting of epithelioid cells with or without giant cells. Phagocytosis of the foreign substance is slight or absent. Substances that in sensitized persons produce an allergic

granulomatous reaction include zirconium, beryllium, and certain dyes used in tattoos. Some substances that at first act as foreign material may later on, after sensitization has occurred, act as allergens, as in the case of sea-urchin spines and silica.

A histologic decision as to whether a granuloma is of the foreign-body type or of the allergic type is not always possible. A granuloma of the allergic type is more likely to show rounded, well-circumscribed collections of epithelioid histiocytes and less likely to have multinucleated histiocytes of the foreign-body type.

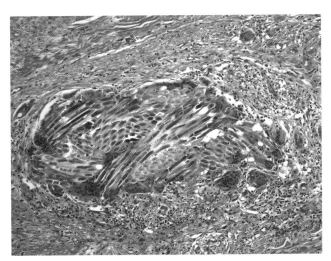

FIGURE 14-20. Foreign body granuloma caused by nylon suture. The suture is composed of blue-gray, linear material, and is surrounded by histiocytes, including many multinucleated foreign body–type giant cells.

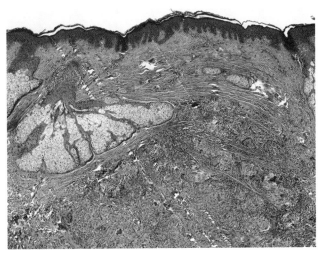

FIGURE 14-22. Foreign body reaction. There are circumscribed, nodular collections of epithelioid histiocytes associated with knife marks (diagonally oriented in this photograph), which serve as a clue to the presence of the foreign material.

Paraffinoma

Foreign-body reactions may occur following injections of oily substances such as mineral oil (paraffin) for cosmetic purposes. These occur as irregular, plaque-like indurations of the skin and subcutaneous tissue (215,216). Ulcers or abscesses may develop. The interval between the time of injection and the development of induration or ulceration may be many years.

The misleading term *sclerosing lipogranuloma* was given to paraffinoma of the male genitalia because of the disproved assumption that it was a local reactive process following injury to adipose tissue (217,218).

Histopathology. Paraffinomas have a "Swiss-cheese" appearance because of the presence of numerous ovoid or round cavities that show great variation in size. These cavities represent spaces occupied by the oily substance (219). The spaces between the cavities are taken up in part by fibrotic connective tissue and in part by an infiltrate of macrophages and lymphocytes. Some of the macrophages have the appearance of foam cells. Variable numbers of multinucleated foreign-body giant cells are present.

In frozen sections of paraffinoma, the foreign material stains orange with Sudan IV or oil red O, although less so than neutral fat (219).

Silicone Granuloma

Reactions to medical-grade silicone have occurred after injection of its liquid form for cosmetic purposes, or from leakage or rupture of silicone gel from breast implants. In the United States, the injection of liquid silicone is now banned, and it is no longer used as the gel in breast implants, in part because of controversy surrounding the unproven hypothesis that silicone leads to autoimmune disease in some individuals. Leakage from silicone breast

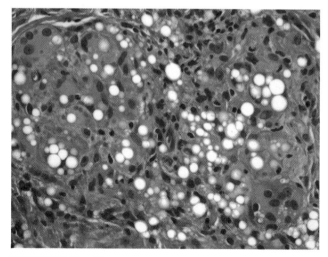

FIGURE 14-23. Silicone granuloma. Silicone used for cosmetic purposes may produce a granulomatous response with a "Swiss cheese" appearance. (Courtesy John Walsh, M.D.)

implants can cause development of subcutaneous nodules and plaques (220). Lesions containing silicone at sites adjacent to and, rarely, distant from areas of injection or implantation may occur (221,222). A localized reaction at injection sites by silicone-coated acupuncture or venepuncture needles has also been reported (223,224).

Histopathology. As in paraffinoma, numerous ovoid or round cavities of varying sizes are seen, resulting in a "Swiss cheese" appearance (Fig. 14-23). These spaces are what remain after the silicone has been removed during processing, although occasionally scant residual silicone is seen as colorless, irregularly shaped, refractile, nonpolarizable material within the spaces. Histiocytes may be present between the cavities; they can be foamy or multinucleated and accompanied by lymphocytes and eosinophils (220, 225). In addition, varying degrees of fibrosis are present. The identification of silicone within a specimen can be facilitated via thick sectioning, dark field microscopy and other techniques (226).

Talc Granuloma

Talc (magnesium silicate) may produce granulomatous inflammation when introduced into open wounds. Historically, talc was used as powder on gloves, but this use has been abandoned for many years, with starch being the currently used surgical dusting powder (227). However, talc may still be introduced into wounds, either because of accidental contamination by a surgeon who uses talcum powder (227) or because talcum may be incorporated into the actual rubber glove during manufacturing (228).

Histopathology. Histologic examination reveals histiocytes and multinucleated giant cells, some of which may contain visible particles of talc. Talc crystals can be needle-shaped with a yellow-brown or blue-green hue, and appear as white birefringent particles with polarized light (228). Their presence can be confirmed by x-ray diffraction studies (229) or energy-dispersive x-ray analysis (228).

Starch Granuloma

Granulomas may result from the contamination of wounds with surgical gloves powdered with cornstarch (227).

Histopathology. A foreign-body reaction with multinucleated giant cells is present. Scattered through the infiltrate, one observes starch granules as ill-defined ovoid basophilic structures measuring 10 to 20 μm in diameter. Most of the granules are seen within foreign-body giant cells. They react with periodic acid-Schiff (PAS) and methenamine silver and, on examination in polarized light, are birefringent, showing a Maltese cross configuration (230).

Cactus Granuloma

Cactus granulomas show, within days or weeks after the injury, tender papules from which cactus spines may still protrude. They may be extruded spontaneously within a few months.

Histopathology. Early papules, a few days after the injury, show fragments of cactus spicules in the dermis that are associated with an intense, perivascular lymphohistiocytic infiltrate containing many eosinophils. After a few weeks, the infiltrate consists of lymphocytes, macrophages, and giant cells (231,232). Sharply marginated spicules are seen within giant cells and lying free in the dermis. The spicules are PAS positive (233).

Interdigital Pilonidal Sinus

In barbers, the implantation of human hair in the interdigital web spaces may cause small, asymptomatic or tender sinus tracts (234,235). Similar lesions are even more common, within web spaces or in other sites in dog groomers and other animal caretakers (236,237).

Histopathology. Histologic examination reveals a sinus tract lined by squamous epithelium containing one or several hairs, thus resembling a hair follicle. Either the sinus tract encases the hair completely, or, if the hair extends deeper than the sinus tract, one finds at the lower end of the hair a foreign-body giant cell reaction intermingled with inflammatory cells (234,238).

Sea-Urchin Granuloma

Injuries from the spines of sea urchins occur most commonly on the hands and feet. Even if the friable spines have been only incompletely removed, the wounds tend to heal after spontaneous extrusion of most of the foreign material (239,240). However, in some persons, violaceous nodules appear at the sites of injury after a latent period of 2 to 12 months (241).

Histopathology. The nodules are composed largely of epithelioid histiocytes and giant cells (239). Doubly refractile material is present in a minority of the granulomas (240). If remnants of a spine are still present, they are surrounded by leukocytes and many large foreign-body giant cells (240). A minority of patients show nongranulomatous findings, the most common of which is a neutrophilic infiltrate (242).

Pathogenesis. The appearance of sarcoid-like granulomas after a latent interval of months in only a small proportion of the injured patients suggests a delayed hypersensitivity reaction (241). The spines of sea urchins, in addition to the calcified material, contain remnants of epithelial cells (241). The double refraction that may be found in the granulomas may be due to the presence of a small amount of silica in the calcified spines (240).

Silica Granuloma

Silica (silicon dioxide) is present in rocks, soil, sand, and glass. It frequently contaminates accidental wounds, in

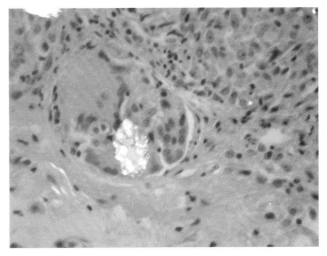

FIGURE 14-24. Silica. Silica, like other foreign materials with a crystalline structure, is doubly refractile when viewed under polarized light.

which it sets up a foreign-body reaction of limited duration followed by fibrosis (243). In the vast majority of cases, silica causes no further sequelae. In exceptional cases, a granulomatous delayed hypersensitivity reaction occurs at the site of the old scar (244). The mean interval for this delayed hypersensitivity reaction is approximately 10 years, but it may be less than a year or more than 50 years after the original injury (245). When this reaction occurs, indurated papules or nodules develop at the site of injury.

Histopathology. In silica granuloma, there are groups of epithelioid histiocytes with a lymphocytic infiltrate that tends to be sparse (244–248). Foreign-body giant cells may be abundant or absent, and Langhans giant cells also may be present. If multinucleated histiocytes are not numerous, a picture resembling sarcoid is produced. However, the diagnosis of sarcoidosis is easily excluded by the presence, especially within giant cells, of crystalline particles varying in size from barely visible to 100μm in length; they represent silica crystals. When examined with polarized light, these particles are doubly refractile (Fig. 14-24). The presence of silicon can be confirmed by x-ray spectrometric or energy dispersive x-ray analysis (245,246).

Pathogenesis. Evidence suggests that the sarcoid-like granulomatous response to silica that occurs long after initial injury represents a delayed-type hypersensitivity reaction (244,245,247,249).

Zirconium Granuloma

Deodorant sticks containing zirconium lactate and creams containing zirconium oxide may cause a persistent eruption composed of soft, red-brown papules in the areas to which they have been applied. Zirconium lactate is no longer present in antiperspirants sold in the United States; however, a granulomatous reaction has also been described in response to roll-on antiperspirant containing aluminum-zirconium complex (250,251).

Histopathology. Histologic examination shows large aggregates of epithelioid cells with a few giant cells and a sparse or moderately dense lymphocytic infiltrate, producing a picture that may be indistinguishable from sarcoidosis (252–254). Because of the small size of the zirconium particles, they cannot be detected on examination with polarized light (252). Their presence, however, can be demonstrated by spectrographic analysis (253) or energy dispersive x-ray analysis (250).

Pathogenesis. Evidence that zirconium granulomas develop on the basis of an allergic sensitization to zirconium includes the following: (a) they occur only in persons sensitized to zirconium (255); (b) the pattern of granulomas inflammation is like that of other granulomatous dermatitides that have been attributed to delayed-type hypersensitivity reactions; and (c) autoradiographic analysis of experimentally induced lesions in sensitized individuals reveals no zirconium within histiocytes (256).

Aluminum Granuloma

Single or multiple persistent subcutaneous nodules may appear several months or even years after the subcutaneous injection of a variety of vaccines or allergen desensitization extracts that are aluminum-adsorbed (257). The aluminum adjuvant is thought to prolong the period of activity of the vaccine or desensitization agent, thus increasing the immunologic response.

Histopathology. The most striking finding is the presence of nodular aggregates of lymphocytes with lymphoid follicles and germinal centers within the dermis and subcutis. There is fibrosis, which may occur in bands that separate the lymphocytic nodules. Eosinophils may be prominent, and the condition may show a pseudolymphomatous appearance (258–260). The granulomatous component consists of histiocytes with ample cytoplasm and, in some cases, a few giant cells or large areas of eosinophilic necrosis surrounded by histiocytes in a palisade (259). PAS staining, with or without diastase digestion, gives the impression of a granular cytoplasm in the macrophages (258). Early lesions tend to show a reaction that is more purely granulomatous (257). Palisading granulomatous reactions have also been reported (261).

Pathogenesis. This condition is believed to represent a delayed hypersensitivity reaction to aluminum. Electron microscopic examination reveals irregular membrane-bound, electron-dense material within macrophages. X-ray microanalysis has shown that the electron-dense material contains aluminum (258).

Zinc-Induced Granuloma

Local allergic reactions to insulin are not uncommon. However, the granulomatous response, which may occur with zinc-containing insulin preparations, is rare. It may begin with sterile furunculoid lesions (262,263).

Histopathology. The early furunculoid lesions show a dense neutrophilic infiltrate and many birefringent rhomboidal crystals of zinc insulin. Later, fibrosis and granulomatous inflammation develop (262).

Berylliosis

Beryllium granulomas are mostly of historical interest. Up to 1949, beryllium-containing compounds were widely used in the manufacture of fluorescent light tubes. Two diseases resulted from this: systemic berylliosis and local beryllium granulomas. Systemic berylliosis developed in some workers in plants manufacturing fluorescent tubes through inhalation of these compounds. Systemic berylliosis primarily shows pulmonary involvement, which results in death in about one-third of patients (264). Beryllium may reach the skin through blood circulation and cause cutaneous granulomas. However, this was a rare event, having been observed in one series in only 4 of 535 patients with systemic berylliosis (264). The granulomas consist of only a few papular lesions over which the skin remains intact.

Purely local beryllium granulomas occurred in persons who cut themselves on broken fluorescent tubes that were coated with a mixture containing zinc-beryllium silicate (265). The cutaneous granulomas after laceration show, as their first sign, incomplete healing of the laceration, followed by swelling, induration, tenderness, and, finally, central ulceration (266).

Histopathology. The cutaneous granulomas of systemic berylliosis, similar to those of sarcoidosis, show very slight or no caseation (264). The cutaneous granulomas following laceration, in contrast to the cutaneous granulomas of systemic berylliosis, show central necrosis, which may be pronounced (265). A moderately dense infiltrate of lymphocytes may be present, resembling the granulomas of tuberculosis. The epidermis shows acanthosis and possibly ulceration. No particles of beryllium are seen in histologic sections, but its presence in the lesions can be demonstrated by spectrographic analysis (266).

Pathogenesis. Systemic berylliosis develops on the basis of a delayed hypersensitivity reaction (267,268).

Tattoo Reactions

Clinically apparent inflammatory reactions to permanent tattoos, while uncommon, are now seen with greater frequency, due to the rise in popularity of tattoos. They have been observed most commonly with red dyes containing mercuric sulfide, such as cinnabar (Chinese red). More recently, there has been a move away from using mercury-containing dyes toward the use of dyes containing other red pigments, such as ferric hydrate (sienna or red ochre), cadmium selenide (cadmium red), and organic dyes, but such mercury-free red dyes may also produce adverse reactions (269,270). Reactions have also been reported with chrome green (271), cobalt blue (272), purple manganese salts (273), yellow cadmium sulfide (274), and iron oxide (275). In some instances, an allergic response to the pigment has been suggested by a positive patch test.

Reactions to "temporary" tattoos are rare. Usually comprised of black commercial henna, these tattoos are painted onto the skin surface. The most common reaction is allergic contact dermatitis, but lichenoid dermatitis, a scarring reaction, and hypopigmentation have been reported (276–280). Tattoos may also occur due to pigmented materials accidentally implanted in the skin, such as graphite, or due to solutions employed for hemostasis (281,282), particularly Monsel's solution (ferric subsulfate).

Histopathology. Permanent tattoos that are not clinically inflamed show irregularly shaped granules of dye that are located within macrophages and extracellularly in the dermis, without an inflammatory reaction (283).

Inflammatory reactions in clinically inflamed permanent tattoos may or may not be granulomatous. Photoexacerbation has been described with reactions to red pigments (269,270) and yellow pigments (274). Nongranulomatous reactions include a perivascular lymphocytic infiltrate with pigment-containing macrophages (269,283); a lichenoid response, which in some instances may resemble lichen planus or hypertrophic lichen planus (269,270,284,285); and a pseudolymphomatous picture with a dense, nodular or diffuse, predominantly lymphocytic infiltrate that also contains histiocytes and coarse tattoo pigment granules (286,287).

Granulomatous reactions may be either of the sarcoidal type (271,288,289) or the foreign-body type (271,275). A tuberculoid pattern has also been described in response to cobalt blue, but this may have been due to a mycobacterial infection (290). The granulomatous responses show tattoo

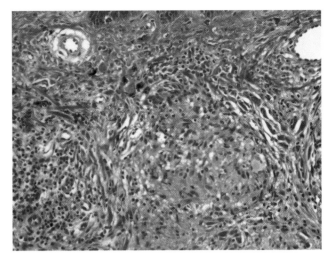

FIGURE 14-26. Decorative tattoo. Granulomatous response to a red tattoo.

granules scattered throughout the infiltrate (Figs. 14-25 and 14-26). In the sarcoidal type, the infiltrate contains nodules of epithelioid histiocytes, and in the foreign-body type, there are obvious multinucleated histiocytes of the foreign-body type. A sparse or dense lymphocytic infiltrate may be present. In the sarcoidal type of reaction, regional lymph nodes may also show tattoo granules (291). There are a few reports of patients with sarcoidal granulomas in their tattoos who also had pulmonary disease (172,288,289,292), uveitis (272,293), or erythema nodosum (288), suggesting a systemic hypersensitivity response to the tattoo, or true sarcoidosis.

Traumatic graphite tattoos show black granules free in the dermis and sometimes within histiocytes (Fig. 14-27). Monsel's tattoos, also typically seen in conjunction with scars, show multinucleate histiocytes containing coarse, brown, refractile pigment (Fig. 14-28), which is positive upon staining for iron. Ferruginization of collagen bundles is typical, and a proliferation of spindled fibrohistiocytic cells may also occur. Aluminum chloride, also used for hemostasis, produces another characteristic histologic appearance, with histiocytes with prominent basophilic stippling within the upper dermis in association with a scar (281) (Fig. 14-29).

Electron microscopic examination of tattoos without an allergic reaction shows that most tattoo granules are located within macrophages, where they often lie within membrane-bound lysosomes. In addition, some tattoo granules are found free in the dermis (294).

Bovine Collagen Implant and Other Tissue Augmentation Materials

Injectable bovine collagen is used for cosmetic purposes, principally on the face to diminish "wrinkles," such as glabellar creases and prominent nasolabial folds. A small

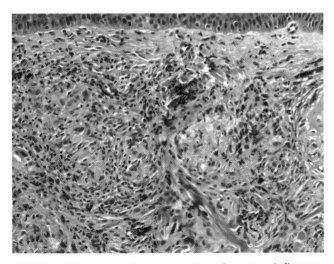

FIGURE 14-25. Decorative tattoo. Granulomatous inflammation in response to pigment used for a tattoo.

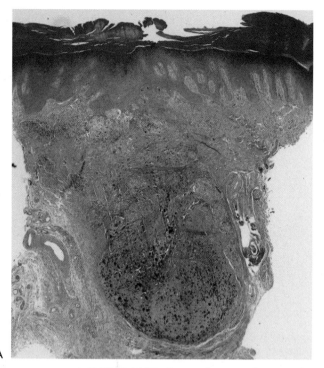

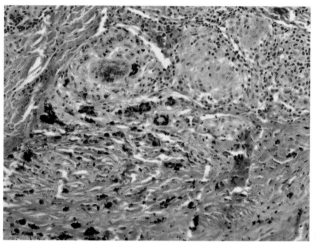

FIGURE 14-27. Traumatic tattoo from graphite. **A:** A circumscribed collection of black material is present in the dermis. **B:** The black material is darker than melanin and the clumps have irregular shapes and sizes; some are intracellular and some are extracellular. There are also knife marks from the foreign material.

minority of patients will develop an allergic granulomatous response at the site of injection. This response usually develops within 1 month of injection, is manifested by induration and erythema, and usually resolves spontaneously in less than a year (225,295). Hyaluronic acid has also been used for similar cosmetic purposes. Though it is less immunogenic, reactions to this injected material have been reported in approximately 3% of patients (296,297). Re-

cent additions to the soft tissue augmentation armamentarium include synthetic substances such as Bioplastique (polydimethylsiloxane) and Artecoll (polymethylmethacrylate), and adverse reactions to these materials have been reported (298–300).

Histopathology. Bovine collagen differs from native collagen by exhibiting a paler, less fibrillar appearance, and by its nonbirefringence when examined with polarized light.

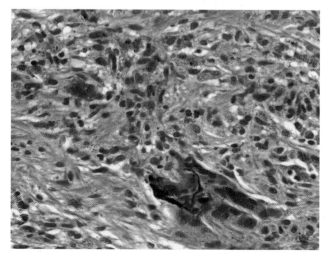

FIGURE 14-28. Monsel's tattoo. Monsel's solution may produce a granulomatous response associated with pigment that is gray-brown, with pigment sometimes in larger clumps.

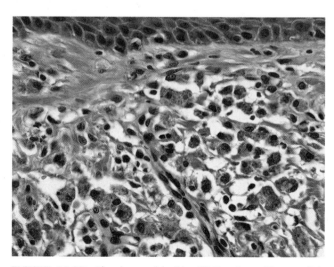

FIGURE 14-29. Aluminum chloride. Histiocytes with purplish granules as a consequence of aluminum chloride used for hemostasis during a previous procedure performed at this site.

It may lie within the center of a palisaded granuloma containing many foreign-body giant cells, or it may be associated with a more diffuse granulomatous reaction. There is a variable associated infiltrate of lymphocytes, eosinophils, plasma cells, and neutrophils that tends to spare the implanted collagen (225).

Biopsies of most patients with erythematous raised areas at sites of hyaluronic acid injections have revealed a granulomatous infiltrate with prominent giant cells. A mild lymphohistiocytic infiltrate without granulomas appears to be less common (296). Bioplastique granuloma exhibits numerous irregularly shaped cystic spaces distributed diffusely throughout a sclerotic stroma (298). At higher power, non-birefringent foreign material is apparent within these irregularly shaped cystic spaces, which are outlined by multinucleate giant cells. Artecoll granuloma shows numerous sharply circumscribed, seemingly empty cystic spaces, uniform in size and shape, mimicking normal adipocytes (298). Epithelioid histiocytes with occasional giant cells surround these spaces. Within them, upon lowering the microscopes' condenser, one notes vaguely visible round, sharply circumscribed, translucent, nonbirefringent foreign bodies.

Corticosteroid Deposits

Corticosteroid preparations for intralesional use are suspensions of insoluble crystalline chemicals; soluble corticosteroids are not effective for intralesional use. These suspensions may be identified histologically after injection of triamcinolone or other steroids. Sites where these deposits have been described include the skin (e.g., in keloids), the nasal mucosa, and Achilles tendon. The material may persist at the site of injection for months or years (225,301).

Histopathology. Corticosteroid deposits are recognizable by their acellular, amphophilic, and granular appearance

in association with clear spaces. The spaces may represent the sites of dissolved crystals. Uncommonly, birefringent crystals can be seen with polarized light. Inflammation tends to be absent or sparse, but a palisaded granuloma may develop (301–304).

CHEILITIS GRANULOMATOSA (MIESCHER–MELKERSSON–ROSENTHAL SYNDROME)

The classic triad of Miescher–Melkersson–Rosenthal syndrome consists of recurrent labial edema, relapsing facial paralysis, and fissured tongue (305). However, not all patients have the classic triad. In a review of 220 patients, labial swelling was seen in 84%, facial palsy in 23%, and fissured tongue in 60% (305). Whereas monosymptomatic labial edema is recognized as part of the syndrome, lingua plicata by itself is not, since this is not uncommon in the general population. One occasionally observes, either in addition to or in place of swelling of the lips, swelling of the forehead, chin, cheeks, eyelids, or tongue (306,307). Submandibular or submental lymph nodes may be enlarged (308). Swelling of the buccal mucosa, gingiva, and pallet also can occur (305). Chronic swelling of the vulva or of the foreskin has been described as a genital counterpart of cheilitis granulomatosa (309,310).

Histopathology. Granulomatous inflammation is not present in all biopsies of clinically involved lips (311). Sections may show simply edema, lymphangiectasia, and a predominately perivascular lymphoplasmacytic infiltrate. The infiltrate is often sparse but may be dense, producing a nodular appearance. If granulomas are present, they are noncaseating and tend to be small and scattered (Fig. 14-30). Collections of epithelioid histiocytes may be poorly

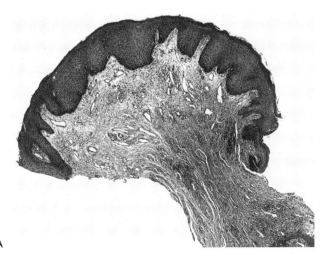
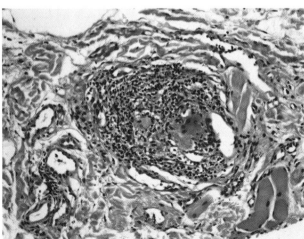

A   B

FIGURE 14-30. Cheilitis granulomatosa. **A:** Biopsy of lip mucosa showing slight vascular ectasia, edema, and a sparse inflammatory infiltrate including lymphocytes. **B:** A subtle granulomatous component.

circumscribed and are often associated with lymphocytes, but occasionally larger and/or "naked" tubercles are present, producing an appearance similar to sarcoidosis (307, 308,311–315). Affected lymph nodes may also show granulomatous inflammation (316).

Pathogenesis. The cause of cheilitis granulomatosa is unknown. Idiosyncratic reactions to exogenous factors, such as food additives, have been postulated to be causal in some cases (317,318). A relationship to sarcoidosis, originally assumed by some authors (316), appears unsubstantiated. Likewise, this syndrome appears to be distinct from Crohn's disease, which may also produce granulomatous inflammation of the lip (317,319).

CHEILITIS GLANDULARIS

Cheilitis glandularis is a rare condition marked by persistent enlargement and eversion of the lower lip. Labial salivary ducts appear to be dilated and exude mucoid material or clear fluid that may be accentuated by gentle squeezing (320,321). A papular component may be present (322). Diagnosis is based primarily on clinical features (320). It has been described mostly in adults but also in children.

Histopathology. Various histologic findings have been reported, none consistently, and this condition may not represent a specific disease (see section on pathogenesis). Salivary gland hyperplasia, duct ectasia, fibrosis, and inflammation comprised of lymphocytes, plasma cells, and histiocytes have been described (321,322). However, any or all of these features may be absent (320). Hyperkeratosis can also occur (320).

Pathogenesis. Cheilitis glandularis is probably caused by several different factors. Marked, chronic sun and wind exposure has been implicated as a common cause, and it has been suggested that this is not truly a disorder of salivary glands, since they may appear histologically normal (320). An atopic diathesis, factitious cheilitis, and hereditary factors have also been implicated (320,322). There are older reports in the literature that describe an increased incidence of squamous cell carcinoma in association with cheilitis glandularis (323). This is probably a consequence of actinic damage, which tends to be associated with this condition and which may be exacerbated by the eversion of the lip (323).

GRANULOMA GLUTEALE INFANTUM

Granuloma gluteale infantum, first described in 1971 (324), shows asymptomatic, round to oval, smooth, papules and nodules, irregularly distributed over regions covered by diapers (324–327). The lesions are typically reddish blue in color, ranging from a few millimeters to a few centimeters in diameter. Although usually seen in infants, this condition has also been described in incontinent adults (327,328). Although clinically this disorder may appear similar to a granulomatous condition, histologically it is not.

Histopathology. Acanthosis is usually present. A dense mixed infiltrate is seen throughout the dermis. Lymphocytes, histiocytes, plasma cells, neutrophils, and eosinophils may all be seen (326). In addition, there may be microabscesses composed of neutrophils and eosinophils, as well as extravasation of erythrocytes together with a proliferation of capillaries (324,329). Multinucleated histiocytes or well-developed granulomas are not a feature of the infiltrate. In a few instances, staining with the PAS reaction has revealed spores and pseudohyphae consistent with the presence of *Candida albicans* in the stratum corneum (330), but fungi are often not detected.

Pathogenesis. In nearly all patients described in the literature, the development of granuloma gluteale infantum has been preceded by diaper dermatitis, which only in some instances has been associated with a *C. albicans* infection (325,329). It appears very likely that exogenous factors are the cause of the eruption (324). Topical applications of fluorinated corticosteroid preparations for a prolonged period of time and prolonged wearing of plastic diapers have been implicated, but a consistent cause has not been identified (331).

REFERENCES

1. Hsu S, Lehner AC, Chang JR. Granuloma annulare localized to the palms. *J Am Acad Dermatol* 1999;41:287.
2. Dicken CH, Carrington SG, Winkelmann RK. Generalized granuloma annulare. *Arch Dermatol* 1969;99:556.
3. Haim S, Friedman-Birnbaum R, Shafrir A. Generalized granuloma annulare: relationship to diabetes mellitus as revealed in 8 cases. *Br J Dermatol* 1970;83:302.
4. Owens DW, Freeman RG. Perforating granuloma annulare. *Arch Dermatol* 1971;83:302.
5. Lucky AW, Prose ND, Bove K, et al. Papular umbilicated granuloma annulare. *Arch Dermatol* 1992;128:1375.
6. Kibarian MA, Mallory SB, Keating J, et al. Papular umbilicated granuloma annulare in association with Alagille syndrome. *Int J Dermatol* 1997;36:207.
7. Duncan WC, Smith JD, Knox JM. Generalized perforating granuloma annulare. *Arch Dermatol* 1973;108:570.
8. Samlaska CP, Sandberg GD, Maggio KL, et al. Generalized perforating granuloma annulare. *J Am Acad Dermatol* 1992;27:319.
9. Penas PF, Jones-Caballero M, Fraga J, et al. Perforating granuloma annulare. *Int J Dermatol* 1997;36:340.
10. Ogino A, Tamaki E. Atypical granuloma annulare. *Dermatologica* 1978;156:97.
11. Mutasim DF, Bridges AG. Patch granuloma annulare: clinicopathologic study of 6 patients. *J Am Acad Dermatol* 2000;42:417.
12. Rubin M, Lynch FW. Subcutaneous granuloma annulare. *Arch Dermatol Syphiligr* 1966;93:416.

13. Kerl H. Knotige rheumatische hautmanifestationen und ihre differential diagnose. *Z Hautkr* 1972;47:193.

14. Lowney ED, Simons HM. "Rheumatoid" nodules of the skin. *Arch Dermatol* 1963;88:853.

15. Felner EI, Steinberg JB, Weinberg AG. Subcutaneous granuloma annulare: a review of 47 cases. *Pediatrics* 1997;100:965.

16. McDermott MB, Lind AC, Marley EF, et al. Deep granuloma annulare (pseudorheumatoid nodule) in children: clinicopathologic study of 35 cases. *Pediatr Dev Pathol* 1998;1:300.

17. Sandwich JT, Davis LS. Granuloma annulare of the eyelid: a case report and review of the literature. *Pediatr Dermatol* 1999;16: 373.

18. Cronquist SD, Stashower ME, Benson PM. Deep dermal granuloma annulare presenting as an eyelid tumor in a child, with review of pediatric eyelid lesions. *Pediatr Dermatol* 1999;16: 377.

19. Moegelin A, Thalmann U, Haas N. Subcutaneous granuloma annulare of the eyelid. A case report. *Int J Oral Maxillofac Surg* 1995;24:236.

20. Salomon RJ, Gardepe SF, Woodley DT. Deep granuloma annulare in adults. *Int J Dermatol* 1986;25:109.

21. Evans MJ, Blessing K, Gray ES. Pseudorheumatoid nodule (deep granuloma annulare) of childhood: clinicopathologic features of twenty patients. *Pediatr Dermatol* 1994;11:6.

22. Dabski K, Winkelmann K. Destructive granuloma annulare of the skin and underlying soft tissues: report of two cases. *Clin Exp Dermatol* 1991;16:218.

23. Bancroft LW, Perniciaro C, Berquist TH. Granuloma annulare: radiographic demonstration of progressive mutilating arthropathy with vanishing bones. *Skeletal Radiol* 1998;27:211.

24. Romaine R, Rudner EJ, Altman J. Papular granuloma annulare and diabetes mellitus. *Arch Dermatol* 1968;98:152.

25. Jelinek JE. Cutaneous manifestations of diabetes mellitus. *Int J Dermatol* 1994;33:605.

26. Calista D, Landi G. Disseminated granuloma annulare in acquired immunodeficiency syndrome: case report and review of the literature. *Cutis* 1995;55:158.

27. Toro JR, Chu P, Yen TS, et al. Granuloma annulare and human immunodeficiency virus infection. *Arch Dermatol* 1999;135: 1341.

28. Cohen PR. Granuloma annulare: a mucocutaneous condition in human immunodeficiency virus-infected patients. *Arch Dermatol* 1999;135:1404.

29. Morris SD, Cerio R, Paige DG. An unusual presentation of diffuse granuloma annulare in an HIV-positive patient—immunohistochemical evidence of predominant CD8 lymphocytes. *Clin Exp Dermatol* 2002;27:205.

30. O'Moore EJ, Nandawni R, Uthayakumar S, et al. HIV-associated granuloma annulare (HAGA): a report of six cases. *Br J Dermatol* 2000;142:1054.

31. Zanolli MD, Powell BL, McCalmont T, et al. Granuloma annulare and disseminated herpes zoster. *Int J Dermatol* 1992;31:55.

32. Friedman JJ, Fox BJ, Albert HL. Granuloma annulare arising in herpes zoster scars. *J Am Acad Dermatol* 1986;14:764.

33. Gradwell E, Evans S. Perforating granuloma annulare complicating tattoos. *Br J Dermatol* 1998;138:360.

34. Crosby DL, Woodley DT, Leonard DD. Concomitant granuloma annulare and necrobiosis lipoidica. *Dermatologica* 1991;183:225.

35. Umbert P, Winkelmann RK. Histologic, ultrastructural, and histochemical studies of granuloma annulare. *Arch Dermatol* 1977; 113:1681.

36. Romero LS, Kantor GR. Eosinophils are not a clue to the pathogenesis of granuloma annulare. *Am J Dermatopathol* 1998;20: 29.

37. Silverman RA, Rabinowitz AD. Eosinophils in the cellular infiltrate of granuloma annulare. *J Cutan Pathol* 1985;12:13.

38. Burket JM, Zelickson AS. Intracellular elastin in generalized granuloma annulare. *J Am Acad Dermatol* 1986;14:975.

39. Gray HR, Graham JH, Johnson WC. Necrobiosis lipoidica: a histopathological and histochemical study. *J Invest Dermatol* 1965;44:369.

40. Trotter MJ, Crawford RI, O'Connell JX, et al. Mitotic granuloma annulare: a clinicopathologic study of 20 cases. *J Cutan Pathol* 1996;23:537.

41. Wood MG, Beerman H. Necrobiosis lipoidica, granuloma annulare, and rheumatoid nodule. *J Invest Dermatol* 1960;34: 139.

42. Dahl MV, Ullman S, Goltz RW. Vasculitis in granuloma annulare. *Arch Dermatol* 1977;113:463.

43. Patterson JW. Rheumatoid nodule and subcutaneous granuloma annulare: a comparative histologic study. *Am J Dermatopathol* 1988;10:1.

44. Kakurai M, Kiyosawa T, Ohtsuki M, et al. Multiple lesions of granuloma annulare following BCG vaccination: case report and review of the literature. *Int J Dermatol* 2001;40:579.

45. Abraham Z, Feuerman EJ, Schafer I, et al. Disseminated granuloma annulare following erythema multiforme minor. *Australas J Dermatol* 2000;41:238.

46. Beer WE, Wayte DM, Morgan GW. Knobbly granuloma annulare (GA) of the fingers of a milkman—a possible relationship to his work. *Clin Exp Dermatol* 1992;17:63.

47. Uenotsuchi T, Imayama S, Furue M. Seasonally recurrent granuloma annulare on sun-exposed areas. *Br J Dermatol* 1999;141: 350.

48. Wolff HH, Maciejewski W. The ultrastructure of granuloma annulare. *Arch Dermatol Res* 1977;259:225.

49. Kallioinen M, Sandberg M, Kinnunen T, et al. Collagen synthesis in granuloma annulare. *J Invest Dermatol* 1992;98:463.

50. Buechner SA, Winkelmann RK, Banks PM. Identification of cells in the cutaneous infiltrate by immunoperoxidase techniques. *Arch Pathol* 1983;108:379.

51. Modlin RL, Vaccaro SA, Gottlieb B, et al. Granuloma annulare: identification of cells in the cutaneous infiltrate by immunoperoxidase techniques. *Arch Pathol* 1984;108:379.

52. Mempel M, Musette P, Flageul B, et al. T-cell receptor repertoire and cytokine pattern in granuloma annulare: defining a particular type of cutaneous granulomatous inflammation. *J Invest Dermatol* 2002;118:957.

53. Mullans E, Helm KF. Granuloma annulare: an immunohistochemical study. *J Cutan Pathol* 1994;21:135.

54. Thyresson HN, Doyle JA, Winkelmann RK. Granuloma annulare: histopathologic and direcct immunofluorescence study. *Acta Derm Venereol (Stockh)* 1980;60:261.

55. Nieboer C, Kalsbeek GL. Direct immunofluorescence studies in granuloma annulare, necrobiosis lipoidica and granulomatosis disciformis Mieschner. *Dermatologica* 1979;158:427.

56. Laymon CW, Fischer I. Necrobiosis lipoidica (diabeticorum?). *Arch Dermatol Syph* 1949;59:150.

57. Alegre VA, Winkelmann RK. A new histopathologic feature of necrobiosis lipoidica diabeticorum: lymphoid nodules. *J Cutan Pathol* 1988;15:75.

58. Shapiro PE, Pinto FJ. The histologic spectrum of mycosis fungoides/Sezary syndrome (cutaneous T-cell lymphoma). *Am J Surg Pathol* 1994;18:645.

59. Su LD, Kim YH, LeBoit PE, et al. Interstitial mycosis fungoides, a variant of mycosis fungoides resembling granuloma annulare and inflammatory morphea. *J Cutan Pathol* 2002;29:135.

60. Cooper PH. Eruptive xanthoma: a microscopic simulant of granuloma annulare. *J Cutan Pathol* 1986;13:207.

61. Magro CM, Crowson AN, Schapiro BL. The interstitial granulomatous drug reaction: a distinctive clinical and pathological entity. *J Cutan Pathol* 1998;25:72.

62. Barr KL, Lowe L, Su LD. Mycobacterium marinum infection simulating interstitial granuloma annulare. A report of two cases. *Am J Dermatopathol* 2003;25:148.

63. Chase DR, Enzinger FM. Epithelioid sarcoma: Diagnosis, prognostic indicators, and treatment. *Am J Surg Pathol* 1985;9:241.

64. Miettinen M, Fanburg-Smith JC, Virolainen M, et al. Epithelioid sarcoma: an immunohistochemical analysis of 112 classical and variant cases and a discussion of the differential diagnosis. *Hum Pathol* 1999;30:934.

65. Dahl MV. Is actinic granuloma really granuloma annulare? *Arch Dermatol* 1986;122:39.

66. Ragaz A, Ackerman AB. Is actinic granuloma a specific condition? *Am J Dermatopathol* 1979;1:43.

67. Hanke CW, Bailin PL, Roenigk HH Jr. Annular elastolytic giant cell granuloma. *J Am Acad Dermatol* 1979;1:413.

68. O'Brien JP. Actinic granuloma. *Arch Dermatol* 1975;111:460.

69. Meadows KP, O'Reilly MA, Harris RM, et al. Erythematous annular plaques in a necklace distribution. Annular elastolytic giant cell granuloma. *Arch Dermatol* 2001;137:1647.

70. Davies MG, Newman P. Actinic granuloma in a young woman following prolonged sunbed usage. *Br J Dermatol* 1997;136:797.

71. Yanagihara M, Kato F, Mori S. Extra- and intra-cellular digestion of elastic fibers by macrophages in annular elastolytic giant cell granuloma. *J Cutan Pathol* 1987;14:303.

72. Sina B, Wood C, Rudo K. Generalized elastophagocytic granuloma. *Cutis* 1992;49:355.

73. Boneschi V, Brambilla L, Fossati S, et al. Annular elastolytic giant cell granuloma. *Am J Dermatopathol* 1988;10:224.

74. Özkaya-Bayazit E, Büyükbabani N, Baykal C, et al. Annular elastolytic giant cell granuloma: sparing of a burn scar and successful treatment with chloroquine. *Br J Dermatol* 1999;140:525.

75. Steffen C. Actinic granuloma (O'Brien). *J Cutan Pathol* 1988;15:66.

76. Mehregan AH, Altman J. Miescher's granuloma of the face. *Arch Dermatol* 1973;107:62.

77. Dowling GB, Wilson Jones E. Atypical (annular) necrobiosis lipoidica of the face and scalp. *Dermatologica* 1967;135:11.

78. Steffen C. Actinic granuloma of the conjunctiva. *Am J Dermatopathol* 1992;14:253.

79. Al-Hoqail IA, Al-Ghamdi AM, Martinka M, et al. Actinic granuloma is a unique and distinct entity: a comparative study with granuloma annulare. *Am J Dermatopathol* 2002;24:209.

80. Muller SA, Winkelmann RK. Necrobiosis lipoidica diabeticorum. *Arch Dermatol* 1966;93:272.

81. O'Toole EA, Kennedy U, Nolan JJ, et al. Necrobiosis lipoidica: only a minority of patients have diabetes mellitus. *Br J Dermatol* 1999;140:283.

82. Verrotti A, Chiarelli F, Amerio P, et al. Necrobiosis lipoidica diabeticorum in children and adolescents: a clue for underlying renal and retinal disease. *Pediatr Dermatol* 1995;12:220.

83. Lowitt MH, Dover JS. Necrobiosis lipoidica. *J Am Acad Dermatol* 1991;25:735.

84. Mehregan AH, Pinkus H. Necrobiosis lipoidica with sarcoid reaction. *Arch Dermatol* 1961;83:143.

85. Mackey JP. Necrobiosis lipoidica diabeticorum involving scalp and face. *Br J Dermatol* 1975;93:729.

86. Gaethe G. Necrobiosis lipoidica diabeticroum of the scalp. *Arch Dermatol* 1964;89:865.

87. Metz G, Metz J. Extracrurale manifestion der necrobiosis lipoidica: isolierter befall des kopfes. *Hautarzt* 1977;28:359.

88. el Sayed F, Elbadir S, Ferrere J, et al. Chronic balanitis: an unusual localisation of necrobiosis lipoidica. *Genitourinary Med* 1997;73:579.

89. Parra CA. Transepithelial elimination in necrobiosis lipoidica. *Br J Dermatol* 1977;96:83.

90. De la Torre C, Losada A, Cruces MJ. Necrobiosis lipoidica: a case with prominent cholesterol clefting and transepithelial elimination. *Am J Dermatopathol* 1999;21:575.

91. Gudmundson K, Smith O, Dervan P, et al. Necrobiosis lipoidica and sarcoidosis. *Clin Exp Dermatol* 1991;16:287.

92. Gudi VS, Campbell S, Gould DJ, et al. Squamous cell carcinoma in an area of necrobiosis lipoidica diabeticorum: a case report. *Clin Exp Dermatol* 2000;25:597.

93. Imtiaz KE, Khaleeli AA. Squamous cell carcinoma developing in necrobiosis lipoidica. *Diabet Med* 2001;18:325.

94. Snow JL, Su WP. Lipomembranous (membranocystic) fat necrosis. Clinicopathologic correlation of 38 cases. *Am J Dermatopathol* 1996;18:151.

95. Requena L, Yus ES. Panniculitis. Part I. Mostly septal panniculitis. *J Am Acad Dermatol* 2001;45:163.

96. Muller SA, Winkelmann RK. Necrobiosis lipoidica diabeticorum. *Arch Dermatol* 1966;94:1.

97. Smith JG Jr, Wansker BA. Asteroid bodies in necrobiosis lipoidica. *Arch Dermatol* 1956;74:276.

98. Nicholas L. Necrobiosis lipoidica diabeticorum with xanthoma cells. *Arch Dermatol* 1943;48:606.

99. Bauer MF, Hirsch P, Bullock WK, et al. Necrobiosis lipoidica diabeticorum: a cutaneous manifestiona of diabetic microangiopathy. *Arch Dermatol* 1964;90:558.

100. Holland C, Givens V, Smoller BR. Expression of the human erythrocyte glucose transporter Glut-1 in areas of sclerotic collagen in necrobiosis lipoidica. *J Cutan Pathol* 2001;28:287.

101. Oikarinen A, Mörtenhumer M, Kallioinen M, et al. Necrobiosis lipoidica: ultrastructural and biochemical demonstration of a collagen defect. *J Invest Dermatol* 1987;88:227.

102. Ullman S, Dahl MV. Necrobiosis lipoidica. *Arch Dermatol* 1977;113:1671.

103. Quimby SR, Muller SA, Schroeter AL. The cutaneous immunopathology of necrobiosis lipoidica diabeticorum. *Arch Dermatol* 1988;124:1364.

104. Laukkanen A, Fraki JA, Vaatainen N, et al. Necrobiosis lipoidica: clinical and immunofluorescent study. *Dermatologica* 1986;172:89.

105. Muller SA, Winkelmann RK. Necrobiosis lipoidica diabeticorum. *Arch Dermatol* 1966;93:1.

106. Veys EM, De Keyser F. Rheumatoid nodules: differential diagnosis and immunohistological findings. *Ann Rheum Dis* 1993;52:625.

107. Chalmers IM, Arneja AS. Rheumatoid nodules on amputation stumps: report of three cases. *Arch Phys Med Rehabil* 1994;75:1151.

108. Moore CP, Willkens RF. The subcutaneous nodule: its significance in the diagnosis of rheumatic disease. *Semin Arthritis Rheum* 1977;7:63.

109. Suliani RJ, Lansman S, Konstadt S. Intracardiac rheumatoid nodule presenting as a left atrial mass. *Am Heart J* 1994;127:463.

110. Horn RT Jr, Goette DK. Perforating rheumatoid nodule. *Arch Dermatol* 1982;118:696.

111. Falcini F, Taccetti G, Ermini M, et al. Methotrexate-associated appearance and rapid progression of rheumatoid nodules in systemic-onset juvenile rheumatoid arthritis. *Arthritis Rheum* 1997;40:175.

112. Williams FM, Cohen PR, Arnett FC. Accelerated cutaneous nodulosis during methotrexate therapy in a patient with rheumatoid arthritis. *J Am Acad Dermatol* 1998;39:359.

113. Dubois EL, Friou GJ, Chandor S. Rheumatoid nodules and rheumatoid granulomas in systemic lupus erythematosus. *JAMA* 1972;220:515.

114. Schofield JK, Cerio R, Grice K. Systemic lupus erythematosus presenting with "rheumatoid nodules." *Clin Exp Dermatol* 1992;17:53.

115. Hahn BH, Yardley HH, Stevens MD. Rheumatoid "nodules" in systemic lupus erythematosus. *Ann Intern Med* 1970; 72:49.

116. Sokoloff L, McCluskey RT, Bunim JJ. Vascularity of the early subcutaneous nodule of rheumatoid arthritis. *Arch Pathol* 1953; 55:475.

117. Elewaut D, De Keyser F, De Wever N, et al. A comparative phenotypical analysis of rheumatoid nodules and rheumatoid synovium with special reference to adhesion molecules and activation markers. *Ann Rheum Dis* 1998;57:480.

118. Alguacil-Garcia A. Necrobiotic palisading suture granulomas simulating rheumatoid nodule. *Am J Surg Pathol* 1993;17: 920.

119. Kuhn C, Lima M, Hood A. Palisading granulomas caused by foreign bodies. *J Cutan Pathol* 1997;24:108.

120. Hayes RM, Gibson S. An evaluation of rheumatic nodules in children. *JAMA* 1942;119:554.

121. Kiel H. The rheumatic subcutaneous nodules and simulating lesions. *Medicine (Baltimore)* 1938;17:261.

122. Finan MC, Winkelmann RK. The cutaneous extravascular necrotizing granuloma (Churg–Strauss granuloma) and systemic disease: a review of 27 cases. *Medicine* 1983;62:142.

123. Smith ML, Jorizzo JL, Semble E, et al. Rheumatoid papules: lesions showing features of vasculitis and palisading granuloma. *J Am Acad Dermatol* 1989;20:348.

124. Higaki Y, Yamashita H, Sato K, et al. Rheumatoid papules: a report on four patients with histopathologic analysis. *J Am Acad Dermatol* 1993;28:406.

125. Jorizzo JL, Olansky AJ, Stanley RJ. Superficial ulcerting necrobiosis in rheumatoid arthritis. *Arch Dermatol* 1982;118:255.

126. Patterson JW, Demos PT. Superficial ulcerating rheumatoid necrobiosis: a perforating rheumatoid nodule. *Cutis* 1985;35: 323.

127. Chu P, Connolly MK, LeBoit PE. The histopathologic spectrum of palisaded neutrophilic and granulomatous dermatitis in patients with collagen vascular disease. *Arch Dermatol* 1994; 130:1278.

128. Dykman CJ, Galen GJ, Good AE. Linear subcutaneous bands in rheumatoid arthritis: an unusual form of rheumatoid granuloma. *Ann Intern Med* 1965;63:134.

129. Gottlieb GJ, Duve RS, Ackerman AB. Interstitial granulomatous dermatitis with cutaneous cords and arthritis: linear subcutaneous bands in rheumatoid arthritis revisited. *Ann Intern Med* 1995;1:3.

130. Long D, Thiboutot DM, Majeski JT, et al. Interstitial granulomatous dermatitis with arthritis. *J Am Acad Dermatol* 1996; 34:957.

131. Aloi F, Tomasini C, Pippione M. Interstitial granulomatous dermatitis with plaques. *Am J Dermatopathol* 1999;21:320.

132. Tomasini C, Pippione M. Interstitial granulomatous dermatitis with plaques. *J Am Acad Dermatol* 2002;46:892.

133. Sangueza OP, Caudell MD, Mengesha YM, et al. Palisaded neutrophilic granulomatous dermatitis in rheumatoid arthritis. *J Am Acad Dermatol* 2002;47:251.

134. DiCaudo DJ, Connolly SM. Interstitial granulomatous dermatitis associated with pulmonary coccidioidomycosis. *J Am Acad Dermatol* 2001;45:840.

135. Perrin C, Lacour JP, Castanet J, et al. Interstitial granulomatous drug reaction with a histological pattern of interstitial granulomatous dermatitis. *Am J Dermatopathol* 2001;23:295.

136. Putkonen T. Symptomenkomplex der beginnenden Sarkoidose. *Dermatol Wochenschr* 1966;152:1455.

137. James DG, Siltzbach LE, Sharma OP, et al. A tale of two cities: a comparison of sarcoidosis in London and New York. *Arch Intern Med* 1969;123:187.

138. Wood BT, Behlen CH III, Weary PE. The association of sarcoidosis, erythema nodosum and arthritis. *Arch Dermatol* 1966; 94:406.

139. Olive KE, Kataria YP. Cutaneous manifestations of sarcoidosis. *Arch Intern Med* 1985;145:1811.

140. Veien NK. Cutaneous sarcoidosis treated with levamisole. *Dermatologica* 1977;154:185.

141. Hanno R, Needelman A, Eiferman RA, et al. Cutaneous sarcoidal granulomas and the development of systemic sarcoidosis. *Arch Dermatol* 1981;117:203.

142. Umbert P, Winkelmann RK. Granuloma annulare and sarcoidosis. *Br J Dermatol* 1977;97:481.

143. Newman LS, Rose CS, Maier LA. Sarcoidosis. *N Engl J Med* 1997;336:1224.

144. Johns CJ, Michele TM. The clinical management of sarcoidosis. A 50-year experience at the Johns Hopkins Hospital. *Medicine* 1999;78:65.

145. Yotsumoto S, Takahashi Y, Takei S, et al. Early onset sarcoidosis masquerading as juvenile rheumatoid arthritis. *J Am Acad Dermatol* 2000;43:969.

146. Seo SK, Yeum JS, Suh JC, et al. Lichenoid sarcoidosis in a 3-year-old girl. *Pediatr Dermatol* 2001;18:384.

147. O'Driscoll JB, Beck MH, Lendon M, et al. Cutaneous presentation of sarcoidosis in an infant. *Clin Exp Dermatol* 1990;15: 60.

148. Scerri L, Cook LJ, Jenkins EA, et al. Familial juvenile systemic granulomatosis (Blau's syndrome). *Clin Exp Dermatol* 1996;21: 445.

149. Manouvrier-Hanu S, Puech B, Piette F, et al. Blau syndrome of granulomatous arthritis, iritis, and skin rash: a new family and review of the literature. *Amer J Med Genet* 1998;76: 217.

150. Mana J, Marcoval J, Graells J, et al. Cutaneous involvement in sarcoidosis. Relationship to systemic disease. *Arch Dermatol* 1997;133:882.

151. Spiteri MA, Matthey F, Gordon T, et al. Lupus pernio: a clinical-radiological study of thirty-five cases. *Br J Dermatol* 1985;112: 315.

152. Jacyk WK. Cutaneous sarcoidosis in black South Africans. *Int J Dermatol* 1999;38:841.

153. Okamoto H, Horio T, Izumi T. Micropapular sarcoidosis simulating lichen nitidus. *Dermatologica* 1985;170:253.

154. Morrison JGL. Sarcoidosis in a child, presenting as an erythroderma with keratotic spines and palmar pits. *Br J Dermatol* 1976;95:93.

155. Lever WF, Freiman DG. Sarcoidosis: a report of a case with erythrodermic lesions, subcutaneous nodes and asteroid inclusion bodies in giant cells. *Arch Dermatol Syph* 1948;57:639.

156. Kelly AP. Ichthyosiform sarcoid. *Arch Dermatol* 1978;114: 1551.

157. Kauh YC, Goody HE, Luscombe HA. Ichthyosiform sarcoidosis. *Arch Dermatol* 1978;114:100.

158. Feind-Koopmans AG, Lucker GPH, van de Kerkhof PCM. Acquired ichthyosiform erythroderma and sarcoidosis. *J Am Acad Dermatol* 1996;35:826.

159. Bazex J, Dupin P, Giordano F. Sarcoidose cutanée et viscérale. *Ann Dermatol Venereol* 1987;114:685.

160. Albertini JG, Tyler W, Miller OF. Ulcerative sarcoidosis. Case report and review of the literature. *Arch Dermatol* 1997;133: 215.

161. Hruza GJ, Kerdel FA. Generalized atrophic sarcoidosis with ulcerations. *Arch Dermatol* 1986;122:320.

162. Schwartz RA, Robertson DB, Tierney LM, et al. Generalized ulcerative sarcoidosis. *Arch Dermatol* 1982;122:320.

163. Rongioletti F, Bellisomi A, Rebora A. Disseminated angiolupoid sarcoidosis. *Cutis* 1987;40:341.

164. Cornelius CE, Stein KM, Hanshaw WJ, et al. Hypopigmentation and sarcoidosis. *Arch Dermatol* 1973;198:249.

165. Darier J, Roussy G. Un cas de tumeurs benignes multiples: sarcoides sous-cutanees ou tuberculides nodulaires hypodermiques. *Ann Dermatol Syph* 1904;2:144.

166. Carriere M, Loche F, Schwarze HP, et al. Nail dystrophy in association with polydactyly and benign familial hypercalcaemia. *Clin Exp Dermatol* 1999;25:256.

167. Vainsencher D, Winkelmann RK. Subcutaneous sarcoidosis. *Arch Dermatol* 1984;120:1028.

168. Mirmirani P, Maurer TA, Herndier B, et al. Sarcoidosis in a patient with AIDS: a manifestation of immune restoration syndrome. *J Am Acad Dermatol* 1999;41:285.

169. Wendling J, Descamps V, Grossin M, et al. Sarcoidosis during combined interferon alfa and ribavirin therapy in 2 patients with chronic hepatitis C. *Arch Dermatol* 2002;138:546.

170. Corazza M, Bacilieri S, Strumia R. Post-herpes zoster scar sarcoidosis. Acta Derm Venereal 1999;79:95.

171. Bisaccia E, Scarborough A, Carr RD. Cutaneous sarcoid granuloma formation in herpes zoster scars. *Arch Dermatol* 1983;119:788.

172. Collins P, Evans AT, Gray W, et al. Pulmonary sarcoidosis presenting as a granulomatous tattoo reaction. *Br J Dermatol* 1994;130:658.

173. Papageorgiou PP, Hongcharu W, Chu AC. Systemic sarcoidosis presenting with multiple tattoo granulomas and an extra-tattoo cutaneous granuloma. *J Eur Acad Dermatol Venerol* 1999;12:51.

174. Jacyk WK. Annular granulomatous lesions in exogenous ochronosis are manifestation of sarcoidosis. *Am J Dermatopathol* 1995;17:18.

175. Walsh NMG, Hanly JG, Tremaine R, et al. Cutaneous sarcoidosis and foreign bodies. *Am J Dermatopathol* 1993;15:203.

176. Marcoval J, Mana J, Moreno A, et al. Foreign bodies in granulomatous cutaneous lesions of patients with systemic sarcoidosis. *Arch Dermatol* 2001;137:427.

177. Kim YC, Triffet MK, Gibson LE. Foreign bodies in sarcoidosis. *Am J Dermatopathol* 2000;22:408.

178. Barrier HJ, Bogoch A. The natural history of the sarcoid granuloma. *Am J Pathol* 1953;29:451.

179. Wigley JEM, Musso LA. A case of sarcoidosis with erythrodemic lesions. *Br J Dermatol* 1951;63:398.

180. Mittag H, Rupec M, Kalbfleisch H, et al. Zur frage der erythrodermischen sarkoidose. *Z Hautkr* 1986;61:673.

181. Okamoto H. Epidermal changes in cutaneous lesions of sarcoidosis. *Am J Dermatopathol* 1999;21:229.

182. Chevrant-Breton J, Revillon L, Pony JC, et al. Sarcoidose à manifestations cutanées extensives ulcéreuses et atrophiantes. *Ann Dermatol Venereol* 1977;104:805.

183. Glass LA, Apisarnthanarax P. Verrucous sarcoidosis simulating hypertrophic lichen planus. *Int J Dermatol* 1989;28:539.

184. Smith HR, Black MM. Verrucous cutaneous sarcoidosis. *Clin Exp Dermatol* 2000;25:96.

185. Alexis JB. Sarcoidosis presenting as cutaneous hypopigmentation with repeatedly negative skin biopsies. *Int J Dermatol* 1994;32:44.

186. Winkelmann RK, Dahl PM, Perniciaro C. Asteroid bodies and other cytoplasmic inclusions in necrobiotic xanthogranuloma with paraproteinemia. *J Am Acad Dermatol* 1998;38:967.

187. Burov EA, Kantor GR, Isaac M. Morpheaform sarcoidosis: report of three cases. *J Am Acad Dermatol* 1998;39:345.

188. Van-Landuyt H, Zultak M, Blanc D, et al. Sarcoidose ostéocutanée chronique multilante. *Ann Dermatol Venereol* 1988;115:587.

189. Bodie BF, Kheir SM, Omura EF. Calvarial sarcoid mimicking metastatic disease. *J Am Acad Dermatol* 1980;3:401.

190. Blinder D, Yahatom R, Taicher S. Oral manifestations of sarcoidosis. *Oral Surg Oral Med Oral Pathol Oral Radiol Endod* 1997;83:458.

191. Maycock RL, Bertrand P, Morison CE, et al. Manifestations of sarcoidosis. *Am J Med* 1963;35:67.

192. Longcope WT, Freiman DG. A study of sarcoidosis. *Medicine (Baltimore)* 1952;31:1.

193. McCoy RC, Fisher CC. Glomerulonephritis associated with sarcoidosis. *Am J Pathol* 1972;68:339.

194. Roberts WC, McAllister HA Jr, Ferrans VJ. Sarcoidosis of the heart. *Am J Med* 1977;63:86.

195. Mistilis SP, Green JR, Schiff L. Hepatic sarcoidosis with portal hypertension. *Am J Med* 1964;36:470.

196. Selenkow HA, Tyler HR, Matson DD, et al. Hypopituitarism due to hypothalamic sarcoidosis. *Am J Med Sci* 1959;238:456.

197. Rupec M, Korb G, Behrend H. Feingewebliche untersuchungen zur entwicklung des positiven Kveim-tests. *Arch Klin Exp Dermatol* 1970;237:811.

198. Steigleder GK, Silva A Jr, Nelson CT. *Histopathology* of the Kveim test. *Arch Dermatol* 1961;84:828.

199. Siltzbach LE, James DG, Neville E, et al. Course and prognosis of sarcoidosis around the world. *Am J Med* 1974;57:847.

200. Koerner SK, Sakowitz AJ, Appelman RI, et al. Transbronchial lung biopsy for the diagnosis of sarcoidosis. *N Engl J Med* 1975;293:268.

201. Shorr AF, Torrington KG, Hnatiuk OW. Endobronchial biopsy for sarcoidosis. A prospective study. *Chest* 2001;120:109.

202. Andonopoulos AP, Papadimitriou C, Melachrinou M, et al. Asymptomatic gastrocnemius muscle biopsy: an extremely sensitive and specific test in the pathologic confirmation of sarcoidosis presenting with hilar adenopathy. *Clin Exp Rheumatol* 2001;19:569.

203. James DG, Williams WJ. Immunology of sarcoidosis. *Am J Med* 1982;72:5.

204. Weissler JC. Southwestern Internal Medicine Conference. Sarcoidosis: immunology and clinical management. *Am J Med Sci* 1994;307:233.

205. Popper HH, Klemen H, Hoefler G, et al. *Presence of mycobacterial DNA in sarcoidosis*. Philadelphia: W.B. Saunders Company, 1997:796.

206. Mitchell DN. Mycobacteria and sarcoidosis. *Lancet* 1996;348:768.

207. Ikonomopoulos JA, Gorgoulis VG, Zacharatos PV, et al. Multiplex polymerase chain reaction for the detection of mycobacterial DNA in cases of tuberculosis and sarcoidosis. *Mod Pathol* 1999;12:854.

208. Li N, Bajoghli A, Kubba A, et al. Identification of mycobacterial DNA in cutaneous lesions of sarcoidosis. *J Cutan Pathol* 1999;26:271.

209. Nilsson K, Pahlson C, Lukinius A, et al. Presence of *Rickettsia helvetica* in granulomatous tissue from patients with sarcoidosis. *J Infect Dis* 2002;185:1128.

210. Azar HA, Lunardelli C. Collagen nature of asteroid bodies of giant cells in sarcoidosis. *Am J Pathol* 1969;57:81.

211. Civatte J. Sarcoidose et infiltrats tuberculoides. *Ann Dermatol Syphiligr* 1963;90:5.

212. Azulay RD. Histopathology of skin lesions in leprosy. *Int J Lepr* 1971;39:244.

213. Wiersema JP, Binford CH. The identification of leprosy among epithelioid cell granulomas of the skin. *Int J Lepr* 1972;40:10.

214. Epstein WL, Shahen JR, Krasnobrod H. The organized epithelioid cell granuloma: differentiation of allergic (zirconium) from colloidal (silica) types. *Am J Pathol* 1963;43:391.
215. Behar TA, Anderson EE, Barwick WJ. Sclerosing lipogranulomatosis: a case report of scrotal injection of automobile transmission fluid and literature review of subcutaneous injection of oils. *Plast Reconstr Surg* 1993;91:352.
216. Cohen JL, Keoleian CM, Krull EA. Penile paraffinoma: self-injection with mineral oil. *J Am Acad Dermatol* 2001;45:s222.
217. Smetana HF, Bernhard W. Sclerosing lipogranuloma. *Arch Pathol* 1950;50:296.
218. Newcomer VD, Graham JH, Schaffert RR, et al. Sclerosing lipogranuloma resulting from exogenous lipids. *Arch Dermatol* 1956;73:361.
219. Oertel VC, Johnson FB. Sclerosing lipogranuloma of male genitalia. *Arch Pathol* 1977;101:321.
220. Mason J, Apisarnthanarax P. Migratory silicone granuloma. *Arch Dermatol* 1981;117:366.
221. Suzuki KAM, Kawana S, Hyakusoku H, et al. Metastatic silicone granuloma: lupus miliaris disseminatus faciei-like facial nodules and sicca complex in a silicone breast implant recipient. *Arch Dermatol* 2002;138:537.
222. Brown SL, Silverman BG, Berg WA. Rupture of silicone-gel breast implants: causes, sequelae, and diagnosis. *Lancet* 1997;350:1531.
223. Yanagihara M, Fujii T, Wakamatu N, et al. Silicone granuloma on the entry points of acupuncture, venepuncture and surgical needles. *J Cutan Pathol* 2000;27:301.
224. Tang L, Eaton JW. Inflammatory responses to biomaterials. *Am J Clin Pathol* 1995;103:466.
225. Morgan AW. Localized reactions to injected therapeutic materials: Part 2. *J Cutan Pathol* 1995;22:289.
226. Raso DS GW, Vesely JJ, Willingham MC. Light microscopy techniques for the demonstration of silicone gel. *Arch Pathol Lab Med* 1994;118:984.
227. Ellis H. Pathological changes produced by surgical dusting powders. *Ann R Coll Surg Engl* 1994;76:5.
228. Kasper CS, Chandler PJ. Talc deposition in skin and tissues surrounding silicone gel-containing prosthetic devices. *Arch Dermatol* 1994;130:48.
229. Tye MJ, Hashimoto K, Fox F. Talc granulomas of the skin. *JAMA* 1966;198:1370.
230. Leonard DD. Starch granulomas. *Arch Dermatol* 1973;107:101.
231. Snyder RA, Schwartz RA. Cactus bristle implantation. *Arch Dermatol* 1983;119:152.
232. Suzuki H, Baba S. Cactus granuloma of the skin. *J Dermatol* 1993;20:424.
233. Winer LH, Zeilenga RH. Cactus granuloma of the skin. *Arch Dermatol* 1955;72:566.
234. Joseph HL, Gifford H. Barber's interdigital pilonidal sinus. *Arch Dermatol* 1954;70:616.
235. Adams CI, Petrie PW, Hooper G. Interdigital pilonidal sinus in the hand. *J Hand Surg [Br]* 2001;26:53.
236. Price SM, Popkin GL. Barber's interdigital hair sinus: a case report in a dog groomer. *Arch Dermatol* 1976;112:523.
237. Mohanna PN, Al-Sam SZ, Flemming AF. Subungual pilonidal sinus of the hand in a dog groomer. *Br J Plast Surg* 2001;54:176.
238. Goebel M, Rupec M. Interdigitaler pilonidaler sinus. *Dermatol Wochenschr* 1967;153:341.
239. Rocha G, Fraga S. Sea urchin granuloma of the skin. *Arch Dermatol* 1962;85:406.
240. Haneke E, Kolsch I. Seeigelgranulome. *Hautarzt* 1980;31:159.
241. Kinmont PDC. Sea-urchin sarcoidal granuloma. *Br J Dermatol* 1965;77:335.
242. De La Torre C, Toribio J. Sea-urchin granuloma: histologic profile. A pathologic study of 50 biopsies. *J Cutan Pathol* 2001;28:223.
243. Epstein E, Gerstl B, Berk M, et al. Silica pregranuloma. *Arch Dermatol* 1955;71:645.
244. Eskeland G, Langmark F, Husby G. Silicon granuloma of the skin and subcutaneous tissue. *Acta Pathol Microbiol Scand Suppl* 1974;248:69.
245. Mowry RG, Sams WM Jr, Caulfield JB. Cutaneous silica granuloma. *Arch Dermatol* 1991;127:692.
246. Schwechat-Millet M, Ziv R, Trau H, et al. Sarcoidosis versus foreign-body granuloma. *Int J Dermatol* 1987;26:582.
247. Rank BK, Hick JD. Pseudotuberculoma granulosum silicoticum. *Br J Plast Surg* 1972;25:42.
248. Arzt L. Foreign body granulomas and Boeck's sarcoid. *J Invest Dermatol* 1955;24:155.
249. Epstein WL. Granulomatous hypersensitivity. *Prog Allergy* 1967;11:38.
250. Skelton HG III, Smith KJ, Johnson FB, et al. Zirconium granuloma resulting from an aluminum zirconium complex: a previously unrecognized agent in the development of hypersensitivity granulomas. *J Am Acad Dermatol* 1993;28:874.
251. Montemarano AD, Sau P, Johnson FB, et al. Cutaneous granulomas caused by an aluminum-zirconium complex: an ingredient of antiperspirants. *J Am Acad Dermatol* 1997;37:496.
252. Williams RM, Skipworth GB. Zirconium granulomas of the glabrous skin following treatment of Rhus dermatitis. *Arch Dermatol* 1959;80:273.
253. Baler GR. Granulomas from topical zirconium in poison ivy dermatitis. *Arch Dermatol* 1965;91:145.
254. Lopresti PJ, Hambrick GW. Zirconium granuloma following treatment of Rhus dermatitis. *Arch Dermatol* 1965;92:188.
255. Shelley WB, Hurley HJ. The allergic orgin of zirconium deodorant granulomas. *Br J Dermatol* 1958;70:75.
256. Epstein WL, Shahen JR, Krasnobrod H. Granulomatous hypersensitivity to zirconium: localization of allergen in tissue and its role in formation of epithelioid cells. *J Invest Dermatol* 1962;38:223.
257. Garcia-Patos V, Pujol RM, Alomar A, et al. Persistent subcutaneous nodules in patients hyposensitized with aluminum-containing allergen extracts. *Arch Dermatol* 1995;131:1421.
258. Slater DN, Underwood JCE, Durrant TE, et al. Aluminum hydroxide granulomas: light and electron microscopic studies and x-ray microanalysis. *Br J Dermatol* 1982;107:103.
259. Fawcett HA, Smith NP. Injection-site granuloma due to aluminum. *Arch Dermatol* 1984;120:1318.
260. Culora GA, Ramsay AD, Theaker JM. Aluminium and injection site reactions. *J Clin Pathol* 1996;49:844.
261. Ajithkumar K, Anand S, Pulimood S, et al. Vaccine-induced necrobiotic granuloma. *Clin Exp Dermatol* 1998;23:222.
262. Morgan AW. Localized reactions to injected therapeutic materials: Part I. *J Cutan Pathol* 1995;22:193.
263. Jordaan HF, Sandler M. Zinc-induced granuloma: a unique complication of insulin therapy. *Clin Exp Dermatol* 1989;14:227.
264. Stoeckle JD, Hardy HL, Weber AL. Chronic beryllium disease. *Am J Med* 1967;46:545.
265. Neave HJ, Frank SB, Tolmach J. Cutaneous granulomas following laceration by fluorescent light bulbs. *Arch Dermatol Syph* 1950;61:401.
266. Dutra FR. Beryllium granulomas of the skin. *Arch Dermatol Syph* 1949;60:1140.
267. Hanifin JM, Epstein WL, Cline MJ. In vitro studies of granulomatous hypersensitivity to beryllium. *J Invest Dermatol* 1970;55:284.

268. Henderson WR, Fukuyama K, Epstein WL, et al. In vitro demonstration of delayed hypersensitivity in patients with berylliosis. *J Invest Dermatol* 1972;58:5.

269. Bendsoe N, Hansson C, Sterner O. Inflammatory reactions from organic pigments in red tattoos. *Acta Derm Venereol (Stockh)* 1991;71:70.

270. Sowden JM, Byrne JPH, Smith AG, et al. Red tattoo reactions: x-ray microanalysis and patch test studies. *Br J Dermatol* 1991; 124:576.

271. Loewenthal LJA. Reactions in green tattoos. *Arch Dermatol* 1960;82:237.

272. Rorsman H, Dahlquist I, Jacobsson S, et al. Tattoo granuloma and uveitis. *Lancet* 1969;2:27.

273. Schwartz RA, Mathias CG, Miller CH, et al. Granulomatous reaction to purple tattoo pigment. *Contact Dermatitis* 1987;16: 198.

274. Bjornberg A. Reactions to light yellow tattoos from cadmium sulfide. *Arch Dermatol* 1963;88:267.

275. Rubinanes EI, Sanchez JL. Granulomatous dermatitis to iron oxide after permanent pigmentation of the eyebrows. *J Dermatol Surg Oncol* 1993;19:14.

276. Lewin PK. Temporary henna tattoo with permanent scarification. *CMAJ* 1999;160:310.

277. Chung WH, Chang YC, Yang LJ, et al. Clinicopathologic features of skin reactions to temporary tattoos and analysis of possible causes. *Arch Dermatol* 2002;138:88.

278. Le Coz CJ, Lefebvre C, Keller F, et al. Allergic contact dermatitis caused by skin painting (pseudotattooing) with black henna, a mixture of henna and p-Phenylenediamine and its derivatives. *Arch Dermatol* 2000;136:1515.

279. Önder M, Atahan CC, Oztas P, et al. Temporary henna tattoo reactions in children. *Int J Dermatol* 2001;40:577.

280. Schultz E, Mahler V. Prolonged lichenoid reaction and cross-sensitivity to para-substituted amino-compounds due to temporary henna tattoo. *Int J Dermatol* 2002;41:301.

281. Elston DM, Bergfeld WF, McMahon JT. Aluminum tatoo: a phenomenon that can resemble parasitized histiocytes. *J Cutan Pathol* 1993;20:326.

282. Wood C, Severin GL. Unusual histiocytic reaction to Monsel's solution. *Am J Dermatopathol* 1980;2:261.

283. Goldstein AP. Histologic reactions to tattoos. *J Dermatol Surg Oncol* 1979;5:896.

284. Winkelmann RK, Harris RB. Lichenoid delayed hypersensitivity reactions in tattoos. *J Cutan Pathol* 1979;6:59.

285. Clarke J, Black MM. Lichenoid tattoo reactions. *Br J Dermatol* 1979;100:451.

286. Blumental G, Okun MR, Ponitch JA. Pseudolymphomatous reaction to tattoos. *J Am Acad Dermatol* 1982;6:485.

287. Zinberg M, Heilman E, Glickman F. Cutaneous pseudolymphoma resulting from a tattoo. *J Dermatol Surg Oncol* 1982;8: 955.

288. Sowden JM, Cartwright PH, Smith AG, et al. Sarcoidosis presenting with a granulomatous reaction confined to red tattoos. *Clin Exp Dermatol* 1992;17:446.

289. Weidman AI, Andrade R, Franks AG. Sarcoidosis. *Arch Dermatol* 1966;94:320.

290. Bjornberg A. Allergic reaction to cobalt in light blue tattoo markings. *Acta Derm Venereol (Stockh)* 1961;41:259.

291. Hanada K, Chiyoya S, Katebira Y. Systemic sarcoidal reaction in tattoo. *Clin Exp Dermatol* 1985;10:479.

292. Dickinson JA. Sarcoidal reactions in tattoos. *Arch Dermatol* 1969;100:315.

293. Mansour AM, Chan CC. Recurrent uveitis preceded by swelling of skin tattoos. *Am J Ophthalmol* 1991;111:515.

294. Abel EA, Silberberg I, Queen D. Studies of chronic inflammation in a red tattoo by electron microscopy and histochemistry. *Acta Derm Venereol (Stockh)* 1972;52:453.

295. Heise H, Zimmermann R, Heise P. Temporary granulomatous inflammation following collagen implantation. *J Craniomaxillofac Surg* 2001;29:238.

296. Micheels P. Human anti-hyaluronic acid antibodies: is it possible? *Dermatol Surg* 2001;27:185.

297. Lupton JR, Alster TS. Cutaneous hypersensitivity reaction to injectable hyaluronic acid gel. *Dermatol Surg* 2000;26:135.

298. Rudolph CM, Soyer HP, Schuller-Petrovic S, et al. Foreign body granulomas due to injectable aesthetic microimplants. *Am J Surg Pathol* 1999;23:113.

299. Reisberger EM, Landthaler M, Weiest L, et al. Foreign body granulomas caused by polymethylmethacrylate microspheres. Successful treatment with Allopurinol. *Arch Dermatol* 2003; 139:17.

300. Hoffman C, Schuller-Petrovic S, Soyer HP, et al. Adverse reactions after cosmetic lip augmentation with permanent biologically inert implant materials. *J Am Acad Dermatol* 1999;40: 100.

301. Balogh K. The histologic appearance of corticosteroid injection sites. *Arch Pathol Lab Med* 1986;110:1168.

302. Bhawan J. Steroid-induced "granulomas" in hypertrophic scar. *Acta Venereol* 1983;63:560.

303. Santa Cruz DJ, Ulbright TM. Mucin-like changes in keloids. *Am J Clin Pathol* 1981;75:18.

304. Weedon D, Gutteridge BH, Hockly RG, et al. Unusual cutaneous reactions to injections of corticosteroids. *Am J Dermatopathol* 1982;4:199.

305. Zimmer WM, Rogers RS III, Reeve CM, et al. Orofacial manifestations of Melkersson–Rosenthal syndrome. *Oral Surg Oral Med Oral Pathol* 1992;74:610.

306. Wagner G, Oberste-Lehn H. Zur kenntnis der symptomatologie der granulomatosis idiopathica. *Z Hautkr* 1963;32:166.

307. Mahler VB, Hornstein OP, et al. Granulomatous glossitis as an unusual manifestation of Melkersson–Rosenthal syndrome. *Cutis* 1995;55:244.

308. Hornstein OP. Melkersson–Rosenthal Syndrome. *Curr Probl Dermatol* 1975;5:117.

309. Westemark P, Henriksson TG. Granulomatous inflammation of the vulva and penis: a genital counterpart to cheilitis granulomatosa. *Dermatologica* 1979;158:269.

310. Hoede N, Heidbückel U, Korting GW. Vulvitis granulomatosa chronica: Melkersson–Rosenthal vulvitis. *Hautarzt* 1982;33: 218.

311. Greene RM, Rogers RS III. Melkersson–Rosenthal syndrome: a review of 36 patients. *J Am Acad Dermatol* 1989;91:57.

312. Miescher G. Über essentielle granulomatöse makrocheilie (cheilitis granulomatosa). *Dermatologica* 1945;91:57.

313. Hornstein O. Uber die pathogenese des sogenannten Melkersson–Rosenthal syndroms (einschliesslich der "cheilitis granulomatosa" Miescher). *Arch Klin Exp Dermatol* 1961; 212:570.

314. Allen CM, Camisa C, Hamzeh S, et al. Cheilitis granulomatosa: report of six cases and review of the literature. *J Am Acad Dermatol* 1990;23:444.

315. Cohen HA, Cohen Z, Ashkenasi A, et al. Melkersson–Rosenthal syndrome. *Cutis* 1994;54:327.

316. Hering H, Scheid P. Kritische bemerkungen zum Melkersson–Rosenthal syndrom als teilbild des Morbus Besnier–Boeck–Schaumann. *Arch Dermatol Syph* (Berlin) 1954;197:344.

317. Lancet. Orofacial granulomatosis [Editorial]. *Lancet* 1991;338: 20.

318. Armstrong DK, Biagioni P, et al. Contact hypersensitivity in patients with orofacial granulomatosis. *Am J Contact Dermat* 1997;8:35.

319. Kano Y, Shiohara T, Yasita A, et al. Granulomatous cheilitis and Crohn's disease. *Br J Dermatol* 1990;123:409.

320. Swerlick RA, Cooper PH. Cheilitis glandularis: a re-evaluation. *J Am Acad Dermatol* 1984;10:466.

321. Rada DC, Koranda FC, Katz FS. Cheilitis glandularis: a disorder of ductal ectasia. *J Dermatol Surg Oncol* 1985;11:372.

322. Weir TW, Johnson WC. Cheilitis glandularis. *Arch Dermatol* 1971;103:433.

323. Michalowski R. Cheilitis glandularis, heterotopic salivary glands and squamous cell carcinoma of the lips. *Br J Dermatol* 1962; 74:445.

324. Tappeiner J, Pfleger L. Granuloma glutaeale infantum. *Hautarzt* 1971;22:383.

325. Uyeda K, Nakayasu K, Takaishi Y. Kaposi sarcoma-like granuloma on diaper dermatitis. *Arch Dermatol* 1973;107:605.

326. Simmons IJ. Granuloma gluteale infantum. *Australas J Dermatol* 1977;18:20.

327. Maekawa Y, Sakazaki Y, Hayashibara T. Diaper area granuloma of the aged. *Arch Dermatol* 1978;114:382.

328. Fujita M, Ohno S, Danno K, et al. Two cases of diaper area granuloma of the adult. *J Dermatol* 1991;18:671.

329. De Zeeuw R, Van Praag MC, Oranje AP. Granuloma gluteale infantum: a case report. *Pediatr Dermatol* 2000;17:141.

330. Delarétaz J, Grigoriu D, De Crousaz H, et al. Candidose nodulaire de la région inguino-génitale et des fesses (granuloma glutaeale infantum). *Dermatologica* 1972;144:144.

331. Sweidan NA, Salman SM, Kibbi AG, et al. Skin nodules over the diaper area. *Arch Dermatol* 1989;125:1703.

15

DEGENERATIVE DISEASES AND PERFORATING DISORDERS

NARAYAN S. NAIK
CARLOS H. NOUSARI
EDWARD R. HEILMAN
ROBERT J. FRIEDMAN

SOLAR (ACTINIC) ELASTOSIS

Senile changes in areas of the skin not regularly exposed to sunlight manifest themselves clinically only in thinning of the skin and a decrease in the amount of subcutaneous fat. In contrast, there are often pronounced changes in the appearance of the exposed skin of elderly persons, especially those with fair complexions. These changes, however, are the result of chronic sun exposure rather than of age. In exposed areas, especially on the face, the skin shows wrinkling, furrowing, and thinning. In addition, there may be an irregular distribution of pigment.

Histopathology. In skin not regularly exposed to sunlight, there is a progressive disappearance of elastic tissue in the papillary dermis with age. It involves the oxytalan fibers, which in young age form a thin, superficial network perpendicular to the dermal-epidermal junction. Electron microscopically, the oxytalan fibers consist solely of microfibrils (Chapter 3). In middle age, the oxytalan fibers in the papillary dermis are split and fewer than at a young age, and in old age they may be absent (1).

In the skin of the face exposed to the sun, especially in persons with fair complexions, hyperplasia of the elastic tissue is usually evident on histologic examination by the age of 30, even though clinically the skin may appear normal. No white person past 40 years of age has normal elastic tissue in the skin of the face (2). The elastic fibers have increased in number, and they are thicker, curled, and tangled.

In patients with clinically evident solar elastosis of the exposed skin, staining with hematoxylin-eosin reveals, in the upper dermis, basophilic degeneration of the collagen separated from a somewhat atrophic epidermis by a narrow band of normal collagen. In the areas of basophilic degeneration, the bundles of eosinophilic collagen have been replaced by amorphous basophilic granular material.

With elastic tissue stains, the areas of basophilic degeneration stain like elastic tissue and therefore are referred to as elastotic material. The elastotic material usually consists of aggregates of thick, interwoven bands in the upper dermis (3) (Fig. 15-1A); but in areas of severe solar degeneration, the elastotic material may have an amorphous rather than a fibrous appearance (Fig. 15-1B), and may extend into the lower portions of the dermis rather than being confined to the upper dermis (4).

On staining with silver nitrate, the distribution of melanin in the basal cell layer may appear irregular, in that areas of hyperpigmentation alternate with areas of hypopigmentation (4).

Histogenesis. Electron microscopic examination of areas of solar elastosis shows elastotic material as the main component. Even though this elastotic material resembles elastic tissue in its chemical composition, it differs significantly in appearance from aged elastic fibers in unexposed, aged skin. Instead of showing amorphous electron-lucent elastin and aggregates of electron-dense microfibrils (Chapter 3), the thick fibers of elastotic material show two structural components: a fine granular matrix of medium electron density and, within this matrix, homogeneous, electron-dense, irregularly shaped inclusions (5). The electron-dense inclusions seem to develop by means of a condensation process in the granular matrix (3). The respective proportion for each of the two components can vary between 30% and 70% of the volume (6). Microfibrils such as those observed in normal or aged elastic fibers are absent. Accordingly, immunoelectron microscopy shows that the elastotic material has retained its antigenicity for elastin but not for microfibrils (7). The number and size of elastotic fibers are greatly increased over the number and size of elastic fibers found in normal or aged skin. Extensive amorphous material can be seen around the elastotic fibers and also among the collagen fibrils. Collagen fibrils are diminished in number, with those present often showing a diminished electron density, a diminished contrast in cross striation, and a splitting up into filaments at their ends (8).

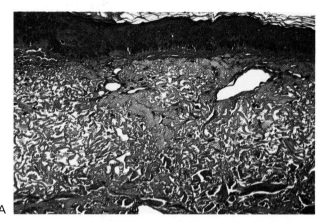
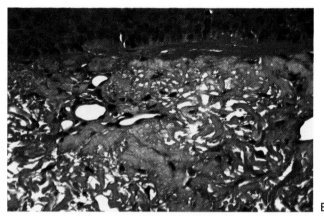

FIGURE 15-1. Solar (actinic) degeneration. **A:** In the upper dermis, separated from the epidermis by a narrow band of normal collagen, there are aggregates of thick, interwoven bands of the elastotic material. **B:** Extensive amorphous material can be seen around and among elastic and collagen fibers.

The fibroblasts show the characteristics of actively synthesizing cells in that they possess an extensive, dilated, rough endoplasmic reticulum containing amorphous or fine granular material that is excreted into the extracellular space (3,9). Often, strands of fine granular material are discernible between the surfaces of active fibroblasts and masses of elastotic material (5).

It can be concluded that the elastotic material is newly formed as the result of an altered function of fibroblasts, which are no longer capable of producing normal elastic fibers or collagen. The elastotic material is not regarded as a degeneration product of preexisting elastic fibers.

The elastotic material that histochemically stains like elastic tissue resembles elastic tissue in its chemical composition and its physical and enzymatic reactions. Thus, the amino acid composition of the elastotic tissue resembles that of elastin and differs significantly from that of collagen. In particular, the elastotic material, like elastic tissue, has a much lower content of hydroxyproline than collagen (10). Moreover, the elastotic material in unfixed sections shows the same brilliant autofluorescence as do elastic fibers on examination with the fluorescence microscope (11), and both the elastotic material and elastic tissue are susceptible to elastase digestion (12). The elastotic material contains a large amount of acid mucopolysaccharides, as indicated by staining with Alcian blue. A significant portion of these acid mucopolysaccharides may be sulfated because prior incubation with hyaluronidase removes only 50% to 75% of the positive-blue-positive staining. The basophilia of the elastotic material, however, is not affected by incubation with hyaluronidase (13).

The irregular distribution of melanin in the epidermis observed in some patients with solar degeneration, when studied by electron microscopy, is found to be caused largely by an impairment of pigment transfer from melano-cytes to keratinocytes. Although some keratinocytes contain many melanosomes, others contain few or no melanosomes. The latter are surrounded by dendrites laden with melanosomes (14).

Differential Diagnosis. For a discussion of differentiation of solar elastosis from pseudoxanthoma elasticum, see Chapter 3.

LOCALIZED SOLAR ELASTOSIS VARIANTS

Several clinically distinct forms of localized solar elastosis have been described. In the nuchal region, the skin, after many years of exposure to the sun, may appear thickened and furrowed. This is referred to as *cutis rhomboidalis nuchae*. *Elastotic nodules of the ears* are localized papular and nodular forms of solar elastosis usually occurring on the antihelix (15–18). Severe solar elastosis may also occur as yellowish plaques associated with small cysts and comedones. *Favre–Racouchot syndrome (nodular elastosis with cysts and comedones)* is an example occurring on facial skin lateral to the eyes (19,20). A similar condition occurring on the arms has been termed *actinic comedonal plaques* (21–23). Two other types of circumscribed solar elastosis occurring on the upper extremities are *solar elastotic bands of the* forearm (3,24), and *collagenous and elastotic marginal plaques of the hands* (25–31).

Elastotic Nodules of the Ears

Elastotic nodules are most often seen on the anterior crus of the antihelix (15,16,18) and occasionally on the helix of the ears (17). They are often bilateral. Clinically, they may mimic basal cell carcinomas, amyloidosis, gouty tophi, or chondrodermatitis nodularis helicis (15–18).

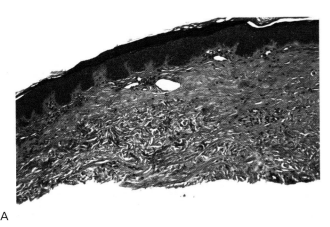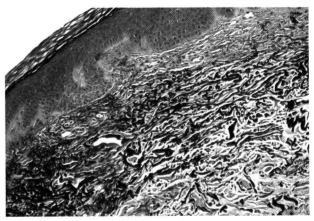

A   B

FIGURE 15-2. Elastotic nodule of the ear. **A:** A dome-shaped papule with marked solar elastosis in the dermis, and clumped and irregular eosinophilic material representing degenerated elastic fibers. **B:** The coarse, clumped material is highlighted with an elastic stain.

Histopathology. Irregular elastotic fibers and clumps of elastotic material are seen in the background of marked dermal solar elastosis (Fig. 15-2A). The fibers and clumps can be highlighted with a Verhoeff-van Gieson elastic stain (17) (Fig. 15-2B).

Favre–Racouchot Syndrome (Nodular Elastosis with Cysts and Comedones)

Favre–Racouchot syndrome is characterized by yellow plaques with multiple open and cystically dilated comedones. The condition typically affects the skin lateral to the eyes in elderly males (19,20). However, a case has also been documented on the shoulder (32). Although the condition is usually bilateral, it may be unilateral (33–35). The condition is thought to be primarily secondary to prolonged solar exposure but smoking may also be a contributing factor in its development (36).

Histopathology. Dilated pilosebaceous openings and large, round, cyst-like spaces are lined by a flattened epithelium and represent greatly distended hair follicles (19, 20). Both the dilated pilosebaceous openings and the cyst-like spaces are filled with layered horny material. Vellus hair shafts and bacteria have been demonstrated within the spaces as well suggesting the cyst-like spaces may represent closed comedones rather than true infundibular cysts (37). The sebaceous glands are atrophic. Solar elastosis often is pronounced (19), but it may be slight or absent (38). Because the comedones are open, they do not tend to become inflamed (39) (see section on acne vulgaris Chapter 18).

Actinic Comedonal Plaques

In actinic comedonal plaques, solitary nodular plaques with a cribriform appearance and comedone-like structures occur on the arms or forearms (21–23). The plaques are composed of confluent erythematous to bluish papules and nodules. The condition has been described in fair skinned individuals with a history of chronic sun exposure.

Histopathology. Dilated corneocyte-filled follicular lumina are present within areas of elastotic, amorphous material (21,22). The overlying epidermis is usually dyskeratotic and atrophic. The histologic findings are quite similar to those seen in Favre–Racouchot syndrome (21,22).

Solar Elastotic Bands of the Forearm

Solar elastotic bands of the forearm consist of soft cordlike plaques across the flexor surface of the forearms (3,24). The bands occur in areas of actinic damage and usually with senile purpura.

Histopathology. Nodular collections of basophilic homogenous amorphous material underlying an atrophic epidermis are conspicuous features. Thickened degenerated elastic fibers within the homogenous material are also observed. Stellate fibroblasts and a perivascular infiltrate of lymphocytes and hemosiderin-laden macrophages are found in close apposition to the elastic fibers. The nodular collections and thickened elastic fibers stain positively with Verhoeff–van Gieson elastic stain (3).

Collagenous and Elastotic Marginal Plaques of the Hands

Collagenous and elastotic marginal plaques of the hands have been described by several names: *degenerative collagenous plaques of the hands* (25,27), *keratoelastoidosis marginalis,* (26), and *digital papular calcific elastosis* (28). This acquired slowly progressive condition is usually seen in elderly males and consists of groups of linear confluent papules along the medial and lateral aspects of the hands at the juncture of the palmar and dorsal surfaces. The medial aspect of the thumb and radial aspect of the index finger are most commonly affected. The condition closely resembles the genodermatosis, *acrokeratoelastoidosis* (29). However, there is no familial predisposition or involvement of the plantar surfaces. Actinic damage and chronic repetitive pressure or trauma has been implicated in its pathogenesis (26,40,41).

Histopathology. The reticular dermis displays an acellular zone of haphazardly arranged collagen with some bundles running perpendicular to the epidermis (27). The bundles of collagen are admixed with fragmented elastic fibers and distinctive angulated amorphous "basophilic elastotic masses" in the upper dermis. These masses can be demonstrated to contain degenerating elastic fibers and calcium (28).

PERFORATING DISORDERS

The perforating disorders comprise a group of unrelated pathologic abnormalities sharing the common characteristic of transepidermal elimination. This phenomenon is characterized by the elimination or extrusion of altered dermal substances and, in some cases, by such material behaving as foreign material.

Traditionally, four diseases have been included in this group: *Kyrle's disease* (hyperkeratosis follicularis et parafollicularis in cutem penetrans), *perforating folliculitis*, *elastosis perforans serpiginosa*, and *reactive perforating collagenosis*. In addition, an important fifth condition known as *perforating disorder of renal failure and/or diabetes* has been added to this group (20,42).

Although transepidermal elimination is a prominent feature in all of these conditions, it has also been described as a secondary phenomenon in other entities, including such inflammatory disorders as granuloma annulare, one variant of pseudoxanthoma elasticum, and chondrodermatitis nodularis helicis. Needless to say, there is a long list of other conditions that can exhibit transepidermal elimination as an associated reaction pattern.

Kyrle's Disease

Kyrle's disease is a rare disorder, described by Kyrle in 1916 (43), which may actually comprise a group of disorders with similar epidermal-dermal reaction patterns associated with chronic renal failure, diabetes, prurigo nodularis, and even keratosis pilaris. Therefore, the discussion of Kyrle's disease and perforating disorders of chronic renal disease and/or diabetes has a very broad overlap in terms of their clinical and pathologic features.

Clinical Features. This eruption presents with a large number of papules, some coalescing into plaques, numbering in the hundreds and often distributed on the extremities.

Although some may appear to involve the follicular units, these lesions are more likely to be extrafollicular. The typical patient is young to middle aged and often has a history of diabetes mellitus. The papules are dome shaped, 2 to 8 mm in diameter, with a central keratotic plug. Excoriations often are found in the vicinity of these lesions. Linear lesions related to possible "Koebnerization" have been described.

Histopathology. The essential histopathologic findings include (a) a follicular or extrafollicular cornified plug with focal parakeratosis embedded in an epidermal invagination; (b) basophilic degenerated material identified in small collections throughout the plug with absence of demonstrable collagen and elastin; (c) abnormal vacuolated and/or dyskeratotic keratinization of the epithelial cells extending to the basal cell zone; (d) irregular epithelial hyperplasia; and (e) an inflammatory component that is typically granulomatous with small foci of suppuration (Fig. 15-3). In most instances, it is important to perform elastic tissue stains and even trichrome stains to exclude perforating elastic fibers as in elastosis perforans serpiginosa or collagen fibers as in reactive perforating collagenosis (44).

Histogenesis. The primary event is claimed to be a disturbance of epidermal keratinization characterized by the formation of dyskeratotic foci and acceleration of the process of keratinization. This leads to the formation of keratotic plugs with areas of parakeratosis (45–47). Because the rapid rate of differentiation and keratinization exceeds the rate of cell proliferation, the parakeratotic column

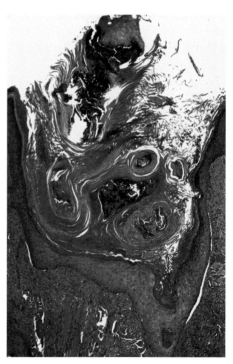

FIGURE 15-3. Kyrle's disease. A large parakeratotic plug containing basophilic debris lies within an invagination of the epidermis. The underlying dermis displays acute and chronic inflammation.

gradually extends deeper into the abnormal epidermis, leading in most cases to perforation of the parakeratotic column into the dermis. Perforation is not the cause of Kyrle's disease, as originally thought (43), but rather represents the consequence or final event of the abnormally sped-up keratinization. This rapid production of abnormal keratin forms a plug that acts as a foreign body, penetrating the epidermis and inciting a granulomatous inflammatory reaction. A certain similarity exists between the parakeratotic column in Kyrle's disease and that observed in porokeratosis of Mibelli (46). In both conditions, a parakeratotic column forms as the result of rapid and faulty keratinization of dyskeratotic cells, but whereas in Kyrle's disease the dyskeratotic cells are often used up so that disruption of the epithelium occurs, the clone of dyskeratotic cells can maintain itself in porokeratosis Mibelli by extending peripherally.

Differential Diagnosis. See Table 15-1.

Perforating Folliculitis

Perforating folliculitis is a perforating disorder that has many features overlapping with Kyrle's disease and perforating disorders of renal disease/diabetes. As described by Mehregan and Coskey (48), this is a relatively uncommon disorder usually observed in the second to fourth decades and is characterized by erythematous follicular papules with central keratotic plugs. The lesions are 2 to 8 mm in diameter and tend to be localized to the extensor surfaces of the extremities and the buttocks. The key to making this diagnosis is the clinical and histologic identification of a follicular unit as the primary site for the inflammatory process.

Histopathology. The main pathologic abnormalities consist of (a) a dilated follicular infundibulum filled with compact ortho and parakeratotic cornified cells (Fig. 15-4A); (b) degenerated basophilic staining material, comprised of granular nuclear debris from nuclear neutrophils, other inflammatory cells, and degenerated collagen bundles (Fig. 15-4B); (c) one or more perforations through the follicular epithelium; and (d) an associated perifollicular inflammatory cell infiltrate composed of lymphocytes, histiocytes, and neutrophils. Additionally, altered collagen and refractile eosinophilically altered elastic fibers are found adjacent to the sites of perforation. When serial sections through the specimen are examined, a remnant of the hair shaft can sometimes be found.

Histogenesis. Perforating folliculitis is the end result of abnormal follicular keratinization most likely caused by irritation, either chemical or physical, and even chronic rubbing. A portion of a curled-up hair is often seen close to or within the area of perforation or even in the dermis, surrounded by a foreign-body granuloma (48).

Differential Diagnosis. In Kyrle's disease, the keratinous plug may be extrafollicular, the perforation usually is present deep in the invagination at the bottom of the keratinous plug, and no eosinophilic degeneration of elastic fibers is found. In addition, in Kyrle's disease, epithelial hyperplasia is a significant feature. For a discussion of the differential diagnosis of perforating folliculitis from elastosis perforans serpiginosa, see the following section

TABLE 15-1. DIFFERENTIAL DIAGNOSES OF PERFORATING DISORDERS

Disease	Primary Defect	Distinctive Features	Histogenesis
Kyrle's disease	Focus of dyskeratotic rapidly proliferating cells in the epidermis	Follicular or extrafollicular cornified plug embedded in an epidermal invagination associated with epithelial hyperplasia and absence of demonstrable collagen and elastin	Disturbance of keratinization, forming a plug that acts as a foreign body penetrating the epidermis and inciting a granulomatous inflammatory reaction
Perforating folliculitis	Hyperkeratotic plug in follicular unit containing a retained hair	Compact ortho and parakeratotic plug with degenerated collagen, altered elastin, and mixed inflammatory cell infiltrate including neutrophils	A primary irritant causing follicular hyperkeratosis resulting in a mechanical breakdown of the follicle wall by the hair shaft
Elastosis perforans serpiginosum	Formation of numerous thickened coarse elastic fibers in the superficial dermis	Formation of narrow channel through an acanthotic epidermis with elimination of eosinophilic elastic fibers	Thickened elastic fibers act as mechanical irritants or "foreign bodies"
Reactive perforating collagenosis	Subepidermal focus of altered collagen caused by trauma	Formation of cup-shaped vertically oriented channel with transepidermal elimination of degenerated collagen	Histochemically altered collagen acts as "foreign body"
Perforating disorder secondary to chronic renal disease and/or diabetes mellitus	Chronic rubbing due to pruritis, resulting in follicular hyperkeratosis and perforation	A combination of features similar to that seen in perforating folliculitis, reactive perforating collagenosis, and prurigo nodularis	Exogenously altered skin in pruritic diabetics and patients with chronic renal disease

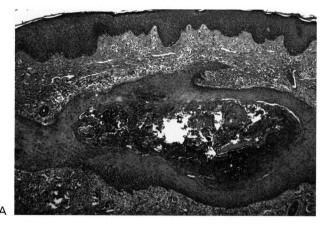
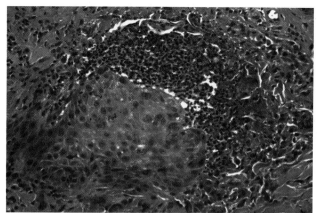

FIGURE 15-4. Perforating folliculitis. **A:** A widely dilated follicular unit contains a mixture of keratin, basophilic debris, inflammatory cells, and degenerated collagen fibers. **B:** An area of disrupted follicular epithelium with adjacent associated perifollicular inflammation and alteration of collagen and elastic fibers.

on differential diagnosis for elastosis perforans serpiginosa, and Table 15-1.

Elastosis Perforans Serpiginosa

Elastosis perforans serpiginosa (EPS) is the most distinctive of the perforating disorders because it demonstrates the best example of transepidermal elimination. In EPS, increased numbers of thickened elastic fibers are present in the upper dermis and altered elastic fibers are extruded through the epidermis. It is a rare disorder that affects young individuals with a peak incidence in the second decade. Men are affected more often than women. EPS is primarily a papular eruption localized to one anatomic site and most commonly affecting the nape of the neck, the face, or the upper extremities. The papules are typically 2 to 5 mm in diameter. These papules are arranged in arcuate or serpiginous groups and may coalesce.

Of particular importance is the association of EPS with systemic diseases. The important associations include Down's syndrome, Ehlers–Danlos syndrome, osteogenesis imperfecta, pseudoxanthoma elasticum, and Marfan's syndrome. In addition, on rare occasions EPS is observed in association with Rothmund–Thompson syndrome or other connective tissue disorders, and as a secondary complication of penicillamine administration.

Histopathology. The essential findings include a narrow transepidermal channel that may be straight, wavy, or of corkscrew shape and thick, coarse elastic fibers in the channel admixed with granular basophilic staining debris (Fig. 15–5A and B). A mixed inflammatory cell infiltrate accompanies the fibers in the channel. Also observed are abnormal elastic fibers in the upper dermis in the vicinity of the channel. In this zone, the elastic fibers are increased in size and number. As these fibers enter the lower portion of the channel, they maintain their normal staining characteristics, but as they approach the epidermal surface they may not stain as expected with elastic stains (49).

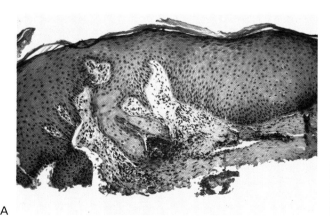
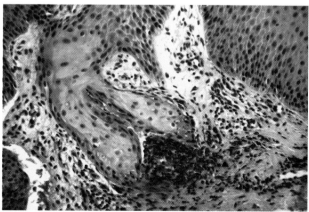

FIGURE 15-5. Elastosis perforans serpiginosa. **A:** A portion of a narrow curved channel through an acanthotic epidermis is shown. **B:** The lower portion of the channel contains coarse elastic fibers and basophilic debris.

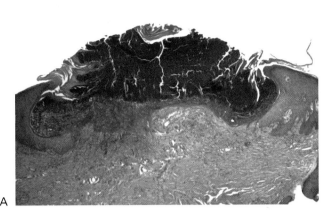

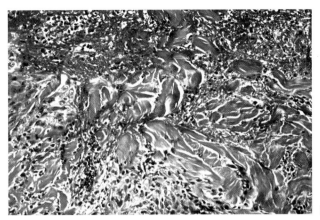

FIGURE 15-6. Reactive perforating collagenosis. **A:** A shallow cup-shaped invagination of the dermis containing a mixture of basophilic material and degenerated collagen bundles. The adjacent epidermis displays acanthosis. **B:** Vertically oriented perforating bundles of collagen are present at the base of the invagination.

Histogenesis. The cause of EPS is not known. Because the elastic fibers show no obvious abnormality within the dermis except hyperplasia, it is conceivable that the thickened elastic fibers act as mechanical irritants or "foreign bodies" and provoke an epidermal response in the form of hyperplasia. The epidermis then envelops the irritating material and eliminates it through transepidermal channels. The degeneration of the elastic fibers within the channels probably is caused by proteolytic enzymes set free by degenerating inflammatory cells (49). The channel is formed as a reactive phenomenon through which the "foreign bodies" are extruded. Because copper metabolism is essential to the formation of elastin (50), and because the administration of penicillamine, a copper-chelating agent, has been found to induce EPS (51), it may be suggested that the primary abnormality begins with a defect in the metabolism of this essential element.

Differential Diagnosis. Both Kyrle's disease and perforating folliculitis have in common with elastosis perforans serpiginosa a central keratotic plug and a perforation through which degenerated material is eliminated. In addition, perforating folliculitis, like elastosis perforans serpiginosa, shows the elimination of degenerated eosinophilic elastic fibers. However, neither of the two diseases shows the great increase in elastic tissue that is observed in elastosis perforans serpiginosa in the uppermost dermis and particularly in the dermal papillae on staining with elastic tissue stains (Table 15-1).

Reactive Perforating Collagenosis

Reactive perforating collagenosis (RPC) is a rare perforating disorder in which altered collagen is extruded by means of transepidermal elimination. True, classic RPC is a genodermatosis that is inherited as an autosomal dominant or recessive trait (52,53). The lesions are precipitated by trauma, arthropod assaults, folliculitis, and even exposure to cold. RPC occurs early in life, and both genders are equally affected.

The primary clinical lesion is a small papule that enlarges to the size of 5 to 10 mm with a hyperkeratotic central umbilication. Often the lesion appears eroded. These lesions spontaneously regress, leaving superficial scars with postinflammatory pigmentary alteration.

An adult, acquired type of RPC has been described in association with diabetes mellitus and chronic renal failure (54–56), but may in fact represent a variant of perforating disorder secondary to chronic renal disease and/or diabetes (see text following).

Histopathology. The classic lesion shows a vertically oriented, shallow, cup-shaped invagination of the epidermis, forming a short channel (Fig. 15-6A). The channel is lined by acanthotic epithelium along the sides. At the base of the invagination there is an attenuated layer of keratinocytes that in some foci appear eroded. Within the channel there are densely packed degenerated basophilic staining material and basophilically altered collagen bundles. Vertically oriented perforating bundles of collagen are present interposed between the keratinocytes of the attenuated bases of the invagination (Fig. 15-6B). It is important that a Masson trichrome stain be done to confirm that the fibers are collagen.

Histogenesis. The basic process in reactive perforating collagenosis consists of the transepidermal elimination of histochemically altered collagen. Nevertheless, as delineated by electron microscopy, the collagen fibrils appear intact, with regular periodicity (57).

Differential Diagnosis. See Table 15-1.

Perforating Disorder Secondary to Chronic Renal Failure and/or Diabetes Mellitus

This dermatosis, which combines clinical features of Kyrle's disease and histologic features of perforating folliculitis, occurs quite commonly in patients with chronic renal failure (42,58). In most instances, the lesions arise within a few months after renal dialysis has been started (59,60). The lesions are usually located mainly on the extensor surfaces of the lower extremities but are often extensive. They consist of follicular papules and often have a central keratotic plug (61). They may coalesce to form verrucous plaques.

Histopathology. Small lesions tend to have the histologic picture of perforating folliculitis, with the perforation, if it occurs, in the infundibular portion of the hair follicle (59,60). In larger lesions, perforations are apt to be at the base of the follicular invagination (62,63). Both types of perforations may be observed in a single biopsy specimen. In some instances, no follicular structure can be identified, and in these cases the lesions can be indistinguishable from reactive perforating collagenosis with superimposed features of prurigo nodularis.

Histogenesis. The usual occurrence of a papular eruption with features of a perforating disorder in association with renal dialysis has led to speculations that this disease may be caused by the accumulation of a poorly dialyzable "uremic" substance (59). In a few instances, however, the disorder has occurred without dialysis (58, 61,63). This condition may have appeared only recently because hemodialysis has been prolonging the lives of chronic renal failure patients, which raises the possibility that this disorder is simply a manifestation of chronically rubbed skin as a result of pruritus with a prominent follicular component.

Differential Diagnosis. See Table 15-1.

PERFORATING CALCIFIC ELASTOSIS (PERIUMBILICAL PERFORATING PSEUDOXANTHOMA ELASTICUM)

In perforating calcific elastosis, also referred to as periumbilical perforating pseudoxanthoma elasticum (PPPXE), a gradually enlarging, well-demarcated, hyperpigmented patch or plaque is usually seen in the periumbilical region in middle-aged, obese, multiparous women with hypertension (64). Most patients described have been African American (65). The patch or plaque is in some instances atrophic with discrete keratotic papules at the periphery (66); in other instances, it has a verrucous border (67), and in still others it has a fissured, verrucous surface throughout (68). Lesions occurring on the breast have also been described (69,70). Perforating calcific elastosis was initially regarded as cases of elastosis perforans serpiginosa coexisting with pseudoxanthoma elasticum (71–75). The disorder was later shown to be distinct from elastosis perforans serpiginosa (67).

Four patients with perforating calcific elastosis associated with renal failure have been described (65,70,76,77). One patient demonstrated regression of the lesions with hemodialysis (65).

Histopathology. Numerous altered elastic fibers are observed in the reticular dermis. They are short, thick, and curled, and are encrusted with calcium salts, as shown by a positive von Kossa stain. They are thus indistinguishable from the elastic fibers seen in pseudoxanthoma elasticum (64). As in pseudoxanthoma elasticum, the elastic fibers are visible even in sections stained with hematoxylin-eosin, owing to their basophilia (66). The altered elastic fibers in perforating calcific elastosis are extruded to the surface either through the epidermis in a wide channel (67) or through a tunnel in the hyperplastic epidermis that ends in a keratin-filled crater (66) (Fig. 15–7A and B).

Histogenesis. Electron microscopic examination reveals electron dense deposits of calcium primarily in the central core of elastic fibers. Calcification of collagen bundles is also seen (69). The etiologic nature of perforating calcific elastosis has been debated. Some have hypothesized that it is an acquired lesion developing as a consequence of local cutaneous trauma from such factors as obesity, multiple pregnancies, ascites, or multiple abdominal surgeries (64,66,69). They cite the characteristic clinical presentation, lack of sys-

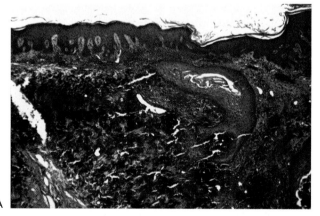
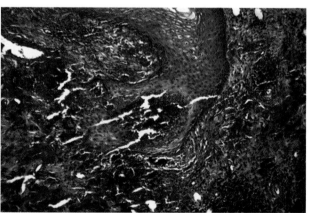

FIGURE 15-7. Perforating calcific elastosis. **A:** Degenerating elastic fibers encrusted with calcium salts in the reticular dermis surround a distorted transepidermal channel. **B:** The calcified fibers are in the process of being extruded through the base of the channel.

temic manifestations, and absence of familial predisposition in most cases. The occurrence of perforating calcific elastosis in patients with renal failure may suggest that conditions resulting in an abnormal calcium phosphate product may produce abnormal calcification of elastic fibers. The occurrence of pseudoxanthoma elasticum-like eruptions in patients exposed to calcium-ammonium nitrate salts (78), and in one patient with chronic idiopathic hyperphosphatasia (79) supports this concept. Others have argued that perforating calcific elastosis may represent a localized cutaneous expression of hereditary pseudoxanthoma elasticum (68). Arguments for the latter theory include a history of hypertension in 75% of reported patients and angioid streaks in 33% of examined patients (65). The presence of perforation is also not distinctive, as the finding has also been noted to occur in lesions of classic hereditary pseudoxanthoma elasticum. The disorder may represent a spectrum ranging from a purely acquired form with no systemic manifestations to an inherited form with limited systemic expression.

LATE-ONSET FOCAL DERMAL ELASTOSIS

Late-onset focal dermal elastosis has been described in a small number of elderly patients with lesions clinically resembling pseudoxanthoma elasticum (80,81).

Histopathology. Focal elastosis along with an increased accumulation of normal-appearing elastic fibers in the mid and deep dermis are seen (80). No pathologic changes of pseudoxanthoma elasticum are present.

Histogenesis. There is an increase in elastin and collagen contents in tested patients as compared with controls. An increase in mRNA for elastin, as well as type I and III collagen from patients' fibroblasts, has been observed. No change in excreted elastin peptides is noted in affected patients. An overexpression of elastin has been postulated (82).

HYPERKERATOSIS LENTICULARIS PERSTANS (FLEGEL'S DISEASE)

A rare dermatosis first described in 1958 (83), hyperkeratosis lenticularis perstans consists of asymptomatic, flat, hyperkeratotic papules from 1 to 5 mm in diameter, located predominantly on the dorsa of the feet and on the lower legs. Removal of the adherent, horny scale causes slight bleeding. In addition to the central horny scale, larger papules often have a peripherally attached collarette of fine scaling. In two reported instances, extensive papular lesions were present on the oral mucosa (84). Other reported sites include the thighs, upper extremities, and ears (85,86).

The disorder starts in late life and persists indefinitely. An autosomal dominant transmission has been noted in several instances (87–89). Unilateral involvement may represent postzygotic mosaicism (90).

Histopathology. In some instances, the histologic picture is nonspecific, showing hyperkeratosis with occasional areas of parakeratosis, irregular acanthosis intermingled with areas of flattening of the stratum malpighii, and vascular dilation with a moderate amount of perivascular round cell infiltration (91). It seems, however, that if the specimen is obtained from a well-developed, markedly hyperkeratotic lesion, a characteristic, although not necessarily diagnostic, histologic picture may be revealed. The lesion shows a greatly thickened, compact, strongly eosinophilic horny layer standing out in sharp contrast to the less heavily stained, basket-weave keratin of the uninvolved epidermis (85). The underlying stratum malpighii appears flattened, with thinning or even absence of the granular layer (Fig. 15-8).

Acanthosis is observed at the periphery. In some instances, bordering on the central depression, the epidermis at the periphery forms a papillomatous elevation resembling a church spire (83,92,93). Vacuolar alteration and apoptotic cells in the basal layer have been seen in some cases (85,94,95). The dermal infiltrate is composed largely of lymphoid cells and is located as a narrow band fairly close to the epidermis with a rather sharp demarcation at its lower border. Immunohistochemical studies have shown the infiltrate to be predominantly T cells (96, 97,98).

Histogenesis. Under electron microscopic examination, the absence of membrane-coating granules was noted in some cases and regarded as the primary lesion of hyperkeratosis lenticularis perstans (84,89).

A defect in the membrane-coating granules seems likely to play a role in Flegel's disease, because in other cases in which membrane-coating granules were present, the granules lacked a lamellar internal structure and appeared vesicular (99,100). In one case, both lamellar and vesicular

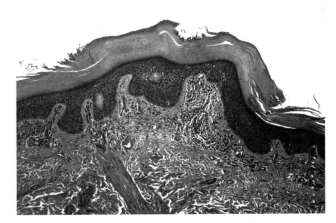

FIGURE 15-8. Hyperkeratosis lenticularis perstans. Dense compact orthokeratosis surmounts an epidermis with focal flattening of the stratum malpighii. A lymphocytic infiltrate is present in the upper dermis.

bodies were observed, with lamellar bodies greatly predominating in uninvolved epidermis and vesicular bodies in lesional epidermis (101). However, one study of lesional skin from four patients found no such abnormalities in lamellar bodies (102).

Other ultrastructural findings in Flegel's disease that have been described in some cases include Sézary cell-like lymphocytes (103), rod-like intracytoplasmic inclusions (104), and worm-like bodies in histiocytes (101). The significance and role of these findings in the etiology of Flegel's disease is unknown.

STRIAE DISTENSAE

Striae distensae occur most commonly on the abdomen and thighs, and in the inguinal region. They consist of bands of thin, wrinkled skin that at first are red, then purple, and finally white.

Histopathology. The epidermis is thin and flattened. There is a decrease in the thickness of the dermis. The upper portion of the dermis shows straight, thin collagen bundles arranged parallel to the skin surface and transverse to the direction of the striae. The elastic fibers are arranged similarly. Fine elastic fibers predominate in early lesions, whereas in older lesions they are thick (105). Within the striae, nuclei are scarce and sweat glands and hair follicles are absent (106).

Histogenesis. The histologic findings support the view that striae distensae are scars. They occur in conditions associated with increased production of glucocorticoids by the adrenal glands. Among these conditions are pregnancy, obesity, adolescence, and especially Cushing's disease (107). In obesity, the increased adrenocortical activity is a consequence of the obesity, and the production of glucocorticoids returns to normal when the body weight is reduced (108). Similarly, the occurrence of striae in nonobese adolescents, as noted in 35% of the girls and 15% of the boys examined, is associated with an increase in 17-kerosteroid excretion (109). Striae may also form in response to prolonged intake of corticosteroids or following the prolonged local application of corticosteroid creams to the skin. The action of the glucocorticoids consists of an antianabolic effect suppressing both fibroblastic and epidermal activity, as tissue culture studies have shown (110).

LINEAR FOCAL ELASTOSIS (ELASTOTIC STRIAE)

Linear focal elastosis (elastotic striae) is an uncommon, but more likely underdiagnosed or under-reported, disorder presenting as palpable striae-like yellow linear bands. The disorder was initially described in the lumbosacral region of elderly males (111). Lesions on the thigh and legs have also been reported (112,113). Occasionally, the

lesions arise in association with striae distensae (114–117). A number of cases have occurred in individuals under 30 years of age (118–120).

Histopathology. Abundant fragmented, clumped, and wavy elastic fibers are present between hypertrophic collagen bundles in the mid-reticular dermis (11,117). Elongated elastic fibers with split ends resembling a "paintbrush" can be seen (121). A decrease in papillary dermal elastic fibers has been demonstrated in the elastotic striae from one patient with coexistent pseudoxanthoma-like papillary dermal elastolysis (113). Unlike striae distensae, there is no decrease in thickness of the dermis or atrophy of the overlying epidermis.

Histogenesis. Electron microscopic examination reveals fragmented elastic tissue throughout the dermis (111). Widespread elastic fiber microfibrils, some occurring in continuity with intracytoplasmic filaments of fibroblasts, along with sequential maturation of elastic fibers have been observed suggesting an elastogenic process (122). An increased number of elastic fibers in lesional skin has also been documented (121). It has been postulated that elastotic striae may represent a regenerative process of striae distensae (114,117). This view is supported by the presence of contiguous striae distensae and elastotic striae in several patients. Accumulations of thin elastic fibers have been observed in late stages of striae distensae (123–125). Thus, linear focal elastosis may represent an excessive "keloidal" repair process occurring in striae distensae (117).

PSEUDOXANTHOMA ELASTICUM-LIKE PAPILLARY DERMAL ELASTOLYSIS

Papillary dermal elastolysis, first described in 1992 (126), is a rare, acquired condition consisting of soft, coalescent yellow-white papules mainly on the lateral neck and supraclavicular regions of elderly women (113,126–133). The clinical appearance of the skin lesions closely resembles that of pseudoxanthoma elasticum (PXE). However, no other systemic features of PXE are seen. A similar and possibly related disorder, *white fibrous papulosis of the neck*, is characterized by more discrete and firm papules (134–140). The term *fibroelastolytic papulosis of the neck* has been suggested to encompass the spectrum of the two disorders (140).

Histopathology. There is a marked decrease to absence of elastic fibers in the papillary dermis (126). Focal elastotic changes in the subpapillary and mid-dermis have also been demonstrated (141). No calcification or fragmentation of elastic fibers is seen. A slight decrease in elastic fibers along with the presence of thickened collagen bundles in the papillary dermis are differentiating features in *white fibrous papulosis of the neck* (136,140).

Histogenesis. Electron microscopic examination confirms the absence of elastic fibers in the papillary dermis along with the presence of immature elastic fibers in the upper reticular dermis. Fibroblasts with prominent rough endoplasmic reticulum with numerous dilatations and elongated dendritic processes are present (126,132). In one patient, formation of loose component fibrils of elastic fibers and elastophagocytosis were seen ultrastructurally (130). Papillary dermal elastolysis has been suggested to be a disorder of intrinsic skin aging due to its histologic similarity (126). However, immunohistochemical studies have shown a decrease in both fibrillin-1 and elastin in affected areas, whereas aged normal-appearing skin demonstrates only a decrease in fibrillin-1. A defect in elastogenesis may contribute to the pathogenesis of the disorder (126,133). The female predominance and the report of a familial occurrence may suggest possible genetic factors (132).

MID-DERMAL ELASTOLYSIS

Mid-dermal elastolysis is a rare disorder, first described in 1977 (142), occurring predominantly on the arms and trunk of middle-aged women. Clinically, two patterns are seen. The type I pattern consists of widespread, large areas of fine wrinkling along skin cleavage lines. The type II pattern consists of small, soft, papular lesions with tiny perifollicular protrusions, leaving the hair follicle itself as an indented center (143,144). These two patterns may coexist in the same patient. Persistent reticulate erythema is a newly described presentation (145). Urticaria (142), erythematous patches (146), or granuloma annulare (147) may precede some of the lesions. These postinflammatory forms of mid-dermal elastolysis have some similarity to a disorder first described in young South African girls termed *postinflammatory elastolysis and cutis laxa* (148–150). In the latter disorder, widespread wrinkling followed an acute phase of firm, erythematous, infiltrated lesions. An overlap with another disorder described as *disseminated nevus anelasticus* is also likely (151).

Histopathology. In this condition there is a selective absence of elastic tissue strictly limited to the mid-dermis of involved areas (142). The perifollicular protrusions around indented hair follicles result from preservation of a thin layer of elastic tissue in the immediate vicinity of the follicles. This causes the hair follicles to appear retracted while the perifollicular skin protrudes (143). A mild perivascular inflammatory infiltrate of mononuclear cells with occasional interstitial multinucleated giant cells exhibiting elastophagocytosis may be seen (152–154). Electron microscopic examination also reveals fragments of normal-appearing elastic fibers within macrophages (152,155).

Histogenesis. The disorder likely represents a postinflammatory process, although in some cases this may be subclinical, or remote. Immunohistochemical evidence of immune activation has been observed in lesional T-lymphocytes and endothelial cells (156). The cytokines and elastases produced by inflammatory cells along with elastophagocytosis by macrophages may contribute to the loss of elastic fibers (152). A possible autoimmune mechanism has been hypothesized based on its associations

with rheumatoid arthritis (157), silicone mammoplasty, elevated autoantibodies, false-positive Lyme titers (158), lupus erythematosus (159), and Hashimoto's thyroiditis (160). An idiosyncratic reaction to ultraviolet light has also been proposed as an etiologic or exacerbating factor (161,162).

MACULAR ATROPHY (ANETODERMA)

Atrophic patches located mainly on the upper trunk characterize macular atrophy, or anetoderma. The skin of the patches is thin and blue-white and bulges slightly. The lesions may give the palpating finger the same sensation as a hernial orifice. Two types of macular atrophy are generally distinguished: the Jadassohn–Pellizzari type, in which the atrophic lesions initially appear red and, on histologic examination, show an inflammatory infiltrate; and the Schweninger–Buzzi type, which clinically is noninflammatory from the beginning. However, not every case can be clearly assigned to one or the other of these two types; many clinically noninflammatory cases show an inflammatory infiltrate when examined histologically (163). The justification for distinguishing between the inflammatory and noninflammatory types has therefore been questioned (164). In many patients, new lesions continue to appear over a period of several years. Rare congenital and familial cases have been reported (165–169).

It appears dubious that a secondary form of macular atrophy occurs in the course of various diseases, such as syphilis, lupus erythematosus, tuberculosis, sarcoidosis, and leprosy (170–173). The macular atrophy then represents the atrophic stage of the preceding disease (174). Other cases of secondary anetoderma have occurred in association with porphyria (175), urticaria pigmentosa (176,177), pilomatricomas (178,179), Down's syndrome (180,181), acrodermatitis chronica atrophicans (182), Takayasu's arteritis (183), Grave's disease (184), Addison's disease (184), autoimmune hemolysis (184), systemic scleroderma (184), varicella (185), anticardiolipin and antiphospholipid antibodies (186–192), HIV (193), Sjögren's syndrome (194,195), alpha-1 antitrypsin deficiency (189), B-cell lymphoma (194,196), plasmacytoma (197,198), cutaneous lymphoid hyperplasia (197), angular cheilitis (199), juvenile xanthogranuloma (200,201), and generalized granuloma annulare (202). Macular atrophy has also been observed after iatrogenic procedures such as leech application (203), monitoring electrode placement in premature infants (204,205), hepatitis B vaccination (206), and after prolonged treatment with penicillamine (207).

Histopathology. Early erythematous lesions usually show a moderately pronounced perivascular infiltrate of mononuclear cells (208). In a few instances, however, the early inflammatory lesions show a perivascular infiltrate in which neutrophils and eosinophils predominate and nuclear dust is present, resulting in a histologic picture of leukocyto-clastic vasculitis (209,210). Microthrombosis has also been noted in patients with anetoderma and associated antiphospholipid antibodies (187–190).

The elastic tissue may still appear normal in the early stage of an erythematous lesion (211). Usually, however, it is already decreased or even absent within the lesion. In cases in which there is a decrease in the amount of elastic tissue, mononuclear cells may be seen adhering to elastic fibers (208). Elastophagocytosis within macrophages and giant cells may be seen (212).

Long-standing, noninflammatory lesions generally show a more or less complete loss of elastic tissue, either in the papillary and upper reticular dermis or in the upper reticular dermis only (Fig. 15-9). A perivascular and periadnexal round-cell infiltrate of varying intensity is invariably present, so that a distinction of an inflammatory and a noninflammatory type is not justified. In some instances, the involved areas show small, normal elastic fibers, which are probably the result of resynthesis, or abnormal, irregular, granular, twisted, fine fibers (163). Immunofluorescence studies of primary anetoderma have revealed immune deposits in a pattern indistinguishable from that of lupus erythematosus (213,214).

Histogenesis. Electron microscopic examination of lesions reveals a few thin, irregular elastic fibers, with more or less complete loss of the amorphous substance elastin but with relative conservation of the microfibrils. Macrophages, lymphocytes, and some plasma cells are observed. It appears possible that partial destruction by elastases originating in the macrophages occurs, because it is known that the elastases preferentially destroy the amorphous substance of the elastic fibers (214). Increased expression of two elastase-type proteinases, gelatinase A and B, has been shown in skin explants from patients with anetoderma (215). Morphometric analysis has demonstrated decreases

in the diameter of oxytalan and dermal elastic fibers, as well as the volume fractions of pre-elastic and dermal elastic fibers (216). This analysis has been used to differentiate anetoderma from other disorders of elastic tissue such as cutis laxa.

There is increasing evidence for an immunologic basis for anetoderma. In support of this hypothesis are the association of numerous autoimmune disorders and the findings of immune deposits at both the dermoepidermal junction and dermal blood vessels (184,213). In particular, the association of antiphospholipid antibodies with anetoderma is intriguing. The exact mechanism by which these antibodies may induce lesions remains to be elucidated. Some authors have postulated that microthrombosis produced by antiphospholipid antibodies with resultant ischemia of dermal tissues may induce elastic fiber degeneration (188,191). Others have hypothesized that the antibodies may alter the inhibitors of elastolytic enzymes, thus allowing the destruction of elastic fibers (217).

PERIFOLLICULAR ELASTOLYSIS

Perifollicular elastolysis is a relatively common condition consisting of small, hypopigmented, follicular papules on the face and upper trunk. The papules may protrude or herniate (218–221). There is a strong association with acne vulgaris and some have suggested the term *papular acne scars* for the disorder (221).

Histopathology. There is an absence of elastic fibers localized to the regions around pilosebaceous units (218).

Histogenesis. Perifollicular elastolysis most likely represents a form of anetoderma related to acne scarring (221). Elastase-producing strains of *Staphylococcus epidermidis* have been found in lesional hair follicles and have been proposed as the causative factor (218,220).

Acro-Osteolysis

The term *acro-osteolysis* refers to destructive lytic changes on the distal phalanges. Three types are recognized: familial; idiopathic, nonfamilial; and occupational, which is associated with exposure to vinyl chloride gas. In addition, acroosteolysis may be a feature of genetic syndromes such as Haim–Munk syndrome, pycnodystosis, Hutchinson–Guilford syndrome, and Hajdu–Cheney syndrome (222–225).

The *familial type* affects mainly the phalanges of the feet and is associated with recurrent ulcers on the soles (226).

The *idiopathic type* affects the hands more severely than the feet. Involvement of the distal phalanges of the fingers causes shortening of the fingers. This variant may be associated with Raynaud's phenomenon. Only one case has been described, with cutaneous lesions consisting of nu-

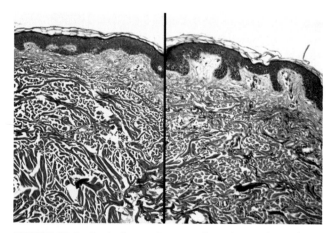

FIGURE 15-9. Anetoderma. Decreased to absent elastic fibers in a case of anetoderma (*left panel*) as compared with a normal control (*right panel*).

merous yellow papules 2 to 4 mm in diameter and showing a linear distribution and coalescence into plaques, mainly on the arms (226).

Occupational acro-osteolysis, like the idiopathic type, causes shortening of the fingers due to osteolysis. This variant is often associated with Raynaud's phenomenon and progressive thickening of the skin of the hands and forearms simulating scleroderma. There may be erythema of the hands, and the thickening may consist of papules and plaques (227). The skin of the face may show diffuse induration (228). In addition, there may be thrombocytopenia, portal fibrosis, and impaired hepatic and pulmonary function (229). A variant of occupational acro-osteolysis has been described in guitar players and is believed to be secondary to mechanical stress (229).

Histopathology. The histologic changes in the papules and plaques of idiopathic and occupational acro-osteolysis consist of thickening of the dermis, with swelling and homogenization of the collagen bundles, indistinguishable from scleroderma. Staining for elastic tissue shows disorganization of the elastic fibers, which appear thin and fragmented (226–228).

Histogenesis. Vinyl chloride disease is an immune-complex disorder associated with hyperimmunoglobulinemia, cryoglobulinemia, and evidence of *in vivo* activation of complement (229). The immunologic nature of the disease explains why it is developed by fewer than 3% of the workers exposed to vinyl chloride gas (227) (Table 15-1).

REFERENCES

1. Frances C, Robert L. Elastin and elastic fibers in normal and pathologic skin. *Int J Dermatol* 1984;23:166.
2. Kligman AM. Early destructive effect of sunlight on human skin. *JAMA* 1969;210:2377.
3. Raimer SS, Sanchez RL, Hubler WR, et al. Solar elastic bands of the forearm: an unusual chronic presentation of actinic elastosis. *J Am Acad Dermatol* 1986;15:650.
4. Mitchell RE. Chronic solar dermatosis: a light and electron microscopic study of the dermis. *J Invest Dermatol* 1967;48:203.
5. Nürnberger F, Schober E, Marsch WC, et al. Actinic elastosis in black skin. *Arch Dermatol Res* 1978;262:7.
6. Marsch WC, Schober E, Nürnberger F. Zur ultrastruktur und morphogenese der elastischen faser und der aktinischen elastose. *Z Hautkr* 1979;54:43.
7. Matsuta M, Izaki S, Ide C, et al. Light and electron microscopic immunohistochemistry of solar elastosis. *J Dermatol* 1987;14:364.
8. Braun-Falco O. Die morphogenese der senil-aktinischen elastose. *Arch Klin Exp Dermatol* 1969;235:138.
9. Ebner H. Über die entstehung des elastotischen materials. *Z Hautkr* 1969;44:889.
10. Smith JG Jr, Davidson E, Sams WM Jr, et al. Alterations in human dermal connective tissue with age and chronic sun damage. *J Invest Dermatol* 1962;39:347.
11. Niebauer G, Stockinger L. Über die senile elastose. *Arch Klin Exp Dermatol* 1965;221:122.
12. Findley GH. On elastase and the elastic dystrophies of the skin. *Br J Dermatol* 1954;66:16.
13. Sams WM Jr, Smith JG Jr. The histochemistry of chronically sun-damaged skin. *J Invest Dermatol* 1961;37:447.
14. Olsen RL, Nordquist J, Everett MA. The role of epidermal lysosomes in melanin physiology. *Br J Dermatol* 1970;83:189.
15. Carter VH, Constantine VS, Poole WL. Elastotic nodules of the antihelix. *Arch Dermatol* 1969;100:282.
16. Kocsard E, Ofner F, Turner B, et al. Elastotic nodules of the antihelix. *Arch Dermatol* 1970;101:370.
17. Weedon D. Elastotic nodules of the ear. *J Cutan Pathol* 1981;8:429.
18. Requena L, Aguilar A, Sanchez Yus E. Elastotic nodules of the ears. *Cutis* 1989;44:45216.
19. Favre M, Racouchot J. L'élastéidose cutanée nodulaire à kystes et à comédons. *Ann Dermatol Syphiligr* 1951;78:681.
20. Helm F. Nodular cutaneous elastosis with cysts and comedones: Favre–Racouchot syndrome. *Arch Dermatol* 1961;84:666.
21. Eastern JS, Martin S. Actinic comedonal plaque. *J Am Acad Dermatol* 1980;3:633.
22. John SM, Hamm H. Actinic comedonal plaque—a rare ectopic form of Favre–Racouchot syndrome. *Clin Exp Dermatol* 1993;18:256.
23. Hauptman G, Kopf A, Rabinovitz HS, et al. The actinic comedonal plaque. *Cutis* 1997;60:145.
24. Stanford DG, Georgouroas KE, Killingsworth M. Raimer's bands: case report with a review of solar elastosis. *Acta Derm Venereol* 1995;75:372.
25. Burks JW, Wise LJ, Clark WH. Degenerative collagenous plaques of the hands. *Arch Dermatol* 1960;82:362.
26. Kocsard E. Keratoelastoidosis marginalis of the hands. *Dermatologica* 1964;131:169.
27. Ritchle EB, Williams HM. Degenerative collagenous plaques of the hands. *Arch Dermatol* 1966;93:202.
28. Jordaan HF, Roussouw DJ. Digital papular calcific elastosis: a histopathological, histochemical and ultrastructural study of 20 patients. *J Cutan Pathol* 1990;17:358.
29. Rahbari H. Acrokeratoelastoidosis and keratoelastoidosis marginalis—any relation? *J Am Acad Dermatol* 1981;5:348.
30. Rahbari H. Collagenous and elastotic marginal plaques of the hands (CEMPH). *J Cutan Pathol* 1991;18:353.
31. Mortimore RJ, Conrad RJ. Collagenous and elastotic marginal plaques of the hands. *Australas J Dermatol* 2001;42:211.
32. Siragusa M, Magliolo E, Batolo D, et al. An unusual location of nodular elastosis with cysts and comedones (Favre–Racouchot's disease). *Acta Derm Venereol* 2000;80:452.
33. Moulin G, Thomas L, Vigneau M, et al. A case of unilateral elastosis with cysts and comedones. Favre–Racouchot syndrome. *Ann Dermatol Venereol* 1994;121:721.
34. Stefanidou M, Ioannidou D, Tosca A. Unilateral nodular elastosis with cysts and comedones (Favre–Racouchot syndrome). *Dermatology* 2001;202:270.
35. Mavilia L, Rossi R, Cannarozzo G, et al. Unilateral nodular elastosis with cysts and comedones (Favre–Racouchot syndrome): report of two cases treated with a new combined therapeutic approach. *Dermatology* 2002;204:251.
36. Keough GC, Laws RA, Elston DM. Favre–Racouchot syndrome: a case for smokers' comedones. *Arch Dermatol* 1997;133:796.
37. Sanchez-Yus E, Del Rio E, Simon P, et al. The histopathology of closed and open comedones of Favre–Racouchot disease. *Arch Dermatol* 1997;133:1592.
38. Hassounah A, Piérard EG. Keratosis and comedos without prominent elastosis in Favre–Racouchot disease. *Am J Dermatopathol* 1987;9:15.
39. Fanta D, Niebauer G. Aktinische (senile) komedonen. *Z Hautkr* 1976;51:791.
40. Sehgal VN, Singh M, Korrane RV, et al. Degenerative collagenous plaque of the hand (linear keratoelastoidosis of the hands). A variant of acrokeratoelastosis. *Dermatologica* 1980;161:200.

41. Todd D. Al-Aboosi M, Hameed O, et al. The role of UV light in the pathogenesis of digital papular calcific elastosis. *Arch Dermatol* 2001:137:379.

42. Sehgal VN, Jain S, Thappa DM, et al. Perforating dermatoses: a review and report of four cases. *J Dermatol* 1993;20:329.

43. Kyrle J. Hyperkeratosis follicularis et parafollicularis in cutem penetrans. *Arch Dermatol Syphilol* 1916;123:466.

44. Carter VH, Constantine VS. Kyrle's disease: I. Clinical findings in five cases and review of literature. *Arch Dermatol* 1968;97:624.

45. Constantine VS, Carter VH. Kyrle's disease: II. Histopathologic findings in five cases and review of the literature. *Arch Dermatol* 1968;97:633.

46. Tappeiner J, Wolff K, Schreiner E. Morbus kyrle. *Hautarzt* 1969;20:296.

47. Bardach H. Dermatosen mit transepithelialer perforation. *Arch Dermatol Res* 1976;257:213.

48. Mehregan AH, Coskey RJ. Perforating folliculitis. *Arch Dermatol* 1968;97:394.

49. Mehregan AH. Elastosis perforans serpiginosa: a review of the literature and report of 11 cases. *Arch Dermatol* 1968;97:381.

50. Tapiero H, Townsend DM, Tew KD. Trace elements in human physiology and pathology. Copper. *Biomed Pharmacother* 2003; 57:386–398.

51. Iozumi K, Nakagawa H, Tamaki K. Penicillamine-induced degenerative dermatoses: report of a case and brief review of such dermatoses. *J Dermatol* 1997;24:458–465.

52. Weiner AL. Reactive perforating collagenosis. *Arch Dermatol* 1970;102:540.

53. Kanan MW. Familial reactive perforating collagenosis and intolerance to cold. *Br J Dermatol* 1974;91:405.

54. Poliak SC, Lebwohl MG, Parris A, et al. Reactive perforating collagenosis associated with diabetes mellitus. *N Engl J Med* 1982;306:81.

55. Cochran RJ, Tucker SB, Wilkin JK. Reactive perforating collagenosis of diabetes mellitus and renal failure. *Cutis* 1983;31:55.

56. Beck HI, Brandrup F, Hagdrup HK, et al. Adult, acquired reactive perforating collagenosis. *J Cutan Pathol* 1988;15:124.

57. Fretzin DF, Beal DW, Jao W. Light and ultrastructural study of reactive perforating collagenosis. *Arch Dermatol* 1980;116:1054.

58. Garcia-Bravo B, Rodriguez-Pichardo A, Camacho F. Uraemic follicular hyperkeratosis. *Clin Exp Dermatol* 1985;10:448.

59. Hurwitz RM, Weiss J, Melton ME, et al. Perforating folliculitis in association with hemodialysis. *Am J Dermatopathol* 1982;4:101.

60. White CR Jr, Heskel NS, Pokorny DJ. Perforating folliculitis of hemodialysis. *Am J Dermatopathol* 1982;4:109.

61. Noble JP, Guillemette J, Eisenmann D, et al. Hyperkératose à type de bouchons kératosiques au cours de l'insuffisance rénale chronique et des maladies métaboliques. *Ann Dermatol Venereol* 1982;109:471.

62. Stone RA. Kyrle-like lesions in two patients with renal failure undergoing dialysis. *J Am Acad Dermatol* 1981;5:707.

63. Hood AF, Hardegen GL, Zarate AR, et al. Kyrle's disease in patients with chronic renal failure. *Arch Dermatol* 1982;118:85.

64. Pruzan D, Rabbin PE, Heilman ER. Periumbilical perforating pseudo-xanthoma elasticum. *J Am Acad Derm* 1992;26:642.

65. Sapadin AN, Lebwohl MG, Teich SA, et al. Periumbilical pseudoxanthoma elasticum associated with chronic renal failure and angioid streaks—apparent regression with hemodialysis. *J Am Acad Dermatol* 1998;39:338.

66. Hicks J, Carpenter CL Jr, Reed PJ. Periumbilical perforating pseudo-xanthoma elasticum. *Arch Dermatol* 1979;115:300.

67. Lund HZ, Gilbert CF. Perforating pseudoxanthoma elasticum: its distinction from elastosis perforans serpiginosa. *Arch Pathol Lab Med* 1976;100:544.

68. Schwartz RA, Richfield DF. Pseudoxanthoma elasticum with transepidermal elimination. *Arch Dermatol* 1978;114:279.

69. Neldner KH, Martinez-Hernandez A. Localized acquired cutaneous pseudoxanthoma elasticum. *J Am Acad Dermatol* 1979;1: 523.

70. Nickoloff BJ, Noodleman R, Abel EA. Perforating pseudoxanthoma elasticum associated with chronic renal failure and hemodialysis. *Arch Dermatol* 1985;121:1321.

71. Smith EW, Malak JA, Goodman RM, et al. Reactive perforating elastosis: a feature of certain genetic disorders. *Bull Johns Hopkins Hosp Med J* 1962;111:235.

72. Schutt DA. Pseudoxanthoma elasticum and elastosis perforans serpiginosa. *Arch Dermatol* 1965;91:151.

73. Caro I, Sher MA, Rippey JJ. Pseudoxanthoma elasticum and elastosis perforans serpiginosa. *Dermatologica* 1975;150:36.

74. Funabashi T, Tsuyuki S. A case of elastosis perforans with pseudoxanthoma elasticum. *Jpn J Dermatol* 1966;75:649.

75. Pai SH, Zak FG. Concurrence of pseudoxanthoma elasticum, elastosis perforans serpiginosa and systemic sclerosis. *Dermatologica* 1970;140:54.

76. Kazakis AM, Parish WR. Periumbilical perforating pseudoxanthoma elasticum. *J Am Acad Dermatol* 1988;19:384.

77. Toporcer MB, Kantor GR. Periumbilical hyperpigmented plaque. Periumbilical perforating pseudoxanthoma elasticum (PPPXE). *Arch Dermatol* 1990;126:1639.

78. Nielsen AO, Christensen OB, Hentzer B, et al. Saltpeter-induced dermal changes electronic-microscopically indistinguishable from pseudoxanthoma elasticum. *Acta Dermato Venereol* 1978;58:323.

79. Mitsudo SM. Chronic idiopathic hyperphosphatasia associated with pseudoxanthoma elasticum. *J Bone Joint Surg* 1971;53A:303.

80. Tajima S, Shimizu K, Izumi T, et al. Late-onset focal dermal elastosis: clinical and histological features. *Br J Dermatol* 1995;133:303.

81. Limas C. Late onset focal dermal elastosis: a distinct clinicopathologic entity? *Am J Dermatopathol* 1999;21:381.

82. Tajima S, Tanaka N, Ohnishi Y, et al. Analysis of elastin metabolism in patients with late-onset focal dermal elastosis. *Acta Derm Venereol* 1999;79:285.

82. Flegel H. Hyperkeratosis lenticularis perstans. *Hautarzt* 1958;9: 362.

83. Van de Staak WJBM, Bergers AMG, Bougaarts P. Hyperkeratosis lenticularis perstans: Flegel. *Dermatologica* 1980;161:340.

84. Price ML, Wilson Jones E, MacDonald DM. A clinicopathological study of Flegel's disease: hyperkeratosis lenticularis perstans. *Br J Dermatol* 1987;116:681.

85. Pearson LH, Smith JG, Chalker DK. Hyperkeratosis lenticularis perstans. *J Am Acad Dermatol* 1987:16:190.

86. Bean SF. The genetics of hyperkeratosis lenticularis perstans. *Arch Dermatol* 1972;106:72.

87. Beveridge GW, Langlands AO. Familial hyperkeratosis lenticularis perstans associated with tumours of the skin. *Br J Dermatol* 1973;88:453.

88. Frenk E, Tapernoux B. Hyperkeratosis lenticularis perstans: Flegel. *Dermatologica* 1976;153:253.

89. Miranda-Romero A, Sanchez Sambucety P, Bajo del Pazo C, et al. Unilateral hyperkeratosis lenticularis perstans (Flegel's disease). *J Am Acad Dermatol* 1998;39:655.

90. Bean SF. Hyperkeratosis lenticularis perstans. *Arch Dermatol* 1969;99:705.

91. Raffle EJ, Rogers J. Hyperkeratosis lenticularis perstans. *Arch Dermatol* 1969;100:423.

92. Krinitz K, Schafer I. Hyperkeratosis lenticularis perstans. *Dermatol Monatsschr* 1971;157:438.

93. Ikada, J. Hyperkeratosis lenticularis perstans. *Arch Dermatol* 1974; 110:464.

94. Hunter GA, Donald GF. Hyperkeratosis lenticularis perstans (Flegel) or dyskeratotic psoriasiform dermatosis. A single dermatosis or two? *Arch Dermatol* 1968;98:239.

95. Jang KA, Choi JH, Sung KJ, et al. Hyperkeratosis lenticularis perstans (Flegel's disease): histologic, immunohistochemical, and ultrastructural features in a case. *Am J Dermatopathol* 1999;21:395.

96. Metze D, Lubke D, Luger T. Hyperkeratosis lenticularis perstans (Flegel's disease)—a complex disorder of epidermal differentiation with good response to synthetic Vitamin D3 derivative. *Hautarzt* 2000;51:31.

97. Blaheta H, Metzler G, Rassner G, Garbe C. Hyperkeratosis lenticularis perstans (Flegel's disease)—lack of response to treatment with tacalcitol and calcipotriol. *Dermatology*; 2001;202:255.

98. Squier CA, Eady RAJ, Hopps RM. The permeability of epidermis lacking normal membrane-coating granules: an ultrastructural tracer study of Kyrle–Flegel disease. *J Invest Dermatol* 1978;70:361.

99. Tezuka T. Dyskeratotic process of hyperkeratosis lenticularis perstans: Flegel. *Dermatologica* 1982;164:379.

100. Kanitakis J, Hermier C, Hokayem D, et al. Hyperkeratosis lenticularis. Flegel's disease: a light and electron microscopic study of involved and uninvolved epidermis. *Dermatologica* 1987;174:96.

101. Tidman MJ, Price ML, MacDonald DM. Lamellar bodies in hyperkeratosis lenticularis perstans. *J Cutan Pathol* 1987;14:207.

102. Langer K, Zonzits E, Konrad K. Hyperkeratosis lenticularis perstans (Flegel's disease): ultrastructural study of lesional and perilesional skin and therapeutic trial of topical tretinoin versus 5-fluorouracil. *J Am Acad Dermatol* 1992;27:812.

103. Ikai K, Murai T, Oguchi M, et al. An ultrastructural study of the epidermis in hyperkeratosis lenticularis perstans. *Acta Derm Venereol* 1978;58:363.

104. Tsuji T, Sawabe M. Elastic fibers in striae distensae. *J Cutan Pathol* 1988;15:215.

105. Zheng P, Lavker RM, Kligman AM. Anatomy of striae. *Br J Dermatol* 1985;112:185.

106. Epstein NW, Epstein WL, Epstein JH. Atrophic striae in patients with inguinal intertrigo. *Arch Dermatol* 1963;87:450.

107. Simkin B, Arce R. Steroid excretion in obese patients with colored abdominal striae. *N Engl J Med* 1962;266:1031.

108. Sisson WR. Colored striae in adolescent children. *J Pediatr* 1954;45:520.

109. Klehr N. Striae cutis atrophicae: Morphokinetic examinations in vitro. *Acta Derm Venereol Suppl (Stockh)* 1979;85:105.

110. Burket JM, Zelickson AS, Padilla RS. Linear focal elastosis (elastotic striae). *J Am Acad Dermatol* 1989;20:633.

111. Ramlogan D, Tan BB, Garrido M. Linear focal elastosis. *Br J Dermatol* 2001;145:188.

112. Akagi A, Tajima S, Kawada A, et al. Coexistence of pseudoxanthoma elasticum-like papillary dermal elastolysis and linear focal dermal elastolysis. *J Am Acad Dermatol* 2002;47:S189.

113. White GM. Linear focal elastosis: a degenerative or regenerative process of striae distensae. *J Am Acad Dermatol* 1992;27:468.

114. Hagari Y, Norimoto M, Mihara M. Linear focal elastosis associated with striae distensae in an elderly woman. *Cutis* 1997;60:246.

115. Chang SE, Park IJ, Moon KC, et al. Two cases of linear focal elastosis (elastotic striae). *J Dermatol* 1998;25:395.

116. Hashimoto K. Linear focal elastosis: keloidal repair of striae distensae *J Am Acad Dermatol* 1998;39:309.

117. Moiin A, Hashimoto K. Linear focal elastosis in a young black man: a new presentation. *J Am Acad Dermatol* 1994;30:874.

118. Trueb RM, Fellas AS. Linear focal elastosis (elastotic striae). *Hautarzt* 1995;46:346.

119. Tamada Y, YokochiK, Ikeya T, et al. Linear focal elastosis: a review of three cases in young Japanese men. *J Am Acad Dermatol* 1997;36:301.

120. Breier F, Trautinger F, Jureck W, et al. Linear focal elastosis (elastotic striae): increased number of elastic fibres determined by a video measuring system. *Br J Dermatol* 1997;137:955.

121. Hagari Y, Mihara M, Morimura T, et al. Linear focal elastosis. An ultrastructural study. *Arch Dermatol* 1991;127:1365.

122. Tsuji T, Sawabe M. Elastic fibers in striae distensae. *J Cutan Pathol* 1988;15:215.

123. Zheng P, Lavker RM, Kligman AM. Anatomy of striae. *Br J Dermatol* 1985;112:185.

124. Pinkus H, Keech MK, Mehregan AH. Histopathology of striae distensae with special reference to striae and wound healing in the Marfan syndrome. *J Invest Dermatol* 1966;46:283.

125. Rongioletti F, Rebora A. Pseudoxanthoma elasticum-like papillary dermal elastolysis. *J Am Acad Dermatol* 1992;26:648.

126. Patrizi A, Neri I, Trevisi P, et al. Pseudoxanthoma elasticum-like papillary dermal elastolysis: another case. *Dermatology* 1994;189:289.

127. Pirard C, Delbrouck-Poot F, Bourlond A. Pseudoxanthoma elasticum-like papillary dermal elastolysis: a new case. *Dermatology* 1994:189:193.

128. El-Charif MA, Mousawi AM, Rubeiz NG, et al. Pseudoxanthoma elasticum-like papillary dermal elastolysis;a report of two cases. *J Cutan Pathol* 1994;21:252.

129. Hashimoto K, Tye MJ. Upper dermal elastolysis: a comparative study with mid-dermal elastolysis. *J Cutan Pathol* 1994; 21:533.

130. Vargaz-Diez E, Penas PF, Fraga J, et al. Pseudoxanthoma elasticum-like papillary dermal elastolysis. A report of two cases and review of the literature. *Acta Derm Venereol* 1997;77:43.

131. Orlandi A, Bianchi L, Nini G, et al. Familial occurrence of pseudoxanthoma elasticum-like papillary dermal elastolysis. *J Eur Acad Dermatol Venereol* 1998;10:175.

132. Ohnishi Y, Tajima S, Ishibashi A, et al. Pseudoxanthoma elasticum-like papillary dermal elastolysis. Report of four Japanese cases and an immunohistochemical study of elastin and fibrillin-1. *Br J Dermatol* 1998;139:141.

133. Shimizu H, Kimura S, Harada T, et al. White fibrous papulosis of the neck: a new clinicopathologic entity? *J Am Acad Dermatol* 1989;20:1073.

134. Vermersch-Langlin A, Delaporte E, Pagniez D, et al. White fibrous papulosis of the neck. *Int J Dermatol* 1993;32:442.

135. Joshi RK, Abanmi A, Hafeen A. White fibrous papulosis of the neck. *Br J Dermatol* 1992;127:295.

136. Cerio R, Gold S, Wilson Jones E. White fibrous papulosis of the neck. *Clin Exp Dermatol* 1991;16:224.

137. Zanca A, Contri MB, Carnevali C, et al. White fibrous papulosis of the neck. *Int J Dermatol* 1996;35:720.

138. Siragusa M, Batolo D, Schepis C. White fibrous papulosis of the neck in three Sicilian patients. *Australas J. Dermatol* 1996; 37:202.

139. Balus L, Amantea A. Donati P, et al. Fibroelastolytic papulosis of the neck: a report of 20 cases. *Br J Dermatol* 1997;137:461.

140. Tajima S, Ohnishi Y, Akagi A, et al. Elastotic change in the subpapillary and mid-dermal layers in papillary dermal elastolysis. *Br J Dermatol* 2000;142:586.

141. Shelley WB, Wood MC. Wrinkles due to idiopathic loss of middermal elastic tissue. *Br J Dermatol* 1977;97:441.

142. Brenner W, Gschnait F, Konrad K, et al. Non-inflammatory dermal elastolysis. *Br J Dermatol* 1979;99:335.

143. Maghraoui S, Grossin M, Crickx B, et al. Mid-dermal elastolyis. Report of a case with a predominant perifollicular pattern. *J Am Acad Dermatol* 1992;26:490.

144. Bannister MJ, Rubel DM, Kossard S. Mid-dermal elastophagocytosis presenting as a persistent reticulate erythema. *Australas J Dermatol* 2001;42:50.

145. Delacrétaz J, Perroud H, Vulliemin JF. Cutis laxa acquise. *Dermatologica* 1977;155:233.

146. Yen A, Tschen J, Raimer SS. Mid-dermal elastolysis in an adolescent subsequent to lesions resembling granuloma annulare. *J Am Acad Dermatol* 1997;37:870.

147. Marshall J, Heyl T, Weber HW. Post inflammatory elastolysis and cutis laxa. *S Afr Med J* 1966;40:1016.

148. Verhagen AR, Woederman MJ. Post-inflammatory elastolysis and cutis laxa. *Br J Dermatol* 1975;95:183.

149. Lewis PG, Hood AF, Barnett NK, et al. Postinflammatory elastolysis and cutis laxa. *J Am Acad Dermatol* 1992;26:882.

150. Crivellato E. Disseminated nevus anelasticus. *Int J Dermatol* 1986;25:171.

151. Heudes AM, Boullie MC, Thomine E, et al. Élastolyse acquise en nappe du derme moyen. *Ann Dermatol Venereol* 1988;115: 1041.

152. Larregue M, Laivre-Mathieu-Thibault M, Titi A, et al. Elastolyse en nappe superficielle acquise et inflammatoire. *J Dermatol (Paris)* 1988;13:38b.

153. Brod BA, Rabkin M, Rhodes AR, et al. Mid-dermal elastolysis with inflammation. *J Am Acad Dermatol* 1992;26:882.

154. Neri I, Patrizi A, Fanti P, et al. Mid-dermal elastolysis: a pathological and ultrastructural study of five cases. *J Cutan Pathol* 1996;23:165.

155. Sterling JC, Coleman N, Pye RJ. Mid-dermal elastolysis. *Br J Dermatol* 1994;130:502.

156. Rudolph RI. Mid dermal elastolysis *J Am Acad Dermatol* 1990; 22:203.

157. Kirsner RS, Falanga V. Features of an autoimmune process in mid-dermal elastolysis. *J Am Acad Dermatol* 1992;27:832.

158. Boyd AS, King LE, Jr. Mid dermal elastolysis in two patients with lupus erythematosus. *Am J Dermatopathol* 2001;23:136.

159. Gambichler T, Linhart C, Wolter M. Mid-dermal elastolysis associated with Hashimoto's thyroiditis. *J Eur Acad Dermatol Venereol* 1999;12:245.

160. Kim JM, Su WPD. Mid dermal elastolysis with wrinkling: report of two cases and review of the literature. *J Am Acad Dermatol* 1992;26:169.

161. Snider RL, Lang PG, Maize JC. The clinical spectrum of mid-dermal elastolysis and the role of UV light in its pathogenesis. *J Am Acad Dermatol* 1993;28:938.

162. Venencie PY, Winkelmann RK. Histopathologic findings in anetoderma. *Arch Dermatol* 1984a;120:1040.

163. Venencie PY, Winkelmann RK, Moore BA. Anetoderma: Clinical findings, association, and long-term follow-up evaluation. *Arch Dermatol* 1984;120:1032.

164. Friedman SJ, Venencie PY, Bradley RR, et al. Familial anetoderma. *J Am Acad Dermatol* 1987;16:341.

165. Aberer E, Weissenbacher G. Congenital anetoderma by intrauterine infection? *Arch Dermatol* 1997;133:526.

166. Peterman A, Scheel M, Sams WM Jr, et al. Hereditary anetoderma. *J Am Acad Dermatol* 1996;35:999.

167. Zellman GL, Levy ML. Congenital anetoderma in twins. *J Am Acad Dermatol* 1997;36:483.

168. Gerritsen MJ, De Rooij MJ, Sybrandy-Fleuren BA, et al. Familial anetoderma. *Dermatology* 1999;198:321.

169. Deluzenne R. Les anétodermies maculeuses. *Ann Dermatol Syphililigr (Paris)* 1956;83:618.

170. Bechelli LM, Valeri V, Pimenta WP, et al. Schweninger–Buzzi anetoderma in women with or without lepromatous leprosy. *Dermatologica* 1967;135:329.

171. Temime P, Baran LR, Friedmann E. Pseudotumoral anetoderma and chronic lupus erythematosus. *Ann Dermatol Syphiligr* 1971; 98:141.

172. Clement M, du Vivier A. Anetoderma secondary to syphilis. *J R Soc Med* 1983;76:223.

173. Edelson Y, Grupper C. Anétodermie maculeuse et lupus érythémateux. *Bull Soc Fr Dermatol Syphiligr* 1970;77:753.

174. Balina LM, Gatti JC, Cardama JE, et al. Congenital poikiloderma and anetoderma in porphyria. *Arch Argent Dermatol* 1966;16:190.

175. Carr RD. Urticaria pigmentosa associated with anetoderma. *Acta Derm Venereol* 1971;51:120.

176. Thivolet J, Cambazard F, Souteyrand P, et al. Mastocytosis evolving into anetoderma. Review of the literature. *Ann Dermatol Venereol* 1981;108:259.

177. Moulin G, Bouchet B, Dos Santos G. Anetodermic cutaneous changes above Malherbe's tumors. *Ann Dermatol Venereol* 1978; 105:43.

178. Shames BS, Nassif A, Bailey CS, et al. Secondary anetoderma involving a pilomatricoma. *Am J Dermatopathol* 1994;16: 557.

179. Kaplan H, Lacentre E, Carabelli S. Changes in the elastic tissue of patients with Down's syndrome. *Med Cutan Ibero Lat Am* 1982;10:79.

180. Schepis C, Siragusa M. Secondary anetoderma in people with Down's syndrome. *Acta Derm Venerol* 1999;79:245.

181. Venencie PY, Winkelmann RK, Moore BA. Anetoderma. Clinical findings, associations, and long-term follow up evaluations. *Arch Dermatol* 1984;120:1032.

182. Taieb A, Dufillot D, Pellegrin-Carloz B, et al. Postgranulomatous anetoderma associated with Takayasu's arteritis in a child. *Arch Dermatol* 1987;12:796.

183. Hodak E, Shamai-Lubovitz O, David M, et al. Immunologic abnormalities associated with primary anetoderma. *Arch Dermatol* 1992;128:799.

184. Tousignant J, Crickx B, Grossin M, et al. Post-varicella anetoderma: 3 cases. *Ann Dermatol Venereol* 1990 ;117:355.

185. Stephansson EA, Niemi KM, Jouhikainen T, et al. Lupus anticoagulant and the skin. A long-term follow-up study of SLE patients with special reference to histopathologic findings. *Acta Derm Venereol* 1991;71:416.

186. Disdier P, Harle JR, Andrac L, et al. Primary anetoderma associated with the antiphospholipid syndrome. *J Am Acad Dermatol* 1994;30:133.

187. Gibson GE, Su WP, Pittelkow MR. Antiphospholipid syndrome and the skin. *J Am Acad Dermaol* 1997;36:970.

188. Stephansson EA, Niemi K-M. Antiphospholipid antibodies and anetoderma: are they associated? *Dermatology* 1995;191:202.

189. Montilla C, Alarcon-Segovia D. Anetoderma in systemic lupus erythematosus: relationship to antiphospholipid antibodies. *Lupus* 2000;9:545.

190. Romani J, Perez F, Llobet M, et al. Anetoderma associated with antiphospholipid antibodies: case report and review of the literature. *J Eur Acad Dermatol Venereol* 2000;15:175.

191. Alvarez-Cuesta CC, Raya-Aguado C, Fernandez-Rippe ML, et al. Anetoderma in a systemic lupus erythematosus patient with anti-PCNA and antiphospholipid antibodies. *Dermatology* 2001;203:348.

192. Ruiz-Rodriguez R, Longaker M, Berger TG. Anetoderma and human immunodeficiency virus infection. *Arch Dermatol* 1992; 128:661.

193. Jubert C, Cosnes A, Clerici T, et al. Sjögren's syndrome and cutaneous B cell lymphoma revealed by anetoderma. *Arthritis Rheum* 1993;36:133.

193. Herrero-Gonzalez JE, Herrero-Mateu C. Primary anetoderma associated with primary Sjögren's syndrome. *Lupus* 2002;11: 124.

194. Kasper RC, Wood GS, Nihal M, et al. Anetoderma arising in cutaneous B cell lymphoproliferative disease. *Am J Dermatopathol* 2001;23:124.

195. Jubert C, Cosnes A, Wechsler J, et al. Anetoderma may reveal cutaneous plasmacytoma and benign lymphoid hyperplasia. *Arch Dermatol* 1995;131:365.

196. Child FJ, Woollons A, Price ML, et al. Multiple cutaneous immunocytoma with secondary anetoderma: a report of two cases. *Br J Dermatol* 2000;143:165.

197. Crone AM, James MP. Acquired linear anetoderma following angular cheilitis. *Br J Dermatol* 1998;138:923.

198. Ang P, Tay YK. Anetoderma in a patient with juvenile xanthogranuloma. *Br J Dermatol* 1999;140;541.

199. Prigent F. Anetoderma secondary to juvenile xanthogranuloma. *Ann Dermatol Venereol* 2001;128:291.

200. Ozkan S, Fetil E, Izler F, et al. Anetoderma secondary to generalized granuloma annulare. *J Am Acad Dermatol* 2000;42:335.

201. Siragusa M, Batolo D, Schepis C. Anetoderma secondary to application of leeches. *Int J Dermatol* 1996;35:226.

202. Prizant TL, Lucky AW, Frieden IJ, et al. Spontaneous atrophic patches in extremely premature infants. Anetoderma of prematurity. *Arch Dermatol* 1996;132;671.

203. Colditz PB, Dunster KR, Joy GJ, et al. Anetoderma of prematurity in association with electrocardiographic electrodes. *J Am Acad Dermatol* 1999;41:479.

204. Daoud MS, Dicken CH. Anetoderma after hepatitis B immunization in two siblings. *J Am Acad Dermatol* 1997;36:779.

205. Davis W. Wilson's disease and penicillamine-induced anetoderma. *Arch Dermatol* 1977;113:976.

206. Kossard S, Kronman KR, Dicken CH, et al. Inflammatory macular atrophy: Immunofluorescent and ultrastructural findings. *J Am Acad Dermatol* 1979;1:325.

207. Cramer HJ. Zur Histopathogenese der dermatitis atrophicans maculosa. *Dermatol Wochenschr* 1963;147:230.

208. Hellwich M, Nickolay-Kiesthardt J. Kasuistischer beitrag zur anetodermia jadassohn. *Z Hautkr* 1986;61:1638.

209. Miller WM, Ruggles CW, Rist TE. Anetoderma. *Int J Dermatol* 1979;18:43.

210. Zaki I, Scerri L, Nelson H. Primary anetoderma: phagocytosis of elastic fibres by macrophages. *Clin Exp Dermatol* 1994;19:388.

211. Bergman R, Friedman-Birnbaum R, Hazaz B, et al. An immunofluorescence study of primary anetoderma. *Clin Exp Dermatol* 1990;15:124.

212. Venencie PY, Winkelmann RK. Ultrastructural findings in the skin lesions of patients with anetoderma .*Arch Dermatol* 1984;120:1084.

213. Venencie PY, Bonnefoy A, Gogly B, et al. Increased expression of gelatinases A and B by skin explants from patients with anetoderma. *Br J Dermatol* 1997;137:517.

214. Ghomrasseni S, Dridi M, Bonnefoix M, et al. Morphometric analysis of elastic skin fibers from patients with: cutis laxa, anetoderma, pseudoxanthoma elasticum, and Buschke Ollendorf and Williams–Beuren syndromes. *J Eur Acad Dermatol Venereol* 2001;15:305.

215. Lindstrom J, Smith KJ, Skelton HG, et al. Increased anticardiolipin antibodies associated with the development of anetoderma in HIV-1 disease. MMCARR. *Int J Dermatol* 1995;34:408.

216. Varadi DP, Saqueton AC. Perifollicular elastolysis. *Br J Dermatol* 1970;83:143.

217. Taafe A, Cunliffe WJ, Clayden AD. Perifollicular elastolysis—a common condition. *Br J Dermatol* 1983;24S:20.

218. Lemarchand-Venencie F, Venencie PY, Foix C, et al. Perifollicular elastolysis. Discussion of the role of secretory elastase from Staphylococcus epidermidis. *Ann Dermatol Venereol* 1985;112:735.

219. Wilson BB, Dent CH, Cooper PH. Papular acne scars. A common cutaneous finding. *Arch Dermatol* 1990;126:797.

220. Haim S, Munk J. Periodontosis a part of an unknown familial congenital disorder. *Refuat Hapeh Vehashinayim* 1969;18:2.

221. Lamy M, Maroteaux P. Pycnodysostosis. *Rev Esp Pediatr* 1965;21:433.

222. Jansen T, Romiti R. Progeria infantum (Hutchinson–Gilford syndrome) associated with scleroderma-like lesions and acroosteolysis: a case report and brief review of the literature. *Pediatr Dermatol* 2000;17:282.

223. Herrmann J, Zugibe FT, Gilbert EF, et al. Arthro-dento-osteo dysplasia (Hajdu-Cheney syndrome). Review of a genetic "acroosteolysis" syndrome. *Z Kinderheilkd* 1973;114:93.

224. Meyerson LB, Meier GC. Cutaneous lesions in acroosteolysis. *Arch Dermatol* 1972;106:224.

225. Markowitz SS, McDonald CJ, Fethiere W, et al. Occupational acroosteolysis. *Arch Dermatol* 1972;106:219.

226. Veltmann G, Lange CE, Stein G. Die Vinyl krankheit *Hautarzt* 1978;29:177.

227. Fine RM. Acro-osteolysis: Vinyl chloride induced "scleroderma." *Int J Dermatol* 1976;15:676.

228. Destouet JM, Murphy WA. Guitar player acro-osteolysis. *Skeletal Radiol* 1981;6:275.

229. Baran R, Tosti A. Occupational acroosteolysis in a guitar player. *Acta Derm Venereol* 1993;73:64.

CUTANEOUS MANIFESTATIONS OF NUTRITIONAL DEFICIENCY STATES AND GASTROINTESTINAL DISEASE

CYNTHIA MAGRO
A. NEIL CROWSON
MARTIN MIHM JR.

DEFICIENCIES OF VITAMINS, OTHER AMINO ACIDS, AND MINERALS

Scurvy

The manifestations of scurvy, due to vitamin C (ascorbic acid) deficiency, have been known for 3,000 years. In 1753, Sir James Lind demonstrated the efficacy of citrus fruits in the prevention of this condition (1,2), which is characterized by follicular purpuric macules with or without follicular hyperkeratosis and cork screw hairs, ecchymoses, particularly in the pretibial areas, and conjunctival and gingival hemorrhages, the latter associated with gingival hyperplasia (3). Subcutaneous hemorrhage with woody edema of the lower extremities and hemarthrosis may occur (4). Nonspecific aches and pains and impaired wound healing are frequent. Anemia, possibly related to decreased amounts of active folate and blood loss, is present in approximately 75% of individuals (4,5). For humans, the principal source of vitamin C, a substance that cannot be synthesized from glucose derivatives, is fruits and vegetables. Scurvy occurs in those such as autistic patients who selectively avoid these foods (6), the elderly, chronic alcoholics, renal dialysis patients, and malnourished displaced refugee populations (7), who also suffer other micronutrient deficiencies when dependent on food aid (8,9).

Histopathology. Follicular hyperkeratosis and perifollicular erythrocyte extravasation without an accompanying vasculopathy are characteristic. Extensive extravasations are usually associated with deposits of hemosiderin within and outside of macrophages. A coiled hair may emanate from the dilated follicular orifice (10).

Differential Diagnosis. Other pauci-inflammatory hyperkeratotic dermatoses that should be considered in the differential diagnosis include keratosis pilaris, vitamin A deficiency, pityriasis rubra pilaris, ichthyosis vulgaris, and a resolving lichenoid follicular hyperkeratotic process such as lichen planopilaris, lichen spinulosus, or lupus erythematosus. Coiled or "corkscrew" hairs are not pathognomonic of scurvy and may be seen in certain ectodermal dysplasia syndromes (11).

Pathogenesis. Most manifestations of scurvy can be attributed to defective collagen synthesis. Lysine and proline hydroxylase enzymes require vitamin C to reduce Fe^{+3} during the reaction. In vitamin C deficiency, the end product, hydroxyproline, which stabilizes the collagenous domain of procollagen, is deficient (3). Ultrastructurally, the dermal fibroblasts appear shrunken and show a decreased amount of rough endoplasmic reticulum (12). Around these fibroblasts, one observes increased amounts of extracellular filamentous or amorphous material that has failed to polymerize into normal collagen fibrils. The extravasation of red cells is caused by vacuolar degeneration and junctional separation of adjoining endothelial cells, and their detachment from the basement membrane in capillaries and small venules (12).

Vitamin A Deficiency (Phrynoderma)

Seen mainly in Asia and Africa, vitamin A deficiency is rare in the United States but may occur following intestinal bypass surgery for obesity (13) or visceral myopathy (14). Dryness and roughness of the skin along with conical follicular keratotic plugs characterize the cutaneous changes. Night blindness, xerophthalmia, and keratomalacia also occur.

Histopathology. The skin shows moderate hyperkeratosis with distension of the upper part of the follicle by large, horny plugs (13). Sebaceous glands are greatly reduced in size and may exhibit epithelial atrophy (15). In severe cases both eccrine and sebaceous glands may exhibit squamous metaplasia (16).

Differential Diagnosis. The other causes of a pauci-inflammatory interfollicular and follicular hyperkeratosis are mentioned in the prior discussion of scurvy. Spotty parakeratosis, hyperplasia of the epidermis, and a superficial dermal infiltrate with basilar vacuolar change are additional histologic features that distinguish pityriasis rubra pilaris from phrynoderma. Superficial dermal fibroplasia with melanophage accumulation is the hallmark of resolved lichen planopilaris and lupus erythematosus. Sebaceous gland atrophy has been described in pellagra. Squamous metaplasia of the eccrine apparatus has been seen with methotrexate therapy and graft-versus-host disease.

Acquired Vitamin B₃ Deficiency (Pellagra)

The word "pellagra" is derived from two Italian words, "pelle" meaning "skin" and "agra" meaning "sharp burning" or "rough." Although primarily ascribed to niacin (vitamin B₃) deficiency, other vitamin deficiencies or protein malnutrition (17) appear integral to the development of the pellagra symptom complex. Presenting as cutaneous lesions, gastrointestinal symptoms, and mental changes, pellagra has been given the acronym of the three Ds: dermatitis, diarrhea, and dementia. In the United States, the enrichment of whole-wheat flour with niacin has almost eliminated pellagra but it is still prevalent in countries such as Mexico and some African nations where cornmeal is the main constituent of the diet, as well as in displaced populations (8,9). Pellagra in the United States and Europe is seen mainly in chronic alcoholics (18) and in patients with anorexia nervosa, malignant gastrointestinal tumors, and intestinal parasitosis (17). Its appearance in carcinoid syndrome is believed to reflect a depression of endogenous niacin production by tumor cell diversion of tryptophan toward serotonin (19). Pellagra has also been reported in patients receiving isoniazid, pyrazinamide, ethionamide, azathioprine, chloramphenicol, and anticonvulsants (20). Isoniazid, a structural analogue of niacin, can cause suppression of endogenous niacin production.

Three basic skin eruptions occur in pellagrins (21,22). The first is a photoinduced eruption that is intensely erythematous and subsequently exfoliates to yield a hyperpigmented residuum. The second eruption comprises painful erythematous erosions in genital and perineal areas possibly induced by pressure, heat, and trauma (17). The increased skin fragility may reflect aberrations in the collagen and elastic fiber content of the skin. Pellagrins may develop a seborrheic dermatitis-like rash involving the face, scalp, and neck. Oral manifestations include beefy, red, cracked lips, and a fissured or smooth, red, sore tongue. Among the neurological symptoms are dementia, psychosis, anxiety, defective memory, burning sensations, sudden attacks of falling, dizziness, and headaches. A cause of sudden death is central pontine myelinolysis (17).

Histopathology. Psoriasiform epidermal hyperplasia with hyperkeratosis, parakeratosis, and a lymphocytic perivascular inflammatory cell infiltrate characterize initial lesions. Additional features include scattered necrotic keratinocytes, granular cell layer loss, and architectural disarray with dysmaturation. Depigmentation of the basal layer with accumulation of fat droplets is described, as is vacuolation of cells within the granular and spinous layers (23). Epidermal atrophy, hypermelanosis, vascular ectasia, and sebaceous atrophy characterize end-stage lesions (23). Seborrheic dermatitis-like lesions may show sebaceous gland hyperplasia with follicular dilatation. Fragmentation, swelling, and thickening of elastic fibers, swelling of collagen fibers, and merging of elastic tissue with collagen have been described. A morphology indistinguishable from necrolytic migratory erythema and acrodermatitis enteropathica has been reported, comprising intracellular edema with vacuolar change of the upper stratum Malpighii and keratinocyte necrosis, sometimes accompanied by neutrophilic infiltration of the upper spinous layers, subcorneal pustulation localized to or in isolation from these areas, and folliculitis (17).

Pathogenesis. A deficiency in urocanic acid caused by a reduction in histidine and histidase activity has been postulated as a possible mechanism of photosensitivity in pellagra; urocanic acid protects the skin from ultraviolet (UV) wavelengths by absorbing light in the ultraviolet-B (UVB) range (17). Kynurenic acid, a metabolic byproduct of the tryptophan-kynurenine-nicotinic pathway, accumulates in pellagra as a result of a deficiency of nicotinamide, which blocks the formation of kynurenic acid. Kynurenic acid induces a phototoxic reaction in skin subjected to long-way UV radiation ranging from 350 to 380 mm (17). Some of the gastrointestinal symptoms may relate to degenerative changes of the dorsal vagal nuclei. The neurological symptoms may be due to chromatolysis of various cortical and brain stem nuclei (17).

Differential Diagnosis. The histopathology is similar to the nutritional dermatoses acrodermatitis enteropathica and necrolytic migratory erythema. In addition, those dermatitides associated with hyperkeratosis, a maturation disarray, and/or scattered degenerating keratinocytes need to be considered as discussed in the differential diagnosis section of necrolytic migratory erythema.

Congenital Vitamin B₃ Deficiency (Hartnup Disease)

Named after the family in which it was first described in 1956, Hartnup disease is a distinctive autosomal recessive syndrome comprising pellagrinous skin (24,25), neurological abnormalities including mental deterioration and cerebellar ataxia, and abnormal aminoaciduria (26). The intermittent skin eruption is seen primarily in the summer at times of maximal sun exposure and at times resembles either poikiloderma vasculare atrophicans (27) or, when vesicles are prominent, hydroa vacciniforme (28). Hartnup disease, in contrast to pellagra, does not respond to treatment with niacin (28).

Histopathology. The histopathology usually resembles pellagra. Poikilodermatous lesions manifest flattening of the epidermis and prominent dermal melanophage accumulation (27).

Pathogenesis. An intestinal and renal tubular defect of tryptophan absorption leads to a deficiency in endogenous niacin, accounting for the pellagra-like symptomatology. The genetic abnormality involves a transporter for monoamino-monocarboxylic acids and maps to chromosome 5p15 (29). Chromatographic studies of urine show persistent aminoaciduria, particularly of tryptophan and of indolic substances derived from tryptophan (25,27).

OTHER FORMS OF NUTRITIONAL DERMATOSES

Necrolytic Migratory Erythema (Glucagonoma Syndrome)

First described in 1942 in a patient with a pancreatic islet cell carcinoma (29), this distinctive dermatosis, which can precede all other symptoms of pancreatic carcinoma by several years (30), is most commonly seen in association with a glucagon-secreting alpha cell tumor of the pancreas. Surgical extirpation of the neoplasm may result in resolution of the eruption, as may amino acid and fatty acid infusion (31,32).

The manifestations of glucagonoma syndrome include cutaneous and mucosal lesions, weight loss, anemia, adult-onset diabetes, glucose intolerance, elevation of serum glucagon levels, and thromboembolism (33). Skin lesions are seen mainly on the face in perioral and perinasal distribution, the perineum, genitals, shins, ankles, and feet, and include erythema, erosions, and flaccid vesicular-pustular lesions that rupture easily and often have a circinate appearance due to peripheral spreading. Rapid healing and the continuous development of new lesions result in daily fluctuations of the eruption. Cheilitis, glossitis, brittle nails, and dyspareunia due to mucosal lesions are also reported (34).

Histopathology. The characteristic acute lesion shows abrupt necrosis of the upper layers of the stratum spinosum, which may detach from the subjacent viable epidermis. Keratinocyte degeneration varies from marked hydropic swelling to cytoplasmic eosinophilia with nuclear pyknosis. Neutrophilic chemotaxis to the necrotic epithelium may eventuate in a subcorneal pustule. Chronic lesions have as their hallmark psoriasiform dermatitis. In both acute and chronic lesions there is architectural disarray, reflecting a maturation defect; it manifests as basal layer hyperplasia, vacuolar change, and a deficient granular

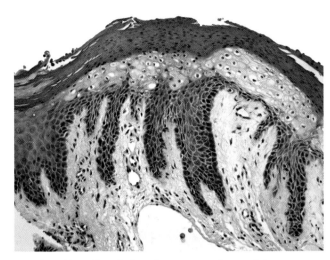

FIGURE 16-1. Necrolytic migratory erythema (glucagonoma syndrome). The lower portion of the stratum malpighii appears viable, whereas the upper portion shows necrolysis or "sudden death." The necrolytic portion manifests cytoplasmic eosinophilic homogenization with pyknotic nuclei.

layer. The epidermis is surmounted by a broad parakeratotic scale (Fig. 16-1). Candida may be noted (35,36).

Pathogenesis. Patients with glucagonoma have sustained gluconeogenesis resulting in a negative nitrogen balance, with protein amino acid degradation, even of epidermal proteins (37). In addition to glucagonoma, necrolytic migratory erythema has been reported with hepatic cirrhosis (39), a jejunal adenocarcinoma with hepatic dysfunction, and malabsorption with villous atrophy (30); glucagon levels may be normal. A comparable syndrome in dogs develops in the setting of diabetes mellitus and hepatic cirrhosis (36). In all of these conditions, malabsorption and diarrhea lead to isolated deficiencies of certain essential fatty acids, zinc, and amino acids. The pathophysiology may reflect in part a phospholipid fatty acid abnormality in cells due to defective delta-6-desaturase enzyme, which is known to be inhibited by zinc deficiency and excess alcohol intake. In patients with unresectable glucagonoma who manifest necrolytic migratory erythema, infusion of amino acids has resulted in rapid clearing of the cutaneous lesions (40).

Differential Diagnosis. The histopathology is similar to other nutritional dermatoses, namely acrodermatitis enteropathica and pellagra. Those dermatitides associated with hyperkeratosis, a maturation disarray, and/or scattered degenerating keratinocytes such as graft-versus-host disease, subacute cutaneous lupus erythematosus, dermatomyositis, pityriasis rubra pilaris, and toxic drug eruptions, particularly those that are photo induced, should also be considered.

Acrodermatitis Enteropathica

Acrodermatitis enteropathica, first described in 1942 (41), is transmitted as an autosomal recessive trait. Caused by defective intestinal absorption of zinc (42), it usually manifests in the first 4 to 10 weeks of life in bottle-fed infants as an acral and periorificial eruption with intractable diarrhea and diffuse partial alopecia. The skin exhibits areas of moist erythema, occasionally associated with vesiculobullous and/or pustular lesions (43). Untreated cases eventuate in death from malnutrition and infection because of immunologic defects reflecting zinc deficiency, the latter including decreased natural killer cell activity, impaired delayed-type hypersensitivity, and thymic atrophy (44). Paronychia, stomatitis, photophobia, blepharitis, conjunctivitis, corneal opacities, and hoarseness are additional manifestations. An acquired form occurs in patients receiving intravenous hyperalimentation with low zinc content (45), in infants who are fed breast milk low in zinc (46), in patients with Crohn's disease, and in the setting of AIDS nephropathy when proteinuria eventuates in excessive loss of protein-bound zinc (44).

Histopathology. The upper part of the epidermis shows pallor due to intracellular edema and is surmounted by a confluent, thick, parakeratotic scale that may contain neutrophils. There is granular cell layer diminution and focal dyskeratosis. As with necrolytic migratory erythema, there may be architectural disarray and dismaturation. Subcorneal vesicles may be present. The epidermis manifests variable psoriasiform hyperplasia and atrophy and, in a few instances, acantholysis (43,46). Superinfection with *Candida* may occur (Fig. 16-2).

Pathogenesis. Defective intestinal absorption of zinc has been demonstrated in children with acrodermatitis enteropathica (47), resulting in plasma zinc levels well below the normal range of 68 to 112 µg/dl. Oral administration of zinc sulfate eventuates in rapid and complete resolution of the

disease. Electron microscopy shows abnormal keratinization with decreased keratohyalin granules and increased numbers of keratinosome-derived lamellae within intercellular spaces. Keratinosomes contain several zinc-dependent enzyme systems, the metabolism of which may be affected (48).

Differential Diagnosis. Pellagra, necrolytic migratory erythema, and acrodermatitis enteropathica share a constellation of histologic features that should suggest a diagnosis of nutritional dermatosis, namely, confluent parakeratosis, granular layer diminution, epidermal pallor and focal dyskeratosis, psoriasiform hyperplasia, and architectural disarray and dismaturation. Other considerations raised in the differential diagnosis of necrolytic migratory erythema should also be entertained.

Kwashiorkor

Kwashiorkor is a form of protein malnutrition coupled to carbohydrate excess resulting in reduction of a patient's weight by 20% to 40%. Primary manifestations include generalized hypopigmentation that begins circumorally and in the pretibial regions. With disease progression, hyperpigmented plaques with a waxy texture develop over the elbows, ankles, and in the intertriginous areas. Dryness, desquamation, and decreased skin elasticity occur. "Crazy pavement" or "flaky-paint dermatosis" describes the extensive desquamation with erosions and fissuring that may be seen in severe cases (49). Hair abnormalities include a diffuse alopecia, alternating bands of normal and hypopigmented hair referred to as the "flag" sign, and an unusual reddish brown discoloration called hypochromotrichia (49). Extracutaneous manifestations include cerebral atrophy secondary to loss of myelin lipid (50), diarrhea, hepatic steatosis, and mucosal abnormalities such as a smooth tongue, angular stomatitis, and perianal and nasal erosions.

Histopathology. The histologic picture of skin lesions is not diagnostic but is said to resemble pellagra (51). The changes include psoriasiform hyperplasia with hyperkeratosis and increased pigmentation throughout the epidermis or atrophy with irregular shortening and flattening of the rete (51).

Pathogenesis. The etiology of the edema includes reduced capillary blood flow, hypoalbuminemia, and increased peripheral vasoconstriction (52).

CUTANEOUS MANIFESTATIONS OF GASTROINTESTINAL DISEASE

Pyoderma Gangrenosum

First described in 1930 (53), pyoderma gangrenosum was once considered pathognomonic of idiopathic ulcerative colitis, but has since been described in association with a wide variety of disorders including roughly 5% of patients with Crohn's disease. Beginning as folliculocentric pustules or fluctuant nodules, the lesions ulcerate and have sharply

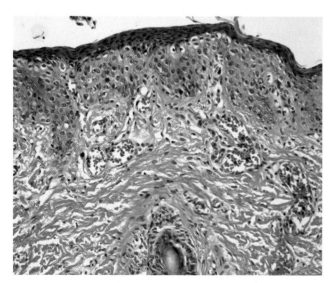

FIGURE 16-2. Acrodermatitis enteropathica. The epidermis demonstrates psoriasiform hyperplasia, dysmaturation, granular cell layer diminution, and vacuolar change. The epidermis is surmounted by a compact parakeratotic scale. Vascular ectasia is also present.

circumscribed violaceous, raised edges in which necrotic pustules may be seen. The disease most commonly occurs in adults who are 30 to 50 years old, on the lower extremities and trunk. Occasionally it occurs in childhood, affecting the buttocks, perineal region, and head and neck area (54). Koebnerization occurs at sites of trauma including intravenous puncture sites, surgical wounds, and peristomal sites (55). Roughly 70% of cases are associated with inflammatory bowel disease, hematological disorders including acute lymphoid and myeloid leukemias and myeloma, rheumatological conditions including rheumatoid arthritis and lupus erythematosus, and hepatopathies (56,57) including chronic active hepatitis, primary biliary cirrhosis, and sclerosing cholangitis (58,59). Both a superficial granulomatous variant (60) and a vesiculopustular variant comprising disseminated vesicles and necrotizing pustules, some follicular-based, have been observed without accompanying systemic disease. The vesiculopustular variant has also been seen in association with ulcerative colitis and/or underlying liver disease (58,61). Pyoderma gangrenosum has been associated with the administration of drugs including interferon (IFN)-α in the setting of chronic granulocytic leukemia, the antipsychotic agent sulpiride (62), and colony-stimulating factors (63).

Histopathology. Pyoderma gangrenosum has a dichotomous tissue reaction, showing central necrotizing suppurative inflammation, usually with ulceration, and a peripheral lymphocytic vascular reaction comprising perivascular and intramural lymphocytic infiltrates, usually without fibrin deposition or mural necrosis (Figs. 16-3 and 16-4). Transitional areas show neutrophils in a loose cuff around the angiocentric lymphocytic infiltrates, defining a mixed lymphocytic and neutrophilic vascular reaction termed a *Sweet's-like*

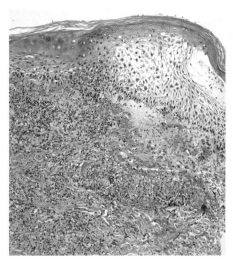

FIGURE 16-4. Pyoderma gangrenosum. The undermined epidermis often shows spongiosis or pustulation.

vascular reaction (64,65). Bullous lesions may also demonstrate a Sweet's-like vascular reaction with perivascular disintegrating neutrophilic infiltrates and hemorrhage without mural necrosis or luminal fibrin deposition. There is marked edema and a more superficially disposed pattern of dermal neutrophilia pathergy (66,67). Although a leukocytoclastic vasculitis may be observed in areas of maximal tissue pathology, pyoderma gangrenosum does not reflect a primary vasculitis (59). In some cases, a necrotizing pustular follicular reaction may be the central nidus of the lesion, particularly in the vesicular pustular variant associated with ulcerative colitis or hepatobiliary disease. In the superficial granulomatous variant, florid pseudoepitheliomatous hyperplasia along with the intraepithelial and superficial dermal suppurative granulomatous inflammation with admixed plasma cells and eosinophils may be observed (60). Cases of pyoderma gangrenosum associated with Crohn's disease may have areas of granulomatous inflammation (68).

Differential Diagnosis. Tissue neutrophilia with epithelial undermining and ulceration in the absence of leukocytoclastic vasculitis, and fungal, bacterial, or mycobacterial organisms (which may if indicated be demonstrable with culture and with special stains, that is, periodic acid-Schiff, Gomori methenamine silver, Brown and Brenn, Gram's, Ziehl–Neelsen and auramine-rhodamine preparations) strongly implicates pyoderma gangrenosum when seen in the appropriate clinical setting (59). An incipient lesion of pyoderma gangrenosum, however, may be indistinguishable from Sweet's syndrome, although the latter is rarely folliculocentric and does not show lysis of dermal collagen or vessel wall necrosis in areas of maximum dermal neutrophilia. In addition, clinical features usually make the distinction possible. Because of prominent follicular involvement, the differential diagnosis should also include other causes of necrotizing pustular follicular reactions with an accompanying vasculopathy such as mixed cryoglobulinemia, Behçet's

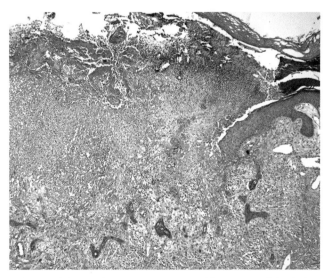

FIGURE 16-3. Pyoderma gangrenosum. The center of the lesion shows a neutrophilic infiltrate with leukocytoclasia and dermolysis. This biopsy is from a patient with Crohn's disease, as evidenced by the presence of multinucleated histiocytes within the infiltrate.

disease, rheumatoid vasculitis, herpetic folliculitis, acute pustular bacterid, and pustular drug reactions (69). These other conditions frequently have a necrotizing mononuclear cell or neutrophil predominant vasculitis in contrast to the non-necrotizing vascular reaction of pyoderma gangrenosum. Other causes of a Sweet's-like vascular reaction include the bowel arthritis dermatosis syndrome, Behçet's disease, idiopathic pustular vasculitis, rheumatoid arthritis, acute pustular bacterid, and Sweet's syndrome (64,65).

Pathogenesis. Direct immunofluorescence testing supports a vasculopathy by virtue of perivascular deposition of immunoreactants, mainly IgM and C3 (70), in more than half of patients. This change occurs in nonspecific vessel injury and does not support a humoral-based pathogenesis. Defective cell-mediated immunity without humoral abnormalities has been implicated in some patients (71). Immunoelectrophoresis has revealed a monoclonal gammopathy, most commonly of the IgA type, in 10% of patients with pyoderma gangrenosum (72).

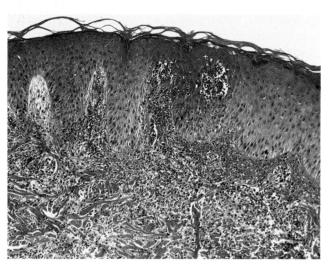

FIGURE 16-5. Bowel arthritis dermatosis syndrome. Pustular vasculitis characterized by dermal papillae micro-abscess formation along with a leukocytoclastic vasculitis involving dermal papillae capillaries.

Bowel-Associated Dermatosis–Arthritis Syndrome (Bowel Bypass Syndrome)

Following intestinal bypass surgery for morbid obesity or after extensive small bowel resection, some patients develop an intermittent eruption, mainly on the extremities, comprising purpuric macules and papules that may evolve into necrotizing vesiculo-pustular lesions. Polyarthritis, malaise, and fever are often associated with and may precede the eruption (73). Although originally called the bowel bypass syndrome, it now bears the more appropriate appellation *bowel arthritis dermatosis syndrome* as a similar picture may develop in patients with diverticulosis, peptic ulcer disease, and idiopathic inflammatory bowel disease (74–77).

Histopathology. Characteristically, there is a perivascular lymphocytic infiltrate with a peripheral cuff of disintegrating neutrophils, erythrocyte extravasation, and absent or minimal fibrin deposition consistent with a Sweet's-like vascular reaction; a leukocytoclastic vasculitis occurs less often (77). Papillary dermal edema may be striking and may lead to subepidermal vesiculation (73). Epidermal pustulation, variable epithelial necrosis, and massive superficial dermal neutrophilia complete the picture (Fig. 16-5) and define pustular vasculitis (73,78).

Pathogenesis. Circulating immune complexes, including those containing cryoproteins, are demonstrable in most patients. The antigenic trigger may be peptidoglycans from intestinal bacteria (74), which are structurally and antigenically similar to the peptidoglycan of *Streptococcus*. The latter exacerbate symptoms in patients with this condition and produce a similar syndrome in animals (74). Direct immunofluorescence testing has shown linear and granular deposits of immunoglobulins and complement along the dermal-epidermal junction and within vessels (74). One study showed *Escherichia coli* antigens in a granular array along the dermal-epidermal junction. Via an indirect methodology, a pemphigus-like pattern of intercellular staining has been reported (74), the significance of which is unclear.

Differential Diagnosis. The differential diagnosis of bowel arthritis dermatosis syndrome includes Sweet's syndrome, incipient pyoderma gangrenosum, and certain of the pustular vasculitides such as acute pustular bacterid related to antecedent streptococcal infection, such as Henoch–Schönlein purpura (78), septic vasculitis due to *Meningococcus* and *Gonococcus*, Behçet's syndrome, and leukocytoclastic vasculitis in patients with a pustular psoriasiform diatheses (79), idiopathic pustular vasculitis, and acute generalized exanthemous pustulosis (65,79). The distinction may be impossible in those conditions that manifest a Sweet's-like vascular reaction—namely, Behçet's disease, Sweet's syndrome, pyoderma gangrenosum, acute pustular bacterid, and idiopathic pustular vasculitis (65).

SPECIFIC DISEASES

Aphthosis (Behçet's Disease)

Behçet's disease is a symptom complex of oral and genital ulceration and iritis that has a worldwide distribution, but is most common in the Pacific Rim and eastern Mediterranean (80,81). The presence of oral ulceration plus any two of genital ulceration, skin lesions (e.g., pustules or nodules), or eye lesions (e.g., uveitis or retinal vasculitis) is held to be diagnostic.

The cutaneous lesions include erythema nodosum-like nodules, vesicles, pustules, pyoderma gangrenosum, Sweet's syndrome, a pustular reaction to needle trauma, superficial migratory thrombophlebitis, ulceration, infiltrative erythema, acral purpuric papulonodular lesions, and acneiform folliculitis (82,83).

The extracutaneous manifestations are categorized as oral and/or genital aphthae, vasculo-, ocular-, entero- or neuro-Behçet's disease, renal disease, and arthritis. Oral aphthosis recurring at least three times over a 12-month period is essential to the diagnosis (81). In vasculo-Behçet's disease, aneurysms and occlusive venous and arterial main vessel lesions occur. The ocular manifestations include uveitis, hypopyon iritis, optic neuritis, and choroiditis. Entero-Behçet's disease manifests as diarrhea, constipation, abdominal pain, vomiting, and melena. Neuro-Behçet's disease presents as brain stem dysfunction, meningoencephalitis, organic psychiatric symptoms, and mononeuritis multiplex (82). Asymptomatic microhematuria and/or proteinuria are among the renal manifestations. An oligoarthritis may involve the wrist, elbow, knee, or ankle joints. Morbidity and mortality in one large series of Turkish patients was greatest in young males; both the onset and the severity of ocular disease was greatest early in the course of disease suggesting that the "disease burden" in Behçet's disease is greatest early on and that it tends to "burn out" over time (84). However, neurological and major vessel disease can occur at any time and can have late onset 5 to 10 years into the course of illness (84).

Histopathology. Cutaneous lesions can be categorized histopathologically into three main groups: vascular, extravascular with or without vasculopathy, and acneiform.

The pathologic spectrum of the cutaneous vasculopathy encompasses a mononuclear cell vasculitis with variable mural and luminal fibrin deposition, a paucicellular thrombogenic vasculopathy (Fig. 16-6), and a neutrophilic vascular reaction involving capillaries and veins of all calibers. The mononuclear cell reaction may be frankly granulo-

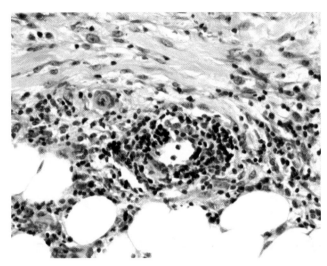

FIGURE 16-7. Behçet's disease. There is a Sweet's-like vascular reaction manifested by angiocentric mononuclear cell and neutrophilic infiltrates with erythrocyte extravasation and leukocytoclasia but without accompanying mural and intraluminal fibrin deposition.

matous or it may be lymphocytic predominant to define a lymphocytic vasculitis. The neutrophilic vascular reaction may resemble that of Sweet's syndrome (Fig. 16-7) (85) or a leukocytoclastic vasculitis. Diffuse extravascular mononuclear cell- and/or neutrophil-predominant inflammation of the dermis, and/or panniculus may occur with or without the aforementioned vascular changes. The histiocytes infiltrating the panniculus may manifest phagocytosis of cellular debris. Suppurative or mixed suppurative and granulomatous folliculitis with or without vasculitis characterizes the acneiform lesions. Acral purpuric papulonodular lesions show lymphocytic interface dermatitis with lymphocytic exocytosis, dyskeratosis, and a perivascular lymphocytic infiltrate, recapitulating the mucosal histopathology (83).

Extracutaneous lesions histologically mirror the skin changes. Oral aphthous ulcers demonstrate a central diffuse neutrophilic infiltrate with necrosis of the epithelium and connective tissue pathergy of the submucosa, and peripherally, a border showing dense lymphocytic infiltration with lymphocytic exocytosis and degenerative epithelial changes. Genital aphthae have the same appearance (82) (Fig. 16-8). The large vessel arteriopathy represents an ischemic sequela of a mononuclear cell vasculitis of the vasa vasorum (86), while venous thrombosis may be due in part to an underlying hypercoagulable state. A lymphocytic vascular reaction with or without mural and intraluminal fibrin deposition is the histopathology of neuro-, entero-, ocular-, and arthritic Behçet's disease, with other organ changes such as demyelination and intestinal ulceration reflecting resultant ischemia (82). The renal histopathology includes IgA nephropathy, focal and diffuse proliferative glomerulonephritis, and amyloidosis (87).

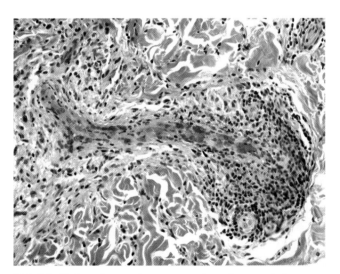

FIGURE 16-6. Behçet's disease. Another characteristic vascular reaction pattern is a pauci-inflammatory thrombogenic vasculopathy.

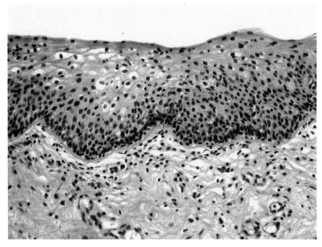

FIGURE 16-8. Behçet's disease. Although the center of an oral or vulvar aphthous ulcer is predominated by a neutrophilic response, biopsies of the periphery typically show a lymphocyte predominate infiltrate both in an extravascular and angiocentric disposition with variable lymphocytic exocytosis.

Differential Diagnosis. The lymphocytic vasculitis observed in Behçet's disease may mimic that seen in association with systemic lupus erythematosus, rheumatoid arthritis (88,89), Sjögren's syndrome, relapsing polychondritis, Degos disease, and paraneoplastic vasculitis in the setting of lymphoproliferative disease. Granulomatous vasculitis may also be observed in Wegener's granulomatosis, allergic granulomatosis of Churg–Strauss, Crohn's disease, sarcoidosis, acquired hypogammaglobulinemia, a postherpetic eruption (90), paraneoplastic syndrome (related to underlying hematological malignancy), rheumatoid arthritis, hypersensitivity reactions to certain infections including syphilis and tuberculosis (91), scleroderma, and late-stage lesions of microscopic polyarteritis nodosa (65,78,89). Other causes of a Sweet's-like vasculopathy include Sweet's syndrome, bowel arthritis dermatosis, pyoderma gangrenosum, and idiopathic pustular vasculitis (64). Conditions that combine a vasculitis with a folliculitis include pyoderma gangrenosum, mixed cryoglobulinemia, rheumatoid vasculitis, and bacterid (69).

Pathogenesis. An immunogenetic basis is likely in view of the association with certain HLA types, namely HLA-B5, HLA-B12, HLA-B27, and HLA-B51 (92). A recurring association in patients of Japanese, Turkish, Korean, and Iranian ethnicities is with HLA-B51 (93,94). Patients have shown a heightened immune response to antigenic components of certain streptococcal species (95,96), *Mycobacterium tuberculosis* (97), herpes simplex (98,99), Epstein–Barr virus, and human immunodeficiency virus (HIV) (100). Underlying abnormalities in T-lymphocyte function may be integral to an aberrant response related to the synthesis by microorganisms and mammalian tissue of a family of polypeptides termed heat shock proteins (HSP) (101,102) produced by cells exposed to stresses such as increased temperature. Sensitized T cells and T-cell clones specific to the 65-kD mycobacterial HSP have

been reported in rheumatoid arthritis (103). T-lymphocytes from patients with Behçet's disease in one study showed a greater stimulation by this HSP compared to normal controls or patients with unrelated disease (104). The gamma-delta T-cell subset has been shown to be the principal populace that responds to the mycobacterial 65-kD HSP, an observation that may account for the increase in circulating gamma-delta T cells in patients with antecedent streptococcal or mycobacterial infections (105) and in those with active Behçet's disease, in whom an exaggerated response to microbial products in mucosal ulcers is postulated (106). The lymphocytes themselves show resistance to Fas-mediated apoptosis, a finding that may promote lymphocyte-mediated tissue destruction in these patients (107).

Tissue neutrophilia may relate to the presence of HLA-B51, which has been associated with neutrophil hyperreactivity (108); neutrophil functions are also increased in Behçet's disease (109).

Vascular thrombosis has been attributed to antibody mediated endothelial injury (110), protein C or S deficiency (111), factor XII deficiency, inhibition of plasminogen activator, and circulating lupus anticoagulant (112–114). A prothrombin gene mutation has recently been described (115). Further evidence of a genetic predisposition to thrombosis is the linkage of HLA-B51 expression and the absence of HLA-B35 as risk factors for venous thrombosis in Turkish patients (93); there is also a statistical linkage between superficial and deep venous thrombosis (116).

INFLAMMATORY BOWEL DISEASE

Crohn's Disease (Regional Enteritis)

First described in 1932, Crohn's disease is an idiopathic disorder of the gastrointestinal tract. The diagnosis is based on a constellation of radiologic, pathologic, and endoscopic data, namely deep mucosal fissures, fistula formation, transmural inflammation, discontinuous colonic, and small bowel disease with preferential right-sided involvement, and sarcoidal granulomatous and fibrosing inflammation of the mucosa and submucosa (117). Extraintestinal manifestations include fever, anemia, lupus anticoagulant, ophthalmic disease such as uveitis and episcleritis, monoarticular large-joint arthritis, polyarthritis, spondylitis, amyloidosis (118), renal lithiasis with resultant hydronephrosis (119), cerebral vascular occlusions, and a spectrum of cutaneous eruptions.

Skin manifestations, principally restricted to patients with colonic disease, occur in 14% to 44% of patients with Crohn's disease depending upon whether or not perianal disease is considered a cutaneous manifestation (117). Ulcers, fissures, sinus tracts, abscesses, and vegetant plaques may extend in continuity from sites of intra-abdominal involvement to the perineum, buttocks, or abdominal wall, ostomy sites, or incisional scars. When sterile granulomatous skin lesions arise at sites discontinuous from the gastrointestinal tract, the appellation "metastatic Crohn's disease" is applied (120). Clinically, metastatic Crohn's disease presents as solitary or multiple nodules, plaques, ulcers, lichenoid lesions, or violaceous perifollicular papules involving extremities, intertriginous areas, abdominal skin folds, or genitalia (121). Erythema nodosum (122), the most common cutaneous manifestation of Crohn's disease (117), and pyoderma gangrenosum develop in 15% and 1.5% of patients, respectively. Palmar erythema, a pustular response to trauma (122), erythema multiforme usually with mucosal involvement (122,123), epidermolysis bullosa acquisita, hidradenitis suppurative, rosacea, secondary cutaneous oxalosis, malabsorption-related acrodermatitis enteropathica (122), vasculitic lesions including benign cutaneous polyarteritis nodosa and digitate hyperkeratosis reminiscent of punctate porokeratosis are described (124). Cutaneous necrosis as a complication of circulating lupus anticoagulant may also occur.

Oral lesions, manifesting as "cobblestone" lesions, aphthous ulcers, lip swelling, and pyostomatitis vegetans, occur in roughly 5% of patients with Crohn's disease (122).

Histopathology. The perianal mucosal lesions and oral lesions of pyostomatitis vegetans show pseudoepitheliomatous hyperplasia in conjunction with suppurative granulomatous inflammation within the epithelium and subjacent corium (Fig. 16-9). The most frequent histologic patterns seen in metastatic Crohn's disease are nonsuppurative granulomata, which may assume a sarcoidal or diffuse pattern, the latter often in close apposition to the epidermis in the fashion of a lichenoid and granulomatous dermatitis (125) and granulomatous vasculitis. Histological examination of the erythema nodosum-like lesion may show one of four patterns: (a) septal panniculitis consistent with clas-

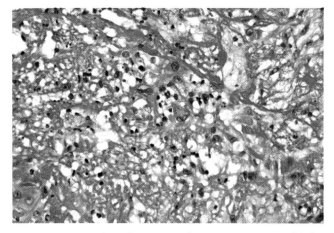

FIGURE 16-9. Crohn's disease: pyoderma gangrenosm. This biopsy shows suppurative granulomatous inflammation with a binucleate histiocyte in the center of the field and a mononuclear cell-predominant vasculopathic reaction pattern; biopsies may show a nerotizing leukocytoclastic and granulomatous vasculitis indistinguishable from cutaneous Wegener's granulomatosis and reminiscent of pyostomatitis vegetans, a prototypic oral lesion of Crohn's disease.

sic erythema nodosum; (b) dermal-based sarcoidal granulomata (126); (c) a dermal-based small-vessel granulomatous (127) or leukocytoclastic vasculitis; or (d) benign cutaneous polyarteritis nodosa (128). The latter shows mural infiltration by histiocytes and neutrophils with variable mural fibrinoid necrosis confined to the muscular arteries of the subcutaneous fat (Fig. 16-12); occasional vessel involvement of the peripheral nerves and skeletal muscle of the affected extremity produce mononeuritis and myositis respectively (100). A pauci-inflammatory thrombogenic vasculopathy characterizes the cutaneous infarcts associated with lupus anticoagulant. Necrobiosis lipoidica-like or granuloma annulare-like foci (129) may also be seen defined by areas of collagen necrobiosis with concomitant mucin or fibrin deposition and a palisading histiocytic infiltrate. Unlike idiopathic granuloma annulare or necrobiosis lipoidica, there usually is an accompanying leukocytoclastic vasculitis, thrombogenic or a granulomatous vasculopathy, and foci of extravascular neutrophilia (129). Dense neutrophilic infiltration of the dermis accompanied by scattered giant cells has been reported (68,130). We have also seen this pattern of suppurative granulomatous inflammation in concert with the aforementioned necrobiosis lipoidica or granuloma annulare tissue reaction. Cases of lip swelling show non-necrotizing granulomatous inflammation (122). The histology of pyoderma gangrenosum has been previously discussed. A suppurative panniculitis may also be seen (131).

Differential Diagnosis. The differential diagnosis of sarcoidal granulomatous inflammation in the skin includes sarcoidosis, id reactions to antecedent streptococcal or mycobacterial infections (91), acquired hypogammaglobulinemia, rosacea, paraneoplastic histiocytopathies such as those associated with low-grade lymphoproliferative disease, rheumatoid arthritis, and granulomatous inflammatory reactions to ingested or inoculated inorganic compounds such as silica, zirconium, and beryllium. The lesions resembling benign cutaneous polyarteritis nodosa differ from systemic polyarteritis nodosa by virtue of confinement of the vasculitis to the subcutaneous fat without dermal involvement (128). The changes of pyostomatitis vegetans also should raise the possibility of Wegener's granulomatosis, mycobacterial infection, blastomycosis, and histoplasmosis. The histopathology of the lip swelling may mimic that of Melkersson–Rosenthal syndrome (122). Lichenoid and granulomatous dermatitis calls into consideration the idiopathic lichenoid disorders such as lichen nitidus, certain microbial id reaction states, and also drug reactions such as those to antibiotic, antihypertensive, lipid-lowering and antihistaminic preparations (125).

Pathogenesis. A common morphology shared by the intestinal and cutaneous disease is one of sarcoidal granulomatous inflammation, suggesting a pathogenetic role for cell-mediated immunity. Circulating immune complexes have been detected in some patients (122) and may play a role in the generation of necrotizing vasculitis; a subset of patients with Crohn's disease has antineutrophil cytoplasmic antibodies. Using *in situ* polymerase chain reaction methods with a probe seeking bacterial 16rsRNA common to a variety of microbial pathogens implicated in Crohn's disease, bacterial RNA has been shown in the vasculature of the gut in active, but not quiescent cases; the skin lesions are uniformly negative. It would seem, therefore, that the skin manifestations of Crohn's disease are not a bacterial id reaction but rather reflect an autoimmune phenomenon, perhaps involving cross reacting antibodies between gut- and skin-based antigens (131).

Ulcerative Colitis

Ulcerative colitis is an idiopathic inflammatory bowel disease involving the large intestine with rectal involvement being almost ubiquitous. It is characterized by glandular destruction and inflammation of variable intensity. Glandular dysplasia eventuating in carcinoma complicates the clinical course, particularly in patients with disease of pediatric onset. Extramucosal associations include chronic active hepatitis, primary sclerosing cholangitis, pulmonary vasculitis (132), chronic fibrosing alveolitis, limited Wegener's granulomatosis of the lung (133), pulmonary apical fibrosis, large-joint monoarticular arthritis, polyarthritis, and ankylosing spondylitis. Cutaneous manifestations may occur, the spectrum of which encompasses vasculitis, erythema nodosum, pyoderma gangrenosum, superficial migratory thrombophlebitis, and cutaneous thrombosis with resultant gangrene (134), the latter two manifestations possibly related to underlying lupus anti-

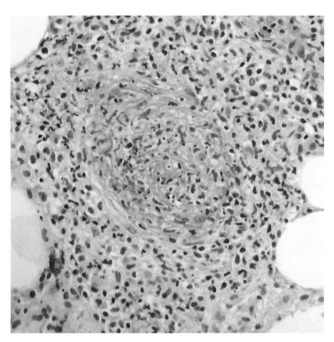

FIGURE 16-11. Polyarteritis nodosa in a patient with ulcerative colitis. Within the subcutaneous fat, the wall of a subcutaneous artery demonstrates striking fibrinoid necrosis and is surrounded and permeated by disintegrating neutrophilic infiltrates unaccompanied by small-vessel involvement. The findings are typical for benign cutaneous polyarteritis nodosa.

coagulant or cryofibrinogenemia (135). Pyoderma gangrenosum is more frequently associated with ulcerative colitis than with Crohn's disease and erythema nodosum more frequently with Crohn's disease (Fig. 16-10). The lesions of pyoderma gangrenosum also include an unusual disseminated vesiculopustular variant (136).

Histopathology. The histology of pyoderma gangrenosum and erythema nodosum is discussed elsewhere. Cutaneous vasculitis in association with ulcerative colitis includes IgA-associated leukocytoclastic vasculitis (78,137) and benign cutaneous polyarteritis nodosa (Fig. 16-11). A pauci-inflammatory thrombogenic vasculopathy involving vessels throughout the dermis and subcutis characterizes the histomorphology of associated lupus anticoagulant and/or cryofibrinogenemia (135).

Celiac Disease

Celiac disease is a malabsorption syndrome with a prevalence of up to 1% of the adult population of Western countries. It reflects small-intestinal mucosal injury caused by a humoral immune response to ingested gluten, and is associated with dermatitis herpetiformis in roughly 25% of cases (138–141). A leukocytoclastic vasculitis has also been described in patients with celiac disease (140). The presence of IgA or IgG antitissue transglutaminase and antiendomysial antibodies is seen in 80% to 90% of pa-

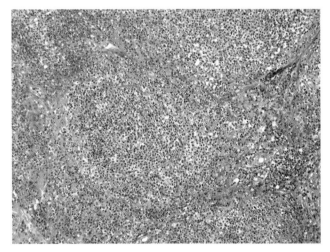

FIGURE 16-10. Ulcerative colitis: pyoderma gangrenosum. The biopsy shows an angiocentric disintegrating neutrophilic infiltrate with accompanying mural fibrin deposition with leukocytoclastic vasculitis. Immunofluorescent studies demonstrated vascular IgA deposition. There is pronounced neutrophilic dermolysis.

tients with active gut mucosal inflammation and has a high specificity for the diagnosis (142). A significant concern with serological confirmation of the diagnosis is the presence in a minority of celiac disease patients of a selective IgA deficiency; in such patients, however, IgG anti-transglutaminase and antiendomysial antibodies are still positive. Underlying mixed cryoglobulinemia may occur, as may mesangial nephritis, the latter a sequela of circulating immune complexes (139,143). Antibodies to transglutaminase may be of pathogenetic significance.

HEPATOBILIARY DISEASE

Sclerosing Cholangitis and Primary Biliary Cirrhosis

Pyoderma gangrenosum, particularly a disseminated superficial vesiculopustular variant (144), and dermatitis herpetiformis have been described in association with sclerosing cholangitis (58). Also, diffuse superficial pyoderma gangrenosum has been described in patients with ulcerative colitis, an associated finding in 70% of patients with sclerosing cholangitis. Isolated case reports of elastosis perforans serpiginosa with coexisting Down's syndrome (145) and disseminated warts along with primary combined immune deficiency and progressive multifocal leukoencephalopathy have been described in association with sclerosing cholangitis. Cutaneous manifestations seen with primary biliary cirrhosis include lichen planus (146), CREST, sarcoidal granulomata (147), and vitiligo (148).

Histopathology. Vesiculopustular pyoderma gangrenosum is characterized by a necrolytic subepithelial blister in which massive papillary edema is accompanied by sheets of neutrophils within the blister cavity, and prominent leukocytoclasia that is often centered on follicles. Peripheral to the areas of neutrophilia, angiocentric mononuclear-cell infiltrates with minimal accompanying vascular injury are observed (Fig. 16-12).

Pathogenesis. Although of unclear pathogenetic significance, antineutrophil cytoplasmic antibodies (ANCAs) in a perinuclear pattern have been detected in 72% of patients with primary sclerosing cholangitis and ulcerative colitis (149,150). An atypical pANCA, termed "xANCA," with a specificity for a 50-kD myeloid envelope protein, is seen in patients with inflammatory bowel disease, autoimmune hepatitis and primary sclerosing cholangitis (151, 152). ANCAs have also been described in Wegener's granulomatosis, microscopic polyarteritis nodosa, and idiopathic crescentic glomerulonephritis. Patients with primary sclerosing cholangitis and concomitant ulcerative colitis (153) have circulating antibodies to colonic epithelial cells (154). An immunogenic basis has also been proposed for primary sclerosing cholangitis in view of the association with HLA-B8 and/or HLA-DR3 antigens.

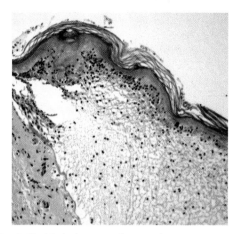

FIGURE 16-12. Vesicular pustular pyoderma gangrenosum. A biopsy of the lesion demonstrated marked subepidermal edema and a subjacent intense neutrophilic and lymphocytic infiltrate with tissue pathergy confined to the superficial dermis.

Hepatitis

Hepatitis can be broadly categorized into infectious and noninfectious causes. Most of the former are viral and are mediated by hepatitis A, B, C, and delta agent, cytomegalovirus, Epstein–Barr virus, and, rarely, varicella, measles, and herpes simplex. Chronic active hepatitis of autoimmune etiology is a necroinflammatory disorder of unknown etiology with a predilection for young women (155). Both the clinical presentation and liver chemistry profile may resemble infectious hepatitis. Hepatitis C antibodies have been demonstrated in patients with classic autoimmune hepatitis, a finding reputed to represent a nonspecific response that disappears during remission. Conversely, an autoantibody profile mimicking chronic active hepatitis may be seen in hepatitis C (155). Other laboratory abnormalities include anemia, hypergammaglobulinemia, positive lupus erythematosus cell preparations, and positive antibodies to non–organ-specific antibodies, such as antinuclear antibodies, ANCAs, and antibodies to smooth muscle and liver/kidney microsomes (155).

The principal cutaneous manifestations of viral and autoimmune hepatitis are lichen planus, leukocytoclastic vasculitis (156), porphyria cutanea tarda (157), erythema multiforme (158), pyoderma gangrenosum (159), and Gianotti–Crosti syndrome (160). Lichen planus has been reported in patients with hepatitis C, chronic active hepatitis of unknown etiology, and primary biliary cirrhosis (161) (Fig. 16-13). The clinical spectrum of skin lesions in patients infected with Hepatitis C comprises photodistributed eruptions, palpable purpura, folliculitis, chilblains-like acral lesions, ulcers, nodules, and urticaria (162). The vasculitis may be on the basis of mixed cryoglobulinemia in the setting of hepatitis C infection (156). Porphyria and erythema multiforme-like eruptions also occur in association with hepatitis C.

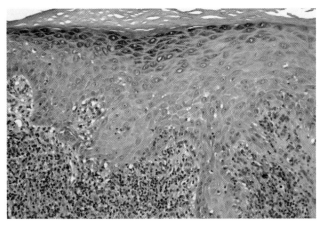

FIGURE 16-13. Lichenoid tissue reaction in the setting of hepatitis C infection. This patient with hepatitis C developed an eruption clinically compatible with lichen planus. The histomorphology confirms the diagnosis by virtue of a dense band-like lymphocytic infiltrate in apposition to an epidermis showing colloid body formation.

Papular acrodermatitis (160) (Gianotti–Crosti syndrome) reflects a primary infection with hepatitis B virus, acquired through the skin or mucous membranes, and comprises a nonpruritic, erythematous, papular eruption on the face, extremities, and buttocks. The eruption usually lasts about 3 weeks and is associated with lymphadenopathy and an acute, usually anicteric hepatitis of at least 2 months' duration that only rarely progresses to chronic liver disease. Hepatitis B surface antigenemia is present (160). A similar eruption may be produced by several other viruses, such as Epstein–Barr virus, coxsackie B virus, and cytomegalovirus (163), in which case there is often no hepatitis or lymphadenopathy.

Histopathology. The histologic appearance of the papules in Gianotti–Crosti syndrome includes a moderately dense infiltrate of lymphocytes and histiocytes in the upper dermis and mid-dermis that is found mainly around capillaries that exhibit endothelial swelling, accompanied by erythrocyte extravasation (163). Focal spongiosis, parakeratosis with mild acanthosis, and a focal interface dermatitis complete the picture (163). The histopathology of lichenoid tissue reactions (Fig. 16-13), pyoderma gangrenosum, erythema multiforme, leukocytoclastic vasculitis, and porphyria cutanea tarda is described in other sections of the book. In the hands, the skin lesions of hepatitis C can be classified by the dominant reaction pattern, the most common being vasculopathies of neutrophilic and lymphocytic vasculitis and pauci-inflammatory subtypes, palisading granulomatous inflammation, sterile neutrophilic folliculitis, neutrophilic lobular panniculitis, benign cutaneous polyarteritis nodosa, neutrophilic dermatoses including neutrophilic urticaria and pyoderma gangrenosum, and interface dermatitis (162). Some patients develop a low-grade lymphoproliferative disease of B-cell lineage cognate to marginal zone lymphoma. Endothelial cell swelling

is common. Mixed cryoglobulinemia differs from conventional leukocytoclastic vasculitis by the presence of intraluminal eosinophilic deposits that are strongly periodic acid-Sciff positive.

Pathogenesis. The sera of all patients with hepatitis B–induced papular acrodermatitis exhibit hepatitis B surface antigens by radioimmunoassay. Antibodies to hepatitis B surface antigens are not detected during the eruptive phase, but only 6 to 12 months after the eruption; patients with antibodies become hepatitis B surface-antigen negative, suggesting a role for humoral immunity in their recovery. As regards the skin lesions of hepatitis C infection, reverse transcriptase in situ polymerase chain reaction studies show expression of viral DNA in endothelia in some cases (162).

Acrokeratosis Neoplastica (Bazex Syndrome)

First described in 1965 (164), this rare but clinically distinctive dermatosis was originally associated with either a primary malignant neoplasm of the upper aerodigestive tract or metastatic cancer to the lymph nodes of the neck. Other associated malignancies have since been described. Thickening of the periungual and subungual skin and of the palms and soles occurs initially when the neoplasm is silent. Subsequently, the skin of the ears, nose, face, and the trunk and extremities becomes involved and shows a violaceous color, peeling, and fissuring (165,166). The palmar lesions may resemble Reiter's disease.

Histopathology. Ill-defined perivascular lymphocytic infiltrates containing a few pyknotic neutrophils in the upper dermis along with mild acanthosis, hyperkeratosis, and scattered parakeratotic foci are described. Eosinophilic and vacuolar degeneration of the spinous layer may be noted (166).

REFERENCES

1. Statters DJ, Asokan VS, Littlewood SM, et al. Carcinoma of the caecum in a scorbutic patient. *Br J Clin Pract* 1990;44:738.
2. Bartholomew M. James Lind's treatise of the scurvy (1753). *Postgrad Med J* 2002;78:695.
3. Levine M. New concepts in the biology and biochemistry of ascorbic acid. *N Engl J Med* 1986;314:892.
4. Haslock I. Hemarthrosis and scurvy [Letter]. *J Rheumatol* 2002; 29:1808.
5. Stokes PL, Melikiah V, Leeming RL, et al. Folate metabolism in scurvy. *Am J Clin Nutr* 1975;28:126.
6. Monks GM, Juracek L, Weigand D, et al. A case of scurvy in an autistic boy. *J Drugs Dermatol* 2002;1:67.
7. Ahmad K. Scurvy outbreak in Afghanistan prompts food aid concerns. *Lancet* 2002;359:1044.
8. Mason JB. Lessons on nutrition of displaced people. *J Nutr* 2002; 132:2096s.
9. Weise Pronzo Z, de Benoist B. Meeting the challenges of micronutrient deficiencies in emergency-affected populations. *Proc Nutr Soc* 2002;61:251.

10. Ellis CN, Vanderveen EE, Rasmussen JE. Scurvy: a case caused by peculiar dietary habits. *Arch Dermatol* 1984;120:1212.
11. Abramovits-Ackerman W, Bustos T, Simosa-Leon V, et al. Cutaneous findings in a new syndrome of autosomal recessive ectodermal dysplasia with corkscrew hairs. *J Am Acad Derm* 1992; 27:917.
12. Hashimoto K, Kitabchi AE, Duckworth WC, et al. Ultrastructure of scorbutic human skin. *Acta Dermatol Venereol (Stockh)* 1970;50:9.
13. Wechsler HL. Vitamin A deficiency following small-bowel bypass surgery for obesity. *Arch Dermatol* 1979;115:73.
14. Bleasel NR, Stapleton KM, Lee MS, et al. Vitamin A deficiency phrynoderma: due to malabsoption and inadequate diet. *J Am Acad Dermatol* 1999;41:322.
15. Frazier CN, Hu C. *Nature* and distribution according to age of cutaneous manifestations of vitamin A deficiency. *Arch Dermatol Syph* 1936;33:825.
16. Bessey OA, Wolbach SB. Vitamin A, physiology and pathology. *JAMA* 1938;110:2072.
17. Hendricks WM. Pellagra and pellagralike dermatoses: etiology, differential diagnosis, dermatopathology, and treatment [review]. *Semin Dermatol* 1991;10:282.
18. Wallengren J, Thelin I. Pellagra-like skin lesions associated with Wernicke's encephalopathy in a heavy wine drinker. *Acta Dermatol Venereol* 2002;82:152.
19. Castiello RJ, Lynch PJ. Pellagra and the carcinoid syndrome. *Arch Dermatol* 1972;105:574.
20. Lyon VB, Fairley JA. Anticonvulsant-induced pellagra. *J Am Acad Dermatol* 2002;46:597.
21. Spivak JL, Jackson DL. Pellagra: An analysis of 18 patients and a review of the literature. *Johns Hopkins Med J* 1977;140:295.
22. Karthikeyan K, Thappa DM. Pellagra and the skin. *Int J Dermatol* 2002;41:476.
23. Montgomery H. Nutritional and vitamin deficiency. In: *Dermatopathology*, vol. 1. New York: Harper and Row, 1967:260.
24. Dent CE. Hartnup disease: an inborn error of metabolism. *Arch Dis Child* 1957;32:363.
25. Halvorsen L, Halvorsen S. Hartnup disease. *Pediatrics* 1963;31: 29.
26. Baron DN, Dent CE, Harris H, et al. Hereditary pellagra-like skin rash with temporary cerebellar ataxia, constant renal aminoaciduria and other bizarre chemical features. *Lancet* 1956; 2:421.
27. Clodi PH, Deutsch E, Niebauer G. Krankheitsbild mit poikilodermieartigen hautveranderungen, aminoacidurie und Indolaceturie. *Arch Klin Exp Dermatol* 1964;218:165.
28. Ashurst PJ. Hydroa vacciniforme occurring in association with Hartnup disease. *Br J Dermatol* 1969;81:486.
29. Nozaki J, Dakeishi M, Ohura T, et al. Homozygosity mapping to chromosome 5p15 of a gene responsible for Hartnup disorder. *Biochem Biophys Res Commun* 2001;284:255.
30. Becker SW, Kahn D, Rothman S. Cutaneous manifestations of internal malignant tumors. *Arch Dermatol Syph* 1942;45:1069.
31. Domen RE, Shaffer MB Jr, Finke J, et al. The glucagonoma syndrome. *Arch Intern Med* 1980;140:262.
32. Alexander EK, Robinson M, Staniec M, et al. Peripheral amino acid and fatty acid infusion for the treatment of necrolytic migratory erythema in the glucagonoma syndrome. *Clin Endocrinol (Oxf)* 2002;57:827.
33. Chastain MA. The glucagonoma syndrome: a review of its features and discussion of new perspectives. *Am J Med Sci* 2001; 321:306.
34. Chao SC, Lee JY. Brittle nails and dyspareunia as first clues to recurrences of malignant glucagonoma. *Br J Dermatol* 2002;146: 1071.

35. Binnick AN, Spencer SK, Dennison WL Jr, et al. Glucagonoma syndrome. *Arch Dermatol* 1977;113:749.
36. Kasper CS, McMurray K. Necrolytic migratory erythema without glucagonoma versus canine superficial necrolytic dermatitis: Is hepatic impairment a clue to pathogenesis? *J Am Acad Dermatol* 1991;25:534.
37. Kaspar CS. Necrolytic migratory erythema: unresolved problems in diagnosis and pathogenesis. A case report and literature review. *Cutis* 1992;49:120.
38. Blackford S, Wright S, Roberts DL. Necrolytic migratory erythema without glucagonoma: the role of dietary essential fatty acids. *Br J Dermatol* 1991;125:460.
39. Goodenberger DM, Lawley TJ, Strober W, et al. Necrolytic migratory erythema without glucagonoma. *Arch Dermatol* 1977; 115:1429.
40. Fujita J, Seino Y, Isida H, et al. A functional study of a case of glucagonoma exhibiting typical glucagonoma syndrome. *Cancer* 1986;57:860.
41. Danbolt N, Closs K. Akrodermatitis enteropathica. *Acta Dermatol Venereol (Stockh)* 1942;23:127.
42. Moynahan EJ. Acrodermatitis enteropathica: a lethal inherited zinc-deficiency disorder. *Lancet* 1974;2:399.
43. Gonzalez JR, Botet MV, Sanchez JL. The histopathology of acrodermatitis enteropathica. *Am J Dermatopathol* 1982;4:303.
44. Reichel M, Mauro TM, Ziboh VA, et al. Acrodermatitis enteropathica in a patient with the acquired immunodeficiency syndrome. *Arch Dermatol* 1992;128:415.
45. Bernstein B, Leyden JL. Zinc deficiency and acrodermatitis enteropathica after intravenous hyperalimentation. *Arch Dermatol* 1978;114:1070.
46. Niemi KM, Anttila PH, Kanerva L, et al. Histopathological study of transient acrodermatitis enteropathica due to decreased zinc in breast milk. *J Cutan Pathol* 1989;16:382.
47. Weissman K, Hoe S, Knudsen L, et al. Zinc absorption in patients suffering from acrodermatitis enteropathica and in normal adults assessed by whole-body counting technique. *Br J Dermatol* 1979;101:573.
48. Ortega SS, Cachaza JA, Tovar IV, et al. Zinc deficiency dermatitis in parenteral nutrition: an electron-microscopic study. *Dermatologica* 1985;171:163.
49. Albers SE, Brozena SJ, Fenske NA. A case of kwashiorkor. *Cutis* 1993;51:445.
50. Househam KC. Computed tomography of the brain in kwashiorkor: a follow-up study. *Arch Dis Child* 1991;66:623.
51. Montgomery H. Nutritional and vitamin deficiency. In: *Dermatopathology*, vol. 1. New York: Harper and Row, 1967:264.
52. Richardson D, Iputo J. Effects of kwashiorkor malnutrition on measured capillary filtration rate in forearm. *Am J Physiol* 1992; 262:H496.
53. Brunsting LA, Goeckerman WE, O'Leary PA. Pyoderma (ecthyma) gangrenosum. *Arch Dermatol* 1930;22:655.
54. Graham JA, Hansen KK, Rabinowitz LG, et al. Pyoderma gangrenosum in infants and children. *Pediatr Dermatol* 1994; 11:10.
55. Cairns BA, Herbst CA, Sartor BR, et al. Peristomal pyoderma gangrenosum and inflammatory bowel disease. *Arch Surg* 1994; 129:769.
56. Schwaegerle SM, Bergfeld WF, Senitzer D, et al. Pyoderma gangrenosum: a review. *J Am Acad Dermatol* 1988;18:559.
57. Callen JP. Pyoderma gangrenosum and related disorders. *Med Clin North Am* 1989;73:1247.
58. Magro CM, Crowson AN. Vesiculopustular lesions in association with liver disease. *Int J Dermatol* 1997;36:837.
59. Crowson AN, Magro CM, Mihm MC Jr. Pyoderma gangrenosum: a review. *J Cutan Pathol* 2003;30:97.

60. Wilson-Jones E, Winkelmann RK. Superficial granulomatous pyoderma: a localized vegetative form of pyoderma gangrenosum. *J Am Acad Dermatol* 1988;18:511.

61. Ayres G. Pyoderma gangrenosum: an unusual syndrome of ulcerative vesicles in arthritis. *Arch Dermatol* 77:269.

62. Srebrnik A, Schachar E, Brenner S. Suspected induction of a pyoderma gangrenosum-like eruption due to sulpride treatment. *Cutis* 2001;67:253.

63. Ross HJ, Moy LA, Kaplan R, et al. Bullous pyoderma gangrenosum after granulocyte colony-stimulating factor treatment. *Cancer* 1991;68:441.

64. Jorizzo JL, Solomon AR, Zanolli M, et al. Neutrophilic vascular reactions. *J Am Acad Dermatol* 1988;19:983.

65. Magro CM, Crowson AN. The cutaneous neutrophilic vascular injury syndromes: a review. *Semin Diagn Pathol* 2001; 18:47.

66. Pye RJ, Choudhury C. Bullous pyoderma as a presentation of acute leukemia. *Clin Exp Dermatol* 1977;2:33.

67. Koester G, Tarnower A, Levisohn D, et al. Bullous pyoderma gangrenosum. *J Am Acad Dermatol* 1993;29:875.

68. Sanders S, Tahan SR, Kwan T, et al. Giant cells in pyoderma gangrenosum. *J Cutan Pathol* 2001;28:98.

69. Magro CM, Crowson AN. Sterile neutrophilic folliculitis with perifollicular vasculopathy: a distinctive cutaneous reaction pattern reflecting systemic disease. *J Cutan Pathol* 1998;25:215.

70. Powell FC, Schroeter AL, Perry HO, et al. Direct immunofluorescence in pyoderma gangrenosum. *Br J Dermatol* 1983;108: 287.

71. Holt PJA, Davies MG, Saunders KC, et al. Pyoderma gangrenosum: clinical and laboratory findings in 15 patients with special reference to polyarthritis. *Medicine (Baltimore)* 1980;59:114.

72. Powell FC, Schroeter AL, Su D, et al. Pyoderma gangrenosum and monoclonal gammopathy. *Arch Dermatol* 1983;119:468.

73. Morrison JGL, Fourie ED. A distinctive skin eruption following small-bowel bypass surgery. *Br J Dermatol* 1980;102:467.

74. Ely PH. The bowel bypass syndrome: a response to bacterial peptidoglycans. *J Am Acad Dermatol* 1980;2:473.

75. Jorizzo JL, Apisarnthanarax P, Subrt P, et al. Bowel-bypass syndrome without bowel bypass: bowel-associated dermatosis-arthritis syndrome. *Arch Intern Med* 1983;143:457.

76. Dicken CH. Bowel-associated dermatosis-arthritis syndrome: bowel bypass syndrome without bowel bypass. *J Am Acad Dermatol* 1986;14:792.

77. Goldman JA, Casey HL, Davidson ED, et al. Vasculitis associated with intestinal bypass surgery. *Arch Dermatol* 1979;115:725.

78. Magro CM, Crowson AN. The clinical and histological spectrum of IgA-associated vasculitis. *Am J Dermatopathol* 1999;21:234.

79. Magro CM, Crowson AN, Peeling R. Vasculitis as the pathogenetic basis of Reiter's disease. *Hum Pathol* 1995;26:633.

80. O'Duffy JD. Behçet's syndrome. *N Engl J Med* 1990;322:326.

81. Main DM, Chamberlain MA. Clinical differentiation of oral ulceration in Behçet's disease. *Br J Rheumatol* 1992;31:767.

82. Magro CM, Crowson AN. Cutaneous manifestations of Behçet's disease. *Int J Dermatol* 1995;34:159.

83. King R, Crowson AN, Murray E, et al. Acral purpuric papulonodular lesions as a manifestation of Behçet's disease. *Int J Dermatol* 1995;34:190.

84. Kural-Seyahi E, Fresko I, Seyahi N, et al. The long-term mortality and morbidity of Behcet syndrome: a 2-decade outcome survey of 387 patients followed at a dedicated center. *Medicine (Baltimore)* 2003;82:60.

85. Oguz O, Serdaroglu S, Turzin Y, et al. Acute febrile neutrophilic dermatosis (Sweet's syndrome) associated with Behçet's disease. *Int J Dermatol* 1992;31:645.

86. Koc Y, Gullu I, Akpek G, et al. Vascular involvement in Behçet's Disease. *J Rheumatol* 1992;19:402.

87. Akutsu Y, Itami N, Tanaka M, et al. IgA nephritis in Behçet's disease: Case report and review of the literature. *Clin Nephrol* 1990;34:52.

88. Sokoloff L, Bunin JJ. Vascular lesions in rheumatoid arthritis. *J Chronic Dis* 1957;5:668.

89. Magro CM, Crowson AN. The spectrum of cutaneous lesions in rheumatoid arthritis: a clinical and pathological study of 43 cases. *J Cutan Pathol* 2003;30:1.

90. Langenberg A, Yen TS, LeBoit PE. Granulomatous vasculitis occurring after cutaneous herpes zoster despite absence of viral genome. *J Am Acad Dermatol* 1991;24:429.

91. Choudhri S, Magro CM, Nicolle L, et al. A unique id reaction to *Mycobacterium leprae*: first documented case. *Cutis* 1994;54:282.

92. Lehner T, Batchelor JR, Challacombe SJ, et al. An immunogenetic basis for the tissue involvement in Behçet's syndrome. *Immunology* 1979;37:895.

93. Kaya Ti, Dura H, Tersen U, et al. Association of class I Hla antigens with the clinical manifestations of Turkish patients with Behcet's disease. *Clin Exp Dermatol* 2002;27:498.

94. Mizuki N, Yabuki K, Ota M, et al. Analysis of microsatellite polymorphism around the hla-B locus in Iranian patients with Behcet's disease. *Tissue Antigens* 2002;60:396.

95. Namba K, Ueno T, Okita M. Behçet's disease and streptococcal infection. *Jpn J Ophthalmol* 1986;30:385.

96. Yokota K, Hayashi S, Fujii N, et al. Antibody response to oral streptococci in Behçet's disease. *Microbiol Immunol* 1992;36:815.

97. Efthimiou J, Hay PE, Spiro SG, et al. Pulmonary tuberculosis in Behçet's syndrome. *Br J Dis Chest* 1988;82:300.

98. Studd M, McCance DJ, Lehner T. Detection of HSV-1 DNA in patients with Behçet's syndrome and in patients with recurrent oral ulcers by the polymerase chain reaction. *J Med Microbiol* 1991;34:39.

99. Hamzaoui K, Kahan A, Ayed K, et al. Cytotoxic T cells against herpes simplex virus in Behçet's disease. *Clin Exp Rheumatol* 1991;9:131.

100. Stein CM, Thomas JE. Behçet's disease associated with HIV infection. *J Rheumatol* 1991;18:1427.

101. Lamb JR, Young DB. T cell recognition of stress proteins: a link between infectious and autoimmune disease. *Mol Biol Med* 1990;7:311.

102. Lehner T, Lavery E, Smith R, et al. Association between the 65 kilodalton heat shock protein, *Streptococcus sangui* and the corresponding antibodies in Behçet's syndrome. *Infect Immun* 1991;59:1424.

103. Holoshitz J, Koning JE, Coligan JE, et al. Isolation of CD4-CD8-mycobacterial reaction T-lymphocyte clones from rheumatoid arthritis synovial fluid. *Nature* 1989;39:226.

104. Pervin K, Childerstone A, Shinnick T, et al. T cell epitope expression of mycobacterial and homologous human 65-kilodalton heat shock protein peptide in short term cell line from patient with Behçet's disease. *J Immunol* 1993;151:2273.

105. Suzuki Y, Hoshi K, Matsuda T, et al. Increased peripheral blood gamma delta+ T cells and natural killer cells in Behçet's disease. *J Rheumatol* 1992;19:588.

106. Bank I, Duvdevani M, Livneh A. Expansion of gammadelta T-cells in Behcet's disease: role of disease activity and microbial flora in oral ulcers. *J Lab Clin Med* 2003;141:33.

107. Yang P, Chen L, Zhou H, et al. Resistance of lymphocytes to FAS-mediated apoptosis in Behcet's diseases and Vogt-Koyangi-Harada syndrome. *Ocul Immunol Inflam* 2002;10:47.

108. Sensi A, Gavioli R, Spisani S, et al. HLA B51 antigen associated with neutrophil hyperactivity. *Dis Markers* 1991;9:327.

109. Pronai L, Ichikawa Y, Nakazawa H, et al. Enhanced superoxide generation and the decreased superoxide scavenging activity of peripheral blood leukocytes in Behçet's disease: effects of colchicine. *Clin Exp Rheumatol* 1991;9:227.

110. Aydintung AO, Tokgoz G, D'Cruz DP, et al. Antibodies to endothelial cells in patients with Behçet's disease. *Clin Immunol Immunopathol* 1993;67:157.
111. Disdier P, Harle JR, Mouly A, et al. Case report: Behçet's syndrome and factor XII deficiency. *Clin Rheumatol* 1992;11:422.
112. Chafa O, Fischer AM, Meriane F, et al. Behçet's syndrome associated with protein S deficiency. *Thromb Haemost* 1992;67:1.
113. Hampton KK, Chamberlain MA, Menon DK, et al. Coagulation and fibrinolytic activity in Behçet's disease. *Thromb Haemost* 1991;66:292.
114. Al-Dalaan A, Al-Ballaa SR, Al-Janadi S, et al. Association of anticardiolipin antibodies with vascular thrombosis and neurological manifestation of Behçet's disease. *Clin Rheumatol* 1993;12:28.
115. Tursen U, Irfan Kaya T, Ikizoglu G. Cardiac complications in Behcet's disease. *Clin Exp Dermatol* 2002;27:651.
116. Tunc R, Keyman E, Melikoglu M, et al. Target organ associations in Turkish patients with Behcet's disease: a cross sectional study by exploratory factor analysis. *J Rheumatol* 2002;29:2393.
117. Greenstein AJ, Janowitz HD, Sachar DB. The extra-intestinal complications of Crohn's disease and ulcerative colitis: a study of 700 patients. *Medicine (Baltimore)* 1976;55:401.
118. Werther JL, Schapira A, Rubenstein O, et al. Amyloidosis in regional enteritis: a report of 5 cases. *Am J Med* 1960;29:416.
119. Present DH, Rabinowitz JC, Bank PA, Janowitz HD. Obstructive hydronephropathy. *N Engl J Med* 1969;280:523.
120. Shum D, Guenther L. Metastatic Crohn's disease: case report and review of the literature. *Arch Dermatol* 1990;126:645.
121. Buckley C, Bayoumi A-HM, Sarkany I. Metastatic Crohn's disease. *Clin Exp Dermatol* 1990;15:131.
122. Burgdorf W. Cutaneous manifestations of Crohn's disease. *J Am Acad Dermatol* 1981;5:689.
123. Lebwohl M, Fleischmajer R, Janowitz H, et al. Metastatic Crohn's disease. *J Am Acad Dermatol* 1984;10:33.
124. Aloi FG, Molinero A, Pippione M. Parakeratotic horns in a patient with Crohn's disease. *Clin Exp Dermatol* 1989;14:79.
125. Magro CM, Crowson AN. Lichenoid and granulomatous dermatitis: a novel cutaneous reaction pattern. *Int J Dermatol* 2000;39:126.
126. Witkowski JA, Parish LC, Lewis JE. Crohn's disease, noncaseating granulomas on the legs. *Acta Dermatol Venereol (Stockh)* 1977;57:181.
127. Burgdorf W, Orken M. Granulomatous perivasculitis in Crohn's disease. *Arch Dermatol* 1981;117:674.
128. Diaz-Perez JL, Winkelmann RK. Cutaneous polyarteritis nodosa. *Arch Dermatol* 1974;110:407.
129. Magro CM, Crowson AN, Regauer S. Granuloma annulare and necrobiosis lipoidica as a manifestation of systemic disease. *Hum Pathol* 1996;27:50.
130. Smoller BR, Weishar M, Gray MH. An unusual cutaneous manifestation of Crohn's disease. *Arch Pathol Lab Med* 1990;114:609.
131. Crowson AN, Nuovo GJ, Mihm MC Jr, et al. Cutaneous manifestations of Crohn's disease, its spectrum, and pathogenesis: intracellular consensus bacterial 16S rRNA is associated with the gastrointestinal but not the cutaneous manifestations of Crohn's disease. *Hum Pathol* 2003 Nov;34(11):1185.
132. Collins WJ, Bendig DW, Taylor WF. Pulmonary vasculitis complicating childhood ulcerative colitis. *Gastroenterology* 1979;77:1091.
133. Kedziora JA, Wolff M, Chang J. Limited forms of Wegener's granulomatosis in ulcerative colitis. *Am J Roentgenol Radium Ther Nucl Med* 1975;125:127.
134. Stapleton SR, Curley RK, Simpson WA. Cutaneous gangrene secondary to focal thrombosis: an important cutaneous manifestation of ulcerative colitis. *Clin Exp Dermatol* 1989;14:387.
135. Ball GV, Goldman LN. Chronic ulcerative colitis, skin necrosis, and cryofibrinogenemia. *Ann Intern Med* 1976;85:464.
136. Barnes L, Lucky AW, Bucuvales JC, et al. Pustular pyoderma gangrenosum associated with ulcerative colitis in childhood. *J Am Acad Dermatol* 1986;15:608.
137. Peters AJ, van de Waal Bake AW, Daha MR, et al. Inflammatory bowel disease and ankylosing spondylitis with cutaneous vasculitis, glomerulonephritis and circulating IgA immune complexes. *Ann Rheum Dis* 1990;49:638.
138. Scott BB, Young S, Raja SM, et al. Celiac disease and dermatitis herpetiformis: Further studies of their relationship. *Gut* 1976;17:759.
139. Moothy AV, Zimmerman SW, Maxim PE. Dermatitis herpetiformis and celiac disease: association with glomerulonephritis, hypocomplementemia and circulating immune complexes. *JAMA* 1978;239:2019.
140. Meyers S, Dikman S, Spiera H, et al. Cutaneous vasculitis complicating celiac disease. *Gut* 1981;22:61.
141. Collin P, Reunala T. Recognition and management of the cutaneous manifestations of celiac disease: a guide for dermatologists. *Am J Clin Dermatol* 2003;4:13.
142. Agardh D, Borulf S, Lernmark A, et al. Tissue tranglutaminase immunoglobulin isotypes in children with untreated and treated celiac disease. *J Pediatr Gastroenterol Nutr* 2003;36:77.
143. Doe WF, Evans D, Hobb JR, et al. Celiac disease, vasculitis and cryoglobulinemia. *Gut* 1972;13:112.
144. Laajam MA, al-Mofarreh MA, al-Zayyani NR. Primary sclerosing cholangitis in chronic ulcerative colitis: report of cases in Arabs and review. *Trop Gastroenterol* 1992;13:106.
145. O'Donnell B, Kelly P, Dervan P, et al. Generalized elastosis perforans serpinginosa in Down's syndrome. *Clin Exp Dermatol* 1992;17:31.
146. Graham-Brown RAC, Sarkany I, Sherlock S. Lichen planus and primary biliary cirrhosis. *Br J Dermatol* 1982;106:699.
147. Harrington AC, Fitzpatrick JE. Cutaneous sarcoidal granulomas in a patient with primary biliary cirrhosis. *Cutis* 1992;49:271.
148. Zauli D, Crespi C, Miserocchi F, et al. Primary biliary cirrhosis and vitiligo. *J Am Acad Dermatol* 1986;15:105.
149. Snook JA, Chapman RW, Fleming K, et al. Anti-neutrophil nuclear antibody in ulcerative colitis, Crohn's disease and primary sclerosing cholangitis. *Clin Exp Immunol* 1989;76:30.
150. Hardarson S, LaBrecque DR, Mitros FA, et al. Antineutrophil cytoplasmic antibody in inflammatory bowel and hepatobiliary diseases: high prevalence in ulcerative colitis, primary sclerosing cholangitis, and autoimmune hepatitis. *Am J Clin Pathol* 1993;99:277.
151. Terjung B, Spengler U, Sauerbruch T, et al. Atypical p-ANCA in IBD and autoimmune liver disorders reacts with a myeloid-specific 50 kD nuclear envelope protein. *Clin Exp Immunol* 2000;120[Suppl 1]:53(abst).
152. Frenzer A, Fierz W, Rundler E, et al. Atypical, cytoplasmic and perinuclear anti-neutrophil cytoplasmic antibodies in patients with inflammatory bowel disease. *J Gastroenterol Hepatol* 1998;13:950.
153. Olsson R, Danielsson A, Jarnerot G, et al. Prevalence of primary sclerosing cholangitis in patients with ulcerative colitis. *Gastroenterology* 1991;100:1319.
154. Chapman RW, Cottone M, Selby WS, et al. Serum autoantibodies, ulcerative colitis and primary sclerosing cholangitis. *Gut* 1990;27:86.
155. Krawitt EL. Autoimmune hepatitis: classification, heterogeneity and treatment. *Am J Med* 1994;96:23S.
156. Durand JM, Lefevre P, Harle JR, et al. Cutaneous vasculitis and cryoglobulinemia type II associated with hepatitis C virus infection. *Lancet* 1991;337:499.

157. Fargion S, Piperno A, Cappellini MD, et al. Hepatitis C virus and porphyria cutanea tarda: Evidence of a strong association. *Hepatology* 1995;21:1754.

158. Antinori S, Esposito R, Aliprandi C, et al. Erythema multiforme and hepatitis C. *Lancet* 1991;337:428.

159. Byrne JP, Hewitt M, Summerly R. Pyoderma gangrenosum associated with active chronic hepatitis. *Arch Dermatol* 1976;112:1297.

160. Gianotti F. Papular acrodermatitis of childhood and other papulovesicular acro-located syndromes [review]. *Br J Dermatol* 1979;100:49.

161. Jubert C, Pawlotsky JM, Pouget F, et al. Lichen planus and hepatitis C virus-related chronic active hepatitis. *Arch Dermatol* 1994;130:73.

162. Crowson AN, Nuovo G, Ferri C, Magro CM. The dermatopathologic manifestations of hepatitis C infection: a clinical, histological, and molecular assessment of 35 cases. *Hum Pathol* 2003 Jun;34(6):573.

163. Spear RL, Winkelman RK. Gianotti–Crosti syndrome: a review of 10 cases not associated with hepatitis B infection. *Arch Dermatol* 1984;120:891.

164. Bazex A, Salvador R, Dupre A, et al. Syndrome paraneoplastique a type d'hyperkeratose des extremities. *Bull Soc Fr Dermatol Syphiligr* 1965;72:182.

165. Pecora AL, Landsman L, Imgrund SP, et al. Acrokeratosis neoplastica (Basex syndrome). *Arch Dermatol* 1983;119:820.

166. Bazex A, Griffith A. Acrokeratosis paraneoplastica: a new cutaneous marker of malignancy. *Br J Dermatol* 1980;103:301.

METABOLIC DISEASES OF THE SKIN

JOHN MAIZE
JOHN MAIZE, JR.
JOHN METCALF

AMYLOIDOSIS

Amyloid

The term "amyloid" is applied to extracellular proteinaceous deposits that are resistant to proteolytic digestion and have distinctive physical properties. Deposits can be localized to a body site or can be "systemic," involving several organs and tissues.

By light microscopy, amyloid appears amorphous, eosinophilic, and hyaline. Characteristic staining qualities distinguish it from other glassy, pink substances. The Congo-red stain results in a brick-red staining reaction and apple-green birefringence, and amyloid stains metachromatically with crystal violet and methyl violet stains. These staining characteristics result from the cross–beta-pleated sheet conformation of the polypeptide backbones of the amyloid fibrils. These fibrils are ultrastructurally 8 to 12 nm in width and of indeterminate length. They are formed of a core of amyloid P component (AP) surrounded by chondroitic sulphate proteoglycan (CSPG), which, in turn, is surrounded by heparin sulphate proteoglycan (HSPG). The outer covering is one of a number of fibril proteins of which more than 20 have been described (1,2).

Chemically, there are more than 16 different amyloids, which, although sharing the physical properties outlined above, are distinguished by having different protein constituents and diverse origins. Thus, it has been recommended that classification of amyloidoses be based on the fibril protein whenever possible (3). Historically, the distinction between AL amyloid (primary systemic amyloidosis resulting from a plasma cell dyscrasia) and AA amyloid (secondary systemic amyloidosis) was made utilizing the latter's sensitivity to permanganate. More recently, immunohistochemistry has been used in the identification of a number of fibril proteins, but this technique also has its limitations. Extraction and chemical analysis have thus been the "gold standard." This, in the past, has required relatively large amounts of fresh tissue. Small-scale extraction, purification, and analysis offer hope that, in the future, identification can be carried out on even small, formalin-fixed, paraffin-embedded tissue biopsies (4).

Cutaneous deposition of amyloid can result from any one of several systemic disease processes. However, cutaneous amyloid deposits can also result from local processes limited to the skin.

Systemic Amyloidoses Involving the Skin: Immunoglobulin Light Chains

In its systemic form, this disease is also known as primary systemic amyloidosis. This uncommon disease results from a plasma cell dyscrasia with production of monoclonal light chains (5). The heart, smooth and skeletal muscle, and other soft tissues, as well as the kidneys, liver, and spleen, are frequently involved. However, deposits can be localized to the skin (and lungs) (2). When they are restricted to the skin, the terms "amyloidosis cutis nodularis atrophicans" and "nodular amyloidosis" have been applied. Heart failure, gastrointestinal bleeding, and renal failure can be fatal complications of the systemic form (6,7). Among cutaneous lesions, petechiae and ecchymoses are most common (7). They are the result of involvement of cutaneous blood vessels and are observed mainly on the face, especially on the eyelids and in the periorbital region. Minor trauma may precipitate these lesions, referred to by some as "pinch purpura." In addition, there may be discrete or coalescing papules or plaques. They usually have a waxy color but may be blue-red as the result of hemorrhage into them (8,9). In rare instances, one observes firm cutaneous or subcutaneous nodules or plaques or areas of induration of the skin resembling morphea (10). Bullae may be induced by minor trauma and may be hemorrhagic occurring occasionally (9,11,12). Among oral lesions, macroglossia is common, occurring in 17% of the patients (6).

Histopathology. Examination of cutaneous lesions in the systemic form of the disease reveals faintly eosinophilic amorphous, often fissured masses of amyloid deposited in the dermis and in the subcutaneous tissues. Quite frequently, accumulations of amyloid are deposited close to the epidermis. They may or may not be separated from the overlying epidermis by a narrow zone of collagen (Fig. 17-1). They are rarely deposited around individual elastic fibers (13). The involvement of the walls of blood vessels is responsible for the frequent presence of extravasated erythrocytes. Inflammatory cells are lacking or scarce (12). Bullous lesions are of uncertain pathogenesis. Several mechanisms have been proposed: (a) the formation of clefts within large dermal amyloid deposits (11,12), or (b) from disruption of basal keratinocytes and the basement membrane zone (14).

In the subcutaneous tissue, there may be large aggregates of amyloid with infiltration of the walls of blood vessels and so-called amyloid rings, which are formed by the deposition of amyloid around individual fat cells (12). The fat cells may then appear as if cemented together by the amyloid.

Even if there are no skin lesions, fine-needle aspirates of the abdominal fat often are of use in documenting the diagnosis (15,16) (Fig. 17-2). Tissue biopsies of normal-appearing skin yield positive results in about 40% of all patients (10,17). These biopsies show small deposits in the walls of small blood vessels in the dermis or the subcutaneous tissue but occasionally also around eccrine glands and lipocytes. The forearm is the recommended area for biopsy (17).

When localized to the skin, the nodular amyloid deposits are surrounded by a dense plasmacytic infiltrate, and production of the immunoglobulin light chains is thought to occur locally (18).

Relationship with Multiple Myeloma. AL amyloidosis results from the production of monoclonal immunoglobulins and/or free light chains, usually eight light chains, by

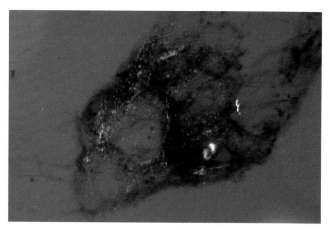

FIGURE 17-2. Primary systemic amyloidosis. Amyloid deposited in subcutaneous fat exhibits green birefringence when stained with Congo red in this aspirate from the abdominal fat pad.

an abnormal population of B cells. The vast majority of the patients (90%) have monoclonal protein in urine or serum (Bence–Jones protein) (19). If overtly malignant plasma cell neoplasia exists, it is referred to as multiple myeloma. Systemic amyloidosis is found in 5% to 15% of multiple myeloma patients. The majority of patients with AL amyloidosis do not have overt multiple myeloma, however. These patients have an underlying B-cell dyscrasia and, despite having no tumor masses, show an increased plasma cell population on bone marrow examination. It is uncertain whether this patient population will inevitably develop multiple myeloma.

Pathogenesis. In the systemic form of AL amyloidosis, the amyloid originates from monoclonal immunoglobulin light chains produced by plasma cells in the bone marrow. In the localized form, the amyloid is thought to be produced by the local plasma cell infiltrate, and, as in the systemic form, the amyloid protein has immunocytochemical characteristics of AL amyloid (18).

Ultrastructurally, amyloid deposits consist of irregularly arranged, straight nonbranching filaments that often appear hollow because their peripheries appear electron dense in comparison with their centers. These filaments are 6 to 7 nm in diameter but are of indeterminate length (20–22).

Serum Amyloid A Amyloidosis

Also known as secondary systemic amyloidosis, serum amyloid A amyloidosis (AA amyloidosis) can result from chronic inflammatory disease or recurring bouts of acute inflammation such as tuberculosis, complications of bronchiectasis, and chronic osteomyelitis. It is now relatively rare in industrialized countries since the development of modern antibiotic therapy, and most cases in the United States and Western Europe are associated with chronic rheumatoid arthritis or related disorders (23). At time of diagnosis, the vast ma-

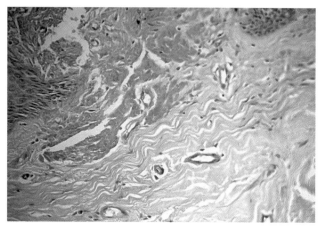

FIGURE 17-1. Primary systemic amyloidosis. PAS stain sharing amorphous, fissured masses of amyloid in the upper dermis. The amyloid material greatly resembles that observed in colloid milium (Fig. 17-4).

jority of patients have renal insufficiency or the nephrotic syndrome. There are no cutaneous lesions.

Histopathology. AA amyloid is deposited in parenchymatous organs such as the kidneys, liver, spleen, and adrenal. These deposits are found first in the interstitium and blood vessel walls; with progression, the deposits gradually replace the parenchyma. Deposits within the glomeruli and peritubular tissues result in renal failure.

Fine-needle aspiration biopsy of the subcutaneous fat and staining of the aspirated material by the Congo-red method is the most sensitive method of diagnosis (15, 16,24,25). Tissue biopsy of skin with underlying subcutaneous fat demonstrates deposits of AA amyloid around lipocytes, in blood vessel walls, around eccrine glands, and sometimes free in the dermis (17).

Pathogenesis. AA amyloid is thought to be derived from serum amyloid A (SAA). SAA proteins are divided into two groups. The first consists of SAA1 and SAA2, acute phase proteins synthesized by the liver, the vast majority of which are bound with high-density lipoproteins. SAA4 (second group) is not an acute phase protein and is synthesized by different organs and tissues (1). Production is stimulated by inflammation via IL-1 and other cytokines. AA protein is then formed when SAA undergoes carboxy terminal cleavage (26–28). This process takes place within lysosomes of macrophages that are receiving antigenic stimulation by a variety of chronic diseases (29). The amyloid is then deposited extracellularly.

Primary Localized Cutaneous Amyloidosis

Lichen Amyloidosis and Macular Amyloidosis

Lichen amyloidosis and macular amyloidosis are best considered as different manifestations of the same disease process. Lichen amyloidosis is characterized by closely set, discrete, brown-red papules that often show some scaling and are most commonly located on the legs, especially the shins, although they may occur elsewhere. Through the coalescence of papules, plaques may form on the legs. These plaques often have verrucous surfaces and then resemble hypertrophic lichen planus or lichen simplex chronicus. Usually the lesions of lichen amyloidosis itch severely. It is assumed by some authors that the pruritis leads to damage of keratinocytes by scratching and to subsequent production of amyloid (30,31).

Macular amyloidosis is characterized by pruritic macules showing pigmentation with a reticulated or rippled pattern. Although macular amyloidosis may occur anywhere on the trunk or extremities, the upper back is a fairly common site (32). In Southeast Asia, where macular amyloidosis is common, prolonged friction from a rough nylon towel or a back scratcher is thought to be its cause (33). The eruption can be easily passed off as postinflammatory hyperpigmentation by physicians unfamiliar with the condition (34).

Macular amyloidosis and lichen amyloidosis sometimes occur together in the same patient, and lichenoid amyloidosis can arise in a setting of macular amyloidosis, presumably due to scratching (35,36). When treated by intralesional injection of steroids, the lichenoid lesions can become macular.

Histopathology. Lichen and macular amyloidosis show deposits of amyloid that are limited to the papillary dermis. Most of the amyloid is situated within the dermal papillae. Although the deposits usually are smaller in macular amyloidosis than in lichen amyloidosis, differentiation of the two on the basis of the amount of amyloid is not possible (34). The two conditions actually differ only in the appearance of the epidermis, which is hyperplastic and hyperkeratotic in lichen amyloidosis. Occasionally, the amount of amyloid in macular amyloidosis is so small that it is missed, even when special stains are used on frozen sections. In such instances, more than one biopsy may be necessary to confirm the diagnosis (37).

In areas in which the entire dermal papilla is filled with amyloid, the amyloid appears homogeneous in both lichen and macular forms. In lesions in which the dermal papillae are only partially filled, as seen more often in macular amyloidosis, the amyloid has a globular appearance and resembles the colloid bodies found in lichen planus (Fig. 17–3A, B, and C). These amyloid bodies in some areas lie in direct contact with the overlying basal cells of the epidermis. Similar colloid bodies are also found in some sections within the epidermis, but in contrast with those located at the epidermal–dermal junction, they do not stain as amyloid. In addition, there often is a striking degree of pigmentary incontinence.

Histogenesis. The light microscopic findings in lichen and macular amyloidosis suggest that degenerating epidermal cells are discharged into the dermis, where they are converted into amyloid. The epidermal origin of the amyloid in lichen and macular amyloidosis is supported by electron microscopy (38,39). Also on electron microscopy, the degenerating epidermal cells resemble the colloid bodies observed in lichen planus. They contain the following components: (a) tonofilaments; (b) degenerated, wavy tonofilaments that are thicker but less electron-dense than normal tonofilaments; (c) lysosomes; and (d) typical filaments of amyloid, 6 to 10 nm thick, that are straight and nonbranching (39). It is postulated that the degenerated wavy tonofilaments are recognized as foreign and are digested by the cell's own lysosomes. Such digestion produces amyloid filaments. A conversion of tonofilaments into amyloid filaments requires that the alpha-pleated sheet configuration of the tonofilaments change into the beta configuration of amyloid (40). However, immunohistochemical studies suggest that components of the lamina densa and anchoring fibrils are also associated with amyloid deposits. Further ultrastructural examination shows disruption of the lamina densa overlying these deposits (41).

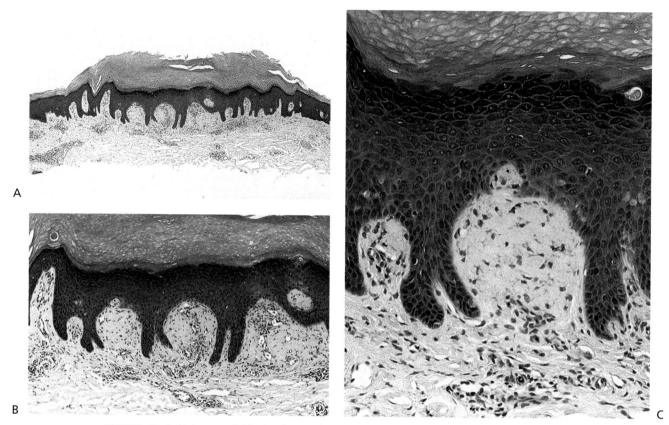

FIGURE 17-3. Lichen amyloidosis. There is hyperkeratosis and epidermal hyperplasia. Dermal papillae are rounded and contain globular deposits of amyloid. **A:** H&E, original magnification ×40. **B:** H&E, original magnification ×100. **C:** H&E, original magnification ×200).

On direct immunofluorescence, all specimens of lichen or macular amyloidosis fluoresce positively for immunoglobulins or complement, particularly immunoglobulin M (IgM) and the third component of complement (C3). Staining for kappa and lambda light chains is positive. The immunofluorescent pattern is globular, and thus is similar to that of lichen planus, except for the absence of fibrin. It suggests that the globular aggregates of lichenoid or macular amyloidosis, like the colloid bodies of lichen planus, act as a filamentous sponge into which immunoglobulins and complement are absorbed (42).

The epidermal derivation of the amyloid in lichen and macular amyloidosis is supported by histochemical and immunologic findings. In contrast to the amyloid of systemic amyloidosis, the amyloid of lichenoid and macular amyloidosis shows fluorescence for disulfide bonds as normally seen in the stratum corneum, suggesting that cross-linking of sulfhydryl groups occurs in amyloidogenesis (43). Furthermore, immunofluorescence studies with an antikeratin antiserum have shown intense staining of the amyloid for the antikeratin antibody (44).

After full agreement apparently had been reached about the keratogenic origin of the amyloid in lichen and macular amyloidosis, some dissenting opinions were expressed.

In one study, amyloid stained negatively for keratin determinants and the positive reactions obtained by previous investigators were regarded as nonimmunologic, because amyloid deposits can easily absorb immunoglobulins (45). Degenerating collagen was regarded as the site of formation of amyloid (46). Other authors found direct amyloid fibril formation at the basal surfaces of living basal cells in lichen amyloidosis (47).

The amyloid that may be found in the stroma or in the adjacent connective tissue of basal cell carcinoma and other epithelial tumors has an appearance on electron microscopy and direct immunofluorescence similar to that of lichen and macular amyloidosis, suggesting that it too is derived from tonofilaments (48). This amyloid also shows positive staining with antikeratin antiserum (44).

Nodular Amyloidosis

Nodular amyloidosis is a rare condition in which nodular deposits of AL amyloid are deposited in the skin, but in which there is no apparent systemic involvement. One or several nodules are encountered, usually on the legs (49) or face (50) but occasionally elsewhere. The nodules commonly measure from 1 to 3 cm in diameter. In their centers, the skin may appear atrophic (51). In exceptional instances, plaques are observed (52).

Histopathology. Beneath an atrophic epidermis are large masses of amyloid that extend through the entire dermis into the subcutaneous fat. Amyloid deposits are also found within the walls of blood vessels, in the membrana propria of the sweat glands, and around fat cells (52). A lymphoplasmacytic infiltrate is scattered through the masses of amyloid and at the periphery (18,50,51,53). In addition to clusters of plasma cells, Russell bodies and amyloid-containing foreign-body giant cells may be seen (54).

Differential Diagnosis. On a histologic basis, differentiation of nodular amyloidosis from primary systemic amyloidosis is not possible.

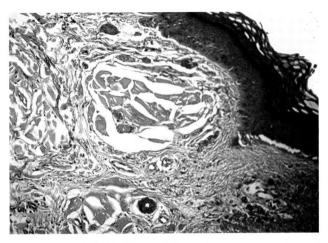

FIGURE 17-4. Colloid milium, adult type. Homogeneous, fissured masses of colloid are present in the uppermost dermis. The colloid material greatly resembles the amyloid material observed in primary systemic amyloidosis (Fig. 17-1).

COLLOID MILIUM AND NODULAR COLLOID DEGENERATION

There are three types of colloid degeneration of the skin: (a) juvenile colloid milium, (b) adult colloid milium, and (c) nodular colloid degeneration. Types a and c are very rare.

Juvenile colloid milium has its onset before puberty and shows numerous round or angular, brownish, waxy papules located mainly on sun-exposed areas, particularly the face (55,56). In nearly half of the reported cases there is a family history, and the possibility of a hereditary defect has been postulated (56).

Adult colloid milium, which starts in adult life, is clinically indistinguishable from the juvenile type, except that in some instances it involves the dorsa of the hands in addition to the face and neck (57,58). Sun exposure often seems to be a precipitating factor (55).

Nodular colloid degeneration shows either a single large nodule on the face (59) or multiple nodules on the face (60) or the chin and scalp (61). Sun exposure does not seem to play a role, because in some instances, the lesions are limited to the trunk (62).

Histopathology. The histologic findings differ in the three types of colloid degeneration, because the colloid in the juvenile form is of epidermal origin, and the colloid in the other two forms is of dermal origin (55,63).

In juvenile colloid milium, fissured colloid masses fill the papillary dermis. The overlying epidermis is flattened, and basal cells show transformation into colloid bodies (64). Ultrastructurally, the colloid material is found within individual basal keratinocytes above an intact basement membrane and in extracellular aggregates in the dermis. These deposits contain remnants of nuclear membrane material, degenerating cell organelles, and desmosomes. The fibrillary structure is similar to that of amyloid ultrastructurally, although staining with Congo red failed to result in birefringence, and other stains for amyloid were negative in the case reported by Handfield-Jones et al. (56).

In adult colloid milium, a narrow zone of connective tissue usually separates the homogeneous masses of colloid located in the papillary dermis from the overlying epidermis (Fig. 17-4). Elastic tissue staining shows some elastic fibers in this narrow zone of connective tissue (55). In addition, solar elastotic fibers are usually seen at the base of the colloid deposits (65).

In nodular colloid degeneration, the epidermis is flattened. The upper three fourths of the dermis are filled with pale pink, homogeneous material; in some lesions, even the entire dermis is filled with this material (61). Scattered nuclei of fibroblasts are present within the colloid (59). There are scattered clefts or fissures, and some dilated capillaries. The hair follicles and sebaceous glands appear well preserved (60).

Pathogenesis. The colloid in all three types shows considerable resemblance to amyloid—not only in its histologic appearance but also in its histochemical reactions (65).

Histochemical staining shows that colloid, like amyloid, is PAS positive and diastase resistant. Staining with Congo red results in green birefringence (sometimes weak), and the colloid fluoresces after staining with thioflavin T (65). However, it does not react with pagoda red and other cotton dyes (66). Serum amyloid P not only is a component of normal and abnormal dermal elastic fibers, but also reportedly can be stained immunocytochemically in colloid milium (67). Juvenile colloid milium exhibits a positive immunostaining reaction to polyclonal antikeratin antibody. This suggests that the histogenesis of this process may differ from that of the adult form in that the colloid in juvenile colloid milium is more likely derived from keratinocytes (68).

Electron microscopy in a case of juvenile colloid milium has shown that the colloid consists of tightly packed bundles of filaments, 8 to 10 nm thick, in a wavy or whorled arrangement (63). The colloid, which forms by filamentous degeneration of tonofilaments, maintains a cytoid configuration in the dermis and may contain nuclear remnants (68,69).

In adult colloid milium, the colloid masses are seen on electron microscopic examination to consist primarily of a granulofibrillar, amorphous substance. On high magnification, very fine filaments, only 2 nm wide, may be seen embedded in the amorphous substance (55,67). There is rather conclusive evidence that colloid is derived from elastic fibers through sequential degenerative changes. This can be observed at the periphery of the lesion, where colloid is being produced, and within the colloid, where one sees fibrils with a tubular structure and a diameter of 10 nm that are strikingly similar to the microfibrils of elastic fibers (57). The colloid in adult colloid milium thus represents a final product of severe solar degeneration (67).

The colloid in nodular colloid degeneration, similar to that in adult colloid milium, consists of an amorphous substance and short, wavy, irregularly arranged filaments (61). The diameter of these filaments is 3 to 4 nm (59). These electron microscopic findings exclude nodular amyloidosis as the diagnosis, because in this condition the filaments have a diameter of about 6 to 7 nm and are long and straight.

LIPOID PROTEINOSIS (HYALINOSIS CUTIS ET MUCOSAE, URBACH–WIETHE DISEASE)

This rare disorder is inherited as an autosomal recessive trait. First described by Siebenmann (70) in 1908, it was established as a distinct clinical and histologic entity by Urbach and Wiethe (71) in 1929. In 1932, Urbach coined the term "lipoid proteinosis" (LP) (72).

Clinically, there are papular and nodular lesions on the face. Areas of diffuse infiltration associated with hyperkeratosis are observed on the elbows, knees, hands, and occasionally elsewhere. The papules and nodules on the face cause pitted scars, giving the skin a pigskin-leather appearance. Verrucous plaques can form in areas of friction (73). Beads of small nodules may be present along the free margins of the eyelids. The tongue is firm because of diffuse infiltration. Extension of the infiltration to the frenulum of the tongue restricts normal movement of the tongue, and infiltration of the vocal cords causes hoarseness, which may be present at birth. Convulsive seizures are not uncommon (74,75).

Histopathology. There is extensive cutaneous deposition of amorphous eosinophilic material surrounding capillaries, sweat coils, and in the thickened papillary dermis (Fig. 17-5). Focal deposits are found in the deeper dermis. In verrucous lesions, the homogeneous bundles often are oriented perpendicular to the skin surface. This hyaline material is PAS positive and resistant to diastase digestion.

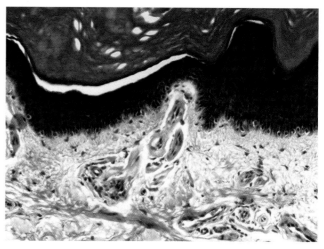

FIGURE 17-5. Lipoid proteinosis. The hyaline material consists of thick mantles surrounding the blood vessels.

Staining with Alcian blue at pH 2.5 is slightly positive and is sensitive to hyaluronidase digestion (76). The presence of lipids is variable and likely results from adherence of lipids to glycoproteins, rather than from abnormal lipid production (77).

Systemic Lesions. Intracranial calcification has been noted quite frequently in x-ray examination of patients with lipoid proteinosis and has been held responsible for convulsive seizures in these patients (74,78). Autopsy findings have established that the calcium is deposited within the walls of capillaries located in the hippocampal gyri of the temporal lobes (79). The fact that, after decalcification, a mantle of PAS-positive material is observed around the endothelium of these vessels indicates that hyalinization precedes calcification of the capillary walls.

The widespread distribution of the pericapillary hyalin deposits has been established by biopsies and autopsies. Deposits have been found in the submucosae of the upper respiratory and digestive tracts, and in the submucosae of the stomach, jejunum, rectum, and vagina; in the retina between the vitreous membrane and the pigment epithelium; and in the testes, pancreas, lungs, kidneys, and elsewhere (75,79).

Pathogenesis. Two different substances present in lesions of lipoid proteinosis have the light microscopic appearance of hyalin because they consist of homogeneous eosinophilic material and are PAS positive and diastase resistant (76,80). Their different appearances and origins, however, become evident on electron microscopy (81,82). One is true hyalin, produced by fibroblasts, and the other represents hyalin-like material consisting of multiplications of basal laminae and is produced by a variety of cells.

Lipids are not an essential feature of the disease. They can be removed with lipid solvents without damage to the protein-carbohydrate complex of the true hyalin. This suggests that the lipids are either free or loosely bound to the hyaline (83).

Although the pathogenesis of LP is not well understood, it may result from one or several enzyme defects leading to abnormal accumulation of glycoproteins (84). There is also evidence to support altered distribution of genetically distinct collagen types (85).

On electron microscopic examination, three major alterations are noted in the dermis: (a) a considerable thickening of basal laminae; (b) massive depositions of amorphous material (hyalin), predominantly in the upper dermis and around blood vessels (86); and (c) a marked reduction in the number and size of collagen fibrils (82,85). The thickening of the basal laminae in multiple layers is evident around small blood vessels, skin appendages, smooth muscle cells, perineuria, and Schwann cells (87). In contrast, there is almost no multiplication of the basal lamina of the epidermis (87). Around capillaries, basal laminae consist of as many as 20 layers, and occasionally even more, arranged in a concentric "onion-skin" arrangement (86). Interspersed between these layers are fine collagen fibrils in an amorphous matrix. The thickened basement membranes stain intensively for laminin and collagen type IV (82).

A unique feature of hyalinosis cutis et mucosae consists of large depositions of amorphous material in the dermis. The exact chemical nature of this hyaline material is not known, but it is a noncollagenous glycoprotein that contains neither laminin nor fibronectin (82).

The collagen within the areas of hyalin deposits appears as fine but otherwise normal fibrils arranged in bundles or in random fashion. Most fibrils have a diameter of less than 50 nm, compared with the usual size of 70 to 140 nm. Involved skin shows a five-fold reduction in collagen type I, the major collagen species of normal skin, and to a lesser extent in collagen type III, as indicated by cell culture studies. As judged by the contents of glycine and hydroxyproline, normal skin contains about 80% collagen, but involved skin in hyalinosis cutis et mucosae contains only 20% collagen as the result of a large accumulation of noncollagenous glycoproteins.

Cultured fibroblasts from lesions of hyalinosis cutis et mucosae have shown an increased synthesis of noncollagenous proteins at the expense of newly synthesized collagens. The hyaline material in hyalinosis cutis et mucosae originates from the overproduction of noncollagenous proteins, most of which are normal constituents of human skin (82).

Differential Diagnosis. Porphyria shows deposits of hyalin-like material around the superficial dermal capillaries indistinguishable from the perivascular deposits of hyalin-like material seen in lipoid proteinosis. However, involvement of the membrana propria of the sweat glands is rare, and no true dermal hyaline is present. In addition, the cutaneous lesions in porphyria are limited to sun-exposed areas.

PORPHYRIA

Seven types of porphyria are recognized (Table 17-1). The light sensitivity in the six types with cutaneous lesions is caused by wavelengths that are absorbed by the porphyrin molecule. These wavelengths lie in the 400-nm range, representing long-wave ultraviolet light (UVA) and visible light (88).

In *erythropoietic porphyria*, a very rare disease that typically develops during infancy or childhood, recurrent vesiculobullous eruptions in sun-exposed areas of the skin gradually result in mutilating ulcerations and scarring. It is inherited in an autosomal recessive pattern (89). Hypertrichosis and brown-stained teeth that fluoresce are additional features (90,91).

In *erythropoietic protoporphyria*, the usual reaction to light is erythema and edema followed by thickening and superficial scarring of the skin (92). In rare instances, vesicles are present that may resemble those seen in hydroa vacciniforme (93–95). It is an autosomal dominant disorder that results from a mutation in the gene that codes for ferrochetalase, the final enzyme in the heme synthesis chain (96). The protoporphyrin is formed in reticulocytes in the bone marrow and is then carried in circulating erythrocytes and in the plasma. When a smear of blood from a patient is examined under a fluorescence microscope, large numbers of red-fluorescing erythrocytes are observed. The protoporphyrin is cleared from the plasma by the liver and excreted into the bile and feces (97). It is not found in the urine. In rare instances, fatal liver disease develops quite suddenly, usually in persons of middle age (98) but occasionally in patients only in the second decade of life (99,100).

In *porphyria variegata*, different members of the same family may have either cutaneous manifestations identical to those of porphyria cutanea tarda or systemic involvement analogous to acute intermittent porphyria, or both, or the condition may remain latent (95,101). The presence of protoporphyrin in the feces distinguishes porphyria variegata from porphyria cutanea tarda (Table 17-1) (102). Also, a sharp fluorescence emission peak at 626 nm is specific for the plasma of porphyria variegata (103,104).

In *porphyria cutanea tarda*, a dominantly inherited disorder, three forms can be distinguished: sporadic, familial, and hepatoerythropoietic (105). In the *sporadic form*, only the hepatic activity of uroporphyrinogen decarboxylase is decreased. Almost all patients are adults, and no clinical evidence of porphyria cutanea tarda is found in other members of the patient's family. Although the sporadic form can

TABLE 17-1. CLASSIFICATION OF THE PORPHYRIAS

Porphyrias	Type; Heredity; Onset	Cutaneous Manifestations	Extra-Cutaneous Manifestations	Urine	Feces	Erythrocytes	Enzymatic Defect
Erythropoietic porphyria	Ery; Rec; Infancy	Blisters, severe scarring	Red teeth; hemolytic anemia	Uro I	Copro I	Uro I, stable fluorescence	Uroporphyrinogen III cosynthase
Erythropoietic protoporphyria	Ery; Dom; Childhood	Burning, edema, thickening, rarely blisters	Rarely fatal liver disease	Negative	Protoporphyrin continuously	Protoporphyrin, transient fluorescence	Ferrochelatase (Heme synthase)
Acute intermittent porphyria (AIP)	Hep; Dom; Young adulthood	Negative	Abdominal pain, neuropathy, psychoses	ALA, PBG continuously	Negative	Negative	Uroporphyrinogen I synthase
Porphyria variegata	Hep; Dom; Young adulthood	Same as PCT	Same as AIP	ALA, PBG during attacks	Protoporphyrin continuously	Negative	Protoporphyrinogen oxidase
Porphyria cutanea tarda (PCT)	Hep; Dom; Middle age	Blisters, scarring, thickening	Decreased liver function, siderosis	Uro III, continuous flourescence		Negative	Uroporphyrinogen decarboxylase
Hepatoerythrocytic porphyria (homozygous form of PCT)	Ery and Hep; Dom; Childhood	Blisters, severe scarring, thickening	Decreased liver function	Uro I, Uro III	Copro I, Copro III	Protoporphyrin	Uroporphyrinogen decarboxylase
Hereditary coproporphyria	Hep; Dom; Young adulthood	Same as PCT	Same as AIP	Copro, ALA, PBG during attacks	Copro continuously	Negative	Coproporphyrinogen oxidase

AIP = acute intermittent porphyria; ALA = delta-aminolevulinic acid; Copro = coproporphyrin; Dom = autosomal dominant; Ery = erythropoietic; Hep = hepatic; PBG = porphobilinogen; PCT = porphyria cutanea tarda; Rec = autosomal recessive; Uro = uroporphyrin.

occur without any precipitating factor (106), in most instances, in addition to the inherited enzymatic defect, an acquired damaging factor to liver function is needed. The damaging agent most commonly is ethanol but may also be estrogens (107).

In the *familial form,* in addition to the hepatic activity, the extrahepatic activity of uroporphyrinogen decarboxylase is decreased to about 50% of normal. The enzymatic activity usually is determined on the erythrocytes. The familial form may occur at any age, including childhood, and often, but not always, there is a family history of overt porphyria cutanea tarda.

In the very rare *hepatoerythropoietic form,* the skin lesions appear in childhood and the activity of uroporphyrinogen decarboxylase in all organs is decreased to less than 10% of normal. Family studies suggest that these patients are homozygous for the gene that causes porphyria cutanea tarda (105).

Clinically, the sporadic form of porphyria cutanea tarda, by far the most common type of porphyria, shows blisters that arise through a combination of sun exposure and minor trauma, mainly on the dorsa of the hands but sometimes also on the face. Mild scarring may result. The skin of the face and the dorsa of the hands often are thickened and sclerotic. Hypertrichosis of the face is common. Evidence of hepatic cirrhosis with siderosis is regularly pres-

ent but generally is mild (108). In rare instances, a malignant hepatoma or a carcinoma metastatic to the liver induces porphyria cutanea tarda (109). In the familial form of porphyria cutanea tarda, the clinical picture is similar to that of the sporadic form, but the changes are more pronounced. In the hepatoerythropoietic form, the manifestations are even more severe. On clinical grounds, the symptoms of most patients resemble those of erythropoietic porphyria, but when symptoms are milder they resemble those of erythropoietic protoporphyria (110). Vesicular eruptions lead to ulceration, severe scarring, partial alopecia, and sclerosis (111). Erythrocytes and teeth may show fluorescence (112). Liver damage develops with increasing age (113).

In *hereditary coproporphyria,* a very rare disorder, there are episodic attacks of abdominal pain and a variety of neurologic and psychiatric disturbances analogous to those observed in acute intermittent porphyria and porphyria variegata (114). In some cases, there are also cutaneous manifestations indistinguishable from those of porphyria cutanea tarda and porphyria variegata (114,115).

Histopathology. The histologic changes in the skin lesions are the same in all six types of porphyria with cutaneous lesions. Differences are based on the severity rather than on the type of porphyria. Homogeneous, eosinophilic material is regularly observed, and bullae are present in some instances. In addition, sclerosis of the collagen is present in old lesions (116,117).

In mild cases, homogeneous, pale, eosinophilic deposits are limited to the immediate vicinity of the blood vessels in the papillary dermis (117). These deposits are best visualized with a PAS stain, because they are PAS positive and diastase resistant.

In severely involved areas, which are most common in erythropoietic protoporphyria, the perivascular mantles of homogeneous material are wide enough in the papillary dermis to coalesce with those of adjoining capillaries. In addition, deeper blood vessels may show homogeneous material around them, and similar homogeneous material may be found occasionally around eccrine glands (118). PAS staining demonstrates this material particularly well. In some instances, it also contains acid mucopolysaccharides, shown with Alcian blue or the colloidal iron stain (117), or lipids, demonstrable with Sudan IV or Sudan black B (93,118). In addition, the PAS-positive epidermal–dermal basement membrane zone may be thickened (117).

In areas of sclerosis, which occur especially in porphyria cutanea tarda, the collagen bundles are thickened. In contrast to scleroderma, PAS-positive, diastase-resistant material is often present in the dermis in perivascular locations (117).

The bullae, which are most common in porphyria cutanea tarda and least common in erythropoietic protoporphyria, arise subepidermally (Fig. 17–6A and B). Some blisters are dermolytic and arise beneath the PAS-positive basement membrane zone (119); others form in the lamina lucida and are situated above the PAS-positive basement membrane zone (120) (Fig. 17-7). It has been suggested that the blisters in porphyria cutanea tarda in mild cases arise within the junctional zone, but that in severe cases they form beneath the PAS-positive basement membrane zone and thus heal with scarring (121). It is quite characteristic of the bullae of porphyria cutanea tarda that the

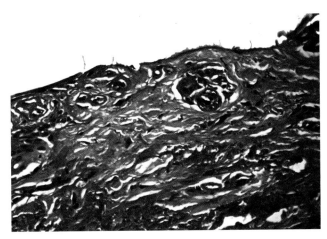

FIGURE 17-7. Porphyria cutanea tarda. On staining with the PAS reaction after diastase digestion, the PAS-positive basement membrane zone is observed at the floor of the blister. PAS-positive hyalin is present in the walls of capillaries in the upper dermis.

dermal papillae often extend irregularly from the floor of the bulla into the bulla cavity (104,122). This phenomenon, referred to as "festooning," is explained by the rigidity of the upper dermis induced by the presence of eosinophilic material within and around the capillary walls in the papillae and the papillary dermis.

The epidermis forming the roof of the blister often contains eosinophilic bodies that are elongated and sometimes segmented (123). These "caterpillar bodies" are PAS positive and diastase resistant. Ultrastructurally, they have been found to contain three components: (a) cellular organelles, including melanosomes, desmosomes, and mitochondria; (b) colloid that may be located intracellularly or extracellularly; and (c) electron-dense material thought to be of basement membrane origin (124).

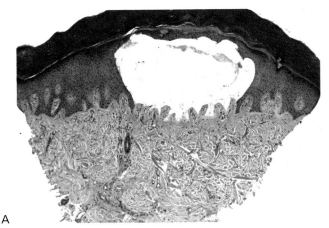
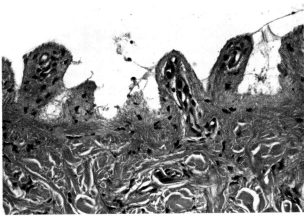

FIGURE 17-6. Porphyria cutanea tarda. **A:** There is a subepidermal blister. The architecture of the dermal papillae remains intact. The dermis contains no significant inflammatory infiltrate (H&E). **B:** Vessels within preserved dermal papillae at the blister base are surrounded by PAS-positive diastase-resistant deposits (D-PAS).

Pathogenesis. The substance around dermal vessels has the appearance of hyalin because it consists of homogeneous, eosinophilic material and is PAS positive and diastase resistant. However, just as the perivascular material in lipoid proteinosis, it is only hyalin-like and consists of multiplications of basal laminae (125). True hyalin, which is present in large amounts in the dermis of lipoid proteinosis, and is produced by fibroblasts as amorphous material, is absent.

On electron microscopic examination, one observes concentric duplications of the basement membrane around the dermal blood vessels. Peripheral to this multilayered basement membrane, one observes a thick mantle of unlayered material with the same filamentous and amorphous composition as that of the basement membrane. Often, a gradual transition from the layered to the unlayered zone can be observed (125,126). Scattered through the thick, unlayered zone are solitary collagen fibrils with an average diameter of only 35 nm, in contrast to the 100 nm of mature collagen (116,125). In cases with severe involvement, intermingled filamentous and amorphous material is seen throughout the upper dermis and even in the mid-dermis.

Proof that the perivascular material in porphyria represents excessively synthesized basement membrane material, and as such contains type IV collagen, is provided by positive immunofluorescence staining with anti–type-IV collagen monospecific antibody (127). The presence of small collagen fibrils analogous to reticulum fibrils suggests the presence also of type III collagen.

Direct immunofluorescence testing has revealed in the majority of patients the presence of immunoglobulins, particularly IgG (117), and occasionally also of complement (128), in the walls of blood vessels and at the epidermal–dermal junction of light-exposed skin. It is unlikely that these deposits indicate an immunologic phenomenon; rather, they are the result of "trapping" of immunoglobulins and complement in the filamentous material.

The *enzymatic defect* that causes each form of porphyria is known (Table 17-1). Enzyme determinations may be carried out on cultured skin fibroblasts, erythrocytes, or liver tissue.

Liver damage is generally mild and chronic in porphyria cutanea tarda. In erythropoietic protoporphyria, however, liver function tests are usually normal, even though microscopic deposits of protoporphyrin in the liver are frequently found (94). Yet, in rare instances, death occurs from liver failure developing swiftly after the initial detection of hepatic dysfunction (98). Patients with liver failure have very high levels of protoporphyrin in the erythrocytes and, at the time of death, show extensive deposits of protoporphyrin in a cirrhotic liver. The protoporphyrin in hepatocytes and Kupffer cells appears as dark brown granules (100). This pigment exhibits birefringence on polariscopic examination and, in unstained sections viewed with ultraviolet light, shows red autofluorescence (98). In patients with normal liver function tests, biopsy of the liver may or may not show portal and periportal fibrosis (99).

Pseudoporphyria Cutanea Tarda

In patients with chronic renal failure who are receiving maintenance hemodialysis, an eruption indistinguishable from that of porphyria cutanea tarda may develop on the dorsa of the hands and fingers during the summer months (129). Rarely, blisters are seen also on the face, and atrophic scarring develops (130). In a series of 180 patients receiving hemodialysis, 28 (16%) showed this type of eruption (131). Normal porphyrin levels in urine, stool, and plasma are the rule in hemodialyzed patients developing clinical signs of porphyria cutanea tarda. However, in a few patients receiving hemodialysis for chronic renal failure, a true porphyria cutanea tarda coexists (132,133). In such patients, if a certain degree of diuresis persists, urinalysis may not be representative of the porphyria metabolism, and the plasma and fecal porphyrins should always be measured (134).

Pseudoporphyria cutanea tarda may also occur following the ingestion of certain drugs, such as furosemide, nalidixic acid, tetracycline hydrochloride, and naproxen (135). Because many patients on hemodialysis for renal failure also are receiving furosemide, withdrawal of the drug can determine whether the dialysis or the medication is the cause of the pseudoporphyria, because in drug-induced cases, withdrawal of the drug is curative (135).

Histopathology. In patients with pseudoporphyria, the histologic picture is indistinguishable from that seen in mild cases of porphyria. The superficial blood vessels show thickened walls, and the PAS-positive basement membrane zone is often thickened as well. Blisters are subepidermal, with festooned dermal papillae. The blisters usually are situated above the PAS-positive basement membrane zone (130,135).

Pathogenesis. Electron microscopic findings are identical to those of porphyria (131). As in porphyria, immunoglobulins are often observed in vessel walls and at the epidermal–dermal junction. Complement is also occasionally present (129,131).

CALCINOSIS CUTIS

There are four forms of calcinosis cutis: metastatic calcinosis cutis, dystrophic calcinosis cutis, idiopathic calcinosis cutis, and subepidermal calcified nodule.

Metastatic Calcinosis Cutis

Metastatic calcification develops as the result of hypercalcemia or hyperphosphatemia. Hypercalcemia may result from (a) primary hyperparathyroidism, (b) excessive intake of vitamin D (136), (c) excessive intake of milk and alkali (137), or (d) extensive destruction of bone through osteomyelitis or metastases of a carcinoma (138). Hyperphosphatemia occurs in chronic renal failure as the result of a decrease in renal clearance of phosphorus and is associated with a compensatory drop in the serum calcium level. The low level of ionized calcium in the serum stimulates parathyroid secretion, leading to secondary hyperparathyroidism and to resorption of calcium and phosphorus from bone. The demineralization of bone causes both osteodystrophy and metastatic calcification (139,140).

Metastatic calcification most commonly affects the media of the arteries and the kidneys. In addition, other visceral organs, such as the myocardium, the stomach, and the lungs (39,141), may be involved.

Metastatic calcification in the subcutaneous tissue is occasionally observed in association with renal hyperparathyroidism (139), in uremia (142), in hypervitaminosis D (136), and as the result of excessive intake of milk and alkali (137), but rarely in primary hyperparathyroidism (138). Palpable, hard nodules, occasionally of considerable size, are located mainly in the vicinity of the large joints (139). With an increase in size, the nodules may become fluctuant (143).

Calciphylaxis is a life-threatening condition in which there is progressive calcification of small and medium-sized vessels of the subcutis often accompanied by necrosis. It most frequently arises in the setting of hyperparathyroidism associated with chronic renal failure (144). Calciphylaxis is often, but not always, associated with an elevated serum calcium/phosphate product (145).

Clinically, the lesions present as panniculitis or vasculitis. Bullae, ulcerations, or a lividoreticulosis-like eruption can be present (144,145). Potential complications of gangrene, sepsis, pancreatitis, and multisystem organ failure contribute to an overall mortality of more than 60% (146).

Instances of *cutaneous metastatic calcinosis* are rare. Most reports have concerned patients with renal hyperparathyroidism and osteodystrophy. The cutaneous lesions may consist of firm, white papules (147), papules in a linear arrangement (143), symmetric, nodular plaques (140), or papules and nodules from which a granular, white substance can be expressed (148).

Mural calcification of arteries and arterioles in the deep dermis or in the subcutaneous tissue occurs rarely in primary hyperparathyroidism (149), but somewhat more frequently in secondary hyperparathyroidism subsequent to renal disease and particularly if subsequent to dialysis for chronic renal disease or to renal allograft (150,151). This may lead to occlusion of these vessels and to infarctive ulcerations, especially on the legs.

Histopathology. Calcium deposits are recognized easily in histologic sections, because they stain deep blue with hematoxylin-eosin. They stain black with the von Kossa stain for calcium. As a rule, the calcium occurs as mas-

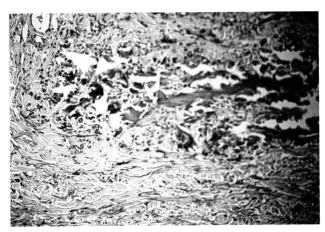

FIGURE 17-8. Metastatic calcinosis cutis. Amorphous deposits of basophilic material are present in the dermis.

sive deposits when located in the subcutaneous fat and usually as granules and small deposits when located in the dermis (Fig. 17-8). Large deposits of calcium often evoke a foreign-body reaction, so that giant cells, an inflammatory infiltrate, and fibrosis may be present around them (140).

In areas of infarctive necrosis, as a result of calcification of dermal or subcutaneous arteries or arterioles, the involved vessels show calcification of their walls and intravascular fibrosis with attempts at recanalization of the obstructed lumina (149). Mural calcification often is most pronounced in the internal elastic membranes of arteries or arterioles (150).

The histologic changes in calciphylaxis include calcium deposits in the subcutis, chiefly within the walls of small and medium-sized vessels (Fig. 17-9). These deposits can be associated with endovascular fibrosis, thrombosis, or global calcific obliteration (152). The fully evolved disease process shows, in addition, areas of necrosis with a clean background or accompanied by neutrophils (146).

It is particularly important that these findings be recognized in order that appropriate therapy, which often includes parathyroidectomy, might be instituted immediately.

Dystrophic Calcinosis Cutis

In dystrophic calcinosis cutis, the calcium is deposited in previously damaged tissue. The values for serum calcium and phosphorus are normal, and the internal organs are spared. There may be numerous large deposits of calcium (calcinosis universalis) or only a few deposits (calcinosis circumscripta).

Calcinosis universalis occurs as a rule in patients with dermatomyositis (Fig. 17-10), but, exceptionally, it has also been observed in patients with systemic scleroderma (153). Large deposits of calcium are found in the skin and subcutaneous tissue and often in muscles and tendons (154).

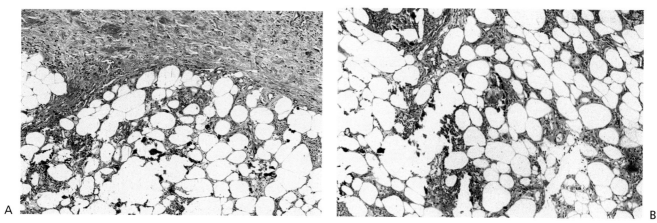

FIGURE 17-9. Calciphylaxis. There is a panniculitis with associated calcification of soft tissues in the walls of small vessels **A:** H&E, original magnification ×20. **B:** H&E, original magnification ×100.

In dermatomyositis, if the patient survives, the nodules of dystrophic calcinosis gradually resolve.

Calcinosis circumscripta occurs as a rule in patients with systemic scleroderma; rarely, however, it may be observed in patients with widespread morphea (155,156). Generally, in the presence of calcinosis, systemic scleroderma manifests itself as acrosclerosis. The association of acrosclerosis and calcinosis is often referred to as the Thibierge–Weissenbach syndrome or as the CREST syndrome, because the manifestations usually consist of calcinosis cutis, Raynaud's phenomenon, esophageal dysfunction, sclerodactyly, and telangiectasia (153,155,157). Patients with this syndrome often have a better prognosis than those with generalized scleroderma or systemic sclerosis. Clinically, calcinosis circumscripta shows successively appearing areas of induration that often break down and extrude white, chalky material.

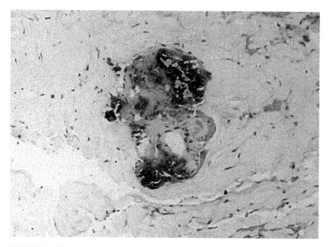

FIGURE 17-10. Dystrophic calcinosis cutis. Granules and globules of calcium are located beneath the epidermis. This biopsy is from the buttock of a child with dermatomyositis who also had extensive calcification of muscles and tendons.

Lupus erythematosus is only rarely associated with dystrophic calcinosis cutis (158).

In addition to occurring in the connective tissue diseases, dystrophic calcinosis is often seen in subcutaneous fat necrosis of the newborn and, rarely, in the subcutaneous nodules occurring in Ehlers–Danlos disease.

Histopathology. As in metastatic calcinosis cutis, the calcium in dystrophic calcinosis cutis usually is present as granules or small deposits in the dermis and as massive deposits in the subcutaneous tissue (156). A foreign-body giant-cell reaction is often found around large deposits of calcium (159). The calcium deposits usually are located in areas in which the collagen or fatty tissue appears degenerated as a result of the disease preceding the calcinosis.

Idiopathic Calcinosis Cutis

Even though the underlying connective tissue disease in some instances of dystrophic calcinosis cutis may be mild and can be overlooked unless specifically searched for, there remain cases of idiopathic calcinosis cutis that resemble dystrophic calcinosis cutis but show no underlying disease (160–162).

One entity is regarded as a special manifestation of idiopathic calcinosis cutis: tumoral calcinosis. It consists of numerous large, subcutaneous, calcified masses that may be associated with papular and nodular skin lesions of calcinosis (163,164). The disease usually is familial and is associated with hyperphosphatemia (164,165). Otherwise, the resemblance of tumoral calcinosis to the dystrophic calcinosis universalis observed with dermatomyositis is great.

Histopathology. Tumoral calcinosis shows in the subcutaneous tissue large masses of calcium surrounded by a foreign-body reaction (159). Intradermal aggregates are present in some cases. Discharge of calcium may take place through areas of ulceration or by means of transepidermal elimination (164).

Pathogenesis. Two authors have studied lesions of idiopathic calcinosis cutis by electron microscopy (160,161). They agree that the deposits consist of pleomorphic calcium phosphate (apatite) crystals. However, according to one opinion the earliest deposits of calcium are situated in the ground substance (160), whereas according to the other the earliest calcium deposits lie within collagen fibrils and subsequently extend into the ground substance as the apatite crystals grow (161).

Idiopathic Calcinosis of the Scrotum

Idiopathic calcinosis of the scrotum consists of multiple asymptomatic nodules of the scrotal skin. The nodules begin to appear in childhood or in early adult life, increase in size and number, and sometimes break down to discharge their chalky contents (166).

Histopathology. At one time the accepted view was that some of the calcific masses in calcinosis of the scrotum were surrounded by a granulomatous foreign-body reaction and others were not (166,167). However, in recent studies in which numerous scrotal nodules were examined, some of the lesions were epidermal cysts, whereas other cystic lesions showed calcification of their keratin contents, and still others showed ruptures of their epithelial walls. The cyst wall was eventually destroyed, leaving only dermal collections of calcium. Thus, according to this view, calcinosis of the scrotum represents the end stage of dystrophic calcification of scrotal epidermal cysts (168,169). Other authors who also had examined either several patients or multiple nodules agreed that the lesions originated from cysts. One author favored eccrine duct milia as the origin because of a positive reaction for carcinoembryonic antigen, a marker of eccrine sweat glands (170). Another author found various types of cysts: epidermal, pilar, and indeterminate cysts showing various degrees of calcification (171). One can assume that early lesions start out as cysts but, as they age and calcify, lose their cyst walls. It is likely that authors who found no cyst walls were examining old lesions.

Subepidermal Calcified Nodule

In subepidermal calcified nodule, also referred to as cutaneous calculi, usually a single small, raised, hard nodule is present. Occasionally, however, there are two or three nodules (172,173), and in some instances there are numerous (174) or even innumerable (175) nodules. Most patients are children, but in some patients a nodule is present at birth (176) or does not appear until adulthood (177). In most instances, the surface of the nodule is verrucous, but it may be smooth. The most common location of the nodule is the face.

Histopathology. The calcified material is located predominantly in the uppermost dermis, although in large nodules it may extend into the deep layers of the dermis. The calcium is present largely as closely aggregated glob-

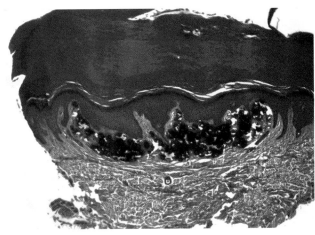

FIGURE 17-11. Subepidermal calcified nodule. A large deposit of calcium in the dermis distorts the overlying epidermis (H&E).

ules (Fig. 17-11). In some instances, however, there are also one or several large, homogeneous masses of calcified material (172,173). Both the globules and the homogeneous masses occasionally contain well-preserved nuclei (172). Macrophages and foreign-body giant cells may be arranged around the large, homogeneous masses (172). The epidermis is often hypertrophic. Calcium granules may be observed within the epidermis, indicative of transepidermal elimination (175,178).

Pathogenesis. The primary event seems to be the formation of large, homogeneous masses that undergo calcification and break up into numerous calcified globules (173). The origin of the homogeneous masses is obscure. It is not likely that they originate from a specific preexisting structure, such as sweat ducts (176) or nevus cells (177), as has been assumed.

GOUT

In the early stage of gout, there usually are irregularly recurring attacks of acute arthritis. In the late stage, deposits of monosodium urate form within and around various joints, leading to chronic arthritis with destruction in the joints and the adjoining bone. During this late stage, urate deposits, called tophi, may occur in the dermis and subcutaneous tissue. The incidence of tophaceous lesions in gout has significantly decreased since 1950, from 14% to 3%, even though the incidence of gout has remained unchanged. Improved methods of treatment account for this decrease (179).

Tophi are observed most commonly on the helix of the ears, over the bursae of the elbows, and on the fingers and toes (180). They may attain a diameter of several centimeters. When large, tophi may discharge a chalky material. In rare instances, gout may present as tophi on the fingertips or as panniculitis on the legs without the coexistence of a gouty arthritis (181–183).

Histopathology. For the histologic examination of tophi, fixation in absolute ethanol or an ethanol-based fixative, such as Carnoy's fluid, is preferable to fixation in formalin; it has been stated that aqueous fixatives such as formalin dissolve the characteristic urate crystals, leaving only amorphous material (184). However, some authors contend that sectioned, formalin-fixed, paraffin-embedded tissue floated in alcohol (as opposed to a water bath) and then placed on a slide without staining will display refractile crystals when examined under polarized light (185). An alternate staining protocol to preserve any urate crystals remaining in formalin-fixed tissue after processing also has been suggested (186).

On fixation in alcohol, tophi can be seen to consist of variously sized, sharply demarcated aggregates of needle-shaped urate crystals lying closely packed in the form of bundles or sheaves (Fig. 17-12). The crystals often have a brownish color and are doubly refractile on polariscopic examination (Fig. 17-13). If a red compensator is used along with polarizing filters in tissue which has been processed to preserve crystals, the crystals will appear yellow when they are parallel to the direction of the compensator and blue when perpendicular to it (187). The aggregates of urate crystals are often surrounded by a palisaded granulomatous infiltrate containing many foreign-body giant cells (Fig. 17-12). The urate crystals appear black and the surrounding tissue yellow when the sections are stained with 20% silver nitrate solution (188).

Even when the specimen has been fixed in formalin, the diagnosis of gout can be made without difficulty because of the characteristic rim of foreign-body giant cells and macrophages surrounding the aggregates of amorphous material. As a secondary phenomenon, calcification, and occasionally ossification, may take place in the sodium urate aggregates.

Histogenesis. Gout, a dominantly inherited disorder, is characterized by hyperuricemia. An asymptomatic stage of hyperuricemia precedes the development of gouty

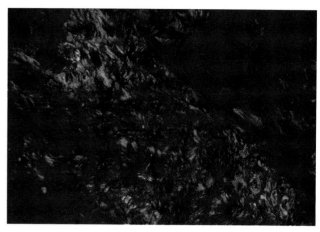

FIGURE 17-13. Gouty tophus. Polarization with a red filter reveals birefringent blue urate crystals in a gouty tophus.

arthritis by many years. Patients with gout are a heterogeneous group. In some patients, diminished renal excretion of uric acid accounts for the hyperuricemia; in others, an excessive production of uric acid from increased purine biosynthesis is found. In other patients with gout, both excessive synthesis of uric acid and decreased renal excretion of uric acid are found (189). The deposits of urate crystals stimulate cytokine production, chiefly interleukin-1 (IL-1). IL-1 is a central mediator of the neutrophil recruitment and activation that are characteristic of joint disease (but not a feature in dermal disease) (190).

OCHRONOSIS

There are two types of ochronosis: endogenous ochronosis (alkaptonuria), which is inherited as an autosomal recessive trait, and localized exogenous ochronosis, which is

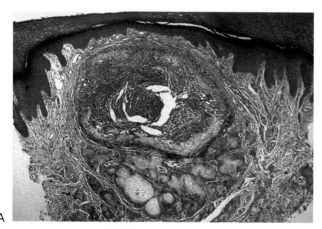

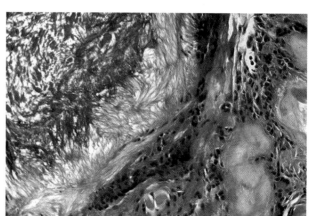

FIGURE 17-12. Gouty tophus. **A:** There are deposits of urate crystals in the reticular dermis that have a radial array. The lucent areas show where some urate crystals were removed during processing of the tissue (H&E). **B:** There are macrophages and multinucleated giant cells surrounding the urate deposits in the dermis (H&E).

prototypically caused by the topical application of a hydro-quinone cream to exposed parts of the skin in order to lighten the color of dark skin.

As the result of the lack of homogentisic acid oxidase in endogenous ochronosis, homogentisic acid accumulates over the course of years in many tissues—especially in the cartilages of the joints, the ears, and the nose; in ligaments and tendons; and in the sclerae. This results in osteoarthritis; in blackening of cartilages, ligaments, and tendons; and in patchy pigmentation of the sclerae. In one unusual case, the presenting complaint was pigmentation of the palms and soles with overlying hyperkeratosis and pitting (191). Intervertebral calcification is a characteristic x-ray finding (191–193). In the course of time, homogentisic acid accumulates in the dermis in sufficient amounts to cause patchy brown pigmentation of the skin. The gene for homogentisic acid oxidase maps to chromosome 3q (193,194).

In localized exogenous ochronosis, there is a macular blue-black hyperpigmentation of portions of the face to which the hydroquinone cream or other responsible agent was applied (195). In more severely involved areas, blue-black papules, milia, and nodules can occur. A condition termed "pseudo-ochronosis" has been recently described as a histopathologic finding in localized angyria occurring primarily in jewelry workers. Clinically, these patients present with blue-black macules ("blue nevus-like") typically on the upper extremities (196).

Histopathology. Involvement of the skin is essentially identical in endogenous and exogenous ochronosis, although it is often more pronounced in exogenous ochronosis (197). The ochronotic pigment, as seen in sections of the dermis stained with hematoxylin-eosin, has a yellow-brown or ochre color; thus, the name ochronosis.

The skin shows ochronotic pigment as fine granules free in the tissue and endothelial cells of blood vessels, in the basement membrane and the secretory cells of sweat glands, and within scattered macrophages (198). The most striking finding, however, is the ochronotic pigment within collagen bundles, causing homogenization and swelling of the bundles. Some collagen bundles assume a bizarre shape; they appear rigid and tend to fracture transversely with jagged or pointed ends (199) (Fig. 17-14). As the result of the breaking up of degenerated collagen bundles, irregular, homogeneous, light brown clumps lie free in the tissue. The altered dermal connective tissue does not stain with silver nitrate as melanin does but becomes black when stained with cresyl violet or methylene blue (200). In addition, ochronotic pigment can be found within elastic fibers (201). In nodular ochronosis, a granulomatous response surrounds this material (202). Transfollicular elimination of ochronotic fibers may occur in patients with severe disease (203).

In pseudo-ochronosis, features similar to ochronosis are present in the form of prominent collagen bundles that are yellow-brown in color. In addition, most cases have shown "ellipsoid black globules" of silver within the dermis (196).

Pathogenesis. In *endogenous ochronosis*, because of an inborn lack of homogentisic acid oxidase, the two amino acids tyrosine and phenylalanine cannot be catabolized beyond homogentisic acid. Most of the homogentisic acid is excreted in the urine. The urine, on standing or after the addition of sodium hydroxide, turns black (alkaptonuria) because, through oxidation and polymerization, homogentisic acid is converted into a dark-colored insoluble product.

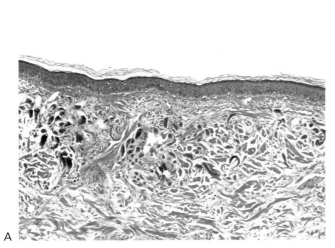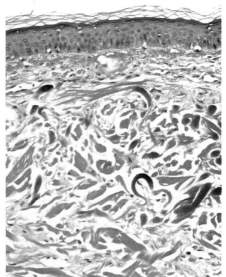

FIGURE 17-14. Exogenous ochronosis. Yellowish orange-colored collagen bundles are present in the superficial reticular dermis. Some are abnormally thickened. **A:** H&E, original magnification ×100. **B:** H&E, original magnification ×200.

However, some of the homogentisic acid gradually accumulates in certain tissues. It is bound irreversibly to collagen fibers as a polymer after oxidation to benzoquinone-acetic acid (190,204).

In *exogenous ochronosis*, a topical agent such as hydroquinone, resorcinol, phenol, mercury, picric acid, or benzene, or a systemic medication such as quinine or antimalarials inhibits the activity of homogentisic acid oxidase in the skin, resulting in the local accumulation of homogentisic acid, which polymerizes to form ochronotic pigment (205, 206). In effect, this process mimics the cutaneous manifestation of endogenous ochronosis (197).

Pseudo-ochronosis appears to be due to deposits of traumatically implanted silver onto collagen bundles (196).

On electron microscopic examination of early lesions, one observes deposition of amorphous, electron-dense ochronotic pigment around individual collagen fibrils within collagen fibers (192). This causes the collagen fibrils to lose their periodicity and to degenerate. Gradually, the collagen fibrils disappear as they are replaced by ochronotic pigment. Ultimately, the ochronotic pigment occupies entire collagen fibers and, by fusion, entire collagen bundles (207). Cross-sections of the bundles then reveal a large, homogeneous, electron-dense aggregate that in some instances shows remnants of collagen fibrils at its periphery, as well as macrophages containing particles of ochronotic pigment (201, 208). Particles of ochronotic pigment can also be found in elastic fibers (201). In pseudo-ochronosis, scanning electron microscopy demonstrates silver deposited on collagen fibers (196).

MUCINOSES

There are six types of cutaneous mucinosis: (a) generalized myxedema; (b) pretibial myxedema; (c) lichen myxedematosus or papular mucinosis; (d) reticular erythematous mucinosis or plaquelike mucinosis; (e) self-healing juvenile cutaneous mucinosis; and (f) scleredema.

Regular demonstration of the presence of mucin in the dermis is possible only in pretibial myxedema, in self-healing juvenile cutaneous mucinosis, and in lichen myxedematosus. In reticular erythematous mucinosis, it is possible in most cases. In generalized myxedema, the amount of mucin usually is too small to be demonstrable, and in scleredema, mucin may be present only in the early stage.

The mucin found in these six diseases represents an increase in the mucin that is normally present in the ground substance of the dermis. It consists of proteins bound to hyaluronic acid (hyaluronan), an acid mucopolysaccharide or glycosaminoglycan. As a result of the great water-binding capacity of hyaluronic acid, dermal mucin contains a considerable amount of water. This water is largely removed during the process of dehydration of the specimen; consequently, in routine sections, the mucin, because of its marked shrinkage, appears largely as threads and granules.

The mucin present in the six types of mucinosis stains a light blue in sections stained with hematoxylin-eosin. It also stains with colloidal iron. It is Alcian-blue–positive at pH 2.5 but negative at pH 0.5 and shows metachromasia with toluidine blue at pH 7.0 and 4.0, but no metachromasia below pH 2.0 (209). It is PAS negative (indicating the absence of neutral mucopolysaccharides) and aldehyde-fuchsin-negative (indicating the absence of sulfated acid mucopolysaccharides). The mucin is completely removed on incubation of histologic sections with testicular hyaluronidase for 1 hr at 37°C (210).

Generalized Myxedema

In generalized myxedema, caused by hypothyroidism, the entire skin appears swollen, dry, pale, and waxy. It is firm to the touch. In spite of its edematous appearance, the skin does not pit on pressure. There is often a characteristic facial appearance: the nose is broad, the lips are swollen, and the eyelids are puffy.

Histopathology. The epidermis may show slight ortho-hyperkeratosis and follicular plugging. Usually, routinely stained sections show no abnormality in the dermis, except in severe cases, in which one may observe swelling of the collagen bundles with splitting up of the bundles into individual fibers with some blue threads and granules of mucin interspersed (211). However, with histochemical stains, such as colloidal iron, Alcian blue, or toluidine blue, it is possible, at least in severe cases, to demonstrate small amounts of mucin, mainly in the vicinity of the blood vessels and hair follicles.

Pretibial Myxedema

Usually, the lesions are limited to the anterior aspects of the legs, but they may extend to the dorsa of the feet. They consist of raised, nodular, yellow, waxy plaques with prominent follicular openings that give a peau d'orange appearance. Similar lesions rarely occur on the radial aspect of the forearms (212).

Pretibial myxedema usually occurs in association with thyrotoxicosis and not infrequently becomes more pronounced after treatment of the thyrotoxicosis. It nearly always occurs in association with exophthalmos, and 15% to 20% also have acropachy (213). Complete remission occurs in about 25% of cases (213). Rarely, pretibial myxedema, with or without exophthalmos, occurs in nonthyrotoxic thyroid disease, such as chronic lymphocytic thyroiditis; the patient is then either euthyroid or hypothyroid (214).

Histopathology. The epidermis and papillary dermis are usually normal. Mucin in large amounts is present in the dermis, particularly in the upper half (Fig. 17-15). As a result, the dermis is greatly thickened. The mucin occurs not only as individual threads and granules but also as extensive deposits resulting in the splitting up of collagen bun-

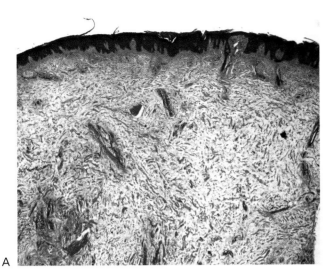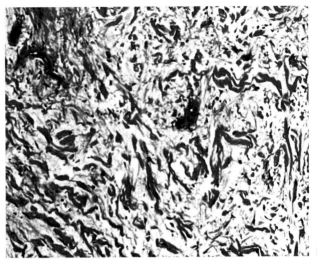

FIGURE 17-15. Pretibial myxedema. **A:** At scanning magnification, the epidermis and papillary dermis are normal. The collagen fibers in the reticular dermis are widely separated by deposits of mucin (H&E). **B:** At higher magnification, stellate fibroblasts are evident among the separated collagen fibers (H&E).

dles into fibers and wide separation of the fibers. As a result of shrinkage of the mucin during the process of fixation and dehydration, there are empty spaces within the mucin deposits. The number of fibroblasts is not increased as a rule, but in areas in which there is much mucin, some fibroblasts have a stellate shape and are then referred to as mucoblasts (213,215). A perivascular infiltrate of lymphocytes may be seen in some cases and mast cells are moderately increased in number (213,215).

Pathogenesis. On electron microscopic examination, the collagen bundles and fibers are separated by wide, electron-lucent, empty spaces. The fibroblasts that produce the mucin are stellate shaped with long, thin cytoplasmic processes and exhibit dilated cisternae of the rough endoplastic reticulum. An amorphous, moderately electron-dense material coats the surface of the fibroblasts. This material is also present in small, irregular clumps within the otherwise empty-appearing spaces (216). At high magnification, the amorphous material appears as a complex of microfibrils and granules, forming a network (217).

Of interest is the almost invariable presence of long-acting thyroid stimulator (LATS) in the serum of patients with pretibial myxedema. There is, however, a rather poor correlation between the severity of the skin lesions and the level of serum LATS; furthermore, LATS is detected in 40% to 60% of patients with an active exophthalmic goiter but without pretibial myxedema. Thus, LATS cannot be regarded as the cause of pretibial myxedema (218). It is likely that the IgG LATS represents an autoantibody that is produced by lymphocytes in thyroid disease, especially in thyrotoxicosis, and is a reflection, rather than a cause, of the underlying disease (214).

The restriction of the myxedema largely to the pretibial area may be explained by the finding that fibro-

blasts from the pretibial area synthesize two to three times more hyaluronic acid than do fibroblasts from other areas when incubated with serum from patients with pretibial myxedema (219). The receptor for thyroid stimulating hormone (TSH-R) is a candidate as the common tissue antigen in Grave's disease, exophthalmos, and pretibial myxedema. TSH-R immunoreactivity has been detected on fibroblasts in the dermis of control patients without thyroid disease (216).

Differential Diagnosis. Pretibial myxedema must be differentiated from pretibial mucinosis associated with venous stasis. In pretibial mucinosis, the excess mucin is localized to the thickened papillary dermis and is accompanied by angioplasia and siderophages (220).

Lichen Myxedematosus

Lichen myxedematosus, or papular mucinosis, is characterized by a more or less extensive eruption of asymptomatic, soft papules, generally 2 to 3 mm in diameter. Although densely grouped, they usually do not coalesce. The face and arms are the most commonly affected areas. In some instances, in addition to papules, large nodules may be present, especially on the face (221). Although the disease is very chronic, spontaneous resolution has been reported (222).

In a variant of lichen myxedematosus called *scleromyxedema*, one finds a generalized eruption of papules as in lichen myxedematosus and, in addition, diffuse thickening of the skin associated with erythema. There is marked accentuation of the skin folds, particularly on the face. Scleromyxedema can be differentiated from scleroderma clinically by the papular component and the absence of telangiectasias. Transitions of lichen myxedematosus to scleromyxedema do occur. Acral persistent papular

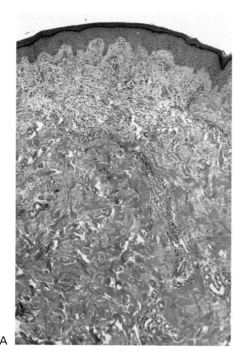
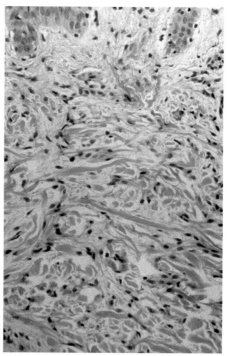

FIGURE 17-16. Lichen myxedematosus. **A:** At scanning power, a dome-shaped papule is evident. The papillary and superficial reticular dermis contain abundant mucin (H&E). **B:** In addition to mucin, there is an increased number of plump fibroblasts in the upper dermis (H&E).

mucinosis presents multiple small papular lesions on the hands and forearms (223). The clinical and histopathologic features resemble the discrete papular form of lichen myxedematosus (224). The detection of IgA monoclonal gammopathy in one case also suggests that it is a localized variant of lichen myxedematosus (225). Cutaneous mucinosis of infancy may also represent a localized form of papular mucinosis on the upper extremities unassociated with monoclonal gammopathy (226). It may remit spontaneously (227).

Multiple dome-shaped papules with histopathologic features suggestive of papular mucinosis have been noted in Birt–Hogg–Dube syndrome (228).

Histopathology. In lichen myxedematosus, fairly large amounts of mucin are present. In contrast with pretibial myxedema, however, the mucinous infiltration is found only in circumscribed areas, is most pronounced in the upper dermis, and is associated with an increase in fibroblasts and collagen (229,230) (Fig. 17-16). The collagen bundles may show a rather irregular arrangement.

Scleromyxedema

The histologic picture found in the papules in scleromyxedema resembles that observed in lichen myxedematosus. In the diffusely thickened skin, there is extensive proliferation of fibroblasts throughout the dermis that are associated with irregularly arranged bundles of collagen. In many areas, the collagen bundles are split into individual fibers by mucin. As a rule, the amount of mucin is greater in the upper half than in the lower half of the dermis (231).

Autopsy examination of patients with lichen myxedematosus and scleromyxedema usually has not shown mucinous deposits in any internal organs (230–232). However, in one case, mucin was detected in renal papillae, and in others it was found in the adventitia and media of blood vessels in several organs (233–235).

Pathogenesis. Electron microscopic examination of scleromyxedema reveals an increase in the number of fibroblasts. They show considerable activity, as indicated by the presence of a markedly dilated, rough endoplasmic reticulum and long cytoplasmic processes. These fibroblasts produce both collagen and ground substance. The presence of many collagen fibrils with reduced diameter, similar to those in scleroderma, indicates that it is young collagen. In many areas, there are small bundles of young collagen fibrils, with each fibril richly coated with ground substance (236).

The presence of a *monoclonal component* (M component) or paraprotein in the sera of patients with lichen myxedematosus and scleromyxedema has been noted in nearly all cases that have been adequately tested. Its absence has been noted in a few cases (237); in another case, it was absent at first but present later on (238).

In nearly all instances, the paraprotein is an IgG, although other immunoglobulin classes occur on rare occasions (232,239). The IgG paraprotein is a very basic protein because of increased lysine content in its light chains (240). Thus, in most instances, it migrates more slowly than gammaglobulin on serum electrophoresis and may even migrate toward the cathode rather than toward the anode (241). In instances in which it migrates with the same speed as gammaglobulin, immunoelectrophoresis is required for its recognition (242). The IgG of lichen myxedematosus differs from the IgG of multiple myeloma not only by usually showing slower electrophoretic migration but also by the fact that its IgG molecules nearly always possess light chains of the lambda type, although light chains of the kappa type have occasionally been found (243,244). In contrast, in multiple myeloma with elevated values for IgG, only about one-third of the reported cases with IgG molecules have lambda light chains, and two-thirds have kappa light chains (245). In addition to showing a monoclonal IgG, many cases of lichen myxedematosus show hyperplasia of plasma cells in the bone marrow (232,233,242, 246). These plasma cells have been shown to synthesize the monoclonal IgG (244). In some cases, the plasma cells in the bone marrow have been regarded as atypical in appearance (247). However, only one case fulfilling the criteria for coexisting multiple myeloma has been documented (248).

The role of the monoclonal IgG in lichen myxedematosus is not clear. Its presence in the dermal mucin has been demonstrated by direct immunofluorescence (247, 249,250). Furthermore, the serum containing the paraprotein stimulates the production of hyaluronic acid and prostaglandin E by fibroblasts *in vitro* (251). However, although the serum from patients with lichen myxedemato-sus stimulates fibroblast proliferation *in vitro*, the purified IgG paraprotein itself has no direct effect on fibroblast proliferation (252).

Reticular Erythematous Mucinosis

Erythematous, reticulated areas with irregular but well-defined margins are present, usually in the center of the chest and of the upper back. This disorder was first described in 1960 as being composed of confluent papules and was called plaque-like mucinosis, but similar cases showing coalescent macules, rather than papules, were designated reticular erythematous mucinosis in 1974 (253, 254). It has since become apparent that macular and papular lesions can coexist (255). In rare instances, lesions spare the trunk and are present on the arms and face (256). The eruption is asymptomatic. It is chronic but usually responds well to small doses of antimalarial drugs of the 4-aminoquinoline group, such as chloroquine. It may be a presenting sign of systemic lupus erythematosus (257).

Histopathology. Two histologic features are usually present: small amounts of dermal mucin and a mild or moderately pronounced mononuclear infiltrate situated predominantly around blood vessels and hair follicles (253,254). The infiltrate is composed of helper T cells (258).

In papular lesions, the mucin usually is fairly conspicuous. As a rule, mucin can be recognized even in routinely stained sections (Fig. 17-17). The mucin stains with Alcian blue and usually also with mucicarmine. In addition, there often is metachromasia on staining with toluidine blue or with the Giemsa stain (253,254). Fibroblasts with bipolar processes are located in the mucinous deposits (259). Immunohistochemistry has revealed a significantly increased number of factor XIIIa dendritic

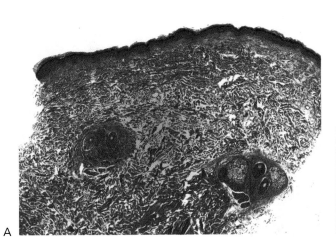
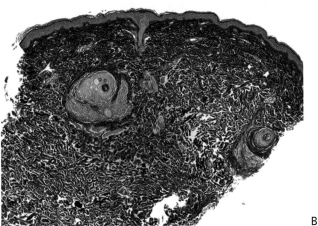

FIGURE 17-17. Reticular erythematous mucinosis. **A:** There is a sparse superficial perivascular and perifollicular infiltrate of lymphocytes around blood vessels in the dermis (H&E). **B:** Colloidal iron staining reveals abundant mucin among collagen fibers.

cells in lesional skin of a patient with reticular erythematous mucinosis but not in the patients uninvolved skin or normal control skin samples (260). These same cells also demonstrated immunoreactivity for one isoform of hyaluronic synthase (260).

In macular lesions, the mucin may be missed in routinely stained sections and become apparent only on staining with Alcian blue. In some instances, no mucin is found, even on staining with Alcian blue (261), but if an Alcian blue stain is negative in paraffin-embedded sections, it may be positive in unfixed, frozen sections (262). If this is negative, too, the diagnosis depends on the presence of the mononuclear infiltrate, clinical appearance, and response of the patient to treatment with antimalarial drugs.

Differential Diagnosis. Reticular erythematous mucinosis, Jessner's lymphocytic infiltrate of skin, and lupus erythematosus may share in common a perivascular and perifollicular lymphocytic infiltrate and increased mucin among collagen bundles. In Jessner's lymphocytic infiltrate, the lymphocytic infiltrate is usually much more dense than that in reticular erythematous mucinosis. Lupus erythematosus almost always shows vacuolar changes in the basal layer of the epidermis and follicular units, but in the rare tumid lesions, vacuolar changes may be inconspicuous. Thus, it may not be possible to distinguish between the tumid lesions of lupus erythematosus and reticular erythematous mucinosis by conventional microscopy. Furthermore, flesh-colored papules and nodules situated on the trunk and demonstrating increased dermal mucin may precede or accompany systemic lupus erythematosus or progressive systemic sclerosis (263). Clinicopathologic correlation is essential in distinguishing these conditions.

Self-Healing Juvenile Cutaneous Mucinosis

This rare dermatosis has been described only in children. It has a sudden onset and undergoes spontaneous resolution within a few months. Infiltrated plaques with a corrugated surface are observed on the torso, and nodules occur on the face and in the periarticular region. There may be associated fever, arthralgias, muscle tenderness, and weakness (264).

Histopathology. Abundant mucinous material, positive-blue-positive at pH 2.5, is present mainly in the upper reticular dermis (265). There may be a superficial perivascular lymphocytic infiltrate and a slight increase in the number of mast cells and fibroblasts in the zone of mucin deposition.

Scleredema

Scleredema, occasionally called scleredema adultorum even though it may occur in children and infants, is characterized by diffuse, nonpitting swelling and induration of the skin (266,267). Three groups can be recognized (268): one with

abrupt onset, one with insidious onset, and one preceded by diabetes. In the first group, the scleredema starts abruptly during or within a few weeks after an upper respiratory tract infection. The skin lesions may clear within a few months or the disease may take a prolonged course. In the second group, the scleredema starts insidiously, for no apparent reason, spreads gradually, and takes a chronic course. The disease in the third group is preceded by diabetes for years, starts insidiously, and persists indefinitely. Usually, the scleredema starts on the face and extends to the neck and upper trunk. Unlike scleroderma, the hands and feet are always spared. In about 75% of the patients, complete resolution takes place within a few months; in the remaining 25%, the disease may persist for as long as 40 years (269). Although visceral lesions may occur, death from scleredema is rare.

Diabetes is commonly associated with persistent scleredema and, in most of these instances, is quite resistant to antidiabetic therapy (269). It has been suggested that the association of persistent scleredema with maturity-onset diabetes be recognized as a special form of scleredema (270).

Histopathology. The dermis in scleredema is about three times thicker than normal (Fig. 17-18). The collagen bundles are thickened and separated by clear spaces, causing "fenestration" of the collagen. The secretory coils of the sweat glands, surrounded by fat tissue, are located in the upper dermis or mid-dermis rather than, as normally, in the lower dermis or at the junction of the dermis and the subcutaneous fat. Because the distance between the epidermis and the sweat glands is unchanged, it can be concluded that much of the subcutaneous fat in scleredema has been replaced by dense collagenous bundles (271). No increase in the number of fibroblasts is noted in association with the hyperplasia of the collagen; in fact, their number may be strikingly decreased (272).

In many instances, especially in early cases, histochemical staining reveals the presence of hyaluronic acid between

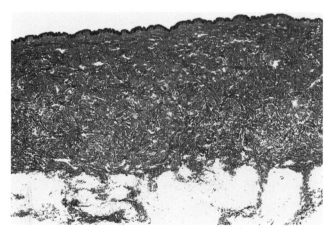

FIGURE 17-18. Scleredema. Panoramic view showing only a greatly thickened reticular dermis. The subcutis is not involved, as in scleroderma (H&E).

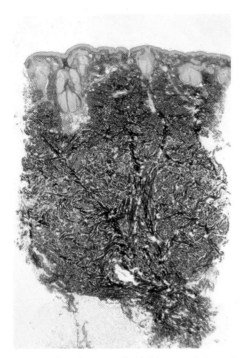

FIGURE 17-19. Scleredema. Colloidal iron staining of an early case reveals increased mucin in the middle and lower dermis.

the bundles of collagen, particularly in the areas of fenestration. Staining with toluidine blue usually reveals metachromasia, which is most evident at pH 7.0, weaker at pH 5.0, and absent at pH 1.5, indicating the presence of only nonsulfated acid mucopolysaccharides (209). Although the hyaluronic acid is usually present throughout the dermis, it may be present only in the deeper portion of the dermis (273) (Fig. 17-19).

In some instances, staining with toluidine blue at pH 7.0 is more intense if unfixed cryostat sections are used in place of formalin-fixed material (274). In some cases, even frozen sections have failed to stain with Alcian blue or toluidine blue (275). It may be postulated that, in cases of long standing in which the disease has reached a steady stage of collagen turnover, staining for hyaluronic acid may give negative results (271). In cases of scleredema in which formaldehyde-fixed specimens fail to show acid mucopolysaccharides, they may show them on fixation in 0.05% cetylpyridinium chloride solution and staining with Alcian blue at pH 2.5 (267). It has been stated that fixation with 1% cetylpyridinium chloride solution in standard formalin fixative combined with colloidal iron staining gives the best results (276).

Systemic Lesions. Occasionally, the tongue and some skeletal muscles are involved, and, on histologic examination, the muscle bundles show edema and loss of striation (275,277). In a few reported cases, pleural and pericardial effusions were present (275,278). In one case, the disease terminated in death, and autopsy revealed, in addi-

tion to pleural and pericardial effusions, diffuse edema of the heart, liver, and spleen (279).

Pathogenesis. In many patients with long-standing scleredema, a monoclonal gammopathy is found in the serum. Usually the paraprotein is either IgG-kappa or IgG-lambda (272). In other cases, it has been IgA-kappa, IgA-lambda, or IgM-lambda (280). There can be coexistence of scleredema with multiple myeloma (281). No immunoglobulin deposits have been found in involved skin sites (272). A marked increase in type 1 collagen gene expression occurs in scleroderma leading to increased collagen synthesis (282).

Differential Diagnosis. It can be difficult to differentiate between end-stage scleroderma in which inflammation is no longer present and scleredema. As a rule, however, in scleroderma, the collagen in the reticular dermis and subcutaneous tissue appears homogenized and hyalinized and stains only lightly with eosin and with the Masson trichrome stain, but in scleredema, the collagen bundles are thickened without being hyalinized and stain normally with eosin and the trichrome stain (271). A marked increase in type I collagen gene expression occurs in scleroderma leading to increased collagen synthesis (282).

MUCOPOLYSACCHARIDOSES

The mucopolysaccharidoses (MPS) comprise a group of storage diseases in which, as the result of a deficiency of specific lysosomal enzymes, there is inadequate degradation of mucopolysaccharides, or glycosaminoglycans. Consequently, this material accumulates within lysosomes of various cells in many organs, including the skin. Greatly elevated levels of mucopolysaccharides are present in the blood, serum, and urine. Ten enzymatically distinct types of mucopolysaccharidosis have been identified, and most appear to have allelic variants (283). Thus, there is marked variation in the manifestations not only from type to type, but also within the same type (284). The most common features, any or all of which may be present or absent, include dwarfism, skeletal deformities, hepatosplenomegaly, corneal clouding, and progressive mental deterioration with premature death from cardiorespiratory complications. In many instances, there is a characteristic facial appearance—thick lips, flattened nose, and hirsutism—referred to as gargoylism. The mode of transmission is autosomal recessive in all types of MPS except type II, the Hunter syndrome, which is X-linked recessive.

Of the ten types of MPS, only types I to III will be discussed here. MPS I presents as three distinctive variants, even though they are all caused by a deficiency of the same enzyme. MPS I H, Hurler's syndrome, causes severe mental retardation and death, usually within the first decade of life (285). In contrast, persons with MPS I S, Scheie's syndrome, have normal intelligence, no dwarfism, and a normal life expectancy (286). MPS I H/S, the Hurler–Scheie syndrome, is intermediate between MPS I H and MPS I S. MPS II, Hunter's syndrome, occurs in a severe form, with mental retardation and early death, and in a mild form, in which mental function is normal and survival to adult life is the rule (287). MPS III, Sanfilippo's syndrome, has mild somatic changes but severe mental retardation (288).

The skin in all ten types of MPS usually appears thickened and inelastic. However, the only type in which distinctive cutaneous lesions are found frequently, although not invariably, is MPS II, Hunter's syndrome. These lesions consist of ivory white papules or small nodules, usually 3 to 4 mm in diameter, that may coalesce to form ridges in a reticular pattern on the upper trunk, especially in the scapular region (287,289). This condition has been referred to as "pebbling" of the skin. Grouped papules on the extensor surfaces at the upper portions of the arms and legs have been noted in one patient with the Hurler–Scheie syndrome (MPS I H/S) (290).

Histopathology. In all ten types of MPS, the normal-appearing or slightly thickened skin, on staining with the Giemsa stain or toluidine blue, shows metachromatic granules within fibroblasts, so that the fibroblasts resemble mast cells (285). The granules also stain with Alcian blue and with colloidal iron (286). Fixation in absolute alcohol in some instances demonstrates the metachromasia better than fixation in formalin (291). In addition, metachromatic granules are occasionally present in some epidermal cells and in the secretory and ductal cells of eccrine glands (285,292,293).

The cutaneous papules observed only in Hunter's syndrome show not only metachromatic granules within dermal fibroblasts but also extracellular deposits of metachromatic material between collagen bundles and fibers (289,291).

In all types of mucopolysaccharidosis, metachromatic granules are visible also in the cytoplasm of circulating lymphocytes when smears of them are stained with toluidine blue after fixation in absolute methanol, a finding that aids in the rapid diagnosis of mucopolysaccharidosis (294).

Histogenesis. Biochemical studies have shown that, in MPS I, as a result of a deficiency in alpha-l-iduronidase, there is an accumulation of heparan sulfate and dermatan sulfate (chondroitin sulfate) (283). Accumulation of dermatan sulfate but not heparan sulfate is linked to impaired elastic fiber assembly, which is thought to contribute to the clinical phenotype in Hurler disease (295). In MPS II, the same two substances are excessively accumulated owing to a deficiency in iduronate sulfatase. In MPS III, there is excessive accumulation of heparan sulfate. Successful bone marrow transplantation in children with Hurler's syndrome can restore the previously deficient alpha-1-iduronidase level (296).

By staining for acid phosphatase and by electron microscopy, the metachromatic granules in the skin and in the lymphocytes have been identified as lysosomes that contain acid mucopolysaccharides, which they are incapable of degrading (293,294).

Electron microscopic examination of the skin reveals in most fibroblasts numerous electron-lucent, greatly dilated, membrane-bound vacuoles representing lysosomes. Some of the vacuoles contain granular material or, less commonly, myelin-like structures representing residual bodies (286). Lysosomes are present also in macrophages, showing the same characteristics as in fibroblasts (288). In addition, from 5% to 20% of the epidermal cells contain lysosomal vacuoles, with acid phosphatase activity, varying from a solitary vacuole to 20 or 30 vacuoles per cell (292).

The dermal Schwann cells also contain electron-lucent lysosomes. In addition, some Schwann cells occasionally show laminated membranous structures ("zebra bodies"). These structures resemble those found in the brains of some patients with mucopolysaccharidosis. In the brain, they contain gangliosides as the result of a deficiency in the lysosomal hydrolase β-d-galactosidase (292). The deposition of gangliosides in the brain leads to mental deterioration through the degeneration and loss of neurons.

ACANTHOSIS NIGRICANS

Acanthosis nigricans can be seen in multiple clinical settings: malignancy-associated, benign, inherited, obesity-associated, syndromic, drug-induced, and mixed (297). The malignant type differs from the benign types by showing more extensive and more pronounced lesions, by its progressiveness, and by its onset usually after the age of 40. The histologic picture is essentially the same in all types.

The *malignant* type is associated with a malignant tumor—most commonly an abdominal, and particularly a gastric, carcinoma (298). However, it may also occur with squamous cell carcinoma, with sarcomas, and with Hodgkin's and non-Hodgkin's lymphomas (297). In some cases, the skin lesions precede the symptoms of malignancy. The sign of Leser-Trélat, which is characterized by the sudden appearance of numerous seborrheic keratoses in association with a malignant tumor, may be an early stage or incomplete form of the malignant type of acanthosis nigricans. The seborrheic keratoses observed in this sign may be accompanied or followed by lesions of acanthosis nigricans (297).

The *benign inherited* type usually has its onset during infancy or early childhood. It is an autosomal dominant trait (299).

Syndromic acanthosis nigricans is especially linked to syndromes associated with insulin resistance (300). In the HAIR-AN syndrome, which affects younger women, there is hyperandrogenism (HA), insulin resistance (IR), and acanthosis nigricans (AN) (297). Another subset links autoimmune states such as lupus erythematosus with uncontrolled diabetes mellitus, acanthosis nigricans, and ovarian hyperandrogenism. These patients have antibodies to the insulin receptor. Acanthosis nigricans has also been associated with insulin resistance in obesity, hypothyroidism, and congenital generalized lipodystrophy (301–303).

Acanthosis nigricans-like lesions have been induced by high dosages of nicotinic acid (304). Acanthosis nigricans has also occurred following use of oral contraceptives, following use of the folic acid antagonist triazinate, and as a localized reaction to insulin (299,305,306).

Clinically, acanthosis nigricans presents papillomatous brown patches, predominantly in the intertriginous areas such as the axillae, the neck, and the genital and submammary regions. In extensive cases of acanthosis nigricans of the malignant type, mucosal surfaces, such as the mouth, vulva, and palpebral conjunctivae, may be involved (298). In the acral type, there is velvety hyperpigmentation of the dorsa of the hands and feet.

Histopathology. Histologic examination reveals hyperkeratosis and papillomatosis but only slight, irregular acanthosis and usually no hyperpigmentation. Thus, the term *acanthosis nigricans* has little histologic justification.

In a typical lesion, the dermal papillae project upward as fingerlike projections. The valleys between the papillae show mild to moderate acanthosis and are filled with keratotic material (Fig. 17-20). Horn pseudocysts can occur in some cases (307). The epidermis at the tips of the papillae and often also on the sides of the protruding papillae appears thinned.

Slight hyperpigmentation of the basal layer is demonstrable with silver nitrate staining in some cases but not in others (308). The brown color of the lesions is caused more by hyperkeratosis than by melanin.

In the acanthosis nigricans lesions of the polycystic ovary syndrome, there are prominent deposits of glycosaminoglycan consisting mostly of hyaluronic acid in the papillary dermis (309).

Histogenesis. The inherited type of acanthosis nigricans can be classified as a type of epidermal nevus. In persons who have acanthosis associated with insulin resistance, high levels of insulin may activate insulin-like growth factor-1 receptors and thereby mediate epidermal proliferation (310). Malignant acanthosis nigricans most likely is mediated by growth factors that are secreted by the associated neoplasm such as transforming growth factor-alpha (311,312). The basal cells from one patient with syndromic acanthosis nigricans demonstrated unusually high expression of the rare keratins 18 and 19 (307).

Differential Diagnosis. Differentiation of acanthosis nigricans from other benign papillomas, particularly from linear epidermal nevi and from the hyperkeratotic type of seborrheic keratosis, may be difficult. As a rule, however, linear epidermal nevi show more marked acanthosis than acanthosis nigricans and have a more compact orthokeratotic stratum corneum. Furthermore, the pilosebaceous units in linear epidermal nevi are rudimentary. Acanthosis nigricans cannot be distinguished histologically from confluent and reticulated papillomatosis.

Confluent and Reticulated Papillomatosis

Confluent and reticulated papillomatosis shows slightly hyperkeratotic and papillomatous-pigmented papules that are confluent in the center and reticulated at the periphery (313). The site of predilection is the sternal region. In the view of some authors, this disorder represents a variant of acanthosis nigricans (314). However, its location and reticulated pattern are distinctive.

Histopathology. Mild hyperkeratosis and papillomatosis are present, as is focal acanthosis, limited largely to the valleys between elongated papillae (314). Thus, the histologic changes are similar to but milder than those of acanthosis nigricans.

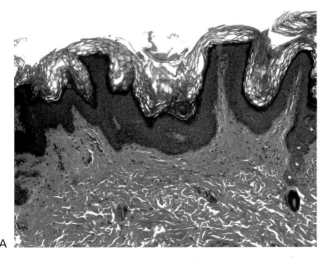 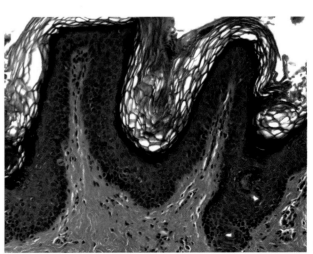

FIGURE 17-20. Acanthosis nigricans. **A:** There are papillomatous projections of the dermis (H&E). **B:** The epidermis is not increased in thickness above the papillomatous projections. The stratum corneum shows loose, basket-weave orthokeratosis (H&E).

Histogenesis. Heavy colonization with *Pityrosporum orbiculare* has been observed in patients with confluent and reticulated papillomatosis, so that this disorder has been regarded as a peculiar host reaction to *P orbiculare* (315,316). However, in a review of the literature, it was found that, even though potassium hydroxide preparations had yielded positive findings for yeast in ten cases, there were positive findings for yeast and hyphae in only one case and negative results in 20 cases (317). Considering the common presence of the yeast phase as a nonpathogen, the role of *Malassezia* (*Pityrosporum*) as the cause of confluent and reticulated papillomatosis can be discounted. Reports of a variety of antibodies that have been used successfully in the treatment of this condition raise the possibility that bacteria play a role in inducing the observed changes, although this is speculative (318).

HEREDITARY HEMOCHROMATOSIS

In hereditary hemochromatosis, large amounts of iron are deposited in various organs of the body, especially in the parenchymal cells of the liver and pancreas and in the myocardial fibers. The classic tetrad of hereditary hemochromatosis consists of hepatic cirrhosis, diabetes, hyperpigmentation of the skin, and cardiac failure.

Unless there is early recognition and adequate treatment by phlebotomy, hemochromatosis is a fatal disorder as the result of liver failure, heart disease, or hepatocellular carcinoma, which occurs in about one-third of the patients with advanced hemochromatosis (319).

Pigmentation of the skin is present in more than 90% of the patients with hereditary hemochromatosis at the time the diagnosis is made, but it is often so mild as to attract little attention (320,321). The pigmentation is most pronounced in exposed areas, especially on the face. Its color usually is brown or bronze but may be blue-gray. The pigmentation is caused largely by melanin and not by iron. In addition to pigmentation, ichthyosis-like changes, koilonychia, and hair loss are common.

Histopathology. Histologic examination of pigmented skin, especially from exposed areas, shows melanin to be present in increased amounts in the basal layer of the epidermis (320,322). Hemosiderin can be demonstrated in the skin of most patients with the aid of an iron stain, such as Perls' stain. It is found as blue-staining granules, mainly around blood vessels, both extracellularly and within macrophages, and in the basement membrane zone of the sweat glands and within cells of the connective tissue surrounding these glands (322). Siderosis around eccrine glands appears specific for hereditary hemochromatosis (320). In rare instances, some iron is present in the epidermis, particularly in the basal cell layer, and in the epithelial cells of the sweat glands (323).

In selecting a site for biopsy, it is not necessary to choose a pigmented area, because if deposits of iron are present in the skin, they are not limited to the areas of pigmentation. It is important, however, not to take a specimen from the legs, where deposits of iron are frequently found in association with even minor venous stasis or as a consequence of a preceding inflammation that may no longer be evident.

A skin biopsy no longer represents an important test for establishing the diagnosis of hereditary hemochromatosis; it is merely of confirmatory value. Determinations in the serum of the level of iron; iron-binding capacity, as measured by the degree of saturation of transferrin with iron; plasma ferritin concentration; and, above all, biopsy of the liver, have replaced the skin biopsy in importance (321). Before liver biopsy, however, genotyping of patients who have abnormal screening exams for iron overload is now being performed. If the person is homozygous for the most common mutation in the hemochromatosis gene (HFE), and has persistently elevated transaminase levels, a biopsy of the liver is considered to evaluate whether fibrosis is present. Phlebotomy can prevent iron overload and development of fibrosis, or can prevent further hepatic injury (324).

Histogenesis. Hereditary hemochromatosis is an autosomal recessive disease caused by mutation in HFE (325). It is the most common genetically inherited disease in people of northern European ancestry (324). About 10% of the U.S. population are carriers of the disease (326). This figure implies a homozygote frequency of 2 or 3 persons per 1,000. The gene for hemochromatosis is located on chromosome 6 and is most commonly altered by a point mutation that results in a cysteine to tyrosine switch at amino acid position 282 of the HFE protein (327). Homozygosity is present in approximately 90% of affected persons (327).

The amino acid substitution responsible for the vast majority of cases results in the inability of HFE to bind to β2 microglobulin, a required step in the shuttling of HFE to the cell surface, the site of interaction of HFE and transferrin. The precise role of HFE in regulating iron stores is not known (324). Although iron absorption through duodenal mucosa is excessive, it is not known if this is the primary event. The degree of saturation of transferrin with iron is very high. Consequently, not all of the iron passing from the intestinal tract can be bound to transferrin, and it is therefore deposited in a variety of organs. Iron accumulates particularly in the parenchyma of the liver and pancreas and in the myocardium, and by damaging the cells in which it accumulates, it causes hepatic cirrhosis, diabetes, and cardiac insufficiency.

Two observations indicate that the cutaneous pigmentation in hereditary hemochromatosis is caused by melanin and not by hemosiderin. The first observation concerns a patient who, in addition to having hemochromatosis, had vitiligo. The areas of vitiligo were fully depigmented despite the finding on histologic examination that they contained just as much iron as deeply pigmented areas (322). The second observation was made in a black patient with idiopathic hemochromatosis who had three epidermal cysts. Although the patient had noticed no change in his skin color, he had observed progressive darkening of the cysts, and histologic examination revealed considerable amounts of melanin both in the walls of the cysts and in their keratinous contents (328). Although pigmented epidermoid cysts have been attributed to hemochromatosis, in a series of 125 epidermal cysts in Indian patients, pigmentation was found in 79 of them, none of which was attributed to hemochromatosis or iron deposition (329).

The increase in the amount of melanin found in the skin of patients with hemochromatosis is brought about by iron in the skin. The iron stimulates melanocytic activity either by increasing oxidative processes or by reacting with epidermal sulfhydryl groups and reducing their inhibitory effect on the enzyme system governing melanin synthesis (330,331).

VITAMIN A DEFICIENCY (PHRYNODERMA)

Deficiency of vitamin A is very rare in the United States, occurring mainly in Asia and Africa. It has been recently described, however, as occurring after small bowel bypass surgery for obesity (332,333). Vitamin A deficiency results in cutaneous changes to which the name *phrynoderma* (toad skin) has been given. These changes consist of dryness and roughness of the skin and the presence of conical, follicular keratotic lesions usually most prominent in the elbows and knees. Clinically, phrynoderma may at times simulate a perforating disorder (334). In addition to causing cutaneous changes, deficiency of vitamin A may cause night blindness, xerophthalmia, and keratomalacia.

Histopathology. The skin shows moderate hyperkeratosis with marked distention of the upper parts of the hair follicles by large, horny plugs (332,335). The horny plugs may perforate the follicular epithelium (333). The sebaceous gland lobules are greatly reduced in size. There may also be atrophy of the sweat glands, such as flattening of the secretory cells (336). In severe cases, the sweat glands and sebaceous glands may undergo keratinizing metaplasia (337).

Differential Diagnosis. Histologic differentiation of phrynoderma from ichthyosis vulgaris and keratosis pilaris is impossible, except in very severe cases of phrynoderma, in which the sweat glands and the sebaceous glands show keratinizing metaplasia. Pityriasis rubra pilaris differs from phrynoderma by showing, in addition to hyperkeratosis and follicular plugging, stuttering parakeratosis, irregular epidermal hyperplasia, and an inflammatory infiltrate in the upper dermis.

PELLAGRA

Pellagra is caused by a deficiency of nicotinic acid (niacin) or its precursor, the essential amino acid tryptophan. As a dietary deficiency disease, it may occur in chronic alcoholics and patients with anorexia nervosa (338). It may also occur

in patients with the carcinoid syndrome; the tumor cells divert tryptophan toward serotonin, thus depressing endogenous niacin production (339). In addition, pellagra is a well-recognized complication of isoniazid therapy for tuberculosis. Because isoniazid is a structural analog of niacin, it can cause the suppression of endogenous niacin production (340). Because 5-fluorouracil inhibits the conversion of tryptophan to nicotinic acid, it also may precipitate pellagra (341). Recently, multiple anticonvulsants have been reported to induce pellagra as well, although the precise mechanism for this is not known (342,343). Deficiencies of other vitamins such as B6 and thiamine that are involved in the synthesis or utilization of niacin, or excess dietary intake of substances (e.g., leucine) that directly inhibit niacin synthesis, can result in clinical symptoms as well (342).

Pellagra presents with cutaneous lesions, gastrointestinal symptoms, and mental changes, resulting in the triad of the three D's: dermatitis, diarrhea, and dementia.

The cutaneous lesions are precipitated by sunlight. A symmetrical photosensitive dermatitis predominantly involves the dorsa of the hands, wrists, and forearms, the face, and the nape of the neck. In the early stage, there is erythema, which usually is sharply demarcated; in severe cases, it may be accompanied by vesicles or bullae. Later, the skin becomes thickened, scaly, and pigmented.

Histopathology. The histologic changes of the skin are nonspecific. Early lesions present a superficial perivascular lymphocytic inflammatory infiltrate in the upper dermis. Vesicles, if present, arise as in erythema multiforme either subepidermally, owing to vacuolar degeneration of the basal layer and edema in the papillary dermis, or intraepidermally, owing to degenerative changes in the epidermis (344). Sometimes there is a distinct pallor of the upper layers of the epidermis with or without an infiltrate of neutrophils. The differential diagnosis of this pattern includes acrodermatitis enteropathica (zinc deficiency), necrolytic migratory erythema of the glucagonoma syndrome and, occasionally, psoriasis (345). There is one report of a contact dermatitis due to topical application of a eutectic mixture of local anesthetics (EMLA), which resembled pellagra microscopically (346).

In older lesions, one observes hyperkeratosis with areas of parakeratosis and prominent but irregular epidermal hyperplasia. The amount of melanin in the basal layer of the epidermis often is increased. Late lesions may show epidermal atrophy, and the dermis may show fibrosis in addition to chronic inflammation (344).

Hartnup Disease

First described in 1956 and named in 1957 after the family in which it was first observed, Hartnup disease is transmitted as an autosomal recessive trait (347,348). It first manifests itself in early childhood and often improves with advancing age. A photosensitivity eruption is present that usually is indistinguishable from pellagra (349). However, in some cases, the cutaneous reaction to sun exposure resembles poikiloderma atrophicans vasculare or, because of the prominence of vesicles, hydroa vacciniforme (350,351). In addition, there may be cerebellar ataxia and mental retardation. Niacin is used to treat Hartnup disease (349).

Histopathology. The cutaneous eruption in Hartnup disease usually shows the same histologic changes observed in pellagra (see earlier). In patients with poikiloderma-like changes, one observes atrophy of the epidermis and the presence of a chronic inflammatory infiltrate and of melanophages in the upper dermis (350).

Histogenesis. The sun-sensitivity eruption with its resemblance to pellagra is caused by an enzymatic defect in the transport of tryptophan and a resultant decrease in the endogenous production of niacin. Specifically, the defective transporter is a transporter of monoamino-monocarboxylic acids, which is encoded by a gene that maps to chromosome 5p (352). The defect in tryptophan transport consists of both an intestinal defect in tryptophan absorption and a renal tubular defect causing inadequate reabsorption of amino acids, including tryptophan. Chromatographic study of the urine shows a constant aminoaciduria, particularly the presence of tryptophan and of indolic substances derived from tryptophan—a finding that establishes the diagnosis (350).

OCULOCUTANEOUS TYROSINOSIS

Oculocutaneous tyrosinosis, also referred to as the Richner–Hanhart syndrome and tyrosinemia type II, is transmitted as an autosomal recessive trait. It is characterized by very tender hyperkeratotic papules and plaques on the palms and soles arising in infancy or childhood; bilateral keratitis, which may lead to corneal opacities; and mental retardation. Palmoplantar lesions may begin as bullae and erosions (353). In some families, however, ocular changes are absent (354). A diet low in tyrosine and phenylalanine increases the disease manifestations.

Histopathology. In most instances, the histologic findings in the keratotic lesions are not diagnostic, showing merely orthokeratotic hyperkeratosis with hypergranulosis and acanthosis (355). In one reported case, vertical parakeratotic columns were present over the openings of the acrosyringia. Multinucleated keratinocytes and dyskeratotic cells were noted in the spinous layer (356). A large intraepidermal bulla seen in another patient probably was also the result of irritation (357).

Histogenesis. Tyrosinemia maps to chromosome 16q 22.1 to 16q 22.2 (349). As a result of a genetic deficiency in hepatic tyrosine aminotransferase, excessive amounts of tyrosine are found in the blood, urine, and tissues. It can be assumed that excessive amounts of intracellular tyrosine enhance cross-links between aggregated tonofilaments. On electron microscopic examination, aggregations of tonofilaments and needle-shaped tyrosine crystalline inclusions are found in keratinocytes (356).

REFERENCES

1. Röcken C, Shakespeare A. Pathology, diagnosis and pathogenesis of AA amyloidosis. *Virchows Arch* 2002;440:111.
2. Sipe JD. Amyloidosis. *Crit Rev Clin Lab Sci* 1994;31:325.
3. Husby G. Nomenclature and classification of amyloid and amyloidosis. *J Intern Med* 1992;232:511.
4. Murphy C, Fulitz M, Hrncic R, et al. Chemical typing of amyloid protein contained in formalin-fixed paraffin-embedded biopsy specimens. *Am J Clin Pathol* 2001;116:135.
5. Glenner GG, Harbaugh J, Ohms JI, et al. An amyloid protein: the amino-terminal variable fragment of an immunoglobulin light chain. *Biochem Biophys Res Commun* 1970;41:1287.
6. Kyle RA, Bayrd ED. Amyloidosis: review of 236 cases. *Medicine (Baltimore)* 1975;54:171.
7. Kyle RA. Amyloidosis. *Int J Dermatol* 1980;19:537, 1981;20:20.
8. Natelson EA, Duncan EC, Macossay CR, et al. Amyloidosis palpebrarum. *Arch Intern Med* 1979;125:304.
9. Beacham BE, Greer KE, Andrews BS, et al. Bullous amyloidosis. *J Am Acad Dermatol* 1980;3:506.
10. Brownstein MH, Helwig EB. The cutaneous amyloidosis. II. Systemic forms. *Arch Dermatol* 1970;102:20.
11. Bluhm JF III, Johnson SC, Norback DH. Bullous amyloidosis. *Arch Dermatol* 1980;116:1164.
12. Westermark P. Amyloidosis of the skin: a comparison between localized and systemic amyloidosis. *Acta Derm Venereol (Stockh)* 1979;59:341.
13. Sepp N, Pichler E, Breathnach SM, et al. Amyloid elastosis: analysis of the role of amyloid P component. *J Am Acad Dermatol* 1990;22:27.
14. Ochiai T, Morishima T, Hao T, et al. Bullous amyloidosis: the mechanism of blister formation revealed by electron microscopy. *J Cutan Pathol* 2001;28:407.
15. Blumenfeld W, Hildebrandt RH. Fine needle aspiration of abdominal fat for the diagnosis of amyloidosis. *Acta Cytol* 1993;37:170.
16. Libbey CA, Skinner M, Cohen AS. Use of abdominal fat tissue aspirate in the diagnosis of systemic amyloidosis. *Arch Intern Med* 1983;143:1549.
17. Rubinow A, Cohen AS. Skin involvement in generalized amyloidosis. *Ann Intern Med* 1978;88:781.
18. Masuda C, Mohri S, Nakajima H. Histopathological and immunohistochemical study of amyloidosis cutis nodularis atrophicans: comparison with systemic amyloidosis. *Br J Dermatol* 1988;119:33.
19. Kyle RA. Amyloidosis: introduction and overview. *J Intern Med* 1992;232:507.
20. Hashimoto K, Kumakiri M. Colloid: amyloid bodies in PUVA-treated human psoriatic patients. *J Invest Dermatol* 1979;72:70.
21. Glenner GG, Page DL. Amyloid, amyloidosis and amyloidogenesis. *Int Rev Exp Pathol* 1976;15:2.
22. Goettler E, Anton-Lamprecht I, Kotzur B. Amyloidosis cutis nodularis. *Hautarzt* 1976;27:16.
23. Gertz MA. Secondary amyloidosis (AA). *J Intern Med* 1992;232:517.
24. Westermark P. Occurrence of amyloid deposits in the skin in secondary systemic amyloidosis. *Acta Pathol Microbiol Scand [A]* 1972;80:718.
25. Orifila C, Giraud P, Modesto A, et al. Abdominal fat tissue aspirate in human amyloidosis: light, electron, and immunofluorescence studies. *Hum Pathol* 1986;17:366.

26. Levin M, Granklin EC, Frangione B, et al. The amino acid sequence of a major nonimmunoglobulin component of some amyloid fibrils. *J Clin Invest* 1972;51:2773.

27. Benditt EP, Eriksen N. Amyloid protein SAA is associated with high density lipoprotein from human serum. *Proc Natl Acad Sci U S A* 1977;74:4025.

28. Skinner M. Protein AA/SAA. *J Intern Med* 1992;232:513.

29. Breathnach SM, Black MM. Systemic amyloidosis and the skin. *Clin Exp Dermatol* 1979;4:517.

30. Jambrosic J, From L, Hanna W. Lichen amyloidosus. *Am J Dermatopathol* 1984;6:151.

31. Leonforte JF. Sur l'origine de l'amyloidose maculeuse. *Ann Dermatol Venereol* 1987;114:801.

32. Shanon J, Sagher F. Interscapular cutaneous amyloidosis. *Arch Dermatol* 1970;102:195.

33. Wong CK, Lin CS. Friction amyloidosis. *Int J Dermatol* 1988; 27:302.

34. Brownstein MH, Hashimoto K. Macular amyloidosis. *Arch Dermatol* 1972;106:50.

35. Brownstein MH, Hashimoto K, Greenwald G. Biphasic amyloidosis: link between macular and lichenoid forms. *Br J Dermatol* 1973;88:25.

36. Bedi TR, Datta BN. Diffuse biphasic cutaneous amyloidosis. *Dermatologica* 1979;158:433.

37. Black MM, Wilson Jones E. Macular amyloidosis. *Br J Dermatol* 1971;84:199.

38. Kumakiri M, Hashimoto K. Histogenesis of primary localized cutaneous amyloidosis: sequential change of epidermal keratinocytes to amyloid via filamentous degeneration. *J Invest Dermatol* 1979;73:150.

39. Hashimoto K, Kobayashi H. Histogenesis of amyloid in the skin. *Am J Dermatopathol* 1980;2:165.

40. Glenner GG. Amyloid deposits and amyloidosis: the betafibrilloses. *N Engl J Med* 1980;302:1283.

41. Horiguchi Y, Fine JD, Leigh IM, et al. Lamina densa malformation involved in histogenesis of primary localized amyloidosis. *J Invest Dermatol* 1992;99:12.

42. MacDonald DM, Black MM, Ramnarain N. Immunofluorescence studies in primary localized cutaneous amyloidosis. *Br J Dermatol* 1977;96:635.

43. Danno K, Horis T. Sulphhydryl and disulphide stainings of amyloid: a comparison with hyaline body. *Acta Derm Venereol (Stockh)* 1981;61:285.

44. Masu S, Hosokawa M, Seiji M. Amyloid in localized cutaneous amyloidosis: immunofluorescence studies with anti-keratin antiserum. *Acta Derm Venereol (Stockh)* 1981;61:381.

45. Ishii M, Asai Y, Hamada T. Evaluation of cutaneous amyloid employing auto-keratin antibodies and the immunoperoxidase technique (PAP method). *Acta Derm Venereol (Stockh)* 1984;64:281.

46. Ishii M, Terao Y, Hamada T. Formation of amyloid from degenerating collagen islands in primary cutaneous amyloidosis. *Clin Exp Dermatol* 1987;12:302(abst).

47. Westermark P, Norén P. Two different pathogenetic pathways in lichen amyloidosus and macular amyloidosis. *Arch Dermatol Res* 1986;278:206.

48. Weedon D, Shand E. Amyloid deposits in the skin in secondary systemic amyloidosis. *Br J Dermatol* 1979;101:141.

49. Potter BA, Johnson WC. Primary localized amyloidosis cutis. *Arch Dermatol* 1971;103:448.

50. Goerttler E, Anton-Lamprecht I, Kotzur B. Amyloidosis cutis nodularis. *Hautarzt* 1976;27:16.

51. Rodermund OE. Zur amyloidosis cutis nodularis atrophicans (Gottron 1950). *Arch Klin Exp Dermatol* 1967;230:153.

52. Lindemayr W, Partsch H. Plattenartig infiltrierte lokalisierte hautamyloidose. *Hautarzt* 1970;21:104.

53. Brownstein MH, Helwig EB. The cutaneous amyloidoses. I. Localized forms. *Arch Dermatol* 1970;102:8.

54. Northcutt AD, Vanover MJ. Nodular cutaneous amyloidosis involving the vulva. *Arch Dermatol* 1985;121:518.

55. Ebner H, Gebhart W. Vergleichende untersuchungen bei juvenilem und adultem Colloid Milium. *Arch Dermatol Res* 1978; 261:231.

56. Handfield-Jones SE, Atherton DJ, Black MM, et al. Juvenile colloid milium: clinical, histological and ultrastructural features. *J Cutan Pathol* 1992;19:434.

57. Kobayashi A, Hashimoto K. Colloid and elastic fibre: Ultrastructural study on the histogenesis of colloid milium. *J Cutan Pathol* 1983;10:111.

58. Stone MS, Tschen JA. Colloid milium. *Arch Dermatol* 1986; 122:711.

59. Dupre A, Bonafe JF, Pieraggi MT, et al. Paracolloid of the skin. *J Cutan Pathol* 1979;6:304.

60. Sullivan M, Ellis FA. Facial colloid degeneration in plaques. *Arch Dermatol* 1961;84:816.

61. Kawashima Y, Matsubara T, Kinbara T, et al. Colloid degeneration of the skin. *J Dermatol* 1977;4:115.

62. Reuter MJ, Becker SW. Colloid degeneration (collagen degeneration) of the skin. *Arch Dermatol Syph* 1942;46:695.

63. Ebner H, Gebhart W. Colloid milium: light and electron microscopic investigations. *Clin Exp Dermatol* 1977;2:217.

64. Percival BH, Duthie DA. Notes on a case of colloid pseudomilium. *Br J Dermatol* 1948;60:399.

65. Graham JH, Marques AS. Colloid milium: a histochemical study. *J Invest Dermatol* 1967;49:497.

66. Yanagihara M, Mehregan AM, Mehregan DR. Staining of amyloid with cotton dyes. *Arch Dermatol* 1984;120:1184.

67. Hashimoto K, Black M. Colloid milium: a final degeneration product of actinic elastoid. *J Cutan Pathol* 1985;12:147.

68. Hashimoto K, Nakayama H, Chimenti S, et al. Juvenile colloid milium: immunohistochemical and ultrastructural studies. *J Cutan Pathol* 1989;16:164.

69. Kumakiri M, Hashimoto K. Histogenesis of primary localized cutaneous amyloidosis: sequential change of epidermal keratinocytes to amyloid via filamentous degeneration. *J Invest Dermatol* 1979;73:150.

70. Siebenmann F. Über mitbeteiligung der schleimhaut bei allgemeiner hyperkeratose der haut. *Arch Laryng Rhin* 1908;20: 101.

71. Urbach E, Wiethe C. Lipoidosis cutis et mucosae. *Virchows Arch A* 1929;273:285.

72. Konstantinov K, Kabakchiev P, Karchev T, et al. Lipoid proteinosis. *J Am Acad Dermatol* 1992;27:293.

73. Paller AS. Histology of lipoid proteinosis. *JAMA* 1994;272: 564.

74. Holtz KH, Schulze W. Beitrag zur klinik und pathogenese der hyalinosis cutis et mucosae (Lipoid-proteinose Urbach-Wiethe). *Arch Dermatol Syph (Berlin)* 1950;192:206.

75. Caplan RM. Visceral involvement in lipoid proteinosis. *Arch Dermatol* 1967;95:149.

76. Fleischmajer R, Nedwich A, Ramos E, et al. Hyalinosis cutis et mucosae. *J Invest Dermatol* 1969;52:495.

77. Shore RN, Howard BV, Howard WJ, et al. Lipoid proteinosis: demonstration of normal lipid metabolism in cultured cells. *Arch Dermatol* 1974;110:591.

78. Laymon CW, Hill EM. An appraisal of hyalinosis cutis et mucosae. *Arch Dermatol* 1957;75:55.

79. Holtz KH. Über gehirn-und augenveränderungen bei hyalinosis cutis et mucosae (lipoid-proteinose) mit autopsiebefund. *Arch Klin Exp Dermatol* 1962;214:289.

80. Van der Walt IJ, Heyl T. Lipoid proteinosis and erythropoietic protoporphyria. *Arch Dermatol* 1971;104:501.

81. Kint A. A comparative electron microscopic study of the perivascular hyaline from porphyria cutanea tarda and from lipoid proteinosis. *Arch Klin Exp Dermatol* 1970;239:203.

82. Fleischmajer R, Krieg T, Dziadek M, et al. Ultrastructure and composition of connective tissue in hyalinosis cutis et mucosae skin. *J Invest Dermatol* 1984;82:252.

83. McCusker JJ, Caplan RM. Lipoid proteinosis (lipoglycoproteinosis). *Am J Pathol* 1962;40:599.

84. Bauer EA, Santa-Cruz DJ, Aisen AL. Lipoid proteinosis: in vivo and in vitro evidence for a lysosomal storage disease. *J Invest Dermatol* 1981;76:119.

85. Harper JI, Duance VC, Sims TJ, et al. Lipoid proteinosis: an inherited disorder of collagen metabolism? *Br J Dermatol* 1985; 113:145.

86. Moy LS, Moy RL, Matsuoka LY, et al. Lipoid proteinosis: ultrastructural and biochemical studies. *J Am Acad Dermatol* 1987; 16:1193.

87. Ishibashi A. Hyalinosis cutis et mucosae. Defective digestion and storage of basal lamina glycoprotein synthesized by smooth muscle cells. *Dermatologica* 1982;165:7.

88. Konrad K, Hönigsmann H, Gschnait F, et al. Mouse model for protoporphyria. I. Cellular and subcellular events in the photosensitivity flare of the skin. *J Invest Dermatol* 1975;65:300.

89. Meola T, Lim HW. The porphyrias. *Dermatol Clin* 1993;11:583.

90. Stretcher GS. Erythropoietic porphyria. *Arch Dermatol* 1977; 113:1553.

91. Murphy GM, Hawk JLM, Nicholson DC, et al. Congenital erythropoietic porphyria. *Clin Exp Dermatol* 1987;12:61.

92. Gschnait F, Wolff K, Konrad K. Erythropoietic protoporphyria: submicroscopic events during the acute photosensitivity flare. *Br J Dermatol* 1975;92:545.

93. Ryan EA. Histochemistry of the skin in erythropoietic protoporphyria. *Br J Dermatol* 1966;78:501.

94. De Leo VA, Mathews-Roth M, Poh-Fitzpatrick M, et al. Erythropoietic protoporphyria: ten years experience. *Am J Med* 1976;60:8.

95. Harber LC, Poh-Fitzpatrick MB, Walther RR. Cutaneous aspects of the porphyrias. *Acta Derm Venereol Suppl (Stockh)* 1982;100:9.

96. Touart D, Sau P. Cutaneous deposition diseases. Part 1. *J Am Acad Dermatol* 1998;39:149.

97. Mathews-Roth MM. Erythropoietic protoporphyria: diagnosis and treatment. *N Engl J Med* 1977;297:98.

98. MacDonald DM, Germain D, Perrot H. The histopathology and ultrastructure of liver disease in erythropoietic protoporphyria. *Br J Dermatol* 1981;104:7.

99. Cripps DJ, Goldfarb SS. Erythropoietic protoporphyria: hepatic cirrhosis. *Br J Dermatol* 1978;98:349.

100. Wells MM, Golitz LE, Bender BJ. Erythropoietic protoporphyria with hepatic cirrhosis. *Arch Dermatol* 1980;116:429.

101. Fromke VL, Bossenmair I, Cardinal R, et al. Porphyria variegata: study of a large kindred in the United States. *Am J Med* 1978;65:80.

102. Mustajoki P. Variegate porphyria. *Ann Intern Med* 1978;89:238.

103. Poh-Fitzpatrick MB. A plasma porphyrin fluorescence marker for variegate porphyria. *Arch Dermatol* 1980;116:543.

104. Corey TJ, De Leo VA, Christianson H, et al. Variegate porphyria: clinical and laboratory features. *J Am Acad Dermatol* 1980;2:36.

105. Elder GH. Recent advances in the identification of enzyme deficiencies in the porphyrias [Comment]. *Br J Dermatol* 1983; 108:729.

106. Köstler E, Seebacher C, Riedel H, et al. Therapeutische und pathogenetische aspekte der porphyria cutanea tarda. *Hautarzt* 1986;37:210.

107. Roenigk HH, Gottlob ME. Estrogen-induced porphyria cutanea tarda. *Arch Dermatol* 1970;102:260.

108. Elder GH, Lee GB, Tovey JA. Decreased activity of hepatic uroporphyrinogen decarboxylase in sporadic porphyria cutanea tarda. *N Engl J Med* 1978;299:274.

109. Keczkes K, Barker DJ. Malignant hepatoma associated with acquired cutaneous porphyria. *Arch Dermatol* 1976;112:78.

110. Czarnecki DB. Hepatoerythropoietic porphyria. *Arch Dermatol* 1980;116:307.

111. Simon N, Berkó G, Schneider I. Hepato-erythropoietic porphyria presenting as scleroderma and acrosclerosis in a sibling pair. *Br J Dermatol* 1977;663.

112. Lim HW, Poh-Fitzpatrick MB. Hepatoerythropoietic porphyria: a variant of childhood-onset porphyria cutanea tarda. *J Am Acad Dermatol* 1984;11:1103.

113. Hönigsmann H, Reichel K. Hepatoerythrozytäre Porphyrie. *Hautarzt* 1979;30:95.

114. Roberts DT, Brodie MJ, Moore MR, et al. Hereditary coproporphyria presenting with photosensitivity induced by the contraceptive pill. *Br J Dermatol* 1977;96:549.

115. Hunter GA. Clinical manifestations of the porphyrias: a review. *Australas J Dermatol* 1979;20:120.

116. Kint A. A comparative electron microscopic study of the perivascular hyaline from porphyria cutanea tarda and from lipoid proteinosis. *Arch Klin Exp Dermatol* 1970;239:203.

117. Epstein JH, Tuffanelli DL, Epstein WL. Cutaneous changes in the porphyrias. *Arch Dermatol* 1973;107:689.

118. Ozasa S, Yamamoto S, Maeda M, et al. Erythropoietic protoporphyria. *J Dermatol* 1977;4:85.

119. Wolff K, Hönigsmann H, Rauschmeier W, et al. Microscopic and fine structural aspects of porphyrias. *Acta Derm Venereol Suppl (Stockh)* 1982;100:17.

120. Klein GF, Hintner H, Schuler G, et al. Junctional blisters in acquired bullous disorders of the dermal-epidermal junction zone. *Br J Dermatol* 1983;109:499.

121. Nagato N, Nonaka S, Ohgami T, et al. Mechanism of blister formation in porphyria cutanea tarda. *J Dermatol* Tokyo 1987; 14:551.

122. Feldaker M, Montgomery H, Brunsting LA. Histopathology of porphyria cutanea tarda. *J Invest Dermatol* 1955;24:131.

123. Egbert BM, LeBoit PE, McCalmont T, et al. Caterpillar bodies: distinctive, basement membrane-containing structures in blisters of porphyria. *Am J Dermatopathol* 1993;15:199.

124. Raso DS, Greene WB, Maize JC, et al. Caterpillar bodies of porphyria cutanea tarda ultrastructurally represent a unique arrangement of colloid and basement membrane bodies. *Am J Dermatopathol* 1996;18:24.

125. Anton-Lamprecht I, Meyer B. Zur ultrastruktur der haut bei protoporphyrinämie. *Dermatologica* 1970;141:76.

126. Ryan EA, Madill GT. Electron microscopy of the skin in erythropoietic protoporphyria. *Br J Dermatol* 1968;80:561.

127. Murphy GM, Hawk JLM, Magnus JA. Late-onset erythropoietic protoporphyria with unusual cutaneous features. *Arch Dermatol* 1985;121:1309.

128. Cormane RH, Szabo E, Tio TY. Histopathology of the skin in acquired and hereditary porphyria cutanea tarda. *Br J Dermatol* 1971;85:531.

129. Gilchrest B, Rowe JW, Mihm MC Jr. Bullous dermatosis in hemodialysis. *Ann Intern Med* 1975;83:480.

130. Thivolet J, Euvrard S, Perrot H, et al. La pseudo-porphyrie cutanée tardive des hémodialyses. *Ann Dermatol Venereol* 1977; 104:12.

131. Perrot H, Germain D, Euvrard S, et al. Porphyria cutanea tardalike dermatosis by hemodialysis. *Arch Dermatol Res* 1977; 259:177.

132. Poh-Fitzpatrick MB, Bellet N, De Leo VA, et al. Porphyria cutanea tarda in two patients treated with hemodialysis for chronic renal failure. *N Engl J Med* 1978;299:292.

133. Poh-Fitzpatrick MB, Masullo AS, Grossman ME. Porphyria cutanea tarda associated with chronic renal failure and hemodialysis. *Arch Dermatol* 1980;116:191.

134. Harlan SL, Winkelmann RK. Porphyria cutanea tarda and chronic renal failure. *Mayo Clin Proc* 1983;58:467.

135. Judd LE, Henderson DW, Hill DC. Naproxen-induced pseudoporphyria. *Arch Dermatol* 1986;122:451.

136. Wilson CW, Wingfield WL, Toone EC Jr. Vitamin D poisoning with metastatic calcification. *Am J Med* 1953;14:116.

137. Wermer P, Kuschner M, Riley EA. Reversible metastatic calcification associated with excessive milk and alkali intake. *Am J Med* 1953;14:108.

138. Mulligan RM. Metastatic calcification. *Arch Pathol* 1947;43:177.

139. Katz AI, Hampers CL, Merrill JP. Secondary hyperparathyroidism and renal osteodystrophy in chronic renal failure [Review]. *Medicine (Baltimore)* 1969;48:333.

140. Kolton B, Pedersen J. Calcinosis cutis and renal failure. *Arch Dermatol* 1974;110:256.

141. Kuzela DC, Huffer WE, Conger JD, et al. Soft tissue calcification in chronic dialysis patients. *Am J Pathol* 1977;86:403.

142. Parfitt AM. Soft tissue calcification in uremia. *Arch Intern Med* 1969;124:544.

143. Putkonen T, Wangel GA. Renal hyperparathyroidism with metastatic calcification of the skin. *Dermatologica* 1959;118:127.

144. Ivker RA, Woosley J, Briggaman RA. Calciphylaxis in three patients with end-stage renal disease. *Arch Dermatol* 1995;131:63.

145. Cockerell CJ, Dolan ET. Widespread cutaneous and systemic calcification (calciphylaxis) in patients with the acquired immuno-deficiency syndrome and renal disease. *J Am Acad Dermatol* 1992;26:559.

146. Essary L, Wick M. Cutaneous calciphylaxis. *Am J Clin Pathol* 2000;113:280.

147. Posey RE, Ritchie EB. Metastatic calcinosis cutis with renal hyperparathyroidism. *Arch Dermatol* 1967;95:505.

148. Eisenberg E, Bartholow PV Jr. Reversible calcinosis cutis. *N Engl J Med* 1963;268:1216.

149. Winkelmann RK, Keating FR Jr. Cutaneous vascular calcification, gangrene and hyperparathyroidism. *Br J Dermatol* 1970;83:263.

150. Chan YL, Mahoney JF, Turner JJ, et al. The vascular lesions associated with skin necrosis in renal disease. *Br J Dermatol* 1983;109:85.

151. Leroy D, Barrellier MT, Zanello D. Purpura réticulé et nécrotique (à type d'angiodermite nécrotique) dû à des calcifications artérielles au cours d'une insuffisance rénale chronique. *Ann Dermatol Venereol* 1984;111:461.

152. Fischer AH, Morris DJ. Pathogenesis of calciphylaxis: study of three cases with literature review. *Hum Pathol* 1995;26:1055.

153. Velayos EE, Masi AT, Stevens MB, et al. The "CREST" syndrome: comparison with systemic sclerosis (scleroderma). *Arch Intern Med* 1979;139:1240.

154. Muller SA, Winkelmann RK, Brunsting LA. Calcinosis in dermatomyositis. *Arch Dermatol* 1959;79:669.

155. Muller SA, Brunsting LA, Winkelmann RK. Calcinosis cutis: its relationship to scleroderma. *Arch Dermatol* 1959;80:15.

156. Holmes R. Morphoea with calcinosis. *Clin Exp Dermatol* 1979;4:125.

157. Carr RD, Heisel EB, Stevenson TD. CREST syndrome. *Arch Dermatol* 1965;92:519.

158. Kabir DJ, Malkinson FD. Lupus erythematosus and calcinosis cutis. *Arch Dermatol* 1969;100:17.

159. Reich H. Das Teutschlaender-Syndrom. *Hautarzt* 1963;14:462.

160. Paegle RD. Ultrastructure of mineral deposits in calcinosis cutis. *Arch Pathol* 1966;2:474.

161. Cornelius CE III, Tenenhouse A, Weber JC. Calcinosis cutis. *Arch Dermatol* 1968;98:219.

162. Haim S, Friedman-Birnbaum R. Two cases of circumscribed calcinosis. *Dermatologica* 1971;143:111.

163. Whiting DA, Simson IW, Kallmeyer JC, et al. Unusual cutaneous lesions in tumoral calcinosis. *Arch Dermatol* 1970;102:465.

164. Pursley TV, Prince MJ, Chausmer AB, et al. Cutaneous manifestations of tumoral calcinosis. *Arch Dermatol* 1979;115:1100.

165. Mozaffarian G, Lafferty FW, Pearson OH. Treatment of tumoral calcinosis with phosphorus deprivation. *Ann Intern Med* 1972;77:741.

166. Shapiro L, Platt N, Torres-Rodriquez VM. Idiopathic calcinosis of the scrotum. *Arch Dermatol* 1970;102:199.

167. Fisher BK, Dvoretzky I. Idiopathic calcinosis of the scrotum. *Arch Dermatol* 1978;114:957.

168. Bode U, Plewig G. Klassifikation follikulärer zysten. *Hautarzt* 1980;31:1.

169. Swinehart JM, Golitz LE. Scrotal calcinosis: dystrophic calcification of epidermoid cysts. *Arch Dermatol* 1982;118:985.

170. Dare AJ, Axelsen RA. Scrotal calcinosis: origin from dystrophic calcification of eccrine duct milia. *J Cutan Pathol* 1988;15:142.

171. Song DH, Lee KH, Kang WH. Idiopathic calcinosis of the scrotum. *J Am Acad Dermatol* 1988;19:1095.

172. Woods B, Kellaway TD. Cutaneous calculi. *Br J Dermatol* 1963;75:1.

173. Tezuka T. Cutaneous calculus: its pathogenesis. *Dermatologica* 1980;161:191.

174. Shmunes E, Wood MG. Subepidermal calcified nodules. *Arch Dermatol* 1972;105:593.

175. Eng AM, Mandrea E. Perforating calcinosis cutis presenting as milia. *J Cutan Pathol* 1981;8:247.

176. Winer LH. Solitary congenital nodular calcification of the skin. *Arch Dermatol Syph* 1952;66:204.

177. Steigleder GK, Elschner H. Lokalisierte calcinosis. *Hautarzt* 1957;8:127.

178. Duperrat B, Goetschel G. Calcification nodulaire solitaire congénitale de la peau (Winer 1952). *Ann Dermatol Syphiligr* 1963;90:283.

179. O'Duffy JD, Hunder GG, Kelly PJ. Decreasing prevalence of tophaceous gout. *Mayo Clin Proc* 1975;50:227.

180. Lichtenstein L, Scott HW, Levin MH. Pathologic changes in gout. *Am J Pathol* 1956;32:871.

181. Lopez Redondo MJ, Requena L, Macia M, et al. Fingertip tophi without gouty arthritis. *Dermatology* 1993;187:140.

182. LeBoit PE, Schneider S. Gout presenting as lobular panniculitis. *Am J Dermatopathol* 1987;9:334.

183. Conejo-Mir J, et al. Panniculitis and ulcers in a young man. *Arch Dermatol* 1998;134:501,504.

184. King DF, King LA. The appropriate processing of tophi for microscopy. *Am J Dermatopathol* 1982;4:239.

185. Darby AJ, Harnes NF, Pritchard MS. Demonstration of urate crystals after formalin fixation. *Hisopathology* 1998;32:382.

186. Shidhan V, Shidham G. Staining method to demonstrate urate crystals after formalin-fixed, paraffin-embedded tissue sections. *Arch Pathol Lab Med* 2000;124:774.

187. Zaharopoulos P, Wong JY. Identification of crystals in joint fluids. *Acta Cytol* 1980;24:197.

188. Cohen PR, Schmidt WA, Rapini RP. Chronic tophaceous gout with severely deforming arthritis: a case report with emphasis on histopathologic considerations. *Cutis* 1991;48:445.

189. Seegmiller JE. Skin manifestations of gout. In: Eisen AZ, et al., eds. *Dermatology in General Medicine*. 4th ed. New York: McGraw-Hill, 1993:1894.

190. Touart DM, Sau P. Cutaneous deposition diseases. Part II. *J Am Acad Dermatol* 1998;39:197.

191. Vijaikumar M, Thappa DM, Srilanth S. Alkaptonuric ochronosis presenting as palmoplantar pigmentation. *Clin Exp Dermatol* 2000;25:305.

192. Nikkels AF, Pierard GE. Medical mystery: the answer. *N Engl J Med* 2001;344:1642.

193. Turiansky GW, Levin SW. Bluish patches on the ears and axillae with dark urine: ochronosis and alkaptonuria. *J Dermatol* 2001;40:333.

194. Janocha S, Wolz W, Srsen S, et al. The human gene for alkaptonuria (AKU) maps to chromosome 3q. *Genomics* 1994;19:5.

195. Snider RL, Thiers BT. Exogenous ochronosis. *J Am Acad Dermatol* 1993;28:662.

196. Robinson-Bostom L, Pomerantz D, Wilkel C. Localized argyria with pseudo-ochronosis. *J Am Acad Dermatol* 2002;46:222.

197. Penneys NS. Ochronosislike pigmentation from hydroquinone bleaching creams. *Arch Dermatol* 1985;121:1239.

198. Lichtenstein L, Kaplan L. Hereditary ochronosis. *Am J Pathol* 1954;30:99.

199. Findlay GH, Morrison JGL, Simson IW. Exogeneous ochronosis and pigmented colloid milium from hydroquinone bleaching creams. *Br J Dermatol* 1975;93:613.

200. Laymon CW. Ochronosis. *Arch Dermatol* 1953;67:553.

201. Teller H, Winkler K. Zur klinik und histopathologie der endogenen ochronose. *Moutarzt* 1973;24:537.

202. Dogliotti M, Leibowitz M. Granulomatous ochronosis: a cosmetic-induced skin disorder in blacks. *Afr Med J* 1979;56:757.

203. Jordaan HF, Van Niekerk DJT. Transepidermal elimination in exogenous ochronosis. *Am J Dermatopathol* 1991;13:418.

204. Zannoni VG, Malawista SE, La Du BN. Studies on ochronosis. II. Studies on benzoquinone-acetic acid, a probable intermediate in the connective tissue pigmentation of alcaptonuria. *Arthritis Rheum* 1962;5:547.

205. Fisher AA. Exogenous ochronosis from hydroquinone bleaching cream. *Cutis* 1998;62:11.

206. Levin CY, Maibach H. Exogenous ochronosis. An update on clinical features, causative agents and treatment options. *Am J Clin Dermatol* 2001;2:213.

207. Atwood HD, Clifton S, Mitchell RE. A histological, histochemical and ultrastructural study of dermal ochronosis. *Pathology* 1971;3:115.

208. Tidman MJ, Horton JJ, Macdonald DM. Hydroquinone-induced ochronosis: light and electron-microscopic features. *Clin Exp Dermatol* 1986;11:224.

209. Holubar K, Mach KW. Scleredema (Buschke). *Acta Derm Venereol (Stockh)* 1967;47:102.

210. Johnson WC, Helwig EB. Cutaneous focal mucinosis. *Arch Dermatol* 1966;93:13.

211. Cawley EP, Lupton CH Jr, Wheeler CE, et al. Examination of normal and myxedematous skin. *Arch Dermatol* 1957;76:537.

212. Wortsman JD, Traycoff RB, Stone S. Preradial myxedema in thyroid disease. *Arch Dermatol* 1981;117:635.

213. Schwartz KM, Fatourechin V, Ahmed DD, et al. Dermopathy of Graves' disease (pretibial myxedema): long-term outcome. *J Clin Endocrinol Metab* 2002;87:438.

214. Lynch PJ, Maize JC, Sisson JC. Pretibial myxedema and nonthyrotoxic thyroid disease. *Arch Dermatol* 1973;107:107.

215. Daumerie C, Ludgate M, Costagliola S, et al. Evidence for thyrotropin receptor immunoreactivity in pretibial connective tissue from patients with thyroid-associated dermopathy. *Eur J Endocrinol* 2002;146:35.

216. Konrad K, Brenner W, Pehamberger H. Ultrastructural and immunological findings in Graves' disease with pretibial myxedema. *J Cutan Pathol* 1980;7:99.

217. Ishii M, Nakagawa M, Hamada T. An ultrastructural study of pretibial myxedema utilizing improved ruthenium red stain. *J Cutan Pathol* 1984;11:125.

218. Schermer DR, Roenigk HH Jr, Schumacher OP, et al. Relationship of long-acting thyroid stimulator to pretibial myxedema. *Arch Dermatol* 1970;102:62.

219. Cheung HS, Nicoloff JT, Kamiel MB, et al. Stimulation of fibroblast biosynthetic activity by serum of patients with pretibial myxedema. *J Invest Dermatol* 1978;71:12.

220. Somach SC, Helm TN, Lawlor KB, et al. Pretibial mucin: Histologic patterns and clinical correlation. *Arch Dermatol* 1993;129:1152.

221. Hill TG, Crawford JN, Rogers CC. Successful management of lichen myxedematosus. *Arch Dermatol* 1976;112:67.

222. Hardie RA, Hunter JAA, Urbaniak S, et al. Spontaneous resolution of lichen myxedematosus. *Br J Dermatol* 1979;100:727.

223. Flowers SL, Cooper PM, Landes HB. Acral persistent papular mucinosis. *J Am Acad Dermatol* 1989;21:293.

224. Stephens CJM, McKee PH, Black MM. The dermal mucinoses. *Adv Dermatol* 1993;8:201.

225. Borradori L, Aractingi S, Blanc F, et al. Acral persistent papular mucinosis and IgA monoclonal gammopathy. *Dermatology* 1992;185:134.

226. Lum D. Cutaneous mucinosis of infancy. *Arch Dermatol* 1980;116:198.

227. Podda M, Rongioletti F, Greiner D, et al. Cutaneous mucinosis of infancy: is it a real entity or the pediatric form of lichen myxoedematosus (papular mucinosis)? *Br J Dermatol* 2001;144:590.

228. Linder NM, Hand J, Burch PA, et al. Birt-Hogg-Dube syndrome: an autosomal dominant disorder with predisposition to cancers of the kidney, fibrofolliculomas, and focal cutaneous minosis. *Int J Dermatol* 2001;40:653.

229. Dalton JE, Seidell MA. Studies on lichen myxedematosus (papular mucinosis). *Arch Dermatol* 1954;67:194.

230. Montgomery H, Underwood LJ. Lichen myxedematosus: differentiation from cutaneous myxedemas or mucoid states. *J Invest Dermatol* 1953;20:213.

231. Rudner EJ, Mehregan A, Pinkus H. Scleromyxedema. *Arch Dermatol* 1966;93:3.

232. Braun-Falco O, Weidner F. Skleromyxödem Arndt-Gottron mit knochenmarks-plasmocytose und myositis. *Arch Belg Dermatol Syphiligr* 1970;26:193.

233. Perry HO, Montgomery H, Stickney JM. Further observations on lichen myxedematosus. *Ann Intern Med* 1960;53:955.

234. McGuiston CH, Schoch EP Jr. Autopsy findings in lichen myxedematosus. *Arch Dermatol* 1956;74:259.

235. Loggini B, Pingitore R, Avvenente A, et al. Lichen myxematosus with systemic involvement: clinical and autopsy findings. *J Am Acad Dermatol* 2001;45:606.

236. Hardemeier T, Vogel A. Elektronenmikroskopische befunde beim sklerömyxodem Arndt–Gottron. *Arch Klin Exp Dermatol* 1970;237:722.

237. Howsden SM, Herndon JH Jr, Freeman RG. Lichen myxedematosus. *Arch Dermatol* 1975;111:1325.

238. Carli-Basset C, Lorette G, Alison Y, et al. Apparition retardée d'une mucinose papuleuse. *Ann Dermatol Venereol* 1979;106:175.

239. Harris RB, Perry HO, Kyle RA, et al. Treatment of scleromyxedema with melphalan. *Arch Dermatol* 1979;115:295.

240. Lawrence DA, Tye MJ, Liss M. Immunochemical analysis of the basic immunoglobulin in papular mucinosis. *Immunochemistry* 1972;9:41.

241. Shapiro CM, Fretzin D, Norris S. Papular mucinosis. *JAMA* 1970;214:2052.

242. Piper W, Hardmeier T, Schäfer E. Das skleromyxödem Arndt–Gottron: Eine paraproteinämische ekrankung. *Schweiz Med Wochenschr* 1967;97:829.

243. Archibald GC, Calvert HT. Hypothyroidism and lichen myxoedematosus. *Arch Dermatol* 1977;113:684.

244. Lai A, Fat RFM, Suurmond D, et al. Scleromyxedema (lichen myxedematosus) associated with a paraprotein, IgG_1 of the type kappa. *Br J Dermatol* 1973;88:107.

245. James K, Fudenberg H, Epstein WL, et al. Studies on a unique diagnostic serum globulin in papular mucinosis (lichen myxedematosus). *Clin Exp Immunol* 1967;2:153.

246. Feldman P, Shapiro L, Pick AI, et al. Scleromyxedema. *Arch Dermatol* 1969;99:51.

247. McCarthy JT, Osserman E, Lombardo PC, et al. An abnormal serum globulin in lichen myxedematosus. *Arch Dermatol* 1964; 89:446.

248. Muldrow ML, Bailin PH. Scleromyxedema associated with IgG lambda multiple myeloma. *Cleve Clin Q* 1983;50:189.

249. Rowell NR, Waite A, Scott DG. Multiple serum protein abnormalities in lichen myxedematosus. *Br J Dermatol* 1969;81:753.

250. Sawada Y, Ohashi M. Scleromyxedema. *J Dermatol (Tokyo)* 1980;7:207.

251. Yaron M, Yaron I, Yust I, et al. Lichen myxedematosus (scleromyxedema) serum stimulates hyaluronic acid and prostaglandin E production by human fibroblasts. *J Rheumatol* 1985;12: 171.

252. Harper RA, Rispler J. Lichen myxedematosus serum stimulates human skin fibroblast proliferation. *Science* 1978;199:545.

253. Perry HO, Kierland RR, Montgomery H. Plaque-like form of cutaneous mucinosis. *Arch Dermatol* 1960;82:980.

254. Steigleder GK, Gartmann H, Linker U. REM-syndrome: reticular erythematous mucinosis (round-cell erythematosis): a new entity? *Br J Dermatol* 1974;91:191.

255. Quimby SR, Perry HO. Plaque-like cutaneous mucinosis: its relationship to reticular erythematous mucinosis. *J Am Acad Dermatol* 1982;6:856.

256. Morison WL, Shea CR, Parrish JA. Reticular erythematous mucinosis syndrome. *Arch Dermatol* 1979;115:1340.

257. Del Pozo J, Pena C, Almagro M, et al. Systemic lupus erythematosus presenting with a reticular erythematous mucinosis-like condition. *Lupus* 2000;9, 144.

258. Braddock SW, Kay HD, Maennle D, et al. Clinical and immunologic studies in reticular erthematous mucinosis and Jessner's lymphocytic infiltrate of skin. *J Am Acad Dermatol* 1993;28:691.

259. Herzberg J. Das REM-Syndrom. *Z Hautkr* 1981;56:1317.

260. Tominga A, Tajima S, Ishibashi A, et al. Reticular erythematous mucinosis syndrome with an infiltration of factor XIIIa+ and hyaluronan synthase 2+ dermal dendrcytes. *Br J Dermatol* 2001;145:141.

261. Stephens CJM, Das AK, Black MM, et al. The dermal mucinoses: a clinicopathologic and ultrastructural study. *J Cutan Pathol* 1990;17:319.

262. Balogh E, Nagy-Vezekényi K, Fórizs E. REM syndrome. *Acta Derm Venereol (Stockh)* 1980;60:173.

263. Van Zomder J, Shaw JC. Papular and nodular mucinosis as a presenting sign of progressive systemic sclerosis. *J Am Acad Dermatol* 2002;46:304.

264. Caputo R, Grima HR, Gelmetti C. Self-healing juvenile cutaneous mucinosis. *Arch Dermatol* 1995;131:459.

265. Pucevich MV, Latour DL, Bale GF, et al. Self-healing juvenile cutaneous mucinosis. *J Am Acad Dermatol* 1984;11:327.

266. Cron RQ, Swetter SM. Scleredema revisited: a post-streptococcal complication. *Clin Pediatr (Phila)* 1994;33:606.

267. Heilbron B, Saxe N. Scleredema in an infant. *Arch Dermatol* 1986;122:1417.

268. Venencie PY, Powell FC, Su WPD, et al. Scleredema: a review of thirty-three cases. *J Am Acad Dermatol* 1984;11:128.

269. Fleischmajer R, Raludi G, Krol S. Scleredema and diabetes mellitus. *Arch Dermatol* 1970;101:21.

270. Krakowski A, Covo J, Berlin C. Diabetic scleredema. *Dermatologica* 1973;146:193.

271. Fleischmajer R, Perlish JS. Glycosaminoglycans in scleroderma and scleredema. *J Invest Dermatol* 1972;58:129.

272. Kövary PM, Vakilzadeh F, Macher E, et al. Monoclonal gammopathy in scleredema. *Arch Dermatol* 1981;117:536.

273. Roupe G, Laurent TC, Malmström A, et al. Biochemical characterization and tissue distribution of the scleredema in a case of Buschke's disease. *Acta Derm Venereol (Stockh)* 1987;67:193.

274. Niebauer G, Ebner H. Skleroedema (Buschke). *Dermatol Monatsschr* 1970;156:940.

275. Curtis AC, Shulak BM. Scleredema adultorum. *Arch Dermatol* 1965;92:526.

276. Matsuoka LY, Wortsman J, Dietrich JG, et al. Glycosaminoglycans in histologic sections. *Arch Dermatol* 1987;123:862.

277. Reichenberger M. Betrachtungen zum Skleroedema adultorum Buschke. *Hautarzt* 1964;15:339.

278. Vallee BL. Scleredema: a systemic disease. *N Engl J Med* 1946; 235:207.

279. Leinwand I. Generalized scleredema: Report with autopsy findings. *Ann Intern Med* 1951;34:226.

280. Ohta A, Uitto J, Oikarinen AI, et al. Paraproteinemia in patients with scleredema. *J Am Acad Dermatol* 1987;16:96.

281. Sansom JE, Sheehan AL, Kennedy CT, et al. A fatal case of scleredema of Buschke. *Br J Dermatol* 1994;130:669.

282. Tasanen K, Palatsi R, Oikarinen A. Demonstration of increased levels of type I collagen in RNA using quantitative polymerase chain reaction in fibrotic and granulomatous skin diseases. *Br J Dermatol* 1998;139:23.

283. Wenstrup RJ, Pinnell SR. The genetic mucopolysaccharides. In: Fitzpatrick TB, Eisen AZ, Wolff K, et al., eds. *Dermatology in General Practice*. 4th ed. New York: McGraw-Hill, 1993:1971.

284. Maire I. Is genotype determination useful in predicting the cinical photype in lysosomal storage diseases? *J Inherit Metab Dis* 2001;24[Suppl 2]:57–61;discussion 45–46.

285. Hambrick GW Jr, Scheie HG. Studies of the skin in Hurler's syndrome. *Arch Dermatol* 1962;85:455.

286. Horiuchi R, Ishikawa H, Ishii Y, et al. Mucopolysaccharidosis with special reference to Scheie syndrome. *J Dermatol* 1976;3: 171.

287. Prystowsky SD, Maumenee IH, Freeman RG, et al. A cutaneous marker in the Hunter syndrome. *Arch Dermatol* 1977;113:602.

288. Lasser A, Carter DM, Mahoney MJ. Ultrastructure of the skin in mucopolysaccharidoses. *Arch Pathol* 1975;99:173.

289. Zivony DI, Spencer DM, Qualman SJ, et al. Ivory colored papules in a young boy. *Arch Dermatol* 1995;131:81.

290. Schiro, JA, Mallory SB, Demmer L, et al. Grouped papules in Hurler–Scheie syndrome. *J Am Acad Dermatol* 1996;35:868.

291. Freeman RG. A pathological basis for the cutaneous papules of mucopolysaccharidosis. II. The Hunter syndrome. *J Cutan Pathol* 1977;4:318.

292. Belcher RW. Ultrastructure of the skin in the genetic mucopolysaccharidoses. *Arch Pathol* 1972;94:511.

293. Belcher RW. Ultrastructure and function of eccrine glands in the mucopolysaccharidoses. *Arch Pathol* 1973;96:339.

294. Belcher RW. Ultrastructure and cytochemistry of lymphocytes in the genetic mucopolysaccharidoses. *Arch Pathol* 1972;93:1.

295. Hinek A, Wilson SE. Impaired elastogenesis in Hurler disease: dermatan sulfate accumulation linked to deficiency in elastin-binding protein and elastic fiber assembly. *Am J Pathol* 2000; 156:925.

296. Whitley CB, Belani KG, Change PN, et al. Long-term outcome of Hurler syndrome following bone marrow transplantation. *Am J Med Genet* 1993;46:209.

297. Schwartz RA. Acanthosis nigricans. *J Am Acad Dermatol* 1994; 31:1.

298. Mikhail GR, Fachnie DM, Drukker BH, et al. Generalized malignant acanthosis nigricans. *Arch Dermatol* 1979;115:201.

299. Curth HO. Classification of acanthosis nigricans. *Int J Dermatol* 1976;15:592.

300. Rendon MI, Cruz PD, Sontheimer RD, et al. Acanthosis nigricans: a cutaneous marker of tissue resistance to insulin. *J Am Acad Dermatol* 1989;21:461.

301. Hud JA Jr, Cohen JB, Wagner JM, et al. Prevalence and significance of acanthosis nigricans in an adult obese population. *Arch Dermatol* 1992;128:941.

302. Ober KP. Acanthosis nigricans and insulin resistance associated with hypothyroidism. *Arch Dermatol* 1985;121:229.

303. Oseid S, Beck-Nielsen H, Pedersen O. Decreased binding of insulin to its receptor in patients with congenital generalized lipodystrophy. *N Engl J Med* 1977;296:245.

304. Stals H, Vercammen C, Peters C, et al. Acanthosis nigricans caused by nicotinic acid. *Dermatology* 1994;189:203.

305. Greenspan AH, Shupack JL, Foo SH, et al. Acanthosis nigricans hyperpigmentation secondary to triazinate therapy. *Arch Dermatol* 1985;121:232.

306. Fleming MG, Simon SI. Cutaneous insulin reaction resembling acanthosis nigricans. *Arch Dermatol* 1986;122:1054.

307. Bonnekuh B, Wevers A, Spangenberger H, et al. Keratin patterns of acanthosis nigricans in syndrome-like association with polythelia, polycystic kidneys, and syndactyly. *Arch Dermatol* 1993;129:1177.

308. Brown J, Winkelmann RK. Acanthosis nigricans: a study of 90 cases [Review]. *Medicine (Baltimore)* 1968;47:33.

309. Wortsman J, Matsuoka LY, Kupchella CE, et al. Glycosaminoglycan deposition in the acanthosis nigricans lesions of the polycystic ovary syndrome. *Arch Intern Med* 1983;143:1145.

310. Cruz PD, Hud JA. Excess insulin binding to insulin-like growth factor receptors: Proposed mechanism for acanthosis nigricans. *J Invest Dermatol* 1992;98:82S.

311. Wilgenbus K, Lentner A, Kuckelkorn R, et al. Further evidence that acanthosis nigricans maligna is linked to enhanced secretion by the tumour of transforming growth factor alpha. *Arch Dermatol Res* 1992;284:266.

312. Haase I, Hunzelmann N. Activation of epidermal growth factor receptor/ERK signaling correlates with suppressed differentiation in malignant acanthosis nigricans. *J Invest Dermatol* 2002;118:891.

313. Gougerot H, Carteaud A. Papillomatose pigmentée innominée. *Bull Soc Fr Dermatol Syphiligr* 1927;34:719.

314. Kesten BM, James HD. Pseudoatrophoderma colli, acanthosis nigricans, and confluent and reticular papillomatosis. *Arch Dermatol* 1957;75:525.

315. Roberts SDB, Lachapelle JM. Confluent and reticulate papillomatosis (Gougerot–Carteaud) and Pityrosporon orbiculare. *Br J Dermatol* 1969;81:841.

316. Yesudian P, Kamalam S, Razack A. Confluent and reticulated papillomatosis (Gougerot–Carteaud). *Acta Derm Venereol (Stockh)* 1973;53:381.

317. Nordby CA, Mitchell AJ. Confluent and reticulated papillomatosis responsive to selenium sulfide. *Int J Dermatol* 1986;25:194.

318. Jang HS, Oh CK, Cha JH. Six cases of confluent and reticulated papillomatosis alleviated by various antibiotics. *J Am Acad Dermatol* 2001;44:652.

319. Fairbanks VF, Baldus WP. Hemochromatosis: the neglected diagnosis. *Mayo Clin Proc* 1986;61:296.

320. Chevrant-Breton J, Simon M, Bourel M, et al. Cutaneous manifestations of idiopathic hemo-chromatosis: study of 100 cases. *Arch Dermatol* 1977;113:161.

321. Milder MS, Cook JD, Stray S, et al. Idiopathic hemochromatosis: an interim report. *Medicine (Baltimore)* 1980;59:34.

322. Perdrup A, Poulsen H. Hemochromatosis and vitiligo. *Arch Dermatol* 1964;90:34.

323. Weintraub LR, Demis DJ, Conrad ME, et al. Iron excretion by the skin: selective localization of iron[59] in epithelial cells. *Am J Pathol* 1965;46:121.

324. Fletcher LM, Halliday JW. Haemochromatosis: understanding the mechanism of disease and implications for diagnosis and patient management following recent cloning of novel genes involved in iron metabolism. *J Intern Med* 2002;251:181.

325. Philpott CC. Molecular aspects of iron absorption: insights into the role of HFE in hemochromatosis. *Hepatology* 2002;35:993.

326. Crosby WH. Hemochromatosis: the missed diagnosis. *Arch Intern Med* 1986;146:1209.

327. Olynyk JK, Cullen DJ, Aquilia S, et al. A population-based study of the clinical expression of the hemochromatosis gene. *N Engl J Med* 1999; 341:719.

328. Leyden JL, Lockshin NA, Kriebel S. The black keratinous cyst: a sign of hemochromatosis. *Arch Dermatol* 1972;106:379.

329. Shet T, Desai S. Pigmented epidermal cysts. *Am J Dermatopathol* 2001;23:477.

330. Robert P, Zürcher H. Pigmentstudien. I. Mitteilung: Über den einfluss von schwermetallverbindungen, hämin, vitaminen, mikrobiellen toxinen, hormonen und weiteren stoffen auf die dopamelaninbildung in vitro und die pigmentbildung in vivo. *Dermatologica* 1950;100:217.

331. Buckley WR. Localized argyria. *Arch Dermatol* 1963;88:531.

332. Wechsler HL. Vitamin A deficiency following small-bowel bypass surgery for obesity. *Arch Dermatol* 1979;115:73.

333. Barr DJ, Riley RJ, Green DJ. Bypass phrynoderma: vitamin A deficiency associated with bowel-bypass surgery. *Arch Dermatol* 1984;120:919.

334. Bleasel NR, Stapleton KM, Lee MS. Vitamin A deficiency phrynoderma: due to malabsorption and inadequate diet. *J Am Acad Dermatol* 1999;41:322.

335. Fasal P. Clinical manifestations of vitamin deficiencies as observed in the Federated Malay States. *Arch Dermatol Syph* 1944;50:160.

336. Frazier CN, Hu C. Nature and distribution according to age of cutaneous manifestations of vitamin A deficiency. *Arch Dermatol Syph* 1936;33:825.

337. Bessey OA, Wolbach SB. Vitamin A: physiology and pathology. *JAMA* 1938;110:2072.

338. Rapaport MJ: Pellagra in a patient with anorexia nervosa. *Arch Dermatol* 1985;121:255.

339. Castiello RJ, Lynch PJ. Pellagra and the carcinoid syndrome. *Arch Dermatol* 1972;105:574.

340. Cohen LK, George W, Smith R. Isoniazid-induced acne and pellagra. *Arch Dermatol* 1974;109:377.

341. Stevens HP, Ostlere LS, Begent RHJ, et al. Pellagra secondary to 5-fluorouracil. *Br J Dermatol* 1993;128:578.

342. Lyon VB, Fairley JA. Anticonvulsant-induced pellagra. *J Am Acad Dermatol* 2002;46:597.

343. Kaur S, Garaya JS and Thami GP. Pellagrous dermatitis induced by phenytoin. *Pediatr Dermatol* 2002;19:93.

344. Moore RA, Spies TD, Cooper ZK. Histopathology of the skin in pellagra. *Arch Dermatol Syph* 1942;46:106.

345. Karthikeyan K, Thappa DM. Pellagra and skin. *Int J Dermatol* 2002;41:476.

346. Dong H, Kerl H, Cerroni L. EMA® cream-induced irritant contact dermatitis. *J Cutan Pathol* 2002;29:190.

347. Baron DN, Dent CE, Harris H, et al. Hereditary pellagra-like skin rash with temporary cerebellar ataxia, constant renal aminoaciduria and other bizarre chemical features. *Lancet* 1956;2:421.

348. Dent CE. Hartnup disease: an inborn error of metabolism. *Arch Dis Child* 1957;32:363.

349. Goldsmith LA. Biochemical diseases. In: Alper JA, ed. *Genetic Disorders of the Skin*. St. Louis: Mosby-Yearbook, 1991:64.

350. Clodi PH, Deutsch E, Niebauer G. Krankheitsbild mit poikilodermieartigen hautveränderungen, aminoacidurie und indolaceturie. *Arch Klin Exp Dermatol* 1964;218:165.

351. Ashurst PJ. Hydroa vacciniforme occurring in association with Hartnup disease. *Br J Dermatol* 1969;81:486.

352. Nozaki J, Dakeishi M, Ohura T. Homozygosity mapping to chromosome 5p15 of a gene responsible for Hartnup disorder. *Biochem Biophys Res Commun* 2001;284:255.

353. Tallab TM. Richner–Hanhart syndrome: importance of early diagnosis and early intervention. *J Am Acad Dermatol* 1996;35:857.

354. Rehák A, Selim MM, Yadav G. Richner–Hanhart syndrome (tyrosinaemia-II): report of four cases without ocular involvement. *Br J Dermatol* 1981;104:469.

355. Larrègue M, De Giacomoni P, Odièvre P, et al. Modification des kératinocytes au cours de la tyrosinose oculo-cutanée: syndrome de Richner-Hanhart. *Ann Dermatol Venereol* 1980; 107:1023.

356. Shimizu N, Ito M, Ito K, et al. Richner–Hanhart's syndrome: Electron microscopic study of the skin lesions. *Arch Dermatol* 1990;126:1342.

357. Zaleski WA, Hill A, Kushniruk W. Skin lesions in tyrosinosis: response to dietary treatment. *Br J Dermatol* 1973;88: 335.

INFLAMMATORY DISEASES OF HAIR FOLLICLES, SWEAT GLANDS, AND CARTILAGE

MICHAEL D. IOFFREDA

INFLAMMATORY DISEASES OF HAIR FOLLICLES

Folliculitis

There are many types of folliculitis, or inflammation of the hair follicle, many of which are covered in other areas of this text. Folliculitis may have an infectious etiology due to bacteria (Chapter 21), viruses such as herpes (Chapter 25), and fungi (Chapter 23), including dermatophytes (tinea capitis, tinea barbae, Majocchi's granuloma) and yeast (*Pityrosporum*). Discussed in Chapter 21 are pseudofolliculitis barbae, folliculitis ("acne") keloidalis nuchae, and the follicular occlusion tetrad. Perforating folliculitis is discussed with the other perforating disorders in Chapter 15. Herein the acneiform folliculitis and miscellaneous follicular disorders will be reviewed.

Acne Vulgaris

Acne vulgaris is a disease of adolescence and early adulthood that only occasionally persists later into adult life—more often in women. Chiefly affecting the face, upper back, and chest, it manifests as two types of lesions: comedones and inflammatory lesions, both follicular based. Comedones may be closed ("whiteheads") or open ("blackheads"). Inflammatory lesions evolve from ruptured comedones or microcomedones, which are not clinically apparent, and originate more frequently from closed than open comedones. Once developed, inflammatory papules may become pustules or nodules, which may subsequently develop into cysts. Cystic acne can result in severe scarring. In acne fulminans, a rare variant occurring mainly in young male patients, lesions rapidly become tender, ulcerated, and crusted, and eventually scar. It may be associated with fever and polyarthralgia (1).

Histopathology. The development of a comedone involves a complex but incompletely understood process that results in infundibular dilatation and thinning of the follicular wall. A plug composed of loosely arranged keratinized cells and sebum forms (Fig. 18-1). Sebum is made up of sebaceous lipids that empty into the follicular lumen and microorganisms. Solvents used in histologic processing remove these lipids.

In closed comedones, the follicular orifice remains more or less normal in size, but when the follicular ostium widens, an open comedone results. Both types of comedones are associated with mild mononuclear inflammation, situated around vessels in the adjacent papillary dermis. Attenuation of the follicular wall may be so extreme as to lead to rupture (2). Release of follicular contents into the dermis generates an inflammatory response initially mediated by neutrophils and later by histiocytes and foreign-body giant cells. When rupture occurs superficially, it tends to lead to the development of a clinical pustule (Fig. 18-2), but when it occurs in the deeper dermis, an inflammatory nodule forms (Fig. 18-3). If the follicular damage is severe, scarring can result.

In severe forms of acne (cystic acne and acne fulminans), inflammation can become extensive, resulting in dermal necrosis with large abscesses (3). Epithelial outgrowths from the damaged follicle may encapsulate and attempt to exteriorize the inflammatory debris, simulating a perforating collagenosis (2).

Pathogenesis. Important advances in the past decade that have impacted our understanding of acne were recently reviewed by Thiboutot (4). Acne is a multifactorial condition, initially requiring sex hormone release during puberty and activation of the sebaceous glands. The major factors contributing to acne development are follicular hyperkeratinization, androgens, sebum, *Propionibacterium acnes*, and inflammation.

Comedone development is associated with increased epithelial cell proliferation in the lower portion of the infundibulum, as measured by tritium labeling techniques (5). Using Ki-67, increased keratinocyte proliferation was demonstrated in normal follicles from acne-affected areas (as compared to areas free of acne), suggesting that some

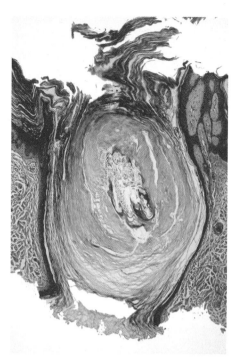

FIGURE 18-1. Comedone, open. A dilated follicular infundibulum is plugged with keratin and sebum. The follicular wall is attenuated, and the orifice is widened.

follicles may be "acne prone" (6). Ki-67 was also increased in comedones.

Comedones exhibit hyperkeratinization, and the keratin is bound more avidly as a result of increased levels of intercellular adhesion materials (7). Although the exact mechanism of follicular hyperkeratinization has yet to be elucidated, there may be a role for follicular linoleic acid deficiency, androgens, and interleukin-1 (4,8). Ultrasturally, follicular keratinocytes in comedones possess increased numbers of desmosomes and tonofilaments, which

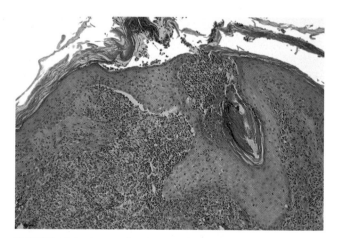

FIGURE 18-2. Acne vulgaris, pustule. Superficial follicular rupture incites suppurative and granulomatous inflammation, with neutrophils predominating in early lesions.

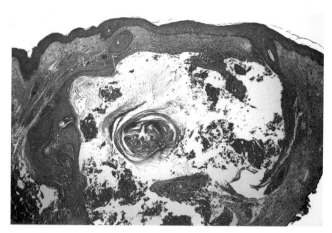

FIGURE 18-3. Acne vulgaris, nodule. Cyst-like follicular dilatation with deep rupture leads to neutrophilic and granulomatous inflammation throughout the dermis.

contribute to hypercornification (9). The black color of open comedones ("blackheads") appears to be related to densely packed keratinocytes, bacteria, and bacterial breakdown products located at the surface (10). If dilatation of the follicular orifice does not occur (closed comedone), continued thinning and ultimate rupture of the infundibular wall becomes more probable.

Generation of inflammation in acne lesions is also a complex process. Potential instigators of inflammation may be derived from the breakdown products of sebaceous lipids, from byproducts derived from *P. acnes*, as well as various immunologic mechanisms directed against this organism (11). The expression of adhesion molecules and inflammatory infiltrates were studied by immunohistochemistry in evolving lesions of acne vulgaris (12). There was vascular expression of ICAM-1, E-selectin, VCAM-1, and HLA-DR, and the inflammatory cells consisted of CD4+ T-lymphocytes.

There is substantial evidence linking the activation of sebum production to androgens, specifically testosterone and dihydrotestosterone (DHT) (13–15). Circulating testosterone is converted in tissues to the more potent DHT by the enzyme 5-α reductase (16). The type I isoform of 5-α reductase is located primarily in sebocytes (but is found also in the epidermis, infundibular hair follicle keratinocytes (17), dermal papilla cells, sweat glands, and fibroblasts). The gene encoding the type I isozyme is found on chromosome 5p (18). Activity of the type I isoform of 5-α reductase was greatest in sebaceous glands from acne-prone areas of the skin as compared to non–acne-prone areas, suggesting that regional differences in pilosebaceous production of DHT may play a role in acne (19).

The precise role of androgenic hormones in the production of acne lesions remains controversial. Androgens are derived from two sources: precursor serum androgens of glandular origin (gonadal and adrenal), and target tissue androgens derived from conversion of circulating precursors. It has been suggested that in patients with mild acne the serum levels of precursor androgens are normal and that in these circumstances only tissue androgen levels are elevated (20). In severe cystic acne, increased serum androgen levels have been found (21), although the majority of acne patients—especially male patients—do not show abnormal levels. Elevated serum androgen levels occur more frequently in women with acne, but similar elevations have been found in hirsute women without acne (22). Another study found significantly higher mean serum androgen levels in females with acne compared to those without, though values were in the range of normal; also, sebaceous glands from the women with acne showed higher mean 5-α reductase type I activity, although the difference was not statistically significant (23). This study suggests that women with acne may have higher serum androgen levels and perhaps a greater capacity to produce DHT within sebaceous glands.

The author emphasized the importance of sebum in acne with a simple statement, "remove sebum and you remove acne" (24). Sebum production in acne is elevated and appears to correlate with disease severity (25). An *in vitro* study of sebaceous gland ultrastructure after exposure to substance P found that this stress-induced neuropeptide promoted the proliferation and differentiation of sebaceous glands, implicating a role for stress in acne (9). The beneficial effect of isotretinoin (13-cis-retinoic acid) appears to result largely from reduction in sebum production, although a substantial decrease in *P. acnes* levels was detected in one study (26), and follicular hyperkeratinization was found to be reduced in another study (27). After two months of treatment with oral isotretinoin, a 70% reduction in sebum excretion is achieved (26), and after four months a reduction of 88% may be attained (28). These changes are associated histologically with a marked reduction in sebaceous gland size (28).

Of all the microorganisms identified in the follicular infundibulum, only *P. acnes* appears to be consistently involved in the pathogenesis of acne lesions. Nevertheless, levels of this organism may not be consistently greater in lesional skin than in normal skin (29,30). Immunologic reactivity to this organism may contribute to the inflammation in acne lesions. In response to *P. acnes*, acne patients may exhibit elevated serum antibody levels, increased immediate hypersensitivity, and augmented cell-mediated immunity (31). A good correlation between delayed skin test reactivity to *P. acnes* and acne lesion severity has been shown (32). The beneficial effects of systemic and topical antibiotics in acne patients are generally attributed to their suppression of *P. acnes* (33), although some studies suggest that oral tetracycline (30) and topical erythromycin (34) may improve acne without reducing the population of *P. acnes*.

Novel acne research involves the study of peroxisomal proliferator activator receptors (PPARs), which, via ligand interaction, modulate various functions of peroxisomes (small organelles that are important in regulating cell proliferation, differentiation, metabolism, and inflammation) (35,36).

Steroid Acne

Steroid acne is a folliculitis caused by the use of corticosteroids, including systemic, topical, inhaled (37), and intranasal (38). Despite its well-known existence (39), steroid acne has become more prevalent with the creation of increasingly potent topical preparations and the introduction of organ transplant surgery and various treatment regimens for cancer (40). Although other medications have been implicated in acneiform eruptions, steroid acne results in a distinctive clinical picture characterized by the sudden appearance of monomorphous papulopustules predominantly on the upper truck and arms, but also on the face (41). Comedones are not apparent. When due to topical steroids, the underlying rash for which it is used initially improves, followed by exacerbation of the underlying rash (42). The exacerbation is controlled only by continued use of topical steroids (physical dependence). Perioral dermatitis may be caused by topical corticosteroids (see the discussion of perioral dermatitis below). Resolution typically occurs without scarring.

Histopathology. Acne due to both topical and systemic corticosteroids shows similar histologic features. Despite the apparent absence of comedones clinically, Hurwitz (40) described histologic features that resembled acne vulgaris (Fig. 18-4), albeit with an accelerated rate of development. In chronological order, biopsied flesh-colored papules that measured 1 mm showed infundibular spongiosis, hyperkeratosis, perifollicular edema, microcomedo formation, and infundibular wall thinning, sometimes with infundibular rupture. It was more common, however, to see only infundibular dilation with compact hyperkeratosis. Biopsied lesions that were ≥2 mm and clinically inflamed frequently showed infundibular rupture, necrotic keratinocytes, and surrounding suppurative and granulomatous inflammation that included multinucleated giant cells amid keratinous debris. Dilated blood vessels were also seen.

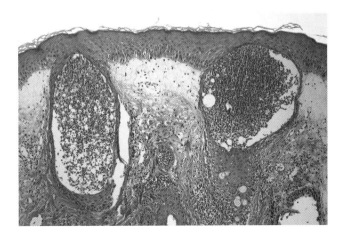

FIGURE 18-4. Steroid acne. Pustules in steroid acne are monomorphous and resemble those in acne vulgaris.

Pathogenesis. Although the exact mechanism of pathogenesis is not known, three phases of lesion development have been described as a result of "addiction" to topical steroids (42): (a) initial improvement of the rash is due to the anti-inflammatory properties of topical corticosteroids; (b) local immunosuppressive effects of the steroids result in bacterial overgrowth; and (c) when steroids are withdrawn, there is rebound and flaring secondary to bacterial overgrowth. In addition to the chronologic sequence described above, some authors have described a pathologic process that is the reverse of acne vulgaris, beginning with folliculitis that proceeds to rupture and concludes with comedone formation (so-called "secondary" comedone) (43). In a study of steroid acne due to systemic therapy, 80% of 125 patients showed significant numbers of *Pityrosporum ovale* in lesional follicles, and itraconazole, an oral antifungal agent, proved more efficacious than other medications (44).

Perioral Dermatitis

Recognition of this relatively common facial eruption is important because of its resemblance to rosacea, seborrheic dermatitis, and occasionally lupus erythematosus (45). Predominantly affecting white women of European extraction ranging in age from the mid-teens into middle age, it results in fine, follicular-based papules periorally, and more rarely, in a periocular distribution (*periocular dermatitis*) (46). The papules are single, grouped, or confluent, with minimal scaling. Pinhead-sized pustules may occur in more severe cases. There is sparing of a 5-mm zone around the vermillion border (41). The condition lacks significant telangiectasia. It is commonly associated with topically applied preparations, especially topical corticosteroids and cosmetics. Perioral dermatitis in children occurs primarily as a result of topical steroid use and is almost identical to the disease in adults (47–49).

Childhood granulomatous periorificial dermatitis is an acneiform facial eruption that shows some similarity to granulomatous rosacea and perioral dermatitis in children, but does have some distinctive features (50,51). It was initially reported in the French literature in 1970 (52). The currently used terminology was first coined in 1989 (50), although other terms have been proposed, such as facial Afro-Caribbean childhood eruption (FACE), reflecting its usual incidence on the face of black children (53). Other features that distinguish childhood granulomatous periorificial dermatitis from childhood perioral dermatitis and acne vulgaris include (a) exclusive incidence in healthy prepubertal children, and (b) absence of pustules and lack of circumoral sparing. Another entity producing clinically similar lesions, lupus miliaris disseminatus faciei, has not been reported in children (53). Clinical lesions may be flesh-colored, hypopigmented, or reddish yellow, and are small (1 to 3 mm), monomorphous, and occur periorally,

perinasally, and periorbitally. Lesions are asymptomatic and self-limited, but may last for years, typically healing without residuals except for some small pitted scars in a small number of patients (52,54). Recently, cases with extrafacial and generalized lesions were reported (54).

Histopathology. Some authors consider perioral dermatitis to be a variant of rosacea, with indistinguishable histologic features (48,55), while others consider the two entities to be distinct (56,57), with some histologic overlap. A proposed clinical classification scheme for rosacea published in 2002 did not classify steroid-induced acneiform eruption or perioral dermatitis as rosacea variants, citing insufficient evidence (57).

The following histologic characteristics of perioral dermatitis have been published (56). Fully developed lesions show spongiosis of the follicular infundibulum with mild mononuclear cell exocytosis (Fig. 18-5), with similar changes sometimes observed in the epidermis adjacent to the involved follicle. The epidermis may show mild acanthosis and parakeratosis, particularly about follicular ostia. The perifollicular dermis shows lymphohistiocytic inflammation around vessels, and in rare cases plasma cells may be prominent. Less developed lesions may exhibit only dermal inflammation. Acute folliculitis is uncommon. Lesions tend to lack the dermal edema and telangiectasias characteristic of rosacea, and show more noticeable epidermal changes.

Lesions of *childhood granulomatous periorificial dermatitis* often resemble granulomatous rosacea, with noncaseating perifollicular granulomas with some giant cells (50,54).

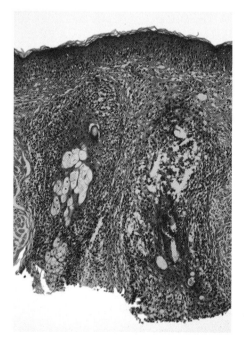

FIGURE 18-5. Perioral dermatitis. There is perifollicular mononuclear inflammation with infundibular spongiosis and exocytosis of lymphocytes.

Other features include epidermal changes consisting of mild hyperkeratosis and spongiosis, and dermal inflammation composed of lymphocytes and histiocytes that is mild to moderate, perivascular, and perifollicular. The granulomatous component is variable; some biopsies lacked granuloma formation or follicular involvement altogether. Some cases showed focal follicular rupture with inflammation to the released contents (50). Special stains for fungi and mycobacteria have been negative (54).

Pathogenesis. Perioral dermatitis was first described as a light-sensitive seborrheid (58), but subsequent investigation has produced a large number of possible etiologies for this condition, including *Candida* organisms, bacteria, particularly of the fusiform type; *Demodex* mites; a wide range of contactants, both irritant and allergic (including cosmetics and fluoride-containing toothpaste); hormones (including birth control pills); topical corticosteroids (particularly potent ones); and emotional as well as systemic conditions. An Australian survey found an increased risk of developing perioral dermatitis with use of foundation makeup along with moisturizer and night cream (59). Periocular dermatitis has been reported with the use of a steroid eye ointment (60).

The etiology of *childhood granulomatous periorificial dermatitis* is not known, but an external contactant has been implicated in some cases, with various agents, including topical fluorinated corticosteroids, reported (54).

Rosacea

Rosacea is an acneiform inflammatory condition that primarily affects the face and is more common after the age of 30. Recently it was noted that the incidence of rosacea is on the rise (61). It is characterized by background erythema within which scattered telangiectasias, papules, and occasional pustules develop. It typically affects the nose, cheeks, glabella, and chin, and is usually bilateral but occasionally unilateral or focal. If it is severe, lesions may spread to the neck and rarely become disseminated (62). Rhinophyma, a bulbous swelling of the soft tissue of the nose, is a late complication that occurs almost exclusively in men. Eye changes—especially blepharitis and conjunctivitis—are quite common in rosacea, and in 5% of the cases a painful keratitis can develop (63). Rosacea can precipitate persistent facial lymphedema.

A recently proposed clinical classification scheme for rosacea delineated four subtypes: (a) erythematotelangiectatic, (b) papulopustular, (c) phymatous, and (d) ocular (57). In this classification, a single rosacea variant was defined, *granulomatous rosacea*, which did not show morphology of one of the subtypes.

Histopathology. Vascular dilatation of upper and middermal vessels with perivascular and perifollicular lymphohistiocytic inflammation (and occasional plasma cells) is generally present in all cases (Fig. 18-6). Lymphatic dilata-

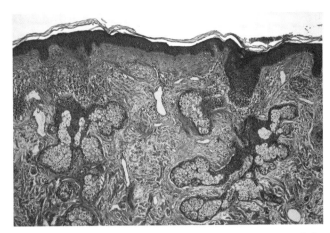

FIGURE 18-6. Rosacea. Lymphocytes surround vellus hair follicles and upper dermal vessels, which are dilated. Solar elastosis is usually prominent, as it is here.

tion is also common and may be prominent. With mild follicular involvement, there is infundibular spongiosis and lymphocyte exocytosis. With more extensive follicular involvement, neutrophils accumulate, resulting in a superficial pustule. Reflecting the clinical presentation, various other pathologic changes can be seen from case to case, including organization of dermal lymphocytes into small nodular aggregates (64,65).

Granulomatous infiltrates are reported to occur in about 10% of all cases of rosacea (65,66), and caseation necrosis has been identified in about 10% of these patients (67). *Granulomatous rosacea* can histologically mimic mycobacterial infections, with epithelioid histiocytes forming a tuberculoid pattern (Fig. 18-7). In such cases, other investigative procedures, including tissue cultures, may be necessary. Less frequently, the changes resemble cutaneous sarcoidosis. Multinucleated giant cells of the foreign-body

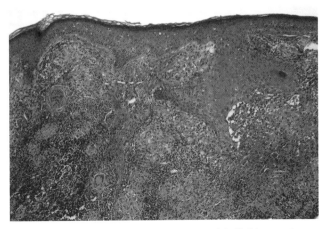

FIGURE 18-7. Granulomatous rosacea. Epithelioid granulomas with moderate lymphocytic inflammation are centered about a disrupted hair follicle. Some multinucleated giant cells are present.

type may aggregate around follicular contents spilled from a ruptured follicle (68).

In a study of rhinophyma, the classic or common type showed histologic features of fully developed rosacea, except for sebaceous gland hyperplasia, which can be prominent (69). The sebaceous ducts become dilated and filled with keratin and sebum. The same study showed that in patients with the severe form of rhinophyma, there is marked dermal thickening with sclerotic collagen bundles and large amounts of mucin, an absence of pilosebaceous structures, sparse inflammation, and telangiectasias (69). Many spindle-shaped and "bizarre" cells staining for factor XIIIa were seen in the interstitium. It was noted that the microscopic findings in the severe form of rhinophyma demonstrate many similarities to elephantiasis nostras caused by chronic lymphedema.

Pathogenesis. Although triggers of rosacea are well known, the pathogenesis of the disease is still unknown. It is probable that the etiology of rosacea is multifactorial (70), but sun damage appears to be a constant feature (71). Rosacea is not associated with an increase in sebum excretion (72). Dahl (73) proposed that the vascular dilatation leads to dermal edema, which in turn promotes the inflammation that is ultimately responsible for the sequelae of rosacea. In this model, warm facial skin from increased blood flow may modify the behavior of bacteria and/or *Demodex*, or change the enzymatic activity of keratinocytes or other skin cells, leading to altered metabolism and inciting inflammation.

The role of *Demodex* organisms has been debated for decades. Some reports claim a significant association of mites in rosacea biopsies (68,74–77), but other studies have not supported this claim (78,79). Although a definitive causative role for *Demodex* in rosacea is uncertain, the mites may represent an important cofactor in heightening disease severity (77).

In recent years, an association with gastrointestinal *Helicobacter pylori* infection has been explored. In one study, a number of rosacea patients had gastrointestinal symptoms related to gastritis; the prevalence of *H. pylori* in those patients with rosacea was 88%, compared to 65% in the control group without rosacea (but with nonulcer dyspepsia) (80). Furthermore, eradication of *H. pylori* with a week of therapy that included oral metronidazole, omeprazole, clarithromycin, and topical intraoral metronidazole resulted in marked improvement or resolution of rosacea symptoms after 2 to 4 weeks. In another report, a man with intractable rosacea for 4 years was treated with a similar treatment regimen directed against *H. pylori* that had been documented by gastroscopy and serologic testing. His skin began to improve with treatment, and cleared completely 2 months later, remaining clear for at least 3 years thereafter (81). Attempts to find *H. pylori* in the skin have been unsuccessful. A proposed pathogenesis is increased flushing due to vasodilators such as NO and gastrin, and inflammatory cytokines such as TNFα and IL-8, all produced by *H. pylori*

(82). Nevertheless, definitive studies validating an association of *H. pylori* with rosacea have yet to be done (83).

Immunoglobulins and complement components have been identified at the dermal–epidermal junction in patients with rosacea (84,85), but others have disputed these findings (86). Immune deposits in the skin of rosacea patients may be a reflection of chronic actinic injury.

Demodicidosis

Demodicidosis is the term for cutaneous disease caused by mites of the genus *Demodex*. Despite more than 65 years of investigation into the role of *Demodex* mites in human skin disease, questions still remain. Aside from their controversial role in rosacea, *Demodex* have been implicated in follicular-based skin eruptions resembling rosacea, albeit with some unique features that warrant consideration as distinct entities (87–89). There are at least three clinical forms of demodicidosis (87). The first, *pityriasis folliculorum*, is characterized by facial erythema with fine follicular plugs and scale producing a "nutmeg-grater" or "sandpaper-like" appearance. It usually affects women and may be associated with itching and burning. The second, *rosacea-like demodicidosis*, resembles rosacea in that there are papules and pustules. In contrast to rosacea, however, there is follicular scaling, sudden onset, rapid progression, and no history of flushing. There may be eyelid involvement (demodectic blepharitis) and poor general health, such as diabetes mellitus (87). Lastly, "*demodicidosis gravis*" resembles severe granulomatous rosacea. These forms may represent a spectrum of disease where the clinical expression depends on the degree of *Demodex* infestation, duration, and the individual's age and overall health (87).

Demodex are obligatory parasites frequently found in mammalian pilosebaceous units, and colonization is usually asymptomatic (76). The mites found in humans are of the species *D. folliculorum* and *D. brevis*. *D. folliculorum*, the predominant mite, has a longer body, inhabits the infundibulum of hair follicles, and is found almost exclusively on the face (90,91). *D. brevis* is smaller and lives exclusively within sebaceous glands on the face and trunk (90,91).

A study of consecutive biopsies submitted to one dermatopathology laboratory showed *Demodex* mites in 10% of all biopsies and 12% of all follicles (90). Their prevalence increased with age, and males were more heavily infested. In another study, there was a nonrandom association between histologic folliculitis and presence of *Demodex* in the follicles (91); mites were found in 42% of inflamed follicles, but in only 10% of noninflamed follicles, while 83% of follicles containing *Demodex* showed inflammation. This demonstrated a strong association, but not cause and effect, for the possibility that *Demodex* could preferentially select inflamed follicles was raised. Additional support for a pathogenic role was provided by reports of sudden facial eruptions in which numerous

Demodex mites were identified and the eruption failed to respond to therapy for rosacea, but cleared quickly with treatments directed against *Demodex*, such as crotamiton (92), or ivermectin and permethrin (93).

Some believe that *Demodex* are pathogenic only in large numbers (92,93), but an individual's overall health also appears to be important, as demonstrated by reports in immunocompromised children (94–96), and multiple reports in patients with HIV and AIDS, where the eruption may also involve the neck, upper trunk, and extremities (95,97–100). It has also been seen in immunocompetent children (101).

Human demodectic alopecia may be a real entity characterized by alopecia, erythema, and scale, with numerous *Demodex* mites in affected follicles (102). It resembles canine demodectic mange, and has been successfully treated with permethrin.

Histopathology. The diagnosis can be made in the clinical setting by examining scale with 40% KOH (103), or by standardized skin surface biopsy (SSSB) where cyanoacrylate glue is used to sample the horny layer and follicular contents (104). The presence of five or more mites in a single low-power field by KOH or more than five per square centimeter by SSSB is considered significant.

Biopsies of *pityriasis folliculorum* show a perivascular and diffuse dermal lymphocytic infiltrate without granuloma formation (87). *Demodex* mites are present within pilosebaceous units. Biopsies of *rosacea-like demodicidosis* (Fig. 18-8) show a primarily perifollicular infiltrate of mononuclear cells with possible granulomatous inflammation (87). The infiltrate is composed predominantly of CD4⁺ T-lymphocytes (77), and perifollicular Langerhans cells may be found. "*Demodicidosis gravis*" shows granulomas with central necrosis (caseation) and foreign-body-type multinucleated giant cells (105).

Pathogenesis. The pathogenesis of *Demodex*-related disease may be related to one of the following: (a) blockage of hair follicles and sebaceous ducts due to reactive epithelial hyperplasia and hyperkeratinization, (b) mites serving as vectors for bacteria, (c) a foreign body reaction to the mite, or (d) induction of host immunity by the mites and their waste (76). Some mite antigen may also elicit a delayed hypersensitivity reaction (77). A mite-derived lipase could potentially release fatty acids from serum triglycerides, producing an irritant reaction (106).

Lupus Miliaris Disseminatus Faciei

Although now considered a variant of rosacea, lupus miliaris disseminatus faciei (acne agminata) has its own distinct clinical presentation. Discrete, flesh-colored, or mildly erythematous papules—arranged singly or in small groups—involve the eyelids and upper lip, areas where rosacea lesions are not commonly found (107). The background erythema and telangiectasias of rosacea are lacking. Papules frequently persist for 12 to 24 months, and are resistant to standard

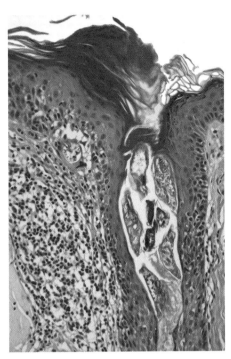

FIGURE 18-8. Demodicidosis. The follicular infundibulum contains multiple Demodex mites, and there is perifollicular lymphohistiocytic inflammation. Where the left side of the follicular epithelium meets the epidermis, an organism appears to be perforating through to the dermis.

rosacea therapy, although spontaneous healing can occur (108). Unusual presentations have included axillary lesions (109), and during pregnancy in a patient with cutaneous lupus erythematosus (110). One group proposed the use of equally cumbersome terminology, "facial idiopathic granulomas with regressive evolution" (111). Clinically similar lesions due to metastatic silicone granuloma were reported in a patient with silicone breast implants (112).

Histopathology. Biopsy specimens sectioned through the central portion of a papular lesion demonstrate one of the most highly characteristic patterns of cutaneous histopathology. Surrounding a usually large area of caseous necrosis, aggregates of epithelioid histiocytes and occasional multinucleate giant cells form a "tubercle" (Fig. 18-9). Sparse lymphoid inflammation is observed peripherally (108,113,114).

Pathogenesis. Despite the histologic picture, no direct relationship with tuberculosis has been documented, including recent testing using polymerase chain reaction with DNA fragments specific for *Mycobacterium tuberculosis* complex (115). Although many consider it to be a subset of rosacea, its exact etiology is unknown.

Eosinophilic Pustular Folliculitis

Ofuji originally described *eosinophilic pustular folliculitis* (EPF) in immunocompetent Japanese patients as itchy follicular papules and pustules arranged in arcuate plaques

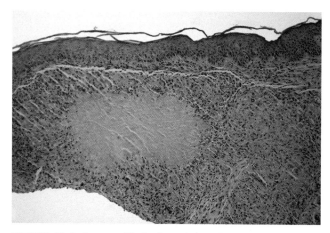

FIGURE 18-9. Lupus miliaris disseminatus faciei. Caseous necrosis is surrounded by epithelioid histiocytes, forming a "tubercle" that mimics *Mycobacterium tuberculosis* infection.

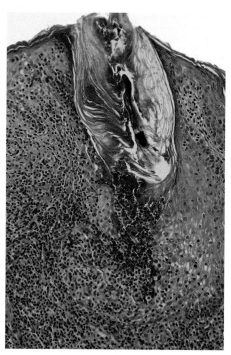

FIGURE 18-10. Eosinophilic pustular folliculitis. Eosinophils and lymphocytes surround and infiltrate the follicle, forming intrafollicular eosinophilic micropustules.

with central healing and peripheral spread (116). Although most reported cases have been from Japan, the condition is now known to be geographically more widespread. Lesions typically involve seborrheic areas, including the face, trunk, and upper arms, with documented reports of extrafollicular lesions of the palms and soles (117). Moderate leukocytosis and eosinophilia in the peripheral blood may be present. There is usually spontaneous healing over months to years (118). There are reports of the eruption in children (119,120), including neonates (121), and in this subset lesions occur predominantly on the scalp. Scarring alopecia of the scalp in an adult has been reported (122). Although a cause has not been identified, rare medication-induced cases have been described, due to carbamazepine (123), after patch testing with minocycline (124) and indeloxazine hydrochloride (125), and after prolonged treatment with oral corticosteroids in a patient with pustulosis palmoplantaris (126). One case was associated with nevoid basal-cell carcinoma syndrome (127).

Lesions with similar histology are well documented in patients with HIV infection (128), including children with HIV (129), and other immunocompromised conditions, such as myelodysplastic syndrome (130), non-Hodgkin's lymphoma (131), B-cell chronic lymphatic leukemia (132), and after bone marrow transplantation (133). There appear to be enough clinical dissimilarities from the disorder described by Ofuji to consider HIV-associated disease a distinct entity, and use of the terms *eosinophilic folliculitis* or *HIV-associated eosinophilic folliculitis* was recommended to reflect this (128). Another classification scheme proposed the designations classical, pediatric, and HIV-associated (134). In HIV patients, lesions tend to be urticarial papules with less tendency to become pustular, and leukocytosis is less common (135). They are most commonly found on the face, scalp, and upper trunk, and are often excoriated.

Histopathology. In Ofuji's disease, there is exocytosis of eosinophils into a spongiotic follicular infundibulum and accompanying sebaceous gland, eventually forming eosinophilic micropustules (122,136,137) (Fig. 18-10). The epidermis adjacent to the affected follicle may contain lymphocytes and eosinophils, with the latter aggregating into small eosinophilic pustules that are subcorneal or intraepidermal; these epidermal changes reflect the histologic picture seen in palmoplantar lesions, where follicles are absent (117,138). In more inflamed lesions, neutrophils may be present (117). In the dermis, there are perivascular and interstitial infiltrates of lymphocytes and numerous eosinophils that may surround sweat glands (139). Associated follicular mucinosis has been reported (140).

A study of 52 biopsies in 50 HIV-positive patients best described the histology of *HIV-associated eosinophilic folliculitis* (135). Perifollicular and intrafollicular lymphocytes and eosinophils are concentrated about the isthmus, and may involve the sebaceous duct. There is spongiosis of the follicular epithelium. Eosinophils and lymphocytes may be seen aggregating in the hair canal, but neutrophils are rare. In early lesions, lymphocytes may predominate and be distributed perifollicularly and interstitially. In more developed lesions, dermal inflammation diminishes and perifollicular/follicular inflammation increases. Less common findings include inflammation of the sebaceous gland, eosinophilic pustules, and follicular rupture (135). Dense eosinophilic infiltrates with degranulation and flame figures, resembling Well's syndrome, may sometimes be seen. A small number of macrophages can be present. Bacteria, yeast, or *Demodex* may be identified, albeit away from the areas of inflammation. Since the disorder is highly pruritic, excoriation is a common secondary finding.

Features that may help to distinguish suppurative folliculitis in HIV-positive patients from *HIV-associated eosinophilic folliculitis* include an infiltrate dominated by neutrophils and macrophages, the presence of microorganisms amid the inflammation, and rupture of the involved follicle. The use of transverse histologic sections has been advocated over vertical sections for increasing diagnostic sensitivity and demonstrating the key pathologic findings in HIV-associated eosinophilic folliculitis (141).

Pathogenesis. The cause of Ofuji's disease (EPF) is not known. Although the prevalence in Japan could not be explained by HLA patterns (122), the occurrence in brothers in the neonatal period hints at some inherited predisposition or possibly an infectious etiology (142).

The perivascular infiltrating cells in EPF were found to be mostly T-lymphocytes, with some CD68+ myelomonocytic cells, and most of the eosinophils were positive for eosinophil cationic protein (143). A moderate increase in the number of tryptase-positive, chymase-negative mast cells, the type predominantly found in the lung and small intestine, was noted around hair follicles and sebaceous glands (136). A study of Ofuji's disease found markers of sebaceous differentiation to be decreased or absent, while follicular differentiation markers were expressed normally (118).

In another study of three patients with EPF, serum levels of interferon γ and interleukins 2, 4, and 6 were measured before and after successful treatment with indomethacin (144). In the EPF patients, investigators found elevated IL-4 that remained unchanged after treatment, and increased interferon γ with disease remission. Decreased expression of IL-5 mRNA in peripheral blood mononuclear cells was demonstrated after the disease was controlled in two EPF patients undergoing treatment with interferon γ (145); IL-5 is responsible for the growth and differentiation of eosinophils.

Ultrastructurally, in EPF lesions characterized by an infundibular pustule, acantholytic outer root sheath keratinocytes showed desmosomal cleavage with microvilli formation, and some contained sebaceous lipid droplets (146). Apposition of T-lymphocytes and Langerhans cells was seen.

In the differential diagnosis, eosinophilic follicular pustules may be seen in erythema toxicum neonatorum, and intraepidermal eosinophilic vesicles can be seen both in acropustulosis and the vesicular phase of incontinentia pigmenti. However, the clinical presentation of these conditions would generally be significantly different than EPF, although it has been suggested that EPF in infants and infantile acropustulosis may be variants of the same disorder (147). Identical eosinophilic pustular eruptions have been described in association with *Pseudomonas* infection (148), and in fungal infections due to dermatophyte (149).

Follicular Mucinosis and Alopecia Mucinosa

Follicular mucinosis is characterized clinically by grouped erythematous papules and/or plaques that may be markedly indurated or nodular, and histologically by mucin accumulation in hair follicles. It is now classified into two types: a primary (idiopathic) type and a secondary variety. The *primary* form tends to have a shorter but benign course. The *secondary* type has been associated with numerous benign and malignant conditions, including lymphomas, of which the majority are mycosis fungoides. A distinct variant of mycosis fungoides, follicular mycosis fungoides, may or may not be associated with follicular mucinosis (150,151).

The *primary* form tends to affect children and young adults more frequently and resolves spontaneously in several months (acute benign type) or several years (chronic benign type) (152). It is often confined to the head and neck, but may be disseminated. The *secondary* type tends to form more widespread plaques and is almost always a disorder of adults.

The secondary type has been found in association with other lympho proliferative disorders including Hodgkin's disease (153–155), cutaneous B-cell lymphoma (156), acute myeloblastic leukemia (157), chronic lymphocytic leukemia (155), and syringolymphoid hyperplasia with cutaneous T-cell lymphoma (158), as well as a number of inflammatory cutaneous disorders such as chronic discoid lupus erythematosus (159), angiolymphoid hyperplasia (160), alopecia areata (161), eosinophilic pustular folliculitis (140), spongiotic dermatitis, lichen striatus, arthropod bites, sarcoidosis, Goodpasture's syndrome (162,163), leprosy (164), and growths such as verrucae (162), melanocytic nevi (165), and squamous cell carcinoma of the tongue (166). The numerous associations with production of follicular mucin certainly suggest that this is a relatively nonspecific reaction pattern.

There has been controversy as to whether the histopathology allows for distinction between the primary and secondary forms. Initially it was considered that the histopathology could be predictive (167). Later, some researchers claimed that transition from the benign form to a lymphomatous type could occur (168–170), while others disputed this finding (162). In 1989 a study of 59 cases concluded that there was no clinical or pathologic pattern by which the ultimate outcome of the condition could be predicted (153).

Others have reported that adults over the age of 40 years with widespread follicular mucinosis are at increased risk for mycosis fungoides or Sézary syndrome (162,169), although Cerroni et al. (170) recently published that criteria purported to differentiate lymphoma-associated follicular mucinosis from the idiopathic type were not effective. A long-term follow-up study (median 10 years) of seven patients aged less than than 40 years with primary follicular mucinosis failed to demonstrate progression to cutaneous T-cell lymphoma, despite the presence of a T-cell clone in five of the patients (171).

In 1957, Pinkus described *alopecia mucinosa,* the term used when follicular mucinosis affects terminal hair-bearing areas and is associated with hair loss (172). Papules and plaques may be present or inconspicuous in this form, which may show only alopecia that is usually complete and well circumscribed (173). Scarring is seen more commonly when the alopecia mucinosa is associated with cutaneous T-cell lymphoma.

Histopathology. Within the outer root sheath and sebaceous gland epithelium, there is reticular epithelial degeneration that sometimes evolves into more extensive cavitation, within which mucin is deposited (174) (Fig. 18-11). Occasionally, little mucin can be detected, perhaps because of removal of this water-soluble material in the processing procedure (175). The deposited mucin is an acid mucopolysaccharide that stains metachromatically with toluidine blue at pH 3.0, as well as with alcian blue in acid pH. The fact that it can be substantially removed by digestion with hyaluronidase demonstrates that the mucin is predominantly hyaluronic acid. Colloidal iron stain may also be used.

Inflammation is composed of lymphocytes and histiocytes, but there may also be eosinophils. There may be exocytosis into the outer root sheath epithelium of the infundibulum and the sebaceous gland epithelium. Although individual pathologic criteria are not absolutely diagnostic of the type of follicular mucinosis (primary or secondary), features that have been proposed as favoring a lymphoma-associated lesion include an atypical lymphocytic infiltrate or increased density of the perifollicular infiltrate with substantial folliculotropism (176) (Fig. 18-12). This study also suggested that a prominent eosinophilic infiltrate and more substantial mucin deposition tend to favor a benign

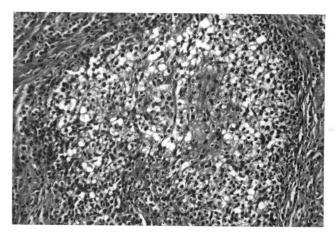

FIGURE 18-12. Follicular mucinosis associated with follicular mycosis fungoides. In addition to changes of follicular mucinosis, there is extensive folliculotropism of lymphocytes with irregularly shaped nuclei.

process, but a more recent study failed to substantiate these findings (153).

Pathogenesis. Electron microscopic studies have shown that the mucin is a product of the outer root-sheath epithelial cells. The cytoplasm shows prominent, dilated, rough-surfaced endoplasmic reticulum containing fine, granular, filamentous material that is secreted into intercellular spaces (177). In two patients with primary, idiopathic alopecia mucinosa with reversible alopecia, I found, using transverse sections, an increased number of resting-phase follicles, mostly catagen, ranging from 46% to 92% of all terminal follicles (unpublished data).

Keratosis Pilaris

This common persistent condition characteristically affects the lateral aspect of the arms, thighs, and buttocks. Keratotic follicular papules, sometimes with surrounding erythema, are present. It is usually asymptomatic and occasionally diffuse. Keratosis pilaris may be seen in association with ichthyosis vulgaris (178), and appears to be more common in patients with atopic dermatitis.

Similar lesions may form as part of a variety of more extensive erythematous keratinizing disorders. Keratosis pilaris atrophicans (179) represents a spectrum of clinical conditions, including keratosis follicularis spinulosa decalvans (180,181), in which the involved follicle becomes atrophic and destroyed, sometimes associated with scarring alopecia of the scalp.

Histopathology. An orthokeratotic keratin plug blocks and dilates the orifice and upper portion of the follicular infundibulum (Fig. 18-13). A twisted hair shaft may be trapped within this keratin material, and mild perivascular mononuclear cell infiltrates are usually present in the adjacent dermis.

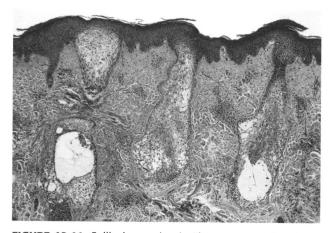

FIGURE 18-11. Follicular mucinosis. The outer root sheath epithelium of several follicles shows reticular degeneration with areas of cavitation that contain strands of bluish-staining mucin.

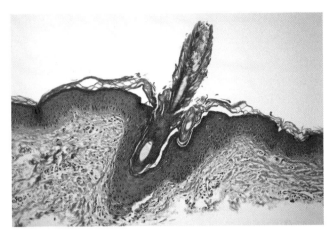

FIGURE 18-13. Keratosis pilaris. The follicle is plugged with compact orthokeratin that protrudes above the skin surface.

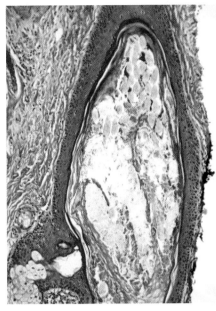

FIGURE 18-14. Trichostasis spinulosa. A dilated follicular infundibulum with retention of multiple vellus hair shafts. The granular grey-blue material is resident bacteria of the follicle.

A similar condition, lichen spinulosus (182), shows a very similar histologic picture except that the keratin plug may protrude more substantially above the follicular orifice and contain one or more hair shafts (183). Lesions similar to keratosis pilaris may also be seen in phrynoderma (see Chapter 16), but the follicular keratin plug is said to be parakeratotic (184).

Pathogenesis. Genetic factors may play a role in this condition. Patients with a generalized form of keratosis pilaris were found to have a chromosome 18p deletion, implicating a gene on the short arm of chromosome 18 (185).

Trichostasis Spinulosa

Trichostasis spinulosa is a fairly common condition that may present clinically as raised follicular spicules, as open comedones, or be inapparent (186). It occurs predominantly on the face, nose, or cheeks of middle-aged and older individuals, but has been reported in a pediatric patient (186). It may be pruritic.

Histopathology. Affected hair follicles demonstrate retention of small hair shafts within a dilated infundibulum, sometimes enveloped in a keratinous sheath (Fig. 18-14). As many as 20 or more hair shafts may be trapped in this way, often projecting above the skin surface (187). A perifollicular mononuclear infiltrate may be present (188). In a clinical setting, the follicular plugs may be easily extracted with fine forceps or a comedone extractor and examined microscopically, demonstrating a cluster of vellus hairs within a keratinous plug.

Pathogenesis. The etiology of trichostasis spinulosa is not known for certain. The retained hairs demonstrate normal telogen club structures, which suggest a normally functioning follicle. Congenital dysplasia of the hair follicles, as well as external factors such as dust, oils, ultraviolet light, heat, and irritants have been proposed (186,188–190). One hypothesis is that hair shaft entrapment is the result of

hyperkeratosis in the follicular infundibulum, thus producing an obstruction to normal hair shedding (189,191,192).

DISEASES OF HAIR FOLLICLES LEADING TO HAIR LOSS—ALOPECIA

A discussion of alopecia generally pertains to loss of hair on the scalp, although other body sites can be affected, as is the case with alopecia areata, trichotillomania, telogen effluvium, and lichen planopilaris, to name a few. A useful way to broadly classify the alopecias is to divide them into nonscarring and scarring types, depending on their (relative) propensity to culminate in permanent hair loss. To take an algorithmic approach to the alopecias, see an excellent paper on the subject by Solomon (193). It is also important to keep in mind that more than one process can contribute to the hair loss; the histology may show features that overlap with various types of alopecia, not allowing it to be put neatly into a single disease category. For example, scarring alopecia can occur in a patient with underlying androgenetic alopecia.

Some types of alopecia are discussed elsewhere in this text, such as lichen planopilaris (Chapter 7), lupus erythematosus (Chapter 10), syphilitic alopecia (Chapter 22), perfolliculitis capitis abscedens et suffodiens (Chapter 21), folliculitis "acne" keloidalis nuchae (Chapter 21), and alopecia neoplastica (Chapter 36). Although hair shaft disorders result in alopecia, a diagnosis is often made on clinical grounds and based on examination of hair shafts rather than biopsy material; therefore, a discussion of hair shaft disorders will not be included here, but can be found in one of several review articles (194,195). Alopecia that is easily diagnosed in the clinical setting based on history, physical examination, and microscopic assessment of gently pulled hairs, thereby negating the need for a scalp biopsy, will also not be discussed; these include postoperative pressure-induced alopecia, temporal triangular alopecia, and loose anagen syndrome. Those forms of alopecia that are more commonly encountered (and more frequently biopsied) will be covered here.

General Considerations in Diagnosing Alopecia: Scalp Biopsy

A punch biopsy or incisional biopsy extending into fat to include terminal hair bulbs is necessary for proper evaluation of alopecia. Punch biopsy is easier for the clinician to perform, and most scalp biopsies are submitted as such. It is generally accepted that at least a 4-mm punch be used in order to obtain a sufficient number of hairs for study. Also, many of the published quantitative parameters for diagnosing different forms of alopecia are based on a 4-mm punch, so this is the one that is generally recommended (196).

Controversy exists regarding the manner in which the punch biopsy should be sectioned: vertically, where the cylinder of tissue is bisected longitudinally, the standard way of sectioning punched specimens procured for other cutaneous disorders, or horizontally (a.k.a. transversely), where the skin cylinder is "bread-loafed," the method pioneered by Headington (197). Horizontal sectioning enables visualization of all the follicles in the specimen (Fig. 18-15), whereas it has been estimated that conventional vertical sections demonstrate only 10% to 15% of the follicles in the sample (197). Dermatopathologists appear to

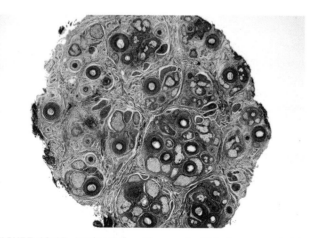

FIGURE 18-15. Horizontal section, scalp. This 4-mm punch biopsy was sectioned horizontally (a.k.a. transversely), enabling visualization of every follicle in the specimen. At this level, through the mid-dermis near the isthmus, arrangement of pilosebaceous structures into "follicular units" is apparent on the right half of the specimen.

be polarized with regard to which method of sectioning is preferable. Of dermatopathologists who favor vertical sections, some feel that they can glean as much information if serial sections are obtained, and some feel uncomfortable interpreting hair follicle anatomy and pathology in a horizontal orientation. A notable disadvantage of transverse sections is the inability to properly evaluate the epidermis (193). However, when a transversely sectioned biopsy is cut through, a portion of the epidermis can usually be seen and evaluated, albeit tangentially.

Some authors have recommended that two 4-mm punch biopsies be performed from the area of disease activity, and that one biopsy be sectioned transversely and the other sectioned vertically. The latter is bisected at the time of the biopsy with one-half sent for routine histology (embedded with the two halves of the transversely sectioned specimen), and the other half processed for direct immunofluorescence (198). In some forms of nonscarring alopecia such as telogen effluvium or early androgenetic alopecia where the histologic findings may be subtle, it may be helpful to take one specimen from the involved vertex of the scalp and one specimen from the occiput; comparing the two, the occipital scalp should be relatively normal in androgenetic alopecia, and equally involved in telogen effluvium. Certainly a single biopsy is preferable from a patient morbidity standpoint, and a single biopsy may be sufficient (199).

For diagnosis of cicatricial alopecia, the recommendation is for one 4-mm punch biopsy specimen from the edge of an involved area where there is new hair loss, a positive hair-pull test, or inflammation as evidenced by clinically apparent erythema (200). The optimal area to sample to assess the potential for hair regrowth (prognosis) is an older, more central area with a "burnt-out" appearance.

In the past, serial horizontal sections would result in numerous sections and multiple slides to review, typically 12 to 20 (199). A proposed method for improving the convenience of transverse processing recommended trisecting or quadrisecting the specimen, inking one side of each resultant disk of tissue in a consistent orientation, then embedding them all in a single cassette so that several microanatomic levels can be viewed on a single slide (199). My experience with this technique, while convenient, is that it would sometimes result in loss of tissue (sometimes critical tissue), as laboratory personnel would significantly efface some of the tissue pieces in order to obtain a "good" slice of *all* of the tissue disks. This can occur particularly when the pieces of tissue are embedded at slightly different levels in the paraffin block.

I have found that a "safer" way to process the punch specimen to avoid loss of tissue is to bisect it once transversely, approximately 1 mm below the epidermal surface, ink the cut surfaces, and embed the two pieces so that the inked surfaces are cut first, a method previously advocated (193,197). Deeper levels from the block will reveal sections that approach the epidermis for one piece of tissue and the subcutis for the other piece of tissue. The ideally obtained punch biopsy for this type of processing would be oriented parallel to the direction of hair growth, decreasing the frequency that hairs are transected by the biopsy procedure. The result is a cylinder of scalp skin in which the sides of the cylinder are not exactly perpendicular to the epidermal surface. With this in mind, when the specimen is bisected 1 mm below the epidermis, the cut should be angled parallel to the epidermal surface (not perpendicular to the sides of the tissue cylinder), so that each histologic section will show all the follicles at roughly the same microanatomic level, which facilitates their interpretation. As a consequence, however, follicles and hair shafts will appear ovoid in shape under the microscope.

Personally, I prefer interpreting transverse sections whenever possible, and this chapter emphasizes this method. Transversely sectioned scalp biopsies offer the following advantages (193): (a) *all* the follicles in the biopsy specimen can be seen and studied, (b) it allows for rapid evaluation of hair density and follicular units, (c) it allows for accurate assessment of follicle size, (d) pathological alterations at different levels of the follicle can easily be evaluated, and (e) it facilitates quantitative interpretation of the biopsy. In my experience, it is a more sensitive technique for detecting tinea capitis when only scattered follicles are involved. Horizontal sections are ideal for evaluating the number of viable follicles and estimating prognosis for hair regrowth. As previously mentioned, interpretation of horizontal sections requires a thorough understanding of hair follicle microanatomy, as well as the normal hair cycle. These are superbly described in Chapter 3, and in other sources (193, 197,201), and will not be reiterated here.

Recently introduced terms include *exogen*, a distinct phase of the hair cycle in which the hair shaft is actively shed, most likely by a proteolytic mechanism (202,203), and *kenogen*, referring to the empty hair follicle after the telogen hair is shed (204). Kenogen is believed to represent a physiologic rest period for the follicle prior to initiation of a new growth phase.

General Considerations in Diagnosing Alopecia: Terminology Defined

Solomon and Templeton (205) note that "working definitions" are "important in the microscopic evaluation of alopecia," although "these definitions are arbitrary and therefore debatable." Although authors have differed in the definitions used to characterize hair follicles, the following definitions are commonly employed. A terminal hair was designated by Headington (197) as having a hair shaft diameter ≥0.06 mm and a vellus hair as having a hair shaft diameter ≤0.03 mm (197). Between terminal and vellus hairs are intermediate hairs (a.k.a. indeterminate), whose shaft diameter, *i*, measures 0.06 mm > *i* > 0.03 mm (Fig.

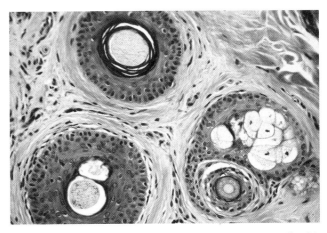

FIGURE 18-16. Normal hairs of varying size (horizontal). This level is through the infundibulum of the terminal follicle (*top*), which shows epidermal-type keratinization with presence of a granular layer. The vellus hair (*right*) is identifiable by a hair shaft diameter that is equal to or less than the thickness of the inner root sheath. An intermediate hair (*lower left*) has a shaft diameter that is between the other two.

18-16). A micrometer is sometimes needed to accurately assess hair shaft diameter, although without actually measuring them, hair follicles can be classified by comparison of the shaft size to the width of the inner root sheath; the diameter of a vellus hair shaft should be less than or equal to the thickness of the inner root sheath (Fig. 18-16). Qualitatively, terminal hairs have their bulbs anchored in the subcutaneous fat, while vellus hair bulbs are in the upper to mid-dermis. *True* vellus hairs lack melanin pigment and are small throughout their existence, while *miniaturized* vellus hairs are terminal hairs that have decreased in size. Since these are histologically identical, it is not necessary to distinguish them for the purpose of diagnosing alopecias; henceforth in this chapter, the term *vellus hairs* will encompass true vellus hairs and miniaturized terminal hairs. While some authors group intermediate hairs with the terminal hair population for the purpose of quantification, I prefer to include them with the vellus group, since more often they represent a transitional follicle undergoing the process of miniaturization to a vellus hair. Reversal of the process via therapy with minoxidil or finasteride can confuse the picture. A cross-section at the lower infundibular level is optimal for visualizing vellus hairs, allowing one to accurately count terminal and vellus hair shafts in order to determine the terminal: vellus hair ratio.

In determining the "telogen" count or anagen to "telogen" ratio, the term *telogen* actually encompasses all phases of the nonanagen follicle, including telogen (characterized by the presence of the club hair), catagen, and telogen germinal unit (Fig. 18-17), since they all represent stages in a continuum—the irreversible process of hair follicle regression and shedding. For instance, a catagen follicle, with an

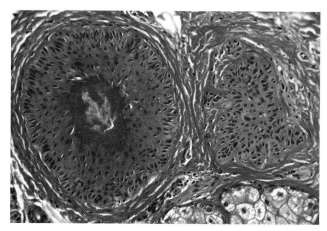

FIGURE 18-17. Normal resting follicles (horizontal). The follicle at *left* shows a telogen club, recognizable by trichilemmal keratinization with a brightly eosinophilic, attached shaft. To the *right* is a telogen germinal unit, a structure found in the mid- to upper-dermis that is characterized by follicular epithelium with radial projections, often reminiscent of the shape of a daisy. In vertical sections, this structure is sometimes visible just beneath the club hair.

epithelial column in the lower dermis, will often show a club structure near the isthmus. Although vellus hairs also cycle, only terminal-sized follicles in catagen and telogen are counted as part of the regressing/resting hair population. The telogen count attained histologically, using these definitions, reflects the count obtained in the clinical setting by forcible hair pluck (using a rubber-tipped hemostat), as this method is unsuccessful at dislodging the smaller, vellus hairs (201,206).

A cross-section through the isthmus is optimal for assessing the number of telogen and catagen hairs, and telogen germinal units. This telogen count should be interpreted in the context of a second count at the infundibular

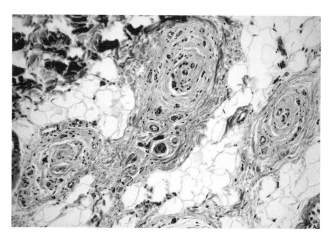

FIGURE 18-18. Fibrous streamers (horizontal). Also known as stellae, these collapsed fibrous sheaths are subcutaneous evidence of hairs that have moved upward through the process of miniaturization or conversion to catagen. They consist of concentrically arranged collagen with numerous capillaries and an increased number of mast cells.

level to assess terminal and vellus hairs, as follicles in telogen or catagen according to their appearance near the isthmus will show a shaft in the infundibulum that looks identical to a terminal anagen follicle; that is, a hair shaft with a diameter ≥0.06 mm "floating" in the infundibular hair canal. Often the infundibular portion of the hair shaft, untethered by the inner root sheath, will be missing, presumably carried away by the microtome blade. In this situation, the pathologist must rely on the caliber of the follicular outer root sheath as well as the diameter of the empty hair canal to extrapolate the size of the hair shaft and obtain more accurate counts.

Miniaturization and conversion to catagen and telogen leave many collapsed fibrous root sheaths in the subcutis (Fig. 18-18). Also known as "stellae" and "fibrous streamers," they are found in all conditions where there is follicular miniaturization, as in androgenetic alopecia, or increased numbers of catagen and telogen hairs, as in telogen effluvium and trichotillomania.

General Considerations in Diagnosing Alopecia: Normal Parameters

Parameters of normal as determined by examination of transversely sectioned scalp biopsies have been published in various sources, and are typically based on a 4-mm punch biopsy. Most were from studies of Caucasian subjects, but ethnic differences in "normal" values have been demonstrated, and this must be taken into consideration when evaluating a scalp biopsy. Caucasians without alopecia should have approximately 40 total hairs in a 4-mm punch biopsy, with roughly 20 to 35 terminal hairs and 5 to 10 vellus hairs (196,197,206,207). The normal terminal: vellus hair ratio for adult scalp is 3 to 4:1 (197), but at least 2:1 (208). In another study, a value of 7:1 was found (207).

Hair density in African Americans was found to be significantly lower than in whites, with an average of 18 terminal and 3 vellus hairs in a 4-mm punch biopsy (209). However, the follicles are typically larger (210). In Koreans, the follicular density was found to be significantly lower than in whites and blacks (211).

Hair follicles on the scalp are arranged in follicular units, bundles of hairs naturally found together. They form hexagonal modules separated from one another by intervening collagen, and are best visualized by transverse sections through the upper dermis near the isthmus (Fig. 18-15) (212). There are typically 10 to 12 follicular units in a 4-mm punch (193). Each follicular unit normally contains two to five terminal hairs and zero to two vellus hairs, along with sebaceous glands and arrector pili muscles (196).

NONSCARRING ALOPECIA

Alopecia that is nonscarring will clinically show intact follicular ostia, and histologically will show a normal density of hair follicles. Despite being categorized as "non-scarring," conditions such as androgenetic alopecia, long-standing alopecia areata, and traction alopecia can lead to irreversible loss of hair follicles. Transverse sections are particularly useful in the histologic diagnosis of nonscarring alopecias, as the anagen to telogen ratio and terminal to vellus hair ratios may be crucial in making an accurate diagnosis. In particular, female patients with a fairly diffuse, nonscarring alopecia can be a diagnostic dilemma based on clinical grounds alone, and a biopsy can help. The main diagnostic possibilities in this setting are (a) female pattern hair loss, (b) acute and chronic telogen effluvium, (c) diffuse alopecia areata, and (d) loose anagen syndrome (213).

Alopecia Areata

Alopecia areata (AA) is characterized clinically by complete or nearly complete absence of hair in one or more circumscribed areas of the scalp. Clinical inflammation, typically manifested by erythema, is not obvious, and the follicular openings are preserved, a clinical finding that allows the examiner to make the assessment of a nonscarring alopecia. In active areas of involvement, hair shedding is seen, as well as some short, fractured hair shafts, including the pathognomonic "exclamation point" hair. Complete scalp involvement (*alopecia totalis*) may occur suddenly or through prolonged, progressive disease. Complete or nearly complete loss of all body hair (*alopecia universalis*) can also occur. Involvement of the eyebrows and eyelashes and regularly spaced pits on the surface of the nails may also be seen. The majority of patients with localized disease undergo spontaneous resolution, but others show persistent disease, and a few patients will have permanent hair loss. "The only predictable thing about the progress of alopecia areata is that it is unpredictable" (214), essentially stating that one cannot reliably predict which patients will have limited disease with spontaneous resolution and which will have recurrent disease or chronic, severe disease.

Histopathology. The diagnostic pathologic feature is peribulbar lymphocytic inflammation ("swarm of bees") affecting anagen follicles (Fig. 18-19) or follicles in early catagen. The inflammatory assault on anagen follicles induces a premature conversion to catagen (Fig. 18-20). Consequently, the number of catagen and telogen follicles found may be marked, approaching 100% (215,216). Follicles may enter a persistent phase of telogen in which the hair shaft has already been shed, manifested by the *telogen germinal unit* (216) (Fig. 18-17). As follicles enter catagen, peribulbar inflammation frequently disappears, but the lymphocytic infiltrate in later catagen may be present around the epithelial remnant of the receding follicle, and also within and surrounding the collapsed follicular sheaths. Telogen hairs show little to no perifollicular inflammation.

Lymphocytes may also be seen sparsely infiltrating the matrix epithelium of anagen follicles, inducing damage to the matrical cells that includes intra- and intercellular

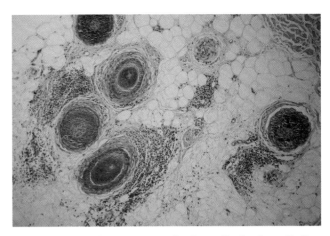

FIGURE 18-19. Alopecia areata (horizontal). Classic peribulbar lymphocytic inflammation likened to a "swarm of bees."

edema, cellular necrosis, and microvesicle formation. As a result of injury to bulbar melanocytes and keratinocytes, pigment casts, which are clumps of melanin pigment, may be found within the dermal papilla, the sheath of miniaturizing or regressing follicles, or in the follicular epithelium (208). Pigment casts are more often found in trichotillomania; one interpretation of their presence in the context of AA is that here, too, they represent external manipulation of the hair (217). Pigment casts have also been found in postoperative pressure-induced alopecia, leading those authors to postulate that they resulted from the sudden conversion of follicles from anagen to catagen, as occurs in trichotillomania and AA (218).

The inflammatory assault may produce dysmorphic follicles and shafts (Fig. 18-21). Anagen hairs not sufficiently damaged so as to enter prematurely into catagen may continue to manufacture a hair shaft, one which may be small, distorted, and often non-pigmented (trichomalacia). The

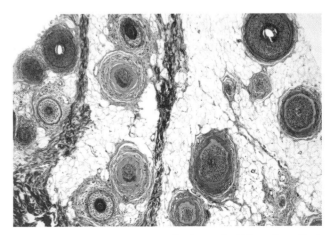

FIGURE 18-20. Alopecia areata (horizontal). Although peribulbar inflammation is not obvious here, the combination of an increased number of resting hairs and miniaturized hairs is characteristic of alopecia areata. Catagen follicles are notable by their eosinophilic "glassy" membrane and lack of a hair shaft.

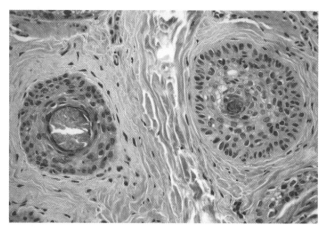

FIGURE 18-21. Alopecia areata (horizontal). Dystrophic hair shafts. The follicle at *left* has no shaft at all; the inner root sheath completely fills the canal. The follicle on the *right* is producing a minute, "pencil-point" hair shaft that will break easily.

hair shaft may taper to a point so tiny and fragile that it fractures. Small, abnormal follicles called *nanogen* hairs are a distinctive finding in long-standing cases (210). They are difficult to categorize as anagen, catagen, or telogen hairs, and in transverse sections they show only a minute, incompletely keratinized hair shaft, or no shaft at all.

As telogen follicles re-enter anagen, they again come under attack from pathogenic lymphocytes which precipitate premature conversion to catagen once again, so that anagen duration becomes shorter and shorter, and the follicles begin to miniaturize (Fig. 18-20). As the follicles decrease in size, they become situated more superficially, though often deeper than normal vellus hairs, with their bulbs situated in the mid to lower dermis (208). With disease chronicity, most of the hairs will become miniaturized. Miniaturization and conversion to catagen and telogen leave many collapsed fibrous root sheaths in the subcutis (Fig. 18-20).

Whiting (219) found that transversely sectioned scalp biopsies showed the diagnostic features of alopecia areata more often than vertically sectioned biopsies. He also published mean quantitative hair counts for horizontally sectioned scalp biopsies of alopecia areata. The mean terminal: vellus hair ratio is similar to that seen in androgenetic alopecia (1.1:1), reflecting extensive miniaturization. The mean anagen to telogen ratio was 73%:27% and the total hair count (mean of 27 hairs) was 33% less than in the control group, with more severely affected patients (alopecia universalis) at the lower end of the spectrum. Others have also found that the follicular density can decrease in severe alopecia totalis and universalis of long duration (a decade or more), with scars replacing some of the follicular sheaths (220).

Whiting and others have emphasized the use of follicular counts to aid in the diagnosis of AA when the characteristic peribulbar inflammation is missing, with a high per-

centage of catagen or telogen hairs and miniaturized hairs as a strong sign of AA (221) (Fig. 18-20). In one study, the presence of eosinophils around the bulb and within fibrous tracts was found to be a helpful diagnostic feature of AA, identifying them in 38 of 71 patients. In biopsies lacking peribulbar lymphocytic inflammation, eosinophils were found approximately 50% of the time (222). Some plasma cells may also be present.

Some authors claim that in long-standing AA, the inflammatory infiltrates appear to diminish (215), while others believe the degree of inflammation found on biopsy does not depend on disease duration, citing cases of long-standing AA that showed a lot of inflammation (208). In a recent reappraisal of the histopathology of AA, Whiting (223) suggested that the key factor in the histologic picture was the duration of the attack, with lymphocytes surrounding mainly terminal hair bulbs in acute episodes and involving mainly miniaturized hair bulbs in chronic, recurrent disease.

In the histologic differential diagnosis, alopecia syphilitica may closely mimic active AA (224). Features that would help to distinguish syphilitic alopecia include lymphocytes situated near the isthmus, the presence of plasma cells, an endothelial reaction, interface dermatitis, or neutrophils in the stratum corneum (224,225). Although androgenetic alopecia shows diminution of follicular size, dermal infiltrates that are present in this condition are usually superficial, perivascular, and peri-infundibular. One paper discussed problematic differential diagnoses with respect to AA using a comparison of clinical and histologic features (226).

Pathogenesis. The exact pathogenesis of AA is not known, but substantial evidence exists to support a role for genetic factors, nonspecific immune and organ-specific autoimmune reactions, and environmental triggers (214,227). The antigenic stimulus for autoimmune attack may be the follicular keratinocyte, melanocyte, or dermal papilla. Advances in the understanding of alopecia in the past decade have benefited from animal models of the disease (228), including the C3H/HeJ mouse (229,230), Dundee experimental bald rat (DEBR) (231), and Smyth chicken (232). Quantitative and qualitative investigational guidelines for the study of AA were proposed in 1999 to facilitate the collaboration between researchers, data comparison, and sharing of tissue specimens (233).

Familial cases of AA are well recognized, suggesting a genetic predisposition (234). A family history of AA reportedly ranges between 10% and 42% (235,236), with higher incidences in patients with disease onset early in life and in identical twins (237). Alopecia areata has been associated with both HLA class I and class II antigens, with different forms and severity of AA found to be associated with certain HLA types (214,238,239). AA has been associated with many conditions, including Down syndrome, atopy, vitiligo, thyroid disease, pernicious anemia, diabetes, myasthenia gravis, lupus erythematosus, rheumatoid arthritis, ulcerative colitis, lichen planus, polymyalgia rheumatica,

Candida endocrinopathy syndrome, and idiopathic thrombocytopenia purpura (214,240).

In a study using indirect immunofluorescence, autoantibodies to various parts of the anagen hair follicle were found in AA patients (241). Most commonly targeted were the outer root sheath, then the matrix, inner root sheath, and hair shaft. Tobin also found serum autoantibodies to pigmented hair follicles in 100% of AA patients, but in only 44% of control patients (242).

Earlier experiments showed the peribulbar infiltrate to be composed predominantly of CD4+ cells (helper T-lymphocytes) (243,244). More recently, CD8+ cells (suppressor-cytotoxic T-lymphocytes) were implicated in the pathogenesis of AA (245,246), with experiments supporting a cooperative role between CD8+ and CD4+ T cells (247). Expression of cell adhesion molecules in the matrix epithelium, dermal papilla, and adjacent vessels has been demonstrated, suggesting a mechanism for leukocyte binding (248,249).

The immune system of the hair follicle is unique, and differs from that of the surrounding skin (250). The epithelial portion of the proximal anagen hair is immune privileged; the inner root sheath and hair matrix do not express MHC class I antigens (250–253). A theory put forth by Paus suggests that in AA, the body's immune system may begin to recognize immune-privileged hair follicle antigens as a result of up-regulated MHC molecules or down-regulation of local immunosuppressive factors (254).

Cytokines may play an important role in AA. When serum cytokine levels were measured, it was found that IL-1α and IL-4 (Th2 cytokines) were elevated in patients with localized AA, while IFN-γ and IL-2 (Th1 cytokines) were significantly increased in AA patients with severe disease (alopecia universalis) (255). IL-1α, IL-1β, and TNF-α have been shown *in vitro* to produce changes in hair follicle morphology that resemble AA (256–258). Also, a role for the peripheral nervous system has been postulated in AA, via neuropeptides with pro- and anti-inflammatory properties released in the vicinity of critical areas of the hair follicle (259–262).

Trichotillomania

Trichotillomania, now commonly referred to as *trichotill* in the name of political correctness, is a condition in which patients pull or manipulate hair from the scalp or other body sites. For example, persistent rubbing of an area of the scalp that may be pruritic, or compulsive avulsion of hair shafts, can lead to zones of alopecia characterized by sparse, ragged, broken stubble. Hair shaft breakage and loss may be associated with damage to the scalp, as evidenced by erosions or crusts. Trichotill occurs most often in children and adolescent females. In children under the age of 6, the disorder may be more benign and self-limited (263). In teens and adults, trichotill is more likely to be associated with psychopathology. It has features in common with obsessive-compulsive disorder (264,265), and in one study a large proportion of patients with trichotill also had comorbid self-injurious habits (266). Trichotill is part of the DSM-IV classification of psychiatric disorders (266). Treatment is often difficult; conventional modalities that may be tried include antidepressant or psychotropic medications, topical adjunctive therapies, and psychotherapy (263). Concomitant alopecia areata has been reported (267).

Histopathology. In horizontally sectioned biopsies of trichotill uncomplicated by the coexistence of other types of alopecia, the density of hair follicles is normal, as is the terminal to vellus hair ratio. The diagnostic finding, when seen, is distorted hair follicle anatomy, without inflammation (208) (Fig. 18-22). Specifically, the pulling of hairs can leave behind empty anagen follicles and "torn away" follicles, the result of plucked hair shafts which retain parts of the hair matrix and root sheaths (208) (Fig. 18-23). Damaged follicles enter the resting phase, leading to an increase in the percentage of catagen and telogen hairs, as high as 75% (268) (Fig. 18-24). Often the hairs do not become normal catagen hairs, appearing distorted and abnormal (208).

Pigment casts, which are clumps of melanin pigment, may be seen in the hair papilla and peribulbar connective tissue. They are also commonly seen in the upper portion of the hair follicle (Fig. 18-22) as a result of pigmented matrical cells being deposited distally as the hair is plucked (208). Pigment casts are due to injury to the hair matrix,

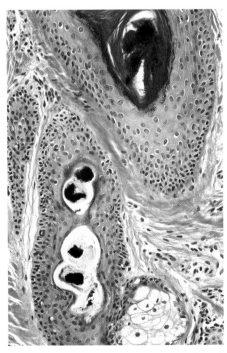

FIGURE 18-22. Trichotillomania. The hair canal is distorted in a spiral configuration, most likely secondary to twisting of the hair. Pigment casts, derived from bulbar or hair shaft melanin, are present.

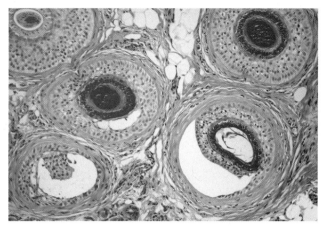

FIGURE 18-23. Trichotillomania (horizontal). At *left* is an empty anagen follicle, where a rim of outer root sheath epithelium remains after the hair was forcefully pulled, taking with it the inner root sheath and part of the outer sheath. At *right*, the follicle is partially avulsed and the shaft, which is normally tightly anchored to the inner root sheath at this level, is gone.

although some authors have theorized that they result from the sudden conversion of anagen to catagen (218). Hair shaft changes, termed *trichomalacia*, may be seen. Characterized by diminished size, distorted and odd shape, and irregular pigmentation of the shaft, trichomalacia is additional evidence of trauma to the matrix (208,268). Traumatized follicles can also show considerable distortion of the bulbar epithelium and conspicuous hemorrhage (268,269).

Since not all follicles in a given area are affected, transversely sectioned scalp biopsies may increase the yield of finding the diagnostic histologic features of trichotill, including increased numbers of catagen and telogen hairs (most cases) and empty or distorted follicles (>50% of cases) (208). The same study found pigment casts and trichomalacia in <50% of cases. When the scalp is also rubbed

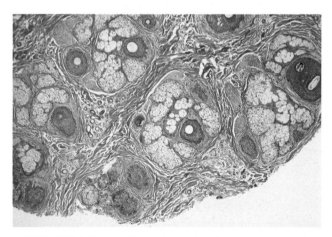

FIGURE 18-24. Trichotillomania (horizontal). Low-power view reveals an increased number of "resting" follicles, with catagen and telogen hairs, and telogen germinal units. A follicle to the *far right* contains a pigment cast.

persistently, epidermal changes of lichen simplex chronicus may be seen in vertical sections (personal observation).

In the histologic differential diagnosis, increased numbers of catagen and telogen hairs that are characteristic of trichotill may also be seen in alopecia areata and telogen effluvium. Trichotill also shares with early alopecia areata the features of a normal hair density and occasional trichomalacia, but trichotill lacks the follicular miniaturization and peribulbar infiltrates. In telogen effluvium, evidence of trauma to follicles, as discussed above, is not seen. The histologic findings in early traction alopecia are said to be identical with those of trichotill, but fewer follicles are involved and the features are less prominent (see below) (208).

Traction Alopecia

Traction alopecia is another type of mechanical alopecia, usually resulting from a variety of hair styling practices, particularly in African Americans, including tight braids, corn rows, straightening, and sponge rollers (270). Hair follicle injury is similar to that produced in trichotill, but in traction alopecia there are differences that relate to the use of less force over a greater period of time (208). Traction alopecia is often classified clinically and histologically as "early" and "late" disease (208). In early disease, tension on hair follicles exists over the course of months to a few years, while in late disease, hair is subject to traction over many years. In early disease, discontinuation of the abnormal forces on the hair will lead to regrowth of hair, but in late disease, follicles are lost, producing a permanent alopecia. Early and late disease are commonly found together in the same patient; as permanently scarred areas develop (late disease), terminal hairs at the periphery are used in styling, becoming the new target of traction (early disease) (208). Occupationally related traction alopecia has been reported due to wearing of a nurse's cap, occurring at the site of pin placement used to secure the cap (271).

Histopathology. In early traction alopecia, the histologic findings are similar to those of trichotill, albeit more subtle (208). For instance, the density of follicles is normal, with a normal number of vellus hairs. Premature conversion of anagen hairs to catagen occurs, resulting in an increased number of catagen and telogen follicles. Pigment casts and trichomalacia are sometimes found, although less often than in trichotillomania. Inflammation is absent.

In late disease, permanent loss of terminal follicles occurs, with replacement of follicular tracts by scar tissue (208). These "follicular scars" resemble columns of fibrous tissue; interfollicular areas are uninvolved. Because vellus hairs are not sufficiently large to be encompassed in the method of styling and affected by tractional forces, these hairs are preserved, and this is reflected in a normal number of vellus follicles, often outnumbering terminal follicles. In late disease, the pathology shows an "end-stage" scarring alopecia, a histologic picture shared by many forms of permanent alopecia in an advanced stage. Pigment casts and trichomalacia are not seen in late traction alopecia.

Anagen Effluvium

Acute loss of actively growing (anagen) hairs occurs as a result of a severe insult that disrupts the mitotic activity of dividing cells in the hair matrix (272), with hair shaft production suffering greatly. The shaft becomes tapered proximally, breaks at the narrowest point, and is shed. The most commonly encountered forms of anagen effluvium are from chemotherapeutic agents and radiation therapy (206), although heavy metal poisoning and other toxins should be considered (272). Rapidly progressing alopecia totalis may present as anagen effluvium.

Microscopic Examination of Hairs. Diagnosis of anagen effluvium is usually made on clinical grounds with the aid of a trichogram or gentle hair pull, so that scalp biopsies are seldom done. Resting (telogen) hairs are immune to the metabolic insult, so that when sufficient anagen hairs are lost through shedding, a forcible hair pluck performed late in the course of disease will show almost all telogen hairs; a telogen count that approaches 100% on trichogram is a clue that a type of anagen effluvium is to blame. Early on, a gentle hair pull will demonstrate "pencil-point" tapered hairs with a pointed or frayed end (206).

In contrast, in loose anagen syndrome, the proximal portion of pulled anagen hairs will show a ruffled hair shaft cuticle, as the inner and outer root sheaths are lost during extraction (206). A recent report described the loss of normal-appearing anagen hairs with an intact inner root sheath and partially intact outer root sheath in the setting of pemphigus vulgaris, where the cleavage plane is in the outer root sheath (273).

Telogen Effluvium

Effluvium is a Latin term meaning "a flowing out" (274). Telogen effluvium results from "outflowing," or shedding, of hair shafts in the telogen phase of the hair growth cycle. The concept was originally delineated by Kligman (275). This condition has many precipitating causes or associated conditions, including giving birth; serious illness, such as HIV infection; high fever; life-threatening trauma; major surgery; restrictive dieting and nutritional deficiencies; hypothyroidism; iron-deficiency anemia; medications, especially hormonal drugs; allergic contact dermatitis; the onset of androgenetic alopecia; and psychological stress (193,208,275–279). The shedding tends to occur diffusely throughout the scalp, and may involve hair over the rest of the body.

Telogen hairs are recognizable by the club structure, often enabling the diagnosis to be made on clinical evidence that includes microscopic examination of shed, pulled, or plucked hairs (trichogram), in conjunction with the history and physical examination of the scalp. In diffi-

cult cases where the differential diagnosis includes androgenetic alopecia and diffuse alopecia areata, a biopsy may be done. A scalp biopsy for horizontal sections is particularly helpful in distinguishing chronic telogen effluvium from androgenetic alopecia (280).

Chronic telogen effluvium was a concept put forth by Whiting in 1996 after studying 355 patients with the disorder (281,282). The patients are usually women aged 30 to 60 with variable shedding that persists for years. Since hairs are replaced as fast as they are shed, patients do not become bald. An obvious cause is not identified (although an initiating factor may exist); hence, the designation "idiopathic." Chronic telogen effluvium has rarely been reported in men (281,283).

Histopathology. Using vertical sectioning of scalp punch-biopsy specimens, only a subjective assessment of the proportion of follicles in telogen can be obtained. More objective analysis can be obtained by examining horizontal sections (Fig. 18-25) (284). There is a normal number of hair follicles and an absence of follicular miniaturization, unless telogen effluvium occurs in patients with established androgenetic or another form of involutional alopecia. Inflammation is generally not seen.

Telogen follicles, also recognizable in histologic sections by the club structure, are increased, but the number of catagen follicles or telogen germinal units may also be increased (Fig. 18-25). Telogen follicles in excess of 15% are considered to be abnormal and suggest a diagnosis of telogen effluvium in the absence of significant inflammation and miniaturization (207,276). Others have suggested that a level of 25% is necessary for a definitive diagnosis of telogen effluvium (208,285), while a telogen count of 20% is "presumptive" evidence (275). According to published data, the telogen count in a normal scalp may range from 0% to 25% (275), with averages of 6% (207) and 13% (275) cited. Kligman (275) also stated that telogen counts

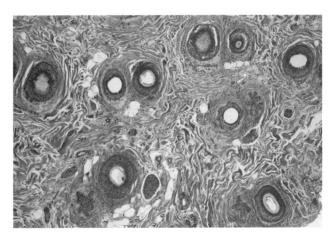

FIGURE 18-25. Telogen effluvium (horizontal). An increased number of telogen hairs is present. Approximately 40% of the 12 follicles in this field are in a stage of telogen; there are two club hairs and three telogen germinal units.

greater than 60% in telogen effluvium are rare. With a telogen count approaching 100% one should consider anagen effluvium or alopecia areata (206,208,216).

Biopsies from the crown/vertex and occiput will yield similar findings since the process is diffuse. Timing of the biopsy clearly affects the pathologic changes observed. Should a biopsy be obtained in the very early stages of recovery, follicles in early anagen will be present in addition to elevated resting follicles. However, if recovery is substantial, the histopathologic assessment may be entirely normal.

In a study of *chronic telogen effluvium*, the average number of hairs in a 4-mm punch biopsy was normal at 39, the terminal to vellus hair ratio was normal, and the average telogen count was 11% (281). In comparison, the average telogen count in androgenetic alopecia was 16.8%, and 6.5% in normal controls. Significant inflammation and fibrosis were present in only 10% to 12% of chronic telogen effluvium and control cases, as compared to 37% of androgenetic alopecia biopsies.

Pathogenesis. In the acute form, increased shedding is noted approximately 3 months after the precipitating factor; this is the timetable for regressing anagen follicles to pass through catagen into telogen. Headington described five different processes by which excessive telogen shedding may occur (276). Briefly, these processes are dependent on changes in the length of the anagen (growth) period, and on the active release of hair shafts in telogen. Teloptosis is the termination of telogen with shedding of the hair, felt to be due to loss of adhesion between the club hair and cells of the surrounding epithelium (286). These authors distinguished two kinds of telogen hairs on trichogram: those with an epithelial sheath, suggesting early telogen, and those devoid of an epithelial sheath, indicating telogen termination or teloptosis. A transcription factor that is involved in physiologic cell death via apoptosis, p53 has been implicated in normal hair follicle regression in mice, and may be important in disorders characterized by premature anagen to telogen conversion, such as telogen effluvium (287).

Androgenetic Alopecia

The hallmark of androgenetic alopecia (AGA) is follicular miniaturization, the process by which hair shafts become progressively finer and shorter. AGA results from an androgenic influence on hair follicles in certain areas of the scalp, and the pattern of involvement in the different sexes has led to use of the terminology *male-pattern* or *female-pattern hair loss*. Some prefer this terminology over AGA because the etiologic role of androgens in women is not fully determined (288–290). AGA is the most common type of hair loss in males, affecting 50% of men by age 50 and almost as many women, according to a few reports (291, 292), leading some to espouse that it is a physiologic pro-

cess, not a pathologic one (293). AGA frequently shows a familial tendency, but inheritance does not follow simple Mendelian genetics and is most likely a polygenic trait (294,295).

In male patients, the process usually begins with bifrontal thinning, often with similar changes over the vertex. In full expression of the condition, there may be almost total baldness of the entire frontal/parietal scalp. The most common pattern seen in women is one of diffuse thinning over the crown and frontal scalp with preservation of the frontal hairline. The process occurs with less severity in women, so that significant balding is unusual.

Histopathology. Satisfactory evaluation of AGA can only be achieved from transverse sectioning of punch biopsy material (207,284,296), allowing for quantitative evaluation. Furthermore, samples smaller than 4 mm in diameter show an insufficient number of follicles for meaningful results.

Diminution of follicular size, or miniaturization, is the histologic hallmark of AGA. To fully appreciate the number of miniaturized follicles, horizontal sections at the level of the lower infundibulum of terminal hair follicles should be examined, as sections below this may miss the vellus hairs whose bulbs are situated in the upper dermis (Fig. 18-26). Cursory inspection at low power reveals random variation in the caliber of hair follicles, consistent with a progressive miniaturization (Fig. 18-27) (297,298), and absence of well-defined follicular units (296). While vellus hairs can be quickly identified by the fact that their shaft diameter is less than or equal to the thickness of their inner root sheath, they are quantitatively defined as having a shaft diameter ≤0.03 mm (197). In his 1984 paper that laid the groundwork for horizontal interpretation of scalp biopsies, Headington (197) also defined terminal hairs as having a shaft diameter ≥0.06 mm, thus recognizing an intermediate/indeterminate category where the shaft diam-

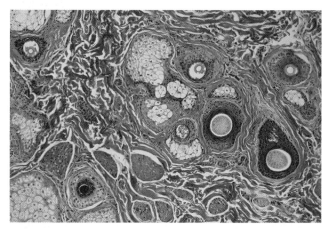

FIGURE 18-26. Androgenetic alopecia (horizontal). At a level through the lower infundibulum of terminal hairs, many vellus hairs become apparent, outnumbering the terminal follicles in this field.

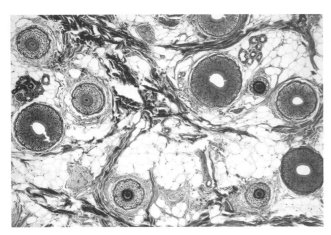

FIGURE 18-27. Androgenetic alopecia (horizontal). Even in the superficial subcutis, variability in the caliber of hair follicles, with an increased number of miniaturized hairs, is apparent. Several fibrous streamers are also seen.

eter, *i*, measures 0.06 mm > *i* > 0.03 mm, between terminal and vellus hairs (see Fig. 18-16). An optical micrometer may be used to measure hair shaft diameter, if necessary.

However, slightly different definitions were used in subsequent articles on AGA, specifically with regard to the intermediate category. For example, Whiting (207) classified terminal hairs as having a "shaft diameter exceeding 0.03 mm . . . thicker than its inner root sheath," thereby grouping intermediate hairs with the terminal hair population (207). He then used a 3:1 (or less) terminal to vellus hair ratio as being diagnostic of male pattern AGA, albeit at other times, he and others quoted a terminal to vellus hair ratio of ≤2:1 to diagnose AGA (207,208,299). Whiting (207) found the *average* terminal to vellus ratio in AGA to be 1.7:1 (207). Using similar definitions of terminal and vellus hairs, Sperling and Winton reported (296) finding an *average* terminal to vellus ratio of 1:6.1, illustrating how in advanced cases, miniaturized hairs will outnumber terminal hairs (208). In my opinion, intermediate hairs should be grouped with the vellus hair population, since more often they represent a transitional follicle undergoing miniaturization to a vellus hair (unless the patient is using agents such as minoxidil or finasteride to reverse the process). Unfortunately, ratios for normal scalp and in AGA where vellus and intermediate hairs are classified together are not available in the literature.

It is easy to undercount the number of vellus hairs, even with horizontal sections (296). Some vellus hairs may be so small as to be mistaken for keratinous debris. The use of toluidine blue stain was reported to be superior to hematoxylin and eosin in identifying the tiniest of hairs, as it stains the inner root sheath intensely blue (296). In subtle cases, comparison with a biopsy from the occipital scalp, which is typically uninvolved, may be helpful.

The onset of AGA may be manifested by a telogen effluvium (300). Whiting found the telogen count in AGA to be

16.8%, as compared to 6.5% in controls (207), with telogen counts as high as 30% reported (296). Since the reduction in follicular size is associated with a shorter anagen phase (the smaller hairs do not grow as long), at a given point in time (for a histologic specimen, this is the moment of biopsy harvest), a greater proportion of follicles will be found in telogen. Telogen hairs may show a normal club, or with increasing severity, telogen germinal units, follicular epithelium that remains after the club hair has been shed (284). Although vellus hairs continue to cycle through anagen and telogen in the papillary dermis, they are not considered to be part of the telogen count (212). Both miniaturization and increased conversion to telogen are associated with the finding of fewer terminal hair bulbs and more fibrous streamers in the deep dermis and subcutis (212). The fibrous streamers in AGA are thicker, more cellular, and possibly more fibrotic than those of normal follicles (208,301,302).

In advanced AGA, there may be a reduced hair density with permanent loss of follicles (207,296). Peri-infundibular fibroplasia, ultimately leading to focal follicular scarring, may be to blame (207,303).

Lymphocytic infiltrates, defined as activated T-cells in one study, are found around superficial vessels and in the vicinity of the lower infundibulum, sebaceous glands, and bulge in follicles transitioning to full miniaturization (301, 304). The presence of inflammation has been reported in as many as 50% (305) to 75% (303) of cases. However, mild perifollicular and upper dermal inflammation can be observed in normal scalp with a similar frequency to AGA (297), and therefore is of no value in diagnosing AGA (208). Moderate inflammation, though, was seen more often in AGA than in normals (207); the infiltrate was composed primarily of lymphocytes and histiocytes, with rare neutrophils, plasma cells, and giant cells. It has been suggested that inflammation in AGA may result from *Demodex*, seborrheic dermatitis, actinic damage, cosmetics, and grooming agents (207), and therefore should not be considered pathogenic (293). Nevertheless, its presence may have a bearing on the potential to respond to treatment. One study found AGA patients with histologic inflammation or fibrosis showed less frequent regrowth upon treatment with 2% minoxidil than AGA patients without inflammation (207), although the figures did not prove to be statistically significant. In conclusion, upper dermal inflammation can be seen in AGA, but it does not support or discount this diagnosis.

Pathogenesis. Androgens are the primary regulators of normal human hair growth. With the arrival of puberty, they transform vellus hairs in many sites, such as the axilla, to terminal hairs, while at the same time mediating the opposite effect on certain scalp follicles in predisposed individuals (306). The effects of androgens on the hair follicle are mediated via androgen receptors in the hair papilla (307). The primary androgen responsible for these effects is dihydrotestosterone (DHT), via androgen receptor binding (308). Within the follicle, the enzyme 5-α reductase produces DHT from serum testosterone. Predisposed scalp displayed high levels of DHT and increased androgen receptor expression in one study (308). In another study, frontal scalp follicles showed higher levels of androgen receptor and 5-α reductase than occipital scalp follicles, and men exhibited higher levels than women (309).

A group of investigators found that the predominant form of 5-α reductase in human scalp is type I, concentrated in sebaceous glands (310). These same investigators found 5-α–reductase type II to be present in the inner layer of the outer root sheath, the proximal inner root sheath, the infundibulum, and some in sebaceous ducts. The type II isozyme is responsible for AGA. It is preferentially inhibited by finasteride, decreasing scalp production of DHT and promoting hair growth in males with AGA (310).

Other serum hormones, such as adrenal-derived dehydroepiandrosterone, may also be converted to DHT by some hair follicles, and steroid sulfatase found in the dermal papilla may be the responsible enzyme (311). This may explain why males affected by X-linked recessive ichthyosis, due to a defect in steroid sulfatase, do not develop AGA, or only mildly (312).

Apoptosis is an important part of hair follicle regression, and therefore, factors that affect apoptosis may play a role in regulating the hair cycle (313). One study of apoptotic mechanisms in AGA suggested that levels of caspases, regulators of programmed cell death, and inhibitors of apoptosis (IAPs) may control hair follicle homeostasis (314,315). Another study found similar expression of bcl-2, p53, and other heat shock proteins in follicles from normal (occipital) scalp and follicles from scalp affected by AGA (frontal), while follicular expression of the proliferation marker Ki67 was decreased in AGA (316). The authors concluded that abnormal regulation of apoptosis was not involved in AGA, but a lower proliferation rate may be. This contradicts an analysis of bcl-2 and TUNEL staining, markers of apoptotic activity, in scalps of cadaveric males with AGA in which significant differences were noted between normal and alopecic scalp follicles (317); the apoptotic "hot spot" was identified in the bulge-isthmus region.

Whiting (212) has postulated that the process of miniaturization cannot be explained simply by shortening of the anagen phase with repeated hair cycles. He suggested that miniaturization of some follicles occurred rapidly, over the course of a single hair cycle, possibly mediated by a change in the size of the dermal papilla, as vellus follicles have smaller papillaa than terminal follicles (300,318). In cell cultures of dermal papillae derived from balding scalp follicles, the cells were smaller and did not grow as well as those derived from nonbalding scalp follicles (319).

There is evidence that fibroplasia of the adventitial sheath surrounding the hair follicle is important to the pathogenesis of AGA (301,302,320). As previously noted, fibrous streamers in AGA may be more fibrotic than those of normal follicles (208,301,302). One study found *Demodex* to be present more frequently in patients with AGA, and postulated that *Demodex*-induced inflammation could contribute to the process, and possibly plays a role in permanence (scarring) (321).

There exists a physiologic rest period during which the post-telogen follicle remains empty. This recently recognized new phase of the hair cycle was termed *kenogen* (204). This phase may last longer and occur with greater frequency in AGA (322).

SCARRING ALOPECIA

Various definitions exist for scarring (cicatricial) alopecia. A clinically relevant definition is the permanent loss of hair follicles, usually manifested on physical examination by absence of follicular ostia, sometimes with a porcelain-white appearance. Histology may or may not reveal true scar formation or inflammation, although most processes leading to permanent hair loss are inflammatory, at least initially. With this definition we can include disorders typically classified as "nonscarring" that in late stages lead to irreversible loss of hair follicles; this biphasic pattern can be seen in androgenetic alopecia, long-standing alopecia areata, and traction alopecia.

Processes that specifically target the hair follicle early in the course of the disease are *primary* scarring alopecias. *Secondary* scarring alopecias result from inflammatory or neoplastic processes that secondarily involve hair follicles. Secondary scarring alopecias will not be discussed here, nor will primary scarring alopecias whose cutaneous manifestations are predominantly non-follicular, such as lichen planopilaris and chronic cutaneous lupus erythematosus. The discussion of scarring alopecias that follows refers to *primary scarring alopecias*, as defined above.

There have been various classification schemes proposed for primary scarring alopecias, including inflammatory versus noninflammatory and neutrophil-mediated versus lymphocyte mediated (323). The usefulness of these schemes is hampered by clinical and histologic overlap between the various types of scarring alopecia, as well as a lack of uniformity in the terminology used by clinicians and dermatopathologists. This is why clinical–pathologic correlation is so important in the interpretation of scarring alopecias. Future proposals for the definitive classification of scarring alopecias will ultimately require incite into pathogenic mechanisms or biologic markers of disease, possibly provided by molecular research (196). A unifying concept of *central centrifugal scarring alopecia*, discussed later, was proposed in 2000 (324). Most recently, from a Workshop on Cicatricial Alopecia sponsored by the North American Hair Research Society, a working classification of scarring alopecia based on clinical and pathologic features was published (200), with hopes for an improved classification scheme pending additional, collaborative investigation. Most importantly, however, this workshop laid the groundwork for meaningful clinical–pathologic correlation, it set guidelines for the study of scarring alopecias in order to uncover etiologic factors, ultimately aiding in treatment, and facilitated collaboration between investigators. Needless to say, the problem of classifying scarring alopecias will not be solved in this chapter. The intent here is to present "classic" features of more commonly encountered disorders and some rarer, more recently described conditions, not to adhere to a particular classification scheme.

In one published algorithm for classifying alopecia, emphasis was placed on the pattern of fibrosis (scarring), with a branch point separating follicular fibrosis from diffuse dermal fibrosis (325). The *pattern* of scarring is important in the permanent alopecias. For example, when a condition produces enough damage to completely destroy the follicle, there is replacement of the pilosebaceous structure by scar tissue (326) (Fig. 18-28). These "follicular scars" may occur without interfollicular fibrosis. Histologically the follicular epithelium is replaced by a column of thickened collagen, sometimes surrounded by a rim of connective tissue that stains faintly blue on H&E-stained sections (Fig. 18-28).

The end stage of many forms of scarring alopecia may look similar, with the "final common pathway" characterized by decreased follicular density, absence of sebaceous glands, replacement of follicles by follicular scars that may extend into the subcutis, and sometimes tufting (see section on tufted folliculitis below). A fairly recent study of elastic tissue in various forms of permanent alopecia showed distinctive staining patterns using the Verhoeff–van Gieson

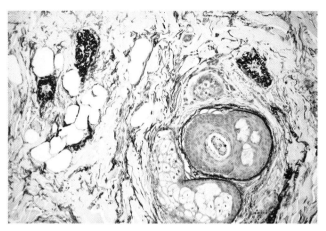

FIGURE 18-29. Pseudopelade of Brocq, elastic stain (horizontal). The elastic fibers that encircle normal follicles stain purple with the Luna stain. Three destroyed follicles have left behind their elastic sheath, characterized by concentric purple fibers with a corrugated appearance.

stain (327). Fibrous tracts of normal follicles show an elastic tissue sheath, which may be destroyed or altered by scarring and inflammation (Fig. 18-29). Cases of end-stage lichen planopilaris showed a wedge-shaped scar involving the upper one-third of the follicle where the elastic sheath was destroyed. Also, in well-developed lesions of lupus erythematosus, a broad pattern of scarring throughout the dermis was characteristic, with destruction of perifollicular elastic sheaths. In cases of "central progressive alopecia in black females" (*follicular degeneration syndrome*), the fibrous tracts were broad ("tree trunk") and outlined by an intact elastic sheath. Thickened elastic fibers were also found throughout the dermis, interpreted to be the result of "recoil" as the dermis became shrunken and hyalinized. "Idiopathic 'ivory white' pseudopelade" showed findings that were identical to this. In morphea, dermal elastic fibers were normal, and the fibrous tracts (with an intact elastic sheath) were narrow.

Although the exact pathogenesis of each type of permanent alopecia may be different, some general pathogenic mechanisms have been proposed. For instance, Headington (328) felt that the basic pathogenesis common to cicatricial alopecias was hair follicle stem cell failure. Massive synchronous apoptosis was suggested in one study (329). And in a commentary on scarring alopecias, the role of the sebaceous gland was emphasized, particularly its importance in the dissociation of the hair shaft from the inner root sheath (330); the asebia mouse is an animal model for scarring alopecia that is based on a sebaceous gland defect (331,332).

Pseudopelade of Brocq

This uncommon condition has arguably generated more controversy and confusion than any other type of alopecia. Many articles have been written about pseudopelade of Brocq (PPB), with some classifying it as a distinct clinical–pathologic entity ("classic" or "idiopathic" PPB), and others

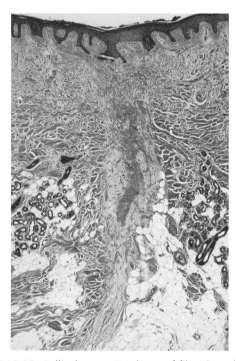

FIGURE 18-28. Follicular scar. A column of fibrosis replaces the hair follicle and extends into the subcutaneous fat.

defining it as an end stage of scarring alopecia resulting from disorders such as lichen planopilaris, discoid lupus erythematosus, scleroderma, folliculitis decalvans, chronic traction, or follicular degeneration syndrome (333,334). Therefore, each time the term is used anew, it must be defined. The salient clinical features that follow are similarly reported by both sides of the debate.

PPB is characterized by asymptomatic, discrete, scattered, or clustered, irregularly shaped, ivory- or porcelain-white patches of alopecia predominantly over the parietal scalp and vertex (323,335), and rarely on nonscalp sites such as the beard (336). The patches are sometimes atrophic, producing an appearance often likened to "footprints in the snow" (328). Late-stage lesions of lichen planopilaris, lupus erythematosus, or scleroderma can produce this same clinical picture (337). Idiopathic PPB is found mostly in Caucasians, women more than men, and occasionally in children (338). Disease progression occurs in "spurts," ultimately running its course and leaving areas of permanent alopecia. The key feature that supposedly makes idiopathic PPB distinctive is the lack of clinical inflammation throughout its course, although some theorize that an inflammatory phase exists but is fleeting (326).

In 1885, Brocq first used the term pseudopelade, which literally means pseudo alopecia areata in French (339). Later, in 1905, Brocq characterized "pseudopelade" as a distinct entity (340). How the concept of PPB subsequently changed over the 20th century was chronicled in an article by Dawber titled, "What Is Pseudopelade?" (341).

A major publication often cited in support of PPB as a separate disorder came from Pinkus (342) in 1978 in which he noted a distinctive pattern of perifollicular and interfollicular elastic tissue in PPB and other forms of scarring alopecia, using acid orcein stain. In 180 cases that satisfied the histologic criteria for idiopathic PPB established by Brocq and others, Pinkus found that the site of destroyed hair follicles (above the level of the bulge) was marked by broad cords of collagenous and elastic fibers (Fig. 18-29). He further subdivided these 180 cases into classic PPB and fibrosing alopecia, the latter characterized by less perifollicular inflammation and, more importantly, the presence of prominent elastic fibers around the lower, cycling portion of the pre-existent hair follicle. The major criticism of Pinkus' work is that his histologic criteria for PPB were not correlated with clinical findings (196).

More recently, elastic tissue staining patterns in various forms of permanent alopecia were examined using Verhoeff–van Gieson stain (327). Two cases of "idiopathic 'ivory white' pseudopelade" showed a hyalinized dermis with thickened elastic fibers, and broad fibrous tracts with an intact elastic sheath, findings indistinguishable from "central progressive alopecia in black females" (*follicular degeneration syndrome*), and similar to the findings of Pinkus.

Braun-Falco et al. (333) subsequently studied 26 cases felt to represent PPB (cases of scarring alopecia due to known, identifiable causes were excluded), and concluded that the clinical and histologic criteria proposed were distinctive enough to warrant designation as a separate disease (337).

On the other hand, many reports support idiopathic PPB as an end-stage scarring alopecia. In the 1950s, Degos et al. (343–346) noted that 70% of the time, a preceding or underlying disease could be found, so the typically described findings were called a "pseudopeladic" state. A recent study (347) used criteria established by Braun-Falco to diagnose PPB in 33 patients. Since two-thirds of these patients showed features of discoid lupus or lichen planopilaris, the authors concluded that PPB could not be considered a distinct entity. Some groups have published evidence that lichen planopilaris and PPB may be variants of the same disease. One of these groups presented four alopecic patients with clinical and histologic features of PPB who also had cutaneous and mucosal findings of lichen planus (348). The authors believed that PPB represented a less inflammatory stage in the disease spectrum of lichen planopilaris. In another study of ten patients who underwent 28 biopsies, the histologic features were not distinctive enough to differentiate PPB from lichen planopilaris (349).

In summary, the diagnosis of idiopathic PPB is one of exclusion. The terminology has become so confusing that for cases where an underlying disorder is not identifiable, Sperling et al. (324) proposes an alternate, more descriptive term: "patchy, scarring alopecia of unknown etiology."

Histopathology. Since the histologic findings of a typical lesion of PPB are those of a "burnt-out" scarring alopecia (196), clinical correlation is always necessary for accurate interpretation. The classic description of PPB is one of predominantly follicular scarring characterized by columns of fibrosis replacing hair follicles (Figs. 18-28 and 18–30), sometimes extending into the subcutaneous fat. This is accompanied by a loss or decrease of sebaceous glands,

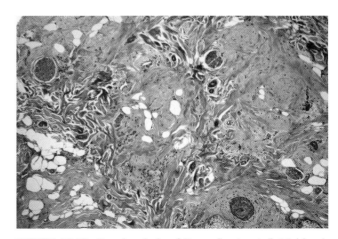

FIGURE 18-30. Pseudopelade of Brocq (horizontal). Viable pilosebaceous follicles are notably absent, replaced by follicular scars. Several unaffected arrector pili muscles remain, marking the site of former follicles.

and absence of widespread (interfollicular) scarring (206, 333). Normal arrector pili muscles remain, isolated in the mid-dermis or inserting on the vertically oriented fibrotic streams (Fig. 18-30). The epidermis may be normal or rarely atrophic, and sweat glands are normal. Marked inflammation is absent.

The apparent lack of inflammation in this disorder may be the result of a short, often missed, inflammatory phase. Such lesions were the targets of one study that found massive folliculocentric lymphocytic infiltration associated with pronounced apoptosis (329). The fact that histologic inflammation exists in some cases has lead some authors to further subdivide PPB into inflammatory and noninflammatory subtypes based on histology (350).

In two sources, the findings of early inflammatory and more developed lesions of PPB are well described (193,328). Early lesions of PPB show variable lymphocytic inflammation in the superficial dermis, which is perivascular or perifollicular, centered about the infundibulum or midpoint of the follicle. The infiltrates may extend into the follicular epithelium and occasionally into sebaceous glands, but deep perifollicular inflammation or interface alteration is not detected. With disease progression there is early loss of sebaceous glands. Inflammation becomes patchy, mild, and perivascular, and eventually disappears. There may be premature disintegration of the inner root sheath and the infundibular epithelium may become eccentrically thinned. Concentric lamellar fibrosis may be present. Fusion of infundibular outer root sheaths ("tufting") may be seen (see section on tufted folliculitis). In time, follicles are destroyed, with naked hair shafts remaining and inciting a granulomatous response. Fibrous tracts mark the site of obliterated follicles. Even features of this often-missed inflammatory phase of PPB are shared by other forms of scarring alopecia (324).

Direct immunofluorescence in PPB is negative, with occasional IgM at the basement membrane zone of the follicular infundibulum (333). Immunofluorescence changes of lupus erythematosus and lichen planopilaris should be absent (351).

Pathogenesis. As a theoretical basis for PPB, Sullivan and Kossard (334) speculated that there could occur a noninflammatory focal loss of follicles, possibly due to premature exhaustion or inhibition of the stem cell compartment to recycle. Headington (328) postulated that the pathogenesis of PPB is probably related to a T-cell mediated inflammatory process involving the bulge region. An autoimmune etiology has also been hypothesized (352,353).

An ultrastructural study of hairs and follicles from scalp affected by pseudopelade found pili torti-like hairs with oblique or longitudinal grooves and ridges, a deformed hair cuticle and cortex, and an asymmetric inner root sheath (354).

Follicular Degeneration Syndrome

Follicular degeneration syndrome (FDS) is a form of scarring alopecia that occurs almost exclusively in African-American patients, usually women, but occasionally in men (355,356). Originally described as "hot comb" alopecia (357), it was subsequently shown that use of a hot comb to straighten the hair was not requisite (355, 356). Controversy exists regarding the concept of FDS as a distinct clinicopathologic entity (358). Headington (328) did not consider it so, noting that premature desquamation of the inner root sheath, considered the pathognomonic histologic finding, was not specific for FDS and could be seen in chronic cutaneous lupus erythematosus and pseudopelade of Brocq. Others have also equated this disorder with pseudopelade of Brocq (323), or classified it under the rubric of central centrifugal scarring alopecia (324).

FDS is usually found in African-American females aged 20 through 49, and is slowly progressive. It primarily involves the crown and vertex of the scalp, expanding outward. The affected scalp becomes soft, shiny, and smooth, without follicular ostia. Clinical erythema, scaling, and induration are absent. Dysesthesia is common (355).

Histopathology. Although premature desquamation of the inner root sheath has been noted in other forms of alopecia, it is a defining feature of FDS, necessary for the diagnosis (355) (Fig. 18-31). Some consider it the earliest observable finding, and the primary event in the pathophysiology. Others consider it a secondary phenomenon (358), arguing that if it were a primary event, hair shaft defects would ensue. The inner root sheath normally degenerates at the isthmus, delimited below by the attachment point of the arrector pili muscle and above by the insertion of the sebaceous duct. "Crumbling" or absence of the inner root sheath below the isthmus, at a level through the deep dermis near the eccrine coils, or in the subcutis, characterizes this finding. Without the inner root sheath, the outer

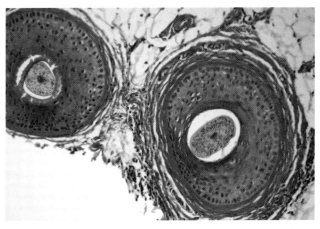

FIGURE 18-31. Follicular degeneration syndrome (horizontal). At a level through the superficial subcutis, the inner root sheath is missing from the follicle on the *right*, and the outer root sheath is eccentrically thinned.

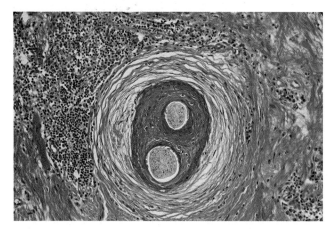

FIGURE 18-32. Follicular degeneration syndrome (horizontal). In the upper dermis, two follicles exhibit fusion of their outer root sheaths along with concentric fibrosis, focal thinning of the outer root sheath, and perifollicular lymphocytic inflammation.

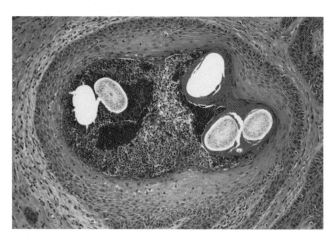

FIGURE 18-33. Folliculitis decalvans (horizontal). Several hairs share an outer root sheath that is filled with neutrophils (follicular-based pustule).

root sheath keratinizes early. Subsequent changes include eccentric thinning of the outer root sheath with migration of the hair shaft through so that it contacts the dermis, concentric lamellar fibroplasia, and perifollicular lymphocytic inflammation, usually concentrated on the side opposite penetration of the shaft through the follicular epithelium (Fig. 18-32). At the infundibular level, inflammation and lamellar fibroplasia decrease. With complete follicular destruction, a column of fibrosis remain at the site, along with arrector pili muscle. Naked hair shaft fragments may be seen, surrounded by granulomatous inflammation. Sebaceous glands are lost. A 4-mm punch biopsy contained an average of only 15 hairs in one study (355). Men with FDS displayed more active inflammation than the previously described women (356). Biopsies of FDS will typically show these changes in only a few follicles.

Pathogenesis. Although the precise etiology is unknown, hair care practices that include heat, bleaching, pomades, and traction, as well as the predominance in African Americans, suggest that environmental, cultural, and genetic factors, as well as possible structural factors unique to hair follicles in blacks, may play a role in the etiology of FDS (355).

Folliculitis Decalvans

Folliculitis decalvans (FD) is typified by a patchy pustular alopecia that recurs (328). Later lesions show areas of scarring with pustules at the periphery (328). Some authors have equated it with erosive pustular dermatosis (359). Cultures from the pustules usually reveal *Staphylococcus aureus*. While some believe the bacteria are pathogenic, others hold that they are the result of superinfection (324). When pustules are absent, the clinical picture resembles pseudopelade of Brocq (360). The finding of tufted hairs is common (361). FD has been reported in a patient with

Darier's disease (362), in other areas besides the scalp, including the beard, face, and nape (363), and in 32-year-old identical twins, suggesting a possible genetic component (364). FD is also discussed in Chapter 21 as part of the chronic deep folliculitides.

Histopathology. Early, pustular lesions will show an abscess centered about the affected follicle at the level of the lower to upper infundibulum (328) (Fig. 18-33), which may show comedonal dilatation (360). Later lesions typically show perifollicular inflammation composed predominantly of lymphocytes (Fig. 18-34), with fewer plasma cells, neutrophils, eosinophils, and giant cells (359,365). There may be hyperkeratosis, follicular plugging, and evidence of tufting (Fig. 18-34). Late-stage lesions will show follicular destruction secondary to diffuse dermal scarring (328). In such lesions the inflammation is less pronounced and is composed of lymphocytes,

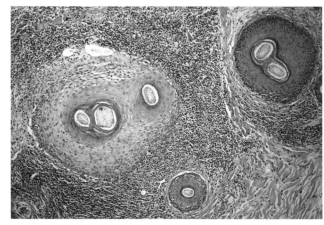

FIGURE 18-34. Folliculitis decalvans (horizontal). There is perifollicular lymphocytic inflammation, tufting, and follicular hyperkeratosis.

macrophages, and some giant cells in response to follicular remnants (365).

Pathogenesis. A number of authors believe that *S. aureus* is somehow involved in the pathogenesis of FD (365), perhaps via bacterial superantigens that stimulate the immune system without intracellular processing (366), or an abnormal host response to *S. aureus* toxins in an otherwise straightforward infection (365). There have been reports of alterations in cell-mediated and humoral immunity, neutrophil chemotaxis, and low serum complement levels (367–369). Other investigators believe the presence of pustules is due to secondary infection with *S. aureus,* or an immune response to disrupted follicles and their contents (324,370).

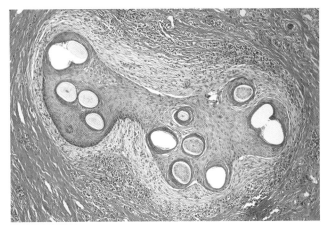

FIGURE 18-35. Tufted folliculitis (horizontal). Also known as polytrichia, multiple hairs share a common outer root sheath and will ultimately exit the scalp through a single opening. Perifollicular fibrosis is present.

Tufted Hair Folliculitis

"Tufted folliculitis" is a finding that may be present in various forms of scarring alopecia, and should not be considered a distinct entity, although some authors feel that it is, specifically characterizing it as a subset of folliculitis decalvans (361,371). Espousing that it is a pattern that occurs in many forms of scarring alopecia, Sperling (196) feels "the term tufted folliculitis should be purged from the lexicon of scarring alopecia." It can be seen as a late process in several conditions, including central centrifugal scarring alopecia, folliculitis decalvans, inflammatory tinea capitis, *Staph. aureus* folliculitis, lichen planopilaris, dissecting cellulitis, follicular degeneration syndrome, and acne keloidalis nuchae (358, 372–374). It has also been reported after traumatic scalp laceration (375), and after years of pemphigus vulgaris involvement of the scalp (376).

"Tufting" corresponds to the clinical finding of "doll's hair deformity," resembling the clustered hairs that are characteristic of a child's doll. Another name for this finding is "polytrichia" (357). It has been reported in a 10-year-old child (377). It should be distinguished from compound hairs, where two to three hairs exit from a single infundibulum, a normal finding on the occipital scalp (378).

Histopathology. Histology shows a single group of three to five follicles, or two to four such groups of follicles, where the infundibular epithelium of the affected hair follicles is fused together (Fig. 18-35), so that the multiple hair shafts are situated in the infundibular hair canal and exit the skin through a shared ostium, which may show hyperkeratosis and parakeratosis (361,379). There is perifollicular fibroplasia superficially, as well as interfollicular fibrosis. The lower segments of the hairs are unaffected. The epidermis may be depressed from contraction of the fibrous tissue, forming a dell from which the hairs emerge. There may be variable infiltrates around the follicles and perivascularly that are composed of lymphocytes, histiocytes, and plasma cells, in addition to neutrophils when pustular lesions are biopsied. The hair tufts may eventually

be destroyed by the process itself, and a foreign body giant cell reaction to free hair shafts may be seen. In one report, hairs were plucked from the tufts, revealing more than one-third telogen hairs (361).

Pathogenesis. Tufting results from injury to the outer root sheath epithelium of hairs in a single follicular unit or in several adjacent follicular units, possibly from a superficial suppurative folliculitis (361,373). There is accompanying perifollicular and interfollicular fibroplasia, leading to contraction of the involved skin and clustering of the follicular units. In healing, the outer root sheaths of the follicles grow together at the infundibular level. Other mechanistic theories include retention of telogen hairs (380), infection by *Staph. aureus* (371), and a congenital lesion, possibly a hair nevus, that became secondarily infected and scarred (379).

Central Centrifugal Scarring Alopecia

Since many forms of scarring alopecia share clinical and histologic features that make them difficult to distinguish with certainty, a unifying concept of *central centrifugal scarring alopecia* (CCSA) was proposed to reflect the overlap (324). CCSA is a category that includes several types of cicatricial hair loss that have in common the following features: (a) alopecia centered on the crown or vertex of the scalp; (b) progressive, chronic disease with eventual "burnout"; (c) fairly symmetrical expansion with the most active areas at the periphery; and (d) clinical and microscopic evidence of inflammation in these active sites (196,324). CCSA encompasses three *patterns* of disease: follicular degeneration syndrome, pseudopelade pattern (a "modern" use of the term, *not* pseudopelade of Brocq), and folliculitis decalvans.

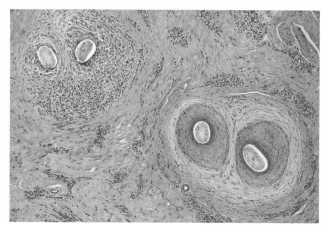

FIGURE 18-36. Central centrifugal scarring alopecia (horizontal). The following features are demonstrated: eccentric thinning of the follicular epithelium, concentric lamellar fibroplasia, lymphoplasmacytic inflammation, dermal fibrosis, and free hair shafts in the dermis inciting a granulomatous response. Many of these changes can be seen in other forms of scarring alopecia.

Histopathology. CCSA displays all of the following histologic features (196,324) (Fig. 18-36): (a) eccentric thinning of the follicular epithelium (outer root sheath), most prominent at the level of the isthmus and lower infundibulum; (b) close apposition of the hair shaft and follicular contents to the dermis; (c) concentric lamellar fibroplasia (resembling "onion skin"); and (d) chronic inflammation composed of lymphocytes and plasma cells surrounding the zone of fibroplasia. In addition, there are (e) eventual migration of the hair shaft into the dermis, inciting more inflammation and additional epithelial destruction, and (f) replacement of the follicle by a vertical band of connective tissue, resulting in a "follicular scar." Singly, these six histologic features may be found in other types of scarring alopecia.

Other features may be present that allow subclassification under one of the three patterns described above. For instance, African-American patients with CCSA who display characteristics of the follicular degeneration syndrome pattern tend to show premature desquamation of the inner root sheath (196). A characteristic histologic feature of the folliculitis decalvans pattern is folliculocentric neutrophilic inflammation, if a pustule from the expanding margin is biopsied.

Postmenopausal Frontal Fibrosing Alopecia

This form of scarring alopecia is considered a frontal variant of lichen planopilaris (381,382). It occurs in older women (mean age, 66.8 years), predominantly postmenopausal, with progressive recession of the frontal hairline (382). Other distinguishing features from lichen planopilaris include a marked decrease or complete loss of the eyebrows in most patients, a focal rather than multifocal

pattern of alopecia that is typically seen in lichen planopilaris, and lack of signs of lichen planus at other sites (382). There are rare exceptions that include one case with oral lichen planus (383), and another with cutaneous lichen planus in a premenopausal female (384). Clinically, the involved areas are pale, without sclerosis or induration, and show loss of follicular orifices (382). At the transition zone, follicles show perifollicular erythema and keratinization. Although frontotemporal recession can occur in postmenopausal women, mostly as a consequence of androgenetic alopecia, the follicular destruction in frontal fibrosing alopecia makes this condition unique (381,382).

Histopathology. Biopsies show histologic features of lichen planopilaris (Fig. 18-37), including perifollicular lymphocytic inflammation affecting the lower infundibulum and isthmus area near the bulge, hydropic degeneration of basal follicular keratinocytes with necrotic cells, concentric fibroplasia around the upper follicle, and absence of interfollicular changes (381,382). Naked hair shafts surrounded by granulomatous inflammation may be seen. Late lesions resemble burnt-out scarring alopecia, with noninflammatory fibrotic tracts replacing follicles and extending into the subcutis (385).

Pathogenesis. The infiltrate is predominantly composed of activated T-helper lymphocytes (381). The possibility that this condition is triggered by androgenetic alopecia was considered, but some patients also displayed androgenetic alopecia over the central scalp that was unaffected by the fibrosing process (381,382). Despite the fact that most

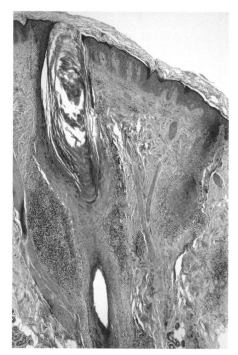

FIGURE 18-37. Postmenopausal frontal fibrosing alopecia. The changes are those of lichen planopilaris, with lichenoid lymphocytic inflammation around the isthmus and lower infundibulum.

patients were postmenopausal, evidence to support a role for hormonal factors has not been demonstrated.

Fibrosing Alopecia in a Pattern Distribution

Fibrosing alopecia in a pattern distribution was described as another lichen planopilaris variant in which the clinically involved areas occur in a distribution characteristic of androgenetic alopecia (386). Both women and men were involved, but women outnumbered men by roughly a 4:1 ratio, and the mean age of affected patients was 59 years. Patients showed progressive fibrosing alopecia of the central scalp in the area of androgenetic alopecia. Affected follicles displayed perifollicular erythema and follicular keratinization. Multifocal lesions typical of lichen planopilaris or other mucocutaneous signs of lichen planus were not seen.

Histopathology. The histology of early and late lesions shows findings identical to those of early and end-stage lichen planopilaris (see the histopathology described above for *postmenopausal frontal fibrosing alopecia*), in conjunction with follicular miniaturization (386). Although both terminal and vellus hairs are affected by the inflammation, the miniaturized follicles appear to be preferentially targeted (324).

MISCELLANEOUS ALOPECIA

Senescent Alopecia

Senescent or senile alopecia refers to the normal hair loss that occurs as a consequence of the aging process, with scalp hair becoming progressively and diffusely thinned starting at age 50, but more typically by age 60 or 70 (304, 334). Both sexes are affected. All elderly individuals will exhibit thinning to some degree, but in severe cases, an individual may seek medical advice (206).

Histopathology. A 4-mm punch biopsy will demonstrate the following: a decrease in the total number of hairs, from a normal of 35 to 45 to 25 to 35, a normal telogen count (<20%), a terminal to vellus hair ratio of at least 2:1, and a lack of deep inflammation (206,208). Horizontal sections are well suited to assess these parameters. The diameter of hairs may be diminished and fibrous tracts may be seen (334). The occiput should show similar findings to other areas of the scalp (206).

Pathogenesis. Presumably, follicles are lost forever. It is tempting to speculate that the regenerative capacity of follicular stem cells is restricted to a finite number of hair cycles.

Lipedematous Alopecia

Lipedematous scalp is localized or diffuse thickening of the scalp without hair loss, a result of thickening of the subcutaneous fat layer (387,388). This finding in association with usually diffuse or patchy alopecia has been termed *lipedematous alopecia* (389–391). It is a rare chronic condition, with only a handful of cases being reported, that occurs most often in African-American females, although it has recently been reported in a white woman (392) and a Japanese man (393). The alopecia is characterized by short hairs that fail to grow longer than 2 cm in length. The scalp feels thick and boggy or spongy upon palpation (391). It is smooth, without furrows, contrary to cutis verticis gyrata. Patients may complain of scalp pruritus, pain, or paresthesias.

Scalp thickness will range from 10 to 15 mm, whereas normal scalp thickness averages 5.8 ± 0.12 mm, according to a study where measurements were made at the bregma using skull x-rays (394). Scalp thickness may also be measured using computed tomography (388), magnetic resonance imaging (393), ultrasound (390), or by introducing a sterile needle into the scalp (389).

Histopathology. The defining abnormality is increased thickness of the subcutaneous fat. To appreciate this on biopsy, the specimen must extend to the galea, and vertical sections are required. Superficial biopsies will not show the diagnostic finding. There is no evidence of adipose tissue hypertrophy or hyperplasia; rather, there is edema, with disruption of the normal subcutaneous architecture of lobules separated by collagenous septae (395). Degeneration of the adipose tissue into loosely associated collagenous strands, vessels, and aggregates of fat cells is also seen (395). Excess mucin deposition is not generally characteristic, but was seen in one case (390). There may be mild hyperkeratosis and acanthosis, as well as a sparse, superficial perivascular, interstitial, and perifollicular mononuclear infiltrate (396) with occasional eosinophils (395).

A good explanation for the associated alopecia has not been found, although some have noted a decrease in the number of follicles and focal bulbar atrophy (395). The hairs are in anagen and appear normal. Scarring in the dermis or subcutis is generally absent, but perifollicular fibrosis has been noted (389,390). Follicular plugging and atrophic follicles have also been reported (389). Microscopic examination of hairs pulled in the clinical setting may show distal loss of the hair cuticle and changes of trichorrhexis nodosa, with hairs that break easily.

Pathogenesis. The etiology is unknown. The approximate doubling in scalp thickness is due entirely to thickening of the adipose layer. Free-floating lipid droplets along with adipocytes in various stages of degeneration were seen using electron microscopy (395). In addition to reduced follicular density, it is postulated that alopecia from aberrant hair shaft production may occur secondary to increased tissue oncotic pressure on hair bulbs (395).

Atrichia with Papular Lesions

Atrichia with papular lesions is a rare autosomal recessive condition characterized by total alopecia involving the scalp and body, and usually the eyebrows (397), although eyelashes may be spared (398). Normal hair is present at birth but is shed within the ensuing months to years of life, never to be replaced (399). At around age 2 years, individuals start to develop generalized cystic papules. Unlike other forms of ectodermal dysplasia, defects in nails, sweat glands, or teeth are not seen (397).

Histopathology. A biopsy from affected scalp will demonstrate an absence of developed hair follicles (Fig. 18-38). Intact sebaceous glands may sometimes be seen (398). Follicular infundibula are present without the lower portion of the follicles, so that hair shafts are not manufactured. Cysts develop from these abnormal follicles, producing clinical papules on the scalp and elsewhere that when biopsied reveal keratinous cysts with differentiation towards the follicular infundibulum (epidermoid) and isthmus (trichilemmal) (398) (Fig. 18-39). The cysts may rupture, leading to foreign body granulomas. Eccrine glands are normal in appearance (400).

Pathogenesis. Mutations in the human hairless (*HR*) gene on chromosome 8p12 produce the clinical phenotype described above (401–403), although a patient with mutations in the vitamin D receptor gene has been reported (404). The hairless gene in humans is a homolog of the murine hairless gene (401,405). The human *HR* gene encodes a zinc finger transcription factor protein that is expressed in the brain and skin (401).

Atrichia with papular lesions is recessively inherited, requiring two defective alleles; while most of the identified mutations have been homozygous within consanguineous families, compound heterozygous mutations have also been found (399). Possession of one allele with a *HR* gene mutation (heterozygous carrier) did not alter the expression of androgenetic alopecia in one study (406), and in a group of men with androgenetic alopecia screened for *HR* gene mutations, a significant association was not found (407).

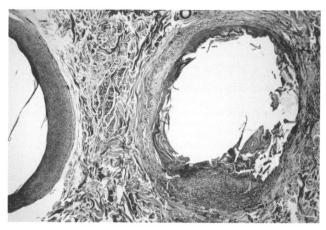

FIGURE 18-39. Atrichia with papular lesions. Biopsy of a papule will show keratinous cysts. The one on the *left* resembles an epidermoid cyst, while the one on the *right* shows trichilemmal differentiation and areas of rupture, inciting inflammation.

INFLAMMATORY DISEASES OF SWEAT GLANDS—ECCRINE

Syringolymphoid Hyperplasia with Alopecia

Thus far, only 11 cases of this rare dermatosis have been reported since the original description in 1969 (158,408). Ten cases involved adult males. Patients present with localized or scattered, erythematous to red-brown patches, plaques, and hyperkeratotic follicular papules. Lesions may cause alopecia, particularly noticeable when located on the scalp, and anhidrosis.

While some cases are idiopathic, others have been associated with cutaneous T-cell lymphoma (CTCL) (409,410). "Idiopathic" cases should be followed closely to monitor for progression to clear-cut CTCL. Additionally, follicular mucinosis may or may not be present (409,411). The cause of the alopecia is unclear, as not all cases with hair loss show follicular mucinosis (158).

Histopathology. There are dense lymphocytic infiltrates surrounding superficial and deep vessels, hair follicles, and eccrine sweat glands. The sweat glands show epithelial hyperplasia, lymphocyte exocytosis, and sometimes obliteration of ductal lumina (409,412) (Fig. 18-40). Follicular mucinosis may be seen in some cases.

In cases associated with CTCL, early lesions may show features more akin to a "precursor" lesion, with psoriasiform epidermal hyperplasia, spongiosis, papillary dermal fibrosis, scattered eosinophils, and a lichenoid infiltrate composed of small lymphocytes and some larger ones with convoluted nuclei, without significant epidermotropism (158). Late lesions show epidermotropism with Pautrier's collections, and denser perivascular and periadnexal infiltrates. Atypical lymphocytes infiltrate the eccrine gland epithelium (syringotropism) and also the follicular outer root sheath. The eccrine glands demonstrate hyperplasia

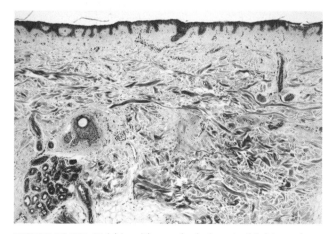

FIGURE 18-38. Atrichia with papular lesions. In this biopsy from the scalp, functional follicles are absent. Only a rudimentary follicle without a hair shaft is seen. Eccrine glands are normal.

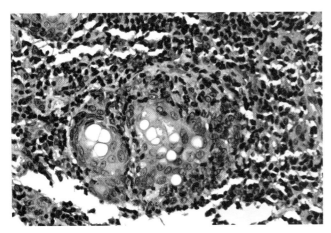

FIGURE 18-40. Syringolymphoid hyperplasia with alopecia. Mildly hyperplastic eccrine sweat glands show partial obliteration of ductal lumina, a dense surrounding lymphocytic infiltrate, and lymphocyte exocytosis (syringotropism).

with formation of complex, sometimes cribiform, structures (158). "Syringotropic variant of mycosis fungoides" was proposed as the preferred term for those cases associated with CTCL (413).

Neutrophilic Eccrine Hidradenitis

Neutrophilic eccrine hidradenitis (NEH) occurs in varied clinical settings (414). *Chemotherapy-associated NEH* is discussed in Chapter 11. NEH has been described in conjunction with infectious agents, including *Serratia marcescens* (415), *Enterobacter cloacae* (416), *Staph. aureus* (417), and HIV-1 (418–421), as well as miscellaneous associations that include granulocyte colony-stimulating factor (422), actinic reticuloid syndrome (423), Behçet's disease (424), acute myelogenous leukemia in the absence of chemotherapy (425), and one case in an otherwise healthy adult (426).

A subset of NEH that occurs in healthy children and young adults, *palmoplantar hidradenitis*, has been reported under many names, including "idiopathic palmoplantar eccrine hidradenitis," "juvenile neutrophilic eccrine hidradenitis," "recurrent eccrine hidradenitis," "idiopathic plantar hidradenitis," "traumatic plantar urticaria," and "plantar erythema nodosum" (427–433). Painful erythematous papules and nodules occur on the palms and soles. Constitutional symptoms are usually absent. In one study of 22 patients, occurrences were most frequent in the spring and fall, and almost half of the patients experienced more than one episode (434). The condition is benign and self-limited. Although the pathogenesis is unclear, temporal association with intense physical activity and exposure to cold, damp footwear have been reported (427,430).

A related condition was recently described, the *Pseudomonas hot-foot syndrome* (435). Painful red to purple nodules developed on weight-bearing sites on the soles of 40 children within 1 to 2 days of using a community wading pool where the floor was covered with an abrasive grit (believed to be important to the pathogenesis). Lesions were cultured from some patients, yielding a strain of *Pseudomonas aeruginosa* identical to that found in the pool, and some of the children had associated *Pseudomonas* folliculitis. Previous reports of hot-tub folliculitis had noted similar plantar lesions (436,437). Nevertheless, one group refuted the existence of the *Pseudomonas* hot-foot syndrome, stating their opinion that the findings were consistent with idiopathic palmoplantar hidradenitis (438).

Histopathology. The histology of *palmoplantar hidradenitis* occurring in children is similar to that of NEH induced by certain forms of chemotherapy (see Chapter 11), except that syringosquamous metaplasia is missing (439). A neutrophilic infiltrate is centered on the eccrine gland coils (Figs. 18-41 and 18–42). There may be mild mixed inflammation surrounding vessels in the deep to mid-dermis, without leukocytoclastic vasculitis. Neutrophilic inflammation may involve the acrosyringium, or assume a nodular pattern in the reticular dermis with abscess formation (429,433). Stains for fungi and bacteria are negative, even in those cases where cultures of lesions are positive for bacteria (414).

In the *Pseudomonas* hot-foot syndrome, biopsies from two of the patients showed superficial and deep perivascular, interstitial, and perieccrine inflammation composed of neutrophils and lymphocytes that extended into subcutaneous fat lobules. One of the cases showed a dermal microabscess with extension into the fat, and focal vasculitis with an intravascular thrombus (435). The authors noted

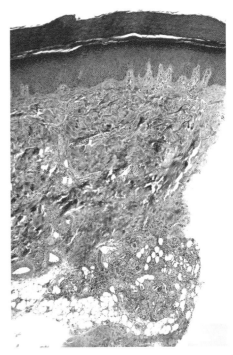

FIGURE 18-41. Palmoplantar hidradenitis. This biopsy from the plantar surface demonstrates an infiltrate around the eccrine gland coil.

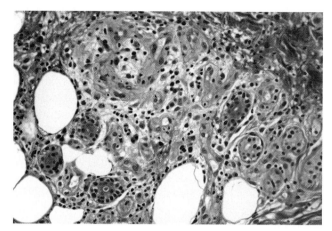

FIGURE 18-42. Palmoplantar hidradenitis. The perieccrine infiltrate is mixed, but predominantly neutrophilic.

that extension into subcutaneous fat lobules was a distinguishing feature from idiopathic NEH in children, a point that others have refuted (438).

INFLAMMATORY DISEASES OF SWEAT GLANDS—APOCRINE

Fox–Fordyce Disease

Fox–Fordyce disease (apocrine miliaria) is a disorder of apocrine sweat glands characterized by firm, itchy, follicular papules in anatomic sites where apocrine glands occur, namely the axillae, areolae, and genitalia (440). It occurs almost exclusively in females after adolescence.

Histopathology. Step sections of a vertically oriented biopsy specimen are usually needed to adequately show the characteristic changes (441,442). There is hyperkeratosis of the follicular infundibulum and excretory duct of the apocrine sweat gland, at the point where the latter inserts into the hair follicle. The apocrine duct behind the obstructing keratin plug becomes dilated (443). A spongiotic vesicle occurs in the follicular infundibulum, possibly representing an apocrine sweat-retention vesicle, with potential to rupture. Lymphocyte exocytosis is seen in the area of spongiosis. There may also be infundibular acanthosis and mild perivascular and periadnexal lymphocytic inflammation in the adjacent upper dermis (444,445). Transverse histological sections facilitated identification of the diagnostic histologic features in one case, and this technique was touted as the most effective way to diagnose Fox–Fordyce disease on biopsy (446).

A third type of sweat gland has been identified in the axillae; it is intermediate in size between the larger apocrine gland and smaller eccrine gland (447). Called the apoeccrine gland, it has a secretory coil like an apocrine gland, but opens directly to the epidermal surface like an eccrine gland. A recent article details a case of Fox–Fordyce disease

characterized by nonfollicular papules that histologically showed blockage of the intraepidermal portion of the apoeccrine sweat duct by cells that were released from the secretory portion via a holocrine mechanism (448).

Pathogenesis. The pathogenesis appears to be related to blockage of the apocrine sweat duct. Apocrine anhidrosis results, as demonstrated by the lack of apocrine secretion following intradermal injections of an epinephrine solution into the affected area (440). There are, however, reports in the literature suggesting that mechanical obstruction alone may not explain Fox–Fordyce disease (444).

INFLAMMATORY DISEASES OF CARTILAGE

Chondrodermatitis Nodularis Helicis

Chondrodermatitis nodularis helicis (CNH) usually presents as a single, small, exquisitely tender, erythematous nodule on the superior rim of the helix of the ear, and less frequently on the antihelix or posterior ear (449,450). The lesion develops a crust and ulceration in the center, producing elevated margins that may mimic basal cell carcinoma. CNH occurs mostly in white men over 40 years of age (451). The lesion tends to persist indefinitely without treatment.

Histopathology. Epidermal ulceration or a wedge-shaped epidermal defect is usually present. The intact adjacent epidermis is hyperplastic and may contain some dyskeratotic keratinocytes. A crust of exudate, parakeratosis, and dermal debris covers the surface of the epidermal defect (452). The dermis directly below shows fibrinoid collagen degeneration which stains more deeply eosinophilic than reticular dermal collagen, is homogeneous, and acellular; it may reach the perichondrial tissue beneath (Fig. 18-43). The stroma adjacent to the zone of

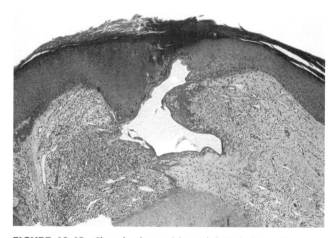

FIGURE 18-43. Chondrodermatitis nodularis helicis. There is a channel through the epidermis with adjacent hyperplasia. The dermis beneath shows fibrinoid degeneration of collagen that stains brightly eosinophilic and extends to the underlying perichondrium. The surrounding dermis shows a proliferation of small vessels, some mononuclear inflammation, and prominent solar elastosis.

degeneration shows vascular proliferation with lympho-histiocytic inflammatory cells. There may also be some fibroplasia and occasional plasma cells and neutrophils (453,454). Glomus cell aggregates have been described in these vascularized granulation tissue-like areas (455). Peripheral solar elastosis is common (452). The underlying perichondrial tissue may be thickened and appear to migrate to the base of the fibrinoid dermal necrosis (456). Degeneration of underlying cartilage with loss of cell nuclei can occur, although it is usually minimal. If cartilaginous degeneration is severe, there may be focal calcification and ossification (457).

Pathogenesis. As the name implies, it was originally thought that this condition begins with cartilaginous degeneration. It is now generally considered to be an attempt at transepidermal elimination of damaged dermal collagen, a type of perforating disorder (452,456, 458,459). The dermal collagen degeneration most likely results from vascular compromise, whether induced by trauma, pressure (during sleep or, more recently, cell phone use (460)), cold, or complications of dermatoheliosis. The limited vasculature at this anatomic site and lack of subcutaneous fat insulation may contribute to the situation. Recently reported was a case of CNH where serum autoantibodies to denatured type II collagen were detected (459).

Relapsing Polychondritis

Relapsing polychondritis (RP) is a rare systemic chondro-malacia that affects cartilage in multiple sites, including the ear, nose, larynx, trachea, bronchi, and joints (461). It also affects proteoglycan-rich tissues, such as the eyes, aorta, heart, kidneys, and skin (461). It usually starts with auricular chondritis, and runs an episodic, progressively destructive course. Mortality of about 25% has been reported, most commonly from damage to the respiratory tract or heart valves (462), although a recent study estimated the survival rate to be 94% at 8 years, a result of improvements in management (461). Disorders commonly associated with RP include rheumatoid arthritis, systemic lupus erythematosus, Sjögren's syndrome, and myelodysplastic syndromes (463,464).

Primary involvement of the ears and nose, consisting of intermittent attacks of painful erythema and swelling, may lead to a dermatology consult. Rarely, only one ear is involved (465). Ultimately, the ears become soft and flabby as a result of cartilage destruction, and the nose assumes a saddle nose deformity (466).

Nonspecific dermatologic findings associated with RP are common, varied, and found most frequently in those RP patients with myelodysplasia (467). They sometimes resemble the skin findings seen in Behçet's disease or inflammatory bowel disease—aphthosis, sterile pustules, limb ulcerations, or distal necrosis (467). Leukocytoclastic vasculitis

is not uncommon (462,468,469), and, indeed, it has been suggested that the cartilaginous damage may be secondary to a primary vasculitis (470). Other associated cutaneous lesions include purpuric or erythema nodosum–like lesions (462,468), chronic dermatitis, superficial phlebitis, livedo reticularis (467), septal and lobular panniculitis with vasculitis (471), erythema elevatum diutinum (472), epidermolysis bullosa acquisita (473), and pseudocyst of the auricle (474).

Histopathology. In early cartilaginous lesions, only the marginal chondrocytes appear degenerate, showing vacuolization, nuclear pyknosis, and loss of basophilia, which has been shown to result from the release of chondroitin sulfate from the cartilage matrix (475). A dense inflammatory infiltrate develops in the perichondrium that is comprised of neutrophils, lymphocytes, eosinophils, plasma cells, and macrophages. Frequently, there is edema or gelatinous cystic degeneration, and with progression, degenerated cartilage blends imperceptibly with the surrounding inflammatory cells, leading to the formation of granulation-type tissue (463). There may be fragmentation of the cartilage with necrosis and lysis of the cartilaginous plates (463). Elastic tissue stain shows clumping and destruction of cartilaginous elastic fibers (476). With successive episodes, fibrosis ensues (477).

Pathogenesis. Circulating antibodies to type II collagen, found exclusively in cartilage, are detected in patients with RP (478,479), and are generally found only in patients with active disease (480). The antibodies are directed against native and undenatured type II collagen, suggesting a primary role for these antibodies in the pathogenesis (rather than a secondary response to injured cartilage) (478). Immunoglobulin and complement components have also been identified in the inflamed cartilage (474,475). RP is strongly associated with HLA-DR4 (481).

Auricle Pseudocyst

In pseudocyst of the auricle, an asymptomatic, fluctuant swelling measuring about 1 cm in diameter is observed on the upper portion of the anterior aspect of the ear, usually in young males (mean age 38.9 years) (482). It is a form of chondromalacia that arises spontaneously or sometimes after minor trauma or infection, relapses frequently, and only rarely involves both ears (483). Pseudocyst is due to cavitation within the auricular cartilage which, when punctured, releases only a few microliters of a clear, deep yellow, viscous fluid. In the differential of cystic swellings of the external ear, this feature aids in the diagnosis, so that if a relatively large amount of liquid is obtained, the cavity must be located outside the cartilage (484).

Histopathology. A small intracartilaginous cavity without an epithelial lining is found on histologic examination. The wall of the pseudocyst consists of auricular cartilage, which is partially degenerated, appearing as faintly

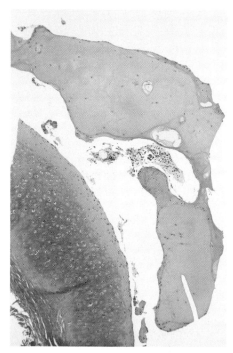

FIGURE 18-44. Pseudocyst of the auricle. There is an intracartilaginous cavity without an epithelial lining. The surrounding auricular cartilage is partially degenerated, appearing faintly eosinophilic and smudgy, with loss of nuclei.

eosinophilic amorphous material (485) (Fig. 18-44). The overlying epidermis, reticular dermis, and perichondrium are all normal (484). Inflammation is not a feature.

Pathogenesis. It has been suggested that the intracartilaginous cavity forms following the release of lysosomal enzymes (486), or overproduction of glycosaminoglycans after repeated trauma or mechanical stimulation (487). As compared to normal serum, aspirated fluid has been found to contain elevated levels of lactate dehydrogenase, especially the LDH-4 and LDH-5 isozymes (488,489), as well as the cytokines IL-6 and IL-1β (490). Investigators hypothesized that these substances were released from the damaged cartilage. Pseudocyst of the auricle has been described in association with relapsing polychondritis (474).

REFERENCES

1. Goldschmidt H, Leyden JJ, Stein KH. Acne fulminans. *Arch Dermatol* 1977;113:444.
2. Strauss JS, Kligman AM. The pathologic dynamics of acne vulgaris. *Arch Dermatol* 1960;82:779.
3. Massa MC, Su WPD. Pyoderma faciale: a clinical study of twenty-nine patients. *J Am Acad Dermatol* 1982;6:84.
4. Thiboutot D. Acne: 1991–2001. *J Am Acad Dermatol* 2002;47:109.
5. Plewig G. Morphologic dynamics of acne vulgaris. *Acta Derm Venereol Suppl (Stockh)* 1980;89:9.
6. Knaggs H, Holland K, Morris C, et al. Quantification of cellular proliferation in acne using the monoclonal antibody Ki-67. *J Invest Dermatol* 1994;102:89.
7. Lavker RM, Leyden JJ. Lamellar inclusions in follicular horny cells: a new aspect of abnormal keratinization. *J Ultrastruct Res* 1979;69:362.
8. Guy R, Green M, Kealey T. Modeling of acne in vitro. *J Invest Dermatol* 1996;106:176.
9. Toyoda M, Morohashi M. Pathogenesis of acne. *Med Electron Microsc* 2001;34:29.
10. Zelickson AS, Mottaz JH. Pigmentation of open comedones. *Arch Dermatol* 1983;119:567.
11. Leyden JJ. New understandings of the pathogenesis of acne. *J Am Acad Dermatol* 1995;32:15S.
12. Layton AM, Morris C, Cunliffe WJ, et al. Immunohistochemical investigation of evolving inflammation in lesions of acne vulgaris. *Exp Dermatol* 1998;7:191.
13. Pochi PE, Strauss JS. Endocrinologic control of the development and activity of the human sebaceous gland. *J Invest Dermatol* 1974;62:191.
14. Thody AJ, Shuster S. Control and function of sebaceous glands. *Physiol Rev* 1989;69:383.
15. Imperato-McGinley J, Gautier T, Cal LQ, et al. The androgen control of sebum production: Studies of subjects with dihydrotestosterone deficiency and complete androgen insensitivity. *J Clin Endocrinol Metab* 1993;76:524.
16. Mercurio MG, Gogstetter DS. Androgen physiology and the cutaneous pilosebaceous unit. *J Gender Spec Med* 2000;3:59.
17. Thiboutot D, Knaggs H, Gilliland K, et al. Activity of the type 1 5-alpha-reductase is greater in the follicular infrainfundibulum compared to the epidermis. *Br J Dermatol* 1997;136:166.
18. Chen W, Zouboulis CC, Orfanos CE. The 5-α-reductase system and its inhibitors. Recent development and its perspective in treating androgen-dependent skin disorders. *Dermatology* 1996;193:177.
19. Thiboutot D, Harris G, Iles V, et al. Activity of the type 1 5-alpha-reductase exhibits regional differences in isolated sebaceous glands and whole skin. *J Invest Dermatol* 1995;105:209.
20. Lookingbill DP, Horton R, Demens LM, et al. Tissue production of androgen in women with acne. *J Am Acad Dermatol* 1985;12:481.
21. Marynick SP, Chakmakjian ZH, McCaffree DL, et al. Androgen excess in cystic acne. *N Engl J Med* 1983;308:981.
22. Lucky AW, McGuire J, Rosenfield RL, et al. Plasma androgens in women with acne vulgaris. *J Invest Dermatol* 1983;81:70.
23. Thiboutot D, Gilliland K, Light J, et al. Androgen metabolism in sebaceous glands from subjects with and without acne. *Arch Dermatol* 1999;135:1041.
24. Shuster S. Acne: the ashes of a burnt out controversy. *Acta Derm Venereol Suppl (Stockh)* 1985;120:34.
25. Strauss JS, Pochi PE, Downing DT. Acne perspectives. *J Invest Dermatol* 1974;62:321.
26. Leyden JJ, McGinley KJ. Effect of 13-cis-retinoic acid on sebum production and Propionibacterium acnes in severe nodulocystic acne. *Arch Dermatol Res* 1982;272:331.
27. Melnik B, Kinner T, Plewig G. Influence of oral isotretinoin treatment on the composition of comedonal lipids. *Arch Dermatol Res* 1988;280:97.
28. Goldstein JA, Comite H, Mescon H, et al. Isotretinoin in the treatment of acne, histologic changes, sebum production, and clinical observations. *Arch Dermatol* 1982;118:555.
29. Leyden JJ, McGinley KJ, Mills OH, et al. Propionibacterium levels in patients with and without acne vulgaris. *J Invest Dermatol* 1975;65:382.
30. Cove JH, Cunliffe WJ, Holland KT. Acne vulgaris: is the bacterial population size significant? *Br J Dermatol* 1980;102:277.

31. Puhvel SM, Amirian D, Weintraub J, et al. Lymphocyte transformation in subjects with nodulo-cystic acne. *Br J Dermatol* 1977;97:205.

32. Kersey P, Sussman M, Dahl M. Delayed skin test reactivity to Propionibacterium acnes correlates with severity of inflammation in acne vulgaris. *Br J Dermatol* 1980;103:651.

33. Akers WA, Allen AM, Burnett JW, et al. Systemic antibiotics for treatment of acne vulgaris. *Arch Dermatol* 1975;111:1630.

34. Resh W, Stoughton RB. Topically applied antibiotics in acne vulgaris. *Arch Dermatol* 1976;112:182.

35. Smith KJ, Dipreta E, Skelton H. Peroxisomes in dermatology. Part I. *J Cutan Med Surg* 2001;5:231.

36. Smith KJ, Dipreta E, Skelton H. Peroxisomes in dermatology. Part II. *J Cutan Med Surg* 2001;5:315.

37. Monk B, Cunliffe WJ, Layton AM, et al. Acne induced by inhaled corticosteroids. *Clin Exp Dermatol* 1993;18:148.

38. Bong JL, Connell JMC, Lever R. Intranasal betamethasone induced acne and adrenal suppression. *Br J Dermatol* 2000;142:579.

39. Leyden JJ, Thew M, Kligman AM. Steroid rosacea. *Arch Dermatol* 1974;110:619.

40. Hurwitz RM. Steroid acne. *J Am Acad Dermatol* 1989;21:1179.

41. Odom RB, James WD, Berger TG. *Andrews' Diseases of the Skin.* Philadelphia: WB Saunders, 2000.

42. Brodell RT, O'Brien MJ Jr. Topical corticosteroid-induced acne. Three treatment strategies to break the 'addiction' cycle. *Postgrad Med* 1999;106:225.

43. Plewig G, Kligman AM. Steroid acne. In: *Acne and Rosacea* by Plewig and Kligman. New York: Springer-Verlag, 1993:415.

44. Yu HJ, Lee SK, Son SJ, et al. Steroid acne vs. Pityrosporum folliculitis: the incidence of Pityrosporum ovale and the effect of antifungal drugs in steroid acne. *Int J Dermatol* 1998;37:772.

45. Mihan R, Ayres S. Perioral dermatitis. *Arch Dermatol* 1964;89:803.

46. Fisher AA. Periocular dermatitis akin to the perioral variety. *J Am Acad Dermatol* 1986;15:642.

47. Manders SM, Lucky AW. Perioral dermatitis in childhood. *J Am Acad Dermatol* 1992;27:688.

48. Laude TA, Salvemini JN. Perioral dermatitis in children. *Semin Cutan Med Surg* 1999;18:206.

49. Boeck K, Abeck D, Werfel S, et al. Perioral dermatitis in children—clinical presentation, pathogenesis-related factors and response to topical metronidazole. *Dermatology* 1997;195:235.

50. Frieden IJ, Prose NS, Fletcher V, et al. Granulomatous perioral dermatitis in children. *Arch Dermatol* 1989;125:369.

51. Knautz MA, Lesher JL. Childhood granulomatous periorificial dermatitis. *Pediatr Dermatol* 1996;13:131.

52. Gianotti F, Ermacora E, Bennelli M-G, et al. Particuliere dermatite peri-orale infantile. Observations sur 5 cas. *Bull Soc Fr Dermatol Syphiligr* 1970;77:341.

53. Williams HC, Ashworth J, Pembroke AC, et al. FACE-Facial Afro-Caribbean childhood eruption. *Clin Exp Dermatol* 1990;15:163.

54. Urbatsch AJ, Frieden I, Williams ML, et al. Extrafacial and generalized granulomatous periorificial dermatitis. *Arch Dermatol* 2002;138:1354.

55. Ackerman AB, Chongchitnant N, Sanchez J, et al. *Histologic Diagnosis of Inflammatory Skin Diseases: An Algorithmic Method Based on Pattern Analysis.* Baltimore: Williams & Wilkins, 1997.

56. Marks R, Black MM. Perioral dermatitis: a histopathological study of 26 cases. *Br J Dermatol* 1971;84:242.

57. Wilkin J, Dahl M, Detmar M, et al. Standard classification of rosacea: report of the National Rosacea Society Expert Committee on the Classification and Staging of Rosacea. *J Am Acad Dermatol* 2002;46:584.

58. Furness GM, Lewis HM. Light sensitive seborrheid. *Arch Dermatol* 1957;75:245.

59. Malik R, Quirk CJ. Topical applications and perioral dermatitis. *Australas J Dermatol* 2000;41:34.

60. Velangi SS, Humphreys F, Beveridge GW. Periocular dermatitis associated with prolonged use of a steroid eye ointment. *Clin Exp Dermatol* 1998;23:297.

61. Silverberg NB, Weinberg JM. Rosacea and adult acne: a worldwide epidemic. *Cutis* 2001;68:85.

62. Marks R, Wilson-Jones E. Disseminated rosacea. *Br J Dermatol* 1969;81:16.

63. Meschig R. Ophthalmological complications of rosacea. In: Plewig G, ed. *Acne and Related Disorders.* London: Dunitz, 1989:321.

64. Ramelet AA. Rosacée: étude histopathologique de 75 cas. *Ann Dermatol Venereol* 1988;115:801.

65. Marks R, Harcourt-Webster JN. Histopathology of rosacea. *Arch Dermatol* 1969;100:683.

66. Rufli T, Cajacob A, Schuppli R. Rosacea granulomatosa, Demodex-granulomatose. *Dermatologica* 1982;165:310.

67. Helm KF, Menz J, Gibson LE, et al. A clinical and histopathologic study of granulomatous rosacea. *J Am Acad Dermatol* 1991;25:1038.

68. Grosshans EM, Kremer M, Maleville J. Demodex folliculorum und die histogenese der granulomatösen rosacea. *Hautarzt* 1974;25:166.

69. Aloi F, Tomasini C, Soro E, et al. The clinicopathologic spectrum of rhinophyma. *J Am Acad Dermatol* 2000;42:468.

70. Wilkin JK. Rosacea, pathophysiology and treatment. *Arch Dermatol* 1994;130:359.

71. Logan RA, Griffiths WAD. Climatic factors and rosacea. In: Plewig G, ed. *Acne and Related Disorders.* London: Dunitz, 1989:311.

72. Burton JL, Pye RJ, Meyrick G, et al. The sebum excretion rate in rosacea. *Br J Dermatol* 1975;92:541.

73. Dahl MV. Pathogenesis of rosacea. In: James WD, ed. *Advanced Dermatology.* Vol. 17. St. Louis: Mosby, 2001:29.

74. Forton F, Seys B. Density of Demodex folliculorum in rosacea: a case-control study using standardized skin surface biopsy. *Br J Dermatol* 1993;128:650.

75. Sibenge S, Gawkrodger DJ. Rosacea: a study of clinical patterns, blood flow, and the role of Demodex folliculorum. *J Am Acad Dermatol* 1992;26:590.

76. Bonnar E, Eustace P, Powell FC. The Demodex mite population in rosacea. *J Am Acad Dermatol* 1993;28:443.

77. Georgala S, Katoulis AC, Kylafis GD, et al. Increased density of Demodex folliculorum and evidence of delayed hypersensitivity reaction in subjects with papulopustular rosacea. *J Eur Acad Dermatol Venereol* 2001;15:441.

78. Erlach E, Gerbart W, Niebauer G. Zur pathogenese der granulomatösen rosacea. *Z Hautkr* 1976;51:459.

79. Ecker RI, Winkelmann RK. Demodex granuloma. *Arch Dermatol* 1979;115:343.

80. Szlachcic A. The link between Helicobacter pylori infection and rosacea. *J Eur Acad Dermatol Venereol* 2002;16:328.

81. Mayr-Kanhauser S, Kranke B, Kaddu S, et al. Resolution of granulomatous rosacea after eradication of Helicobacter pylori with clarithromycin, metronidazole and pantoprazole. *Eur J Gastroenterol Hepatol* 2001;13:1379.

82. Rebora A, Drago F, Picciotto A. Helicobacter pylori in patients with rosacea. *Am J Gastroenterol* 1994;89:1603.

83. Strauss JS. Some thoughts on rosacea. *J Eur Acad Dermatol Venereol* 2000;14:345.

84. Jablonska S, Chorzelski T, Maciejowska E. The scope and limitations of the immunofluorescence method in the diagnosis of lupus erythematosus. *Br J Dermatol* 1970;83:242.

85. Gajewska M. Rosacea in common male baldness. *Br J Dermatol* 1975;93:63.

86. Abell E, Black MM, Marks R. Immunoglobulin and complement deposits in the skin in inflammatory facial dermatoses. *Br J Dermatol* 1974;91:281.

87. Baima B, Sticherling M. Demodicidosis revisited. *Acta Derm Venereol* 2002;82:3.

88. Ayres SJ, Ayres S. Demodectic eruptions (Democidosis) in the human. *Arch Dermatol* 1960;83:816.

89. Purcell SM, Hayes TJ, Dixon SL. Pustular folliculitis associated with Demodex folliculorum. *J Am Acad Dermatol* 1986;15:1159.

90. Aylesworth R, Vance JC. Demodex folliculorum and Demodex brevis in cutaneous biopsies. *J Am Acad Dermatol* 1982;7:583.

91. Vollmer RT. Demodex-associated folliculitis. *Am J Dermatopathol* 1996;18:589.

92. Shelley WB, Shelley ED, Burmeister V. Unilateral demodectic rosacea. *J Am Acad Dermatol* 1989;20:915.

93. Forstinger C, Kittler H, Binder M. Treatment of rosacea-like demodicidosis with oral ivermectin and topical permethrin cream. *J Am Acad Dermatol* 1999;41:775.

94. Castanet J, Monpoux F, Mariani R, et al. Demodicidosis in an immunodeficient child. *Pediatr Dermatol* 1997;14.

95. Barrio J, Lecona M, Hernanz JM, et al. Rosacea-like demodicidosis in an HIV-positive child. *Dermatology* 1996;192:143.

96. Sahn EE, Sheridan DM. Demodicidosis in a child with leukemia. *J Am Acad Dermatol* 1992;27:799.

97. Redondo MJ, Soto GO, Fernandez RE, et al. Demodex-attributed rosacea-like lesions in AIDS. *Acta Derm Venereol* 1993;73:437.

98. Jansen T, Kastner U, Kreuter A, et al. Rosacea-like demodicidosis associated with aquired immunodeficiency syndrome. *Br J Dermatol* 2001;144:139.

99. Ashack RJ, Frost ML, Norins AL. Papular pruritic eruption of Demodex folliculitis in patients with acquired immunodeficiency syndrome. *J Am Acad Dermatol* 1989;21:306.

100. Dominey A, Rosen T, Tschen J. Papulonodular demodicidosis associated with acquired immunodeficiency syndrome. *J Am Acad Dermatol* 1989;20:197.

101. Patrizi A, Neri I, Chieregato C. Demodicidosis in immunocompetent young children: report of eight cases. *Dermatology* 1997;195:239.

102. Elston DM, Lawler KB, Iddins BO. What's eating you? Demodex folliculorum. *Cutis* 2001;68:93.

103. Ayres SJ. Rosacea and rosacea-like demodicidosis. *Int J Dermatol* 1987;26:198.

104. Forton F, Seys B, Marchall JL, et al. Demodex folliculorum and topical treatment: acaricidal action evaluated by standardized skin surface biopsy. *Br J Dermatol* 1998;138:461.

105. De Dulanto F, Camacho-Martinez. Demodicose 'gravis'. *Ann Dermatol Venerol* 1979;106:699.

106. Jimenez-Acosta F, Planas L, Penneys N. Demodex mites contain immunoreactive lipase. *Arch Dermatol* 1989;125:1436.

107. Ukei H, Masuda T. Lupus miliaris disseminatus faciei. *Hautarzt* 1979;30:553.

108. Kumano K, Tani M, Murata Y. Dapsone in the treatment of miliary lupus of the face. *Br J Dermatol* 1983;109:57.

109. Bedlow AJ, Otter M, Marsden RA. Axillary acne agminata (acne miliaris disseminatus faciei). *Clin Exp Dermatol* 1998;23:125.

110. Walchner M, Plewig G, Messer G. Lupus miliaris disseminatus faciei evoked during pregnancy in a patient with cutaneous lupus erythematosus. *Int J Dermatol* 1998;37:864.

111. Skowron F, Causeret AS, Pabion C, et al. F.I.GU.R.E.: facial idiopathic granulomas with regressive evolution. Is 'lupus miliaris disseminatus faciei' still an acceptable diagnosis in the third millenium? *Dermatology* 2000;201:287.

112. Suzuki K, Aoki M, Kawana S, et al. Metastatic silicone granuloma: lupus miliaris disseminatus faciei-like facial nodules and

sicca complex in a silicone breast implant recipient. *Arch Dermatol* 2002;138:537.

113. Scott KW, Calnan CD. Acne agminata. *Trans St Johns Hosp Dermatol Soc* 1967;53:60.

114. Simon N. Ist der Lupus miliaris disseminatus tuberkulöser ätiologie? *Hautarzt* 1975;26:625.

115. Hodak E, Trattner A, Feuerman H, et al. Lupus miliaris disseminatus faciei-the DNA of Mycobacterium tuberculosis is not detectable in active lesions by polymerase chain reaction. *Br J Dermatol* 1997;137:614.

116. Ofuji S, Ogino A, Horio T, et al. Eosinophilic pustular folliculitis. *Acta Derm Venereol Suppl (Stockh)* 1970;50:195.

117. Ishibashi A, Nishiyama Y, Miyata C, et al. Eosinophilic pustular folliculitis (Ofuji). *Dermatologica* 1974;149:240.

118. Blume-Peytavi U, Chen W, Djemadji N, et al. Eosinophilic pustular folliculitis (Ofuji's disease). *J Am Acad Dermatol* 1997;37:259.

119. Lucky AW, Esterly NS, Heskel N, et al. Eosinophilic pustular folliculitis in infancy. *Pediatr Dermatol* 1984;1:202.

120. Duarte AM, Kramer J, Yusk JW, et al. Eosinophilic pustular folliculitis in infancy and childhood. *Am J Dis Child* 1993;147:197.

121. Buckley DA, Munn SE, Higgins EM. Neonatal eosinophilic pustular folliculitis. *Clin Exp Dermatol* 2001;26:251.

122. Orfanos CE, Sterry W. Sterile eosinophile pustulose. *Dermatologica* 1978;157:193.

123. Mizoguchi S, Setoyama M, Higashi Y, et al. Eosinophilic pustular folliculitis induced by carbamazepine. *J Am Acad Dermatol* 1998;38:641.

124. Andreano JM, Kantor GR, Bergfeld WF, et al. Eosinophilic cellulitis and eosinophilic pustular folliculitis. *J Am Acad Dermatol* 1989;20:934.

125. Kimura k, Ezoe K, Yokozeki H, et al. A case of eosinophilic pustular folliculitis (Ofuji's disease) induced by patch and challenge tests with indeloxazine hydrochloride. *J Dermatol* 1996;23:479.

126. Mizukawa Y, Shiohara T. Eosinophilic pustular folliculitis induced after prolonged treatment with systemic corticosteroids in a patient with pustulosis palmoplantaris. *Acta Derm Venereol* 1998;78:221.

127. Kishimoto S, Yamamoto M, Nomiyama T, et al. Eosinophilic pustular folliculitis in association with nevoid basal cell carcinoma syndrome. *Acta Derm Venereol* 2001;81:202.

128. Rosenthal D, LeBoit PE, Klumpp L, et al. Human immunodeficiency virus associated eosinophilic folliculitis. *Arch Dermatol* 1991;127:206.

129. Ramdial PK, Morar N, Dlova NC, et al. HIV-associated eosinophilic folliculitis in an infant. *Am J Dermatopathol* 1999;21:241.

130. Jang KA, Chung ST, Choi JH, et al. Eosinophilic pustular folliculitis (Ofuji's disease) in myelodysplastic syndrome. *J Dermatol* 1998;25:742.

131. Parizi A, di Lernia V, Neri I, et al. Eosinophilic pustular folliculitis (Ofuji disease) and non-Hodgkin lymphoma. *Acta Derm Venereol* 1992;72:146.

132. Lambert J, Berneman Z, Dockx P, et al. Eosinophilic pustular folliculitis and B-cell chronic lymphatic leukaemia. *Dermatology* 1994;189:58.

133. Evans TR, Mansi JL, Bull R, et al. Eosinophilic pustular folliculitis occurring after bone marrow autograft in a patient with non-Hodgkin's lymphoma. *Cancer* 1994;73:2512.

134. Moritz DL, Elmets CA. Eosinophilic pustular folliculitis. *J Am Acad Dermatol* 1991;24:903.

135. McCalmont TH, Altemus O, Maurer T, et al. Eosinophilic folliculitis. *Am J Dermatopathol* 1995;17:439.

136. Ishiguro N, Shishido E, Okamoto R, et al. Ofuji's disease: a report on 20 patients with clinical and histopathologic analysis. *J Am Acad Dermatol* 2002;46:827.

137. Ofuji S. Eosinophilic pustular folliculitis. *Dermatologica* 1987; 174:53.

138. Holst R. Eosinophilic pustular folliculitis. *Br J Dermatol* 1976; 95:661.

139. Guillaume JC, Dubertret L, Cosnes A, et al. Folliculite à éosinophiles (maladie d'Ofuji). *Ann Dermatol Venereol* 1979; 106:347.

140. Basarab T, Jones RR. Ofuji's disease with unusual histological features. *Clin Exp Dermatol* 1996;21:67.

141. Piantanida EW, Turiansky GW, Kenner JR, et al. HIV-associated eosinophilic folliculitis: diagnosis by transverse histologic sections. *J Am Acad Dermatol* 1998;38:124.

142. Dupond AS, Aubin F, Bourezane Y, et al. Eosinophilic pustular folliculitis in infancy: report of two affected brothers. *Br J Dermatol* 1995;132:296.

143. Selvagg E, Thune P, Larsen TE, et al. Eosinophil cationic protein in eosinophilic pustular folliculitis: an immunohistochemical investigation. *Clin Exp Dermatol* 1997;22:255.

144. Teraki Y, Imanishi K, Shiohara T. Ofuji's disease and cytokines: remission of eosinophilic pustular folliculitis associated with increased serum concentrations of interferon gamma. *Dermatology* 1996;192:16.

145. Fushimi M, Tokura Y, Sachi Y, et al. Eosinophilic pustular folliculitis effectively treated with recombinant interferon gamma: suppression of mRNA expression of interleukin 5 in peripheral blood mononuclear cells. *Br J Dermatol* 1996;134: 766.

146. Horiguchi Y, Mitani T, Ofuji S. The ultrastructural histopathology of eosinophilic pustular folliculitis. *J Dermatol* 1992;19:201.

147. Vicente J, Espana A, Idoate M, et al. Are eosinophilic pustular folliculitis of infancy and infantile acropustulosis the same entity? *Br J Dermatol* 1996;135:807.

148. Brenner S, Wolf R, Ophir J. Eosinophilic pustular folliculitis of unknown cause? *J Am Acad Dermatol* 1994;31:210.

149. Haupt HM, Stern JB, Weber CB. Eosinophilic pustular folliculitis: fungal folliculitis? *J Am Acad Dermatol* 1990;23:1012.

150. van Doorn R, Scheffer E, Willemze R. Follicular mycosis fungoides, a distinct disease entity with or without associated follicular mucinosis: a clinicopathologic and follow-up study of 51 patients. *Arch Dermatol* 2002;138:191.

151. Bonta MD, Tannous ZS, Demierre MF, et al. Rapidly progressing mycosis fungoides presenting as follicular mucinosis. *J Am Acad Dermatol* 2000;43:635.

152. Dawber R. *Diseases of the Hair and Scalp*. Oxford: Blackwell Science, 1997.

153. Gibson LE, Muller SA, Leiferman KM, et al. Follicular mucinosis: clinical and histopathologic study. *J Am Acad Dermatol* 1989;20:441.

154. Stewart M, Smoller BR. Follicular mucinosis in Hodgkin's disease: a poor prognostic sign? *J Am Acad Dermatol* 1991;24: 784.

155. Mehregan AD, Gibson EL, Muller AS. Follicular mucinosis: histopathologic review in 33 cases. *Mayo Clin Proc* 1991;66:387.

156. Benchikhi H, Wechsler J, Rethers L, et al. Cutaneous B-cell lymphoma associated with follicular mucinosis. *J Am Acad Dermatol* 1995;33:673.

157. Sumner WT, Grichnik JM, Shea CR, et al. Follicular mucinosis as a presenting sign of acute myeloblastic leukemia. *J Am Acad Dermatol* 1998;38:803.

158. Tannous Z, Baldassano MF, Li VW, et al. Syringolymphoid hyperplasia and follicular mucinosis in a patient with cutaneous T-cell lymphoma. *J Am Acad Dermatol* 1999;41:303.

159. Cabré J, Korting GW. Zum symptomatischen charakter der "Mucinosis follicularis": Ihr Vorkommen beim Lupus erythematodes chronicus. *Dermatol Wochenschr* 1964;149:513.

160. Wolff HH, Kinney J, Ackerman AB. Angiolymphoid hyperplasia with follicular mucinosis. *Arch Dermatol* 1978;114:229.

161. Fanti PA, Tosti A, Morelli R, et al. Follicular mucinosis in alopecia areata. *Am J Dermatopathol* 1992;14:542.

162. Hempstead RW, Ackerman AB. Follicular mucinosis: a reaction pattern in follicular epithelium. *Am J Dermatopathol* 1985; 7:245.

163. Ackerman AB. Histopathologic concept of epidermolytic hyperkeratosis. *Arch Dermatol* 1970;102:253.

164. Lazaro-Medina A, Tianco EA, Avila JM. Additional markers for the type I reactional states in borderline leprosy. *Am J Dermatol* 1990;12:417.

165. Jordaan HF. Follicular mucinosis in association with a melanocytic nevus: a report of two cases. *J Cutan Pathol* 1987;14:122.

166. Walchner M, Messer G, Rust A, et al. Follicular mucinosis in association with squamous cell carcinoma of the tongue. *J Am Acad Dermatol* 1998;38:622.

167. Emmerson RW. Follicular mucinosis: a study of forty-seven patients. *Br J Dermatol* 1969;81:395.

168. Pinkus H. Commentary: alopecia mucinosa. *Arch Dermatol* 1983;119:698.

169. Sentis HJ, Willemze R, Scheffer E. Alopecia mucinosa progressing into mycosis fungoides: a long-term follow-up of two patients. *Am J Dermatopathol* 1988;10:478.

170. Cerroni L, Fink-Puches R, Back B, et al. Follicular mucinosis: a critical reappraisal of clinicopathologic features and association with mycosis fungoides and Sezary syndrome. *Arch Dermatol* 2002;138:182; [Comment] *Arch Dermatol* 2002;138:244.

171. Brown HA, Gibson LE, Pujol RM, et al. Primary follicular mucinosis: long-term follow-up of patients younger than 40 years with and without clonal T-cell receptor gene rearrangement. *J Am Acad Dermatol* 2002;47:856.

172. Pinkus H. Alopecia mucinosa: inflammatory plaques with alopecia characterized by root sheath mucinosis. *Arch Dermatol* 1957;76:419.

173. Snyder RA, Crain WR, McNutt S. Alopecia mucinosa: report of a case with diffuse alopecia and normal-appearing scalp skin. *Arch Dermatol* 1984;120:496.

174. Johnson WC, Higdon RS, Helwig EB. Alopecia mucinosa. *Arch Dermatol* 1969;79:395.

175. Braun–Falco O. In the discussion of Zambal Z: ablagerungen in der Haut bei Alopecia mucinosa. *Arch Klin Exp Dermatol* 1970;237:155.

176. Logan RA, Headington JT. Follicular mucinosis: a histologic review of 80 cases. *J Cutan Pathol* 1988;15(abstr):324.

177. Ishibashi A. Histogenesis of mucin in follicular mucinosis: an electron microscopic study. *Acta Derm Venereol Suppl (Stockh)* 1976;56:163.

178. Mevorah B, Marazzi A, Frenk E. The prevalence of accentuated palmoplantar markings and keratosis pilaris in atopic dermatitis, autosomal dominant ichthyosis vulgaris and control dermatological patients. *Br J Dermatol* 1985;112:679.

179. Arndt KA, Rand RE. Follicular syndromes with inflammation and atrophy. In: Fitzpatrick TB, et al., eds. *Dermatology in General Medicine*. 4th ed. New York: McGraw-Hill, 1993:766.

180. Alfadley A, Al Hawsawi K, Hainau B, et al. Two brothers with keratosis follicularis spinulosa decalvans. *J Am Acad Dermatol* 2002;47:S275.

181. Romaine KA, Rothschild JG, Hansen RC. Cicatricial alopecia and keratois pilaris. Keratosis follicularis spinulosa decalvans. *Arch Dermatol* 1997;133:381.

182. Friedman SJ. Lichen spinulosus. A clinicopathologic review of thirty-five cases. *J Am Acad Dermatol* 1990;22:261.

183. Boyd AS. Lichen spinulosus: case report and overview. *Cutis* 1989;43:557.

184. Nakjang Y, Yuttanavivat T. Phrynoderma: a review of 105 cases. *J Dermatol (Tokyo)* 1988;15:531.

185. Nazarenko SA, Ostroverkhova NV, Vasiljeva EO, et al. Keratosis pilaris and ulerythema ophryogenes associated with an 18p deletion caused by a Y/18 translocation. *Am J Med Genet* 1999; 85:179.

186. Harford RR, Cobb MW, Miller ML. Trichostasis spinulosa: a clinical simulant of acne open comedones. *Pediatr Dermatol* 1996;13:490.

187. Sarkany J, Gaylarde PM. Trichostasis spinulosa and its management. *Br J Dermatol* 1971;84:311.

188. Young MC, Jorizzo JL, Sanchez RL, et al. Trichostasis spinulosa. *Int J Dermatol* 1985;24:575.

189. Ladany E. Trichostasis spinulosa. *J Invest Dermatol* 1954;23:33.

190. Kailasam V, Kamakam A, Thambiah AS. Trichostasis spinulosa. *Int J Dermatol* 1979;18:297.

191. Pinkus H. Multiple hairs (Flemming–Giovannini). *J Invest Dermatol* 1951;17:291.

192. Goldschmidt H, Hojyo-Tomoka MT, Kligman AM. Trichostasis spinulosa. *Hautarzt* 1975;26:299.

193. Solomon AR. The transversely sectioned scalp biopsy specimen: the technique and an algorithm for its use in the diagnosis of alopecia. *Adv Dermatol* 1994;9:127.

194. Whiting DA. Structural abnormalities of the hair shaft. *J Am Acad Dermatol* 1987;16:1.

195. Dawber RPR. An update of hair shaft disorders. In: Whiting DA, ed. *Dermatologic Clinics.* Vol. 14. Philadelphia: WB Saunders, 1996:753.

196. Sperling LC. Scarring alopecia and the dermatopathologist. *J Cutan Pathol* 2001;28:333.

197. Headington JT. Transverse microscopic anatomy of the human scalp. *Arch Dermatol* 1984;120:449.

198. Elston DM, McCollough ML, Angeloni VL. Vertical and transverse sections of alopecia biopsy specimens: combining the two to maximize diagnostic yield. *J Am Acad Dermatol* 1995;32:454.

199. Frishberg DP, Sperling LC, Guthrie VM. Transverse scalp sections: a proposed method for laboratory processing. *J Am Acad Dermatol* 1996;35:220.

200. Olsen EA, Bergfeld WF, Cotsarelis G, et al. Summary of North American Hair Research Society (NAHRS)–sponsored Workshop on Cicatricial Alopecia, Duke University Medical Center, February 10 and 11, 2001. *J Am Acad Dermatol* 2003;48:103.

201. Sperling LC. Hair anatomy for the clinician. *J Am Acad Dermatol* 1991;25:1.

202. Milner Y, Sudnik J, Filippi M, et al. Exogen, shedding phase of the hair growth cycle: characterization of a mouse model. *J Invest Dermatol* 2002;119:639.

203. Paus R. Principles of hair cycle control. *J Dermatol* 1998;25:793.

204. Rebora A, Guarrera M. Kenogen. A new phase of the hair cycle? *Dermatology* 2002;205:108.

205. Solomon AR, Templeton SF. Alopecia. In: Farmer ER, Hood AF, eds. *Pathology of the Skin.* New York: McGraw-Hill, 2000; 833.

206. Sperling LC. Evaluation of hair loss. *Curr Probl Dermatol* 1996; 8:97.

207. Whiting DA. Diagnostic and predictive value of horizontal sections of scalp biopsy specimens in male pattern androgenetic alopecia. *J Am Acad Dermatol* 1993;28:755.

208. Sperling LL, Lupton GP. Histopathology of non-scarring alopecia. *J Cutan Pathol* 1995;22:97.

209. Sperling LC. Hair density in African Americans. *Arch Dermatol* 1999;135:656.

210. Sperling LC. *An Atlas of Hair Pathology with Clinical Correlations.* New York: Parthenon Publishing Group, 2003.

211. Lee HJ, Ha SJ, Lee JH, et al. Hair counts from scalp biopsy specimens in Asians. *J Am Acad Dermatol* 2002;46:218.

212. Whiting DA. Possible mechanisms of miniaturization during androgenetic alopecia or pattern hair loss. *J Am Acad Dermatol* 2001;45:S81.

213. Chartier MB, Hoss DM, Grant-Kels JM. Approach to the adult female patient with diffuse nonscarring alopecia. *J Am Acad Dermatol* 2002;47:809.

214. Madani S, Shapiro J. Alopecia areata update. *J Am Acad Dermatol* 2000;42:549.

215. Messenger AG, Slater DN, Bleehen SS. Alopecia areata: alterations in the hair growth cycle and correlation with the follicular pathology. *Br J Dermatol* 1986;114:337.

216. Headington JT, Mitchell A, Swanson N. New histopathologic findings in alopecia areata studied in transverse section. *J Invest Dermatol* 1981;76:325.

217. Ackerman AB. *Histologic Diagnosis of Inflammatory Skin Diseases.* Baltimore: Williams & Wilkins, 1997.

218. Hanly AJ, Jorda M, Badiavas E, et al. Postoperative pressure-induced alopecia: report of a case and discussion of the role of apoptosis in non-scarring alopecia. *J Cutan Pathol* 1999;26: 357.

219. Whiting DA. Histopathology of alopecia areata in horizontal sections of scalp biopsies. *J Invest Dermatol* 1995;104:27S.

220. Abell E, Gruber HM. A histopathologic reappraisal of alopecia areata. *J Cutan Pathol* 1987;14:347.

221. Kim IH, Jo HY, Cho CG, et al. Quantitative image analysis of hair follicles in alopecia areata. *Acta Derm Venereol* 1999;79: 214.

222. Elston DM, McCollough ML, Bergfeld WF, et al. Eosinophils in fibrous tracts and near hair bulbs: a helpful diagnostic feature of alopecia areata. *J Am Acad Dermatol* 1997;37:101.

223. Whiting DA. The histopathologic features of alopecia areata: a new look. 2003;139:1555.

224. Lee JYY, Hsu ML. Alopecia syphilitica, a simulator of alopecia areata: histopathology and differential diagnosis. *J Cutan Pathol* 1991;18:87.

225. Elston DM, McCollough ML, Bergfeld WF. Eosinophils in fibrous tracts and near hair bulbs: a helpful diagnostic feature of alopecia areata [Comment]. *J Am Acad Dermatol* 2000;42:305.

226. Hoss DM, Grant-Kels JM. Diagnosis: alopecia areata or not? *Semin Cutan Med Surg* 1999;18:84.

227. McElwee KJ, Tobin DJ, Bystryn JC, et al. Alopecia areata: an autoimmune disease? *Exp Dermatol* 1999;8:371.

228. McElwee KJ, Hoffmann R. Alopecia areata—animal models. *Clin Exp Dermatol* 2002;27:410.

229. Sundberg JP, Cordy WR, King LE. Alopecia areata in aging C3H/HeJ mice. *J Invest Dermatol* 1994;102:847.

230. McElwee KJ, Boggess D, King LE Jr, et al. Experimental induction of alopecia areata-like hair loss in C3H/HeJ mice using full-thickness skin grafts. *J Invest Dermatol* 1998;111: 797.

231. Michie HJ, Jahoda CAB, Oliver RF, et al. The DEBR rat: an animal model of human alopecia areata. *Br J Dermatol* 1991; 125:94.

232. Smyth JR Jr, McNeil M. Alopecia areata and universalis in the Smyth chicken model for spontaneous autoimmune vitiligo. *J Invest Dermatol* 1999;4:211.

233. Olsen E, Hordinsky M, McDonald-Hull S, et al. Alopecia areata investigational assessment guidelines. National Alopecia Areata Foundation. *J Am Acad Dermatol* 1999;40:242.

234. Duvic M, Nelson A, de Andrade M. The genetics of alopecia areata. *Clin Dermatol* 2001;19:135.

235. Muller SA, Winkelmann RK. Alopecia areata: an evaluation of 736 patients. *Arch Dermatol* 1963;88:290.

236. Shellow WV, Edwards JE, Koo JY. Profile of alopecia areata: a questionnaire analysis of patient and family. *Int J Dermatol* 1992;31:186.

237. Scerri L, Pace JL. Identical twins with identical alopecia areata. *J Am Acad Dermatol* 1992;27:766.

238. Colombe BW, Price VH, Khoury EL, et al. HLA class II antigen associations help to define two types of alopecia areata. *J Am Acad Dermatol* 1995;33:757.

239. de Andrade M, Jackow CM, Dahm N, et al. Alopecia areata in families: association with the HLA locus. *J Invest Dermatol* 1999;4:220.

240. Levin RM, Travis SF, Heymann WR. Simultaneous onset of alopecia areata and idiopathic thrombocytopenic purpura: a potential association? *Pediatr Dermatol* 1999;16:31.

241. Tobin DJ, Hann SK, Song MS, et al. Hair follicle structures targeted by antibodies in patients with alopecia areata. *Arch Dermatol* 1997;133:57.

242. Tobin DJ, Orentreich N, Fenton DA, et al. Antibodies to hair follicles in alopecia areata. *J Invest Dermatol* 1994;102:166.

243. Todes-Taylor N, Turner R, Wood GS, et al. T cell subpopulations in alopecia areata. *J Am Acad Dermatol* 1984;11:216.

244. Khoury EL, Price VH, Abdel-Salam MM, et al. Topical minoxidil in alopecia areata: no effect on the perifollicular lymphoid infiltration. *J Invest Dermatol* 1992;99:40.

245. McElwee KJ, Spiers EM, Oliver RF. In vivo depletion of CD8+ T cells restores hair growth in the DEBR model for alopecia areata. *Br J Dermatol* 1996;135:211.

246. Gilhar A, Ullmann Y, Berkutzki T, et al. Autoimmune hair loss (alopecia areata) transferred by T-lymphocytes to human scalp explants on SCID mice. *J Clin Invest* 1998;101:62.

247. Gilhar A, Landau M, Assy B, et al. Mediation of alopecia areata by cooperation between CD4+ and CD8+ T lymphocytes: transfer to human scalp explants on Prkdc(scid) mice. *Arch Dermatol* 2002;138:916.

248. Nickoloff BJ, Griffiths CEM. Aberrant intercellular adhesion molecule-1 (ICAM-1) expression by hair follicle epithelial cells and endothelial leukocyte adhesion molecule-1 (ELAM-1) by vascular cells are important adhesion molecule alterations in alopecia areata. *J Invest Dermatol* 1991;96:91S.

249. McDonagh AJG, Snowden JA, Stierle C, et al. HLA and ICAM-1 expression in alopecia areata in vivo and in vitro: the role of cytokines. *Br J Dermatol* 1993;129:250.

250. Paus R. Immunology of the hair follicle. In: Bos JD, ed. *The Skin Immune System*. Boca Raton, FL: CRC Press, 1997:377.

251. Christoph T, Muller-Rover S, Audring H, et al. The human hair follicle immune system: cellular composition and immune privilege. *Br J Dermatol* 2000;142:862.

252. Westgate GE, Craggs RI, Gibson WT. Immune privilege in hair growth. *J Invest Dermatol* 1991;97:417.

253. Paus R, Eichmuller S, Hofmann U, et al. Expression of classical and nonclassical MHC class I antigens in murine hair follicles. *Br J Dermatol* 1994;131:177.

254. Paus R. Immunology of the hair follicle. The National Alopecia Areata Foundation and the National Institute of Arthritis and Musculoskeletal and Skin Diseases. Washington, DC, November 5, 1998.

255. Teraki Y, Imanishi K, Shiohara T. Cytokines in alopecia areata: contrasting cytokine profiles in localized form and extensive form (alopecia universalis). *Acta Derm Venereol* 1996;76:421.

256. Philpott MP, Sanders DA, Bowen J, et al. Effects of interleukins, colony-stimulating factor and tumour necrosis factor on human hair follicle growth in vitro: a possible role for interleukin-1 and tumour necrosis factor-alpha in alopecia areata. *Br J Dermatol* 1996;135:942.

257. Hoffmann R. The potential role of cytokines and T cells in alopecia areata. *J Invest Dermatol* 1999;4:235.

258. Bodemer C, Peuchmaur M, Fraitaig S, et al. Role of cytotoxic T cells in chronic alopecia areata. *J Invest Dermatol* 2000;114:112.

259. Hordinsky M, Kennedy W, Wendelschafer-Crabb G, et al. Structure and function of cutaneous nerves in alopecia areata. *J Invest Dermatol* 1995;104[Suppl]:28S.

260. Raud J, Lundeberg T, Brodda-Jansen G, et al. Potent anti-inflammatory action of calcitonin gene-related peptide. *Biochem Biophys Res Commun* 1991;180:1429.

261. Ericson M, Binstock K, Guanche A, et al. Differential expression of substance P in perifollicular scalp blood vessels and nerves after topical therapy with capsaicin 0.075% (Zostrix HP) in controls and patients with extensive alopecia areata. *J Invest Dermatol* 1999;112:653.

262. Rossi R, Del Bianco E, Isolani D, et al. Possible involvement of neuropeptidergic sensory nerves in alopecia areata. *Neuroreport* 1997;8:1135.

263. Walsh KH, McDougle CJ. Trichotillomania. Presentation, etiology, diagnosis and therapy. Am J *Clin Dermatol* 2001;2:327.

264. Hautmann G, Hercogova J, Lotti T. Trichotillomania. *J Am Acad Dermatol* 2002;46:807.

265. Keuthen NJ, O'Sullivan RL, Sprich-Buckminster S. Trichotillomania: current issues in conceptualization and treatment. *Psychother Psychosom* 1998;67:202.

266. du Toit PL, van Kradenburg J, Niehaus DJ, et al. Characteristics and phenomenology of hair-pulling: an exploration of subtypes. *Compr Psychiatry* 2001;42:247.

267. Trueb RM, Cavegn B. Trichotillomania in connection with alopecia areata. *Cutis* 1996;58:67.

268. Muller SA. Trichotillomania: a histopathologic study in sixty-six patients. *J Am Acad Dermatol* 1990;23:56.

269. Mehregan AH. Trichotillomania. *Arch Dermatol* 1970;102:129.

270. Olsen EA. Androgenetic alopecia. In: Olsen EA, ed. *Disorders of Hair Growth*. New York: McGraw-Hill, 1994:400.

271. Hwang SM, Lee WS, Choi EH, et al. Nurse's cap alopecia. *Int J Dermatol* 1999;38:187.

272. Grossman KL, Kvedar JC. Anagen hair loss. In: Olsen EA, ed. *Disorders of Hair Growth*. New York: McGraw-Hill, 1994:223.

273. Delmonte S, Semino MT, Parodi A, et al. Normal anagen effluvium: a sign of pemphigus vulgaris. *Br J Dermatol* 2000;142:1244.

274. *Dorland's Illustrated Medical Dictionary*. Philadelphia: WB Saunders, 1985.

275. Kligman AM. Pathologic dynamics of human hair loss. I. Telogen effluvium. *Arch Dermatol* 1961;83:175.

276. Headington JT. Telogen effluvium. *Arch Dermatol* 1993;129:356.

277. Fiedler VC, Hafeez A. Diffuse alopecia: telogen hair loss. In: Olsen E, ed. *Disorders of Hair Growth*. New York: McGraw-Hill, 1994:241.

278. Almagro M, del Pozo J, Garcia-Silva J, et al. Telogen effluvium as a clinical presentation of human immunodeficiency virus infection. *Am J Med* 2002;112:508.

279. Tosti A, Piraccini BM, van Neste DJ. Telogen effluvium after allergic contact dermatitis of the scalp. *Arch Dermatol* 2001;137:187.

280. Rand S. Chronic telogen effluvium: potential complication for clinical trials in female androgenetic alopecia? [Comment] *J Am Acad Dermatol* 1997;37:1021.

281. Whiting DA. Chronic telogen effluvium: increased scalp hair shedding in middle-aged women. *J Am Acad Dermatol* 1996;35:899.

282. Whiting DA. Chronic telogen effluvium. *Dermatol Clin* 1996;14:723.

283. Thai KE, Sinclair RD. Chronic telogen effluvium in a man. *J Am Acad Dermatol* 2002;47:605.
284. Headington JT. Transverse microscopic anatomy of the human scalp. *Arch Dermatol* 1984;120:449.
285. Kligman AM. Pathologic dynamics of human hair loss. I. Telogen effluvium. *Arch Dermatol* 1961;83:175.
286. Pierard-Franchimont C, Pierard GE. Teloptosis, a turning point in hair shedding biorhythms. *Dermatology* 2001;203:115.
287. Botchkarev VA, Komarova EA, Siebenhaar F, et al. p53 Involvement in the control of murine hair follicle regression. *Am J Pathol* 2001;158:1913.
288. Birch MP, Lalla SC, Messenger AG. Female pattern hair loss. *Clin Exp Dermatol* 2002;27:383.
289. Olsen EA. Female pattern hair loss. *J Am Acad Dermatol* 2001;45:S70.
290. Orme S, Cullen DR, Messenger AG. Diffuse female hair loss: are androgens necessary? *Br J Dermatol* 1999;141:521.
291. Bolduc C, Shapiro J. Management of androgenetic alopecia. *Am J Clin Dermatol* 2000;1:151.
292. Hoffmann R, Happle R. Current understanding of androgenetic alopecia. Part II: clinical aspects and treatment. *Eur J Dermatol* 2000;10:410.
293. Rocahel MC, Ackerman AB. Common baldness an inflammatory disease? *Dermatopathol Pract Concept* 1999;5:319.
294. Hoffmann R. Male androgenetic alopecia. *Clin Exp Dermatol* 2002;27:373.
295. Ellis JA, Harrap SB. The genetics of androgenetic alopecia. *Clin Dermatol* 2001;19:149.
296. Sperling LC, Winton GB. The transverse anatomy of androgenetic alopecia. *J Dermatol Surg Oncol* 1990;16:1127.
297. Headington JT, Novak E. Clinical and histologic studies of male pattern baldness treated with topical minoxidil. *Curr Ther Res* 1984;36:1098.
298. Abell E. Histologic response to topically applied minoxidil in male-pattern alopecia. *Clin Dermatol* 1988;6:191.
299. Whiting DA. Diagnostic and predictive value of horizontal sections of scalp biopsies in male pattern androgenetic alopecia. *J Cutan Pathol* 1990;17:325.
300. Paus R, Cotsarelis G. The biology of hair follicles. *N Engl J Med* 1999;341:491.
301. Jaworsky C, Kligman AM. Characterization of inflammatory infiltrates in male pattern alopecia: implications for pathogenesis. *Br J Dermatol* 1992;127:239.
302. Mahe YF, Michelet JF, Billoni N, et al. Androgenetic alopecia and microinflammation. *Int J Dermatol* 2000;39:576.
303. Abell E. Pathology of male pattern alopecia. *Arch Dermatol* 1984;120:1607.
304. Kligman AM. The comparative histopathology of male-pattern baldness and senescent baldness. *Clin Dermatol* 1988;6:108.
305. Lattanand A, Johnson WC. Male pattern alopecia. A histopathological and histochemical study. *J Cutan Pathol* 1975;2:58.
306. Oliveira I, Messenger AG. The hair follicle: a paradoxical androgen target organ. *Horm Res* 2000;54:243.
307. Randall VA, Thornton MJ, Hamada K, et al. Mechanism of androgen action in cultured dermal papilla cells derived from human hair follicles with varying responses to androgens in vivo. *J Invest Dermatol* 1992;98:86S.
308. Trueb RM. Molecular mechanisms of androgenetic alopecia. *Exp Gastroenterol* 2002;37:981.
309. Sawaya ME, Price VH. Different levels of 5alpha-reductase type I and II, aromatase, and androgen receptor in hair follicles of women and men with androgenetic alopecia. *J Invest Dermatol* 1997;109:296.
310. Bayne EK, Flanagan J, Einstein M, et al. Immunohistochemical localization of types 1 and 2 5alpha-reductase in human scalp. *Br J Dermatol* 1999;141:481.
311. Hoffmann R, Rot A, Niiyama S, et al. Steroid sulfatase in the human hair follicle concentrates in the dermal papilla. *J Invest Dermatol* 2001;117:1342.
312. Happle R, Hoffmann R. Absence of male-pattern baldness in men with X-linked recessive ichthyosis? A hypothesis to be challenged. *Dermatology* 1999;198:231.
313. Seiberg M, Marthinuss J, Stenn KS. Changes in expression of apoptosis-associated genes in skin mark early catagen. *J Invest Dermatol* 1995;104:78.
314. Sawaya ME, Blume-Peytavi U, Mullins DL, et al. Effects of finasteride on apoptosis and regulation of the human hair cycle. *J Cutan Med Surg* 2002;6:1.
315. Sawaya ME, Keane RW, Blume-Peytavi U, et al. Androgen responsive genes as they affect hair growth. *Eur J Dermatol* 2001;11:304.
316. Prieto VG, Sadick NS, Shea CR. Androgenetic alopecia: analysis of proliferation and apoptosis. *Arch Dermatol* 2002;138:1101.
317. Cowper SE, Rosenberg AS, Morgan MB. An investigation of apoptosis in androgenetic alopecia. *Am J Dermatopathol* 2002;24:204.
318. Jahoda CA. Cellular and developmental aspects of androgenetic alopecia. *Exp Dermatol* 1998;7:235.
319. Randall VA, Hibberts NA, Hamada K. A comparison of the culture and growth of dermal papilla cells from hair follicles from non-balding and balding (androgenetic alopecia) scalp. *Br J Dermatol* 1996;134:437.
320. Whiting DA. Chronic telogen effluvium: increased scalp hair shedding in middle-aged women [Comment]. *J Am Acad Dermatol* 1997;37:1021.
321. Millikan LE. Androgenetic alopecia: the role of inflammation and Demodex. *Int J Dermatol* 2001;40:475.
322. Guarrera M, Rebora A. Anagen hairs may fail to replace telogen hairs in early androgenic female alopecia. *Dermatology* 1996;192:28.
323. Wiseman MC, Shapiro J. Scarring alopecia. *J Cutan Med Surg* 1999;3:S45.
324. Sperling LC, Solomon AR, Whiting DA. A new look at scarring alopecia. *Arch Dermatol* 2000;136:205–211; [Comment] *Arch Dermatol* 2000;136:235.
325. Modly CE, Wood CM, Burnett JW. Evaluation of alopecia: a new algorithm. *Cutis* 1989;43:148.
326. Elston DM, Bergfeld WF. Cicatricial alopecia (and other causes of permanent alopecia). In: Olsen EA, ed. *Disorders of Hair Growth.* New York: McGraw-Hill, 1994:285.
327. Elston DM, McCollough ML, Warschaw KE, et al. Elastic tissue in scars and alopecia. *J Cutan Pathol* 2000;27:147.
328. Headington JT. Cicatricial alopecia. *Dermatol Clin* 1996;14:773.
329. Pierard-Franchimont C, Pierard GE. Massive lymphocyte-mediated apoptosis during the early stage of pseudopelade. *Dermatologica* 1986;172:254.
330. Stenn KS, Sundberg JP, Sperling LC. Hair follicle biology, the sebaceous gland, and scarring alopecias. *Arch Dermatol* 1999;135:973.
331. Sundberg JP, Boggess D, Sundberg BA, et al. Asebia-2J (Scd1(ab2J)): a new allele and a model for scarring alopecia. *Am J Pathol* 2000;156:2067.
332. Stenn KS. Insights from the asebia mouse: a molecular sebaceous gland defect leading to cicatricial alopecia. *J Cutan Pathol* 2001;28:445.
333. Braun-Falco O, Imai S, Schmoeckel C, et al. Pseudopelade of Brocq. *Dermatologica* 1986;172:18.

334. Sullivan JR, Kossard S. Acquired scalp alopecia. Part I: a review. *Australas J Dermatol* 1998;39:207.

335. Ioannides G. Alopecia: a pathologist's view. *Int J Dermatol* 1982;21:316.

336. Madani S, Trotter MJ, Shapiro J. Pseudopelade of Brocq in beard area. *J Am Acad Dermatol* 2000;42:895.

337. Braun-Falco O, Bergner T, Heilgemeir GP. Pseudopelade Brocq-krankheitsbild oder krankheitsentität. *Hautarzt* 1989; 40:77.

338. Bulengo-Ransby SM, Headington JT. Pseudopelade of Brocq in a child. *J Am Acad Dermatol* 1990;23:944.

339. Brocq L. Alopecia. *J Cutan Vener Dis* 1885;3:49.

340. Brocq L, Lenglet E, Ayrignac J. Recherches sur l'alopecie atrophiante, variete pseudopelade. *Ann Dermatol Syphilol (France)* 1905;6:209.

341. Dawber R. What is pseudopelade? *Clin Exp Dermatol* 1992; 17:305.

342. Pinkus H. Differential patterns of elastic fibers in scarring and non-scarring alopecias. *J Cutan Pathol* 1978;5:93.

343. Degos R, Rabut R, Duperrat B. Alopecie en petit aires. Reticulose lymphocytaire benigne. *Bull Soc Fr Dermatol Syphiligr* 1955;62:134.

344. Degos R, Rabut R, Duperrat B, et al. Apropos de III cas d'alopecies cicatricielles en petit aires (teignes eexclues). L'etat pseudopeladique. *Bull Soc Fr Dermatol Syphiligr* 1951;58: 451.

345. Degos R, Rabut R, Duperrat B, et al. L'etat pseudopeladique. *Ann Dermatol Syphilol (France)* 1954;81:5.

346. Degos R, Rabut R, Hewitt J. Etat pseudopeladique du a des metastases cacinomateuses alopeiantes. *Bull Soc Fr Dermatol Syphiligr* 1954;61:509.

347. Amato L, Mei S, Massi D, et al. Cicatricial alopecia; a dermatopathologic and immunopathologic study of 33 patients (pseudopelade of Brocq is not a specific clinico-pathologic entity). *Int J Dermatol* 2002;41:8.

348. Silvers DN, Katz BE, Young AW. Pseudopelade of Brocq is lichen planopilaris: report of four cases that support this nosology. *Cutis* 1993;51:99.

349. Nayar M, Schomberg K, Dawber RPR, et al. A clinicopathological study of scarring alopecia. *Br J Dermatol* 1993;128:533.

350. Olsen EA. Pseudopelade of Brocq. In: Olsen EA, ed. *Disorders of Hair Growth.* New York: McGraw-Hill, 1994:294.

351. Jordon RE. Subtle clues to diagnosis by immunopathology: scarring alopecia. *Am J Dermatopathol* 1980;2:157.

352. Pincelli C, Girolomoni G, Benassi L. Pseudopelade of Brocq: an immunologically mediated disease? *Dermatologica* 1987;176:49.

353. Whiting DA. Cicatricial alopecia: clinico-pathological findings and treatment. *Clin Dermatol* 2001;19:211.

354. Sakamoto F, Ito M, Saito R. Ultrastructural study of acquired pili torti-like hair defects accompanying pseudopelade. *J Dermatol* 2002;29:197.

355. Sperling LC, Sau P. The follicular degeneration syndrome in black patients. "Hot comb alopecia" revisited and revised. *Arch Dermatol* 1992;128:68.

356. Sperling LC, Skelton HG, Smith KJ, et al. Follicular degeneration syndrome in men. *Arch Dermatol* 1994;130:763.

357. LoPresti P, Papa C, Kligman A. Hot comb alopecia. *Arch Dermatol* 1968;98:234.

358. Sullivan JR, Kossard S. Acquired scalp alopecia. Part II. A review. *Australas J Dermatol* 1999;40:61.

359. Olsen EA. Erosive pustular dermatosis and folliculitis decalvans. In: Olsen EA, ed. *Disorders of Hair Growth.* New York: McGraw-Hill, 1994:296.

360. Templeton SF, Solomon AR. Scarring alopecia: a classification based upon microscopic criteria. *J Cutan Pathol* 1994;21:97.

361. Annessi G. Tufted folliculitis of the scalp: a distinctive clinicohistological variant of folliculitis decalvans. *Br J Dermatol* 1998;138:799.

362. Choudry K, Charles-Holmes R, Vella EJ, et al. Scarring alopecia due to folliculitis decalvans in a patient with Darier's disease. *Clin Exp Dermatol* 2001;26:307.

363. Karakuzu A, Erdem T, Aktas A, et al. A case of folliculitis decalvans involving the beard, face and nape. *J Dermatol* 2001;28:329.

364. Douwes KE, Landthaler M, Szeimies RM. Simultaneous occurrence of folliculitis decalvans capillitii in identical twins. *Br J Dermatol* 2000;143:195.

365. Powell JJ, Dawber RPR, Gatter K. Folliculitis decalvans including tufted folliculitis: clinical, histological and therapeutic findings. *Br J Dermatol* 1999;140:328.

366. Brooke RCC, Griffiths CEM. Folliculitis decalvans. *Clin Exp Dermatol* 2001;26:120.

367. Frazer NG, Grant PW. Folliculitis decalvans with hypocomplementemia. *Br J Dermatol* 1982;107[Suppl 22]:88.

368. Shitara A, Igareshi R, Morohashi M. Folliculitis decalvans and cellular immunity-two brothers with oral candidiasis. *Jpn J Dermatol* 1974;28:113.

369. Wheeland RG, Thurmond RD, Gilmore WA, et al. Chronic blepharitis and pyoderma of the scalp: an immune deficiency state in a father and son with hypercalcemia and decreased intracellular killing. *Pediatr Dermatol* 1983;1:134.

370. Sperling LC, Whiting D, Solomon A. Folliculitis decalvans and tufted folliculitis are specific infective diseases that may lead to scarring, but are not a subset of central centrifugal scarring alopecia [Reply to Comment] *Arch Dermatol* 2001;137:373.

371. Powell J, Dawber RP. Folliculitis decalvans and tufted folliculitis are specific infective diseases that may lead to scarring, but are not a subset of central centrifugal scarring alopecia. [Comment] *Arch Dermatol* 2001; 137:373.

372. Ramos ML, Munoz-Perez MA, Pons A, et al. Acne keloidalis nuchae and tufted hair folliculitis. *Dermatology* 1997;194:71.

373. Smith NP, Sanderson KV. Tufted folliculitis of the scalp. *J R Soc Med* 1978;71:606.

374. Pujol RM, Garcia-Patos V, Ravella-Mateu A, et al. Tufted hair folliculitis. A specific disease? *Br J Dermatol* 1994;130:259.

375. Fernandes JC, Correia TM, Azevedo F, et al. Tufted hair folliculitis after scalp injury. *Cutis* 2001;67:243.

376. Petroni-Rosi V, Kruni A, Mijuskovi M, et al. Tufted hair folliculitis: a pattern of scarring alopecia? *J Am Acad Dermatol* 1999;41:112.

377. Grabczynska SA, Holden CA. Tufted folliculitis in a 10-year-old child. *Br J Dermatol* 1999;140:975.

378. Loewenthal LJA. "Compound" and grouped hairs of the human scalp: their possible connection with follicular infections. *J Invest Dermatol* 1947;8:263.

379. Tong AKF, Baden HP. Tufted hair folliculitis. *J Am Acad Dermatol* 1989;21:1096.

380. Dalziel KL, Telfer NR, Wilson CL, et al. Tufted folliculitis. A specific bacterial disease? *Am J Dermatopathol* 1990;12:37.

381. Kossard S. Postmenopausal frontal fibrosing alopecia. Scarring alopecia in a pattern distribution. *Arch Dermatol* 1994;130: 770.

382. Kossard S, Lee MS, Wilkinson B. Postmenopausal frontal fibrosing alopecia: a frontal variant of lichen planopilaris. *J Am Acad Dermatol* 1997;36:59.

383. Trueb RM, Torriceli R. Lichen planopilaris unter dem bild einer postmenopausalen frontalen fibrosierenden alopezie. *Hautarzt* 1998;49:388.

384. Faulkner CF, Wilson NJ, Jones SK. Frontal fibrosing alopecia associated with cutaneous lichen planus in a premenopausal woman. *Australas J Dermatol* 2002;43:65.

385. Lee WS, Hwang SM, Ahn SK. Frontal fibrosing alopecia in a postmenopausal woman. *Cutis* 1997;60:299.

386. Zinkernagel MS, Trueb RM. Fibrosing alopecia in a pattern distribution: patterned lichen planopilaris or androgenetic alopecia with a lichenoid tissue reaction pattern? *Arch Dermatol* 2000; 136:205.

387. Cornbleet T. Cutis verticis gyrata? Lipoma? *Arch Dermatol Syph* 1935;32:688.

388. Lee JH, Sung YH, Yoon JS, et al. Lipedematous scalp. *Arch Dermatol* 1994;130:802.

389. Coskey RJ, Fosnaugh RP, Fine G. Lipedematous alopecia. *Arch Dermatol* 1961;84:619.

390. Kane KS, Kwan T, Baden HP, et al. Women with new-onset boggy scalp. *Arch Dermatol* 1998;134:499.

391. Bridges AG, von Kuster LC, Estes SA. Lipedematous alopecia. *Cutis* 2000;64:199.

392. Tiscornia JE, Molezzi A, Hernandez MI, et al. Lipedematous alopecia in a white woman. *Arch Dermatol* 2002;138:1517.

393. Ikejima A, Yamashits M, Ikeda S, et al. A case of lipedematous alopecia occurring in a male patient. *Dermatology* 2000;210: 168.

394. Garn MS, Selby S, Young R. Scalp thickness and fat-loss theory of balding. *Arch Dermatol Syph* 1954;70:601.

395. Fair KP, Knoell KA, Patterson JW, et al. Lipedematous alopecia: a clinicopathologic, histologic and ultrastrucutral study. *J Cutan Pathol* 2000;27:49.

396. Curtis JW, Heising RA. Lipedematous alopecia associated with skin hyperelasticity. *Arch Dermatol* 1964;84:619.

397. Damste J, Prakken JR. Atrichia with papular lesions: a variant of congenital ectodermal dysplasia. *Dermatologica* 1954;108: 114.

398. Kanzler MH, Rasmussen JE. Atrichia with papular lesions. *Arch Dermatol* 1986;122:565.

399. Henn W, Zlotogorski A, Lam H, et al. Atrichia with papular lesions resulting from compound heterozygous mutations in the hairless gene: a lesson for differential diagnosis of alopecia universalis. *J Am Acad Dermatol* 2002;47:519.

400. Ishii Y, Kusuhara T, Nagata T. Atrichia with papular lesions associated with gastrointestinal polyposis. *J Dermatol* 1979;6: 111.

401. Ahmad M, ul Haque MF, Brancolini V, et al. Alopecia universalis associated with a mutation in the human hairless gene. *Science* 1998;279:720.

402. Nothen MM, Cichon S, Vogt IR, et al. A gene for universal congenital alopecia maps to chromosome 8p21–22. *Am J Hum Genet* 1998;62:386.

403. Sprecher E, Bergman R, Szargel R, et al. Atrichia with papular lesions maps to 8p in the region containing the human hairless gene. *Am J Med Genet* 1998;80:546.

404. Miller J, Djabali K, Chen T, et al. Atrichia caused by mutations in the vitamin D receptor gene is a phenocopy of generalized atrichia caused by mutations in the Hairless gene. *J Invest Dermatol* 2001;117:612.

405. Panteleyev AA, Paus R, Ahmad W, et al. Molecular and functional aspects of the hairless (hr) gene in laboratory rodents and humans. *Exp Dermatol* 1998;7:249.

406. Sprecher E, Shalata A, Dabhah K, et al. Androgenetic alopecia in heterozygous carriers of a mutation in the human hairless gene. *J Am Acad Dermatol* 2000;42:978.

407. Hillmer AM, Kruse R, Macciardi F, et al. The hairless gene in androgenetic alopecia: results of a systematic mutation screening and a family-based association approach. *Br J Dermatol* 2002;146:601.

408. Sarkany I. Patchy alopecia, anhidrosis, eccrine gland wall hypertrophy and vasculitis. *Proc R Soc Med* 1969;62:157.

409. Tomaszewski MM, Lupton GP, Krishnan J, et al. Syringolymphoid hyperplasia with alopecia. *J Cutan Pathol* 1994;21: 520.

410. Esche C, Sander CA, Zumdick M, et al. Further evidence that syringolymphoid hyperplasia with alopecia is a cutaneous T-cell lymphoma. *Arch Dermatol* 1998;134:753.

411. Berger TG, Goette DK. Eccrine proliferation with follicular mucinosis. *J Cutan Pathol* 1987;14:188.

412. Vaklizadeh F, Brocker EB. Syringolymphoid hyperplasia with alopecia. *Br J Dermatol* 1984;110:95.

413. Burg G, Schmockel C. Syringolymphoid hyperplasia with alopecia-a syringotropic cutaneous T-cell lymphoma? *Dermatology* 1992;184:306.

414. Wenzel FG, Horn TD. Nonneoplastic disorders of the eccrine glands. *J Am Acad Dermatol* 1998;38:1.

415. Combemale P, Faisant M, Azoulay-Petit C, et al. Neutrophilic eccrine hidradenitis secondary to infection with Serratia marcescens. *Br J Dermatol* 2000;142:784.

416. Allegue F, Rocamora A, Martin-Gonzalez M, et al. Infectious eccrine hidradenitis. *J Am Acad Dermatol* 1990;22:1119.

417. Taira JW, Gerber HB. Eccrine hidradenitis. *Int J Dermatol* 1992;31:433.

418. Smith KJ, Skelton HG, James WD, et al. Neutrophilic eccrine hidradentiis in HIV-infected patients. *J Am Acad Dermatol* 1990;23:945.

419. Bachmeyer C, Reygagne P, Aractingi S. Recurrent neutrophilic eccrine hidradenitis in an HIV-1 infected patient. *Dermatology* 2000;200:328.

420. Krischer J, Rutschmann O, Roten SV, et al. Neutrophilic eccrine hidradenitis in a patient with AIDS. *J Dermatol* 1998; 25:199.

421. Sevila A, Morell A, Banuls J, et al. Neutrophilic eccrine hidradenitis in an HIV-infected patient. *Int J Dermatol* 1996; 35:651.

422. Bachmeyer C, Chaibi P, Aractingi S. Neutrophilic eccrine hidradenitis induced by granulocyte colony-stimulating factor. *Br J Dermatol* 1998;139:354.

423. Tojo M, Iwatsuki K, Furukawa H, et al. Neutrophilic eccrine hidradenitis in actinic reticuloid syndrome. *Eur J Dermatol* 2002;12:198.

424. Bilic M, Mutasim DF. Neutrophilic eccrine hidradenitis in a patient with Behcet's disease. *Cutis* 2001;68:107.

425. Roustan G, Salas C, Cabrera R, et al. Neutrophilic eccrine hidradenitis unassociated with chemotherapy in a patient with acute myelogenous leukemia. *Int J Dermatol* 2001;40: 144.

426. Kuttner BJ, Kurban RS. Neutrophilic eccrine hidradenitis in the absence of an underlying malignancy. *Cutis* 1988;41: 403.

427. Naimer SA, Zvulunov A, Ben-Amitai D, et al. Plantar hidradenitis in children induced by exposure to wet footwear. *Pediatr Emerg Care* 2000;16:182.

428. Drake M, Sanchez-Burson JM, Dona-Naranjo MA, et al. Juvenile neutrophilic eccrine hidradenitis: a vasculitis-like plantar dermatosis. *Clin Rheumatol* 2000;19:481.

429. Stahr BJ, Cooper PH, Caputo RV. Idiopathic plantar hidradenitis occurring primarily in children. *J Cutan Pathol* 1994;21:289.

430. Ben-Amitai D, Hodak E, Landau M, et al. Idiopathic palmoplantar eccrine hidradenitis in children. *Eur J Pediatr* 2001; 160:189.

431. Hern AE, Shwayder TA. Unilateral plantar erythema nodosum. *J Am Acad Dermatol* 1992;26:259.

432. Metzker A, Brodsky F. Traumatic plantar urticaria: an unrecognized entity? *J Am Acad Dermatol* 1988;18:144.

433. Rabinowitz LG, Cintra ML, Hood AF, et al. Recurrent palmo-plantar hidradenitis in children. *Arch Dermatol* 1995;131:817.

434. Simon M, Cremer H, von den Driesch P. Idiopathic recurrent palmplantar hidradenitis in children. *Arch Dermatol* 1998;134:76.

435. Fiorillo L, Zucker M, Sawyer D, et al. The Pseudomonas hot-foot syndrome. *N Engl J Med* 2001;345:335.

436. Rasmussen JE, Graves WHI. Pseudomonas aeruginosa, hot tubs, and skin infections. *Am J Dis Child* 1982;136:553.

437. Kosatsky T, Kleeman J. Superficial and systemic illness related to a hot tub. *Am J Med* 1985;79:10.

438. Zvulunov A, Trattner A, Naimer S. Pseudomonas hot-foot syndrome. *N Engl J Med* 2001;345:1643.

439. Buezo GF, Requena L, Fraga Fernandez J, et al. Idiopathic palmoplantar hidradenitis. *Am J Dermatopathol* 1996;18:413.

440. Shelley WB, Levy EJ. Apocrine sweat retention in man. II. Fox–Fordyce disease (apocrine miliaria). *Arch Dermatol* 1956;73:38.

441. MacMillan DC, Vickers HR. Fox–Fordyce disease. *Br J Dermatol* 1971;84:181.

442. Mevorah B, Duboff GS, Wass RW. Fox–Fordyce disease in pre-pubescent girls. *Dermatologica* 1968;136:43.

443. Helm TN, Chen PW. Fox–Fordyce disease. *Cutis* 2002;69:335.

444. Ghislain PD, van Der Endt JD, Delescluse J. Itchy papules of the axillae. *Arch Dermatol* 2002;138:259.

445. Ranalletta M, Rositto A, Drut R. Fox–Fordyce disease in two prepubertal girls: histopathologic demonstration of eccrine sweat gland involvement. *Pediatr Dermatol* 1996;13:294.

446. Stashower ME, Krivda SJ, Turiansky GW. Fox–Fordyce disease: diagnosis with transverse histologic sections. *J Am Acad Dermatol* 2000;42:89.

447. Sato K, Leidal R, Sato F. Morphology and development of an apoeccrine sweat gland in human axillae. *Am J Physiol* 1987;252:R166.

448. Kamada A, Saga K, Jimbow K. Apoeccrine sweat duct obstruction as a cause for Fox–Fordyce disease. *J Am Acad Dermatol* 2003;48:453.

449. Cox NH. Posterior auricular chondrodermatitis nodularis. *Clin Exp Dermatol* 2002;27:324.

450. Tatnall FM, Sarkany I. Bilateral chondrodermatitis nodularis antihelicis. *Clin Exp Dermatol* 1984;9:322.

451. Zuber TJ, Jackson E. Chondrodermatitis nodularis chronica helicis. *Arch Fam Med* 1999;8:445.

452. Goette DK. Chondrodermatitis nodularis chronica helicis: a perforating necrobiotic granuloma. *J Am Acad Dermatol* 1980;2:148.

453. Newcomer VD, Steffen CG, Sternberg TH, et al. Chondrodermatitis nodularis chronica helicis. *Arch Dermatol* 1953;68:241.

454. Shuman R, Helwig EB. Chrondrodermatitis helicis. *Am J Clin Pathol* 1954;24:126.

455. Haber H. Chondrodermatitis nodularis chronica helicis. *Hautarzt* 1960;11:122.

456. Leonforte JE. Le nodule douloureux de l'oreille: Hyperplasie épidermique avec élimination transépithéliale. *Ann Dermatol Venereol* 1979;106:577.

457. Garcia E, Silva L, Martins O, et al. Bone formation in chondrodermatitis nodularis helicis. *J Dermatol Surg Oncol* 1980;6:582.

458. Santa Cruz DJ. Chondrodermatitis nodularis helicis: a trans-epidermal perforating disorder. *J Cutan Pathol* 1980;7:70.

459. Yoshinaga E, Enomoto U, Fujimoto N, et al. A case of chondrodermatitis nodularis chronica helicis with an autoantibody to denatured type II collagen. *Acta Derm Venereol* 2001;81:137.

460. Elgart ML. Cell phone chondrodermatitis. *Arch Dermatol* 2000;136:1568.

461. Letko E, Zafirakis P, Baltatzis S, et al. Relapsing polychondritis: a clinical review. Semin *Arthritis Rheum* 2002;31:384.

462. McAdam LP, O'Hanlan MA, Bluestone R, et al. Relapsing polychondritis: prospective study of 23 patients and a review of the literature. *Medicine (Baltimore)* 1976;55:193.

463. Thompson LD. Relapsing polychondritis. *Ear Nose Throat J* 2002;81:705.

464. Enright H, Miller W. Autoimmune phenomena in patients with myelodysplastic syndromes. *Leuk Lymphoma* 1997;24:483.

465. Case records of the Massachusetts General Hospital: relapsing polychondritis. *N Engl J Med* 1982;307:1631.

466. Thurston CS, Curtis AC. Relapsing polychondritis. *Arch Dermatol* 1966;93:664.

467. Frances C, el Rassi R, Laporte JL, et al. Dermatologic manifestations of relapsing polychondritis. A study of 200 cases at a single center. *Medicine* 2001;80:173.

468. Weinberger A, Myers AR. Relapsing polychondritis associated with cutaneous vasculitis. *Arch Dermatol* 1979;115:980.

469. Michet CJ, McKenna CH, Luthra HS, et al. Relapsing polychondritis: survival and predictive role of early disease manifestations. *Ann Intern Med* 1986;104:74.

470. Handrock K, Gross W. Relapsing polychondritis as a secondary phenomenon of primary systemic vasculitis. *Ann Rheum Dis* 1993;52:895.

471. Disdier P, Andrac L, Swiader L, et al. Cutaneous panniculitis and relapsing polychondritis: two cases. *Dermatology* 1996;193:266.

472. Bernard P, Bedane C, Delrous JL, et al. Erythema elevatum diutinum in a patient with relapsing polychondritis. *J Am Acad Dermatol* 1992;26:312.

473. Papa CA, Maroon MS, Tyler WB. Epidermolysis bullosa acquisita associated with relapsing polychondritis: an association with eosinophilia? *Cutis* 2000;66:65.

474. Helm TN, Valenzuela R, Glanz S, et al. Relapsing polychondritis: a case diagnosed by direct immunofluorescence and coexisting with pseudocyst of the auricle. *J Am Acad Dermatol* 1992;26:315.

475. Valenzuela R, Cooperrider PA, Gogate P, et al. Relapsing polychondritis. *Hum Pathol* 1980;11:19.

476. Feinerman LK, Johnson WC, Weiner J, et al. Relapsing polychondritis. *Dermatologica* 1970;140:369.

477. Barranco VP, Minor DP, Solomon H. Treatment of polychondritis with dapsone. *Arch Dermatol* 1976;112:1286.

478. Foidart JM, Abe S, Martin GR, et al. Antibodies to type II collagen in relapsing polychondritis. *N Engl J Med* 1978;299:1203.

479. Terato K, Shimozuru Y, Katayama K, et al. Specificity of antibodies to type II collagen in rheumatoid arthritis. *Arthritis Rheum* 1990;33:1493.

480. Foidart JM, Katz SI. Relapsing polychondritis. *Am J Dermatopathol* 1979;1:257.

481. Zeuner M, Straub RH, Rauh G, et al. Relapsing polychondritis: clinical and immunogenetic analysis of 62 patients. *J Rheumatol* 1997;24:96.

482. Lim CM, Goh YH, Chao SS, et al. Pseudocyst of the auricle. *Laryngoscope* 2002;112:2033.

483. Fukamizu H, Imaizumi S. Bilateral pseudocysts of the auricles. *Arch Dermatol* 1984;120:1238.

484. Kopera D, Soyer HP, Smolle J, et al. "Pseudocyst of the auricle," othematoma and otoseroma: three faces of the same coin? *Eur J Dermatol* 2000;10:451.

485. Glamb R, Kim R. Pseudocyst of the auricle. *J Am Acad Dermatol* 1984;11:58.

486. Cohen PR, Grossman ME. Pseudocyst of the auricle: case report and world literature review. *Arch Otolaryngol Head Neck Surg* 1990;116:1202.

487. Choi S, Lam K, Chan K, et al. Endochondral pseudocyst of the auricle in Chinese. *Arch Otolaryngol* 1984;110:792.

488. Ichioka S, Yamada A, Ueda K, et al. Pseudocyst of the auricle: case reports and its biochemical characteristics. *Ann Plast Surg* 1993;31:471.

489. Miyamoto H, Okajima M, Takahashi I. Lactate dehydrogenase isozymes in and intralesional steroid injection therapy for pseudocyst of the auricle. *Int J Dermatol* 2001;40:380.

490. Yamamoto T, Yokoyama A, Umeda T. Cytokine profile of bilateral pseudocyst of the auricle. *Acta Derm Venereol* 1996; 76:92.

INFLAMMATORY DISEASES OF THE NAIL

THOMAS D. GRIFFIN

An understanding of the normal anatomy and histology of the nail unit precedes understanding the pathology that may occur there (see Chapter 3). Inflammatory pathologic processes in the nail unit affect mainly the matrix, nail bed, hyponychium, and nail folds. Changes in the nail plate occur secondarily. A basic understanding of where pathologic processes affect the nail unit will guide the practitioner in choosing a site of biopsy. As in other clinical situations, understanding the location and type of pathology leads to more effective diagnosis and treatment of the disease process.

Because of the unique anatomy of the nail unit, there is a limited number of possible reaction patterns to inflammatory processes. These reaction patterns may have different features from those seen in the skin. Because the nail unit produces a product, the nail plate, some inflammatory processes of the nail matrix may lead to irreversible damage resulting in an abnormal or absent plate, much akin to processes affecting the hair unit that lead to scarring alopecia. On the other hand, processes affecting the nail bed and hyponychium that do not affect the formation of the plate may affect its shape or adhesiveness. The nail bed responds to injury by becoming metaplastic, that is, by switching from onycholemmal keratinization (without keratohyalin granules) to epidermoid keratinization. It becomes hyperplastic, showing hyperkeratosis, parakeratosis, hypergranulosis, marked spongiosis, and exudative scale crust formation. The products of this reaction build up between the nail bed and plate. This process leads to the altered shape and shedding patterns of the nail plate that are common to several diseases affecting the nail bed, such as psoriasis and onychomycosis.

Inflammatory diseases may also affect the nail folds. When the ventral surface of the proximal nail fold is affected, one may see inflammation of the cuticle and alterations of the dorsal surface of the nail plate. Eczema and contact dermatitis of the fingers may affect both the proximal and lateral nail folds.

Inflammatory processes affecting the nail may have many overlapping features. Although a specific diagnosis may be made in many cases, such as in lichen planus affecting the matrix, often it may be difficult to distinguish between, for example, psoriasis and eczema affecting the nail bed.

BIOPSY OF NAIL UNIT

Biopsy of the nail unit is recommended in many cases when the diagnosis is in doubt or when definitive histopathologic diagnosis is needed before beginning therapy. Nail matrix biopsy is best performed after reflecting back the proximal nail fold (1). The nail plate may remain intact or may be avulsed before the biopsy. It is of utmost importance to avoid bisecting the matrix. One should obtain a 2- to 3-mm punch biopsy from the center of the matrix so that the excision is entirely within and surrounded by matrix. It is also important to avoid both the curvilinear portion of the lunula and the most proximal portion of the matrix, since interruption of these areas may lead to defects in the nail plate.

The nail bed may be sampled using a punch biopsy through the nail plate down to the periosteum (2). Longitudinal incisional biopsies may also be done. In this procedure, the lateral nail fold, matrix, bed, and hyponychium are removed en bloc. This procedure is excellent for defining disease processes of the nail unit. It is probably too extensive for routine nail biopsies, and is not necessary for making a histopathologic diagnosis in most cases.

The proximal nail fold region may be sampled by a punch biopsy or a transverse excisional biopsy (2). Care must be taken to avoid going so deep in this area as to transect the tendon of the extensor digitorum communis, which inserts into the proximal dorsal portion of the terminal phalanx. Transection of this tendon will result in a drop deformity of the distal phalanx. The distal free margin of the proximal nail fold must also be avoided to prevent notching.

ECZEMATOUS DERMATITIS

Most forms of eczematous dermatitis affect the nail unit, with atopic dermatitis being most common. Contact dermatitis due to nail cosmetics or occupational exposure

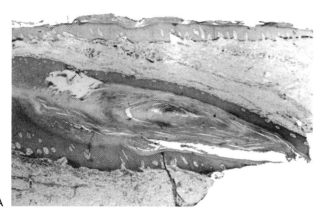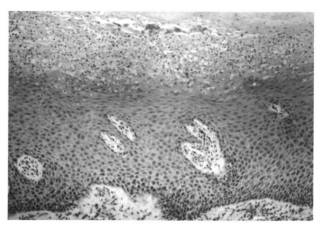

FIGURE 19-1. Psoriasis of the nail matrix. **A:** There is absence of the granular layer, acanthosis of the epidermis and vascular proliferation in the underlying papillary dermis. **B:** A spongiotic pustule is seen in the epidermis.

may affect all areas of the nail unit. Nail plate changes usually result from matrix or proximal nail fold involvement. Onycholysis may be due to nail bed involvement that begins distally at the hyponychium and spreads inward to involve the nail bed. Secondary chronic paronychial infection may occur. The biopsy should be focused on the site of involvement, usually the nail bed or nail matrix. The histologic changes include spongiosis and exocytosis of mononuclear cells, and an acanthotic epidermis. Stains for fungal organisms should be performed to rule out onychomycosis.

PSORIASIS

Nail involvement in psoriasis may occur in up to 50% of patients. Nail changes may occur in up to 80% of patients with psoriatic arthritis. In 10% of patients with psoriasis, nail involvement may be the only manifestation.

Psoriasis may involve any part of the nail unit, including the matrix, nail bed, hyponychium, and nail folds. Biopsy through the nail plate and nail bed is preferred for diagnosis of psoriasis involving the nail. Sections should be stained with hematoxylin-eosin and also with periodic acid–Schiff (PAS) stain or silver methenamine stain to rule out fungal infection. Because psoriasis and onychomycosis share many clinical and histologic features, a positive fungal stain is the only reliable way of distinguishing histologically between psoriasis and onychomycosis (3).

Psoriatic involvement of the proximal nail matrix causes clinical pitting and roughening of the surface of the nail plate. Histologically, one sees foci of parakeratosis on the surface of the plate, which, when shed, leave pits in the plate. Involvement of the mid-matrix and distal matrix leads to clinical leukonychia. Once again, the histology is that of foci of parakeratosis in the nail plate; however, in leukonychia, the parakeratotic cells are located in the deeper portions of the plate.

The "oil drop sign" of psoriatic nails is a reddish-brown discoloration of the nail bed and hyponychium (4). It represents an early, acute focus of psoriasis involving the nail bed or nail matrix. One sees hyperkeratosis and parakeratosis with collections of neutrophils in the stratum corneum representing a Munro microabscess (Fig. 19-1). The nail epidermis may show hypergranulosis with focal hypogranulosis. There is elongation of the dermal papillae with dilatation and proliferation of capillaries surrounded by lymphocytes, histiocytes, and occasional neutrophils. Distal nail onycholysis shows a similar histology and therefore has a similar histogenesis. The split in psoriatic onycholysis occurs between where neutrophils and parakeratotic foci are located within the plate and the underlying hyponychium (5). The yellow leading edge of onycholytic nail correlates with the presence of neutrophils in the nail plate keratin.

Ultimately, well-developed psoriasis of the nail bed leads to subungual hyperkeratosis and exudate, which lift the nail plate off the bed. The nail bed epithelium shows psoriasiform acanthosis with elongated rete ridges and capillary proliferation. Neutrophils may be present in the superficial epidermis and within the keratin. Late or chronically traumatized psoriatic nails may develop features of lichen simplex chronicus (6), including marked compact orthokeratosis, hypergranulosis, and fibrosis of the papillary dermis, characterized by vertical streaks of coarse collagen fibers.

LICHEN PLANUS

The incidence of nail involvement occurring in association with disseminated lichen planus ranges from 1% to 10% (7). Lichen planus may develop in the absence of cutaneous involvement and is most common in the fifth and sixth decade. Fingernails are more commonly affected than toenails (8). Lichen planus may involve the nail matrix, nail bed, and hyponychium. Examination and understanding of the pathogenesis of clinical changes will aid the clinician in determining where to sample the nail unit.

Involvement of the proximal nail matrix leads to longitudinal grooves and ridges (onychorrhexis) of the nail plate. As in lichen planus of the skin, one sees hyperkeratosis, hypergranulosis, vacuolar degeneration, necrotic keratinocytes, Civatte bodies, and a band-like infiltrate of lymphocytes and histiocytes accompanied by melanophages (Fig. 19-2). Hyperpigmentation of the nail (melanonychia) may result. If lichen planus of the proximal nail matrix is treated early in its course, onychorrhexis may be reversible. As with other skin appendages, such as hair, if the process progresses, fibrosis and scarring may result, leading to permanent deformity.

If the nail matrix is involved diffusely, onychoschizia (lamellar changes with fragility and brittleness) results. Once again, if treated before scarring occurs, the changes are reversible. When severe, unchecked lichen planus of the matrix occurs and pterygia form. The matrix is replaced by fibrosis connecting the proximal nail fold to the nail bed. As a result, the two epithelia adhere and grow distally together, constituting a pterygium.

Occasionally, lichen planus of the nail bed alone may occur. Proximal onycholysis, to be differentiated from distal onycholysis in psoriasis, occurs because of involvement of the proximal nail bed. The nail plate is otherwise normal. Papular lesions of lichen planus may occur in various locations of the nail bed and lead to focal atrophy. As a result, the overlying nail plate will be focally dimpled or spooned (koilonychia). In some cases, complete shedding of the nail plate due to diffuse nail bed involvement may occur.

BULLOUS DISEASES

Several vesiculobullous diseases may affect the nail unit. In Darier–White disease, nail changes usually occur in association with other clinical findings. Rarely, involvement may be limited to the nail alone. Nail changes may occur in the proximal nail fold, matrix, nail bed, and hyponychium. The proximal nail fold may show keratotic papules that are histologically similar to those of acrokeratosis verruciformis of Hopf. However, in addition to papillary epidermal hyperplasia, focal areas of suprabasilar acantholysis may be seen (9).

Involvement of the nail matrix in Darier–White disease is usually located in the distal lunula and manifests clinically as a white longitudinal streak. Histologically, this leukonychia is due to foci of persistent parakeratosis in the lower nail plate related to the usual histology of Darier–White disease of the distal matrix.

The nail bed and hyponychium are commonly involved in Darier–White disease. Involvement may be mild, leading to red and white longitudinal streaks. More severe involvement leads to wedge-shaped, distal, subungual keratosis, accompanied by nail fragility. In time, the nail plate may become markedly thickened. The nail bed epithelium becomes hyperplastic with parakeratosis between the nail bed and nail plate. Suprabasilar clefts are absent in the nail bed (9). An interesting finding is the presence of atypical keratinocytes in the nail bed epidermis, many of which may be multinucleated (9).

Nail involvement in pemphigus vulgaris is uncommon but may affect the proximal and lateral nail folds, leading to chronic paronychia and superficial nail plate changes

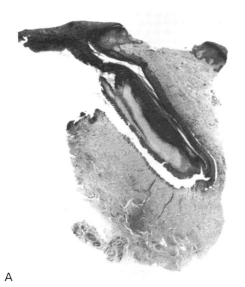
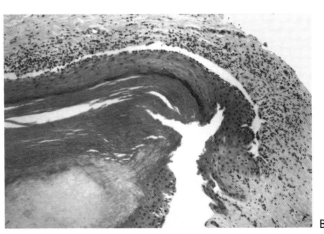

A   B

FIGURE 19-2. Lichen planus of the dorsal nail matrix epidermis. **A:** Hyperkeratosis and a superficial lymphocytic infiltrate are apparent at scanning magnification. **B:** At higher magnification, one sees vacuolar degeneration at the dermoepidermal junction with flattening of the rete pattern and an interface infiltrate of lymphocytes at the dermoepidermal junction.

(10). Biopsy of the involved nail fold reveals suprabasilar acantholysis and positive direct immunofluorescence with IgG and C3 in the intercellular spaces of the epidermis. Involvement of the matrix causes onychomadesis (proximal separation of the nail plate) (11). Pemphigus foliaceus may also affect the nail unit.

Bullous and cicatricial pemphigoid have been reported to involve the nail unit, with clinical effects implicating involvement of both matrix and nail bed, including longitudinal splits and pterygium formation (12). Erythema multiforme and toxic epidermolysis may affect the nail matrix, resulting in either sloughing of the nail or, in some cases, scarring, leading to anonychia or pterygium formation (13). Epidermolysis bullosa in many of its manifestations affects the nail unit. Epidermolysis bullosa simplex may cause onycholysis or onychogryphosis. In epidermolysis bullosa simplex–herpetiformis, nail dystrophy or anonychia may result from subungual blister formation. Junctional epidermolysis bullosa may lead to dystrophy and anonychia in all of its forms. Nail changes have been described for the Cockayne–Touraine, albopapuloid, and Hallopeau–Siemens varieties of dystrophic epidermolysis bullosa (14).

CONNECTIVE TISSUE DISEASE

The nail unit is affected by most types of connective tissue disease, primarily in the microvasculature of the proximal nail fold (15). *In vivo* capillary microscopy reveals dilated capillary loops with adjacent hemorrhage and avascularity. This pattern is present in 80% to 95% of patients with progressive systemic sclerosis. However, an identical clinical pattern may be seen in patients with dermatomyositis, other connective tissue disease, and idiopathic Raynaud phenomenon. A crescent-shaped biopsy of the proximal nail fold reveals deposits of eosinophilic PAS-positive material in the keratin of the cuticle (15). These deposits tend to be more extensive in patients with connective tissue disease and in patients with more severe *in vivo* capillary microscopy abnormalities. More data are needed to evaluate whether proximal nail fold biopsy for the presence and degree of PAS-positive deposits is of value in predicting the development of connective tissue disease in patients with idiopathic Raynaud phenomenon.

INFECTION

Fungal infection of the nails may be the most common nail disorder (16). There are four main types: distal subungual onychomycosis, proximal subungual onychomycosis, white superficial onychomycosis, and candidal onychomy-

cosis. Distal subungual onychomycosis is the most common form and is usually caused by *Trichophyton rubrum*. The fungus initially invades the hyponychium and lateral nail folds, causing yellowing, onycholysis, and eventual subungual hyperkeratosis. Biopsy of the nail bed shows hyperkeratosis. A PAS with diastase stain should be performed on all nail biopsies. This stain reveals fungal organisms that are usually located in the lower stratum corneum near the nail bed epidermis. A PAS with diastase stain performed on clippings of infected nail plate or scrapings of subungual debris will yield a diagnosis of onychomycosis more quickly than fungal culture, but will not identify the organism (Fig. 19-3). The nail bed epidermis shows acanthosis, spongiosis, and exocytosis of lymphocytes and histiocytes. In proximal subungual onychomycosis, infection initially involves the area of the proximal nail fold. Proximal white subungual onychomycosis is rare in the general population, but common in patients affected with the human immunodeficiency virus (HIV) (17). In these patients, proximal white subungual onychomycosis is caused by *Trichophyton rubrum*. On the other hand, superficial white onychomycosis is caused by *Trichophyton mentagrophytes*, located on the superficial nail plate only (16). In HIV-infected persons, superficial white onychomycosis is usually caused by *T. rubrum* (17). *Candida* species are a common cause of chronic paronychia. *Candida* may involve the nail plate and nail bed in patients with chronic mucocutaneous candidiasis and in HIV-infected patients. *Candida albicans* is the major fungus affecting the nail in pediatric patients with AIDS and may cause hypertrophic nail bed infection (17).

Bacterial infections caused by *Staphylococcus aureus* and *Pseudomonas aeruginosa* occur mainly in the nail folds and lead to acute paronychia. Bacteria may also be involved along with *Candida* in chronic paronychia. Pseudomonas organisms may colonize onycholytic nail plates, leading to green discoloration (16).

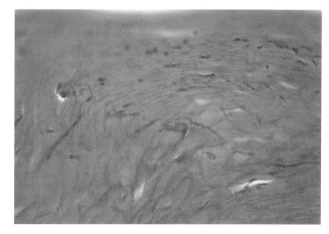

FIGURE 19-3. Onychomycosis of the nail plate. Nail clippings stained using PAS with diastase showing septate hyphal elements within the nail plate keratin.

Sarcoptes scabiei may involve the nail unit. Organisms are often present in distal subungual hyperkeratotic debris found in the hyponychium and may be a cause of persistent epidemics of scabies. Norwegian scabies may cause severe involvement of the nail folds (18).

Herpes simplex type I or II may cause herpetic whitlow or herpetic paronychia involving the nail folds.

REFERENCES

1. Scher RK. Surgical gems: biopsy of the matrix of nail. *J Dermatol Surg Oncol* 1980;6:19.
2. Scher RK. Punch biopsies of the nails: a simple, valuable procedure. *J Dermatol Surg Oncol* 1978;4:528.
3. Kouskoukis CE, Scher RK, Ackerman AB. What histologic finding distinguishes onychomycosis and psoriasis? *Am J Dermatopathol* 1983;5:501.
4. Kouskoukis CE, Scher RK, Ackerman AB. The "oil drop" sign of psoriatic nails: a clinical finding specific for psoriasis. *Am J Dermatopathol* 1983;5:259.
5. Robbins TO, Kouskoukis CE, Ackerman AB. Onycholysis in psoriatic nails. *Am J Dermatopathol* 1983;5:39.
6. Kouskoukis CE, Scher RK, Ackerman AB. The problem of features of lichen simplex chronicus complicating the histology of diseases of the nail. *Am J Dermatopathol* 1984;6:45.
7. Scher RK, Ackerman AB. Lichen planus. *Am J Dermatopathol* 1983;5:375.
8. Tosti A, Peluso AM, Fanti PA, et al. Nail lichen planus: clinical and pathologic study of 24 patients. *J Am Acad Dermatol* 1993; 28:724.
9. Zaias N, Ackerman AB. The nail in Darier–White disease. *Arch Dermatol* 1973;107:193.
10. Dhawan SS, Zaias N, Pena J. The nail fold in pemphigus vulgaris [Letter]. *Arch Dermatol* 1990;126:1374.
11. Parameswara VR, Chinnappaiah Naik RP. Onychomedesis associated with pemphigus vulgaris. *Arch Dermatol* 1981;117: 759.
12. Burge SM, Powell SM, Ryan TJ. Cicatricial pemphigoid with nail dystrophy. *Clin Exp Dermatol* 1985;10:472.
13. Wancher B, Thornmann J. Permanent anonychia after Stevens–Johnson syndrome. *Arch Dermatol* 1977;113:970.
14. Pearson RW. Clinical pathologic types of epidermolysis bullosa in nondermatological complications. *Arch Dermatol* 1988;124: 718.
15. Scher RK, Tom DWK, Lally EV, et al. The clinical significance of periodic acid-Schiff-positive deposits in cuticle-proximal nail fold biopsy specimens. *Arch Dermatol* 1985;121:1406.
16. Cowen PR, Scher RK. Geriatric nail disorders: diagnosis and treatment. *J Am Acad Dermatol* 1992;26:521.
17. Daniel CR, Norton LA, Scher RK. The spectrum of nail disease in patients with human immunodeficiency virus infection. *J Am Acad Dermatol* 1992;27:93.
18. Scher RK. Subungual scabies. *Am J Dermatopathol* 1983;5: 187.

INFLAMMATORY DISEASES OF THE SUBCUTANEOUS FAT

N. SCOTT MCNUTT
ABELARDO MORENO
FÉLIX CONTRERAS

CLASSIFICATION OF PANNICULITIS

A histopathologic classification of panniculitis is based on the microscopic and macroscopic changes in the subcutaneous fat. The diseases presented in this chapter are divided into groups based on their patterns of involvement of the anatomic structures in the subcutis (1–3) (Table 20-1). However, for definite diagnoses, it is important to consider whether there are associated changes, such as in the overlying dermis and epidermis, as well as what types of inflammatory cells are involved (4). Clinical history and distribution of lesions often are important. The subcutaneous fat can be divided into the following anatomic regions: the septa between fat lobules, the fat lobules themselves, the blood vessels, and the nerves. When the septa are involved by inflammation, the histologic changes include septal widening due to edema, hemorrhage, fibrosis, or inflammatory infiltration by neutrophils, eosinophils, and macrophages, with or without granuloma formation. Involvement of the fat lobules includes necrosis, cellular infiltration, and fibrosis. Necrosis of fat is common and the different types of necrosis have been classified by etiology as ischemic, traumatic, enzymatic, metabolic, inflammatory, and infectious. The cellular infiltrate associated with necrosis can be composed predominantly of polymorphonuclear leukocytes (neutrophils and eosinophils), lymphocytes (occasionally with germinal centers), and macrophages (with or without granulomas). Fibrosis of the fat lobules is a late event, which is the end result of multiple causes of lobular panniculitis ranging from that due to simple trauma to that due to complex connective tissue diseases. By analysis of the patterns of involvement of these regions, it is possible to make a specific diagnosis in a patient with panniculitis even when the interactions between inflammatory cells and target cells in panniculitis show considerable overlap in their basic mechanisms at the cellular and molecular levels.

Although the classification of panniculitis stresses the differences between the lobules of fat and the interlobular septa, there is an intimate relationship between the two. The septa contain the major blood vessels and nerves that supply the delicate plexus of vessels within the fat lobules and also contain the major vessels that pass on to the overlying dermis. When blood vessels are the target of inflammation, the various sizes of the blood vessels and their wall structures can cause certain diseases to be localized in the fat. Inflammation of the walls of large vessels often involves only the fat lobules immediately adjacent to the vessels. The medium-sized vessels are in the septa and inflammation of their walls leads to septal panniculitis and in some cases also leads to secondary ischemic destruction of the fat lobules. Inflammation of the small vessels can affect the septa, lobules, or both. The relatively sluggish blood flow through the small vessels in the fat facilitates the exudation of substances and the emigration of inflammatory cells into the panniculus. For example, immune complexes or medications can be deposited in the walls of these vessels. Moreover, the subcutaneous fat cells, or adipocytes, form a closely regulated metabolic reserve, on which certain chemical compounds interact preferentially; for example, pancreatic lipases that have been released into the circulating blood or fat-soluble chemicals and medications can localize in the fat and cause metabolic or inflammatory changes. Hereditary and gender differences exist in fat metabolism and these can be expressed in metabolic differences in different anatomic sites in the same individual. For example, *in vivo* and *in vitro*, abdominal subcutaneous adipose tissue is more responsive metabolically to beta-adrenergic stimulation than is the subcutaneous fat of the thigh. The thickness and orientation of the septa differ in normal males versus females and hypoandrogenized males, which suggest that this is under hormonal control (5). The septa are thicker in areas of the skin that are subjected to greater weight bearing, suggesting that genetic programming and mechanical forces both influence the thickness of the normal septa.

In the upper portion of the panniculus are the secretory coils of eccrine and apocrine glands and the lower portion of

TABLE 20-1. CLASSIFICATION OF PANNICULITIS

I. With prominent vasculitis (septal or lobular)
   A. Neutrophilic
      Leukocytoclastic immune-complex vasculitis
      Subcutaneous polyarteritis nodosa
      Thrombophlebitis
      Type 2 leprosy reaction (erythema nodosum leprosum; Lucio's phenomenon)
      Behçet's syndrome
   B. Lymphocytic
      Nodular vasculitis
      Perniosis
      Angiocentric lymphomas
      Lupus erythematosus
   C. Granulomatous
      Nodular vasculitis/erythema induratum of Bazin
      Type 2 leprosy reaction
      Wegener's granulomatosis
      Churg–Strauss allergic granulomatosis

II. Without prominent vasculitis
   A. Septal inflammation
      1. Lymphocytic and mixed
         Erythema nodosum
         Variants of erythema nodosum
      2. Granulomatous
         Palisaded granulomatous diseases
         Sarcoidosis
         Subcutaneous infection
         Tuberculosis
         Syphilis
         Necrobiosis lipoidica
         Necrobiotic xanthogranuloma
      3. Sclerotic
         Scleroderma/ morphea
         Eosinophilic fasciitis
         Ischemic liposclerosis
         Toxins, particularly injected ones
         Postirradiation panniculitis
   B. Lobular inflammation
      1. Neutrophilic
         Infection
         Ruptured folliculitis and cysts
         Pancreatic fat necrosis
         Alpha-1-antitrypsin deficiency
      2. Lymphocytic
         Lupus panniculitis (lupus profundus)
         Poststeroid panniculitis
         Ischemic lipomembranous panniculitis
         Localized lipedema (minimal infiltration)
         Lymphoma/leukemia
      3. Macrophagic
         Rosai–Dorfman disease
         Histiocytic cytophagic panniculitis
         Ischemic lipomembranous panniculitis
      4. Granulomatous
         Erythema induratum/nodular vasculitis
         Palisaded granulomatous diseases
         Sarcoidosis
         Crohn's disease
         Ruptured follicular cyst

5. Mixed inflammation, with many foam cells
   Alpha-1-antitrypsin deficiency
   Weber–Christian disease
   Traumatic fat necrosis
   Factitial panniculitis (foreign body panniculitis)
6. Eosinophilic
   Eosinophilic panniculitis
   Arthropod bite reaction
   Hypersensitivity reaction to internal parasites, or medications
7. Enzymatic fat necrosis
   Pancreatic enzyme panniculitis
   Alpha-1-antitrypsin deficiency panniculitis
8. Crystal deposits
   Sclerema neonatorum
   Subcutaneous fat necrosis of the newborn
   Gout
   Oxalosis
   Calcific panniculitis/calciphylaxis
   Cold panniculitis
   Poststeroid panniculitis
9. Embryonic fat pattern
   Lipoatrophy
   Lipodystrophy
10. Sclerotic
   Ischemic lipodermatosclerosis
   Membranous panniculitis (lipomenbranous panniculitis)
   Postirradiation panniculitis
   Eosinophilic fasciitis, late stage
   Morphea and scleroderma

hair follicles. Consequently, diseases of the skin appendages can involve the panniculus secondarily. The subcutis also has a lower border on the fascia, and inflammatory diseases that affect the fascia can penetrate upward into the septa and lobules.

Unfortunately, a significant problem is that the clinical appearance of the lesions of panniculitis is not very specific since most patients have deep erythematous nodules. A consideration of the clinical distribution, number of lesions, and whether they are ulcerated help in the formulation of a clinical differential diagnosis. Some early clinical studies led to the description of clinical "entities," such as Weber–Christian disease or panniculitis of Rothmann

and Makai, which unfortunately exhibit nonspecific histopathologic changes, that occur in a variety of actual diseases that cause panniculitis.

Another major problem in the classification of panniculitis is that often the size of the biopsy is inadequate. The individual lobules of fat may be more than 1 mm in diameter and several lobules and septa are needed to discern accurately a pattern of involvement. Consequently, an adequate biopsy should be an elliptical, excisional, or incisional one that gives at least a specimen of fat 6 mm in greatest dimension, and should include deep subcutis as well as the overlying skin. Only a few diagnoses can be made on a specimen of aspirated fat or a needle or punch biopsy of a nodule in the subcutis; the use of these biopsy modalities is to be discouraged for purposes of histologic classification of panniculitis.

A third problem is that most of the lesions have a time course in which there occurs a early form of inflammation with varying degrees of vascular changes, followed by a stage of phagocytosis of fat and a more or less pronounced granulomatous reaction, and by a final stage of fibrosis. Such a time course is evident in the overall lesion and may also be different in various areas of the lesion. With small biopsies or with a nonspecific pattern of inflammation, a simple categorical diagnosis of "panniculitis" may be necessary until further studies and clinical follow-up information allows the placement of the disease into a more exact category (6–8).

Table 20-1 presents a summary of the classification of panniculitis. Not all of the disease entities are presented in detail in this chapter and some can be found elsewhere in this book: leukocytoclastic vasculitis (Chapter 8), systemic polyarteritis nodosa (Chapter 8), sarcoidosis (Chapter 14), granuloma annulare (Chapter 14), rheumatoid nodule (Chapter 14), necrobiosis lipoidica (Chapter 1), scleroderma (Chapter 10), necrobiotic xanthogranuloma (Chapter 27), and gummatous tertiary syphilis (Chapter 22).

In the natural progression of lesions of vasculopathic panniculitis, as well as in septal or lobular panniculitis, a complex mixture of patterns can result depending on the stage of evolution of the disease. For example, factitial panniculitis can exhibit a mixed pattern with microscopic features (hematoma, foreign bodies, dermal lesions, and fibrosis) that fit into more than one category. Subcutaneous panniculitic T-cell lymphoma may present with patterns of leukemic infiltration, lupus erythematosus-like lesions, granulomatous lesions, and angiodestructive vasculitic lesions.

ERYTHEMA NODOSUM

Clinical Presentation. An acute form and a chronic form of erythema nodosum exist, which differ in their clinical manifestations but do not have uniformly recognized differences in their histologic characteristics (2,9).

In the *acute form* of erythema nodosum, there is a sudden appearance of tender, bright red, or dusky red-purple nodules to plaques that only slightly elevate the level of the skin surface (Fig. 20-1). The lesions vary from 1 to 5 cm in diameter and have a strong predilection for the anterior surfaces of the lower legs, although they may occur elsewhere, especially on the calves, thighs, and, in severe cases, on the forearms, hands, and even the face. They occur mostly on the dependent regions of the body, and tend to be distributed symmetrically. The lesions do not ulcerate and generally involute within a few weeks without leaving a depressed scar. As a result of the intermittent appearance of new lesions, the disease may persist for several months.

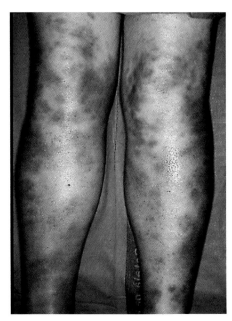

FIGURE 20-1. Erythema nodosum. Erythematous nodules are abundant on the anterior shins bilaterally.

The acute disease often is accompanied by fever, malaise, leukocytosis, and arthropathy (10). The lesions are tender and warm. Lesions near a joint can mimic arthritis. Focal hemorrhages are common and can cause the lesions to resemble bruises (erythema contusiforme), even to changing in color from red to purple, and on to green and blue, as they age and resolve. Bilateral hilar adenopathy can be present in patients with acute erythema nodosum with or without sarcoidosis since a number of pulmonary infections can produce both hilar adenopathy and erythema nodosum. Erythema nodosum occurs in 10% to 20% of patients with sarcoidosis and is thought to portend a good prognosis (10).

The *chronic form* of erythema nodosum is also known as *erythema nodosum migrans* (11) or subacute nodular migratory panniculitis of Vilanova and Piñol Aguade (12). There are one or several red, subcutaneous nodules that are found, usually unilaterally, on the lower leg. Vilanova and Piñol Aguade observed that almost all of the patients were women (16 to 65 years of age) with a solitary lesion and a recent history of sore throat and arthralgia. Tenderness is slight or absent. The nodules enlarge by peripheral extension into plaques, often with central clearing. The duration may be from a few months to a few years.

Histopathology. The histologic changes are present mainly in and near the septa of the subcutaneous tissue (Fig. 20-2). The overlying dermis often has only a minimal to moderate, superficial and deep, perivascular lymphocytic infiltrate.

In *early lesions of acute erythema nodosum*, there is edema of the septa with a lymphohistiocytic infiltrate, having a

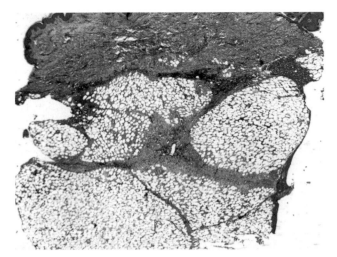

FIGURE 20-2. Acute erythema nodosum. Most of the inflammation is in the subcutis, in and near the septa. The septa at the bottom of the figure are almost normal in thickness whereas the upper portion of the subcutis has thickened septa.

slight admixture of neutrophils and eosinophils (13) (Fig. 20-3A1, A2, B, and C). Focal fibrin deposition and extravasation of erythrocytes occur frequently (6) and can be revealed by spectral microscopy (Fig. 20-3A2). Often the inflammation is most intense at the periphery of the edematous septa and extends into the periphery of the fat lobules between the individual fat cells in a lace-like fashion. Necrosis of the fat is not prominent. Rarely, clusters of neutrophils are present or the infiltrate is predominantly neutrophilic (14) (Fig. 20-4). Clusters of macrophages around small blood vessels, or a slit-like space, occur in early lesions and are known as Miescher's radial nodules (15,16) (Fig. 20-5). Some authors have failed to find central vessels (2) and have considered Miescher's nodules to be characteristic of erythema nodosum, stating that they can be found in all stages of erythema nodosum (16). The degree of vascular involvement is variable (6,17) (Fig. 20-6A, B, and C). There is usually edema of the walls of

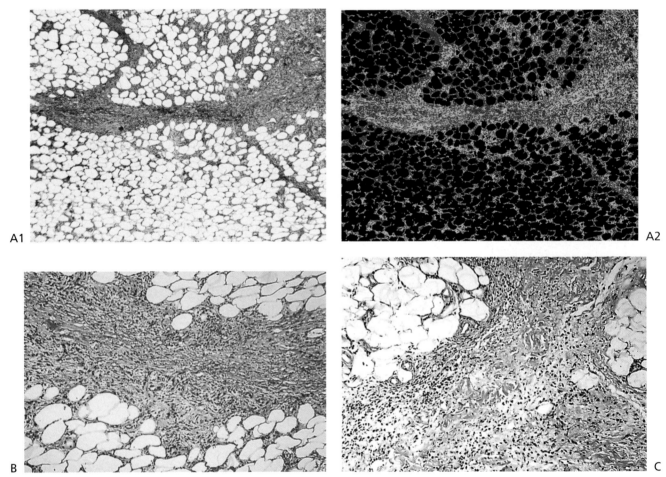

FIGURE 20-3. Acute erythema nodosum. Part **(A1)** shows acute erythema nodosum with inflammation at the junction of the septa and lobules with some hemorrhages. Part **(A2)** is a matching spectral image showing the spectral domains of red blood cells in the hemorrhages in red, as distinguished from the spectral domain of the eosin-stained collagen here shown in green. Hematoxylin in nuclei is shown in blue. Part **(B)** is a higher magnification of a septal region showing the paraseptal inflammation, and **(C)** shows early fibrosis of the edematous septa in acute erythema nodosum.

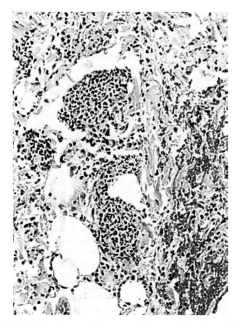

FIGURE 20-4. Acute erythema nodosum. Clusters of neutrophils can be found in the paraseptal region, without evidence of intact bacteria.

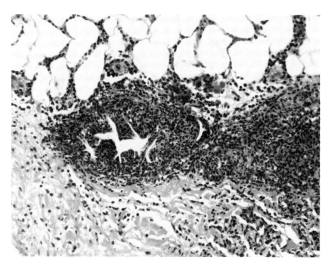

FIGURE 20-5. Acute erythema nodosum. Miescher's radial granulomas are characteristic findings and are formed by macrophages and neutrophils.

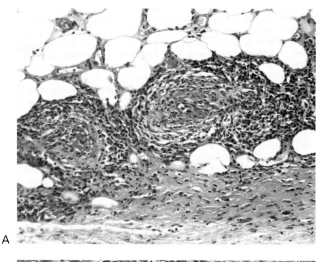

A

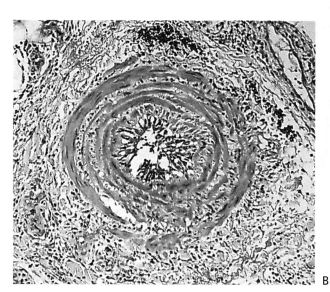

B

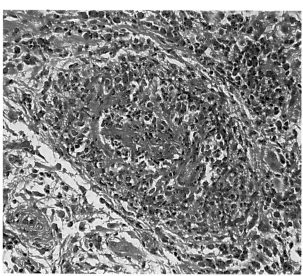

C

FIGURE 20-6. Acute erythema nodosum. Vasculitis is uncommon but can be found in the paraseptal and septal blood vessels. Part (A) shows vascular damage with a mixed neutrophil and macrophage infiltrate and thrombosis; (B) demonstrates edema and inflammation in the wall of a small vein in the septa; and (C) shows more advanced inflammation of the wall of a vein in erythema nodosum.

veins with separation of the muscular layers (Fig. 20-6B). Infiltration by lymphocytes is common, but neutrophils and eosinophils can be present also. Necrosis of the vessel walls is very rare but has been observed in a few patients with lesions clinically indistinguishable from erythema nodosum (18,19). For example, focal vasculitis has been found in a few patients with acute erythema nodosum secondary to infections, and in a few cases of recurrent erythema nodosum that is secondary to medications or estrogenic oral contraceptives (Fig. 20-6C).

Later lesions of acute erythema nodosum show widening of the septa, often with fibrosis and with inflammation at the edges of the septa and involving the periphery of the fat lobules (Fig. 20-7). Neutrophils usually are absent and the vascular changes are less prominent than in early lesions. There are more macrophages in the infiltrate. Macrophages at the edges of the fat lobules show phagocytosis of lipid from damaged adipocytes and the small droplets of lipid in their cytoplasm give them a "foam cell" appearance. Granulomas formed by macrophages, without lipid deposition, are more frequent when late lesions are compared to early ones (Fig. 20-8). The granulomas often are loosely formed with macrophages predominating in a focus with multinucleated giant cells. Occasionally, well-formed, discrete sarcoidal granulomas occur in small numbers in the septa. The multinucleated cells usually have an irregular distribution of the nuclei in the cytoplasm. The oldest lesions have septal widening and fibrosis with a decrease in all of the inflammatory cells.

In *chronic erythema nodosum*, the histologic findings are generally the same as those of the late stages of acute erythema nodosum. However, granulomas and lipogranulomas often are more pronounced. There is vascular proliferation and thickening of the endothelium with extrava-

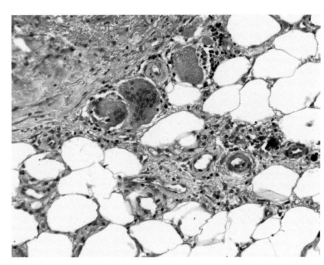

FIGURE 20-8. Late erythema nodosum. Multinucleated giant cells are common in the septa of late lesions. Tuberculoid granulomas can also be found.

sation of erythrocytes (20). In some instances numerous well-formed granulomas can be found and consist of epithelioid macrophages and giant cells without caseous necrosis (6). Although significant degrees of vasculitis have been observed by some authors (12,21), others have found vascular changes to be slight or absent (22,23). The presence of thickened fibrotic septa with marked capillary proliferation and massive granulomatous reaction have lead several authors to consider *erythema nodosum migrans* as an entity separate from the late lesions of acute erythema nodosum (24). Other authors consider all of these histologic patterns to be included within the spectrum of chronic erythema nodosum (2,9).

Pathogenesis. Although the cause of erythema nodosum cannot always be determined in an individual patient, streptococcal infection is the most common among the known causes, especially in children, as evidenced by elevation of antistreptolysin O titers. The diseases that can be associated with erythema nodosum are numerous and have been reviewed recently (2,25). In short, they may be divided into: infections with bacteria, fungi, or protozoa; viral diseases; malignancies; medications; and miscellaneous conditions. The most frequent bacterial infections are streptococcal infection, tuberculosis, *Yersinia enterocolitica* infection (26), brucellosis, leptospirosis, tularemia, *Chlamydia* infection, and *Mycoplasma pneumoniae* infection. The most frequently associated fungal infections are coccidioidomycosis, histoplasmosis (27), dermatophytosis, aspergillosis, and blastomycosis, depending on the geographic location and immune status of the patient. Protozoal infections, such as toxoplasmosis, amoebiasis, and *Giardia* infection can cause erythema nodosum. Among the associated viral and rickettsial infections are herpes simplex, infectious mononucleosis (due to Epstein–Barr virus infection), lymphogranuloma venereum, ornitho-

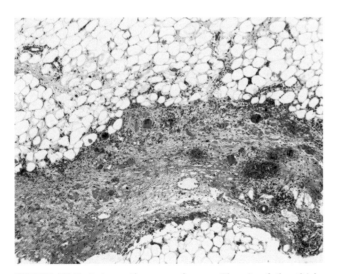

FIGURE 20-7. Late erythema nodosum. Fibrosis of the thickened septa is advanced and accompanied mainly by a lymphocytic infiltrate, often with a few eosinophils.

sis, and psittacosis. Erythema nodosum occurs with some cases of leukemia, Hodgkin's disease, non-Hodgkin's lymphomas, as well as with some other cancers, particularly after irradiation or other treatment releases antigens into the circulation by tumor necrosis. Among the miscellaneous associations are several diseases that can cause considerable difficulty in diagnosis, particularly acute sarcoidosis, which can have erythema nodosum as part of a symptom complex along with slight hilar adenopathy, fever, arthralgias, and occasionally acute iritis, uveitis and parotid swelling (*uveoparotid fever*). The sarcoidal granulomas that can occur in erythema nodosum are less frequent, are septal in location, and are associated with edema, in contrast to the abundant granulomas that occur in subcutaneous sarcoidosis, without much edema and mostly in the lobules of the subcutaneous fat. Likewise, Crohn's disease can be associated with erythema nodosum (10) and the two diseases can be difficult to distinguish from each other histologically in the skin involvement unless there is ulceration, which does not occur in erythema nodosum (28). Other associated conditions are ulcerative colitis, and Behçet's disease (29). The panniculitis in Behçet's disease may resemble erythema nodosum clinically, but often is different histologically in having neutrophilic and lymphocytic vasculitis which is septal or lobular in distribution (30). Erythema nodosum and Sweet's syndrome have been reported in the same patient (31). Among the many medications that can cause erythema nodosum, the most common ones are sulfonamides, estrogens, and oral contraceptives (32). Rare associations are with aminopyrine, antimony compounds, arsphenamine, bromides, iodides, phenacetin, salicylates, immunizations, and vaccinations (2). Such a great diversity in inciting agents and circumstances suggests that several mechanisms may be capable of triggering the clinical and histopathologic changes that are classified as erythema nodosum.

Direct immunofluorescence studies have shown deposits of immunoglobulins only very rarely in the blood vessel walls in erythema nodosum (7). Small amounts of complement in the vessel walls and abundant fibrin around the vessels are frequent but nonspecific findings. On electron microscopic examination, nonspecific vascular changes consisting of damage to endothelial cells and lymphocytic infiltration have been described (33).

The occurrence of erythema nodosum as a response to medications and to tuberculin skin testing in patients with a positive reaction suggest that a type IV delayed hypersensitivity reaction may play an important role, especially given the paucity of reports of immunoglobulin deposition and the usual failure to detect circulating immune complexes (34). However, in some patients a type III immune complex reaction could be responsible. Circulating immune complexes and rheumatoid factors have been detected in some patients with sarcoidosis and erythema nodosum (35). In approximately 50% of cases, there is no cause identified (36). The predilection for the anterior shins and for dependent parts of the body suggests that trauma or sluggish blood flow plays a role in the localization of the lesions.

Differential Diagnosis. Erythema nodosum needs to be distinguished from *erythema induratum* and *nodular vasculitis*. Vasculitis and zones of fat necrosis are absent in erythema nodosum and frequent in erythema induratum. In patients suspected to have erythema nodosum but with necrotizing vasculitis, the possibility of *cutaneous polyarteritis nodosa* must be considered. In the latter disease, medium-sized arteries rather than veins or small-caliber blood vessels are affected, with necrosis of the walls of affected arteries. In contrast, *nodular vasculitis* has mainly lymphocytic infiltration with fibrous thickening and obliteration of vascular lumens. *Superficial migratory thrombophlebitis*, unlike erythema nodosum, has a large vein containing thrombus in the center of the lumen. *Syphilitic gummas* are ulcerative irregular granulomatous lesions that produce depressed scars. *Subcutaneous tuberculosis* can mimic erythema nodosum in lesions that are extending from underlying organs, soft tissues, or bone. Stains for acid-fast organisms and cultures are needed. Subcutaneous tuberculosis can spare the upper portion of the panniculus, whereas erythema nodosum does not. Erythema nodosum does not have granulomas or sclerosis in the overlying dermis, and in this way can be distinguished from most cases of sarcoidosis, scleroderma, necrobiosis lipoidica diabeticorum, ruptured follicular cysts, and factitial traumatic panniculitis.

EOSINOPHILIC PANNICULITIS AND FASCIITIS

Clinical Features. The diagnosis of eosinophilic panniculitis is based on the histologic appearance of numerous eosinophils in the fat, which can be found as a reaction pattern in the following clinical diseases or conditions: erythema nodosum, vasculitis, arthropod bites, parasitic infection, drug injections, Well's syndrome, eosinophilic fasciitis, hypereosinophilic syndrome, and eosinophilic leukemia (37–41).

Histopathology. Usually there is a mixed inflammatory infiltrate of lymphocytes, macrophages, and numerous eosinophils, involving both septa and lobules of the subcutis (Fig. 20-9). A pure infiltrate of normal eosinophils indicates the hypereosinophilic syndrome, in contrast to eosinophilic leukemia, in which the eosinophils are cytologically atypical. The overlying dermis should be studied carefully for important findings as well. The eosinophils aggregate often on dermal collagen fibers and degranulate to form masses of eosinophilic granules, which are called "flame figures" in Well's syndrome. The histologic sections should be searched for parasites, but they may be at a site distant from the skin, such as in the gastrointestinal tract or other sites, in which case the panniculitis is a reaction to circulating antigens.

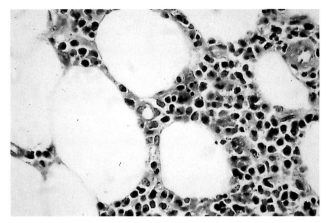

FIGURE 20-9. Eosinophilic panniculitis. Eosinophils in abundance in the fat lobules is not a specific finding, which can be seen in a variety of disorders, most commonly in arthropod bite reactions.

Differential Diagnosis. The differential diagnosis includes reactions to foreign bodies (need to test for polarizable material in the sections), reactions to parasites, deep arthropod bite reactions, or drug injections. Peripheral blood studies will rule in or out eosinophilic leukemia, which also has eosinophilic precursor cells in the infiltrate in the subcutis. Macrophages can ingest eosinophil granules from degranulated eosinophils in a variety of hypersensitivity reactions and should be distinguished from true eosinophilic myelocytes and metamyelocytes. Several patients have been reported to have a hypereosinophilic syndrome with lymphoid abnormalities that are clonal T-cell proliferations (42,43). In eosinophilic fasciitis, the involvement of the overlying subcutis can produce dense hyalinized sclerosis resembling scleroderma, even with plasma cells. However, if the biopsy includes the fascia itself, the fascia contains eosinophils, which is the finding that separates eosinophilic fasciitis from morphea and scleroderma. Eosinophilic fasciitis may present as Shulman's syndrome, characterized by the sudden onset of thickened, bound-down skin, which follows in some cases a clear episode of intense exercise. Eosinophilic fasciitis also can be a presentation of a reaction to a drug, such as L-tryptophan, a toxic oil, or infection (2,44,45).

PANNICULITIS ASSOCIATED WITH SEVERE ALPHA-1–ANTITRYPSIN DEFICIENCY

Clinical Features. Patients born with a severe deficiency of alpha-1 antitrypsin (AAT) have exaggerated damage due to inflammation in the skin, such as after trauma to the subcutis. AAT deficiency is estimated to be present in one out of every 3,500 live births in the white population (46). This enzyme is the major component of the alpha-1 peak on serum electrophoresis and is an inhibitor of the serine

proteases trypsin, chymotrypsin, plasmin, thrombin, and neutrophil-produced elastase. The antitrypsin proenzyme is produced in the liver but is not secreted in most of the affected individuals. Liver disease is often the presenting problem, including hepatomegaly, neonatal cholestatic jaundice, and cirrhosis in children (47,48). Large PAS-positive, diastase-resistant globules of proenzyme can be seen in hepatocytes, especially near the fibrous septa. Inflammation in the lung leads to unopposed release of neutrophil elastase that produces panacinar emphysema, involving destruction of respiratory bronchioles, alveolar ducts and alveoli. The pulmonary disease usually becomes evident in young to middle-aged adults. Skin lesions present after trauma as recurrent nodules that can drain a yellow fluid derived from the enzymatic breakdown of the fibrous tissue and fat (49–51) (Fig. 20-10).

Histopathology. Biopsies of well-developed lesions show a mixed pattern of septal and lobular inflammation characterized by many neutrophils and destruction of the fat and the fibrous septa (Fig. 20-11). Sterile abscesses surround and isolate fat lobules (52) (Fig. 20-12). Late lesions have an infiltrate of macrophages and lymphocytes with many foam cells and fibrosis (51,53). The macrophages can exhibit cytophagic activity and particularly can ingest neutrophil fragments and extravasated erythrocytes. Biopsies of early lesions have not been studied in a series of cases, but in some patients, the early manifestations are neutrophilic infiltrates between collagen bundles in the dermis, with scattered solitary neutrophils and small collections of neutrophils in the septa and lobules of the subcutaneous fat (54). Depending on the size of the lesion, the subcutaneous involvement can be patchy with necrotic foci contrasting with the normal fat lobules in the vicinity (51,53).

Differential Diagnosis. The histopathologic changes are not specific for AAT deficiency, but rather are shared by a number of diseases than can be responsible for *necrotizing panniculitis.* A biopsy of a subcutaneous nodule occasionally shows a nonspecific pattern of necrotizing acute

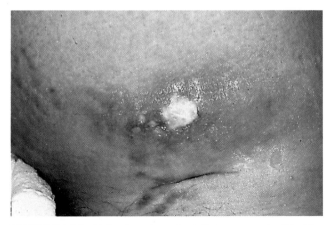

FIGURE 20-10. Alpha-1 antitrypsin deficiency panniculitis. The inflammatory lesions in the subcutis are often accompanied by dermal inflammation and can perforate through the epidermis.

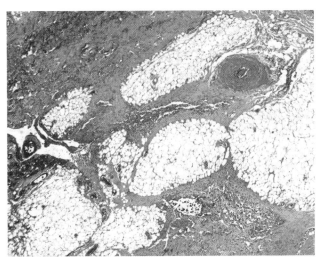

FIGURE 20-11. Alpha-1 antitrypsin deficiency panniculitis. Abscesses dissect between the fat lobules and involve the lower dermis.

inflammation characterized by fat necrosis and a massive neutrophilic infiltrate, often accompanied by karyorrhexis, fibrin deposition, focal vasculitis, and histiocytic reparative reaction. These changes also can be produced by very acute necrosis (liquefaction necrosis) in cases of *nodular vasculitis*, pyoderma gangrenosum, inflammatory reaction near ulcers from a variety of causes, and can represent changes due to infection by pyogenic bacteria, including mycobacteria (55). If a meticulous study, including cultures and enzymatic studies, fails to reveal a satisfactory final diagnosis, then the term "necrotizing panniculitis" can be a suitable histologic diagnosis until other methods or information become available.

The clinical features of AAT deficiency overlap with those of Weber–Christian disease to the extent that a determination of serum levels of the enzyme should be performed on all cases clinically suspected of having Weber–Christian

disease or any patient with ulcerating and necrotizing panniculitis. Weber–Christian disease is more restricted to the fat lobules than AAT deficiency panniculitis, which involves septa, lobules, and overlying dermis (54). Histiocytic cytophagic panniculitis (often a form of subcutaneous T-cell lymphoma with reactive histiocytosis) is in the differential diagnosis due to the fact that macrophage cytophagic activity also can occur in AAT deficiency. The prominence of neutrophils in AAT deficiency is in contrast to the lymphocytes in histiocytic cytophagic panniculitis. In the early lesions, infection needs to be ruled out since erysipelas and even some mycobacterial infections can have a similar histology (55). Serum electrophoresis is important in detecting carriers and affected individuals with AAT deficiency.

SUPERFICIAL MIGRATORY THROMBOPHLEBITIS

Clinical Presentation. Multiple tender, erythematous nodules are found usually on the lower legs but occasionally on the arms and trunk (56,57). After several days, a cord-like induration a few centimeters long can be felt along the course of the inflamed vein (58). As the old lesions resolve, usually within a few weeks, new nodules may erupt. Recurrent migratory thrombophlebitis can occur as a manifestation of Behçet's syndrome. It is also part of Trousseau's syndrome, in which there is an associated visceral carcinoma. Hypercoagulability and stasis are precipitating factors (56,57).

Histopathology. The lesion is centered around a large vein in the subcutis, usually in a septal location and occasionally in the deep vascular plexus, at the junction of deep dermis and subcutis (Fig. 20-13). The affected vein has a thick wall with the smooth muscle distributed in fascicles in the wall. The lumen often is completely occluded by thrombus. An inflammatory infiltrate extends between the muscle bundles and only a short distance into the tissue

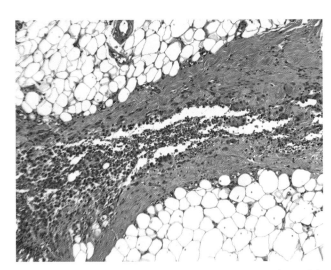

FIGURE 20-12. Alpha-1 antitrypsin deficiency panniculitis. High magnification of an abscess showing the neutrophils in the septa.

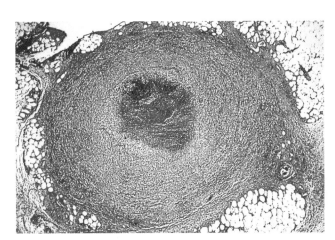

FIGURE 20-13. Superficial migratory thrombophlebitis. A vein is filled with thrombus, and the inflammation involves the adjacent septa and lobules.

surrounding the vein (2,59). In early lesions, the infiltrate is composed of many neutrophils, but later it consists mainly of lymphocytes, macrophages, and a few giant cells (56,57). If recanalization of the lumen of the vein takes place, granulomas with giant cells can be found even in the lumen of the affected vessel. These granulomas participate in the resorption of the thrombus (58).

Differential Diagnosis. Owing to the elevated hydrostatic pressure in the veins of the lower legs in ambulatory patients, the walls of the veins have an increased amount of elastic fibers and smooth muscle in their walls. They can be distinguished from arteries when there is minimal inflammation and when elastic tissue stains show an absence of an internal elastic lamina. Thrombus usually occludes the lumen of veins in superficial migratory thrombophlebitis. Polyarteritis nodosa affects arteries and is recognized if the affected vessels can be identified as arteries based on lumen diameter, wall thickness, internal elastic lamina, and location.

SUBCUTANEOUS POLYARTERITIS NODOSA

Clinical Presentation. Systemic polyarteritis nodosa can affect the skin by several types of presentations. The affected arteries are deeply located in the deep dermal vascular plexus at the junction of dermis and subcutis or in the deep subcutis itself. A common clinical manifestation is a region of net-like erythema (*livedo reticularis*), with some tenderness to palpation. This livedo is fixed and not transient or altered by the temperature of the environment. To obtain a biopsy of the affected deep artery, it has been shown that the exact site and depth are important. The affected artery may lie deep beneath the center of the pale area, which is surrounded by a rim of redness due to vasodilation at the periphery of the ischemic region. Biopsies into those red net-like lines visible at the skin surface often miss or show very little of the affected artery. Systemic manifestations can be reflected in hypertension, proteinuria, elevated circulating immune complexes, decreased complement levels, deep muscle tenderness and pain, and cerebral infarcts. In *Sneddon's syndrome*, the combination of livedo reticularis and cerebral infarcts can be due to polyarteritis nodosa, hypercoagulable states, or lupus erythematosus. Cutaneous manifestations of polyarteritis nodosa are common in hepatitis C infection. Superficial biopsies may show only telangiectasia and extravasation of erythrocytes, or occasionally a mild leukocytoclastic vasculitis, probably depending of the sizes of the circulating immune complexes. Some patients with histologically demonstrated polyarteritis nodosa on skin biopsy have a form of polyarteritis that tends to remain limited to the skin for prolonged time periods. Some cases have not shown involvement other than in the skin and subcutaneous tissue for as long as 15 years, which has given dermatologists the impression that there is a distinct entity of skin-limited polyarteritis nodosa, often

named *cutaneous polyarteritis nodosa*. Follow-up studies of such patients have shown that, despite being initially limited to the skin histologically and clinically, cutaneous polyarteritis nodosa may show signs of systemic disease at variable time periods after initial diagnosis in a large proportion of the patients. Hypertension, hematuria, testicular and muscle biopsies showing polyarteritis, and serum tests indicative of hepatitis B or C infection all point to systemic rather than localized cutaneous polyarteritis (60). Perhaps the exact nature and sizes of the circulating immune complexes could explain the overlapping features, and why the disease is limited to the skin for a long time in some patients. Polyarteritis nodosa can lead to deep ulceration of the skin into the subcutis. Some authors have analyzed the same information and have presented the entity of cutaneous polyarteritis as a special distinct condition by discounting the overlap with systemic disease and the importance of following the patients over time (2).

Histopathology. The inflammatory infiltration into the walls of arteries and arterioles tends to be focal. Segments along the length of the artery are involved differently and may have only a portion of its cross-sectioned profile involved by the destructive inflammation (Fig. 20-14). The focal areas have fibrin deposition in the vessel wall with necrosis of the intimal and medial portions of the vessel. Early lesions have mostly neutrophilic infiltration, with destruction of them to produce fragmented segments of the nuclei, *nuclear dust*. Later lesions have more lymphocytic infiltrate into the vessel as well as around it. Macrophage infiltration is also part of the process of resolution of the lesion. Immunofluorescence has shown immune complexes in the vessel walls (IgG, IgM, and C3). The vascular destruction often does not completely occlude the lumen, which is in part a consequence of the tendency of derma-

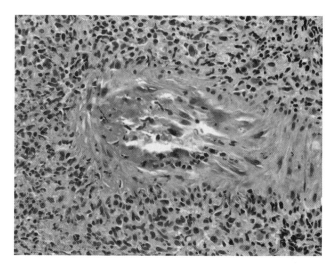

FIGURE 20-14. Subcutaneous polyarteritis nodosa. The small arteries in the septa have focal inflammation of their walls, with neutrophils and fibrin deposition.

tologists to biopsy early lesions rather than ulcerated ones. Some authors have stressed a difference in the localization of lesions to artery bifurcations in systemic polyarteritis and not in cutaneous polyarteritis (2). Such differences, if they are present, may be related to hydrostatic shear stress forces being greater at bifurcations and in patients with hypertension. Since the arteries tend to be in the deep dermal plexus and in the septa, the inflammatory process in the subcutis is classified as a septal panniculitis with vasculitis.

Differential Diagnosis. The distinction between polyarteritis and thrombophlebitis has been discussed previously in the section on thrombophlebitis. The distinction between systemic versus localized cutaneous polyarteritis depends heavily on the degree of investigation of the systemic factors, including the presence of proteinuria or hematuria (the glomeruli filter out circulating immune complexes). Elevations in muscle enzymes and muscle tenderness could lead to muscle biopsy as part of the investigation. Hypertension may also be a related systemic phenomenon. Investigation into the possible circulating viral antigens, such as hepatitis B or C, could also be revealing of systemic disease. It is most unlikely that arteritis will remain localized only to the skin when it is due to circulating immune complexes. Hypercoagulable states and lupus erythematosus need to be excluded.

ERYTHEMA INDURATUM (NODULAR VASCULITIS)

Clinical Presentation. The lesions of *erythema induratum*, also sometimes referred to as "nodular vasculitis," consist of painless to tender, deep-seated, circumscribed nodules to plaques, usually on the lower legs with a predilection for the posterior calves. Gradually the lesions extend toward the surface, forming blue-red plaques that can ulcerate before healing with atrophy and scarring (Fig. 20-15). Recurrences are common and often are precipitated by the onset of cold weather. Women are more commonly affected than men. *Erythema induratum of Bazin* refers to erythema induratum associated with tuberculosis. *Nodular vasculitis* was the name proposed by Montgomery for those cases with erythema induratum-like lesions that were not associated with tuberculosis (20,59).

Histopathology. In contrast to erythema nodosum, which is mainly a septal panniculitis, erythema induratum (nodular vasculitis) initially is mainly a lobular panniculitis due to vasculitis that produces ischemic necrosis of the fat lobule with relatively less involvement of the structures of the septa. The fat necrosis can be extensive, caseous as well as coagulative, and elicits granulomatous inflammation (Fig. 20-16A, B). Epithelioid cells and giant cells form broad zones of inflammation surrounding the necrosis but also can form well-delimited granulomas of the tuberculoid type (Fig. 20-17A, B). Ziehl–

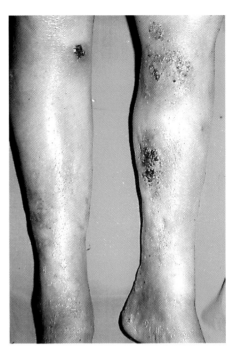

FIGURE 20-15. Nodular vasculitis/erythema induratum. Advanced disease presents as hemorrhagic ulcers and depressed lesions with a predilection for the posterior calf region.

Neelsen stains do not reveal intact mycobacteria (61). In approximately one-third of cases, granulomas are sparse or absent, and lymphocytes and plasma cells predominate (61). Both the tuberculoid granulomas and lymphoid infiltrate extend between the fat cells, largely replacing them.

Vascular changes are extensive and severe. Small- and medium-sized arteries and veins show infiltration of their walls by a dense lymphoid or granulomatous inflammatory infiltrate (Fig. 20-18A), associated with endothelial swelling, edema of the vessel walls, and fibrous thickening of the intima (59). Thrombosis and occlusion, or just compromise, of the lumen can produce extensive ischemic and caseous necrosis of the fat in about half of the cases (Fig. 20-18B and C). Extensive necrosis leads to involvement of the overlying dermis and subsequent ulceration. The necrotic fat has fat cysts, with surrounding amorphous, finely granular, eosinophilic material containing some pyknotic nuclei. Later lesions contain many foamy histiocytes surrounding areas of fat necrosis.

Pathogenesis. The primary event in erythema induratum is a vasculitis of the subcutaneous arteries and veins. If fat necrosis develops, it is the result of ischemia following vascular damage. Erythema induratum in the past usually has been caused by a hypersensitivity reaction to tuberculosis, which is a "tuberculid" reaction (62–64). However, neither inoculation of lesional tissue into guinea pigs nor cultures of such tissue have yielded isolates of tubercle bacilli. Also, erythema induratum responds to

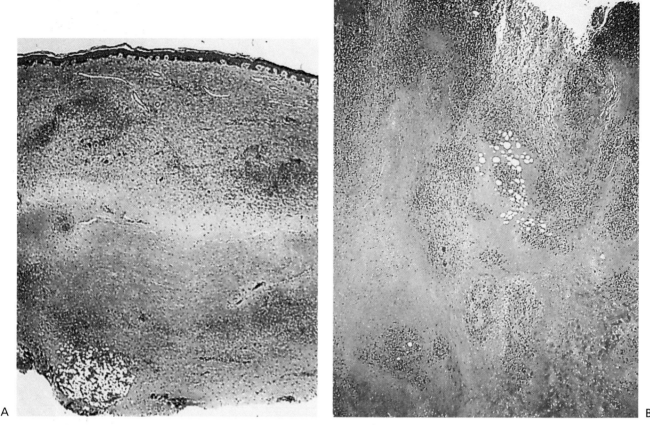

FIGURE 20-16. Erythema induratum. Part **(A)** shows large areas of caseous necrosis replacing the subcutaneous fat, septa and portions of the overlying dermis; and part **(B)** is a region of perforation of the inflammation through the skin surface.

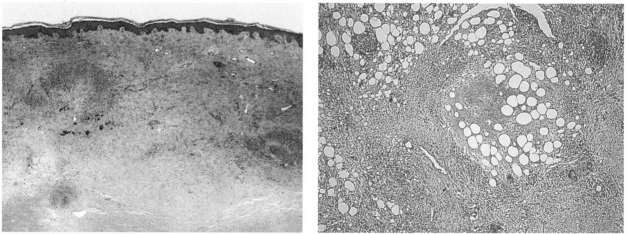

FIGURE 20-17. Erythema induratum. Part **(A)** is a region of caseous necrosis at lower magnification, with mainly lymphocytic infiltrates around remaining subcutaneous and dermal blood vessels; and part **(B)** is from a smaller region of lobular fat necrosis with surrounding lymphocytes, macrophages, and multinucleated cells.

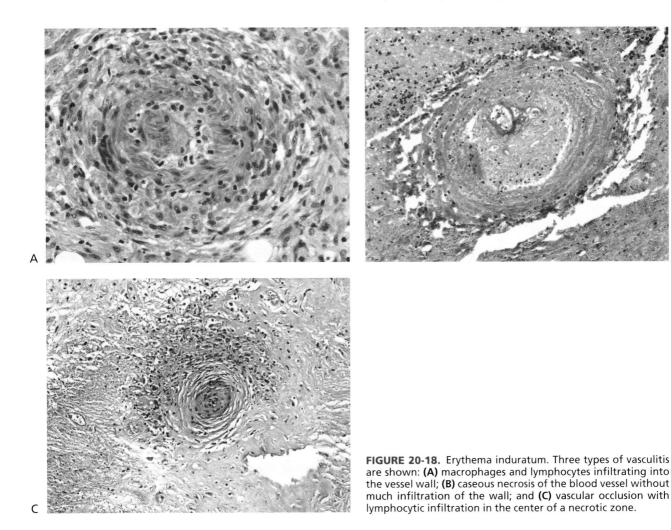

FIGURE 20-18. Erythema induratum. Three types of vasculitis are shown: **(A)** macrophages and lymphocytes infiltrating into the vessel wall; **(B)** caseous necrosis of the blood vessel without much infiltration of the wall; and **(C)** vascular occlusion with lymphocytic infiltration in the center of a necrotic zone.

treatment with corticosteroids (65). In contrast, evidence against erythema induratum being a tuberculid consists of the finding that active tuberculosis is no more frequent in patients with erythema induratum than in the general population. In addition, patients with tuberculosis can develop erythema nodosum (66). A delayed hypersensitivity reaction seems likely to be the basis of nodular vasculitis in nontuberculous patients, since S100-positive dendritic cells are increased in number within granulomas near the vessels in nodular vasculitis and not in polyarteritis nodosa (67). These dendritic cells could present antigens to T cells.

Differential Diagnosis. Erythema induratum can be distinguished from erythema nodosum by the prominent lymphohistiocytic vasculitis in erythema induratum, which can be found only very rarely in erythema nodosum. When caseation necrosis is present, it clearly separates erythema induratum from erythema nodosum. Direct cutaneous mycobacterial infection lacks the vasculitis of erythema induratum. Mycobacteria can be difficult to find in subcutaneous lesions of tuberculosis and are absent from erythema induratum with the Ziehl–

Neelsen method for acid-fast staining. Detection of DNA from *M. tuberculosis* in lesions of erythema induratum by polymerase chain reaction (68) but with negative cultures suggests a hypersensitivity reaction to fragments of tubercle bacilli (63).

The difficult distinctions are between *erythema induratum*, *thrombophlebitis*, and *subcutaneous polyarteritis nodosa*, all of which can produce the clinical picture of nodules on the legs with vasculitis. Polyarteritis nodosa has neutrophilic infiltrates and fibrinoid necrosis of arterial vessel walls, whereas erythema induratum and nodular vasculitis have lymphohistiocytic infiltrates of the vessel walls with intimal proliferation and thrombosis. Elastic tissue stains are helpful in some lesions for distinguishing small arteries affected by polyarteritis from small veins affected by thrombophlebitis. However, the anatomic distinction between arteries and veins can be difficult when the inflammation destroys the elastic fibers or when the elastic tissue is increased in the walls of veins due to venous hypertension that is commonly present in patients with stasis in the lower legs. Deep biopsies and step sections in the tissue blocks may be necessary to demonstrate the focal necrotizing vasculitis in polyarteritis nodosa since thrombosis and reactive changes near these foci can closely resemble nodular vasculitis in routine sections. At times only a general diagnosis of "panniculitis with vasculitis" can be given until other biopsies or additional clinical information clarify the nature of the disorder.

LUPUS ERYTHEMATOSUS PANNICULITIS

Clinical Features. In patients with chronic cutaneous lupus erythematosus, the lesions can be deep and can involve the dermis and subcutis or just the panniculus alone (69–71). The patients can have either chronic discoid lupus erythematosus or systemic lupus erythematosus. In about two-thirds to half of the patients with these uncommon lesions, there are firm, indurated subcutaneous nodules with no specific clinical changes in the overlying skin. Histology is more sensitive and detects changes of discoid lupus erythematosus in 67% of these patients (72).

The lesions are deep nodules and plaques that tend to involve the skin of the trunk and proximal extremities, particularly the lateral aspects of the upper arms, thighs, and buttocks. Symmetrical lesions on the anterior chest or upper arms can suggest a traumatic or factitial etiology, and indeed trauma may play a role in the localization of the lupus inflammation to these sites. Approximately 70% of these patients also have other lesions that are typical of discoid lupus erythematosus, and 50% have evidence of mild systemic lupus erythematosus (71). The lesions are painful and have a tendency to ulcerate and to heal leaving depressed scars. When the overlying skin is involved, there is loss of hair, erythema, poikiloderma, and epidermal atrophy. Some patients present with localized depressions without erythema, clinically resembling lipoatrophy (73). The term "lupus profundus" has been used for both lupus panniculitis and discoid lupus erythematosus lesions that involve the dermis and extend deeply into the subcutis. Over time, lesions that begin as pure panniculitis can develop dermal sclerosis and leave deep depressions in the skin surface.

Histopathology. The histologic sections reveal a deep lymphocytic infiltration in the fat lobules and in the septa (69). Lymphoid aggregates, nodules, and germinal centers, also known as follicular centers, are common (69,74). The dermis can have just a superficial and deep perivascular lymphocytic infiltrate with plasma cells or can have all of the changes of lesions of discoid lupus erythematosus. A distinctive feature is the so-called "hyaline necrosis" of the fat, in which portions of the fat lobule have lost nuclear staining of the fat cells and have an accumulation of fibrin and other proteins in a homogeneous eosinophilic matrix between the residual fat cells and extracellular fat globules (Fig. 20-19) (69). Blood vessels are infiltrated by lymphoid cells and their lumen diameter may be restricted

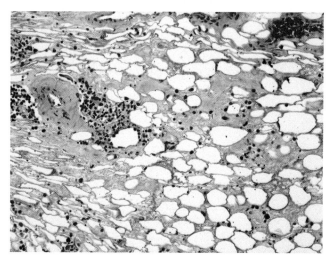

FIGURE 20-19. Lupus erythematosus panniculitis. Fat necrosis is accompanied in the lobules by the deposition of hyaline material and a lymphocytic infiltrate.

(Fig. 20-20A). Usually there is mucinous edema of the septa and the overlying dermis (Fig. 20-20B). Calcification may be present in older lesions.

Pathogenesis. Approximately 50% of patients with lupus profundus have positive immunofluorescence findings at the dermal-epidermal junction and at hair follicle basement membranes. Usually there is granular deposition of IgM and C3 and linear deposition of fibrin. Granular deposits of IgG and IgA may be present also in active lupus cases. Many patients have similar deposits in deep dermal and subcutaneous blood vessel walls. Fibrin is distributed diffusely in the panniculus, both in the lobules and in the septa in areas with hyaline necrosis. It seems likely that trauma is involved in the localization of lesions, perhaps through increased vascular permeability and leakage of circulating antinuclear antibodies or immune complexes into the fat lobules. A few patients with lupus panniculitis have a partial genetic deficiency of C2 and C4 (75). A lupus-like syndrome has been reported in approximately one-third of patients with C2 deficiency (76,77). In patients with complement at the dermal–epidermal junction, deposition of the so-called membrane-attack complex, composed of C5b-9, can be demonstrated as well.

Differential Diagnosis. Patients with lupus panniculitis have been given the diagnosis of *Weber–Christian disease* in the past. The overlap in appearances may prevent any distinction between these two diseases by routine histology. However, Weber–Christian disease can be sharply localized just to the fat lobules; in contrast, lupus panniculitis causes mucinous edema (detectable with Alcian blue stains) and inflammation around the blood vessels of the dermis. Immunofluorescence and serologic studies allow a positive diagnosis of lupus erythematosus in many instances.

A particularly troublesome differential diagnosis is between lupus panniculitis and *subcutaneous T-cell lymphoma*

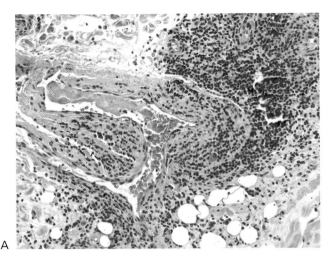
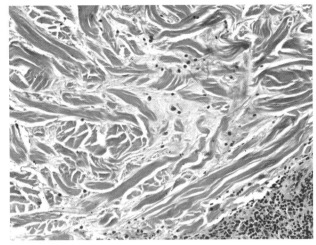

A   B

FIGURE 20-20. Lupus erythematosus panniculitis. Part **(A)** shows distinctive lymphocytic infiltration through blood vessel walls that can be concentric and induce fibrosis. Part **(B)** demonstrates the frequently abundant blue-gray mucinous change between collagen bundles in the dermis and septa of the panniculus.

(78). Although each of these two entities may have dense lymphoid infiltrates in the fat, usually the lymphoma has cytologically atypical lymphocytes. However, some cases of subcutaneous T-cell lymphoma are composed of small cells that lack obvious cytologic atypia in routine sections. A mixed population of CD4 and CD8-positive T-cells may be found, making T-cell receptor gene rearrangement studies necessary for showing clonality in the lymphoid infiltrate. After these studies, there remain a few indeterminate cases on a spectrum from lupus panniculitis to subcutaneous T-cell lymphoma because they have been classified as lupus panniculitis, responsive to chloroquine and/or prednisone therapy, but have atypical cells, with CD5 and CD7 diminution, and DNA analysis showing clonal lymphocytes in the population (78).

Erythema induratum, like lupus panniculitis, also shows hyaline necrosis and vasculitis, but has more granulomatous inflammation than in most cases of lupus panniculitis. Erythema induratum lacks the mucinous edema of the dermis.

RELAPSING FEBRILE NODULAR NONSUPPURATIVE PANNICULITIS (WEBER–CHRISTIAN DISEASE)

Clinical Presentation. The diagnosis of Weber–Christian disease is exclusionary. It is made much less frequently now than in 1950 to 1970, probably due to the greater power of current laboratory testing to reveal lupus erythematosus panniculitis, AAT panniculitis, or histiocytic cytophagic panniculitis in cases that might have been classified as Weber–Christian disease in the past. The classical clinical description is a disease characterized by the appearance of crops of tender nodules and plaques in the subcutaneous

fat, usually associated with mild fever. The lower extremities are favored sites but lesions may occur elsewhere and may ulcerate (Fig. 20-21). The disease occurs mostly in middle-aged women but has been described in all ages and in both sexes. In general, the disease has a good prognosis. However, if internal fat necrosis also is present, it may be fatal (79–81).

Histopathology. The histopathologic appearance itself is not sufficiently specific to exclude other diseases (Fig. 20-22A and B). The classical description of the disease is that it evolves through three stages. In the first phase, there is only erythema and induration clinically. Histologically, acute inflammation is found in the fat lobules with degeneration of fat cells and an infiltrate of neutrophils, lymphocytes, and macrophages. The second phase has an infiltrate discretely localized to the fat lobules, consisting mainly

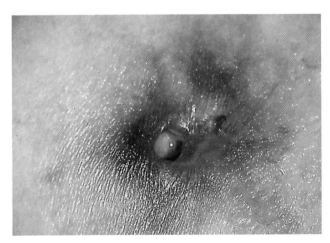

FIGURE 20-21. Weber–Christian disease. An indurated nodule on the leg has developed a perforation and drains a turbid, sterile, oily fluid with some necrotic tissue.

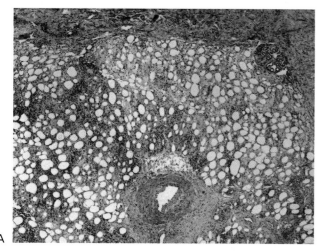
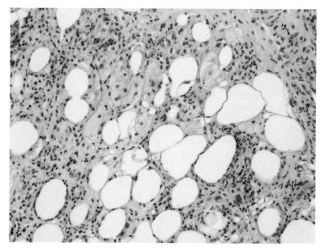

FIGURE 20-22. Weber–Christian disease: sharp localization of the inflammation in the fat lobules that is a distinctive but nonspecific finding **(A)**; higher magnification showing fat-laden macrophages and lymphocytes in the lobules **(B)**.

of macrophages, foam cells, and extracellular lipid called "microcysts." In some cases, the lesions perforate the skin surface and discharge a sterile, oily liquid. The third phase has depressed and indurated clinical lesions. Fibroblasts, collagen, and scattered lymphocytes, and a few plasma cells replace the fat. Vascular changes are mild (79–85).

Systemic lesions occur in some cases of Weber–Christian disease and serve to distinguish this disease from most other types of panniculitis, except for histiocytic cytophagic panniculitis and AAT deficiency panniculitis. In autopsy studies, inflammatory changes have been found in perivisceral fat, and intravisceral fat in the liver, spleen, bone marrow, or near the pleural or peritoneal cavity. A large amount of oily fluid may accumulate in the pleural or peritoneal cavity (81,85–87).

Pathogenesis. If Weber–Christian disease exists as a distinct disease, the cause is unknown, but circulating immune complexes have been found in some cases (14, 81,88).

Differential Diagnosis. The histologic appearance of Weber–Christian disease is most distinctive in the second phase when there is an infiltration by lymphocytes and macrophages between fat cells that is discretely localized to the fat lobules. *Erythema nodosum* with unusual predominance of neutrophils can resemble the early phase of Weber–Christian disease, except for the localization of erythema nodosum primarily in the septa and Weber–Christian mainly in the lobules. Likewise, *AAT deficiency* can resemble early Weber–Christian disease except that the neutrophilic infiltrate in AAT deficiency usually affects the dermis and septa as well as the lobules. *Subcutaneous fat necrosis of pancreatic disease* can produce some of these findings but usually can be recognized by the extensive necrosis and deposition of bluish calcium precipitates with fatty acids. *Histiocytic cytophagic panniculitis* has some of the clin-

ical features but histologically has a lymphoid infiltrate with macrophages that have ingested lymphocytes, neutrophils, and eosinophils to be called "beanbag cells" (89). *Subcutaneous panniculitic T-cell lymphoma* can underlie a histiocytic cytophagic panniculitis reaction and may also need to be excluded. After removal of all these other diseases, very few unexplained cases remain to be classified as Weber–Christian disease.

PANNICULITIS ROTHMANN–MAKAI

The term "panniculitis Rothmann–Makai" was proposed in 1945 as a designation for a "heterogeneous group of cases of idiopathic panniculitis that do not fit into any of the distinctly defined syndromes, such as Weber–Christian disease, erythema nodosum, or erythema induratum" (90). This diagnosis is based entirely on negative criteria (91) and consequently should be avoided. It seems preferable to refer to such cases as "unclassified panniculitis" until more definitive studies are available.

PALISADED GRANULOMATOUS PANNICULITIS

Clinical Features. Several granulomatous disorders that usually affect the dermis can also produce deep subcutaneous nodules. Some of these disorders can present in the subcutis without granulomas in the overlying dermis. In the subcutis these diseases may form lesions that differ clinically and histologically in some aspects from their counterpart dermal lesions. *Subcutaneous granuloma annulare*, for example, is more frequent in young children and young adults, whereas the dermal form is more frequent in adults. The subcutaneous nodules may not produce erythema of the overlying skin. The lesions are most frequent on the head, hands, buttocks, and shins, but can occur at other sites. Approximately 25% of patients with subcutaneous granuloma annulare also have dermal lesions. *Rheumatoid nodule* most typically is a deep subcutaneous nodule, but can also involve the overlying dermis. Rheumatoid nodules tend to be on the elbows, fingers, and knees, and are present in approximately 20% of patients with rheumatoid arthritis. Although they usually occur in patients with severe deforming joint disease, rheumatoid nodules can be the initial presentation of rheumatoid arthritis. The subcutaneous lesions of granuloma annulare and rheumatoid nodule rarely perforate through the skin without associated trauma. Magro et al. (92–94) have emphasized the occurrence of *granuloma annulare-like lesions in association with systemic disease*. The list of systemic diseases is long, but rheumatoid arthritis is one of the main associated diseases. Other causes include thyroid disease, collagen-vascular diseases, viral infections (such as with parvovirus B19), and medications. One of the clinical clues that these are granuloma annulare-like reactions to systemic disease is that the lesions often occur in anatomic sites that are unusual for true granuloma annulare.

Histopathology. Both subcutaneous granuloma annulare and rheumatoid nodules produce necrosis of the fat lobules and any involved septa with a palisade of histiocytic cells around the focal areas of necrosis, which can be relatively large when compared to the size of typical dermal lesions (Fig. 20-23). Typically subcutaneous granuloma annulare has abundant mucin in the necrotic centers of the lesions. The mucin is so abundant as to be visible in routine hematoxylin and eosin stained sections. The presence of mucin can be confirmed on Alcian blue or colloidal iron stains.

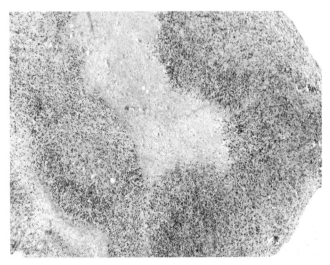

FIGURE 20-23. Subcutaneous granuloma annulare. This is different from the dermal lesions of granuloma annulare in that larger palisaded granulomas with central mucinous deposition and fibrosis are common in the subcutis.

However, the detection of small amounts by these sensitive special stains can be less specific for granuloma annulare. In contrast, rheumatoid nodules have more fibrin in the routine sections of necrotic centers of the lesions. Immunofluorescence is so sensitive that it can detect fibrin in the centers of both granuloma annulare and rheumatoid nodules. When both mucin and fibrin are visible in the routine sections of the necrotic centers, a granuloma annulare-like lesion associated with a systemic disease should be suspected. In all of these instances, the macrophages appear similar in that they are enlarged, have abundant eosinophilic cytoplasm, and are aggregated closely together to give them an "epithelioid" appearance. Multinucleated giant cells may be present. Neutrophils may be found in the small vessels in the necrotic centers of the granuloma annulare-like lesions. Neutrophilic infiltrates in the vessels and in the interstitium around collagen bundles are more typical of rheumatoid nodules and papules.

Pathogenesis. The etiology of granuloma annulare is unknown, even in the ordinary dermal form, and certainly in the subcutaneous form. With the recognition of the granuloma annulare-like lesions in systemic diseases, multiple etiologies could produce granuloma annulare. If this is true, then granuloma annulare becomes a reaction pattern of the dermis and/or subcutis. Studies of patients with granuloma annulare by routine immunofluorescence showed deposition of immune complexes (IgG, IgM, C3, with fibrin) in the small blood vessel walls in the centers of some lesions. These findings were only present in biopsies of early lesions (95). It is recognized now that the binding of certain types of IgG to the surface of fibroblasts in culture can cause overproduction of mucin by these fibroblasts (96). Therefore, it seems a reasonable hypothesis that the mucin production in granuloma annulare relates to the deposition of IgG on the surface of collagen bundles and fibroblasts. In rheumatoid nodules, the deposition of rheumatoid factor (IgM/IgG complexes) locally in the tissue might stimulate the fibroblasts in some patients to produce sufficient mucin to give the morphology that we call granuloma annulare-like lesions in systemic disease. Further studies are needed on the pathogenesis of these reactions. The presence of anti-Ro and anticardiolipin antibodies in some patients may produce vasculitis and pauci-inflammatory vascular thrombosis in association with rheumatoid arthritis lesions (97).

Differential Diagnosis. The distinction between subcutaneous granuloma annulare (mucin deposition) and rheumatoid nodule (fibrin deposition) can be made in many cases in the routine histology. When the lesions exhibit an unusual clinical distribution of lesions for granuloma annulare, and when the lesions have both mucin and fibrin in the necrotic centers, then the diagnosis of granuloma annulare-like lesion in systemic disease can be offered but it needs further investigation and correlation with the clinical findings in the patient. *Necrobiotic xanthogranuloma* is usually a dermal lesion, but the lesions can be large and involve the subcutis as well. It can have some histologic features in common with the palisaded granulomas, but the necrotic centers contain cholesterol clefts and are surrounded by macrophages with abundant lipid-filled, pale cytoplasm. *Crohn's disease* can produce subcutaneous granulomas with necrosis but the granulomas usually do not have a palisaded appearance. Most subcutaneous lesions of Crohn's disease are around the perineum or oral sites. They tend to occur near areas of rectal involvement or ileostomy sites. *Sarcoidosis* may produce granulomas in the septa or in the lobules or both. The lesions tend to remain as discrete granulomas, and usually lack necrosis. In large granulomas, the centers may have fibrin deposition, but without the granular debris of necrosis. Treatment of sarcoidosis with systemic steroids can produce central necrosis in the granulomas. The lesions lack palisading but may have slight mucin deposition in the stroma around the periphery but not in the centers of the granulomas. Small polarizable crystals have been found in some lesions of sarcoidosis but not in the other disorders in this subsection (98,99). The presence of other polarizable material raises the question of possible factitial panniculitis.

PANNICULITIS DUE TO PHYSICAL OR CHEMICAL AGENTS

Clinical Features. Trauma may be due to physical injury or to chemical injury, such as that produced by the injection of noxious substances. Physical injury can be produced by blunt pressure or impact, cold or excessive heat, or electrical injury. All of these factors can produce firm nodules in the subcutaneous fat. In many instances, these various inciting agents can be distinguished best by the clinical history and distribution of the lesions. Surreptitious injections of noxious substances can produce bizarre clinical and histologic patterns of lesions, but can be suspected clinically by the distribution of lesions only in areas easily reached by the patient (*factitial panniculitis*). Drug injections by nurses usually are located in the deltoid region or on the buttocks. Self-injection of insulin often involves the thigh or lower abdomen and can produce subcutaneous lesions. Meperidine hydrochloride or Demerol (100) and pentazocine or Talwin (101) injections are known to produce traumatic panniculitis. The injection of oily substances such as hydrocarbons or silicone has been common in the past for certain cosmetic effects, but reactions to these substances or to contaminants in them produce a panniculitis with varying degrees of inflammatory infiltration (102,103). The long-term effects of injection of buttock fat autotransplants to sites, such as the backs of hands, for cosmesis have yet to be studied. Mentally ill persons and drug addicts may purposely or inadvertently inject themselves with foreign substances, such as feces or milk, sometimes used to dilute or cut narcotics. These various physical and chemical traumas lead to indurated subcu-

taneous nodules that may undergo liquefaction, ulcerate, and discharge pus or a thick oily fluid. Healing leaves depressed scars (104). Lesions produced by extreme cold usually do not ulcerate unless associated with pernio or vasculitis with cryoglobulinemia. Cold injury may occur in children after eating an iced food such as a popsicle (105–107). The cold injury produces nodules or plaques that appear from 1 to 3 days after exposure and that subside spontaneously within 2 weeks. Excessive heat and electrical injury usually are accompanied by ulceration and eschar formation.

Histopathology. The injection of the various toxic agents will produce a variable histologic picture of acute inflammation, with aggregation of neutrophils and focal fat necrosis with hemorrhage (104). Older lesions have infiltrates of lymphocytes and macrophages (Fig. 20-24A) with fibrosis (Fig. 20-24B). Vasculitis usually is absent with injections, but can be present with heat-induced injury and with perniosis associated with cold, damp conditions. Polarized light reveals certain types of foreign material in injection sites, but polarizable crystals have been found in some lesions of sarcoidosis (98,99). The injection of oily liquids leads to the formation of many pockets of fatty material ("fat cysts"), often with a surrounding fibrous reaction containing foamy macrophages, that overall impart a "Swiss-cheese appearance" to the tissue after the fat has been extracted by routine histologic processing (102,103). Fixation of the tissue in osmium tetroxide may be useful since endogenous lipids (but not most exogenous lipids) contain many unsaturated double bonds that react readily with osmium tetroxide to produce a black deposit of reduced osmium oxides. Injections of granulocyte-monocyte-colony-stimulating factor (GMCSF) or interleukin-2 can produce nodules at the sites of injections in the skin and subcutis that mimic leukemic or lymphoma infiltration due to their content of very highly stimulated monocytes or lymphocytes (108).

Trauma due to cold injury initially has an infiltrate of lymphocytes and macrophages near the blood vessels of the deep plexus at the junction of dermis and subcutis. Such changes have also been described in perniosis. Biopsies at the 3rd day, at the height of reaction, show rupture of the fat cells with fat pockets in the tissue surrounded by an infiltrate of lymphocytes, macrophages, neutrophils, and occasional eosinophils (106).

Pathogenesis. The subcutaneous fat of children is more sensitive to cold injury than that of older children and adults. In all newborn infants and in 40% of infants 6 months of age, the application of an ice cube to the skin produces nodules of cold panniculitis. By 9 months of age, such cold reactivity in infants is rare (107). The greater degree of saturation of the lipids in newborns raises the crystallization temperature of the fat and produces greater susceptibility to cold injury (109,110). This mechanism of injury is involved also in *sclerema neonatorum.*

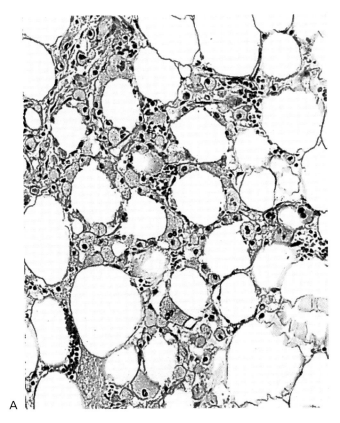

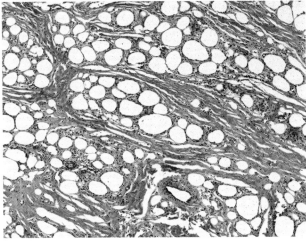

FIGURE 20-24. Traumatic fat necrosis: acute area of fat necrosis with lymphocytes and macrophages in the fat lobules **(A)**; and late lesion in which the fat lobules and septa have been replaced by dense fibrosis **(B)**.

LOCALIZED LIPOATROPHY AND LIPODYSTROPHY

Clinical Features. Both localized lipoatrophy and lipodystrophy can have lesions with a similar clinical appearance; however, lipoatrophy usually involves one or several circumscribed, round, depressed areas, from one to several centimeters in diameter. In contrast, lipodystrophy produces the loss of large areas of subcutaneous fat, particularly in *acquired generalized lipodystrophy* (111). Most cases of lipodystrophy are of the cephalothoracic type and involve the face, neck, upper extremities, and upper trunk. Some cases have been noted that extend downward from the iliac crest. Lipodystrophy has been reported with diabetes (112) and with glomerulonephritis (113). Lipoatrophic panniculitis also occurs in *connective tissue panniculitis* (114). In HIV-positive patients on highly active antiretroviral therapy (HAART) including protease inhibitors, their prolonged life span has revealed that this therapy can produce a striking lipodystrophy syndrome. Loss of subcutaneous fat on the face and extremities can be severe and is accompanied by redistribution of fat to produce a "buffalo hump" and an increase in visceral fat deposits. This syndrome includes insulin resistance, diabetes mellitus/carbohydrate intolerance, hypertriglyceridemia, reduced high-density lipoprotein cholesterol, elevated low-density lipoprotein cholesterol, and reduced levels of the adipocyte cytokine *adiponectin* and the adipocyte hormone *leptin* (115,116).

Histopathology. Lesions of lipodystrophy are described with total loss of the subcutaneous fat producing dermis adjacent to the fascia (112). However, localized lipoatrophy has been described as having two types: inflammatory and non-inflammatory or "involutional" types. In the *inflammatory type*, multiple lesions are common and have a lymphocytic infiltrate around the blood vessels and scattered diffusely in the fat lobules (73). Areas of fat necrosis can be present with infiltration by macrophages.

In the *involutional type*, usually there is only a solitary lesion that exhibits a decrease in size of the individual adipocytes. They are separated from each other by abundant eosinophilic, hyaline material, or in some instances by mucoid material (117).

Pathogenesis. Adipose tissue in adult mammals is under complex hormonal control. Insulin receptors on the surface of the fat cells inhibit lipolysis and stimulate lipogenesis. This contributes to increased fat deposition, whereas stimulation of beta-adrenergic receptor sites on the plasma membrane of fat cells increases lipolysis. Glucagon can also increase lipolysis. Although the fat cells themselves in the subcutis receive no direct innervation, innervation of the small blood vessels of the fat may produce noradrenergic stimuli for lipolysis. When normal adult adipose tissue is subjected to lipolysis by such stimuli or by fasting for

72 hours, significant changes in the morphology of the fat take place. Unilocular fat cells can become multilocular in sensitive fat regions after only 48 hours of fasting. With prolonged fasting, the unilocular engorged fat cells lose their fat droplets and become more spindle-shaped cells indistinguishable from fibroblasts or undifferentiated perivascular mesenchymal cells (118,119).

LIPEDEMA

Clinical Features. Lipedema is an entity that is relatively poorly recognized by pathologists but more prominent in the literature of surgeons and radiologists. In its localized tumefactive form it presents as localized swelling, sometimes affecting both buttocks, thighs, or the legs in middle-aged women (120–125). The swelling persists despite elevation of the extremities, and is a nonpitting edema. In the tumefactive form, the swelling is not uniform and may have deep depressions in it. More commonly the swelling is not tumefactive but is more diffuse, painless, bilateral, and symmetrical, and involves the thighs and lower legs, but not the feet (120).

Histopathology. In a localized area, there are increased interspaces between fat cells, without dilation of blood vessels or evident dilation of lymphatic spaces, without increased mucin on Alcian blue or colloidal iron stains, and without much inflammation. In some cases, trauma to these protuberant masses can result in deep depressions in the lesions that correspond histologically to zones of loose fibrous tissue that lack fat cells, and have slight amounts of hemosiderin in macrophages. Mast cells may be slightly increased in the lesions but are probably reactive. There is no collagenous capsule at the periphery of the tumefactive form. There is no atypia of the adipocyte nuclei.

Pathogenesis. The result of the lipedema is great thickening of the subcutaneous tissues without much evidence of classical lymphedema. However, careful studies have shown microaneurysms of the lymphatic vessels localized to the areas of lipedema (126). It is different from *cellulite*, which produces a diffuse peau d'orange pebbly appearance to the skin of the thighs and buttocks regions of women. The cellular basis of cellulite is extension of adipose tissue from the subcutis up into the reticular dermis and not edema of the fat lobules. The anatomic construction of the border between reticular dermis and subcutis is more densely collagenous in males than in females, predisposing women to the development of cellulite (5). Another possible relationship is to *Dercum's disease* or *adiposis dolorosa*, which differs in being painful clinically and in having inflammation of nerves. Further careful histologic and clinical studies of these cases are needed.

Differential Diagnosis. The tumefactive nature of the swelling in some cases of lipedema leads toward a differential diagnosis that includes lipoma with edema or mucinous change, lymphedema, scleredema, or scleromyxedema. The lack of a delicate capsule makes lipedema different from lipoma. The lack of increased mucin on Alcian blue stains separates lipedema from scleredema, scleromyxedema, or myxoid lipoma.

SUBCUTANEOUS NODULAR FAT NECROSIS IN PANCREATIC DISEASE

Clinical Features. In patients with pancreatitis or pancreatic neoplasms, the release of lipase enzymes into the blood can lead to nodules of fat necrosis in the subcutis. The pretibial region is the most common site of the nodules, but they may occur on the thighs, buttocks, and elsewhere (Fig. 20-25). The nodules usually are tender and red and may be fluctuant (127), but they only rarely discharge oily fluid through fistulae (128).

Histopathology. The histologic appearance of the subcutaneous nodules in pancreatic disease is characteristic in most instances (129). In the foci of fat necrosis, there are ghost-like fat cells having thick, faintly stained cell peripheries and no nuclear staining (Fig. 20-26). Calcification forms basophilic granules in the cytoplasm of the necrotic fat cells, and sometimes lamellar deposits around individual fat cells or patchy basophilic deposits at the periphery of the fat necrosis (127) (Fig. 20-27). A polymorphous infiltrate surrounds the foci of fat necrosis and consists of neutrophils, lymphoid cells, macrophages, foam cells, and foreign-body giant cells (130). There can be extensive hemorrhage into the lesions. Old lesions have macrophages, foam cells, lymphocytes, and fibroblasts, with fibrosis and hemosiderin deposition (127). In some cases with pancreatic enzyme panniculitis, possibly with early lesions, biopsies of subcutaneous nodules show only a nonspecific pattern of necrotizing panniculitis with a neutrophilic inflammatory response. Multiple biopsies and deep biopsies or biopsies of lesions of different ages may allow a definitive diagnosis.

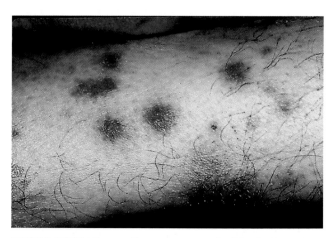

FIGURE 20-25. Pancreatic enzyme panniculitis. Erythematous nodules appear most commonly on the lower legs.

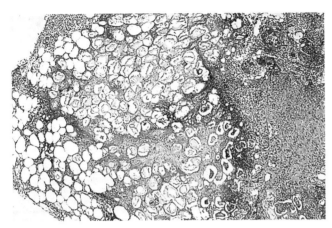

FIGURE 20-26. Pancreatic enzyme panniculitis. Necrotic fat cells contain eosinophilic deposits of partially hydrolyzed fat. Calcification forms granular basophilic material. Focal hemorrhage is frequent.

Systemic Lesions. Fat necrosis also occurs in internal organs. The symptoms of arthralgia can be due to periarticular fat necrosis (130). Fat necrosis is common also in the pancreas and surrounding fat tissue and in the fat of the omentum, mesentery, pericardial, and perirenal regions, as well as in the mediastinum and bone marrow (127). Calcium precipitation with the released fatty acids can be extensive enough to produce life-threatening hypocalcemia.

Pathogenesis. The damaged or tumorous pancreatic acinar cells release lipase, phospholipase, trypsin, and amylase into the surrounding tissues and blood. The serum values for amylase and lipase usually are elevated transiently and may not be detected in all cases. Amylase levels often peak 2 to 3 days after the appearance of the subcutaneous nodules (129). Lipase can be detected in the regions of fat necrosis and in ascitic fluid (131). It is not clear how the pancreatic proenzymes become activated in the tissues to produce fat necrosis. Local changes in vascular permeability due to

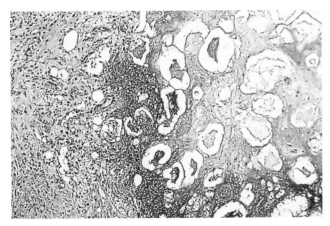

FIGURE 20-27. Pancreatic enzyme panniculitis. Many neutrophils are present in the margin of the zone of calcification and of fat necrosis.

trauma or other circulating enzymes, such as trypsin or phospholipase A2, may allow the pancreatic lipase to enter the interstitial compartment of the fat lobules and produce fat necrosis. Free fatty acids released by the lipolysis combine with calcium to form the soapy basophilic deposits in the tissue (132). Enzymatic damage to the integrity of the vascular wall can produce extensive hemorrhage.

Differential Diagnosis. The usual diagnostic distinction histologically is whether the fat necrosis is due to pancreatic disease or to physical trauma. Clinically other considerations may also include erythema nodosum, erythema induratum, nodular vasculitis, AAT deficiency, disseminated infection, or Weber–Christian disease. Only pancreatic enzyme fat necrosis produces the basophilic deposits of calcium precipitated with abundant free fatty acids. All of the entities can have neutrophils in the fat. Basophilic DNA debris from neutrophil nuclei must be distinguished from calcium deposits. Von Kossa stains for calcium phosphate are positive on the calcium deposits in pancreatic enzyme fat necrosis. Septic foci of bacterial or fungal infection can require special stains to detect these organisms. Despite vascular damage and hemorrhage, neutrophilic vasculitis usually is absent in fat necrosis due to pancreatic disease. Old lesions that have resorbed the calcium soaps cannot be distinguished easily from the other entities.

SCLEREMA NEONATORUM

Clinical Features. Sclerema neonatorum is a very rare disorder, usually in premature infants, that is characterized by a diffuse, rapidly spreading, nonpitting hardening of the subcutaneous fat of neonates in the first few days of life. The skin seems wax-like, tight, cold, and indurated. Death usually supervenes in a few weeks, if untreated. On autopsy, the subcutis is greatly thickened, hardened, and lard-like. Most infants with sclerema neonatorum are cyanotic at birth, have difficulty maintaining their body temperature, and have a major debilitating illness (110).

Histopathology. The subcutaneous tissue owes its thickening to the increase in the size of the fat cells and to the presence of wide, intersecting fibrous bands (109,110). The lipid crystals inside the fat cells produce rosettes of fine needle-like clefts after lipid extraction in routine processing. In frozen sections, the crystals are not extracted and are visible in polarized light (133). In most instances there is very little evidence of any inflammatory reaction to the fat necrosis, but very rarely an inflammatory reaction containing giant cells can be found (133,134). Characteristically, the changes develop rapidly, are extensive, and elicit less inflammatory reaction than those of subcutaneous fat necrosis of the newborn or of localized cold panniculitis in young children.

Systemic Lesions. In most cases of sclerema neonatorum, the changes are limited to the subcutaneous fat (110). However, in two cases, autopsy revealed lesions in the visceral fat that were identical to those in the subcutis. In one case the lesions were widespread (133), while in the other the systemic lesions were limited to the perirenal and retroperitoneal fat (134).

Pathogenesis. Compared to the fat of the adult, the subcutaneous fat of the newborn has a greater ratio of saturated to unsaturated fatty acids, which raises the solidification point of the fat closer to room temperature. In sclerema neonatorum these changes are exaggerated so that the neutral fat (triglyceride) crystallizes at room temperature. The increased ratio of saturated (palmitic or stearic acid) to unsaturated fatty acids (such as oleic acid) may be produced by defective enzyme pathways that lead to an excess of saturated fatty acids (110). X-ray diffraction studies have shown that the crystals in the fat cells are due to triglycerides (135). It is likely that the use of thermally controlled incubators for premature infants has caused this disease to be extremely rare. This same mechanism of injury is operative in localized cold panniculitis in infants.

Differential Diagnosis. Generalized edema due to an immature renal system can mimic some aspects of sclerema neonatorum clinically, but in renal failure the generalized edema is pitting, while in sclerema it is not. Lymphedema (Milroy's disease) can produce nonpitting edema, particularly of the legs, in an otherwise healthy infant. Biopsies are not advised but show dilation of lymphatics. Erysipelas is more demarcated, warm, and tender than sclerema.

SUBCUTANEOUS FAT NECROSIS OF THE NEWBORN

Clinical Features. Subcutaneous fat necrosis of the newborn usually occurs in premature or full-term infants often after a complicated delivery by forceps or cesarean section (136). Indurated erythematous to violaceous nodules and plaques appear in the subcutis a few days to a week after birth. Rarely, in cases with numerous nodules, the lesions may discharge a caseous material (137). The patient's health generally is good and the nodules resolve spontaneously after a few weeks or months. On rare occasions, infants are severely ill and die (137). In 16 reported cases, the subcutaneous fat necrosis was associated with hypercalcemia, and three patients died (138). Thrombocytopenia, hypertriglyceridemia, and hypoglycemia have also been reported (139). The development of extensive fat necrosis has been reported in infants following induced hypothermia used in cardiac surgery (140) or after surface hypothermic treatment of birth asphyxia, with hypercalcemia 7 weeks later. An underlying defect in composition and metabolism of fat has been assumed in such cases. The cases need to be followed for the development of hypercalcemia, which may occur in approximately one-third of cases (136). Subcutaneous fat necrosis has been reported also in a number of rare associations (3), including with maternal cocaine use and intrapartum administration of calcium channel blockers.

Histopathology. Focal areas of fat necrosis are present in the fat lobules and are infiltrated by macrophages and foreign-body–type giant cells (Fig. 20-28A and B). Fat deposits in the macrophages and giant cells contain crystalline fat, which after lipid extraction appears as needle-shaped clefts in a radial arrangement (141) (Fig. 20-29). In frozen sections, the radial clefts contain doubly refractile crystals. Calcium deposits usually are small and are scattered in the necrotic fat. If the necrosis is extensive, calcium deposits may be large and require several years to be resorbed.

Pathogenesis. Electron microscopic examination shows that the phagocytosis of fat crystals starts with the invasion of fat cells by cytoplasmic projections of macrophages. Subsequently, fat crystals are seen within the cytoplasm of macrophages and of foreign-body–type giant cells, which result from fusion of the macrophages (141).

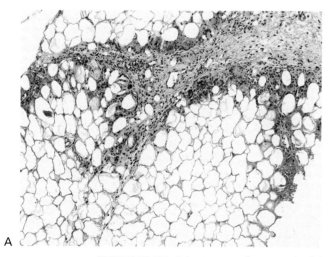
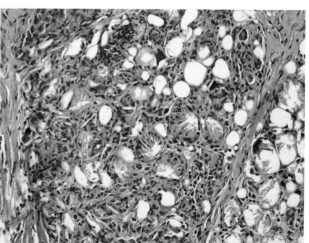

A   B

FIGURE 20-28. Subcutaneous fat necrosis of the newborn. Early lesion with many macrophages and multinucleated cells at the periphery of the damaged fat lobule **(A)**. Later lesion with replacement of the fat lobules by macrophages and multinucleated cells **(B)**.

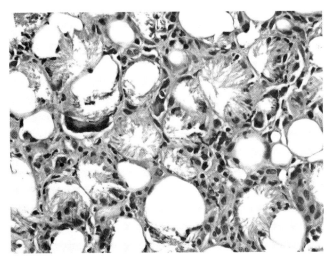

FIGURE 20-29. Subcutaneous fat necrosis of the newborn. A higher magnification shows that the radial arrays of crystalline fat leave clefts in the cytoplasm of the macrophages and damaged adipocytes.

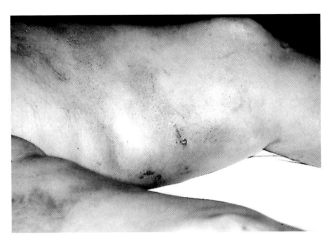

FIGURE 20-30. Calcifying panniculitis. This patient with hyperparathyroidism developed erythematous, hemorrhagic, indurated plaques that were cold to touch.

The cause of subcutaneous fat necrosis of the newborn is not known. There is debate about the role of trauma since many of the patients have been premature infants who were born by forceps delivery or who otherwise endured a difficult delivery. However, lesions were reported in children delivered by cesarean section (3,136).

Differential Diagnosis. Both subcutaneous fat necrosis of the newborn and sclerema neonatorum have crystalline arrays of needle-like clefts in the fat. Sclerema is a catastrophic diffuse illness that gives little time for extensive inflammation so that in sclerema there is an absence of focal areas of fat necrosis with macrophages and giant cells. In sclerema, there is also an absence of calcifications and the presence of wide bands of fibrous tissue in the subcutis (110). Treatment of children with high doses of steroids—for example, as was done for rheumatic fever—can produce poststeroid panniculitis with subcutaneous lesions very similar histologically to those of subcutaneous fat necrosis of the newborn (142). The deep nodules usually occur within 1 to 30 days after the cessation of high-dose steroid treatment. Traumatic fat necrosis has focal areas of necrosis and inflammation but lacks the crystals in the fat. Localized infection can be difficult to exclude clinically, but the infants with subcutaneous fat necrosis are generally rather healthy and are not septic.

CALCIFYING PANNICULITIS

Clinical Features. Patients with end-stage renal disease or hyperparathyroidism may develop indurated, erythematous, cold, subcutaneous, and dermal nodules and plaques (Fig. 20-30). The lesions can progress to extensive dry gangrenous necrosis of the skin and subcutis. The lesions can be related to the prior administration of medications containing cal-

cium or phosphates, so that the balance of calcium to phosphate is so disturbed as to favor precipitation of calcium phosphate salts in the tissue. Plaques often are localized at usual sites of subcutaneous injection such as the thighs and abdomen.

Histopathology. The early or minimal lesions of patients with this disorder often have calcification of the media of the medium-sized blood vessels and of the walls of small capillaries in the subcutis (Fig. 20-31). In *calciphylaxis* associated with chronic renal failure, calcification and fibrointimal hyperplasia occludes the lumen of small arteries (143). In severe cases, calcium phosphate crystals form in the small vessels and interspaces between fat cells in the lobules of subcutaneous fat. The affected vessels can undergo thrombosis producing ischemic necrosis of the subcutaneous fat and even the overlying dermis and epidermis.

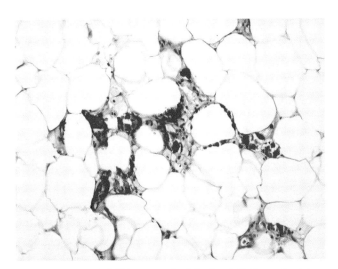

FIGURE 20-31. Calcifying panniculitis. Precipitation of calcium phosphate salts in the blood vessel walls produces a purple-stained deposit. These deposits lead to thrombosis and ischemic necrosis of the adjacent fat and overlying skin.

Pathogenesis. Calciphylaxis is a condition in which the balance of calcium and phosphate favors precipitation of calcium phosphate at the sites of trauma, cold injury, injection of medications containing calcium or phosphate compounds, or in vessel walls. The patients usually have end-stage renal disease or primary hyperparathyroidism. Case reports indicate that the phenomenon of calcium precipitation can be induced locally by injections of an anticoagulant drug such as calcium heparinate (144), by infusions containing excess phosphate, or for unknown reasons during hemodialysis (145). In young children, extensive subcutaneous calcifications can result from subcutaneous fat necrosis of the newborn. In adults, the differential diagnosis also includes a prior episode of pancreatic fat necrosis or traumatic fat necrosis. Radiologic findings in traumatic fat necrosis are generally a central lucent fat cyst with surrounding curvilinear calcifications, or coarse or microcalcifications (146). The extensive calcification of the media of small arterioles is distinctive for calciphylaxis. The concept of calciphylaxis, as introduced by Seyle, was reviewed recently and was presented as involving challenge by agents in a setting of hypersensitivity that led to local calcification. The metastatic calcification in renal disease is due to elevated calcium and phosphate levels, and is only vaguely related to the Seyle's presentation of calciphylaxis (147).

LIPOMEMBRANOUS CHANGE OR LIPOMEMBRANOUS PANNICULITIS

Clinical Features. Patients with severe stasis, diabetes, and other causes of arterial vascular insufficiency to the lower legs can develop indurated plaques in the subcutis. They are depressed and painful, but rarely ulcerate (148–151). The lesions are named lipomembranous panniculitis based on the microscopic finding of lipomembranes around fat deposits or "cysts," more properly termed pseudocysts. Lipomembranous change has been found also in a number of primary disorders including lupus erythematosus panniculitis, morphea, erythema nodosum, erysipelas, necrobiosis lipoidica, and traumatic panniculitis (152,153). Ischemia and/or stasis can lead to extensive, depressed, hard areas of skin, often on the lower legs and accompanied by hemosiderosis, or epidermal and dermal atrophy, a condition named *lipodermatosclerosis* (154).

Histopathology. Biopsies deep into the fat show a lobular panniculitis with focal macrophage infiltration and fibrosis around shrunken lobules. Within the lobules, there are fat pseudocysts that are lined by a thin eosinophilic layer, called a lipomembrane, which has fine, feathery projections into the fat cavity (Fig. 20-32A). Spectral imaging shows that the lipomembranes are spectrally distinct from the periphery of surrounding fat cells (Fig. 20-32B). The lipomembrane is positive on PAS stain (Fig. 20-33), and in late lesions with elastic tissue stains (153). The lipomembranes are positive for CD68 and lysozyme indicating a contribution of these enzymes from the macrophages in the production of lipomembranes. Late or older lesions are only weakly positive or become negative for CD68 and lysozyme (153). Early lesions also have focal areas of fat necrosis, such as those produced by partial ischemia. Lipomembranes often can be found in the remaining small fat lobules in late stages of *lipodermatosclerosis*, in which there also is dermal fibrosis with loss of epidermal appendages, and fibrous tissue replacement of much of the subcutaneous fat (154).

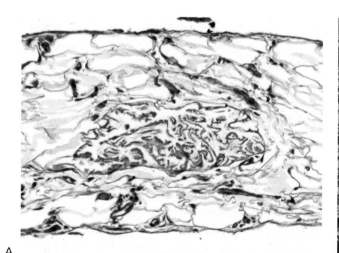
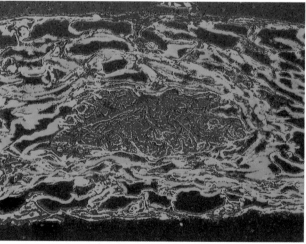

A   B

FIGURE 20-32. Lipomembranous panniculitis. Necrosis of the fat has produced a layer of pale amphoteric to eosinophilic material, a "lipomembrane" around the periphery of the fat globules **(A)**. Spectral image demonstrating in red that the distinctive spectrum of the lipomembranes is similar to hematoxylin staining of nuclear material. The cytoplasm of adjacent damaged fat cells is shown in green, and the collagen of the septa is in blue **(B)**.

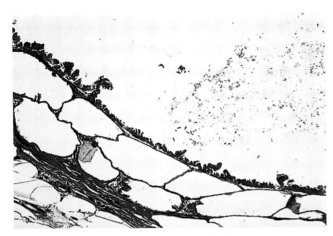

FIGURE 20-33. Lipomembranous panniculitis. Lipomembranes have feathery projections into the fat globules and are PAS positive (PAS stain).

Differential Diagnosis. This is not a very specific entity and probably reflects the tendency of necrotic fat to accumulate fibrin and lysosomal enzyme–containing material from macrophages at the surface of the exposed fat. Although extensive lipomembranous change is rare in uncomplicated traumatic fat necrosis when compared to ischemic panniculitis, a few cases of extensive lipomembranous change have followed minor surgical trauma, possibly related to medications the patient received.

HISTIOCYTIC CYTOPHAGIC PANNICULITIS (SUBCUTANEOUS T-CELL LYMPHOMA WITH HEMOPHAGOCYTIC SYNDROME)

Clinical Features. Histiocytic cytophagic panniculitis is frquently a fatal systemic disease that is characterized by recurrent, widely distributed, painful subcutaneous nodules associated with malaise and fever (89,155–157). The nodules can be hemorrhagic (Fig. 20-34). Ulcers may be present (158). Hepatosplenomegaly, pancytopenia, and progressive liver dysfunction develop in most cases (159). Patients may follow a long chronic course or the disease can be fulminant; patients usually die a hemorrhagic death due to depletion of blood coagulation factors. Aggressive chemotherapeutic intervention, analogous to that used for malignant histiocytosis, has resulted in remission in one patient (160). In some patients, the disease seems limited to the skin and subcutaneous tissue and follows a more benign course (155).

Histopathology. In the subcutis the inflammation is both septal and lobular (Fig. 20-34). A deep biopsy usually shows both subcutaneous and dermal nodules composed of macrophages and a mixed inflammatory infiltrate. Often there is necrosis and hemorrhage (Fig. 20-35). The nuclei of the macrophages are within the range of sizes and shapes seen in

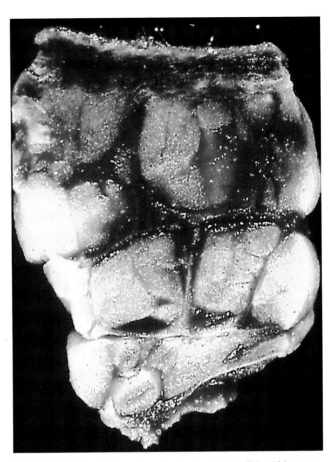

FIGURE 20-34. Histiocytic cytophagic panniculitis. This cross-sectioned skin nodule shows both septal and lobular infiltration and hemorrhage. Note also the dermal hemorrhage.

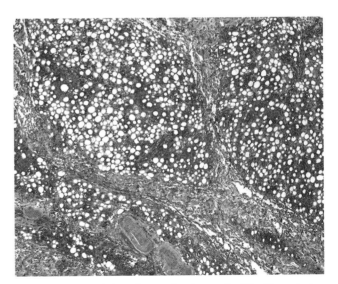

FIGURE 20-35. Histiocytic cytophagic panniculitis. There is hemorrhagic necrosis of the fat with an infiltrate of lymphocytes and macrophages.

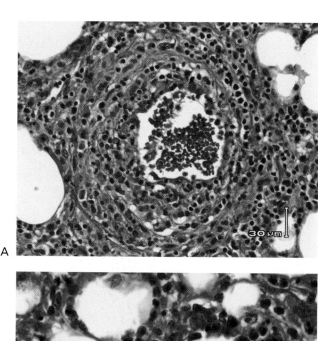

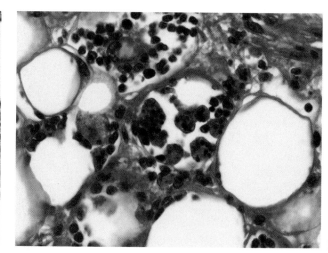

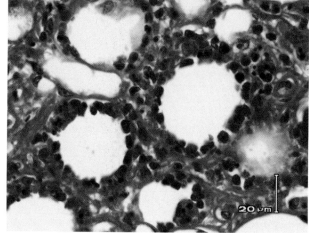

FIGURE 20-36. Histiocytic cytophagic panniculitis. Extensive infiltration of blood vessel walls by lymphocytes **(A)**. Characteristic cytophagic histiocytes that have engulfed lymphocytes and erythrocytes to form so-called "bean bag cells" **(B)**. Distinctive rings of atypical lymphocytes around fat cells in subcutaneous T-cell lymphoma, which is often a trigger for the cytophagic histiocytic activity **(C)**.

benign inflammatory disorders. In some cases, lymphocytes infiltrate medium-sized blood vessel walls (Fig. 20-36A). In some areas, the macrophages become so engorged by phagocytosis of erythrocytes, lymphocytes, and cell fragments that they have been called "beanbag cells" (89) (Fig. 20-36B). In some patients, early lesions contain a rather dense infiltrate of small lymphocytes and only a few focal areas with cytophagic histiocytes. In some of the cases due to subcutaneous T-cell lymphoma, atypical lymphocytes can be found in rosettes around fat cells (Fig. 20-36C).

The involvement of other organs by similar cytophagic macrophages leads to diffuse infiltration of the liver, bone marrow, spleen, lymph nodes, myocardium, lungs, and gastrointestinal tract (161). Cytophagic macrophages can deplete almost all bone marrow elements.

Pathogenesis. When originally described, the disease was differentiated from malignant histiocytosis by the fact that the nuclei of the macrophages in the cytophagic panniculitis were not cytologically atypical. Due to the fulminant course in some patients, the disease was considered by some authors to be a variant form of malignant histiocytosis that can remain confined to the skin and subcutis for a protracted pe-

riod (162). However, more recently the similarity to terminal hemophagocytic syndromes associated with lymphomas (163,164) has led to consideration that most cases of cytophagic panniculitis result from an abnormal lymphocyte population that has stimulated benign macrophages to engage in fulminant hemophagocytosis (165–169). Some of these patients begin with a CD56-positive subcutaneous panniculitic T-cell lymphoma that terminates in a hemophagocytic syndrome (170). Viral infections associated with hemophagocytic syndromes, without lymphoma, usually do not have panniculitis. Benign cytophagic histiocytes can be found in some cases of alpha-1–antitrypsin deficiency panniculitis, ruptured cysts, infections, and can be mimicked by emperipolesis in Rosai–Dorfman disease (4).

MISCELLANEOUS PANNICULITIS

The administration of bromide and iodide compounds can produce a panniculitis, usually in association with changes in the overlying epidermis and dermis. Due to the decrease in therapeutic use of bromide and iodide compounds, the

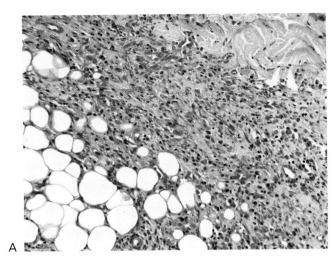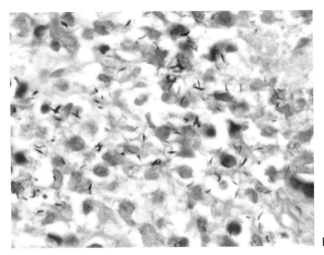

FIGURE 20-37. Mycobacterial panniculitis. Direct mycobacterium tuberculosis infection of the panniculus in an HIV+ patient that has produced primarily a paraseptal panniculitis with many eosinophils and macrophages adjacent to the septa. Erythema nodosum can be mimicked **(A)**. Staining for mycobacteria shows that numerous red, acid-fast bacilli (*arrow*) are present in this example (AFB stain) **(B)**.

number of patients with this disorder has decreased dramatically. In reactions to bromides and iodides, there is epidermal hyperplasia that can develop pseudoepitheliomatus features with intraepidermal abscesses of neutrophils and eosinophils. Allergy to potassium bromide has been demonstrated in some patients by a lymphocyte-transformation test (171).

Painful lipomatous masses can develop in severely obese patients with histologic evidence of inflammation of nerves and endocrine abnormalities. This disease, called adiposis dolorosa or Dercum's disease, is rare, occurs in middle age, and affects females more than males (172,173).

Mycobacterial infection of the fat can produce a *mycobacterial panniculitis* that can mimic erythema nodosum (Fig. 20-37A) as well as erythema induratum (174). Special stains for acid-fast bacteria and cultures are important for the identification of the mycobacteria that are responsible (Fig. 20-37B). Often nontuberculous mycobacteria are involved in countries with a low incidence of tuberculosis.

Morphea or scleroderma can produce a panniculitis that has dense infiltrates of lymphocytes and plasma cells at the periphery of the fat lobules, particularly at the junction of deep reticular dermis and the subcutis. Characteristically, the septa are widened and have hyalinized sclerotic collagen. Similar changes in the collagen are noted in the overlying dermis in most cases. Some of the changes are similar to those of lupus panniculitis so that immunofluorescence and serologic tests are needed to distinguish them (175–177). Discoid lupus erythematosus with panniculitis has more fibrinoid necrosis of the dermis, which stains more brightly eosinophilic than the staining of the pale sclerotic collagen bundles of morphea or scleroderma panniculitis.

Pyoderma gangrenosum can produce ulcers that are difficult to distinguish from those of an ulcerating primary panniculitis (31,178). However the gross appearance of pyoderma gangrenosum is characteristic in the irregularity of the ulcers, the usual shallowness, and the undermined violaceous borders. Biopsies taken at the edges of the ulceration may show pustules and lymphocytic inflammation in the dermis with extension of the lymphoid cells into the septa and lobules of the panniculus. The lesions do not have the extensive necrosis of the fat that is present in erythema induratum or the macrophage infiltration into the lobules in Weber–Christian disease. The sterile abscesses of alpha-1–antitrypsin deficiency panniculitis resemble those of pyoderma gangrenosum, but extend deeper than pyoderma gangrenosum, which lacks abscesses in the fat.

REFERENCES

1. Ackerman AB. *Histologic Diagnosis of Inflammatory Skin Diseases: A Method by Pattern Analysis.* Philadelphia: Lea and Febiger, 1978.
2. Requena L, Sanchez Yus E. Panniculitis. Part I. Mostly septal panniculitis. *J Am Acad Dermatol* 2001;45:163–183.
3. Requena L, Sanchez Yus E. Panniculitis. Part II. Mostly lobular panniculitis. *J Am Acad Dermatol* 2001;45:325–361.
4. Diaz-Cascajo C, Borghi S, Weyers W. Panniculitis. Definition of terms and diagnostic strategy. *Am J Dermatopathol* 2000;22:530–549.
5. Rosenbaum M, Prieto V, Hellmer J, et al. An exploratory investigation of the morphology and biochemistry of cellulite. *Plast Reconstruct Surg* 1998;101:1934–1939.
6. Winkelmann RK, Forstrom L. New observations in the histopathology of erythema nodosum. *J Invest Dermatol* 1975;65:441–446.
7. Niemi KM, Forstrom L, Hannuksela M, et al. Nodules on the legs. *Acta Derm Venereol (Stockh)* 1977;57:145–154.
8. Pierini LE, Abulafia J, Wainfeld S. Idiopathic lipogranulomatous hypodermitis. *Arch Dermatol* 1969;98:290–298.

9. White WL, Hitchcock MG. Diagnosis: erythema nodosum or not? *Semin Cutan Med Surg* 1999;18:47–55.

10. Braverman IM. *Skin Signs of Systemic Disease.* 2 ed. Philadelphia: WB Saunders, 1981.

11. Bafverstedt B. Erythema nodosum migrans. *Acta Derm Venereol (Stockh)* 1968;48:381–384.

12. Vilanova X, Piñol Aguade J. Subacute nodular migratory panniculitis. *Br J Dermatol* 1959;71:45–50.

13. Ackerman AB, Ragaz A. *The Lives of Lesions: Chronology in Dermatopathology.* New York: Masson Publishing, 1984.

14. Forstrom L, Winkelmann RK. Acute panniculitis. *Arch Dermatol* 1977;113:909–917.

15. Miescher G. Zur Histolgie des Erythema nodosum. *Acta Derm Venereol (Stockh)* 1947;27:447–468.

16. Sanchez Yus E, Sanz Vico MD, de Diego V. Miescher's radial granuloma. A characteristic marker of erythema nodosum. *Am J Dermatopathol* 1989;11:434–442.

17. Zabel M. Zur Histopathologie des Erythema nodosum. *Z Hautkr* 1977;52:1253–1258.

18. Ackerman AB. In answer to "Questions to the Editorial Board". *Am J Dermatopathol* 1983;5:409–410.

19. Whitton T, Smith AG. Erythema nodosum secondary to meningococcal septicaemia. *Clin Epp Dermatol* 1999;97–98.

20. Montgomery H. *Dermatopathology.* New York: Harper & Row, 1967.

21. Fine RM, Meltzer HD. Chronic erythema multiforme. *Arch Dermatol* 1969;100:33–38.

22. Hannuksela M. Erythema nodosum migrans. *Acta Derm Venereol (Stockh)* 1973;53:313–317.

23. Forstrom L, Winkelmann RK. Granulomatous panniculitis in erythema nodosum. *Arch Dermatol* 1975;111:335–340.

24. Prestes C, Winkelmann RK, Su WPD. Septal granulomatous panniculitis: comparison of the pathology of erythema nodosum migrans (migratory panniculitis) and chronic erythema nodosum. *J Am Acad Dermatol* 1990;22:477–483.

25. Weedon D. *Skin Pathology.* 2nd ed. London: Churchill Livingstone, 2002.

26. DeBois J, van de Pitte J, de Greef H. Yersinia enterocolitica as a cause of erythema nodosum. *Dermatologica* 1978;156:65–78.

27. Medeiros AA, Marty SD, Tosh FE, et al. Erythema nodosum and erythema multiforme as clinical manifestations of histoplasmosis in a community outbreak. *N Engl J Med* 1966;274:415–420.

28. Gellert A, Green ES, Beck ER, et al. Erythema nodosum progressing to pyoderma gangrenosum as a complication of Crohn's disease. *Postgrad Med J* 1983;59:791–793.

29. Chun SI, Su WPD, Lee S, Rogers RS. Erythema nodosum-like lesions in Behçet's syndrome. *J Cutan Pathol* 1989;16:259–265.

30. Kim B, LeBoit PE. Histopathologic features of erythema nodosum-like lesions in Bechet disease. Comparison with erythema nodosum focusing on the role of vasculitis. *Am J Dermatopathol* 2000;22:379–390.

31. Blaustein A, Moreno A, Noguera J, et al. Septal granulomatous panniculitis in Sweet's syndrome. *Arch Dermatol* 1985;121:785–788.

32. Salvatore MA, Lynch PJ. Erythema nodosum, estrogens, and pregnancy. *Arch Dermatol* 1980;116:557–558.

33. Haustein UF, Klug H. Ultrastrukturelle Untersuchungen der Blutgefasse beim Erythema nodosum. *Dermatol Monatsschr* 1977;163:13–22.

34. Nunnery E, Persellin RH, Pope RM. Lack of circulating immune complexes in uncomplicated erythema nodosum. *J Rheumatol* 1983;10:991–994.

35. Verrier Jones J, Cummings RH, Asplin CM, et al. Evidence of circulating immune complexes in erythema nodosum and early sarcoidosis. *Ann N Y Acad Sci* 1976;278:212–219.

36. Alvarez-Lario B, Piney E, Rodriguez-Valverde V, et al. Eritema nodoso: estudio de 103 casos. *Med Clin (Barc)* 1987;88:5–8.

37. Winkelmann RK, Frigas E. Eosinophilic panniculitis: a clinicopathologic study. *J Cutan Pathol* 1986;13:1–12.

38. Burket JM, Burket BJ. Eosinophilic panniculitis. *J Am Acad Dermatol* 1985;12:161–164.

39. Glass LA, Zaghloul AB, Solomon AR. Eosinophilic panniculitis associated with recurrent parotitis. *Am J Dermatopathol* 1989;11:555–559.

40. Ollague W, Ollague J, Guevara de Veliz A, et al. Human gnathostomiasis in Ecuador (nodular migratory eosinophilic panniculitis). *Int J Dermatol* 1984;23:647–651.

41. Kato N. Eosinophilic panniculitis. *J Dermatol* 1993;20:185–187.

42. Whittaker SJ, Jones RR, Spry CJF. Lymphomatoid papulosis and its relationship to "idiopathic" hypereosinophilic syndrome. *J Am Acad Dermatol* 1988;18:339–344.

43. Cogan E, Schandene L, Crusiaux A, et al. Clonal proliferation of type 2 helper T cells in a man with the hypereosinophilic syndrome. *N Engl J Med* 1994;330:535–538.

44. Varga J, Kahari VM. Eosinophilia-myalgia syndrome, eosinophilic fasciitis, and related fibrosing disorders. *Curr Opin Rheumatol* 1997;9:562–570.

45. Fonseca Capdevila E. Sindrome toxico por aceite de colza adulterado: 10 anos despues [Editorial]. *Piel* 1993;8:7–10.

46. Fagerhol MK, Cox DW. The Pi polymorphism: genetic, biochemical and clinical aspects of human alpha-1-antitrypsin. *Adv Hum Genet* 1981;11:1–62.

47. Eriksson S, Carlson J, Velez R. Risk of cirrhosis and primary liver cancer in alpha-1-antitrypsin deficiency. *N Engl J Med* 1986;314:736–739.

48. Sveger T. Alpha-1-antitrypsin deficiency in early childhood. *Pediatrics* 1978;62:22–25.

49. Breit SN, Clark P, Robinson JPea. Familial occurrence of alpha-1-antitrypsin deficiency and Weber–Christian disease. *Arch Dermatol* 1983;119:198–202.

50. Bleumink E, Klokke HA. Protease-inhibitor deficiencies in a patient with Weber–Christian panniculitis. *Arch Dermatol* 1984;120:936–940.

51. Smith KC, Su WP, Pittelkow MR, et al. Clinical and pathologic correlations in 96 patients with panniculitis, including 15 patients with deficient levels of alpha 1-antitrypsin. *J Am Acad Dermatol* 1989;21:1192–1196.

52. Hendrick SJ, Silverman AK, Solomon AR, et al. Alpha 1-antitrypsin deficiency associated with panniculitis. *J Am Acad Dermatol* 1988;18:684–692.

53. Smith KC, Pittelkow MR, Su WPD. Panniculitis associated with severe alpha 1-antitrypsin deficiency. Treatment and review of the literature. *Arch Dermatol* 1987;123:1655–1661.

54. Geller JD, Su WPD. A subtle clue to the histopathologic diagnosis of early alpha-1-antitrypsin deficiency panniculitis. *J Am Acad Dermatol* 1994;31:241–245.

55. Langenberg A, Egbert B. Neutrophilic tuberculous panniculitis in a patient with polymyositis. *J Cutan Pathol* 1993;20:177–179.

56. Samlaska CP, James WD. Superficial thrombophlebitis I. Primary hypercoagulable states. *J Am Acad Dermatol* 1990;22:975–989.

57. Samlaska CP, James WD. Superficial thrombophlebitis II. Secondary hypercoagulable states. *J Am Acad Dermatol* 1990;23:1–18.

58. Schuppli R. Zur Atiologie der Phlebitis saltans. *Hautarzt* 1959;10:466–467.

59. Montgomery H, O'Leary PA, Barker NW. Nodular vascular diseases of the legs: Erythema induratum and allied conditions. *JAMA* 1945;128:335–341.

60. Minkowitz G, Smoller BR, McNutt NS. Benign cutaneous polyarteritis nodosa. Relationship to systemic polyarteritis nodosa and to hepatitis B infection. *Arch Dermatol* 1991;127:1520–1523.

61. Rademaker M, Lowe DG, Munro DD. Erythema induratum (Bazin's disease). *J Am Acad Dermatol* 1989;21:740–745.
62. Schneider JW, Jordaan HF. The histopathologic spectrum of erythema induratum of Bazin. *Am J Dermatopathol* 1997;19:323–333.
63. Ollert MW, Thomas P, Korting HC, et al. Erythema induratum of Bazin. Evidence of T-lymphocyte hyperresponsiveness to purified protein derivative of tuberculin: report of two cases and treatment. *Arch Dermatol* 1993;129:469–473.
64. Schneider JW, Jordaan HF, Geiger DH, et al. Erythema induratum of Bazin. A clinicopathological study of 20 cases and detection of Mycobacterium tuberculosis DNA in skin lesions by polymerase chain reaction. *Am J Dermatopathol* 1995;17:350–356.
65. van der Lugt L. Some remarks about tuberculosis of the skin and tuberculids. *Dermatologica* 1965;131:26–275.
66. Thompson R, Urbach F. Erythema induratum. *Int J Dermatol* 1987;26:402–405.
67. Cribier B. Etude immunohistochimique de la vasculite nodulaire. Role possible d'une hypersensibilite retardee cellulaire. *Ann Dermatol Venereol* 1992;119:958–963.
68. Penneys NS, Leonardi CL, Cook S, et al. Identification of Mycobacterium tuberculosis DNA in five different types of cutaneous lesions by the polymerase chain reaction. *Arch Dermatol* 1993;129:1594–1598.
69. Sanchez NP, Peters MS, Winkelmann RK. The histopathology of lupus erythematosus panniculitis. *J Am Acad Dermatol* 1981;5:673–680.
70. Izumi AK, Takiguchi P. Lupus erythematosus panniculitis. *Arch Dermatol* 1983;119:61–64.
71. Tuffanelli DL. Lupus panniculitis. *Semin Dermatol* 1985;4:79–81.
72. Ng PP, Tan SH, Tan T. Lupus erythematosus panniculitis: a clinicopathologic study. *Int J Dermatol* 2002;41:488–490.
73. Peters MS, Winkelmann RK. Localized lipoatrophy (atrophic connective tissue disease panniculitis). *Arch Dermatol* 1980;116:1363–1368.
74. Harris RB, Duncan SC, Ecker RI, et al. Lymphoid follicles in subcutaneous inflammatory disease. *Arch Dermatol* 1979;115:442–443.
75. Taieb A, Hehunstre JP, Goetz J, et al. Lupus erythematosus panniculitis with partial genetic deficiency of C2 and C4 in a child. *Arch Dermatol* 1986;122:576–582.
76. Meyer O, Hauptmann G, Tappeiner G, et al. Genetic deficiency of C4, C2 or C1q and lupus syndromes. Association with anti-Ro(SS-A) antibodies. *Clin Exp Immunol* 1985;62:678–684.
77. Provost TT, Arnett FC, Reichlin M. C2 deficiency, lupus erythematosus and anticytoplasmic Ro(SS-A) antibodies. *Arthitis Rheum* 1983;26:1533–1535.
78. Magro CM, Crowson AN, Kovatich AJ, et al. Lupus profundus, indeterminate lymphocytic lobular panniculitis and subcutaneous T-cell lymphoma: a spectrum of subcuticular T-cell lymphoid dyscrasia. *J Cutan Pathol* 2001;28:235–247.
79. Hendricks WM, Ahmad M, Gratz E. Weber–Christian syndrome in infancy. *Br J Dermatol* 1978;98:175–186.
80. Albrectsen B. The Weber–Christian syndrome, with particular reference to etiology. *Acta Derm Venereol (Stockh)* 1960;40:474–484.
81. Ciclitira PJ, Wight DGD, Dick AP. Systemic Weber–Christian disease. *Br J Dermatol* 1980;103:685–692.
82. Thiers BH. Relapsing febrile nonsuppurative nodular panniculitis (Weber–Christian disease). In: Demis DJ, McGuire J, eds. *Clinical Dermatology*. Philadelphia: Harper & Row, 1984:1–7.
83. Lever WF. Nodular nonsuppurative panniculitis (Weber–Christian disease). *Arch Dermatol* 1949;59:31–35.
84. Cummins LJ, Lever WF. Relapsing febrile nodular nonsuppurative panniculitis (Weber–Christian disease). *Arch Dermatol Syphilol* 1938;38:415–426.
85. Steinberg B. Systemic nodular panniculitis. *Am J Pathol* 1953;29:1059–1073.
86. Miller JL, Kritzler RA. Nodular nonsuppurative panniculitis. *Arch Dermatol Syphilol* 1943;47:82–96.
87. Pinals RS. Nodular panniculitis associated with an inflammatory bone lesion. *Arch Dermatol* 1970;101:359–363.
88. MacDonald A, Feiwel M. A review of the concept of Weber–Christian panniculitis with a report of five cases. *Br J Dermatol* 1968;80:355–361.
89. Winkelmann RK, Bowie EJW. Hemorrhagic diathesis associated with benign histiocytic, cytophagic panniculitis and systemic histiocytosis. *Arch Intern Med* 1980;140:1460–1463.
90. Baumgartner W, Riva G. Panniculitis, die herdformige Fettgewebsentzundung. *Helv Med Acta* 1945;12[Suppl 14]:3–69.
91. Schuppli R. Die Panniculitis Typus Rothmann-Makai. In: Marchionini A, ed. *Handbuch der Haut- und Geschlectskrankheiten*. Vol. 2. Berlin: Springer-Verlag, 1965:2–127.
92. Crowson AN, Magro CM, Dawood MR. A causal role for parvovirus B19 infection in adult dermatomyositis and other autoimmune syndromes. *J Cutan Pathol* 2000;27:505–515.
93. Magro CM, Crowson AN, Regauer S. Granuloma annulare and necrobiosis lipoidica tissue reactions as a manifestation of systemic disease. *Hum Pathol* 1996;27:50–56.
94. Magro CM, Crowson AN, Shapiro BL. The interstitial granulomatous drug reaction: a distinctive clinical and pathological entity. *J Cutan Pathol* 1998;25:72–78.
95. Umbert P, Winkelmann RK. Granuloma annulare: direct immunofluorescence study. *Br J Dermatol* 1976;95:487–492.
96. Truhan AP, Roenigk HH Jr. The cutaneous mucinoses. *J Am Acad Dermatol* 1986;14:1–18.
97. Magro CM, Crowson AN. The spectrum of cutaneous lesions in rheumatoid arthritis: a clinical and pathological study of 43 patients. *J Cutan Pathol* 2003;30:1–10.
98. Marcoval J, Mana J, Moreno A, et al. Foreign bodies in granulomatous cutaneous lesions of patients with systemic sarcoidosis. *Arch Dermatol* 2001;137:427–430.
99. Kim YC, Triffet MK, Gibson LE. Foreign in sarcoidosis. *Am J Dermatopathol* 2000;22:408–412.
100. Forstrom L, Winkelmann RK. Factitial panniculitis. *Arch Dermatol* 1974;110:747–750.
101. Parks DL, Perry HO, Muller SA. Cutaneous complications of pentazocine injections. *Arch Dermatol* 1971;104:231–235.
102. Oertel YC, Johnson FB. Sclerosing lipogranuloma of the male genitalia. *Arch Pathol* 1977;101:321–326.
103. Winer LH, Steinberg TH, Lehman R, et al. Tissue reactions to injected silicone liquids. *Arch Dermatol* 1964;90:588–593.
104. Ackerman AB, Mosher DT, Schwamm HA. Factitial Weber–Christian syndrome. *JAMA* 1966;198:731–736.
105. Rotman H. Cold panniculitis in children. *Arch Dermatol* 1966;94:720–721.
106. Duncan WC, Freeman RG, Heaton CL. Cold panniculitis. *Arch Dermatol* 1966;94:722–724.
107. Epstein EH Jr, Oren ME. Popsicle panniculitis. *N Engl J Med* 1970;282:966–967.
108. Assmann K, Nashan D, Grabbe S, et al. Persistent inflammatory reaction at the injection site of Il-2 with lymphoma-like inflammatory infiltrates. *Hautarzt* 2002;53:554–557.
109. Pasyk K. Sclerema neonatorum. Light and electron microscopic studies. *Virchows Arch Pathol Anat* 1980;338:87–103.
110. Kellum RE, Ray TL, Brown GR. Sclerema neonatorum. *Arch Dermatol* 1968;97:372–380.

111. Misra A, Garg A. Clinical features and metabolic derangements in acquired generalized lipodystrophy: case reports and review of the literature. *Medicine* 2003;82:129.

112. Taylor WB, Honeycutt WM. Progressive lipodystrophy and lipoatrophic diabetes. *Arch Dermatol* 1961;84:31–36.

113. Chartier S, Buzzanga JB, Paquin F. Partial lipodystrophy associated with a type 3 form of membranoproliferative glomerulonephritis. *J Am Acad Dermatol* 1987;16:201–205.

114. Handfield-Jones SE, Stephens CJ, Mayou BJ, et al. The clinical spectrum of lipoatrophic panniculitis encompasses connective tissue panniculitis. *Br J Dermatol* 1993;129:619–624.

115. Tong Q, Sankale JL, Hadigan CM, et al. Regulation of adiponectin in human immunodeficiency virus-infected patients: relationship to body composition and metabolic indices. *J Clin Endocrinol Metab* 2003;88:1559–1564.

116. Nagy GS, Tsiodras S, Martin LD, et al. Human immunodeficiency virus type-1 related lipoatrophy and lipohypertrophy are associated with serum concentrations of leptin. *Clin Infect Dis* 2003;36:795–802.

117. Peters MS, Winkelmann RK. The histopathology of localized lipoatrophy. *Br J Dermatol* 1986;114:27–36.

118. Greenwood MRC, Johnson PR. The adipose tissue. In: Weiss L, Greep RO, eds. *Histology.* 4th ed. New York: McGraw-Hill, 1977:179–203.

119. Brooks JSJ, Perosio PM. Adipose tissue. In: Sternberg SS, ed. *Histology for Pathologists.* 2nd ed. Philadelphia: Lippincott-Raven, 1997:167–196.

120. Rudkin GH, Miller TA. Lipedema: a clinical entity distinct from lymphedema. *Plast Reconstr Surg* 1994;94:841–849.

121. Bilancini S, Lucci M, Tucci S. Lipedema: clinical and diagnostic criteria. *Angiologia* 1990;42:133–137.

122. Bilancini S, Lucci M, Tucci S, et al. Functional lymphatic alterations in patients suffering from lipedema. *Angiology* 1995;46:333–339.

123. Lee JH, Sung YH, Yoon JS, et al. Lipedematous scalp. *Arch Dermatol* 1994;130:802–803.

124. Fair KP, Knoell KA, Patterson JW, et al. Lipedematous alopecia: a clinicopathologic, histologic, and ultrastructural study. *J Cutan Pathol* 2000;27:49–53.

125. Wienert V, Leeman S. Lipedema. *Hautarzt* 1991;42:484–486.

126. Amann-Vesti BR, Franzeck UK, Bollinger A. Microlymphatic aneurysms in patients with lipedema. *Lymphology* 2001;34:170–175.

127. Cannon JR, Pitha JV, Everett MA. Subcutaneous fat necrosis in pancreatitis. *J Cutan Pathol* 1979;6:501–506.

128. De Graciansky P. Weber–Christian syndrome of pancreatic origin. *Br J Dermatol* 1967;79:278–283.

129. Hughes PSH, Apisarnthanarax P, Mullins JF. Subcutaneous fat necrosis associated with pancreatic disease. *Arch Dermatol* 1975;111:506–509.

130. Mullin GT, Caperton EM Jr, Crespin SR, et al. Arthritis and skin lesions resembling erythema nodosum in pancreatic disease. *Ann Intern Med* 1968;68:75–87.

131. Millns JL, Evans HL, Winkelmann RK. Association of islet cell carcinoma of the pancreas with subcutaneous fat necrosis. *Am J Dermatopathol* 1979;1:273–280.

132. Levine N, Lazarus GS. Subcutaneous fat necrosis after paracentesis. Report of a case in a patient with acute pancreatitis. *Arch Dermatol* 1976;112:993–994.

133. Zeek P, Madden EM. Sclerema adiposum neonatorum of both internal and external adipose tissue. *Arch Pathol* 1946;41:166–174.

134. Flory CM. Fat necrosis of the newborn. *Arch Pathol* 1948;45:278–288.

135. Horsfield GI, Yardley HJ. Sclerema neonatorum. *J Invest Dermatol* 1965;44:326–332.

136. Burden AD, Krafchik BR. Subcutaneous fat necrosis of the newborn: a review of 11 cases. *Pediatr Dermatol* 1999;16:384–387.

137. Oswalt GC Jr, Montes LF, Cassady G. Subcutaneous fat necrosis of the newborn. *J Cutan Pathol* 1978;5:193–199.

138. Norwood-Galloway A, Lebwohl M, Phelps RG, et al. Subcutaneous fat necrosis of the newborn with hypercalcemia. *J Am Acad Dermatol* 1987;16:435–439.

139. Tran JT, Sheth AP. Complications of subcutaneous fat necrosis of the newborn: a case report and review of the literature. *Pediatr Dermatol* 2003;20:257–261.

140. Silverman AK, Michels EH, Rasmussen JE. Subcutaneous fat necrosis in an infant, occurring after hypothermic cardiac surgery. *J Am Acad Dermatol* 1986;15:331–336.

141. Tsuji T. Subcutaneous fat necrosis of the newborn. Light and electron microscopic studies. *Br J Dermatol* 1976;95:407–416.

142. Roenigk HH Jr, Haserick JR, Arundell FD. Poststeroid panniculitis. *Arch Dermatol* 1964;90:387–391.

143. Fischer AH, Morris DJ. Pathogenesis of calciphylaxis: study of three cases with literature review. *Hum Pathol* 1995;26:1055–1064.

144. Buchet S, Blanc D, Humbert P, et al. La panniculite calcifiante. *Ann Dermatol Venereol* 1992;119:659–666.

145. Lowry LR, Tschen JA, Wolf JE, et al. Calcifying panniculitis and systemic calciphylaxis in an end-stage renal patient. *Cutis* 1993;51:245–247.

146. Bilgen IG, Ustun EE, Memis A. Fat necrosis of the breast: clinical, mammographic and sonographic features. *Eur J Radiol* 2001;39:92–99.

147. Smoller BR, Horn TD. *Dermatopathology in Systemic Disease.* New York: Oxford University Press, 2001.

148. Alegre VA, Winkelmann RK, Aliaga A. Lipomembranous changes in chronic panniculitis. *J Am Acad Dermatol* 1988;19:39–46.

149. Jorizzo JL, White WL, Zanolli MD, et al. Sclerosing panniculitis. *Arch Dermatol* 1991;127:554–558.

150. Kirsner RS, Pardes JB, Eaglstein WH, et al. The clinical spectrum of lipodermatosclerosis. *J Am Acad Dermatol* 1993;28:623–627.

151. Demitsu T, Okada O, Yoneda K, et al. Lipodermatosclerosis—report of three cases and review of the literature. *Dermatology* 1999;199:271–273.

152. Snow JL, Su WPD, Gibson LE. Lipomembranous (membranocystic) changes associated with morphea: a clinicopathologic review of three cases. *J Am Acad Dermatol* 1994;31:246–250.

153. Diaz-Cascajo C, Borghi S. Subcutaneous pseudomembranous fat necrosis: new observations. *J Cutan Pathol* 2002;29:5–10.

154. Weedon D. Panniculitis. In: Weedon D, ed. *Skin Pathology.* 2nd ed. London: Churchill Livingstone, 2002:521–541.

155. White JW Jr, Winkelmann RK. Cytophagic histiocytic panniculitis is not always fatal. *J Cutan Pathol* 1989;16:137–144.

156. Garcia Consuegra J, Barrio MI, Fonseca E, et al. Histiocytic cytophagic panniculitis: report of a case in a 12 year old girl. *Eur J Pediatr* 1991;150:468–469.

157. Peters MS, Su WPD. Panniculitis. *Dermatol Clin* 1992;10:37–57.

158. Willis SM, Opal SM, Fitzpatrick JE. Cytophagic histiocytic panniculitis. Systemic histiocytosis presenting as chronic, non-healing, ulcerative skin lesions. *Arch Dermatol* 1985;121:910–913.

159. Alegre VA, Winkelmann RK. Histiocytic cytophagic panniculitis. *J Am Acad Dermatol* 1989;20:177–185.

160. Alegre VA, Fortea JM, Camps C, et al. Cytophagic histiocytic panniculitis. Case report with resolution after treatment. *J Am Acad Dermatol* 1989;20:875–878.

161. Crotty CP, Winkelmann RK. Cytophagic histiocytic panniculitis with fever, cytopenia, liver failure, and terminal hemorrhagic diathesis. *J Am Acad Dermatol* 1981;4:181–194.

162. Ducatman BS, Wick MR, Morgan TW, et al. Malignant histiocytosis: a clinical, histologic, and immunohistochemical study of 20 cases. *Hum Pathol* 1984;15:368–377.

163. Jaffe ES, Costa J, Fauci AS, et al. Malignant lymphoma and erythrophagocytosis simulating malignant histiocytosis. *Am J Med* 1983;75:741–749.

164. Avinoach I, Halevy S, Argov S, et al. Gamma/delta T-cell lymphoma involving the subcutaneous tissue and associated with a hemophagocytic syndrome. *Am J Dermatopathol* 1994;16:426–433.

165. Gonzalez CL, Medeiros LJ, Braziel RM, et al. T-cell lymphoma involving subcutaneous tissue. A clinicopathologic entity commonly associated with hemophagocytic syndrome. *Am J Surg Pathol* 1991;15:17–27.

166. Peters MS, Winkelmann RK. Cytophagic panniculitis and B cell lymphoma. *J Am Acad Dermatol* 1985;13:882–885.

167. Aronson IK, West DP, Variakojis D, et al. Panniculitis associated with cutaneous T-cell lymphoma and cytophagic histiocytosis. *Br J Dermatol* 1985;112:87–96.

168. Perniciaro C, Zalla MJ, White JW Jr, et al. Subcutaneous T-cell lymphoma. Report of two additional cases and further observations. *Arch Dermatol* 1993;129:1171–1176.

169. Hytiroglou P, Phelps RG, Wattenberg DJ, et al. Histiocytic cytophagic panniculitis: molecular evidence for a clonal T-cell disorder. *J Am Acad Dermatol* 1992;27:333–336.

170. Hoque SR, Child FJ, Whittaker SJ, et al. Subcutaneous panniculitis-like T-cell lymphoma: a clinicopathological, immunophenotypic and molecular analysis of six patients. *Br J Dermatol* 2003;148:516–525.

171. Diener W, Kruse R, Berg P. Halogenpannikulitis auf Kaliumbromid. *Monatsschr Kinderheild* 1993;141:705–707.

172. Dercum FX. Adiposis dolorosa. *Am J Med Sci* 1892;104:521.

173. Winkelman NW, Eckel JL. Adiposis dolorosa (Dercum's disease). A clinicopathologic study. *JAMA* 1925;85:1935–1940.

174. Santa Cruz DJ, Strayer DS. The histologic spectrum of the cutaneous mycobacterioses. *Hum Pathol* 1982;13:485–495.

175. Su WPD, Person JR. Morphea profunda. A new concept and a histopathologic study of 23 cases. *Am J Dermatopathol* 1981;3:251–260.

176. Winkelmann RK. Panniculitis in connective tissue disease. *Arch Dermatol* 1983;119:336–344.

177. Winkelmann RK, Padilha-Goncalves A. Connective tissue panniculitis. *Arch Dermatol* 1980;116:291–294.

178. Powell FC, Schroeter AL, Su WPD, et al. Pyoderma gangrenosum and monoclonal gammopathy. *Arch Dermatol* 1983;119:468–472.

BACTERIAL DISEASES

SEBASTIAN LUCAS

A wide range of bacteria, including mycobacteria and rickettsia, affect the skin and subcutis. In the ensuing descriptions of the histopathology of most of the cutaneous bacterial infections that may be encountered by the diagnostic pathologists, reference is also made to some epidemiology, clinical features, and pathophysiology. The pathogenesis of the skin lesions is multifactorial, including toxin production, pyogenic and granulation tissue chemo-attractants, immunopathology (complement activation and cell-mediated immunity), and vasculitis.

IMPETIGO

Two types of impetigo occur: impetigo contagiosa, or nonbullous impetigo, usually caused by group A streptococci; and bullous impetigo, including the staphylococcal scalded-skin syndrome, which is caused by *Staphylococcus aureus* (1).

Impetigo Contagiosa

Impetigo contagiosa is primarily an endemic disease of preschool-age children that may occur in epidemics. Very early lesions consist of vesicopustules that rupture quickly, and are followed by heavy, yellow crusts. Most of the lesions are located in exposed areas. An occasional sequela is acute glomerulonephritis.

Histopathology. The vesicopustule arises in the upper layers of the epidermis above, within, or below the granular layer. It contains numerous neutrophils (Fig. 21-1). Not infrequently, a few acantholytic cells can be observed at the floor of the vesicopustule. Occasionally, Gram-positive cocci can also be found within the vesicopustule, both within neutrophils and extracellularly (2).

The stratum malpighii underlying the bulla is spongiotic, and neutrophils often can be seen migrating through it. The upper dermis contains a moderately severe inflammatory infiltrate of neutrophils and lymphoid cells.

At a later stage, when the bulla has ruptured, the horny layer is absent, and a crust composed of serous exudate and the nuclear debris of neutrophils may be seen covering the stratum malpighii.

Pathogenesis. In the United States, group A streptococci used to be the most frequently recovered organisms in patients with impetigo contagiosa, either alone or in association with *Streptococcus aureus*. However, the predominant pathogen responsible for impetigo has changed, and *S. aureus* is the most common organism in the United States and United Kingdom (3).

Differential Diagnosis. Histologic differentiation of impetigo contagiosa from subcorneal pustular dermatosis and from pemphigus foliaceus can be difficult. However, only impetigo shows Gram-positive cocci in the bulla cavity. In addition, pemphigus foliaceus usually shows fewer neutrophils, more acantholytic cells, and occasionally some dyskeratotic granular cells.

Bullous Impetigo and Staphylococcal Scalded-Skin Syndrome

Phage group II staphylococci may produce bullous impetigo and the staphylococcal scalded-skin syndrome. Bullous impetigo occurs mainly in newborns, infants, and young children. Occasionally, it is observed in adults, particularly in those with deficiencies in cell-mediated immunity (4,5). It is characterized by vesicles that rapidly progress to flaccid bullae with little or no surrounding erythema. The contents of the bullae are clear at first; later on, they may be turbid. Bullous impetigo may spread and become generalized, so that clinical distinction from staphylococcal scalded-skin syndrome may be impossible (6). An important difference, however, is that cultures from intact bullae of bullous impetigo, unlike those of the staphylococcal scalded-skin syndrome, grow phage group II *S. aureus*.

Staphylococcal scalded-skin syndrome, first described more than 100 years ago and also known as Ritter's disease, occurs largely in the newborn and in children younger than 5 years. It rarely occurs in adults or in older children (7–9), except in the presence of a severe underlying disease (10).

The disease begins abruptly with diffuse erythema and fever. Large, flaccid bullae filled with clear fluid form and

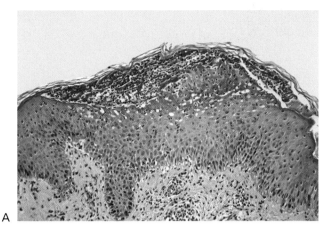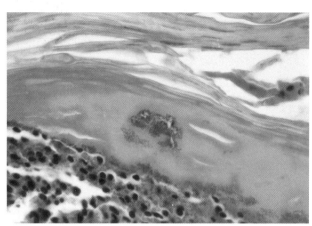

A   B

FIGURE 21-1. Impetigo contagiosa. **A:** A subcorneal pustule containing numerous neutrophils is present. **B:** The underlying stratum malpighii shows spongiosis, and neutrophils are seen migrating through it (H&E stain).

rupture almost immediately. Large sheets of superficial epidermis separate and exfoliate. The disease runs an acute course and is fatal in less than 4% of all cases in children (11). Most fatalities occur in neonates with generalized lesions. In contrast, in the rare cases of staphylococcal scalded-skin syndrome occurring in adults, the prognosis is much worse, with a mortality rate exceeding 50%. Death is usually related to the coexistent disease or to immunosuppressive therapy given for it. Both bullous impetigo and staphylococcal scalded-skin syndrome are transmissible, and can cause epidemics in nurseries, where they may occur together (12).

An important difference between the two diseases is that no phage group II staphylococci can be grown from the bullae of the staphylococcal scalded-skin syndrome, in contrast to the bullae of bullous impetigo. The absence of phage group II staphylococci from the bullae of staphylococcal scalded-skin syndrome results from the fact that these staphylococci are present at a distant focus. Usually, the distant focus is extracutaneous and consists of a purulent conjunctivitis, rhinitis, or pharyngitis. Rarely, the distant focus consists of a cutaneous infection or a septicemia.

Histopathology. In both bullous impetigo and staphylococcal scalded-skin syndrome, the cleavage plane of the bulla, like that in impetigo contagiosa, lies in the uppermost epidermis either below or, less commonly, within the granular layer. A few acantholytic cells are often seen adjoining the cleavage plane. In contrast to impetigo contagiosa, however, there are few or no inflammatory cells within the bulla cavity. In bullous impetigo, the upper dermis may show a polymorphous infiltrate, whereas in the staphylococcal scalded-skin syndrome the dermis is usually free of inflammation.

Pathogenesis. The causative epidermolysins are the exfoliative toxins (ET) produced by *S. aureus.* There are many strains of these serine protease enzymes. Their target is

desmoglein-1, a desmosomal glycoprotein, which has a role in cell-to-cell adhesion in the superficial epidermis (13).

Electron microscopy shows that the cleavage plane of lesions in humans as well as in mice is at the interface between the spinous and granular layers, with some upward extension into the lower granular layer. Splitting occurs without damage to adjacent acantholytic keratinocytes. ET appears to act primarily on the intercellular substance, because in studies carried out on newborn mice, the intercellular spaces widen and microvilli form before the desmosomes separate within their interdesmosomal contact zone (14).

Differential Diagnosis. Both staphylococcal scalded-skin syndrome and severe erythema multiforme of the toxic epidermal necrolysis or Lyell type show clinically extensive detachment of the epidermis and thus may clinically resemble one another. This has resulted in confusion in the past, so that at one time both diseases were referred to as Lyell's disease or toxic epidermal necrolysis. However, the two diseases can be easily differentiated histologically; in severe erythema multiforme, the entire, or nearly the entire, epidermis detaches itself, with considerable necrosis of the epidermal cells, whereas in staphylococcal scalded-skin syndrome only the uppermost portion of the epidermis becomes detached, with relatively slight damage to the underlying epidermal cells.

ECTHYMA

Ecthyma is essentially ulcerated impetigo contagiosa. It occurs chiefly below the knees as multiple crusted ulcers. It is clearly streptococcal in origin, because skin cultures are nearly always positive for group A streptococci. In addition, coagulase-positive staphylococci as secondary invaders can frequently be cultured from lesions (15).

Histopathology. A nonspecific ulcer is observed with numerous neutrophils both in the dermis and in the serous exudate at the floor of the ulcer.

ERYSIPELAS

Erysipelas is an acute superficial cellulitis of the skin caused by group A streptococci. It is characterized by the presence of a well-demarcated, slightly indurated, dusky red area with an advancing, palpable border. In some patients, erysipelas has a tendency to recur periodically in the same areas. In the early antibiotic era, the incidence of erysipelas appeared to be on the decline and most cases occurred on the face. More recently, however, there appears to have been an increase in the incidence, and facial sites are now less common whereas erysipelas of the legs is predominant. Potential complications in patients with poor resistance or after inadequate therapy may include abscess formation, spreading necrosis of the soft tissue, infrequently necrotizing fasciitis, and septicemia (16). Nephritic and cardiac complications are rare because erysipelas is usually produced by non-nephritogenic and nonrheumatogenic strains of streptococci.

Histopathology. The dermis shows marked edema and dilatation of the lymphatics and capillaries. There is a diffuse infiltrate, composed chiefly of neutrophils, that extends throughout the dermis and occasionally into the subcutaneous fat. It shows a loose arrangement around dilated blood and lymph vessels. If sections are stained with the Giemsa or Gram stain, streptococci are found in the tissue and within lymphatics.

In cases of recurring erysipelas, the lymph vessels of the dermis and subcutaneous tissue show fibrotic thickening of their walls with partial or complete occlusion of the lumen.

NECROTIZING FASCIITIS

Necrotizing fasciitis, like erysipelas, is caused by group A β-hemolytic streptococci and it shows rapidly spreading erythema. However, the erythema is ill-defined and progresses to painless ulceration and necrosis along fascial planes. Whereas erysipelas involves the more superficial layers of the skin, cellulitis extends more deeply into the subcutaneous tissues (17). Although virtually all cases of erysipelas are caused by β-hemolytic streptococci, primarily group A, the differential diagnosis of cellulitis is much more extensive. In addition to group A streptococci, possible etiologic agents include *Staphylococcus aureus* and, less frequently, *Streptococcus pneumoniae*, *Haemophilus influenzae*, and (rarely) a laundry list of other organisms, including vibrios, Gram-negative bacteria such as *Pseudomonas*, *Aeromonas*, clostridia, and other anaerobes, legionella, *Erysipelothrix rhusiopathiae*, and *Helicobacter cinaedi*. Minor trauma is fre-

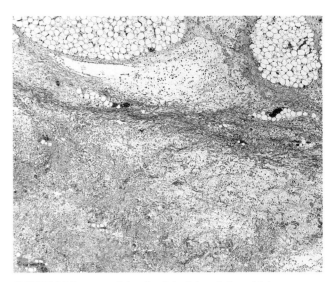

FIGURE 21-2. Necrotizing fasciitis. Subcutis fat with lower-zone necrosis and mild inflammatory cells in upper zone (H&E stain).

quently a predisposing factor, and there is a significant association with chicken pox in children (18). In these and other patients with necrotizing fasciitis due to group A streptococci, there may be onset of shock and organ failure, which are manifestations of the streptococcal toxic shock syndrome. Unless treated by wide surgical debridement, necrotizing fasciitis is often fatal (19). Probing of the subcutaneous tissue discloses extensive undermining and a serosanguineous exudate (20).

Histopathology. The histologic picture is characterized by necrosis and variable acute and chronic inflammation (Figs. 21-2 and 21-3). Sometimes there is minimal inflammation, with necrosis and clusters of bacteria (21). Clumps

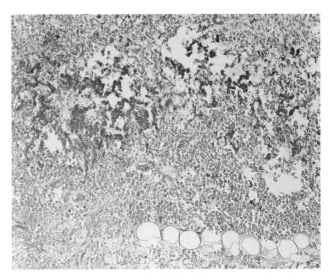

FIGURE 21-3. Necrotizing fasciitis. Higher-power view of necrotic subcutis (H&E stain).

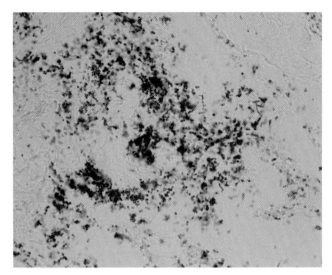

FIGURE 21-4. Necrotizing fasciitis. Clusters of Gram-positive streptococci—note the chains of cocci (Gram stain).

of Gram-positive bacteria are usually present (Fig. 21-4). Often there is thrombosis of blood vessels as the result of damage to vessel walls from the inflammatory process. The key feature in distinguishing necrotizing fasciitis from a less-threatening superficial cellulitis is the location of the inflammation. In the former, the inflammation involves the subcutaneous fat, fascia, and muscle in addition to the dermis. A biopsy may be submitted at the time of surgical debridement for frozen section examination. In an appropriate setting, the presence of edema and neutrophils in these deep locations supports the diagnosis; frank necrosis may not be demonstrable, and bacteria are frequently not evident in an initial biopsy (22).

ACUTE SUPERFICIAL FOLLICULITIS

Impetigo Bockhart

Impetigo Bockhart, caused by staphylococci, is characterized by an eruption of small pustules, many of which are pierced by hairs.

Histopathology. Impetigo Bockhart presents a subcorneal pustule situated in the opening of a hair follicle. The upper portion of the hair follicle is surrounded by a considerable inflammatory infiltrate composed predominantly of neutrophils.

Pseudomonas Folliculitis

In recent years, patients have exhibited outbreaks of pruritic macules, papules, and follicular pustules after using heated swimming pools, whirlpools, or "hot tubs." The eruption usually starts 8 to 48 hours after exposure in a contaminated facility and usually resolves spontaneously within 7 to 10 days (23).

Histopathology. There is distension and disruption of a hair follicle, the pilar canal of which is filled with a dense infiltrate of neutrophils. There also is a perifolliculitis, and the epithelium of the hair follicle may be disrupted (24).

Pathogenesis. The causative organism is *Pseudomonas aeruginosa*, which is ubiquitous in nature and may be found in soil, in fresh water, and on human skin. Proper chlorination and maintenance of pools decrease the population of *Pseudomonas.*

ACUTE DEEP FOLLICULITIS (FURUNCLE)

A furuncle is caused by staphylococci and consists of a tender, red, perifollicular swelling terminating in the discharge of pus and of a necrotic plug.

Histopathology. A furuncle shows an area of perifollicular necrosis containing fibrinoid material and many neutrophils. At the deep end of the necrotic plug, in the subcutaneous tissue, is a large abscess. A Gram stain shows small clusters of staphylococci in the center of the abscess (25).

CHRONIC SUPERFICIAL FOLLICULITIS

Acne varioliformis, or acne necrotica, is characterized by recurrent, small, indolent, follicular papules on the forehead and scalp. The lesions undergo central necrosis and usually heal with small, pitted scars (26).

Histopathology. Early lesions show a marked perifollicular lymphocytic infiltrate with exocytosis of lymphocytes into the external root sheath. This is followed by necrosis of the hair follicle and of the perifollicular epidermis. Late lesions have central cores of necrotic tissue.

CHRONIC DEEP FOLLICULITIS

Folliculitis barbae is a deep-seated infection of the bearded region in men. There are follicular papules and pustules followed by erythema, crusting, and boggy infiltration of the skin. Abscesses may or may not be present. Scarring and permanent hair loss usually ensue.

Folliculitis decalvans occurs predominantly in men. Scattered through the scalp are bald, atrophic areas showing follicular pustules at their peripheries. In some instances, other hairy areas, such as the bearded and pubic regions and the axillae and the eyebrows and eyelashes, are also involved. Through peripheral spreading, the atrophic areas gradually increase in size (27).

Folliculitis keloidalis nuchae represents a chronic folliculitis on the nape of the neck in men that causes hypertrophic scarring. In early cases, there are follicular papules, pustules, and occasionally abscesses. The lesions are replaced gradually by indurated fibrous nodules.

Histopathology. In early lesions of all three forms of chronic deep folliculitis, one observes a perifollicular infiltrate composed largely of neutrophils but also containing lymphoid cells, histiocytes, and plasma cells. The infiltrate develops into a perifollicular abscess leading to destruction of the hair and hair follicles. Older lesions show chronic granulation tissue containing numerous plasma cells, as well as lymphoid cells and fibroblasts. Often, foreign-body giant cells are present around remnants of hair follicles, and particles of keratin may be located near the giant cells. As healing takes place, fibrosis is observed. If there is hypertrophic scar formation, as in folliculitis keloidalis nuchae, numerous thick bundles of sclerotic collagen are present.

PSEUDOFOLLICULITIS OF THE BEARD

Pseudofolliculitis of the beard represents a foreign-body inflammatory reaction surrounding an ingrown beard hair. It occurs in men with curly hair, especially blacks, who shave closely. Clinically, one observes follicular papules and pustules resembling those of a bacterial folliculitis.

Histopathology. As a result of its curvature, the advancing sharp free end of the hair, as it approaches the skin, causes an invagination of the epidermis accompanied by inflammation, and often an intraepidermal microabscess. As the hair enters the dermis, a more severe inflammatory reaction develops with down-growth of the epidermis in an attempt to ensheath the hair. This is accompanied by abscess formation within the pseudofollicle and a foreign-body giant cell reaction at the tip of the invading hair (28).

Follicular Occlusion Triad (Hidradenitis Suppurativa, Acne Conglobata, and Perifolliculitis Capitis Abscedens et Suffodiens)

The three diseases included in the follicular occlusion triad have similar pathogeneses and similar histopathologic findings. Quite frequently, two of the three diseases, and occasionally all three diseases, are encountered in the same patient (29). All three diseases represent a chronic, recurrent, deep-seated folliculitis resulting in abscesses, and followed by the formation of sinus tracts and scarring. Although the primary etiology of these conditions is not bacterial, they are discussed in this chapter because the differential diagnosis includes the deep bacterial folliculitides.

In hidradenitis suppurativa, the axillary and anogenital regions are affected. Acute and chronic forms can be distinguished (30). The acute form exhibits red, tender nodules that become fluctuant, and heal after discharging pus. In the chronic form, deep-seated abscesses lead to

the discharge of pus through sinus tracts. Severe scarring results (31).

Acne conglobata, an entity different from acne vulgaris, occurs mainly on the back, buttocks, and chest, and only rarely on the face or the extremities. In addition to comedones, fluctuant nodules discharging pus or a mucoid material occur, as well as deep-seated abscesses that discharge through interconnecting sinus tracts.

In perifolliculitis capitis abscedens et suffodiens, nodules and abscesses as described for acne conglobata occur in the scalp.

Pilonidal sinus is often considered to be a part of this group of disorders ("follicular occlusion tetrad"). Its pathogenesis appears to be similar, and it is often present in patients with one or more of the other members of the group.

Histopathology. Early lesions in all three diseases of the follicular occlusion triad show follicular hyperkeratosis with plugging and dilatation of the follicle. The follicular epithelium may proliferate or may be destroyed (Figs. 21-5 to 21-9). At first, there is little inflammation, but eventually a perifolliculitis develops with an extensive infiltrate composed of neutrophils, lymphocytes, and histiocytes. Abscess formation results and leads to the destruction first of the pilosebaceous structures and later also of the other cutaneous appendages. Apocrine glands in hidradenitis suppurativa of the axillae or groin regions may be secondarily involved by the inflammatory process. In response to this destruction, granulation tissue containing lymphoid and plasma cells, and foreign-body giant cells related to fragments of keratin and to embedded hairs, infiltrates the area near the remnants of hair follicles. As the abscesses extend deeper into the subcutaneous tissue, draining sinus tracts develop that are lined with epidermis. In areas of healing, extensive fibrosis may be observed (29).

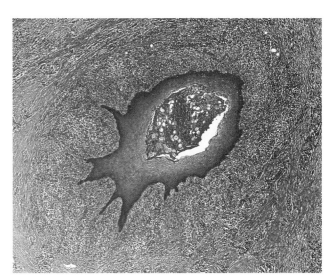

FIGURE 21-5. Acute folliculitis. Hair shaft with early internal inflammation and perifolliculitis (H&E stain).

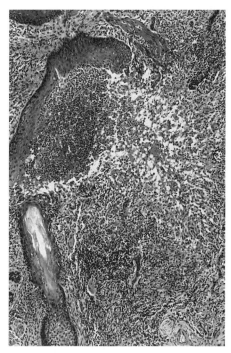

FIGURE 21-6. Acute folliculitis. Hair shaft disrupted by acute inflammation that spreads into the dermis (H&E stain, medium power).

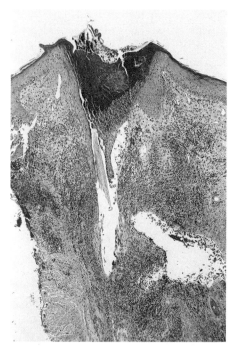

FIGURE 21-8. Follicular occlusion disorder. In an end-stage region, there is scarring with patchy inflammation, which tracks down a healed sinus at the site of a destroyed hair follicle.

Pathogenesis. The common initiating event in the three diseases of the follicular occlusion triad appears to be follicular hyperkeratosis leading to retention of follicular products. Thus, the designation hidradenitis suppurativa is a misnomer, because involvement of apocrine as well as of eccrine glands represents a secondary phenomenon and is the result of extension of the inflammatory process into deep structures.

It appears doubtful that the diseases comprising the follicular occlusion triad are caused primarily by bacterial infection, because cultures from unopened abscesses often are negative (32).

The beneficial effect of the internal administration of corticosteroid suggests that the three diseases represent antigen-antibody reactions resulting in tissue breakdown. Defects in cell-mediated immunity exist in some patients with hidradenitis suppurativa.

BLASTOMYCOSIS-LIKE PYODERMA (PYODERMA VEGETANS)

Two entirely different diseases have been described under the terms *pyoderma vegetans* or *pyodermite végétante of Hallopeau.* One disease, now referred to as pemphigus vegetans of Hallopeau, shows the typical intercellular immunofluorescence of the pemphigus group on direct immunofluorescence testing. The other disease represents a vegetating tissue reaction, possibly secondary to bacterial infection (33). In order to emphasize the difference between it and pemphigus vegetans of Hallopeau, it is preferable to refer to this disease as blastomycosis-like pyoderma rather than as pyoderma vegetans (34).

Blastomycosis-like pyoderma shows one or multiple large, verrucous, vegetating plaques with scattered pustules

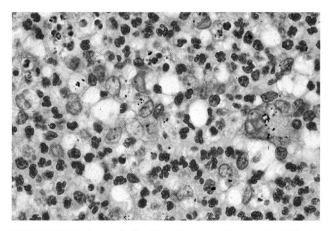

FIGURE 21-7. Acute folliculitis. Gram-positive cocci visible in the inflammation (Gram stain).

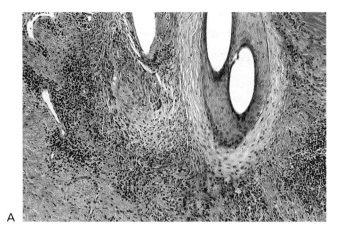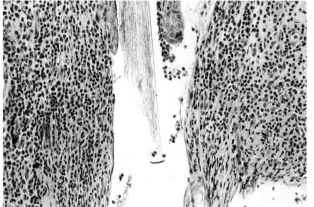

A　　　　　　　　　　　　　　　　　　　　　　　　　　　　B

FIGURE 21-9. A,B: Follicular occlusion disorder. An actively inflamed sinus contains hairs surrounded by neutrophils, granulation tissue, and scar tissue.

and elevated borders. The plaques show considerable resemblance to those observed in fungal blastomycosis. The location of the plaques varies considerably from case to case. In some instances, the face and legs are affected; in others it is the intertriginous areas. Some authors have observed an association with ulcerative colitis (35).

Histopathology. The two major features of blastomycosis-like pyoderma are pseudocarcinomatous hyperplasia and multiple abscesses in the dermis as well as in the hyperplastic epidermis. The abscesses are composed of neutrophils in some cases and of eosinophils in others (33–35).

Pathogenesis. Bacteria, most commonly *S. aureus*, can be regularly found in blastomycosis-like pyoderma; however, the presence of several different strains and the variable response of patients to antibiotic therapy suggest that the bacteria are secondary invaders, although they may be responsible for the vegetating tissue reaction. A deficiency in cellular immunity (36) and a decrease in the chemotactic activity of the neutrophils have also been observed.

Differential Diagnosis. In cases with largely eosinophils in the abscesses, pemphigus vegetans must be excluded by direct immunofluorescence. If there is marked pseudocarcinomatous hyperplasia, multiple biopsies may be necessary for differentiation from true squamous cell carcinoma.

TOXIC SHOCK SYNDROME

Toxic shock syndrome (TSS) is an acute febrile illness usually caused by certain toxin-producing strains of *S. aureus.* Occasionally, however, group A beta-hemolytic *Streptococcus* can cause this illness (37). In the initial report in 1978, the disease was described in a series of seven children (38). Although many cases have been associated in recent years with the use of superabsorbent vaginal tampons by men-

struating women, additional reported settings for TSS have included surgical wound infections of the skin (39), empyema, fasciitis, osteomyelitis, peritonsillar abscesses, and other infections (40). Fever, hypotension, or shock, an extensive rash resembling scarlet fever or sunburn, and involvement of three or more organ systems are the initial defining manifestations, whereas desquamation occurs 1 to 2 weeks after the onset. In rare instances, bullae are also present (41). In addition, there may be conjunctivitis and oropharyngitis. Internal organs may be affected by toxic encephalopathy, thrombocytopenia, renal failure, or hepatic damage. Mortality has been estimated at 5% to 10% (42).

Histopathology. Although in some cases the findings in the skin are not specific, in most instances the histologic findings are quite characteristic, consisting of a superficial perivascular and interstitial mixed-cell infiltrate containing neutrophils and sometimes eosinophils, foci of spongiosis containing neutrophils, and scattered necrotic keratinocytes that sometimes are arranged in clusters within the epidermis (43). If bullae are present, they are subepidermal in location.

Pathogenesis. Even though in rare cases *S. aureus* bacteremia occurs, the cause of TSS is a toxin that is produced locally at the site of a toxigenic staphylococcal infection. Several toxins have been implicated in TSS, including TSS toxin-1 (TSST-1) and the staphylococcal enterotoxins B, C, and F (44). Susceptibility to disease correlates with absence of protective antibodies to the toxin, and cytokine activation may be involved in some aspects of its pathogenesis. Streptococcal TSS has been associated with bacteriemia and extensive necrotizing fasciitis, unlike the staphylococcal syndrome usually associated with occult or minor focal infections. Streptococcal TSS appears to be caused also by toxins produced by the bacteria, including pyrogenic exotoxin A, which shares some homologies with TSST-1 (45).

ACUTE SEPTICEMIA

Three types of acute fulminating septicemia have cutaneous manifestations that are diagnostically significant. They are those caused by *Neisseria meningitidis*, *Pseudomonas*, and *Vibrio vulnificus*.

Acute Meningococcemia

Fulminating septicemic infections with *N. meningitidis* exhibit extensive purpura consisting of both petechiae and ecchymoses. The centers of the petechiae may show small pustules. In addition, shock, cyanosis, and severe consumption coagulopathy occur (46). Without treatment, death may result within 12 to 24 hours. On autopsy, extensive hemorrhaging is found in many internal organs, especially the lungs, kidneys, and adrenals.

On rare occasions, acute septicemia with purpura can be produced by other organisms, such as *Diplococcus pneumoniae*, *Streptococcus*, or *S. aureus* (47).

Histopathology. The cutaneous petechiae and ecchymoses show, in many dermal vessels, thrombi composed of neutrophils, platelets, and fibrin. In addition, there is an acute vasculitis with considerable damage to the vascular walls resulting in large and small areas of hemorrhaging into the tissue. Neutrophils and nuclear dust are present within and around the damaged vessels. In most instances, many meningococci can be demonstrated in the luminal thrombi, within vessel walls, and around vessels as Gram-negative diplococci. They are present in the cytoplasm of endothelial cells and neutrophils and also extracellularly. Intraepidermal and subepidermal pustules filled with neutrophils may also be observed (48).

Pathogenesis. In the past, vascular collapse and death were attributed to massive bilateral hemorrhaging into the adrenal glands and were known as the Waterhouse–Friderichsen syndrome. However, it was then learned that death can occur without significant damage to the adrenals. Therefore, it was assumed that the generalized hemorrhagic diathesis was caused by the consumptive depletion of plasma clotting factors and the resulting disseminated intravascular coagulation (49). It seems likely, however, that there are two distinct pathogenic mechanisms operating in acute meningococcemia (46). First, a shocklike terminal phase is associated with the development of widespread thrombosis of the pulmonary microcirculation. These thrombi, which are caused by meningococcal toxins, are composed of leukocytes and fibrin and often also contain meningococci. They produce severe cor pulmonale, which cannot be prevented by treatment with heparin. Similar microthrombi are found also in the skin, spleen, heart, and liver. Second, a meningococcal endotoxin produces disseminated intravascular coagulation resulting in thrombi composed of fibrin only. These thrombi are found in the capillaries of the adrenal cortex and the kidneys and may cause hemorrhagic infarction of the adrenal glands and renal cortical necrosis. This secondary phase of the disease can be modified with heparin therapy, but its control does not improve survival, because the adrenal and renal lesions are not immediately life-threatening, in contrast to the pulmonary lesions, which result in shock and death.

Pseudomonas Septicemia

The classic and diagnostic cutaneous lesions of *P. aeruginosa* or *Pseudomonas cepacia* septicemia are referred to as ecthyma gangrenosum. *Pseudomonas* septicemia usually occurs in debilitated, leukemic, or severely burned patients, particularly after they have received treatment with several antibiotics. The cutaneous lesions may be single but usually are multiple. They consist of punched-out ulcers about 1 cm in diameter that have hemorrhagic borders. They usually are preceded by hemorrhagic bullae (50). In Tzanck smears prepared from the bases of the lesions, Gram-negative rods can be identified, confirming the diagnosis. In rare instances of *Pseudomonas* septicemia, multiple large, indurated, subcutaneous nodules are observed in addition to the cutaneous ulcers (51,52).

Occasionally, lesions of ecthyma gangrenosum have been observed in immunocompromised patients without bacteremia; these cases have better prognoses (53).

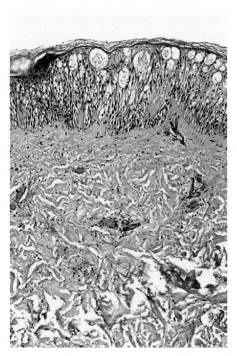

FIGURE 21-10. Pseudomonas septicemia. Skin showing infarction of epidermis, with abnormal mid-dermal vessels (H&E stain). In later lesions, a "punched-out" ulcer typically develops.

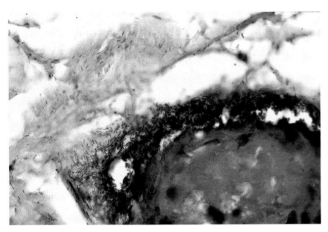

FIGURE 21-11. Pseudomonas septicemia. Bacilli infiltrating the deep vessel wall and into the surrounding dermis. The lumen is thrombosed. There is no inflammation (H&E stain).

Histopathology. The ulcers show at their bases a necrotizing vasculitis with only scant neutrophilic infiltration and little nuclear dust. There is, however, extensive bacillary infiltration of the perivascular region and the adventitia and media of blood vessels. Nevertheless, the intima and the lumen usually are spared (54). *Pseudomonas* bacilli first invade the walls of the deep subcutaneous vessels and then spread along the surfaces of the vessels to the dermis (55). By causing perivascular and vascular necrosis, the bacilli cause extravasation of erythrocytes and the formation of ulcers (Figs. 21-10 and 21-11).

The subcutaneous nodules are the result of cellulitis caused by the presence of large numbers of *Pseudomonas* bacilli (51).

Vibrio vulnificus Septicemia

V. vulnificus infections occur in coastal regions of the United States. Raw seafood consumption, particularly raw oysters, or wounds acquired in marine environments can cause the infection. *V. vulnificus* is a virulent pathogen, producing significant morbidity and, unless treated, mortality, especially in patients with cirrhosis of the liver.

Striking skin lesions are an early sign of septicemic infection. Indurated plaques show blue discoloration, vesicles, and bullae. Large ulcers may develop (56).

Histopathology. Noninflammatory bullae form as the result of dermal necrosis, which is caused by the extracellular toxin produced by the bacterium. Clusters of bacteria may be seen in dermal vessels without associated dermal infiltrate (57).

Pathogenesis. V. vulnificus is a Gram-negative rod that is motile by means of a single polar flagellum. It can be isolated from the blood and bullae of patients with this infection.

CHRONIC SEPTICEMIA

Meningococcemia and gonococcemia can occur in association with a chronic intermittent, benign eruption.

Chronic Meningococcemia

In patients with partial immunity to *N. meningitidis*, an infection with this organism produces chronic meningococcemia. This disease is characterized by recurrent attacks of fever, each lasting about 12 hours, associated with migratory joint pains and a papular and petechial eruption. Positive blood cultures are obtained during the febrile attacks.

Histopathology. The cutaneous lesions of chronic meningococcemia, in contrast to those of acute meningococcemia, show no bacteria and no vascular thrombosis or necrosis. Instead, one observes in papular lesions a perivascular infiltrate composed largely of lymphoid cells and only a few neutrophils (58,59). In petechial lesions, one may find, in addition to a limited area of perivascular hemorrhage, a fairly high percentage of neutrophils and fibrinoid material in the walls of the vessels, so that the histologic picture resembles that of a leukocytoclastic vasculitis (59). The presence of meningococci cannot be demonstrated, not even through direct immunofluorescence testing (58).

Chronic Gonococcemia

Patients with chronic gonococcemia, also referred to as disseminated gonococcal infection (60), like those with chronic meningococcemia, have intermittent attacks of fever and polyarthralgia. The cutaneous lesions of the two diseases are also similar, except that those of chronic gonococcemia are few in number and have a predominantly acral distribution. In contrast to chronic meningococcemia, there are often, in addition to papules and petechiae, vesicopustules with hemorrhagic halos and, rarely, hemorrhagic bullae. Blood cultures often are positive for *Neisseria gonorrhoeae*, but only during attacks of fever. A search for gonococci should also be made in possible sites of primary infection.

Histopathology. The capillaries in the upper dermis and mid-dermis are surrounded by an infiltrate of neutrophils and a variable admixture of mononuclear cells and red cells. There often is nuclear dust, as in leukocytoclastic vasculitis. Fibrinoid material may be present in the walls of some vessels, and fibrin thrombi in some lumina (61). Pustular lesions are usually observed in intraepidermal locations with neutrophils both within them and in the underlying dermis (62). Bullae are subepidermal in location (63).

Gram-negative diplococci are observed in tissue sections only on rare occasions in the walls of blood vessels (64). They are found more readily in direct smears of pus from freshly opened pustules. It is of interest that direct smears reveal gonococci more commonly than cultures (65). However, *N. gonorrhoeae* can frequently be identified in tissue sections by use of fluorescent-antibody techniques (66). For this purpose, fluorescein-labeled antigonococcus globulin is used. Diplococci, as well as single cocci and disintegrated antigenic material, are then observed, largely in perivascular locations. The reason that direct smears are more apt to show diplococci than cultures and that the fluorescent-antibody technique is particularly effective in demonstrating gonococci is that smears and the fluorescent-antibody technique are not dependent on living organisms, as are cultures.

Pathogenesis. Whereas most strains of gonococci are susceptible to the bactericidal action of normal serum, those causing disseminated gonococcal infection are resistant (60).

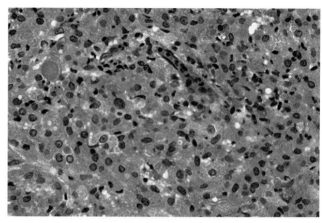

FIGURE 21-12. Malakoplakia. Sheets of macrophages with eosinophilic cytoplasm; several in the center contain Michaelis–Gutmann inclusion bodies (H&E stain).

MALAKOPLAKIA

Malakoplakia may affect various organs, most commonly the urinary tract and the gastrointestinal tract (67). In rare instances, it involves the skin (68,69). The lesions are the result of an inability of macrophages to phagocytose bacteria adequately. The most common organism grown in cultures of tissue material is *Escherichia coli* (70), but in some instances other bacteria such as *S. aureus, Rhodococcus equi,* and nontuberculosis mycobacteria (71) are cultured. Some patients with lesions of malakoplakia have altered immune responsiveness as a result of carcinoma, autoimmune systemic diseases such as systemic lupus erythematosus, or immunosuppressive therapy for lymphoma or for renal transplantation (72).

Cutaneous malakoplakia lesions are chronic, and may be associated with internal lesions. The appearance of the cutaneous lesions is nonspecific and variable. Most commonly, one observes a fluctuant area, a draining abscess, draining sinuses, or an ulcer; however, in some patients, a solitary, tender nodule or a cluster of tender papules is observed. The cutaneous disease is benign and self-limited.

Histopathology. There are sheets of large histiocytes containing fine, eosinophilic granules in their cytoplasm. Many of them contain, in addition to the granules, ovoid or round basophilic inclusions, referred to as Michaelis–Gutmann bodies, that vary in size from 5 to 15 μm (69) (Fig. 21-12). These bodies either are homogeneous or have a "target" appearance by showing concentric laminations. The infiltrate may also contain lymphocytes, plasma cells, and polymorphs.

The Michaelis–Gutmann inclusion bodies and the cytoplasmic granules are PAS-positive, diastase-resistant, and Alcian-blue-positive. In addition, the Michaelis–Gutmann bodies stain with the von Kossa stain for calcium and contain small amounts of iron that may be demonstrated by Perls' stain. With the Gram stain, Gram-negative bacteria may be seen in some of the histiocytes, and, in the rare case

caused by mycobacteria, Ziehl–Neelsen stain reveals the organisms. The bodies may be observed in skin scrapings of lesions (73).

Pathogenesis. Electron microscopic examination reveals that the cytoplasm of the granular cells contains numerous phagolysosomes corresponding to the PAS-positive granules. Some phagolysosomes contain lamellae in a concentric arrangement (69). The Michaelis–Gutmann bodies develop within phagolysosomes by the progressive deposition of electron-dense calcific material on the whorled or concentric lamellae until they are ultimately completely calcified. Bacteria may be observed in the cytoplasm of the granular cells and in various stages of digestion within phagolysosomes (71).

Malakoplakia represents an acquired defect in the lysosomal killing and digestion of phagocytized bacteria. Deficiencies of β-glucuronidase and of 3',5' guanosine monophosphate dehydrogenase have been documented (70,74).

MYCOBACTERIAL INFECTIONS

Taxonomically, the mycobacteria are divided into two major groups: the rapid growers and the slow growers in culture. *Mycobacterium leprae* lies outside this scheme because it cannot be cultured *in vitro.* Within each group the species are organized in subgroups according to certain culture (growth requirement) and biochemical characteristics. Among the infections to be considered in this chapter, the important slow growers are *Mycobacterium tuberculosis* complex, including BCG; the *Mycobacterium avium* complex, including *M. avium* and *Mycobacterium intracellulare*; the *Mycobacterium kansasii* complex; the complex that includes *Mycobacterium marinum* and *Mycobacterium ulcerans*; and mycobacteria with special growth requirements, such as *Mycobacterium haemophilum*. Rapid growers that affect the skin include *Mycobacterium fortuitum* complex, which also includes *Mycobacterium chelonei* (75). Many other mycobacteria can occasionally cause skin lesions (76–78).

Tuberculosis and leprosy bacilli are intracellular parasites that are found in the tissues of humans (and occasionally animals). Transmission requires exposure to infected people. The other mycobacteria are abundant in nature in both soil and water, and exposure to infection occurs throughout life, although usually without significant clinical disease.

Mycobacteria are bacilli that are weakly Gram-positive and are classically identified in histologic sections by stains that exploit their resistance to decoloration by acid—that is, acid-fast bacilli (79). All mycobacteria apart from the leprosy bacillus (see below) are well stained by the standard Ziehl–Neelsen technique.

TUBERCULOSIS

Tuberculosis was until recently considered to be a diminishing clinical problem in industrialized nations, while remaining a dominant public health problem in resource-poor countries. However, there is a global resurgence of tuberculosis because of a combination of factors, including immigration from endemic countries (particularly in Asia and Africa), increased movement of refugees, the HIV pandemic, and poverty (80). As a result, cutaneous tuberculosis remains a clinical and diagnostic problem (81,82).

Infection of the skin and subcutis by *M. tuberculosis* occurs by three routes: (a) direct inoculation into the skin (causing a primary chancre, or tuberculosis verrucosa cutis, or tuberculosis cutis orificialis lesions); (b) hematogenous spread from an internal lesion (causing lupus vulgaris, miliary tuberculosis, and tuberculous gumma lesions); and (c) an underlying tuberculous lymph node by direct extension (causing scrofuloderma). For descriptive purposes, these different tuberculous dermatitides are delineated (a modified "Beyt classification" is used) (77). But in clinical practice, many cases do not readily fit into these clinical and histologic categories (78,83,84).

The basic reaction of human tissues to tuberculous bacilli is a sequence, first of acute nonspecific inflammation during which the bacilli multiply, and cannot be phagocytosed and killed by neutrophil polymorphs. Macrophages then phagocytose the organisms, but their efficacy in killing them depends crucially on enhanced activation. T-cell allergy to tuberculous antigens induces secretion of cytokines that recruit and activate macrophages, which become epithelioid cells. Some will fuse to form giant cells, the typical form of which in tuberculosis is the Langhans giant cell with the nuclei arranged around the periphery of the cytoplasm. As delayed hypersensitivity

increases, there is caseation necrosis within the granuloma, caseation being a homogeneous eosinophilic infarct-like necrotic process whereby the macrophages die. It is probably mediated by cytokines (such as tumor necrosis factor) and the macrophage proteases. This necrotic process inactivates or kills many of the mycobacteria in the lesion, but it does not eliminate them (85,86).

The necrotic granuloma is thus typical of tuberculosis and other mycobacterial infections, but it is not specific, being seen in numerous other infections that involve this type of cell-mediated immunity (e.g., histoplasmosis, syphilis, and leishmaniasis).

The determinants of what happens in tuberculosis infection therefore include the virulence of the organism (tuberculosis is more virulent than most of the nontuberculosis mycobacteria), the size of the inoculum, the route of infection, and the immune status of the patient. It is evident that if cell-mediated immunity is impaired, the T-cell/macrophage system will not operate to contain the infection. The resulting pathology is generally less granulomatous (fewer activated macrophages) and has a higher density of mycobacteria. Such conditions are HIV infection with its sequel of AIDS, steroid therapy, and cytotoxic drugs.

Primary Tuberculosis

Primary infection with tuberculosis occurs only rarely on the skin. Children or adults may acquire it following minor trauma or contact with infected material—as a result, for instance, of mouth-to-mouth artificial respiration (87), inoculation during autopsy (88), needle-stick injury (89), or inoculation during tattooing (90). Usually, the cutaneous lesion arises within 2 to 4 weeks after the inoculation. It consists of an asymptomatic crust-covered ulcer referred to as tuberculous chancre. The regional lymph nodes become enlarged and tender and may suppurate and produce draining sinuses.

Histopathology. The histologic development of the lesion is very much like that observed in experimental cutaneous inoculation of the guinea pig. In the earliest phase, the histologic picture is that of an acute neutrophilic reaction, with areas of necrosis resulting in ulceration. Numerous tubercle bacilli are present, particularly in the areas of necrosis (88). After 2 weeks, monocytes and macrophages predominate. Three to 6 weeks after onset, epithelioid cells and giant-cell granulomas develop, followed by caseation necrosis within the granuloma mass (Fig. 21-13). In time, the necrosis lessens, and the number of tubercle bacilli decreases until it is so greatly reduced that the bacilli may be impossible to demonstrate in histologic sections. Simultaneous with the decrease in the number of tubercle bacilli in the lesion, the tuberculin test with purified protein derivative (PPD), previously negative, becomes positive. The draining lymph nodes receive tubercle bacilli and enlarge

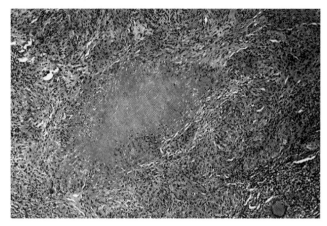

FIGURE 21-13. Tuberculosis. A prosector's wart following inoculation of the finger from a tuberculous cadaver. There is central caseation necrosis with dense macrophage and lymphocyte surround (H&E stain).

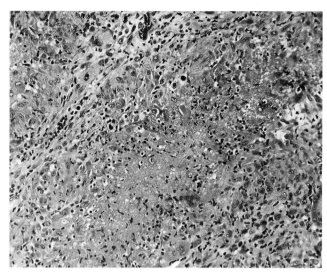

FIGURE 21-14. Tuberculosis. An epithelioid cell granuloma and caseation (H&E stain).

through developing caseating granulomas, parallel to a primary infection in the lung.

Tuberculosis Verrucosa Cutis

Tuberculosis verrucosa cutis represents an inoculated exogenous infection of the skin in persons with a degree of immunity—that is, previous exposure to tuberculosis. In tuberculosis verrucosa cutis, one usually observes a single lesion presenting as a verrucous plaque with an inflammatory border and showing gradual peripheral extension. The verrucous surface exhibits fissures from which pus often can be expressed. The most common sites are the hands and, in children, the knees, buttocks, and thighs.

Histopathology. The histologic picture includes hyperkeratosis and acanthosis. Beneath the epidermis, there is an acute inflammatory infiltrate. Abscess formation may be observed in the upper dermis or within downward extensions of the epidermis. In the mid-dermis, tuberculoid granulomas with a moderate amount of necrosis are usually present (Fig. 21-14). Tubercle bacilli are more numerous in this disease than in lupus vulgaris and occasionally can be demonstrated histologically.

Miliary Tuberculosis of the Skin

Involvement of the skin with miliary tuberculosis is rare in the immunocompetent, occurring mostly in infants and only occasionally in adults. Usually, internal involvement is widespread as a result of hematogenous dissemination, and the cutaneous eruption is generalized, consisting of erythematous papules and pustules 2 to 5 mm in diameter (91). The tuberculin test generally is negative. The disease has a high fatality rate.

There exists, however, a milder form of hematogenous dissemination of tubercle bacilli in neonates born of tuberculous mothers. This form shows limited visceral involvement and only a few scattered erythematous papules with central crusts (92).

Histopathology. In severe cases, the center of the papule shows a microabscess containing neutrophils, cellular debris, and numerous tubercle bacilli. This is surrounded by a zone of macrophages with occasional giant cells. In the milder form, the histologic picture in the skin is similar, except that the Ziehl–Neelsen stain is negative for acid-fast organisms.

Lupus Vulgaris

The lesions of lupus vulgaris are usually found on the head or neck. The skin of and around the nose is frequently involved (93). The lesions consist of one or a few well-demarcated, reddish brown patches containing deep-seated nodules, each about 1 mm in diameter. If the blood is pressed out of the skin with a glass slide, these nodules stand out clearly as yellow-brown macules, referred to, because of their color, as apple-jelly nodules. The disease is very chronic, with slow, peripheral extension of the lesions. In the course of time, the affected areas become atrophic, with contraction of the tissue. It is a characteristic feature of lupus vulgaris that new lesions may appear in areas of atrophy. Superficial ulceration or verrucous thickening of the skin occurs occasionally. Squamous cell carcinoma develops at the margins of ulcers in rare instances.

Histopathology. Tuberculoid granulomas composed of epithelioid cells and giant cells are present. Caseation necrosis within the tubercles is slight or absent (94). Although the giant cells usually are of the Langhans type, with peripheral arrangement of the nuclei, some can be of the foreign-body type, with irregular arrangement of the

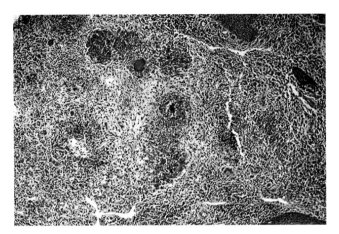

FIGURE 21-15. Tuberculosis. Epithelioid cell granulomas with central acute inflammation ("mixed" granuloma). Scanty acid-fast bacilli were seen in this case (H&E stain).

nuclei. There is an associated infiltrate of lymphocytes (Figs. 21-15 and 21-16). Sometimes this may be so prominent that the granulomatous component is obscured. The inflammation is most pronounced in the upper dermis, but in some areas it may extend into the subcutaneous layer. Tuberculoid granulomas cause destruction of the cutaneous appendages. In areas of healing, extensive fibrosis may be present.

Secondary changes in the epidermis are common. The epidermis may undergo atrophy and subsequent destruction, causing ulceration, or it may become hyperplastic, showing acanthosis, hyperkeratosis, and papillomatosis. At the margins of ulcers, pseudoepitheliomatous hyperplasia often exists. Unless a deep biopsy is done in such cases, one may see only the epithelial hyperplasia and a nonspecific inflammation, and the diagnosis may be missed (93). In rare instances, squamous cell carcinoma supervenes (95).

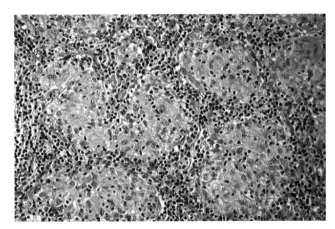

FIGURE 21-16. Lupus vulgaris. Near-confluent nonnecrotizing epithelioid cell granulomas in the dermis (H&E stain).

Tubercle bacilli are present in such small numbers that they can very rarely be demonstrated by staining methods. Polymerase chain reaction (PCR) detection of mycobacterial DNA is more often positive (96). In some instances of lupus vulgaris when an old focus of primary infection cannot be detected, a positive tuberculin test and the response to antituberculous therapy must suffice as proof of a tuberculous etiology.

Pathogenesis. Lupus vulgaris is a form of secondary or reactivation tuberculosis developing in previously infected and sensitized persons. Hypersensitivity to PPD tuberculin is high. Although the mode of infection is often not apparent, the disease rarely seems to be the result of an exogenous reinfection of the skin; usually it results from hematogenous spread from an old, reactivated focus in the lung or from lymphatic extension from a tuberculous cervical lymphadenitis (77).

Scrofuloderma

Scrofuloderma represents a direct extension to the skin of an underlying tuberculous infection present most commonly in a lymph node or a bone. The lesion first manifests as a blue-red, painless swelling that breaks open and then forms an ulcer with irregular, undermined, blue borders.

Histopathology. The center of the lesion usually exhibits nonspecific changes, such as abscess formation or ulceration. In the deeper portions and at the periphery of the lesion, if the biopsy specimen is adequate, one usually sees tuberculoid granulomas with a considerable amount of necrosis and a pronounced inflammatory reaction. Usually, the number of tubercle bacilli is sufficient for them to be found in histologic sections.

Tuberculous Gumma

Hematogenous infection of the skin from an internal lesion may result in a large dermal or subcutaneous nodule that is necrotic and ultimately ulcerates the epidermis.

Histopathology. Most of the lesion is caseation necrosis with a rim of epithelioid cells and giant cells (Figs. 21-17 and 21-18). Acid-fast bacilli are scanty.

Tuberculosis Cutis Orificialis

The lesions of tuberculosis cutis orificialis are shallow ulcers with a granulating base occurring singly or in small numbers on or near the mucosal orifices of patients with advanced internal tuberculosis. The infection has spread by direct contamination from an internal lesion that is excreting bacilli. Most patients have a low degree of immunity. The ulcers, which are often very tender, may occur inside the mouth, on the lips, around the anus, or on the perineum (97). In the case of genitourinary tuberculosis, ulcers may occur on the vulva.

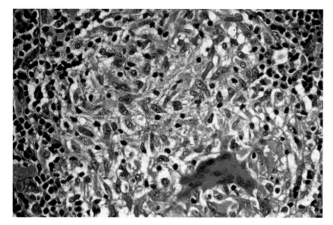

FIGURE 21-17. Lupus vulgaris. Same lesion as in Fig. 21-18, showing an epithelioid cell granuloma and Langhans giant cell (H&E stain).

Histopathology. The histologic picture may show merely an ulcer surrounded by a nonspecific inflammatory infiltrate. In most instances, tuberculoid granulomas with pronounced necrosis are found deep in the dermis (97). Tubercle bacilli are usually readily demonstrated in the sections, even when the histologic appearance is nonspecific.

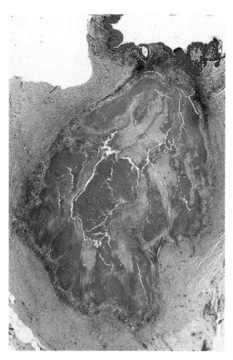

FIGURE 21-18. Tuberculosis. A tuberculoma-like appearance with much caseation necrosis in the dermis (H&E stain).

Differential Diagnosis of Cutaneous Tuberculosis

Because tuberculosis can produce such a wide variety of inflammatory reactions—non-necrotic granulomas, necrotic granulomas, nonspecific acute inflammation, and epithelial hyperplasia (83)—it is not surprising that many other lesions have similar histologic appearances. These other lesions include sarcoidosis, mycoses, leishmaniasis, nontuberculosis mycobacterioses and leprosy, syphilis, foreign-body implantation reactions, Wegener's granulomatosis, and rosacea.

Sarcoidosis usually has little lymphocytic reaction around the granulomas, unlike most forms of granulomatous tuberculosis. When necrosis occurs in a sarcoid, it is usually fibrinoid in type rather than caseating. A thorough search for acid-fast bacilli, a search for fungal infection with PAS and Grocott stains, and the use of polarizing light to exclude foreign material are obviously important in arriving at a diagnosis. Clinical data and the result of a tuberculin test are also significant. Culture of a lesion should establish the diagnosis in most cases. Recently, the use of PCR technology on paraffin sections to detect specific mycobacterial DNA has proved useful in confirming tuberculosis in the absence of evident organisms in sections (98).

Tuberculids

According to some authors, the tuberculids (a term first proposed in 1896 [99]) comprise two types of dermatoses: papulonecrotic tuberculids and lichen scrofulosorum (100,101). Cases of nodular vasculitis, when associated with tuberculosis, are included within the group of tuberculids and are called erythema induratum (Bazin's disease) (see Chapter 8).

Tuberculids are skin lesions in patients with tuberculosis, often occult, elsewhere in the body. The most common sites of infection are lymph nodes (102). By definition, stains for acid-fast bacilli and culture for mycobacteria are negative; delayed hypersensitivity skin tests for tuberculosis are positive, and the lesions heal on antituberculous therapy. Recently, using the PCR technique, mycobacterial DNA has been identified in some lesions (103). This supports the concept of tuberculids as immunologic reactions to degenerate dead bacilli or antigenic fragments thereof that have been deposited in the skin and subcutis.

Papulonecrotic Tuberculids

Papulonecrotic lesions are erythematous papules that usually develop on the limbs in a symmetrical distribution (104). They ulcerate and heal, leaving depressed scars. These tuberculids often recur until treated. Occasionally they may develop into lupus vulgaris.

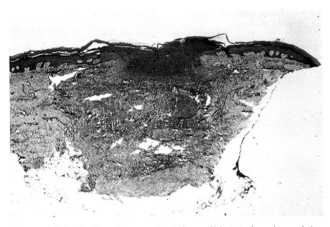

FIGURE 21-19. Papulonecrotic tuberculid. Wedge-shaped infarction of the dermis and epidermis, caused by vasculitis (H&E stain).

Histopathology. Vascular involvement is observed in early lesions. It may consist of a leukocytoclastic vasculitis (90) or a lymphocytic vasculitis. In either case, it is associated with fibrinoid necrosis and thrombotic occlusion of individual vessels (105). Subsequently, a wedge-shaped area of necrosis forms, with its broad base toward the epidermis (104) (Figs. 21-19 and 21-20). As this wedge is gradually cast off, epithelioid and giant cells gather around its periphery, although focal granuloma formation is poor. Follicular necrosis or suppuration may occur, although diffuse acute inflammatory cells are infrequent. Ziehl–Neelsen stains are, of course, negative.

Differential Diagnosis. Numerous conditions may be confused clinically or histopathologically with papulonecrotic tuberculids. They include pityriasis lichenoides acuta, syphilides, miliary tuberculosis, perforating granuloma annulare, and suppurative folliculitis (104).

Lichen Scrofulosorum

This lesion consists of yellow or brown follicular papules, 0.5 to 3.0 mm in diameter, on the trunk. They heal without scarring.

Histopathology. Superficial dermal granulomas are observed, usually in the vicinity of hair follicles or sweat ducts. The granulomas are composed of epithelioid cells, with some Langhans giant cells and a narrow margin of lymphoid cells at the periphery (Fig. 21-21). Generally, caseation necrosis is absent.

Differential Diagnosis. Distinction of lichen scrofulosorum from sarcoidosis may be impossible on histologic grounds alone.

Pathogenesis. The histogenesis of tuberculids is still unclear. Tubercle bacilli are absent in tuberculids, either because they have arrived hematogenously in fragmented form or because they have been destroyed at the sites of the tuberculids by immunologic mechanisms. Mycobacterial DNA is, however, demonstrable in many cases (103,106). The reaction in the papulonecrotic tuberculid consists of an Arthus reaction with vasculitis followed by a delayed hypersensitivity response with granuloma formation (90). In the case of lichen scrofulosorum, there is only a delayed hypersensitivity reaction resulting in granuloma formation (101).

Tuberculid-type reactions are also described with nontuberculosis mycobacteria (*Mycobacterium bovis* and *M. avium*) (107,108).

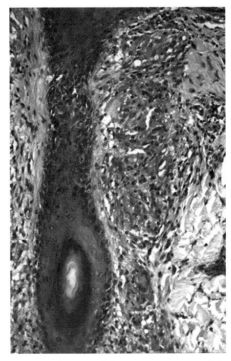

FIGURE 21-21. Lichen scrofulosorum. Nonnecrotizing epithelioid cell granulomas alongside a hair shaft (H&E stain).

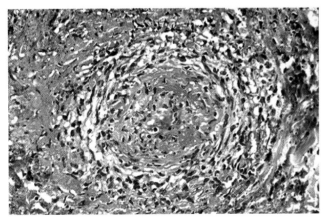

FIGURE 21-20. Papulonecrotic tuberculid. Necrotizing vasculitis of a dermal artery, with granulomatous surround (H&E stain).

INFECTIONS WITH NONTUBERCULOSIS MYCOBACTERIA

Among the nontuberculosis, nonleprosy mycobacterial infections of the skin, those caused by *M. marinum* are the most common among nonimmunosuppressed people (109). Unlike *M. tuberculosis*, which is transmitted from person to person, nontuberculosis mycobacteria are abundant in nature, in soil and water, and contact is frequent in most zones of the world (76,110).

These skin infections may be acquired by direct inoculation into the skin or by hematogenous spread from a visceral focus. Increased use of immunosuppression in medicine (e.g., for transplantation and cancer chemotherapy) and the pandemic of HIV/AIDS have resulted in many more mycobacterial skin infections. The cell-mediated immune system is a major defense against such organisms and is affected or destroyed during the course of these immunosuppressive conditions. The clinical and histopathologic patterns are also altered, with organisms being found in greater density than in immunocompetent persons.

The histopathologic picture in nontuberculosis mycobacterioses is just as variable as the clinical picture and may present nonspecific acute and chronic inflammation, suppuration and abscess formation, or tuberculoid granulomas with or without caseation (83,111). In some instances, both tissue reactions occur concurrently. The presence or absence of acid-fast bacilli depends on the tissue reaction. In suppurative lesions, numerous acid-fast bacilli often can be found.

Infection with *Mycobacterium kansasii*

M. kansasii is usually a lymph node and pulmonary infection (112), and skin lesions are unusual. Implantation causes a chronic cutaneous nodule and sometimes ulceration (113).

The lesions are often crusted. There may be sporotrichosis spread up the extremity (109,114). In immunocompromised patients such as those with HIV infection, there may be multiple visceral lesions (lung and bone) with hematogenous dissemination to skin. The skin lesions are acute abscesses with large numbers of acid-fast bacilli (Fig. 21-22).

Infection with *M. avium-intracellulare*

M. avium complex infection is a common cause of cervical lymph node mycobacteriosis in normal children, and of pulmonary disease in previously damaged lungs (76). Prior to the HIV pandemic, skin infections were rare, with hematogenously borne lesions in skin and subcutis observed in patients usually with immunosuppressing diseases (78).

Severely immunocompromised patients such as those with HIV infection have a very high prevalence of *M. avium-intracellulare* bacteremia (115) and many show one or more cutaneous papules and nodules (116,117). Steroid therapy also predisposes to skin lesions. The histology may be granulomatous or mixed acute and chronically inflammatory, as with tuberculosis (76). Sometimes there is a histology resembling that of lepromatous leprosy (Figs. 21-23, 21-24, and 21-25). Macrophages contain large numbers of bacilli without necrosis, and a spindle cell transformation of macrophages, forming a histoid-like lesion (as in leprosy), can occur (118,119).

Infection with *Mycobacterium marinum*

Infections with *M. marinum* can be contracted through minor abrasions incurred while bathing in swimming pools or in ocean or lake water or while cleaning home aquariums (120). Infected swimming pools have caused epidemics, the largest of which affected 290 persons (121). The period of incubation usually is about 3 weeks, but may be longer (109).

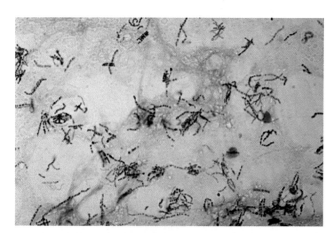

FIGURE 21-22. Mycobacterium kansasii infection. Needle aspirate of a skin lesion on an immunocompromised patient. Abundant elongated and beaded acid-fast bacilli typical of *Mycobacterium kansasii* (Ziehl–Neelsen stain).

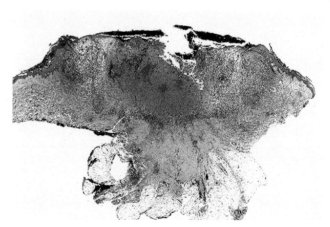

FIGURE 21-23. *Mycobacterium avium* intracellular infection. Discrete inflammatory lesion in an elderly female (H&E stain).

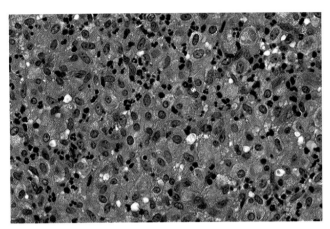

FIGURE 21-24. *Mycobacterium avium* intracellular infection. Same lesion as in Fig. 21.23. Unactivated macrophages with eosinophilic cytoplasm (H&E stain).

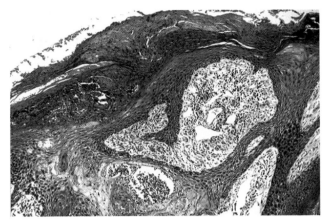

FIGURE 21-26. *Mycobacterium marinum* infection. A marked pseudoepitheliomatous epidermal hyperplasia, with acute inflammatory foci within the epidermis (H&E stain).

Clinically, most of the lesions caused by *M. marinum* are solitary and consist of indolent, dusky red, hyperkeratotic, papillomatous papules, nodules, or plaques. Superficial ulceration is occasionally observed. The fingers, knees, elbows, and feet are most commonly affected. In some instances, satellite papules arise and ascending sporotrichosis spread occurs (122). Lesions may form at different sites in the case of multiple injuries. Although spontaneous healing usually takes place within a year, the lesions persist in some patients for many years. A few HIV-associated cases have been reported (123). Fatal disseminated *M. marinum* infection is rare (124).

Histopathology. Early lesions no more than 2 or 3 months old show a nonspecific inflammatory infiltrate composed of neutrophils, monocytes, and macrophages. In lesions about 4 months old, a few multinucleated giant cells and a few small epithelioid cell granulomas usually are present, and in lesions 6 months old or older, typical tubercles or tuberculoid structures may be seen (125). Areas of necrosis are only

occasionally present in the centers of the granulomas. The epidermis often shows marked hyperkeratosis with an acute inflammatory infiltrate and ulceration (Fig. 21-26).

Acid-fast bacilli usually can be identified in histologic sections of early lesions that show a nonspecific inflammatory infiltrate. In contrast, tuberculoid granulomas generally no longer show acid-fast organisms unless areas of central necrosis are present. Although primary lesions usually require a few months for the formation of tuberculoid granulomas, the sporotrichosis nodules that arise later show tuberculoid granulomas and a lack of acid-fast bacilli even when they have been present for only a few weeks.

Differential Diagnosis. The granulomatous reaction produced by *M. marinum* is similar to that observed in tuberculosis verrucosa cutis or lupus vulgaris. The pattern of pseudoepitheliomatous hyperplasia with granulomas and polymorphonuclear neutrophil infiltrate is also seen in several cutaneous mycoses (e.g., sporotrichosis and chromoblastomycosis), so fungal stains need to be examined alongside Ziehl–Neelsen stains. For definitive identification, culture may be necessary.

Buruli Ulcer (*M. ulcerans*)

Buruli ulceration, an infection caused by a nontuberculosis mycobacterium, *M. ulcerans*, is endemic in West and Central Africa, Central America, and South Australia (126–128). The organism is now identified in nature, near inland water and rivers, and is directly implanted or follows an aquatic insect bite. The infection commences as a palpable cutaneous nodule. This may, in some cases heal, but probably more usually progresses to ulceration of the skin with extensive undermining of the epidermis, and extension of the necrosis down to fascia and even bone (129). These painless ulcers are usually located on extremities and buttocks, but trunk and facial ulcers also occur (128).

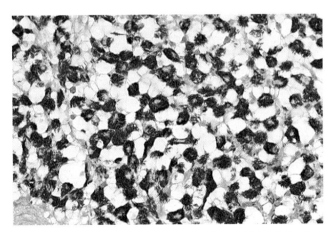

FIGURE 21-25. *Mycobacterium avium* intracellular infection. Same lesion as in Fig. 21–23. showing abundant acid-fast bacilli, similar to lepromatous leprosy (Ziehl–Neelsen stain).

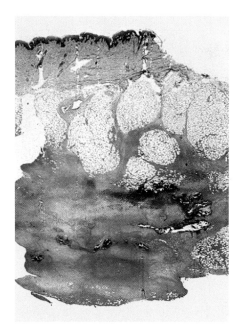

FIGURE 21-27. Buruli ulcer (*Mycobacterium ulcerans* infection). Early preulcerating lesion, with deep dermal and subcutaneous fat necrosis (H&E stain).

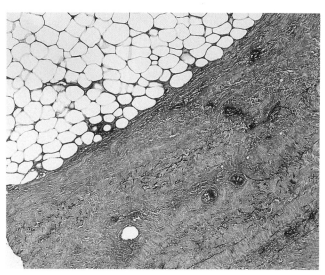

FIGURE 21-28. Buruli ulcer. The ischemic-type fat and collagen necrosis, without cellular reaction; the hematoxyphilic clusters are mycobacteria (H&E stain).

Histopathology. The infection begins as a subcutaneous nodule exhibiting "ghost" ischemic-type dermal collagen and fat necrosis with deposition of fibrin, and hematoxyphilic extra-cellular clumps of mycobacteria. Ulceration proceeds as the epidermis loses its vascular supply. Ziehl–Neelsen stains reveal vast numbers of acid-fast bacilli in the necrotic fat (Figs. 21-27, 21-28, and 21-29); their distribution is often irregular. A variable degree of neutrophil infiltration and thrombosis of vessels are also observed. In time, a nonspecific granulation tissue or a granulomatous reaction commences from the depth and sides of the ulcer; healing and re-epithelialization take place with considerable scarring. Acid-fast bacilli decline rapidly in number during healing (127,130). The histopathologic case definition for Buruli ulcer, useful for research studies, is (a) the typical pattern of infarctive-like necrosis of deep dermal collagen and fat, and (ideally, but not always found in limited samples), (b) nearby clusters of acid-fast bacilli.

Pathogenesis. The widespread necrosis of subcutaneous tissue is caused by a toxin secreted by *M. ulcerans*, a pathogenesis unique to this species of mycobacteria. It is polyketide mycolactone, and strain and geographical differences in mycolactone virulence are already described (the disease is less severe in Australia than in central Africa, related to different mycolactone strains). This toxin causes necrosis when inoculated into guinea pig skin and into macrophages in tissue culture (126). Like *M. marinum*, *M. ulcerans* shows optimal cultural growth at 30 to 33°C.

Healing of Buruli ulcer coincides with development of delayed hypersensitivity to the mycobacterium, possibly contingent on the cessation of mycolactone production.

Other Nontuberculosis Mycobacterioses

Infections in the skin and subcutis caused by the rapid growers, *M. chelonei*, *M. fortuitum*, and *Mycobacterium abscessus* are associated with medical injections through unsterile contaminated needles and cannulae (76,131). Sporotrichosis spread can occur with *M. chelonei* (132). The inflammatory reaction is usually a mixed acute (neutrophilic) and chronic (granulomatous) response, with acid-fast bacilli visible on sections (76) (Figs. 21-30 and 21-31). Localized and disseminated *M. haemophilum* infection is reported in patients with HIV and other causes of immunosuppression (106,133–135).

Bacille Calmette-Guérin (BCG) is the most commonly used vaccine, yet it rarely results in significant cutaneous lesions. Persisting ulcerating lesions may be observed. Histologically, these lesions are caseating granulomas in the

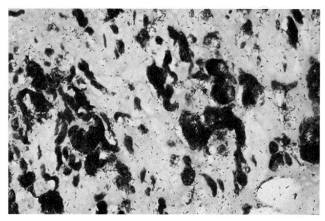

FIGURE 21-29. Buruli ulcer. Clumps of acid-fast bacilli within the fat necrosis (Ziehl–Neelsen stain).

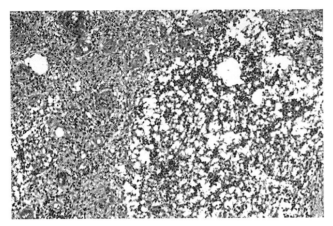

FIGURE 21-30. *Mycobacterium fortuitum* injection abscess. Dermal mixed granulomatous and acute inflammation (H&E stain).

dermis, as seen in tuberculosis, but acid-fast bacilli are rarely observed. In immunocompromised patients, there may be generalized cutaneous nodules, and histology shows abundant bacilli, poorly formed bacilli, and variable or no necrosis (136).

LEPROSY

Leprosy is caused by *M. leprae* and predominantly affects the skin and peripheral nerves. The disease is endemic in many tropical and subtropical countries but is declining in prevalence as a result of multidrug therapy. The Indian subcontinent, Southeast Asia, sub-Saharan countries in Africa, and Brazil comprise the areas most affected at present (137,138). The mode of transmission of leprosy is unknown, but it is probably inhalation of bacilli (76), which may be excreted from the nasal passages of a multibacillary patient, or possibly implanted from organisms in the soil.

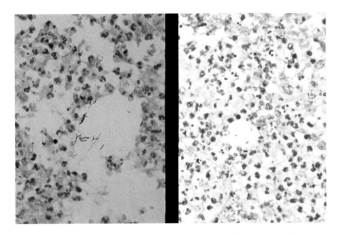

FIGURE 21-31. *Mycobacterium fortuitum* injection abscess. Clusters of acid-fast bacilli within a fat vacuole (Ziehl–Neelsen stain).

Direct person-to-person infection by means of the skin occurs rarely if at all. After inhalation, it is likely that bacilli pass through the blood to peripheral and cutaneous nerves, where infection and host reaction commence.

Immunopathologic Spectrum of Leprosy

The sequence of disease pathogenesis is complex and very chronic, and depends on host–parasite immunologic responses. The leprosy bacillus is nontoxic, and clinicopathologic manifestations are the result of immunopathology and/or the progressive accumulation of infected cells. Leprosy is the best example of a disease showing an immunopathologic spectrum whereby the host immune reaction to the infective agent ranges from apparently none to marked, with a consequent range of clinicopathologic manifestations (139,140). Tuberculoid leprosy indicates a high cellular immune response (i.e., T cells and macrophage activation) and few bacilli in tissues; at the opposite pole, lepromatous leprosy indicates an absent cellular immune response to *M. leprae* antigens, with no macrophage activation and abundant bacilli in tissues. The spectrum of leprosy is a continuum, and patients may move in either direction according to host response and treatment. The standard delineation follows that of Ridley and Jopling, with categories defined along the spectrum by a combination of clinical, microbiological, histopathologic, and immunologic indices: TT (tuberculoid), BT (borderline tuberculoid), BB (midborderline), BL (borderline lepromatous), and LL (lepromatous). The term "borderline" is used to denote patterns that share some features of both tuberculoid and lepromatous leprosy (138,139).

TT and LL patients are stable, the former often self-healing and the latter remaining heavily infected unless given appropriate chemotherapy. Patients presenting at the BT point will often downgrade toward BL leprosy in the absence of treatment. The central point of the spectrum (BB) is the most unstable, with most patients downgrading to LL if not treated. The term "indeterminate leprosy" is used to describe patients presenting with very early leprosy lesions that cannot be categorized definitely along the immunopathologic spectrum (e.g., cannot be determined as BT or LL).

It is likely that in endemic zones, a high proportion of people are infected by *M. leprae*, but either have full immunity and no disease, or have developed one or a few lesions that have self-healed without significant morbidity. The progression of infection and disease is summarized in Fig. 21-32. Patients with determined leprosy are most numerous at the BT and LL points of the spectrum.

Staining of *Mycobacterium leprae* Bacilli

The classical method for demonstrating leprosy bacilli in lesions is a modified Ziehl–Neelsen stain, where the degree of acid and alcohol removal of carbol fuchsin is less than in the

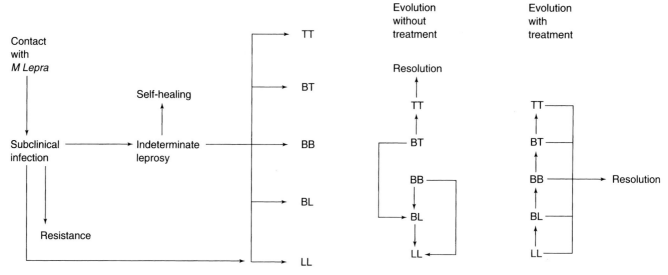

FIGURE 21-32. Leprosy. The sequence of events that may follow infection with *Mycobacterium leprae.*

methods used for identifying other mycobacteria. The Fite methods are the most commonly used (140,141). Methenamine silver stains are also useful in detecting fragmented acid-fast bacilli. The sensitivity of detection of acid-fast bacilli by histologic means remains poor, because about 1000 bacilli per cubic centimeter of tissue must be present in order to detect one bacillus in a section. For lesions where bacilli are scanty, it is recommended that at least six sections be examined before declaring them negative. The standard enumeration of leprosy bacilli in lesions—the bacterial index (BI)—follows Ridley's logarithmic scale (which applies to both skin biopsies and slit skin smears):

BI = 0: no bacilli observed
BI = 1: 1 to 10 bacilli in 10 to 100 high-power fields (hpf, oil immersion)
BI = 2: 1 to 10 bacilli in 1 to 10 hpf
BI = 3: 1 to 10 bacilli per hpf
BI = 4: 10 to 100 bacilli per hpf
BI = 5: 100 to 1000 bacilli per hpf
BI = 6: >1000 bacilli per hpf

Solid-staining bacilli indicate that the organisms are capable of multiplication. Fragmented (beaded) and granular acid-fast bacilli indicate that they are dead. Patients with no bacilli detectable in lesions are termed paucibacillary; those with some or many bacilli are multibacillary (this distinction is important in determining the duration of chemotherapy) (142).

Immunocytochemical methods for demonstrating mycobacterial antigens have a limited role. The most frequently used is a polyclonal anti-BCG antibody (143). In untreated lesions, it will not detect small numbers of bacilli if ordinary histochemical methods have proved negative. However, im-

munocytochemistry does have a role in demonstrating the presence of leprosy antigen after the bacilli have fragmented, been partly digested by macrophage enzymes, and lost their acid-fast staining quality (see below).

Clinical Pathology of Leprosy

For general discussions of clinical leprosy and leprosy pathology, see Job (144) and Britton and Lockwood (138).

Early, Indeterminate Leprosy

Many patients present with obvious or advanced skin and peripheral nerve lesions (the latter are primarily nerve enlargement and the consequences of anesthesia): these patients have "determined leprosy." However, the earliest detectable skin lesion comprises one or a few hypopigmented macules with variable loss of sensation. Any part of the body may be affected.

Histopathology. There is mild lymphocytic and macrophage accumulation around neurovascular bundles, the superficial and deep dermal vessels, sweat glands, and erector pili muscle; focal lymphocytic invasion into the lower epidermis and into the dermal nerves may be observed. No formed epithelioid cell granulomas are present (if they were, it would not be indeterminate leprosy but a tuberculoid leprosy). Schwann cell hyperplasia is a feature, but it is highly subjective. Not all these features are present in every case. The diagnosis hinges on finding one or more acid-fast bacilli in the sites of predilection: in nerve, in erector pili muscle, just under the epidermis, or in a macrophage about a vessel. Without demonstrating bacilli, the diagnosis can only be presumptive (Figs. 21-33 and 21-34).

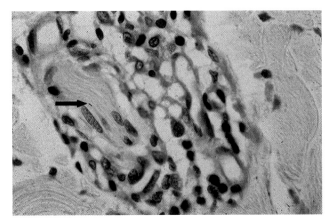

FIGURE 21-34. Indeterminate leprosy. High-power view of a small dermal nerve with surrounding lymphocytes and an arrowed intraneural acid-fast bacillus. There is no granuloma formation (Wade–Fite stain).

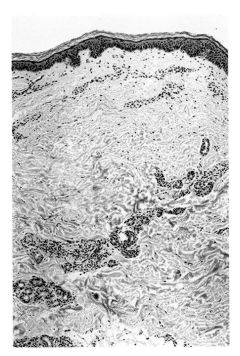

FIGURE 21-33. Indeterminate leprosy. Slight pandermal perineurovascular and periappendageal chronic inflammation (H&E stain).

Lepromatous Leprosy

Lepromatous (LL) leprosy initially has cutaneous and mucosal lesions, with neural changes occurring later. The lesions usually are numerous and are symmetrically arranged. There are three clinical types: macular, infiltrative nodular, and diffuse. In the macular type, numerous ill-defined, confluent, either hypopigmented or erythematous macules are observed. They are frequently slightly infiltrated. The infiltrative-nodular type, the classical and most common variety, may develop from the macular type or arise as such. It is characterized by papules, nodules, and diffuse infiltrates that are often dull red. Involvement of the eyebrows and forehead often results in a leonine facies, with a loss of eyebrows and eyelashes. The lesions themselves are not notably hypoesthetic, although, through involvement of the large peripheral nerves, disturbances of sensation and nerve paralyses develop. The nerves that are most commonly involved are the ulnar, radial, and common peroneal nerves.

The diffuse type of leprosy, called Lucio leprosy, which is most common in Mexico and also in Central America, shows diffuse infiltration of the skin without nodules. This infiltration may be quite inconspicuous except for the alopecia of the eyebrows and eyelashes it produces. Acral, symmetric anesthesia is generally present (145).

A distinctive variant of lepromatous leprosy, the histoid type, first described in 1963 (146), is characterized by the occurrence of well-demarcated cutaneous and subcuta-

neous nodules resembling dermatofibromas. It frequently follows incomplete chemotherapy or acquired drug resistance, leading to bacterial relapse.

Rarely, lepromatous leprosy can present as a single lesion, rather than as multiple lesions (147).

Histopathology. Lepromatous leprosy, in the usual macular or infiltrative nodular lesions, exhibits an extensive cellular infiltrate that is almost invariably separated from the flattened epidermis by a narrow grenz zone of normal collagen (Fig. 21-35 and 21-36). The infiltrate causes the

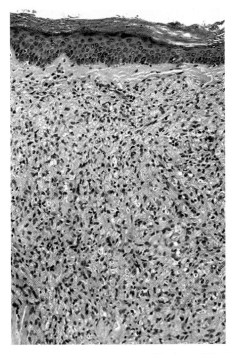

FIGURE 21-35. Lepromatous leprosy. Skin in multibacillary leprosy with a mass of macrophages in the dermis (no granuloma formation), leaving a clear grenz zone under the epidermis (H&E stain).

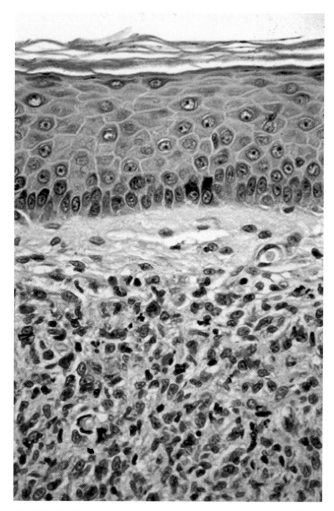

FIGURE 21-36. Lepromatous leprosy. Same case as in Fig. 21.35. Acid-fast bacilli, mostly solid, in large numbers (Wade–Fite stain).

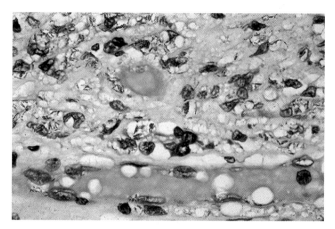

FIGURE 21-37. Lepromatous leprosy. Macrophages and endothelial cells of the capillary contain solid acid-fast bacilli (Wade–Fite stain).

destruction of the cutaneous appendages and extends into the subcutaneous fat. In florid early lesions, the macrophages have abundant eosinophilic cytoplasm and contain a mixed population of solid and fragmented bacilli (BI = 4 or 5) (Fig. 21-33). The bacilli, on Wade–Fite staining, can be seen to measure about 5.0 by 0.5 µm, and if solid may be packed like cigars. Bacilli are commonly observed in endothelial cells also (Fig. 21-37). There is no macrophage activation to form epithelioid cell granulomas. Lymphocyte infiltration is not prominent, but there may be many plasma cells.

In time, and with antimycobacterial chemotherapy, degenerate bacilli accumulate in the macrophages—the so-called lepra cells or Virchow cells—which then have foamy or vacuolated cytoplasm (Fig. 21-38). They resemble xanthoma cells and, on staining with fat stains, are shown to contain lipid—largely neutral fat and phospholipids—rather than cholesterol. The Wade–Fite stain reveals that the bacilli are fragmented or granular and, especially in

very chronic lesions, disposed in large basophilic clumps called globi. In lepromatous leprosy, in contrast to tuberculoid leprosy, the nerves in the skin may contain considerable numbers of leprosy bacilli, but remain well preserved for a long time and slowly become fibrotic.

When lepromatous leprosy is treated, the bacilli die rapidly and become fragmented within weeks or months. However, it can take several years for the bacterial debris to be cleared by host macrophages. The *M. leprae* antigen may persist even longer, and can be demonstrated by immunocytochemical stains (Wade–Fite or silver) even when no bacilli are evident (Fig. 21-39).

The histopathology of Lucio (diffuse) leprosy is similar, but with a characteristic heavy bacillation of the small blood vessels in the skin (145).

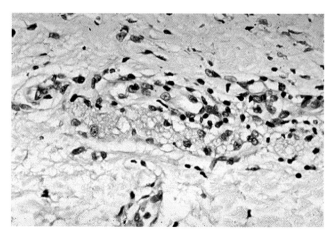

FIGURE 21-38. Lepromatous leprosy. Old treated lesion, with large foamy macrophages and no identifiable bacilli (Wade–Fite stain).

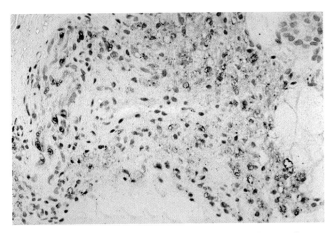

FIGURE 21-39. Lepromatous leprosy. Old treated lesion; foamy macrophages remain, but no acid-fast bacilli visible. However, an antimycobacterial immunocytochemical stain reveals persistent leprosy antigen (anti-BCG stain).

Histoid Leprosy

Histoid leprosy shows the highest loads of bacilli (the BI is frequently 6), and the majority are solid staining, arranged in clumps like sheaves of wheat. The macrophage reaction is unusual in that the cells frequently become spindle-shaped and oriented in a storiform pattern, similar to those of a fibrohistiocytoma (Fig. 21-40). The epidermis may be stretched over such dermal expansile nodules.

Borderline Lepromatous Leprosy

The lesions of borderline lepromatous (BL) leprosy are less numerous and less symmetrical than LL lesions and often display some central dimples.

Histopathology. The important difference between LL and BL leprosy histology is that in BL the lymphocytes are more prominent and there is a tendency for some activa-

tion of macrophages to form poorly to moderately defined granulomas. Perineural fibroblast proliferation, forming an "onion skin" in cross-section, is typical. Foamy cells are not prominent, and globi do not usually accumulate; the BI ranges from 4 to 5.

Midborderline Leprosy

The skin lesions in midborderline (BB) leprosy are irregularly dispersed and shaped erythematous plaques with punched-out centers. There may be small satellite lesions. Edema is prominent in the lesions.

Histopathology. In BB leprosy, the macrophages are uniformly activated to epithelioid cells but are not focalized into distinct granulomas, and lymphocytes are scanty. There are no Langhans giant cells. The BI ranges from 3 to 4. Dermal edema is prominent between the inflammatory cells.

Borderline Tuberculoid Leprosy

Borderline tuberculoid (BT) lesions are asymmetrical and may be scanty. They are dry, hairless plaques with central hypopigmentation. Nerve enlargement is usually found, and the lesions are usually anesthetic.

Histopathology. Granulomas with peripheral lymphocytes follow the neurovascular bundles and infiltrate sweat glands and erector pili muscles. Langhans giant cells are variable in number and are not large in size. Granulomas along the superficial vascular plexus are frequent, but they do not infiltrate up into the epidermis. Nerve erosion and obliteration are typical (Figs. 21-41, 21-42, and 21-43).

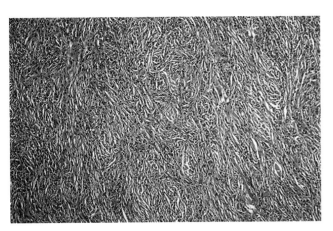

FIGURE 21-40. Lepromatous leprosy. A histoid lesion, with spindle cell proliferation of macrophages, resembling a storiform tumor. The acid-fast bacillus stain showed larger numbers of bacilli (H&E stain).

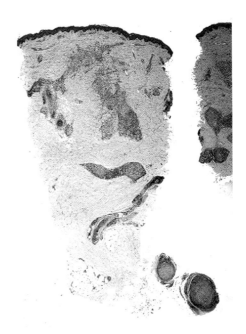

FIGURE 21-41. Tuberculoid leprosy. A typical lesion, showing pandermal perineurovascular granulomas and lymphocytes (H&E stain).

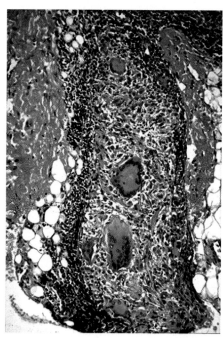

FIGURE 21-42. Tuberculoid leprosy. Granulomatous neuritis; dense lymphocytosis surrounding and eroding into the deep dermal nerve, with giant cells (H&E stain).

Acid-fast bacilli are scanty (BI ranges from 0 to 2) and are most readily found in the Schwann cells of nerves. Immunocytochemical staining for S-100 protein often demonstrates the perineural and intraneural granuloma well (Fig. 21-44).

Tuberculoid Leprosy

The skin lesions of tuberculoid (TT) leprosy are scanty, dry, erythematous, hypopigmented papules, or plaques with sharply defined edges. Anesthesia is prominent (ex-

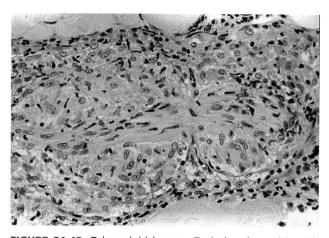

FIGURE 21-43. Tuberculoid leprosy. Typical endoneuritis with granulomas eroding into the nerve (H&E stain).

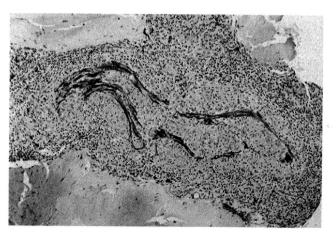

FIGURE 21-44. Tuberculoid leprosy. Granulomatous neuritis; granulomas within the dermal nerve disrupting the Schwann cells and axons (S-100 immunoperoxidase stain).

cept on the face). The number of lesions ranges from one to five. Thickened local peripheral nerves may be found. The lesions heal rapidly on chemotherapy.

Histopathology. Primary TT leprosy has large epithelioid cells arranged in compact granulomas along with neurovascular bundles, with dense peripheral lymphocyte accumulation. Langhans giant cells are typically absent. Dermal nerves may be absent (obliterated) or surrounded and eroded by dense lymphocyte cuffs. Acid-fast bacilli are rarely found, even in nerves. A second pattern of TT leprosy is found in certain reactional states (see below).

Peripheral Nerves

In all these patterns of leprosy, the major peripheral nerves are often undergoing parallel pathologies. The inflammation is similar, and the same classification system is applied. However, the density of acid-fast bacilli is often a logarithm higher than in the nearby skin (148).

Leprosy Reactions

Leprosy reactions are classified into two main types (1 and 2). A third reaction is specific to Lucio multibacillary leprosy (149).

Type 1 Reactions

Because the immunopathologic spectrum of leprosy is a continuum, patients may move along it in both directions. Should such shifts be rapid, they induce an inflammatory reaction with edema that results in enlargement of lesions with more erythema. Shifts toward the tuberculoid pole are called upgrading or reversal reactions; shifts toward the lepromatous pole are termed downgrading reactions. Both are aspects of delayed hypersensitivity, or type 1, leprosy reactions. TT patients are stable. BT patients may downgrade without treatment. Multibacillary patients, particularly those at the BL point, frequently upgrade on chemotherapy, and about one-quarter of them will exhibit significant reactions. BB patients are most unstable and will move either way depending on therapy, often with reactions. The most important aspect of type 1 reactions is not the skin but the condition of the peripheral nerves, in which a similar inflammatory process is going on. Reaction induces increased intraneural inflammation and edema, which is damaging. At worst, there is caseous necrosis of large peripheral nerves resulting from upgrading reactions.

Histopathology. The histopathology of type 1 reactions has still not been well evaluated (150). The distinction between upgrading and downgrading reactions is difficult to make and may require serial examinations. Typically, there is edema within and about the granulomas, and proliferation of fibrocytes in the dermis. In upgrading reactions, the granuloma becomes more epithelioid and activated, and Langhans giant cells are larger (Fig. 21-45); there may be erosion of granulomas into the lower epidermis, and there may be fibrinoid necrosis within granulomas and even within dermal nerves. In downgrading reactions, necrosis is much less common, and over time the density of bacilli increases. Multibacillary leprosy patients who upgrade on therapy show old foamy macrophages and degenerate bacilli admixed with new epithelioid cell granulomas.

Type 2 Reaction: Erythema Nodosum Leprosum

Erythema nodosum leprosum (ENL) occurs most commonly in LL leprosy and less frequently in borderline lepromatous (BL) leprosy. It may be observed not only in patients under treatment but also in untreated patients. Clinically, the reaction has a greater resemblance to erythema multiforme than to erythema nodosum. On the

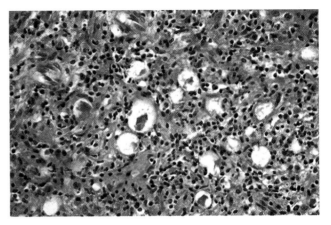

FIGURE 21-46. Leprosy, erythema nodosum leprosum (erythema nodosum leprosum, type 2 reaction). Macrophages with vacuoles and globi, and a polymorphonuclear cell infiltrate (H&E stain).

skin one observes tender, red plaques and nodules together with areas of erythema and occasionally also purpura and vesicles. Ulceration, however, is rare. The eruption is widespread and is accompanied by fever, malaise, arthralgia, and leukocytosis. New lesions appear for only a few days in some cases but for weeks and even years in others. This is the only type of reactional leprosy that responds to treatment with thalidomide.

Histopathology. In erythema nodosum leprosum, the lesions are foci of acute inflammation superimposed on chronic multibacillary leprosy (Fig. 21-46). Polymorph neutrophils may be scanty or so abundant as to form a dermal abscess with ulceration (151). Whereas foamy macrophages containing fragmented bacilli are usual, in some patients no bacilli remain and macrophages have a granular pink hue on Wade–Fite staining, indicating mycobacterial debris. An antimycobacterial immunocytochemical stain (e.g., anti-BCG) will indicate abundant antigen. A necrotizing vasculitis affecting arterioles, venules, and capillaries occurs in some cases of ENL; these patients may have superficial ulceration.

Lucio Reaction

The Lucio reaction occurs exclusively in diffuse lepromatous leprosy, in which it is a fairly common complication. It usually occurs in patients who have received either no treatment or inadequate treatment. In contrast to erythema nodosum leprosum, fever, tenderness, and leukocytosis are absent. The lesions consist of barely palpable, hemorrhagic, sharply marginated, irregular plaques. They develop into crusted lesions and, particularly on the legs, into ulcers. There may be repeated attacks or continuous appearance of new lesions for years.

Histopathology. In the Lucio reaction, vascular changes are critical (145). Endothelial proliferation leading to lu-

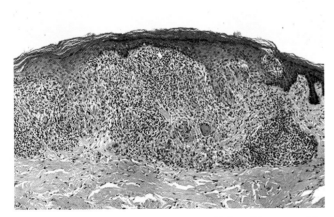

FIGURE 21-45. Leprosy, type 1 reaction (delayed hypersensitivity). Granulomatous erosion of the epidermis; this feature is not usually encountered in nonreacting leprosy (H&E stain).

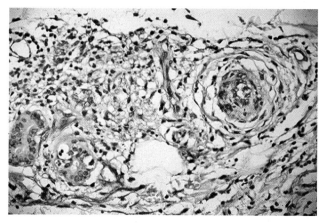

FIGURE 21-47. Leprosy, lucio reaction. Dermal vessels showing endarteritis obliterans and abundant bacilli within endothelial cells (Wade–Fite stain).

minal obliteration is observed in association with thrombosis in the medium-sized vessels of the dermis and subcutis. There is a sparse, largely mononuclear infiltrate. Dense aggregates of acid-fast bacilli are found in the walls and the endothelium of normal-appearing vessels, as well as in vessels with proliferative changes (Fig. 21-47). Ischemic necrosis, brought on by the vascular occlusion, leads to hemorrhagic infarcts and results in crusted erosions or frank ulcers.

Electron Microscopy. Under electron microscopy, *M. leprae* can be seen to consist of an electron-dense cytoplasm lined by a trilaminar plasma membrane. Outside of this membrane lies the bacterial cell wall surrounded by a radiolucent area, the waxy coating typical of mycobacteria (79). Lepra bacilli are found in the skin, predominantly in macrophages and in Schwann cells.

Pathogenesis. With respect to immunologic reactivity, patients with lepromatous leprosy have a defect in cell-mediated immune responses to the lepra bacilli, which therefore cannot be eradicated from the body spontaneously (138,152,153). The primary defect lies in the T-lymphocytes, which can be stimulated only slightly or not at all to react against the lepra bacilli and thus do not adequately activate macrophages to destroy phagocytosed bacilli. This defect is specific for *M. leprae* because patients with lepromatous leprosy show normal immunologic responses to antigens other than lepromin in both *in vivo* and *in vitro* testing.

The specific inability of T-lymphocytes obtained from patients with lepromatous leprosy to react against lepromin is shown by the fact that, when these lymphocytes are incubated with lepromin, they show little or no production of macrophage migration inhibiting factor (MIF). In contrast, the lymphocytes of patients with tuberculoid leprosy produce significant amounts of MIF on exposure to lepromin. One modern view is that in tuberculoid patients,

exposure to leprosy antigens results in a predominant T-helper 1 (Th-1) cytokine secretion profile, which results in macrophage activation. Conversely, in lepromatous patients, the cytokine profile (Th-2) inhibits cell-mediated immunity, and promotes humoral immunity, which does not contribute to host defense (152,154). In reversal reactions, there is an increase in the lymphocyte response to lepromin during the reaction and a decrease during the postreaction phase.

Analysis of T-cell subsets in lesions have shown that in tuberculoid leprosy, with its high degree of resistance to the leprosy bacilli, the T-helper lymphocytes are distributed evenly throughout the epithelioid cell aggregates, and the suppressor T-lymphocytes are restricted to the peripheries of the granulomas. In lepromatous leprosy, both helper and suppressor T-lymphocytes are distributed diffusely throughout the lesions (155,156). It is noteworthy that the distribution of helper and suppressor T cells in tuberculoid leprosy is similar to that observed in sarcoidosis.

In patients with either erythema nodosum leprosum or the Lucio reaction, deposits of IgG and the third component of complement (C3), as well as circulating immune complexes, have been found in the vessel walls of the dermal lesions. This suggests that both reactions are mediated by immune complexes (Gell and Coombes type III reaction) (143).

The lepromin skin test, or Mitsuda test, consists of the intradermal injection of a preparation of *M. leprae* derived from autoclaved infected human tissue. A positive reaction consists of the formation of a nodule measuring 5 mm or more in diameter after 2 to 4 weeks. On histologic examination, the nodule shows an epithelioid cell granuloma. The reaction is positive only in the high-resistance (tuberculoid and borderline tuberculoid) forms of the disease. In indeterminate leprosy, it may be positive or negative. The test reveals the inability of patients at the lepromatous end of the spectrum to react to the injection of *M. leprae* with an epithelioid cell granuloma, and its main value is therefore as a marker of specific cell-mediated immunity to this organism, which varies continuously along the immunopathologic spectrum.

HIV Infection and Leprosy

Because HIV induces a generalized immunosuppressive state, and because a wide range of intracellular infectious agents normally controlled by the T-cell/macrophage system may proliferate to cause significant disease, it was expected that leprosy might also be affected. Specifically, the disease might become more prevalent in HIV and leprosy co-endemic areas, and individual patients might downgrade toward lepromatous disease as their HIV disease progresses. However, epidemiologic studies have shown no effect of HIV infection on the incidence of leprosy in properly controlled studies (157,158) nor has a change in the proportions of tuberculoid versus lepromatous patients been noted (159). At present, the only clinicopathologic difference between HIV-infected and noninfected leprosy patients that is suggested is an increased likelihood of HIV-positive patients undergoing type 1 upgrading reactions (159,160). This rather paradoxical phenomenon awaits further evaluation.

Histopathologic Differential Diagnosis

The leprosy bacillus cannot yet be grown *in vitro*. Tuberculoid (granulomatous) leprosy needs to be distinguished from the many other granulomatous dermatitides. The presence of acid-fast bacilli in nerves is conclusive proof of leprosy, as is the demonstration of an intraneural granuloma. The S-100 stain may highlight this phenomenon (161), although in practice, if the diagnosis is in doubt after investigation with ordinary stains, this immunocytochemical method is not usually diagnostic either. In leprosy, naked granulomas are found only in BB leprosy, and acid-fast bacilli will be found in the lesions. Sarcoidosis may rarely cause granulomas to form within peripheral nerves (162), but does not appear to do so in dermal nerves. The general vertical perineurovascular distribution of granulomatous inflammation and involvement of sweat glands in tuberculoid leprosy are helpful. The presence or absence of plasma cells or of intraepidermal lymphocytes is not helpful. Unlike other mycobacterial skin infections such as tuberculosis, and unlike granulomatous leishmaniasis, the epidermis in tuberculoid leprosy is usually flat and non-hyperplastic. Late secondary and tertiary cutaneous syphilis is characterized by epithelioid and giant cell granulomas in the dermis, not directly involving nerves, and the epithelium is usually hyperplastic. Intragranuloma necrosis (fibrinoid or caseating) occurs in leprosy in type 1 reactions—sometimes spontaneously. This can be confused with necrobiotic lesions such as granuloma annulare. Necrosis within a nerve that is granulomatous is diagnostic of leprosy.

Early, indeterminate leprosy overlaps with many specific and nonspecific dermatitides manifesting perineurovascular lymphocytic infiltrates. Finding bacilli in critical sites (in nerves, under the epidermis, in erector pili muscle, or in macrophages) is critical. In the absence of bacilli and the presence of a pandermal infiltrate, leprosy can only be suspected. Problems may arise from contaminant mycobacteria in staining solutions and in the water baths used for floating out sections. Such organisms are usually above the plane of the section, overlap the cell nuclei, and usually stain darker than *M. leprae*. The use of PCR for identifying paucibacillary leprosy in skin sections and tissues has not been as successful as it once was thought to be (163).

Ultimately, there is a proportion of suspect paucibacillary leprosy lesions for which the histopathologist cannot make a firm diagnosis either way, and intra- and interobserver variation may be considerable (164). Clinical diagnosis of single-lesion leprosy is also imperfect (147).

Lepromatous leprosy infiltrates can resemble xanthoma, although the cytoplasmic granularity is coarser in the latter disease. The presence of acid-fast bacilli is obviously important, and in long-treated lesions that may cause confusion, antimycobacterial immunocytochemistry is helpful. Erythema nodosum leprosum may be overlooked because it is a combined chronic and acute inflammatory infiltrate, but once thought of, the presence of bacilli or antigen is diagnostic. Certain other mycobacterioses in immunosuppressed patients, such as *M. avium-intracellulare*, may produce histoid-like multibacillary lesions (118) (see Figs. 21-23 and 21-24); however, nerves are not involved in this infection.

ANTHRAX

Anthrax, caused by *Bacillus anthracis*, is enzootic in many countries (165). It occurs occasionally among workers in tanneries and wool-scouring mills through the handling of infected hides, wool, or hair imported from Asia. The lesion starts as a papule. The papule enlarges, and a hemorrhagic pustule forms (166). After the pustule has ruptured, a thick, black eschar covers the area. Marked erythema and edema surround the lesion. Characteristically, pain is slight or absent.

Histopathology. At the site of the eschar, the epidermis is destroyed, and the ulcerated surface is covered with necrotic tissue. There is marked edema of the dermis. Vasculitis, hemorrhage, and variable acute and chronic inflammatory infiltrate are observed (Figs. 21-48 and 21-49).

Anthrax bacilli are present in large numbers and can be recognized in sections stained with the Gram stain. The bacillus is large, rod-shaped, encapsulated, Gram-positive, 6 to 10 µm long, and 1 to 2 µm thick. Anthrax bacilli are found particularly in the necrotic tissue toward the surface of the ulcer but also in the dermis (Fig. 21-50). Phagocytosis of the bacilli by either neutrophils or histiocytes is absent.

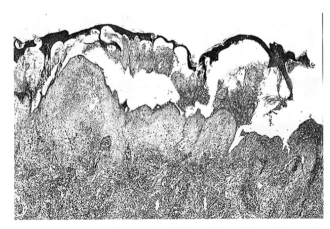

FIGURE 21-48. Anthrax. Acute lesion with epidermal necrosis and pandermal inflammation (H&E stain).

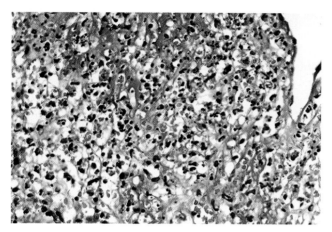

FIGURE 21-49. Anthrax. Acute inflammation and dermal edema (H&E stain).

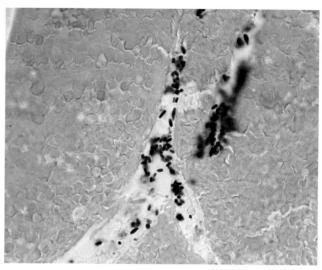

FIGURE 21-51. *Clostridium perfringens* injection abscess. Cluster of wide Gram-positive rods, typical of Clostridium organisms (Gram stain).

Injection Abscesses

The pandemic of injection drug abuse has resulted in numerous patients presenting with dermal and subcutaneous abscesses, having used contaminated syringes and needles. Similar abscesses have also been frequently noted in healthcare settings, where injection solutions may also be contaminated (167). Numerous bacterial and mycobacterial species may be found on culture, including staphylococci and streptococci. A recent epidemic in the United Kingdom involved *Clostridium perfringens* and *Clostridium novyi* infections (168). These infections may progress to necrotizing fasciitis, myositis, bacteriemia, and septic shock with fatalities.

A standard panel of Gram, silver stain (e.g., Grocott) and Ziehl–Neelsen is useful in identifying the organisms, although culture is required for specific diagnosis (Fig. 21-51). The histopathology is not usually specific. Acute inflamma-

tion, edema, and tissue necrosis are usual. In chronic lesions, much granulation tissue, fibrosis, and sinuses develop. In mycobacterial injection lesions, there may also be granulomas.

TULAREMIA

Tularemia is caused by *Francisella tularensis*, a small, Gram-negative, pleomorphic coccobacillus. It is usually acquired by humans through direct contact with rodents, but it may be transmitted from rodents to humans by insects, such as mosquitoes, ticks, or deer flies (169). The disease often occurs in small epidemics. There are two types: ulceroglandular, the more common type, and typhoidal. These types reflect differences in host response. In ulceroglandular tularemia, there is a vigorous inflammatory reaction, pneumonia is less common, and the patient's prognosis is good. In the typhoidal form, there are few localizing signs, pneumonia is more common, and mortality without therapy is much higher.

In the ulceroglandular type, one or several painful ulcers occur as primary lesions at the site of infection, usually on the hands. Tender subcutaneous nodes may form along the lymph vessels that drain the primary lesion or lesions. There is considerable swelling of the regional lymph nodes, and the infection is associated with marked constitutional symptoms. Healing of the lesions takes place in 2 to 5 weeks (170,171).

Histopathology. The primary ulcer shows at its base a nonspecific inflammatory infiltrate associated with a granulomatous reaction. In some cases, only a moderate number of epithelioid cells and a few giant cells are observed

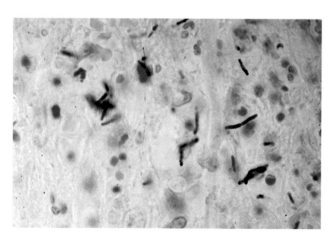

FIGURE 21-50. Anthrax. Numerous Gram-positive thick bacilli within the acute inflammation (Gram).

(170). In others, however, large, well-developed tuberculoid granulomas are apparent. These granulomas may show central necrosis with the presence of nuclear dust. Late lesions may show epithelioid cell tubercles that have no central necrosis and are surrounded by only a slightly inflammatory reaction, and they may thus have an appearance resembling that of sarcoidosis (172).

The tender nodes that may be found along lymph vessels show multiple granulomas deep in the dermis and extending into the subcutaneous tissue. The central zones of necrosis in the granulomas may attain a much greater size than in the primary ulcer. Similarly, the regional lymph nodes show multiple granulomas with centrally located abscess necrosis or caseous necrosis (170,173).

RICKETTSIAL INFECTIONS

These are acquired by tick bites, the natural reservoir being infected animals. Rocky Mountain spotted fever is caused by *Rickettsia rickettsii*, a small, pleomorphic coccobacillus that is an obligate intracellular parasite. Contrary to its name, the disease is encountered most commonly in the Southeast of the United States and has been acquired even within New York City (174,175). Boutonneuse fever (Mediterranean spotted fever) is caused by *Rickettsia conorii*, and is widespread in Africa as well.

In *R. rickettsii* infection, after an incubation period of 1 to 2 weeks, chills and fever develop, and a few days later, a rash appears that begins on the extremities and spreads to the trunk. The lesions at first are macular to papular but become purpuric within 2 to 3 days. There may be only petechiae, but in fatal cases widespread ecchymoses are common. Gangrene may result from small vessel occlusion (176). Because the diagnosis may not be made in the beginning and the course may be rapid, mortality exceeds 10%, despite the effectiveness of antibiotics such as tetracycline and chloramphenicol if given in time. Whenever a diagnosis of Rocky Mountain spotted fever is suspected, a search should be made for an eschar indicating the site of a tick bite. One may find a hemorrhagic crust 8 to 10 mm in diameter surrounded by an erythematous ring. In some severe systemic cases, there are no obvious skin lesions (177,178).

In boutonneuse fever, characteristic "tache noire" eschars develop. The histopathology is similar in both infections (179).

Histopathology. In the advanced lesion there is dermal an epidermal necrosis. The small vessels of the dermis and of the subcutaneous fat exhibit a necrotizing vasculitis with a perivascular infiltrate consisting mostly of lymphocytes and macrophages (Figs. 21-52 and 21-53). There is extravasation of erythrocytes. As a result of injury to the endothelial cells, luminal thrombosis and microinfarcts occur. The causative organism, which measures 0.3 by 1

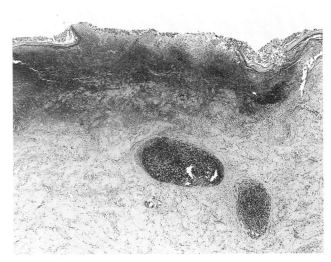

FIGURE 21-52. *Rickettsia conorii* infection. Typical eschar necrosis of superficial dermis and epithelium (H&E stain).

μm, is too small to be visible by light microscopy using ordinary stains. However, rickettsial antigen can be identified in sections of skin lesions by immunocytochemistry (178), and PCR on skin samples is specific. Coccal and bacillary forms are observed in endothelial cells in association with perivascular lymphocytic infiltration. Electron microscopic examination of the tick bite site demonstrates rickettsial organisms within the cytoplasm and the nuclei of endothelial cells. These organisms appear as electron-dense, round or oval structures surrounded by an electron-lucent halo. The entire organism is bounded by a limiting cell wall. The organisms range in size from 0.3 to 0.5 μm in greatest diameter.

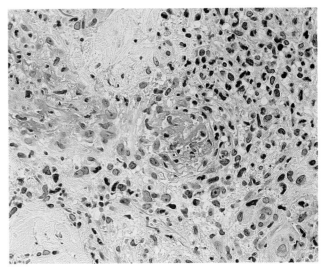

FIGURE 21-53. *Rickettsia conorii* infection. Dermal arteriole with arteritis and fibrin thrombosis (H&E stain).

CHANCROID

Chancroid, caused by *Haemophilus ducreyi*, is a sexually transmitted disease leading to one or several ulcers, chiefly in the genital region (180,181). The ulcers exhibit little if any induration and often have undermined borders. They are usually tender. Inguinal lymphadenitis, either unilateral or bilateral, is common and, unless treated, often results in an inguinal abscess.

Histopathology. The histologic changes observed beneath the ulcer are sufficiently distinct to permit a presumptive diagnosis of chancroid in many instances. The lesion consists of three zones overlying each other and shows characteristic vascular changes (181,182) (Fig. 21-54). The surface zone at the floor of the ulcer is rather narrow and consists of neutrophils, fibrin, erythrocytes, and necrotic tissue. The next zone is fairly wide and contains many newly formed blood vessels showing marked proliferation of their endothelial cells. As a result of the endothelial proliferation, the lumina of the vessels are often occluded, leading to thrombosis. In addition, there are degenerative changes in the walls of the vessels. The deep zone is composed of a dense infiltrate of plasma cells and lymphoid cells.

Demonstration of bacilli in tissue sections stained with Giemsa stain or Gram stain is occasionally possible (Fig. 21-55). The bacilli are most apt to be found between the cells of the surface zone (182). However, in smears of

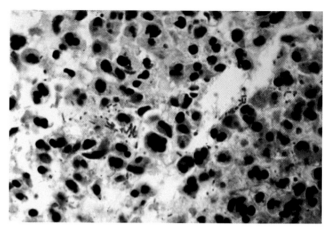

FIGURE 21-55. Chancroid. Bacilli (in the superficial zone) lying in parallel chains (Giemsa stain).

serous exudate obtained from the undermined edge of the ulcer, the bacilli usually can be seen on staining with the Giemsa or Gram stain. *H. ducreyi* is a fine, short, Gram-negative coccobacillus, measuring about 1.5 by 0.2 μm, often arranged in parallel chains. *In situ* hybridization may also specify chancroid organisms (183). Electron microscopy reveals that the bacilli are extracellular, and thus rarely visible in phagosomes of macrophages (184).

The diagnosis of chancroid is confirmed by culture on selective blood-enriched agar (185). Chancroid may clinically resemble donovanosis by showing nontender or only slightly tender, indurated ulcers without undermined margins (186). On the other hand, particularly in the presence of several lesions, herpes simplex has to be excluded, although in herpes simplex the ulcerations usually are not as deep as those in chancroid.

GRANULOMA INGUINALE (DONOVANOSIS)

Granuloma inguinale, also called donovanosis, is a sexually transmitted disease caused by *Calymmatobacterium granulomatis* (187). The organism is a Gram-negative short bacillus, about 2 to 3 μm long, with bipolar staining. The disease is endemic, but relatively uncommon, in the tropics (188).

Granuloma inguinale occurs in the genital or perianal region either as a single lesion or as several lesions (189). The lesions consist of ulcers filled with exuberant granulation tissue that bleeds easily (the characteristic beefy appearance). The borders of the ulcers are elevated and often have serpiginous outlines. Because the lesions spread by peripheral extension, they may attain a large size. In some instances, ulceration leads to mutilation resulting from destruction of tissue (190). In others, excessive granulation tissue causes vegetating lesions. Occasionally, squamous

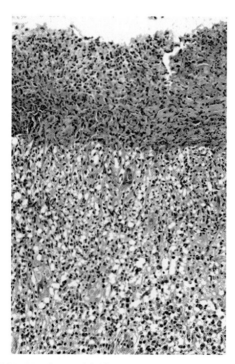

FIGURE 21-54. Chancroid. Three-zone pattern of ulcer and inflammation: superficial necrotic zone, underlying granulation tissue, and deeper fibrosis with plasma cells (H&E stain).

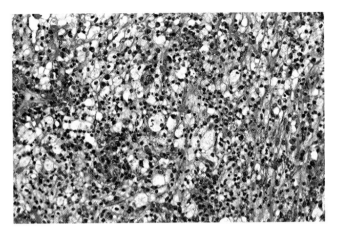

FIGURE 21-56. Donovanosis. Acute inflammation intermixed with foamy macrophages (H&E stain).

cell carcinoma supervenes (191). Local lymphadenopathy occurs through secondary infection of ulcerated skin.

Histopathology. At the edge of the ulcer, the epidermis exhibits acanthosis that may reach the proportions of pseudocarcinomatous hyperplasia. Present in the dermis is a dense infiltrate that is composed predominantly of histiocytes and plasma cells (Fig. 21-56). Scattered throughout this infiltrate are small abscesses composed of neutrophils. The number of lymphoid cells is conspicuously small (192).

The macrophages, which may be large, have a typical vacuolated appearance; these vacuoles contain bacilli and comprise the so-called "Donovan bodies." *C. granulomatis* does not stain with hematoxylin-eosin stains, but is well delineated by the Warthin–Starry method as short bacilli, either singly or in clumps (182,192) (Fig. 21-57). Giemsa stain shows bipolar condensations of stain. Electron microscopy reveals that the bacteria reside in phagosomes (193).

Differential Diagnosis. Overdiagnosis of carcinoma is possible because of epithelial hyperplasia. The inflammatory pattern is similar to that observed in rhinoscleroma.

RHINOSCLEROMA

Rhinoscleroma is a chronic infectious but only mildly contagious disease caused by *Klebsiella rhinoscleromatis*, a Gram-negative bacillus. The nose, pharynx, larynx, trachea, and occasionally also the skin of the upper lip are distorted and infiltrated with hard, granulomatous masses. The disorder always begins in the nose. Although formerly endemic in Central Europe, it is now encountered mainly in Central America and Africa (194–196).

Histopathology. The cellular infiltrate is a chronic granulation tissue with abundant plasma cells and Mikulicz cells. Polymorphs may be present (but they cannot kill the bacteria). Russell bodies (plasma cells with retained globules of immunoglobulins) are frequently observed. The characteristic cell is the Mikulicz cell, a large histiocyte measuring from 10 to 100 μm in diameter (Fig. 21-58). It has a pale, vacuolated cytoplasm. Within the cytoplasm of the Mikulicz cells, one finds many bacilli (Fig. 21-59). They can be seen faintly in sections stained with hematoxylin and eosin but are better visualized with the Giemsa stain or a Warthin–Starry silver stain (197). They are also stained red by the PAS technique. They are Gram-negative rods that measure 2 to 3 μm in length and appear round or ovoid in cross-section. Immunocytochemistry can also be used to confirm rhinoscleroma (195,198).

In long-standing lesions, marked fibrosis is present. The mucosal epithelium overlying the cellular infiltrate often exhibits hyperplasia, which may be so pronounced as to give rise to a mistaken diagnosis of squamous cell carcinoma.

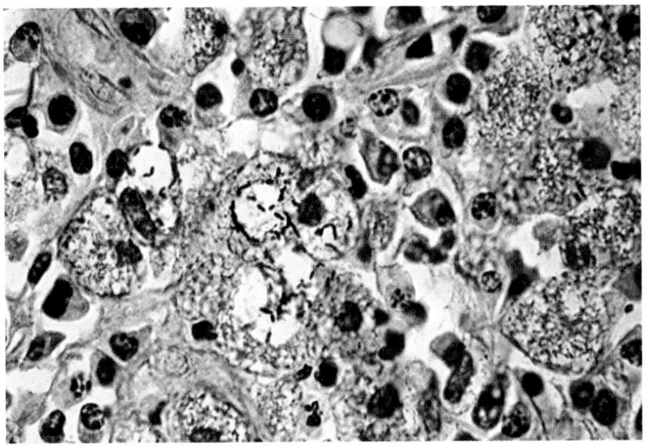

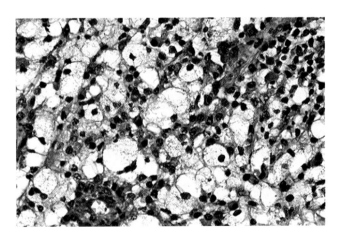

FIGURE 21-57. Donovanosis. Silver-positive bacilli within macrophages (Warthin–Starry stain).

FIGURE 21-58. Rhinoscleroma. Foamy macrophages (Mikulicz cells) and plasma cells; the bacilli are faintly visible within the macrophages (H&E stain).

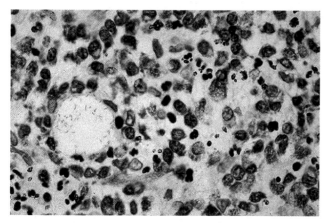

FIGURE 21-59. Rhinoscleroma. Bacilli within the macrophages (Giemsa stain).

Electron microscopy reveals numerous phagosome vacuoles of varying size within the Mikulicz cells. Some vacuoles contain one or a few bacilli up to 4 μm in length. They are surrounded by a characteristic coat of finely granular, filamentous material arranged in a radial fashion. This coating material contains mucopolysaccharides and is responsible for the positive PAS reaction of the bacteria (196).

Differential Diagnosis. The histopathology of rhinoscleroma is essentially similar to that of donovanosis (granuloma inguinale). Foamy, vacuolated macrophages are also observed in many other chronic inflammatory conditions (e.g., leprosy, chronic staphylococcal abscess, mycoses, and leishmaniasis), but special stains and associated clinicopathologic features usually enable their distinction. Plasma cells and Russell bodies, similarly, correlate with chronicity in many diverse infections, such as treponematoses, amoebiasis, leishmaniasis, and tuberculosis.

LYMPHOGRANULOMA VENEREUM

Lymphogranuloma venereum is a sexually transmitted disease caused by *Chlamydiae trachomatis*. *Chlamydiae* are obligate intracellular parasites with a unique biphasic life cycle (199).

The incubation period of lymphogranuloma venereum varies from 3 to 30 days but averages 7 days. The primary lesion is a small erosion or papule 5 to 8 mm in size. This lesion heals within a few days and may pass unnoticed. Within 1 to 2 weeks after the appearance of the primary lesion, enlargement of the inguinal lymph nodes begins. Inguinal lymphadenopathy occurs in most men infected with this disease but in only some women. The involved inguinal lymph nodes at first are firm but subsequently develop multiple areas of suppuration, resulting in draining sinuses. The lymphadenopathy usually subsides within

2 to 3 months. Rarely, elephantiasis of the penis and scrotum or chronic penile ulcerations arise as a late complication (200).

In women in whom the infection begins in the lower portion of the vagina, drainage is to the iliac and anorectal lymph nodes rather than to the inguinal lymph nodes, and may result in proctitis (189). Rectal stricture and perineal ulcerations are fairly common late complications in these women. Lymph stasis may lead to marked vulvar edema, referred to as esthiomene. Proctitis and rectal stricture also occur in homosexual men (201).

Histopathology. The changes in the initial papule are nonspecific. There is ulceration and a nonspecific granulation tissue. In the lymph nodes, stellate abscesses with surrounding epithelioid cells and macrophage giant cells represent the characteristic lesion. A similar pathology is seen in cat-scratch disease nodes. Ordinary histologic stains do not demonstrate the infecting organisms in skin or node. The diagnosis may be confirmed by culture of a skin lesion or lymph node, and serology is useful (202).

Chlamydiae undergo a developmental cycle and, as can be seen by electron microscopy, occur in two forms: elementary body and initial body (199). The elementary body is adapted to an extracellular environment and is infective for other cells. It measures about 0.3 μm in diameter and consists of a round, electron-dense inner body surrounded by an electron-lucid halo and a membrane. After entering a host cell by means of phagocytosis, it develops into a metabolically active initial body 0.5 to 1 μm in diameter. Multiplication takes place by division of the nucleus. This division results in two elementary bodies, which on leaving the host cell can infect other cells.

CAT-SCRATCH DISEASE

Bartonella henselae (previously *Rochalimaea henselae*) causes cat-scratch disease, and the organism is carried in the blood and oral cavities of cats (203). The skin lesion develops 2 to 4 days after a scratch or bite from a cat. It may be macular, papular, or a nodule, usually on the arm or hand. Two to 3 weeks later, a large, tender swelling of a group of lymph nodes develops in the drainage area of the scratch. The cat scratch heals in a normal fashion, but the affected lymph nodes become fluctuant as a result of suppuration. The average duration of lymph node enlargement is 2 months (204,204a,205).

Histopathology. The primary papules at the site of the scratch show one or several acellular areas of necrobiosis in the dermis. These areas are of various shapes, including round, triangular, and stellate. Surrounding them are several layers of histiocytic and epithelioid cells, with the innermost layer exhibiting a palisading arrangement. A few giant cells may be present. The periphery of the epithelioid cell reaction is surrounded by a zone of lymphoid cells.

The reaction in the lymph nodes is similar to that observed in the skin, except that the central areas of necrosis in the epithelioid cell granulomas undergo abscess formation through the accumulation of numerous neutrophils. Macrophage giant cells are also present. As the abscesses enlarge, they become confluent.

The delicate, pleomorphic, Gram-negative bacilli can be demonstrated with the Warthin–Starry silver-impregnation stain peripheral to the necrosis of involved lymph nodes (205) and in the skin at the primary site of inoculation (206). Immunocytochemistry also reveals the bacilli, and serodiagnostic tests are available. For specific identification (see below), PCR techniques and *in vitro* culture may be used (203).

Electron microscopic examination reveals that the bacteria are invariably extracellular and form small clusters. They are 0.8 to 1.5 μm long and 0.3 to 0.5 μm wide, with homogeneous bacterial walls (207).

BACILLARY ANGIOMATOSIS

Bacillary angiomatosis is a new disease, first described in 1983 (208) as a skin or disseminated infection in patients' immunosuppressed by HIV infection. It is also rarely encountered in patients with other immunocompromising conditions and even in immunocompetent people (209). The agents are Gram-negative bacilli: *Bacillus quintana* and *Bacillus henselae* (210). The pathology is similar to that of the late cutaneous stage of bartonellosis, caused by *Bacillus bacilliformis* (211). As with cat-scratch disease, exposure to cats is a major risk factor for acquiring this infection (212).

The skin lesions are reddish or brown papules on any part of the body, usually in large numbers, that resemble Kaposi's sarcoma. They may also present as subcutaneous lumps without skin involvement (213,214).

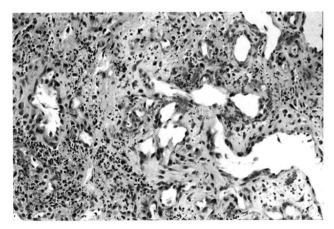

FIGURE 21-60. Bacillary angiomatosis. Dermis shows vascular proliferation, leukocytoclasia and oedema (H&E stain).

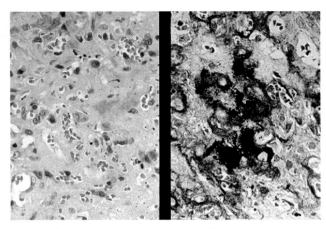

FIGURE 21-61. Bacillary angiomatosis. **Left:** clumps and smudges of basophilic extracellular material, the bacteria (H&E stain). **Right:** the silver-positive bacilli (Warthin–Starry stain).

Histopathology. The epidermis may be flat or hyperplastic. In the dermis there are single or multinodular proliferations of capillaries accompanied by an inflammatory infiltrate that includes variable numbers of neutrophil polymorphs and mononuclear cells, as well as edema. Leukocytoclasia is frequently observed (215). Characteristic of bacillary angiomatosis are extracellular deposits of palely hematoxyphilic granular material (Fig. 21-60). Warthin–Starry staining reveals these deposits to be dense masses of short bacilli (Fig. 21-61). The Grocott–Gomori methenamine silver method also demonstrates the argyrophilic bacilli. These bacilli may also be delineated by modified Gram stains such as the Brown–Hopps stain.

Differential Diagnosis. The major differential diagnoses are Kaposi's sarcoma, pyogenic granuloma, and epithelioid hemangioma (215). The presence of clumps of bacilli is obviously important. The capillary proliferation does not have the organized arborizing quality of that in pyogenic granuloma. Spindle cell proliferation and intracellular hyaline globules as seen in Kaposi's sarcoma are not features of bacillary angiomatosis, and Kaposi's sarcoma does not include polymorphs; however, the two conditions may be difficult to distinguish, and many pathologists have learned about bacillary angiomatosis from being informed that the lesions of "Kaposi's sarcoma" disappeared on treatment with antibiotics. Epithelioid hemangioma has plumper (histiocytoid) endothelial cell proliferation and no acute inflammation.

BOTRYOMYCOSIS

Botryomycosis, despite its name, is not a fungal infection but a chronic suppurative infection of skin (and other organs such as lungs and meninges) in which pyogenic bacteria form granules similar to those seen in mycetoma (216).

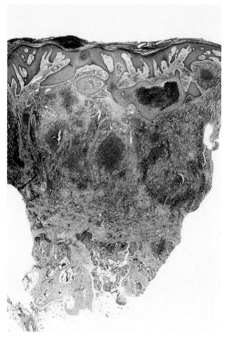

FIGURE 21-62. Botryomycosis. There is pseudoepitheliomatous hyperplasia, and small abscesses in the dermis containing clumps of bacteria (H&E stain).

Although immunosuppressed patients, including those with HIV infection, may acquire botryomycosis (217), most patients have no known immune defect. Occasionally the lesion is associated with another dermatosis such as follicular mucinosis (218).

The skin lesions are local nodules, ulcers, or sinuses communicating with deep abscesses. They occur mainly on the extremities.

Histopathology. The dermal inflammation is predominantly that of neutrophil polymorph abscesses with surrounding granulation tissue and fibrosis (Fig. 21-62).

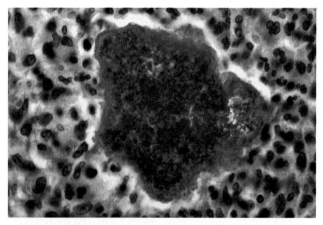

FIGURE 21-63. Botryomycosis. An abscess within which is a basophilic bacterial clump with an eosinophilic surrounding Hoeppli–Splendore reaction (H&E stain, high power).

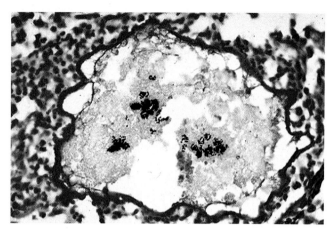

FIGURE 21-64. Botryomycosis. A staphylococcal lesion showing Gram-positive cocci (the majority are degenerate and nonstaining) (Gram stain).

Within the abscesses are granules (grains) shaped like a bunch of grapes, hence the name of the disease (Fig. 21-63). The grains may vary from 20 μm to 2 mm in diameter. They are composed of closely aggregated nonfilamentous bacteria with a peripheral, radial deposition of intensely eosinophilic material—a Hoeppli–Splendore (HS) reaction. The bacteria are usually *S. aureus*, but streptococci and certain Gram-negative bacilli such as *Proteus*, *Pseudomonas*, and *E. coli* are sometimes found. Gram stains delineate these broad categories of infection, although sometimes the organisms in Gram-positive infections are degenerate and lose their Gram-positive staining reaction (Fig. 21-64). The HS reaction material comprises antibody and fibrin.

The overlying epithelium often exhibits pseudoepitheliomatous hyperplasia. Transepithelial elimination of grains may be observed (as with mycetoma) (219).

Pathogenesis. Local implantation of infection may be a factor in some cases, with persistence of a foreign body. Bacteremia is documented in many patients, but in others the lesions appear *de novo*. The characteristic formation of the peribacterial HS reaction probably prevents phagocytosis and intracellular killing of the bacteria, leading to chronicity.

NOCARDIOSIS

Nocardia organisms are Gram-positive, weakly acid-fast, filamentous, branching bacilli that are ubiquitous in the soil. The main species are *Nocardia asteroides*, which is global in distribution, and *Nocardia brasiliensis*, which is found mainly in the Americas (220,221).

N. asteroides is an opportunist agent, and immunocompromised patients, such as those with HIV infection (222,223) and organ transplant recipients, are liable to nocardiosis. Infection of the skin follows direct implantation

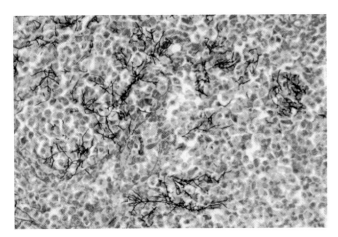

FIGURE 21-65. Nocardiosis. Fine, filamentous branching bacilli of Nocardia asteriodes (Grocott silver stain).

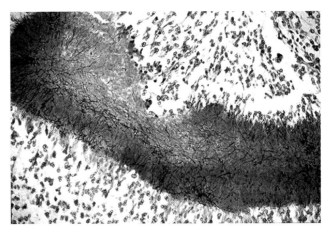

FIGURE 21-66. Actinomycosis. Part of a bacterial colony, with hematoxyphilic filamentous bacteria (H&E stain).

from the environment, hematogenous spread from pulmonary infection, or direct spread through the chest wall from a lung lesion. The skin lesions include erythematous nodules, pustular ulcers, and sinuses. They may be single or multiple.

N. brasiliensis affects immunocompetent as well as immunosuppressed people. The primary and secondary skin lesions are similar to those of *N. asteroides*. Sporotrichosis spread up a limb, with lymphatic involvement, may occur (224). Both species may produce a chronic mycetoma-like lesion with much fibrosis and tissue destruction.

Histopathology. The bacteria induce a mixed acute abscess and granulomatous response in the skin, with fibrosis. Occasionally the bacteria are clumped together with a surrounding Hoeppli–Splendore reaction (see sections on botryomycosis and mycetoma). More often they are more loosely dispersed and resemble *Actinomycosis* spp. Hematoxylin-eosin stains demonstrate the bacilli poorly. They are 1 μm in diameter, filamentous, branching, beaded, Gram-positive, Grocott silver–positive, and usually weakly acid-fast so that a modified Ziehl–Neelsen stain appropriate for leprosy bacilli stains them (Fig. 21-65). This latter feature assists in the distinction of *Nocardia* from *Actinomyces* and related bacilli; specific antisera with immunocytochemistry are also helpful (222), and culture is definitive. The shape of the organisms distinguishes them from mycobacteria. The Grocott silver method is the most sensitive screening stain for nocardiosis.

ACTINOMYCOSIS

Actinomyces israelii is a Gram-positive, branching, filamentous bacterium. It resides as a commensal organism in the oral cavity and tonsillar crypts. The main clinicopathologic manifestations are cervicofacial, thoracic, and intestinal actinomycosis (225). In the first of these, skin lesions result

from extension of suppuration from the oral mucosa through to the facial skin, with sinus formation and discharge of pus and sulfur granules (see below). Thoracic and intestinal infections may produce discharging sinuses onto the skin from infection tracking outward from lung and gut (226). On rare occasions, purely cutaneous actinomycotic infection occurs, and hematogenous dissemination can produce multiple skin sinuses. An infected pilonidal sinus of the penis has been reported (227).

Histopathology. The inflammatory reaction to actinomycotic infection is typically a chronic abscess with polymorphs, surrounding granulation tissue, and fibrosis (228). The organisms are usually tangled together in a matted colony, forming a granule or grain (like botryomycosis and mycetoma). These grains, commonly termed "sulfur granules," may be 20 μm to 4 mm in diameter. The bacilli within are 1-μm diameter filaments that are hematoxyphilic and Gram-positive (Figs. 21-66 and 21-67). They stain with the Grocott silver method. Often only the pe-

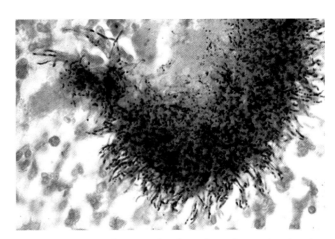

FIGURE 21-67. Actinomycosis. The edge of a grain, showing beaded Gram-positive filaments (Gram stain).

ripheral filaments stain with the Gram method, because of degeneration of the inner bacteria. The peripheral filaments often terminate in a club. A Hoeppli–Splendore reaction may be found peripheral to the bacteria in the grain. The histologic differentiation from nocardiosis is discussed previously.

Further detailed descriptions of these bacterial infections of the skin may be found in Connor and Chandler (229).

REFERENCES

1. Dagan R. Impetigo in childhood: changing epidemiology and new treatments. *Pediatr Ann* 1993;22:235.
2. Kouskoukis CE, Ackerman AB. What histologic finding distinguishes superficial pemphigus and bullous impetigo? *Am J Dermatopathol* 1984;66:179.
3. Peter G, Smith AL. Group A streptococcal infections of the skin and pharynx. *N Engl J Med* 1977;297:311.
4. Levine J, Norden CW. Staphylococcal scalded-skin syndrome in an adult. *N Engl J Med* 1972;287:1339.
5. Reid LH, Weston WL, Humbert JR. Staphylococcal scalded skin syndrome. *Arch Dermatol* 1974;109:239.
6. Elias PM, Levy SW. Bullous impetigo: occurrence of localized scalded skin syndrome in an adult. *Arch Dermatol* 1976;112:856.
7. Ridgway HB, Lowe NJ. Staphylococcal syndrome in an adult with Hodgkin's disease. *Arch Dermatol* 1979;115:589.
8. Diem E, Konrad K, Graninger W. Staphylococcal scalded-skin syndrome in an adult with fatal disseminated staphylococcal sepsis. *Acta Derm Venereol (Stockh)* 1982;62:295.
9. Borchers SL, Gomez EC, Isseroff RR. Generalized staphylococcal scalded skin syndrome in an anephric boy undergoing hemodialysis. *Arch Dermatol* 1984;120:912.
10. Hardwick N, Parry CM, Sharpe GR. Staphylococcal scalded skin syndrome in an adult: influence of immune and renal factors. *Br J Dermatol* 1995;132:468.
11. Elias PM, Fritsch P, Epstein EH Jr. Staphylococcal scalded skin syndrome [review]. *Arch Dermatol* 1977;113:207.
12. Melish ME, Glasgow LA. The staphylococcal scalded-skin syndrome. *N Engl J Med* 1970;282:1114.
13. Ladhani S. Understanding the mechanism of action of the exfoliative toxin of Staphylococcus aureus. *FEMS Immunol Med Microbiol* 2003;39:181–189.
14. Dimond RL, Wolff HH, Braun-Falco O. The staphylococcal scalded skin syndrome. *Br J Dermatol* 1977;96:483.
15. Kelly C, Taplin D, Allen AM. Streptococcal ecthyma. *Arch Dermatol* 1971;103:306.
16. Grosshans E. The red face: erysipelas. *Clin Dermatol* 1993;11:307.
17. Bisno AL, Stevens DL. Streptococcal infections of skin and soft tissues. *N Engl J Med* 1996;334:240.
18. Laupland KB, et al. Invasive group A streptococcal disease in children in association with varicella-zoster virus infection. *Pediatrics* 2000;105:E60
19. Buchanan CS, Haserick JR. Necrotizing fasciitis due to group A beta-hemolytic streptococci. *Arch Dermatol* 1970;101:664.
20. Koehn GS. Necrotizing fasciitis. *Arch Dermatol* 1978;114:581.
21. Hidalgo-Grass C, et al. Effect of a bavterial pheromone peptide on host chemokine degredation in group A streptococcal necrotizing soft-tissue infections. *Lancet* 2004;363:696–703.
22. Stamenkovic I, Lew PD. Early recognition of potentially fatal necrotizing fasciitis: the use of frozen section biopsy. *N Engl J Med* 1984;310:1689.
23. Silverman AR, Nieland ML. Hot tub dermatitis: a familial outbreak of Pseudomonas folliculitis. *J Am Acad Dermatol* 1983;8:153.
24. Fox AB, Hambrick GW JR. Recreationally associated Pseudomonas aeruginosa folliculitis. *Arch Dermatol* 1984;120:1304.
25. Pinkus H. Furuncle. *J Cutan Pathol* 1979;6:517.
26. Kossard S, Collins A, McCrossin J. Necrotizing lymphocytic folliculitis. *J Am Acad Dermatol* 1987;16:1007.
27. Laymon CW, Murphy RJ. The cicatricial alopecias. *J Invest Dermatol* 1947;8:99.
28. Strauss JS, Kligman AM. Pseudofolliculitis of the beard. *Arch Dermatol* 1956;74:533.
29. Hyland CH, Kheir SM. Follicular occlusion disease with elimination of abnormal elastic tissue. *Arch Dermatol* 1980;116:925.
30. Dvorak VC, Root RK, MacGregor RR. Host-defensive mechanisms in hidradenitis suppurative. *Arch Dermatol* 1977;113:450.
31. Brunsting HA. Hidradenitis suppurativa: abscess of the apocrine sweat glands. *Arch Deramatol Syphilol* 1939;39:108.
32. Djawari D, Hornstein OP. Recurrent chronic pyoderma with cellular immunodeficiency. *Dermatologica* 1980;116:116.
33. Su WPD, Duncan SC, Perry HO. Blastomycosis-like pyoderma. *Arch Dermatol* 1979;115:170–173.
34. Williams HM Jr, Stone OJ. Blastomycosis-like pyoderma. *Arch Dermatol* 1966;93:226–228.
35. Brunsting LA, Underwood LJ. Pyoderma vegetans in association with chronic ulcerative colitis. *Arch Deramatol Syphilol* 1949;60:161.
36. Djawari D, Hornstein OP. In vitro studies on microphage functions in chronic pyoderma vegetans. *Arch Dermatol Res* 1978;263:97.
37. Bartter T, Dascal A, Carrol K, et al. Toxic strep syndrome. *Arch Intern Med* 1988;148:1421.
38. Todd J, Fishaut M, Kapral F, et al. Toxic shock syndrome caused by phage group I Staphylococci. *Lancet* 1978;2:1116.
39. Huntley AC, Tanabe JL. Toxic shock syndrome as a complication of dermatologic surgery. *J Am Acad Dermatol* 1987;16:227.
40. Rheingold AL, Hargrett NT, Dan BB, et al. Non-menstrual toxic shock syndrome: a review of 130 cases. *Ann Intern Med* 1992;96:871.
41. Elbaum DJ, Wood C, Abuabara F, et al. Bullae in a patient with toxic shock syndrome. *J Am Acad Dermatol* 1984;10:267.
42. Findley RF, Odom RB. Toxic shock syndrome [review]. *Int J Dermatol* 1982;21:117.
43. Hurwitz RM, Ackerman AB. Cutaneous pathology of the toxic shock syndrome. *Am J Dermatopathol* 1985;7:563.
44. Smith JH, Krull F, Cohen GH, et al. A variant of toxic shock syndrome: clinical, microbiologic, and autopsy findings. *Arch Pathol* 1983;107:351.
45. Stevens DL, Tanner MH, Winship J, et al. Severe group A streptococcal infections associated with a toxic shock-like syndrome and scarlet fever toxin A. *N Engl J Med* 1989;321:1.
46. Dalldorf FG, Jennette JC. Fatal meningococcal septicemia. *Arch Pathol* 1977;101:6.
47. Plaut ME. Staphylococcal septicemia and pustular purpura. *Arch Dermatol* 1969;99:82.
48. Shapiro L, Teisch JA, Brownstein MH. Dermatohistopathology of chronic gonococcal sepsis. *Arch Dermatol* 1973;107:403.
49. Winkelstein A, Songster CL, Caras TS, et al. Fulminant meningococcemia and disseminated intravascular coagulation. *Arch Intern Med* 1969;124:55.
50. Hall JH, Callaway JL, Tindall JP, et al. Pseudomonas aeruginosa in dermatology. *Arch Dermatol* 1968;97:312.

51. Schlossberg D. Multiple erythematous nodules as a manifestation of Pseudomonas aeruginosa septicemia. *Arch Dermatol* 1980; 116:446.

52. Bazel J, Grossman ME. Subcutaneous nodules in pseudomonas sepsis. *Am J Med* 1986;80:528.

53. Huminer D, Siegman-Igra Y, Morduchowicz G, et al. Ecthyma gangrenosum without bacteremia: report of six cases and review of the literature. *Arch Intern Med* 1987;147:299.

54. Mandell JN, Feiner HP, Price NM, et al. Pseudomonas cepacia endocarditis and ecthyma gangrenosum. *Arch Dermatol* 1977; 113:199.

55. Dorff GI, Geimer NF, Rosenthal DR, et al. Pseudomonas septicemia: illustrated evolution of its skin lesion. *Arch Intern Med* 1971;128:591.

56. Wickboldt LG, Sanders CV. Vibrio vulnificus infection: case report and update since 1970. *J Am Acad Dermatol* 1983;9: 243.

57. Tyring SK, Lee PC. Hemorrhagic bullae associated with Vibrio vulnificus septicemia. *Arch Dermatol* 1986;122:818.

58. Ognibene AJ, Ditto MR. Chronic meningococcemia. *Arch Intern Med* 1964;114:29.

59. Nielsen LT. Chronic meningococcemia. *Arch Dermatol* 1970; 102:97.

60. Schoolnik GK, Buchanan TM, Holmes KK, et al. Gonococci causing disseminated gonococcal infection are resistant to the bactericidal action of normal human sera. *J Clin Invest* 1976;58: 163.

61. Shapiro L, Teisch JA, Brownstein MR. Dermatohistopathology of chronic gonococcal sepsis. *Arch Dermatol* 1973;107:403.

62. Björnberg A. Benign gonococcal sepsis. *Acta Derm Venereol (Stockh)* 1970;50:313.

63. Ackerman AB. Hemorrhagic bullae in gonococcemia. *N Engl J Med* 1970;282:793.

64. Ackerman AB, Miller RC, Shapiro L. Gonococcemia and its cutaneous manifestations. *Arch Dermatol* 1965;91:227.

65. Abu-Nassar H, Fred HL, Yow EM. Cutaneous manifestations of gonococcemia. *Arch Intern Med* 1963;112:731.

66. Kahn G, Danielson D. Septic gonococcal dermatitis. *Arch Dermatol* 1969;99:421.

67. Stanton MJ, Maxted W. Malakoplakia: a study of the literature and current concepts of pathogenesis, diagnosis and treatment. *J Urol* 1981;125:139.

68. McClure J. Malakoplakia. *J Pathol* 1983;140:275.

69. Palou J, Torras H, Baradad M, et al. Cutaneous malakoplakia. *Dermatologica* 1988;176:288.

70. Abou NI, Pombejara C, Sagawa A, et al. Malakoplakia: Evidence for monocyte lysosomal abnormality correctable by cholinergic agonist in vitro and in vivo. *N Engl J Med* 1973;297:1413.

71. Sencer O, Sencer H, Uluoglu O, et al. Malakoplakia of the skin. *Arch Pathol* 1979;103:446.

72. Sian CS, McCabe RE, Lattes CG. Malakoplakia of skin and subcutaneous tissue in a renal transplant recipient. *Arch Dermatol* 1981;117:654.

73. Kumar PV, Tabbei SZ. Cutaneous malakoplakia diagnosed by scraping cytology. *Acta Cytol* 1988;32:125.

74. Schwartz DA, Ogden PO, Blumberg HM, et al. Pulmonary malakoplakia in a patient with the acquired immunodeficiency syndrome: differential diagnostic considerations. *Arch Pathol Lab Med* 1990;114:1267.

75. Goodfellow M, Wayne LG. Taxonomy and nomenclature. In: Ratledge C, Stanford J, eds. *The biology of the mycobacteria*. London: Academic Press, 1982:470.

76. Lucas SB. Mycobacteria and the tissues of man. In: Ratledge C, Stanford J, eds. *The biology of the mycobacteria*, vol. 3. London: Academic Press, 1988:107.

77. Beyt BE, Ortbals DW, Santa Cruz DJ, et al. Cutaneous mycobacteriosis: analysis of 34 cases with a new classification of disease. *Medicine (Baltimore)* 1980;60:95.

78. Saxe N. Mycobacterial skin infections. *J Cutan Pathol* 1985;12: 300.

79. Draper P. The anatomy of mycobacteria. In: Ratledge C, Stanford J, eds. *The biology of the mycobacteria*. London: Academic Press, 1982:9.

80. World Health Organization. Global epidemiology of tuberculosis. Available at: www.who.int/mediacentre/factsheets/fs104/en/.

81. Farina MC, Gegundez MI, Pique E, et al. Cutaneous tuberculosis: a clinical, histopathologic, and bacteriologic study. *J Am Acad Dermatol* 1995;33:433.

82. Sehgal VN, Jain MK, Srivastava G. Changing pattern of cutaneous tuberculosis: a prospective study. *Int J Dermatol* 1989; 28: 231.

83. Santa Cruz DJ, Strayer DS. The histopathologic spectrum of the cutaneous mycobacteriosis. *Hum Pathol* 1982;13:485.

84. Kakakhel K, Fritsch P. Cutaneous tuberculosis. *Int J Dermatol* 1989;28:355.

85. Dannenberg AM. Immune mechanisms in the pathogenesis of pulmonary tuberculosis. *Rev Infect Dis* 1989;11:S369.

86. Rook GAW, Bloom BR. Mechanisms of pathogenesis of tuberculosis. In: Bloom BR, ed. *Tuberculosis: pathogenesis, protection and control*. Washington, DC: American Society for Microbiology Press, 1994:485.

87. Helman KM, Muschenheim C. Primary cutaneous tuberculosis resulting from mouth-to-mouth respiration. *N Engl J Med* 1965; 273:1035.

88. Goette DK, Jacobson KW, Doty RD. Primary inoculation tuberculosis of the skin. *Arch Dermatol* 1978;114:567.

89. Kramer F, Sasse SA, Simms JC, Leedom JM. Primary cutaneous tuberculosis after a needle-stick injury from a patient with AIDS and undiagnosed tuberculosis. *Ann Intern Med* 1993;119:594.

90. Horney DA, Gaither JM, Lauer R, et al. Cutaneous inoculation tuberculosis secondary to "jailhouse tattooing." *Arch Dermatol* 1985;121:648.

91. Rietbroek RC, Dahlmans RPM, Smedts F, et al. Tuberculosis cutis miliaris disseminata as a manifestation of miliary tuberculosis: Literature review and report of a case of recurrent skin lesions. *Rev Infect Dis* 1991;13:265.

92. McCray MK, Esterly NB. Cutaneous eruption in congenital tuberculosis. *Arch Dermatol* 1981;117:460.

93. Warin AP, Wilson-Jones E. Cutaneous tuberculosis of the nose with unusual clinical and histologic features leading to a delay in diagnosis. *Clin Exp Dermatol* 1977;2:235.

94. Marcoral J, Servitje O, Moreno A, et al. Lupus vulgaris: clinical, histologic, and bacteriologic study of 10 cases. *J Am Acad Dermatol* 1992;26:404.

95. Haim S, Friedman-Birnbaum R. Cutaneous tuberculosis and malignancy. *Cutis* 1978;21:643.

96. Serfling U, Penneys NS, Loenardi CL. Identification of Mycobacterium tuberculosis DNA in a case of lupus vulgaris. *J Am Acad Dermatol* 1993;28:318.

97. Regan W, Harley W. Orificial and pulmonary tuberculosis. *Australas J Dermatol* 1979;20:88.

98. Penneys NS, Leonardi CL, Cook S, et al. Identification of Mycobacterium tuberculosis DNA in five different types of cutaneous lesions by PCR. *Arch Dermatol* 1993;129:1594.

99. Darier MJ. Des "tuberculides" cutanees. *Arch Dermatol Syph* 1896;7:1431.

100. Morrison JGL, Furie ED. The papulonecrotic tuberculide. *Br J Dermatol* 1974;91:263.

101. Smith NP, Ryan TJ, Sanderson RV, et al. Lichen scrofulosorum: a report of four cases. *Br J Dermatol* 1976;94:319.

102. Breathnach SM, Black MM. Atypical tuberculide (acne scrofulosorum) secondary to tuberculous lymphadenitis. *Clin Exp Dermatol* 1981;6:339.

103. Victor T, Jordaan HF, van Niekerk DJ, et al. Papulonecrotic tuberculid. Identification of Mycobacterium tuberculosis DNA by polymerase chain reaction. *Am J Dermatopathol* 1992;14:491.

104. Jordaan HF, van Niekerk DJ, Louw M. Papulonecrotic tuberculid: a clinical, histopatholological and immunohistochemical study of 15 patients. *Am J Dermatopathol* 1994;16:474.

105. Wilson-Jones E, Winkelmann RK. Papulonecrotic tuberculid: a neglected disease in Western countries. *J Am Acad Dermatol* 1986;14:815.

106. Degitz K, Steidl M, Thomas P, et al. Aetiology of tuberculids. *Lancet* 1993;341:239.

107. Iden DL, Rogers RS, Schroeter AL. Papulonecrotic tuberculid secondary to Mycobacterium bovis. *Arch Dermatol* 1978;114:564.

108. Williams JT, Pulitzer DR, DeVillez RL. Papulonecrotic tuberculid secondary to disseminated Mycobacterium avium complex. *Int J Dermatol* 1994;33:109.

109. Brown BA, Wallace RJ. Infections due to non-tuberculous mycobacteria. In: Mandell GL, Bennett JE, Dolin R, eds. *Principles and practice of infectious diseases*, 5th ed. Edinburgh: Churchill Livingstone, 2000:2630–2636.

110. von Reyn CF, Barber TW, Arbeit RD, et al. Evidence of previous infection with Mycobacterium avium-Mycobacterium intracellulare complex among healthy subjects: an international study of dominant mycobacterial skin test reactions. *J Infect Dis* 1993;168:1553.

111. Inwald D, Nelson M, Cramp M, et al. Cutaneous manifestations of mycobacterial infection in patients with AIDS. *Br J Dermatol* 1994;130:111.

112. Kennedy C, Chin A, Lien RAM, et al. Leprosy and human immunodeficiency virus infection: a closer look at the lesions. *Int J Dermatol* 1990;29:130.

113. Hanke CW, Temofeew RK, Slama SL. Mycobacterium kansasii infection with multiple cutaneous lesions. *J Am Acad Dermatol* 1987;16:1122.

114. Owens DW, McBride ME. Sporotrichoid cutaneous infection with Mycobacterium kansasii. *Arch Dermatol* 1969;100:54.

115. Nightingale SD, Byrd LT, Southern PM, et al. Incidence of Mycobacterium avium-intracellulare complex bacteremia in human immuno-deficiency virus-positive patients. *J Infect Dis* 1992;165:1082.

116. Havlir DV, Ellner JJ. Mycobacterium avium complex. In: Mandell GL, Bennett JE, Dolin R, eds. *Principles and practice of infectious diseases*, 5th ed. Edinburgh: Churchill Livingstone, 2000:2616–2629.

117. Barbaro DJ, Orcutt VL, Coldiron BM. Mycobacterium avium–Mycobacterium intracellulare infection limited to the skin and lymph nodes in patients with AIDS. *Rev Infect Dis* 1989;11:625.

118. Wood C, Nickoloff BJ, Todes-Taylor NR. Pseudotumour resulting from atypical mycobacterial infection: a "histoid" variety of Mycobacterium avium-intracellulare complex infection. *Am J Clin Pathol* 1985;83:524.

119. Cole GW, Gebhard J. Mycobacterium avium infection of the skin resembling lepromatous leprosy. *Br J Dermatol* 1979;101:71.

120. Huminer D, Pitlik SD, Block C, et al. Aquarium-borne Mycobacterium marinum skin infection. *Arch Dermatol* 1986;122:698.

121. Philpott JA, Woodburne AR, Philpott OS, et al. Swimming pool granuloma. *Arch Dermatol* 1963;88:158.

122. Dickey RF. Sprotrichoid mycobacteriosis caused by M marinum (balnei). *Arch Dermatol* 1969;98:385.

123. Debat-Zoguereh D, Bonnet E, Mars ME, et al. Mycobactériose cutanée à Mycobacterium marinum au cours de l'infection par le VIH. *Med Mal Infect* 1993;23:37.

124. Tchornobay AM, Claudy AL, Perrot JL, et al. Fatal disseminated Mycobacterium infection. *Int J Dermatol* 1992;31:286.

125. Travis WD, Travis LB, Roberts GD, et al. The histopathologic spectrum in Mycobacterium marinum infection. *Arch Pathol Lab Med* 1985;109:1109.

126. van der Werf T, Stinear T, Stienstra Y, van der Graaf WTA, Small PL. Mycolactones and Mycobacterium ulcerans disease. *Lancet* 2003;362:1062–1064.

127. Heyman J. Out of Africa: observations on the histopathology of Mycobacterium ulcerans. *J Clin Pathol* 1993;46:5.

128. Marston BJ, Diallo MO, Horsburgh CR, et al. Emergence of Buruli ulcer disease in the Daloa region of Côte d'Ivoire. *Am J Trop Med Hyg* 1995;52:219.

129. Uganda Buruli Group. Clinical features and treatment of pre-ulcerative Buruli lesions: Myucobacterium ulcerans infection. *BMJ* 1970;2:390.

130. Hayman J, McQueen A. The pathology of Mycobacterium ulcerans infection. *Pathology* 1983;17:594.

131. Wallace RJ, Swenson JM, Silcox VA, et al. Spectrum of disease due to rapidly growing mycobacteria. *Rev Infect Dis* 1983;5:657.

132. Murdoch ME, Leigh IM. Spirotrichoid spread of cutaneous Mycobacterium chelonei infection. *Clin Exp Dermatol* 1989;14:309.

133. McGovern J, Bix BC, Webster G. Mycobacterium haemophilium skin disease successfully treated with excision. *J Am Acad Dermatol* 1994;30:269.

134. Rogers PL, Walker RE, Lane HC, et al. Disseminated Mycobacterium haemophilum infection in two patients with the acquired immunodeficiency syndrome. *Am J Med* 1988;84:640.

135. Kristjansson M, Bieluch VM, Byeff PD. Mycobacterium haemophilum infection in immunocompromised patients: case report and review of the literature. *Rev Infect Dis* 1991;13:906.

136. Abramowsky C, Gonzalez B, Sorensen RU. Disseminated BCG infections with primary immunodeficiencies. *Am J Clin Pathol* 1993;100:52.

137. Noordeen SK. Eliminating leprosy as a public health problem. *Int J Lepr* 1995;63:559.

138. Britton WJ, Lockwood DNJ. Leprosy. *Lancet* 2004;363:1209–1219.

139. Ridley DS, Jopling WH. Classification of leprosy according to immunity: a five-group system. *Int J Lepr* 1966;34:255.

140. Ridley DS. Histological classification and the immunological spectrum of leprosy. *Bull World Health Organization* 1974;51:451.

141. Lowy L. Processing of biopsies for leprosy bacilli. *J Med Lab Technol* 1956;13:558.

142. van Brakel WH, de Soldenhoff R, McDougall AC. The allocation of leprosy patients into paucibacillary and multibacillary groups for multidrug therapy, taking into account the number of body areas affected by skin, or skin and nerve lesions. *Lepr Rev* 1992;63:231.

143. Ridley MJ, Ridley DS. The immunopathology of erythema nodosum leprosum: the role of extravascular complexes. *Lepr Rev* 1983;54:95.

144. Job CK. Pathology of leprosy. In: Hastings RC, ed. *Leprosy*. Edinburgh: Churchill Livingstone, 1994:193.

145. Rea TH, Ridley DS. Lucio's pheonomenon: a comparative histological study. *Int J Lepr* 1979;47:161.

146. Wade HW. The histoid variety of lepromatous leprosy. *Int J Lepr* 1963;31:129.

147. Pönnighaus JM. Diagnosis and management of single lesions in leprosy. *Lepr Rev* 1996;67:89.

148. Ridley DS, Ridley MJ. The classification of nerves is modified by delayed recognition of M leprae. *Int J Lepr* 1986;54:596.

149. Ridley DS. *Pathogenesis of leprosy and related diseases*. London: Wright, 1988.

150. Ridley DS, Radia KB. The histological course of reactions in borderline leprosy and their outcome. *Int J Lepr* 1981;49:383.

151. Hussain R, Lucas SB, Kifayet A, et al. Clinical and histological discrepancies in diagnosis of ENL reactions classified by assessment of acute phase proteins SAA and CRP. *Int J Lepr* 1995; 63:222.

152. Ottenhoff THM. Immunology of leprosy: lessons from and for leprosy. *Int J Lepr* 1994;62:108.

153. Choudhuri K. The immunology of leprosy: unravelling an enigma. *Int J Lepr* 1995;63:430.

154. Salgame P, Abrams JS, Clayberger C, et al. Differing lymphokine profiles of functional subsets of human CD4 and CD8 T cell clones. *Science* 1991;254:279.

155. Modlin RL, Hofman FM, Meyer PR, et al. In situ demonstration of T lymphocyte subsets in granulomatous inflammation: leprosy, rhinoscleroma and sarcoidosis. *Clin Exp Immunol* 1983;51:430.

156. Modlin RL, Rea TH. Immunopathology of leprosy. In: Hastings RC, ed. *Leprosy*. Edinburgh: Churchill Livingstone, 1994:225.

157. Orege PA, Fine PEM, Lucas SB, et al. A case control study of human immunodeficiency virus-1 (HIV-1) infection as a risk factor for tuberculosis and leprosy in western Kenya. *Tubercle Lung Dis* 1993;74:377.

158. Pönnighaus JM, Mwanjasi LJ, Fine PEM, et al. Is HIV infection a risk factor for leprosy? *Int J Lepr* 1991;59:221.

159. Lucas SB. HIV and leprosy [Editorial]. *Lepr Rev* 1993;64:97.

160. Blum L, Flageul B, Sow S, et al. Leprosy reversal reaction in HIV-positive patients. *Int J Lepr* 1993;61:214.

161. Fleury RN, Bacchi CE. S-100 protein and immunoperoxidase technique as an aid in the histopathologic diagnosis of leprosy. *Int J Lepr* 1987;55:338.

162. Gainsborough N, Hall SM, Hughes RAC, et al. Sarcoid neuropathy. *J Neurol* 1991;238:177.

163. De Wit MYL, Faber WR, Krieg SR, et al. Application of a polymerase chain reaction for the detection of Mycobacterium leprae in skin tissues. *J Clin Microbiol* 1991;29:906.

164. Fine PEM, Job CK, Lucas SB, et al. The extent, origin and implications of observer variation in the histopathological diagnosis of leprosy. *Int J Lepr* 1993;61:270.

165. Lew D. Bacillus anthracis: anthrax. In: Mandell GL, Bennett JE, Dolin R, eds. *Principles and practice of infectious disease*, 5th ed. Edinburgh: Churchill Livingstone, 2000:2215–2219.

166. Breathnach AF, Turnbull PCB, Eykyn SJ, et al. A labourer with a spot on his chest. *Lancet* 1996;347:96.

167. Rodriguez G, Ortegon M, Camargo D, et al. Iatrogenic Mycobacterium abscessus infection: histopathology of 71 patients. *Br J Dermatol* 1997;137:214–218.

168. Ebright JR, Peiper B. Skin and soft tissue infections in injection drug users. *Infect Dis Clin North Am* 2002;16:697–712.

169. Cross J, Penn RL. Francisella tularensis: tularemia. In: Mandell GL, Bennett JE, Dolin R, eds. *Principles and practice of infectious disease*, 5th ed. Edinburgh: Churchill Livingstone, 2000: 2393–2401.

170. Kodama BF, Fitzpatrick JE, Gentry RH. Tularemia. *Cutis* 1994; 54:279.

171. Myers SA, Sexton DJ. Dermatologic manifestations of arthropod-borne diseases. *Infect Dis Clin North Am* 1994;8:689.

172. Cerny Z. Skin manifestations of tularaemia. *Int J Dermatol* 1994;33:468.

173. von Schroeder HP, McDougall EP. Ulceroglandular and pulmonary tularemia: a case resulting from a cat bite to the hand. *J Hand Surg* 1993;18:132.

174. Salgo MP, Telzak EE, Carrie B, et al. A focus of Rocky Mountain spotted fever within New York City. *N Engl J Med* 1985; 318:1345.

175. Walker DH, Raoult D. Rickettsia rickettsii and other spotted fever group rickettsiae. In: Mandell GL, Bennett JE, Dolin R, eds. *Principles and practice of infectious disease*, 5th ed. Edinburgh: Churchill Livingstone, 2000:2035–2041.

176. Kirkland KB, Marcom P, Sexton DJ, et al. Rocky mountain spotted fever complicated by gangrene: report of six cases and review. *Clin Infect Dis* 1993;16:629.

177. Sexton DJ, Corey GR. Rocky mountain "spotless" and "almost spotless" fever: a wolf in sheep's clothing. *Clin Infect Dis* 1992; 15:439.

178. White WL, Patrick JD, Miller LR. Evaluation of immunoperoxidase techniques to detect Rickettsia rickettsii in fixed tissue sections. *Am J Clin Pathol* 1994;101:747.

179. Dujella J, Morovic M, Dzelalija B, et al. Histopathology and immunopathology of skin biopsy specimens in Mediterranean spotted fever. *Acta Virol* 1991;35:566–572.

180. Morse SA. Chancroid and Haemophilus ducreyi. *Clin Microbiol Rev* 1989;2:137.

181. Hand WL. Haemophilus spp including chancroid. In: Mandell GL, Bennett JE, Dolin R, eds. *Principles and practice of infectious disease*, 5th ed. Edinburgh: Churchill Livingstone, 2000: 2378–2382.

182. Freinkel AL. Histological aspects of sexually transmitted genital lesions. *Histopathology* 1987;11:819.

183. Parsons LM, Shayegani M, Waring AL, et al. DNA probe for the identification of Haemophilus ducreyi. *J Clin Microbiol* 1989;27:1441.

184. Marsch WC, Haas N, Stuttgen G. Ultrastructural detection of Haemophilus ducreyi in biopsies of chancroid. *Arch Dermatol Res* 1978;263:153.

185. Fiumara NJ, Rothman K, Tang S. The diagnosis and treatment of chancroid. *J Am Acad Dermatol* 1986;15:939.

186. Werman BS, Herskowitz LJ, Olansky S, et al. A clinical variant of chancroid resembling granuloma inguinale. *Arch Dermatol* 1983;119:890.

187. Ballard RC. Calymmatobacterium granulomatis. Donovanosis, granuloma inguinale. In: Mandell GL, Bennett JE, Dolin R, eds. *Principles and practice of infectious disease*, 5th ed. Edinburgh: Churchill Livingstone, 2000:2457–2458.

188. Sehgal VN, Shyam Prasad AL. Donovanosis: current concepts. *Int J Dermatol* 1986;25:8.

189. Lucas SB. Tropical pathology of the female genital tract and ovaries. In: Fox H, ed. *Haines and Taylor obstetrical and gynaecological pathology*, 5th ed. Edinburgh: Churchill Livingstone, 2003:1133–1156.

190. Spagnolo DV, Coburn PR, Cream JJ, et al. Extragenital granuloma inguinale (donovanosis) diagnosed in the United Kingdom: a clinical, histological, and electron microscopical study. *J Clin Pathol* 1984;37:945.

191. McKay CR, Binch WI. Carcinoma of the vulva following granuloma inguinale. *Am J Syph* 1952;36:511.

192. Hirsch BC, Johnson WC. Pathology of granulomatous disease: mixed inflammatory granulomas. *Int J Dermatol* 1984;23:585.

193. Davis CM, Collins C. Granuloma inguinale: an ultrastructural study of Calymmatobacterium granulomatis. *J Invest Dermatol* 1969;53:315.

194. Okoth-Olende CA, Bjerregaard B. Scleroma in Africa: a review of cases from Kenya. *East Afr Med J* 1990;67:231.

195. Meyer PR, Shum TK, Becker TS, et al. Scleroma (rhinoscleroma): a histologic immunohistochemical study with bacteriologic correlates. *Arch Pathol Lab Med* 1983;107:377.

196. Shum TK, Whitaker CW, Meyer PR. Clinical update on rhinoscleroma. *Laryngoscope* 1982;92:1149.

197. Hoffman E, Loose LD, Harkin JC. The Mikulicz cell in rhinoscleroma. *Am J Pathol* 1973;73:47.

198. Gumprecht TF, Nichols PW, Meyer PR. Identification of rhinoscleroma by immunoperoxidase technique. *Laryngoscope* 1983; 93:627.

199. Jones RE, Batteiger BE. Chlamydia trachomatis. In: Mandell GL, Bennett JE, Dolin R, eds. *Principles and practice of infectious diseases*, 5th ed. Edinburgh: Churchill Livingstone, 2000: 1989–2003.

200. Hopsu-Havu VK, Sonck CE. Infiltrative, ulcerative and fistular lesions of the penis due to lymphogranuloma venereum. *Br J Vener Dis* 1973;49:193.

201. Bolan RK, Sands M, Schachter J, et al. Lymphogranuloma venereum and acute ulcerative proctitis. *Am J Med* 1982;72:703.

202. Barnes RC. Laboratory diagnosis of human chlamydial infections. *Clin Microbiol Rev* 1989;2:119.

203. Clarridge JE, Raich TJ, Pirwani D, et al. Strategy to detect and identify Bartonella species in routine clinical laboratory yields Bartonella henselae from HIV-positive patients and unique Bartonella strain from his cat. *J Clin Microbiol* 1995;33:2107.

204. Carithers HA. Cat scratch disease: an overview based on a study of 1,200 patients. *Am J Dis Child* 1985;139:1124.

204a. Lucas SB. Cat scratch disease [Editorial]. *J Pathol* 1991;163:93.

205. Wear DJ, Margileth AM, Hadfield TL, et al. Cat scratch disease: a bacterial infection. *Science* 1983;221:1403.

206. Margileth AM. Dermatologic manifestations and update of cat scratch disease. *Pediatr Dermatol* 1988;5:1.

207. Kudo E, Sakaki A, Sumitomo M, et al. An epidemiological and ultrastructural study of lymphadenitis caused by Warthin–Starry positive bacteria. *Virchows Arch [A]* 1988;412:563.

208. Stoler MH, Bonfiglio TA, Steigbigel RT, et al. An atypical subcutaneous infection associated with AIDS. *Am J Clin Pathol* 1983;80:714.

209. Milde P, Brunner M, Borchard F, et al. Cutaneous bacillary angiomatosis in a patient with chronic lymphocytic leukaemia. *Arch Dermatol* 1995;131:933.

210. Chian CA, Arrese JE, Peirrard GE. Skin manifestations of Bartonella infections. *Int J Dermatol* 2002;41:461–466.

211. Cottell SL, Noskin GA. Bacillary angiomatosis: clinical and histologic features, diagnosis and treatment. *Arch Intern Med* 1994;154:524.

212. Tappero JW, Mohle-Boetani J, Koehler JE, et al. The epidemiology of bacillary angiomatosis and bacillary peliosis. *JAMA* 1993;269:770.

213. Cockerell CJ. The clinico-pathologic spectrum of bacillary (epithelioid) angiomatosis. In: Rotterdam H, Racz P, Greco MA, et al, eds. *Progress in AIDS pathology*, vol. 2. New York: Field & Wood, 1990:111.

214. Schinella RA, Greco MA. Bacillary angiomatosis presenting as a soft-tissue tumour without skin involvement. *Hum Pathol* 1990;21:567.

215. LeBoit PE, Berger TG, Egbert BM, et al. Bacillary angiomatosis: the histopathology and differential diagnosis of a pseudoneoplastic infection in patients with HIV disease. *Am J Surg Pathol* 1989;13:909.

216. Hacker P. Botryomycosis. *Int J Dermatol* 1983;22:455.

217. Toth IR, Kazal HL. Botryomycosis in acquired immunodeficiency syndrome. *Arch Pathol Lab Med* 1987;111:246.

218. Harman RR, English MP, Halford M, et al. Botryomycosis: a complication of extensive follicular mucinosis. *Br J Dermatol* 1980;102:215.

219. Goette DK. Transepithelial elimination in botryomycosis. *Int J Dermatol* 1981;20:198.

220. Curry WA. Human nocardiosis: a clinical review with selected case reports. *Arch Intern Med* 1980;140:818.

221. Berd D. Nocardia brasiliensis infection in the United States: a report of nine cases and a review of the literature. *Am J Clin Pathol* 1973;59:254.

222. Lucas SB, Hounnou A, Peacock CS, et al. Nocardiosis in HIV-positive patients: an autopsy study in West Africa. *Tubercle Lung Dis* 1994;75:301.

223. Uttamchandari RB, Daikos GL, Reyes RR, et al. Nocardiosis in 30 patients with advanced human immunodeficiency virus infection: clinical features and outcome. *Clin Infect Dis* 1994;18: 348.

224. Tsuboi R, Takamori K, Ogawa H, et al. Lymphocutaneous nocardiosis caused by Nocardia asteriodes: case report and review of the literature. *Arch Dermatol* 1986;122:1183.

225. Russo TA. Agents of actinomycosis. In: Mandell GL, Bennett JE, Dolin R, eds. *Principles and practice of infectious diseases*, 5th ed. Edinburgh: Churchill Livingstone, 2000:2645–2654.

226. Brown JR. Human actinomycosis: a study of 181 subjects. *Hum Pathol* 1973;4:319.

227. Rashid AM, Williams RM, Parry D, Malone PR. Actinomycosis associated with a pilonidal sinus of the penis. *J Urol* 1992; 148:405.

228. Behberhani MJ, Heeley JD, Jordan HV. Comparative histopathology of lesions produced by Actinomyces israelii, A. naeslundii, and A. viscosus in mice. *Am J Pathol* 1983;110:267.

229. Connor DH, Chandler FW, eds. Bacterial infections, vol. 1, part 111 of *Pathology of infectious diseases*. Stamford, CT: Appleton & Lange, 1996.

TREPONEMAL DISEASES

A. NEIL CROWSON
CYNTHIA MAGRO
MARTIN MIHM JR.

The venereal and nonvenereal treponemal diseases are caused by motile bacteria of the family *Spirochaetaceae*, which also includes the genera *Borrelia* and *Leptospira*. Accurate recognition of spirochetal infection requires correlation of a given patient's travel and medical history to a detailed knowledge of the clinical and histologic expression of each pathogen. The pathogenic treponemes resemble each other in dark-field and biopsy preparations, being coiled, silver-staining organisms 6 to 20 μm by 0.10 to 0.18 μm, and have a high degree of DNA sequence homology (1,2). A single genetic difference in the 5' and 3' flanking regions of the 15-kDa lipoprotein gene tpp15 was described for venereal and nonvenereal treponematoses in one study (3), evidence that suggests that these organisms evolved from a common ancestor to cause different diseases (4). Size and sequence heterogeneity is demonstrated by other treponeme genes such as those controlling expression of the tprK antigen, a target of opsonizing antibodies that is important to host immune protection, variance in which may play a role in evasion of the host response (5). The nonvenereal treponematoses include yaws, pinta, and endemic syphilis.

VENEREAL SYPHILIS

Acquired syphilis, caused by *Treponema pallidum*, has afflicted humanity since at least the 15th century (6). Although it was a major cause of morbidity and mortality in the early 20th century, public health programs and the advent of penicillin so reduced its incidence in First World countries that many physicians became unfamiliar with its signs and symptoms (1). The incidence of acquired syphilis is increasing; in 1990, the incidence was 20 per 100,000 in the United States and 360 per 100,000 in parts of Africa, in part reflecting the epidemic of human immunodeficiency virus infection, with which acquired syphilis is linked epidemiologically and with which co-infection is common (7). *T. pallidum* is generally spread through contact between in-

fectious lesions and disrupted epithelium at sites of minor trauma incurred during sexual intercourse. The transmission rate is between 10% and 60%.

Primary syphilis is defined by a skin lesion, or chancre, in which organisms are identified; it typically arises 21 days after exposure at the inoculation site, and is classically a painless, brown-red, indurated, round papule, nodule, or plaque 1 to 2 cm in diameter. Lesions may be multiple or ulcerative, and the regional lymph nodes may be enlarged.

Secondary syphilis results from the hematogenous dissemination of organisms, yielding widespread clinical signs accompanied by constitutional symptoms inclusive of fever, malaise, and generalized lymphadenopathy. A generalized eruption occurs, comprising of brown-red macules and papules, papulosquamous lesions resembling guttate psoriasis, and, rarely, pustules (8). Lesions may be follicular-based, annular, or serpiginous, particularly in recurrent attacks of secondary syphilis. Other skin signs include alopecia and condylomata lata, the latter comprising broad, raised, gray, confluent papular lesions arising in anogenital areas, pitted hyperkeratotic palmoplantar papules termed "syphilis cornée," and, in rare severe cases, ulcerating lesions that define "lues maligna." Some patients develop shallow, painless ulcers in the mucosae.

Meningovascular syphilis is usually seen in tertiary syphilis after 7 to 12 years of disease (9), but can occur in the secondary stage and be symptomatic; usually, it manifests as basilar meningitis and can be associated with cranial nerve palsies (10). Acute transverse myelitis (11), glomerulonephritis, and self-limited hepatitis are other uncommon manifestations.

Primary- and secondary-stage lesions may resolve without therapy or go unnoticed by the patient, who then passes into a latent phase. The latter may be subdivided into early and late stages, an arbitrary distinction that may help to guide the therapeutic approach. The Center for Disease Control bases its distinction of the early (infectious) latent stage from the late (noninfectious) latent stage on whether the duration of the infection is less or more than 1 year, respectively. The World Health Organization uses a 2-year period to make this distinction. After a variable latent period, the patient enters the *tertiary stage*.

Tertiary syphilis comprises gummatous skin and mucosal lesions ("benign tertiary syphilis"), cardiovascular manifestations, and neurologic manifestations. The skin lesions may be solitary or multiple, and can be divided into superficial nodular and deep gummatous types. The nodular type has a smooth, atrophic center with a raised, serpiginous border. The gummatous lesions present as subcutaneous swellings that ulcerate (12).

Congenital syphilis, on the rise since the mid-1980s (13), is a diagnosis rendered when organisms are identified in dark-field, immunofluorescent, or conventionally stained tissues or smears of lesional skin, placenta, or umbilical cord (14). A presumptive case is an infant born to a mother with inadequately treated syphilis at the time of delivery, or when an infant or child with a reactive treponemal test for syphilis exhibits evidence of congenital syphilis by virtue of physical or long-bone radiologic examination, a reactive cerebrospinal fluid (CSF) VDRL, an elevated CSF protein or white blood cell count of unknown cause, or quantitative treponemal titers four times higher than the mother's at the time of birth (14). Clinical signs include rhinitis, chancres, or a maculopapular desquamative rash (13). Transplacental infection occurs in more than 50% of infants born to mothers with primary or secondary syphilis, roughly 40% of those born to mothers in the early latent stage, and only 10% of those born to mothers with late latent infections (14).

Histopathology of Syphilis. The two fundamental pathologic changes in syphilis are (a) swelling and proliferation of endothelial cells; and (b) a perivascular infiltrate of lymphoid cells and often of plasma cells. In late secondary and tertiary syphilis, there are also granulomatous infiltrates comprising epithelioid histiocytes and giant cells. Newborns with congenital syphilis have shown at autopsy multiorgan involvement by an angioinvasive CD68+ mononuclear cell infiltrate that imparts an "onion-skin" morphology to involved vessels with numerous demonstrable spirochetes (15).

Primary Syphilis

The epidermis at the periphery of the syphilitic chancre reveals changes comparable to those observed in lesions of secondary syphilis, namely, acanthosis, spongiosis, and exocytosis of lymphocytes and neutrophils. Toward the center, the epidermis becomes thinned, edematous, and permeated by inflammatory cells. In the center, the epidermis may be absent. The papillary dermis is edematous. A dense perivascular and interstitial lymphohistiocytic and plasmacellular infiltrate spans the entire thickness of the dermis (Fig. 22-1); the lymphocytes are principally of T-helper

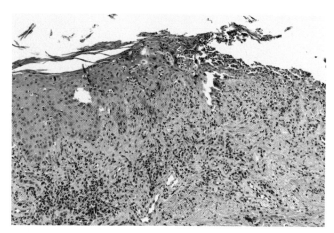

FIGURE 22-1. Primary syphilitic chancre. The epithelium is eroded and the corium contains a dense plasma-cell-rich infiltrate. There is neovascularization with secondary necrotizing vasculitic changes manifested by mural fibrin deposition.

phenotype. Neutrophils are often admixed. Endarteritis obliterans characterized by endothelial swelling and mural edema is observed (Fig. 22-2).

By silver staining with the Levaditi stain or the Warthin–Starry stain and by immunofluorescent techniques, spirochetes are usually identified along the dermal–epidermal junction and within and around blood vessels. If seen in their full length, which is rare, spirochetes generally show 8 to 12 spiral convolutions, each measuring from 1 to 1.2 μm in length (Fig. 22-3). It should be remembered that silver also stains melanin and reticulum fibers. Differentiation may cause some difficulties, but should be possible based on the fact that the melanin in the dendritic processes of melanocytes has a granular appearance, the granules being thicker and more heavily stained than *T. pallidum* (16). Reticulin fibers, although wavy, do not exhibit a spiral ap-

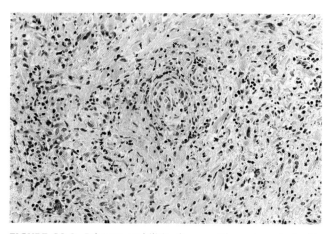

FIGURE 22-2. Primary syphilitic chancre. There is endarteritis obliterans manifested by endothelial cell swelling, endothelial hyperplasia, and expansion of vessel walls by edema and a lymphohistiocytic infiltrate with resultant lumenal attenuation. A diffuse extravascular plasma-cell-rich infiltrate is present.

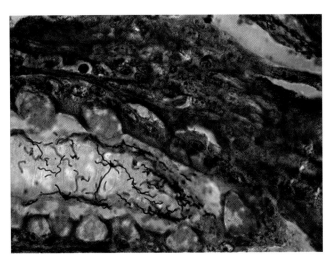

FIGURE 22-3. Treponeme morphology. A silver stain reveals numerous elongate coiled spirochetes ranging in length from 8 to 12 μm.

pearance. Correlation with serology is always prudent in our opinion.

Histologic examination of enlarged regional lymph nodes in primary syphilis most commonly reveals a chronic inflammatory infiltrate containing many plasma cells with endothelial hyperplasia and follicular hyperplasia. Spirochetes are numerous and can nearly always be identified with the Warthin–Starry stain. In some cases, non-necrotizing granulomas resembling those of sarcoidosis are found in the lymph nodes (17).

Histogenesis. T. pallidum can be demonstrated by histochemistry or by immunohistochemistry. The latter comprises immunofluorescent methods in frozen (18) or fresh specimens and immunoperoxidase methods employable in fixed tissues (19). By electron microscopy, the organism can be seen in both intra- and extra-cellular dispositions in the epidermis and dermis (20), within keratinocyte nuclei (21), fibroblasts (21,22), nerve fibers (23), blood vessel endothelia, and the lumina of lymphatic channels (21). Phagocytic vacuoles of macrophages and neutrophils may contain organisms (24), as may the cytoplasms of plasma cells. Ultrastructurally, the organism is 8 to 16 μm in length with regular spirals, a wavelength of 0.9 μm, with an amplitude of 0.2 μm, and a cytoplasmic body 0.13 μm in diameter with tapering ends, all enveloped by a 7-nm trilaminar cytoplasmic membrane (25). The organisms attach to host cells by means of acorn-shaped nosepieces. The contractile motility of the spirochete is mediated by three or four axial filaments that course the length of the cytoplasmic body (26). A paraplastic membrane surrounds these axial filaments in young organisms, but is replaced by an electron-dense amorphous substance produced by the host cell as an immunologic response in older spirochetes (23).

Differential Diagnosis. Lesions of chancroid are the most difficult to differentiate clinically from a syphilitic chancre. The characteristic histopathology of chancroid is one of dense lymphohistiocytic infiltrates with a paucity of plasma cells and a granulomatous vasculitis. An epidermal reaction pattern similar to the syphilitic chancre is observed, namely, psoriasiform epidermal hyperplasia and spongiform pustulation. A Giemsa or Alcian blue stain reveals coccobacillary forms between keratinocytes and along the dermal–epidermal junction. The infiltrate is composed mainly of T-helper lymphocytes and histiocytes including Langerhans cells (27).

Secondary Syphilis

There is considerable histologic overlap among the various clinical forms of secondary syphilis, such as the macular, papular, and papulosquamous types (28,29). Nevertheless, epidermal changes are least pronounced in the macular type and most pronounced in papulosquamous lesions.

Biopsies generally reveal psoriasiform hyperplasia, often with spongiosis and basilar vacuolar alteration, and often with edema of the papillary dermis (Fig. 22-4). Exocytosis of lymphocytes, spongiform pustulation, and parakeratosis also may be observed (16,28). The parakeratosis may be patchy or broad, with or without intracorneal neutrophilic abscesses. Although lesions may mimic psoriasis, attenuation of the suprapapillary plate is uncommon. Scattered necrotic keratinocytes may be observed. Ulceration is not a feature of macular, papular, or papulosquamous lesions of secondary syphilis. The dermal changes include marked papillary dermal edema and a perivascular and/or periadnexal infiltrate that may be lymphocyte predominant, lymphohistiocytic, histiocytic predominant, or frankly granulomatous, and that is of greatest intensity in the papillary

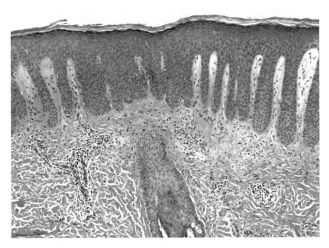

FIGURE 22-4. Secondary syphilis. There is striking psoriasiform hyperplasia of an epidermis surmounted by an orthohyperkeratotic and parakeratotic scale, and prominent papillary dermal edema.

dermis and extends as loose perivascular aggregates into the reticular dermis. Obscuration of the superficial vasculature and lichenoid morphology is observed in some cases, and a cell-poor infiltrate is seen in others. In a few cases, when the infiltrate is heavy, atypical nuclei may be present and may then suggest the possibility of mycosis fungoides (30) or non-Hodgkin's lymphoma. Neutrophils may permeate the eccrine coil to produce a neutrophilic eccrine hidradenitis or manifest as a neutrophil-imbued scale-crust (16) (Fig. 22-5). Granulomatous inflammation is almost invariable in lesions of more than 4 months duration (29), and may be present in some cases of early syphilis (31). A plasma cell component is inconspicuous or absent in 25% of the cases (28) (Fig. 22-6). Eosinophils are not usually observed. Vascular changes such as endothelial swelling and mural edema accompany the angiocentric infiltrates in half of the cases (28). Necrotizing vascular injury is distinctly unusual. A silver stain is recommended in all cases that are suspected of being secondary syphilis; it shows spirochetes in about a third of the cases of secondary syphilis, mainly within the epidermis and less commonly around the blood vessels of the superficial plexus. In some instances, the silver stain is positive even when dark-field examination of the patient's lesions is negative (16). By the immunofluorescent technique, all cases are positive. Phenotypic analysis of the infiltrate reveals a lymphoid populace composed mainly of T cells with an equal proportion of cytotoxic and T-helper cells.

There are several histologic variants of secondary syphilis—namely, condylomata lata, syphilitic alopecia, pustular lesions (Fig. 22-5), syphilis cornée, and lues maligna. Lesions of condylomata lata show all of the aforementioned changes observed in macular, papular, and papulosquamous lesions, but more florid epithelial hyper-

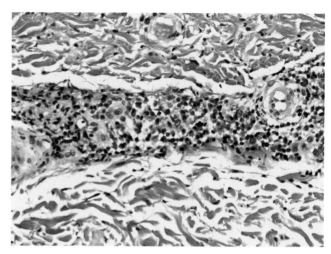

FIGURE 22-6. Secondary syphilis. A dense, lymphocytic and often plasma cell-rich infiltrate surrounds the cutaneous vessels of the dermis.

plasia and intraepithelial microabscess formation are observed (16,32). A Warthin–Starry stain shows numerous treponemes (23).

Biopsies of syphilitic alopecia may demonstrate a superficial and deep perivascular and perifollicular lymphocytic and plasmacellular infiltrate that permeates the outer root sheath epithelium with a concomitant perifollicular fibrosing reaction (16). An involutional tendency characterized by increased numbers of telogen hairs is observed. A concomitant necrotizing pustular follicular reaction may also be seen (8).

An unusual variant of secondary syphilis is lues maligna (33,34), an ulcerative form characterized by severe thrombotic endarteritis obliterans involving vessels at the dermal-subcutaneous junction with resultant ischemic necrosis. A concomitant dense plasmacellular infiltrate with a variable admixture of histiocytes may be observed. Defective cell–mediated immunity may play an integral role in the pathogenesis of lues maligna, particularly in cases where vascular alterations are minimal (35,36). Several cases of lues maligna arising in the setting of HIV disease have been described with involvement of the oral cavity as the principal manifestation. A case of secondary syphilis resembling bullous pemphigoid by both light microscopy and immunofluorescent studies has been described (37).

Syphilis cornée/keratoderma punctatum associated with secondary syphilis manifests an epidermal invagination containing a horny plug composed of laminated layers of parakeratotic cells with loss of the granular cell layer and thinning of the stratum spinosum (38). A moderately dense perivascular plasmacellular infiltrate with concomitant capillary wall thickening involves the cutaneous vasculature.

In the rare pustular lesions of secondary syphilis, a necrotizing pustular follicular reaction accompanied by noncaseating granulomata and a perivascular lympho-

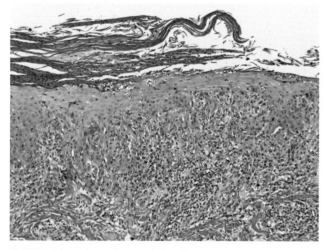

FIGURE 22-5. Secondary syphilis. There is psoriasiform epidermal hyperplasia with basilar vacuolopathy and a lymphocytic interface dermatitis. The epidermis is surmounted by a parakeratotic scale rich in neutrophils. Plasma cells may be inconspicuous, as in this example.

plasmacellular infiltrate typically characterizes the histopathology (8). A pustular psoriasiform process with an absent granular cell layer and a strikingly thickened cornified layer laced with neutrophils may be seen (Fig. 22-5); if the clinical correlate is rugose or elephantine skin thickening, the designation *rupial syphilis* may be applied (8).

In addition to small, sarcoidal granulomata in papular lesions of early secondary syphilis, late secondary syphilis may show extensive lymphoplasmacellular and histiocytic infiltrates resembling nodular tertiary syphilis (39). Conversely, lesions of early tertiary syphilis may lack granulomata (40).

Although often nonspecific, the hepatitis of secondary syphilis may produce a granulomatous or cholestatic morphology on liver biopsy; hepatic necrosis and spirochetes may also be observed (41). The nephrosis or glomerulonephritis of secondary syphilis shows proliferative changes in the glomeruli (42).

Histogenesis. The renal changes in secondary syphilis relate to immune complexes containing treponemal antigen. Not only has direct immunofluorescence shown granular deposits of immunoglobulin and complement along the glomerular basement membrane (42,43), but indirect immunofluorescence antibody studies employing rabbit treponemal antibody and sheep antirabbit globulin conjugate have demonstrated treponemal antigen in the glomerular deposits (42).

Differential Diagnosis. The differential diagnosis of lesions of secondary syphilis includes other causes of lichenoid dermatitis including lichen planus, a lichenoid hypersensitivity reaction, pityriasis lichenoides and connective tissue disease, sarcoidosis, psoriasis, and psoriasiform drug eruptions (16). Prominent spongiosis, suprabasilar dyskeratosis, a mid and deep perivascular component, and the presence of plasma cells are not histologic features of lichen planus or psoriasis. Although a mid-dermal perivascular infiltrate, keratinocyte necrosis, and prominent lymphocytic exocytosis are present in pityriasis lichenoides, the infiltrate is purely mononuclear in nature and neither of spongiform pustulation nor plasmacellular infiltration is observed (44). Although lichenoid hypersensitivity reactions and psoriasiform drug reactions may also demonstrate a perivascular infiltrate of plasma cells, tissue eosinophilia is typically observed as well.

Tertiary Syphilis

Tertiary syphilis is categorized into nodular tertiary syphilis confined to the skin; benign gummatous syphilis principally affecting skin, bone, and liver; cardiovascular syphilis; syphilitic hepatic cirrhosis; and neurosyphilis. In the first variant, the granulomas are small and may be absent in rare cases (40). The granulomatous process is limited to the dermis, with scattered islands of epithelioid cells admixed with

a few multinucleated giant cells, lymphocytes and plasma cells. As a rule, necrosis is not conspicuous. The vessels may show endothelial swelling (36).

In benign gummatous syphilis, the main pathology, irrespective of the organ involved, is one of granulomatous inflammation with central zones of acellular necrosis. In cutaneous lesions, the blood vessels throughout the dermis and subcutaneous fat exhibit endarteritis obliterans along with angiocentric plasmacellular infiltrates of variable density. The skin lesions involve the subcutaneous fat as well as the dermis (45).

In cardiovascular syphilis, elastic tissue fragmentation and reduplication with neovascularization and fibrosis of main arteries occurs. Neurosyphilis includes an asymptomatic form—meningovascular syphilis—and parenchymatous syphilis, which is divided into generalized paresis of the insane and tabes dorsalis (46). In meningovascular syphilis, an inflammatory endarteritis involves the leptomeningeal vessels. In generalized paresis of the insane, gliosis with ventricular dilatation is observed; spirochetes are identified in the cortex in 50% of the cases. In tabes dorsalis, there is demyelinization of the posterior columns of the spinal cord, atrophy of the posterior spinal roots, and lymphoplasmacellular leptomeningitis (9,46).

NONVENEREAL TREPONEMATOSES

Yaws (Frambesia Tropica)

Yaws is caused by *T. pallidum*, subspecies *pertenue*, which is indistinguishable microscopically from *T. pallidum* subspecies *pallidum*, but has been shown to be distinctive by virtue of the substitution of a single nucleotide coding for a 19-kD polypeptide demonstrable by Southern blot analysis (47). Other molecular methodologies confirm distinctive DNA sequences (2,4). Yaws is spread by casual contact between first- or second-degree lesions and abraded skin, and is most prevalent in warm, moist, tropical climates; 95% of the studied population in one province of Ecuador proved seropositive in one series (48). Children are particularly afflicted (49). Sites of involvement include buttocks, legs, and feet. Unlike syphilis, yaws does not manifest transplacental spread to neonates (4).

Primary Yaws

The initial primary stage lesion, or "mother yaw," begins as an erythematous papule roughly 21 days postinoculation, which enlarges peripherally to form a 1- to 5-cm nodule surrounded by satellite pustules covered by an amber crust. A red, crusted appearance prompted German physicians to lend the appellation "frambesia" to the disease. Lesions may heal as pitted, hypopigmented scars. Fever, arthralgia, and lymphadenopathy may coexist.

Secondary Yaws

Similar constitutional symptoms weeks to months later may herald progression to the secondary stage, characterized by involvement of any or all of skin, bones, joints, and cerebrospinal fluid. *Skin lesions* resemble the "mother yaw" but tend to be smaller and more numerous, hence the designation "daughter yaws." Periorificial lesions may mimic venereal syphilis. A circinate appearance ("tinea yaws") may be observed, as may a morbilliform eruption and/or condylomatous vegetations involving the axillae and groin. Macular, hyperkeratotic, and papillomatous lesions may be present on palmoplantar surfaces, and may cause the patient to walk with a painful, crab-like gait ("crab yaws"). Papillomatous nail-fold lesions may give rise to "piannic onychia." Relapsing cutaneous disease occurs up to 5 years later, tending to involve periorificial and periaxillary sites. A lifelong noninfectious latent state may then eventuate. *Bone lesions* consist of painful, sometimes palpable periosteal thickening of arms and legs, occasionally accompanied by soft tissue swellings around the involved small bones of the hands and feet.

Tertiary Yaws

Roughly 10% of cases progress to *tertiary yaws*, the skin manifestations of which comprise subcutaneous abscesses, ulcers that may coalesce to form serpiginous tracts, keloids, keratoderma, and palmoplantar hyperkeratosis. The bone and joint lesions of this stage include osteomyelitis, hypertrophic or gummatous periostitis, and chronic tibial osteitis, which may lead to "saber shin" deformities. Bilateral hypertrophy of the nasal processes of the maxilla produces the rare but characteristic "goundou," which obstructs the nasal passages and, if not treated with early antibiotic therapy, may require surgery. Another otorhinolaryngologic complication is "gangosa," characterized by nasal septal or palatal perforation. Although neurologic and ophthalmologic involvement is not a universally accepted phenomenon, reports of macular atrophy and culture-positive aqueous humor suggest that yaws may exhibit neurophthalmologic manifestations similar to those of venereal syphilis. A less virulent form of the disease, observed in lower-prevalence areas, is termed "attenuated yaws," the cutaneous manifestations of which comprise greasy gray lesions in the skin folds.

Histopathology. *Primary lesions* show acanthosis, papillomatosis, spongiosis, and neutrophilic exocytosis with intraepidermal microabscess formation. A heavy, diffuse, dermal infiltrate of plasma cells, lymphocytes, histiocytes, and granulocytes is observed; unlike syphilis, blood vessels manifest little or no endothelial proliferation (50,51) (Figs. 22-7 and 22-8). The *secondary lesions* show the same histologic appearance, resembling condylomata lata in their epidermal changes, but differing by virtue of the dermal infiltrate being in a diffuse, as opposed to a perivascular, disposition. The ulcerative lesions of *tertiary yaws* greatly resemble those

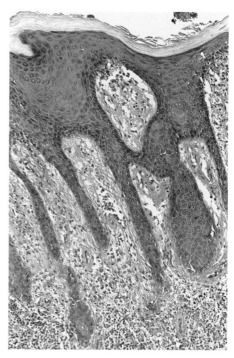

FIGURE 22-7. Yaws, the primary lesion. The biopsy shows a psoriasiform hyperplasia of the epidermis, accompanied by slight spongiosis and an intense lymphohistiocytic and plasmacellular infiltrate in the subjacent corium.

observed in late syphilis in histologic appearance (51). The spirochetes can be demonstrated in primary and secondary lesions by dark-field examination. Silver stains demonstrate numerous organisms between keratinocytes. Unlike *T. pallidum*, which is found in both epidermis and dermis, *T. pertenue* is almost entirely epidermotropic (51).

Differential Diagnosis. The distinction between yaws and syphilis is based on clinical features. Although the location of the organism in a skin biopsy may be helpful, no

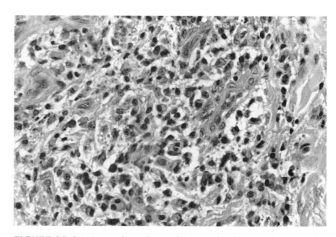

FIGURE 22-8. Yaws, the primary lesion. The biopsy shows an intense angiocentric lymphohistiocytic and plasmacellular infiltrate without the characteristic endarteritis obliterans vascular alterations observed in syphilis.

histologic feature or laboratory test absolutely distinguishes the two diseases (52).

Pinta

Unique among the treponematoses, pinta, caused by *T. carateum*, demonstrates only skin manifestations (53). The disorder is endemic to Central America and restricted to the Western Hemisphere. It affects no age group preferentially, and is the mildest of the treponematoses, with hypopigmentation being the only significant sequel. The incidence of pinta is declining precipitously for reasons unknown. Transmission appears to be from lesion to skin, classically between family members; the ritualistic whipping of diseased adults and unaffected youths is the putative mode of transmission in one aboriginal tribe in the Amazon basin (53).

The *primary lesion* is characterized by an erythematous papule surrounded by a halo, and occurs 1 to 8 weeks postinoculation. By direct extension or through fusion of satellite lesions, the primary site may grow to a diameter of 12 cm, forming an ill-defined erythematous plaque on the legs or other exposed sites. In infants, the primary lesion classically occurs at the sites where the baby was most closely held to the affected mother. The *secondary lesions*, or "pintids," manifest months after inoculation as small, erythematous, scaly papules that coalesce to form psoriasiform plaques. Both primary and secondary lesions are highly infectious. In the tertiary stage, hypopigmented macules are present over bony prominences such as wrists, ankles, and elbows. Symmetrical areas of achromia, alternating with areas of normal or hyperpigmented skin, may result in a mottled appearance. Atrophy and/or hyperkeratosis may be present. An attenuated variant is not described.

Histopathology. Primary and secondary lesions show a similar morphology—namely, acanthosis with spongiosis and a sparse dermal infiltrate of lymphocytes, plasma cells, and neutrophils disposed about dilated blood vessels (54). Endothelial swelling in the dermal vasculature is inconspicuous (55). Lichenoid inflammation may be present, accompanied by hyperkeratosis, hypergranulosis, basal layer vacuolopathy, and pigmentary incontinence. Increased numbers of Langerhans cells are present in the epidermis (56). Lesions of the *tertiary stage* are hyperpigmented, characterized by large numbers of melanophages within the dermis, or depigmented, manifesting complete absence of epidermal melanin. Both lesions show epidermal atrophy and perivascular lymphocytic infiltrates. Organisms are present in all but late, long-standing lesions.

Histogenesis. Electron microscopy reveals absent melanocytes in depigmented lesions of tertiary or late pinta (56).

Endemic Syphilis (Bejel)

Unlike yaws, endemic syphilis, caused by *T. pallidum* subspecies *endemicum*, is largely confined to the arid climates of the Arabian Peninsula and the southern border of the Sahara Desert (53), whose seminomadic populations term the disease "bejel." Children 2 to 15 years of age constitute the principal reservoir. Infection occurs by skin-to-skin contact or by means of fomites such as communal pipes or drinking vessels.

Primary stage skin lesions are rare and are characterized by erythematous papules or ulcers of the oropharyngeal mucosa or the skin of the nipple of an uninfected mother nursing an infected infant.

More commonly, the initial manifestation is the *secondary stage* lesions, characteristically multiple, shallow, rather painless ulcers involving lips, buccal mucosa, tongue, fauces, or tonsils. Such lesions may be accompanied by hoarseness due to treponemal laryngitis and/or regional lymphadenopathy. Condylomata lata involving the axillae and anogenital regions are also observed. Rarely, the secondary stage manifests as erythematous, crusted papules, macules, or an annular papulosquamous eruption, which may be accompanied by generalized lymphadenopathy or periostitis.

The *tertiary stage* comprises gummatous lesions of nasopharynx, larynx, skin, and bone, which may progress to ulcers that heal as depigmented, sometimes geographic scars with peripheral hyperpigmentation. Bone and joint involvement may manifest as tibial periostitis, which mimics that of yaws, or as mutilating lesions involving the nasal septum and palate. Ophthalmologic involvement comprises uveitis, chorioretinitis, choroiditis, and optic atrophy; *T. pallidum* has been cultured from intraocular fluid.

Histopathology. Although the pathology of early lesions of endemic syphilis is not well characterized, late lesions are said to show parakeratosis, acanthosis, spongiosis, pigmentary incontinence, and a dermal lymphohistiocytic and plasma cell infiltrate.

Lyme Disease

Background

First described in patients from Lyme, Connecticut in 1975 (57), Lyme disease is a systemic spirochetosis caused by *Borrelia burgdorferi* and transmitted by the soft ticks of the species *Ornithodoros* (58). The disease in the index cases manifested as inflammatory arthritis and central nervous system and cardiac symptoms (59) preceded by cutaneous erythema.

Although the tick *Ixodes dammini* is the prototypic vector (58,60), other species of ticks from the genus *Ixodes* can also be infected—namely, *I. ricinus* (61), *I. pacificus,* and *I. scapularis* (62,63). Lyme disease is the most common tick-borne disease in the United States (64), and has been reported in 43 states and elsewhere in North America, and in Europe, Africa, and Asia (62). Infection by multiple different bacterial species transmitted by the same infected tick may occur. Co-infection of ticks and humans by *Ehrlichia chaffeensis*, the etiologic agent of human granulocytic ehrlichiosis, and by *B. burgdorferi* is demonstrable in areas where the two diseases are endemic (65–69). Babesiosis is another tick-borne infection that can be co-expressed with Lyme disease (67,70).

There are three phases of Lyme disease. In stage I disease, hematogenous dissemination from lesions of erythema chronicum migrans to other organs may occur, the effects of which are usually self-limited (71) and include orchitis, splenomegaly, lymphadenopathy, and mild pneumonitis. The two main systems involved in stage II are neural and cardiac (71). The triad of meningitis, cranial neuritis, and radiculoneuritis is characteristic for neural involvement; Lyme cerebritis may also occur. Cardiac involvement manifests mainly as tachycardia and heart blocks, the basis of which is epi- and trans-myocarditis. A biopsy of myocardium may show interstitial lymphoplasmacellular infiltrates, with a band-like endocardial disposition said to be characteristic. A non-neutrophilic myocardial vasculitis has been described. Chronic disease at organ sites where spirochetes persist, most commonly the skin and nervous system in Europe and the musculoskeletal system in North America, constitutes stage III. Lyme arthritis and synovitis are characterized by a migratory oligoarthritis that usually involves the knee joint, with the shoulder, wrist, temporomandibular, and ankle joints involved in some cases.

Erythema Chronicum Migrans

First described by Arvid Afzelius in 1909 (62), erythema chronicum migrans is the distinctive cutaneous manifestation of stage I Lyme disease in both Europe and America, and represents the site of primary tick inoculation. Patients may not be aware of the often painless tick bite. The lesion starts as an area of scaly erythema or a distinct red papule within 3 to 30 days after the tick bite, before spreading centrifugally with central clearing after a few weeks, occasionally reaching a diameter of 25 centimeters (72). The clinical presentation may be atypical by virtue of purpuric, vesicular, or linear lesions. Average lesional duration is 10 weeks in the European variant and 4 weeks in the American variant; in some cases, lesions persist for as long as 12 months. Females are affected more frequently in the European variant than in the American variant. The lesions may be solitary or multiple, the latter reflecting hematogenous dissemination of the spirochete, which may be accompanied by fever, fatigue, headaches, cough, and arthralgias (58).

Histopathology. An intense superficial and deep angiocentric, neurotropic, and eccrinotropic infiltrate predominated by lymphocytes with a variable admixture of plasma cells and eosinophils is the principal histopathology (Fig. 22-9). Plasma cells have been identified most frequently in the peripheries of lesions of erythema chronicum migrans, whereas eosinophils are identified in the centers of the lesions (73). Not infrequently, these florid dermal alterations are accompanied by eczematous epithelial alterations, and some cases exhibit edema of blood vessels with transmural migration of

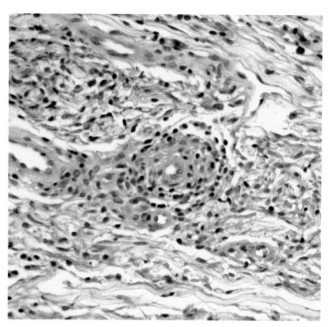

FIGURE 22-9. Erythema chronicum migrans. The central nidus at the inoculation site demonstrates a necrotizing granulomatous vasculitis, whereas the periphery is predominated by an angiocentric lymphohistiocytic vasculopathy, shown here.

lymphocytes, histiocytes and plasma cells (Fig. 22-9), granulomatous neuritis or vasculitis with luminal thrombosis (unpublished data), and interstitial infiltration of the reticular dermis with a concomitant incipient sclerosing reaction. A Warthin–Starry stain may be positive; one study demonstrated spirochetes by this technique in 41% of the cases, with approximately one to two spirochetes, measuring 10 to 25 μm by 0.2 to 0.3 μm per section (73). Spirochetes have been identified primarily from the advancing border of the lesion. Most patients have elevated IgM antibody titers (71).

Differential Diagnosis. The differential diagnosis includes other causes of delayed hypersensitivity where potential antigenic stimuli include other forms of arthropod assaults, drugs, and contactants. A similar distribution of the dermal infiltrate is observed in connective tissue disease; however, tissue eosinophilia along with concomitant eczematous changes are not features of the latter. Differentiation from erythema annulare centrifugum may be impossible.

Dermal Atrophying and Sclerosing Lesions as Manifestations of Lyme Disease (Acrodermatitis Chronica Atrophicans)

First described in 1883 in Germany and subsequently named by Herxheimer in 1902 (74), acrodermatitis chronica atrophicans usually begins as a diffuse or localized erythema on one extremity with the underlying dermis having a doughy consistency. After several months, the lesions become atrophic. The skin is frequently so thin that vessels and subcutaneous tissue can be easily visualized (74). Appendageal structures disappear, resulting in hair loss and decreased sweat and sebum production. The lesions are located mainly on the upper and lower extremities, frequently around joints, and spare the palms, soles, face, and trunk (75). Sclerosis may predominate in late-stage lesions and take several distinct forms—namely, pseudosclerodermatous plaques over the dorsa of the feet; dense, fibrotic linear bands over ulnar and tibial areas; or localized fibromas overlying joint surfaces (74). Antibodies against *B. burgdorferi* are present in 100% of cases. Patients frequently have an elevated erythrocyte sedimentation rate and hypergammaglobulinemia. Either at the peripheries of lesions or distant from them, anetoderma, lymphocytoma, and morphea have also been described (75).

Histopathology. Within a few months to a year, the epidermis appears atrophic with loss of the rete ridges. There is granular layer diminution, and the epidermis is surmounted by a hyperkeratotic scale. In one study, a sparse interface dermatitis characterized by lymphocyte tagging along the dermal–epidermal junction, as well as basal layer cytolysis, was seen in 41% of cases (76) (Fig. 22-10), resulting in variable postinflammatory pigmentary alterations ranging from leukoderma to hyperpigmentation (74). The papillary dermis appears edematous, with a grenz zone of collagen fibers oriented parallel to the epidermis (77) ranging from a few strands to a wide zone (78), with subsequent eosinophilic homogenization (77). A band-like lymphocytic infiltrate is found in the mid- and upper dermis, and in some cases may produce a lichenoid morphology, obscuring the dermal–epidermal junction. Occasionally it extends throughout the cutis and subcutis (76,77). The infiltrate is predominantly in an angiocentric, eccri-

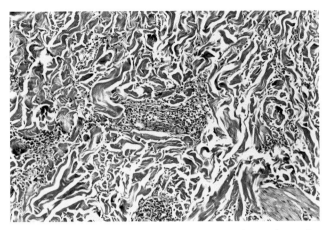

FIGURE 22-11. *Borrelia burgdorferi*–associated morphea. The dermis exhibits a sclerodermoid tissue reaction characterized by widened hypereosinophilic collagen fibers with loss of the normal fibrillar architecture and an interstitial lymphohistiocytic infiltrate in close apposition to the altered collagen fibers. Special stains reveal spirochetal forms amid the inflammatory infiltrate.

notropic, and folliculotropic disposition, and comprises mainly lymphocytes and histiocytes (77). Eosinophils, neutrophils, and plasma cells form a minor cell populace (77). The vessels amid the superficial infiltrate appear destroyed (76). Within the infiltrate, there is piecemeal fragmentation of collagen, and elastic tissue is lacking. Beneath the infiltrate, disorganization and destruction of the collagen, along with hyperplasia, fragmentation, and basophilia of the elastic fibers (76) are observed. An end-stage lesion exhibits a characteristic constellation of epidermal atrophy, large dilated dermal vessels, and an attenuated dermis composed of damaged and degenerated collagen and elastic fibers with lipoid phanerosis (77). The collagen may appear homogenized and hypereosinophilic (77) (Fig. 22-11). There is ultimately marked atrophy of adnexae with periadnexal fibrosis.

Histogenesis. Acrodermatitis chronica atrophicans is mainly a stage III (late) cutaneous manifestation of the European variant of Lyme disease; the major vector is *I. ricinus* (74) and hence the distribution of the lesion is worldwide, with middle Europe being the epicenter (74). Most North American cases occur in European immigrants; *I. ricinus* is not an inhabitant of North America (74). Immunophenotyping reveals that most of the lymphocytes are of T-cell phenotype and that the elastic fibers express HLA-DR (76), suggesting a role for cell-mediated immunity in lesional development.

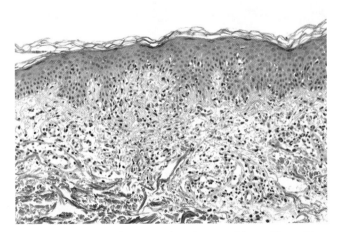

FIGURE 22-10. Acrodermatitis chronica atrophicans. The epidermis shows basketweave orthokeratosis with a sparse interface dermatitis with lymphocyte tagging along the dermal-epidermal junction. The papillary dermis is edematous and the reticular dermal collagen fibers exhibit an orientation parallel to the epidermis. A concomitant interstitial lymphohistiocytic infiltrate is found in intimate apposition to the attenuated collagen fibers. This is an incipient or evolving lesion; atrophy will follow with loss of the retiform pattern.

Other Atrophying and Sclerosing Disorders Associated with Lyme Disease

Atrophoderma of Pasini and Pierini, facial hemiatrophy of Perry–Romberg, lichen sclerosus et atrophicus, eosinophilic fasciitis, and morphea (Fig. 22-11) are among the atrophying and sclerosing disorders of connective tissue that have been associated with *B. burgdorferi* infection based on the positive serology for *B. burgdorferi* in patients with these conditions, the isolation of spirochetal organisms in cultures of the respective skin lesions, and/or their identification in histologic sections (62,63,78,79). In addition, acrodermatitis chronica atrophicans and morphea may coexist in the same patient. A possible etiologic basis of the sclerosis in all five entities—either as the inciting event (in morphea and eosinophilic fasciitis) or as an end-stage phenomenon (in atrophoderma, facial hemiatrophy, and lichen sclerosus)—may relate to increased production of interleukin I mediated by the *B. burgdorferi* spirochete resulting in enhanced fibroblast production (77). Only progressive facial hemiatrophy will be considered further, because all the conditions are covered elsewhere in this volume (Chapter 10).

Facial hemiatrophy is an apposite term for an atrophying condition of the skin, subcutaneous fat, muscle, and bone involving either one division of the trigeminal nerve or half of the face. Occasionally the entire ipsilateral side of the body may be affected or the atrophy may first manifest on the trunk or extremities.

Histopathology. A sclerodermoid tissue reaction mimicking morphea is observed, including the presence of adnexal atrophy and subcutaneous fibrosis. The muscles are atrophic, with loss of striations, edema, and vacuolation. Ocular and neurologic complications including iritis, keratitis, optic nerve atrophy, trigeminal neuralgia, and facial palsy may occur (62).

Borrelial Lymphocytoma Cutis

Lymphocytoma cutis is a benign cutaneous lymphoid hyperplasia first described by Spiegler before the end of the 19th century and subsequently named lymphocytoma cutis in 1921 by Kaufmann–Wolff. Various triggering factors have been isolated, such as drugs, contactants, and infections, suggesting that an excessive immune response to antigen may be its etiologic basis. The *B. burgdorferi* spirochete transmitted by *I. ricinus* has been implicated among the infectious agents. Evidence supportive of a spirochetal etiology of some cases of lymphocytoma cutis includes the identification of spirochete-like structures in mercury- and silver-stained sections of skin biopsies from patients with lymphocytoma cutis in whom increased serum titers of antibodies against *Borrelia* spirochetes are observed (80). The term *borrelioma* has been coined to describe such lesions. Lymphocytoma cutis in association with *B. burgdorferi* infection has the same clinical appearance as lesions arising in other settings—namely, as isolated or multiple violaceous, firm nodules, and infiltrative plaques (62). Sites of predilection for the solitary lesions are the earlobes, nipples, and areolae mammae. Lesions of lymphocytoma cutis may occur at sites of erythema chronicum migrans or in patients with stage II Lyme disease. Jessner's lymphocytic infiltrate of the skin is considered by some authors to be a

form of lymphocytoma cutis, and has been reported in one patient whose biopsy showed spirochetes (62).

Histopathology. Skin biopsies show superficial and deep angiocentric, neurotropic and eccrinotropic lymphocytic infiltrates, often accompanied by plasma cells and eosinophils, the former at the periphery and the latter in the center of lesions (73). The dermal alterations may be accompanied by epidermal spongiosis, and some cases show edema of blood vessels, transmural migration of lymphocytes and plasma cells, granulomatous vasculitis with luminal thrombosis, lymphohistiocytic neuritis, and interstitial reticular dermal infiltrates with a sclerosing reaction. Germinal centers may be observed. A florid inflammatory cell infiltrate with granulomatous vasculitis and neuritis will be seen at the tick bite punctum, whereas a biopsy taken within 1 cm of the edge will show a pauci-inflammatory process with only sparse mononuclear cells, no eosinophils or plasma cells, and a vasculopathy comprising endothelial swelling and hyperplasia and mural edema accompanied by mucinosis (81). Biopsies taken between the center and edge show superficial and deep perivascular lymphocytic, plasmacellular, and eosinophilic infiltrates with variable eczematous alterations. Although spirochetes have been identified in the lesional border in only 40% of cases (73), most patients manifest elevated IgM antibody titers (63), and we therefore rely heavily on serology to make the diagnosis. Others hold that the diagnosis at this stage is largely a clinical one due to the incidence of false-positive and false-negative results (82); the sensitivity and specificity of confirmatory molecular tests is not optimal and culture is insensitive (83). The background high seropositivity rates in healthy patients in endemic and nonendemic areas has prompted a two-tiered approach through which seropositive patients undergo a subsequent and more specific Western blot analysis (84,85). Meta-analysis of available molecular methods shows that assays of skin and synovial fluid have the highest sensitivities and specificities; plasma and cerebrospinal fluid assays are less accurate (83). Quantitative polymerase chain reaction of erythema chronicum migrans lesions shows positivity in up to 80% of cases with the mean number of spirochetes in a 2-mm biopsy specimen ranging from 10 to 11,000; larger numbers of spirochetes correlate to smaller lesions and to shorter duration of skin symptomatology (86). Molecular tests for Lyme disease are reserved as complementary or confirmatory tools for cases where the index of suspicion is high (83).

Differential Diagnosis. The clinical differential diagnosis encompasses other forms of annular erythema (87). Other causes of lymphocytoma cutis should be considered, such as drug therapy (88) or other infections (i.e., herpetic or mycobacterial). A well-differentiated lymphocytic lymphoma and chronic lymphocytic leukemia should be excluded, because both may mimic the diffuse type of lymphocytoma cutis. When eosinophils and plasma cells are present and when there are germinal centers, the distinction from malignant lymphoma (apart from marginal zone lymphoma) is less challenging.

Other arthropod assaults, drug hypersensitivity, contact reactions, and connective tissue diseases such as lupus erythematosus, scleroderma, morphea, Sjögren's syndrome, mixed connective tissue disease, and relapsing polychondritis can mimic Lyme disease. Tissue eosinophilia and epidermal changes help to discriminate Lyme disease from connective tissue disease, but differentiation from erythema annulare centrifugum is more problematic. Tissue necrosis at the primary inoculation site of Lyme disease can mimic a brown recluse spider bite (89).

Histogenesis. Most ticks become infected with *B. burgdorferi* by feeding on small animals, in particular the whitefooted mouse. *B. burgdorferi* is a long, narrow spirochete with flagella (90). It has at least 30 different proteins, including two major outer-surface proteins—Osp A and Osp B, which elicit antibody responses late in the course of the disease (90). It has been suggested that phagocytosis of the spirochete by macrophages leads to two different mechanisms of degradation: a phagolysosomal process, which may lead to MHC-class II–restricted antigen processing, and cytosolic degradation, which leads to MHC-class I–restricted antigen presentation. This disparity may in part explain the variable immunologic aspects of Lyme disease (91).

REFERENCES

1. Hook EW, Marra CM. Acquired syphilis in adults. *N Engl J Med* 1992;326:1060.
2. Stamm LV, Greene SR, Bergen HL, et al. Identification and sequence analysis of Treponema pallidum tprJ, a member of a polymorphic multigene family. *FEMS Microbiol Lett* 1998;169:155.
3. Centurion-Lara A, Castro C, Castillo R, et al. The flanking region sequence of the 15kDa lipoprotein gene differentiate pathogenic treponemes. *J Infect Dis* 1998;177:1036.
4. Wicher K, Wicher V, Abbruscato F, et al. Treponema pallidum subsp. Pertenue displays pathogenetic properties different from those of T. pallidum subsp. Pallidum. *Infect Immunol* 2000;68:3219.
5. Centurion-Lara A, Godornes C, Castro C, et al. The tprK gene is heterogeneous among Treponema pallidum strains and has multiple alleles. *Infect Immunol* 2000;68:824.
6. Sparling PF. Natural history of syphilis. In: Homes KK, Mardh P-A, Sparling PF, et al. *Sexually Transmitted Diseases.* 2nd ed. New York: McGraw-Hill, 1990:213.
7. Kamali A, Nunn AJ, Mulder DW, et al. Seroprevalence and incidence of genital ulcer infections in a rural Ugandan population. *Sex Transm Infect* 1999;75:98.
8. Noppakun N, Dinerart SM, Solomon AR. Pustular secondary syphilis. *Int J Dermatol* 1987;26:112.
9. Stockli HR. Neurosyphilis heute. *Dermatologica* 1982;165:232.
10. Moskovitz BL, Klimek JJ, Goldman RL, et al. Meningovascular syphilis after "appropriate" treatment of primary syphilis. *Arch Intern Med* 1982;142:139.
11. Janier M, Pertuiset EF, Poisson M, et al. Manifestations precoces de 1a syphilis neuro-meningee. *Ann Derm Venereol (Stockh)* 1985;112:133.
12. Tanabe JL, Huntley AC. Granulomatous tertiary syphilis. *J Am Acad Dermatol* 1986;15:341.
13. Johnson PC, Farnie MA. Testing for syphilis. *Dermatol Clin* 1994;12:9.
14. Sanchez PJ. Congenital syphilis. *Adv Pediatr Infect Dis* 1992;7:161.
15. Guarner J, Greer PW, Bartlett J, et al. Congenital syphilis in a newborn: an immunopathologic study. *Mod Pathol* 1999;12:82.
16. Jeerapaet P, Ackerman AS. Histologic patterns of secondary syphilis. *Arch Dermatol* 1973;107:373.
17. Hartsock RJ, Halling LW, King FM. Luetic lymphadenitis. *Am J Clin Pathol* 1970;53:304.
18. Yobs AR, Brown L, Hunter EF. Fluorescent antibody technique in early syphilis. *Arch Pathol* 1964;77:220.
19. Beckett JR, Bigbee JW. Immunoperoxidase localization of Treponema pallidum. *Arch Pathol* 1979;103:135.
20. Metz J, Metz G. Elektronenmikroskopischer nachweis von Treponema pallidum in hautefflorescenzen der unbehandelten lues I und II. *Arch Dermatol Forsch* 1972;243:241.
21. Sykes JA, Miller JN, Kalan AJ. Treponema pallidum within cells of a primary chancre from a human female. *Br J Vener Dis* 1974;50:40.
22. Wecke J, Bartunek J, Stuttgen G. Treponema pallidum in early syphilitic lesions in humans during high-dosage penicillin therapy: an electron microscopical study. *Arch Dermatol Res* 1976;257:1.
23. Poulsen A, Kobayasi T, Secher L et al. Treponema pallidum in macular and papular secondary syphilis skin eruptions. *Acta Derm Venereol (Stockh)* 1986;66:251.
24. Azar RH, Pham TD, Kurban AK. An electron microscopic study of a syphilitic chancre. *Arch Pathol* 1970;90:143.
25. Poulsen A, Kobayasi T, Secher L et al. The ultrastructure of Treponema pallidum isolated from human chancres. *Acta Derm Venereol (Stockh)* 1985;65:367.
26. Klingmuller G, Ishibashi Y, Radke K. Der elektronenmikroskopische Aufbau des Treponema pallidum. *Arch Klin Exp Dermatol* 1968;233:197.
27. Magro CM, Crowson AN, Alfa M, et al. A comparative histomorphological analysis of chancroid in seronegative and HIV positive African patients. *Hum Pathol* 1996;27:1066.
28. Abell E, Marks R, Wilson Jones E. Secondary syphilis. A clinicopathological review. *Br J Dermatol* 1975;93:53.
29. Paterou M, Stavrianeas N, Civatte J, et al. Histologie de 1a syphilis secondaire. *Ann Dermatol Venereol* 1979;106:923.
30. Cochran RIE, Thomson J, Fleming KA, et al. Histology simulating reticulosis in secondary syphilis. *Br J Dermatol* 1976;95:251.
31. Kahn LE, Gordon W. Sarcoid-like granulomas in secondary syphilis. *Arch Pathol* 1971;92:334.
32. Montgomery H. *Dermatopathology.* New York: Harper & Row, 1967:417.
33. Fisher DA, Chang LW, Tuffanelli DL. Lues maligna. *Arch Dermatol* 1979;99:70.
34. Degos R, Touraine R, Collart P, et al. Syphilis maligne precoce d'evolution mortelle (avec examen anatomique). *Bull Soc Fr Dermatol Syphiligr* 1970;77:10.
35. Adam W, Korting GW. Lues maligna. *Arch Klin Exp Dermatol* 1960;210:14.
36. Petrozzi JW, Lockshin NA, Berger RI. Malignant syphilis. *Arch Dermatol* 1974;109:387.
37. Lawrence T, Saxe N. Bullous secondary syphilis. *Clin Exp Dermatol* 1992;17:44.
38. Kerdel-Vegas F, Kopf AW, Tolmach JA. Keratoderma punctatum syphiliticum: Report of a case. *Br J Dermatol* 1954;66:449.
39. Lantis LR, Petrozzi JW, Hurley HJ. Sarcoid granuloma in secondary syphilis. *Arch Dermatol* 1969;99:748.
40. Matsuda-John SS, McElgunn PST, Ellis CN. Nodular late syphilis. *J Am Acad Dermatol* 1983;9:269.
41. Longstreth P, Hoke AQ, McElroy C. Hepatitis and bone destruction as uncommon manifestations of early syphilis. *Arch Dermatol* 1976;112:1451.

42. Tourville DR, Byrd LR, Kim DU, et al. Treponemal antigen in immunopathogenesis of syphilitic glomerulonephritis. *Am J Pathol* 1976;82:479.

43. Bansal RC, Cohn H, Fani K, et al. Nephrotic syndrome and granulomatous hepatitis. *Arch Dermatol* 1978;114:1228.

44. Magro CM, Morrison C, Kovatich A, et al. Pityriasis lichenoides is a cutaneous T-cell dyscrasia: a clinical, genotypic, and phenotypic study. *Hum Pathol* 2002;33:788.

45. Holtzmann H, Hassenpflug K. Tertiarsyphilitische lymphknotenbeteiligung vom granulierenden typ bei einem kranken mit plattenartigen gummen der haut. *Arch Klin Exp Dermatol* 1962;215:230.

46. Luxon LM. Neurosyphilis [Review]. *Int J Dermatol* 1980;19:310.

47. Noordhoek GT, Hermans PWM, Paul AN, et al. Treponema pallidum subspecies pallidum (Nichols) and Treponema pallidum subspecies pertenue (CDC 2575) differ in at least one nucleotide: comparison of two homologous antigens. *Microb Pathog* 1989;6:29.

48. Guderian RH, Guzman JR, Calvopina M, et al. Studies on a focus of yaws in the Santiago Basin, province of Esmeraldas, Ecuador. *Trop Geogr Med* 1991;43:142.

49. Engelkens HJH, Judanarso J, Oranje AP, et al. Endemic treponematoses. Part 1. Yaws. *Int J Dermatol* 1992;30:77.

50. Williams HU. Pathology of yaws. *Arch Pathol* 1935;20:596.

51. Hasselmann CM. Comparative studies on the histopathology of syphilis, yaws and pinta. *Br J Vener Dis* 1957;33:5.

52. Greene CA, Harman RRM. Yaws truly: a survey of patients indexed under "Yaws" and a review of the clinical and laboratory problems of diagnosis. *Clin Exp Dermatol* 1986;11:41.

53. Engelkens HJH, Niemel PLA, van der Sluis JL, et al. Endemic treponematoses. Part II. Pinta and endemic syphilis. *Int J Dermatol* 1991;30:231.

54. Pardo-Castello V, Ferrer I. Pinta. *Arch Dermatol Syph* 1942;45:843.

55. Hasselmann CM. Studien uber die histopathologie von pinta, frambosie und syphilis. *Arch Klin Exp Dermatol* 1955;201:1.

56. Rodriguez HA, Albores-Saavedra J, Lozano MM, et al. Langerhans' cells in late pinta. *Arch Pathol* 1971;91:302.

57. Steere AC, Grodzicki RL, Kornblatt AN, et al. The spirochetal etiology of Lyme disease. *N Engl J Med* 1983;308:733.

58. Duray PH. Histopathology of clinical phases of human Lyme disease. *Rheum Dis Clin North Am* 1989;15:691.

59. Steere AC, Malawista SE, Snydman DR, et al. Lyme arthritis: An epidemic of oligoarticular arthritis in children and adults in three Connecticut communities. *Arthritis Rheum* 1977;20:7.

60. Benach JL, Bosler EM, Hanrahan JP, et al. Spirochetes isolated from the blood of two patients with Lyme disease. *N Engl J Med* 1983;308:740.

61. Barbour AB, Tessier SL, Todd WJ. Lyme disease spirochetes in Ixodid tick spirochetes share a common surface antigenic determinant defined by a monoclonal antibody. *Infect Immunol* 1983;41:795.

62. Abele DC, Anders KH. The many faces and phases of borreliosis. I. Lyme disease. *J Am Acad Dermatol* 1990;23:167.

63. Asbrink E, Hovmark A. Cutaneous manifestations in Ixodesborne Borrelia spirochetosis. *Int J Dermatol* 1987;26:215.

64. Lebech AM. Polymerase chain reaction in diagnosis of Borrelia burgdorferi infections and studies on taxonomic classification. *APMIS Suppl* 2002;105:1.

65. Christova I, Schouls L, van de Pol I, et al. High prevalence of granulocytic Ehrlichiae and Borrelia burgdorferi sensu lato in Ixodes ricinus ticks from Bulgaria. *J Clin Microbiol* 2001;39:4172.

66. Cao WC, Zhao QM, Zhang PH, et al. Granulocytic Ehrlichiae in Ixodes persulcatus ticks from an areas in China where Lyme disease is endemic. *J Clin Microbiol* 2000;38:4208.

67. Hilton E, deVoit J, Benach JL, et al. Seroprevalence and seroconversion for tick-borne diseases in a high-risk population in the northeast United States. *Am J Med* 1999;106:404.

68. Bakken JS, Dumler JS. Human granulocytic ehrlichiosis. *Clin Infect Dis* 2002;31:554.

69. Wormser GP, Horowitz HW, Nowakowski J, et al. Positive Lyme disease serology in patients with clinical and laboratory evidence of human granulocytic ehrlichiosis. *Am J Clin Pathol* 1997;107:142.

70. Krause PJ, MacKay K, Thompson CA, et al. Disease-specific diagnosis of coinfecting tickborne zoonoses: babesiosis, human granulocytic ehrlichiosis, and Lyme disease. *Clin Infect Dis* 2002;34:1184.

71. Sigel LH, Curran AS. Lyme disease: A multifocal worldwide disease. *Ann Rev Public Health* 1991;12:85.

72. Cote J. Lyme disease. *Int J Dermatol* 1991;30:500.

73. Berger BW. Erythema chronicum migrans of Lyme disease. *Arch Dermatol* 1984;120:1017.

74. Burgdorf WHS, Woret WI, Schultes O. Acrodermatitis chronica atrophicans. *Int J Dermatol* 1979;595.

75. Kaufman L, Gruber BL, Philips ME, et al. Late cutaneous Lyme disease: acrodermatitis chronica atrophicans. *Am J Med* 1989;86:828.

76. Aberer E, Klade H, Hobisch G. A clinical, histological, and immunohistochemical comparison of acrodermatitis chronica atrophicans and morphea. *Am J Dermatopathol* 1991;13:334.

77. Montgomery H. *Dermatopathology*. New York: Harper & Row, 1967:766.

78. Aberer E, Klade H, Stanek G, et al. Borrelia burgdorferi and different types of morphea. *Dermatologica* 1991;182:145.

79. Aberer E, Stanek G, Ertl M, et al. Evidence for spirochetal origin of circumscribed scleroderma (morphea). *Acta Derm Venereol (Stockh)* 1987;67:225.

80. Hovmark A, Asbrink E, Olsson I. The spirochetal etiology of lymphadenosis benign cutis solitaria. *Acta Derm Venereol (Stockh)* 1986;66:479.

81. Shulman KJ, Melski JW, Reed KD, et al. The characteristic histologic features of erythema chronicum migrans. *Lab Invest* 1996;74:46A(abst).

82. Edlow JA. Erythema migrans. *Med Clin North Am* 2002;86:239.

83. Dumler JS. Molecular diagnosis of Lyme disease: review and meta-analysis. *Mol Diagn* 2001;6:1.

84. Bunikis J, Barbour AG. Laboratory testing for suspected Lyme disease. *Med Clin North Am* 2002;86:311.

85. Pinto DS. Cardiac manifestations of Lyme disease. *Med Clin North Am* 2002;86:285.

86. Liveris D, Wang G, Girao G, et al. Quantitative detection of Borrelia burgdorferi in 2-millimeter skin samples of erythema chronicum migrans lesions: correlation of results with clinical and laboratory findings. *J Clin Microbiol* 2002;40:1249.

87. Grau RH, Allen PS, Cornelison RL Jr. Erythema migrans and the differential diagnosis of annular erythema. *J Okla State Med Assoc* 2002;95:257.

88. Magro CM, Crowson AN. Drug-induced immune dysregulation as a cause of atypical cutaneous lymphoid infiltrates: a hypothesis. *Hum Pathol* 1996;27:125.

89. Oosterhoudt KC, Zaoutis T, Zorc JJ. Lyme disease masquerading as brown recluse spider bite. *Ann Emerg Med* 2002;39:558.

90. Jantausch BA. Lyme disease, Rocky Mountain spotted fever, ehrlichiosis: emerging and established challenges for the clinician. *Ann Allergy* 1994;73:4.

91. Rittig MG, Haupl T, Krause A, et al. Borrelia burgdorferi-induced ultrastructural alterations in human phagocytes: a clue to pathogenicity? *J Pathol* 1994;173:269.

23

FUNGAL DISEASES

MOLLY HINSHAW
B. JACK LONGLEY

Phylogenetically, fungi are eukaryotic protists that are distinguished from plants by their lack of chlorophyll (1). The Greek word *mycoses* means fungus and was first penned by R. Virchow in 1856 to describe infections by this group of organisms. In the past, bacterial infections, lymphoma, and other disorders have also been termed "mycoses," despite a lack of relation to fungi. We will discuss fungal infections and protothecosis here. Protothecosis is a cutaneous infection by algae of the genus *Prototheca* and will continue to be included in this chapter because there is no separate chapter for infections by algae. Actinomycosis, botryomycosis, and erythrasma are bacterial diseases that have historically been included with the fungal diseases. In the interest of clarity, these will be discussed in the chapter on bacterial diseases.

Terminology in fungal infections must be consistent. Given the confusing ways in which fungal definitions have been used, we have defined our terms here (Table 23-1). *Hyphae* are elongated filamentous forms of fungi that usually form an intertwining mass called a *mycelium*. Septate hyphae give rise to arthrospores by asexual reproduction. Rounded, box-like, or short cylindrical arthrospores can often be identified. *Yeasts* are single-celled, usually rounded fungi that reproduce by budding (blastospore formation). Yeast cells and their progeny may adhere to one another, form chains or "pseudohyphae," and may also form mycelia; thus, they may be difficult to distinguish from true hyphae by light microscopy. *Dematiaceous fungi* are fungi that bear melanin-like pigment on their walls. *Tinea* is a clinical term that describes superficial fungal infections of the skin; it is usually modified with an anatomic or other term to describe the location or color of the infection. The *dermatophytes* are fungi that were originally classified by Sabouraud (2), redefined by Emmons (3), and include the three genera *Microsporum*, *Trichophyton*, and *Epidermophyton*. Therefore, *dermatophytosis* is not an appropriate histologic diagnostic term unless a definite assignment of an organism to one of these three genera of dermatophytes can be made. *Dermatomycosis* refers to any fungal infection of the skin and may be caused by dermatophytes, yeast, or other fungi, including those that do not usually cause cutaneous disease.

The primary cutaneous fungal pathogens fall into two groups: those that tend to cause superficial infections and those that cause deep infections. A third group of cutaneous fungal pathogens are those that usually cause systemic disease and only secondarily involve the skin. The basic pattern of cutaneous infection is relatively uniform within each of these three groups. The degree of inflammatory response to these three categories of fungal infection, however, varies based on a number of factors, particularly host immune status. For example, infections with organisms causing superficial dermatomycoses, such as the dermatophytes, *Candida* species, *Malassezia* (*Pityrosporum*) *furfur*, and *Cladosporium* (*Exophiala* or *Phaeoannellomyces*) *werneckii*, are generally characterized by hyphae or pseudohyphae and sometimes yeast cells in the keratin layer of the epidermis and in follicles. The variable intensity of the tissue reaction in the epidermis and follicular epithelium ranges from almost no response to a very mild focal spongiosis to a more exuberant or chronic spongiotic-psoriasiform pattern. Superficial fungal infections may provoke a superficial lymphocytic or a mixed dermal inflammatory infiltrate. Organisms causing superficial dermatomycosis are not found in the dermis except in the case of follicular rupture.

Deep cutaneous fungal infections typically show a mixed dermal inflammatory cell infiltrate that is often associated with pseudoepitheliomatous hyperplasia and occasionally with dermal fibrosis. Primary cutaneous aspergillosis, chromomycoses, phaeohyphomycosis, phaeomycetoma, rhinosporidiosis, and lobomycosis are fungi that infect the deeper cutaneous tissues.

Incidental cutaneous infections by fungi that usually primarily involve other organs, such as blastomycosis or coccidioidomycosis, typically show a pattern similar to that seen with the deep primary cutaneous fungi: a mixed dermal infiltrate with multinucleated giant cells associated with pseudoepitheliomatous hyperplasia. However, a few organisms such as *Histoplasma* and *Loboa loboi* are more

TABLE 23-1. TERMINOLOGY OF FUNGI

Term	Definition	Example
Dermatophyte	Imperfect fungi	*Trichophyton, Microsporum, Epidermophyton*
Dermatomycosis	Any fungal infection of the skin caused by dermatophytes, yeast, or fungi including those that do not usually cause disease	
Arthrospores	Asexual fungal spore formed by hyphal segmentation	*Coccidioides immitis*
Hyphae	The fine branching tubes that make up the body (or mycelium) of a multicellular fungus	Dermatophytes
Mycelium	Intertwining mass of hyphae	
Yeast	Round to oval fungal forms that reproduce by budding or blastogenesis	*Candida, Cryptococcus, Malassezia*
Blastoconidia	Daughter cells of parent yeast	
Pseudohyphae	A chain of easily disrupted fungal cells with constrictions rather than depth at the junctions	*Candida* spp.
Dematiaceous fungi	Mold or yeast with melanin pigment in their walls	*Phaeohyphomycosis, Chromomycosis*
Sporangia	Spherule containing endospores	*Coccidioides imitis*
Sporangioblasts	Another term for endospores	*Rhinosporidium seeberi*
Grains	Dense accumulations (microcolonies) of fungi or bacteria	Eumycetoma
Tinea	Clinical term to describe superficial fungal infections of the skin	Faciei, cruris, pedis, manus
Dimorphic	Fungus that grows in more than one form (mold, yeast, sclerotic body, sulfur grains, spherules with endospores, etc.)	Histoplasmosis, coccidiomycosis, blastomycosis, paracoccidiomycosis

likely to be associated with epidermal thinning than with hyperplasia. Other systemic fungal infections show characteristic tissue reaction patterns. For example, disseminated candidiasis has prominent microabscess formation, cryptococcosis has a gelatinous or granulomatous reaction pattern, and zygomycosis and aspergillosis have a tendency for vascular invasion and infarction.

Multiple special stains highlight certain fungal elements. These techniques can be helpful especially when the overall histologic pattern is suspicious for a fungal infection but fungi are not apparent on hematoxylin and eosin (H&E) stained sections. The periodic acid-Schiff (PAS) reaction stains fungi red and can be used with diastase (PAS-D). Fungi stain positively with PAS-D because of two substances rich in neutral polysaccharides cellulose and chitin that are contained in their cell walls. Both cellulose and chitin are diastase resistant. Adding diastase to the PAS reaction clears the tissue of glycogen granules that may be mistaken for fungal spores. Gomori methenamine silver nitrate (GMS) stains fungi black and is also useful. Giemsa and Gram stains, silver stains, Fontana–Masson, mucicarmine, Alcian blue, India ink, and acid-fast stain also highlight various fungal elements in other primary or secondary cutaneous fungal infections.

DERMATOPHYTOSIS

Dermatophytes are a group of molds that invade and consume keratin by their generation of proteases (4). They originally came from soil where they lived on keratinaceous debris. Ultimately, these organisms were picked up by animals and humans to become the pathogens that we know today (5).

Three genera of imperfect fungi comprise the dermatophytes: *Trichophyton, Microsporum,* and *Epidermophyton.* More than 40 species exist, although many are not pathogenic to humans. Dermatophytes are grouped according to their natural habitat as anthropophilic, zoophilic, and geophilic with primary reservoirs of infection in humans, animals, and soil, respectively (5). Fungi in all three categories may cause human infections. In immunocompetent hosts, the dermatophytes cause only superficial infections of the epidermis, hair, and nails. *Epidermophyton* species, as the name suggests, infect mainly the epidermis, although occasionally the nails are involved. *Microsporum* species infect the epidermis and hair, while *Trichophyton* species may infect the epidermis, hair, and nails (6).

Clinically, fungal infections of seven anatomical regions are commonly recognized: *tinea capitis* (including *tinea favosa* or *favus of the scalp*), *tinea barbae, tinea faciei, tinea corporis* (including *tinea imbricata*), *tinea cruris, tinea of the hands and feet,* and *tinea unguium* (Table 23-2).

Tinea capitis is dermatophytosis of the skin and hair of the scalp. Clinically, one often sees scale crust and hairs that are broken off either at the level of the scalp or slightly above it. In the United States, *T. tonsurans* is the most common pathogen of this anatomic site where one sees broken-off hairs (black-dot ringworm) in some patients and a marked inflammatory reaction in others (7). *T.*

TABLE 23-2. COMMON CAUSAL DERMATOPHYTES BY ANATOMIC REGIONS

Clinical Diagnosis	Causal Organisms
Tinea capitis	*Trichophyton tonsurans* (black dot), *T. violaceum* (black dot), *T. schoenleinii* (favus), *Microsporum canis*
Tinea faciei	*T. verrucosum, T. mentagrophytes, T. rubrum*
Tinea corporis	*T. rubrum, T. mentagrophytes, E. floccosum, T. concentricum*
Tinea manus	*T. rubrum*
Tinea pedis	*T. rubrum, T. mentagrophytes, Epidermophyton floccosum*
Tinea unguium	*T. rubrum, T. mentagrophytes* (vesicobullous), *E. floccosum*

schoenleinii causes *favus*, but cases caused by other *Trichophyton* species are rare. *M. audouinii, M. canis,* and much less commonly other *Microsporum* species may also cause tinea capitis. *M. canis* is zoophilic and therefore tends to cause a more inflammatory response than *M. audouinii,* which is anthropophilic; both show a band of bright green fluorescence in the hair under a Wood light (8). A severe inflammatory boggy plaque, the so-called kerion Celsi, may result from infection with zoophilic dermatophytes such as *M. canis. Trichophyton* species other than *T. schoenleinii,* which shows subtle pale green fluorescence along the length of the hair, do not fluoresce in a Wood light.

Favus, a severe tinea capitis rarely seen in the United States, is usually caused by *T. schoenleinii,* although a similar clinical picture may occasionally be seen with other fungi. Favus affects mainly the scalp, where it produces inflammation with formation of perifollicular hyperkeratotic crusts called scutula. Destruction of the hair occurs relatively late in the infection. The lesions may heal with scarring and permanent alopecia.

Tinea faciei is a fungal infection of the glabrous skin of the face characterized by a persistent eruption of red macules, papules, and patches, the latter of which may show an arcuate border. It is caused usually by *T. rubrum* and occasionally by *T. mentagrophytes* or *T. tonsurans* (9).

Tinea barbae, which is rare in the United States, is a fungal infection limited to the coarse hair-bearing beard and mustache areas of men. Tinea barbae may be caused by *T. mentagrophytes,* but usually is due to *T. verrucosum (faviform),* an infection also often referred to as "cattle ringworm" because it is usually contracted from cattle. Both *T. mentagrophytes* and *T. verrucosum* are zoophilic and typically cause a kerion-like, boggy, nodular inflammatory infiltration (10).

Tinea corporis is a dermatophytosis of glabrous skin most commonly caused by *T. rubrum* followed by *M. canis* and *T. mentagrophytes.* In cases caused by *T. rubrum,* one sees

large erythematous patches with central clearing and an arcuate or polycyclic scaly border. In infections with *M. canis,* tinea corporis is more inflammatory and annular lesions with raised papulovesicular borders and central clearing are common. *T. mentagrophytes* typically produces a few annular lesions with little or no central clearing. *T. verrucosum* may occasionally cause tinea corporis appearing as grouped follicular pustules referred to as *agminate folliculitis* (10). Majocchi's granuloma, caused by *T. rubrum,* is a nodular granulomatous perifolliculitis caused by rupture of an affected follicle, typically of the lower extremity. Majocchi's granuloma often occurs in association with tinea pedis or onychomycosis. KO*H.* examination of extracted hairs reveals the ectothrix infection as a sheath of arthrospores on the outside of the shaft and arthrospores inside the shaft.

Tinea cruris, usually caused by *T. rubrum* and occasionally by *T. mentagrophytes* or *Epidermophyton floccosum,* shows sharply demarcated erythematous patches or thin plaques in the groin. The infection may spread to the perineal and/or perianal regions as well as the scrotum.

Tinea of the feet and hands (tinea pedis et manus) is the most common form of dermatophyte infection and is usually caused by *T. rubrum, E. floccosum,* or *T. mentagrophytes.* Tinea pedis may present clinically as interdigital maceration, plantar (i.e., "moccasin" scale), or vesiculobullous lesions. *T. rubrum* is anthropophilic and causes relatively noninflammatory scaling on the plantar feet. Infections with *T. mentagrophytes* tend to cause inflammatory, vesiculobullous tinea pedis.

Tinea unguium specifically refers to a dermatophyte infection of the nail whereas onychomycosis is a nail infection due to any fungi including dermatophytes, *Candida* species, or a nondermatophyte (11). Up to 90% of mycotic toenail infections and 50% of fingernail infections are caused by dermatophytes, but yeasts (especially *Candida albicans*) and nondermatophyte molds are also implicated (12). Criteria for diagnosing nondermatophyte onychomycosis have been offered as (a) the presence of hyphae in the infected subungual debris; (b) persistent failure to culture recognized dermatophytes; and (c) positive cultures of a nondermatophyte (13).

Four clinical types of onychomycosis include distal and lateral subungual onychomycosis (DLSO), superficial white onychomycosis (SWO), proximal subungual onychomycosis (PSO), and *Candida* infections of the nail. In general, hyperkeratosis and onycholysis are common clinical presentations of onychomycosis. DLSO is the most common form found in all patients including those with HIV and is caused by dermatophytes, usually *T. rubrum* (14). SWO is caused primarily by *T. mentagrophytes* and is more commonly seen in HIV. PSO is typically caused by *T. rubrum* and is rare in the general population, but can be a presenting sign of HIV. PSO in AIDS is often caused by *T. mentagrophytes* (15). *Candida* nail infections present as paronychia, hyperkeratosis, or onycholysis. Nondermato-

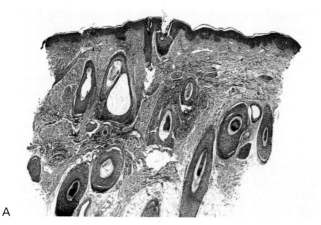

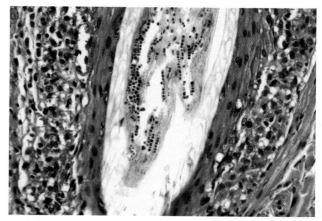

A   B

FIGURE 23-1. Tinea capitis. **A:** H&E stain shows arthrospores and hyphal elements in most follicles. A lymphohistiocytic, perifollicular infiltrate is present. **B:** H&E stain shows arthrospores in
endothrix infection.

phytes implicated in onychomycosis include *Candida*
species, *Scytalidium (Hendersonula)*, and *Aspergillus* (most
commonly niger). Fungi thought to be contaminants in
nail cultures in all but the immunosuppressed include *Cladosporium*, *Alternaria*, *Fusarium*, *Acremonium*, and *Scopu-
lariopsis* (16). There is considerable controversy about the
clinical significance of nondermatophyte fungi in nail cultures when a dermatophyte is also identified on culture.

Histopathology. In tinea capitis and tinea barbae, infection of follicles usually starts with colonization of the stratum corneum of the perifollicular epidermis (Fig. 23-1).
Hyphae extend down the follicle, growing on the surface of
the hair shaft. Hyphae then invade the hair, penetrate the
cuticle and invade inward, first in the subcuticular portion
of the cortex, just under the hair surface, and then more
deeply in the hair cortex, extending to the upper limit of
the zone of keratinization (17). Rounded and box-like
arthrospores may be found mainly within the hair shaft in
endothrix infections or penetrating the surface of the hair
shaft and forming a sheath around it in ectothrix infections. Endothrix infections are caused by *T. tonsurans* or *T.
violaceum*. Except for *T. schoenleinii*, which causes favus, all
other dermatophytes infecting hair shafts cause *ectothrix*
infections. Although hyphae invade the shafts in both
types of infections, they may not be evident in a hair
plucked from an endothrix infection because the more superficial hyphae rapidly break up into arthrospores and destroy the keratin of the hair shaft. When plucked, the
weakened shaft typically breaks at a relatively superficial
point so that only the arthrospores are seen. The dermis,
which almost never contains fungi, shows a perifollicular
mononuclear cell infiltrate of varying intensity. In addition
to a chronic inflammatory infiltrate, multinucleated giant
cells may be present in the vicinity of disrupted or degenerated hair follicles (18). In kerion Celsi, there is a pronounced inflammatory tissue reaction to the fungi with

follicular pustule formation and interfollicular neutrophilic infiltration, as well as a marked chronic inflammatory
infiltrate surrounding the hair follicles. In cases with a severe inflammatory reaction, fungi may be difficult to identify either by microscopic examination or by culture, but
may be demonstrated using fluorescein-labeled *T. mentagrophytes* antiserum that cross-reacts with antigens of all
dermatophyte species (19).

In tinea of the glabrous skin, which includes tinea faciei,
tinea corporis, tinea cruris, and tinea of the feet and hands,
fungi occur only in the horny layers of the epidermis and
do not invade hairs and hair follicles. Two exceptions to
this are *T. rubrum* and with *T. verrucosum*, both of which
may invade hairs and hair follicles causing subsequent perifolliculitis.

The number of fungi seen in the horny layer usually is
small so that they may be easily missed even when treated
with the PAS reaction or stained with GMS. Occasionally,
they are present in sufficient numbers that, even in sections
stained with hematoxylin-eosin, they can be recognized as
faintly basophilic, refractile structures (Fig. 23-2). Their
identification in hematoxylin-eosin–stained sections may
be aided by lowering the microscope condenser, which enhances the refractivity of the fungal elements. In infections
with *Microsporum* or *Trichophyton*, only hyphae are seen,
and, in infections with *E. floccosum*, chains of spores are
present. If fungi are present in the horny layer, they usually
are "sandwiched" between two zones of cornified cells, the
upper being orthokeratotic and the lower consisting partially of parakeratotic cells. This "sandwich sign" should
prompt the performance of a stain for fungi for verifica-
tion. The presence of neutrophils in the stratum corneum
is another valuable diagnostic clue (20). In the absence of
demonstrable fungi, the histologic picture of fungal infections of the glabrous skin is not diagnostic. Depending on
the degree of reaction of the skin to the presence of fungi,

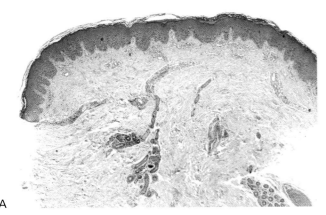

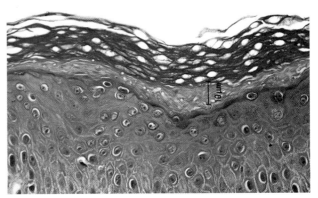

A

B

FIGURE 23-2. Tinea corporis. **A:** H&E stain shows a superficial perivascular, predominantly lymphoid infiltrate with mild psoriasiform epidermal hyperplasia and compact hyperkeratosis. **B:** Cross-sections of refractile hyphae are visible as clear spaces in parakeratotic stratum corneum (H&E stain).

one sees the histologic features of an acute, a subacute, or a chronic, spongiotic dermatitis (Chapter 9).

The nodular perifolliculitis, "Majocchi granuloma," caused by *T. rubrum* shows numerous hyphae and spores within hairs and hair follicles and in the inflammatory infiltrate of the dermis on staining with the PAS reaction or with GMS stain. Fungal elements may also reach the dermis through a break in the follicular wall. Although the spores present within hairs or hair follicles measure about 2 μm in diameter, those located in the dermis, especially within multinucleated giant cells, may be larger, measuring up to 6 μm (21). The dermal process shows an inflammatory infiltrate of lymphoid cells, macrophages, epithelioid cells, and multinucleated giant cells as well as central necrosis and occasionally suppuration.

The agminate folliculitis caused by *T. verrucosum* (*faviform*) shows hyphae and spores within hairs and hair follicles in PAS-stained sections (10). The dermis around the hair follicles, however, contains no fungi. Depending on the severity and on the stage of the inflammatory reaction, either an acute or a chronic inflammatory infiltrate is predominant around the hair follicles in the dermis. In well-established lesions, the inflammatory infiltrate contains many plasma cells, microabscesses, and small aggregates of foreign-body giant cells (10).

In tinea unguium, nail plate biopsy is potentially the method of choice for diagnosis. Although microscopic examination of potassium hydroxide mounts or cultures of nail fragments often establish a diagnosis of onychomycosis, false-negative results may occur if the infection is in the nail bed or is situated in the lower portion of the nail plate. Nail clippings or nail biopsy taken by punch technique or scalpel under local anesthesia will often reveal the fungi on PAS-D stained sections (22). *T. rubrum* is by far the most common causal fungus; occasionally *T. mentagrophytes* is present.

Three histologic patterns are common in nail plate biopsies of onychomycosis (23). In superficial infections, mycelial elements, best visualized with PAS or GMS, are seen in the outer layer of the nail plate. Routine histologic examination of nail plate with PAS staining is a simple, rapid, and sensitive test for fungal elements (24). The second histologic pattern is seen in clinical onycholysis when PAS stained sections of nail plate reveal slender, uniform mycelial elements invading the undersurface of the nail plate (Fig. 23-3). In this pattern, there may also be an inflammatory infiltrate of lymphocytes and neutrophils as well as serum and keratotic debris on the undersurface of the nail plate. Biopsies of nail bed or nail fold epithelium may reveal psoriasiform hyperplasia, spongiosis, and hyperkeratosis making the identification of fungal elements critical to the correct diagnosis. The third common histologic pattern is seen in *Candida* infections where hyphal forms

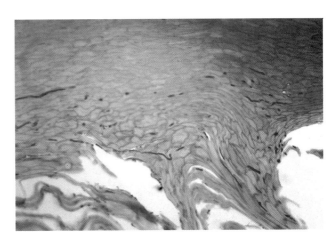

FIGURE 23-3. Tinea unguium. Slender, uniform mycelial elements can be seen within this parakeratotic nail plate (PAS-D stain).

are seen on the undersurface of the nail plate; this will be discussed in a later section. Other less typical morphologic patterns of onychomycosis may signal an infection with unusual fungi or partial treatment with antimycotics.

PCR of nail plate biopsies has been studied for the diagnosis of onychomycosis but is not routinely used (25). PCR is very sensitive and ubiquitous contaminant fungi may cause false positive results. Fungal cultures and histologic confirmation of true hyphal or yeast forms would add to the utility of PCR for identification of specific named fungi. Alone, however, PCR is not yet specific enough to be widely used.

Pathogenesis. Debate exists regarding factors that predispose individuals to onychomycosis. Trauma is thought to facilitate the entry of fungus into the nail. Epidemiologic data suggest that the incidence increases with age, but other factors such as humidity, local trauma, and common living/bathing sites have been variably significant predictors (26).

In favus, mainly hyphae and only a few spores of *T. schoenleinii* are present in the stratum corneum of the epidermis around and within hairs. The scutula consist of compact hyperkeratosis as well as parakeratotic cells, exudate, and inflammatory cells intermingled with segmented hyphae and spores that are well preserved at the periphery but appear degenerated and granular in the center of the scutula (27). In active areas, the dermis shows a pronounced inflammatory infiltrate containing multinucleated giant cells and many plasma cells in association with degenerating hair follicles. In old areas, there is fibrosis and an absence of pilosebaceous structures (18).

DISEASES CAUSED BY *MALASSEZIA FURFUR*

Malassezia is a genus of lipophilic yeast and is the only cutaneous commensal fungal species in humans (28). Two dermatoses, pityriasis versicolor and *Malassezia* (*Pityrosporum*) folliculitis, are generally accepted as being caused by the genus *Malassezia*. The frequently used term "tinea versicolor" is not accurate since *Malassezia* are not dermatophytes. In pityriasis versicolor, multiple round to oval pink to light brown patches with fine white scale are seen primarily on the trunk and upper extremities. Gentle scraping of the patches will induce the scale that can be examined for spores and short hyphae. *Malassezia* (*Pityrosporum*) folliculitis is a pruritic eruption of 2- to 4-mm acneiform follicular papules and pustules on the trunk and arms of otherwise healthy hosts (29). KOH examination of the lesions will reveal only yeast forms.

In addition to these two diseases, *Malassezia* has been found in lesions of seborrheic dermatitis, atopic dermatitis, neonatal cephalic pustulosis, and confluent and reticulated

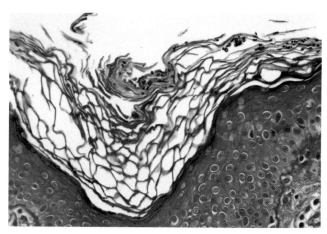

FIGURE 23-4. Pityriasis (tinea) versicolor. A slightly hyperkeratotic stratum corneum contains numerous hyphae and spores (H&E stain).

papillomatosis of Gougerot and Carteaud (30,31). Seborrheic dermatitis, for example, has been reported to respond to antifungal therapy and has been associated with heavy colonization by *M. furfur*. These observations and their interpretation are controversial, however, and it has not been established that *M. furfur* contributes to the pathogenesis of seborrheic dermatitis (32,33).

Histopathology. In contrast to other fungal infections of the glabrous skin, the horny layer in lesions of pityriasis (tinea) versicolor contains abundant amounts of fungal elements, which can often be visualized in sections stained with hematoxylin-eosin as faintly basophilic structures. *Malassezia* (*Pityrosporum*) is present as a combination of both hyphae and spores (Fig. 23-4), the light microscopic appearance of which is often referred to as "spaghetti and meatballs." The inflammatory response in pityriasis versicolor is usually minimal, although there may occasionally be slight hyperkeratosis (34), slight spongiosis, or a minimal superficial perivascular lymphocytic infiltrate.

Histogenesis. The names *M. furfur*, *P. orbiculare*, and *P. ovale* are often used interchangeably probably because these are culturally identical (35). In patients with pityriasis versicolor, *M. furfur* becomes dimorphous by forming numerous true septate hyphae in addition to spores. The organism then becomes pathogenic (28).

Several theories exist to explain the characteristic pigmentary alterations in pityriasis versicolor, although none have been convincingly proven. Hypopigmentation may be caused by filtering of UV light by the organism, a block in melanosome transfer to keratinocytes (36), the inhibition of melanin synthesis by azelaic acid (37), or lipoxygenase produced by *Malassezia* (38). Hyperpigmentation is thought by some to be secondary to inflammation, hyperkeratosis, or greater numbers of organisms in the skin (39).

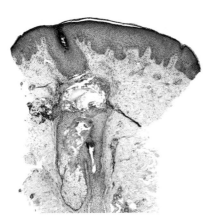
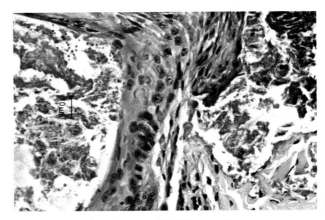

A

B

FIGURE 23-5. *Malassezia (Pityrosporum)* folliculitis. **A:** A plugged and ruptured follicle contains numerous round yeast forms (H&E stain). **B:** H&E stain shows round and budding yeast forms in follicle and surrounding dermis.

Malassezia (*Pityrosporum*) Folliculitis

The involved pilosebaceous follicles show hyperkeratosis with dilatation resulting from plugging of the infundibulum with keratinous material. Inflammatory cells are present both within and around the follicular infundibulum (40). In some instances, the follicular epithelium is disrupted with development of a peri-infundibular abscess (41) (Fig. 23-5). In every instance, PAS-stained sections show PAS-positive, diastase-resistant, spherical to oval, singly budding yeast organisms 2 to 4 μm in diameter. They are located predominantly within the infundibulum and at the dilated orifice of the follicular lumen but are occasionally observed also in the perifollicular dermis. No hyphae are seen.

Histogenesis. It has been assumed that *Malassezia* organisms cause hyperkeratosis in the follicular ostium, thereby preventing the normal flow of sebum and causing the follicular, acne-like lesions (40).

CANDIDIASIS

Candida albicans is a dimorphous fungus growing in both yeast and filamentous forms on the skin. It exists in a commensal relationship with man. The spectrum of infection may be divided into four groups: acute mucocutaneous candidiasis, chronic mucocutaneous candidiasis, disseminated candidiasis, and *Candida* onychomycosis.

Acute Mucocutaneous Candidiasis

Acute mucocutaneous candidiasis is the benign, self-limited form of candidiasis and is caused by environmental changes that are local, as in hot, humid conditions, or that are systemic, as in antibiotic or corticosteroid therapy.

Clinical variants of acute mucocutaneous candidiasis include erosio interdigitalis blastomycetica, *Candida* vaginitis, paronychia, *Candida* intertrigo and thrush. Intertriginous lesions show erythematous, often-eroded patches, and thin plaques often with peripheral erythematous macules and papules, the so-called satellite lesions. *Candida* infections of the mucous membranes are noted as erythematous patches or white plaques that reveal a glistening, erythematous undersurface when scraped.

Candida infection is associated with specific host and environmental factors. *Candida* is the most common pathogen in patients having had a solid organ transplant, and tends to occur within the first 6 months after transplant. Age (infancy, old age), antibiotic use, malignancy, chemotherapy, endocrinopathies (diabetes, Cushing's syndrome), and immune system disorders including HIV/AIDS are risk factors for *Candida* infection (42,43). More effective treatment of AIDS has led to a decline in the incidence of clinically apparent candidiasis in these patients.

Congenital cutaneous candidiasis is a result of ascending intrauterine infection from vaginal candidiasis. There are widely scattered macules, papulovesicles, and pustules at birth or in a few days thereafter. *Neonatal candidiasis*, on the other hand, manifests as oral candidiasis or diaper dermatitis after the first week of life and is acquired during passage through the birth canal (44).

Histopathology. Cutaneous and mucous membrane infection with *Candida* show similar features. If the primary lesion is a vesicle or pustule, it is usually subcorneal as in impetigo (Fig. 23-6). In some instances, the pustules have a spongiform appearance, so that they are indistinguishable from the spongiform pustules of Kogoj seen in pustular psoriasis (45) (Chapter 7).

The fungal organisms are present, usually in small amounts only, in the stratum corneum. They are predominantly pseudohyphae and ovoid spores some of the latter in

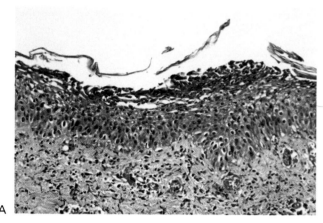
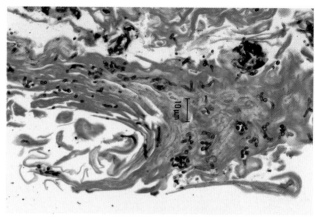

FIGURE 23-6. Candidiasis. **A:** H&E stain shows a subcorneal pustule with an underlying mixed dermal infiltrate. **B:** GMS stain shows pseudohyphae and ovoid yeast in hyperkeratotic stratum corneum.

the budding stage. These septate pseudohyphae show branching at a 90-degree angle and measure from 2 to 4 μm in diameter. The pseudohyphae tend to be constricted at their septa and to have septa at their branch points (46). The ovoid spores vary from 3 to 6 μm in size (Table 23-3).

Pathogenesis. On electron microscopy, the majority of the mycelia and spores are situated inside the cells of the stratum corneum, many of which are parakeratotic (47).

Chronic Mucocutaneous Candidiasis

Chronic mucocutaneous candidiasis (CMC) is a heterogeneous group of conditions in which patients have chronic and recurrent *Candida* infections of the skin, nails, and mucous membranes. CMC may be inherited as an autosomal dominant or recessive condition. It may also be due to endocrinopathies or immunodeficiency. By definition, systemic involvement does not occur in CMC (48). The individual lesions of CMC are similar clinically and histologically to those seen in acute mucocutaneous candidiasis and must be distinguished by their clinical course (48). The ex-

ception is seen in CMC beginning in childhood when a rare clinical variant called "*Candida* granuloma" may develop. *Candida* granuloma presents clinically as numerous hyperkeratotic, crusted plaques on the face and scalp, which occasionally occur elsewhere (49).

Currently, the type of chronic mucocutaneous candidiasis most commonly seen is probably seen in patients with AIDS who often have recurrent *Candida* infections of the mouth and perianal area. Oral candidiasis may occur as an early sign of immunosuppression, before other symptoms have appeared (50), and if persistent, may be an indication of esophageal candidiasis (51). In addition, *Candida* organisms are frequently observed on the surface of lesions of oral hairy leukoplakia, which is a viral leukoplakia caused by Epstein–Barr virus, perhaps in combination with human papillomavirus (Chapter 25).

Histopathology. The histologic findings are identical with those of acute mucocutaneous candidiasis, except in cases of *Candida* granuloma. *Candida granuloma* shows pronounced papillomatosis and hyperkeratosis and a dense infiltrate in the dermis composed of lymphoid cells, neu-

TABLE 23-3. HISTOLOGIC APPEARANCE OF TISSUE AND FUNGI IN SUPERFICIAL DERMATOMYCOSES

Disease	Histologic appearance	Fungal size and morphology
Dermatophytosis	Minimal to spongiotic-psoriasiform, pustular, or folliculitis pattern with mixed dermal infiltrate.	Refractile, 1–2 μm septate hyaline hyphae in stratum corneum, occasional chains of spores.
Pityriasis (tinea) versicolor	Slight hyperkeratosis.	2–8 μm round spores, 2–3 μm thick, short, sometimes curved hyphae.
Mallassezia (Pityrosporum) folliculitis	Plugged, sometimes ruptured follicle with follicular and perifollicular mixed infiltrate.	2–8 μm round spores within follicle, rarely in perifollicular tissue. Usually no hyphae.
Candidiasis	Spongiotic or subcorneal pustular dermatitis with mixed dermal infiltrate. Erosions may be present.	3–6 μm round to oval, sometimes budding spores, 2–4 μm thick pseudohyphae.

trophils, plasma cells, and multinucleated giant cells. The infiltrate may extend into the subcutis (52). *Candida albicans* usually is present only in the stratum corneum (45,49). In some instances, however, fungal elements are found also within hairs, in the viable epidermis, and in the dermis.

Disseminated Candidiasis

Candida is the fourth leading cause of hospital-acquired bloodstream infection in the United States, but cutaneous involvement is only seen in 13% of cases (53,54). It primarily affects those with impaired host-defense mechanisms, particularly those with hematologic malignancies. *C. albicans* accounts for just over half of the cases of *Candida* fungemia and *C. glabrata* ranks number two, the incidence of the latter increasing directly with age (53,55). Cutaneous lesions of disseminated candidiasis are erythematous or violaceous papulonodules with central clearing that measure 0.5 to 1.0 cm in diameter. They are distributed singly or, more commonly, grouped on the trunk and proximal extremities. The triad of fever, rash, and diffuse muscle tenderness in an immunocompromised host is presumptive for disseminated candidiasis (56). However, the clinical diagnosis may be difficult as patients often present with nonspecific symptoms and current methods for diagnosing candidemia rely on blood cultures that require several days. In addition, the speciation of *Candida* by culture is problematic given that all yeast cultures that form germ tubes and chlamydospores are, by generalization, designated *C. albicans* in many labs (57). Thus, a skin biopsy may be critical to the early diagnosis of disseminated candidiasis. Because the diffuse muscle tenderness is caused by infiltration of muscle tissue by yeast organisms, biopsy of a tender muscle area may also aid in establishing the diagnosis of disseminate candidiasis (58).

Histopathology. Histologic examination reveals one or several aggregates of hyphae and spores focally within the dermis, often at sites of vascular damage and generally visible only in sections stained with the PAS reaction or the GMS stain. Some of the spores, which are 3 to 6 µm in diameter, show budding (54). The aggregates of hyphae and spores may lie in an area of leukocytoclastic vasculitis (59), within a microabscess (57), or in an area of only mild inflammation (54). The aggregates of *Candida* often are small, and step sections through the biopsy specimen may be necessary to find them. The epidermis is usually unaffected.

Candida Onychomycosis

Candida onychomycosis is a form of nail infection characterized by separation of the nail plate from the nail bed. Paronychia and loss of the proximal nail fold are not uncommon in *Candida* infections of the nail unit.

Histopathology. *Candida* commonly causes onycholysis but distinguishes itself histologically from the dermatophytes by its lack of nail plate invasion (23). Yeast forms may be seen along the undersurface of the nail plate. *Candida* may mimic the psoriasiform changes and inflammatory response of onychomycosis caused by dermatophytes. *Candida* species occur as ovoid yeast that measure 3 to 6 µm in diameter, and as pseudohyphae that measure 2 to 4 µm in diameter. These pseudohyphae may be thick, bulbous, and have an irregular caliber compared with the smooth, thin, and regular hyphae of dermatophytes.

ASPERGILLOSIS

Aspergillus species are ubiquitous in the environment. Humans are constantly exposed to and frequently colonized by these organisms, although they rarely cause disease. Severe, invasive aspergillosis typically involves the lungs and is usually seen only in immunocompromised hosts, particularly those with neutropenia, hematologic malignancy, or a history of chronic corticosteroid or antibiotic therapy (60). *Aspergillus fumigatus* is the most common cause of both colonization and invasive aspergillosis, followed in frequency by *A. flavus* and *A. niger* (61). Cutaneous aspergillosis may occur as a primary infection or may be secondary to disseminated aspergillosis (Table 23-4). The lesions of primary cutaneous aspergillosis are usually found at an intravenous infusion site, either at the actual access site (62, 63) or where the unit has been secured with a colonized board or tape (63,64). There may be one or more macules, papules, plaques, or hemorrhagic bullae that may rapidly progress into necrotic ulcers with a surface-heavy black eschar. In immunocompromised patients, dissemination may follow and is often fatal if untreated with amphotericin B, itraconazole, or newer antifungals such as caspofungin (60).

Primary cutaneous infection has been seen in patients with AIDS, but dissemination is not typical in these patients unless they have one or more of the previously mentioned risk factors (65). Umbilicated papules resembling lesions of molluscum contagiosum, and representing "dermatophyte-like" involvement of follicles, has been described in AIDS-related cases (64). In addition, *Aspergillus* may colonize burn or surgical wounds and subsequently invade viable tissue; in these cases the prognosis is generally good (66,67).

Secondary cutaneous aspergillosis, usually associated with invasive lung disease, shows multiple scattered lesions as a result of embolic, hematogenous spread, and has a poor prognosis (60,68).

Histopathology. Unlike most deep cutaneous fungal infections, pseudoepitheliomatous epidermal hyperplasia is not characteristic of cutaneous aspergillosis. In the more serious primary forms and in the secondary disseminated

TABLE 23-4. HISTOLOGIC APPEARANCE OF TISSUE AND FUNGI IN DEEP AND SECONDARY DERMATOMYCOSES

Disease	Histologic appearance	Fungal size and morphology
Aspergillosis	Primary infection: granulomatous infiltrate. Immunocompromised host (primary and secondary infection): angioinvasion, ischemic necrosis, and hemorrhage.	2–4 μm septate hyphae with dichotomous branching at 45-degree angle.
Zygomycosis (mucormycosis, phycomycosis)	Angioinvasion with thrombosis and infarction, necrosis, and variable, mild, neutrophilic infiltrate.	7–30 μm hyphae with branching at irregular angles and intervals. Variably thin, often collapsed or twisted walls.
Subcutaneous phaeohyphomycosis (phaeohyphomycotic cyst)	Deep, coalescing, suppurative granulomatous foci surrounded by fibrous capsule.	Loosely arranged, septate, occasionally branching pigmented hyphae varying from 2 to 25 μm diameter.
Alternariosis	Pseudocarcinomatous epithelial hyperplasia with intraepidermal microabscesses and suppurative granulomatous dermal infiltrate.	5–7 μm septate hyphae with variable branching and brown pigmentation. 3–10 μm round to oval spores, often with double contours.
North American blastomycosis	Pseudocarcinomatous epithelial hyperplasia with intraepidermal microabscesses. Suppurative granulomatous dermal infiltrate with giant cells.	8–15 μm thick-walled spores with single broad-based buds.
Paracoccidioidomycosis	Like North American blastomycosis.	6–20 μm spores with narrow-necked, single or multiple buds. "Mariner's wheels" up to 60 μm in diameter.
Lobomycosis	Atrophic epidermis with dermal macrophage and giant cell infiltrate. Unstained organisms give sievelike appearance to dermis.	9–10 μm "lemon-shaped" spores with single budding, often in chains.
Chromoblastomycosis	Like North American blastomycosis.	6–12 μm thick-walled, dark brown spores, often in clusters. Some cells possess cross walls.
Coccidioidomycosis	Primary inoculation: mixed dermal infiltrate with granulocytes, lymphocytes, and occasional histiocytic giant cells. Systemic: like North American blastomycosis, but granulomas may be more tuberculoid in nature.	10–80 μm thick-walled spores with granular cytoplasm. The larger spores contain endospores.
Cryptococcosis	"Gelatinous reaction" with many spores; "granulomatous reaction" with fewer spores.	4–12 μm spore with wide capsule in "gelatinous reaction"; 2–4 μm spore in "granulomatous reaction."
Histoplasmosis var. *capsulatum*	Suppurative granulomatous infiltrate in ulcerative skin lesions, neutrophils and eosinophils in oral lesions. Histiocytes contain variable numbers of organisms.	2–4 μm round, narrow-necked budding spores with clear halo (pseudocapsule) in the cytoplasm of large histiocytes.
var. *duboisii* (African)	Granulomatous dermal infiltrate with focal suppuration.	8–15 μm ovoid spores in macrophages and free in tissue.
Sporotrichosis	Cutaneous lesions: epidermal hyperplasia with intraepidermal abscesses, suppurative granulomatous dermal infiltrate, occasional asteroid bodies. Subcutaneous nodules: central zone of neutrophils surrounded by zones of epithelioid macrophages and round cells.	4–6 μm round to oval spores.
Eumycetoma	Abscess in granulation tissue, fibrosis, and sinus tracts.	0.5–2.0 mm sulfur granules composed of 4–5 μm thick septate hyphae.
Rhinosporidiosis	Hyperplastic epithelium with papillomatosis, deep invagination with pseudocysts, and "Swiss cheese" corium.	7–12 μm spores, sporangia up to 300 μm.

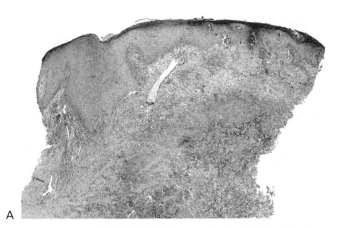

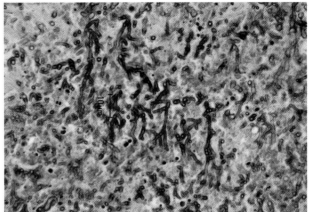

FIGURE 23-7. Aspergillosis. **A:** H&E stain shows a central area of dermal necrosis with branching hyphae. **B:** H&E stain shows septate hyphae branching at an acute angle in a background of necrotic tissue.

form, numerous *Aspergillus* hyphae are seen in the dermis (Fig. 23-7). Hyphae may be seen in hematoxylin-eosin–stained sections, but PAS or silver methenamine staining may be required. The hyphae, which measure 2 to 4 μm in diameter (60), are often arranged in a radiate fashion, are septate, and show branching at an acute angle. Spores are absent. Hyphae may be seen invading blood vessels (60), and may be seen around areas of ischemic necrosis with very little inflammation in some instances. In other cases, there may be an acute inflammatory reaction with polymorphonuclear leukocytes in addition to lymphocytes and histiocytes.

In patients with primary cutaneous or subcutaneous aspergillosis who are otherwise in good health, the number of hyphae present is relatively small, and there may be a well-developed granulomatous reaction (69).

ZYGOMYCOSIS (MUCORMYCOSIS, PHYCOMYCOSIS)

Zygomycosis describes infections by ubiquitous molds of two orders: Mucorales and Entomophthorales. The term mucormycoses describes infection with *Rhizopus* or *Mucor*, the two medically significant genera of the order Mucorales (70). Infections with these organisms are aggressive and often occur in ketotic diabetics but infections may also be seen in other settings such as burns, iatrogenic immunosuppression, chronic renal failure, hematopoietic malignancy, and AIDS (71). Entomophthoraceae may cause chronic cutaneous and subcutaneous infections in otherwise healthy hosts.

Cutaneous zygomycosis occurs by implantation of fungi or by hematogenous dissemination. Three main forms exist: rhinocerebral, primary cutaneous, and chronic subcutaneous zygomycosis.

Rhinocerebral zygomycosis is a fulminant infection of the paranasal sinuses that quickly spreads to contiguous structures such as the skin, nose, orbit, and the brain (70). Clinical findings include nasal discharge, swelling, mucocutaneous ulceration, and eschar formation.

Primary cutaneous zygomycosis may occur following burns, major trauma, or following minor trauma in immunosuppressed patients or those with diabetes (70). It has also been reported after the use of infected tape (72,73). Individual lesions occur early as pustules or blisters that soon ulcerate and form eschars. Depending on the host status, the ulcers either heal or lead to fatal systemic spread (74). These molds may cause acute, rapidly developing, often lethal infections of immunocompromised patients. Cutaneous lesions may also be seen as a result of embolization and infarction in patients with systemic zygomycosis. The lesions may begin as erythematous macules that blister and ulcerate, or may occur as an indurated nodule (75).

Chronic subcutaneous zygomycosis occurs in tropical and subtropical areas in otherwise healthy people. Lesions most commonly occur on the face and are slowly enlarging, painless, firm swellings in the dermis (70).

Histopathology. The histologic changes in zygomycosis are primarily dermal. The hallmark of zygomycosis is vascular invasion by very large, long, nonseptate hyphae with thrombosis and infarction (70,75) (Fig. 23-8A). Hyphae branch at 90-degree angles and may also be found in the surrounding tissue (76). The hyphae are thin-walled, so that they may be twisted or collapsed and often appear ring-shaped or oval in cross-sections or tangential sections (Fig. 23-8B) (70). They are often easily located even in routinely stained sections because of their very large size, up to 30 μm in diameter, although they may be visualized even better in PAS- or GMS-stained sections. Spores are rarely seen.

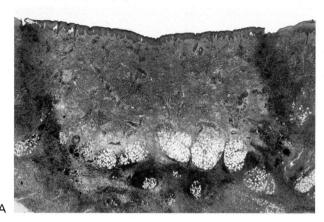
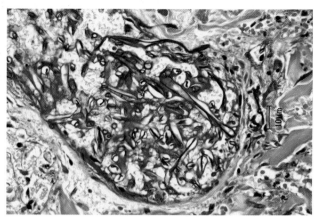

FIGURE 23-8. Zygomycosis (mucormycosis). **A:** H&E stain shows infarction of dermis, epidermis, and subcutaneous fat with lymphohistiocytic and neutrophilic infiltrate, and angioinvasion by broad nonseptate hyphae. **B:** H&E stain shows irregularly branching, twisted, and collapsed hyphae.

SUBCUTANEOUS PHAEOHYPHOMYCOSIS

Phaeohyphomycosis is a subcutaneous or systemic infection caused by dematiaceous, mycelia-forming fungi (77). This is a histopathologic definition of a disease process that can be caused by many different organisms and that can have multiple different clinical presentations. *Bipolaris*, *Phialophora*, *Alternaria*, and *Exophiala* are fungi responsible for phaeohyphomycosis (78,79). Phaeohyphomycosis has been labeled a "chronic mycosis" in the past, but is distinct from chromomycosis, which is characterized by pigmented spores without hyphal forms. Although eumycetoma caused by dematiaceous fungi could be included under this definition, that has not generally been the case, probably since eumycetoma is such a distinctive clinical entity (80).

Phaeohyphomycetes often infect people who are not overtly immunosuppressed. However, immunosuppression does increase the risk of infection with less commonly pathogenic phaeohyphomycetes, such as *Alternaria infectoria*, as well as the risk for disseminated disease (81,82).

Subcutaneous phaeohyphomycosis typically presents as a solitary abscess or nodule on the extremity of an adult male. A history of trauma or a splinter can sometimes be elicited. The other major clinical forms of phaeohyphomycosis are infections of the paranasal sinuses and of the central nervous system.

Histopathology. Lesions of subcutaneous phaeohyphomycosis start as small, often stellate foci of suppurative granulomatous inflammation. The area of inflammation gradually enlarges and usually forms a single large cavity with a surrounding fibrous capsule, the so-called phaeohyphomycotic cyst (83) (Fig. 23-9A). The central space is filled with pus formed of polymorphonuclear leukocytes and fibrin. There is a surrounding granulomatous reaction composed of histiocytes, including epithelioid cells and

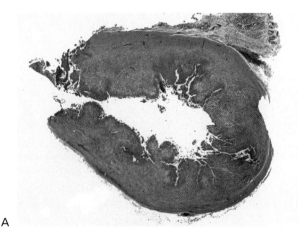
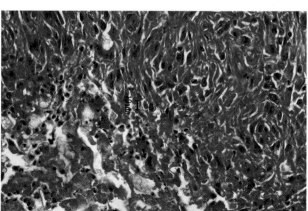

FIGURE 23-9. Phaeohyphomycosis. **A:** H&E stain shows a pseudocyst with a large central cavity and a fibrous capsule. **B:** H&E stain shows pigmented hyphal forms at edge of cavity.

multinucleated giant cells, lymphocytes, and plasma cells. Diligent searching may identify an associated splinter in the tissue or liquid pus. The organisms are found within the cavity and at its edge, often within histiocytes (Fig. 23-9B). The hyphae often have irregularly placed branches and show constrictions around their septae that may cause them to resemble pseudohyphae or yeast forms, but true yeast forms are rare. Mycelia, if present, are more loosely arranged than the compact masses of hyphae seen in eumycetoma. Pigment is not always obvious, and may be highlighted using the Fontana–Masson stain (78).

Pathogenesis. The subcutaneous cystic type of phaeohyphomycosis is usually caused by *Phialophora gougerotii* (formerly called *Sporotrichum gougerotii*) (84). In rare instances, it is due to *Exophiala* (*Fonsecaea*, *Wangiella*) dermatitidis (85). Melanin is directly involved in the virulence of phaeohyphomycetes. Strains of these fungi that lack pigment demonstrate reduced virulence in mouse models (86,87). Nondematiaceous strains have decreased resistance to fungicidal effects of the phagolysosome (88). Melanin is able to scavenge free radicals used by phagocytic cells to kill fungi. Melanin may also bind the hydrolytic enzymes used by phagocytic cells to lyse fungal cell membranes. These factors may help explain the virulence of phaeohyphomycetes in immunocompetent patients.

Differential Diagnosis. The organisms of phaeohyphomycosis can be distinguished from *Aspergillus* species because the latter have hyphae with relatively uniform diameter and regular dichotomous branching (89). Furthermore, disseminated aspergillosis is associated with vascular invasion, ischemic necrosis, and relatively less inflammation.

CUTANEOUS ALTERNARIOSIS

Because the hyphae of *Alternaria* species are pigmented, alternariosis may also be considered a phaeohyphomycosis. *Alternaria* species commonly colonize human skin (90), but

are generally nonpathogenic for humans. Cutaneous alternariosis may occur following trauma (91) via colonization of a preexisting lesion, which usually consists of dermatitis of the face that has been treated topically with corticosteroids (92), or rarely, by hematologic spread, most likely from pulmonary infection caused by inhalation of the organism. Patients with cutaneous alternariosis are often debilitated or immunocompromised or receiving immunosuppressive therapy (89,93). Despite the increasing prevalence of HIV infection, however, the disease is rare in patients with AIDS (94). Morphologically, the lesions of cutaneous alternariosis are so variable as to be nonspecific, and include crusted ulcers, verrucous or granulomatous and multilocular lesions, (92), and subcutaneous nodules (91).

Histopathology. Although fungi are found mainly in the deeper layers of the dermis. In the subcutaneous region in the hematogenous and the traumatogenic forms, they are localized predominantly in the epidermis in cases in which *Alternaria* colonizes preexisting lesions (92). The dermis shows a suppurative granulomatous reaction associated with variable pseudoepitheliomatous epidermal hyperplasia and ulceration. Organisms may be present both as broad, branching, brown septate hyphae, 5 to 7 μm thick (80) (Fig. 23-10), and as large, round to oval, often doubly contoured spores measuring 3 to 10 μm in diameter (92). The spores may be seen both lying free in the tissue (90), and within macrophages and giant cells (95). There may be intraepidermal microabscesses with hyphae in the stratum corneum and stratum spinosum (90). The hyphae and spores stain deeply with PAS or silver methenamine.

NORTH AMERICAN BLASTOMYCOSIS

North American blastomycosis, caused by *Blastomyces dermatitidis*, occurs in three forms: primary cutaneous inoculation blastomycosis, pulmonary blastomycosis, and systemic blastomycosis (96).

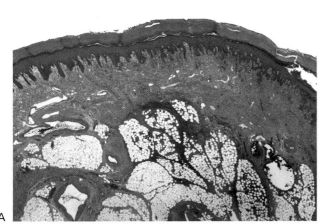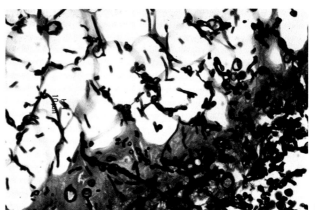

FIGURE 23-10. Alternariosis. **A:** H&E stain shows a mixed inflammatory infiltrate in the deep dermis and subcutaneous fat. **B:** GMS stain shows broad branching hyphae.

Primary cutaneous inoculation blastomycosis is very rare and occurs almost exclusively as a laboratory or autopsy room infection. It starts at the site of injury on a hand or wrist as an indurated, ulcerated, chancriform solitary lesion. Lymphangitis and lymphadenitis may develop in the affected arm. Small nodules may be present along the involved lymph vessel. Spontaneous healing takes place within a few weeks or months (97).

Pulmonary blastomycosis, the usual route of acquisition of the infection, may be asymptomatic or may produce mild to moderately severe, acute pulmonary signs, such as fever, chest pain, cough, and hemoptysis. The pulmonary lesions either resolve or progress to chronic pulmonary blastomycosis with cavity formation. In rare instances, acute pulmonary blastomycosis is accompanied by erythema nodosum (98). Occasionally, however, cutaneous lesions are the only clinical manifestation after pulmonary infection (99). This phenomenon of a benign systemic disease presenting with cutaneous lesions may also be seen rarely after infection with coccidioidomycosis, cryptococcosis, histoplasmosis, and sporotrichosis. In the benign systemic form of blastomycosis with only cutaneous lesions, the lesions usually are on the face and are of the verrucous type (100).

In systemic blastomycosis, the lungs are the primary sites of infection. Granulomatous and suppurative lesions may occur in many different organs, but aside from the lungs, they are most commonly found in the skin, followed by the bones, the male genital system, the oral and nasal mucosa, and the central nervous system. Untreated systemic blastomycosis has a mortality rate in excess of 80% (101). Antimycotic therapy can reduce mortality to 10% in otherwise uncomplicated cases, but systemic blastomycosis has a particularly aggressive course in immunosuppressed patients and carries at least a 30% mortality rate even with treatment (102,103).

Cutaneous lesions are very common in systemic blastomycosis, occurring in about 70% of patients. They may be solitary or numerous. They occur either as verrucous lesions, the more common type, or as ulcerative lesions. Verrucous lesions show central healing with scarring and a slowly advancing, raised, verrucous border that is beset by a large number of pustules or small, crusted abscesses. Ulcerative lesions begin as pustules and rapidly develop into ulcers with a granulating base. In addition, subcutaneous abscesses may occur; they usually develop as an extension of bone lesions. Lesions of the oral or nasal mucosa may present either as ulcers or as heaped-up masses of friable tissue. In some instances, they are contiguous with cutaneous lesions (101). An unusual early cutaneous manifestation of systemic blastomycosis is a pustular eruption that may be widespread (104) or largely acral in distribution (105).

Histopathology. Early lesions of blastomycosis demonstrate a dermal inflammatory infiltrate of polymorphonuclear leukocytes with numerous organisms. After a few weeks, occasional giant cells may be seen. Later, a verrucous histologic pattern with pseudoepitheliomatous hyperplasia similar to that seen in skin lesions of systemic blastomycosis is characteristic (Fig. 23-11A). The regional lymph nodes show a granulomatous reaction with numerous giant cells, in which the organisms are predominantly located (106).

A biopsy from the active border of a verrucous lesion will best demonstrate diagnostic histopathology. There is considerable downward proliferation of the epidermis, often amounting to pseudocarcinomatous hyperplasia. Intraepidermal abscesses often are present. Occasionally, multinucleated giant cells are completely enclosed by the proliferating epidermis. The dermis is permeated by a polymorphous infiltrate. Neutrophils usually are present in large numbers and form small abscesses. Multinucleated giant cells are scattered throughout the dermis. Usually they lie alone and not within groups of epithelioid cells.

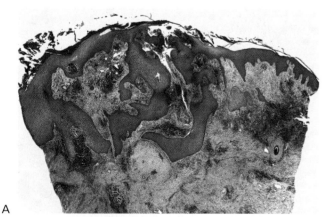

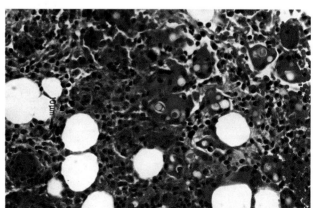

FIGURE 23-11. North American blastomycosis. **A:** H&E stain shows marked, pseudoepitheliomatous hyperplasia with intraepidermal microabscess formation. **B:** H&E stain shows broad-based budding spore (*arrow*) in multinucleated giant cell.

Occasionally, there are tuberculoid formations, although without evidence of caseation necrosis (107). In the ulcerative lesions, the dermal changes are the same as in the verrucous lesions, but the epidermis is absent.

The spores of *B. dermatitidis* are found in histologic sections often only after a diligent search, usually in clusters of neutrophils or within giant cells (Fig. 23-11B). One or several spores may lie within a giant cell where they are easily spotted even in hematoxylin- and eosin-stained sections. Unstained, the spores resemble small, round holes punched out of the cytoplasm of the giant cells. On high magnification, the spores are seen to have a thick wall, which gives them a double-contoured appearance. They measure 8 to 15 µm in diameter (average 10 µm). Occasionally, spores show a single broad-based bud. As in most fungal infections, many more spores are visualized in sections stained with the PAS reaction or with methenamine silver than in routinely stained sections.

Pathogenesis. The diagnosis of *B. dermatitidis* is based on finding physical evidence of the organism because reliable serologic tests are not available and clinical examinations are nonspecific. Fine needle aspiration or wet prep of wound fluid fixed in 95% alcohol and stained with Papanicolaou and H& E stain is a rapid means to find diagnostic broad-based budding forms (108,109). Also of great value is the demonstration of the spores of *B. dermatitidis* in tissue sections either by direct immunofluorescence (110) or by immunoperoxidase (111). The required antiserum is prepared in rabbits with pure cultures of fungi and is conjugated either with fluorescein isothiocyanate or with horseradish peroxide. The antiserum can be applied to fresh as well as to formalin-fixed, paraffin-embedded tissue sections. Prior staining with hematoxylin-eosin does not interfere with the procedure.

Corresponding antisera are valuable also for the demonstration of the spores of *Sporothrix schenckii*, *Cryptococcus neoformans* (111), *C. albicans*, *C. tropicalis*, *C. krausei*, *Aspergillus*, and *Histoplasma capsulatum* (112).

Differential Diagnosis. The verrucous lesions of systemic blastomycosis must be differentiated from other deep fungal infections, tuberculosis verrucosa cutis, halogenodermas, and squamous cell carcinoma. Mucicarmine staining, which highlights the capsule of *Cryptococcus neoformans*, allows its differentiation from the spores of *B. dermatitidis*, and the narrow-necked budding forms of *H. capsulatum* can be distinguished from the broader-based buds of *B. dermatitidis* without special stains. Tuberculosis verrucosa cutis shows no spores in the tissue, the number of neutrophils is smaller, and areas of caseation necrosis usually are present. Halogenodermas may be difficult to differentiate from a deep fungal infection without obvious organisms, but the presence of intraepidermal abscesses, a mixed dermal inflammatory infiltrate, and multinucleated giant cells is usually sufficient to rule out squamous cell carcinoma. Keratoacanthoma shares morphologic features with blastomycosis including a verrucous architecture and intraepidermal abscesses. However, keratoacanthoma has a high degree of keratinization, a glassy appearance of the keratinocytes, and an abrupt cut-off between the central crater and adjacent epidermis.

PARACOCCIDIOIDOMYCOSIS

Paracoccidioidomycosis, also called *South American blastomycosis* because it occurs almost exclusively in South and Central America, is a chronic granulomatous disease caused by *Paracoccidioides brasiliensis*.

P. brasiliensis almost always gains entrance into the human body through inhalation and infects the lungs, where there is a subclinical infection that can be recognized only through a positive paracoccidioidin skin test (113). The typical patient with clinical disease is an adult male with an indolent, slowly progressive course. The first clinical manifestation is usually lesions in the oropharynx and on the gingivae. The lesions in the mouth begin as papules and nodules that then ulcerate. Subsequently, extensive granulomatous, ulcerated lesions develop in the mouth, nose, larynx, and pharynx. Extensive cervical lymphadenopathy develops, with suppuration of some of the lymph nodes. The oral lesions may extend to the neighboring skin, with formation of similar granulomatous, ulcerated lesions around the mouth and nose (113).

Through both lymphatic and hematogenous spread, the disease may subsequently involve many lymph nodes, both subcutaneous and visceral, and the lower gastrointestinal tract. In cases with wide dissemination, the lungs are clinically involved, presenting a picture greatly resembling chronic pulmonary tuberculosis (114). Adrenal insufficiency due to destruction of the adrenal glands, uncommon in other systemic mycoses except histoplasmosis, is not infrequent (115). Rarely, widely scattered cutaneous lesions resulting from hematogenous spread are observed during the stage of dissemination. The lesions may be papular, pustular, nodular, papillomatous, or ulcerated (116).

The disease develops and disseminates more rapidly in children, the so-called subacute progressive juvenile form (117). Although experience is limited, it appears that there is little effect on the course of paracoccidioidomycosis in early HIV infection, but that HIV patients with severe immunosuppression are at risk for a more fulminant course (118).

Histopathology. Examination of cutaneous or mucosal lesions reveals a granulomatous infiltrate showing epithelioid and giant cells in association with an acute inflammatory infiltrate and abscess formation (119). Spores may lie within giant cells or free in the infiltrate, especially in the abscesses. They are best demonstrated with the PAS reaction or with methenamine silver. Pseudoepitheliomatous hyperplasia may be marked (Fig. 23-12A).

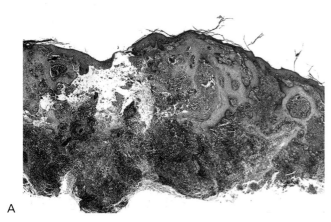

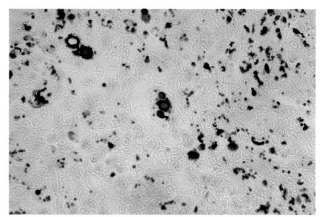

A   B

FIGURE 23-12. Paracoccidioidomycosis. **A:** H&E stain shows marked pseudoepitheliomatous epidermal hyperplasia with microabscess formation and a mixed dermal infiltrate. **B:** GMS stain shows variably sized yeast, some with multiple buds.

Many of the spores present in the tissue show only single, usually narrow-based buds or no buds at all (116). In the rare spores with multiple budding, peripheral buds are distributed over the whole surface of the ball-shaped fungus cell (Fig. 23-12B). Because of protrusion of the peripheral buds, such yeast cells in cross sections have the appearance of a marine pilot's wheel. Whereas nonbudding or singly budding spores measure from 6 to 20 μm in diameter, spores with multiple budding may measure up to 60 μm in size.

Differential Diagnosis. B. dermatitides and *Cryptococcus neoformans* may be difficult to distinguish from *Paracoccidioides* when only single budding organisms are seen. North American blastomycosis is distinguished by its thick refractile wall and broad-based blastospores. The capsule of *C. neoformans* stains with mucicarmine, and is thus specifically identified.

LOBOMYCOSIS

Lobomycosis is an extremely indolent fungal infection characterized by asymptomatic, usually smooth, nodular lesions that resemble keloids on the ear, face, or extremity. The lesions may coalesce to form plaques, but generally are limited to one area. Although the lesions persist, the condition is limited to the skin, except for occasional involvement of a regional lymph node (120). The infection, which is probably caused by a minor local injury, occurs sporadically in the South American tropics and in Panama (121). The causative fungus is designated *Loboa loboi*.

Histopathology. The dermis shows an extensive infiltrate of macrophages and large giant cells separated from a usually atrophic epidermis by a Grenz zone. Scattered lymphocytes and plasma cells are present, but neutrophils are not typically present. Numerous fungus spores lie both within

these cells and outside of them, and because the fungus does not stain with hematoxylin-eosin, there may be so many unstained areas that the section may have a sieve-like appearance (122) (Fig. 23-13).

On staining with the PAS reaction or with methenamine silver, the fungus spores are on average 10 μm in diameter. They possess a thick capsule, about 1 μm in thickness, with a tip that gives the organisms a distinctive "lemon-like" appearance. The spores occasionally show single budding, and often form single chains joined together by small, tubular bridges (123).

Pathogenesis. The macrophages contain abundant PAS-positive granular material that appears to consist of fragments of fungal capsules, indicating that the host macrophages are unable to digest the glycoproteins in the capsules (124).

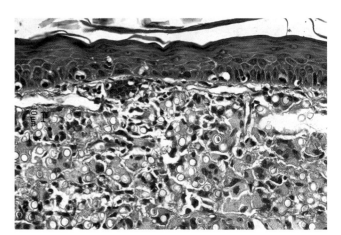

FIGURE 23-13. Lobomycosis. A diffuse dermal infiltrate of multinucleated giant cells containing spores is present beneath a flattened epidermis (H&E stain).

CHROMOBLASTOMYCOSIS

Chromoblastomycosis is a slowly progressive cutaneous mycosis caused by pigmented (dematiaceous) fungi that occur as round, nonbudding forms in tissue sections. Inasmuch as budding is absent, the designation chromo*blasto*mycosis is somewhat inappropriate. In the past, the related term *chromomycosis* has been used for these infections as well as for subcutaneous and cerebral infections by dematiaceous fungi in which hyphal forms almost always predominate. These two latter types of infections are clinically and histologically distinct and are usually classified as phaeohyphomycoses (125).

Chromoblastomycosis is most often caused by one of five closely related species: *Phialophora verrucosa, Fonsecaea pedrosoi, F. compactum, Exophiala (Fonsecaea, Wangiella) jeanselmei, E. spinifera, Rhinocladiella aquaspera,* and *Cladosporium carrionii* may each produce chromoblastomycosis (126). These fungi are saprophytes and thus can be found growing in soil, decaying vegetation, or rotten wood in subtropical and tropical countries. The primary lesion is thought to develop as a result of traumatic implantation of the fungus into the skin (127).

The cutaneous lesions generally arise on the lower extremities and are variably pruritic papular, nodular, verrucous, or plaque-like lesions (126,127). While some of the lesions heal with scarring, new ones may appear in the vicinity as a result of spreading of the fungus along superficial lymphatic vessels (128), or autoinoculation (125). Lymphatic disruption with elephantiasis may occur.

Hematogenous dissemination may cause extensive cutaneous lesions (129), but it is a rare event, even in immunocompromised persons, and the disease is not as aggressive as other systemic fungal infections that secondarily involve the skin (130).

Histopathology. Cutaneous chromoblastomycosis resembles North American blastomycosis in that both demonstrate a lichenoid-granulomatous inflammatory pattern. In chromoblastomycosis, there is pseudoepitheliomatous epidermal hyperplasia and an extensive dermal infiltrate composed of many epithelioid histiocytes (131). Other components of the infiltrate include multinucleated giant cells, small abscesses and clusters of neutrophils, and variable numbers of lymphocytes, plasma cells, and eosinophils. Tuberculoid formations may be present, but caseation necrosis is absent (132,133).

Fungi are found within giant cells as well as free in the tissue, especially in the abscesses. They appear as conspicuous, dark brown, thick-walled, ovoid or spheric spores varying in size from 6 to 12 μm, and may lie either singly or in chains or clusters (125) (Fig. 23-14). Because of their brown pigmentation, the spores can be easily seen without the use of special stains. Reproduction is by intracellular wall formation and septation, not by budding, and in some of the spores cross walls can be seen. In cases demonstrating marked hyperplasia of the epidermis, fungal spores can be seen within microabscesses or giant cells as in North American blastomycosis. Transepidermal elimination of fungal spores may be observed, resulting in clinically visible black dots (134,135).

Pathogenesis. Although percutaneous inoculation of the fungus is widely accepted as the mode of infection, the fact that the cutaneous manifestations show no chancriform syndrome but rather a granulomatous infiltrate resembling that of North American blastomycosis suggests that the cutaneous lesions of chromomycosis may arise by hematogenous dissemination from a silent primary pulmonary focus. Though this view is supported by occasional reports of hematogenous dissemination and by the observation of multiple areas of calcification in the chest x-ray film of a

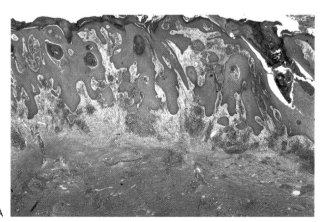
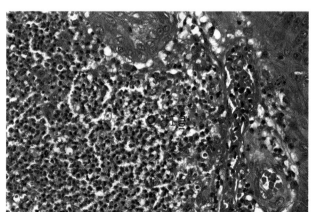

FIGURE 23-14. Chromoblastomycosis. **A:** H&E stain shows pseudoepitheliomatous epidermal hyperplasia with microabscess formation and a mixed inflammatory infiltrate. **B:** Pigmented spores (adjacent to scale marker) resembling "copper pennies" are surrounded by a neutrophilic infiltrate (H&E stain).

patient with chromoblastomycosis (136), convincing evidence is lacking. In support of the concept that cutaneous inoculation may cause cutaneous chromoblastomycosis, pigmented fungal elements were found on embedded wood splinters associated with a foreign-body reaction and in direct contact with the surrounding dermis in two patients (137), and one patient developed classic cutaneous chromoblastomycosis caused by *F. pedrosoi* after trauma with a tree branch containing the same organisms (138).

COCCIDIOIDOMYCOSIS

Coccidioidomycosis, also known as Valley fever, is caused by the dimorphic fungus *Coccidioides immitis*. Like blastomycosis, it occurs in three forms: primary cutaneous inoculation coccidioidomycosis, pulmonary coccidioidomycosis, and systemic coccidioidomycosis. This soil-dwelling organism is endemic in the Southwestern United States, especially in the San Joaquin and Sacramento Valleys, in southern Arizona, and in Mexico (139). Inhalation of aerosolized arthrospores accounts for the vast majority of infections with *coccidioides*. Approximately 60% of those infected are asymptomatic and of the symptomatic patients, 90% to 99% experience only mild flu-like symptoms (139).

Primary cutaneous inoculation coccidioidomycosis is very rare. In a few instances, as in primary cutaneous inoculation blastomycosis, it has occurred as a laboratory or an autopsy room infection (140–142); but, unlike primary cutaneous inoculation blastomycosis, it has also been found as a naturally occurring infection through injuries by contaminated thorns or splinters (143,144). A tender, ulcerated nodule forms within 1 to 3 weeks at the site of inoculation and may enlarge into a granulomatous, ulcerated plaque. This is followed, as in the case of accidental inoculation with *B. dermatitidis*, by regional lymphangitis and lymphadenitis. Healing usually takes place within a few months, but in one reported patient, meningitis developed, requiring prolonged intrathecal treatment with amphotericin B (144).

Pulmonary coccidioidomycosis is the most common form of the infection; epidemiologic skin test studies suggest that between 30% and 90% of the population in the Southwestern United States have been infected (145–147). The fungus is resident in the soil of these arid or semiarid areas and arthrospores are inhaled by the host when the soil is disturbed. Most immunocompetent infected individuals are asymptomatic, although about 40% will develop transient symptoms of an acute respiratory infection. The development of erythema nodosum is not uncommon, but most individuals recover without serious sequelae (148). In 2% to 8% of the cases, however, the pulmonary lesions progress to chronic disease with cavity formation before finally healing (149).

Systemic coccidioidomycosis follows the primary pulmonary infection in only about 1 of 10,000 cases in otherwise immunocompetent Caucasians. However, Mexicans are about 5 times, blacks 25 times, and Filipinos 175 times more likely to acquire systemic disease than whites, which has a mortality rate of about 50% when untreated (139, 150). Studies of this difference have focused on human leukocyte antigen (HLA) genes that produce molecules responsible for antigen presentation to T cells, the portion of the immune system important in elimination of fungi. Some studies have shown HLA subtypes A9 and B5 as well as ABO blood group B to be associated with disseminated coccidioidomycosis, and each occurs with greater frequency in African Americans and Filipinos than Caucasians. The risk of dissemination and a fatal outcome is also greater in HIV-infected patients, particularly those with AIDS (151,152). Disseminated coccidioidomycosis may occasionally represent the first manifestation of AIDS (151). Immunosuppressive therapy may cause activation of a latent pulmonary infection of coccidioidomycosis. Dissemination of the infection after iatrogenic immunosuppression is frequently explosive and may be fatal (150). Therefore, all patients with a history of travel or residence in endemic areas should receive a coccidioidin skin test and have a chest roentgenogram before immunosuppressive therapy is initiated (153). In systemic coccidioidomycosis, many organs, especially the meninges, lungs, bones, and lymph nodes, may be involved. Coccidioidal fungemia often occurs in severe, acute forms of systemic coccidioidomycosis and is associated with a high mortality (151).

Cutaneous lesions occur in 15% to 20% of the cases of systemic coccidioidomycosis (154). They may consist of verrucous papules, nodules, or plaques, or of subcutaneous abscesses, which may break through the skin to form draining sinuses. One or a few cutaneous nodules or plaques may occasionally be the only clinical manifestation of systemic coccidioidomycosis, heralding a relatively good prognosis (153,154). A rare manifestation is the sudden widespread appearance of small pustules on an erythematous base (155), just as has been described in North American blastomycosis.

Histopathology. In primary cutaneous inoculation coccidioidomycosis, one observes a dense dermal inflammatory infiltrate of neutrophils, eosinophils, lymphoid cells, and plasma cells with an occasional giant cell. Small abscesses may be seen (140). Spores, and in some cases also hyphae, are present (154). The regional lymph nodes show a well-developed granulomatous reaction consisting of epithelioid and giant cells. Spores are found within and outside the giant cells.

The verrucous nodules and plaques of the skin in systemic coccidioidomycosis histologically resemble those of North American blastomycosis (Fig. 23-15A). However, they show less of a tendency toward abscess formation, and caseation necrosis may occur (107). The causative organ-

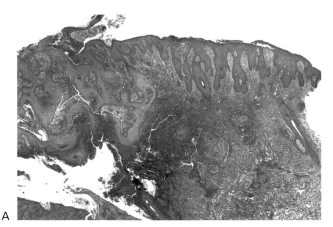
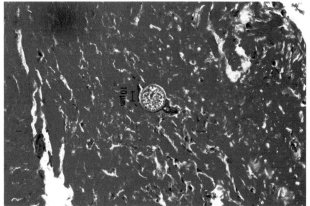

A
B

FIGURE 23-15. Coccidioidomycosis. **A:** The low-power pattern is similar to that of North American blastomycosis with pseudoepitheliomatous epidermal hyperplasia and a mixed inflammatory infiltrate (H&E stain). **B:** A large round thick-walled spore with granular cytoplasm is present in a background of necrotic tissue (H&E stain).

isms are found as spores, free in the tissue and within multinucleated giant cells, and as a rule, they are present in large numbers.

The subcutaneous abscesses show a central area of necrosis surrounded by a granulomatous infiltrate that is tuberculoid in type and composed of lymphoid cells, plasma cells, epithelioid cells, and some giant cells. Numerous spores are present extracellularly as well as intracellularly in the giant cells (107). The pustules seen in a few cases show the presence of spores within them (156).

The nodose skin lesions occurring in primary pulmonary coccidioidomycosis have the same histologic appearance as those in idiopathic erythema nodosum (156).

The spores of *Coccidioides immitis* vary in size from 10 to 80 μm (Fig. 23-15B), the average size being about 40 μm. Thus, the fungi of *Coccidioides* are much larger than those of *Blastomyces*, *Cryptococcus*, or *Phialophora*. The spores are round and thick-walled and have a granular cytoplasm. Multiplication takes place by the formation of endospores, which may be seen lying inside the larger spores. The endospores are released into the tissue by rupture of the spore wall. Endospores may measure up to 10 μm in diameter.

Pathogenesis. The coccidioidin skin test, which consists of the intradermal injection of 0.1 ml of a 1:100 dilution of coccidioidin, is of value in distinguishing between primary pulmonary infection and systemic infection. The test converts from negative to positive within a few weeks of the primary pulmonary infection and remains positive in patients with adequate immunity. Patients with erythema multiforme or nodose lesions are exquisitely sensitive to coccidioidin, and even higher dilutions have been recommended for use in such cases (157). In contrast, patients with disseminated disease tend to have a persistently negative skin test (142).

CRYPTOCOCCOSIS

Cryptococcosis is an infection caused by the yeast *Cryptococcus neoformans* that occurs throughout much of the world. *C. neoformans* is found in the excreta of birds, mainly pigeons and chickens, and in soil contaminated by them. The yeast is spread by aerosol, and transient colonization of the respiratory tract and skin of humans is not rare (158). Primary cutaneous (inoculation) cryptococcosis is extremely rare (159,160). The organism generally enters the body through the respiratory tract, where it can cause symptomatic or asymptomatic infection, either of which may be followed by hematogenous spread (161). Although clinical disease occurs in some apparently normal individuals, it usually develops in immunocompromised hosts, especially those with AIDS (162), but also in patients taking corticosteroids (163,164), and in patients with hematopoietic malignancies (165,166) or sarcoidosis (166–168).

Meningitis is the most common clinical manifestation of systemic infection. Symptom onset is insidious. Patients report a dull headache most commonly with little fever until late in the disease. Other signs of meningeal irritation such as nuchal rigidity are absent (161). In addition, there may be osseous lesions and involvement of the kidneys and prostate. Cutaneous lesions are found in 10% to 15% of the cases of systemic cryptococcosis (169). In rare instances, lesions of the oral mucosa also occur (165). Without adequate treatment, mortality with the systemic form is 70% to 80%; untreated cerebromeningeal cryptococcosis is almost invariably fatal. Cryptococcemia is an extremely grave prognostic sign (161,170).

In some instances of systemic cryptococcosis, central nervous system involvement is not seen, and there are only one or a few lesions in the skin, lymph nodes, bones, or eyes. In cases in which only cutaneous lesions are present, the disease may take a benign course, ending with healing of the lesions, even without treatment (171,172). However, cutaneous lesions may be the presenting sign of systemic cryptococcosis, and may be followed by wide dissemination of the disease with a fatal ending (161,170).

Cutaneous lesions are variable and may consist of papules, pustules, herpetiform vesicles, nodules, infiltrated plaques, subcutaneous swellings or abscesses, or ulcers (169). Lesions resembling those of molluscum contagiosum, Kaposi's sarcoma, or acne have been described in patients with AIDS (173–175). In infections limited to the skin, generally only one or possibly two lesions are present, but in cases with widespread systemic infection, there are often multiple cutaneous lesions (163,169).

Cryptococcal cellulitis is a variant form that may occasionally be limited to the skin. This form has an abrupt onset and spreads rapidly. There may be multiple sites of involvement (176). It is seen only in markedly immunosuppressed hosts, especially in renal transplant patients (177).

Histopathology. Two types of histologic reaction to infection with *C. neoformans* may occur in the skin as well as elsewhere: gelatinous and granulomatous. Both types may be seen in the same skin lesion (161,164). Gelatinous lesions show numerous organisms in aggregates and only very little tissue reaction (Fig. 23-16A). In contrast, granulomatous lesions show a pronounced tissue reaction consisting of histiocytes, giant cells, lymphoid cells, and fibroblasts. Areas of necrosis may also be seen and the organisms are present in a much smaller number than in gelatinous lesions, found mainly within giant cells and histiocytes or occasionally free in the tissue (178).

C. neoformans, a round to ovoid spore, measures from 4 to 12 μm in diameter in the gelatinous reaction but often only 2 to 4 μm in the granulomatous reaction (178) (Fig. 23-16B). The spore stains with the PAS reaction, the methenamine silver stain and shows a dark brown or black color with the Fontana–Masson stain, which completely disappears with melanin bleach (179). Like *Blastomyces dermatitidis*, it multiplies by budding. In the gelatinous reaction pattern, a broad capsule surrounds the fungus and there is very little infiltration of inflammatory cells. The capsule does not stain with hematoxylin-eosin or with the PAS reaction, but because of the presence of acid mucopolysaccharides, it stains metachromatically purple with methylene blue (180), blue with Alcian blue (181), and red with mucicarmine (182). When the Alcian blue stain and the PAS reaction are combined, the yeast cell stains red and the surrounding capsule blue. However, when the yeast cells do not form a capsule, an intense granulomatous inflammatory reaction of histiocytes, giant cells, lymphocytes, and fibroblasts is elicited (179).

Cryptococcal cellulitis shows nonspecific acute and chronic inflammation in which cryptococcal organisms can be demonstrated with the PAS and mucicarmine stains (177).

Pathogenesis. Cryptococcus neoformans is inhaled as a relatively small, nonencapsulated organism measuring approximately 3 μm in diameter. Under favorable nutrient conditions in the human host, the size of the organism increases up to 12 μm, and a wide gelatinous capsule forms. The lack of tissue reaction to encapsulated *C. neoformans* is best explained by the fact that the thick capsule prevents organism contact with the host tissue, and thus inhibits phagocytosis of the organism (178). Failure of the organism to form a capsule probably is the result of a defect in one of its metabolic pathways (179).

On electron microscopy, the mucinous capsule of *C. neoformans* is seen to consist of radially arranged fibrillary material, with the fibrils intertwining and having a beaded appearance (183).

Ever since cases of cryptococcosis with only one or a few cutaneous lesions have been described, some authors have

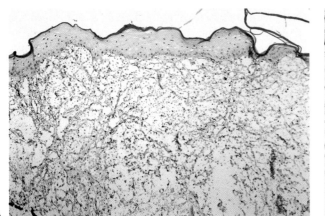
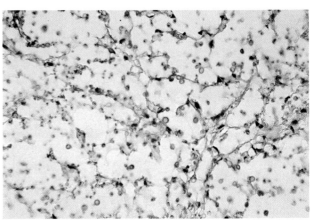

FIGURE 23-16. Cryptococcosis. **A:** H&E stain shows spores surrounded by wide capsules with relatively little inflammatory reaction. **B:** Spores, but not their capsules, can be visualized in routine stained sections (H&E stain).

assumed that a purely cutaneous form of cryptococcosis produced by cutaneous inoculation exists (184,185). However, the fact that purely cutaneous lesions show no chancriform syndrome with regional lymphadenopathy speaks against the theory of primary inoculation of the skin (163). It has been recommended that all cases that seem to be purely cutaneous cryptococcosis should be considered potentially disseminated (186). Cultural studies should include the spinal fluid, sputum, prostatic fluid, and urine to rule out disseminated disease (187). Of note, there are multiple reports of cross-reactivity of *Cryptococcus* with unrelated fungi with the use of agglutination kits (188,189). Confirmation of a positive capsular antigen test with a second test helps limit false positives.

Differential Diagnosis. In the granulomatous type of reaction, *C. neoformans* may have no capsule, may be small, with an average diameter of only 3 μm, and is found largely within macrophages and giant cells. Histologic differentiation from *B. dermatitidis*, which also reproduces by budding, *H. capsulatum*, and other fungi, may then be difficult. However, only *C. neoformans* stains black with the Fontana–Masson stain (179).

HISTOPLASMOSIS

Histoplasmosis is found throughout the world, but the largest endemic focus is in the central eastern United States, especially the Ohio and lower Mississippi river valleys, where 85% to 90% of the population has positive skin tests for histoplasmin (190). It has been estimated that 40 million persons have undergone pulmonary infection with *H. capsulatum*, and that there are 200,000 new cases annually in the United States (191,192).

Like blastomycosis and coccidioidomycosis, histoplasmosis may occur in three forms: primary cutaneous inoculation histoplasmosis, primary pulmonary histoplasmosis caused by inhalation, and disseminated histoplasmosis.

Primary cutaneous inoculation histoplasmosis, a very rare event, is benign and self-limited in duration. It generally occurs as a laboratory infection and presents as a chancriform syndrome, with a nodule or ulcer at the site of inoculation and associated lymphangitis and lymphadenitis (193,194).

Primary pulmonary histoplasmosis, the common form of infection, is usually asymptomatic, although acute pulmonary histoplasmosis with symptoms resembling those of influenza may develop in a minority of patients. Chronic pulmonary histoplasmosis usually occurs in patients with preexisting lung disease and may result in the formation of cavities (190). It develops in about 1 of 2,000 infections, resembles pulmonary tuberculosis in its symptoms, and may end fatally unless treated. Reactivation of pulmonary histoplasmosis following treatment with infliximab (Remicade) has been reported, and should be considered when fever and pulmonary symptoms develop in these patients (195).

Before the advent of HIV, disseminated histoplasmosis developed in only 1 of 50,000 infections (196), and was usually found in infants, in patients with lymphoma (197,198), or in those receiving immunosuppressive treatment (199). Although not as frequent in the general AIDS population as coccidioidomycosis and cryptococcosis (200), disseminated histoplasmosis can be the most frequent opportunistic infection in AIDS patients living in highly endemic areas (201,202).

Disseminated histoplasmosis presents a variable clinical picture, depending on the degree of parasitization. Cases with severe degrees of parasitization (acute disseminated disease) occur principally in infants and immunosuppressed patients, and may be fatal. There is often high, persistent fever and extensive involvement of the reticuloendothelial system with hepatosplenomegaly; anemia, leukocytopenia, and thrombocytopenia may also be seen. Cases with moderate degrees of parasitization (subacute disseminated disease) occur in both adults and infants, who, if adequately treated, may survive. Fever, hepatosplenomegaly, and bone marrow depression are mild or moderate. Adrenal involvement leading to adrenal insufficiency, as well as gastrointestinal ulceration, meningitis, and endocarditis, are common. Cases with mild degrees of parasitization (chronic disseminated disease) are associated with destructive focal lesions in a number of organs, and occur almost exclusively in adults. There may or may not be fever, hepatosplenomegaly, bone marrow depression, adrenal insufficiency, meningitis, or endocarditis. In the chronic disseminated form, the response to treatment generally is good (193). If no cutaneous or oral lesions are present, the most useful diagnostic method is a bone marrow biopsy and occasionally also biopsy of the liver or of a palpable lymph node (199).

Cutaneous lesions occur in only 6% of patients with disseminated histoplasmosis, but may rarely be the presenting sign (203–205). Cutaneous lesions occur in a wide variety of forms, none of which can be said to be characteristic. Most commonly they consist of primary ulcers, often with annular, heaped-up borders (204,206). They may also consist of papules, nodules, or large plaque-like lesions (203,207). Papules may umbilicate, causing a resemblance to lesions of molluscum contagiosum (208). Lesions may be purpuric or crusted, or may develop pustular caps and ulcerate. There may be tender, red nodules due to panniculitis (209). A rare cutaneous manifestation is a generalized pruritic erythroderma (210,211). In addition, there may be a number of nonspecific cutaneous manifestations associated with histoplasmosis, including erythema nodosum and erythema multiforme (212).

In contrast to the rarity of cutaneous lesions, lesions of the oral mucosa occur in about half of all cases of disseminated histoplasmosis and are not infrequently the presenting sign of the disease (203). Lesions of the oral mucosa often start as painless papular swellings and usually ulcer-

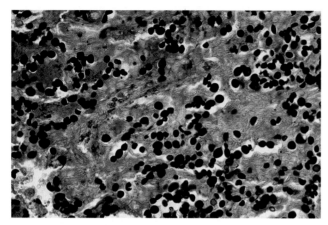

FIGURE 23-17. Histoplasmosis. Large spores of *Histoplasma capsulatum* var. *duboisii* are seen extracellularly and in giant cells (GMS stain).

ate. The contiguous skin may also be involved. Biopsy of a mucosal or cutaneous lesion may be the most rapid method of arriving at a specific diagnosis of disseminated histoplasmosis, and may allow for the rapid institution of lifesaving therapy as culture may require up to a 4-week incubation period (213).

Histopathology. The diagnostic feature in all types of cutaneous histoplasmosis is the presence of tiny 2- to 4-µm spores within the cytoplasm of macrophages and variably within giant cells (207,214). The spores of *H. capsulatum* are visualized in sections stained with hematoxylin and eosin, Gram stain, or Giemsa stain (Fig. 23-17). They appear as round or oval bodies surrounded by a clear space that was originally interpreted as a capsule, giving rise to the name *H. capsulatum*. The spores, not including the clear space surrounding them, measure from 2 to 4 µm in diameter. Silver impregnation stains and electron microscopic studies show that *H. capsulatum* does not possess a capsule and that the inner portion of the clear space represents the cell wall of the fungus and the clear space itself is filled with granular material that separates the cell wall of the fungus from the cytoplasm of the macrophage (214). On electron microscopy, it can be seen that each spore of *H. capsulatum*, including its halo, is located within a phagosome that is lined by a trilaminar membrane (214).

In acute disseminated histoplasmosis, lesions consist mostly of heavily parasitized histiocytes with relatively little surrounding tissue reaction. Cutaneous lesions in the chronic form of the disease tend to be composed of better-differentiated macrophages with fewer organisms (203). A suppurative granulomatous pattern may develop, especially in ulcerated lesions. There may be foci of necrosis, and giant cells may also be present. Although well-developed tubercles are characteristic of pulmonary histoplasmosis, they are unusual in the skin. Oral lesions, especially when

ulcerated, may show a more mixed infiltrate with neutrophils and eosinophils (215).

Pathogenesis. H. capsulatum is a dimorphous fungus that grows in culture at temperatures below 35°C, and on natural substrates in soil as a mycelial fungus elaborating macroaleuriospores (8 to 16 µm) and microaleuriospores (2 to 5 µm). When inhaled, the latter sprout and transform into small budding yeasts that are 2 to 5 µm in diameter. In cultures at a temperature of 37°C, the organism also grows in the yeastlike form (216).

Differential Diagnosis. The histologic appearance of histoplasmosis, characterized by the presence of parasitized macrophages within a chronic inflammatory infiltrate, is much like that of rhinoscleroma, granuloma inguinale, and cutaneous leishmaniasis. For their differential diagnosis, see Table 24-1. *H. capsulatum* is the only pathogen to parasitize macrophages that stains with the usual fungal stains, such as the PAS reaction and methenamine silver. Histoplasmosis does not possess a true capsule and can thus be distinguished from *C. neoformans*, particularly when the capsule of the latter is noted to stain black with Fontana–Masson stain.

African Histoplasmosis

In addition to classic histoplasmosis caused by *H. capsulatum*, there is a form of histoplasmosis that is caused by *H. capsulatum* var. *duboisia*, and that has been called African histoplasmosis because it occurs almost exclusively in Central Africa. The portal of entry is not known. It usually occurs as a relatively indolent form involving the skin as well as the subcutaneous tissue, bones, and lymph nodes (217,218). This organism relatively rarely causes a disseminated form of disease that involves many internal organs and that may be fatal, thus resembling more classical disseminated histoplasmosis (219).

The cutaneous lesions may be one, a few, or many. They consist of papules, nodules, and plaques that often ulcerate (220). There may be large, subcutaneous granulomas that develop into fluctuant, nontender abscesses (216). Purulent bone lesions may result in draining sinus tracts extending through the skin (218).

Histopathology. The cutaneous lesions show a dense, mixed cellular infiltrate containing numerous giant cells and scattered histiocytes, lymphocytes, and plasma cells. There are focal aggregates of neutrophils forming small abscesses (220). Numerous yeast cells, 8 to 15 µm in diameter, are present mainly in the giant cells but also in histiocytes and extracellularly (218).

Pathogenesis. In spite of the fact that African histoplasmosis differs in its clinical character and in the size of the organism from classic histoplasmosis, it is clear that *H. capsulatum* and *H. duboisia* are variants of the same species, since, after prolonged *in vitro* growth at 37°C, the small yeast cells of *H. capsulatum* can assume the same size as those of *H. duboisia* (218).

SPOROTRICHOSIS

Surveys with the sporotrichin skin test, showing a positive reaction in up to 10% of the population in certain areas, suggest that many infections with *Sporothrix schenckii* are minor or asymptomatic, and not recognized clinically (221,222). Clinical sporotrichosis usually occurs as one of two primary cutaneous forms, either the fixed cutaneous or the lymphocutaneous form. Both result from direct inoculation at a site of minor trauma. Although the infection may rarely disseminate from either form by autoinoculation to other skin sites or by hematogenous spread (223–225), systemic sporotrichosis more commonly follows pulmonary infection. Development of systemic sporotrichosis, although rare, occurs particularly in persons with a depressed immune response, such as patients with lymphoma or persons receiving long-term systemic corticosteroids (226). *S. schenckii* is not a common opportunist in HIV-infected individuals, but disseminated sporotrichosis has been seen in a few patients with AIDS (227).

The lymphocutaneous form of sporotrichosis starts with a painless papule that grows into an ulcer, usually on a finger or hand. Subsequently, a chain of asymptomatic nodules appears along the lymph vessel draining the area. These lymphatic nodules may undergo suppuration with subsequent ulceration.

In the fixed cutaneous form, a solitary plaque or occasionally a group of lesions is seen, most commonly on an arm or the face. It may show superficial crusting or a verrucous surface (228–230). There is no tendency toward lymphatic spread.

Systemic sporotrichosis may be unifocal or multifocal, and usually develops subsequent to pulmonary infection. Unifocal systemic sporotrichosis may affect the lungs, a single joint or symmetric joints, the genitourinary tract, or, rarely, the brain (231). Chronic pulmonary sporotrichosis resembles pulmonary tuberculosis (232). Multifocal systemic sporotrichosis nearly always shows widely scattered cutaneous lesions, which start as nodules or as subcutaneous abscesses and undergo ulceration (233). In addition, one usually observes involvement of the lungs (225), or of several joints of the extremities (233). The predilection of *S. schenckii* for cooler parts of the body, such as the skin, lungs, and joints of the extremities has been attributed to the fact that the organism grows best at temperatures less than 37°C.

Histopathology. Early primary cutaneous lesions of sporotrichosis usually show a nonspecific inflammatory infiltrate composed of neutrophils, lymphoid cells, plasma cells, and histiocytes (234). Longer-standing, clinically verrucous lesions show a hyperplastic epidermis with small, intraepidermal and a dermal lymphoplasmacytic infiltrate with small abscesses, eosinophils, giant cells, and small granulomas often associated with asteroid bodies (229, 234). Later, through coalescence, a characteristic arrangement of the infiltrate in three zones may develop. These include a central "suppurative" zone composed of neutrophils; surrounding it, a "tuberculoid" zone with epithelioid cells and multinucleated histiocytes; and peripheral to it, a "round-cell" zone of lymphoid cells and plasma cells (229,233).

The lymphatic nodules of lymphocutaneous sporotrichosis, as well as the cutaneous nodules of multifocal systemic sporotrichosis, at first show scattered granulomas within an inflammatory infiltrate, predominantly in the deep dermis and subcutaneous fat (229,235). These enlarge and coalesce to form irregularly shaped suppurative granulomata, and eventually a large abscess surrounded by zones of histiocytes and lymphocytes as described for primary lesions (229).

In many instances, it is not possible to recognize the causative organisms of *S. schenckii* in tissue sections, particularly in the two common forms, the lymphocutaneous and fixed cutaneous. This seems to be true especially in cases of sporotrichosis reported in the United States (236) and Europe (235). In these areas, negative findings are common even with diastase digestion of glycogen granules prior to staining of sections with the PAS reaction. Nor has staining with methenamine silver increased the frequency of positive findings (235). Even in cases with positive findings, numerous sections often have to be examined before one or a few organisms are visualized (237). Immunohistochemical staining using primary antibodies directed against *S. schenckii* may increase the percentage of cases in which the organism can be demonstrated to 83%, more than double that achieved with ordinary histochemical methods (238). In addition, there are apparently significant geographic differences, since, in a series of cutaneous sporotrichosis reported from Japan, 98% of the cases showed spores in tissue sections on staining with the PAS reaction (239). If present, the spores of *S. schenckii* appear as round to oval bodies 4 to 6 μm in diameter that stain more strongly at the periphery than in the center (235) (Fig. 23-18). Single or occasionally multiple buds are present. In some instances, small, cigar-shaped bodies up to 8 μm long are also present (224,233). In only very few cases can clumps of branching, nonseptate hyphae be demonstrated (224,233).

Asteroid bodies may be seen in sporotrichosis as well as in a number of other infectious processes, and in sarcoidosis. Asteroid bodies are visible in sections stained with hematoxylin-eosin, and in sporotrichosis consist a central spore 5 to 10 μm in diameter surrounded by radiating elongations of a homogeneous eosinophilic material. The

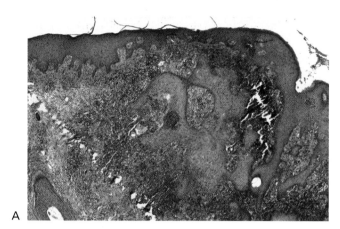
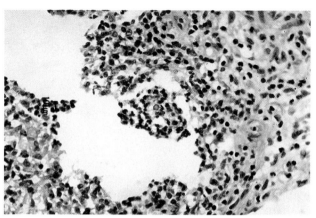

FIGURE 23-18. Sporotrichosis. **A:** H&E stain shows pseudoepitheliomatous epidermal hyperplasia with microabscess formation. **B:** H&E stain. A round spore, staining more darkly at the periphery than centrally, is surrounded by a neutrophilic infiltrate.

Splendore–Hoeppli phenomenon of radiating eosinophilic material found around infectious agents, described in sporotrichosis by Splendore (240) and in schistosomiasis by Hoeppli (241), has been thought to represent deposition of antigen–antibody complexes and debris from host inflammatory cells (242). Measurements of the greatest diameter of asteroid bodies in sporotrichosis vary from 7 to 25 μm, with a mean of 20 μm (229). Asteroid bodies have been observed in only a few cases of sporotrichosis occurring in the United States, and it may be difficult to demonstrate the central spore. However, asteroid bodies are found frequently in cases of sporotrichosis from South Africa, Japan, and Australia with an incidence varying from 39% to 65% (243).

Pathogenesis. S. schenckii occurs throughout the world and is commonly contracted through exposure to vegetal matter, often a splinter or thorn, although transmission by insects and animals has been reported (244). In nearly all cases of sporotrichosis, even in those without demonstrable fungi in the tissue, *S. schenckii* can be grown easily on Sabouraud medium. The fungus is dimorphic: at room temperature, it grows in a mycelial form with conidiophores bearing conidia as a "bouquet" at the tip; at 37°C, it grows in a yeast form (236). At 39°C, there is no growth, a fact that has led to the use of local thermotherapy (235,239).

Differential Diagnosis. If the fungus is not found in sections, a diagnosis of sporotrichosis can only be suspected; however, it can be excluded in dubious cases by a negative cutaneous sporotrichin test, which is almost always positive except in cases of disseminated disease (235). The subcutaneous abscesses of tularemia and of infections with *Mycobacterium marinum* may have the same histologic appearance as the cutaneous and subcutaneous nodules and abscesses of sporotrichosis, and must be excluded.

EUMYCETOMA (FUNGAL MYCETOMA)

A number of fungi and filamentous bacteria may cause an indolent local infection, characterized by induration associated with draining sinuses. These diverse agents may have clinically identical presentations that have been collectively called mycetoma (245). The term *actinomycetoma* refers to such infections when filamentous bacteria cause them; they are discussed further in Chapter 21. *Eumycetoma*, however, is caused by a group of true fungi with thick septate hyphae, including *Petriellidum boydii* (*Allescheria boydii*, *Pseudoallescheria boydii*), *Madurella grisea*, and *M. mycetomatis* (246). Although much more common in tropical regions, eumycetoma is seen occasionally in the United States, where the most common cause is *Petriellidum boydii* (247). Differentiation between actinomycetoma and eumycetoma is important because they respond to different treatments.

Eumycetoma is a persistent, invariably progressive local infection without a tendency for systemic spread. There is no obvious association with immunosuppression. The infection starts as a subcutaneous nodule(s) usually on the foot at a site of trauma; thus the term *Madura foot* has been used synonymously with mycetoma (246). The nodules eventuate in abscesses and draining sinuses. Gradually, the muscles and tendons are damaged, and osteomyelitis develops. Grossly visible "sulfur granules" or "grains," which are tightly knit clusters of organisms, are discharged from the draining sinuses. These granules are black in cases of eumycetoma caused by the dematiaceous fungi *M. grisea* and *M. mycetomatis* (248,249), whereas they are colorless in eumycetoma caused by *Petriellidum boydii* (250).

Histopathology. Histologic examination of the indurated skin shows extensive granulation tissue containing abscesses that may lead into sinuses. The granulation tissue is

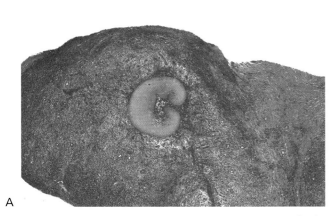

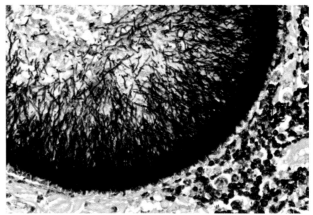

A B

FIGURE 23-19. Eumycetoma. **A:** H&E stain shows a "sulfur granule" in a purulent area of granulation tissue. **B:** The sulfur granule is composed largely of septate hyphae of *Petriellidium boydii* (GMS stain).

nonspecific in appearance. In the early phase of the disease, the tissue surrounding the abscesses is composed of lymphoid cells, plasma cells, histiocytes, and fibroblasts, whereas in the late phase fibroblasts may predominate. The diagnosis can be established only by finding the "sulfur granules" (Fig. 23-19A). Because they occur almost exclusively in abscesses or sinuses, an area containing purulent material should be chosen as the site for biopsy.

Most granules measure between 0.5 and 2.0 mm in diameter, and are thus large enough to be visible macroscopically (248). The granules of both eumycetoma and actinomycetoma stain with the PAS reaction and with methenamine silver (Fig. 23-19B). Granules of eumycetoma are composed of septate hyphae 4 to 5 μm thick, whereas the granules of actinomycetoma usually consist of fine, branching filaments or bacillary forms that are only about 1 μm thick (249). A Gram stain aids in differentiating bacterial from fungal causes of mycetoma; the filaments of actinomycetoma are Gram positive, whereas the hyphae in grains of eumycetoma are Gram negative (251). The study of discharged granules crushed on a slide and stained with lactophenol blue also allows differentiation between the thin filaments of actinomycetoma and the thicker hyphae of eumycetoma (251).

RHINOSPORIDIOSIS

Rhinosporidiosis is a chronic infection that is caused by *Rhinosporidium seeberi*. Rhinosporidiosis typically involves mucosal surfaces, most frequently the nasal mucosa, and may involve contiguous skin. This disease is seen primarily in India and Ceylon, but a number of cases have been seen in South America and a few in the United States (252).

The mode of transmission is not known. Lesions start as a papule, which is often pruritic, that grows into an erythe-matous polypoid mass that may cause obstruction of the nose and nasopharynx. Small cysts and pseudocysts develop and may discharge a combination of mucus, pus, and organisms, creating tiny white dots and giving lesions a characteristic "strawberry-like" appearance (253). Lesions of the ocular mucosa tend to be flatter, and skin lesions have a warty shape (252). Involvement of the genital mucosa has also been reported (254). Dissemination of the organism is extremely rare (255).

Histopathology. The epithelium is hyperplastic with papillomatosis and deep invaginations, some of which form pseudocysts (Fig. 23-20A). Numerous globular cysts of varying shape, representing sporangia in different stages of development, give the corium a distinctive "Swiss cheese" appearance. There is a surrounding dense, mixed inflammatory infiltrate with lymphocytes and histiocytes, including occasional giant cells, plasma cells, neutrophils, and eosinophils.

R. seeberi is a large, endosporulating organism with a distinctive morphology that can usually be recognized in hematoxylin- and eosin-stained sections (Fig. 23-20B). Sporangia develop from individual spores about the size of an erythrocyte (256). The spores develop into small uninucleate cysts that enlarge and develop a chitinous, eosinophilic wall. With increasing size, nuclear divisions lead to the development of up to 16,000 spores in a sporangium. These distinctive structures may be 300 μm in diameter. Rupture of the cyst or release of the spores through a pore in the cyst wall results in individual spores into the surrounding tissue. The organisms stain with the PAS reaction at all stages, but GMS and mucicarmine stains are not effective for organisms less than 100 μm in diameter (257).

Differential Diagnosis. The different clinical presentation of coccidioidomycoses and the smaller size of the spherical coccidioidal sporangia (less than 60 μm in diameter) allow for an easy distinction of that disease from rhinosporidiosis.

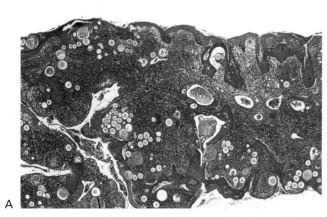

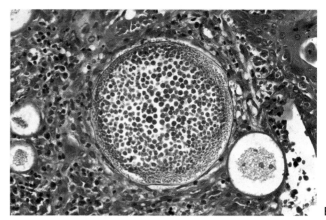

FIGURE 23-20. Rhinosporidiosis. **A:** H&E stain shows marked papillomatosis and deep invaginations of the nasal mucosa. **B:** A sporangium contains many individual spores (H&E stain).

CUTANEOUS PROTOTHECOSIS

Prototheca is a genus of algae that causes cutaneous infections in humans. Discussion of *Prototheca* is included in this chapter because this organism may be isolated on Sabouraud's medium and has traditionally been discussed in mycology texts, and because this text has no separate chapter for diseases caused by algae. Although there is one report of cutaneous infection in a patient also infected with HIV (258), cutaneous protothecosis usually occurs in otherwise healthy persons following trauma and wound contamination with water (259). Lesions develop very slowly and may be single or multiple papules, plaques, or nodules with smooth, verrucous, or ulcerated surfaces (259–263).

Histopathology. The histologic appearance, like the clinical appearance, is not characteristic, so that the diagnosis depends on the finding of the organisms. Usually there is a mixed inflammatory infiltrate with areas of necrosis and fairly numerous giant cells (Fig. 23-21). In sections stained with hematoxylin-eosin, the organisms stain faintly or not at all. On staining with PAS or silver methenamine, however, the organisms stain well and are seen both within giant cells and free in the tissue (260).

Individual organisms are spheric and measure 6 to 10 μm in diameter (263). However, as the result of septation, many contain endospores and then are considerably larger. Further subdivision of daughter cells within the parent cell leads to the formation of "sporangia" containing as many as 50 cells lying clustered together as morula-like structures (259). Ultimately, such a sporangium breaks down into individual organisms.

Pathogenesis. *Prototheca* is a genus of saprophytic, achloric (nonpigmented) algae. These organisms reproduce asexually by way of internal septation, producing autospores identical to the parent cell. *Prototheca* forms creamy, yeast-like colonies on Sabouraud's medium between 25°C and 37°C. These colonies become visible within 48 hours (260).

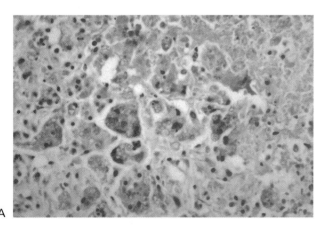

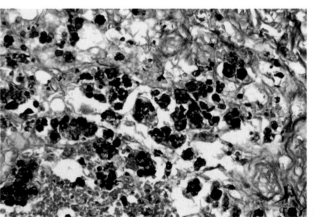

FIGURE 23-21. Protothecosis. **A:** H&E stain shows individual cells and clusters of organisms within giant cells. **B:** The morula-like clusters in multinucleated giant cells are highlighted by silver impregnation (GMS stain).

REFERENCES

1. Hawksworth DL, Sutton BC, Ainsworth GC, eds. *Ainsworth & Biby's dictionary of the fungi*, 7th ed. London: Commonwealth Mycological Institute, 1983.
2. Sabouraud R. *Les teignes*. Paris: Masson et Cie, 1910.
3. Emmons CW. Dermatophytes: natural groupings based on the form of spores and accessory organs. *Arch Dermatol Syphilol* 1934;30:337.
4. Okafor JI, Ada N. Keratinolytic activity of five human isolates of the dermatophytes. *J Commun Dis* 1999;32:300–305.
5. Lesher JL. *An atlas of microbiology of the skin*. New York: Parthenon Publishing Group, 2000.
6. Weitzman I, Summerbell RC. The Dermatophytes. *Clin Microbiol Rev* 1995;8:240–259.
7. Rasmussen JE, Ahmed AR. Trichophytin reactions in children with tinea capitis. *Arch Dermatol* 1978;114:371.
8. Goldstein AO, Smith KM, Ives TJ, et al. Effective Management of conditions involving the skin, hair, and nails. *Geriatrics* 2000;55:41–52.
9. Pravda DJ, Pugliese MM. Tinea faciei. *Arch Dermatol* 1978; 114:250.
10. Birt AR, Wilt JC. Mycology, bacteriology, and histopathology of suppurative ring-worm. *Arch Dermatol* 1954;69:441.
11. Ellis DH. Diagnosis of onychomycosis made simple. *J Am Acad Dermatol* 1999;40:S3–8.
12. Ellis DH, Watson AB, Marley JE, et al. Non-dermatophytes in onychomycosis of the toenails. *Br J Dermatol* 1997;136:490–493.
13. Zaias N. *The nail in health and disease*, 2nd ed. Norwalk, CT: Appleton & Lange, 1990.
14. Gupta AK, Taborda P, Taborda V, et al. Epidemiology and prevalence of onychomycosis in HIV-positive individuals. *Intern J Dermatol* 2000;39:746–753.
15. Garcia HP, DeLucas R, Gonzalez J, et al. Toenail onychomycosis in patients with acquired immune deficiency syndrome: treatment with terbinafine. *Br J Dermatol* 1997;137:577–580.
16. Gupta AK, Jain HC, Lynde CW, et al. Prevalence and epidemiology of unsuspected onychomycosis in patients visiting dermatologists' offices in Ontario, Canada—a multicenter survey of 2001 patients. *Intern J Dermatol* 1997;36:783–787.
17. Kligman AM, Mescon H, DeLamater ED. The Hotchkiss–McManus stain for the histopathologic diagnosis of fungus diseases. *Am J Clin Pathol*, 1951;21:86.
18. Graham JH, Johnson WC, Burgoon CF Jr, et al. Tinea capitis. *Arch Dermatol* 1964;89:528.
19. Imamura S, Tanaka M, Watanabe S. Use of immunofluorescence staining in kerion. *Arch Dermatol* 1975;111:906.
20. Gottlieb GJ, Ackerman AB. The "sandwich sign" of dermatophytosis. *Am J Dermatopathol* 1986;8:347.
21. Mikhail GR. *Trichophyton rubrum* granuloma. *Int J Dermatol* 1970;9:41.
22. Scher RK, Ackerman AB. The value of nail biopsy for demonstrating fungi not demonstrable by microbiologic techniques. *Am J Dermatopathol* 1980;2:55.
23. Longley BJ, Scher RK. Anatomy and growth of the normal nail. In: *Pathology of the skin*, 3rd ed. Mosby–Year Book. In press.
24. Machler BC, Kirsner RS, Elgart GW. Routine histologic examination for the diagnosis of onychomycosis: an evaluation of sensitivity and specificity. *Cutis* 1998;61:217–219.
25. Baek S, Chae H, Houh D, et al. Detection and differentiation of causative fungi of onychomycosis using PCR amplification and restriction enzyme analysis. *Int J Dermatol* 1998;37:682–686.
26. Tosti A, Piraccini BM, Mariani R, et al. Are local and systemic conditions important for the development of onychomycosis? *Eur J Dermatol* 1998;1:41–44.

27. Dvoretzky I, Fisher BK, Movshovitz M, et al. Favus. *Int J Dermatol* 1980;19:89.
28. Ashbee HR, Evans EGV. Immunology of diseases associated with Malessezia species. *Clin Microbiol Rev* 2002;15:21–57.
29. Bäck O, Faergemann J, Hörnqvist R. *Pityrosporum* folliculitis: a common disease of the young and middle-aged. *J Am Acad Dermatol* 1985;12:56.
30. Broberg A, Faergemann J. Infantile seborrhoeic dermatitis and *Pityrosporum ovale*. *Br J Dermatol* 1989;120:359–362.
31. Sugita T, Takashima M, Shinoda T, et al. New yeast species, Malassezia dermati, isolated from patients with atopic dermatitis. *J Clin Microbiol* 2002;40:1363–1367.
32. Heng MCY, Henderson CL, Barker DC, et al. Correlation of *Pityrosporum ovale* density with clinical severity of seborrheic dermatitis as assessed by a simplified technique. *J Am Acad Dermatol* 1990;23:82.
33. Leyden JJ, McGinley KJ, Kligman AM. Role of microorganisms in dandruff. *Arch Dermatol* 1976;112:333.
34. Galadari I, El Komy M, Mousa A, et al. Tinea versicolor: histologic and ultrastructural investigation of pigmentary changes. *Int J Dermatol* 1992;31:253.
35. Porro MN, Passi S, Caprilli F, et al. Induction of hyphae in cultures of *Pityrosporum* by cholesterol and cholesterol esters. *J Invest Dermatol* 1977;69:531.
36. Charles CR, Sire DJ, Johnson BL, et al. Hypopigmentation in tinea versicolor: a histochemical and electron microscopic study. *Int J Dermatol* 1972;12:48–58.
37. Nazzaro-Porro M, Passi S. Identification of tyrosinase inhibitor in cultures of *Pityrosporum*. *J Investig Dermatol* 1978;71:205–208.
38. Nazzaro-Porro M, Passi S, Picardo M, et al. Lipoxygenase activity of *Pityrosporum* in vitro and in vivo. *J Investig Dermatol* 1986;87:108–112.
39. Dotz WI, Henrikson DM, Yu GSM. Tinea versicolor: a light a electron microscopic study of hyperpigmented skin. *J Am Acad Dermatol* 1985;12:37–44.
40. Berretty P, Neumann M, Hausman R, et al. Follikulitis, verursacht durch *Pityrosporum*. *Hautarzt* 1980;31:613.
41. Potter BS, Burgoon CFJ, Johnson WC. *Pityrosporum* folliculitis: report of seven cases and review of the *Pityrosporum* organism relative to cutaneous disease. *Arch Dermatol* 1973;107:388.
42. Jautova J, Baloghova J, DorkoE, et al. Cutaneous candidosis in immunosuppressed patients. *Folia Microbiol* 2001;46:359–360.
43. Jautova J, Viragova S, Ondrasovic M, et al. Incidence of Candida species from human skin and nails: a survey. *Folia Microbiol* 2001;46:333–337.
44. Chapel TA, Gagliardi C, Nichols W. Congenital cutaneous candidiasis. *J Am Acad Dermatol* 1982;6:926.
45. Degos R, Garnier G, Civatte J. Pustulose par *Candida albicans* avec lésions psoriasiformes rappelant le psoriasis pustuleux. *Bull Soc Fr Dermatol Syphiligr* 1962;69:231.
46. Kwon-Chung KJ, Bennett JE. Candidiasis. In: Kwong-Chung KJ, Bennett JE. *Medical mycology*. Philadelphia: Lea & Febiger, 1992:280.
47. Scherwitz C. Ultrastructure of human cutaneous candidosis. *J Invest Dermatol* 1982;78:200.
48. Kirkpatrick CH. Chronic mucocutaneous candidiasis. *J Am Acad Dermatol* 1994;31:S14.
49. Kugelman TP, Cripps DJ, Harrell ER Jr. *Candida* granulom with epidermophytosis: report of a case and review of the lite ture. *Arch Dermatol* 1963;88:150.
50. Conant MA. Hairy leukoplakia: a new disease of the oral cosa. *Arch Dermatol* 1987;123:585.
51. Tavitian A, Raufman J-P, Rosenthal LE. Oral candidias marker for esophageal candidiasis in the acquired immu ciency syndrome. *Ann Intern Med* 1986;104:54.

52. Hauser FV, Rothman S. Monilial granuloma: report of a case and review of the literature. *Arch Dermatol Syphil* 1950;61:297.

53. Edmond MB, Wallace SE, McClish DK, et al. Nosocomial bloodstream infections in United States hospitals: a three-year analysis. *Clin Infect Dis* 1999;29:239–244.

54. Bodey GP, Luna M. Skin lesions associated with disseminated candidiasis. *JAMA* 1974;229:1466.

55. Kao AS, Brandt ME, Pruitt WR, et al. The epidemiology of candidemia in two United States cities: results of a population-based active surveillance. *Clin Infect Dis* 1999;29:1164–1170.

56. Jarowski CI, Fialk MA, Murray HW, et al. Fever, rash, and muscle tenderness: a distinctive clinical presentation of disseminated candidiasis. *Arch Intern Med* 1978;138:544.

57. Jacobs MI, Magid MS, Jarowski CI. Disseminated candidiasis: newer approaches to early recognition and treatment. *Arch Dermatol* 1980;116:1277.

58. Kressel B, Szewczyk C, Tuazon CU. Early clinical recognition of disseminated candidiasis by muscle and skin biopsy. *Arch Intern Med* 1978;138:429.

59. Grossman ME, Silvers DN, Walther RR. Cutaneous manifestations of disseminated candidiasis. *J Am Acad Dermatol* 1980;2:111.

60. Kontoyiannis DP, Bodey GP. Invasive aspergillosis in 2002: an update. *J Clin Microbiol Infect Dis* 2002;21:161–72.

61. Kwon-Chung KJ, Bennett JE. Aspergillosis. In: Kwong-Chung KJ, Bennett JE, eds. *Medical mycology*. Philadelphia: Lea & Febiger, 1992:201.

62. Allo MD, Miller J, Townsend T, et al. Primary cutaneous aspergillosis associated with Hickman intravenous catheters. *N Engl J Med* 1987;317:1105.

63. Grossman ME, Fithian EC, Behrens C, et al. Primary cutaneous aspergillosis in six leukemic children. *J Am Acad Dermatol* 1985;12:313.

64. Hunt SJ, Nagi C, Gross KG, et al. Primary cutaneous aspergillosis near central venous catheters in patients with the acquired immunodeficiency syndrome. *Arch Dermatol* 1992;128:1229.

65. Pursell KJ, Telzak EE, Armstrong D. *Aspergillus* species colonization and invasive disease in patients with AIDS. *Clin Infect Dis* 1992;14:141.

66. Panke TW, McManus AT, Spebar MJ. Infection of a burn wound by *Aspergillus niger*: gross appearance simulating ecthyma gangrenosa. *Am J Clin Pathol* 1979;72:230.

67. Lai C-S, Lin S-D, Chou C-K, et al. Aspergillosis complicating the grafted skin and free muscle flap in a diabetic. *Plast Reconstr Surg* 1993;92:532.

68. Findlay GH, Roux HF, Simson IW. Skin manifestations in disseminated aspergillosis. *Br J Dermatol* 1971;85:94.

69. Caro I, Dogliotti M. Aspergillosis of the skin: report of a case. *Dermatologica* 1973;146:244.

70. Kwon-Chung KJ, Bennett JE. Mucormycosis. In: Kwon-Chung KJ, Bennett JE. *Medical mycology*. Philadelphia: Lea & Febiger, 1992:524.

71. Adam RD, Hunter G, DiTomasso J, et al. Mucormycosis: emerging prominence of cutaneous infections. *Clin Inf Dis* 1994;19:67.

Hammond DE, Winkelmann RK. Cutaneous phycomycosis: report of three cases with identification of *Rhizopus*. *Arch Dermatol* 1979;115:990.

Stenberg G, Bottone EJ, Keusch GT, et al. Hospital-acquired mucormycosis (*Rhizopus rhizopodiformis*) of skin and subcutaneous tissue. *N Engl J Med* 1978;299:1115.

AJ, Rao R, Prabhu MR, et al. Cutaneous phycomycosis (mucosis) with fatal pulmonary dissemination. *Arch Dermatol* 1976;112:509.

Kaplan MH, Ong M, et al. Cutaneous lesions in disseminated mucormycosis. *JAMA* 1973;225:737.

76. Rabin ER, Lundberg GD, Mitchell ET. Mucormycosis in severely burned patients: report of two cases with extensive destruction of the face and nasal cavity. *N Engl J Med* 1961;264:1286.

77. Ajello L. The gamut of human infections caused by dematiaceous fungi. *Jpn J Med Mycol* 1981;22:1.

78. Fothergill AW. Identification of dematiaceous fungi and their role in human disease. *Clin Infect Dis* 1996;22[Suppl 2]:S179–184.

79. Pec J, Palencarova E, Plank L, et al. Phaeohyphomycosis due to *Alternaria* spp, and Phaeosclera dermatioides: a histopathological study. *Mycoses* 1996;39:217–221.

80. McGinnis MR. Chromoblastomycosis and phaeohyphomycosis: new concepts, diagnosis, and mycology. *J Am Acad Dermatol* 1983;8:1.

81. Gerdsen R, Uerlich M, DeHoog GS, et al. Sporotrichoid phaeohyphomycosis due to *Alternaria infectoria*. *Br J Dermatol* 2001; 145:484–486.

82. Revankar SG, Patterson JE, Sutton DA, et al. Disseminated phaeohyphomycosis: review of an emerging mycosis. *Clin Infect Dis* 2002;34:467–476.

83. Ziefer A, Connor DH. Phaeomycotic cyst: a clinicopathologic study of twenty-five patients. *Am J Trop Med Hyg* 1980;29:901.

84. Young JM, Ulrich E. Sporotrichosis produced by *Sporotrichum gougeroti*. *Arch Dermatol* 1953;67:44.

85. Greer KE, Gross GP, Cooper PH, et al. Cystic chromomycosis due to Wangiella dermatitidis. *Arch Dermatol* 1979;115:1433.

86. Jacobson ES. Pathogenic roles for fungal melanins. *Clin Microbiol Rev* 2000;13:708–713.

87. Feng B, Wang X, Hauser M, et al. Molecular cloning and characterization of WdPKS1, a gene involved in dihydroxynaphthalene melanin biosynthesis and virulence in Wangiella (Exophiala) dermatitidis. *Infect Immun* 2001;69:1781–1794.

88. Schnitzler N, Peltroche-Llacsahuanga H, Bestier N, et al. Effect of melanin and carotenoids of Exophilia (Wangiella) dermatitis on phagocytosis, oxidative burst, and killing by human neutrophils. *Infect Immun* 1999;67:94–101.

89. Kwon-Chung KJ, Bennett JE. Phaeohyphomycosis. In: Kwon-Chung KJ, Bennett JE. *Medical mycology*. Philadelphia: Lea & Febiger, 1992:620.

90. Pedersen NB, Mardh PA, Hallberg T, et al. Cutaneous alternariosis. *Br J Dermatol* 1976;94:201.

91. Mitchell AJ, Solomon AR, Beneke ES, et al. Subcutaneous alternariosis. *J Am Acad Dermatol* 1983;8:673.

92. Male O, Pehamberger H. Sekundäre kutanmykosen durch alternariaarten. *Hautarzt* 1986;37:94.

93. Chevrant-Breton J, Boisseau-Lebreuil M, Fréour E, et al. Les alternarioses cutanées humaines: a propos de 3 cas. Revue de la littérature. *Ann Dermatol Venereol* 1981;108:653.

94. Woolrich A, Koestenblatt E, Don P, et al. Cutaneous protothecosis and AIDS. *J Am Acad Dermatol* 1994;31:920.

95. Bourlond A, Alexandre G. Dermal alternariosis in a kidney transplant recipient. *Dermatologica* 1984;168:152.

96. Lemos LB, Guo M, Baliga M. Blastomycosis: Organ involvement and etiologic diagnosis. A review of 123 patients from Mississippi. *Ann Diag Pathol* 2000;4:391–406.

97. Larson DM, Eckman MR, Alber RL, et al. Primary cutaneous (inoculation) blastomycosis: an occupational hazard to pathologists. *Am J Clin Pathol* 1983;79:253.

98. Miller DD, Davies SF, Sarosi GA. Erythema nodosum and blastomycosis. *Arch Intern Med* 1982;142:1839.

99. Mercurio MG, Elewski BE. Cutaneous blastomycosis. *Cutis* 1992; 50:422.

100. Klapman MH, Superfon NP, Solomon LM. North American blastomycosis. *Arch Dermatol* 1970;101:653.

101. Witorsch P, Utz JP. North American blastomycosis: a study of 40 patients. *Medicine (Baltimore)* 1968;47:169.

102. Witzig RS, Hoadley DJ, Greer DL, et al. Blastomycosis and human immunodeficiency virus: three new cases and review. *South Med J* 1994;87:715.
103. Pappas PG, Threlkeld MG, Bedsole GD, et al. Blastomycosis in immunocompromised patients. *Medicine (Baltimore)* 1993;72:311.
104. Hashimoto K, Kaplan RJ, Daman LA, et al. Pustular blastomycosis. *Int J Dermatol* 1977;16:277.
105. Henchy FP III, Daniel CR III, Omura EF, et al. North American blastomycosis: an unusual clinical manifestation. *Arch Dermatol* 1982;118:287.
106. Wilson JW, Cawley EP, Weidman FD, et al. Primary cutaneous North American blastomycosis. *Arch Dermatol* 1955;71:39.
107. Moore M. Mycotic granulomata and cutaneous tuberculosis: a comparison of the histopathologic response. *J Invest Dermatol* 1945;6:149.
108. Desai AP, Pandit AA, Gupte PD. Cutaneous blastomycosis: report of a case with diagnosis by fine needle aspiration cytology. *Acta Cytologica* 1997;41:1317–1319.
109. Sen SK, Talley P, Zua M. Blastomycosis: report of a case with noninvasive, rapid diagnosis of dermal lesions by the papanicolaou technique. *Acta Cytologica* 1997;41:1399–1401.
110. Kaplan W, Kraft DE. Demonstration of pathogenic fungi in formalin-fixed tissues by immunofluorescence. *Am J Clin Pathol* 1969;52:420.
111. Russell B, Beckett JH, Jacobs PH. Immunoperoxidase localization of *Sporothrix schenckii* and *Cryptococcus neoformans*. *Arch Dermatol* 1979;115:433.
112. Moskowitz LB, Ganjei P, Ziegels-Weissman J, et al. Immunohistologic identification of fungi in systemic and cutaneous mycoses. *Arch Pathol Lab Med* 1986;110:433.
113. Londero AT, Ramos CD. Paracoccidioidomycosis: a clinical and mycologic study of forty-one cases observed in Santa Maria, RS, Brazil. *Am J Med* 1972;52:771.
114. Salfelder K, Doehnert G, Doehnert H-R. Paracoccidioidomycosis: anatomic study with complete autopsies. *Virchows Arch* 1969;348:51.
115. Murray HW, Littman ML, Roberts RB. Disseminated paracoccidioidomycosis (South American blastomycosis) in the United States. *Am J Med* 1974;56:209.
116. Hirsh BC, Johnson WC. Pathology of granulomatous diseases: mixed inflammatory granulomas. *Int J Dermatol* 1984;23:585–598.
117. Borges-Walmsley IM, Chen D, Shu X, et al. The pathobiology of paracoccidiodes brasiliensis. *Trends Microbiol* 2002;10:80–87.
118. Bakos L, Kronfeld M, Hampe S, et al. Disseminated paracoccidioidomycosis with skin lesions in a patient with acquired immunodeficiency syndrome. *J Am Acad Dermatol* 1989;20:854.
119. Götz H. Klinische und experimentelle studien über das granuloma paracoccidioides. *Arch Dermatol Syphiligr* 1954;198:507.
120. Azulay RD, Carneiro JA, Cunha MDG, et al. Keloidal blastomycosis (Lobo's disease) with lymphatic involvement: a case report. *Int J Dermatol* 1976;15:40.
121. Tapia A, Torres-Calcindo A, Arosemena R. Keloidal blastomycosis (Lobo's disease) in Panama. *Int J Dermatol* 1978;17:572.
122. Woodard JC. Electron microscopic study of lobomycosis (*Loboa loboi*). *Lab Invest* 1972;27:606–612.
123. Bhawan J, Bain RW, Purtilo DT, et al. Lobomycosis: an electron microscopic, histochemical and immunologic study. *J Cutan Pathol* 1976;3:5.
124. Burns RA, Roy JS, Woods C, et al. Report of the first human case of lobomycosis in the United States. *J Clin Microbiol* 2000;38:1283–1285.
125. Milam CP, Fenske NA. Chromoblastomycosis. *Systemic Mycoses Parasitic Dis* 1989;7:219–225.
126. Bayer C, Fuhrmann E, Coelho CC, et al. Expression of heat shock protein 27 in chromomycosis. *Mycosis* 1998;41:447–452.
127. Bansal AS, Prabhakar P. Chromomycosis: a twenty-year analysis of histologically confirmed cases in Jamaica. *Trop Geograph Med* 1987;41:222–226.
128. Derbes VJ, Friedman I. Chromoblastomycosis. *Dermatol Tropica* 1964;3:201.
129. Azulay RD, Serruya J. Hematogenous dissemination in chromoblastomycosis. *Arch Dermatol* 1967;95:57.
130. Wackym PA, Gray GF Jr, Richie RE, et al. Cutaneous chromomycosis in renal transplant recipients: Successful management in two cases. *Arch Intern Med* 1985;145:1036.
131. Nödl F. Zue histologie der chromomykose. *Z Hautkr* 1963;35:305.
132. Moore M, Cooper ZK, Weiss RS. Chromomycosis (chromoblastomycosis). *JAMA* 1943;122:1237.
133. French AJ, Russell SR. Chromoblastomycosis: report of first case recognized in Michigan, apparently conducted in South Carolina. *Arch Dermatol Syphil* 1953;67:129.
134. Batres E, Wolf JE Jr, Rudolph AH, et al. Transepithelial elimination of cutaneous chromomycosis. *Arch Dermatol* 1978;114:1231.
135. Goette DK, Robertson D. Transepithelial elimination in chromomycosis. *Arch Dermatol* 1984;120:400.
136. Caplan RM. Epidermoid carcinoma arising in extensive chromoblastomycosis. *Arch Dermatol* 1968;97:38.
137. Tschen JA, Knox JM, McGavran MH, et al. Chromomycosis: the association of fungal elements and wood splinters. *Arch Dermatol* 1984;120:107.
138. Rubin HA, Bruce S, Rosen T, et al. Evidence for percutaneous inoculation as the mode of transmission for chromoblastomycosis. *J Am Acad Dermatol* 1991;25:951.
139. Louie L, Ng S, Hajjeh R, et al. Influence of host genetics on the severity of coccidioidomycosis. *Emerg Infect Dis* 2000;5:1–15.
140. Trimble JR, Doucette J. Primary cutaneous coccidioidomycosis: report of a case of a laboratory infection. *Arch Dermatol* 1956;74:405.
141. Overholt EL, Hornick RB. Primary cutaneous coccidioidomycosis. *Arch Intern Med* 1964;114:149.
142. Carroll GF, Haley LD, Brown JM. Primary cutaneous coccidioidomycosis. *Arch Dermatol* 1977;113:933.
143. Levan NE, Huntington RW Jr. Primary cutaneous coccidioidomycosis in agricultural workers. *Arch Dermatol* 1965;92:215.
144. Winn WA. Primary cutaneous coccidioidomycosis: reevaluation of its potentiality based on study of three new cases. *Arch Dermatol* 1965;92:221.
145. Drutz DJ, Catanzaro A. Coccidioidomycosis. Part I. *Am Rev Respir Dis* 1978;117:559.
146. Drutz DJ, Catanzaro A. Coccidioidomycosis. Part II. *Am Rev Respir Dis* 1978;117:727.
147. Dodge RR, Lebowitz MD, Barbee R, et al. Estimates of *C. immitis* infection by skin test reactivity in an endemic community. *Am J Public Health* 1985;75:863.
148. Medoff G, Kobayashi GS. Strategies in the treatment of systemic fungal infections. *N Engl J Med* 1980;302:145.
149. Harrell ER, Honeycutt WM. Coccidioidomycosis: a traveling fungus disease. *Arch Dermatol* 1963;87:188.
150. Deresinski SC, Stevens DA. Coccidioidomycosis in compromised hosts: experience at Stanford University Hospital. *Medicine (Baltimore)* 1974;54:377.
151. Ampel NM, Dols CL, Galgiani JN. Coccidioidomycosis during human immunodeficiency virus infection: results of a prospective study in a coccidioidal endemic area. *Am J Med* 1993;94:235.

152. Wheat J. Histoplasmosis and coccidioidomycosis in individuals with AIDS: a clinical review. *Infect Dis Clin North Am* 1994; 8:467.

153. Schwartz RA, Lamberts RJ. Isolated nodular cutaneous coccidioidomycosis: the initial manifestation of disseminated disease. *J Am Acad Dermatol* 1981;4:38.

154. Levan NE, Kwong MQ. Coccidioidomycosis: persistent pulmonary lesion, solitary "disseminated" lesion of face, occupational aspects. *Arch Dermatol* 1963;87:511.

155. Bayer AS, Yoshikawa TT, Galpin JE, et al. Unusual syndromes of coccidioidomycosis: diagnostic and therapeutic considerations. *Medicine (Baltimore)* 1976;55:131.

156. Winer LH. Histopathology of the nodose lesion of acute coccidioidomycosis. *Arch Dermatol Syphil* 1950;61:1010.

157. Kwon-Chung KJ, Bennett JE. Coccidioidomycosis. In: Kwon-Chung KJ, Bennett JE. *Medical mycology*. Philadelphia: Lea & Febiger, 1992:356.

158. Randhawa HS, Paliwal DK. Occurrence and significance of *Cryptococcus neoformans* in the oropharynx and on the skin of a healthy human population. *J Clin Microbiol* 1977;6:325.

159. Glaser JB, Garden A. Inoculation of cryptococcosis without transmission of the acquired immunodeficiency syndrome. *N Engl J Med* 1985;313:266.

160. Ng WF, Loo KT. Cutaneous cryptococcosis—primary versus secondary disease: report of two cases with review of literature. *Am J Dermatopathol* 1993;15:372.

161. Hajjeh RA, Brandt ME, Pinner RW. Emergence of Cryptococcal disease: epidemiologic perspectives 100 years after its discovery. *Epidem Rev* 1995;17:303–320.

162. Dismukes WE. Cryptococcal meningitis in patients with AIDS. *J Infect Dis* 1988;157:624.

163. Schupbach CW, Wheeler CE Jr, Briggaman RA, et al. Cutaneous manifestations of disseminated cryptococcosis. *Arch Dermatol* 1976;112:1734.

164. Chu AC, Hay RJ, MacDonald DM. Cutaneous cryptococcosis. *Br J Dermatol* 1980;103:95.

165. Cawley EP, Grekin RH, Curtis AC. Torulosis: a review of the cutaneous and adjoining mucous membrane manifestations. *J Invest Dermatol* 1950;14:327.

166. Frieden TR, Bia FJ, Heald PW, et al. Cutaneous cryptococcosis in a patient with cutaneous T cell lymphoma receiving therapy with photopheresis and methotrexate. *Clin Infect Dis* 1993;17:776.

167. Diamond RD, Bennett JE. Prognostic factors in cryptococcal meningitis: a study of 111 cases. *Ann Intern Med* 1974;80:176.

168. Kaplan MH, Rosen PP, Armstrong D. Cryptococcosis in a cancer hospital: clinical and pathological correlates in forty-six patients. *Cancer* 1977;39:2265.

169. Pema K, Diaz J, Guerra LG, et al. Disseminated cutaneous cryptococcosis: comparison of clinical manifestations in the pre-AIDS and AIDS eras. *Arch Intern Med* 1994;154:1032.

170. Perfect JR, Durack DT, Gallis HA. Cryptococcemia. *Medicine (Baltimore)* 1983;62:98.

171. Sussman EJ, McMahon F, Wright D, et al. Cutaneous cryptococcosis without evidence of systemic involvement. *J Am Acad Dermatol* 1984;11:371.

172. Gordon PM, Ormerod AD, Harvey G, et al. Cutaneous cryptococcal infection without immunodeficiency. *Clin Exp Dermatol* 1993;19:181.

173. Penneys NS, Hicks B. Unusual cutaneous lesions associated with acquired immunodeficiency syndrome. *J Am Acad Dermatol* 1985;13:845.

174. Manrique P, Mayo J, Alvarez JA, et al. Polymorphous cutaneous cryptococcosis: nodular, herpes-like, and molluscum-like lesions in a patient with the acquired immunodeficiency syndrome. *J Am Acad Dermatol* 1992;26:122.

175. Blauvelt A, Kerdel FA. Cutaneous cryptococcosis mimicking Kaposi's sarcoma as the initial manifestation of disseminated disease. *Int J Dermatol* 1992;31:279.

176. Hall JC, Brewer JH, Crouch TT, et al. Cryptococcal cellulitis with multiple sites of involvement. *J Am Acad Dermatol* 1987; 17:329.

177. Carlson KC, Mehlmauer M, Evans S, et al. Cryptococcal cellulitis in renal transplant recipients. *J Am Acad Dermatol* 1987; 17:469.

178. Gutierrez F, Fu YS, Lurie HI. Cryptococcosis histologically resembling histoplasmosis: a light and electron microscopical study. *Arch Pathol* 1975;99:347.

179. Ro JY, Lee SS, Ayala AG. Advantage of Fontana–Masson stain in capsule-deficient cryptococcal infection. *Arch Pathol Lab Med* 1987;111:53.

180. Linell F, Magnusson B, Nordén Å. Cryptococcosis: review and report of a case. *Acta Derm Venereol (Stockh)* 1953;33:103.

181. Ruiter M, Ensink GJ. Acute primary cutaneous cryptococcosis. *Dermatologica* 1964;128:185.

182. Littman ML, Walter JE. Cryptococcosis: current status. *Am J Med* 1968;45:922.

183. Collins DN, Oppenheim IA, Edwards MR. Cryptococcosis associated with systemic lupus erythematosus: light and electron microscopic observations on a morphologic variant. *Arch Pathol* 1971;91:78.

184. Brier RL, Mopper C, Stone J. Cutaneous cryptococcosis: presentation of a case and a review of previously reported cases. *Arch Dermatol* 1957;75:262.

185. Miura T, Akiba H, Saito N, et al. Primary cutaneous cryptococcosis. *Dermatologica* 1971;142:374.

186. Noble RC, Fajardo LF. Primary cutaneous cryptococcosis: review and morphologic study. *Am J Clin Pathol* 1972;57:13.

187. Sarosi GA, Silberfarb PM, Tosh FE. Cutaneous cryptococcosis: a sentinel of disseminated disease. *Arch Dermatol* 1971; 104:1.

188. Ruchel R. False-positive reaction of a Cryptococcus antigen test owing to Pseudallescheria mycosis. *Mycoses* 1994;37:69.

189. Hamilton JR, Noble A, Denning DW, et al. Performance of cryptococcal antigen latex agglutination kits on serum and cerebrospinal fluid specimens of AIDS patients before and after pronase treatment. *J Clin Microbiol* 1991;29:333–339.

190. Goodwin RA Jr, Des Prez RM. Histoplasmosis. *Am Rev Respir Dis* 1978;117:929.

191. Kwon-Chung KJ, Bennett JE. Histoplasmosis. In: Kwon-Chung KJ, Bennett JE. *Medical mycology*. Philadelphia: Lea & Febiger, 1992:464.

192. U.S. National Communicable Disease Center. Morbidity and mortality weekly report annual supplement: Summary 1968. *MMWR* 1969;17.

193. Tosh FE, Balhuizen J, Yates JL, et al. Primary cutaneous histoplasmosis. *Arch Intern Med* 1964;114:118.

194. Tesh RB, Schneidau JD Jr. Primary cutaneous histoplasmosis. *N Engl J Med* 1966;275:597.

195. Nakelchik M, Mangino JE. Reactivation of histoplasmosis after treatment with infliximab. *Am J Med* 2002;112:78.

196. Goodwin RA Jr, Owens FT, Snell JD, et al. Chronic pulmonary histoplasmosis. *Medicine* (Baltimore) 1976;55(6):413–452.

197. Cawley EP, Curtis AC. Histoplasmosis and lymphoblastoma: are these diseases related? *J Invest Dermatol* 1948;11:443.

198. Ende N, Pizzolato P, Ziskind J. Hodgkin's disease associated with histoplasmosis. *Cancer* 1952;5:763.

199. Kauffman CA, Israel KS, Smith JW, et al. Histoplasmosis in immunosuppressed patients. *Am J Med* 1978;64:923.

200. Bonner JR, Alexander WJ, Dismukes WE, et al. Disseminated histoplasmosis in patients with the acquired immune deficiency syndrome. *Arch Intern Med* 1984;144:2178.

201. Wheat LJ. Histoplasmosis in Indianapolis. *Clin Infect Dis* 1992;14:S91.

202. Neubauer MA, Bodensteiner DC. Disseminated histoplasmosis in patients with AIDS. *South Med J* 1992;85:1166.

203. Goodwin RA Jr, Shapiro JL, Thurman GH, et al. Disseminated histoplasmosis: clinical and pathologic correlations. *Medicine (Baltimore)* 1980;59:1.

204. Studdard J, Sneed WF, Taylor MR Jr, et al. Cutaneous histoplasmosis. *Am Rev Respir Dis* 1976;113:689.

205. Curtis AC, Grekin JN. Histoplasmosis: a review of the cutaneous and adjacent mucous membrane manifestations with a report of three cases. *JAMA* 1947;134:1217.

206. Miller HE, Keddie FM, Johnstone HG, et al. Histoplasmosis: cutaneous and mucomembranous lesions, mycologic and pathologic observations. *Arch Dermatol Syphil* 1947;56:715.

207. Chanda JJ, Callen JP. Isolated nodular cutaneous histoplasmosis: the initial manifestation of recurrent disseminated disease. *Arch Dermatol* 1978;114:1197.

208. Barton EN, Ince RWE, Patrick AL, et al. Cutaneous histoplasmosis in the acquired immune deficiency syndrome: a report of three cases from Trinidad. *Trop Geogr Med* 1988;40:153.

209. Abildgaard WH Jr, Hargrove RH, Kalivas J. *Histoplasma* panniculitis. *Arch Dermatol* 1985;121:914.

210. Samovitz M, Dillon TK. Disseminated histoplasmosis presenting as exfoliative erythroderma. *Arch Dermatol* 1970;101:216.

211. Cramer HJ. Erythrodermatische hauthistoplasmose. *Dermatologica* 1973;146:249.

212. Sellers TF Jr, Price WN Jr, Newberry WM Jr. An epidemic of erythema multiforme and erythema nodosum caused by histoplasmosis. *Ann Intern Med* 1965;62:1244.

213. Zarabi CM, Thomas R, Adesokan A. Diagnosis of systemic histoplasmosis in patients with AIDS. *South Med J* 1992;85:1171.

214. Dumont A, Piché C. Electron microscopic study of human histoplasmosis. *Arch Pathol* 1969;87:168.

215. Nejedly RF, Baker LA. Treatment of localized histoplasmosis with 2-hydroxstilbamidine. *Arch Intern Med* 1955;95:37.

216. Rippon JW. *Medical mycology*. Philadelphia: Saunders, 1974.

217. Lucas AO. Cutaneous manifestations of African histoplasmosis. *Br J Dermatol* 1970;82:435.

218. Nethercott JR, Schachter RK, Givan KF, et al. Histoplasmosis due to *Histoplasma capsulatum* var *duboisii* in a Canadian immigrant. *Arch Dermatol* 1978;114:595.

219. Williams AO, Lawson EA, Lucas AO. African histoplasmosis due to *Histoplasma duboisii*. *Arch Pathol* 1971;92:306.

220. Flegel H, Kaben U, Westphal H-J. Afrikanische histoplasmose. *Hautarzt* 1980;31:50.

221. Schneidau JD Jr, Lamar LM, Hairston MA Jr. Cutaneous hypersensitivity to sporotrichin in Louisiana. *JAMA* 1964;188:371.

222. Ingrish FM, Schneidau JD Jr. Cutaneous hypersensitivity to sporotrichin in Maricopa county, Arizona. *J Invest Dermatol* 1967;49:146.

223. Urabe H, Honbo S. Sporotrichosis. *Int J Dermatol* 1986;25:255.

224. Shelley WB, Sica PA Jr. Disseminate sporotrichosis of skin and bone cured with 5-fluorocytosine: photosensitivity as a complication. *J Am Acad Dermatol* 1983;8:229.

225. Smith PW, Loomis GW, Luckasen JL, et al. Disseminated cutaneous sporotrichosis: three illustrated cases. *Arch Dermatol* 1981;117:143.

226. Lynch PJ, Voorhees JJ, Harrell ER. Systemic sporotrichosis. *Ann Intern Med* 1970;73:23.

227. Shaw JC, Levinson W, Montanaro A. Sporotrichosis in the acquired immunodeficiency syndrome. *J Am Acad Dermatol* 1989;21:1145.

228. Dellatorre DL, Lattanand A, Buckley HR, et al. Fixed cutaneous sporotrichosis of the face: successful treatment of a case and review of the literature. *J Am Acad Dermatol* 1982;6:97.

229. Lurie HI. Histopathology of sporotrichosis: notes on the nature of the asteroid body. *Arch Pathol* 1963;75:421.

230. Carr RD, Storkan MA, Wilson JW, et al. Extensive verrucous sporotrichosis of long duration: report of a case resembling cutaneous blastomycosis. *Arch Dermatol* 1964;89:124.

231. Wilson DE, Mann JJ, Bennett JE, et al. Clinical features of extracutaneous sporotrichosis. *Medicine (Baltimore)* 1967;46:265.

232. Baum GL, Donnerberg RL, Stewart D, et al. Pulmonary sporotrichosis. *N Engl J Med* 1969;280:410.

233. Stroud JD. Sporotrichosis presenting as pyoderma gangrenosum. *Arch Dermatol* 1968;97:667.

234. Fetter BF. Human cutaneous sporotrichosis due to *Sporotrichum schenckii*: technique for demonstration of organisms in tissues. *Arch Pathol* 1961;71:416.

235. Male O. Diagnostische und therapeutische probleme bei der kutanen sporotrichose. *Z Hautkr* 1974;49:505.

236. Segal RJ, Jacobs PH. Sporotrichosis. *Int J Dermatol* 1979;18:639.

237. Fetter BF, Tindall JP. Cutaneous sporotrichosis: clinical study of nine cases utilizing an improved technique for demonstration of organisms. *Arch Pathol* 1964;78:613.

238. Marques MEA, Coelho KIR, Sotto MN, et al. Comparison between histochemical and immunohistochemical methods for diagnosis of sporotrichosis. *J Clin Pathol* 1992;45:1089.

239. Kariya H, Iwatsu T. Statistical survey of 100 cases of sporotrichosis. *J Dermatol* 1979;6:211.

240. Splendore A. Sobre a cultura d'uma nova especiale de cogumello pathogenico (sporotrichose de Splendore). *Rev Soc Sci São Paulo* 1908;3:62.

241. Hoeppli R. Histological observations in experimental schistosomiasis Japonica. *Chin Med J* 1932;46:1179.

242. Hiruma M, Kawada A, Ishibashi A. Ultrastructure of asteroid bodies in sporotrichosis. *Mycoses* 1991;34:103.

243. Auld JC, Beardsmore GL. Sporotrichosis in Queensland: a review of 37 cases at the Royal Brisbane Hospital. *Australas J Dermatol* 1979;20:14.

244. Reed KD, Moore FM, Geiger GE, et al. Zoonotic transmission of sporotrichosis: case report and review. *Clin Infect Dis* 1993;16:384.

245. Palestine RF, Rogers RS III. Diagnosis and treatment of mycetoma. *J Am Acad Dermatol* 1982;6:107.

246. Hay RJ, MacKenzie DWR. Mycetoma (Madura foot) in the United Kingdom: a survey of forty-four cases. *Clin Exp Dermatol* 1983;8:553.

247. Green WO Jr, Adams TE. Mycetoma in the United States: a review and report of seven additional cases. *Am J Clin Pathol* 1964;42:75.

248. Butz WC, Ajello L. Black grain mycetoma: a case due to *Madurella grisea*. *Arch Dermatol* 1971;104:197.

249. Taralakshmi VV, Pankajalakshmi VV, Arumugam S, et al. Mycetoma caused by *Madurella mycetomii* in Madras. *Australas J Dermatol* 1978;19:125.

250. Barnetson RSC, Milne LJR. Mycetoma. *Br J Dermatol* 1978;99:227.

251. Zaias N, Taplin D, Rebell G. Mycetoma. *Arch Dermatol* 1969;99:215.

252. Karunaratne WAE. *Rhinosporidiosis in man*. London: Athlone Press of University of London, 1964.

253. Prins LC, Tange RA, Dingemans KP. Rhinosporidiosis in the Netherlands: a case report including ultramicroscopic features. *J Otorhinolaryngol Relat Spec* 1983;45:237.

254. Kwon-Chung KJ, Bennett JE. Rhinosporidiosis. In: Kwon-Chung KJ, Bennett JE. *Medical mycology*. Philadelphia: Lea & Febiger, 1992:695.

255. Rajam RV, Viswanathan GS, Rao A, et al. Rhinosporidiosis: a study with report of a fatal case of systemic dissemination. *Indian J Surg* 1955;17:269.

256. Mayhall CG, Miller CW, Eisen AZ, et al. Cutaneous protothecosis: successful treatment with amphotericin B. *Arch Dermatol* 1976;112:1749.

257. Easley JR, Meuten DJ, Levy MG, et al. Nasal rhinosporidiosis in the dog. *Vet Pathol* 1986;23:50.

258. Woolrich A, Koestenblatt E, Don P, et al. Cutaneous protothecosis and AIDS. *J Am Acad Dermatol* 1994;31:920.

259. Nabai H, Mehregan AH. Cutaneous protothecosis: report of a case from Iran. *J Cutan Pathol* 1974;1:180.

260. Wolfe ID, Sacks HG, Samorodin CS, et al. Cutaneous protothecosis in a patient receiving immunosuppressive therapy. *Arch Dermatol* 1976;112:829.

261. Venezio FR, Lavoo E, Williams JE, et al. Progressive cutaneous protothecosis. *Am J Clin Pathol* 1982;77:485.

262. Tindall JP, Fetter BF. Infections caused by achloric algae: protothecosis. *Arch Dermatol* 1971;104:490.

262. Mars PW, Rabson AR, Rippey JJ, et al. Cutaneous protothecosis. *Br J Dermatol* 1971;85:76.

263. Nelson AM, Neafie RC, Connor DH. Cutaneous protothecosis and chlorellosis, extraordinary "aquatic-borne" algal infections. *Clin Dermatol* 1987;5:76.

PROTOZOAN DISEASES AND PARASITIC INFESTATIONS

KLAUS SELLHEYER
ECKART HANEKE

The increase in international travel from endemic regions has brought diseases to North America and Europe that were once thought of being confined to tropical countries only. Furthermore, HIV infection has become an important co-factor in acquiring diseases that are normally rare in the developed world. Leishmaniasis for that matter was recently considered an emerging infection, as it has been recognized as an opportunistic disease, particularly in HIV-infected individuals (1). Immigrants from Asia, Africa, and South America represent another contingent afflicted by diseases that are normally not prevalent in the United States and Western Europe.

LEISHMANIASIS

Leishmaniasis is a protozoan disease with a prevalence of 12 million cases and an annual incidence of almost 2 million new cases worldwide, making it one of the most common infectious diseases globally (along with malaria, helminthic infestations of the gastrointestinal tract, and HIV infection) (2). The inciting organism belongs to the order Trypanosomatidae, which comprises two genera pathogenic to humans: *Trypanosoma* and *Leishmania* (3).

Leishmania spp. primarily affect cells of monocyte-macrophage lineage; these organisms have both flagellar (promastigote) and aflagellar (amastigote) stages during their life cycle. The former is found in the intestines of sandflies, which function as the arthropod vector for *Leishmania* spp. In the Old World, the sandflies belong to the genus *Phlebotomus*, and in the New World to the genera *Lutzomyia* and *Psychodopygus* (3). After the promastigotes have entered the skin of the human host via the bite of infected sandflies, they transform into amastigotes within histiocytes. If the histiocytic response to *Leishmania* spp. remains confined to the skin, cutaneous lesions develop; if dissemination of the protozoa occurs, internal organs become involved.

At the center stage of all different forms of leishmaniasis is a disruption of macrophage activation with the subsequent avoidance of intracellular killing mechanisms (4). The parasites do so by inhibiting lysosomal phosphatases and protein kinase C. Substrates of protein kinase C are involved in cytoskeletal rearrangements and vacuolar trafficking, and are thus important in cellular signaling. *Leishmania* spp. also inhibit the synthesis of proinflammatory cytokines and increase the production of antiinflammatory cytokines, thereby preventing their elimination from the human host.

Classification of Leishmaniasis

The former simplistic classification dividing leishmaniasis into a cutaneous, mucocutaneous, and visceral form has been abandoned in favor of a classification that recognizes the overlap in the clinical spectrum of various types of leishmaniasis (1,5–8):

- Localized (acute) cutaneous leishmaniasis
- Diffuse (acute) cutaneous leishmaniasis (disseminated anergic cutaneous leishmaniasis)
- Chronic cutaneous leishmaniasis (including leishmaniasis recidivans or lupoid leishmaniasis)
- Post–kala-azar dermal leishmaniasis
- Mucocutaneous leishmaniasis
- Visceral leishmaniasis
- Viscerotropic leishmaniasis

Each form of leishmaniasis is associated with a different type of *Leishmania* spp., and has a specific predilection for a geographic location (Table 24-1).

Localized (Acute) Cutaneous Leishmaniasis

Representing the most common form of skin involvement, localized acute cutaneous leishmaniasis affects primarily the exposed parts of the body, such as face, scalp, and arms (9–11). It appears initially as a painless, erythematous

TABLE 24-1. *LEISHMANIA* SPECIES[a] AND GEOGRAPHIC LOCATIONS ASSOCIATED WITH DIFFERENT CLINICAL FORMS OF LEISHMANIASIS

Form of disease	New World Parasite	Old World Parasite	Geographic location
Localized (acute) cutaneous leishmaniasis	*L. b. braziliensis* *L. b. guyanensis* *L. b. panamensis* *L. m. mexicana* *L. m. amazonensis* *L. donovani chagasi*	*L. major* *L. tropica* *L. aethiopica* *L. infantum*	North Africa, India, Middle East, China, South Russia, Pakistan, Mediterranean, Central and South America, Texas, Caribbean
Localized (acute) cutaneous leishmaniasis	*L. m. amazonensis* *L. mexicana* *L. m. pifanoi*	*L. aethiopica*	Venezuela, Bolivia, Mexico, Dominican Republic, Brazil, Ethiopia
Leishmaniasis recidivans	*L. braziliensis*	*L. tropica*	Central and South America, Middle East
Post kala-azar dermal leishmaniasis	*L. donovani chagasi*	*L. donovani* *L. tropica* *L. infantum*	India, Bangladesh, East Africa, Sudan
Mucocutaneous leishmaniasis	*L. b. braziliensis*		Brazil, Venezuela, Peru, Equador, Colombia
Visceral leishmaniasis	*L. donovani chagasi*	*L. donovani* *L. infantum* *L. tropica*	China, India, Bangladesh, Asia, Sudan, Africa, East Russia, Mediterranean, South America
Viscerotropic leishmaniasis		*L. tropica*	Iraq, Kuwait

[a]New World parasites have species and subspecies names; Old World parasites have only a species name.
L. b. braziliensis, *Leishmania braziliensis braziliensis*; *L. m. mexicana*, *Leishmania mexicana mexicana*.
Source: Adapted and slightly modified from Grevelink SA, Lerner EA. Leishmaniasis. *J Am Acad Dermatol* 1996;34:257.

papule which enlarges over a period of 4 to 12 weeks to a nodule or a plaque measuring up to 2 cm in diameter (Fig. 24-1A). Ulceration is common. After several months the lesion spontaneously regresses, starting from the center and progressing outwards. The end stage is represented by a scar accompanied by hypo- or hyper pigmentation (1,5, 8,12). New World leishmaniasis commonly presents with a single lesion, and Old World leishmaniasis with multiple lesions (1,5).

Histopathology. The characteristic changes are noted throughout the dermis and consist of a dense, diffuse infiltrate of histiocytes admixed with lymphocytes and few plasma cells (1,5,7–13) (Fig. 24-1B). Eosinophils and neutrophils are rare; the latter are more numerous if the lesion is ulcerated (12). The cytoplasm of the histiocytes is filled with numerous dull blue-grey, round to oval bodies measuring 2 to 4 μm in diameter exhibiting a round basophilic nucleus, and a rod-shaped paranuclear kinetoplast, a specialized mitochondrial structure containing extracellular DNA (Fig. 24-1C). These intracellular bodies stain red or dark blue with Giemsa but not with periodic acid-Schiff (PAS) and Gomori's methenamine silver (GMS) because they lack a capsule. They represent amastigotes, known as Leishman–Donovan bodies. When numerous, they can also be seen extracellularly.

The epidermal changes are nonspecific and consist of hyperkeratosis, parakeratosis, and epidermal atrophy or hyperplasia (1,5,7,9,11,13). Ulceration is also noted. The basal cell layer may show hydropic degeneration, and the

follicular ostia may display plugging with compact orthokeratotic material (13).

Differential Diagnosis. The organisms of histoplasmosis do not exhibit a kinetoplast and do stain with PAS and GMS. *Klebsiella rhinoscleromatis*, the inciting agent of rhinoscleroma, also resides in macrophages and measures 2 to 3 μm in diameter. In contrast to leishmaniasis, rhinoscleroma reveals a large number of plasma cells with formation of Russell bodies. Granuloma inguinale, caused by *Calymmatobacterium granulomatis*, displays numerous small abscesses throughout the inflammatory infiltrate (see Chapters 21 and 23).

Diffuse (Acute) Cutaneous Leishmaniasis

Diffuse acute cutaneous leishmaniasis, also known as disseminated anergic cutaneous leishmaniasis, is a rare variant of localized cutaneous leishmaniasis, and is due to a lack of a *Leishmania*-specific cellular immune response (14). It begins as a single lesion and then spreads diffusely all over the body, characteristically as nonulcerated nodules, often involving upper and lower extremities, buttocks, and face (1,5,14) (Fig. 24-2). In atypical cases, ulceration of the nodules is noted (15).

Histopathology. The histopathological changes of the individual lesions are the same as those seen in localized acute cutaneous leishmaniasis except for a larger number of Leishman–Donovan bodies and a relative lack of accompanying lymphocytes (1,5,14,16). In the rare ulcerated

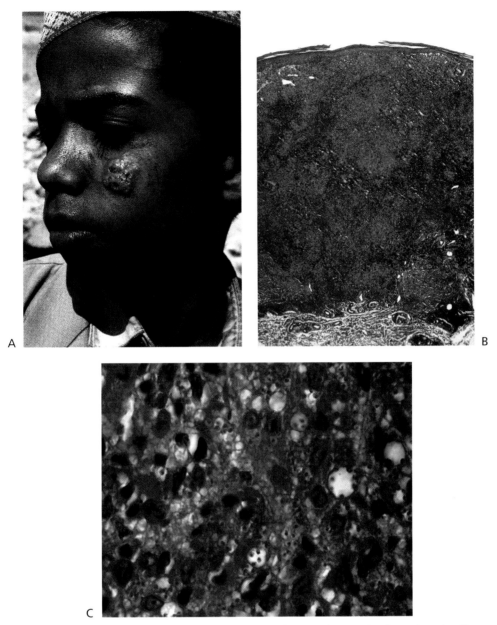

A

B

C

FIGURE 24-1. Localized acute cutaneous leishmaniasis. **A:** Lesion on the face of a schoolboy from Yemen (From Schaller KF, ed. *Colour Atlas of Tropical Dermatology and Venerology.* New York: Springer, 1994:109, with permission.) **B:** A dense, diffuse infiltrate of histiocytes and lymphocytes is noted throughout most of the dermis. **C:** On high magnification the amastigotes with their kinetoplasts can be identified.

lesions of diffuse cutaneous leishmaniasis, eosinophils are predominant within the inflammatory infiltrate and reveal ultrastructural characteristics of parasiticidal activity (15).

Chronic Cutaneous Leishmaniasis

If the lesions do not resolve within 1 to 2 years, the condition is termed chronic cutaneous leishmaniasis (8,17). Two subtypes are noted: nonhealing chronic cutaneous leishmaniasis and leishmaniasis recidivans (the latter also called lupoid leishmaniasis, relapsing chronic cutaneous leishma-

niasis or recurrent cutaneous leishmaniasis) (17–19). In the former, the original lesion of localized (acute) cutaneous leishmaniasis persists, clinically presenting as an erythematous plaque of several years duration and no evidence of healing (17). Leishmaniasis recidivans refers to the appearance of new lesions in the center or at the periphery of an atrophic scar derived from a previous lesion of localized (acute) cutaneous leishmaniasis (5,17,18). It carries great clinical resemblance to lupus vulgaris and presents with erythematous papules, often coalescing into crust-covered plaques, in association with a scar. The face is the area of

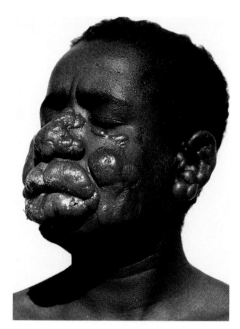

FIGURE 24-2. Diffuse acute cutaneous leishmaniasis. Ethiopian patient with pseudolepromatous appearance. (From Schaller KF, ed. *Colour Atlas of Tropical Dermatology and Venerology.* New York: Springer, 1994:113, with permission.)

predilection (18,19). It is either due to reactivation of persistent organisms or exogenous reinfection (5).

Histopathology. Both subtypes of chronic cutaneous leishmaniasis reveal essentially the same histopathological changes, except for the presence of scar tissue in leishmaniasis recidivans in contrast to nonhealing chronic cutaneous leishmaniasis (18).

The histopathologic hallmark of chronic cutaneous leishmaniasis is a dense, diffuse, or nodular infiltrate composed of epithelioid cell granulomas within the superficial and deep dermis (7,13,19–21). The granulomas are tuberculoid in nature, made up of epithelioid histiocytes and Langerhans giant cells surrounded by lymphocytes and plasma cells. Necrosis at the center of the granulomas is exceedingly rare (7,13,19,21), however, occasionally documented (20). Leishman–Donovan bodies are either absent or very small in number. There is an inverse relationship between the number of organisms and the age of the lesion (22). The epidermal changes are nonspecific.

Differential Diagnosis. Other granulomatous dermatitides, especially lupus vulgaris, have to be differentiated from chronic cutaneous leishmaniasis (19,20). This may require the employment of ancillary techniques such as immunohistochemistry with *Leishmania*-specific antibodies (23) or the polymerase chain reaction (24).

Post–Kala-azar Dermal Leishmaniasis

Post–kala-azar dermal leishmaniasis occurs 1 to 5 years after successful treatment of visceral leishmaniasis (1,5,8,17). It

presents initially as hypopigmented macules over the trunk and extremities. The macules become progressively erythematous and evolve into nonulcerated papules and nodules with marked involvement of the face, clinically resembling lepromatous leprosy (1,5,8,17,25,26). The human host is apparently able to confine *Leishmania* to the skin but cannot eradicate the organisms from the body (25).

Histopathology. Reports on the histopathology of post–kala-azar dermal leishmaniasis are sparse. Hypopigmented macules display a superficial perivascular lymphocytic infiltrate with admixed plasma cells without evidence of granuloma formation (25). The amount of epidermal melanin is decreased (7).

The nonulcerated papules and nodules show a dense, diffuse infiltrate composed of histiocytes, lymphocytes, and plasma cells within the dermis with sharply defined margins and a narrow Grenz zone (25,26). Granulomas are not reported and organisms are sparse. This is in contradistinction to earlier studies that describe the presence of well-formed epithelioid cell granulomas in nodular lesions of post–kala-azar dermal leishmaniasis (27,28). The overlying epidermis is often atrophic, and the hair follicles show prominent keratotic plugging (26).

Mucocutaneous Leishmaniasis

Mucocutaneous leishmaniasis, most commonly seen in South America, affects the upper respiratory tract and usually develops subsequently to healed localized (acute) cutaneous leishmaniasis (1,5,17,22). The mucosal lesions usually appear within 2 years of the initial skin involvement but may take as long as 30 years to develop (22). They often begin in the nasal septum that becomes inflamed and later perforates. The lips (especially the upper lip), oral cavity, pharynx, and even the trachea and bronchi can become involved, imposing a severe life-threatening condition on the patient. South American mucocutaneous leishmaniasis probably develops secondary to hematogenous or lymphatic dissemination from primary cutaneous lesions or occasionally from direct extension of nearby skin lesions (5).

Histopathology. The histopathologic changes of mucocutaneous leishmaniasis are subdivided into edematous, granulomatous proliferative, and granulomatous necrotizing stages (29). In the early edematous stage, parasites are scanty, a lymphohistiocytic infiltrate with admixed plasma cells in the superficial and deep dermis is noted, and the overlying epidermis is thin. When the patient develops proliferative lesions, parasites become obvious, tuberculoid granulomas can be seen, and pseudocarcinomatous epidermal hyperplasia develops. These changes characterize the granulomatous proliferative phase. In clinically destructive lesions, areas of necrosis with numerous neutrophils and abundant Leishman–Donovan bodies constitute the granulomatous necrotizing phase.

Visceral Leishmaniasis

Visceral leishmaniasis is a systemic disease characterized by fever, lymphadenopathy, hepatosplenomegaly, ascites, pancytopenia, and emaciation (1,5,17). The Indian name *kala-azar* (meaning "black fever") refers to the diffuse darkening of the skin, most pronounced on the face, hands, and feet, but is seen only in a small proportion of patients and is peculiarly confined to people from the Indian subcontinent (17). The initial cutaneous lesion of visceral leishmaniasis, the leishmanioma, is rarely seen. While generally being devoid of cutaneous involvement during the course of the active visceral disease, patients co-infected with HIV can present with skin lesions. The lesions comprise erythematous papules, often confluent to plaques, and, less often, hypo- and hyper-pigmented macules with a tendency to localize symmetrically on acral zones (30). These lesions have to be differentiated from those seen in post–kala-azar dermal leishmaniasis, which appear after the patient has been successfully treated for visceral leishmaniasis.

Histopathology. The cutaneous lesions in HIV-infected patients are histopathologically nonspecific and consist of a perivascular infiltrate within the superficial dermis composed of lymphocytes and histiocytes with numerous intracytoplasmic organisms within the latter (30). Leishman–Donovan bodies are also found extracellularly (30,31), and in one case in eccrine sweat glands, suggesting transepithelial elimination (31). Parasitization of Kaposi's sarcoma by *Leishmania* spp. (31,32), as well as a leishmanial cutaneous spindle cell pseudotumor (31,33), are also reported.

Viscerotropic Leishmaniasis

Originally thought of as causing cutaneous lesions only, *L. tropica* was recently found as the inciting agent of a visceral form of leishmaniasis in veterans of Operation Desert Storm (34). The condition was termed viscerotropic leishmaniasis. No skin involvement is documented.

ACANTHAMOEBIASIS

Among the three free-living genera of amoebae capable of producing cutaneous lesions (*Acanthamoeba* spp., *Entamoeba histolytica* and *Balamuthia mandrillaris*) acanthamoebiasis recently surfaced as the most common one, seen mostly in conjunction with the AIDS epidemic. It also causes keratitis in nonimmunocompromised individuals wearing soft contact lenses. Granulomatous amebic encephalitis, a fatal disease, is another manifestation of *Acanthamoeba* spp. infection; like cutaneous acanthamoebiasis it affects primarily immunoincompetent patients (35–37). In disseminated acanthamoebiasis, other organ systems such as bones (causing osteomyelitis) can be affected (38).

Acanthamoeba spp. exist in two forms. The amebic cysts, measuring 13 to 19 μm in diameter (35), are resistant to desiccation and excyst to trophozoites only in a favorable environment such as the human host. The latter, between 10 and 20 μm in size (39), reveal slender acanthopodia for slow movement and represent the infectious and invasive form of *Acanthamoeba* spp. (36).

The cutaneous lesions in acanthamoebiasis are nonspecific and consist of papules, nodules, and chronic, non-healing ulcers, tender or nontender, ranging from 0.5 to 3 cm in diameter with the ulcers being sometimes larger (36–42). The skin may serve either as the initial port of entry or may become secondarily involved via hematogenous spread (41,42).

Histopathology. Depending on the number of organisms a nodular or diffuse inflammatory infiltrate composed mostly of neutrophils and histiocytes admixed with extensive tissue necrosis is noted, sometimes evolving into abscess formation (35,38,41). Cutaneous lesions can also present under the histopathologic picture of a leukocytoclastic vasculitis with fibrin deposits within the vessel wall and leukocytoclasis (35,39–41). Lobular panniculitis with necrotizing vasculitis is another form of presentation (37).

Mixed within the inflammatory infiltrate are the round trophozoites projecting acanthopodia and revealing a vacuolated cytoplasm with a centrally placed nucleus and a single prominent nucleolus (Fig. 24-3). Despite often being numerous, the trophozoite forms are inconspicuous and can be missed easily, closely resembling macrophages (8,36,41). The cyst forms, also being present, display a double wall, the outer wall wavy and wrinkled in appearance and the inner wall shallow and scalloped surrounding the cytoplasm. The cyst walls stain with PAS and GMS (38,41).

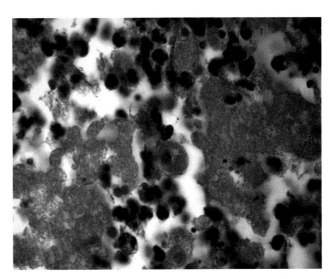

FIGURE 24-3. Acanthamoebiasis. In the center the trophozoite with a large nucleus and basophilic cytoplasm is noted among necrotic debris. (Specimen courtesy of Khalil G. Ghanem, M.D., John Hopkins Hospital, Baltimore, MD.)

Differential Diagnosis. The yeast forms of *Blastomyces dermatitidis* are slightly smaller and have characteristically thick cell walls and broad-based buds; often an overlying epidermal hyperplasia with neutrophilic microabscesses is present (38,41). The cysts of *Entamoeba histolytica* are negative for GMS and do not display an undulating double membrane (41).

SCABIES

Acarid mites produce several skin manifestations in humans, the most common one represented by scabies, which is caused by the eight-legged itch mite *Sarcoptes scabiei* var. *hominis*, also referred to as *Satcoptes sarcoptes scabiei*. Animal pathogenic mites also affect the skin, but only transiently, since the mites do not survive for an extended period of time (3).

Burrows are the pathognomonic lesions of scabies and are found mostly in the florid, papulovesicular type of sarcoptic acariasis (Fig. 24-4A). They are produced by female mites and occur mainly on the palms, the palmar and lateral aspects of the fingers, the interdigital spaces, the flexor surfaces of the wrists, the nipples of women, the genitals of men, and, to a lesser extent, on the buttocks and axillae. Characteristically the head is spared, except in newborns and infants (43). The burrows appear as fine, tortuous,

blackish threads a few millimeters long. A vesicle may be visible near the blind end of the burrow. The mite is situated in this vesicle and may be visible as a tiny gray speck by dermatoscopy. Although pathognomonic, the burrow is not the most common lesion seen in scabies. Small, erythematous, often excoriated papules are more frequent (43).

In some patients, itching nodules persist for several months after successful treatment, and is therefore named nodular scabies or persistent scabietic nodules. They are found most commonly on the scrotum and are thought to result from a prolonged response to persistent scabies antigens (44).

In a third, rare variant, the so-called Norwegian scabies or crusted scabies, innumerable mites are present. Patients with this variant show widespread erythema, hyperkeratosis, and crusting, but no obvious burrows.

Histopathology. A definitive diagnosis of scabies can be made only by demonstration of the mite or its products. A very superficial epidermal shave biopsy of an early papule or, preferably, of an entire burrow may be carried out with a #15 scalpel blade (45). Local anesthesia is not required. The biopsy specimen is placed on a glass slide, and a drop of immersion oil and then a cover slip are placed on top of it (Fig. 24-4B). This technique yields a higher percentage of positive preparations than the often performed mere scraping of a suspicious lesion with a scalpel blade.

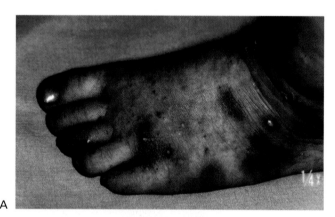

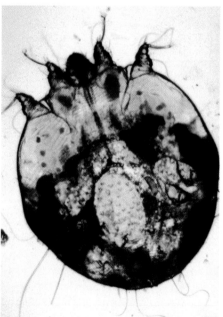

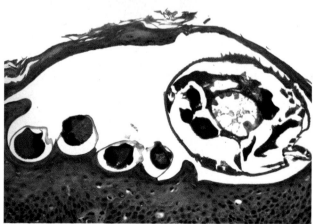

FIGURE 24-4. Scabies. **A:** Numerous pustules and papules are noted on the back of the foot and the toes of this infected child. **B:** Adult female mite found in skin scrapings. **C:** The female mite is located in a burrow within the stratum corneum. The smaller organisms on the left represent developing mite embryos within eggshells.

Histologic examination of a specimen containing a burrow reveals that the burrow in almost its entire length is located within the horny layer (46). Only the extreme, blind end of the burrow, where the female mite is situated, extends into the stratum malpighii (47). The mite has a rounded body and measures about 350 to 450 μm in length and 250 to 350 μm in width (3) (Fig. 24-4C).

In the papulovesicular form of scabies, spongiosis is present in the stratum malpighii near the mite to such an extent that formation of a vesicle is often the result. Even if no mite is found in the sections, the presence of eggs containing larvae, eggshells, or fecal deposits (scybala) within the stratum corneum is indicative of scabies (46,48). The dermal infiltrate in sections containing mites shows varying numbers of eosinophils.

In nodular or persistent nodular scabies, there is a dense, chronic inflammatory, often pseudolymphomatous, infiltrate in which many eosinophils may be present. Vasculitis is considered by some as being frequent (48), but by others as representing a rather uncommon event (44). These diverse findings may be related to the duration of the scabietic nodules and the timing of the biopsy (44). The nodules are rich in indeterminate cells, sometimes misleading to the diagnosis of Langerhans cell histiocytosis based on light microscopy and immunophenotyping alone (49). Atypical mononuclear, CD30+ cells may be found (50), and in some instances, the nodules show, as in persistent arthropod bites or stings (see later), a histologic picture resembling lymphoma (51). Viable mites are hardly ever found in the nodules. However, mite parts are seen in up to 22% (44).

In Norwegian scabies, the thickened horny layer is riddled with innumerable mites, so that nearly every section shows several parasites (48).

Pathogenesis. Earlier scanning electron microscopical studies reveal the keratinocytes around the burrow to be compacted, indicating that the mite physically forces its way in between the keratinocytes, rather than chewing a passage (47). More recent studies, however, employing also transmission electron microscopy, find the secretion of cytolytic substances by the mite as a contributing factor in advancing the parasite body through the skin in addition to mere compression (52). The cellular damage was greatest around the body, especially the mite capitulum.

Both cell-mediated and humoral immune responses are activated in scabies. The acute eczematoid reaction in the epidermis is indicative of cell-mediated hypersensitivity. A role for humoral hypersensitivity is suggested by the presence of immunoglobulin M (IgM) and the third component of complement (C3) in vessel walls (44,53). In addition to being reported in the mentally deficient and the physically debilitated, Norwegian scabies is observed generally in patients who are severely compromised in their immune responses, including those with leukemia, lymphoma, and AIDS (54).

CUTANEOUS LARVA MIGRANS

Cutaneous larva migrans is caused by skin-penetrating larvae of nematodes, most commonly of the cat and dog hookworm *Ancylostoma braziliense*. *A. caninum*, *A. tubaeformis*, *Uncinaria stenocephala*, *Bunostomum phlebotomum*, and *Gnathostomum spinigerum*; other hookworms parasitic to dogs, cats, cattle, and other mammals, are also linked to the condition (55,56). The infestation occurs through contact with soil contaminated with the larvae. The exposed parts of the body, most commonly the feet but also the buttocks in travelers who lie nude in the sand, are most commonly involved. Creeping eruption represents the clinical manifestation of cutaneous larva migrans and is

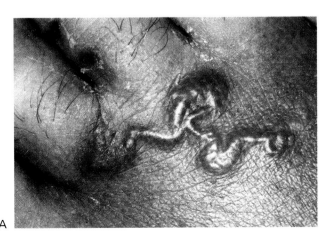 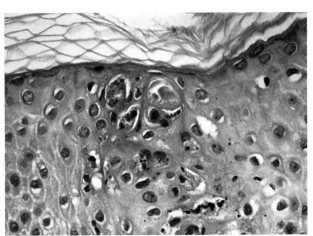

FIGURE 24-5. Cutaneous larva migrans. **A:** This curvilinear superficial burrow is the prototypical clinical manifestation (From Schaller KF, ed. *Colour Atlas of Tropical Dermatology and Venerology.* New York: Springer, 1994:116, with permission.) **B:** The organism is found within the epidermis. (Photograph courtesy of Jae-Sook Ryu, M.D., Hanyang University College of Medicine, Seoul, Korea.)

manifested by an irregularly linear, thin, raised, serpiginous burrow, 2 to 3 mm wide (Fig. 24-5A). The larva moves a few millimeters per day. The eruption is self-limited because humans are accidental hosts, leaving the hookworm incapable of sexually maturing.

Histopathology. The visible track does not correlate with the exact location of the larva and represents an inflammatory response composed of lymphocytes admixed with many eosinophils in the epidermis and upper dermis (56). The parasite is found 1 to 2 cm ahead of the visible track within a burrow located in the epidermis (55) (Fig. 24-5B). The lesion, aside from the larva, which is often not observed in the biopsies, shows spongiosis and intraepidermal vesicles in which necrotic keratinocytes can be seen.

Pathogenesis. The tissue penetration and the movements of the hookworm larvae within the epidermis are at least in part due to active production and secretion of proteases by the parasite (57).

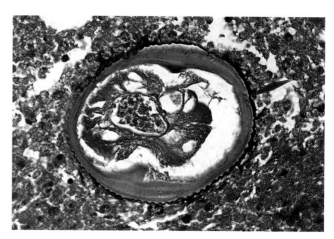

FIGURE 24-6. Dirofilariasis. The helminth is surrounded by necrotic debris within the subcutis. This organism represented *Dirofilaria tenuis.* (Photograph courtesy of Yezid Gutierrez, M.D., Ph.D., Cleveland Clinic Foundation, Cleveland, OH.)

SUBCUTANEOUS DIROFILARIASIS

Dirofilariasis is a zoonosis most commonly seen on the North American continent in the southeastern United States, with 75% of almost all cases being reported from Florida, thereby representing the epicenter of the infestation (58). The definitive hosts of *Dirofilaria* spp. are dogs, cats, and raccoons, as well as bears and porcupines (the latter two seen in the northern United States and in Canada, where dirofilariasis cases have also occasionally been reported).

Subcutaneous infection of humans by *Dirofilaria* spp. is rare and usually caused in North America by *D. tenuis*, *D. ursi*, or *D. subdermata*, and in Europe, Africa, and Asia by *D. repens* (59,60). Mosquitoes transmit microfilariae from infected animals to humans, the terminal hosts. In humans, the parasite never reaches the sexually mature adult stage capable of producing microfilariae, thereby rendering human-to-human transmission impossible (61).

Over the course of the infestation, one or, occasionally, several well-defined, firm, slightly red, tender nodules, measuring 1 to 2 cm in diameter and clinically often mistaken for lipomas (59), develop in areas not covered by clothes, especially the head. Multiple lesions usually result from migration of a single worm (58).

Histopathology. At the center of the subcutaneous nodule, there is a tightly convoluted worm seen in multiple transverse and diagonal sections. Transverse sections measure from 50 to 300 μm in diameter with the male worms being smaller than the female ones (58). The parasite possesses a thick, laminated cuticle displaying longitudinal ridges and transversal striae in *D. repens* and *D. tenuis* (Fig. 24-6), and a smooth cuticle in the dog heartworm *D. immitis*, the cause of pulmonary dirofilariasis in humans, allowing for species identification on histologic sections (59). It is imperative to thoroughly section the tissue block in order not to miss

the helminth (62). The worm is embedded in eosinophilic material and surrounded by an inflammatory reaction that includes many eosinophils, mononuclear cells, and often foreign-body giant cells. Unlike fungal infections, fat necrosis is conspicuously absent (62). The extent of fibrosis in the surrounding tissue correlates with the extent to which the parasite is degenerated (58).

Differential Diagnosis. Although the dermatological manifestation of subcutaneous sparganosis are identical to the infestation with *D. tenuis*, the former which is caused by the larval stage of the tapeworm *Spirometra* spp., can affect any organ system. The larva has the typical histology of a pseudophyllidean tapeworm consisting of a tegument, a cellular subtegument, and mesenchymal tissues with numerous large, longitudinal muscle cells and excretory canals (58). However, it still can be histologically mistaken for *Dirofilaria* spp. (58,62).

ONCHOCERCIASIS

Onchocerciasis is common in certain regions of Central America, Venezuela, and tropical Africa. It is transmitted by black flies of the genus *Simulium*, which breed in fast-flowing rivers; through their proboscis, the infective larvae of *Onchocerca volvulus*, a filarial nematode, enter the human skin. They mature to the adult stage in the subcutaneous tissue. The adult worms live in the deep dermis and subcutis and become clinically apparent as asymptomatic subcutaneous nodules called onchocercomas, of which there are usually only a few, ranging in size from 0.5 to 2.0 cm (Fig. 24-7A). The adult worms do not cause any harm; however, their progeny, consisting of millions of microfilariae, live in the dermis and the aqueous humor of the eyes, where they provoke inflammatory changes after several

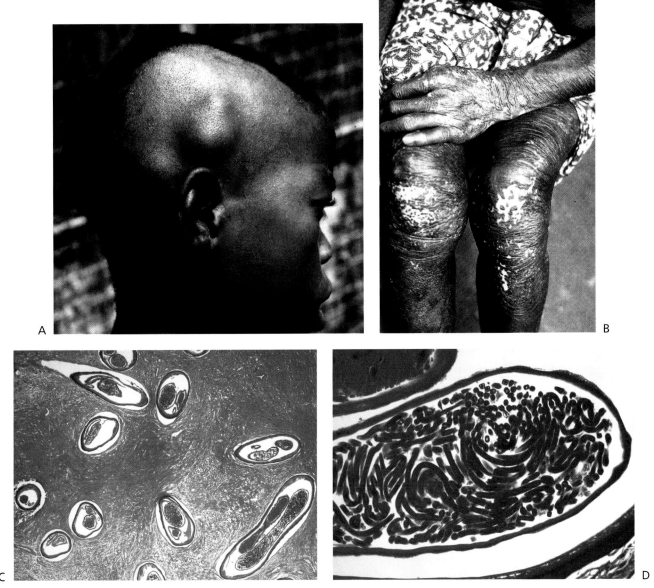

FIGURE 24-7. Onchocerciasis. **A:** African patient with onchocercoma on the head. **B:** African patient with oncocercal dermatitis. (From Schaller KF, ed. *Colour Atlas of Tropical Dermatology and Venerology.* New York: Springer, 1994:127, with permission.) **C:** In an onchocercoma multiple cross and transverse sections of the adult organism can be seen surrounded by dense fibrosis. **D:** On high magnification, the microfilariae within the female adult worm become obvious. When released by the female worm, the microfilariae evoke the changes seen in onchocercal dermatitis. (C and D specimen courtesy of Yezid Gutierrez, M.D., Ph.D., Cleveland Clinic Foundation, Cleveland, OH.)

years. In the eyes, keratitis, iridocyclitis, chorioretinitis, and optic atrophy, ultimately result in blindness (63). On slit lamp examination, the microfilariae in the anterior chamber of the eyes may be seen to be moving actively (63). Clinically, onchocercal dermatitis is characterized by itching, edema, lichenification, and pigment shifting ("leopard skin") (64–66) (Fig. 24-7B). Later on, the skin becomes atrophic. A clinical classification and grading system of the cutaneous changes in onchocerciasis has been proposed but is not universally accepted yet (64). *Onchocerca volvulus,* like *Wuchereria bancrofti,* may also be a cause of lymphatic

filariasis, in which massive numbers of microfilariae may occlude lymphatics and result in elephantiasis (67). Lymphadenopathy and so-called hanging groins (adenolymphoceles) are other manifestations of the disease (64).

Histopathology. The onchocercomas show a chronic inflammatory infiltrate and fibrosis at their peripheries. Their centers consist of dense fibrous tissue containing transverse and diagonal sections of adult worms measuring from 125 to 450 μm in transverse diameter and up to 500 mm in length in females and 42 mm in males (68) (Fig. 24-7C and D). Some of them are alive at the time of biopsy. Dead worms are surrounded by an inflammatory reaction containing foreign-body giant cells. Microfilariae, hatched by female worms, are occasionally observed within lymphatic vessels of the onchocercomas, through which they are disseminated in the skin. They are from 5 to 9 μm in diameter and from 220 to 360 μm in length (68).

In early, untreated onchocercal dermatitis, many undulating microfilariae are present within the dermis, mainly close to the epidermis (65). Their number decreases greatly with time, and thus they may be difficult to find in old lesions (66). In early infections, reactive changes in the dermis are minimal, but, in the course of years, chronic inflammatory cells including eosinophils accumulate around the vessels, and, ultimately, fibrosis of the dermis, especially perivascularly, results (65). Hyperorthokeratosis, parakeratosis, epidermal hyperplasia (in the late-stage flattening of the epidermis), tortuosity of dermal vessels, and pigment incontinence are other features of long-standing onchocercal dermatitis (65).

Pathogenesis. The slow development of the cutaneous changes and also of the ocular changes suggests that microfilariae, as they gradually disintegrate, act as a source of foreign protein and that the dermatitis and the various forms of eye involvement are the result of a coordinated response by the cellular and humoral immune system (65,66,68). Indeed, while alive, microfilariae do not evoke a strong inflammatory response. Only when dying or dead, either during the natural course of their life span or therapeutically induced, microfilariae produce a prominent inflammatory reaction, with eosinophils being essential in the process (65,66,68).

STRONGYLOIDIASIS

Strongyloides stercoralis is a small intestinal nematode that is endemic in the southeastern United States (especially eastern Kentucky, rural Tennessee, southern Virginia, and the western Carolinas), and that in addition to gastrointestinal symptoms produces cutaneous manifestations (69). The latter include linear or serpiginous urticarial lesions moving at a rate of 5 to 15 cm/h caused by rapidly migrating larvae (*larva currens*), progressive petechial and purpuric eruptions, chronic urticaria, prurigo nodularis, and lichen simplex chronicus (69–71). A fatal disseminated infestation with *Strongyloides stercoralis* is seen primarily in patients receiving long-term corticosteroid therapy and presents clinically with extensive purpura (71,72).

Histopathology. The serpiginous urticarial lesions thought to represent the migrating path of larvae are consistently negative for organisms (71). In disseminated infestations, *S. stercoralis* filariform larvae, measuring from 9 to 15 μm in diameter, are seen at all levels of the dermis and are associated with vascular damage producing purpura and petechiae (71,72). These changes often do not provoke an inflammatory response, probably because these patients are severely immunocompromised (71).

SCHISTOSOMIASIS

Schistosomiasis is caused by trematodes of the genus *Schistosoma* and affects 180 to 200 million people in 71 countries, thereby making it the most important trematode pathogenic to humans worldwide (73). It is acquired through exposure to skin-penetrating cercariae, a stage in the life cycle of the parasite. The cercariae emerge from a freshwater snail which functions as an obligate intermediate host to the fluke. The cercariae burrow through the skin and migrate to venous plexuses, where they mature.

Three species of *Schistosoma* are pathogenic to humans. *S. mansoni* is common in the Caribbean islands and in northeastern South America; *S. japonicum* is found in Eastern Asia; and *S. haematobium* is common in the Middle East and in Africa. The usual habitats of *S. mansoni* are the portal circulation and mesenteric venules of the large intestines, with discharge of the eggs in the stool. The usual habitat of *S. japonicum* is the small gut, also resulting in discharge of the eggs with the stool. The usual habitats of *S. haematobium* are the pelvic and vesical venules, with passage of the eggs with the urine. *S. mansoni* and *S. japonicum*, through granulomas in the liver, may cause portal hypertension and esophageal varices, and *S. haematobium*, through granulomas in the bladder, may lead to hematuria and hydronephrosis (74). In Africa, mixed infections with both *S. mansoni* and *S. haematobium* are not uncommon (75,76).

The cutaneous manifestations of schistosomiasis can be divided into three types depending on the life cycle of the trematode (73,77).

Dermatitis schistosomica (swimmer's itch) is caused by the initial penetration of the skin by human or nonhuman cercariae and manifests as a pruritic maculopapular eruption usually lasting several hours, sometimes days and, rarely, weeks depending upon previous sensitization. Cercariae of nonhuman species of *Schistosoma* spp. (usually avian species primarily affecting ducks or other water birds) can penetrate the skin but subsequently die. The dermatitis produced by anthropophilic *Schistosoma* is milder than that caused by nonhuman species (73).

The second cutaneous manifestation of schistosomiasis, also transitory, is comprised of the *bilharzides* or *schistosomides*. Several weeks after penetration, the cercariae have matured into worms 15 to 25 mm in length. The female then releases thousands of eggs into the blood stream. Their release may be accompanied by anaphylactoid reactions manifested by a combination of fever, urticaria, and sometimes purpura known in Japan as Katayama syndrome and in China as Yangtze fever (73,77).

A specific cutaneous involvement (known as *bilharziasis cutanea tarda*) represents the third cutaneous manifestation of schistosomiasis, and is caused by ectopic deposition of eggs within the dermis when ova have become dislodged from their natural habitat in the venous circulation. Most commonly seen in *S. haematobium*, it is still a rare event and presents as papular, verrucous, ulcerative, or granulomatous lesions usually of the genital or perianal skin (73,77,78). In rare instances, the thorax, abdomen and, even less commonly, the face or scalp are involved (75,79–81).

Histopathology. Bilharziasis cutanea tarda represents the main persistent cutaneous lesion of schistosomiasis. Its pathologic hallmark is a palisading, necrotizing granulomatous inflammation within the dermis consisting of histiocytes, lymphocytes, plasma cells, and rare multinucleated giant cells surrounding complete or degenerated schistosomal ova located in the central area of necrosis (75,78,79) (Fig. 24-8). A predominant population of eosinophils as part of the inflammation is also described (78,81). In older lesions the eggs are calcified and surrounded by fibrosis; the inflammatory infiltrate is sparse or absent (73). The overlying epidermis often reveals pseudocarcinomatous hyperplasia (78,79,82,83). Transepithelial elimination of the ova is described (83).

The ova measure up to 1 mm in greatest dimension and possess a chitinous outer shell that stains positively with PAS. However, only *S. mansoni* but not *S. haematobium* or *S. japonicum* are acid fast-positive (75,79,81). The presence and position of a spine on the shell of the ova permit their classification within the tissue. *S. haematobium* ova have a spine in the apical position, whereas the spine of *S. mansoni* ova is on the lateral aspect, and *S. japonicum* ova have no spine. In rare instances, one may also see adult worms inside distended blood vessels in the dermis (79).

Pathogenesis. The eggs and embryos are said to release soluble substances that act as antigens sensitizing T-lymphocytes. These, in turn, release lymphokines leading to migration of macrophages and eosinophils, and to granuloma formation (73).

SUBCUTANEOUS CYSTICERCOSIS

The pork tapeworm *Taenia solium* develops in the human intestinal tract following the ingestion of inadequately cooked pork containing *T. solium* larvae. The tapeworm discharges its eggs in the feces. When eggs with the encysted larvae are ingested by humans, usually through contamination of hands and food by the subject's own feces but also by regurgitation of eggs from the intestinal tract into the stomach by reverse peristalsis (84), they hatch, and larvae entering the bloodstream invade various tissues, where they develop into cysticerci. Whereas the infestation with an egg-producing adult tapeworm confined to the intestines (taeniasis) imposes little harm to the patient, cysticerci can have deleterious effects by evoking cerebral cysticercosis, the most common parasitic infestation of the central nervous system worldwide (85). More than 1,000 cases per year are reported in the United States (86).

Subcutaneous cysticercosis is considerably less common. Clinically, one or several, or, rarely, numerous firm, asymptomatic nodules are present in the subcutaneous tissue. They usually measure 1 to 2 cm in diameter and can persist for many years (84,87,88). The subcutaneously located cysts of cysticercosis do not carry any risk to the patient's health but are of great value in the diagnosis of cerebral cysticercosis, which causes seizures (85).

Histopathology. A thick, fibrous capsule covered by several layers of epithelioid cells admixed with a few Langerhans giant cells but without caseous necrosis surrounds a cystic cavity containing clear fluid and a white, irregularly shaped membranous structure representing a cysticercus larva (89). Eosinophilic infiltration of the capsule is present (89). Step sections reveal the scolex of the larva with suckers and hooks (84,87) (Fig. 24-9).

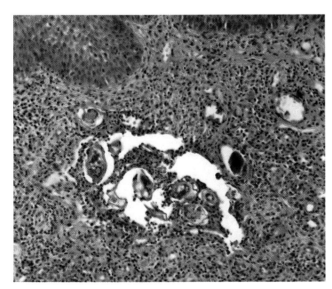

FIGURE 24-8. Schistosomiasis. In bilharziasis cutanea tarda, the schistosomal eggs provoke a granulomatous reaction within the dermis. (Photograph courtesy of Yezid Gutierrez, M.D., Ph.D., Cleveland Clinic Foundation, Cleveland, OH.)

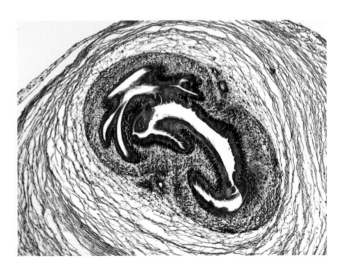

FIGURE 24-9. Subcutaneous cysticercosis. This cysticercus larva was found in a cavity within the subcutis surrounded by granulation tissue and necrotic debris. (Specimen courtesy of Dieter Krahl, M.D., Institut für Dermatohistologie, Heidelberg, Germany.)

MYIASIS

The order Diptera (having two wings) includes flies, gnats, and mosquitoes. When fly larvae inhabit the human body, the condition is called myiasis (from the Greek word for fly, *myia*). The distribution of myiasis is worldwide, with greater abundance of cases and of causative species in the tropics.

The cutaneous manifestations of myiasis can be subdivided into three clinically recognized subcategories: wound myiasis, furuncular myiasis, and creeping myiasis (not to be mistaken with the creeping eruption caused by cutaneous larva migrans) (90–92).

In wound myiasis, which may be caused by many different fly species including the common housefly *Musca domestica*, the fly larvae (maggots) are deposited on necrotic flesh.

Furuncular myiasis occurs mostly in the tropics and is caused in Africa by the tumbu fly *Cordylobia anthropophaga*, and in the American tropics by the human botfly *Dermatobia hominis*. The latter has a unique life cycle. The female fly captures blood-sucking insects such as mosquitoes or other flies in the air and deposits a number of eggs on their abdomen. When these vectors come in contact with a human host, the *Dermatobia* larvae hatch and enter the skin where they cause a furuncular lesion known as a "warble." Within 6 to 12 weeks, an adult fly develops and leaves the human host through the breathing orifice of the warble.

In creeping myiasis, larvae of *Gasterophilus* spp. or *Hypoderma* spp., flies parasitic to horses or cattle, burrow into the skin and cause a migratory pattern. In contrast to the creeping eruption seen in larva migrans, the movements are more restricted and proceed more slowly.

Histopathology. In wound myiasis, the larvae generally remain superficial, are usually alive, and can be recognized grossly at the time of biopsy (91). In furuncular myiasis,

there is an intense, mixed inflammatory infiltrate composed of neutrophils, eosinophils, lymphocytes, plasma cells, and Langerhans giant cells surrounding the cavity, which is occupied by the larva (90,93,94) (Fig. 24-10). In creeping myiasis due to *Hypoderma* spp., the inflammatory response is very minimal (91).

Pathogenesis. Both *Dermatobia hominis* and *Cordylobia anthropophaga* secrete a bacteriostatic fluid that prevents secondary bacterial infection of the larval cavity (90,95,96).

TUNGIASIS

Tungiasis is a cutaneous infestation by the gravid female sand flea *Tunga penetrans* that is endemic in the Caribbean, Central and South America, sub-Saharan Africa, and on the Indian subcontinent (97,98).

Only the female fleas are capable of penetrating the skin. They burrow a cavity with the head turned toward the dermis feeding on the host. The gravid female eliminates its eggs through an apical opening of the cavity to the outside, and dies soon thereafter, exhibiting a total life span of approximately 1 month (97).

The condition is acquired by walking barefoot. Characteristically, the lesions are located on the toes, the interdigital spaces, and the soles and heels. They are mostly single and consist of a tender nodule 5 to 6 mm in diameter, with a black to brown central tip representing the posterior end of the parasite.

Histopathology. The flea is located in the epidermis and upper dermis inside a cavity (Fig. 24-11A and B). In its apical portion, it is surrounded by a hyperplastic epidermis. In the absence of bacterial superinfection, any perilesional inflammatory infiltrate is usually minimal and consists of lymphocytes, neutrophils, and eosinophils (97). Inside the cavity, portions of the exoskeleton, hypodermal layer, trachea, and digestive tract identify the organism as an arthropod. The uniformly present developing eggs are likely the most useful to differentiate *T. penetrans* from other organisms (99).

ARTHROPOD ASSAULT REACTIONS

Arthropod bites and stings are common afflictions in humans. They induce a localized or widespread and often systemic reaction, depending on the type of the assaulting species and the capacity of the body to react.

Most stings evoked by mosquitoes, bees, wasps, hornets, or bedbugs are characterized initially by a localized urticarial reaction, often followed by the development of a papule and papulovesicle associated with intense pruritus. Frequently, a central punctum can be recognized. In more intense reactions, most commonly seen on the legs, the lesions are bullous (100) (Fig. 24-12A). Typically, they re-

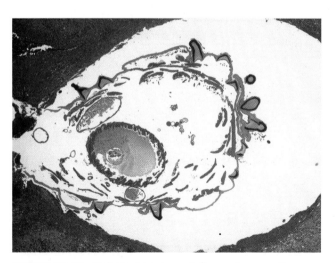

FIGURE 24-10. Myiasis. An intense inflammatory reaction surrounded this larva seen in a case of furuncular myiasis. (Specimen courtesy of Dieter Krahl, M.D., Institut für Dermatohistologie, Heidelberg, Germany.)

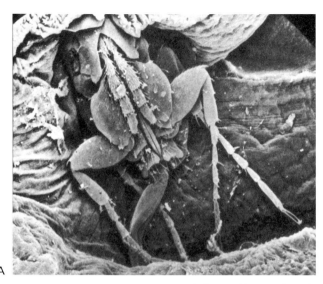

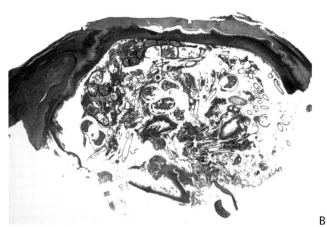

A   B

FIGURE 24-11. Tungiasis. **A:** This scanning electron micrograph shows the swollen abdomen of the female sand flea feeding on human blood. (Reprinted with permission from Schuller-Petrović S et al. Tungiasis—eine immer häufigere Urlaubsdermatose. *Hautarzt* 1987;38:162–164). **B:** On H&E-stained section, the typical superficial intradermal location of the flea is noted.

solve without sequelae within days. In rare cases, however, they may persist for weeks or months and are then referred to as a persistent arthropod assault reaction (101,102).

Bites by the brown recluse spider *Loxosceles reclusa* are common in the south central United States. Often painless initially, they are capable of inducing significant skin necrosis (necrotic arachnidism) (103).

Hypersensitivity to insect bites, especially from fleas, gnats, mosquitoes, or bedbugs, may result in papular urticaria, also known as lichen urticatus or strophulus infantum. It is characterized by grouped urticarial papules and papulovesicles with a tendency to spread. Spontaneous res-

olution within several days is usual (104). The condition cannot be reliably distinguished from arthropod bites (105).

Histopathology. The classical histopathologic hallmark of an arthropod bite is a wedge-shaped, superficial and deep, perivascular and interstitial inflammatory dermal infiltrate composed of lymphocytes and eosinophils, often in association with an overlying focus of spongiosis, which sometimes evolves into a vesicle or even progresses to epidermal necrosis (106) (Fig. 24-12B). These changes are indistinguishable from papular urticaria (105).

Mosquito bites initially show mainly neutrophils, mostly vasculocentric, and later a predominantly mononuclear in-

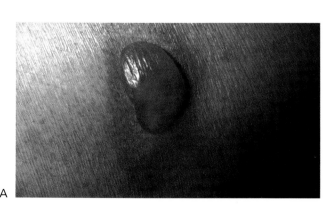

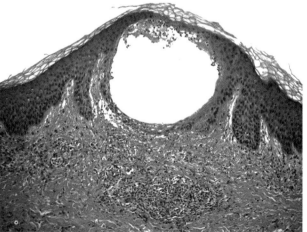

A   B

FIGURE 24-12. Arthropod assault reaction. **A:** Sometimes the clinical reaction to an arthropod assault is intense and results in a blister (so-called *culicosis bullosa*). **B:** On histological sections in the center of the arthropod assault, an intraepidermal vesicle can often be seen.

filtrate of lymphocytes and plasma cells. Eosinophils are few or absent (107,108).

Bites of the brown recluse spider initially show a neutrophilic perivasculitis with hemorrhage. Later on, in cases of necrotic ulcers, one finds arterial wall necrosis and an infiltrate containing many eosinophils (109).

Some persistent arthropod assault reactions produce a dense lymphoid infiltrate, often with formation of lymphoid follicles that has to be differentiated from lymphoma (110). In contrast to lymphomas, the lymphoid follicles in persistent arthropod reactions frequently show germinal centers and do not show evidence of clonality. Large transformed, CD30+ lymphoid cells with hyperchromatic nuclei may also be found but do not represent a sign of malignancy (102).

Occasionally parts of the sting apparatus may be retained within the dermis inducing a chronic inflammatory response, often with associated eosinophils, accompanied by pseudocarcinomatous epidermal hyperplasia (111).

Pathogenesis. The primary toxin in the brown recluse envenomation is sphingomyelinase D, which interacts with the outer plasma membrane of erythrocytes, endothelial cells, and platelets. The severe skin necrosis seen in this spider bite is a consequence of vascular damage (112).

Acknowledgment. The excellent technical assistance of Lisa Wierzbicki is greatly appreciated. Issa Issa provided invaluable assistance with the microphotography.

REFERENCES

1. Choi CM, Lerner EA. Leishmaniasis as an emerging infection. *J Invest Dermatol Symp Proc* 2001;6:175.
2. World Health Organization. Leishmania/HIV Co-infection in Southwestern Europe 1990–98: Retrospective Analysis of 965 Cases. Geneva: World Health Organization, 2000.
3. Guiterrez Y. Diagnostic Pathology of Parasitic Infections with Clinical Correlations. 2nd ed. New York and Oxford: Oxford University Press, 2000.
4. Kane MM, Mosser DM. *Leishmania* parasites and their ploys to disrupt macrophage activation. *Curr Opin Hematol* 2000;7:26.
5. Grevelink SA. Lerner EA. Leishmaniasis. *J Am Acad Dermatol* 1996;34:257.
6. Pearson RD, Sousa A de Q. Clinical spectrum of leishmaniasis. *Clin Infect Dis* 1996;22:1–13.
7. Mehregan DR, Mehregan AH, Mehregan DA. Histologic diagnosis of cutaneous leishmaniasis. *Clin Dermatol* 1999;17:297.
8. Salman SM, Rubeiz NG, Kibbi A-G. Cutaneous leishmaniasis: clinical features and diagnosis. *Clin Dermatol* 1999;17:291.
9. Amin M, Manisali M. Cutaneous leishmaniasis affecting the face: report of a case. *J Oral Maxillofac Surg* 2000;58:1066.
10. Maloney DM, Maloney JE, Dotson D, et al. Cutaneous leishmaniasis: Texas case diagnosed by electron microscopy. *J Am Acad Dermatol* 2002;47:614.
11. Royer M, Crowe M. American cutaneous leishmaniasis: a cluster of 3 cases during military training in Panama. *Arch Pathol Lab Med* 2002;126:471.
12. El-Hassan AM, Zijlstra EE. Leishmaniasis in Sudan. 1. Cutaneous leishmaniasis. *Trans R Soc Trop Med Hyg* 2001;95[Suppl 1]:S1.
13. Kurban AK, Malak JA, Farah FS, et al. Histopathology of cutaneous leishmaniasis. *Arch Dermatol* 1966;93:396.
14. Simpson MH, Mullins JF, Stone OJ. Disseminated anergic cutaneous leishmaniasis. An autochthonous case in Texas and the Mexican States of Tamaulipas and Nuevo Leon. *Arch Dermatol* 1968;97:301.
15. Bittencourt AL, Barral A, Costa JML, et al. Diffuse cutaneous leishmaniasis with atypical aspects. *Int J Dermatol* 1992;31:568.
16. Goihman-Yahr M. American mucocutaneous leishmaniasis. *Dermatol Clin* 1994;12:703.
17. Kubba R, Al-Gindan Y. Leishmaniasis. *Dermatol Clin* 1989;7:331.
18. Momeni AZ, Yotsumoto S, Mehregan DR, et al. Chronic lupoid leishmaniasis. Evaluation by polymerase chain reaction. *Arch Dermatol* 1996;132:198.
19. Strick RA, Borok M, Gasiorowski HC. Recurrent cutaneous leishmaniasis. *J Am Acad Dermatol* 1983: 9:437.
20. Peltier E, Wolkenstein P, Deniau M, et al. Caseous necrosis in cutaneous leishmaniasis. *J Clin Pathol* 1996;49:517.
21. Hill PA. A case of granulomatous dermatitis: cutaneous leishmaniasis. *Pathology* 1997;29:434.
22. Samady JA, Janniger CK, Schwartz RA. Cutaneous and mucocutaneous leishmaniasis. *Cutis* 1996;57:13.
23. Kenner JR, Aronson NE, Bratthauer GL, et al. Immunohistochemistry to identify *Leishmania* parasites in fixed tissues. *J Cutan Pathol* 1999;26:130.
24. Safaei A, Motazedian MH, Vasei M. Polymerase chain reaction for diagnosis of cutaneous leishmaniasis in histologically positive, suspicious and negative skin biopsies. *Dermatology* 2002;205:18.
25. Mukherjee A, Ramesh V, Misra RS. Post-kala-azar dermal leishmaniasis: a light and electron microscopic study of 18 cases. *J Cutan Pathol* 1993;20:320.
26. Singh N, Ramesh V, Arora VK, et al. Nodular post-kala-azar dermal leishmaniasis: a distinct histopathological entity. *J Cutan Pathol* 1998;25:95.
27. Sen Gupta PC, Bhattacharjee B. Histopathology of post-kala-azar dermal leishmaniasis. *J Trop Med Hyg* 1953;56:110.
28. Yawalkar SJ, Mardhekar BV, Mahabir BS. Post-kala-azar dermal leishmaniasis. *J Trop Med Hyg* 1966;69:140.
29. Sangueza OP, Sangueza JM, Stiller MJ, et al. Mucocutaneous leishmaniasis: a clinicopathologic classification. *J Am Acad Dermatol* 1993;28:927.
30. Postigo C, Llamos R, Zarco C, et al. Cutaneous lesions in patients with visceral leishmaniasis and HIV infection. *J Infect* 1997;35:265.
31. Perrin C, Taillan B, Hofman P, et al. Atypical cutaneous histological features of visceral leishmaniasis in acquired immunodeficiency syndrome. *Am J Dermatopathol* 1995;17:145.
32. Taillan B, Marty P, Schneider S, et al. Visceral leishmaniasis involving a cutaneous Kaposi's sarcoma lesion and free areas of skin. *Eur J Med* 1992;4:255.
33. Perrin C, Michiels JF, Bernard E, et al. Cutaneous spindle cell pseudotumors due to *Mycobacterium gordonae* and *Leishmania infantum*. An immunophenotypic study. *Am J Dermatopathol* 1993;15:553.
34. Magill AJ, Grögl M, Gasser RA Jr, et al. Visceral infection by *Leishmania tropica* in veterans of Operation Desert Storm. *N Engl J Med* 1993;328:1383.
35. Tan B, Weldon-Linne CM, Rhone DP, et al. *Acanthamoeba* infection presenting as skin lesions in patients with the acquired immunodeficiency syndrome. *Arch Pathol Lab Med* 1993;117:1043.
36. Wortman PD. Acanthamoeba infection. *Int J Dermatol* 1996;35:48.
37. Rosenberg AS, Morgan MB. Disseminated acanthamoebiasis presenting as lobular panniculitis with necrotizing vasculitis in a patient with *AIDS*. *J Cutan Pathol* 2001:28:307.

38. Steinberg JP, Galindo RL, Kraus ES, et al. Disseminated acanthamebiasis in a renal transplant recipient with osteomyelitis and cutaneous lesions: case report and literature review. *Clin Infect Dis* 2002;35:e43.
39. Deluol A-M, Teilhac M-F, Poirot J-L, et al. Cutaneous lesions due to *Acanthamoeba sp* in a patient with *AIDS*. *J Eukaryot Microbiol* 1996;43:130S.
40. Helton J, Loveless M, White CR Jr. Cutaneous acanthamoeba infection associated with leukocytoclastic vasculitis in an *AIDS* patient. *Am J Dermatopathol* 1993;15:146.
41. Murakawa GJ, McCalmont T, Altman J, et al. Disseminated acanthamebiasis in patients with *AIDS*. A report of five cases and a review of the literature. *Arch Dermatol* 1995;131:1291.
42. Torno MS Jr, Babapour R, Gurevitch A, et al. Cutaneous acanthamoebiasis in *AIDS*. *J Am Acad Dermatol* 2000;42:351.
43. Orkin M, Maibach HI. This scabies pandemic. *N Engl J Med* 1978;298:496.
44. Liu H-N, Sheu W-J, Chu T-L. Scabietic nodules: a dermatopathologic and immunofluorescent study. *J Cutan Pathol* 1992;19:124.
45. Martin WE, Wheeler CE Jr. Diagnosis of human scabies by epidermal shave biopsy. *J Am Acad Dermatol* 1979;1:335.
46. Head ES, Macdonald EM, Ewert A, et al. *Sarcoptes scabiei* in histopathologic sections of skin in human scabies. *Arch Dermatol* 1990;126:1475.
47. Shelley WB, Shelley ED. Scanning electron microscopy of the scabies burrow and its contents, with special reference to the *Sarcoptes scabiei* egg. *J Am Acad Dermatol* 1983;9:673.
48. Fernandez N, Torres A, Ackerman AB. Pathological findings in human scabies. *Arch Dermatol* 1977;113:320.
49. Hashimoto K, Fujiwara K, Punwaney J, et al. Post-scabietic nodules: a lymphohistiocytic reaction rich in indeterminate cells. *J Dermatol* 2000;27:181.
50. Gallardo F, Barranco C, Toll A, Pujol RM. CD30 antigen expression in cutaneous inflammatory infiltrates of scabies: a dynamic immunophenotypic pattern that should be distinguished from lymphomatoid papulosis. *J Cutan Pathol* 2002;29:368.
51. Thomson J, Cochrane T, Cochran R, et al. Histology simulating reticulosis in persistent nodular scabies. *Br J Dermatol* 1974;90:421.
52. Fimiani M, Mazzatenta C, Alessandrini C, et al. The behaviour of *Sarcoptes scabiei* var. *hominis* in human skin: an ultrastructural study. *J Submicrosc Cytol Pathol* 1997;29:105.
53. Hoefling KK, Schroeter AL. Dermatoimmunopathology of scabies. *J Am Acad Dermatol* 1980;3:237.
54. Brites C, Weyll M, Pedroso C, et al. Severe and Norwegian scabies are strongly associated with retroviral (HIV-1/HTLV-1) infection in Bahia, Brazil. *AIDS* 2002;16:1292.
55. Jelinek T, Maiwald H, Nothdurft HD, et al. Cutaneous larva migrans in travelers: synopsis of histories, symptoms, and treatment of 98 patients. *Clin Infect Dis* 1994;19:1062.
56. Park J-W, Kwonh S-J, Ryu J-S, et al. Two imported cases of cutaneous larva migrans. *Korean J Parasitol* 2001;39:77.
57. Hawdon JM, Jones BF, Perregaux MA, et al. Ancylostoma caninum: metalloprotease release coincides with activation of infective larvae in vitro. *Exp Parasitol* 1995;80:205.
58. Herzberg AJ, Boyd PR, Guiterrez Y. Subcutaneous dirofilariasis in Collier County, Florida, U.S.A. *Am J Surg Pathol* 1995;19:934.
59. Jelinek T, Schulte-Hillen J, Löscher T. Human dirofilariasis. *Int J Dermatol* 1996;35:872.
60. Shenefelt PD, Esperanza L, Lynn A. Elusive migratory subcutaneous dirofilariasis. *J Am Acad Dermatol* 1996;35:260.
61. Van den Ende J, Kumar V, Van Gompel A, et al. Subcutaneous dirofilariasis caused by *Dirofilaria (Nochtiella) repens* in a Belgian patient. *Int J Dermatol* 1995;34:274.
62. Ratnatunga N, Wijesundera MS. Histopathological diagnosis of subcutaneous *Dirofilaria repens* infection in humans. *Southeast Asian J Trop Med Public Health* 1999;30:375.
63. Font RL, Guiterrez Y, Semba RD, et al. Ocular onchocerciasis. In: Meyers WM, Neafie RC, Marty AM, et al., eds. *Helminthiases*, vol. 1 of *Pathology of Infectious Diseases*. Washington, DC: Armed Forces Institute of Pathology, 2000:307.
64. Murdoch ME, Hay RJ, Mackenzie CD, et al. A clinical classification and grading system of the cutaneous changes in onchocerciasis. *Br J Dermatol* 1993;129:260.
65. Stingl P. Onchocerciasis: clinical presentation and host parasite interactions in patients of Southern Sudan. *Int J Dermatol* 1997;36:23.
66. Vernick W, Turner SE, Burov E, et al. Onchocerciasis presenting with lower extremity, hypopigmented macules. *Cutis* 2000;65:293.
67. Routh HB, Bhowmik KR. Filariasis. *Dermatol Clin* 1994;12:719.
68. Neafie RC, Marty AM, Duke BOL. Onchocerciasis. In: Meyers WM, Neafie RC, Marty AM, et al., eds. *Helminthiases*, vol. 1 of *Pathology of Infectious Diseases*. Washington, DC: Armed Forces Institute of Pathology, 2000:287.
69. Jacob CI, Patten SF. *Strongyloides stercoralis* infection presenting as generalized prurigo nodularis and lichen simplex chronicus. *J Am Acad Dermatol* 1999;41:357.
70. Boeckers M, Bork K. Prurigo und weitere diagnostisch bedeutsame Hautsymptome bei Strongyloidose. *Hautarzt* 1988;39:34.
71. Von Kuster LC, Genta RM. Cutaneous manifestations of strongyloidiasis. *Arch Dermatol* 1988;124:1826.
72. Chaudhary K, Smith RJ, Himelright IM, et al. Case report: purpura in disseminated strongyloidiasis. *Am J Med Sci* 1994;308:186.
73. Amer M. Cutaneous schistosomiasis. *Dermatol Clin* 1994;12:713.
74. Mahmoud AA. Schistosomiasis. *N Engl J Med* 1977;297:1329.
75. Wood MG, Srolovitz H, Schetman D. Schistosomiasis: paraplegia and ectopic skin lesions as admission symptoms. *Arch Dermatol* 1976;112:690.
76. Harries AD, Fryatt R, Walker J, et al. Schistosomiasis in expatriates returning to Britain from the tropics: a controlled study. *Lancet* 1986;1:86.
77. Farrell AM, Woodrow D, Bryceson ADB, et al. Ectopic cutaneous schistosomiasis: extragenital involvement with progressive upward spread. *Br J Dermatol* 1996;135:110.
78. Uthman MAE, Mostafa WZ, Satti MB. Cutaneous schistosomal granuloma. *Int J Dermatol* 1990;29:659.
79. Torres VM. Dermatologic manifestations of schistosomiasis mansoni. *Arch Dermatol* 1976;112:1539.
80. Andrade Filho J de S, Lopes MS, Corgozinho Filho AA, Pena GP. Ectopic cutaneous schistosomiasis: report of two cases and a review of the literature. *Rev Inst Med Trop São Paulo* 1998;40:253.
81. Jacyk WK, Lawande RV, Tulpule SS. Unusual presentation of extragenital cutaneous Schistosomiasis mansoni. *Br J Dermatol* 1980;103:205.
82. Kick G, Schaller M, Korting HC. Late cutaneous schistosomiasis representing an isolated skin manifestation of *Schistosoma mansoni* infection. *Dermatology* 2000;200:144.
83. Ramdial PK. Transepithelial elimination of late cutaneous vulvar schistosomiasis. *Int J Gynecol Pathol* 2001;20:166.
84. Matsushima H, Hatamochi A, Shinkai H, et al. A case of subcutaneous cysticercosis. *J Dermatol* 1998;25:438.
85. Falanga V, Kapoor W. Cerebral cysticercosis: diagnostic value of subcutaneous nodules. *J Am Acad Dermatol* 1985;12:304.
86. Evans C, Garcia HH, Robert H, et al. Controversies in the management of cysticercosis. *Emerg Infect Dis* 1997;3:403.
87. Miura H, Itoh Y, Kozuka T. A case of subcutaneous cysticercosis (*Cysticercus cellulosae* cutis). *J Am Acad Dermatol* 2000;43:538.

88. Pönnighaus JM, Nkhosa P, Baum H-P. Kutane Manisfestation der Zystizerkose. *Hautarzt* 2001;52:1098.

89. Amatya BM, Kimula Y. Cysticercosis in Nepal: a histopathologic study of sixty-two cases. *Am J Surg Pathol* 1999;23:1276.

90. Hausdörfer-Scheiff S, Bourlond A, Pirard C. Histopathological aspects of myiasis. *Dermatology* 1993;186:298.

91. Noutsis C, Millikan LE. Myiasis. *Dermatol Clin* 1994;12:729.

92. Guse ST, Tieszen ME. Cutaneous myiasis from *Dermatobia hominis*. *Wilderness Environ Med* 1997;8:156.

93. Grogan TM, Payne CM, Payne TB, et al. Cutaneous myiasis: immunohistologic and ultrastructural morphometric features of a human botfly lesion. *Am J Dermatopathol* 1987;9:232.

94. Norwood C, Smith KJ, Neafie R, et al. Are cutaneous reactions to fly larvae mediated by CD4+, TIA+ NK1.1 T cells? *J Cutan Med Surg* 2001;5:400.

95. Lane RP, Lovell CR, Griffiths WAD, et al. Human cutaneous myiasis: a report of three cases due to *Dermatobia hominis*. *Clin Exp Dermatol* 1987;12:40.

96. Götz M. Tropenaufenthalt und furunkuloide Myiasis. *Pathologe* 1995;16:285.

97. Veraldi S, Schianchi R. Guess what? Tungiasis. *Eur J Dermatol* 1999;9:57.

98. Grunwald MH, Shai A, Mosovich B, et al. Tungiasis. *Australas J Dermatol* 2000;41:46.

99. Smith MD, Procop GW. Typical histologic features of *Tunga penetrans* in skin biopsies. *Arch Pathol Lab Med* 2002;126:714.

100. Blum RR, Phelps RG, Wei H. Arthropod bites manifesting as recurrent bullae in a patient with chronic lymphocytic leukemia. *J Cutan Med Surg* 2001;5:312.

101. Rantanen T, Reunala T, Vuojohlahti P, et al. Persistent pruritic papules from deer ked bites. *Acta Derm Venereol* 1982;62:307.

102. Hwong H, Jones D, Prieto VG, et al. Persistent atypical lymphocytic hyperplasia following tick bite in a child: report of a case and review of the literature. *Pediatr Dermatol* 2001;18:481.

103. Blackman JR. Spider bites. *J Am Board Fam Pract* 1995;8:288.

104. Heng MCY, Loss SG, Haberfelde GC. Pathogenesis of papular urticaria. *J Am Acad Dermatol* 1984;10:1030.

105. Jordaan HF, Schneider JW. Papular urticaria: a histopathologic study of 30 patients. *Am J Dermatopathol* 1997;19:119.

106. Ackerman AB, Chongchitnant N, Sanchez J, et al. Histologic Diagnosis of Inflammatory Skin Diseases: An Algorithmic Method Based on Pattern Analysis. 2nd ed. Baltimore, Philadelphia, London: Williams & Wilkins, 1997:202.

107. Bandmann H-J, Bosse K. Histologie des Mückenstiches (Aedes aegypti). *Arch Klin Exp Dermatol* 1967;231:59.

108. Künzig M, Steigleder GK. Histopathologische Untersuchungen des Mückenstich infiltrates bei Patienten mit verschiedenen Grunderkrankungen und unterschiedlicher Medikation. *Z Hautkr* 1977;52:37.

109. Pucevich MV, Chesney TMcC. Histopathologic analysis of human bites by the brown recluse spider. *Arch Dermatol* 1983;119:851.

110. Gilliam AC, Wood GS. Cutaneous lymphoid hyperplasias. *Semin Cutan Med Surg* 2000;19:133.

111. Hur W, Ahn SK, Lee SH, Kang WH. Cutaneous reaction induced by retained bee stinger. *J Dermatol* 1991;18:736.

112. Rees RS, Nanney LB, Yates RA, et al. Interaction of brown recluse spider venom on cell membranes: the inciting mechanism? *J Invest Dermatol* 1984;83:270.

DISEASES CAUSED BY VIRUSES

XIAOWEI XU
LORI A. ERICKSON
DAVID E. ELDER

Many viral infections have prominent skin manifestations. Characteristic skin lesions suggest a specific viral illness, the diagnosis of which can be confirmed by appropriate procedures. Viral infections of the skin are of increased significance in immunocompromised patients. Viruses are complexes of nucleic acids and proteins that have the capacity for replication in animal, plant and bacterial cells. They are obligatory intracellular organisms that lack organelles, such as ribosomes and mitochondria. To replicate themselves, viruses use the metabolic machinery of the host cells. Virally induced alterations in cell function and antigenicity, cell death, and host responses to the presence of viruses are factors that lead to the manifestations of viral disease (1). Before viruses can enter a cell, they must attach themselves to specific receptors on the cell surface. Thus, virus infection is a receptor-mediated, species- and cell-type–specific process (2). Viruses enter the cytoplasm of a cell by a process called endocytosis, acquiring an outer coat of plasma membrane. Once inside the cell, uncoating is triggered by pH changes in endosomes. As the outer coat and the capsid are being digested, the exposed nucleoids lose their characteristic structure (3). The viruses now are in "eclipse phase" and do not become apparent until replication has taken place and new virions or viruses appear. During the replication process, the viral proteins that are produced follow the genetic code of the specific virus nucleic acid, and the proteins formed are characteristic of the virus rather than of the host cells. Viral particles are assembled in the infected cells and released either by lysis of the cell or by budding from the cell surface.

The diameters of viruses infecting skin vary from 20 nm for the echoviruses to 300 nm for the poxviruses. Under favorable conditions, poxviruses may be recognizable under a light microscope—for example, variola viruses as Paschen bodies. As a rule, however, viruses can be resolved by light microscopy only when aggregated into inclusion bodies. *Inclusion bodies* are roughly spherical. Their average size is about 7 μm, the size of an erythrocyte. Electron microscopy has shown that inclusion bodies represent sites at which virus replication is occurring or has occurred. They are ob-

served in three groups of viruses: the herpesvirus and papillomavirus groups, where they are found within the nuclei of cells, and in the poxvirus group, where they occur within the cytoplasm. In the nucleus, they are surrounded by a clear halo as a result of margination of the nuclear chromatin. In some viral infections, such as molluscum contagiosum, inclusion bodies contain masses of virions and are basophilic and Feulgen positive. In contrast, in other infections such as herpesvirus infection, the viruses have left the inclusion bodies, except for a few residual nucleoids, and the inclusion bodies are then eosinophilic and Feulgen negative.

There are five families of viruses that commonly affect the skin or adjoining mucous surfaces: (a) the Herpesviridae, DNA viruses that multiply within the nucleus of the host cell, including herpes simplex types 1 and 2, varicella-zoster virus, cytomegalovirus, Roseolovirus (human herpes virus 6), Epstein–Barr virus (lymphocryptovirus), HHV-7, and HHV-8; (b) the Poxviridae, which are DNA viruses that multiply within the cytoplasm, including smallpox, milkers' nodules, orf, and molluscum contagiosum; (c) the Papovaviridae, which contain DNA and replicate in the nucleus, including the various types of verrucae; (d) the Picornaviridae, which contain RNA in their nucleoids, including coxsackievirus group A, causing hand-foot-and-mouth disease; and (e) the Retroviridae, whose genetic material is RNA, including human immunodeficiency virus (HIV), the cause of acquired immunodeficiency syndrome (AIDS). In addition to these five families, exanthems can occur following infection with many other virus families, such as Adenoviridae, Togaviridae, Reoviridae, Parvoviridae, Paramyxoviridae, Flaviviridae and Hepadnaviridae. Lesions from the first three DNA virus family infections contain diagnostic viral inclusions. Infections from the other virus families often produce rather histologically nonspecific changes with superficial perivascular dermatitis and occasional apoptotic cells in the epidermis.

Besides histologic examination, two other laboratory approaches can be used: virologic and serologic approaches. The virologic approach includes isolation of virus in cell culture, detection of viral particles by immunoassays or electron microscopy, and detection of viral nucleic acid by PCR-based assays or labeled complementary DNA probes. The serologic approach includes demonstration of a fourfold or greater rise in antiviral IgG antibody using acute and convalescent sera, or demonstration of virus-specific IgM antibody in a single late acute or early recovery phase serum. A serologic approach is still used today for certain viral infections, such as infectious mononucleosis and hepatitis. However, the virologic approach is used more frequently than before. The timing, quality, and handling of the specimen are critical for an accurate diagnosis using the virologic approach. It is important to obtain specimens during the acute phase of a virus infection from the site of the infection. The optimal temperature for storage and transport of specimen for viral culture is 40°C in a refrigerator or on wet ice. Most of the viruses are stable at this temperature for 3 to 5 days. If a specimen needs to be stored longer than 3 to 4 days, a 700°C freezer should be used and the specimen should be transported on dry ice. With the development of molecular biology, PCR-based rapid viral detection assays have been developed and are used in clinical diagnostic laboratories.

The Herpesviridae are double-stranded DNA viruses with three subfamilies. Herpes virus infections of humans include herpes simplex virus (type 1 and 2), varicellovirus, cytomegalovirus, roseolovirus (human herpes virus 6), Epstein–Barr virus (lymphocryptovirus), HHV-7, and HHV-8.

HERPES SIMPLEX

Two immunologically distinct viruses can cause herpes simplex: herpes simplex virus type 1 (orofacial type) and herpes simplex virus type 2 (genital type), often referred to as HSV-1 and HSV-2, respectively (4). HSV are transmitted through the exchange of saliva, semen, cervical fluid or vesicle fluid from active lesions. Primary infection with HSV-1 is often subclinical in childhood. In about 10% of the cases, acute gingivostomatitis occurs, usually in childhood and only rarely in early adult life. Primary infection may also occur in rare instances as a respiratory infection, or Kaposi's varicelliform eruption, or keratoconjunctivitis, or as a fatal visceral disease of the newborn. Recurrent HSV-1 infections occur most commonly on or near the vermilion border of the lips (herpes labialis, or "cold sores"). Recurrences may be triggered by sunlight, physical or emotional stress, immunosuppression, menses, hot or cold, or febrile illness (5). Besides the lips, any parts of the skin or oral mucosa can be affected by HSV-1. Herpes genitalis is one of the most common sexually transmitted diseases worldwide (6). Seroconversion for HSV-2, the most common cause of genital herpes rarely occurs before

the onset of sexual activity. Occasionally, an infant contracts HSV-2 *in utero* or by direct contact in the birth canal (7). Even though most infections of the genitalia and adjoining skin are caused by HSV-2, some infections in this area are caused by HSV-1. Genital HSV-1 infections are less likely to recur than HSV-2 infections: the rate of recurrence was 14% for HSV-1 infections compared with 60% for HSV-2 infections (8). Only 10% to 25% of individuals who are HSV-2 seropositive report a history of genital herpes (9).

Both primary and recurrent herpes simplex, in their earliest stages, show one or several groups of tiny clear vesicles on an edematous red base. If located on a mucous surface, the vesicles erode quickly, whereas, if located on the skin, they may become pustular before crusting. The lesions usually heal without scarring, except in cases where secondary bacterial infection occurs. The following are special forms of cutaneous herpes simplex: eczema herpeticum (Kaposi's varicelliform eruption), herpetic folliculitis, and herpetic whitlow.

Eczema herpeticum is a potentially life-threatening herpetic infection of a pre-existing skin disease (10). It occurs most commonly in patients with atopic eczema, although it may also occur in other skin diseases such as seborrheic dermatitis, pityriasis rubra pilaris, pemphigus foliaceus, Darier's disease, and postperioral dermabrasion (11). An extensive rash with small vesicles filled with yellow pus and high fever is the common presentation of eczema herpeticum, which has been linked to increased interleukin-4 and decreased natural killer cells and IL-2 receptor in patients with atopic eczema (12,13). *Herpetic folliculitis* presents as painful, grouped erythematous, perifollicular vesicles that do not respond to antibacterial or antifungal agents, usually occurring in the bearded region and scalp (14). The characteristic vesiculofollicular lesions usually heal within a few weeks. *Herpetic whitlow* manifests as painful, deep-seated vesicles limited to the paronychial or volar aspects of the distal phalanx of a finger. Herpetic whitlow occurs largely in medical and dental personnel following minor injuries and may be caused by either HSV-1 or HSV-2 (15). Other forms of HSV infections include HSV keratoconjunctivitis, which is the number-one cause of corneal blindness in the United States (16), and a rare necrotizing balanitis (17). Noncutaneous forms of herpes simplex infection include herpetic oropharyngitis, pneumonia, encephalitis, esophagitis, and proctitis.

Recurrent Infection. Recurrent infections of the oral cavity, skin, or genitals can result either from reactivation of a latent infection or from a new infection. Primary infection with either HSV-1 or HSV-2 is often subclinical and is followed by emergence of specific circulating antibodies and latency of the infection. In some persons infected with either HSV-1 or HSV-2, the virus can become activated intermittently and give rise to recurrent lesions. Although recurrences, particularly of HSV-2, can be due to reinfection, they are often caused by reactivation of a latent infection of the regional sensory ganglia, where the virus exists in a latent, nonreplicative state.

Herpes Simplex in Compromised Hosts

Severe primary or secondary herpetic infection with systemic involvement may occur in immunocompromised patients. Co-infection with HSV and HIV frequently occurs, probably because they potentiate each other's transmission. About 70% of HIV-positive patients are seropositive for HSV-2 (18). Three forms of herpes simplex are characteristically found in children or adults with impairment of the cellular immune system. The most common of the three forms is *chronic ulcerative herpes simplex*, and the other two are *generalized acute mucocutaneous herpes simplex* and *systemic herpes simplex*.

Chronic ulcerative herpes simplex exhibits persistent ulcers and erosions, usually starting on the face or in the perineal region (19). Without treatment, gradual widespread extension is the rule. The infection may progress into systemic herpes simplex. *Generalized acute mucocutaneous herpes simplex* follows an initial localized vesicular eruption. Dissemination associated with fever takes place, suggestive of smallpox or varicella infection (20). In some instances, death results without the presence of visceral lesions. *Systemic herpes simplex* usually follows oral or genital lesions of herpes simplex. Areas of necrosis, particularly in the liver, adrenals, pancreas, and brain, lead rapidly to death. In some patients, a few cutaneous lesions of herpes simplex also exist.

Congenital Herpes Simplex

Because almost 1% of patients in prenatal clinics have HSV-2 infections by culture of the vagina, and one-third of these have active lesions, the potential of congenital herpes simplex infection exists. It is important, however, to distinguish primary HSV-2 infection of the mother from recurrent infection. In recurrent infection, the presence of neutralizing antibody to HSV-2 results in a low rate of attack of the fetus (21). In maternal HSV-2 *primary infection*, the mode of infection of the infant is important. Transplacental infection of the fetus occurring during the first 8 weeks of gestation produces severe congenital malformations. If infection occurs at a later time, malformations are less severe and consist of growth and psychomotor retardation, microcephaly, and a widespread, recurrent vesicular eruption that can mimic a mechanobullous disorder.

Localized herpetic lesions several days after delivery are the initial manifestation if infection is acquired in the birth canal. In vertex deliveries, the scalp is a common site for the development of initial herpetic vesicles. It is rare for transplacental or neonatal infection to remain limited to the skin. It can be followed by systemic herpetic infection, such as encephalitis, hepatoadrenal necrosis, and pneumonia (22).

Herpes Simplex Associated with Erythema Multiforme

Herpes simplex virus is the most common identified etiologic agent in recurrent erythema multiforme (23). Molecular diagnostic methods, primarily the polymerase chain reaction, have been used to detect herpetic DNA in the skin lesions of recurrent erythema multiforme in both adults and children (24). The association is further supported by suppression of recurrent lesions in this group by therapy directed at herpes simplex virus.

Histopathology of Herpes Simplex

The earliest changes of herpes simplex lesions include nuclear swelling of keratinocytes. With hematoxylin and eosin stains, these nuclei appear slate gray and homogeneous with margination of the nuclear chromatin. A few necrotic keratinocytes in the epidermis may also be seen. The changes usually begin along the basal layer keratinocytes and then involve the entire epidermis. Later, skin herpes simplex produces profound degeneration of keratinocytes, resulting in acantholysis. Degeneration of epidermal keratinocytes occurs in two forms: ballooning degeneration and reticular degeneration. Ballooning degeneration consists of swelling of epidermal keratinocytes. Balloon cells have a homogeneous, eosinophilic cytoplasm (Figs. 25-1 and 25-2), and they may be multinucleated (Tzanck cells). Balloon cells lose their intercellular bridges and become separated from one another (secondary acantholysis), and unilocular vesicles result. Ballooning degeneration occurs mainly at the bases of viral vesicles, so that the vesicle

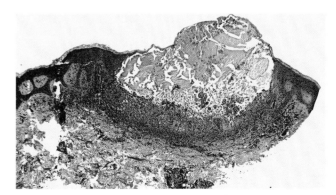

FIGURE 25-1. Herpes simplex. A vesicular lesion with marked acanthosis and ballooning degeneration of the cells at the floor of the vesicle (low magnification).

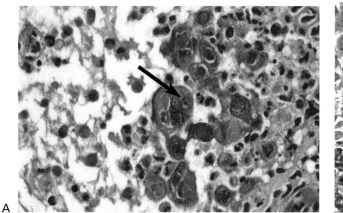
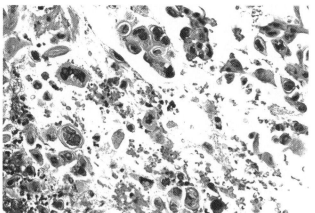

FIGURE 25-2. Herpes simplex. **A:** Same as Fig. 25-1, but at high magnification. Balloon cells at the floor of a vesicle. In the center, eosinophilic inclusion bodies surrounded by a halo lies in the nuclei of balloon cells (*arrow* points to the intranuclear inclusion). Other cells exhibit the more characteristic pattern of homogeneous pale chromatin without inclusion bodies. **B:** High magnification, balloon cells at the floor of a vesicle. These cells exhibit characteristic homogeneous pale chromatin and nuclei molding.

formed intraepidermally ultimately may be subepidermal. Ballooning degeneration can affect epithelial cells of hair follicles, sebaceous glands, and rarely eccrine duct cells. Reticular degeneration is the result of rupture of ballooning cells due to progressive hydropic swelling of the epidermal cells. Reticular degeneration occurs in the upper portions and at the peripheries of viral vesicles. Reticular degeneration is not specific for viral vesicles, because it also occurs in the vesicles of contact dermatitis. Through coalescence of cells with reticular degeneration, a multilocular vesicle may result, the septa of which are formed by residual cell membrane. In older vesicles, the cellular walls disappear. The originally multilocular portions of the vesicle may become unilocular.

Inclusion bodies are frequently observed in the centers of enlarged, round nuclei of balloon cells. The inclusion bodies are eosinophilic and surrounded by a clear space or halo (Fig. 25-2). They measure from 3 to 8 μm in diameter. Neutrophils are often present within established vesicles. Neutrophils may be prominent in the lesions of herpetic whitlow. The upper dermis beneath viral vesicles contains an inflammatory infiltrate of variable density. In some cases of herpes simplex, vascular damage is present, showing necrosis of vessel walls, microthrombi, and hemorrhage. In addition, eosinophilic inclusions may be found in endothelial cells and fibroblasts. As in all vesiculobullous diseases, an early lesion should be selected for biopsy; otherwise, secondary changes, especially invasion of inflammatory cells, may obscure the diagnostic features.

In later lesions, necrosis of epidermis is often present with abundant neutrophils. A dense mixed cell infiltrate in the upper dermis with ghosts of necrotic multinucleated acantholytic cells with slate gray nuclei may still be seen.

Herpetic involvement of hair follicle and pilosebaceous units is not uncommon in recurrent lesions (25). In fact,

necrosis of a pilosebaceous unit is a clue to search for multinucleated cells with characteristic slate gray nuclei. In herpetic folliculitis, pilosebaceous involvement is a predominant feature. Rarely, the eccrine ducts and glands are involved by the virus. The histology of eczema herpeticum is similar to vesicles of herpes simplex, but usually with denser neutrophilic infiltrates.

Chronic ulcerative herpes simplex may be difficult to recognize as being of viral genesis if the epidermis is absent. However, viral cytopathic changes may be observed in keratinocytes at the margin of the ulcer. Viral cultures or typing of HSV-1 and HSV-2 by direct immunofluorescence or immunoperoxidase technique can be used to prove the diagnosis. However, the most rapid and accurate method may be the use of molecular diagnostic methods such as the polymerase chain reaction (26).

Tzanck Smear. Cytologic examination of a Giemsa-stained smear taken from the floor of a freshly opened early vesicle is often useful. The presence of many balloon cells results from the fact that the smear is taken from the floor of the blister, where ballooning degeneration is most pronounced. Many acantholytic balloon cells with one or several nuclei may be seen in herpes simplex, varicella and zoster. The Tzanck smear cannot distinguish among HSV-1, HSV-2, and varicella zoster virus.

Histogenesis and viral identification. The herpes simplex virus can be directly identified by culture, direct immunofluorescence testing, or molecular diagnostic tests. The gold standard for diagnosis is a viral culture. For culture, material from the floor of a blister or other infected material is inoculated onto HeLa cells, human amnion cells, or fibroblasts. The virus has cytopathic effects on the cultured cells. Direct immunofluorescence examination for the presence of the viral antigen in cells infected with herpes simplex virus is then performed. Herpes simplex DNA can be extracted and amplified by PCR from stained and unstained Tzanck smears, crusts, fresh tissue, and paraffin sections of suspected lesions. With appropriate primers, each herpes-type virus can be specifically identified from the amplified product.

For distinction between the two types of HSV, immunoperoxidase staining may be performed on sections of the lesions using two monoclonal antibodies, one directed against HSV-1 and the other against HSV-2. *In situ* hybridization can also be used for visual demonstration of viral genomic material in tissue (27). For determination of the antibody titer in the patient's serum, a complement fixation reaction is usually used. The serologic test for HSV is useful to confirm HSV infection in persons with a questionable history of herpetic disease and in those who have unrecognized or subclinical infection, so they may be aware of their potential to transmit the virus.

On electron microscopy, the herpes simplex virus is spherical. Its DNA-containing core measures approximately 40 nm in diameter. The virion has a diameter of about 100 nm and together with its outer coat measures around 135 nm (28). Ultrastructurally, the virion of herpes simplex is indistinguishable from that of varicella.

Differential Diagnosis. Viral vesicles produced by the herpes simplex virus and by the varicella-zoster virus are identical. Furthermore, an incompletely developed case of herpes zoster can mimic herpes simplex infection, both clinically and histologically. In the context of immunosuppression, chronic cutaneous forms of both viruses exist and their specific identification may not be possible by clinical morphology or light microscopy. Molecular diagnostic methods are the quickest and most reliable way to separate and identify the specific viruses in these situations.

KAPOSI'S VARICELLIFORM ERUPTION

Kaposi varicelliform eruption is the name given to a distinct cutaneous eruption caused by HSV-1 and HSV-2, vaccinia virus, and Coxsackie A16 virus superimposed on a preexisting dermatosis (29), usually atopic dermatitis (30). Occasionally, seborrheic dermatitis or other dermatosis, such as Darier's disease, benign familial pemphigus, pemphigus foliaceus, mycosis fungoides, Sézary's syndrome, or ichthyosis vulgaris, provide the "soil" in which Kaposi's varicelliform eruption develops (11).

Eczema herpeticum is usually caused by HSV-1 and on rare occasions by HSV-2. Eczema herpeticum can occur as either a primary or a recurrent type of infection. A primary infection with HSV-1 occurs in persons without circulating HSV-1 antibodies. The great majority of patients with the primary type of eczema herpeticum are infants and children. The recurrent type of eczema herpeticum occurs in patients with circulating HSV-1 antibodies. The first attack of eczema herpeticum, whether of the primary or the recurrent type, may be the result of exogenous infection, whereas subsequent attacks may result from either reinfection or reactivation. The primary type of eczema herpeticum can be a serious disease with viremia and potential internal organ involvement resulting in death. In contrast, the recurrent type of eczema herpeticum generally shows no viremia and internal organ involvement except in immunologically compromised patients. Occasionally, secondary bacterial infection with subsequent septicemia may cause death. The mortality of eczema herpeticum is approximately 10%, with most fatalities occurring in infants and children with a primary type of herpetic infection and in adults with inadequate cellular immunity.

Clinically, all forms of eczema herpeticum and eczema vaccinatum look alike, but eczema vaccinatum has not been seen in modern practice because vaccinia virus has not been used, until recently for smallpox prevention (31). Both show a more or less extensive eruption composed of vesicles and pustules that may be umbilicated. These vesicles and pustules occur chiefly in the areas of the preexisting dermatosis but also on normal skin. The face is usually severely affected and may be edematous. There may be fever and prostration.

Histopathology. Both eczema herpeticum and eczema vaccinatum show vesicles and pustules of the viral type. Even though the pustules exhibit only necrotic epidermis in their centers, one may still see reticular and ballooning degeneration at their peripheries. In eczema herpeticum, but not in eczema vaccinatum, multinucleated epithelial giant cells often are present.

Differential Diagnosis. Because eczema herpeticum and eczema vaccinatum look alike clinically, and because the histologic similarity is great in the absence of inclusion bodies and of multinucleated epithelial cells, differentiation of the two diseases may have to depend on nonhistologic means, such as a history of possible exposure to the vaccinia virus. The most efficient and rapid means of identifying the viral agent is to use DNA amplification methods and appropriate probes.

VARICELLA AND HERPES ZOSTER

Varicella (chickenpox) and herpes zoster (shingles) are produced by the same virus, the varicella zoster virus. Varicella zoster virus (VZV) is endemic in the population but becomes epidemic during late winter and early spring (32). Varicella results from contact of a nonimmune person with this virus, whereas herpes zoster occurs in persons who have had previous varicella, either clinically or subclinically. Herpes zoster is caused by reactivation of a latent infection in either a spinal or a cranial sensory ganglion. On reactivation, the virus spreads from the ganglion along the corresponding sensory nerve or nerves to the skin.

Varicella

In varicella, a generalized eruption develops after an incubation period of about 2 weeks. Varicella is primarily a disease of childhood; 90% of cases occur in children aged 14 years or younger (33). The transmission rate of acute varicella to susceptible household contacts is estimated to be as high as 80% to 90%, making it one of the most infectious viral diseases in humans. VZV is acquired from patients with primary varicella or herpes zoster through either direct contact with infected vesicular fluid or inhalation of aerosolized respiratory secretions. Recent experiments suggest that the VZV is lymphotropic, especially to T cells. After the initial viremia and a period of viral replication, a second, higher-titer viremic phase results in widespread dissemination of the virus. The rash develops as VZV-infected mononuclear cells invade vascular endothelial cells, gaining access to cutaneous tissue. After the primary varicella infection resolves, the VZV enters a latent phase in the dorsal root ganglia (34). Pruritic rash of chickenpox, the hallmark of the disease, typically begins on the head and spreads to the trunk and finally the extremities; proximal involvement is greater than distal. The skin lesions of varicella begin as erythematous macules to small papules, which develop into vesicles. In mild cases, most vesicles become crusted without changing into pustules. In severe cases, the vesicles may have slightly hemorrhagic bases ("dew drops on rose petals"). New lesions continue to develop for several days, and so lesions in different stages, papules, vesicles, pustules, and crusted lesions can be observed. Typically, varicella lesions heal without scarring as new epithelium forms at the base; however, hypopigmentation, skin pitting, and keloid formation may result, especially among darker-skinned individuals. Varicella in adults is generally associated with a greater number of skin lesions, more systemic complaints, and a higher risk of such serious complications as pneumonia, encephalitis, and death. Subclinical varicella, documented by increases in antibody titer after exposure to the virus, has been estimated to occur in as much as 5% of the population (35).

Three systemic complications can occur in varicella without the existence of immunosuppression: primary varicella pneumonia, Reye's syndrome, and varicella of the fetus and newborn. Primary varicella pneumonia occurs in approximately 14% of adults with varicella and carries a significant mortality. Reye's syndrome is an acute, severe, and usually fatal encephalopathy associated with fatty degeneration of the viscera, particularly of the liver. It follows mainly varicella but also other viral infections. Although usually observed in children, it also may occur in adults (36). Varicella in the first 20 weeks of pregnancy has a 2% risk of producing embryopathy or other congenital malformations (37). Maternal varicella late in pregnancy may be transmitted to the fetus transplacentally or may contaminate the baby during passage through the birth canal, resulting in neonatal varicella.

Varicella in Compromised Hosts

In patients with impairment of the cellular immune system, continued viral replication may lead to a prolonged course and to dissemination to various organs. Varicella pneumonia is not uncommon, even in children, and death may result from dissemination. The varicella-zoster virus may produce particularly severe problems for patients with AIDS. There may be continuous dissemination of vesicular lesions, formation of chronic vegetative lesions, and large necrotic lesions (38).

Herpes Zoster

It is known that VZV establishes latency in ganglia following the primary infection causing varicella (chickenpox), and that the virus may reactivate after years of dormancy to produce herpes zoster (shingles). It is now widely accepted that the virus is mainly latent in neuronal cells, with only a small proportion of non-neuronal cells infected. The ganglia most often involved are those of the lumbar and thoracic nerves. When the virus is reactivated, newly synthesized VZV visions are transported along the sensory nerve and released into the skin. Trigger mechanisms include trauma, stress, old age, and immunosuppression. The incidence of herpes zoster (shingles) increases with age (39). Although herpes zoster occurs largely in adults, particularly in those of advanced age, about 5% of patients with herpes zoster are children less than 15 years of age. The course in children without immune defects usually is mild. The eruption in herpes zoster consists of grouped vesicles on inflammatory bases and arranged along the course of a sensory nerve. The bases of the lesions frequently are hemorrhagic, and some may become necrotic and ulcerate. Not infrequently, there are a few scattered nondermatomal lesions, and rarely there is a generalized eruption, including mucosal lesions, indistinguishable from that of varicella. The most common places of involvement include the thoracolumbar (T3-L2) and facial (V1) dermatomes. Severe neuritis with acute pain, dysesthesia, and skin hypersensitivity is common and more severe in people older than 50 and in immunocompromised patients. Zoster sine herpete, or "pain without the rash," is a rare presentation of herpes zoster; dermatomal pain is present with failure to develop a rash, likely because of neural inflammation and damage caused by viral reactivation. Herpes zoster during pregnancy is not as serious a problem as primary varicella during pregnancy; it does not result in serious morbidity or intrauterine VZV infection. Transplacental transmission of the virus does not occur with maternal herpes zoster; pre-existing normal immunity is thought to protect the fetus.

Herpes Zoster in Compromised Hosts

Both the incidence and the severity of herpes zoster are greater in patients with impaired cellular immunity. The incidence of herpes zoster is particularly high in patients with advanced Hodgkin's disease who are receiving chemotherapy or radiation, and in persons infected with HIV. In the context of HIV infection, herpes zoster may fail to resolve, may disseminate, or may produce atypical vegetative and ulcerative lesions (40). Although patients with disseminated herpes zoster but without associated serious illness have good prognoses, patients with impaired cellular immunity may develop widespread, fatal systemic manifestations, such as pneumonia, gastroenteritis, or encephalitis.

Histopathology. Lesions of varicella and herpes zoster are histologically indistinguishable from those of herpes simplex (Fig. 25-3). Frequently, however, the degree of vessel damage, microthrombi, and hemorrhage are more pronounced in varicella and, particularly, in herpes zoster than in herpes simplex. Herpes zoster vasculitis may mimic giant cell arteritis (41). In severe cases of varicella and in disseminated herpes zoster, eosinophilic inclusion bodies have also been observed in the dermis within the nuclei of capillary endothelial cells and of fibroblasts bordering the affected vessels. In contrast, in localized herpes zoster, in which the virus reaches the epidermis by way of the cutaneous nerves rather than the capillaries, inclusion bodies have been demonstrated within neurilemmal cells of the small nerves in the dermis underlying the vesicles. Immunohistochemical methods using specific monoclonal antibodies may have some utility in separating VZV from herpes simplex virus. Using an antibody specific for a envelope glycoprotein, Nikkels et al. (42) demonstrated VZV reactivity in sebaceous cells, endothelial cells, mononuclear phagocytes, and factor XIIIa–positive dendrocytes (42).

Tzanck Smear. Cytologic examination of the contents of vesicles is carried out for varicella and herpes zoster in the same way as for herpes simplex. It is a very useful diagnostic test, confirming the diagnosis in 80% to 100% of the cases, whereas viral cultures can confirm in only 60% to 64% (43).

Histogenesis and Viral Identification. Cultures remain the gold standard for virologic confirmation, and the virus can be cultured easily from vesicular fluid within 5 days of the onset of symptoms or before the crusting of lesions. However, culture is not very sensitive and in contrast with herpes simplex, the VZV does not grow in ordinary tissue cultures, it only grows in human fetal diploid kidney cells or human foreskin fibroblasts. Specific antibodies are available for serologic or immunohistochemical viral identification. Electron microscopic examination of the cutaneous lesions of varicella and herpes zoster reveals virus particles in the capillary endothelium in varicella and sporadically in the axons of dermal nerves in herpes zoster. The herpes simplex virus and the VZV are indistinguishable by electron microscopy.

CYTOMEGALOVIRUS

Cytomegalovirus (CMV) is a herpes virus that is ubiquitous in human populations. It has been estimated that 1% of newborns are infected transplacentally, and about 5% more acquire the infection at the time of birth. There is a steady increase with age in the number of individuals with antibodies in the serum, and this number takes a significant jump at the time of adolescence, presumably due to transfer of virus through the oral route (44). CMV may also be sexually transmitted. Owing to its ability to remain latent in peripheral leukocytes, CMV can be transmitted via transfusion. Most individuals have a mild flu-like episode upon initial infection; however, the virus subsequently becomes latent and persists in many tissues in the body. In immunocompromised individuals, reactivation and involvement of almost any organ of the body can

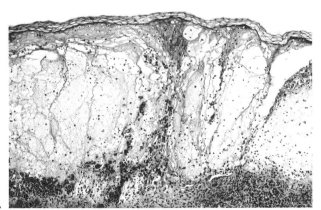
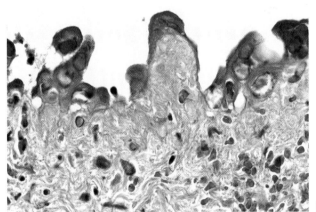

FIGURE 25-3. Varicella and herpes zoster. **A:** Reticular degeneration is present, especially at the top of the vesicle, resulting in a multilocular vesicle. In addition, ballooning degeneration can be seen at the floor of the vesicle. **B:** High magnification; balloon cells exhibit characteristic homogeneous pale chromatin and nuclei molding. Dermal hemorrhage is common.

take place and produce a widespread, potentially fatal, systemic infection (45).

Skin manifestation of CMV infection is rare in immunocompetent persons. Cutaneous lesions reported in the immunocompromised patients vary greatly: a more or less widespread maculopapular rash that may become purpuric, urticaria, vesiculobullous lesions, keratotic lesions, genital ulceration, ulceration of the chest, sharply punched-out ulcers, and epidermolysis have been reported (46). In the context of HIV infection, CMV-associated viral cytopathic changes can be observed as epiphenomena in skin biopsies in that they do not appear to be the primary pathogen in the specimen and the cause of the skin eruption.

Neonates with congenital CMV infection may exhibit the clinical picture of the "blueberry muffin baby" at delivery, which is manifested by petechiae and purpuric, magenta-colored macules, papules, and plaques, as well as blueberry-colored ecchymoses. The apparent hemorrhagic-purpuric skin lesions are thought to reflect extramedullary hematopoiesis. Ultrastructural study demonstrates that complexes of red cells in various stages of maturation occur in the skin of these patients, similar to the erythroblastic islands in the bone marrow (47). Transplacental transfer of CMV is one of the causes of TORCH, which represents an acronym of congenital infections by TOxoplasma, Rubella, Cytomegalovirus, and Herpesvirus, and may result in extensive damage to the developing brain, chorioretinitis and pneumonitis (48).

Histopathology. Dilated dermal vessels exhibit, among normal endothelial cells, large, irregularly shaped endothelial cells with large, hyperchromatic, basophilic, intranuclear inclusions that are around 10 μm in size, as well as small intracytoplasmic inclusions (around 3 μm in size) (Fig. 25-4). Some of the inclusions are surrounded by clear halos. A mixed inflammatory infiltrate with focal leukocytoclastic changes may also be present. In the context of HIV infection, other pathologic processes may also be present in the same tissue section.

Histogenesis and viral identification. CMV culture can be performed using human fibroblasts. PP65 is a CMV viral protein that is detectable in infected peripheral mononuclear cells, which is a sensitive method to estimate the systemic viral load (49). Immunohistochemical studies using monoclonal or polyclonal antibodies to CMV antigens can be used in paraffin-embedded sections to reveal viral proteins and confirm the presence of the virus. CMV DNA can also be amplified from skin biopsy specimens with PCR using specific primers for CMV, or can be identified by *in situ* hybridization. Electron microscopy shows in-

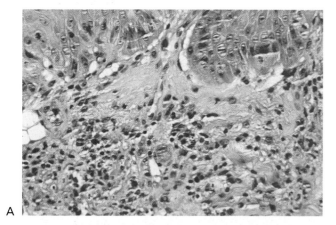

A

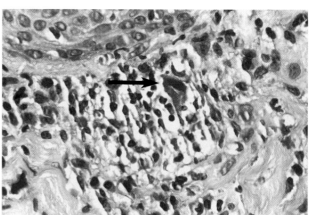

B

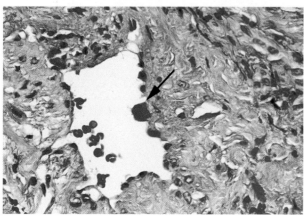

C

FIGURE 25-4. Cytomegalic inclusion disease. Scanning magnification shows superficial perivascular and diffuse inflammation with prominent vessels. Enlarged endothelial cells may be apparent at this magnification. **B:** High magnification; one infected dermal cell in the center shows enlarged, hyperchromatic, basophilic, intranuclear inclusions. There is a mixed inflammatory infiltrate in the dermis. **C:** Dilated dermal vessel with large, irregularly shaped endothelial cells. The enlarged endothelial cells contain hyperchromatic, basophilic, intranuclear inclusions (*arrow* points to inclusions). There may also be basophilic cytoplasmic inclusions.

tranuclear viral particles approximately 110 nm in diameter. The virus greatly resembles herpes simplex.

Epstein–Barr Virus

The Epstein–Barr virus (EBV) is thought to be responsible for a number of diseases such as infectious mononucleosis, oral hairy leukoplakia, and cutaneous lymphoproliferative disorders as well as Burkett's lymphoma and nasopharyngeal carcinoma (50). Infection with the EBV develops first in the salivary gland. Large amounts of the virus are released in the saliva, enabling it to spread from one person to another. People infected with EBV will retain it for life and most are asymptomatic. It has been estimated that the virus infects almost everyone in developing countries and more than 80% of people in developed countries. Most people are infected with the virus during childhood, and are usually not noticeably affected. On the other hand, people infected for the first time during or after adolescence (10% to 20% of people living in developed countries) have a 50% chance of developing infectious mononucleosis (IM). The main site of viral persistence is within latently infected lymphocytes, although infectious virus is also released into saliva from infected cells in the oropharynx (51).

IM is a self-limited manifestation of acute EBV infection. The transient rash that occurs quite commonly in patients with IM who have received antibiotic therapy is an erythematous, maculopapular eruption, usually located on the trunk and upper extremities. The palms, soles, and oral mucosa also have been reported to be occasionally involved. The pathogenesis of the rash is believed to be secondary to polyclonal B-cell activation that occurs during EBV infection with production of polyclonal antibodies that form immune complexes capable of fixing complement (52). Oral hairy leukoplakia is another manifestation of EBV infection that occurs in immunosuppressed HIV-positive and HIV-negative individuals. In HIV-positive individuals, it serves as an indicator of disease severity and rapid progression to AIDS. The presence of oral hairy leukoplakia in an individual should prompt the clinician to perform a thorough history taking and investigation of immune status. These lesions characteristically resemble whitish patches with a verrucous or filiform irregular surface that cannot be scraped off and are located primarily on the lateral surfaces of the tongue unilaterally or bilaterally. The condition is usually asymptomatic, but in some cases a burning sensation can occur, which is most likely secondary to co-infection by *Candida* (53). Lymphoproliferative disorders associated with EBV are well documented in the literature. EBV has recently been demonstrated to be associated with cutaneous T-cell lymphoma (CTCL) (54). EBV genome has also been detected in post-renal transplant cutaneous lymphoma, recurrent necrotic papulovesicles of the face (55) and cutaneous angiocentric lymphoma (56).

Histopathology. The histology of the macular lesion associated with infectious mononucleosis is non-specific and usually shows superficial perivascular lymphohistiocytic infiltrates. The histologic features that typify oral hairy leukoplakia include irregular epithelial hyperplasia with associated parakeratosis and acanthosis. Ballooning of keratinocytes occurs, and there are small pyknotic nuclei with intranuclear inclusions and a clear perinuclear halo. The cytoplasm may adopt a ground-glass appearance. There is also a mild inflammatory infiltrate observed in the superficial dermis. Langerhans cells are noted to be absent in the epithelium. Hyphae of *Candida* are observed within the superficial epithelium of a majority of the patients with oral hairy leukoplakia and may play a role in the development of the epithelial hyperplasia observed in oral hairy leukoplakia. A leukocytoclastic vasculitis and neuropathy associated with chronic EBV infection have also been reported.

Human Herpesviruses 6, 7, and 8

Human herpesviruses 6, 7, and 8 are newly discovered viruses in the past few years. These ubiquitous viruses may cause primary or chronic persistent infection or remain in a state of latency for many years, until a decrease in the immunologic state of the host leads to reactivation of infection (57). HHV-6 was first isolated in 1986 from patients with lymphoproliferative disorders and was classified into two variants as HHV-6A and HHV-6B. HHV-6B is the causative agent of exanthem subitum. Children start to be infected with HHV-6 at 6 months of age and almost all have antibodies by 2 years of age. The transmission of HHV-6 is essentially by a salivary route (58). HHV-6 infects latently after the primary infection and reactivates especially under immunosuppressive conditions. Skin rash in the first month after allogeneic bone marrow transplant (59), generalized vesiculobullous eruptions after allogeneic bone marrow transplantation (60), papular-purpuric "gloves and socks" syndrome (61), Gianotti–Crosti syndrome (62) and a serious systemic reaction to a limited number of drugs called hypersensitivity syndrome, have all been associated with HHV-6 (63). HHV-6 has also been detected in skin biopsy samples of patients with graft-versus-host disease, pityriasis rosea, and lymphoproliferative malignancies.

HHV-7, isolated from CD4+ T-lymphocytes from the peripheral blood of a healthy individual, has been recognized as a new lymphotropic herpesvirus. Healthy adults frequently shed the virus into saliva, and children are infected at a young age but somewhat later than HHV-6B. Latency is established in peripheral blood T cells, and a persistent infection in the salivary glands is believed to be the most likely mode of transmission. The primary infection with HHV-7 is linked to febrile illness with or without rash that resembles exanthema subitum. Pityriasis rosea is thought to be associated with HHV-7, however the association is still controversial (64).

HHV-8 was first identified in tissue samples of patients with Kaposi's sarcoma (KS) associated with AIDS in 1994. Serologic studies have demonstrated that, unlike other human herpesviruses, HHV-8 is not ubiquitous; instead, its infection rates parallel the incidence of Kaposi's sarcoma in the region. HHV-8 spreads through exchange of saliva and other sexual activities. HHV-8 can be found in all types of KS, whether related to HIV or not. HHV-8 seems to resemble EBV in its possible transforming properties, and HHV-8 is clearly associated with KS, multicentric Castleman disease, and primary effusion lymphoma (65). There may be a synergistic relationship between the HIV-1 Tat protein and HHV-8 infection. Tat promotes the growth of the Kaposi's sarcoma spindle cells. Like other herpes viruses, HHV-8 establishes latent and persistent infection. Only a minority of infected cells yields infectious viral particles, and their role in the development of KS and other associated diseases has not been clearly established. Presence of virus can be established in mononuclear cells of peripheral blood, endothelial cells, and spindle cells within skin lesions.

Histopathology. Exanthem subitum is linked to HHV-6 infection. It is a form of superficial perivascular dermatitis with papillary dermal edema. Exocytosis of lymphocytes is often present. Inclusions similar to those in herpes simplex infection are not seen. KS is described in Chapter 33.

POXVIRIDAE

The Poxviridae are double-stranded DNA viruses with two subfamilies and 11 genera. Poxvirus infections of humans include variola (smallpox), cowpox, vaccinia, molluscum contagiosum, paravaccinia (Milker's nodule), and orf (ecthyma contagiosum).

Variola (Smallpox)

Smallpox was one of the most infectious and deadly diseases in the world, afflicting millions of people each year regardless of age, race, or socioeconomic status before it was eradicated in 1977 (66). There were two forms of smallpox: variola major and variola minor. Variola major had a case fatality rate of approximately 25%, while variola minor, a less virulent form, had a case fatality rate below 1%. Although the two forms cause disease of different severity, they are indistinguishable from one another. Smallpox was spread through respiratory transmission of the virus found in the oropharyngeal secretions of infected individuals. Penetration is usually through the respiratory tract and local lymph nodes and then the virus enters the blood (primary viremia). Internal organs are infected; then the virus re-enters the blood (secondary viremia) and spreads to the skin. The onset of smallpox was acute, with fever, malaise, headaches, and backaches. The initial toxemia phase lasted 4 to 5 days. On about the 3rd or 4th day, the characteristic rash appeared. First, it appeared on the buccal and pharyngeal mucosa, face, and forearms. Within a day, it spread to the trunk and lower limbs. The lesions of the rash began first as macules, which soon became papules, and then developed into pustular vesicles. The lesions usually protruded from the skin and they were firm to touch. The lesions dried up and often became crusted by day 14. By the end of the 3rd week, most crusts had fallen off, with the exception of the palms and the soles (67). This entire process took 3 to 4 weeks, and the areas affected by the rash can be permanently scarred. The rare hemorrhagic type of smallpox that appeared in immunocompromised individuals was associated with bleeding from the conjunctiva and mucous membranes, very severe toxemia, and early death, usually before the lesions of the skin had developed. Modified-type smallpox was seen in persons who had been vaccinated, usually many years earlier. In these cases, the skin lesions evolved quickly and they were more variable in size.

Histopathology. There is prominent ballooning and reticular degeneration. Under light microscopy, aggregations of variola virus particles, called Guarnieri bodies, may be found in cytoplasm; occasional intranuclear inclusions can also be found. However, similar changes can be seen in vaccinia, monkeypox, or cowpox.

Vaccinia

Vaccinia virus was used for smallpox vaccination via inoculation into the superficial layers of the skin of the upper arm. However, with the eradication of smallpox, routine vaccination with vaccinia virus ceased for many years, but may soon become more common because of security concerns. Four to five days following vaccination with vaccinia virus, a papule appears at the site of vaccination. Two or three days later the papular lesion becomes vesicular, growing until it reaches its maximum diameter on the 9th or 10th day. The lesion dries from the center outward, and the brown scab falls off after about 3 weeks, leaving a scar–a mark by which previous vaccinees can be recognized (68). Complications of vaccination can occur but are very rare, including the following conditions: progressive vaccinia (vaccinia necrosum), which is a severe, potentially fatal illness characterized by progressive necrosis at the site of vaccination; eczema vaccinatum, which is similar to eczema herpeticum in patients with chronic eczema; generalized vaccinia which is characterized by a vesicular rash that sometimes covers the entire body, and postvaccinial encephalitis (69). Other localized lesions such as keloid, dermatofibrosarcoma protuberans, and malignant fibrous histiocytoma have been reported at the site of inoculation. These complications are extremely rare.

Histopathology. The histologic changes are similar to those of herpes simplex and zoster and varicella. However, intracytoplasmic inclusions are seen in vaccinia, unlike in herpes infection.

HUMAN COWPOX INFECTION

Despite its name, the reservoir hosts of cowpox virus are rodents, from which it can occasionally spread to cats, cows, humans, and zoo animals, including large cats and elephants. Infection in these animals is usually manifested as a single, small, crusted ulcer. Transmission to humans has traditionally occurred via contact with the infected teats of milking cows. However, currently, infection is seen more commonly among domestic cats, from which it can be transmitted to humans. Patients present with painful, hemorrhagic pustules or black eschars, usually on the hand or face, accompanied by edema, erythema, lymphadenopathy, and systemic involvement (70). Crusted lesions resembling anthrax and sporotrichosis infection have been reported.

Histopathology. The pathology of the skin lesions caused by cowpox virus is similar to that of smallpox. However, there is greater epithelial thickening and less rapid cell necrosis. Early lesions of human cowpox infection show prominent reticular degeneration. Eosinophilic, intracytoplasmic inclusion bodies are present, a valuable feature in distinguishing poxvirus from herpesvirus infections. Under electron microscopic examination, it is rectangular and morphologically indistinguishable from the variola virus.

PARAPOX VIRUS INFECTIONS (MILKERS' NODULES AND ORF)

Milkers' nodules, orf, and bovine papular stomatitis pox are clinically identical in humans and are induced by indistinguishable paravaccinia viruses. *Milkers' nodules* are acquired from udders infected with pseudocowpox or paravaccinia (parapox). This disease is called bovine papular stomatitis pox when the source of the infection is calves with oral sores contracted through sucking infected udders. *Orf* (ecthyma contagiosum) is acquired from infected sheep or goats with crusted lesions on the lips and in the mouth.

The most common presentation of Orf is a circumscribed solitary nodule or papule on the fingers or hands (71). Milkers' nodules usually presents with multiple lesions. After an incubation period of 3 to 7 days, parapox

virus infections produce one to three (rarely more) painful lesions measuring 1 to 2 cm in diameter on the fingers, or occasionally elsewhere as a result of autoinoculation. During a period of approximately 6 weeks, they pass through six clinical stages, each lasting about 1 week:

1. Maculopapular stage
2. Target stage, during which the lesions have red centers, white rings, and red halos
3. Acute weeping stage
4. Nodular stage, which shows hard, nontender nodules
5. Papillomatous stage, in which the nodules have irregular surfaces
6. Regressive stage, during which the lesions involute without scarring

Histopathology. During the maculopapular and target stages, there is vacuolization of cells in the upper third of the stratum malpighii, leading to multilocular vesicles. Eosinophilic inclusion bodies are in the cytoplasm of vacuolated epidermal cells, a distinguishing feature from herpes virus infections. Intranuclear eosinophilic inclusion bodies are also present in some cases. During the target stage, vacuolated epidermal cells with inclusion bodies are only in the surrounding white ring. Ballooning degeneration occurs, the affected keratinocytes rupture, and the resulting defects have a tendency to coalesce and to produce reticulated vesicles (Fig. 25-5). The epidermis shows elongation of the rete ridges, and the dermis contains many newly formed, dilated capillaries and a mononuclear infiltrate.

In the acute weeping stage, the epidermis is necrotic throughout. A massive infiltrate of mononuclear cells extends throughout the dermis. In some lesions, the mononuclear cell infiltrates may be comprised mainly of large, transformed lymphoblasts. Such lesions might be misdiagnosed as a lymphoid neoplasm, if careful attention is not given to the changes in the keratinocytes. A lichenoid reaction with a high percentage of histiocytes, a common response to viral infections of the skin, can also be seen.

In the later stages, the epidermis shows acanthosis with fingerlike downward projections, and the dermis shows vasodilatation and chronic inflammation, followed by resolution. The histology of orf and milkers' nodule is identical.

Histogenesis and viral identification. In lesions less than 2 weeks old, the virus can be grown in tissue cultures of various cell types, including bovine or rhesus monkey kidney cells and human amnion cells or fibroblasts. In older lesions, one has to rely on serologic changes or on viral antigen demonstration in lesional material. Electron microscopy reveals that the parapox virus is cylindrical in shape and has convex ends. It consists of a dense DNA core surrounded by a less dense, wide capsid and by two narrow,

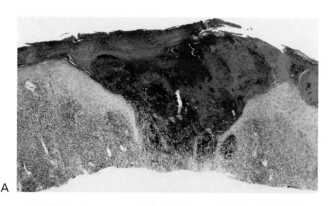

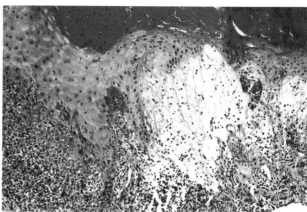

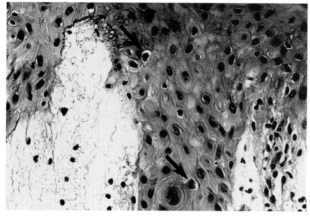

FIGURE 25-5. Orf. **A:** Scanning magnification; in target stage, central hemorrhage and tissue necrosis with peripheral reticulated degeneration and dense inflammatory infiltrates. **B:** Reticulated vesicles are a characteristic feature of a viral infection affecting the epidermis, and the dermis contains many newly formed, dilated capillaries and a mononuclear infiltrate. **C:** Eosinophilic inclusion bodies in the cytoplasm of vacuolated epidermal cells (*arrow* points to the inclusions) distinguish orf from herpesvirus infections. Intranuclear eosinophilic inclusion bodies are also present in some cases.

electron-dense outer layers. On the average, the virion measures 140 by 310 nm.

MOLLUSCUM CONTAGIOSUM

Molluscum contagiosum occurs worldwide. It is seen most commonly in children, but it may be found in persons of all ages. The virus is transmitted by direct bodily contact, through minor abrasions, or indirectly via fomites. Among young adults, it is usually a sexually transmitted disease. The incubation period for this virus, as determined by human volunteers who underwent inoculation, ranges from 14 to 50 days.

Molluscum contagiosum may be found anywhere on the body, but rarely occurs on the palms or soles. It consists of a variable number of small, discrete, waxy, skin-colored, delled, dome-shaped papules, usually 2 to 5 mm in size. A papule of molluscum contagiosum may appear inflamed. In immunocompetent patients, the lesions involute spontaneously. During involution, there may be mild inflammation and tenderness.

Since 1980, there have been reports in the United States of greater severity of molluscum contagiosum in patients infected with HIV. In the setting of immunosuppression,

molluscum contagiosum can attain considerable size and be widely disseminated. In immunocompromised patients, particularly those with AIDS, hundreds of lesions of molluscum contagiosum may be observed, showing little tendency toward involution. Furthermore, clinically normal skin in the vicinity of molluscum lesions in HIV-infected persons may be infected by molluscum virus (72). Infection with molluscum contagiosum produces little immunity, with reinfection being relatively common among immunocompromised individuals. In the context of AIDS, a variety of systemic fungal diseases, including cryptococcosis, histoplasmosis, and penicillium marnefei, can disseminate and produce skin lesions that resemble molluscum contagiosum.

Histopathology. In molluscum contagiosum, the epidermis is acanthotic. Many epidermal cells contain large, intracytoplasmic inclusion bodies—the so-called molluscum bodies (Fig. 25-6). These bodies first appear as single, minute, ovoid eosinophilic structures in the lower cells of the stratum malpighii at a level one or two layers above the basal cell layer. The molluscum bodies increase in size as infected cells move toward the surface. The molluscum bodies in the upper layers of the epidermis displace and compress the nucleus so that it appears as a thin crescent at the periphery of the cell. At the level of the granular layer,

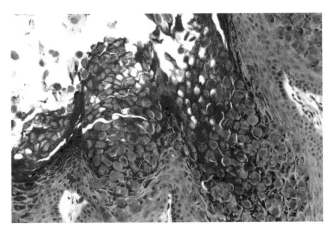

FIGURE 25-6. Molluscum contagiosum. Numerous intracyto-plasmic inclusion bodies, so-called molluscum bodies, can be seen forming in the lower epidermis. They increase in size as they move toward the surface.

the staining reaction of the molluscum bodies changes from eosinophilic to basophilic. In the horny layer, basophilic molluscum bodies measuring up to 35 μm in diameter lie enmeshed in a network of eosinophilic horny fibers. In the center of the lesion, the stratum corneum ultimately disintegrates, releasing the molluscum bodies. Thus, a central crater forms. Secondary infection and ulceration can occur.

The surrounding dermis usually shows little or no inflammatory reaction, except in instances in which the lesion of molluscum contagiosum ruptures and discharges molluscum bodies and horny material into the dermis. During the period of spontaneous involution, a mononuclear infiltrate may be observed in close apposition to the lesion infiltrating between the infected epidermal cells.

Electron microscopic examination reveals that the molluscum inclusion bodies contain, embedded in a protein matrix, large numbers of molluscum contagiosum viruses. The virus of molluscum contagiosum belongs to the poxvirus group. Like the viruses of variola, vaccinia, and cowpox, it is "brick shaped" and measures approximately 300 by 240 nm. The virus of molluscum contagiosum has not been grown in tissue culture. Molluscum contagiosum virus can be detected directly in tissue specimens using *in situ* hybridization (73).

PAPILLOMAVIRIDAE

Human papilloma viruses belong to the family Papovairidae. Human papillomaviruses are nonenveloped double-stranded DNA viruses. An infectious origin for skin warts was first recognized in 1891, and viral particles were isolated from human skin papillomatous lesions in 1949. Since that time, over 80 fully sequenced human papillomavirus genotypes have been identified with another 70

additional genotypes suggested through polymerase chain reaction analysis (74). The genetic heterogeneity is reflected in the differing clinical presentations of HPV infection. The cutaneous and mucosal manifestations of HPV infection include the common wart verruca vulgaris, the genital wart condyloma acuminatum, and less common entities, including epidermodysplasia verruciformis and oral focal epithelial hyperplasia (Heck's disease). Human papillomavirus is regarded as an oncogenic virus and is well known to be association with cervical and anogenital cancers (75). Recently HPV has been implicated in oropharyngeal squamous cell carcinoma (76), lung cancer (77), esophageal cancer (78), and in nonmelanoma skin cancers (79), particularly in immunosuppressed patients (80). Specific viral genotypes showing fairly good association with various clinical presentations are listed below, although considerable overlap exists.

Verruca vulgaris: 1, 2, 4, 7, 49
Verruca plana: 3, 10, 28, 49
Palmoplantar wart: 1, 2, 3, 4, 27, 29, 57
Condyloma acuminatum (high cancer risk): 16, 18, 31, 33, 51
Focal epithelial hyperplasia (Heck's disease): 13, 32
Bowenoid papulosis: 16, 18, 31, 33, 51
Butcher's warts: 7
Epidermodysplasia verruciformis: 3, 5, 8 to 10, 12, 14, 17, 19 to 29, 36, 38, 47, 50
Laryngeal carcinoma: 30
Head and neck (oropharyngeal) squamous cell carcinoma: 16
Giant condyloma of Bushke and Loewenstein: 6
Cervical and vulvar dysplasia: 16, 18, 31, 33, 51

The association of particular HPV types with specific groups of warts, however, is not absolute. The value of HPV typing in the clinical setting is not clear. Definitive HPV typing can be obtained through DNA hybridization or amplification of HPV genomic material by the polymerase chain reaction. However, positive results cannot be considered definitive in predicting outcome. High-risk HPV types can be missed through sampling errors. In the end, close follow-up is important in the management of HPV infection, particularly when the patient has clinical exposure to potentially high-risk HPV types (81).

All HPV types target squamous epithelial cells. Entry of HPV into squamous epithelium results in three different type of infections: latent infection, in which there is no gross or microscopic evidence of disease; subclinical infection, in which colposcopy or microscopy reveals disease in the absence of clinical disease; and clinical disease. Early HPV genes are expressed in basal epithelial cells. Clinical and histologic evidence of HPV infection usually develops 1 to 8 months after initial exposure. Untreated, these lesions may regress spontaneously, persist as benign lesions, or progress to precancerous lesions and eventually, cancer (82).

Verruca Vulgaris

Verruca vulgaris, the common wart, most commonly presents singly or in groups on the dorsal aspects of the fingers and hands as painless, circumscribed, firm elevated papules with papillomatous ("verrucous") hyperkeratotic surfaces. The palms and soles are less common sites and present at these sites as mosaic warts. Verruca vulgaris is rarely identified on the oral mucosa. The face and scalp are the most common sites for filiform warts, variants of verruca vulgaris that show threadlike, keratinous projections arising from horny bases.

Verrucae vulgares are circumscribed, firm, elevated papules with papillomatous ("verrucous") hyperkeratotic surfaces. They occur singly or in groups. Generally, they are associated with little or no tenderness. Verrucae vulgares occur most commonly on the dorsal aspects of the fingers and hands. They are also found on the soles of the feet and less often on the palms as mosaic warts. Rarely, verrucae vulgares occur on the oral mucosa. Filiform warts, variants of verruca vulgaris, show threadlike, keratinous projections arising from horny bases. New warts may form at sites of trauma (Koebner phenomenon). Verrucae vulgares are often associated with HPV-2, but may be induced by HPV-1, -4, -7 and -49.

Histopathology. Verrucae vulgares show acanthosis, papillomatosis, and hyperkeratosis. The rete ridges are elongated and, at the periphery of the verruca, are often bent inward so that they appear to point radially toward the center (arborization). The characteristic features that distinguish verruca vulgaris from other papillomas are foci of vacuolated cells, referred to as koilocytotic cells, vertical tiers of parakeratotic cells, and foci of clumped keratohyaline granules. These three changes are quite pronounced in young verrucae vulgares. The foci of koilocytes are located in the upper stratum malpighii and in the granular layer (Fig. 25-7). The koilocytes possess small, round, deeply basophilic nuclei surrounded by a clear halo and pale-staining cytoplasm. These cells contain few or no keratohyaline granules, even when they are located in the granular layer. The vertical tiers of parakeratotic cells are often located at the crests of papillomatous elevations of the rete malpighii overlying a focus of vacuolated cells. Compared with ordinary parakeratotic nuclei, the nuclei of the parakeratotic cells in verrucae vulgares are larger and more deeply basophilic, and many of them appear rounded rather than elongated. Although no granular cells are seen overlying the papillomatous crests, they are increased in number and size in the intervening valleys and contain heavy, irregular clumps of keratohyaline granules (Fig. 25-7).

In filiform warts, the papillae are more elongated than in verrucae vulgares (Fig. 25-7C). They contain dilated capillaries, and small areas of hemorrhage may be seen in the thickened horny layer at the tip of the filiform wart.

Although warts are very common, especially in children and adolescents, defective cell-mediated immunity predisposes to the development of some types of warts. The frequency of warts in persons with renal transplants receiving immunosuppressive therapy is greater than that of the general population (83). In the context of HIV infection, a variety of papillomavirus infections have been reported. Eradication of cutaneous infection becomes increasingly difficult as the degree of immunosuppression becomes more profound.

Histogenesis and viral identification. No difference has been noted in electron microscopic appearance among the virus particles in the various types of HPV. However, the quantity varies with the different types. Frequently, virus particles are absent in verrucae vulgares on electron microscopic examination. Negative results of electron microscopic examination do not exclude the presence of HPV. Viral antigens, such as papillomavirus common antigen, can be detected using immunohistochemistry, and HPV DNA can be amplified from lesions using the polymerase chain reaction and appropriate primers. Viral genomic material can also be identified by *in situ* hybridization. Viral DNA replication occurs in proliferating basal cells, but structural capsid protein forms in the midepidermis, so that mature HPV viral structures, if present, are observed only in the upper epidermis.

The virus particles are spherical bodies with a diameter of about 50 nm. Each particle consists of an electron-dense nucleoid with a stippled appearance surrounded by a less dense capsid. The wart virus replicates in the nucleus, where the viral particles are located as dense aggregates in a crystalloid arrangement. Eosinophilic intranuclear bodies are very rare in verrucae vulgares. The wart virus does not grow in tissue cultures and is not pathogenic for any animals.

Deep Palmoplantar Warts

Deep palmoplantar warts can be tender and occasionally swollen and red. Although they may be multiple, they do not coalesce as do mosaic warts, which are verrucae vulgares. Deep palmoplantar warts occur not only on the palms and soles but also on the lateral aspects and tips of the fingers and toes. Unlike superficial, mosaic-type palmoplantar warts, deep palmoplantar warts usually are covered with a thick callus. When the callus is removed with a scalpel, the wart becomes apparent.

A plantar wart associated with HPV-60 may appear as a nodule on the weight-bearing surface of the sole. The nodule usually is smooth with visible rete ridges but may become hyperkeratotic. If the lesion is incised, cheesy material may be expressed. A pigmented verrucous variant associated with HPV-65, and a whitish keratotic wart associated with HPV-63 have been reported.

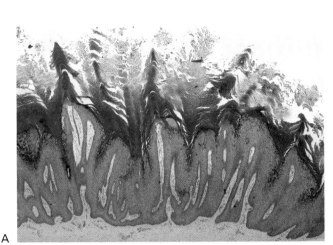

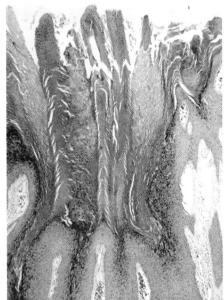

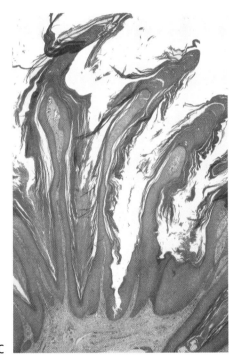

FIGURE 25-7. Verruca vulgaris. Low magnification; hyperkeratosis, acanthosis, and papillomatosis. The rete ridges are elongated and bent inward at both margins and thus appear to point radially to the center. **A:** Groups of large, vacuolated cells lie in the upper stratum malpighii and in the granular layer. **B:** Same as *(A)*, but at high magnification. **C:** Verruca vulgaris of filiform type; there is marked papillomatosis.

Histopathology. Whereas superficial, mosaic-type palmoplantar warts have a histologic appearance analogous to that of verruca vulgaris and represent HPV-2 or HPV-4 infection, deep palmoplantar warts are commonly associated with HPV-1 infection, but can also be seen with HPV-60, -63 and -65. These lesions, also known as myrmecia ("anthill") or inclusion warts, are characterized by abundant keratohyalin, which differs from normal keratohyalin by being eosinophilic. There is prominent hyperkeratosis. Starting in the lower epidermis, the cytoplasm of many cells contains numerous eosinophilic granules, which en-

large in the upper stratum malpighii and coalesce to form large, irregularly shaped, homogeneous "inclusion bodies." They either encase the vacuolated nucleus or are separated from it by perinuclear vacuolization. The nuclei in the stratum corneum persist, appearing as deeply basophilic round bodies surrounded by a wide, clear zone (Fig. 25-8). In addition to the large intracytoplasmic eosinophilic inclusion bodies, some of the cells in the upper stratum malpighii with vacuolated nuclei contain a small intranuclear eosinophilic "inclusion body." It is round and of about the same size as the nucleolus, which, however, is basophilic (Fig.

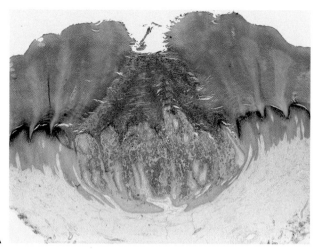

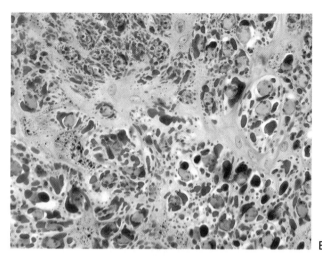

A   B

FIGURE 25-8. Deep palmoplantar wart (myrmecia). **A:** Virally induced proliferation of keratinocytes results of the lesion. The elongated retia are displaced laterally while their tips point to the center in the deep portion. The lesion is covered by thickened keratin, resulting in a tendency to grow inward rather than outward from the surface. **B:** The epidermal squamous cells contain polygonal, refractile-appearing, eosinophilic, cytoplasmic inclusions. Nuclei also contain round eosinophilic bodies.

25-8). Regression of plantar warts is often associated with thrombosis of superficial vessels, hemorrhage, and necrosis of the epidermis.

Histogenesis and viral identification. Under electron microscopic examination, viral particles are first observed in the upper portion of the stratum malpighii within and around the nucleolus. Their number increases, and in cells just beneath the stratum corneum, nucleoli are no longer detected. In many instances, the material of the nucleus appears to be entirely replaced by virus particles except for a thin rim of chromatin closely applied to the nuclear membrane. The particles tend to be arranged in regular or crystalline formations. In the stratum corneum, no normal cell structures are recognizable, but there remain large, compact aggregates of virus particles surrounded by keratinous matter.

Verruca Plana

Verrucae planae are slightly elevated, flat, smooth papules. They may be hyperpigmented. The face and the dorsa of the hands are affected most commonly. In rare instances, there is extensive involvement, with lesions also on the extremities and trunk. If starting in childhood and occurring in several members of the family, such disseminate cases of verruca plana have been mistakenly held to be instances of epidermodysplasia verruciformis, from which they differ by the absence of red, "tinea versicolor-like" patches and lack of malignant transformation of some of the exposed lesions.

Histopathology. Verrucae planae show hyperkeratosis and acanthosis but, unlike verrucae vulgares, have no papillo-

matosis, only slight elongation of the rete ridges, and no areas of parakeratosis. In the upper stratum malpighii, including the granular layer, there is diffuse vacuolization of the cells (Fig. 25-9). Some of the vacuolated cells are enlarged to about twice their normal size. The nuclei of the vacuolated cells lie at the centers of the cells, and some of them appear deeply basophilic. The granular layer is uniformly thickened, and the stratum corneum has a pronounced basket-weave appearance resulting from vacuolization of the horny cells. The dermis appears normal. In spontaneously regressing warts there is often a superficial lymphocytic infiltrate in the dermis with exocytosis and apoptosis of cells in the epidermis.

Histogenesis. Verrucae planae are induced by HPV-3 and HPV-10. Electron microscopic examination reveals marked cytoplasmic edema. The tonofilaments are dislodged to the periphery of the cell. The keratohyaline granules appear normal. Viral particles are numerous in the nuclei of vacuolated cells.

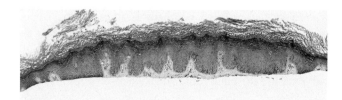

FIGURE 25-9. Verruca plana. One observes hyperkeratosis and acanthosis but no papillomatosis or parakeratosis. Numerous vacuolated cells lie in the upper stratum malpighii, including the granular layer. The horny layer has a pronounced basket-weave appearance resulting from the vacuolization of the horny cells.

Epidermodysplasia Verruciformis

Epidermodysplasia verruciformis (EV) is a genetic disease characterized by HPV infection with types not seen in otherwise healthy individuals. It usually begins in childhood and is characterized by a generalized infection by HPV, frequent association with cutaneous carcinomas, and abnormalities of cell-mediated immunity (84). Two forms of EV are recognized. One is induced by HPV-3 and HPV-10 and characterized by a persistent widespread eruption resembling verrucae planae with a tendency toward confluence into plaques. Some of the cases are familial. There is no tendency to malignant transformation in this form. The second form is primarily related to HPV-5. There is often a familial history with an autosomal recessive or X-linked recessive inheritance. In addition to the plane warts, irregularly outlined, slightly scaling macules of various shades of brown, red, and white, tinea versicolor-like lesion, seborrheic keratosis-like lesions have been noted (85). The eruption usually begins in childhood. Development of Bowen's disease (squamous cell carcinoma *in situ*) within lesions in exposed areas is a common occurrence, and invasive lesions of squamous cell carcinoma are occasionally found. Malignant transformation occurs in about 25% of patients with EV. The oncogenic potential is highest for HPV-5, followed by HPV-8. EV-like lesions can develop in renal transplant patients (86) and in HIV-infected persons (87).

Histopathology. The epidermal changes, although similar to those observed in verruca plana, often differ by being more pronounced and more extensive (Fig. 25-10). Affected keratinocytes are swollen and irregularly shaped. They show abundant, slightly basophilic cytoplasm and contain numerous round, basophilic keratohyalin granules. A few dyskeratotic cells may be seen in the lower part of the epidermis. Although some nuclei appear pyknotic, others appear large, round, and empty owing to marginal distribution of the chromatin. In immunocompromised patients, EV often lack the histologic features of verruca planae, a focally thickened granular layer is a marker for viral detection, and the risk for dysplasia in such lesions is much higher than in epidermodysplasia verruciformis not associated with acquired immunosuppression (88).

Histogenesis. In epidermodysplasia verruciformis skin lesions, many HPV types have been found, and in some individual patients, several types have been identified (89). Electron microscopic examination shows viral particles, often in a semicrystalline pattern within nuclei located in the stratum granulosum. In contrast, the swollen cells in the stratum malpighii show virions in their nuclei in small aggregates only in some cases but none at all in others.

Viral particles are absent in lesions of Bowen's disease or squamous cell carcinoma arising from EV, but rarely these can be observed in the upper layers of the epidermis overlying malignant lesions. However, HPV-5–specific DNA or HPV-8–specific DNA has been demonstrated on several occasions in squamous cell carcinomas arising in lesions of EV. The underlying defect in EV is not clear but may involve oncogene or immunologic dysfunction.

Condyloma Acuminatum

Condylomata acuminata, or anogenital warts, can occur on the penis, female genitals, and in the anal region. Condylomata acuminate are transmitted sexually, and HPV infection is one of the most common viral sexually transmitted diseases in the world, with an estimated 1% prevalence in the

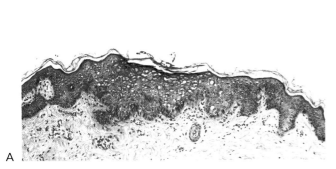
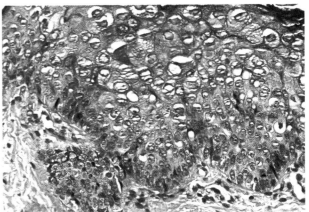

FIGURE 25-10. Epidermodysplasia verruciformis. **A:** The epidermis is hyperkeratotic and slightly acanthotic. Vacuolated cells are present in the upper stratum malpighii and granular layer. **B:** Affected keratinocytes have abundant, slightly basophilic cytoplasm. Keratohyalin granules may be prominent, although not in this example. Some nuclei may appear pyknotic, others appear large, round, and empty.

sexually active population in the United States. The estimated prevalence of HPV DNA or HPV antigens in young women may be as high as 10% to 11%. Recent studies show that HPV DNA is detectable by PCR in more than 99.7% of cervical cancers, making HPV infection the most important risk factor in the development of this disease (90). Malignant progression is associated with infection by certain HPV types. Anogenital HPV types 6 and 11 rarely progress to invasive disease and are considered low risk. HPV types 16, 18, 31, 33, and 51 have been associated with both *in situ* and invasive processes of the male and female genital regions as well as the vagina and cervix in women. Additional types associated with malignancy include 35, 39, 42 through 45, 52, and 56. However, even with infection by high-risk types, these lesions most often spontaneously regress with no long-term adverse effects (91). Progression includes a spectrum from Bowen's disease to squamous cell carcinoma, potentially with extension to metastasis.

Condylomata acuminata usually are found on the penis and around the anus in men. In women, frequent areas of infection include the vulva, vaginal introitus, perineal area, perianal area, and cervix. Lesions of the skin consist of fairly soft, verrucous papules that occasionally coalesce into cauliflower-like masses. Condylomas are flatter on mucosal surfaces.

Histopathology. In condyloma acuminatum, the stratum corneum is only slightly thickened. Lesions located on mucosal surfaces show parakeratosis. The stratum malpighii shows papillomatosis and considerable acanthosis, with thickening and elongation of the rete ridges. Mitotic figures may be present. Usually, invasive squamous cell carcinoma can be ruled out because the epithelial cells show an orderly arrangement and the border between the epithelial proliferations and the dermis is sharp, with a single basal layer (Fig. 25-11). The most characteristic feature, impor-

tant for the diagnosis, is the presence of areas in which the epithelial cells show distinct perinuclear vacuolization. These vacuolated epithelial cells are relatively large and possess hyperchromatic, round nuclei resembling the nuclei seen in the upper portion of the epidermis in verrucae vulgares. It must be kept in mind, however, that vacuolization is a normal occurrence in the upper portions of all mucosal surfaces, so that vacuolization in condylomata acuminata can be regarded as being possibly of viral genesis only if it extends into the deeper portions of the stratum malpighii. Koilocytotic ("raisin") nuclei, double nuclei, and apoptotic keratinocytes may be present, but are often less prominent than in uterine cervical lesions.

The diagnosis of HPV infections of the vulva can be complicated by the frequent absence of koilocytosis, and there are reports of HPV detection in lesions that depart from the typical morphology of condyloma. In one study, HPV-DNA—principally HPV6—was detected in 18 of 25 vulvar seborrheic keratoses (72%), while 15% of nongenital seborrheic keratoses were positive for this virus. Therefore, a majority of vulvar seborrheic keratoses may represent senescent condylomas (92).

Giant Condylomata Acuminata of Buschke and Loewenstein

The Buschke–Loewenstein tumor, also called giant condyloma acuminatum, is generally observed in males. The most frequent location is the glans penis and foreskin (where urethral fistulae may result), but they may occur also on the vulva and in the anal region. Clinically, it is a cauliflower-like tumor with resemblance to a large aggregate of condylomata acuminata, especially in the early stage. It is characterized by its large size with the propensity to ulcerate and infiltrate into deeper tissues, contrasting with a microscopically benign pattern. The hallmark of the disease is the high rate of recurrence (66%) and of malignant transformation (56%). Distant metastases are extremely rare. Overall mortality is 20%, all occurring in patients with recurrences (93).

Histopathology. The lesion shows a benign papillomatous growth characterized predominantly by epithelial hyperplasia, hyperacanthosis, and hyperkeratosis. Generally, vacuolization of keratinocytes is mild or absent, in contrast to condyloma acuminatum. There is tremendous proliferation of the epidermis with displacement of the underlying tissue, but the ratio of nucleus to cytoplasm is low. The invasive strands of tumor usually possess a well-developed basal cell layer. (For further discussion of verrucous carcinoma, see Chapter 28.)

Histogenesis. Papillomaviruses induce a variety of proliferative lesions in humans. Of the many types of human papillomaviruses that have been identified, a subset that includes types 16, 18, 31, 33, and 51 is associated with anogenital cancers (94). These cancers develop from pre-

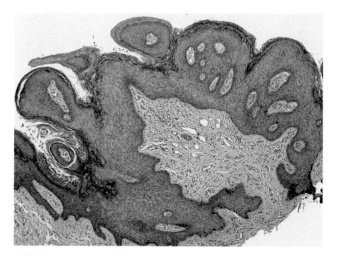

FIGURE 25-11. Condyloma acuminatum. There is pronounced acanthosis. Many cells of the stratum malpighii appear vacuolated and have round, hyperchromatic nuclei.

cursor lesions, such as condylomata acuminata on the external genitalia, vulvar intraepithelial neoplasia (VIN), vaginal intraepithelial neoplasia in the vagina (VAIN), and cervical intraepithelial neoplasia on the cervix (CIN). Viral production occurs in low-grade lesions that are only slightly altered in their pattern of differentiation from normal cells, but the concentration of mature virions in condylomata acuminata is low. The production of viral particles, genome amplification, capsid protein synthesis, and virion assembly is dependent on differentiation, and is restricted to suprabasal cells. In more atypical lesions, viral DNA is usually found integrated into host chromosomes and no viral production is noted. The viral DNA encodes nine overlapping genes, early (E1-E7) and late (L1–2). Early genes are involved in oncogenic transformation in high-risk HPV types, especially E6 and E7 which enable HPV to use cellular proteins for continued viral replication by arresting the process of keratinocyte differentiation and inactivation of cell cycle regulators, such as p53 and retinoblastoma protein, thus providing the initial step in progression to malignancy (95).

BOWENOID PAPULOSIS OF THE GENITALIA

Bowenoid papuloses are small, red papules of the genitalia. Some lesions are distinctly verrucous in appearance. The lesions are located in men on the glans and shaft of the penis and in women in the perineal and vulvar areas. Generally, the lesions are diagnosed clinically as genital warts, and the histologic finding of "Bowen's disease" appears incongruous.

The lesions have a definite tendency toward spontaneous resolution; some lesions regress, but others may appear and in turn also regress. Still, in some patients, lesions have persisted for prolonged periods. In rare cases, invasive squamous cell carcinoma has been described as arising in a Bowenoid papule.

Some authors regard the disorder as benign and, in particular, as different from Bowen's disease (57), but others have found that Bowenoid papulosis presents a premalignant lesion with a high risk for cervical neoplasia both for female patients and for sexual partners of male patients (96). Invasive squamous cell carcinoma develops in a small number of cases and it seems that women over 40 have the greatest risk.

Histopathology. Bowenoid papulosis shows the typical features of Bowen's disease. These features consist of full thickness epidermal atypia with crowding and an irregular, "windblown" arrangement of the nuclei, many of which are large, hyperchromatic, and pleomorphic (Fig. 25-12). Dyskeratotic and multinucleated keratinocytes are also present, as are atypical mitoses. The basement membrane is intact. True koilocytes are uncommon. Bowenoid papulosis may be histologically indistinguishable from vulvar intraepithelial neoplasia (VIN III), a term that is synonymous with squamous cell carcinoma *in situ* or Bowen's disease. Some researchers believe that Bowenoid papulosis differs from Bowen's disease by virtue of a lesser degree of cytologic atypia. In a few instances, Bowenoid papulosis and condylomata acuminata have been found coexisting in the same patient.

Histogenesis. Bowenoid papulosis represents infection by HPV types associated with high risk of malignancy evolution, such as HPV types 16, 18, 31, 33, and 51. As noted above, these types elaborate oncoproteins that interfere with normal cellular homeostasis.

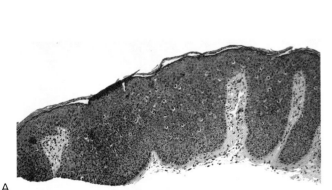
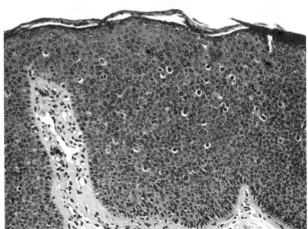

FIGURE 25-12. Bowenoid papulosis. **A:** The epithelium is irregularly thickened with disorderly maturation, which may impart a "windblown" look at scanning or intermediate magnification. **B:** The keratinocytic nuclei are crowded and there is partial arrest of maturation. Mitoses are present above the basal layers, and the nuclei tend to be hyperchromatic and irregular, sometimes with nucleoli.

Differential Diagnosis. Bowenoid papulosis of the genitalia in most instances is differentiated from Bowen's disease on the basis of clinical data, such as onset at an earlier average age, multiplicity of lesions, smaller size of lesions, verrucoid appearance of some lesions, and tendency toward spontaneous regression. Thus, Bowen's disease or squamous cell carcinoma *in situ* (VIN III) cannot be ruled out by biopsy alone in most cases.

Changes induced by recent application of podophyllum resin need to be considered. The changes induced by podophyllum resin consist of necrotic keratinocytes and bizarre mitotic figures and are most pronounced during the first 72 hours after application.

ORAL FOCAL EPITHELIAL HYPERPLASIA

A rare condition, oral focal epithelial hyperplasia (Heck's disease) has since been found to occur in many countries and races, but most commonly among the Eskimos of Greenland (97). It primarily occurs in children, often in small endemic foci, but lesions may occur in young and middle-aged adults. There is no gender predilection. Sites of greatest involvement include the labial, buccal, and lingual mucosa, but gingival and tonsillar lesions have also been reported.

There are numerous soft, white papules 2 to 10 mm in diameter. Individual lesions are broad based or slightly elevated as well as demarcated plaques. Papules and plaques are usually the color of normal mucosa, but may be pale or, rarely, white. Most are discrete, but some are confluent. The lesions are asymptomatic. Although the disease is chronic, spontaneous remissions occur. Oral focal hyperplasia has been described in the context of HIV infection (98).

Histopathology. The oral epithelium shows acanthosis with thickening and elongation of the rete ridges. The thickened mucosa extends upward, not down into underlying connective tissues, hence, the lesional rete ridges are at the same depth as the adjacent normal rete ridges. The ridges themselves are widened, often confluent and sometimes club-shaped; they are not long and thin as in *psoriasis* and other diseases. Throughout the epithelium, there are areas where the cells show marked vacuolization and stain only faintly. Vacuolization is most pronounced in the upper portion of the epithelium, but it may extend into the broadened rete ridges (Fig. 25-13).

Histogenesis. Electron microscopic examination reveals viral particles with the size of the human papillomavirus arranged in a crystalline pattern. HPV types 13 and 32 are typical for oral focal epithelial hyperplasia (99).

Differential Diagnosis. The histologic appearance of the affected oral epithelium in focal epithelial hyperplasia is

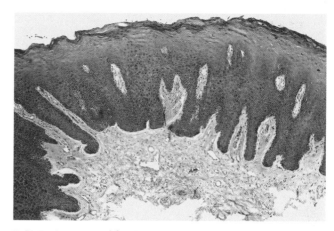

FIGURE 25-13. Oral focal epithelial hyperplasia. The oral epithelium shows acanthosis with thickening and elongation of the rete ridges. The ridges are widened, often confluent and sometimes club shaped. Vacuolization is most pronounced in the upper portion of the epithelium.

identical to that of oral epithelial nevus, or white sponge nevus.

Picornaviridae

Picornaviridae consists of single-stranded RNA viruses that are 10 to 30 nm, naked, icosahedral, and contain only four to six genes. They are the smallest of the RNA viruses and are very important in human disease. Picornaviridae infections of humans have been classified into five groups: Enterovirus (polio), Hepadnaviridae (hepatitis A), Cardiovirus (encephalomyocarditis), Rhinovirus (common cold), and Aphthovirus (foot-and-mouth diseases). Picornaviridae infection is one of the most common causes of viral exanthem. In addition to nonspecific findings, enterovirus infection also causes distinct syndromes, such as hand-foot-mouth disease, herpangina, and hemorrhagic conjunctivitis (100).

HAND-FOOT-AND-MOUTH DISEASE

Hand-foot-and-mouth disease is caused by a coxsackievirus, an Enterovirus. In most instances, coxsackievirus type A16 has been isolated; only rarely has another type, such as A5 or A9, been found (101). Hand-foot-and-mouth disease occurs in small epidemics, affecting mainly children and having a mild course that usually lasts less than a week. Transmission is mainly via fecal-oral contact and less commonly by respiratory droplets (102). Symptoms usually appear 3 to 5 days after exposure. After a 1-to 2-day mild prodrome of low-grade fever, sore throat, and malaise, small red macules present on the oral mu-

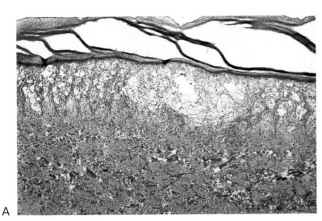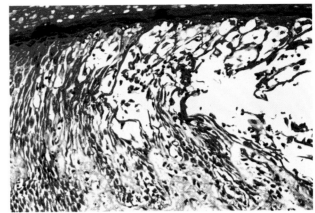

A   B

FIGURE 25-14. Hand-foot-and-mouth disease. **A:** Scanning magnification shows intraepidermal vesicles (early lesion) with pronounced reticular degeneration. **B:** Pronounced reticular degeneration and balloon degeneration. Neither inclusion bodies nor multinucleated cells are present.

cosal, and progress to 1- to 3-mm vesicles, where they evolve into small ulcers. Between 25% to 65% of patients may have the classic vesicular lesions on the hand and feet, which presented as scattered small vesicles surrounded by an erythematous halo on the palms of the hands, soles of the feet, and ventral surfaces and sides of the fingers and toes (103). Similar lesions may develop on the rest of the skin.

Histopathology. Early vesicles are intraepidermal, whereas old vesicles may be subepidermal in location. There is pronounced reticular degeneration of the epidermis, resulting in multilocular vesiculation. In the deep layers of the epidermis, some ballooning degeneration may be found. Neither inclusion bodies nor multinucleated giant cells are present (Fig. 25-14).

Histogenesis and Diagnosis. Viral culture has been the gold standard until recently, when PCR has become the diagnostic test for rapid and accurate enterovirus infection. The sensitivity of PCR is almost double that of viral culture (104). Electron microscopic examination reveals that some keratinocytes contain within their cytoplasm aggregates of virus particles exhibiting a crystalloid pattern (105). The coxsackievirus can be cultured from stool and occasionally from skin vesicles. The virus grows well on human epithelial cell and monkey kidney cell cultures.

Hepatitis A Virus

The hepatitis A virus is a common cause of hepatitis worldwide. Spread of infection is through the fecal-oral route. Hepatitis A is endemic in developing countries, and most residents are exposed in childhood. In contrast, the adult population in developed countries demonstrates falling rates of exposure with improvements in hygiene and sanitation. Hepatitis A usually presents as fever, jaundice, and hepatomegaly. Extrahepatic manifestations are rarely found in hepatitis A viral infection. Urticaria and scarlatiniform eruption and rare cases of cutaneous vasculitis and cryoglobulinemia have been reported (106).

Retroviridae

Retroviridae are RNA retroviruses and are currently classified into seven genera, including human immunodeficiency virus (HIV), the cause of acquired immunodeficiency syndrome (AIDS), and human T-lymphotropic virus (HTLV).

ACQUIRED IMMUNODEFICIENCY SYNDROME

HIV infects predominantly CD4$^+$ cells, most notably T-helper cells, and leads to a profound alteration of immune system function that predisposes patients to numerous opportunistic infections, malignancies, and neurologic diseases. The virus is spread almost exclusively through blood and semen.

Cutaneous findings in HIV disease are frequent and include viral, bacterial, fungal, and noninfectious etiologies (107). Some infections occur in clinically obscure forms because they do not have recognizable morphologic features. In addition, systemic infectious diseases can produce skin lesions, even though the classic organs of involvement for that agent may not include the skin. Dermatologic diseases common to the general population, such as *seborrheic dermatitis*, often have an increased prevalence or severity in these individuals (108). Several skin diseases occur nearly exclusively in HIV-infected individuals, such as oral hairy leukoplakia, bacillary angiomatosis, and Kaposi's sarcoma.

HIV itself produces cutaneous findings shortly after exposure. In addition, gradual deterioration of the immune system renders HIV-infected patients susceptible to numerous cutaneous viral diseases, including herpesviruses, human papillomavirus, and molluscum contagiosum (109). Approximately 2 to 6 weeks following HIV exposure, patients may present with a transient illness related to HIV replication and host response. More than 50% of patients report symptoms of acute HIV infection: a macular or morbilliform rash usually involving the trunk is present in 40% to 80% of patents with acute HIV infection (110). Because the standard immunoassay and Western blot are often negative with acute infection, additional tests may be needed when there is a high index of suspicion. P24 antigen assay has fewer false positives and may be a more cost-effective way to diagnose primary HIV infection (111).

Pruritic papular eruption (PPE) is the most common cutaneous manifestation in HIV-infected patients. Opportunistic viral infections affecting the skin and mucous membranes are also common (40). Herpetic infections are one of the most important causes of opportunistic infections in patients with HIV and frequently include cutaneous manifestations. Unlike in the healthy individual, in which case the lesions are often self-limited, herpetic infections cause significant chronic morbidity in immunocompromised patients. As immune function declines, the herpetic lesions may become chronic and progress to painful ulceration. Herpes zoster may be complicated by repeated bouts, involvement of multiple dermatomes, chronic verrucous zoster, and rarely, herpes zoster may disseminate. CMV infection is associated with CD4+ cell counts of less than 100 and has a spectrum of presentations including pulmonary, ocular, gastrointestinal, and neurologic involvement, although CMV skin lesions are uncommon (112). While a majority of adults harbor EBV in latent phase, oral hairy leukoplakia is a rare disorder found almost exclusively in HIV-infected individuals. Approximately 25% of HIV-infected individuals may be affected. White, verrucous, confluent plaques that are most commonly located on the lateral aspects of the tongue characterize oral hairy leukoplakia, which do not scrape off with a tongue depressor (113). EBV appears to be necessary for production of this lesion, although HPV and *Candida* are also frequently present. The condition is a result of EBV infection of epithelial cells that leads to hyperkeratotic thickening. Molluscum contagiosum generally presents as CD4+ counts fall below 100/mm³. While the lesions spontaneously resolve in immunocompetent hosts, the lesions are often extensive and progressive in HIV-infected individuals, who are also subject to so-called giant molluscum contagiosum with lesions ranging from 1 to 6 cm in diameter (114).

Bacterial infections are also common in AIDS. Staphylococcus aureus is the most common cutaneous bacterial pathogen in HIV-seropositive patients. HIV-infected patients are also prone to streptococcal impetigo and axillary lymphadenitis. Another unique infectious disease first recognized in the context of HIV infection is bacillary angiomatosis. Bacillary angiomatosis is a systemic infectious disease caused by gram-negative *Bartonella henselae* or *B. quintana* (115). Patients may have palpable subcutaneous nodules, which may resemble Kaposi's sarcoma or hemangioma but resolve with appropriate antibiotic therapy. The lesions often are painful, unlike those of Kaposi's sarcoma. HIV-infected patients are susceptible to mycobacterial infections that can sometimes produce unusual skin manifestations. Syphilis is common in these individuals and often the presenting infection of HIV disease (116). Secondary syphilis assumes a variety of manifestations in HIV-infected patients, including oral erosions, nodules, papules, vesicles, hyperkeratotic plaques, and papulosquamous or maculopapular eruptions.

Patients with HIV are subject to fungal, protozoa and arthropod infections that produce mucocutaneous findings. Oral candidiasis is often an early clinical manifestation of AIDS and in progressing may cause painful esophagitis. Other infections such as *Cryptococcus, Histoplasma, Coccidioidomycosis*, tinea versicolor, phaeohyphomycosis, nocardiosis, and mucormycosis are not uncommonly seen in these patients (117). The *scabies* mite is the most common parasitic infestation of HIV-infected individuals (118). Scabies is highly contagious in HIV-infected patients via direct contact. Demodicidosis involves the proliferation of *Demodex* mites within the pilosebaceous unit, and is reported in association with HIV infection (119). Disseminated acanthamebiasis has been reported in these patients and often presents skin manifestations such as pustules, subcutaneous and deep dermal nodules, and ulcers, most often seen on the extremities and face.

Noninfectious cutaneous disorders are also common in HIV infection and can occur at all stages of disease. An explosive episode of psoriasis or severe seborrheic dermatitis can be the presenting symptom of HIV disease. Seborrheic dermatitis is a common disease affecting 2%-4% of the general population, but up to 85% of HIV-positive individuals experience seborrheic dermatitis at some point during their disease. It can be quite severe, with the severity correlating with the patient's clinical status and CD4 count (120). Less common areas such as the chest, back, axilla, and groin are often involved in HIV-seropositive patients. The histology of this eruption is similar to that of idiopathic seborrheic dermatitis, although some feel that distinctive histologic patterns are present (121). While the incidence of psoriasis in HIV disease is similar to the general population, it is often more severe, refractory to treatment, and has a higher prevalence of psoriatic arthritis. Reiter's syndrome, characterized by arthritis, urethritis, and conjunctivitis, may be associated with psoriasis in HIV-infected individuals (122). As many as 30% of HIV-infected individuals experience xerosis or acquired ichthyosis with fine white scales and cracking skin without erythema, which may be diffuse or preferentially affect the anterior tibia, dorsal hand, and forearm (123). Whereas xerosis reveals minimal inflammation microscopically, acquired ichthyosis is histologically similar to ichthyosis vulgaris, often with hyperkeratosis and diminished or absence of the granular cell layer. A nonspecific follicular eruption, named eosinophilic pustular folliculitis, is present in a significant number of patients with HIV infection (124). The eruption is chronic and pruritic. An interface dermatitis associated with HIV, observed in a series of 25 patients with AIDS, presents as a more or less widespread eruption of pink or red macules, papules, or plaques. It resembles and may represent a form of drug eruption or erythema multiforme (125).

Adverse cutaneous drug reactions are common in HIV-positive individuals, and they are prone to side effects associated with antimicrobial and antiviral medications (126). For example, after 1 to 2 weeks of Trimethoprim-sulfamethoxazole treatment for *Pneumocystis carinii* infection, up to 50% to 60% of HIV-infected patients may develop a morbilliform rash. HIV-infected individuals also have an increased incidence of photosensitivity reactions. Chronic actinic dermatitis, a rare photosensitivity reaction is sometimes the presenting manifestation of HIV seropositivity (127). Porphyria cutanea tarda is reported more frequently in HIV-infected individuals compared to the general population. Other lesions, such as pityriasis rubra pilaris, porokeratosis, yellow nail syndrome, alopecia, asteatosis, vasculitis, acrodermatitis enteropathica, and neutrophilic eccrine hidradenitis have been reported.

Kaposi's sarcoma is the most common AIDS-associated cancer in the United States. Over 95% of all Kaposi's sarcoma lesions have been associated with HHV-8 (128). Skin lesions of Kaposi's sarcoma typically present with asymptomatic reddish-purple patches that sometimes progress to raised plaques or nodules. One-third of patients experience oral cavity lesions characterized by red-to-purple plaques or nodules. Other tumors such as melanoma (129) and squamous and basal cell carcinoma have been reported in these patients.

Histopathology. The histology of the acute exanthema of HIV infection is rather nonspecific with a tight perivascular infiltrate of lymphocytes in the dermis. Epidermal changes are usually mild, but may include spongiosis, vacuolar change, and/or keratinocyte apoptosis (130,131); or there may be nonspecific lymphocytic infiltrates with mild epidermal changes, primarily spongiosis (110).

The lesions of oral hairy leukoplakia show irregular keratin projections, parakeratosis, and acanthosis. A characteristic finding within the epithelium is vacuolar change of superficial keratinocytes (Fig. 25-15). *Candida* organisms may be demonstrable. Seborrheic dermatitis in patients with AIDS may show nonspecific changes, including spotty keratinocytic necrosis, leukocytoclasis, and plasma cells in a superficial perivascular infiltrate (121). The papular eruption of AIDS may exhibit nonspecific perivascular eosinophils with mild folliculitis, although epithelioid cell granulomas have also been reported (132). The interface dermatitis shows, as the name implies, vacuolar alteration of the basal cell layer, scattered necrotic keratinocytes, and a superficial perivascular lymphohistiocytic infiltrate. The vacuolar alteration and number of necrotic keratinocytes tend to be more pronounced than in drug eruptions (125). The changes found are nonspecific but are suggestive of features described in graft-versus-host disease and become more prominent in late-stage disease. Eosinophilic pustular folliculitis shows folliculitis with transmigration of eosinophils into the follicular epithelium, mimicking the changes observed in Ofuji's disease. However, in many cases, the

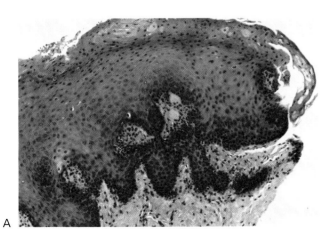 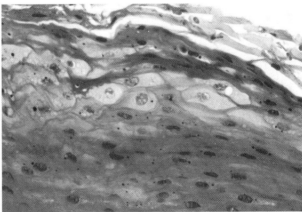

FIGURE 25-15. Oral hairy leukoplakia. **A:** Scanning magnification shows the characteristic complex rete pattern of lingual epithelium. There is hyperkeratosis and parakeratosis, and there may be neutrophils in the stratum corneum. Pallor of superficial keratinocytes is focally apparent. **B:** Detail of swollen, pale superficial keratinocytes, with open pale nuclei, but without specific viral cytopathic changes and scant inflammation in the superficial lamina propria.

histologic picture is less specific, showing only a polymorphous inflammatory response and mild folliculitis (131, 133). Cutaneous acanthamebiasis shows both pustular and vasculitis changes; the microscopic identification of organisms is difficult because of the macrophage-like appearance of the microbes in routine sections (134). A PAS stain can be used to highlight the organisms.

DISEASES CAUSED BY OTHER VIRUSES

Hepatitis B Virus

Hepatitis B virus (HBV) is a double-stranded DNA virus belonging to the hepadnavirus family. Transmission of the virus is frequently through IV drug use, sexual activity, and mother-to-fetus transmission (135). During the acute phase, 15% of the patients will develop urticaria, fever, and malaise (136). Polyarteritis nodosum (PAN) is one of the more serious and common complications of HBV infection (137). About 2 in 500 people with HBV develop PAN, but up to 50% of people with PAN test positive for HBsAg. Cutaneous involvement occurs in 10% to 20% of people with PAN, which presents as palpable purpura that progress to large ulcers. Tender, purple, subcutaneous nodules can occur as well as livedo vasculitis (138). There is fibrinoid necrosis of medium size vessel wall with a cellular infiltrate composed mainly of $CD8^+$ T cells and macrophages. Depositions of immune complex, IgM, C3, and HBsAg in the vessel walls are observed.

Papular acrodermatitis of childhood (Gianotti–Crosti syndrome) occurs in children infected with HBV, and is not common in adults (139). The clinical presentation includes a non-relapsing erythematous popular eruption localized to the face and limbs, with lymphadenopathy and acute hepatitis (mostly anicteric). The lesions do not affect mucosal surfaces. Papular acrodermatitis of childhood is common in Southern Europe and Japan, but rare in the United States. This condition can also be associated with CMV, EBV, respiratory syncytial virus, and enterovirus infection (140). The histology is characterized by a mixture of spongiotic and lichenoid dermatitis with a dense perivascular infiltrate.

Serum sickness-like syndrome is considered the most common dermatologic manifestation associated with HBV, which occurs in 20% to 30% of patients during the prodromal phase of the HBV infection. The skin manifestation includes urticaria, angioedema, and rashes. The urticaria lesions show erythrocyte extravasation, endothelial cell swelling, and various degrees of fibrinoid change of postcapillary venules (141). The pathology is induced by deposition of immune complexes, which are composed of HBsAg, IgG, IgM, and C3.

HBV has also been associated with mixed cryoglobulinemia (142), however, it is much less common than that associated with hepatitis C virus infection. A recurrent papular rash on the trunk and extremities (143) and lichen planus have been reported as complications of hepatitis B vaccination in both adults and children (144).

Hepatitis C Virus

Hepatitis C virus (HCV) is a single-stranded RNA virus that belongs to *Hepacivirus*, the third genus of the Flaviviridae family. Individuals with exposure to blood or blood products are at risk of infection with HCV. The prevalence in the United States ranges from 0.5% to 2%. Mixed cryoglobulinemia (MC) is the most documented extrahepatic manifestation of HCV infection (145). It presents cutaneously as inflammatory palpable purpura that are usually confined to the lower extremities, which progress to ulceration. It is established that the majority (80%) of what was previously known as essential MC is now known to be related to chronic HCV infection (146). Despite a high prevalence of HCV markers in patients with MC, only an estimated 13% to 54% of patients with chronic HCV will develop MC. It is believed that HCV-IgG and HCV-lipoprotein complexes may act as B-cell superantigens inducing the synthesis of non-HCV reactive IgM with rheumatoid factor-like activity that leads to immune complex formation. Because of the high prevalence of liver abnormalities seen in patients with MC, hepatotropic viruses should be ruled out as causative agents. Histologic features for MC are those of an acute vasculitis involving small- and/or mid-size dermal vessels. Intravascular hyaline deposits are generally not seen except in the areas beneath the ulcer.

Lichen planus (LP) is common in patients with HCV. The prevalence of HCV ranges from 16% to 55% and 0.17% to 4.8% in LP patients and control groups, respectively (147). The lesions of HCV-related LP are similar to those of classic LP. However, a majority of reported HCV-related LP cases have oral involvement. Histologically, LP is characterized by a subepidermal, band-like lymphohistiocytic infiltrate with interface change, sawtooth rete ridges, and pigmentary continence.

Recent reports documented a high but variable prevalence of HCV infection in patients with porphyria cutanea tarda (PCT). The prevalence is higher in Southern Europe (67% to 91%) and lower in Northern Europe (8% to 10%). The prevalence in the United States is reported to be between 50% and 75% (148). In most cases, the HCV exposure and associated liver dysfunction precede the onset of PCT, suggesting that a viral infection can reveal a porphyrin metabolism defect in susceptible patients. Histologically, PCT is characterized by a cell-poor subepidermal bulla with increased PAS-positive, diastase-resistant hyaline material in the vessel walls and basement membrane.

Other lesions associated with HCV infection include erythema multiforme and erythema nodosum (149), Henoch–Schönlein purpura (150), Behçet's syndrome (151), necrolytic acral erythema (152), PAN (153), prurigo nodularis (154), pyoderma gangrenosum (155), and urticarial vasculitis (156).

Parvovirus B19

Parvovirus, a single-stranded DNA virus, belongs to the family Parvoviridae. Parvovirus B19 is the only parvovirus that clearly causes human disease (157). The virus is highly tropic for erythroid progenitor cells, and thus is classified as an erythrovirus. The cellular receptor for B19 is a globoside, also known as blood group P antigen (40). Parvovirus infection is ubiquitous and occurs worldwide. Transmission of the virus occurs through the respiratory route in most cases. Two dermatologic conditions have been linked to Parvovirus B19 infection, erythema infectiosum and papular purpuric gloves-and-socks syndrome (157,158). Infection may also result in nonspecific findings, such as reticular erythema, maculopapular eruptions, purpuric eruptions, palpable purpura, and angioedema. Other dermatologic entities, such as erythema multiforme (159), Gianotti–Crosti syndrome (160), and recently various vasculitic syndromes including Henoch-Schönlein purpura (HSP), Wegener's granulomatosis, and microscopic polyarteritis have been linked to B19 infection (161).

The most well-known dermatologic manifestation of parvovirus B19 is erythema infectiosum. This well-recognized exanthema also is called fifth disease, with a distinctive "slapped-cheek" appearance. Less widely recognized and described only a decade ago, papular purpuric gloves-and-socks syndrome is also associated with parvovirus B19. Clinically, the rash consists of symmetric erythema and edema of the hands and feet, with gradual progression to petechiae and purpura. One of the clinical hallmarks of the rash is the sharp demarcation on the wrists and ankles. Resolution occurs within 1 to 2 weeks, with no permanent sequelae. However, in immunocompromised patients, papular purpuric gloves-and-socks syndrome may lead to more serious complications, such as persistent anemia. The histology is not entirely specific. Most cases have revealed interstitial histiocytic infiltrates with piecemeal fragmentation of collagen and a mononuclear cell–predominant vascular injury pattern, showing dilated and irregular shaped dermal vessels with swelling of endothelial cells. Mild to moderate perivascular infiltrates of mononuclear cells were noted (162).

Measles

Measles virus is a single-stranded RNA virus that belongs to the family Paramyxoviridae. Measles is an epidemic disease with worldwide distribution. Measles virus is transmitted via respiratory secretions, predominantly as aerosols but also by direct contact. The symptoms usually last for 10 days and resolve without consequence. However, there is an increased risk of more severe diseases, such as severe pneumonitis or encephalitis, in immunocompromised individuals (163). A biopsy of the rash shows nonspecific histologic change with epidermal spongiosis and mild vesiculation with scattered degenerated keratinocytes (164). Biopsies from AIDS patients with measles show necrosis of clusters of keratinocytes in the upper spinous layer and granular layer of the epidermis. Unlike in erythema multiforme the necrosis occurs in the basal layer keratinocytes. Multinucleated keratinocytes may or may not be prominent in the measles biopsy. Cytoplasmic swelling of the keratinocytes in the granular layer may be present even when multinucleated cells are sparse (165).

Rubella

Rubella, an enveloped, single-stranded RNA virus, is a member of the Togaviridae family. Rubella, also known as German measles, is a viral exanthema of childhood that is generally subclinical and inconsequential. Viremia occurs approximately 1 week before the rash; the rash is seen when circulating antibodies appear. The rash is maculopapular, erythematous, discrete, and pruritic. The face is usually the first area of devolvement and then spreads to extremities. The entire body may be involved within 1 day. On the 2nd day, there is clearing of the face and the rash is commonly cleared by the 3rd day. Histologically, the change is not specific with a mild, perivascular lymphocytic infiltrate (166,167).

REFERENCES

1. Murray N, McMichael A. Antigen presentation in virus infection. *Curr Opin Immunol* 1992;4:401.
2. Poranen MM, Daugelavicius R, Bamford DH. Common principles in viral entry. *Annu Rev Microbiol* 2002;56:521.
3. Sieczkarski SB, Whittaker GR. Dissecting virus entry via endocytosis. *J Gen Virol* 2002;83:1535.
4. Riley LE. Herpes simplex virus. *Semin Perinatol* 1998;22:284.
5. Whitley RJ, Roizman B. Herpes simplex virus infections. *Lancet* 2001;357:1513.
6. Nahmias AJ, Lee FK, Beckman-Nahmias S. Sero-epidemiological and -sociological patterns of herpes simplex virus infection in the world. *Scand J Infect Dis Suppl* 1990;69:19.
7. Kohl S. Neonatal herpes simplex virus infection. *Clin Perinatol* 1997;24:129.
8. Reeves WC, Corey L, Adams HG, et al. Risk of recurrence after first episodes of genital herpes. Relation to HSV type and antibody response. *N Engl J Med* 1981;305:315.
9. Wald A, Zeh J, Selke S, et al. Reactivation of genital herpes simplex virus type 2 infection in asymptomatic seropositive persons. *N Engl J Med* 2000;342:844.
10. Mackley CL, Adams DR, Anderson B, et al. Eczema herpeticum: a dermatologic emergency. *Dermatol Nurs* 2002;14:307.
11. Yeung-Yue KA, Brentjens MH, Lee PC, et al. Herpes simplex viruses 1 and 2. *Dermatol Clin* 2002;20:249.

12. Raychaudhuri SP, Raychaudhuri SK. Revisit to Kaposi's varicelliform eruption: role of IL-4. *Int J Dermatol* 1995;34:854.

13. Goodyear HM, McLeish P, Randall S, et al. Immunological studies of herpes simplex virus infection in children with atopic eczema. *Br J Dermatol* 1996;134:85.

14. Jang KA, Kim SH, Choi JH, et al. Viral folliculitis on the face. *Br J Dermatol* 2000;142:555.

15. Giacobetti R. Herpetic whitlow. *Int J Dermatol* 1979;18:55.

16. Sieczkarski SB, Whittaker GR. Dissecting virus entry via endocytosis. *J Gen Virol* 2002;83:1535.

17. Powers RD, Rein MF, Hayden FG. Necrotizing balanitis due to herpes simplex type 1. *JAMA* 1982;248:215.

18. Hook EW, III, Cannon RO, Nahmias AJ, et al. Herpes simplex virus infection as a risk factor for human immunodeficiency virus infection in heterosexuals. *J Infect Dis* 1992;165:251.

19. Salvini F, Carminati G, Pinzani R, et al. Chronic ulcerative herpes simplex virus infection in HIV-infected children. *AIDS Patient Care STDS* 1997;11:421.

20. Lopyan L, Young AW Jr, Menegus M. Generalized acute mucocutaneous herpes simplex type 2 with fatal outcome. *Arch Dermatol* 1977;113:816.

21. Prober CG, Hensleigh PA, Boucher FD, et al. Use of routine viral cultures at delivery to identify neonates exposed to herpes simplex virus. *N Engl J Med* 1988;318:887.

22. Kohl S. Neonatal herpes simplex virus infection. *Clin Perinatol* 1997;24:129.

23. Schofield JK, Tatnall FM, Leigh IM. Recurrent erythema multiforme: clinical features and treatment in a large series of patients. *Br J Dermatol* 1993;128:542.

24. Darragh TM, Egbert BM, Berger TG, et al. Identification of herpes simplex virus DNA in lesions of erythema multiforme by the polymerase chain reaction. *J Am Acad Dermatol* 1991;24:23.

25. Weinberg JM, Mysliwiec A, Turiansky GW, et al. Viral folliculitis. Atypical presentations of herpes simplex, herpes zoster, and molluscum contagiosum. *Arch Dermatol* 1997;133:983.

26. Nahass GT, Goldstein BA, Zhu WY, et al. Comparison of Tzanck smear, viral culture, and DNA diagnostic methods in detection of herpes simplex and varicella-zoster infection. *JAMA* 1992;268:2541.

27. Wang JY, Montone KT. A rapid simple in situ hybridization method for herpes simplex virus employing a synthetic biotin-labeled oligonucleotide probe: a comparison with immunohistochemical methods for HSV detection. *J Clin Lab Anal* 1994;8:105.

28. Morecki R, Becker NH. Human herpesvirus infection: its fine structure identification in paraffin-embedded tissue. *Arch Pathol* 1968;86:292.

29. Mooney MA, Janniger CK, Schwartz RA. Kaposi's varicelliform eruption. *Cutis* 1994;53:243.

30. Moss EM. Atopic dermatitis. *Pediatr Clin North Am* 1978;25:225.

31. Moses AE, Cohen-Poradosu R. Images in clinical medicine. Eczema vaccinatum—a timely reminder. *N Engl J Med* 2002;346:1287.

32. Lin F, Hadler JL. Epidemiology of primary varicella and herpes zoster hospitalizations: the pre-varicella vaccine era. *J Infect Dis* 2000;181:1897.

33. Preblud SR. Varicella: complications and costs. *Pediatrics* 1986;78:728.

34. McCrary ML, Severson J, Tyring SK. Varicella zoster virus. *J Am Acad Dermatol* 1999;41:1.

35. Pitel PA, McCormick KL, Fitzgerald E, et al. Subclinical hepatic changes in varicella infection. *Pediatrics* 1980;65:631.

36. Meythaler JM, Varma RR. Reye's syndrome in adults: diagnostic considerations. *Arch Intern Med* 1987;147:61.

37. Pastuszak AL, Levy M, Schick B, et al. Outcome after maternal varicella infection in the first 20 weeks of pregnancy. *N Engl J Med* 1994;330:901.

38. Gnann JW, Jr. Varicella-zoster virus: atypical presentations and unusual complications. *J Infect Dis* 2002;186[Suppl 1]:S91.

39. Schmader K. Herpes zoster in older adults. *Clin Infect Dis* 2001;32:1481.

40. Garman ME, Tyring SK. The cutaneous manifestations of HIV infection. *Dermatol Clin* 2002;20:193.

41. Al Abdulla NA, Rismondo V, Minkowski JS, et al. Herpes zoster vasculitis presenting as giant cell arteritis with bilateral internuclear ophthalmoplegia. *Am J Ophthalmol* 2002;134:912.

42. Nikkels AF, Debrus S, Sadzot-Delvaux C, et al. Comparative immunohistochemical study of herpes simplex and varicella-zoster infections. *Virchows Arch A Pathol Anat Histopathol* 1993;422:121.

43. Solomon AR, Rasmussen JE, Weiss JS. A comparison of the Tzanck smear and viral isolation in varicella and herpes zoster. *Arch Dermatol* 1986;122:282.

44. Khoshnevis M, Tyring SK. Cytomegalovirus infections. *Dermatol Clin* 2002;20:291.

45. Vancikova Z, Dvorak P. Cytomegalovirus infection in immunocompetent and immunocompromised individuals—a review. *Curr Drug Targets Immune Endocr Metabol Disord* 2001;1:179.

46. Lee JY. Cytomegalovirus infection involving the skin in immunocompromised hosts: a clinicopathologic study. *Am J Clin Pathol* 1989;92:96.

47. Hodl S, Aubock L, Reiterer F, et al. [Blueberry muffin baby: the pathogenesis of cutaneous extramedullary hematopoiesis]. *Hautarzt* 2001;52:1035.

48. Stegmann BJ, Carey JC. TORCH Infections: toxoplasmosis, other (syphilis, varicella-zoster, parvovirus B19), rubella, cytomegalovirus (CMV), and herpes infections. *Curr Womens Health Rep* 2002;2:253.

49. Arribas JR, Arrizabalaga J, Mallolas J, et al. [Advances in the diagnosis and treatment of infections caused by herpesvirus and JC virus]. *Enferm Infecc Microbiol Clin* 1998;16[Suppl 1]:11.

50. Iwatsuki K, Xu Z, Ohtsuka M, et al. Cutaneous lymphoproliferative disorders associated with Epstein–Barr virus infection: a clinical overview. *J Dermatol Sci* 2000;22:181.

51. Steven NM. Epstein–Barr virus latent infection in vivo. *Rev Med Virol* 1997;7:97.

52. Cohen JI. Epstein–Barr virus infection. *J Virol* 1999;2458.

53. Ikediobi NI, Tyring SK. Cutaneous manifestations of Epstein–Barr virus infection. *Dermatol Clin* 2002;20:283.

54. Su IJ, Tsai TF, Cheng AL, et al. Cutaneous manifestations of Epstein–Barr virus-associated T-cell lymphoma. *J Am Acad Dermatol* 1993;29:685.

55. Jung DY, Kim JW, Lee SK, et al. Epstein–Barr virus–associated lymphoproliferative skin lesion with recurrent necrotic papulovesicles of the face. *J Dermatol* 1999;26:448.

56. Iwatsuki K, Ohtsuka M, Harada H, et al. Clinicopathologic manifestations of Epstein–Barr virus–associated cutaneous lymphoproliferative disorders. *Arch Dermatol* 1997;133:1081.

57. De Araujo T, Berman B, Weinstein A. Human herpesviruses 6 and 7. *Dermatol Clin* 2002;20:301.

58. Ranger-Rogez S, Venot C, Denis F. [Human herpesviruses 6 and 7 (HHV-6 and HHV-7)]. *Rev Prat* 1999;49:2227.

59. Yoshikawa T, Ihira M, Ohashi M, et al. Correlation between HHV-6 infection and skin rash after allogeneic bone marrow transplantation. *Bone Marrow Transplant* 2001;28:77.

60. Yokote T, Muroi K, Kawano C, et al. Human herpesvirus-6–associated generalized vesiculobullous eruptions after allogeneic bone marrow transplantation. *Leuk Lymphoma* 2002;43:927.

61. Ruzicka T, Kalka K, Diercks K, et al. Papular-purpuric 'gloves and socks' syndrome associated with human herpesvirus 6 infection. *Arch Dermatol* 1998;134:242.

62. Yasumoto S, Tsujita J, Imayama S, et al. Case report: Gianotti–Crosti syndrome associated with human herpesvirus-6 infection. *J Dermatol* 1996;23:499.

63. Fujino Y, Nakajima M, Inoue H, et al. Human herpesvirus 6 encephalitis associated with hypersensitivity syndrome. *Ann Neurol* 2002;51:771.

64. De Araujo T, Berman B, Weinstein A. Human herpesviruses 6 and 7. *Dermatol Clin* 2002;20:301.

65. Hengge UR, Ruzicka T, Tyring SK, et al. Update on Kaposi's sarcoma and other HHV8 associated diseases. Part 1: epidemiology, environmental predispositions, clinical manifestations, and therapy. *Lancet Infect Dis* 2002;2:281.

66. Breman JG, Henderson DA. Diagnosis and management of smallpox. *N Engl J Med* 2002;346:1300.

67. Klainer AS. Smallpox. *Clin Dermatol* 1989;7:19.

68. Copeman PW, Banatvala JE. The skin and vaccination against smallpox. *Br J Dermatol* 1971;84:169.

69. Goldstein JA, Neff JM, Lane JM, et al. Smallpox vaccination reactions, prophylaxis, and therapy of complications. *Pediatrics* 1975;55:342.

70. Baxby D, Bennett M, Getty B. Human cowpox 1969–93: a review based on 54 cases. *Br J Dermatol* 1994;131:598.

71. Leavell UW Jr, McNamara MJ, Muelling R, et al. Orf: report of 19 human cases with clinical and pathological observations. *JAMA* 1968;203:657.

72. Smith KJ, Skelton HG III, Yeager J, et al. Molluscum contagiosum: ultrastructural evidence for its presence in skin adjacent to clinical lesions in patients infected with human immunodeficiency virus type 1. Military Medical Consortium for Applied Retroviral Research. *Arch Dermatol* 1992;128:223.

73. Forghani B, Oshiro LS, Chan CS, et al. Direct detection of Molluscum contagiosum virus in clinical specimens by in situ hybridization using biotinylated probe. *Mol Cell Probes* 1992;6:67.

74. Jenkins D. Diagnosing human papillomaviruses: recent advances. *Curr Opin Infect Dis* 2001;14:53.

75. Crum CP. Contemporary theories of cervical carcinogenesis: the virus, the host, and the stem cell. *Mod Pathol* 2000;13:243.

76. Mork J, Lie AK, Glattre E, et al. Human papillomavirus infection as a risk factor for squamous-cell carcinoma of the head and neck. *N Engl J Med* 2001;344:1125.

77. Syrjanen KJ. HPV infections and lung cancer. *J Clin Pathol* 2002;55:885.

78. Astori G, Merluzzi S, Arzese A, et al. Detection of human papillomavirus DNA and p53 gene mutations in esophageal cancer samples and adjacent normal mucosa. *Digestion* 2001;64:9.

79. Jenson AB, Geyer S, Sundberg JP, Ghim S. Human papillomavirus and skin cancer. *J Invest Dermatol Symp Proc* 2001;6:203.

80. Meyer T, Arndt R, Nindl I, et al. Association of human papillomavirus infections with cutaneous tumors in immunosuppressed patients. *Transpl Int* 2003;16:146.

81. Rock B, Shah KV, Farmer ER. A morphologic, pathologic, and virologic study of anogenital warts in men. *Arch Dermatol* 1992;128:495.

82. Brentjens MH, Yeung-Yue KA, Lee PC, et al. Human papillomavirus: a review. *Dermatol Clin* 2002;20:315.

83. Leigh IM, Glover MT. Skin cancer and warts in immunosuppressed renal transplant recipients. *Recent Results Cancer Res* 1995;139:69.

84. Pereira De Oliveira WR, Carrasco S, Neto CF, et al. Nonspecific cell-mediated immunity in patients with epidermodysplasia verruciformis. *J Dermatol* 2003;30:203.

85. Tomasini C, Aloi F, Pippione M. Seborrheic keratosis-like lesions in epidermodysplasia verruciformis. *J Cutan Pathol* 1993;20:237.

86. Tieben LM, Berkhout RJ, Smits HL, et al. Detection of epidermodysplasia verruciformis-like human papillomavirus types in malignant and premalignant skin lesions of renal transplant recipients. *Br J Dermatol* 1994;131:226.

87. Berger TG, Sawchuk WS, Leonardi C, et al. Epidermodysplasia verruciformis-associated papillomavirus infection complicating human immunodeficiency virus disease. *Br J Dermatol* 1991;124:79.

88. Morrison C, Eliezri Y, Magro C, et al. The histologic spectrum of epidermodysplasia verruciformis in transplant and AIDS patients. *J Cutan Pathol* 2002;29:480.

89. Nuovo GJ, Ishag M. The histologic spectrum of epidermodysplasia verruciformis. *Am J Surg Pathol* 2000;24:1400.

90. Munoz N. Human papillomavirus and cancer: the epidemiological evidence. *J Clin Virol* 2000;19:1.

91. Nobbenhuis MA, Helmerhorst TJ, van den Brule AJ, et al. Cytological regression and clearance of high-risk human papillomavirus in women with an abnormal cervical smear. *Lancet* 2001;358:1782.

92. Bei H, Cviko A, Yuan L, et al. Seborrheic Keratosis of the Vulva: A Unique Subset of Vulvar Condyloma Distinct from Cutaneous Seborrheic Keratosis and Fibroepithelial Stromal Polyp. United States and Canadian Academy of Pathology annual meeting, Washington DC, 2003.

93. Watanabe T, Kawamura T, Jacob SE, et al. Pityriasis rosea is associated with systemic active infection with both human herpesvirus-7 and human herpesvirus-6. *J Invest Dermatol* 2002;119:793.

94. Della TG, Donghi R, Longoni A, et al. HPV DNA in intraepithelial neoplasia and carcinoma of the vulva and penis. *Diagn Mol Pathol* 1992;1:25.

95. Munger K, Howley PM. Human papillomavirus immortalization and transformation functions. *Virus Res* 2002;89:213.

96. von Krogh G, Horenblas S. Diagnosis and clinical presentation of premalignant lesions of the penis. *Scand J Urol Nephrol Suppl* 2000;201.

97. Archard HO, Heck JW, Stanley JR. Focal epithelial hyperplasia. *Oral Surg* 1965;20:201.

98. Viraben R, Aquilina C, Brousset P, et al. Focal epithelial hyperplasia (Heck disease) associated with AIDS. *Dermatology* 1996;193:261.

99. Henke RP, Guerin-Reverchon I, Milde-Langosch K, et al. In situ detection of human papillomavirus types 13 and 32 in focal epithelial hyperplasia of the oral mucosa. *J Oral Pathol Med* 1989;18:419.

100. Lopez-Sanchez AF, Guijarro-Guijarro B, Hernandez-Vallejo G. Human repercusions of foot and mouth disease and other similar viral diseases. *Med Oral* 2003;8:26.

101. Ellis AW, Kennett ML, Lewis FA, et al. Hand, foot and mouth disease: an outbreak with interesting virological features. *Pathology* 1973;5:189.

102. Potbart HA, Kirkegarrd K. Picornavirus pathogenesis: viral access, attachement, and entry into susceptible cells. *Semin Virol* 1992;3:483.

103. Fields JP, Mihm MC Jr, Hellreich PD, et al. Hand, foot, and mouth disease. *Arch Dermatol* 1969;99:243.

104. Tsao KC, Chang PY, Ning HC, et al. Use of molecular assay in diagnosis of hand, foot and mouth disease caused by enterovirus 71 or coxsackievirus A 16. *J Virol Methods* 2002;102:9.

105. Haneke E. Electron microscopic demonstration of virus particles in hand, foot and mouth disease. *Dermatologica* 1985;171:321.

106. Schiff ER. Atypical clinical manifestations of hepatitis A. *Vaccine* 1992;10[Suppl 1]:S18.

107. Nunley JR. Cutaneous manifestations of HIV and HCV. *Dermatol Nurs* 2000;12:163.

108. Kaplan MH, Sadick N, McNutt NS, et al. Dermatologic findings and manifestations of acquired immunodeficiency syndrome (AIDS). *J Am Acad Dermatol* 1987;16:485.

109. Costner M, Cockerell CJ. The changing spectrum of the cutaneous manifestations of HIV disease. *Arch Dermatol* 1998;134:1290.

110. Hulsebosch HJ, Claessen FA, van Ginkel CJ, et al. Human immunodeficiency virus exanthem. *J Am Acad Dermatol* 1990;23:483.

111. Chandwani S, Moore T, Kaul A, et al. Early diagnosis of human immunodeficiency virus type 1-infected infants by plasma p24 antigen assay after immune complex dissociation. *Pediatr Infect Dis J* 1993;12:96.

112. Cavert W. Viral infections in human immunodeficiency virus disease. *Med Clin North Am* 1997;81:411.

113. Birnbaum W, Hodgson TA, Reichart PA, et al. Prognostic significance of HIV-associated oral lesions and their relation to therapy. *Oral Dis* 2002;8[Suppl 2]:110.

114. Williams LR, Webster G. Warts and molluscum contagiosum. *Clin Dermatol* 1991;9:87.

115. Koehler JE, Tappero JW. Bacillary angiomatosis and bacillary peliosis in patients infected with human immunodeficiency virus. *Clin Infect Dis* 1993;17:612.

116. Blocker ME, Levine WC, St Louis ME. HIV prevalence in patients with syphilis, United States. *Sex Transm Dis* 2000;27:53.

117. Cohen PR, Grossman ME. Recognizing skin lesions of systemic fungal infections in patients with AIDS. *Am Fam Physician* 1994;49:1627.

118. Czelusta A, Yen-Moore A, Van der SM, et al. An overview of sexually transmitted diseases. Part III. Sexually transmitted diseases in HIV-infected patients. *J Am Acad Dermatol* 2000;43:409.

119. Patrizi A, Neri I, Chieregato C, et al. Demodicidosis in immunocompetent young children: report of eight cases. *Dermatology* 1997;195:239.

120. Lifson AR, Hessol NA, Buchbinder SP, et al. The association of clinical conditions and serologic tests with CD4+ lymphocyte counts in HIV-infected subjects without AIDS. *AIDS* 1991;5:1209.

121. Soeprono FF, Schinella RA, Cockerell CJ, et al. Seborrheic-like dermatitis of acquired immunodeficiency syndrome: a clinicopathologic study. *J Am Acad Dermatol* 1986;14:242.

122. Smith KJ, Skelton HG, Yeager J, et al. Cutaneous findings in HIV-1-positive patients: a 42-month prospective study. Military Medical Consortium for the Advancement of Retroviral Research (MMCARR). *J Am Acad Dermatol* 1994;31:746.

123. Farthing CF, Staughton RC, Rowland Payne CM. Skin disease in homosexual patients with acquired immune deficiency syndrome (AIDS) and lesser forms of human T cell leukaemia virus (HTLV III) disease. *Clin Exp Dermatol* 1985;10:3.

124. Buchness MR, Lim HW, Hatcher VA, et al. Eosinophilic pustular folliculitis in the acquired immunodeficiency syndrome: treatment with ultraviolet B phototherapy. *N Engl J Med* 1988;318:1183.

125. Rico MJ, Kory WP, Gould EW, et al. Interface dermatitis in patients with the acquired immunodeficiency syndrome. *J Am Acad Dermatol* 1987;16:1209.

126. Coopman SA, Stern RS. Cutaneous drug reactions in human immunodeficiency virus infection. *Arch Dermatol* 1991;127:714.

127. Gregory N, DeLeo VA. Clinical manifestations of photosensitivity in patients with human immunodeficiency virus infection. *Arch Dermatol* 1994;130:630.

128. Martinelli PT, Tyring SK. Human herpesvirus 8. *Dermatol Clin* 2002;20:307.

129. McGregor JM, Newell M, Ross J, et al. Cutaneous malignant melanoma and human immunodeficiency virus (HIV) infection: a report of three cases. *Br J Dermatol* 1992;126:516.

130. Smith KJ, Skelton HG, III, Angritt P. Histopathologic features of HIV-associated skin disease. *Dermatol Clin* 1991;9:551.

131. Hevia O, Jimenez-Acosta F, Ceballos PI, et al. Pruritic papular eruption of the acquired immunodeficiency syndrome: a clinicopathologic study. *J Am Acad Dermatol* 1991;24:231.

132. Goodman DS, Teplitz ED, Wishner A, et al. Prevalence of cutaneous disease in patients with acquired immunodeficiency syndrome (AIDS) or AIDS-related complex. *J Am Acad Dermatol* 1987;17:210.

133. Holmes RB, Martins C, Horn T. The histopathology of folliculitis in HIV-infected patients. *J Cutan Pathol* 2002;29:93.

134. Murakawa GJ, McCalmont T, Altman J, et al. Disseminated acanthamebiasis in patients with AIDS: a report of five cases and a review of the literature. *Arch Dermatol* 1995;131:1291.

135. Holland PV, Alter HJ. The clinical significance of hepatitis B virus antigens and antibodies. *Med Clin North Am* 1975;59:849.

136. Befeler AS, Di Bisceglie AM. Hepatitis B. *Infect Dis Clin North Am* 2000;14:617.

137. Willson RA. Extrahepatic manifestations of chronic viral hepatitis. *Am J Gastroenterol* 1997;92:3.

138. Parsons ME, Russo GG, Millikan LE. Dermatologic disorders associated with viral hepatitis infections. *Int J Dermatol* 1996;35:77.

139. Gianotti F. HBsAg and papular acrodermatitis of childhood. *N Engl J Med* 1978;298:460.

140. Nelson JS, Stone MS. Update on selected viral exanthems. *Curr Opin Pediatr* 2000;12:359.

141. Rosen LB, Rywlin AM, Resnick L. Hepatitis B surface antigen positive skin lesions: two case reports with an immunoperoxidase study. *Am J Dermatopathol* 1985;7:507.

142. Gower RG, Sausker WF, Kohler PF, et al. Small vessel vasculitis caused by hepatitis B virus immune complexes: small vessel vasculitis and HBsAG. *J Allergy Clin Immunol* 1978;62:222.

143. Pyrsopoulos NT, Reddy K. Extrahepatic manifestations of chronic viral hepatitis. *Curr Gastroenterol Rep* 2001;3:71.

144. Limas C, Limas CJ. Lichen planus in children: a possible complication of hepatitis B vaccines. *Pediatr Dermatol* 2002;19:204.

145. Jackson JM. Hepatitis C and the skin. *Dermatol Clin* 2002;20:449.

146. Jones AM, Warken K, Tyring SK. The cutaneous manifestations of viral hepatitis. *Dermatol Clin* 2002;20:233.

147. Pawlotsky JM, Dhumeaux D, Bagot M. Hepatitis C virus in dermatology: a review. *Arch Dermatol* 1995;131:1185.

148. Chuang TY, Brashear R, Lewis C. Porphyria cutanea tarda and hepatitis C virus: a case-control study and meta-analysis of the literature. *J Am Acad Dermatol* 1999;41:31.

149. Calista D, Landi G. Lichen planus, erythema nodosum, and erythema multiforme in a patient with chronic hepatitis C. *Cutis* 2001;67:454.

150. Madison DL, Allen E, Deodhar A, et al. Henoch–Schonlein purpura: a possible complication of hepatitis C related liver cirrhosis. *Ann Rheum Dis* 2002;61:281.

151. Akaogi J, Yotsuyanagi H, Sugata F, et al. Hepatitis viral infection in Behçet's disease. *Hepatol Res* 2000;17:126.

152. Khanna VJ, Shieh S, Benjamin J, et al. Necrolytic acral erythema associated with hepatitis C: effective treatment with interferon alfa and zinc. *Arch Dermatol* 2000;136:755.

153. Cacoub P, Maisonobe T, Thibault V, et al. Systemic vasculitis in patients with hepatitis C. *J Rheumatol* 2001;28:109.

154. Neri S, Raciti C, D'Angelo G, et al. Hyde's prurigo nodularis and chronic HCV hepatitis. *J Hepatol* 1998;28:161.

155. Keane FM, MacFarlane CS, Munn SE, et al. Pyoderma gangrenosum and hepatitis C virus infection. *Br J Dermatol* 1998;139:924.

156. Daoud MS, Gibson LE, Daoud S, et al. Chronic hepatitis C and skin diseases: a review. *Mayo Clin Proc* 1995;70:559.

157. Katta R. Parvovirus B19: a review. *Dermatol Clin* 2002;20:333.

158. Grilli R, Izquierdo MJ, Farina MC, et al. Papular-purpuric "gloves and socks" syndrome: polymerase chain reaction demonstration of parvovirus B19 DNA in cutaneous lesions and sera. *J Am Acad Dermatol* 1999;41:793.

159. Garcia-Tapia AM, Fernandez-Gutierrez DA, Giron JA, et al. Spectrum of parvovirus B19 infection: analysis of an outbreak of 43 cases in Cadiz, Spain. *Clin Infect Dis* 1995;21:1424.

160. Boeck K, Mempel M, Schmidt T, et al. Gianotti–Crosti syndrome: clinical, serologic, and therapeutic data from nine children. *Cutis* 1998;62:271.

161. Cioc AM, Sedmak DD, Nuovo GJ, et al. Parvovirus B19 associated adult Henoch Schonlein purpura. *J Cutan Pathol* 2002;29:602.

162. Magro CM, Dawood MR, Crowson AN. The cutaneous manifestations of human parvovirus B19 infection. *Hum Pathol* 2000;31:488.

163. Stalkup JR. A review of measles virus. *Dermatol Clin* 2002;20:209.

164. Ackerman AB, Suringa DW. Multinucleate epidermal cells in measles. *Arch Dermatol* 1971;103:180.

165. McNutt NS, Kindel S, Lugo J. Cutaneous manifestations of measles in AIDS. *J Cutan Pathol* 1992;19:315.

166. Vander Straten MR, Tyring SK. Rubella. *Dermatol Clin* 2002;20:225.

167. Cherry JD. Viral exanthems. *Dis Mon* 1982;28:1.

THE HISTIOCYTOSES

WALTER H. C. BURGDORF
BERNHARD ZELGER

The histiocytic disorders cover a wide range of primary and secondary, solitary and multiple, benign and malignant disorders unified only by being for the most part uncommon and poorly understood. The "X" in histiocytosis X as originally proposed by Liechtenstein (1) was designed to reflect the unknown; even though we have drifted away from the designation, it to some degree still reflects our knowledge. As Headington pointed out in an oft-cited obituary, the concept of the histiocyte has hindered our approach to many diseases (2). The word "histiocyte" itself is not particularly helpful. Loosely translated, it means a "cell of the tissue." Medical dictionaries tend to define the histiocyte as a "macrophage" or a "tissue macrophage," but many of diseases known as histiocytoses are clearly not disorders of macrophages, but instead involve dendritic cells (Langerhans cell disease) or less often lymphocytes (most cases of malignant histiocytosis) or keratinocytes (some examples of atypical fibroxanthoma). Despite these misgivings, we have retained the term histiocytosis both as a chapter heading and in the text, in order to avoid creating more confusion.

There are two major cell lines responsible for the spectrum of diseases considered as histiocytoses (3,4):

1. The bone marrow-derived monocytes, which migrate to tissue, where they differentiate into macrophages or professional phagocytes, known by many names based on their site, such as Kupffer cells in the liver. They are active metabolically and rich in lysosomes. There are a number of monoclonal antibodies available to identify macrophages; the most important and useful are directed against CD68. Perhaps the most specific is PG-M1 as it is most restricted to monocyte/macrophage epitopes; others include KP1 and KiM1P which are more likely to also stain neutrophils and mast cells. Lysozyme is also often employed but is not as specific.
2. The dendritic cells are for the most part bone marrow-derived and reside in the skin, lymph nodes or other organs. In the skin, the prominent dendritic cell is the Langerhans cell (LC), characterized by Birbeck granules, S-100, and CD1a positivity. Melanocytes also have a dendritic appearance but are not included in this group. LC initially take up antigens in the epidermis,

migrate through the dermis to lymphatics and then lymph nodes and there present processed antigens in association with MHC molecules to T cells. The migrating LC is known as a veiled cell, while the antigen-presenting form is the interdigitating dendritic cell (IDC). Veiled cells no longer express Birbeck granules, while IDC also fail to express CD1a.

Other dendritic cells include:

- Follicular dendritic cells (FDCs), which interact with B cells in the germinal centers. They express CD21 and CD35 and have desmosomes, suggesting they arise from mesenchymal stem cell.
- Dermal dendrocyte, a perivascular cell recognized by factor XIIIa positivity and a failure to stain for S-100 or CD1a (5). FXIIIa can also be expressed by activated macrophages. FXIIIa is the rate-limiting enzyme in the formation of fibrin thrombi and is most prominent in the superficial dermis. It is more likely to be positive in acute and early lesions. The dermal dendrocyte appears to be the major cell in dermatofibromas. In contrast, the monoclonal antibody CD34 identifies a stem cell antigen; a variety of spindled dermal cells such as immature fibroblasts, endothelial cells and perhaps dendritic cells stain positive with this marker, but dermatofibromas are negative. Table 26-1 summarizes the immunohistochemical staining patterns of these cells and their related tumors.
- Plasmacytoid dendritic cells are closely related to macrophages; when stimulated by viral infections, they undergo a maturation process and then drive a prominent Th1 polarization. The markers used to identify them include IL-3 receptor-α, CD40 and CLA/HECA452.

A source of confusion is the indeterminate cell, whose vague name accurately reflects the current situation (6). No single definition is agreed upon; possibilities cited in the recent literature include:

- Veiled cell, that is, an LC migrating to the dermis
- LC precursor (exactly the opposite of a veiled cell)
- Abnormal or dysregulated LC
- Cell with features of both a macrophage and LC

TABLE 26-1. IMMUNOPHENOTYPES OF MACROPHAGES AND DENDRITIC CELLS

Cell/Marker	S100	CD1a	BG	CD21	CD35	CD68	Lys
Langerhans cell	+	+	+	−	−	−	−/+
Macrophage	−/+	−	−	−	−	+	+
Follicular dendritic cell	−	−	−	+	+	−/+	−
Interdigitating dendritic cell	+	−	−	−	−	−/+	−/+

The immunophenotype depends on what definition one chooses; it is generally agreed that S-100 and CD1a are positive and no Birbeck granules are found.

A number of cautions are required. A diagnosis is rarely if ever based on the presence or absence of a single antigen, but instead on the clinicopathologic picture. Both macrophages and dendritic cells go through a maturation process, so their profiles may change. In addition, since monocytes and most dendritic cells arise from a similar bone marrow–derived stem cell, there may be overlaps with macrophages expressing S100 or even CD1a (7).

The "histiocytoses" can be classified based on the light microscopic pattern and in a more refined way using a limited number of special stains. Table 26-2 shows a simplified immunohistochemical and electron microscopic classification. Our detailed classification (8) is presented in Table 26-3. Caputo's classification as presented in his monograph is also quite workable (9). Notable by their absence from this discussion are the classifications of the Histiocyte Society (10), which approach cutaneous dendritic cell and macrophage disorders in a manner completely different from that we favor.

In addition to the diseases to be discussed in this chapter, a wide array of disorders can display similar histologic patterns. Most are discussed elsewhere in this book.

1. *Metabolic disorders.* In addition to hyperlipoproteinemias and other disorders of fat metabolism, many lysosomal disorders and other storage diseases may feature cutaneous xanthomas or other infiltrates. In previous editions of this text, diseases such as Farber disease (lipogranulomatosis), Gaucher disease, Niemann–Pick disease, and Tangier disease were covered in detail. They may present with normal skin, pigmentary changes, or nodules in which the abnormal metabolic accumulations can be identified, usually by electron microscopy.

The diagnosis of these disorders is not a practical question for the dermatopathologist, and they will not be further considered.

2. *Infectious diseases.* Tuberculosis, lepromatous leprosy (especially the histiocytoid variant), other mycobacterial infections, and leishmaniasis may produce granulomas. Malakoplakia is a chronic granulomatous response presumably to an infectious agent, which occurs occasionally in the skin. The key histologic finding is the presence of intracellular Michaelis–Gutmann bodies.

3. *Tumors.* Some lymphomas present with cutaneous granulomatous infiltrates; included in this group are Hodgkin lymphoma and some forms of peripheral T-cell lymphoma (Lennert lymphoma). Most diseases diagnosed in the past as histiocytic malignancies are lymphomas. Malignant fibrous histiocytoma and its more superficial cutaneous variant, atypical fibroxanthoma, are established diagnoses, but their line of differentiation remains controversial.

Melanocytic tumors can be confused with macrophage disorders, both clinically and histologically. The red-brown color of xanthogranulomas is similar to that of Spitz nevi. Balloon cell nevi and melanoma are occasionally mistaken histologically for xanthomatous lesions (11). Touton giant cells can sometimes be confused with multinucleated rosette cells in melanocytic nevi. Fortunately, immunohistochemical studies readily resolve these potential difficulties (12,13).

4. *Trauma.* Most dermatofibromas and some verruciform xanthomas are the result of trauma, be it an insect bite, folliculitis, or another insult. Some xanthomas arise secondary to cutaneous damage from light or following marked inflammation. External objects, such as glass fragments, silica, and many others, may produce cutaneous granulomas, often of the sarcoidal type. A ruptured follicular cyst is also accompanied by a macrophage response.

TABLE 26-2. SIMPLIFIED APPROACH TO HISTIOCYTOSES

Disorder	S-100	CD1a	Birbeck Granules	Macrophage Markers
Langerhans cell disease	+	+	+	−
Xanthogranuloma family	− (+ rare)	−	−	+
Indeterminate cell histiocytosis	+	+/−	−	+
Sinus histiocytosis with massive lymphadenopathy	+	−	−	+

TABLE 26-3. DETAILED CLASSIFICATION OF HISTIOCYTOSES

Langerhans cell disease	**S-100⁺, CD1a⁺, BG⁺, CD68⁻**
Xanthogranuloma family	**S-100⁻, CD1a⁻, BG⁻, CD68⁺**
Juvenile xanthogranuloma	
Papular xanthoma	
Scalloped cell xanthogranuloma	
Xanthoma disseminatum	
Reticulohistiocytoma	
Multicentric reticulohistiocytosis	
Spindle cell xanthogranuloma	
Progressive nodular histiocytosis	
Benign cephalic histiocytosis	
Generalized eruptive histiocytosis	
Xanthelasma	
Indeterminate cell histiocytosis	**S-100⁺, CD1a⁺, BG⁻, CD68 ⁺**
Sinus histiocytosis with massive lymphadenopathy	**S-100⁺, CD1a⁻, BG⁻, CD68⁺**
Histiocytic sarcoma	**CD68⁺; diagnosis of exclusion (exclude lymphoma, leukemia, melanoma)**
Xanthomas associated with lipid abnormalities	
Eruptive	
Tuberous	
Tendon	
Plane	
Xanthelasma (some)	
Normolipemic xanthomas	
Paraneoplastic	
Necrobiotic xanthogranuloma	
Diffuse normolipemic plane xanthoma	
Verruciform xanthoma	
Miscellaneous	

BG, Birbeck granules.

5. *Idiopathic.* Unfortunately, most "histiocytic" diseases fit here, and there is little logic to what has been considered a macrophage disorder and what has been cubbyholed elsewhere. For example, granuloma annulare has a macrophage infiltrate but is considered a necrobiotic disorder. Both rheumatoid arthritis and sarcoidosis may feature infiltrates of macrophages in the skin and other organs; nonetheless, they are not considered "histiocytoses."

LANGERHANS CELL DISEASE

Langerhans cell disease (LCD) is characterized by a proliferation of Langerhans cells. The clinical spectrum of LCD is broad, with skin involvement a common finding. While LCD has been subdivided into several clinical types, overlaps are the rule—not the exception—and lumping appears more appropriate than splitting. Acute disseminated LCD (Abt–Letterer–Siwe disease) usually occurs in infants, but can be seen in older children or adults. The most common manifestations are fever, anemia, thrombocytopenia, enlargement of the liver and spleen, lymphadenopathy, and pulmonary infiltrates. Osteolytic lesions are uncommon except in the mastoid region of the temporal bone, resulting in a clinical picture of otitis media. Cutaneous lesions are found in about 80% of cases, often as a presenting sign.

Numerous grouped, red-brown papules covered with scales or crusts may be accompanied by petechiae. This type of eruption may be extensive, involving particularly the scalp, face, and trunk, with a striking resemblance to seborrheic dermatitis or Darier disease. Cutaneous LCD is very pleomorphic; lesions may be vesicular (14), ulcerated, urticarial (15), or xanthomatous (16). Nail bed involvement is not uncommon (17). If there is a diffuse cutaneous eruption, one must anticipate multiorgan involvement. In rare instances, a widespread cutaneous eruption is the only clinical manifestation in infants and even in the elderly (18). The prognosis in such cases is good. Other adults may have similar cutaneous findings but also multisystem disease and do poorly (19).

Congenital self-healing reticulohistiocytosis (CSHRH) (Hashimoto–Pritzker disease) (20) is another variant of LCD, not a distinct disorder (21). It is usually present at birth but may not appear until several days or weeks after delivery. Affected infants have scattered papules and nodules. Large nodules tend to break down in the center and form crater-shaped ulcers. Usually, the number of lesions varies from several to a dozen; on rare occasions, numerous lesions are widely scattered over the entire skin. In about 25% of cases, a solitary nodule is present (22). The lesions begin to involute within 2 to 3 months and usually have completely regressed within 12 months. But the patients should be carefully followed; relapses may occur, including bone involvement, and the occasional case may advance to acute disseminated disease (23). While acute disseminated LCD may also be present at birth, it is rarely nodular.

In chronic multifocal LCD, diabetes insipidus, exophthalmos, and multiple defects of the bones, especially of the cranium, represent the classic triad of Hand–Schüller–Christian disease. Any one or even all three of the cardinal symptoms may be absent, and entirely different organs may be involved. For example, enlargement of the liver, spleen, lungs, or lymph nodes may be found. Osteolytic lesions of the long bones may result in spontaneous fractures. Cutaneous lesions occur in about one third of the cases. Three types of skin lesions may occur. Most common are infiltrated nodules and plaques undergoing ulceration, especially in the axillae, the anogenital region, and the mouth. Next in frequency is an extensive eruption identical to that in infants but usually less severe. Finally, in rare instances yellow xanthomas are seen. Patients with LCD also tend to develop more juvenile xanthogranulomas than expected.

Chronic focal LCD or eosinophilic granuloma represents the fourth and, along with CSHR, the least severe variant. The lesions are either solitary or few. Most common are lesions of the bones, but the skin or the oral mucosa is occasionally involved, either with or without osseous lesions. Involvement of the jaw leading to a loose or floating tooth is a fairly typical occurrence. Eosinophilic ulcer of the oral mucosa has a similar name but is not otherwise related; it usually involves the tongue, is often triggered by trauma, resolves spontaneously, and does not contain LC. Although the lesions are usually chronic, there is a tendency toward spontaneous healing, and simple surgery is generally curative. In rare instances, cases originally diagnosed as chronic focal disease may progress into multifocal or even disseminated disease.

The clinical course and the prognosis of LCD are difficult to predict. The most important parameters in prognosis are those recommended for staging: age of patient, number of organs involved, and degree of organ dysfunction. Abnormalities of the bone marrow, spleen, liver, or lungs indicate a poor prognosis. Skin involvement alone suggests a favorable outcome. Paradoxically, the presence of skin disease at birth (the nodules of CSHRH) is a good sign, but involvement before age 2 (Letterer–Siwe disease) is a bad one. Histologic features correlate poorly with outcome (24). Patients with disseminated LCD seem to be at risk for a variety of systemic tumors, including lymphomas, leukemias, and lung tumors (25). In general, about 10% of patients with multifocal disease die, 30% undergo complete remission, and the remaining 60% embark upon a chronic, shifting course (26,27).

Histopathology. The histologic picture unites the many varied forms of LCD. The key to diagnosis is identifying the typical LCD cell in the appropriate surroundings. The cell has a distinct folded or lobulated, often kidney-shaped, nucleus. Nucleoli are not prominent, and the slightly eosinophilic cytoplasm is unremarkable. A variety of methods can be employed to confirm the identity of such cells. For years the gold standard has been to employ electron microscopy searching for the typical Birbeck or Langerhans cell granules. Today using paraffin-fixed tissue, both the S-100 and CD1a antigens can be identified. While demonstration of Birbeck granules is no longer considered necessary, this approach may miss variant forms such as indeterminate cell histiocytosis.

Although Lever emphasized three kinds of histologic reactions in LCD—proliferative, granulomatous, and xanthomatous—only the first two are commonly seen. A relationship exists between the type of histologic reaction and the clinical type of disease. In general, the proliferative reaction with its almost pure LC infiltrate is typical of acute disseminated LCD and the granulomatous reaction of chronic focal or multifocal LCD, as the name eosinophilic granuloma suggests. The xanthomatous reaction is seen in Hand–Schüller–Christian disease but primarily in other organs, especially the meninges and bones. Xanthomatous lesions in the skin are decidedly rare (16).

The proliferative reaction is encountered in the skin in petechiae, as well as in almost translucent, hemorrhagic or crusted papules. It is characterized by the presence of an extensive infiltrate of LC. The infiltrate usually lies close to or involves the epidermis, resulting in ulceration and crusting (Fig. 26-1A). Large kidney-shaped tumor cells can be seen just below or even impinging upon the epidermis (Fig. 26-1B). Staining with S-100 or CD1a shows both the normal and abnormal LC (Fig. 26-1C). The cytology is quite distinctive, and a touch preparation from an ulcerated or weeping lesion, stained with a hematologic stain, can often provide a preliminary diagnosis (28).

The nodules of CSHRH show densely aggregated LC with abundant eosinophilic cytoplasm (Fig. 26-1D). Some of the LC are large and form giant cells, with diameters up to 50 μm. In some cells, the cytoplasm has a "ground-glass" appearance responsible for the term "reticulohistiocyte," a morphologic pattern seen occasionally in LCD and commonly in macrophage disorders. Although qualitative ultrastructural differences have been reported for CSHRH, such as fewer Birbeck granules and the presence of laminated dense bodies, the bottom line is that CSHRH cannot be distinguished with certainty from other types of LCD by histologic criteria alone (21,23).

The granulomatous reaction is found most commonly in infiltrated plaques and nodules in the genital area, in the axillary region, or on the scalp, as well as in the soft tissue and bone lesions. Extensive aggregates of LC often extend deep into the dermis. Eosinophils are present in various

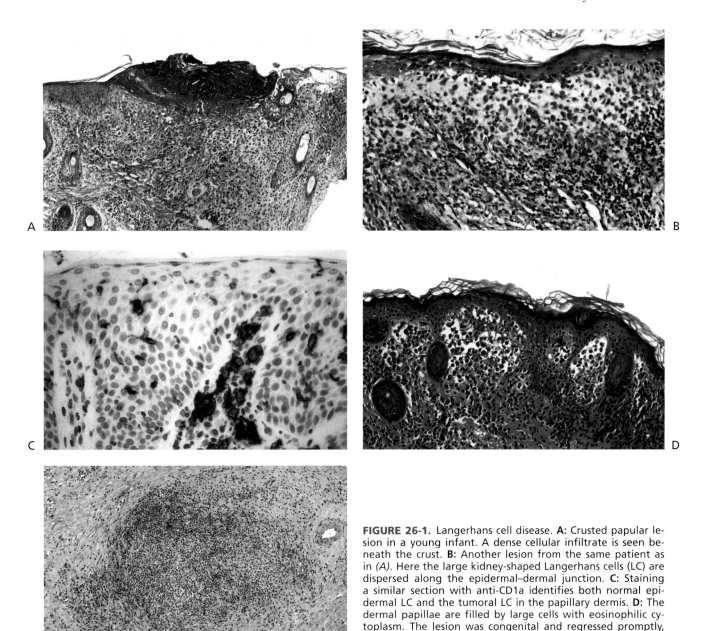

FIGURE 26-1. Langerhans cell disease. **A:** Crusted papular lesion in a young infant. A dense cellular infiltrate is seen beneath the crust. **B:** Another lesion from the same patient as in *(A)*. Here the large kidney-shaped Langerhans cells (LC) are dispersed along the epidermal–dermal junction. **C:** Staining a similar section with anti-CD1a identifies both normal epidermal LC and the tumoral LC in the papillary dermis. **D:** The dermal papillae are filled by large cells with eosinophilic cytoplasm. The lesion was congenital and regressed promptly, confirming the diagnosis of congenital self-healing reticulohistiocytosis. **E:** A deep nodular cutaneous infiltrate rich in eosinophils with clusters of typical large LC.

quantities (Fig. 26-1E). Generally, they lie in clusters instead of being diffusely scattered, and may develop into microabscesses. Irregularly shaped, multinucleated giant cells are occasionally seen. Various numbers of macrophages, neutrophils, lymphocytes, and plasma cells may be present. Frequently, extravasation of erythrocytes is found.

The uncommon xanthomatous reaction reveals in the dermis numerous foamy cells, as well as varying numbers of LC and some eosinophils. Multinucleated giant cells are frequently present. They are mainly of the foreign-body type but occasionally have the appearance of Touton giant

cells. The S-100 and CD1a staining is likely to be weak or even negative in the foamy cells.

A final question is that of malignant LCD ("malignant histiocytosis X"; not to be confused with malignant histiocytosis). The International Lymphoma Study group identified several examples of Langerhans cell sarcoma (29). In such instances, there may be nodal, extranodal, or systemic involvement by highly atypical LC with frequent mitoses and marked pleomorphism (30). Acute disseminated LCD can reasonably be argued to be a malignancy because it is progressive, destructive, potentially fatal, and shows clonality. Some cases have been identified with marked cytologic atypia, including mitoses, and a poor clinical outcome (31,32). Unfortunately, most often the diagnosis has been made retrospectively. It must be reemphasized that cellular morphology is a poor way to predict the course of LCD, except in the case of nodular frankly anaplastic sarcomas or lymphomas, both of which are rare.

Other dendritic cells may also produce tumors and sarcomas. Follicular dendritic cell tumor/sarcoma can present in the skin where it is usually an indolent process. It may be associated with Castleman disease. Epstein–Barr virus induces a proliferation of benign FDC, which contain viral DNA; this possibility should be excluded. Tumors and sarcomas of interdigitating dendritic cells also occur and may on rare occasion involve the skin (29).

Visceral Lesions. The visceral lesions seen in LCD show the same three types of reactions just described for the skin. The organs most commonly affected are the spleen, liver, lungs, lymph nodes, and bones. In Hand–Schüller–Christian disease, the diabetes insipidus is caused by granulomatous infiltration of the posterior pituitary gland, the tuber cinereum, or the hypothalamus; the exophthalmos, by retro-orbital accumulations of granulomatous tissue; and the multiple defects in the skull, by the osteolytic effect of granulomatous infiltrates. Pulmonary LCD typically occurs in adult smokers, and has so many different features that many suspect it is a separate disease (33).

Pathogenesis. Although the key cell of LCD is very similar to a normal Langerhans cell, there may be subtle differences (34,35). Birbeck granules are convincing proof of the relationship, but they are present in varying amounts in LCD. Particularly when dealing with a sparsely infiltrated dermatitic picture, the search can be frustrating. In larger infiltrates, one can usually readily find the characteristic organelles. In addition to the S-100 and CD1a stains, which are part of the diagnostic approach to LCD, many other special stains have been employed, such as peanut agglutinin (PNA) and proliferating-cell nuclear antigen (PCNA) (36), which may have prognostic value. Other indicators of proliferation may also be positive.

LCD is most often a clonal process. Different groups have studied female patients with the disease and used a variety of X-linked polymorphisms to demonstrate clonality (37,38). Despite these studies, many view LCD as a reactive process because of its tendency toward spontaneous remissions and its good response to mild, nontoxic therapeutic regimens. In a fascinating historical review, Nezelof and Basset (30), who identified the cell of then "histiocytosis X" as an LC, lament the fact that discovering this association has provided few clues as to what causes the disease.

Differential Diagnosis. The differential diagnosis for LCD varies with the histologic pattern. The most difficult situation is an early proliferative dermatitic lesion with little epidermotropism and few characteristic cells. Without adequate clinical background, it is easy to make the mistaken diagnosis of superficial perivascular dermatitis. One should keep LCD in mind in all biopsies of dermatitis from infants and freely employ the S-100 stain for screening. When a nodule or tumor is present, the presence of eosinophils and the sheets of characteristic cells usually lead to the diagnosis. The cutaneous xanthomas are not distinctive and while the foamy cells may stain weakly with S-100 or CD1a, usually the surrounding infiltrate has enough positive cells to allow a diagnosis. Some cases of CSHRH may be clinically confused with the blueberry muffin syndrome, congenital leukemic infiltrates, or mast cell disease, but the microscopic picture brings clarity.

XANTHOGRANULOMA FAMILY

Macrophages may have a variety of morphologic characteristics, including vacuolated, xanthomatized, spindle-shaped, scalloped, and oncocytic cells (40) (Table 26-4). A xanthogranuloma is a lesion in which there is a heterogeneous population of macrophages including several of these cell types, often with giant cells. The xanthogranuloma family refers to the largest group of cutaneous macrophage disorders. There are some disorders in which one macrophage variant predominates; these disorders may be further divided into solitary and multiple forms, as shown in Figure 26-2.

JUVENILE XANTHOGRANULOMA

Juvenile xanthogranuloma (JXG) is a benign disorder in which one, several, or occasionally numerous, red to yellow nodules are present (41). Because the lesions are also seen in adults, JXG is admittedly an imperfect term. Since we have used xanthogranuloma to describe a type of lesion and family of disorders, we prefer to retain the designation JXG for these specific lesions.

The papules and nodules are usually 0.5 to 1.0 cm in diameter. Most lesions appear during the first year of life; 20% are present at birth. In children the lesions may grow rapidly but almost always regress within a year. Lesions in

TABLE 26-4. PATTERNS OF CUTANEOUS MACROPHAGES

Type of Macrophage	Associated Giant Cells
Foamy	Touton
Scalloped	Foreign body
Oncocytic	Ground glass
Spindle	Rarely seen
Vacuolated	Few

UNIFYING CONCEPT OF
XANTHOGRANULOMA FAMILY

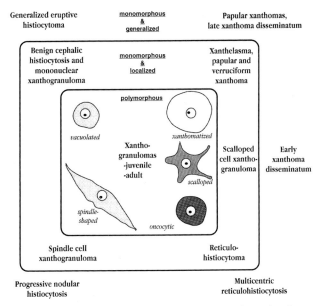

FIGURE 26-2. Unifying concept of xanthogranuloma family.

adults are not uncommon but are usually solitary and persistent (42).

JXG may be clinically subdivided into several forms. The micronodular variant is most common; patients are infants with many small nodules. Occasionally a macronodular form is seen with only a few lesions, but these are often several centimeters in diameter. The solitary giant xanthogranuloma may be larger than 5 cm (43). There are frequently clinical overlaps between the micro- and macronodular forms. Plaques may also be seen, as well as prominent nasal involvement (the Cyrano sign) (44). A lichenoid variant has also been reported (45). There are also subcutaneous or deep JXG (46–48). On occasion JXG develop in LCD; this probably reflects the similar bone marrow origin of macrophages and LC (49).

A number of systemic complications are associated with JXG. Ocular involvement including glaucoma and bleeding into the anterior chamber is the most common; it occurs in less than 10% of young patients (50). Oral lesions may occur. An association between JXG, cafe-au-lait macules, neurofibromatosis I, and juvenile chronic myelogenous leukemia has been reported (51), but must be rare. We have seen macrophage lesions misdiagnosed clinically as cafe au lait macules and histologically as both neural tumors and myelomonocytic leukemia; thus, to suggest this association, one should genetically document the neurofibromatosis and accurately classify the leukemia. JXG have also been identified in many other organ systems (52), including the central nervous system (CNS) (53), kidney, lungs, liver, testes, and pericardium. This systemic involvement is one of the strongest arguments against the dermal dendrocyte being the precursor cell for xanthogranulomas (54).

Bone involvement with JXG is most confusing. Erdheim–Chester disease is a rare macrophage disorder featuring sclerotic bone lesions associated with soft tissue xanthogranulomatous inflammation (55) and occasional skin involvement including periorbital disease (56). It is almost always seen in adults. Thus, when soft tissue JXG is diagnosed, the skeletal system should be surveyed and the diagnosis of Erdheim–Chester disease considered. The combination of a "histiocytic" skin lesion and radiologic evidence of bone lesions does not always mean LCD.

Histopathology. The typical JXG contains macrophages with a variety of cellular features (57). On low power, a well-circumscribed nodule, often exophytic and with a epidermal collarette is found (Fig. 26-3A). Typically many of the stylized morphologic variants of macrophages can be seen. There is usually a characteristic progression as the lesions mature (58). Early lesions may show large accumulations of vacuolated cells without significant lipid infiltration intermingled with only a few lymphocytes and eosinophils (Fig. 26-3B). When no foamy cells or giant cells are seen, the possibility of JXG is often overlooked (59,60). This mononuclear variant of JXG is identical to lesions found in benign cephalic histiocytosis and generalized eruptive histiocytosis. Usually some degree of lipidization is present, even in very early lesions, manifested by pale cells. In mature lesions, a granulomatous infiltrate is usually present containing foamy cells, foreign-body giant cells, and Touton giant cells as well as macrophages, lymphocytes, and eosinophils. The presence of giant cells, most of them Touton giant cells, showing a wreath of nuclei surrounded by foamy cytoplasm is quite typical for JXG (Fig. 26-3C), but not diagnostic as wreath-shaped giant cells can be seen in other disorders including some melanocytic nevi. Occasionally, Touton giant cells are absent even in mature lesions. Older, regressing lesions show proliferation of fibroblasts and fibrosis replacing part of the infiltrate. Two types of spindle cells may be identified; the spindle-cell or fusiform macrophages are dispersed throughout the lesion and are S-100 negative. LC may be found as bystanders, generally at the periphery of the lesion.

Pathogenesis. The cause of JXG is unknown. S-100 positivity is not uncommon and should not prompt the reflex diagnosis of LCD. CD1a positivity has also been reported but is much less common (47). Some suggest that the dermal dendrocyte is the precursor cell for JXG and its variants, based on occasional FXIIIa positivity; others implicate the plasmacytoid dendritic cell (54). Passenger dendritic cells are present in many dermal inflammatory processes and this may be all the explanation that is needed. We feel many more histologic features speak for a macrophage origin.

Differential Diagnosis. The clinical differential diagnosis includes Spitz nevi, mastocytomas, and dermatofibromas.

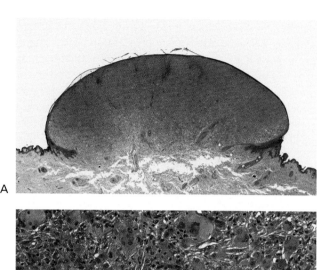

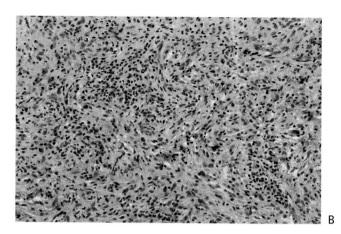

FIGURE 26-3. Juvenile xanthogranuloma. **A:** Elevated nodule with epidermal collarette. At scanning magnification, a pale pink color and a few giant cells can be identified. **B:** Numerous mononuclear macrophages admixed with eosinophils. **C:** Numerous Touton giant cells; cytoplasm within the wreath of macrophages is slightly more eosinophilic than that at the periphery.

The typical histologic picture of JXG is unmistakable. The many variants lead to a baffling array of diagnostic possibilities that are considered under the individual variants.

PAPULAR XANTHOMA

Papular xanthomas (PX) are small red-brown papules often with a yellowish hue. Patients present with one, several, or many papules (61,62). Although the lesions may be generalized, they have neither the distribution pattern of xanthoma disseminatum nor the confluence of diffuse normolipemic plane xanthoma. Plaques are not seen. The patients show no abnormalities of lipid metabolism. Most patients are adults, but occasional cases have been seen in children (63). The oral mucosa may be involved.

Cases of eruptive normolipemic xanthomas have also been described (64). Here the lesions appear suddenly, as in eruptive xanthoma associated with chylomicronemia, but with a more random distribution not favoring the extremities. They are usually macules and small papules with some confluence.

Histopathology. Nodules containing foamy cells with numerous Touton giant cells are seen in the dermis. Extracellular lipids are not seen. Even when early lesions are biopsied, xanthomatized cells dominate with only a small component of mononuclear vacuolated macrophages or other cell types. There may be central sclerosis as well as peripheral thickening of collagen bundles (62,65) (Fig. 26-4A and B).

Pathogenesis. Why some macrophages become xanthomatized in the presence of normal serum lipid levels is not known. Despite the early definition of papular xanthoma as a macrophage disorder without a macrophage precursor phase (66), there clearly must be macrophages present initially that rapidly become xanthomatized. Neutrophilic papular xanthomas have been described in normolipemic patients with HIV/AIDS (67). They may develop following similar pathways to the paraneoplastic xanthomas secondary to the massive changes in lymphocyte proliferation. These xanthomas contain neutrophils and nuclear dust in addition to foamy cells.

Differential Diagnosis. Papules containing foamy cells and extracellular lipids may also be associated with elevated lipid levels or be a paraneoplastic marker, as in diffuse normolipemic plane xanthoma. Solitary lesions may be mistaken

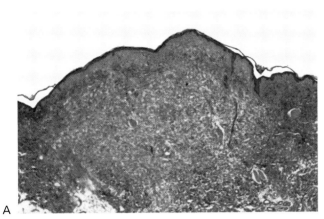
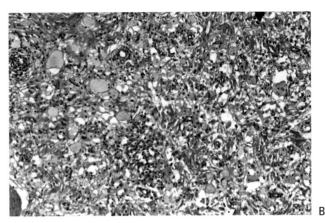

FIGURE 26-4. Papular xanthoma. **A:** Pale papule without epidermal reaction or clefting. **B:** Numerous foamy macrophages, some with multiple nuclei, are seen along with inflammatory cells. Extracellular lipids are not present.

clinically for dermatofibroma, Spitz nevus, and a variety of other benign proliferations.

SCALLOPED CELL XANTHOGRANULOMA

Scalloped cell xanthogranuloma is not clinically distinct. We identified a number of lesions in which the predominant macrophage is scalloped, once we had become aware of this morphologic variant in xanthoma disseminatum and began searching for solitary lesions to fill in our unifying concept scheme (68). The lesions are typically on the head, neck, or back of young men and may be diagnosed as juvenile xanthogranuloma, or less often melanocytic nevus or basal cell carcinoma. Histologically, scalloped macrophages predominate although a melange of other macrophage types may be found (Fig. 26-5A and B).

XANTHOMA DISSEMINATUM

In the rare condition of xanthoma disseminatum (XD), numerous widely disseminated but often closely set and even coalescing, round to oval, orange, or yellow-brown papules and nodules are found mainly on the flexor surfaces, such as the neck, axillae, antecubital fossae, groin, and perianal region. Peculiar target lesions may be seen. Often there are lesions around the eyes (69). The mucous membranes are affected in 40% to 60% of cases. In addition to oral lesions, there may be pharyngeal and laryngeal involvement. Three patterns have been identified (70); the most typical is the persistent form; rarely lesions may regress spontaneously, and even more infrequently in the progressive form there may be significant internal organ involvement. Although the largest review suggests that most cases begin in childhood (70), we have only seen the disease in adults.

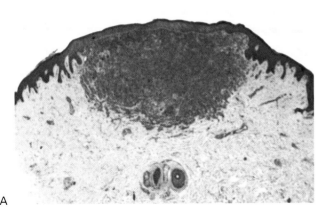
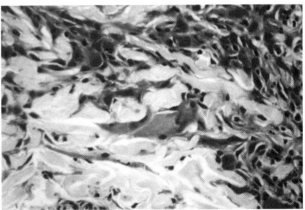

FIGURE 26-5. Scalloped cell xanthogranuloma. **A:** Small well-circumscribed dermal nodule without obvious giant cells or pale areas. **B:** Pale scalloped macrophage seen at base of infiltrate. Such cells can also be found in the early lesions of xanthoma disseminatum.

Diabetes insipidus is encountered in about 40% of cases but usually is mild and transitory, in contrast to that seen with LCD. It results from the infiltration of the hypothalamic-pituitary axis by xanthomatous cells. Characteristically, internal lesions other than diabetes insipidus are absent. In a few instances multiple osteolytic lesions have been found, especially in the long bones, as well as lung and CNS infiltrates.

A possible variant of XD, disseminated xanthosiderohistiocytosis, has been described in patients with hematologic malignancies (71). This disorder may also be related to disseminated dermal dendrocytomas (72), since the clinical photographs are almost interchangeable, with multiple papules and nodules on the chest and highly distinctive keloidal lesions on the extremities. The lesions are not truly xanthomatous but instead contain spindle cells, staining positively with FXIIIa with varying degrees of fibrosis. These unique patients also very much resemble the spindle cell variant of juvenile xanthogranuloma and its disseminated form, progressive nodular histiocytosis.

Histopathology. In early lesions, scalloped macrophages dominate the histologic picture. In contrast, papular xanthoma and diffuse plane xanthoma show only a minority of nonfoamy cells. More developed lesions may still show scalloped cells, but xanthomatization occurs in most cases. Most well-developed lesions contain a mixture of scalloped cells, foamy cells, and inflammatory cells, as well as Touton and foreign-body giant cells (73).

Pathogenesis. In the past, some authors have assumed a relationship between XD and LCD. Although in both conditions xanthomatous lesions and diabetes insipidus may occur, XD occurs in older patients, often has mucosal involvement, and only rarely involves bone. In addition, the pituitary involvement is different. Finally, xanthomatous lesions are expected in XD and rare in LCD. Immunohistochemistry also supports this clinical view, since the macrophages in XD fail to stain with S-100 and CD1a, and Birbeck granules are not present. Most cells are positive for macrophage markers, especially the foamy and giant cells, whereas others show FXIIIa positivity (73).

RETICULOHISTIOCYTOSIS

We divide what has traditionally been called reticulohistiocytosis into giant cell reticulohistiocytoma (GCRH) and multicentric reticulohistiocytosis (MRH). Both disorders occur almost exclusively in adults. The histologic picture is very similar in the two types but everything else is different.

GCRH is simply a xanthogranuloma in which the oncocytic macrophages and ground class giant cells dominate (74,75). It is never clinically unique but diagnosed as a JXG or dermatofibroma. The clinical features, distribu-

tion, and course are identical to JXG (76). In over 90% of cases, the lesion is single but occasionally multiple lesions are seen (77). Even patients with multiple lesions show no sign of systemic involvement.

In multicentric reticulohistiocytosis, a name first coined by Goltz and Laymon (78), the patients tend to be female, usually in the fifth or sixth decade of life, with widespread cutaneous involvement and a destructive arthritis (79,80). Nodules ranging in size from a few millimeters to several centimeters are most common on the extremities. Multiple papules on the face may coalesce, producing a leonine facies (81). Many small papules along the nail fold create the "coral bead sign." In about half of the patients, nodules are present also on the oral or nasal mucosa. Finally, about 25% also have xanthelasmata.

The polyarthritis may be mild or severe, but is almost always present. If severe, it may be mutilating, especially on the hands, through destruction of articular cartilage and subarticular bone. In addition, there is an association with hyperlipidemia (30% to 50%), a variety of internal malignancies (15% to 30%) (82,83), and autoimmune diseases (5% to 15%). The disease tends to wax and wane over many years, with mutilating arthritis and disfigurement real possibilities.

Histopathology. The characteristic histologic feature in both GCRH and MRH is the presence of numerous multinucleate giant cells and oncocytic macrophages showing abundant eosinophilic, finely granular cytoplasm, often with a "ground-glass" appearance (Fig. 26-6A and B). In older lesions, giant cells and fibrosis are more common. There may be subtle differences between the two lesions (76).

The polyarthritis present in nearly all instances of MRH is caused by the same type of infiltrate as found in the cutaneous lesions. In early or mild cases, the granulomatous infiltrate is confined to the synovial membrane. In patients with mutilating arthritis, the granulomatous infiltrate is also found in the subarticular cartilage and bone, leading to fragmentation and degeneration. Although similar infiltrates have been described in other organs, their clinical significance is unclear.

Pathogenesis. Ultrastructural examination shows abundant mitochondria and lysosomes, which correlate with the ground-glass appearance. Similar changes are found in oncocytic thyroid and renal tumors.

The cause of the solitary lesions is unknown, just as with JXG. In MRH, the concept of superantigen stimulation has been brought forward; a cytokine may selectively stimulate the oncocytic macrophages, resulting in their proliferation and subsequent tissue destruction.

Differential Diagnosis. It is futile to try and distinguish between a solitary GCRH and JXG. The two lesions are part of a spectrum and overlaps occur. A single macrophage lesion with ground-glass cytoplasm does not make the diagnosis of MRH, but instead should simply be viewed as

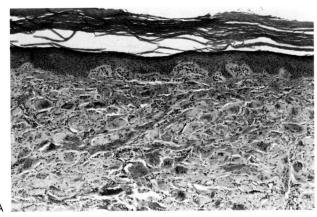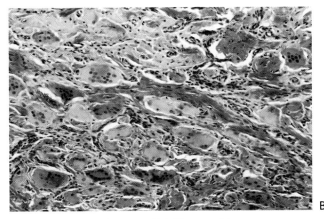

FIGURE 26-6. Multicentric reticulohistiocytosis. **A:** A diffuse dermal giant cell infiltrate with sparse inflammation and a thinned epidermis. **B:** Oncocytic giant cells with ground glass cytoplasm filling the upper dermis. The giant cells are large and irregular, containing many haphazardly arranged nuclei.

having the same clinical significance as JXG. The clinical differential diagnosis of MRH is lengthy, but a skin biopsy is quite helpful in pointing one in the right direction. Gout, rheumatoid arthritis, sarcoidosis, and even lepromatous leprosy may be considered.

SPINDLE CELL XANTHOGRANULOMA

Spindle cell xanthogranulomas are not clinically distinct (84). They are usually on the head or neck of young adults and identified as JXG or dermatofibromas. Histologically they are even more likely to be misdiagnosed, usually as dermatofibromas or blue nevi. Microscopically they lack melanin and do not have reactive changes in the overlying epidermis or lateral entrapment of collagen so typical of dermatofibromas (Fig. 26-7A and B). They stain with the

typical macrophage stains, but also for FXIIIa and smooth muscle actin.

PROGRESSIVE NODULAR HISTIOCYTOSIS

Progressive nodular histiocytosis is a rare clinically distinct disorder (85,86). Patients typically have hundreds of lesions of two types: superficial xanthomatous papules 2 to 10 mm in diameter and deep fibrous nodules 1 to 3 cm in diameter. The key to diagnosis is these two unique lesions. Conjunctival, oral, or laryngeal lesions may occur. Lesions rarely if ever regress. Familial or congenital cases have not been reported.

Histopathology. Two patterns can be recognized that correlate with the clinical lesions. The smaller papules are xanthomatous with foamy cells and occasional Touton giant

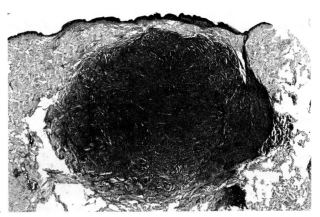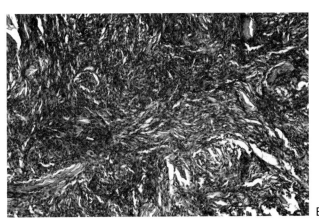

FIGURE 26-7. Spindle cell xanthogranuloma. **A:** Dermal nodule with storiform pattern. No evidence of epidermal reaction or peripheral entrapment of collagen. **B:** Spindled macrophages at higher magnification. The lesion was from a patient with progressive nodular histiocytosis.

cells; they are papular xanthomas. The larger nodules are the classic distinctive lesions; they are spindle cell xanthogranulomas (84).

Differential Diagnosis. When the distinctive clinical picture is present, the diagnosis of progressive nodular histiocytosis should be considered, but no harm is done if the patient is diagnosed with multiple JXG. Hereditary progressive mucinous histiocytosis is a rare disorder inherited in autosomal dominant fashion and seen only in women (87). While it sounds similar to progressive nodular histiocytosis, the lesions histologically resemble dermatofibromas with unexplained mucin deposits.

BENIGN CEPHALIC HISTIOCYTOSIS

Benign cephalic histiocytosis is a self-healing eruption usually limited to the skin (88). The eruption usually starts during the first 3 years of life and is almost always on the face, although it may become generalized. The lesions consist of red to yellow papules, which after a few years become flat and pigmented and finally resolve (89). In at least one instance, systemic involvement (pituitary gland) has been described (90).

Histopathology. The infiltrate tends to be sparse and consists of macrophages with regularly shaped nuclei and sparse cytoplasm. Three patterns have been observed: papillary dermal, lichenoid, and diffuse (91). The papillary dermal pattern is most common; there is a cohesive infiltrate of macrophages in the upper dermis. The cells tend to be large and have an eosinophilic cytoplasm. Foamy cells and epidermotropism are rare; eosinophils are often seen. The diffuse pattern is a minor variant in which the macrophages are sparser and spread throughout the dermis. The lichenoid pattern is easily confused with LCD,

but the nuclear changes seen in the latter are not present; crusting and ulceration are also uncommon (Fig. 26-8A and B).

Pathogenesis. The cause of BCH is unknown.

Differential Diagnosis. It is most important to exclude LCD with S-100 and CD1a staining, as clinical distinction can on occasion be difficult. Benign cephalic histiocytosis overlaps with generalized eruptive histiocytosis, progressive nodular histiocytosis, papular xanthomas, and multiple JXG (43). In an instructive case, a child with BCH developed typical JXG following varicella infection with facial involvement (92). If the lesions are clinically typical, the diagnosis can be made with some confidence.

GENERALIZED ERUPTIVE HISTIOCYTOSIS

Generalized eruptive histiocytosis (GEH) may represent the initial stage of a variety of macrophage disorders including JXG, xanthoma disseminatum, multicentric reticulohistiocytosis and progressive nodular histiocytosis. Clinically, it is characterized by the presence of innumerable flesh-colored to red macules and papules that develop in crops and that may involute spontaneously (93,94). The disease takes a variable course; it may persist, remit, or relapse. As the infiltrates regress, the lesions may evolve into hyperpigmented macules. Although most patients are adults, the condition may arise already in infancy (95,96). In rare instances, oral lesions have been observed. There may be an associated underlying disorder, such as a malignancy; the eruption may improve when the malignancy is treated (97).

Histopathology. Histologic examination reveals an infiltrate composed of various types of macrophages; most often small vacuolated cells are seen in a perivascular

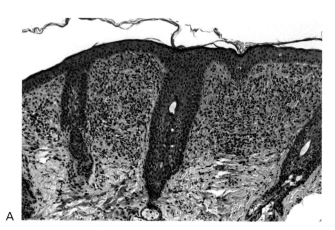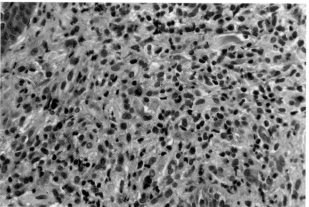

FIGURE 26-8. Benign cephalic histiocytosis. **A:** A modest lichenoid infiltrate without foamy cells. The epidermis is normal. **B:** The macrophages are smaller and rounder than in Langerhans cell disease. No eosinophils are present. This histologic picture is not specific; it is the prototype of an early macrophage infiltrate as seen in eruptive histiocytoma, early juvenile xanthogranuloma, and benign cephalic histiocytosis.

arrangement, but other morphologic variants may be represented or even dominate. Multinucleated giant cells are usually absent.

Pathogenesis. The etiology is unknown. As a matter of definition, one is dealing with a proliferation of macrophages that are not markedly phagocytic. These cells appear so rapidly that it is not surprising that they are often undifferentiated. Older lesions may show fibrosis or giant cells. The macrophages may in some cases appear in response to cytokines released by tumors, but in general their appearance remains unexplained.

Differential Diagnosis. The sudden onset and the lack of foamy cells or giant cells should suggest the diagnosis.

INDETERMINATE CELL HISTIOCYTOSIS

The diagnosis of indeterminate cell histiocytosis (ICH) was first proposed by Wood et al. (98) when they reassessed a previously reported case. Clinically, most patients present with numerous persistent red-brown papules or nodules that may coalesce (6,99). Solitary lesions may also occur, including congenital regressing nodules, clinically identical to CSHRH (100). A possible association with B cell lymphoma has been suggested (101), but other systemic lesions have not been found.

Histopathology. A monomorphous infiltrate of mononuclear cells intermingled with some giant cells and foamy cells is found. In our hands, these cases are positive for S-100 and CD68, as well as showing focal CD1a reactivity. The presence of macrophage markers and S-100 positivity does not exclude the presence of a xanthogranuloma variant.

Pathogenesis. We do not consider ICH as a single specific entity. In addition, we are certain that most cases described as ICH have little to do with the several different cells described as indeterminate cells. We feel most cases are macrophage disorders variants of xanthogranuloma where the predominant cell is derived from an earlier or aberrant lineage. Other cases, such as those resembling CSHRH, are clearly variants on LCD and we suspect that the veiled cell (migrating LC) is the other cell most often described as an indeterminate cell. Some examples of ICH may be reactive; such infiltrates have been described in nodular scabies and following pityriasis rosea (102). A spindle-cell variant has also been described (103), perhaps representing a variant of IDC tumor.

SINUS HISTIOCYTOSIS WITH MASSIVE LYMPHADENOPATHY (ROSAI–DORFMAN DISEASE)

Sinus histiocytosis with massive lymphadenopathy (SHML) was first described by Rosai and Dorfman in 1969 (104), although Destombes (104a) had previously described the

disorder in Africa. Massive cervical lymphadenopathy, usually bilateral and painless, is the most common manifestation. SHML is generally a benign disorder in spite of its propensity to form large masses and to disseminate to both nodal and extranodal sites. In most patients the disease resolves spontaneously, others have persistent problems, and very few die (105). About 10% of patients with nodal disease have cutaneous involvement (106). The lesions are typically papules or nodules. The skin and subcutaneous soft tissue are also the most common sites of involvement when patients present with extranodal disease (107,108). Such individuals may represent a separate but closely related disorder as very few advance to nodal or systemic disease (109). Occasionally the soft tissue lesion may present as a breast mass (110) or panniculitis.

Histopathology. The skin lesions contain a polymorphous infiltrate in which lymphocytes and macrophages with clear cytoplasm are most prominent. The low-power view has been compared to that of a "lymph node in the skin" (Fig. 26-9A and B). Occasionally they may be multinucleated or have a foamy cytoplasm. The hallmark histologic feature is emperipolesis of lymphocytes (105) (Fig. 26-9C). Emperipolesis differs slightly from phagocytosis in that the lymphocytes are taken up but seem not to be attacked and digested by enzymes. Thus, they appear intact. On occasion, red cells can also be taken up.

In the lymph nodes, the sinuses are greatly dilated and crowded with inflammatory cells, particularly macrophages.

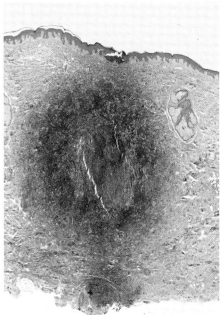

A

FIGURE 26-9. Sinus histiocytosis with massive lymphadenopathy. **A:** Nodular infiltrate rich in pale-staining cells centrally. *(continued)*

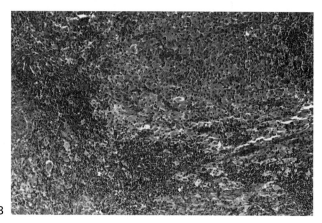
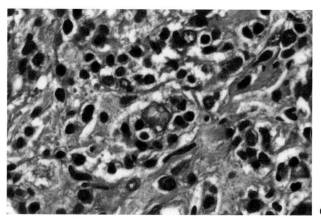

FIGURE 26-9. *(continued)* **B:** Typical pattern of pale sinusoidal macrophages admixed with darker-staining lymphocytes. **C:** Numerous large macrophages, several of which have ingested lymphocytes, demonstrating emperipolesis.

Here they tend to have an abundant foamy cytoplasm and also display emperipolesis.

Pathogenesis. The cells are S-100 positive but CD1a negative, and do not contain Birbeck granules. They tend to have a variety of macrophage markers and the responsible cell is felt to be an activated macrophage, which for unknown reasons also expresses S-100 (111,112).

HISTIOCYTIC SARCOMA

Even though malignant tumors of macrophage lineage are rare, they are occasionally encountered in the skin (113). The large International Lymphoma Study Group identified 18 such cases with three involving the skin, both with solitary and multiple lesions (29). There were also three cases of widespread systemic disease, corresponding to the old term of malignant histiocytosis. The tumors consist of large cells with frequent mitoses and varying degrees of pleomorphism. Multinucleate giant cells, foamy cells, and spindle-shaped cells may be encountered. Erythrophagocytosis is absent or inconspicuous, while emperipolesis is even more rare. The diagnosis must be supported by CD68 positivity, which is also accompanied by positive lysozyme staining in 90% of cases. Other macrophage markers may also be positive as well as S-100. Markers for dendritic cells, T cells and B cells must be negative. On electron microscopy, lysosomes are found, but Birbeck granules and desmosomes are absent. Histiocytic sarcoma remains an aggressive disease; only patients with solitary extranodal disease such as a single skin lesion are occasionally cured.

XANTHOMAS ASSOCIATED WITH LIPID ABNORMALITIES

Even though we place xanthomas among the macrophage disorders, we have left those associated with lipid abnor-

malities as a separate category as they are generally viewed as such by both clinicians and pathologists. Xanthomas are a cutaneous clue to the possible presence of hyperlipidemia, traditionally defined as an elevated fasting cholesterol level of over 200 mg/dl or a triglyceride level of over 180 mg/dl. Today HDL cholesterol is also measured and used to calculate the LDL-cholesterol level. The desirable LDL-cholesterol level is less than 130 mg/dl. If abnormalities are detected, lipoprotein analysis is also usually performed. Hyperlipidemia may be unexpectedly identified during routine evaluations or searched for because of a family history of lipid abnormalities, cardiovascular disease, or the presence of one of its many secondary causes.

Once hyperlipidemia is identified, one must first exclude these secondary causes, which include diabetes mellitus, hypothyroidism, nephrotic syndrome, biliary disease, alcohol abuse, and a variety of medications, including estrogens, corticosteroids, and retinoids. In the 1960s, Frederickson (113a) classified the primary hyperlipidemias on the basis of their electrophoretic lipoprotein phenotype. They considered not just cholesterol and triglycerides, but the main lipoprotein classes in which they were transported throughout the body—chylomicrons, very-low-density lipoproteins (VLDL), low-density lipoproteins (LDL), and high-density lipoproteins (HDL). This traditional scheme is still used for a first diagnostic orientation but does not allow pathophysiologic classification of the lipoprotein disorder for two reasons:

1. The protein component of lipoproteins, known as apoproteins, has been extensively characterized and subdivided. The various apoproteins serve to bind lipids, regulate enzymes, and identify cell receptors. For example, a patient may have normal amounts of cholesterol but decreased levels of HDL, which is essential for the removal of intracellular cholesterol.
2. The specific genetic defect has been identified for a number of disorders, the best known of which is famil-

ial hypercholesterolemia, in which there is an absent or functionally defective LDL receptor.

Most patients with lipoprotein abnormalities do not have xanthomas, but the presence of xanthomas and especially the identification of extracellular lipids on histologic examination of the lesion should alert the clinician to the need for an internal evaluation. Table 26.5 gives an algorithmic approach to patients with cutaneous xanthomas. The type of xanthoma is primarily a clinical diagnosis and correlates poorly with the exact lipid abnormality. With these limitations in mind, Table 26-5 gives a brief overview of the relationship between xanthomas and hyperlipidemias (114).

The xanthomas may clinically be divided into eruptive xanthomas, tuberous xanthomas, tendon xanthomas, and plane xanthomas. We view xanthelasma as a morphologic variant of plane xanthoma more closely related to the macrophage disorders, but have discussed it here for the sake of continuity. Eruptive xanthomas are almost always associated with chylomicronemia and are most commonly seen in secondary forms of hyperlipoproteinemia. Eruptive xanthomas consist of small, soft, yellow papules with a predilection for the buttocks and the posterior aspects of the thighs. They come and go with fluctuations in the chylomicron level in the plasma. The lipid in these lesions is primarily triglycerides. Triglycerides are more rapidly metabolized than cholesterol. This may explain the more transient nature of eruptive xanthomas as compared to other xanthomas.

Tuberous and tuberoeruptive xanthomas are found predominantly in cases with an increase in LDL and VLDL remnants. They are large nodes or plaques located most commonly on the elbows, knees, fingers, and buttocks. Most of the lipid in these xanthomas is in the form of cholesterol. Atypical VLDL remnants (β-VLDL) accumulate in type III hyperlipoproteinemia.

Tendon xanthomas occur in patients with excessive plasma LDL levels, such as familial hypercholesterolemia and familial apolipoprotein B-100 defect, as well as in phytosterolemia and cholestanolemia (cerebrotendinous xan-

thomatosis). The Achilles tendons and the extensor tendons of the fingers are most frequently affected.

Plane xanthomas typically develop in skin folds and especially in the palmar creases, where they are diagnostic for dysbetalipoproteinemia. Diffuse plane xanthomas are typically seen as multiple grouped papules and poorly defined yellowish plaques in normolipemic patients, often with paraproteinemia, lymphoma, or leukemia. On the other hand, intertriginous plane xanthomas suggest homozygous familial hypercholesterolemia. The palmar xanthomas associated with cholestasis (primary biliary cirrhosis and biliary atresia) are plaque-like and tend to extend past the creases.

Xanthelasmata consist of slightly raised, yellow, soft plaques on the eyelids. Although xanthelasmata are the commonest of the cutaneous xanthomas, they are also the least specific because they most frequently occur in persons with normal lipoprotein levels. We argue that xanthelasma belong in the family of macrophage disorders, as they rarely show extracellular lipids, frequently have giant cells, and do not typically disappear with appropriate lipid-lowering therapy.

Histopathology. The histologic appearance of xanthomas of the skin and the tendons is characterized by foamy cells, macrophages that have engulfed lipid droplets (115). Most of the xanthoma cells are mononuclear, but giant cells, especially of the Touton type with a wreath of nuclei, may be found. The most diagnostic finding suggesting that a xanthomatous lesion reflects an underlying lipid abnormality is the presence of free lipids that have not yet been taken up by macrophages. The lipid droplets can be better seen if frozen or formalin-fixed sections are stained with fat stains such as scarlet red or Sudan red. There may be varying degrees of fibrosis, giant cells, and clefts, depending on the type and site of xanthoma sampled, but most are surprisingly similar. All xanthomas are characterized by a degree of fixation artifact. Formalin fixation and paraffin embedding remove lipids so that only their shadows are left behind. Larger extracellular deposits of cholesterol and other sterols leave behind clefts.

In the past, much emphasis was placed on the refractile nature of xanthomatous deposits. Frozen or formalin-fixed frozen sections can be examined under polarized light. Cholesterol esters are doubly refractile, whereas other lipids are not. Thus, tendon and tuberous xanthomas tend to be doubly refractile, whereas other xanthomas are not. Chronic lesions are far more likely to show fibrosis.

Some differences exist in the histologic appearance of the various types of xanthoma. Eruptive xanthomas, when of recent origin, often show a considerable admixture of nonfoamy cells, among them lymphocytes, macrophages, and neutrophils, whereas the number of well-developed foamy cells may still be small. Because the rapid transport of lipid, especially triglycerides, into the tissue overwhelms the capacity of the macrophages, extracellular lipids are usually found (Fig. 26-10A and B). These pools of lipid surrounded by macrophages mimic granuloma annulare histologically (116). Fully developed eruptive xanthomas

TABLE 26-5. ALGORITHM FOR CUTANEOUS XANTHOMAS

When an infiltrate with foamy cells is found . . . .
1. Is extracellular lipid present?
   If YES, marker for underlying hyperlipidemia
2. Check serum lipid levels
   2.1. If abnormal, diagnosis confirmed
   2.2. If normal, consider
      2.2.1. Xanthogranulomas (papular xanthoma, xanthoma disseminatum)
      2.2.2. Noncholesterol lipid disorders (sitosterolemia, cholestanolemia)
      2.2.3. Paraneoplastic disorders
      2.2.4. Postinflammatory, posttraumatic lesions
      2.2.5. Storage disorders and other rare syndromes

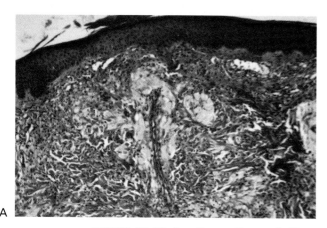

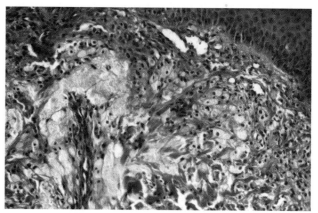

FIGURE 26-10. Eruptive xanthoma. **A:** Numerous pale areas containing foamy cells are dispersed throughout the dermis. **B:** At higher magnification the extracellular lipids can be appreciated. They offer a reliable indication that this xanthoma is relatively recent in origin and associated with a lipid abnormality.

are rich in foamy cells. Some may show crystals, causing confusion with gout (117).

Tuberous xanthomas consist of large and small aggregates of foamy cells. In early lesions, there usually is a slight admixture of nonfoamy cells, among them lymphocytes, macrophages, and neutrophils. In well-developed lesions, the infiltrate is composed almost entirely of foamy cells. Ultimately, collagen bundles replace many of these cells. Cholesterol clefts may be found (Fig. 26-11). Tendon xanthomas are identical to tuberous xanthomas in histologic appearance but may be even larger and are often submitted without their overlying skin.

Plane xanthomas should be suspected when the overlying epidermis is thickened with hyperkeratosis and a stratum lucidum, indicating a palmar location (Fig. 26-12 A and B). Plane xanthomas from other sites have no unique features.

Xanthelasmata located on the eyelids differ from tuberous xanthomas by the fairly superficial location of the foamy cells and the nearly complete absence of fibrosis. Superficial striated muscles, vellus hairs, small vessels, and a thinned epi-

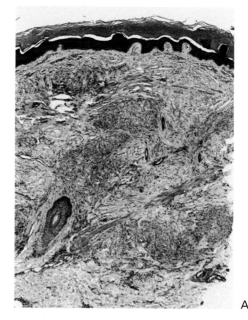

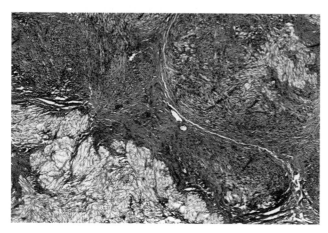

FIGURE 26-11. Tuberous xanthoma. Diffuse deposits of cholesterol probably occupied the pale area at the lower left, while in the upper right side, clefts are more prominent.

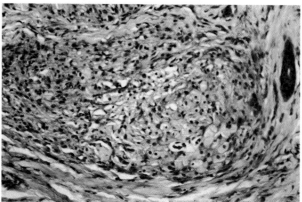

FIGURE 26-12. Plane xanthoma. **A:** Acral skin with dermis replaced by multiple pale bulbous infiltrates. **B:** At higher power, numerous foamy macrophages with their nuclei displaced to the cell periphery can be seen.

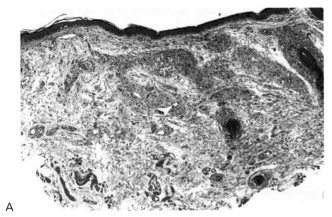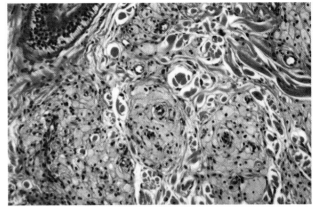

A

B

FIGURE 26-13. Xanthelasma. **A:** The thin epidermis and muscle fibers at base are a clue to the eyelid location. **B:** Lobules of foamy cells in this location allow the specific diagnosis of xanthelasma.

dermis all suggest location on the eyelid, and serve as clues to the histologic diagnosis of xanthelasma (Fig. 26-13A and B). Metastatic adenocarcinoma to the eyelids, most often of breast origin, and primary adnexal carcinomas (sebaceous and signet ring) can be mistaken for xanthelasmata.

Pathogenesis. Whereas the pathogenesis of many forms of hyperlipidemia is well understood, the formation of xanthomas is a complex process of dysregulation of macrophage sterol flux. Elevated levels of cholesterol-rich LDL and VLDL remnants tend to predispose to xanthomas. Under physiologic conditions, about 80% of LDL-cholesterol is taken up by specific LDL-receptor mediated endocytosis. The remaining LDLs are removed from the circulation by the scavenger receptor pathways of macrophages. In familial hypercholesterolemia and familial dysbetalipoproteinemia, the accumulating LDLs and VLDL remnants are predominantly scavenged by macrophages, a pathway without feedback regulation, leading to continuous cellular lipid accumulation and foamy cells. Thus, these xanthomas are caused by an increased load of altered sterol-rich lipoproteins.

On the other hand, xanthomas can also be caused by disturbed mechanisms of macrophage cholesterol reflux. Specific ATP-binding cassette (ABC) transporters play the key role in macrophage sterol efflux, regulation of HDL metabolism, and reverse cholesterol transport. Defective ABCA1 transporter has been shown to be the molecular cause of Tangier disease and familial HDL deficiency. Thus, both overload of macrophages with altered and aged lipoproteins (increased scavenger pathway) and defective cholesterol efflux from macrophages (abnormal transporters) appear to play a crucial role in xanthoma formation.

NORMOLIPEMIC XANTHOMAS

A wide number of disorders must be considered if xanthomas are identified in a normolipemic patient. Parker has divided this group into the following categories (118):

Type IA: a lipoprotein containing another source of excess sterol (such as cholestanol in cerebrotendinous xanthomatosis or sitosterol in phytosterolemia). In both cases, tuberous and tendon xanthomas are most common, with marked amounts of extracellular lipids.

Type IB: a lipoprotein containing abnormal apoprotein, which selectively binds cholesterol or triglyceride that is present nonetheless in normal amounts. These disorders are for convenience grouped with the traditional lipid-related xanthomas.

Type II: associated with lymphoproliferative disease (diffuse plane xanthomas and necrobiotic xanthogranuloma).

Type III: no lipoprotein abnormality or associated lymphoproliferative disease; many are idiopathic and others post-traumatic. In addition to those xanthomas in the xanthogranuloma family (xanthoma disseminatum and papular xanthoma) and rarely in LCD, one must consider verruciform xanthoma, post-inflammatory and post-traumatic xanthomas and a variety of rare syndromes.

PARANEOPLASTIC DISORDERS

Necrobiotic Xanthogranuloma with Paraproteinemia

A rare disorder, necrobiotic xanthogranuloma with paraproteinemia (NXG) can usually be recognized histologically but may overlap with diffuse normolipemic plane xanthoma. Large, often yellow, indurated plaques are found with atrophy, telangiectasia, and occasionally also ulceration (119). The most common location is periorbital; in one review, 21 of 22 patients had skin findings in this area (120). The thorax is also commonly involved. Systemic involvement includes a cardiac myopathy with giant cell infiltrates and hematologic malignancies (121).

Histopathology. Infiltrates containing macrophages, foamy cells, and often also an admixture of other inflammatory

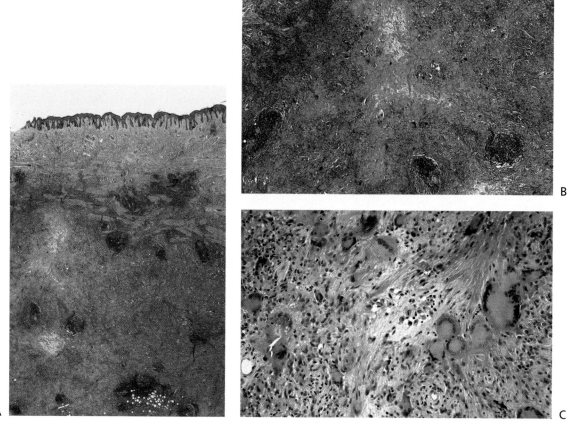

FIGURE 26-14. Necrobiotic xanthogranuloma. **A:** Low-power view showing a diffuse infiltrate with amorphous necrobiotic areas, cellular regions rich in giant cells, and a nodular lymphocytic infiltrate. **B:** Higher magnification showing prominent lymphoid follicles and pale necrobiotic regions. **C:** Another view showing numerous Touton giant cells and extensive necrobiosis.

cells are present either as focal aggregates or as large, intersecting bands occupying the dermis and subcutaneous tissue (Fig. 26-14A). The intervening tissue shows extensive necrobiosis (degeneration of collagen imparting unique staining characteristics) (Fig. 26-14B). Other characteristic findings are numerous lumonoid follicles and giant cells, both of the Touton type with a peripheral rim of foamy cytoplasm and of the foreign-body type (Fig. 26-14C). Cholesterol clefts are also common (122).

Pathogenesis. In most patients, serum protein electrophoresis shows an IgG monoclonal gammopathy that usually consists of kappa light chains. Bone marrow examination has revealed multiple myeloma. The xanthomas seen in POEMS syndrome may have a similar etiology (123).

Differential Diagnosis. Other necrobiotic disorders, especially necrobiosis lipoidica diabeticorum and subcutaneous granuloma annulare or rheumatoid nodule, may be considered. In necrobiotic xanthogranuloma, the necrobiosis is far more extensive and often occurs in broad bands, associated with extensive infiltrates of Touton giant cells, foamy macrophages, and lymphocytes. Vascular involvement is rare,

but panniculitis is common. Thus, the cellularity and extent of necrobiosis usually serve as reliable clues, as does the usual periorbital location.

Diffuse Normolipemic Plane Xanthoma

In diffuse normolipemic plane xanthoma (DNPX), another rare disorder, one observes papules, patches, or, most commonly, even larger diffuse areas of orange-yellow discoloration of the skin. Whereas the smaller lesions are distinct, the diffuse areas have a poorly defined border. The face, particularly the periorbital areas, and the upper trunk are sites of predilection. The disorder may mimic xanthelasma initially but progresses to involve wide areas of skin. The lesions usually persist indefinitely. By definition, the patient has no lipid abnormalities (124,125).

Many but not all cases of diffuse normolipemic plane xanthoma are associated with hematologic disorders, most commonly paraproteinemias, including multiple myeloma, benign monoclonal gammopathy (often IgA), Castleman disease, and cryoglobulinemia (126). The skin disorder may precede the hematologic problem by many years.

Generalized papular xanthomas and eruptive normolipemic xanthomas are probably variations on the same theme; both have been reported in association with many of the conditions associated with diffuse normolipemic plane xanthomas. There are also cases that begin as papular xanthomas, but the lesions evolve and coalesce into diffuse plane xanthomas (127). In addition, DNPX has many features in common with necrobiotic xanthogranuloma (128), including the presence of large patches and plaques, periorbital involvement, and association with paraproteinemias.

Histopathology. Histologic examination reveals large sheets and clusters of foamy cells, as well as singly and in small groups, diffusely scattered throughout the dermis. In some areas, the foamy cells lie in thin streaks between collagen bundles, and occasionally a perivascular arrangement is noted. There may be an admixture of macrophages and lymphocytes; rarely, Touton giant cells are seen. Scattered foamy cells have been observed even in clinically normal skin.

Pathogenesis. The mechanism of xanthoma formation is unclear. Possible explanations include the secretion of cytokines or immunoglobulins by the underlying lymphocytic proliferation, which in turn could stimulate macrophages or alter lipoprotein activity. This theory fails to explain why the skin involvement so often occurs first. The immunohistochemical phenotyping of the macrophages has yielded variable results.

Differential Diagnosis. A single lesion cannot be distinguished from other small xanthomas. If marked necro-

biosis or giant cell formation is present, necrobiotic xanthogranuloma should be considered.

Verruciform Xanthoma

Verruciform xanthoma (VX) occurs most commonly in the oral cavity, where it was first described by Shafer (129). Lesions are typically solitary, asymptomatic hyperkeratotic papillomatous nodules. Most cases involve the gingival or alveolar mucosa, although other oral sites may be affected (130). Although the process is usually benign, it has been associated with carcinoma in situ (131).

In addition, VX may occur in the skin in several settings (132). The most predictable situation is as part of a CHILD (congenital hemidysplasia, ichthyosiform erythroderma, and limb defects) nevus, one type of epidermal nevus. Idiopathic cutaneous VX is usually anogenital or perioral; trauma is probably the triggering agent. Similar changes have been seen in sun-damaged skin, again associated with carcinoma in situ (133). VX has been reported secondary to a variety of inflammatory lesions, including discoid lupus erythematosus (134), lichen planus, bullous diseases, and following psoriasiform inflammation in AIDS (135).

Histopathology. The low-power picture is that of a verruca, often leading to a mistaken diagnosis. There is marked elongation of the rete ridges extending to a uniform level in the dermis (Fig. 26-15A). An infiltrate of foamy cells is confined to the elongated dermal papillae located between the rete ridges (Fig. 26-15B). Sometimes

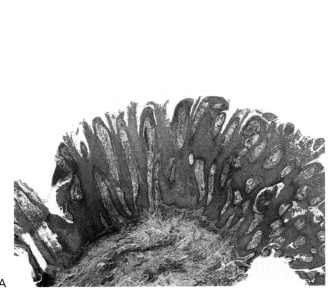
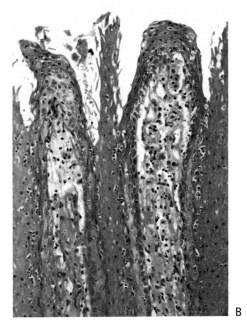

FIGURE 26-15. Verruciform xanthoma. **A:** Papilloma with marked elongation and thinning of the dermal papillae. There is prominent hyperkeratosis with a modest lymphocytic infiltrate at base. **B:** Higher magnification showing foamy cells in the papillae with inflammatory cells in the adjacent crust.

the xanthomatous cells may appear granular. The vessels in the papillae are also more prominent. The overlying epithelium is parakeratotic, and candidal hyphae or bacteria may be found.

Pathogenesis. Degenerating keratinocytes or perhaps even melanocytes (136) are felt to be the source of the lipid material. While human papillomavirus has been searched for, it has not been unequivocally identified in more than a few scattered cases (132). Trauma and inflammation are the two best-established triggers. The foamy cells are positive for macrophage markers and express scavenger receptors similar to those found in xanthomas associated with hyperlipidemia (137).

Miscellaneous Xanthomas

It is difficult to make rhyme or reason of the many other causes of normolipemic xanthomas. One recurrent theme is trauma, as in VX. Xanthomas have developed in areas of chronic inflammation, such as atopic dermatitis (138), persistent light eruption, mycosis fungoides (139), or even contact dermatitis (140), although we find the illustrations in many of these reports fail to convincingly demonstrate a nodule made up of foamy cells.

Acknowledgments. Drs. Bodo Melnik, George Murphy, Stefano Pileri, and Arno Rütten provided us with advice and histologic material essential for the preparation of this chapter.

REFERENCES

1. Lichtenstein L. Histiocytosis X. Integration of eosinophilic granuloma, Letterer-Siwe disease and Hand–Schüller–Christian disease as related manifestations of a single nosologic entity. *Arch Pathol* 1953;56:84.
2. Headington JT. The histiocyte. In memoriam. *Arch Dermatol* 1986;122:532.
3. Foucar K, Foucar E. The mononuclear phagocyte and immunoregulatory effector (M-PIRE) system: evolving concepts. *Semin Diagn Pathol* 1990;7:4.
4. Ben-Ezra JM, Koo CH. Langerhans' cell histiocytosis and malignancies of the M-PIRE system. *Am J Clin Pathol* 1993;99:464.
5. Murphy GF, Liu V. The dermal immune system. In: Bos JD, ed. *Skin Immune System*, 2nd ed. Boca Raton, FL: CRC Press, 1997:347.
6. Sidoroff A, Zelger B, Steiner H, et al. Indeterminate cell histiocytosis—a clinicopathological entity with features of both X- and non-X histiocytosis. *Br J Dermatol* 1996;134:525.
7. Tomaszewski MM, Lupton GP. Unusual expression of S-100 protein in histiocytic neoplasms. *J Cutan Pathol* 1998;25:129.
8. Zelger B, Burgdorf WH. The cutaneous "histiocytoses." *Adv Dermatol* 2001;17:77.
9. Caputo R. *Text Atlas of Histiocytic Syndromes.* London: Martin Dunitz Ltd., 1998.
10. Favara BE, Feller AC, Pauli M, et al. Contemporary classification of histiocytic disorders. The WHO Committee On Histiocytic/Reticulum Cell Proliferations. Reclassification Working Group of the Histiocyte Society. *Med Pediatr Oncol* 1997;29:157.
11. Northcutt AD. Epidermotropic xanthoma mimicking balloon cell melanoma. *Am J Dermatopathol* 2000;22:176.
12. Busam KJ, Rosai J, Iversen K, et al. Xanthogranulomas with inconspicuous foam cells and giant cells mimicking malignant melanoma: a clinical, histologic, and immunohistochemical study of three cases. *Am J Surg Pathol* 2000;24:864.
13. Busam KJ, Granter SR, Iversen K, et al. Immunohistochemical distinction of epithelioid histiocytic proliferations from epithelioid melanocytic nevi. *Am J Dermatopathol* 2000;22:237.
14. Higgins CR, Tatnall FM, Leigh IM. Vesicular Langerhans cell histiocytosis—an uncommon variant. *Clin Exp Dermatol* 1994;19:350.
15. Butler DF, Ranatunge BD, Rapini RP. Urticating Hashimoto–Pritzker Langerhans cell histiocytosis. *Pediatr Dermatol* 2001;18:41.
16. Chi DH, Sung KJ, Koh JK. Eruptive xanthoma-like cutaneous Langerhans cell histiocytosis in an adult. *J Am Acad Dermatol* 1996;34:688.
17. Jain S, Sehgal VN, Bajaj P. Nail changes in Langerhans cell histiocytosis. *J Eur Acad Dermatol Venereol* 2000;14:212.
18. Novice FM, Collison DW, Kleinsmith DM, et al. Letterer–Siwe disease in adults. *Cancer* 1989;63:166.
19. Mejia R, Dano JA, Roberts R, et al. Langerhans' cell histiocytosis in adults. *J Am Acad Dermatol* 1997;37:314.
20. Hashimoto K, Pritzker MS. Electron microscopic study of reticulohistiocytoma. An unusual case of congenital, self-healing reticulohistiocytosis. *Arch Dermatol* 1973;107:263.
21. Schaumburg-Lever G, Rechowicz E, Fehrenbacher B, et al. Congenital self-healing reticulohistiocytosis—a benign Langerhans cell disease. *J Cutan Pathol* 1994;21:59.
22. Bernstein EF, Resnik KS, Loose JH, et al. Solitary congenital self-healing reticulohistiocytosis. *Br J Dermatol* 1993;129:449.
23. Longaker MA, Frieden IJ, LeBoit PE, et al. Congenital "self-healing" Langerhans cell histiocytosis: the need for long-term follow-up. *J Am Acad Dermatol* 1994;31:910.
24. Risdall RJ, Dehner LP, Duray P, et al. Histiocytosis X (Langerhans' cell histiocytosis). Prognostic role of histopathology. *Arch Pathol* Lab Med 1983;107:59.
25. Egeler MR, Neglia JP, Puccetti DM, et al. Association of Langerhans cell histiocytosis with malignant neoplasms. *Cancer* 1993;71:865.
26. Lieberman PH, Jones CR, Steinman RM, et al. Langerhans cell (eosinophilic) granulomatosis. A clinicopathologic study encompassing 50 years. *Am J Surg Pathol* 1996;20:519.
27. Howarth DM, Gilchrist GS, Mullan BP, et al. Langerhans cell histiocytosis: diagnosis, natural history, management, and outcome. *Cancer* 1999;85:2278.
28. Colon-Fontanez F, Eichenfield LE, Krous HF, et al. Congenital Langerhans cell histiocytosis: the utility of the Tzanck test as a diagnostic screening tool. *Arch Dermatol* 1998;134:1039.
29. Pileri SA, Grogan TM, Harris NL, et al. Tumours of histiocytes and accessory dendritic cells: an immunohistochemical approach to classification from the International Lymphoma Study Group based on 61 cases. *Histopathology* 2002;41:1.
30. Itoh H, Miyaguni H, Kataoka H, et al. Primary cutaneous Langerhans cell histiocytosis showing malignant phenotype in an elderly woman: report of a fatal case. *J Cutan Pathol* 2001;28:371.
31. Wood C, Wood GS, Deneau DG, et al. Malignant histiocytosis X. Report of a rapidly fatal case in an elderly man. *Cancer* 1984;54:347.
32. Ben-Ezra J, Bailey A, Azumi N, et al. Malignant histiocytosis X. A distinct clinicopathologic entity. *Cancer* 1991;68:1050.
33. Vassallo R, Ryu JH, Colby TV, et al. Pulmonary Langerhans'-cell histiocytosis. *N Engl J Med* 2000;342:1969.

34. Hage C, Willman CL, Favara BE, et al. Langerhans' cell histiocytosis (histiocytosis X): immunophenotype and growth fraction. *Hum Pathol* 1993;24:840.

35. Yu RC, Alaibac M, Chu AC. Functional defect in cells involved in Langerhans cell histiocytosis. *Arch Dermatol Res* 1995;287:627.

36. Helm KF, Lookingbill DP, Marks JG Jr A clinical and pathologic study of histiocytosis X in adults. *J Am Acad Dermatol* 1993;29:166.

37. Willman CL, Busque L, Griffith BB, et al. Langerhans'-cell histiocytosis (histiocytosis X)—a clonal proliferative disease. *N Engl J Med* 1994;331:154.

38. Yu RC, Chu C, Buluwela L, et al. Clonal proliferation of Langerhans cells in Langerhans cell histiocytosis. *Lancet* 1994;343:767.

39. Nezelof C, Basset F. From histiocytosis X to Langerhans cell histiocytosis: a personal account. *Int J Surg Pathol* 2001;9:137.

40. Zelger BW, Sidoroff A, Orchard G, et al. Non-Langerhans cell histiocytoses. A new unifying concept. *Am J Dermatopathol* 1996;18:490.

41. Sangueza OP, Salmon JK, White CR Jr, et al. Juvenile xanthogranuloma: a clinical, histopathologic and immunohistochemical study. *J Cutan Pathol* 1995;22:327.

42. Whitmore SE. Multiple xanthogranulomas in an adult: case report and literature review. *Br J Dermatol* 1992;127:177.

43. Zelger BG, Zelger B, Steiner H, et al. Solitary giant xanthogranuloma and benign cephalic histiocytosis—variants of juvenile xanthogranuloma. *Br J Dermatol* 1995;133:598.

44. Caputo R, Grimalt R, Gelmetti C, et al. Unusual aspects of juvenile xanthogranuloma. *J Am Acad Dermatol* 1993;29:868.

45. Kolde G, Bonsmann G. Generalized lichenoid juvenile xanthogranuloma. *Br J Dermatol* 1992;126:66.

46. Janney CG, Hurt MA, Santa Cruz DJ. Deep juvenile xanthogranuloma. Subcutaneous and intramuscular forms. *Am J Surg Pathol* 1991;15:150.

47. de Graaf JH, Timens W, Tamminga RY, et al. Deep juvenile xanthogranuloma: a lesion related to dermal indeterminate cells. *Hum Pathol* 1992;23:905.

48. Sanchez Yus E, Requena L, Villegas C, et al. Subcutaneous juvenile xanthogranuloma. *J Cutan Pathol* 1995;22:460.

49. Hoeger PH, Diaz C, Malone M, et al. Juvenile xanthogranuloma as a sequel to Langerhans cell histiocytosis: a report of three cases. *Clin Exp Dermatol* 2001;26:391.

50. Chang MW, Frieden IJ, Good W. The risk of intraocular juvenile xanthogranuloma: survey of current practices and assessment of risk. *J Am Acad Dermatol* 1996;34:445.

51. Zvulunov A, Barak Y, Metzker A. Juvenile xanthogranuloma, neurofibromatosis, and juvenile chronic myelogenous leukemia. World statistical analysis. *Arch Dermatol* 1995;131:904.

52. Freyer DR, Kennedy R, Bostrom BC, et al. Juvenile xanthogranuloma: forms of systemic disease and their clinical implications. *J Pediatr* 1996;129:227.

53. Botella-Estrada R, Sanmartin O, Grau M, et al. Juvenile xanthogranuloma with central nervous system involvement. *Pediatr Dermatol* 1993;10:64.

54. Kraus MD, Haley JC, Ruiz R, et al. "Juvenile" xanthogranuloma: an immunophenotypic study with a reappraisal of histogenesis. *Am J Dermatopathol* 2001;23:104.

55. Shamburek RD, Brewer HB Jr, Gochuico BR. Erdheim–Chester disease: a rare multisystem histiocytic disorder associated with interstitial lung disease. *Am J Med Sci* 2001;321:66.

56. Valmaggia C, Neuweiler J, Fretz C, et al. A case of Erdheim–Chester disease with orbital involvement. *Arch Ophthalmol* 1997;115:1467.

57. Zelger B, Cerio R, Orchard G, et al. Juvenile and adult xanthogranuloma. A histological and immunohistochemical comparison. *Am J Surg Pathol* 1994;18:126.

58. Kubota Y, Kiryu H, Nakayama J, et al. Histopathologic maturation of juvenile xanthogranuloma in a short period. *Pediatr Dermatol* 2001;18:127.

59. Shapiro PE, Silvers DN, Treiber RK, et al. Juvenile xanthogranulomas with inconspicuous or absent foam cells and giant cells. *J Am Acad Dermatol* 1991;24:1005.

60. Newman CC, Raimer SS, Sanchez RL. Nonlipidized juvenile xanthogranuloma: a histologic and immunohistochemical study. *Pediatr Dermatol* 1997;14:98.

61. Sanchez RL, Raimer SS, Peltier F, et al. Papular xanthoma. A clinical, histologic, and ultrastructural study. *Arch Dermatol* 1985;121:626.

62. Breier F, Zelger B, Reiter H, et al. Papular xanthoma: a clinicopathological study of 10 cases. *J Cutan Pathol* 2002;29:200.

63. Caputo R, Gianni E, Imondi D, et al. Papular xanthoma in children. *J Am Acad Dermatol* 1990;22:1052.

64. Caputo R, Monti M, Berti E, et al. Normolipemic eruptive cutaneous xanthomatosis. *Arch Dermatol* 1986;122:1294.

65. Chen CG, Chen CL, Liu HN. Primary papular xanthoma of children: a clinicopathologic, immunohistopathologic and ultrastructural study. *Am J Dermatopathol* 1997;19:596.

66. Winkelmann RK. Cutaneous syndromes of non-X histiocytosis. A review of the macrophage-histiocyte diseases of the skin. *Arch Dermatol* 1981;117:667.

67. Smith KJ, Yeager J, Skelton HG. Histologically distinctive papular neutrophilic xanthomas in HIV-1+ patients. *Am J Surg Pathol* 1997;21:545.

68. Zelger BG, Orchard G, Rudolph P, et al. Scalloped cell xanthogranuloma. *Histopathology* 1998;32:368.

69. Ferrando J, Campo-Voegeli A, Soler-Carrillo J, et al. Systemic xanthohistiocytoma: a variant of xanthoma disseminatum? *Br J Dermatol* 1998;138:155.

70. Caputo R, Veraldi S, Grimalt R, et al. The various clinical patterns of xanthoma disseminatum. Considerations on seven cases and review of the literature. *Dermatology* 1995;190:19.

71. Battaglini J, Olsen TG. Disseminated xanthosiderohistiocytosis, a variant of xanthoma disseminatum, in a patient with a plasma cell dyscrasia. *J Am Acad Dermatol* 1984;11:750.

72. Nickoloff BJ, Wood GS, Chu M, et al. Disseminated dermal dendrocytomas. A new cutaneous fibrohistiocytic proliferative disorder? *Am J Surg Pathol* 1990;14:867.

73. Zelger B, Cerio R, Orchard G, et al. Histologic and immunohistochemical study comparing xanthoma disseminatum and histiocytosis X. *Arch Dermatol* 1992;128:1207.

74. Purvis WEI, Helwig EB. Reticulohistiocytic granuloma ("reticulohistiocytoma") of the skin. *Am J Clin Pathol* 1954;24:1005.

75. Hunt SJ, Shin SS. Solitary reticulohistiocytoma in pregnancy: immunohistochemical and ultrastructural study of a case with unusual immunophenotype. *J Cutan Pathol* 1995;22:177.

76. Zelger B, Cerio R, Soyer HP, et al. Reticulohistiocytoma and multicentric reticulohistiocytosis. Histopathologic and immunophenotypic distinct entities. *Am J Dermatopathol* 1994;16:577.

77. Toporcer MB, Kantor GR, Benedetto AV. Multiple cutaneous reticulohistiocytomas (reticulohistiocytic granulomas). *J Am Acad Dermatol* 1991;25:948.

78. Goltz RW, Laymon CW. Multicentric reticulohistiocytosis of the skin and synovia. *Arch Dermatol* 1954;69:717.

79. Barrow MV, Holubar K. Multicentric reticulohistiocytosis. A review of 33 patients. *Medicine (Baltimore)* 1969;48:287.

80. Campbell DA, Edwards NL. Multicentric reticulohistiocytosis: systemic macrophage disorder. *Baillieres Clin Rheumatol* 1991;5:301.

81. Torres L, Sanchez JL, Rivera A, et al. Progressive nodular histiocytosis. *J Am Acad Dermatol* 1993;29:278.

82. Snow JL, Muller SA. Malignancy-associated multicentric reticulohistiocytosis: a clinical, histological and immunophenotypic study. *Br J Dermatol* 1995;133:71.

83. Valencia IC, Colsky A, Berman B. Multicentric reticulohistiocytosis associated with recurrent breast carcinoma. *J Am Acad Dermatol* 1998;39:864.

84. Zelger BW, Staudacher C, Orchard G, et al. Solitary and generalized variants of spindle cell xanthogranuloma (progressive nodular histiocytosis). *Histopathology* 1995;27:11.

85. Taunton OD, Yeshurun D, Jarratt M. Progressive nodular histiocytoma. *Arch Dermatol* 1978;114:1505.

86. Burgdorf WH, Kusch SL, Nix TE Jr, et al. Progressive nodular histiocytoma. *Arch Dermatol* 1981;117:644.

87. Bork K, Hoede N. Hereditary progressive mucinous histiocytosis in women. Report of three members in a family. *Arch Dermatol* 1988;124:1225.

88. Gianotti F, Caputo R, Ermacora E, et al. Benign cephalic histiocytosis. *Arch Dermatol* 1986;122:1038.

89. Pena-Penabad C, Unamuno P, Garcia-Silva J, et al. Benign cephalic histiocytosis: case report and literature review. *Pediatr Dermatol* 1994;11:164.

90. Weston WL, Travers SH, Mierau GW, et al. Benign cephalic histiocytosis with diabetes insipidus. *Pediatr Dermatol* 2000; 17:296.

91. Gianotti R, Alessi E, Caputo R. Benign cephalic histiocytosis: a distinct entity or a part of a wide spectrum of histiocytic proliferative disorders of children? A histopathological study. *Am J Dermatopathol* 1993;15:315.

92. Rodriguez-Jurado R, Duran-McKinster C, Ruiz-Maldonado R. Benign cephalic histiocytosis progressing into juvenile xanthogranuloma: a non-Langerhans cell histiocytosis transforming under the influence of a virus? *Am J Dermatopathol* 2000;22:70.

93. Winkelmann RK, Muller SA. Generalized eruptive histiocytoma. *Arch Dermatol* 1963;88:586.

94. Caputo R, Alessi E, Allegra F. Generalized eruptive histiocytoma. A clinical, histologic, and ultrastructural study. *Arch Dermatol* 1981;117:216.

95. Caputo R, Ermacora E, Gelmetti C, et al. Generalized eruptive histiocytoma in children. *J Am Acad Dermatol* 1987;17:449.

96. Jang KA, Lee HJ, Choi JH, et al. Generalized eruptive histiocytoma of childhood. *Br J Dermatol* 1999;140:174.

97. Arnold ML, Anton-Lamprecht I. Multiple eruptive cephalic histiocytomas in a case of T-cell lymphoma. A xanthomatous stage of benign cephalic histiocytosis in an adult patient? *Am J Dermatopathol* 1993;15:581.

98. Wood GS, Hu CH, Beckstead JH, et al. The indeterminate cell proliferative disorder: report of a case manifesting as an unusual cutaneous histiocytosis. *J Dermatol Surg Oncol* 1985;11:1111.

99. Manente L, Cotellessa C, Schmitt I, et al. Indeterminate cell histiocytosis: a rare histiocytic disorder. *Am J Dermatopathol* 1997;19:276.

100. Levisohn D, Seidel D, Phelps A, et al. Solitary congenital indeterminate cell histiocytoma. *Arch Dermatol* 1993;129:81.

101. Vasef MA, Zaatari GS, Chan WC, et al. Dendritic cell tumors associated with low-grade B-cell malignancies. Report of three cases. *Am J Clin Pathol* 1995;104:696.

102. Wollenberg A, Burgdorf WH, Schaller M, et al. Long-lasting "christmas tree rash" in an adolescent: isotopic response of indeterminate cell histiocytosis in pityriasis rosea? *Acta Derm Venereol* 2002;82:288.

103. Rosenberg AS, Morgan MB. Cutaneous indeterminate cell histiocytosis: a new spindle cell variant resembling dendritic cell sarcoma. *J Cutan Pathol* 2001;28:531.

104. Rosai J, Dorfman RF. Sinus histiocytosis with massive lymphadenopathy. A newly recognized benign clinicopathological entity. *Arch Pathol* 1969;87:63.

104a. Destombes P. Adenites avec surcharge lipidique de l'enfant ou de l'adulte jeune, observées aux Antilles et au Malie (quatre observations) *Bull Soc Pathol Exot* 1965;58:1169.

105. Foucar E, Rosai J, Dorfman R. Sinus histiocytosis with massive lymphadenopathy (Rosai–Dorfman disease): review of the entity. *Semin Diagn Pathol* 1990;7:19.

106. Thawerani H, Sanchez RL, Rosai J, et al. The cutaneous manifestations of sinus histiocytosis with massive lymphadenopathy. *Arch Dermatol* 1978;114:191.

107. Perez A, Rodriguez M, Febrer I, et al. Sinus histiocytosis confined to the skin. Case report and review of the literature. *Am J Dermatopathol* 1995;17:384.

108. Annessi G, Giannetti A. Purely cutaneous Rosai–Dorfman disease. *Br J Dermatol* 1996;134:749.

109. Brenn T, Calonje E, Granter SR, et al. Cutaneous rosai-dorfman disease is a distinct clinical entity. *Am J Dermatopathol* 2002;24: 385.

110. Mac-Moune Lai F, Lam WY, Chin CW, et al. Cutaneous Rosai–Dorfman disease presenting as a suspicious breast mass. *J Cutan Pathol* 1994;21:377.

111. Innocenzi D, Silipo V, Giombini S, et al. Sinus histiocytosis with massive lymphadenopathy (Rosai–Dorfman disease): case report with nodal and diffuse muco-cutaneous involvement. *J Cutan Pathol* 1998;25:563.

112. Middel P, Hemmerlein B, Fayyazi A, et al. Sinus histiocytosis with massive lymphadenopathy: evidence for its relationship to macrophages and for a cytokine-related disorder. *Histopathology* 1999;35:525.

113. Boisseau-Garsaud AM, Vergier B, Beylot-Barry M, et al. Histiocytic sarcoma that mimics benign histiocytosis. *J Cutan Pathol* 1996;23:275.

113a. Frederickson DS, Levy RI, Lees RS. Fat transport in lipoproteins—an integrated approach to mechanisms and disorders. *N Engl J Med* 1967;276:32.

114. Cruz PD Jr, East C, Bergstresser PR. Dermal, subcutaneous, and tendon xanthomas: diagnostic markers for specific lipoprotein disorders. *J Am Acad Dermatol* 1988;19:95.

115. Braun-Falco O, Eckert F. Macroscopic and microscopic structure of xanthomatous eruptions. *Curr Probl Dermatol* 1991;20:54.

116. Cooper PH. Eruptive xanthoma: a microscopic simulant of granuloma annulare. *J Cutan Pathol* 1986;13:207.

117. Walsh NM, Murray S, D'Intino Y. Eruptive xanthomata with urate-like crystals. *J Cutan Pathol* 1994;21:350.

118. Parker F. Normocholesterolemic xanthomatosis. *Arch Dermatol* 1986;122:1253.

119. Kossard S, Winkelmann RK. Necrobiotic xanthogranuloma with paraproteinemia. *J Am Acad Dermatol* 1980;3:257.

120. Finan MC, Winkelmann RK. Necrobiotic xanthogranuloma with paraproteinemia. A review of 22 cases. *Medicine (Baltimore)* 1986;65:376.

121. Umbert I, Winkelmann RK. Necrobiotic xanthogranuloma with cardiac involvement. *Br J Dermatol* 1995;133:438.

122. Finan MC, Winkelmann RK. Histopathology of necrobiotic xanthogranuloma with paraproteinemia. *J Cutan Pathol* 1987; 14:92.

123. Chang SE, Choi JH, Sung KJ, et al. POEMS syndrome with xanthomatous cells. Polyneuropathy organomegaly endocrinopathy M-protein skin changes. *Am J Dermatopathol* 1999;21: 567.

124. Altmann J, Winkelmann RK. Diffuse normolipemic plane xanthoma. *Arch Dermatol* 1962;85:633.

125. Lynch PJ, Winkelmann RK. Generalized plane xanthoma and systemic disease. *Arch Dermatol* 1966;93:639.

126. Marcoval J, Moreno A, Bordas X, et al. Diffuse plane xanthoma: clinicopathologic study of 8 cases. *J Am Acad Dermatol* 1998; 39:439.

127. Horiuchi Y, Ito A. Normolipemic papuloeruptive Xanthomatosis in an infant. *J Dermatol* 1991;18:235.

128. Williford PM, White WL, Jorizzo JL, et al. The spectrum of normolipemic plane xanthoma. *Am J Dermatopathol* 1993;15:572.

129. Shafer WG. Verruciform xanthoma. *Oral Surg Oral Med Oral Pathol* 1971;31:784.

130. Mostafa KA, Takata T, Ogawa I, et al. Verruciform xanthoma of the oral mucosa: a clinicopathological study with immunohistochemical findings relating to pathogenesis. *Virchows Arch A Pathol Anat Histopathol* 1993;423:243.

131. Drummond JF, White DK, Damm DD, et al. Verruciform xanthoma within carcinoma in situ. *J Oral Maxillofac Surg* 1989;47:398.

132. Mohsin SK, Lee MW, Amin MB, et al. Cutaneous verruciform xanthoma: a report of five cases investigating the etiology and nature of xanthomatous cells. *Am J Surg Pathol* 1998;22:479.

133. Jensen JL, Liao SY, Jeffes EW 3rd. Verruciform xanthoma of the ear with coexisting epidermal dysplasia. *Am J Dermatopathol* 1992;14:426.

134. Meyers DC, Woosley JT, Reddick RL. Verruciform xanthoma in association with discoid lupus erythematosus. *J Cutan Pathol* 1992;19:156.

135. Smith KJ, Skelton HG, Angritt P. Changes of verruciform xanthoma in an HIV-1+ patient with diffuse psoriasiform skin disease. *Am J Dermatopathol* 1995;17:185.

136. Balus S, Breathnach AS, O'Grady AJ. Ultrastructural observations on "foam cells" and the source of their lipid in verruciform xanthoma. *J Am Acad Dermatol* 1991;24:760.

137. Furue M, Suzuki H, Kodama T, et al. Colocalization of scavenger receptor in CD68 positive foam cells in verruciform xanthoma. *J Dermatol Sci* 1995;10:213.

138. Goerdt S, Kretzschmar L, Bonsmann G, et al. Normolipemic papular xanthomatosis in erythrodermic atopic dermatitis. *J Am Acad Dermatol* 1995;32:326.

139. Darwin BS, Herzberg AJ, Murray JC, et al. Generalized papular xanthomatosis in mycosis fungoides. *J Am Acad Dermatol* 1992;26:828.

140. Parsad D, Saini R, Verma N. Xanthomatous reaction following contact dermatitis from vitamin E. *Contact Dermatitis* 1997;37:294.

27

PIGMENTARY DISORDERS OF THE SKIN

RICHARD L. SPIELVOGEL
GARY R. KANTOR

CONGENITAL DIFFUSE MELANOSIS

This condition, also termed *melanosis diffusa congenita* (1) or *generalized cutaneous melanosis* (2,3) is thought to be recessively inherited, appears at or shortly after birth, and demonstrates progressive diffuse hyperpigmentation. The pigmentation is most intense on the abdomen and back and may be reticulate in the axillae and groin. Thin nails (3) and yellow-white hair (1) have been noted.

Histopathology. Increased melanization is seen in both the basalar and midepidermal keratinocytes, along with melanophages in the superficial dermis.

Histogenesis. On electron microscopic examination, Braun–Falco et al. (1) noted increased numbers of single melanosomes in the keratinocytes and Klint et al. (3) described dispersion of melanosomes throughout the keratinocyte cytoplasm.

RETICULATE PIGMENTARY ANOMALIES

Numerous cutaneous disorders have been documented that are characterized by hyperpigmentation that is clinically seen in a reticulate, retiform, or fishnet-like pattern. These disorders are unified by increased melanin in the epidermis and exclude postinflammatory pigmentary alterations and conditions displaying reticulation secondary to vascular phenomena such as livedo reticularis.

Dyskeratosis congenita characteristically demonstrates an acquired reticulated brown hyperpigmentation, beginning in the first decade of life, and spreading across the neck, upper chest, and arms. The pigmentation is commonly associated with nail dystrophy, leukoplakia, bone marrow dysfunction, and a predisposition to malignancy (4).

Macular amyloidosis in the interscapular region may demonstrate a reticulate pattern (5). Progressive cribriform and zosteriform hyperpigmentation begins in the second decade of life with reticulate pigmentation of the lower half of the trunk or thighs in a dermatomal distribution (6). *Acropigmentation symmetrica of Dohi* (dyschromatosis symmetrica hereditaria) is a progressive autosomal dominant disorder that appears as hyperpigmented and hypopigmented macules on the face and dorsa of the hands and feet, progressing to cover the acral areas (7,8). *Reticulate acropigmentation of Kitamura* presents as slightly depressed hyperpigmented macules on the dorsal hands and feet that evolve to a reticulate pattern as the individual ages. There is progression to involve the extremities, lateral neck, and occasionally the trunk and face. There has been an association with palmar and plantar pits (9). Reticulate acropigmentation of Kitamura and *Dowling–Degos disease* (reticulate pigmented anomaly of the flexures) may appear together (10), supporting the concept that they are different expressions of a single disorder. In Dowling–Degos disease, a dominantly inherited dermatosis, heavily pigmented macules arranged in a reticulate pattern with a tendency to coalesce appear on flexural skin, axillae, lateral neck, inframammary and inguinal folds, antecubital and popliteal fossae, and intergluteal cleft, but may also be seen on the genitalia, inner thighs, chest, face, and abdomen (11). Extensive areas of the skin may be affected. Pitted perioral scars, hyperpigmented comedones, hidradenitis suppurativa, multiple cysts and abscesses, keratoacanthomas and squamous cell carcinomas have been associated.

The *Naegeli–Franceschetti–Jadassohn syndrome* (Naegeli's reticular pigmented dermatosis) is an autosomal-dominant inherited disorder with reticulate pigmentation involving the neck and flexural skin along with perioral and periocular skin (12). There are numerous associated findings including hypohidrosis, keratoderma, hypoplasia of finger-pad dermatoglyphics, and teeth and nail abnormalities. *Dermatopathia pigmentosa reticularis* (13) is similar to Naegeli's reticular pigmented dermatosis and the X-linked recessive syndrome of dyskeratosis congenita may also demonstrate reticulate hyperpigmentation.

Histopathology. The histologic findings in these conditions are quite similar. There is hyperpigmentation of the basalar keratinocytes with either a normal or slightly increased number of melanocytes. Dyskeratosis congenita demonstrates mild interface vacuolization with melanophages in the upper dermis (14). Reticulate acropigmentation of Kitamura and to a greater degree, Dowling–Degos disease, demonstrate digitated elongations of the hyperpigmented rete ridges with a tendency to spare the suprapapillary epithelium. In Dowling–Degos disease these thin, branching, heavily pigmented downward proliferations also involve the infundibula of follicles and in some instances horn cysts may be seen (11). Although there is no preceding inflammatory dermatosis in dermatopathia pigmentosa reticularis, clumps of melanin-laden melanophages are seen in the papillary dermis in a patchy distribution without overlying epidermal hyperpigmentation (15). Finally, reticulate macular amyloidosis demonstrates a patchy distribution of melanin within the amyloid globules, which are seen in the dermal papillae.

Histogenesis. These conditions are thought to be inherited, although the genes responsible for their expression have not been definitively identified. The majority of cases of dyskeratosis congenita demonstrate X-linked recessive inheritance mapped to the distal long arm of the X chromosome (16).

LINEAR AND WHORLED NEVOID HYPERMELANOSIS

This congenital or early-life disorder, occasionally familial, presents with multiple hyperpigmented linear streaks and whorls composed of small homogeneous tan to brown macules that frequently follow the lines of Blaschko (17,18). The pattern is the inverse of that found in hypomelanosis of Ito (18), and must be differentiated from resembling conditions including incontinentia pigmenti, epidermal nevus, and zebra-like hyperpigmentation (18,19).

Histopathology. There is hyperpigmentation of the basalar keratinocytes with prominent melanocytes (18,19). Pigmentary incontinence with melanophages in the papillary dermis is variably present (19,20).

Histogenesis. The genetic abnormality has not been defined, but developmental somatic mosaicism has been proposed as an explanation for this patterned hypermelanosis (17,18).

MELASMA

Melasma is an acquired, localized, usually symmetrical hyperpigmentation of the face occurring in women. The forehead, cheeks, upper lip, and chin are affected. It often is associated with pregnancy or the ingestion of oral contraceptives and is aggravated by sunlight.

Histopathology. An epidermal and a dermal type can be recognized, although frequently there is a combination of the two types. Melanin is significantly increased in all epidermal layers. Light and histochemical (dopa) studies reveal an increase in the number and activity of melanocytes that are engaged in increased formation, melanization, and transfer of pigment granules to keratinocytes and melanophages (21,22).

ADDISON'S DISEASE

Addison's disease represents a hypofunction of the adrenal cortex and is characterized by progressive weakness, hypotension, and hyperpigmentation of the skin and oral mucous membranes. In some cases hyperpigmentation is the initial clinical manifestation (23). The hyperpigmentation is generalized but is most pronounced on sun-exposed skin, at sites of pressure, and on the genitalia. Patchy oral mucosal pigmentation is often present.

Histopathology. The histologic findings simulate the normal findings in patients with naturally dark skin and are therefore not diagnostic. Increased amounts of melanin are seen in the basalar keratinocytes and often in the keratinocytes in the upper spinous layer. The number of melanocytes is not increased. Variable numbers of melanophages may be seen in the papillary dermis (24).

Histogenesis. Most commonly, Addison's disease is the result of an idiopathic atrophy of the adrenal glands on an autoimmune basis, with subsequent inadequate production of cortisol and aldosterone.

Addison's disease is often associated with other autoimmune diseases. Other causes of adrenal hypofunction include damage of adrenal glands by tuberculosis, metastatic carcinoma, and deep fungal infections.

The hyperpigmentation in Addison's disease is caused by an increased release of melanocyte-stimulating hormone (MSH) from the pituitary gland. Adrenocorticotropic hormone (ACTH) and MSH synthesis and secretion in the pituitary gland are linked. The increased production of ACTH and MSH in Addison's disease is a compensatory, feedback-controlled response to low adrenal gland activity.

POSTINFLAMMATORY PIGMENTARY ALTERATION

Pigment alteration in the skin from a preceding inflammatory disorder can produce clinical hypopigmentation, hyperpigmentation, or both. It occurs commonly in processes that affect the dermal–epidermal interface such as fixed drug eruptions, lichen planus, benign lichenoid keratosis, and erythema multiforme. In some individuals the alteration can be dramatic, producing dark pigmentation resembling primary melanocytic lesions or marked hypopigmentation resembling vitiligo. Wood's light accentuates epidermal melanin and is useful as a clinical tool in defining the nature and extent of pigmentary alteration.

Histopathology. Epidermal melanin is increased in clinical hyperpigmentation and decreased in clinical hypopigmentation. In both clinical forms of pigmentary alteration, melanophages are present in the superficial dermis, along with a variably dense infiltrate of lymphohistiocytes around superficial blood vessels and in dermal papillae (25) (Fig. 27-1). Necrotic keratinocytes and coarse collagen bundles in the papillary dermis are occasionally seen (25,26).

BERLOQUE DERMATITIS AND PHYTOPHOTODERMATITIS

Localized hyperpigmented patches produced by furocoumarin-containing oil of bergamot found in perfumes have a distinctive clinical presentation. The patches assume drop-like shapes resembling pendants (French: *berloque*), and are usually located on the sides of the neck or retroauricular areas. Plants containing furocoumarin produce a postinflammatory hyperpigmentation and include lime, wild and cow parsnip, wild carrot, bergamot orange, and fig (27). The dermatitis produced by celery results from a furocoumarin produced by a fungus infecting the celery.

Histopathology. Features identical to postinflammatory hyperpigmentation are found, including increased epidermal melanin and melanophages in the superficial dermis. Variable chronic inflammation is present.

CHEMICAL DEPIGMENTATION

Chemicals are capable of producing depigmentation that resembles vitiligo. Hydroquinones and phenols are the most common causes and are found in bleaching agents,

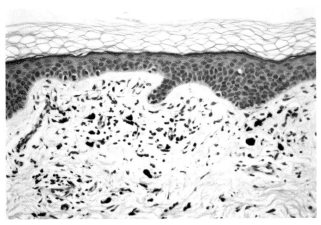

FIGURE 27-1. Postinflammatory hyperpigmentation. There are numerous melanophages in the papillary dermis along with a mild perivascular lymphocytic infiltrate. The epidermis is normal.

adhesives, cosmetics, photographic processing materials, and antioxidants used in the manufacture of rubber (28, 29). Depigmentation may also occur in body sites remote from chemical contact, presumably from systemic absorption or inhalation.

Histopathology. Features indistinguishable from vitiligo are found (28). Decreased or absent melanocytes are present with a variable superficial perivascular lymphocytic infiltrate.

IDIOPATHIC GUTTATE HYPOMELANOSIS

This common disorder of unknown cause produces a few or numerous sharply circumscribed white macules predominantly on the sun-exposed extensor surfaces of the extremities in persons over 30 years of age. They measure 2 to 6 mm in diameter and, once formed, do not enlarge (30).

Histopathology. In sections stained with the Fontana–Masson method, the melanin content in lesional skin is markedly reduced and there is either a significant reduction or an absence of dopa-positive melanocytes. The lesional borders are sharply demarcated. Within the hypomelanotic epidermis, the melanin granules are irregularly distributed (31). Immunoperoxidase studies confirm an absolute decrease in the number of melanocytes rather than a block in melanocyte differentiation (32).

Histogenesis. On electron microscopic examination, the scattered residual melanocytes in lesional skin are round and less dendritic with fewer melanosomes that are incompletely melanized (33).

PUVA-INDUCED PIGMENT ALTERATIONS

PUVA therapy consists of the oral ingestion or topical application of a furocoumarin-containing psoralen compound followed by patient exposure to high-intensity UVA radiation in a controlled-light-box setting. It is widely used for treating psoriasis and cutaneous T-cell lymphoma and less commonly used for a variety of other dermatoses including repigmentation therapy of vitiligo.

A spectrum of clinical and histologic changes is seen during and after PUVA therapy. Acutely, the phototoxic erythema peaks at 48 to 72 hours. Hyperpigmentation (tanning) is delayed for several days and is more pronounced and longer lasting than that induced by UVB exposure (34). Prolonged therapy leads to photoaging with cutaneous atrophy, fine wrinkling, mottled hyperpigmentation and hypopigmentation, telangiectasias, and loss of elasticity (35). Stellate lentigines or PUVA freckles often develop after prolonged therapy (36). There is also a dose-dependent increase in the risk of squamous cell carcinoma (37), especially in the genital areas (38).

Histopathology. The histologic changes of PUVA-induced acute phytotoxicity are similar to sunburn with numerous pink apoptotic cells ("sunburn cells") scattered throughout the epidermis. Early in the therapeutic course, the melanocytes in the basalar epidermis and keratinocytes in the mid spinous layer are heavily melanized. Prolonged therapy leads to gradual flattening of the rete ridges, telangiectasias, increased papillary dermal acid mucopolysaccharide deposition, thinning and basophilic degeneration of elastic fibers, and hyperplasia and fragmentation of elastic fibers (39). Hyperpigmented skin without other clinical changes frequently demonstrates small foci of keratinocytic nuclear atypia and loss of the normal maturation pattern (40). Actinic keratoses, Bowen's disease, and squamous cell carcinomas may develop. PUVA freckles or lentigines show increased numbers of melanocytes and elongation of the rete ridges with focal atypical melanocytes (41).

Histogenesis. On election microscopy, melanosomes are diffusely distributed throughout the epidermis (42). There is basement membrane thickening with focal dissolution. Elastic fibers in the dermis appear homogenized and fragmented (43). In the deep dermis, there is reduplication of the basal layer of capillaries and increased pinocytosis of endothelial cells (44).

DRUG-INDUCED PIGMENTARY ALTERATIONS

Drug-induced pigmentary alterations are quite common. Implicated agents include nonsteroidal anti-inflammatory drugs, antimalarials, tetracyclines, psychotropics including phenothiazines, antineoplastic agents including cytotoxics, heavy metals including gold, amiodarone, amitriptyline, and clofazimine (45,46). A variety of pathogenic mechanisms are seen including increased production of melanin leading to hyperpigmentation of basilar keratinocytes, vacuolar change at the dermoepidermal junction with pigmentary incontinence and dermal melanophages, binding of the drug to melanin and deposition of stable complexes, and deposition of the drug itself as granules in the dermal extracellular matrix or in macrophages. In addition, drugs may induce the synthesis of special pigments, such as lipofuscin, or damage blood vessels leading to red blood cell extravasation and hemosiderophages (45,46). Clinical features vary from generalized hyperpigmentation to specific patterns attributed to individual drugs such as the flagellated streaks attributed to bleomycin (47).

Histopathology. Minocycline may cause generalized bluish-brown pigmentation in a photodistribution due to increased basilar keratinocytic melanin, blue-black pigmentation of acne and other scars due to hemosiderin deposition in dermal macrophages, gray-blue pigmentation

of the anterior legs and arms due to deposition of drug complexes and protein extracellularly in the dermis and deposition on elastic fibers.

Antimalarial agents deposit pigment granules in dermal macrophages and extracellularly (45). Phenothiazines commonly deposit electron dense granules in dermal macrophages. The granules are composed of a drug metabolite and melanin leading to progressive blue pigmentation on sun-exposed skin (48). Amiodarone may provoke a photoallergic reaction with blue-gray pigmentation due to the deposition of lipofuscin granules in macrophages around superficial dermal blood vessels. These are accentuated by PAS staining. Lipofuscinosis may also be caused by antibiotics (45).

Chemotherapy agents commonly produce both generalized and localized hyperpigmentation of the basalar keratinocytes. Bleomycin, busulfan, doxorubicin, daunorubicin, flourouracil, cyclophosphamide, and carmustine additionally may demonstrate melanophages in the superficial dermis (47). Globules of mercury have been found in dermal and subcutaneous abscesses after oral ingestion (49).

PIGMENTARY PRESENTATIONS OF CUTANEOUS AND SYSTEMIC DISEASES

Mycosis fungoides may present with hypopigmented (50,51) or hyperpigmented (52) lesions. The former occurs in children and young adults, is slowly progressive, and often is present for many years before diagnosed. Sarcoidosis (53) may display hypopigmented skin lesions, but usually demonstrates some degree of clinical induration. Darier's (54) disease may also present with hypopigmentation. Although pigmented variants of basal cell carcinoma are not uncommon, pigmented Bowen's disease (55), pigmented Paget's disease (56), and depigmented extramammary Paget's disease (57) can be difficult to recognize clinically. Skin metastases from breast carcinoma may be pigmented and can even simulate malignant melanoma (58). Lastly, generalized hyperpigmentation may be the presenting sign of metastatic malignant melanoma and primary pituitary tumors (see also Addison's disease above).

Histopathology. The histologic changes are those of the primary dermatosis. In hypopigmented mycosis fungoides, variable melanin pigmentary incontinence occurs (51), whereas hyperpigmented mycosis fungoides shows striking melanin pigment in the basal layer and giant melanin pigment granules throughout the spinous layer (52). No alteration of melanocytes is present in hypopigmented sarcoidosis and no appreciable change in melanin pigment is noted (53). Decreased melanin pigment is seen in the basal layer of hypopigmented Darier's disease (54). Pigmented

Bowen's disease shows abundant melanin pigment in basal keratinocytes, highly dendritic melanocytes, and numerous melanophages (55). Pigmented Paget's disease and pigmented epidermotropic metastatic breast carcinoma demonstrate dendritic melanocytes at the dermoepidermal junction with variable melanin pigment in the cytoplasm of tumor cells (56). Normal numbers of melanocytes are present in depigmented extramammary Paget's disease, but epidermal melanization is markedly reduced (57). In generalized hyperpigmentation from metastatic melanoma or endocrinopathy, variable epidermal pigment and melanophages are present.

Histogenesis. Election microscopy of hypopigmented mycosis fungoides shows degenerative changes in melanocytes. The melanocytes demonstrate dilatation of rough endoplasmic reticulum, mitochondrial swelling, incompletely melanized melanosomes, and vacuolization and disintegration of the cytoplasm (59). Giant melanosomes are seen in keratinocytes of hyperpigmented mycosis fungoides and melanin granules are also present in the cytoplasm of mycosis and Langerhans cells (52). Fewer melanosomes are present within keratinocytes in hypopigmented sarcoidosis, and melanocytes feature variable degenerative changes (53).

ALBINISM

Albinism is a heritable disorder causing a generalized lack of pigmentation of the skin, hair, and eyes. Involvement of the eyes only is called ocular albinism and is X-linked recessive. Oculocutaneous albinism (OCA) affects both eyes and skin and is autosomal recessive.

There are at least ten types of OCA based on the degree of tyrosinase activity, hair color, and associated systemic disorders. Tyrosinase is a copper-containing enzyme responsible for the biosynthesis of melanin. Mutations to the tyrosinase gene result in inactivity of the enzyme (tyrosinase-negative OCA) and cause the most severe subtype (60). Tyrosinase activity can be detected in plucked anagen hair bulbs by radioisotope assay (61), or by incubation in tyrosine solution and examination for pigment formation. In tyrosinase-positive OCA, synthesis of melanin pigment is reduced but present and patients acquire some melanin pigment in hair, skin, and eyes beginning in childhood. Hair color varies from yellow (yellow-mutant OCA) to red (rufous OCA) to platinum (pt OCA) to brown (brown OCA) to black (black locks-albinism-deafness syndrome [BADS]). Associated systemic disorders include platelet defect and ceroid storage (Hermansky–Pudlak syndrome), defects in immunity (Chédiak–Higashi and Griscelli syndromes), and microphthalmia and mental retardation (Cross syndrome). Cutaneous malignancies, particularly squamous cell carcinoma, are frequent in all forms of albinism.

Prenatal diagnosis of OCA can be made by analysis of fetal skin biopsy for the tyrosinase gene in fetal cells obtained by amniocentesis (62).

Histopathology. Histologic examination shows the presence of basal melanocytes in skin and hair bulb; however, Fontana–Masson's stain fails to show any melanin. In patients with the tyrosinase-positive type of albinism, the epidermal melanocytes form pigment if sections of skin are incubated with dopa.

In the Hermansky–Pudlak syndrome, giant melanosomes are present along with melanophages in the dermis (63).

Histogenesis. Electron microscopic examination in OCA shows normally structured melanocytes in the epidermis (64). However, there is a reduction in the melanization of melanosomes. For instance, in tyrosinase-positive albinism, there are fewer melanized stage III and IV melanosomes, whereas in tyrosinase-negative albinism, the melanosomes contain no melanin and represent stage I and II melanosomes. Melanosome transfer to keratinocytes is not altered.

The tyrosinase gene has been localized in the long arm of chromosome 11 (65). Mutations in the protein-coding region of the gene are responsible for the tyrosinase-negative OCA. In contrast, tyrosinase-positive OCA has been mapped to the P gene on chromosome 15 and mutations of this gene are associated with a wide range of clinical manifestations (66).

PIEBALDISM (PATTERNED LEUKODERMA)

Piebaldism is an autosomally dominant disorder characterized by irregularly shaped depigmented patches that are present from birth and are associated in about 85% of the cases with a white forelock arising from a depigmented area in the center of the forehead. Depigmentation has a predilection for the ventral skin, that is, the center of the face, the ventral chest, and the abdomen. Small islands of hyperpigmentation, 1 to 5 cm in diameter are usually present within the depigmented areas. The condition used to be called partial albinism, but this term is no longer used because of the difference in pathogenesis between oculocutaneous albinism and piebaldism.

A variant of piebaldism is *Klein–Waardenburg syndrome*, also dominantly inherited, characterized by lateral displacement of the inner canthi of the eyes, heterochromia of the irides, and congenital deafness. About half of the patients have a white forelock, and about 12% have patches of depigmentation from birth.

Histopathology. The depigmented skin and hair usually have no melanocytes (67). Also, hair from the white forelock does not show darkening of the hair bulb on incubation in tyrosinase solution. In some cases, the forelock epidermis may show a few melanocytes that are dopa positive (68).

Histogenesis. Electron microscopic examination of the depigmented skin usually reveals a complete absence of melanocytes (68). In contrast, Langerhans cells are normal in appearance and distribution. In some instances, an occasional melanocyte is seen with unmelanized ellipsoidal or spherical melanosomes. Electron microscopy of plucked forelock hair reveals absence of melanin in the cortex, cuticle, and inner root sheath (68). The small hyperpigmented islands show many abnormal spherical, granular melanosomes.

A mutation of the gene that encodes melanocytic migration into the hair follicle and epidermis during embryonic development has been implicated (65).

VITILIGO

Vitiligo is an acquired, disfiguring, patchy, total loss of skin pigment. Stable patches often have an irregular border but are sharply demarcated from the surrounding skin. There may be surrounding hyperpigmented skin. In expanding lesions, there may rarely be a slight rim of erythema at the border and a thin zone of transitory partial depigmentation. Hairs in patches of vitiligo are white. The scalp and eyelashes are rarely affected. In generalized vitiligo, the face, upper trunk, dorsal hands, periorificial areas, and genitals are most commonly affected in a symmetrical fashion. Localized disease occurs as a linear, dermatomal patch (segmental vitiligo). Induction with trauma (Koebner phenomenon) and association with halo nevi occurs with generalized, but not segmental vitiligo.

In *Vogt–Koyanagi–Harada syndrome,* aseptic meningitis is often the initial symptom, followed by uveitis and dysacousia. Patches of vitiligo involving the skin and frequently also the eyelashes and scalp develop. There is often an association with alopecia areata.

Histopathology. The most prominent feature in vitiligo is the alteration of melanocytes at the dermoepidermal junction. With silver stains or the dopa reaction, well-established lesions of vitiligo are totally devoid of melanocytes. The periphery of expanding lesions, which are hypopigmented rather than completely depigmented, still show a few dopa-positive melanocytes and some melanin granules in the basal layer (69). In the outer border of patches of vitiligo, melanocytes are often prominent and demonstrate long dendritic processes filled with melanin granules. Early lesions show a superficial perivascular and occasionally lichenoid mononuclear cell infiltrate at the border. Focal areas of vacuolar change at the dermal–epidermal junction in association with a mild mononuclear cell infiltrate have been seen in the normal-appearing skin adjacent to vitiliginous areas (70,71). In long-standing lesions, degenerative changes in cutaneous nerves and adnexal structures have been reported (72).

Histogenesis. Electron microscopic studies (71,73) and immunohistochemistry studies using a panel of 17 monoclonal antibodies directed against melanocytes (74) confirm the complete absence of melanocytes in areas of long-standing vitiligo (Fig. 27-2). In the hypopigmented zone of expanding lesions, most melanocytes show signs of degeneration. Some studies have demonstrated peripheral damage to keratinocytes and melanocytes (75). A combination of hair follicle split-dopa stains and hair follicle split-scanning electron microscopy showed inactive, dopa-negative melanocytes in the outer root sheaths of normal hair follicles. These inactive melanocytes are also present in the outer root sheaths of hair follicle from vitiliginous patches. Treatment of vitiligo stimulates these inactive melanocytes in the middle and lower parts of the outer root sheaths to divide, proliferate, and migrate upward to the dermal–epidermal junction of overlying skin. Melanocytes then radiate to form the pigmented islands clinically visible in repigmented lesions (76,77).

Autoimmune mechanisms with an underlying genetic predisposition are the most likely cause of vitiligo, although neurohumoral and autocytotoxic hypotheses are al-

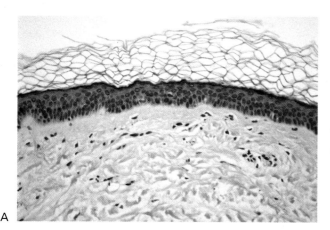
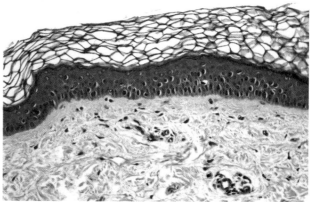

A   B

FIGURE 27-2. Vitiligo. **A:** There is a total loss of melanocytes in the depigmented skin near the border of this patch. **B:** S-100 protein immunoperoxidase staining confirms the loss of melanocytes although Langerhans and dermal dendritic cells stain positively.

ternative theories or contributing mechanisms. Antibodies to melanocytes have been found by immunoprecipitation in the sera of patients with vitiligo but not in normal sera (78). Also, sera from patients with vitiligo causes damage to melanocytes in cell cultures, suggesting that the antibodies present in these sera may be involved in the pathogenesis of vitiligo (79). Vitiligo patients have an increased association of known autoimmune disorders including thyroiditis, pernicious anemia, Addison's disease, diabetes, and alopecia areata. Lastly, patients with metastatic malignant melanoma may develop vitiligo (80). Evidence of cellular mechanisms in the pathogenesis include the finding of T cells expressing a cutaneous lymphocyte-associated antigen typical of skin-homing T cells are found at the edge of vitiligo patches. This finding is consistent with a hypothesis that lesional T cells rather than circulating antimelanocytic antibodies may be responsible for the patchy destruction of cutaneous melanocytes in vitiligo (81). Another study showed striking aberrations of T-cell subtypes in active areas of vitiligo when compared to static patches of disease (82).

CHÉDIAK–HIGASHI SYNDROME

The Chédiak–Higashi syndrome is a rare autosomally recessive disorder characterized by cutaneous, ocular, neurologic, and hematologic abnormalities. There is a greatly increased susceptibility to bacterial infections and a unique "accelerated phase" that often leads to death (83). The accelerated phase is manifested by fever, jaundice, hepatosplenomegaly, lymphadenopathy, pancytopenia, and widespread lymphohistiocytic organ infiltrates. Viruses, particularly Epstein–Barr virus, have been associated with triggering the accelerated phase. Giant lysosomal granules in the cytoplasm of circulating white blood cells are typical.

The Chédiak–Higashi syndrome is a subtype of oculocutaneous albinism (see earlier), and patients demonstrate fair skin with susceptibility to severe sunburn, silvery colored hair, and pale irides with photophobia and nystagmus. Severe and recurrent infections of the respiratory tract and skin are common.

Histopathology. Light microscopic features of skin sections show normal findings (84). Fontana–Masson's stain shows sparse melanin granules, some of which are grouped and others of which are larger than normal (84). Similar large, irregularly shaped melanin granules are scattered in the upper dermis within melanophages. Hair shafts also demonstrate abnormal aggregates of melanin (85).

The giant lysosomal granules can be demonstrated in peripheral blood, in skin (melanocytes or Langerhans cells), and other organs. A blood smear stained with Giemsa or Wright's stain shows the granules are azurophilic. They are found in all white blood cell lines but are most easily seen in neutrophils.

Histogenesis. Electron microscopic examination reveals within melanocytes giant melanosomes of irregular shape surrounded by a limiting membrane. They further increase in size by fusing with other giant particles. Within the giant melanosomes, one observes a granular matrix and filaments showing periodicity and varying degrees of pigmentation. The largest melanosomes show signs of degeneration leading to vacuolization and the formation of residual bodies. In addition, normal melanosomes are present in the melanocytes and are transferred to keratinocytes; however, they are packaged into abnormally large lysosomes. Similar abnormally large, membrane-bound lysosomes are found in the hair. The giant melanosomes in melanocytes and the giant lysosomes in keratinocytes form because of a defect in membrane or microtubule function. Hypopigmentation occurs because the melanosomes within keratinocytes are found within a relatively few large lysosomes rather than dispersed throughout the cell cytoplasm.

The giant granules in the cytoplasm of white blood cells develop by the fusion of primary lysosomes with one another and with cytoplasmic material. Even though microorganisms are phagocytized into phagocytic vacuoles in a normal fashion, their intracellular killing is delayed because of the unavailability of primary lysosomes to discharge their bacterial enzymes into the phagocytic vacuoles. Also, cathepsin G, a potent antimicrobial protease in neutrophils, is absent in Chédiak–Higashi syndrome.

Prenatal diagnosis of Chédiak–Higashi syndrome may be made by fetal blood sampling or study of amniotic fluid or chorionic villous cells (86).

REFERENCES

1. Braun-Falco O, Burg G, Selzle D, et al. Melanosis diffusa congenita. *Hautarzt* 1980;31:324.
2. Platin P, Sassolas B, Garanov J, et al. What is your diagnosis? Generalized cutaneous melanosis. *Ann Dermatol Venereol* 1990; 117:739.
3. Klint A, Oomen C, Geerts ML, et al. Congenital diffuse melanosis. *Ann Dermatol Venereol* 1987;114:11.
4. Schnur RE, Heymann WR. Reticulate hyperpigmentation. *Semin Cutan Med Surg* 1997;16:72–80.
5. Brownstein MH, Hashimoto K. Macular amyloidosis. *Arch Dermatol* 1972;106:50.
6. Rower JM, Carr RD, Lowney ED. Progressive cribriform and zosteriform hyperpigmentation. *Arch Dermatol* 1978;114:98.
7. Kim NI, Park SY, Youn JI, et al. Dyschromatosis symmetrica hereditaria affecting two families. *Korean J Dermatol* 1980;18: 585.
8. Oyama M, Shimizu H, Tajima S, et al. Dyschromatosis symmetrica hereditaria (reticulate acropigmentation of Dohi): report of a Japanese family with the condition and a literature review of 185 cases. *Br J Dermatol* 1999;140:491–496.
9. Kanwar AJ, Kaur S, Rajagopalan M. Reticulate acropigmentation of Kitamura. *Int J Dermatol* 1990;29:219.
10. Tappero JW, Kershenovich J, Berger TG. Combined acral and flexural reticulate pigmentary anomaly. *Arch Dermatol* 1992; 128:1411.

11. Wilson Jones E, Grice K. Reticulate pigmented anomaly of the flexures: Dowling–Degos disease, a new genodermatosis. *Arch Dermatol* 1978;114:1150.

12. Whiting DA. Naegeli's reticular pigmented dermatosis. *Br J Dermatol* 1971;85:71.

13. Maso MJ, Schwartz RA, Lambert C. Dermatopathia pigmentosa reticularis. *Arch Dermatol* 1990;126:935.

14. Costello MJ, Bunke CM. Dyskeratosis congenita. *Arch Dermatol* 1956;73:123–132.

15. Rycroft RG, Calnan CD, Allenby CF. Dermatopathia pigmentosa reticularis. *Clin Exp Dermatol* 1977;2:39.

16. Arngrimsson R, Dokai L, Luzatto L. Dyskeratosis congenita: three additional families show linkage to a locus in Xq28. *J Med Genet* 1993;30:618–619.

17. Kalter DC, Griffiths WA, Atherton DJ. Linear and whorled nevoid hypermelanosis. *J Am Acad Dermatol* 1988;19:1037–1044.

18. Akiyama M, Aranami A, Sasaki Y, et al. Familial linear and whorled nevoid hypermelanosis. *J Am Acad Dermatol* 1994;30:831–833.

19. Mendiratta V, Sharman RC, Arya L, et al. Linear and whorled nevoid hypermelanosis. *J Dermatol* 2001;28:58–59.

20. Hofmann U, Wagner N, Grimm T, et al. Linear and whorled nevoid hypermelanosis. Case report and review of the literature. *Hautarzt* 1998;49:408–412.

21. Sanchez NP, Pathuk MA, Sato S, et al. Melasma: a clinical, light microscopic, ultrastructural and immunofluorescence study. *J Am Acad Dermatol* 1981;4:698.

22. Koon WH, Yoon KH, Lee ES, et al. Melasma: histopathological characteristics in 56 Korean patients. *Br J Dermatol* 2002;146:228–237.

23. Clerkin EP, Sayegh S. Melanosis as the initial symptom of Addison's disease. *Lahey Clin Foundation Bull* 1966;15:173.

24. Montgomery H, O'Leary PA. Pigmentation of the skin in Addison's disease, acanthosis nigricans, and hemochromatosis. *Arch Dermatol* 1930;21:970.

25. Ackerman AB. *Histologic Diagnosis of Inflammatory Skin Diseases.* Philadelphia: Lea & Febiger, 1978:178.

26. Murphy GF. *Dermatopathology: A Practical Guide to Common Disorders.* Philadelphia: Saunders, 1995:322.

27. Storer JG, Rasmussen JE. Plant dermatitis. *J Am Acad Dermatol* 1983;9:1.

28. Fisher AA. Differential diagnosis of idiopathic vitiligo. Part III. Occupational leukoderma. *Cutis* 1994;53:278.

29. Fisher AA. Differential diagnosis of idiopathic vitiligo from contact leukoderma: Part II. Leukoderma due to cosmetics and bleaching creams. *Cutis* 1994;53:232.

30. Cummings KI, Cottel WI. Idiopathic guttate hypomelanosis. *Arch Dermatol* 1966;93:184.

31. Ortonne JP, Perrot H. Idiopathic guttate hypomelanosis: Ultrastructural study. *Arch Dermatol* 1980;116:664.

32. Wallace ML, Grichnik JM, Prieto VG, et al. Numbers and differentiation status of melanocytes in idiopathic guttate hypomelanosis. *J Cutan Pathol* 1998;25:375–379.

33. Ploysangam T, Dee-Ananlap S, Suvanprakorn P. Treatment of idiopathic guttate hypomelanosis with liquid nitrogen: light and electron microscopic studies. *J Am Acad Dermatol* 1990;23:681.

34. Abel EA. Acute and chronic side effects of PUVA therapy: clinical and histologic changes. In Abel EA, ed. *Photochemotherapy in Psoriasis.* New York: Igaku-Shoin, 1992:.

35. Pfau RG, Hood AF, Morrison WC. Photoaging: the role of UVB, solar-simulated UVB, visible, and psoralen UVA radiation. *Br J Dermatol* 1986;114:318.

36. Miller RA. Psoralens and UVA-indicated stellate hyperpigmented freckling. *Arch Dermatol* 1982;118:619.

37. Stern RS, Laird N, Melski J, et al. Cutaneous squamous cell carcinoma in patients treated with PUVA. *N Engl J Med* 1984;310:1156.

38. Stern RS, Members of Photo Chemotherapy Follow-up Study. Genital tumors among men with psoriasis exposed to psoralens and ultraviolet A radiation (PUVA) and ultraviolet B radiation. *N Engl J Med* 1990;322:1093.

39. Bergfeld WF. Histologic changes in skin after photo chemotherapy. *Cutis* 1977;20:504.

40. Abel EA, Cox AJ, Farber EM. Epidermal dystrophy and actinic keratoses in psoriasis patients following oral psoralen photo chemotherapy (PUVA). *J Am Acad Dermatol* 1982;7:333.

41. Rhodes AR, Harrist TJ, Momtaz TK. The PUVA-induced pigmented macule: a lentiginous proliferation of large, sometimes cytologically atypical melanocytes. *J Am Acad Dermatol* 1983;9:47.

42. Hashimoto K. Psoralen-UVA treated psoriatic lesions: ultrastructural changes. *Arch Dermatol* 1978;114:711.

43. Zelickson AS, Mottaz JH, Zelickson BD, et al. Elastic tissue changes in skin following PUVA therapy. *J Am Acad Dermatol* 1980;3:186.

44. Torras H, Bombi JA. PUVA therapy: long term degenerative effects. II. Study of ultrastructural changes in the skin induced by PUVA therapy. *Med Cutan Ibero Lat Am* 1987;15:179.

45. Crowson NA, Magro CM. The dermatopathology of drug eruptions. *Curr Prob Dermatol* 2002;14:117–146.

46. Dereure O. Drug-induced skin pigmentation. *Am J Clin Dermatol* 2001;2:253–262.

47. Weedon D. *Skin Pathology.* London: Churchill Livingstone, 1997.

48. MacMorran WS, Krahn LE. Adverse reactions to psychotropic drugs. *Psychosomatics* 1997;38:413–422.

49. Jun JB, Min PK, Kim DW, et al. Cutaneous nodular reaction to mercury. *J Am Acad Dermatol* 1997;37:858–862.

50. Zackheim HS, Epstein EH, Grekin DA, et al. Mycosis fungoides presenting as areas of hypopigmentation. *J Am Acad Dermatol* 1982;6:340–345.

51. Whitmore SE, Simmons-O'Brien E, Rotter FS. Hypopigmented mycosis fungoides. *Arch Dermatol* 1994;130:476–480.

52. David M, Shanon A, Hazaz B, et al. Diffuse, progressive hyperpigmentation: an unusual skin manifestation of mycosis fungoides. *J Am Acad Dermatol* 1987;16:257–260.

53. Clayton R, Breatnach A, Martin B, et al. Hypopigmented sarcoidosis in the negro. *Br J Dermatol* 1977;96:119–125.

54. Peterson CM, Lesher JL, Sangueza OP. A unique variant of Darier's disease. *Int J Dermatol* 2001;40:278–280.

55. Krishnan R, Lewis A, Orengo IF, et al. Pigmented Bowen's disease (squamous cell carcinoma in situ): a mimic of malignant melanoma. *Dermatol Surg* 2001;27:673–674.

56. Requena L, Sangueza M, Sangueza OP, et al. Pigmented mammary Paget disease and pigmented epidermotropic metastases from breast carcinoma. *Am J Dermatopathol* 2002;24:189–198.

57. Chen Y, Wong T, Lee JY. Depigmented genital extramammary Paget's disease: a possible histogenetic link to Toker's clear cells and clear cell papulosis. *J Cutan Pathol* 2001;28:105–108.

58. Shamal-Lubovitz O, Rothem A, Ben-David E, et al. Cutaneous metastatic carcinoma of the breast mimicking malignant melanoma, clinically and histologically. *J Am Acad Dermatol* 1994;31:1058–1060.

59. Breathnach SM, McKee PH, Smith MP. Hypopigmented mycosis fungoides: report of 5 cases with ultrastructural observations. *Br J Dermatol* 1982;106:643–659.

60. Spritz RA, Strunk KM, Biebel LB, et al. Detection of mutations in the tyrosinase gene in a patient with type IA oculocutaneous albinism. *N Engl J Med* 1990;322:1724–1728.

61. King RA, Olds DP. Hair bulb tyrosinase activity in oculocutaneous albinism: suggestions for pathway control and block location. *Am J Med Genet* 1985;20:49–55.

62. Shimizu H, Nizeki H, Suzumori K, et al. Prenatal diagnosis of oculocutaneous albinism by analysis of the fetal tyrosinase gene. *J Invest Dermatol* 1994;103:104–106.

63. Biswas S, Lloyd IC. Oculocutaneous albinism. *Arch Dis Child* 1999;80:565–569.

64. Hishida H. Electron microscopic studies of melanosomes in oculo-cutaneous albinism. *Jpn J Dermatol [A]* 1973;83:119.

65. Tomita Y. The molecular genetics of albinism and piebaldism. *Arch Dermatol* 1994;130:355–358.

66. Lee S, Nicholls RD, Bundey S, et al. Mutations of the P gene in oculocutaneous albinism, ocular albinism, and Prader–Willi syndrome plus albinism. *N Engl J Med* 1994;330:529–534.

67. Winship I, Young K, Martell R. Piebaldism: an autonomous autosomal dominant entity. *Clin Genet* 1991;39:330–337.

68. Chang T, McGrae JD, Hashimoto K. Ultrastructural study of two patients with both piebaldism and neurofibromatosis I. *Pediatr Dermatol* 1993;10:224–234.

69. Brown J, Winkelmann RK, Wolfe K. Langerhans' cells in vitiligo. *J Invest Dermatol* 1967;49:386–390.

70. Moellmann G, Klein-Angerer S, Scollay DA, et al. Extra cellular granular material and degeneration of keratinocytes in the normally pigmented epidermis of patients with vitiligo. *J Invest Dermatol* 1982;79:321–330.

71. Galadari E, Mehregan AH, Hashimoto K. Ultrastructural study of vitiligo. *Int J Dermatol* 1993;32: 269–271.

72. Gokhale BB, Mehta LN. Histopathology of vitiliginous skin. *Int J Dermatol* 1983;22:477–480.

73. Birbeck MS, Breathnach AS, Everall JD. An electron microscope study of basal melanocytes and high-level clear cells (Langerhans' cells) in vitiligo. *J Invest Dermatol* 1961;37:51–64.

74. LePoole IC, van den Wijngaard RM, Westerhof W, et al. Presence or absence of melanocytes in vitiligo lesions: an immunohistochemical investigation. *J Invest Dermatol* 1993;100:816–822.

75. Bhawan J, Bhutani LK. Keratinocyte damage in vitiligo. *J Cutan Pathol* 1983;10:207–212.

76. Cui J, Shen LY, Wang GC. Role of hair follicles in the repigmentation of vitiligo. *J Invest Dermatol* 1991;97:410–416.

77. Arrunategui A, Arroyo C, Garcia L, et al. Melanocyte reservoir in vitiligo. *Int J Dermatol* 1994;33: 484–487.

78. Naughton GK, Eisinger M, Bystryn J. Detection of antibodies to melanocytes in vitiligo by specific immunoprecipitation. *J Invest Dermatol* 1983;81:540–542.

79. Norris DA, Kissinger RM, Naughton GM, et al. Evidence for immunologic mechanisms in human vitiligo: patients' sera induce damage to human melanocytes in vitro. *J Invest Dermatol* 1988;90:783–789.

80. Nordlund JJ, Kirkwood JM, Forget BM, et al. Vitiligo in patients with metastatic melanoma: a good prognostic sign. *J Am Acad Dermatol* 1983;9:689–696.

81. Badri AM, Todd PM, Garioch JJ, et al. An immunohistological study of cutaneous lymphocytes in vitiligo. *J Pathol* 1993;170: 149–155.

82. Mozzanica N, Frigerio V, Finzi AF, et al. T-cell subpopulations in vitiligo: a chronobiologic study. *J Am Acad Dermatol* 1990;22: 223–230.

83. Barak Y, Nir E. Chédiak–Higashi syndrome. *Am J Pediatr Hematol Oncol* 1987;9:42–55.

84. Carillo-Farga J, Gutierrez-Palomera G, Ruiz-Maldonado R, et al. Giant cytoplasmic granules in Langerhans' cells of Chédiak–Higashi syndrome. *Am J Dermatopathol* 1990;12:81–87.

85. Anderson LL, Paller AS, Malpass D, et al. Chédiak–Higashi syndrome in a black child. *Pediatr Dermatol* 1992;9:31–36.

86. Diukman R, Tanigawara A, Cowan MJ, et al. Prenatal diagnosis of Chédiak–Higashi syndrome. *Prenat Diagn* 1992;12:877–885.

BENIGN PIGMENTED LESIONS AND MALIGNANT MELANOMA

DAVID E. ELDER
ROSALIE ELENITSAS
GEORGE F. MURPHY
XIAOWEI XU

Melanocytic proliferations are composed of one or more of three related types of cells: melanocytes, nevus cells, or melanoma cells, each of which may be located in the epidermis or in the dermis. Melanocytes are solitary dendritic cells that generally are separated from one another by other cells (keratinocytes or fibroblasts). Localized proliferation of melanocytes may occur, giving rise to benign or malignant melanocytic neoplasms, characterized by melanocytes that lie in contiguity with one another to form a tumor. Benign tumors of melanocytes are generally called "melanocytic nevi," while malignant tumors are called "malignant melanomas," and the cells of these lesions are called "nevus cells" or "melanoma cells," respectively. Although the term "melanoma" was at one time taken to include benign pigmented lesions, this is now considered to be synonymous with "malignant melanoma," and the two terms will be used interchangeably in this chapter. Major morphologic differences among melanocytes, nevus cells, and melanoma cells are summarized in Table 28-1.

Melanocytic lesions are of importance primarily because of malignant melanoma, which is the single most common potentially lethal neoplasm of the skin. The incidence of melanoma has risen dramatically over the last several decades. However, the mortality has risen less dramatically than the incidence, likely due to earlier diagnosis. There is considerable geographic variation in the incidence of melanoma, related to exposure to sunlight and the susceptibility of the population. Thus, the global incidence is highest in the Australian tropics, but very low in most other tropical countries with their less susceptible populations.

Benign melanocytic nevi occur in all ethnic groups, although there is evidence for shared etiologic factors with melanoma, with a greater incidence in susceptible populations living in sunny climates. Nevi and other benign pigmented lesions are occasionally of cosmetic significance, especially in the case of giant or so-called "garment" congenital nevi. Other than cosmetically, nevi are of impor-tance primarily in relation to melanoma. Thus, nevi are important as simulants of melanoma, as potential precursors of melanoma, and as markers of individuals at increased risk for melanoma. Because nevi are simulants of melanoma both clinically and histologically, criteria that distinguish between nevus and melanoma are of critical importance. This differential diagnosis, especially at the histologic level, is the primary topic of this chapter.

BENIGN PIGMENTED LESIONS

Benign pigmented lesions composed of epidermal melanocytes include freckles, solar lentigines ("actinic" or formerly senile lentigo), the melanotic macules of Albright's syndrome, and Becker's melanosis. The cafe-au-lait patches of neurofibromatosis have been described elsewhere. Benign pigmented lesions derived from dermal melanocytes include the Mongolian spot, the nevi of Ota and of Ito, and the blue nevus. Benign tumors of nevus cells are called melanocytic nevi. They can be divided into junctional nevi including lentigo simplex, compound nevi, and intradermal nevi. There are special variants of melanocytic nevi, the more important of which include the Spitz nevus, pigmented spindle-cell nevus, congenital melanocytic nevus, and dysplastic nevus.

DERMAL MELANOCYTOSES AND HAMARTOMAS

It is important to distinguish dermal melanoses caused by the presence of melanocytes in the dermis from those produced by the presence of melanin free within the dermis. Clinically, the two different processes may have very similar appearances (1). In this section we consider the former condition. Dermal melanosis associated with metastatic

TABLE 28-1. MELANOCYTES, NEVUS CELLS, AND MELANOMA CELLS

Melanocytes	Nevus Cells	Melanoma Cells
Cytoplasm is dendritic	Rounded or spindle	Rounded or spindle
Cells are solitary	Arranged in clusters	In clusters and large sheets
Nuclei are small and regular	Nuclei of most cells are small and regular	Most nuclei are large, irregular, and hyperchromatic
Mitoses are rare	Mitoses are rare	Mitoses are usually present

melanoma is discussed in a later section of this chapter, while inflammatory disorders associated with pigmentary alterations are discussed in Chapter 27.

Mongolian Spot

The typical Mongolian spot occurs in the sacrococcygeal region as a uniformly blue discoloration resembling a bruise. It consists of a noninfiltrated, round or ovoid, rather ill-defined patch of varying size. It is found very frequently in Mongoloid and Negroid infants, but it also occurs occasionally in Caucasoid infants. It is present at birth and usually disappears spontaneously within 3 to 4 years (2).

Occasionally, Mongolian spots occur outside the lumbosacral region as aberrant Mongolian spots, such as on the middle or upper part of the back; they may then be multiple and bilateral and persist. Extensive and persistent Mongolian spots are commonly seen in patients with bilateral nevus of Ota (3).

Histopathology. In the Mongolian spot, the dermis shows in its lower half or two thirds greatly elongated, slender, often slightly wavy dendritic cells containing melanin granules. These cells are present in a low concentration and lie widely scattered between the collagen bundles, and like the collagen bundles, they generally lie parallel to the skin surface. No melanophages are seen.

Nevi of Ota and of Ito and Dermal Melanocyte Hamartoma

Nevi of Ota and Ito and dermal melanocyte hamartoma are types of dermal melanocytosis that differ from the Mongolian spot by usually having a speckled rather than a uniform blue appearance and by showing a greater concentration of dermal melanocytes, with location in the upper rather than in the lower portion of the dermis (3–6).

The *nevus of Ota* represents a usually unilateral discoloration of the face composed of blue and brown, partially confluent macules. The periorbital region, temple, forehead, malar area, and nose are usually involved. Because of this usual distribution, Ota called the lesion *nevus fusco-ceruleus ophthalmomaxillaris.* There is frequently also a patchy blue discoloration of the sclera of the ipsilateral eye and occasionally also of the conjunctiva, cornea, and retina. In some instances, the oral and nasal mucosa is similarly af-

fected. In about 10% of the cases, the lesions of the nevus of Ota are bilateral rather than unilateral. They may be present at birth; they may also appear during the first year of life or during adolescence but only rarely in childhood. They have a tendency toward gradual extension. Malignant change in the cutaneous lesions of a nevus of Ota is extremely rare (3).

In the nevus of Ota, the involved areas of the skin show a brown to slate blue uniform or mottled discoloration, usually without any infiltration. Occasionally, some areas are slightly raised. In some patients, discrete nodules varying in size from a few millimeters to a few centimeters and having the appearance of blue nevi are found within the areas of discoloration. Persistent Mongolian spots are quite common in association with the nevus of Ota. Extensive Mongolian spots are typically found in bilateral cases of nevus of Ota (3).

The *nevus of Ito* differs from the nevus of Ota by its location in the supraclavicular, scapular, and deltoid regions. It may occur alone or in association with an ipsilateral or bilateral nevus of Ota (4,6). Like the nevus of Ota, it has a mottled, macular appearance.

In the *dermal melanocyte hamartoma,* there may be a single, very extensive area of gray-blue pigmentation present from the time of birth. Histologic and ultrastructural examinations reveal numerous dermal melanocytes (5). The involvement may be nearly generalized (7). In other instances, there are several coalescing blue macules that have gradually extended within a circumscribed area from the time of childhood (8).

Histopathology. The noninfiltrated areas of the nevus of Ota, as well as the nevus of Ito and the dermal melanocyte hamartoma, show, like the Mongolian spot, elongated, dendritic melanocytes scattered among the collagen bundles. However, in these three forms of dermal melanocytosis, the melanocytes generally are more numerous and more superficially located than in the Mongolian spot. Although most of the fusiform melanocytes lie in the upper third of the reticular dermis, melanocytes may also occur in the papillary layer, and may extend as far down as the subcutaneous tissue. Melanophages are seen in only few lesions (5,7). A histologic classification of Ota's nevus has been proposed according to the distribution of the dermal melanocytes from superficial to deep. This correlates with the color and location of the nevus, and probably with response to therapy (9).

Slightly raised and infiltrated areas show a larger number of elongated, dendritic melanocytes than do noninfiltrated areas, thus approaching the histologic picture of a blue nevus, and nodular areas are indistinguishable histologically from a blue nevus (10).

Malignant changes in lesions of nevus of Ota have been reported in a handful of cases (11). The histologic appearance of the tumors may be that of a malignant or cellular blue nevus (12). In a few instances, a primary melanoma of the choroid, iris, orbit, or brain has developed in patients with a nevus of Ota involving an eye (13,14). A benign or low-grade lesion termed a melanocytoma of the meninges may also occur (15).

Histogenesis of the Dermal Melanocytoses

The blue color of the dermal melanocytoses depends on the phenomenon whereby light passing through the skin is scattered as it strikes dark particles, such as melanin. Owing to the Tyndall effect, the colors of light that have a longer wavelength, such as red, orange, and yellow, tend to be less scattered and therefore continue to travel in a forward direction, but the colors of shorter wavelength, such as blue, indigo, and violet, are scattered to the side and backward to the skin surface. This phenomenon is also responsible for the distinctive color of blue nevi.

The Mongolian spot is a result of the delayed disappearance of dermal melanocytes. On electron microscopy, the dermal melanocytes are seen to contain numerous fully melanized melanosomes. Only a few melanocytes show premelanosomes as evidence of ongoing melanoneogenesis (2).

Because the concentration of melanocytes in the nevi of Ota and Ito and in the dermal melanocyte hamartoma is greater than in the Mongolian spot, it has been suggested that these lesions are nevoid or hamartomatous, analogous to the blue nevus. Although the lesional cells are considered to be melanocytes, the DOPA reaction may be negative, likely due to all melanogenic enzyme having been consumed in heavily pigmented melanocytes (5).

BLUE NEVI

Blue nevi generally occur on the skin, although in rare instances, they have been observed in mucous membranes (16). On the skin, three types of benign blue nevi are recognized: the common blue nevus, the cellular blue nevus, and the combined nevus. In addition, there are malignant blue nevi, discussed in a later section.

Histologically, the common feature of blue nevi is the presence of pigmented spindle and dendritic melanocytes in a focal area of the reticular dermis, associated unlike the dermal melanocytoses with alterations in the dermal collagen architecture.

In a recent study, persistence and recurrence of blue nevi was discussed, demonstrating that blue nevi of all histologic types and combinations are capable of persistence with clinical recurrence (17). The persistence usually is histologically similar to the original, but in some cases is more "cellular" and/or atypical. Limited follow-up of these cases has not demonstrated frankly malignant behavior. Clinical recurrence may also be associated with malignancy of a blue nevus-like lesion, but this study demonstrates that malignant tumor progression is not necessarily the case. In the absence of necrosis en masse, marked cytologic atypia, and frequent mitotic figures, recurrence of a blue nevus or a cellular blue nevus is likely to be a benign phenomenon (17). However, we would recommend complete excision and follow-up for such lesions.

Common Blue Nevus

The *common blue nevus* occurs as a small, well-circumscribed, dome-shaped nodule of slate blue or blue-black color (Fig. 28-1A). The lesion rarely exceeds 1 cm in diameter. Common blue nevi are frequently found on or near the dorsa of the hands and feet, as well as on the scalp. Usually, there is only one lesion, but there may be several. A rare manifestation is the plaque type of blue nevus, which shows within a circumscribed area numerous macules and papules. This type of lesion may be present at birth (18) or may become clinically apparent later in life (19). Malignant degeneration has not been reported in the common blue nevus.

Histopathology. In the common blue nevus, the melanocytes have a similar appearance to those seen in the Mongolian spot and in the nevus of Ota, but they are typically larger and their density is much greater. Greatly elongated, slender, often slightly wavy melanocytes with long, occasionally branching dendritic processes lie grouped in irregular bundles in the dermis (Fig. 28-1B, C, and D). The bundles of cells may extend into the subcutaneous tissue or lie close to the epidermis. However, the epidermis is normal, except in the combined nevus. The greatly elongated melanocytes lie predominantly with their long axis parallel to the epidermis. Most of them are filled with numerous fine granules of melanin, often so completely that their nuclei cannot be visualized. The melanin granules also characteristically fill the long, often wavy, occasionally branching dendritic processes. Wavy fiber bundles similar to nerves may be present, indicative of Schwannian differentiation (20). Occasionally, lesional cells are seen in the perineurium of authentic nerves, a finding that is not indicative of malignancy. Melanophages are frequently seen near the bundles of melanocytes, but are usually not numerous or dense. The melanophages differ from the melanocytes by being shorter and thicker, by showing no dendritic processes, and by containing larger granules. In contrast to the melanocytes, the melanophages are DOPA negative. The

malignancy and recurrences tend to be more cellular than the original lesions, the behavior may be benign in the absence of compelling indicators of malignancy, such as necrosis, high-grade atypia, and mitoses (17).

Cellular Blue Nevus

The *cellular blue nevus* (CBN) consists of a blue nodule that is usually larger than the common blue nevus. It generally measures 1 to 3 cm in diameter, but it may be larger. It shows either a smooth or an irregular surface. About half of all cellular blue nevi have been located over the buttocks or in the sacrococcygeal region (27–29). Although rare, malignant degeneration of cellular blue nevi can occur (28).

Histopathology. The profile of a CBN is often distinctive at scanning magnification, with an often bulky, heavily pigmented cellular tumor often spanning the reticular dermis, and not associated with an overlying *in situ* melanoma (Figs. 28-2A through E). In lesions that enter the subcutis there is often a cellular nodule at the base, connected to the overlying tumor in a "dumbbell" pattern. Areas of deeply pigmented dendritic melanocytes, as seen also in the common type of blue nevus, are admixed with cellular islands composed of closely aggregated, rather large spindle-shaped or more epithelioid cells with ovoid nuclei and abundant pale cytoplasm often containing little or no melanin. Melanophages with abundant melanin may be present between the islands. Although pigment is usually prominent, amelanotic CBN have been described (30). Four histologic subtypes have been recognized: mixed biphasic, alveolar, fascicular or neuronevoid (also known as the monophasic spindle-cell type), and atypical varieties (28). In the common mixed-

biphasic type, there are clusters of epithelioid cells with somewhat clear cytoplasm, between which there are fascicles of spindle cells (Fig. 28-2E). Pigment is usually more prominent in the latter. The monophasic spindle-cell type is somewhat more problematic and may overlap with spindle-cell tumorigenic melanomas and with malignant blue nevi. The absence of an overlying *in situ* component may help to rule out the former. Attributes that may suggest malignancy in a CBN are discussed in the Malignant Blue Nevus section. They include frequent mitoses, high-grade cytologic atypia, and spontaneous tumor necrosis or ulceration.

Larger islands composed of spindle-shaped cells may consist of many intersecting bundles of cells extending in various directions and resembling the storiform pattern seen in a neurofibroma. In some of the intersecting bundles, the cells appear round, perhaps as a result of cross-sectioning. Not infrequently, the cellular islands penetrate into the subcutaneous fat, often forming a bulbous expansion there that is highly characteristic of cellular blue nevi (the dumbbell pattern).

Lesions termed "atypical" blue nevi have become recognized as a rare but distinct variant of cellular blue nevi, characterized by unusual features including architectural atypia (infiltrative margin and/or asymmetry) and/or cytologic atypia (hypercellularity, nuclear pleomorphism, hyperchromasia, occasional mitotic figures, and/or subtle necrosis) (27,28,31). Although most of these lesions have a benign course, a few cellular blue nevi (not necessarily all "atypical") have been locally aggressive (32,33) or have metastasized at least to regional lymph nodes (34,35), and a guarded prognosis is appropriate in the presence of more than a few mitoses (see Melanocytic Tumors of Uncertain

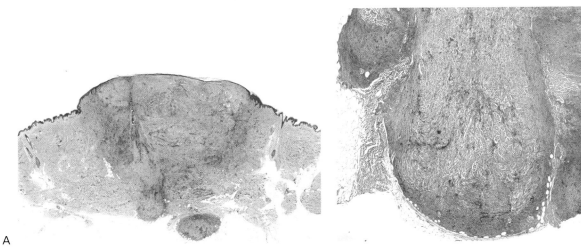

A

B

FIGURE 28-2. (A) Cellular blue nevus. Usually broader at its surface than its base, the cellular blue nevus spans the reticular dermis, usually involving the superficial panniculus. There is often a region of increased cellularity that may form a bulbous expansion at the base. A small satellite lesion, as seen here, is an unusual finding. **(B)** The bulbous expansion where the lesion meets the panniculus at the base is a characteristic but not an invariable finding. *(continued)*

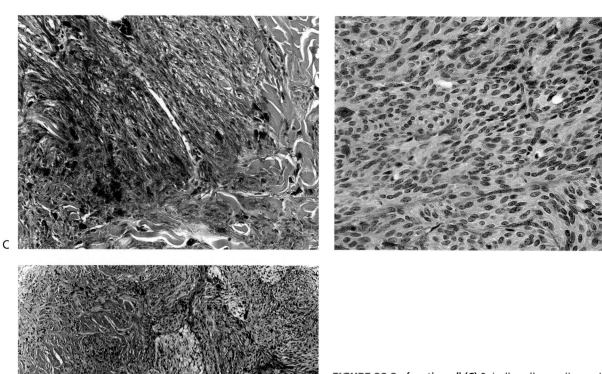

FIGURE 28-2. *(continued)* **(C)** Spindle cells usually predominate in cellular blue nevi. They lie in contiguity with one another, unlike the cells of common blue nevi, most of which are separated from one another by collagen bundles. **(D)** In other areas, it is common to find sheets of cuboidal cells with pale cytoplasm in a cellular blue nevus. **(E)** This mixed biphasic pattern is a distinctive feature of many cellular blue nevi, with ovoid islands of polygonal cells with somewhat clear cytoplasm alternating with spindle cells, the latter often pigmented. Mitoses are very rare in most examples. Changes at the periphery may be indistinguishable from those of a common blue nevus.

Potential section near end of chapter). The absence or scarcity of mitotic figures and the absence of areas of necrosis or of high-grade atypia are evidence against a diagnosis of malignant blue nevus, and the presence of areas of dendritic, blue nevus type cells elsewhere in the tumor as well as the lack of a characteristic intraepidermal component argue against a diagnosis of melanoma.

In several instances, in which cellular blue nevi were excised with regional lymph nodes under the mistaken diagnosis of melanoma, moderately pleomorphic cells of cellular nevus have been found in the regional lymph nodes, often in the marginal sinuses or in the capsule (36), but sometimes more massively involving the node (35). It is sometimes assumed that these cells do not represent true metastases but were passively transported to the lymph nodes and lodged there as inert deposits. However, some examples of this phenomenon in our experience have shown high-grade uniform atypia, necrosis, and fairly numerous mitoses, apparently indicative of an active neoplasm. Some of these lesions may best be interpreted as "metastatic tumors of uncertain potential."

Combined Nevus

The term *combined nevus* is applied to the association of a blue nevus with an overlying melanocytic nevus (37), or to other combinations of benign nevi (38). Clinically, combined nevi often present with a focal area of deep pigmentation.

Histopathology. In a combined nevus, one component is often a congenital pattern nevus in which pigmented spindle cells form a focal collection of fascicles among nests of ordinary nevus cells. The fascicles tend to be organized along the lines of a blue nevus that may be either a common or a cellular blue nevus. The other component may be an overlying nevus of the junctional, compound, intradermal or, rarely, Spitz nevus types (38). Such lesions may simulate melanoma clinically, because of the appearance of a very darkly pigmented spot within a background nevus. Histologically, the pigmented spindle cells of the blue nevus component may give rise to suspicion based on apparent asymmetry of pigment distribution, but mitoses and high-grade atypia are absent, and the pigmented cells often blend with the background nevus rather than displacing or destroying it. Further, it is extremely unusual for a melanoma to arise in the dermal component of a nevus in the absence of a characteristic intraepidermal component.

Histogenesis of Blue Nevi

There is general agreement that the cells of the common blue nevus are melanocytes, which may show evidence of Schwannian differentiation. This occasional resemblance to neural tumors had led in the past to suggestions of neural origin for blue nevi (39). However, the lesional cells of blue nevi and their variants react positively with antibodies to the S-100 and HMB-45 antigens, the latter in this context being quite specific for melanocytic differentiation (40). Also, melanosomes are present by electron microscopy (EM 48), and the electron microscopic DOPA reaction indicates that the spindle-shaped cells of the cellular blue nevus have melanogenic potential (41).

FRECKLES AND HYPERPIGMENTATIONS

By definition, a freckle (ephelis) is a small flat tan or brown lesion that histologically shows increased pigment in keratinocytes, but no increase in the number of melanocytes. Hyperpigmentations may be described as larger, macular pigmented lesions that show increased melanin pigment in keratinocytes without melanocytic proliferation. Lentigines are macular hyperpigmentations that differ from freckles and hyperpigmentations in that the number of epidermal melanocytes is increased within the basal cell layer. However, in common parlance, the term "freckle" is often used to refer both to ephelides and to solar lentigines, as well as other forms of macular hyperpigmentations. Ephelides appear early in childhood and are associated with fair skin type and red hair. Solar lentigines appear with age and are a sign of photodamage. Both lesions are strong risk indicators for melanoma and nonmelanoma skin cancer. Melanocortin-1-receptor (MC1R) gene variants are also associated with fair skin, red hair, and melanoma and nonmelanoma skin cancer. In a large case-control study, carriers of MC1R gene variants had a markedly increased risk of developing ephelides, whereas the risk of developing severe solar lentigines was moderately increased, suggesting that MC1R is a major gene controlling susceptibility to the development of these forms of macular hyperpigmentations (42).

Ephelides (Freckles)

Freckles, or ephelides, are small, red-brown, macules scattered over skin exposed to the sun. Exposure to the sun deepens the pigmentation of freckles, in contrast to lentigo simplex whose already deep pigment does not change.

Ephelides, simple lentigines, and solar lentigines are difficult to distinguish from one another clinically, and are considered together in most clinical and epidemiologic studies. Taken together, these lesions constitute a significant risk factor for the development of melanoma (43).

Histopathology. Freckles show hyperpigmentation of the basal cell layer, but in contrast to lentigo simplex, there is no elongation of the rete ridges and, by definition, no obvious increase in the concentration of melanocytes. However, in a study of lesions from children using DOPA preparations, melanocyte frequencies in freckles were significantly greater than in adjacent nonpigmented skin. Cellular atypia of melanocytes was noticed in four of six freckles. Reactivity of melanocytes for HMB-45 was noticed in two freckles, compared with no reactivity in adjacent skin (44). It is likely that freckles represent a hyperplastic and hyperactive response of melanocytes to UV light.

Histogenesis. On electron microscopy, the melanocytes within freckles are found to be essentially similar to those of dark-skinned persons. Melanocytes of the surrounding epidermis, by contrast, show constitutionally fewer and minimally melanized melanosomes, many of which are rounded rather than elongated (45). Such round melanosomes are characteristic of the lightly pigmented skin of individuals with red hair and/or blue eyes and a cutaneous phenotype that is prone to freckles.

Melanotic Macules of Albright's Syndrome

Albright's syndrome usually is characterized by unilateral polyostotic fibrous dysplasia, precocious puberty in females, and melanotic patches. The patches generally are large in size and few in number, are located on only one side of the midline, often on the same side as the bone lesions, and have a jagged, irregular border, like the "coast of Maine," in contrast to the smooth "coast of California" type of border of the cafe-au-lait patches of neurofibromatosis.

Histopathology. Except for hyperpigmentation of the basal layer, there is no abnormality, and both the number and size of the melanocytes are normal (46).

Differential Diagnosis. The melanotic macules of Albright's syndrome only rarely show the "giant" melanin granules that are commonly seen in some of the melanocytes and keratinocytes within the cafe-au-lait patches of neurofibromatosis. Histologically, the melanotic macules may be indistinguishable from ephelides without correlative clinical information.

Mucosal Melanotic Macules (Mucosal Lentigines)

These benign lesions present as a pigmented patch on a mucous membrane. Common locations include vermilion border of the lower lip, the oral cavity, the vulva and, less often, the penis. These lesions may simulate melanoma clinically but histologically there is no contiguous melanocytic proliferation and no significant atypia. Because there may be a slight increase in number of melanocytes, though there is no nest formation, the term "genital lentiginosis" has proposed for those lesions affecting genital paramucosae (47). The lesions may be synonymously referred to as "mucosal lentigo" or "mucosal melanotic macule."

In the common location on the vulva ("vulvar lentigo"), this process may appear quite alarming clinically, presenting as a broad, irregular and asymmetric patch of brown to blue-black hyperpigmentation, often meeting the "ABCD" criteria for melanoma discussed below (48). Similar lesions may also be seen on penile skin (47). The lesions may be multicentric with alternating areas of normal and pigmented mucosa resembling areas of partial regression of a melanoma. The lesions are entirely macular, which would be unusual in an invasive melanoma. The so-called "labial lentigo" ("labial melanotic macule" [49]), a hyperpigmented macule of the lip, is closely related to the lesions of genital skin. It is rarely biopsied because the clinical appearances are characteristic and do not suggest malignancy. These lesions are uniformly pigmented light brown, usually completely macular, and usually about <6 mm in diameter. These macules are biologically indolent (50).

Histopathology. Upon initial inspection, a biopsy specimen may appear normal. The findings include mild acanthosis without elongation of rete ridges, and hyperpigmentation of basal keratinocytes, often best recognized in comparison with surrounding epithelium, in association with scattered melanophages in the dermis. Although melanocytes may be normal in number, in most instances they are slightly increased (47,51). Because of this slight increase in number, the lesions are termed lentigines by strict histologic criteria (47). In contrast to true melanocytic neoplasms (nevi or melanomas), the cell bodies of the lesional melanocytes are separated by those of keratinocytes, that is, there is no contiguous proliferation of melanocytes. Occasionally, especially in the penile and vulvar lesions, there are prominent dendrites of melanocytes ramifying among the hyperpigmented keratinocytes. There may be associated mild keratinocytic hyperplasia, and scattered melanophages in the papillary dermis, resulting from pigmentary incontinence, may account for the blue-black color and the pigmentary variegation that may simulate melanoma clinically.

Differential Diagnosis. The histologic distinction from radial growth phase melanoma is easy because of the absence of neoplastic (contiguous) melanocytic proliferation and cytologic atypia of melanocytes.

Pathobiology. The process appears likely to be one of reactive hyperplasia with some features of post-inflammatory hyperpigmentation, rather than a neoplasm (52). The phenomenon is benign with associated lesional growth stabilization over time.

Becker's Melanosis

Becker's melanosis, also called Becker's pigmented hairy nevus, occurs most commonly as a large, unilateral patch showing hyperpigmentation and hypertrichosis on the shoulder, back, or chest of an adult male (53). Usually, the patch is sharply but irregularly demarcated, but occasionally the lesion presents as coalescing macules instead of a solitary patch. The lesion commonly appears during the second decade of life. In some instances, Becker's melanosis affects areas other than the shoulder and chest. Also, it may be multiple and bilateral, and may occasionally be found in women.

In one report, nine cases of melanoma in association with Becker's nevus were described (54). Five of these were on the same body site as the nevus. It remains to be determined whether these reports represent a greater incidence than chance would suggest.

The hairiness always appears after the pigmentation, and, quite frequently, no hypertrichosis is seen. It is therefore possible that cases described as progressive cribriform and zosteriform hyperpigmentation represent a variant of Becker's melanosis without hypertrichosis (55).

Of interest is the association of a pilar smooth muscle hamartoma with Becker's melanosis. In such cases, the area of Becker's melanosis may show slight perifollicular papular elevations or slight induration (56).

Histopathology. The epidermis shows slight acanthosis and regular elongation of the rete ridges. There is hyperpigmentation of the basal layer, and melanophages are seen in the upper dermis. The number of melanocytes is increased. This increase is particularly evident when melanocytes are stained for dopaoxidase activity in both involved and uninvolved skin nearby (57). The hair structures appear normal or increased in number.

An increase in smooth muscle fibers exists in nearly all cases, although it may be slight (58). In cases with an associated smooth muscle hamartoma, irregularly arranged, thick bundles of smooth muscle are present in the dermis (56). The term Becker nevus syndrome has been proposed for a phenotype characterized by the presence of a particular type of organoid epithelial nevus showing hyperpigmentation, increased hairiness and hamartomatous augmentation of smooth muscle fibers (smooth muscle hamartoma), and other developmental defects such as ipsilateral hypoplasia of breast and skeletal anomalies including scoliosis, spina bifida occulta, or ipsilateral hypoplasia of a limb (59).

The melanomas that have been described in association with Becker's nevus have been of the superficial spreading type, originating in the epidermis (54).

LENTIGINES

Lentigines are macular hyperpigmentations in which the number of epidermal melanocytes is increased and there are no nests of melanocytes as are present, by definition, in nevi. The term "lentigo" is derived from the Latin "lenz" meaning lens or lentil (60). Thus, the term in its original usage is clinical, referring to a small ovoid or lens-shaped pigmented spot. The term has come to be applied to larger pigmented lesions, especially those that recapitulate to a greater or lesser extent the histologic features of a lentigo simplex: basal proliferation of melanocytes arranged as single cells rather than in nests, typically but not always associated with elongation of the rete ridges. This pattern of melanocytic proliferation is termed "lentiginous." Lentiginous melanocytic proliferation is seen in the macules of solar lentigo and lentigo simplex, and in the macular or plaque components of lentiginous junctional and compound nevi, of lentiginous dysplastic nevi, and of melanomas of the lentigo maligna, acral, and mucosal-lentiginous types.

Solar Lentigo (Actinic Lentigo)

Solar lentigines commonly occur as multiple lesions in areas exposed to the sun, such as the face and extensor surfaces of the forearms, but most commonly on the dorsa of the hands. The lesions rarely occur before the fifth decade and, therefore, were often referred to as senile lentigo (61). However, sun exposure, rather than age, is the eliciting factor. Thus, the lesions do not occur on sun-protected skin, even in the elderly. Solar lentigines are commonly seen in sun-exposed Caucasoids. They are not indurated, possess a uniform dark brown color, and have an irregular outline. They vary in diameter from minute to >1 cm, and may coalesce. Solar lentigines, like ephelides, are risk markers for the development of melanoma (62), and are commonly numerous in the skin around melanomas, as seen in melanoma re-excision specimens. Lesions termed "sunburn freckles" by some clinicians may overlap clinically and his-

tologically with actinic lentigines. They are blotchy macular areas of tan hyperpigmentation, often of the order of one centimeter in diameter, that often appear on the shoulders or other sun-exposed areas of a young person after a severe sunburn (63). Other potentially related lesions are intensely dark, perfectly macular reticulated lesions that have been called "reticulated lentigo" (64) or "ink spot lentigo" (65).

Solar lentigines differ from ephelides in that they are more prevalent, increase in prevalence and number with higher age (ephelides which tend to decline in number), and are most prevalent on the trunk and occur more frequently in males than in females, unlike ephelides, which are more evenly distributed (66).

Solar lentigines and relatively flat seborrheic keratoses may resemble each other in clinical appearance, and both are commonly referred to as "liver spots" or "age spots." Seborrheic keratoses in general show more hyperkeratosis clinically. In contrast, lentigo maligna differs from solar lentigo in clinical appearance by its irregular distribution of pigment, often in a finely reticulated pattern, and by its greater asymmetry and border irregularity.

Prolonged treatment with psoralen and ultraviolet light A (PUVA) can induce formation of pigmented macules ("PUVA lentigines") in the irradiated areas. These are similar to solar lentigines but their color is darker and their pigment is more irregularly distributed (67).

Histopathology. The rete ridges are significantly elongated. They either appear club-shaped or are tortuous and show small, bud-like extensions. The elongated rete ridges are composed, especially in their lower portion, of deeply pigmented basaloid cells intermingled with melanocytes. The melanocytes appear significantly increased in number in some cases, but only slightly or not at all increased in others (68) (Fig. 28-3). They possess a heightened capacity

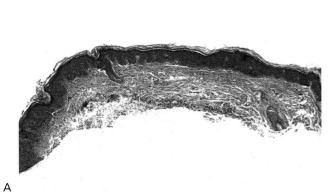
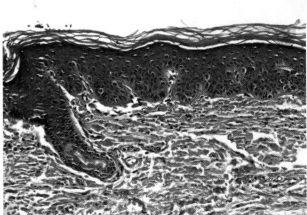

FIGURE 28-3. Actinic lentigo. **(A)** Scanning magnification shows a localized area of elongated rete ridges in elastotic actinically damaged skin. **(B)** Higher magnification shows basal hyperpigmentation, and slight to moderate prominence of melanocytes, without contiguous proliferation. Sometimes there is slight atypia of randomly scattered melanocytes (mild random atypia).

for melanin production, as shown by the fact that, on staining with DOPA, they display more numerous as well as longer and thicker dendritic processes than the melanocytes of control skin (69). The upper dermis shows elastosis and often contains scattered melanophages and occasionally a mild, perivascular lymphoid infiltrate.

Solar lentigines differ histologically from ephelides by definition, in having an increased number of epidermal melanocytes. However, in some lesions, the proliferation may be demonstrable only by formal counting (70). In contrast to lentigo simplex, lentiginous nevi, and lentiginous melanomas, the melanocytic proliferation is noncontiguous.

In some lesions, the rete ridges are elongated to such an extent that strands of basaloid cells form anastomosing branches, resulting in a reticulated pattern closely resembling that seen in the reticulated pigmented type of seborrheic keratosis from which they differ by the absence of horn cysts (68).

PUVA-induced pigmented macules represent solar lentigines on the basis of irregular elongation of their rete ridges. They show an increased number of large melanocytes that may appear slightly atypical (71).

The lesion called large-cell acanthoma, which presents as a slightly scaly tan macule on photodamaged skin, is identified histologically by having epidermal keratinocytes with nuclei roughly twice the size of adjacent keratinocytes, with minimal nuclear pleomorphism. There are clinical, histologic, and immunohistochemical overlapping characteristics with solar lentigo, suggesting that large-cell acanthoma should be considered as a related condition (72).

In the reticulated or "ink-spot" lentigo, histologic evaluation, including electron microscopy and DOPA-incubated vertical sections, demonstrated lentiginous hyperplasia of the epidermis, marked hyperpigmentation of the basal layer with "skip" areas that involved the rete ridges, and a minimal increase in the number of melanocytes (65).

Histogenesis. By electron microscopy, the basal layer of keratinocytes contains increased melanosomes and melanosome complexes, and the melanosome complexes within keratinocytes appear larger than those found in uninvolved skin (68). Even in the upper layers of the epidermis, including the horny layer, numerous melanosomes are present largely in a dispersed state rather than as complexes.

Differential Diagnosis. In lentigo simplex as in solar lentigo, the rete ridges are elongated, but in contrast, the lesional melanocytes are more obviously increased in number and focally lie in contiguity with one another. Lentigo maligna shows flattening or absence of the rete ridges together with continuous contiguous proliferation and uniform atypia of its melanocytes; like lentigo simplex, however, it may be associated with a dermal lymphocytic infiltrate. In actinic lentigo, the lesional melanocytes do not lie in contiguity with one another, even though they may be increased in number. There is only slight cytologic

atypia, and no pagetoid melanocytosis of melanocytes above the basal layer.

Lentigo Simplex and Related Lesions

Lentigines are macular hyperpigmentations in which the number of epidermal melanocytes is increased. In solar lentigines, as described above, the cell bodies are separated from one another by those of keratinocytes, and the proliferation may be termed "noncontiguous." The proliferation may be described as "contiguous" if the cell bodies at least focally touch one another, as in lentigo simplex (and also in lentiginous nevi and in lentiginous melanomas).

Lentigo simplex most frequently arises in childhood, but it may appear at any age (73). Usually in lentigo simplex, there are only a few scattered lesions without predilection to areas of sun exposure. They are small, symmetrical, and well-circumscribed macules that are evenly pigmented but vary individually from brown to black (Fig. 28-4A). They are not indurated and usually measure only a few millimeters in diameter. Clinically a lentigo simplex is indistinguishable from a junctional nevus. Special forms of lentigo simplex are lentiginosis profusa, the multiple lentigines syndrome or leopard syndrome, and speckled lentiginous nevus, also referred to as nevus spilus.

Lentiginosis profusa shows innumerable small, pigmented macules either from birth or starting in childhood or early adulthood without any other abnormalities. The mucous membranes are spared. There may be a family history (74,75). *Agminated* or *segmental lentigines* have been defined as a circumscribed group of small, pigmented macules arranged in a small or large group, often in a segmental pattern, each macule consisting of a lentiginous intraepidermal proliferation of melanocytes (76,77). The *speckled lentiginous nevus*, or *nevus spilus*, consists of a light brown patch or band present from the time of birth that in childhood becomes dotted with small, dark brown macules (78,79).

The *multiple lentigines syndrome*, a dominant trait, is characterized by the presence of thousands of flat, dark brown macules on the skin but not on the mucous surfaces. The lentigines begin to appear in infancy and gradually increase in number. Although most macules vary from pinpoint dots to 5 mm in diameter, some dark spots are much larger, up to 5 cm in diameter. Features of this rare syndrome known also by the mnemonic *leopard syndrome,* in addition to the lentigines (L), may include electrocardiographic conduction defects (E), ocular hypertelorism (O), pulmonary stenosis (P), and abnormalities of the genitalia (A) consisting of gonadal or ovarian hypoplasia, retardation of growth (R), and neural deafness (D). Not all of these manifestations are present in every case. Cardiomyopathy may also be present and associated with significant mortality (80). Another syndrome associated with lentigines is known under the acronyms *NAME* or *LAMB* or

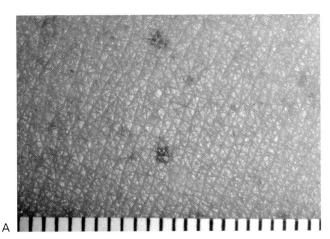
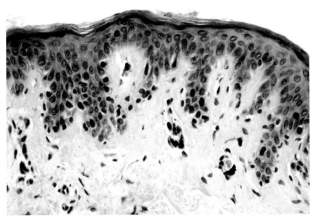

A

B

FIGURE 28-4. Lentigo simplex. **(A)** Clinically, the lesions are small, usually <2mm, fairly symmetrical, and well circumscribed. It is not possible to distinguish clinically among ephelides, simple lentigines, and lentiginous junctional nevi. (Clinical photograph courtesy of Peter Wilson.) **(B)** Melanocytes are present in contiguity near the tips and sides of elongated rete ridges, or lentiginous proliferation. There is no continuous proliferation between the rete. The presence of at least a single nest would define a *lentiginous junctional nevus* (*jentigo*).

myxoma syndrome (lentiginous nevi, atrial and/or mucocutaneous myxomas, myxoid neurofibromas, ephelides, blue nevi). It has been proposed that these mnemonics be dropped because the particular features encompassed within this syndrome are unclear, and the term "cutaneous lentiginosis with atrial myxomas" is an adequate description of this syndrome (81). The Carney complex, a familial multitumoral syndrome, comprises spotty skin pigmentation (lentigines and blue nevi), myxomas (heart, skin, and breast), endocrine "overactivity" usually manifested by endocrine tumors (adrenal cortex, pituitary, testis, and thyroid), schwannomas, and two unusual pigmented tumors, epithelioid blue nevus (skin), and psammomatous melanotic schwannoma (skin, viscera or nerve tissue). Carney complex has been linked to chromosome 2p16 and the PRKAR1A gene at 17q22–24 (82).

The *Peutz–Jeghers syndrome* shows dark brown macules clinically resembling lentigines in the perioral region. Similar macules are seen on the vermilion border and the oral mucosa and, often, the dorsa of the fingers. Although a few cases of this dominantly inherited disorder have shown only the pigmentary anomaly, there are usually multiple polyps in the gastrointestinal tract, mainly in the small intestine (83,84). Although early reports did not demonstrate a predisposition to cancer in patients with this syndrome, more recent studies have described an increased risk for both gastrointestinal and extra-gastrointestinal cancers. Women with the Peutz–Jeghers syndrome have an extremely high risk for breast and gynecologic cancer. Recently, a Peutz–Jeghers syndrome susceptibility gene, encoding the serine threonine kinase

STK11 (also called LKB1), was identified in this syndrome (85). A complex of PJS-like pigmentation without polyposis, designated as isolated mucocutaneous melanotic pigmentation (IMMP), has recently been described, and also appears to be associated with increased risk of cancer in diverse organs (86).

Histopathology. Lentigines, in general, show a slight or moderate elongation of the rete ridges, an increase in the concentration of melanocytes in the basal layer, an increase in the amount of melanin in both the melanocytes and the basal keratinocytes, and melanophages in the upper dermis. The melanocytes in the epidermis lie in focal contiguity with one another near the tips and sides of the elongated rete, but the proliferation is not continuous between the rete (Fig. 28-4B). There are no nests by definition. In some instances, melanin is also seen in the upper layers of the epidermis, including the stratum corneum. A mild inflammatory infiltrate may be intermingled with the melanophages within the underlying papillary dermis. In lesions otherwise clinically characteristic of lentigo simplex, small nests of nevus cells are commonly seen at the epidermal–dermal junction, especially at the lowest pole of rete ridges. The lesions then combine features of a lentigo simplex and a junctional nevus, leading to their descriptive diagnosis as "jentigo" (76), or "lentiginous junctional nevus." Because of the existence of these transitional forms, the lentigo simplex is regarded as a potential precursor of what may become a melanocytic nevus, and is discussed as such in a later section.

In *lentiginosis profusa* and the *multiple lentiginosis syndromes,* as a rule, the lesions are "pure" lentigines without the formation of nevus cell nests. In larger macules, however, there may be junctional nevus cell nests, and there may even be nevus cell nests in the upper dermis (87).

In *speckled lentiginous nevus*, or nevus spilus, the light brown patch or band shows the histologic features of lentigo simplex. The speckled areas show junctional nests of nevus cells at the lowest pole of some of the rete ridges, diffuse lentiginous melanocytic proliferation, as well as dermal aggregates of nevus cells. Various types of nevi (e.g., junctional nevi, blue nevi, and Spitz nevi) may present in the same lesion over time, and histologic features of congenital melanocytic nevi may be present within the spots, suggesting that these lesions may be considered as variants of congenital nevi (79).

In the lesions of *Peutz–Jeghers syndrome*, the basal cell layer shows marked hyperpigmentation. Although the number of melanocytes may appear to be slightly increased, no increase has been found in DOPA-stained sections (88). The intestinal polyps appear to be hamartomas, because glands are intermingled with smooth muscle bundles (85).

The presence of occasional giant melanin granules has been described in various forms of lentigines and lentiginous nevi, as well as in other conditions associated with hyperpigmentation, including the cafe-au-lait spots of neurofibromatosis and, less commonly, in cafe-au-lait spots without neurofibromatosis, and, on occasion, even in normal skin of healthy persons (89,90). Thus, they have no diagnostic specificity. Giant melanin granules vary in size from 1 to 6 μm. Because of their size and heavy melaniza-

tion, the larger granules are readily recognized by light microscopy. Although seen largely within melanocytes, they also occur in keratinocytes and melanophages to which they have been transferred, although many are too large for conventional donation by affected melanocytes to keratinocytes. On electron microscopy, the giant melanin granules have been termed macromelanosomes, and are regarded as autolysosomes referred to as "melanin macroglobules" and representing lysosome-mediated accumulation of melanosomes to form massive rounded to ellipsoid melanized bodies (91).

Table 28-2 summarizes some of the salient clinical and histologic features observed in the various forms of hyperpigmentations and lentigines.

MELANOCYTIC NEVI

Common Melanocytic Nevus

Although the term "nevus" may refer to a variety of hamartomatous and/or neoplastic lesions in the skin, the unqualified term in common usage and in this chapter refers to a *melanocytic nevus,* which is generally considered to be a benign neoplastic proliferation of melanocytes. Nevi vary considerably in their clinical appearance. In addition to the pathologic variants, which will be discussed separately, five clinical types may be recognized: (a) flat lesions, (b) slightly elevated lesions often with a raised center and a flat periphery, (c) papillomatous lesions, (d) dome-shaped lesions,

TABLE 28-2. HYPERPIGMENTATIONS AND LENTIGINES

	Clinical	Basal Layer	Melanocytes	Features
Ephelid	Sun-exposed skin, decrease with age, darker with exposure	Increased melanin	No increase by routine histology	HMB-45 reactivity, rounded melanosomes
Melanotic macule, Albright's syndrome	Fibrous dysplasia, precocious puberty Albright's syndrome	Increased melanin	Normal in number and size	
Mucosal lentigines	Lower lip, genital skin	Increased melanin	Appear normal to slightly increased	Mild acanthosis, pigment incontinence
Becker's melanosis	Unilateral, hypertrichosis	Increased melanin	Increased	Elongation of rete, smooth muscle fibers in dermis
Solar lentigo	Sun-exposed skin, increase with age	Increased melanin	Appear normal to increased, no contiguity	Elongated rete, solar elastosis
Lentigo simplex	Early onset, not related to sun-exposure	Increased melanin	Increased, in focal contiguity	Elongated rete
Lentiginosis profusa	Many lesions at birth or childhood	Increased melanin	Increased, in focal contiguity	Elongated rete, nevus nests in some lesions
Multiple lentiginosis syndromes (leopard, LAMB)	Many lesions, dominant trait	Increased melanin	Increased, in focal contiguity	Elongated rete, nevus nests in some lesions
Speckled lentiginous nevus	Macule at birth, becomes speckled	Increased melanin	Increased, in focal contiguity	Elongated rete, nevus nests in speckled areas
Peutz–Jegher lentigines	Perioral, dominant trait, GI polyps	Increased melanin (marked)	No increase by DOPA stain	

and (e) pedunculated lesions. The first three types are always pigmented; the latter two may or may not be pigmented. Any of the elevated lesions may be surrounded by a flat periphery, within which changes of melanocytic dysplasia may be seen histologically ("nevus with dysplasia"). Dome-shaped lesions often contain several coarse hairs. Although exceptions occur, one can predict to a certain degree from the clinical appearance of a nevus whether on histologic examination it will prove to be a junctional nevus (confined to the epidermis), a compound nevus (epidermal and dermal), or an intradermal nevus. Most small flat lesions represent either a lentigo simplex or a junctional nevus. Flat lesions or lesions with a flat periphery >5 mm in diameter with irregular indefinite borders and pigment variegation are clinically dysplastic nevi, although if these changes are severe, melanoma may need to be ruled out. Most slightly elevated lesions and some papillomatous lesions represent compound nevi (especially if they are pigmented). Finally, most papillomatous lesions and nearly all dome-shaped and pedunculated lesions that are not pigmented represent intradermal nevi (92).

Melanocytic nevi are only rarely present at birth. Most nevi appear in adolescence and early adulthood. In this age period, they may occur episodically and, rarely, as widespread eruptive nevi (93–95). Occasionally, new nevi arise in midlife and rarely in later life. Except for occasional cosmetic significance, nevi are important only in relation to melanoma, for which they are risk markers, simulants, and potential precursors (62,96,97).

A general concept of clinical importance for melanocytic nevi is that, unlike melanoma that inexorably progresses over time, nevi enlarge to a point, stabilize, and then involute. This clinical attribute is directly related to the importance of heightened suspicion that is aroused when a previously stable nevus undergoes change in size or pigmentation.

Histopathology. Melanocytic nevi are defined and recognized by the presence of nevus cells, which, even though they are melanocytes, differ from ordinary melanocytes by being arranged at least partially in clusters or "nests." Other defining characteristics of nevus cells include a tendency to round rather than dendritic cell shape, and a propensity to retain pigment in their cytoplasm rather than to transfer it to neighboring keratinocytes (98). Nevus cells show considerable variation in their appearance, and often are not pigmented, so that they are often recognizable as nevus cells more by their arrangement in clusters or nests than by their cellular characteristics. As the result of a shrinkage artifact, nevus cell nests often appear partially separated from their surrounding stroma, and in some nevi such as the spindle and epithelioid cell variant, from surrounding epithelium.

Although a histologic subdivision of nevi into junctional, compound, and intradermal nevi is generally accepted, it should be realized that these are transitional

stages in the "life cycle" of nevi, which are believed to start out as junctional nevi and, after having become intradermal nevi, undergo involution.

Lentigo Simplex

The lentigo simplex, described above, may be regarded as an early or evolving form of melanocytic nevus. Histologically, these are small (usually <2 mm), and characterized by an increased number of nevoid melanocytes, present in contiguity with one another near the tips and sides of elongated rete ridges. This pattern, characteristic of lentigines, is therefore described as "lentiginous melanocytic proliferation." The lack of nests at the histologic level distinguishes the lentigo from a nevus, by definition. However, transitional forms between a simple lentigo and a lentiginous junctional nevus (a lentigo with a few nests) are commonly observed, and the two histologic "entities" are indistinguishable clinically, giving rise to the term "nevoid lentigo" (78), or "jentigo" (76). The former term has been misused more or less synonymously with "lentigo maligna" (73,99), and therefore we prefer the term "lentiginous junctional nevus" for these very common lesions (64) (Fig. 28-5).

Junctional Nevus

In a junctional nevus, nevus cells may lie in well-circumscribed nests either entirely within the lower epidermis or bulging downward into the dermis but still in contact with the epidermis, perhaps in the process of "dropping off" to form a compound nevus. The nevus cells in these nests generally have a regular, cuboidal appearance, although they are occasionally spindle-shaped. In addition, varying numbers of diffusely arranged single nevus cells are seen in the lowermost epidermis, especially in the basal cell layer. In many lesions, single cells are about as common as nests, recapitulating the histology of a simple lentigo. Such lesions in our practice are termed "lentiginous junctional nevi" (Fig. 28-5). Varying amounts of melanin granules are seen in the nevus cells. Some of the nevus cells, on staining with silver, show dendritic processes containing melanin granules, making them indistinguishable from melanocytes, but in general the degree of dendritic differentiation is reduced compared to melanocytes. The nested and single melanocytes are arranged mainly at the tips and sides of rete ridges; "continuous" proliferation of single cells between the rete, confluence of nests, or pagetoid extension of cells into the suprabasal epidermal layers, may be indicators of dysplasia or evolving *in situ* melanoma.

Although nevus cells only occasionally penetrate into the upper layers of the epidermis ("pagetoid extension"), aggregates of melanin granules may be seen in the stratum corneum in deeply pigmented junctional nevi. Often, the rete ridges are elongated as in lentigo simplex and single cells as well as nests of nevus cells are seen at the bases of

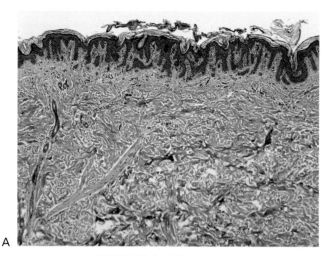 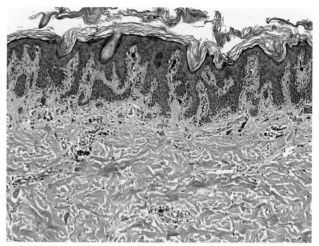

FIGURE 28-5. (A) Lentiginous junctional nevus. Most examples are <4 mm, usually about 2 to 3 mm in diameter. A dermal component, if present in a lentiginous nevus, lies in the center of the lesion and the epidermal component extends beyond its "shoulder." **(B)** In the epidermis, single cells and nests of nevi are arranged near the dermal–epidermal junction near the tips and sides of elongated rete ridges (a "lentiginous" pattern). There is minimal or no atypia. There is no "continuous" proliferation of melanocytes in the suprapapillary regions of the epidermis between the rete ridges. These architectural features are repeated but exaggerated in dysplastic nevi, which in addition exhibit mild to moderate random cytologic atypia, and more conspicuous stromal reactions.

the rete ridges. Not infrequently, as in lentigo simplex, the upper dermis contains an infiltrate of melanophages and mononuclear cells. These lesions that combine features of lentigo simplex and junctional nevus are exceedingly common, and may be termed "lentiginous junctional nevi." Lesions with these features larger than 5 mm clinically or 4 to 5 mm in a histologic section often prove to be dysplastic nevi.

In children, some junctional nevi may show considerable cellularity with some pleomorphism and with some pagetoid cells above the basal layer. They may also often show fine dusty melanin particles and a dense inflammatory infiltrate (84,100). Some of these lesions may represent Spitz nevi or dysplastic nevi. Others may correlate with a tendency for ordinary junctional nevus cells to be enlarged, or epithelioid, in younger individuals. The small size of the lesion, the sharp lateral demarcation, the lack of severe or uniform atypia and of mitoses, and the fact that in children melanomas are very rare help in the distinction from melanoma. However, if the criteria mentioned above are present, the diagnosis of melanoma should be considered, even in a child.

Compound Nevus

Clinically, a compound nevus is a pigmented papule (Fig. 28-6A) or a plaque. In a nondysplastic compound nevus, there is no adjacent macular component. Histologically, a compound nevus possesses features of both a junctional and

an intradermal nevus. Nevus cell nests are present in the epidermis, as well as appearing to "drop off" from the epidermis into the superficial dermis and in the dermis Fig. 28-6B). This time-honored theory of "abtropfung" or dropping off of nevus cells proposed by Unna has been recently challenged by the finding that junctional nevi are more common in adults than in children (101). Nevus cells in the upper, middle, and lower dermis may present characteristic morphologic variations called *types A, B,* and *C,* respectively (39,102). Usually, the *type A* nevus cells in the upper dermis are round to cuboidal and show abundant cytoplasm containing varying amounts of melanin granules. Type A cells with especially abundant cytoplasm, as may occur in children and young adults, may be termed "epithelioid cells" (Fig. 28-6C). Melanophages are occasionally seen in the surrounding stroma. The cells in the mid-dermis usually are *type B cells*; they are distinctly smaller than the type A cells, display less cytoplasm and less melanin, and generally lie in well-defined aggregates or cords. They may to some extent resemble lymphoid cells (Fig. 28-6D). *Type C nevus cells* in the lower dermis tend to resemble fibroblasts or Schwann cells, because they are usually elongated and possess a spindle-shaped nucleus. They often lie in strands and only rarely contain melanin (Fig. 28-6E). Occasional nevi show abnormal stratification within the deeper dermis of otherwise benign type A nevus cells, resulting in the designation of "inverted type A nevus."

The decrease in size and progression from nests to cords to more neuroid spindle cells with dermal descent seen in nevi is often referred to as maturation and is regarded as evidence of benignity, because the size of the cells in a melanoma usually does not decrease with depth. The process of nevus cell maturation has alternatively been regarded as one of senescence or atrophy (103). If dermal nevus cells are confined to the papillary dermis, they often retain a discrete or "pushing" border with the stroma. However, nevus cells that enter the reticular dermis tend to disperse among collagen fiber bundles as single cells or attenuated single files of cells. This pattern of infiltration of the dermis differs from that in melanomas, where groups of cells tend to dissect and displace the collagen bundles in a more "expansive" pattern (104). Lesions where nevus cells extend into the lower reticular dermis and the subcutaneous fat or are located within nerves, hair follicles, sweat ducts, and sebaceous glands, may be termed "congenital pattern nevi" (105).

Intradermal Nevus

Intradermal nevi show essentially no junctional activity. The upper dermis contains nests and cords of nevus cells. Multinucleated nevus cells may be seen, in which small nuclei lie either in a rosette-like arrangement or close together in the center of the cell. These nevus giant cells differ significantly in appearance from the irregularly and even

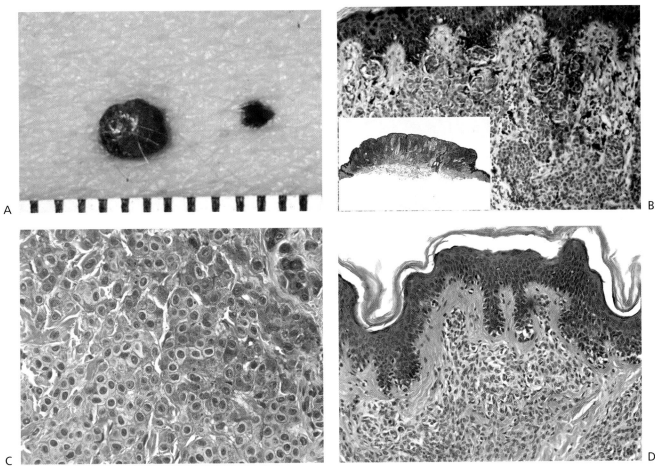

FIGURE 28-6. (A) Compound nevi. Each lesion is a true papule without any adjacent macular component. The lesion on the right is a pigmented compound nevus. The lesion on the left has little pigment, and clinically is a predominantly dermal nevus. **(B)** Histologically, the lesion is a true papule without an adjacent junctional component (*inset*). Nests of nevus cells are present at the dermal–epidermal junction. It is believed that these nests become separated from the epidermis, to lie in the dermis, piling up on one another in an "accretive" pattern of growth, and resulting in gradual elevation of the epidermis above its original position to form the papule. Pigment is present mostly in junctional and superficial dermal nevus cells. **(C)** Dermal nevus with type A nevus cells. The type A cells have visible cytoplasm that is in contact with cytoplasm of neighboring nevus cells. The nuclei are small, without atypia or prominent nucleoli. There are no mitoses. **(D)** Lentiginous compound nevus. In this as in many nevi, nests are admixed with single cells in the junctional component, a lentiginous pattern. The cells in the dermis are small lymphocyte-like type B cells. *(continued)*

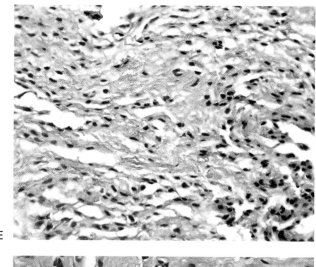

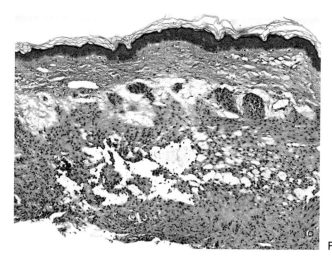

E

F

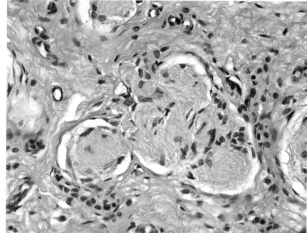

G

FIGURE 28-6. *(continued)* **(E)** Type C dermal nevus cells at the base of a nevus. The cells at the base of a nevus tend to be spindled in shape and to have collagen between the individual cells. If they extend into the reticular dermis, they tend to "disperse" as individual cells among the superficial collagen fibers, a pattern that is also characteristic of Spitz nevi. **(F)** Dermal nevus with "pseudolymphatic spaces." The type B nevus cells at the top of the lesion have small nuclei and scant cytoplasm, reminiscent of lymphocytes. The spaces are a common artifact in dermal or compound nevi. They may simulate lymphatic invasion of a melanoma, but are completely benign. The cells at the base of the lesion are predominantly type C cells. **(G)** Neurotized dermal nevus cells at the base of a dermal nevus. The structures at the base of a "neurotized" dermal nevus may be reminiscent of nerve fibers or neural organs such as Wagner–Meissner corpuscles.

bizarrely shaped giant cells that are seen frequently in Spitz nevus and occasionally also in melanoma. As a result of shrinkage during tissue processing, clefts may form between some nests of nevus cells and the surrounding epidermis as well as stroma, the latter leaving a defect that simulates a lymphatic space and thus mimics lymphatic invasion (106) (Fig. 28-6F).

Whereas the nevus cell nests located in the upper dermis often contain a moderate amount of melanin (particularly type A cells), the type C nevus cells in the midportion and lower dermis rarely contain melanin. These type C cells appear spindle-shaped, are arranged in bundles, and are embedded in collagenous fibers having a loose, pale, wavy appearance similar to that of the fibers in a neurofibroma ("neurotized nevus"). Such formations have been referred to as neuroid tubes. In other areas, the nevus cells lie within concentrically arranged, loosely layered filamentous tissue, forming so-called nevic corpuscles that resemble Meissner's tactile bodies (Fig. 28-6G). Neurotized nevus cells express the marker S-100A6 protein, a form of S-100 found in Schwann cells, supporting the hypothesis that

maturation in these lesions recapitulates some features of Schwann cell differentiation (107).

Occasional intradermal nevi are devoid of nevus cell nests in the upper dermis and contain only spindle-shaped nevus cells embedded in abundant, loosely arranged collagenous tissue. These nevi may be referred to as neural nevi. The differentiation from a solitary neurofibroma may be difficult in routinely stained sections, but distinction might be possible with an immunohistochemical technique employing myelin basic protein, which is positive only in neurofibroma (108) (see Histogenesis section). Neurofibromas also tend to contain small nerve twigs and axons, a feature not typical of neurotized nevi.

Some intradermal and, less commonly, compound nevi show hyperkeratosis and papillomatosis, which may be associated with a lacelike, downward growth of epidermal strands and with horn cysts. Such nevi resemble seborrheic keratoses in their epidermal architecture. In other instances, large hair follicles are observed. Rupture of a large hair follicle may manifest itself clinically in an increase in the size of the nevus associated with an inflammatory reaction, leading to clinical suspicion of a melanoma. Histologic examination in such instances shows a partially destroyed epidermal follicular lining with a pronounced inflammatory infiltrate containing foreign body giant cells as a reaction to the presence of keratin in the dermis. Occasionally, intradermal nevi contain scattered, large fat cells within the aggregates of nevus cells. This is likely to be a regressive phenomenon in which fat cells replace involuting nevus cells (109), or alternatively true adipocyte metaplasia within the stroma of the nevus.

Some intradermal nevi, including variants of spindle and epithelioid cell nevi, induce marked deposition of coarse, sometimes hyalinized collagen. Such nevi are described as sclerosing variants. This change occasionally may confound diagnosis, but is not of biological significance.

In occasional otherwise typical dermal nevi (or in the dermal component of compound nevi), rare mitoses are found in the dermis. This phenomenon has been described in children (100), and in association with pregnancy (110). If there are no other indicators of malignancy, we report these cases as "nevi with mitoses," and generally recommend complete excision. The possibility of nevoid melanoma (see Nevoid Melanoma section) should be seriously considered in such lesions (111).

Pathogenesis of Acquired Melanocytic Nevi

For many years, Masson's theory of the dual origin of nevus cells was widely accepted (39). He believed that the nevus cells in the upper dermis developed from epidermal melanocytes, while the nevus cells in the lower dermis developed from Schwann cells, as suggested by the frequent presence of nerve-like structures in the latter. The fact that both melanocytes and Schwann cells are derived from the neural crest seemed to support Masson's view, as did the presence of a nonspecific cholinesterase reaction in both deep nevus cells and Schwann cells, and the absence of melanin in the deep nevus cells (112). However, in favor of a melanocytic origin of these deep dermal nevus cells was the presence of melanosomes with dopaoxidase activity even in nevus cells deep in the dermis that had a neuroid appearance on light microscopy (113). An electron microscopic examination of neuroid structures in nevi revealed that these "nevic corpuscles" contained no Schwann cells or axons, but were instead composed exclusively of cells that contain premelanosome-like dense bodies in their perikaryon (114). Furthermore, myelin basic protein has been found to be regularly present by immunoperoxidase in Schwann cells and absent in all types of melanocytic nevi (108).

Another important point in favor of a single origin of the nevus cell is to be found in the life cycle of nevi. Although there are exceptions, most nevi appear in childhood, adolescence, and early adulthood, and, with advanc-

ing age, there is a progressive decrease in the number of nevi (115). The evolution and regression of nevi correlate with their histologic appearance. Junctional proliferation of nevus cells is present in almost every nevus in children, but decreases with age. Intradermal nevi, by contrast, are most unusual in the first decade of life, and their proportion increases progressively with age. The incidence of fibrosis, fatty infiltration, and neuroid changes increases with age. Thus, the formation of cylindrical neuroid structures represents the end stage of differentiation and not a source of origin of intradermal nevi (115,116).

Concerning the relationship between epidermal melanocytes and nevus cells, some authors believe that these two types of cells have a different embryologic genesis, the nevus cell originating from a neural crest precursor cell referred to as a nevoblast (117). Most authors regard the two cell types as identical (118). It would seem that the morphologic features by which nevus cells differ from melanocytes, such as the absence of dendrites as seen by light microscopy, their arrangement in cell nests, their larger size, and their tendency to retain pigment, are secondary adjustments of the cells. Electron microscopy has shown that the fine structure of nevus cells is comparable to that of epidermal melanocytes (119). Cultured nevus cells, whether derived from congenital or acquired lesions, have been found to be highly dendritic, as are epidermal melanocytes (118). In conclusion, it seems established that nevus cells differ from Schwann cells and are benign neoplastic variants of melanocytes.

The molecular pathology of nevi is beginning to be understood. In a recent study of the BRAF oncogene, which had previously been found to be mutated in a high percentage of metastatic melanomas (120), mutations resulting in the V599E amino-acid substitution were found in 68% of melanoma metastases, 80% of primary melanomas and, unexpectedly, in 82% of nevi (121). Activating mutations of the oncogene nRAS have also been described in melanoma-associated nevi and in congenital nevi (122–125). These data suggest that mutational activation of the RAS/RAF/MAPK mitogenic pathway in nevi is a critical step in the initiation of melanocytic neoplasia but alone is insufficient for melanoma tumorigenesis (121). High levels of the tumor suppressor gene product p16INK4 in benign nevi may represent the mechanism whereby the cell cycle remains regulated in nevi, even in the presence of activating oncogene mutations (126–128).

Balloon Cell Nevus

Balloon cell nevi are histologic curiosities that possess no clinical features by which they can be differentiated from other nevi. They are quite rare (129).

Histopathology. Balloon cells may be seen within the epidermis singly or in groups, or may be absent from the epidermis. In the dermis, they lie arranged in lobules of vary-

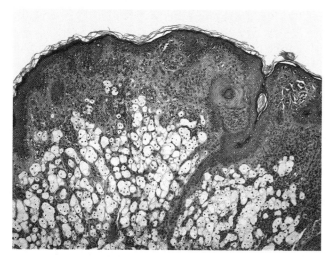

FIGURE 28-7. Balloon cell nevus. Large cells with pale cytoplasm are admixed with mature nevus cells. There is no high-grade atypia or mitotic activity.

ing size often with an admixture of ordinary nevus cells, and often with transitional forms between the ordinary and ballooned nevus cells (Fig. 28-7). The balloon cells may be multinucleated, and are considerably larger than ordinary nevus cells. Their nuclei are small, round, and usually centrally placed. Their cytoplasm appears either empty or finely granular, often with a few small melanin granules. There may be melanophages that are solidly packed with pigment. Stains for lipids, glycogen, and acid or neutral mucopolysaccharides are negative in the balloon cells. *Electron microscopic examination* reveals in balloon cells numerous large vacuoles formed by enlargement and coalescence of melanosomes (130,131). Balloon cell nevus is differentiated from balloon cell melanoma by the usual criteria. The large adipocytes present in some intradermal nevi as a result of fatty infiltration or stromal metaplasia differ from balloon cells by routine histology by having a flattened nucleus located at the periphery of the cell. In the differentiation from clear cell hidradenoma and other clear cell tumors the absence of PAS-positive glycogen and keratin in balloon cell nevus might be helpful; balloon nevus cells also stain for S-100 protein, although eccrine neoplasms (and adipocytes) may also express this marker.

Nevi of Special Sites

There is variation in the morphology of common nevi by site. In a study of Australian schoolchildren, gender differences in nevus density on the back and lower limbs were similar to gender differences for melanoma, with back lesions favoring males, and lower extremity lesions favoring females. Small nevi (2 to 4 mm) were most dense on the arms, whereas large nevi (≥5 mm) were most dense on the posterior trunk where they were related to age, male sex,

and freckling. The findings were considered to support the hypothesis of site-specific differences in nevus proliferative potential (132). Nevi in certain locations may exhibit features that are unusual in the vast majority of common nevi on the trunk, limbs, or face and scalp. These "special site nevi" have been best defined in acral locations (palmar and plantar, and subungual nevi), and in genital skin. Nevi in skin flexural areas (ear lobe, axilla, umbilicus, inguinal creases, pubis, scrotum and perianal area) may also show unusual features, similar to those to be described below for acral nevi (133).

Nevi of Acral Skin

Melanocytic nevi are present on the skin of the palms or soles in as many as 4% to 9% of the population (134). Clinically, they are usually small, symmetrical, well circumscribed brown macules, with a tendency to dark ridging along dermoglyphics that can be clinically striking and may impart a seemingly irregular border. They are usually stable, and are more often junctional than are nevi of the trunk.

Histopathology. Acral nevi tend to be more cellular than most common nevi, and the nevus cells may be arranged in predominantly lentiginous rather than nested patterns in the epidermis. Recently, pagetoid proliferation ("pagetoid melanocytosis") of lesional nevus cells in the epidermis above the basal layer was described in benign acral nevi (135–138). These features may perhaps account for recommendations in the older literature to remove acral nevi because of suspicion of melanoma. However, there is no evidence that these lesions, when devoid of true dysplasia, are common precursors or risk markers for acral melanomas.

Acral nevi may simulate and must be differentiated from melanoma, and this may be difficult especially in small biopsies. Clemente et al. (136) studied a series of acral nevi and identified a subset that they termed acral-lentiginous nevi. The distinctive features of these nevi compared to other acral nonlentiginous nevi included several features also seen in acral-lentiginous melanomas: poor lateral circumscription, elongation of rete ridges, continuous junctional proliferation of melanocytes, the presence of scattered melanocytes within the upper epidermis, and the presence of junctional melanocytes with abundant pale cytoplasm and round to oval, sometimes hyperchromatic, nuclei with prominent nucleoli. In lentiginous compound acral nevi, the nevus cells in the dermis, unlike melanoma cells, mature to the lesional base. There is no high-grade uniform cytologic atypia, no extensive and high-level pagetoid melanocytosis in the epidermis, and there are no mitoses (Fig. 28-8). There may be patchy lymphocytes and occasional melanophages in the dermis. Some of these features may suggest dysplastic nevus. However, the rete ridge pattern of keratinocytes in most acral nevi does not show the uniform elongation with occasional accentuation of

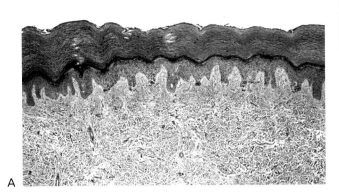

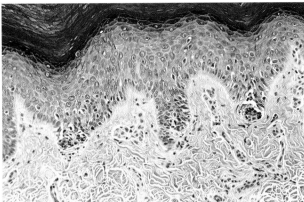

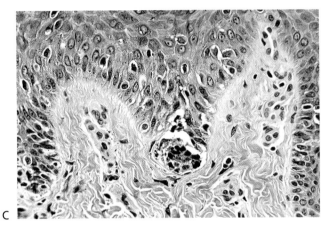

FIGURE 28-8. **(A)** Acral lentiginous nevus. The lesion is small, quite well circumscribed, and entirely contained within the biopsy specimen. **(B)** Acral lentiginous nevus. Nests of nevoid to small epithelioid melanocytes predominate near the dermal epidermal junction. They tend to be small, evenly spaced, and discrete. **(C)** Acral lentiginous nevus. Although a few lesional cells may be present above the junction in a "pagetoid" pattern, there is no severe uniform atypia or mitotic activity, and there is no continuous proliferation of single cells between the nests.

anastomosing rete that characterizes dysplastic nevi, the complete array of stromal changes of dysplastic nevi are not observed in most acral nevi, and atypia of melanocytes, as a rule, is minimal or absent. In case of doubt, it may be appropriate to evaluate the patient's other nevi, especially if there is a family or personal history of melanoma. An acral lentiginous lesion that extends to specimen borders should be evaluated carefully, and clinicopathologic correlation should be obtained to ensure that the specimen does not represent the periphery of a larger lesion. In such cases it may be judicious to recommend complete excision, to rule out additional pathology, and to preclude persistence or recurrence of the lesion. Finally, because a nevus is acral does not preclude the unusual possibility that it is also dysplastic, but this diagnosis must rely on the presence of cytologic and stromal criteria for dysplastic nevus in addition to those commonly encountered in nevi of acral sites.

Melanonychia Striata (Longitudinal Melanonychia)

Melanonychia striata refers to a pigmented band extending in the long axis of the nail. Such bands are common in blacks and Asians and therefore regarded as normal (139,140). However, the sudden appearance of melanony-chia striata is cause for concern, particularly in whites, requiring a punch biopsy of the nail matrix (141). An exception is the melanonychia striata seen in the Laugier–Hunziker syndrome, which may affect one, several, or all fingernails in association with pigmented macules of the lips or the buccal mucosa. This type of melanonychia is always benign (139,142).

For carrying out the biopsy, longitudinal bilateral releasing incisions are made along the medial and lateral sides of the posterior nail fold. Next, the entire posterior nail fold is reflected proximally in order to expose and make visible the very end of the pigmented streak, which is usually within the matrix of the nail. Then the biopsy specimen is taken with a 3- or 4-mm punch through the nail plate and matrix down to the phalangeal bone (143,144).

Histopathology. Histologic examination in most instances shows merely basal cell layer hyperpigmentation without an obvious increase in the number of melanocytes. Such lesions have been termed "melanotic macules" (145). In a recent study of 18 cases, 10 were melanotic macules, 1 was melanoma *in situ*, 1 showed keratinocytic atypia, and 3 were subungual hemorrhages (146). In other cases, a junctional nevus or a compound nevus of acral type as described above, or an acral lentiginous melanoma, either *in situ* or invasive, may be found. The junctional or compound nevi tend to be of the lentiginous acral nevus pattern described above. Longitudinal melanonychia may also be associated with pigmented Bowen's disease (141). Longitudinal melanonychia in children is almost always benign: in a study of 40 cases in children under the age of 16, the histologic diagnosis was nevus in 19 cases (junctional in 17 cases and compound in 2), lentigo in 12 cases, and simple hyperpigmentation ("functional melanonychia) in 9. None of the patients in this series had melanoma (147). Subungual melanomas, although very rare, do however occasionally occur in children (148).

Nevus of Genital Skin

Some clinically unremarkable nevi located on or near genital skin may present with histologic features that simulate some aspects of melanomas. The lesions have no clinical significance except the possibility of diagnostic error. They have been termed "atypical melanocytic nevi of the genital type (AMNGT)," and are most often seen on the vulva of young (premenopausal) women, but may also been seen on perineal skin (149–151). Similar lesions also occur uncommonly on the male genitalia (152). The lesions are often removed incidentally. They are typically symmetrical papular lesions, usually <1 cm in diameter, and uniformly pigmented with discrete well-circumscribed borders. The atypical features appear to represent a histologic curiosity seen in a minority of vulvar nevi. In a comparative histologic study of vulvar and common nevi most of the vulvar lesions were unremarkable (153). Vulvar nevi themselves are quite uncommon; in patients in a gynecology practice, the prevalence was only 2.3% (154). An interesting variant

pattern of nevi has been described in association with lichen sclerosus et atrophicus, most commonly on skin of the vulva, perineum, or rarely elsewhere. These nevi had features in common with persistent ("recurrent") melanocytic nevi and can mimic malignant melanoma. This "activated" melanocytic phenotype seen in lichen sclerosus-associated melanocytic nevi suggests a stromal-induced change (150). The clinical differential diagnosis for atypical genital nevi also includes early "genital lentigines," as described above.

Histopathology. The scanning magnification impression is typically that of a small, well-circumscribed papular lesion composed of nevus cells arranged in clusters in the papillary dermis, and arranged mainly in nests in the epidermis where the cells do not extend beyond the shoulder of the dermal component, as typically occurs in compound dysplastic nevi (Fig. 28-9). The nevus cells may be large, with prominent nucleoli, and abundant cytoplasm containing finely-divided melanin pigment. The epidermal nests may vary considerably in size and shape, tending to become confluent. The nests tend to be variable in size, shape and position, originating from the sides as well as the tips of rete, and often oriented parallel to the surface. The melanocytes within the nests are often dyshesive. Single cells and nests of nevus cells may occasionally be seen within the epithelia of skin adnexa. The epidermis occasionally is irregularly thickened, resulting in an asymmetrical silhouette. Some of the features seen in atypical vulvar nevi may arouse a suspicion of melanoma. However, the lesions are comparatively small and well circumscribed, without significant junctional proliferation of atypical melanocytes beyond the major dermal component, as is

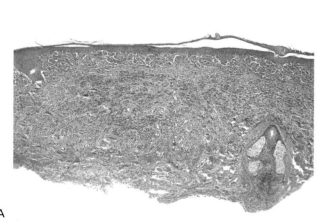
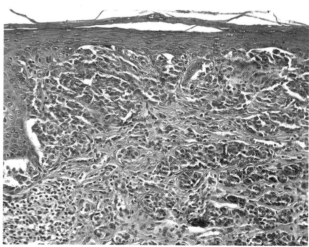

A

B

FIGURE 28-9. (A) Nevus of genital skin. Nevi on genital skin may exhibit atypical features at high power, but are usually relatively small and symmetrical and thus benign in their appearance at scanning magnification, and also clinically. **(B)** Atypical features in genital nevi may include nests that tend to be large and confluent, and to vary a good deal in size and shape, and cells that tend to be large, with macronucleoli, and dyshesive from one another. Mitoses are rare or absent, and there is no adjacent *in situ* or microinvasive radial growth phase component.

seen in most mucosal melanomas. Moreover, there is little or no pagetoid spread of single or nested melanocytes into the epidermis, there is no necrosis and usually no ulcer, and importantly there is no mitotic activity in the dermis (153). Stromal patterns more characteristic of melanoma (diffuse fibroplasia) or dysplasia (concentric fibroplasia) are generally lacking in these lesions (151). The diagnosis of melanoma in vulvar skin should be made with caution in a premenopausal woman.

In an apparently unrelated phenomenon, atypical nevi have been described in association with lichen sclerosus et atrophicus. These lesions resembled persistent or recurrent melanocytic nevi (150).

Nevi of Flexural Sites

Based on histologic findings, it has been suggested that nevi in flexural sites may differ histologically from those at other sites, in general resembling the appearances of nevi of genital skin, and potentially simulating melanoma. In a study of 40 melanocytic nevi of flexural sites (axilla, umbilicus, inguinal creases, pubis, scrotum, and perianal area), 22 of them had "a nested and dyshesive pattern" similar to the genital pattern nevi. This pattern was characterized by the confluence of enlarged nests with variation in size, shape and position at the dermo–epidermal junction and by the diminished cohesion of melanocytes. Nevi of breast skin in our experience may show similar features. These changes in flexural nevi should not be overinterpreted as indicative of melanoma (133).

Spitz Nevus

The Spitz nevus, named after Sophie Spitz, who first described it in 1948 (155), is known also as *benign juvenile melanoma* (a term that should be discouraged) and as *spindle and epithelioid cell nevus*. The lesion was originally thought to occur largely in children, but it is now well recognized in young to early middle-aged adults (156,157). Rarely, it is present at birth (158).

The lesion usually is solitary and is encountered most commonly on the lower extremities and face (159). In most instances, it consists of a dome-shaped, hairless, small pink nodule. Most Spitz nevi are small: in 95% of the patients, the size of the tumor is <1 cm, and in 75% it is ≤6 mm (160). The color is usually pink because of a scarcity of melanin and in some lesions associated vascularization of the stroma, and it is then often diagnosed clinically as granuloma pyogenicum, angioma, or dermal nevus. However, it may be tan and, in some cases, brown or even black. Ulceration is seen only rarely. After an initial period of growth, most Spitz nevi are stable.

In rare instances, multiple tumors are encountered either agminated (grouped) in one area (161), or widely disseminated (162) (Fig. 28-10A). In a case of agminated

Spitz nevi, a mosaic pattern of chromosomal translocation was demonstrated in lesional fibroblasts, suggesting a local event in embryogenesis (161).

Histopathology. Spitz nevi are usually compound, but they can be intradermal or entirely junctional. Ackerman's term "nevus of large spindle and/or epithelioid cells" reflects the characteristic cytologic appearances that provide the essential definition for the lesion (157). Because of the large size of the lesional cells often with considerable nuclear and cytoplasmic pleomorphism, and the frequent presence of an inflammatory infiltrate, the histologic picture often resembles that of a nodular melanoma. There is no doubt that, before the recognition of Spitz nevi as an entity, many cases were misdiagnosed as melanoma. Even today, differentiation from a melanoma can often be very difficult and occasionally even impossible. Features that aid in the distinction may be summarized as *architectural pattern* and *cytologic features* (Fig. 28-10A through G).

Architectural Pattern

Spitz nevi resemble common nevi. They are usually compound, but as stated above, they can be intradermal or entirely junctional. They are small, symmetrical, and well circumscribed. It is somewhat unusual for the intraepidermal component to extend beyond the dermal component, and such a finding should prompt consideration of melanoma (163). The epidermal component is arranged in nests that tend to be oriented vertically and, though large, do not show significant variation in size and shape or tend to become confluent. In Spitz nevi with junctional activity, there are often artifactual semilunar clefts separating nests of nevus cells at the epidermal–dermal junction from overlying epidermal cells. Not so commonly seen in melanoma, this feature represents a useful diagnostic feature (163).

Although there may be diffuse junctional activity, permeation of the epidermis by tumor cells (pagetoid melanocytosis) is relatively slight. If present, it usually consists of single nevus cells or small groups of cells and is generally limited to the lower half of the epidermis (157) (Fig. 28-10G). In a few Spitz nevi, however, pagetoid migration of lesional cells into the epidermis may be quite marked, especially in young children. These "pagetoid Spitz nevi" appear clinically as a small (<0.4 cm) pigmented macule in young patients. Features favoring nevus over melanoma include small size, circumscription, symmetry, even distribution of cells, and lack of marked cytologic atypia (164). Pagetoid involvement of the suprabasal epidermis is not a common feature of Spitz nevi in adults; in such a case the diagnosis of melanoma should be considered (165). Occasionally, nests of lesional cells are seen in transit through the epidermis, described as transepidermal elimination of nevus cells (166,167).

The epidermis involved by Spitz nevi is often hyperplastic with elongated rete ridges. Occasionally, this hyperpla-

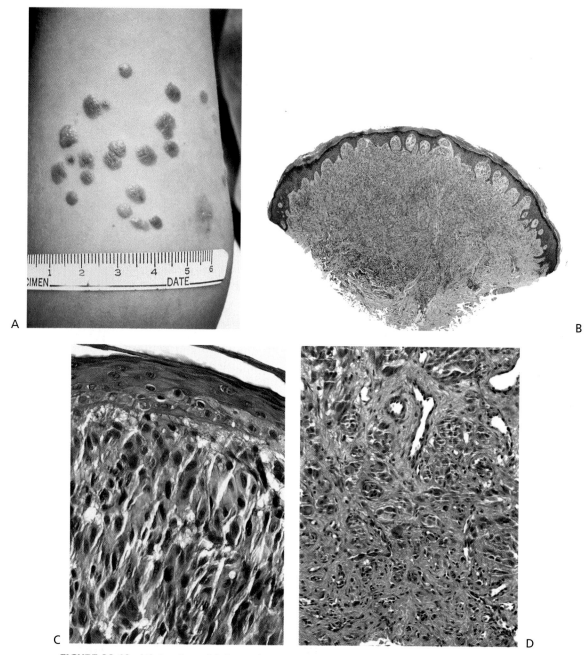

FIGURE 28-10. (A) Agminated Spitz nevi. Most Spitz nevi are single lesions. In this example of agminated, or grouped Spitz nevi, each individual lesion is a characteristic Spitz nevus: relatively small, symmetrical, well-circumscribed tan papules. **(B)** Most Spitz nevi are small, circumscribed, symmetrical papules, at scanning magnification and clinically. This lesion is somewhat larger than most examples. **(C)** Spitz nevi are defined by the presence of large cells, with abundant amphophilic cytoplasm, which may be spindled or polygonal in shape (large spindle and/or epithelioid melanocytes). The nuclei in a given Spitz nevus are more homogenous than in most melanomas, usually large but with open chromatin and smooth nuclear membranes, and with prominent nucleoli. **(D)** "Maturation" from larger cells near the surface to smaller cells at the base is an important feature of Spitz nevi. *(continued)*

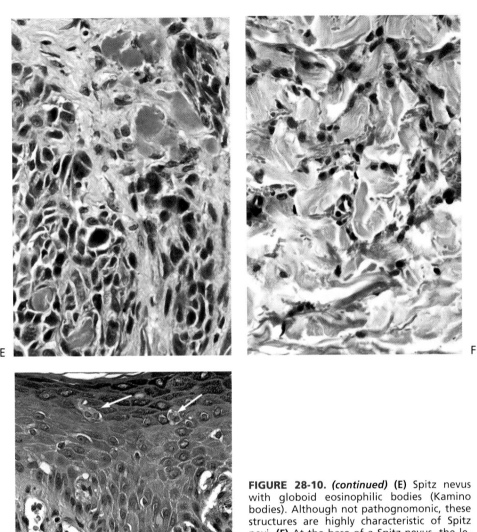

FIGURE 28-10. *(continued)* **(E)** Spitz nevus with globoid eosinophilic bodies (Kamino bodies). Although not pathognomonic, these structures are highly characteristic of Spitz nevi. **(F)** At the base of a Spitz nevus, the lesional cells become smaller, and become "dispersed" among the reticular dermis collagen fibers. This is the same lesion shown in Fig. 28–10D. Note the reduction in size ("maturation") of the lesional cells at the base. **(G)** Pagetoid extension of some cells of a Spitz nevus into the epidermis, as seen here, is not diagnostic of a melanoma if other attributes of melanoma are not observed. This pagetoid melanocytosis is not uncommon, at least focally, in lesions of young children.

sia is sufficiently florid to be termed pseudoepitheliomatous, representing a possible source of confusion with squamous cell carcinoma especially in a superficial biopsy (168). However, the epidermis may be thinned and even ulcerated, especially in very young children. Found in fewer than half of the patients, diffuse edema and telangiectasia in the papillary dermis, if present, are of slight diagnostic importance. The edema may cause a loose arrangement of the nevus cell nests (163).

Cytologic Features

Important cytologic features of Spitz nevi include the presence of large spindle cells and epithelioid cells (Fig. 28-10C). Spindle cells or epithelioid cells may predominate, or the two types of cells may be intermingled ("large spindle and/or epithelioid cells") (157). Apart from the shape of their cell bodies, the spindle cells and the epithelioid cells in any given Spitz nevus resemble one another in nuclear and in cytoplasmic consistency, suggesting that they may represent dimorphic expression of a single cell type. The cells are large, with abundant amphophilic cytoplasm that may contain scant finely divided melanin pigment although in most of the cells, pigment is typically absent. The nuclei are large, with pale, delicate chromatin and regular, smooth nuclear membranes, and prominent eosinophilic or amphophilic nucleoli. The size of the lesional cells, more than any other feature, sets the Spitz nevus apart from the common nevus (169), and also from most melanomas. Bizarre giant cells may be seen in both melanoma and Spitz nevi, the difference being that, in the latter, they usually have regular nuclei of similar size, whereas in melanoma the nuclei are usually more pleomorphic. Mitoses are absent in about half of the cases. This is helpful in ruling out melanoma in these lesions. Usually, there are only a few mitoses, but occasionally, they are quite numerous in the epidermal compartment. A dermal mitotic rate of greater than two mitoses per square millimeter (170) or mitoses within the lower half of the dermal component are unusual in Spitz nevi and may warrant a diagnosis of melanoma or a descriptive diagnosis of "melanocytic tumor of uncertain potential." Atypical mitoses are uncommon, and, if they are found, the lesion should be interpreted with great caution (163). The complete absence of mitoses in 50% of Spitz nevi is very helpful in ruling out melanoma in these cases.

Of special importance is *maturation* of the cells with increasing depth, so that they become smaller and look more like the cells of a common nevus (163) (Fig. 28-10D, E, and F). Also important is the *uniformity* of the lesional cells from one side of the lesion to the other: at any given level of the lesion from the epidermis to its base, the lesional cells look the same. Although large superficially, the cells at the base of most Spitz nevi are small, and they tend to disperse as single cells or files of single cells among reticular dermis collagen bundles. Involvement of the reticular dermis is highly characteristic of Spitz nevi, and as they descend into this part of the dermis, some of the cells become separated from the apparent border of the lesion to form "outlier cells" (160) that can be revealed by a stain for S-100 antigen. Other benign nevi also tend to infiltrate in this way if they involve the reticular dermis (170). Melanomas, in contrast, tend to form solid tongues or fascicles of tumor cells that separate and displace the collagen bundles in the reticular dermis, without forming outlier cells.

A useful though not pathognomonic cytologic criterion for Spitz nevi is the presence within the epidermis of red globules resembling colloid bodies in 60% to 80% of cases. They may form larger bodies through coalescence. These "Kamino bodies" are most commonly seen in the basal layer above the tips of dermal papillae (Fig. 28-10E). Similar-appearing eosinophilic globules have been noted in the epidermis in only 2% of melanomas and 0.9% of ordinary nevi, in which they are, however, less conspicuous because

they do not coalesce (171,172). Although often these bodies may resemble apoptotic cells, formal studies have found no evidence of active apoptosis, and have related the eosinophilic material to hyalinized collagen or basement membrane-like material (173).

Melanin is in many instances completely or nearly absent in Spitz nevi. In a few cases, melanin is moderate or dense. Some of these "pigmented Spitz nevi" are better classified as pigmented spindle-cell nevi, related lesions that are discussed in the next section. An inflammatory infiltrate is found in many Spitz nevi and may be quite heavy. Its distribution can be band-like, mainly at the base, as in some melanomas. Often, however, the infiltrate is patchy around blood vessels and is seen throughout the lesion (156,160,163).

On comparing Spitz nevi occurring in adults with those of children, it appears that pure epithelioid cell Spitz nevi are rare in adults. Also, lesions in adults often are more pigmented than in children (174). Furthermore, desmoplastic Spitz nevi occur predominantly in adults (157).

Desmoplastic Spitz Nevi

In some examples of Spitz nevi (and also in some nevi with smaller cells that may not meet criteria for Spitz nevi), diffuse fibrosis is present (175–177). These desmoplastic Spitz nevi generally show no junctional activity, nesting, or pigmentation. The nevus cells are predominantly spindle-shaped and compressed by a desmoplastic stroma. However, they differ from a dermatofibroma by the presence of epithelioid and often also multinucleated cells. Desmoplastic melanoma almost always shows an associated lentiginous *in situ* component, in contrast to the rarity of junctional activity in desmoplastic Spitz nevi. Furthermore, desmoplastic melanomas are almost invariably negative (in their spindle cell component) for the HMB-45 and Melan-A (MART-1) melanocytic markers, which in contrast are usually positive in Spitz nevi (178,79).

Hyalinizing Spitz Nevi

These nevi are related lesions that present with spindle or epithelioid nevus cells embedded in a paucicellular hyalinized collagenous stroma. Some of these lesions have been mistaken histologically for metastatic carcinomas (180).

Angiomatoid Spitz Nevi

These nevi present histologically with large spindle and/or epithelioid nevus placed among angiomatoid densely arranged, small blood vessels lined by plump endothelial cells embedded in a collagenous stroma. The Spitz nevus cells may be quite inconspicuous among the vessels in some cases. There have been no reported cases of recurrence or metastases (181).

Histogenesis. On electron microscopic examination, Spitz nevi show in their upper portion melanocytes with numerous melanosomes; in their lower portion, the number of melanosomes in the melanocytes decreases. Melanization is incomplete in most melanosomes, and there is evidence of lysosomal degradation of melanosome complexes (182). The paucity of melanin in most Spitz nevi is thus explained. Biological marker studies have shed little or no light on the mechanisms whereby Spitz nevi appear to have the capacities for relatively rapid invasive and tumorigenic proliferation in the dermis, but to lack the capacity for metastasis.

Diagnostic and Prognostic Markers

Morphometric and immunohistochemical studies have shown differences between Spitz nevi and melanomas, but none of these adjuncts to histologic diagnosis is in standard use. By immunohistochemistry, Spitz nevi react not only with differentiation markers for melanocytes such as S-100 antigen, but also with HMB-45 and Melan-A/MART-1, melanosomal antigens often expressed in proliferating melanocytic lesions (178,179,183). Spitz nevi tend to show a more orderly pattern of stratification of HMB-45 reactivity from superficial to deep compared to melanomas (178). A recent study demonstrated interesting differences in S-100A6 protein expression between Spitz nevi and melanomas (184). Like nevi and unlike melanomas, Spitz nevi show a tendency toward diminution of nuclear size and/or DNA content (185,186), as well as for reactivity with certain antigens, from the superficial to the deep portions of the nevus (178). This stratification may be regarded as an expression of maturation, which is diagnostically and no doubt also biologically important in the distinction between Spitz nevi and melanomas.

Nuclear size or volume assessed morphometrically has provided fairly good discrimination in some hands, especially when measured at the base of the tumor or when combined with a "maturation parameter," namely the ratio of nuclear area between the deep and superficial portions (187). Cell proliferation marker studies using PCNA or cyclin antibodies have in general shown Spitz nevi to be intermediate between common nevi and melanomas, but the specificity has been insufficient for diagnostic use (188–190). Perhaps of some potential practical utility is the absence of aneuploidy as judged by cytofluorometry (191,192) or DNA *in situ* hybridization (FISH) (193,194), a feature that is specifically associated with Spitz nevi compared to melanomas in several studies. However, these methods have not been applied to a sufficiently large and well-characterized series of difficult cases for which they are most needed, but also for which their utility is likely to be most limited. In one such study, de Wit et al. using FISH were able to identify only three of five lesions that had been originally diagnosed as Spitz nevi but later reclassified as

melanoma because of the occurrence of metastasis (195). In another recent study, 5 of 22 Spitz nevi had an aneuploid cell population, so that the presence of aneuploidy cannot be considered diagnostic of melanoma (196).

In a recent study by Bastian et al. using fluorescence *in situ* hybridization (FISH) on tissue arrays, copy number increases often associated with oncogenic mutations involving the HRAS gene on chromosome 11p have been found in about 10% of cases. Tumors with 11p copy number increases were larger, predominantly intradermal, had marked desmoplasia, characteristic cytologic features, and had an infiltrating growth pattern. HRAS activation by either mutation or copy number increase alone could explain several of the histologic features that overlap with those of melanoma. It is speculated that HRAS activation in the absence of cooperating additional genetic alterations may drive the partially transformed melanocytes of these "atypical" Spitz nevi into senescence or a stable growth arrest (197). There are no data to suggest that Spitz nevi with HRAS activation are at risk for progression to melanoma, however the biological potential of these lesions is not completely understood.

Differential Diagnosis. The distinction between Spitz and other benign nevi is usually trivial except for dysplastic nevi, which may be indicators of an individual at increased risk for melanoma. In cases of doubt in this regard, we add a note to the effect that the differential diagnosis may include a dysplastic nevus, and recommend that the patient be evaluated for other risk factors, such as multiple dysplastic nevi, and a family or personal history of melanoma. Occasional examples of histiocytic tumors such as epithelioid histiocytomas or juvenile xanthogranulomas may be confused with epithelioid Spitz nevi or with melanomas, especially when foam cells or Touton giant cells are inconspicuous (198). It has been demonstrated that Melan-A and tyrosinase markers are sensitive and specific in making the diagnosis of a melanocytic lesion while histiocytic markers such as CD68 and Factor XIIIa are likely to be positive in the histiocytic lesions (199,200).

The differential diagnosis with melanoma is of course of much greater importance. Differentiation of a Spitz nevus from a nodular melanoma can be difficult and even impossible in some cases, because all of the changes seen in the Spitz nevus may also be observed in melanoma. This differential has been discussed extensively above. Crotty et al. consider that that the presence of symmetry, Kamino bodies, and uniformity of cell nests or sheets from side-to-side favor a Spitz nevus, while the presence of abnormal mitoses, a dermal mitotic rate of >2/mm², and mitotic figures within 0.25 mm of the deep border of the lesion favor a melanoma (201). To this list we would add the characteristic dispersion pattern of single cells at the base, which favors a Spitz or other benign nevus.

There are cases on record that were diagnosed as instances of Spitz nevus but later proved to be melanoma

TABLE 28-3. SPITZ NEVUS VERSUS MELANOMA

Spitz Nevus	Melanoma
Pattern Features	
Usually <6 mm in diameter	Usually >6 mm in diameter
Usually symmetrical	Often but not always asymmetrical
Single attenuated cells between reticular dermis collagen bundles at base	Nests and fascicles rather than single cells in the reticular dermis
Epidermal hyperplasia, hyperkeratosis, and hypergranulosis may be prominent	Epidermal reaction is often minimal
Usually little or no pagetoid spread of lesional cells into epidermis	Usually obvious pagetoid spread into epidermis
Epidermal component usually does not extend beyond lateral border	Lateral extension (radial growth phase) is common except in nodular melanoma
Ovoid nests of lesional cells oriented perpendicular to epidermis	Nests variable in size, shape, and orientation
Discontinuous junctional proliferation	May be continuous proliferation
Little or no pigment	Often heavily pigmented, or irregularly scattered pigmented cells within lesion
Small uniform nests in dermis at base	Larger variable nests at base
Cytologic Features	
Nuclear chromatin is open, with prominent nucleoli.	Nuclei may be hyperchromatic and clumped
Nuclear membranes are regular	Irregular nuclear membranes.
Single and confluent eosinophilic globoid bodies in epidermis and superficial dermis	If present, globoid Kamino bodies are inconspicuous and usually single
Mitoses absent or low mitotic rate	Mitoses rarely absent, rate often high
Atypical mitoses rare or absent	Atypical mitoses common
Mitoses rare in lower third of lesion	Mitoses common in lower third
Cells uniform from side to side	Greater tendency to cellular variability
Cells mature with descent to base	Little or no maturation

(195). Other cases, regarded by some as "malignant Spitz nevi," have metastasized to regional lymph nodes but not beyond (202). These lesions, often large, ulcerated, deeply infiltrative, and mitotically active, can alternatively be signed out descriptively as "melanocytic tumors of uncertain potential." The diagnosis of a Spitz nevus depends on an assessment of multiple morphologic features, which are summarized above and in Table 28-3. Given that so-called metastasizing Spitz nevi have been associated with long-term survival, it may be appropriate to regard the metastases as "metastatic melanocytic tumors of uncertain potential," rather than unqualified metastatic malignant melanoma. However, in our practice, such individuals would be offered a consideration of adjuvant protocols for metastatic melanoma.

Because of the difficulty of making an absolutely certain differentiation from melanoma, it is advisable as a precautionary measure in our opinion that lesions diagnosed as Spitz nevi be excised completely, especially in persons at or beyond puberty, particularly since such lesions are usually small in size. Although the issue is debatable (203), exceptions to this general rule might include those lesions where there are cosmetic or other contraindications to excision, and where the diagnosis of Spitz nevus is certain despite the partial nature of the biopsy (204). Also, one should never exclude a diagnosis of melanoma based on age alone, because melanomas may arise in children, although this is rare.

Pigmented Spindle Cell Nevus

This tumor, first described by Richard Reed in 1973 (205), may be regarded as a variant of the Spitz nevus (152,157), or as a distinctive clinicopathologic entity (206). In our experience and that of others, most cases differ significantly from classical Spitz nevi, but some present with overlapping features, indicative of a close relationship between the two entities (207,208). Although this distinction has no clinical significance in that each is a benign lesion, it is important to rule out melanoma, and this is facilitated by an understanding of the differences between these two common melanoma simulants.

The lesions are usually 3 to 6 mm in diameter, deeply pigmented, and either flat or slightly raised. Most patients are young adults, and the most common location is on the lower extremities. Pigmented spindle-cell nevi are uncommon after the age of 35. A classical presentation is that of a newly evolved black plaque on the thigh of a young woman. Because of the heavy pigment and the history of sudden appearance, a diagnosis of melanoma is often suspected clinically. In contrast, Spitz nevi are usually submitted with a benign clinical diagnosis, such as an angioma or a dermal nevus. Like Spitz nevi, the lesions are generally stable after a relatively sudden appearance and a short-lived period of growth.

Histopathology. The pigmented spindle-cell nevus is characterized by its relatively small size and its symmetry, and by a proliferation of uniform, narrow elongated spindle-shaped, often heavily pigmented melanocytes at the dermal–epidermal junction (206–209). The nests of spindle cells are vertically oriented, and tend to blend with adjacent keratinocytes rather than forming clefts as in Spitz nevi. Eosinophilic globules ("Kamino bodies") may be present (210) (Fig. 28-11). The tumor cells often form bundles that are separated by elongated rete ridges. In the papillary dermis, the nevus cells lie in compact clusters, pushing the connective tissue aside. Numerous melanophages may be diffusely present within the underlying papillary dermis. Involvement of the reticular dermis, common in Spitz nevi, is unusual in pigmented spindle-cell nevus. Some lesions show upward epidermal extension of junctional nests of melanocytes. Single-cell upward invasion of the epidermis in a pagetoid pattern may be present but is usually not prominent (138,207). Features that may lead to a diagnosis qualified as "atypical pigmented spindle-cell nevus" include architectural abnormalities including poor circumscription and pagetoid melanocytosis, prominent cytologic atypia, or a prominent epithelioid cell component (207). There may also be considerable overlap with dysplastic nevi (207). The significance of these "atypi-

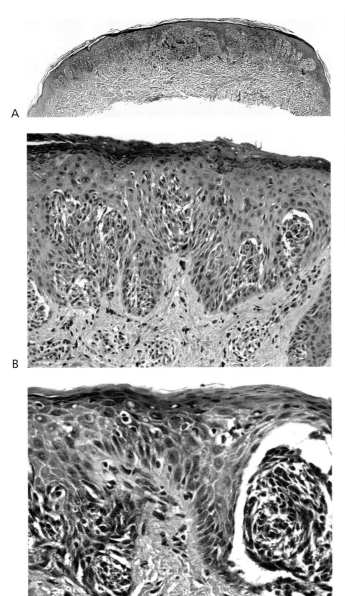

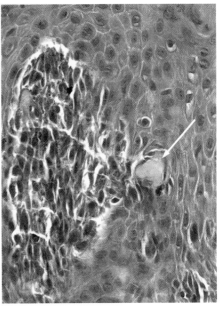

FIGURE 28-11. (A) Pigmented spindle cell nevus. The typical configuration of this lesion is that of a plaque whose breadth is considerably greater than its height. The lesional cells are typically junctional or confined to the epidermis and papillary dermis. **(B)** As in the classic Spitz nevus, lesional cells are arranged in nests that tend to be vertically oriented. Unlike those of the Spitz nevus, the cells are narrow elongated spindle cells without epithelioid cells, and they contain abundant, usually coarse melanin pigment. **(C)** As in Spitz nevi, some (usually slight) degree of pagetoid melanocytosis is not unexpected. Mitoses may be numerous in the epidermis, but the lesional cells in the dermis tend to be mature, with few if any mitoses. Clefting artifact between the nests and the adjacent keratinocytes tends to be less prominent than in Spitz nevi, but may be present, as seen here. **(D)** Kamino bodies in a pigmented spindle cell nevus. This nevus has prominent eosinophilic globoid Kamino bodies in its epidermal compartment.

cal" variants appears to lie in their greater chance of being misdiagnosed as melanoma, since all reports of pigmented spindle-cell nevi emphasize their benign behavior after excision.

Differential Diagnosis. The most important differential is with melanoma of the superficial spreading type. In contrast to these melanomas, pigmented spindle-cell nevi are smaller, symmetrical, and show sharply demarcated lateral margins. The tumor cells appear strikingly uniform "from side to side." If lesional cells of pigmented spindle-cell nevi descend into the papillary dermis, they mature along nevus lines, in contrast to melanomas. Mitoses may be present in the epidermis in either lesion, but are uncommon in the dermis in pigmented spindle-cell nevi. Abnormal mitoses are exceedingly uncommon. Pagetoid melanocytosis is usually not prominent, and the spindle cell cytology differs from that of the epithelioid cells that predominate in most superficial spreading melanomas. Lentigo maligna melanomas may have spindle cells in their vertical growth phase component, but the epidermal component is usually composed of smaller, nevoid albeit atypical cells. Some rare examples of lesions with larger expansile nodules may be difficult to distinguish from melanoma and a descriptive diagnosis may be appropriate ("melanocytic tumor of uncertain potential"). Some cases may present overlapping features with dysplastic nevi, but may usually be distinguished on the basis of their irregularly thickened epidermis, their vertically oriented nests, and their uniformity of cell type. In some cases, this distinction may be more difficult. Such lesions can be signed out descriptively, with a recommendation for additional clinical assessment of the patient to rule out other melanoma risk factors. If these are absent, the significance of an isolated lesion is likely to be minimal.

Congenital Melanocytic Nevus

A congenital melanocytic nevus may be defined as a lesion present at birth and containing nevus cells. Congenital nevi are found in about 1% to 2% of newborn infants (211, 212). In many instances, congenital nevi are larger than acquired nevi, measuring >1.5 cm in diameter (213). However, only a few are of considerable size. Those measuring >20 cm in greatest diameter are referred to as giant congenital melanocytic nevi (214) (Fig. 28-12A). *Nongiant congenital melanocytic nevi* are usually slightly raised and often pigmented, and they may show a moderate growth of hair. They may be classified as "small" (<1.5 cm in diameter) or "intermediate" (>1.5 cm and <20 cm, or amenable to local excision) (214,215). Special forms are the *cerebriform congenital nevus*, which is found on the scalp as a skin-colored, convoluted mass (216); the *spotted grouped pigmented nevi*, showing closely set brown to black papules (217); the *congenital acral melanocytic nevus*, which consists of a blue black patch on the sole or the distal portion of a finger clinically resembling an acral lentiginous melanoma (218); and the *desmoplastic hairless hypopigmented nevus*, which presents clinically as a hard, ligneous, progressively hypopigmented and alopecic giant congenital nevus and is characterized histologically by intense dermal fibrosis, scarce nevus cells, and hypotrophic or absent hair follicles (219). *Giant congenital melanocytic nevi* often have the distribution of a garment ("garment nevi"). They usually are deeply pigmented and are covered with a moderate growth of hair. Often, there are

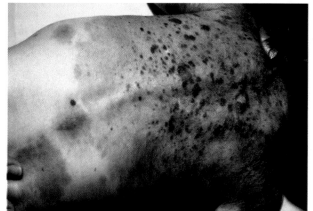
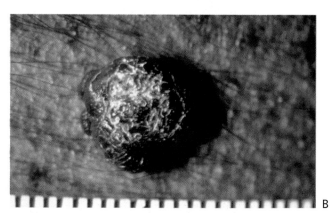

FIGURE 28-12. **(A)** Giant congenital nevus (clinical). These lesions have also been called *garment nevi* because of their coverage of such large areas of skin. Focal areas of increased pigmentation, sometimes associated with palpable nodularity, are not uncommon in giant congenital nevi. Such foci should be followed carefully, and any lesions showing evidence of progressive changes should be excised to rule out melanoma. **(B)** Melanoma in a giant congenital nevus. This nodule developed on the back of the patient illustrated in *(A)*, at the age of 4 years. The patient died within about 2 years of metastatic melanoma.

many scattered "satellite" lesions of a similar appearance (220). These satellite nevi are benign, in contrast to the satellite metastases that may be associated with melanomas. Leptomeningeal melanocytosis is occasionally found in cases in which the giant congenital nevus involves the neck and scalp. There may be not only epilepsy and mental retardation but also a primary leptomeningeal melanoma (221). In a recent study, magnetic resonance findings of meningeal melanosis were identified in 14 of 43 asymptomatic children with giant congenital melanocytic nevi. These findings are consistent with an increased lifetime risk of central nervous system melanoma (222).

Incidence of Cutaneous Melanoma

The lifetime incidence of melanoma arising either in a giant congenital nevus or, as seen rarely, in one of the many smaller satellite nevi, is estimated to lie between about 6% and 12% (223–238). Thus, the majority of patients with congenital nevi will never develop melanoma. The melanoma may be present at birth, or it may arise in infancy or any time later in life (Fig. 28-12B). The mortality of such melanomas is substantial. In a recent cohort study in which 33 patents with giant congenital nevi were followed, two fatal melanomas developed, representing a relative risk approximately 1,000-fold greater than that in the general population (226). In another study of 92 cases, the relative risk for melanoma was increased 239-fold (230), and in a third study of 80 pediatric cases, four melanomas (three of them fatal) occurred after an average follow-up of about 5 years (227). In follow-up data on 160 patients in the New York University Registry of Large Congenital Melanocytic

Nevi (median age at entry: 14 months) followed prospectively for an average of 5.5 years, three extracutaneous melanomas developed: 2 were in the central nervous system (CNS) and 1 was retroperitoneal (237). In reviews of the literature, approximately 70% of the melanomas that occurred in patients with giant congenital nevi have occurred before puberty; some of these melanomas have occurred in extracutaneous sites, especially the central nervous system (226). It is therefore generally agreed that it would be desirable for giant melanocytic nevi to be excised, if feasible. However, complete excision is often not possible, and melanomas may develop in extra-cutaneous sites. Thus, clinical surveillance is considered to be an acceptable alternative in such situations (230,237).

The incidence of melanoma in nongiant congenital nevi, that is, in those <20 cm in greatest diameter, is unknown, but probably greater than that in a comparable area of normal skin. It is likely that the risk is related to the lesion's size (224). The excision of all nongiant congenital nevi, where feasible, is advised by many (224, 239), although not by all authors (214,240). Most of the melanomas observed in these nongiant lesions have occurred after puberty (225).

Histopathology. The histologic appearance of giant congenital nevi differs from that of acquired nevi in terms of their greater size and depth, and in the involvement of skin appendages (Fig. 28-13). Nongiant congenital nevi may have the same histologic appearance as acquired nevi, or may show features of congenital nevi (Fig. 28-14). (105,241,242). The features in nongiant congenital nevi are neither sensitive nor specific for truly congenital origin of a nevus. A recent histologic study with comparison with

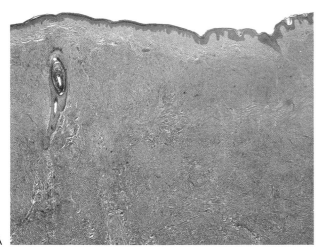
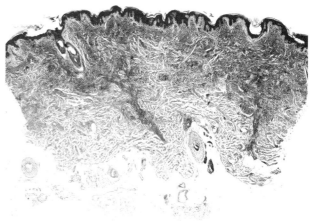

FIGURE 28-13. (A) This nevus is very broad (many centimeters, extending well beyond the borders of the image), and deep, that is, the lesional cells extend from the epidermis through the reticular dermis and into the fat. **(B)** In another giant congenital nevus, sheets of nevus cells are placed among reticular dermis collagen bundles. The dermal component of giant congenital nevi is often variably cellular, and in addition to nevi differentiation there may be evidence of Schwannian or even heterotopic elements.

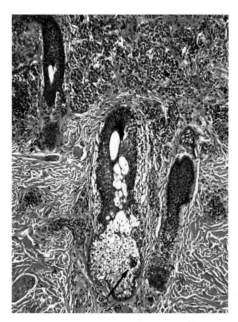

FIGURE 28-14. Compound nevus with congenital pattern features. Nevus cells extend around skin appendages and between fibers of the reticular dermis. The presence of nevus cells within skin appendages (as here in the sebaceous unit) is a quite specific feature indicating true congenital onset of a nevus. The extension of nevus cells into the upper reticular dermis and around skin appendages is quite characteristic of congenital nevi. However, acquired nevi may also exhibit this deep pattern, and conversely, congenital nevi are not always deep.

clinical data showed that 32 nevi with the histologic criteria of congenital nevi were actually acquired, and that 179 nevi present at birth did not fulfill these criteria. In the case of deep and large (giant) congenital nevi, in contrast, the clinicopathologic correlation was 100% (243). Cytologically, the cells of congenital nevi are similar to those of acquired nevi. The nevus cells are typically positive for the melanocytic markers S-100, HMB-45 and Melan-A, the latter of which has the best combination of sensitivity and specificity (183).

Nongiant (Small and Intermediate) Congenital Melanocytic Nevi

At one time these were thought to be superficial at birth and to show deep involvement later (213). However, a serial study showed no change in pattern in follow-up biopsies (244). This and other studies have shown various patterns in the distribution of the nevus cells independent of the age of the patient. Thus, nongiant congenital nevi may be junctional, compound, or intradermal nevi, and their location in the dermis may be either superficial, which may include junctional involvement, or superficial and deep (244,245). They may differ from acquired nevi by one or more features: (a) presence of melanocytes around and within hair follicles, in sweat ducts and glands, in sebaceous glands, in or in intimate association with vessel walls,

in arrector pili muscles, and in the perineurium of nerves; (b) extension of melanocytes between collagen bundles singly or in double rows; and (c) extension into the deepest reticular dermis and into the subcutis (213) (Fig. 28-14). However, many nongiant congenital nevi show none of these features. For example, some documented congenital nevi have been entirely junctional (244), while the likelihood of deep dermal involvement appears to increase with the size of the lesion (246) and is actually uncommon in lesions <3 cm in diameter (242). Conversely, the presence of most of the features mentioned above has been documented in nevi that were indubitably clinically apparent after birth ("tardive" congenital nevi) (247). Thus, nevi with the constellation of features described above may be characterized as "nevi with congenital pattern features," but not all of these lesions are truly congenital in origin. It remains to be seen whether such nevi have any special significance as risk markers or potential precursors of melanoma (236).

Among the special forms of nongiant congenital nevi, the *cerebriform congenital nevus* usually presents as an intradermal nevus with neuroid changes simulating those seen in neurofibroma (216). Lesions called *spotted grouped pigmented nevi* also are intradermal nevi. They are either eccrine- or follicle-centered. If they are eccrine-centered, each eccrine sweat duct is tightly enveloped by nevus cells, whereas hair follicles are involved only slightly (217). If they are follicle-centered, nevus cell nests are found mainly around the hair follicles. In the *acral nevus*, a compound nevus is seen with considerable pigmentation in the upper dermis, and aggregates of nonpigmented nevus cells are seen around blood vessels and eccrine glands in the lower dermis (218). In a lesion called desmoplastic hairless hypopigmented nevus, there is intense dermal fibrosis, scarce nevus cells, and hypotrophic or absent hair follicles. Follow-up biopsies have documented the progressive nature of the fibrosis and nevus cell depletion (219).

In some congenital melanocytic nevi, changes are observed that may simulate a melanoma. In a recent study, features that could simulate malignant melanoma in a congenital nevus included (a) asymmetry and poor circumscription; (b) an increased number of single melanocytes which predominated over nests of melanocytes in some high power fields; (c) single melanocytes not equidistant from one another; (d) scattered single melanocytes present above the dermoepidermal junction; and (e) confluence of nests of melanocytes, all features in common with malignant melanoma (248). In our experience, such changes are generally slight in degree, and severe uniform cytologic atypia or frequent mitoses are not observed.

Giant Congenital Melanocytic Nevi

These are often more complex than nongiant congenital nevi. Three patterns may be found within them: a compound or intradermal nevus, a "neural nevus," and a blue nevus pattern (221). In most instances, the compound or intradermal nevus component predominates, whereas, in others, the "neural nevus" component predominates. In the latter case, formations such as neuroid tubes and nevic corpuscles are present. These areas may show considerable similarity to a neurofibroma. A component resembling a blue nevus or a cellular blue nevus is found in some of the giant pigmented nevi, usually as a minor component. In rare instances, however, the entire congenital lesion consists of a giant blue nevus, which, in one patient with a lesion of the scalp was reported to extend to the dura (32) and in another had infiltrated the brain (33). Nevus cells may be present in lymph nodes draining skin containing a giant congenital nevus; this phenomenon should not be mistaken for involvement by a melanoma. In general, the nodal nevus cells lie in capsular or sinusoidal septal collagen, and the cells lack atypia (249).

The pattern of occurrence of *melanoma in giant congenital nevi* was studied in a review of 34 patients who had primary cutaneous melanomas within their nevi; in two additional patients, melanoma developed at cutaneous sites other than within their nevi. All patients in whom melanoma developed within the nevi had nevi in axial locations; however, 91% of the nevi were axial. No melanoma was found that had arisen in any of the 26 nevi confined to the extremities. In addition, no melanoma was found that had arisen in thousands of satellite nevi (232). If a melanoma arises in a congenital nevus, it usually originates at the epidermal–dermal junction and the appearances are those of ordinary forms of melanoma, usually of the superficial spreading or nodular types. Most of the congenital nevi associated with such melanomas are small and superficial (250). Occasionally, however, a melanoma in a giant congenital nevus, in contrast with nearly all other cutaneous melanomas, arises deep in the dermis or subcutis (251–254).

Histologically, in our experience, some of the melanomas in giant congenital nevi have consisted largely of undifferentiated "blastic" cells resembling lymphoblasts and containing little or no melanin, while others are comprised of large epithelioid cells similar to those of many melanomas. Other patterns of malignancy that have been described in congenital nevi have included neoplasms with the appearance of a neurosarcoma (255), lesions that have been termed malignant blue nevus (256–258), neoplasms with heterologous mesenchymal elements including rhabdomyoblasts (259) and lipoblasts, undifferentiated spindle-cell cancers, and well-differentiated neoplasms termed minimal deviation melanomas (258). It has been emphasized that peculiar differentiation is to be expected in neoplasms of giant congenital nevi, and that alarmingly cellular neoplasms may not behave aggressively (258). Thus, pathology does not always readily predict outcome. This is especially true in our experience when melanomas arise in the first few months of life.

Cytological and architectural atypia may occasionally be seen in congenital nevi, and criteria for the distinction of these lesions from melanoma are similar to those discussed in the differential diagnosis of dysplastic nevi and superficial spreading melanomas in later sections. In an interesting study, abnormal DNA content was found to correlate with cytologic atypia in giant congenital nevi (260). It is possible that the presence of atypical foci could increase the risk of malignant transformation.

Melanomas in small congenital nevi are typically of the usual superficial spreading type. In a recent study, 40 of 190 cases of melanoma were associated with preexisting nevi; of these, 15 had congenital features with a largest diameter of 1.5 cm, that is, "small" congenital nevi. These 15 cases were melanomas of the superficial type with a mean tumor thickness lower than that of melanomas not associated with nevi (0.33 vs. 1.50 cm). Thus, a relatively high percentage of small congenital nevi were found to be associated with melanomas, indicating that they may be considered as potential melanomas precursor. Nevertheless, the risk of progression of any given lesion is very low (236).

Although melanomas may occur in the dermal component of congenital nevi, cellular *proliferative nodules in congenital nevi* often do not behave in a clinically aggressive fashion (261). In a clinical pathologic study of a cohort of 26 cases, with a mean of 5-year follow-up on 16 patients, the lesions had an invariably benign clinical course. The features that are useful to differentiate cellular proliferative nodule from melanoma include (a) lack of high-grade uniform cellular atypia; (b) lack of necrosis within the nodule; (c) rarity of mitoses; (d) evidence of maturation in the form of blending or transitional forms between the cells in the nodule and the adjacent nevus cells; (e) lack of pagetoid spread into the overlying epidermis; and (f) no destructive expansile growth (262). If some of these features are present in slight degree, the descriptive diagnosis of "melanocytic tumor of uncertain potential" may be appropriate. Bastian et al. recently studied different types of proliferations arising in congenital nevi by comparative genomic hybridization. Cases of congenital nevi with foci of increased cellularity showed no aberrations, whereas lesions with cellular nodules had aberrations of whole chromosomes exclusively, a pattern that in turn differed significantly from the findings in frank melanomas, in which only 5% showed numerical changes only. This difference might explain the more benign clinical behavior of these nodules and may be of diagnostic value in ambiguous cases (263).

Leptomeningeal Melanocytosis

There is a diffuse infiltration of the leptomeninges with pigmented melanocytes. Also, the blood vessels entering the brain and spinal cord may be surrounded by melanocytes, and there may be areas of infiltration of the brain or spinal cord with melanocytes. Leptomeningeal melanoma can infiltrate the leptomeninx and form multiple nodules in the brain (264,265).

Deep Penetrating Nevus (Plexiform Spindle Cell Nevus)

This is a distinctive entity that has some features of combined nevus, blue nevus, and Spitz nevus (266,267). In the first report of 70 cases from a referral center, many cases had previously been misdiagnosed histologically as melanomas. Similar lesions have also been described as plexiform spindle-cell nevi (38,268,269). Most of the lesions occurred in the second and third decades (range 3 to 63 years). The head, neck and shoulder were the most frequent sites of involvement, with no occurrences on the hands or feet. The lesions ranged from 2 to 9 mm, and were darkly pigmented papules and nodules, often diagnosed clinically as blue nevi or cellular blue nevi. In a mean follow-up of 7 years, none recurred or metastasized. However, a prospective follow-up series has not been reported. On cross-section, the lesions extended at least halfway into the dermis, with a smooth, dome-shaped elevation of the epidermis.

Histopathology. At scanning magnification, the lesions are circumscribed and pyramidal in shape, with a broad base abutting the epidermis, and an apex extending into or towards the fat (Fig. 28-15). Nests of nevus cells at the dermal–epidermal junction are usually present. The dermal component is composed of loosely arranged nests or plexiform fascicles of large pigmented spindle and epithelioid cells interspersed with melanophages. In many cases there is an admixture of smaller, more conventional nevus cells. The lesional cell nests tend to surround skin appendages, and to infiltrate the collagen at the periphery of the lesion. The cells do not tend to "mature" with descent into the dermis. Some lesions have a patchy mild lymphocytic infiltrate.

At higher magnification, nuclear pleomorphism may be striking in some lesions, with variation in size and shape, hyperchromasia, and nuclear pseudoinclusions. Nucleoli are usually inconspicuous but a few large eosinophilic nucleoli may be observed. Importantly, mitoses are absent or very rare, with no more than one or two in multiple sections of any given lesion. The cytoplasm is abundant, and contains finely divided brown melanin pigment. The lesional cells react positively for S-100 protein and HMB-45 antigen (269).

Differential Diagnosis. Deep penetrating nevi can be distinguished from *nodular melanoma* by architectural and cytologic features. Most bulky tumorigenic melanomas exhibit a more striking pattern of epidermal involvement with spread of atypical cells into the epidermis and, often, with ulceration. Melanomas are likely to be more broad than deep, while deep penetrating nevi tend to be vertically oriented like Spitz nevi. Tumorigenic melanomas usually exhibit a more destructive pattern of infiltration, with displacement and compression of the stroma, and often with necrosis. Most also display marked nuclear atypia with frequent and often abnormal mitoses. A few nodular spindle-cell melanomas have lower-grade nuclear atypia, and in these cases the presence of more than a few mitoses may be decisive. A study found rates of expression of the cell cycle proliferation marker PCNA to be somewhat higher in deep penetrating nevi than in ordinary banal nevi, but considerably lower than in melanomas (270).

Benign lesions that may show some tendency to overlapping features with deep penetrating nevi include *com-*

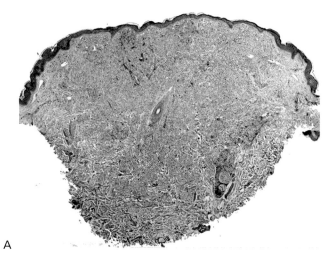

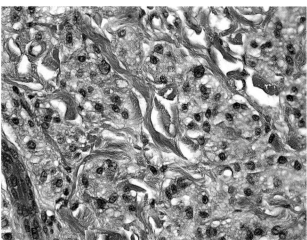

A · B

FIGURE 28-15. (A) Deep penetrating nevus. At scanning magnification, the lesion is pyramidal, with its base applied to the epidermis, and its apex in the reticular dermis. **(B)** The lesional cells in the dermis are arranged in clusters. They may be heavily pigmented and there may be scattered large, hyperchromatic, and pleomorphic nuclei, constituting *random* cytologic atypia. Mitoses are absent or very rare.

mon and cellular blue nevi, as well as *spindle and epithelioid cell nevi.* Although deep penetrating nevi can usually be distinguished from these benign lesions, the distinction from melanoma is of greatest importance. Neural involvement is not an indicator of malignancy in these lesions.

Halo Nevus

A halo nevus, also known as Sutton's nevus or nevus depigmentosa centrifugum, represents a pigmented nevus surrounded by a depigmented zone, or halo (Fig. 28-16A). The nevus may be of almost any of the types described in the preceding sections, and a similar halo reaction may be seen rarely in relation to primary or metastatic melanoma (271). In the common type of halo nevus, which is characterized histologically by an inflammatory infiltrate and is therefore referred to as *inflammatory halo nevus,* the central nevus only rarely shows erythema or crusting; however, it undergoes involution in most instances, a process that extends over a period of

several months. The area of depigmentation shows no clinical signs of inflammation and, even though it may persist for many months and even years, ultimately repigments in most cases. Halo nevi tend to progress through several clinical stages. The classic lesion is a brown nevus with a surrounding rim of depigmentation, and may be referred to as a stage I halo nevus. The central nevus may lose its pigment and appear pink with a surrounding halo (stage II), the central papule may disappear leading to a circular area of macular depigmentation (stage III) or the depigmented area may repigment (stage IV), leaving no trace of its prior existence. In unusual lesions, darkening of the central nevus rather than lightening has been described (272). There are well-documented examples in which a halo nevus fails to involute, even though an inflammatory infiltrate is present, and repigmentation of the halo takes place (273). Most persons with halo nevi are children or young adults, and the back is the most common site. Not infrequently, halo nevi are multiple, occurring either simultaneously or successively.

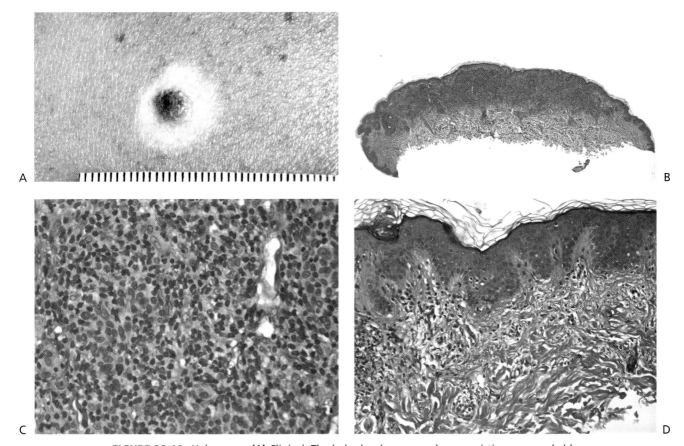

FIGURE 28-16. Halo nevus. **(A)** Clinical. The halo develops around a pre-existing unremarkable compound nevus. **(B)** A dense infiltrative lymphocytic response blurs the silhouette of the lesional nevus cells in the dermis at scanning magnification. **(C)** Small lymphocytes are diffusely placed among the dermal nevus cells, which may appear swollen and slightly atypical (*reactive* atypia). Severe or uniform atypia or mitotic activity should suggest the possibility of melanoma. **(D)** At the periphery of the nevus, the halo is a region where pigment and melanocytes are reduced or absent, and there may be a subtle lymphocytic infiltrate at the dermal–epidermal junction, as here.

Besides the more common inflammatory halo nevus with histologically apparent inflammation, there also are cases of *noninflammatory halo nevi* in which histologic examination shows no inflammatory infiltrate (274). In such instances, the nevus does not involute. In addition, there is the so-called *halo nevus phenomenon*, also referred to as *halo nevus without halo*. In these instances, the nevus shows histologic signs of inflammation analogous to a halo nevus but without presenting a halo clinically (275). Such nevi may involute.

Halo dermatitis around a melanocytic nevus refers to a temporary inflammatory reaction surrounding a nevus (*Meyerson's eczematous nevus*) (276). There is a papular compound nevus that becomes surrounded by an eczematous halo. Histologically, the epidermis adjacent to the nevus is spongiotic. An analogous phenomenon of "nevocentric" erythema multiforme has also been described where cytotoxic/interface alterations predominate (277). Similar changes may be seen around atypical or dysplastic nevi (278).

Histopathology. An inflammatory halo nevus in its early stage shows nests of nevus cells embedded in a dense inflammatory infiltrate, in the upper dermis and at the epidermal–dermal junction (Fig. 28-16B, C, and D). Later, scattered nevus cells tend to predominate over nests. Even when melanin is still present in the nevus cells, these cells often show evidence of damage to their nucleus and cytoplasm, and some frankly apoptotic nevus cells are commonly observed. Some cells, especially superficially, may have enlarged ovoid nucleoli, changes that may be regarded as a form of "reactive atypia." High-grade nuclear atypia is not observed. Importantly, the lesional cells tend to show evidence of "maturation," becoming smaller with descent from superficial to deep within the lesion. Nevus cell mitoses are rare, and if present should prompt consideration of the possibility of melanoma. Most of the cells in the dense inflammatory infiltrate are lymphocytes. However, some of them are macrophages, in which varying amounts of melanin are contained. As the infiltrate invades the nevus cell nests, it often is difficult to distinguish between the lymphoid cells of the infiltrate and the type B nevus cells in the mid-dermis, because they, too, may have the appearance of lymphoid cells. Immunohistochemical studies using S-100 or a more specific marker such as Melan-A may be very helpful in identifying the nevus cells in the infiltrate (279). The infiltrate tends to extend upward into the lower portion of the epidermis. In most instances, the infiltrate is characterized by dense cellular packing without vasodilatation or intercellular edema and by sharp demarcation along its lower border.

At a later stage, only a few, and finally no distinct nevus cells can be identified. Gradually, after all nevus cells have disappeared, the inflammatory infiltrate subsides.

In both the inflammatory and the noninflammatory halo nevus, the epidermis of the halo at first shows a reduction in the amount of melanin on staining with silver and fewer dopapositive melanocytes than are seen in the normal epidermis. Ultimately, there is complete absence of melanin and also a negative dopa reaction. Especially in early lesions, lymphocytes may be seen rosetting around damaged melanocytes in the halo.

Histogenesis. Immunohistochemical staining for S-100 protein helps in the identification of nevus cells within the inflammatory infiltrate, because their number may be small and it may be difficult to differentiate them from the lymphocytes of the infiltrate (279). However, Langerhans cells and some histiocytes also react with S-100 protein, and therefore a more specific marker such as Melan-A is preferable. Electron microscopic study reveals that, under the influence of the lymphocytic infiltrate, all nevus cells and melanocytes within reach of the infiltrate at first are damaged and ultimately disappear. In the nevus, many nevus cells appear vacuolated and contain only few melanosomes, but large aggregates of melanosomes are seen within macrophages (280,281).

In the depigmenting halo, the melanocytes show various kinds of degeneration, such as vacuolization and coagulation of the cytoplasm and autophagocytosis of melanosomes. The melanocytes are seen partially in the upper layers of the epidermis and are apparently shed from the epidermis (282). In early stage lesions, few melanocytes and some Langerhans cells are seen, while at a more advanced clinical stage, only Langerhans cells are present in the basal layer. It has been suggested that an initial noncellular stage of inhibition of both the melanocytes and the nevus cells may be responsible for the development of the depigmented halo, preceding the appearance of a dermal lympho-macrophagic infiltrate that ultimately leads to the destruction of the nevus (280). Both in halo nevi and in vitiligo, the depigmentation takes place through disappearance of the melanocytes. However, the association of vitiligo and halo nevus is not sufficiently common for halo nevus to be regarded as a form of vitiligo. The abundance of potential antigen-presenting cells and lymphocytes (including CD8+ T cells) in the regressing nevus at the site of depigmentation suggests that these cells participate in the destruction of nevus cells and melanocytes in the halo phenomenon (283). In an interesting study of the lymphoid elements infiltrating halo nevi, oligoclonal expansion of T cells was observed in all patients, and in one patient, T cells using the same TCR β-chain were observed in distinct halo nevi, demonstrating a local expansion of common clones that are most likely activated by shared antigens within the nevi (284).

Differential Diagnosis. It can be difficult to differentiate early lesions of inflammatory halo nevus from a melanoma; both types of lesions may have a dense cellular infiltrate in the dermis, and, in halo nevi, the nevus cell nests, as a result of having been invaded by the cellular infiltrate, may appear atypical. The danger of misinterpretation is greatest in halo nevi without a halo, the so-called halo nevus phenomenon. However, the inflammatory infiltrate in halo nevi is more pronounced than in melanoma and extends diffusely through the lesion, rather than being concentrated at the periphery as in most examples of tumorigenic melanoma. The diagnosis of melanoma rather than halo nevus is likely in a complex lesion that has an adjacent *in situ* or microinvasive component. Whether or not such an adjacent component is present, attributes of the nodule itself that should prompt consideration of melanoma include larger size, asymmetry, lack of lesional cell maturation, uniform high-grade nuclear atypia, and mitotic activity.

If no identifiable nevus cells are present, the diagnosis of halo nevus is suggested by the presence of melanophages in the dense cellular infiltrate and by the absence of melanin in the epidermis on staining with silver.

Recurrent Nevus (Pseudomelanoma)

Recurrence of a nevus may show clinical hyperpigmentation, which in turn on biopsy may show histologic changes suggestive of melanoma (285–289). Recurrence may follow incomplete removal of a nevus, particularly by a shave biopsy or electrodesiccation, or the nevus may apparently have been completely excised. Clinical recurrence is common. In a prospective follow-up study, twenty-eight percent of all nevi, and 41% of hairy nevi, were reported to have recurred within 12 months after shave excision (290). The pigmentation in recurrent nevi is confined to the region of the scar, and typically presents within a few weeks of the surgical procedure. After this rapid appearance, the pigment is stable. In contrast, recurrent melanoma does not respect the border of the scar, and extends over time into the adjacent skin. Paradoxically, recurrent melanoma occurs more slowly, over months or years, but progresses inexorably.

Histopathology. Although most recurrent nevi are not cytologically atypical, in a few instances they contain atypical melanocytes, both singly and in nests, arranged mainly along the epidermal–dermal junction, but occasionally also extending into the upper dermis and also into the epidermis in a pagetoid pattern (138) (Fig. 28-17). The junctional nests are often composed of pigmented epithelioid melanocytes forming irregular nests possibly the result of their growth within an atrophic epidermal layer that interfaces with scar tissue. Deep remnants of the nevus may be seen in the reticular dermis beneath the scar (289). A lymphocytic infiltrate with melanophages may be seen in the upper dermis. Nevus cells in the dermis tend to show evidence of maturation, and the Ki-67 proliferation rate is low (291). Distinction from melanoma may be difficult without a pertinent history. However, the presence of fibrosis in the upper dermis and often of remnants of a melanocytic nevus beneath the zone of fibrosis, as well as the sharp lateral demarcation, usually makes a correct diagnosis possible. As is true clinically, the recurrent nevus is confined to the epidermis above the scar, while recurrent melanoma may extend into the adjacent epidermis. However, persistent nevus, after a partial biopsy, may also in-

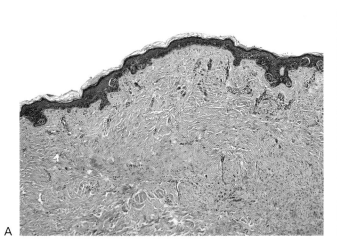
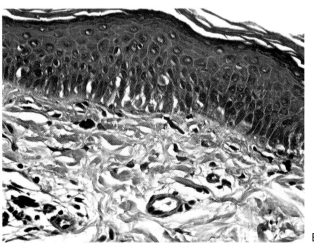

FIGURE 28-17. (A) Recurrent and persistent melanocytic nevus. Recurrent pigmentation may occur after complete excision of a nevus, or may occur in the scar of a partial removal, as in this example where the pathology of the recurrent nevus is seen only above the scar, and residual dermal nevus cells of the persistent original nevus are present to the right of the scar and beneath it. **(B)** The cells of the recurrent nevus in the epidermis are variably enlarged, and they may be arranged with single cells predominating in foci and extending up into the epidermis in a pagetoid pattern, which is usually, as here, relatively subtle. Severe uniform atypia with extensive pagetoid proliferation should suggest the possibility of recurrent melanoma. The prior biopsy should be reviewed, if possible.

volve skin adjacent to a scar. In this instance, ordinary criteria for the distinction between melanomas and nevi apply, as discussed below. In any problematic case in which the diagnosis is in doubt, the original biopsy should be obtained for review.

Histogenesis. The nevus cells in some recurrent lesions may originate from residual nevus cells located either at the periphery of the lesion or along the outer root sheath of hairs. Recurrences that follow complete excision may be due to activation of melanocytes. The confinement of these reactive changes to the regenerating epidermis above the biopsy scar suggests that the process may be related to growth factors involved in wound healing. Some of these, such as fibroblast growth factors and c-kit ligand, are known to be trophic for melanocytes *in vitro* (292).

Dysplastic Nevus

Dysplastic nevi were first described under the designations of *B–K mole syndrome* or *atypical mole syndrome* as multiple lesions occurring in patients with one or several melanomas and in some of their relatives (293,294). It soon became apparent that multiple moles, in addition to their familial occurrence, can occur as a sporadic phenomenon in patients with a melanoma. This was referred to as the *dysplastic nevus syndrome* (295). Subsequently, cases of multiple dysplastic nevi without melanoma were reported (296). This was followed by the recognition that dysplastic nevi frequently occur as solitary lesions, and are quite common, being found in 5% to 20% of various populations, depending on the criteria used (297). Dysplastic nevi do not constitute a single gene-related genetic syndrome, and in today's usage, it is more common to simply characterize individuals as having dysplastic nevi, with some estimate of their number and degree of clinical atypia, rather than as having a particular form of dysplastic nevus syndrome.

Dysplastic nevi form, clinically and histologically, a continuum extending from a common nevus to a superficial spreading melanoma (298). They may be located anywhere on the body but are found most commonly on the trunk. A suitable rigorous definition of a clinically dysplastic nevus includes (a) the presence of a macular component either as the entire lesion or surrounding a papular center; (b) large size, exceeding 5 mm; (c) irregular or ill-defined "fuzzy" border; and (d) irregular pigmentation within the lesion (62,299) (Figs. 28-18A and B). When defined in this manner, clinically recognized dysplastic nevi are a central risk factor for cutaneous melanoma; in a large case-control study, one clinically dysplastic nevus was associated with a twofold risk for melanoma, while ten or more conferred a 12-fold increased risk (62).

Histopathology. When dysplastic nevi were first described in association with melanoma, it was considered that dysplastic nevi by definition always contained cytologically atypical melanocytes (297). Later, it was argued by

some that an abnormal pattern of lentiginous melanocytic growth was a sufficient criterion without requiring atypia (300). It was even stated that "most compound nevi that are confined to the epidermis and the papillary dermis are dysplastic nevi" (300). Subsequently, the term "Clark's nevus" was coined to encompass all nevi with lentiginous junctional components (either alone or adjacent to a dermal component), irrespective of lesional size or of the presence or absence of cytologic atypia (301). This definition would include the very common small lentiginous junctional and compound nevi. Thus, the term "Clark's nevus" is not synonymous with the term "dysplastic nevus." Because of controversy regarding its use and definition, use of the term "dysplastic nevus" was discouraged by another National Institutes of Health (NIH) panel, which proposed the synonymous term "nevus with architectural disorder and melanocytic atypia" (302). This clumsy term has not been widely used. Specificity in distinguishing dysplastic from nondysplastic nevi is likely to be increased by the inclusion of size and cytologic atypia as criteria, as was done in the original reports. In our practice, small lesions or lesions with architectural features of dysplastic nevi but without cytologic atypia may be reported as "compound nevi," as "lentiginous compound nevi," or the NIH descriptive terminology may be used. Criteria for assessing melanocytic dysplasia may be summarized in two categories: *architectural features*, and *cytologic features* (297). These features are closely but not perfectly correlated (303) (Fig. 28-18).

Architectural Pattern

In the architectural pattern of melanocytic dysplasia, the lesions are either entirely junctional, or there is a prominent junctional component which is symmetrically distributed at the "shoulders" or junctional edges that extend laterally beyond a central dermal component (Fig. 28-18C). At higher magnification, lentiginous proliferation of nevus cells in the epidermis is the dominant feature in the junctional component. There is elongation of the rete ridges, and an increase in the number of melanocytes, arranged in nests whose long axes tend to lie parallel to the epidermal surface, and which tend to lie near the tips and sides of elongated rete ridges, and to form "bridges" via apparent fusion of nests between adjacent rete (Fig. 28-18D). There may be scattered single cells as well, but these do not predominate and there is no continuous lentiginous proliferation of single cells between the rete. The melanocytes in the junctional nests are frequently spindle-shaped, but they may be large and epithelioid and show abundant cytoplasm with fine, dusty melanin particles. If the lesion is compound, nests of melanocytes in the papillary dermis show a uniform appearance and evidence of maturation with descent into the dermis, as seen in an ordinary compound nevus. In these compound dysplastic nevi, the in-

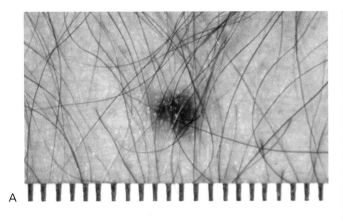

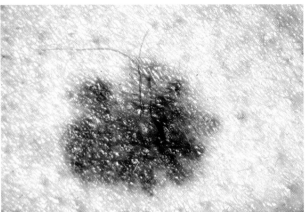

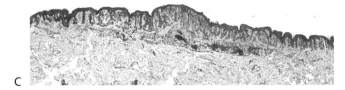

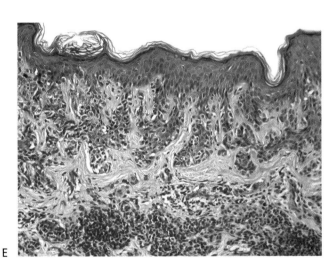

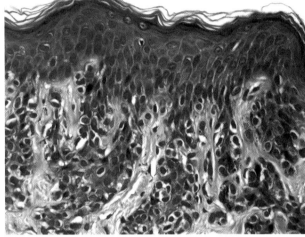

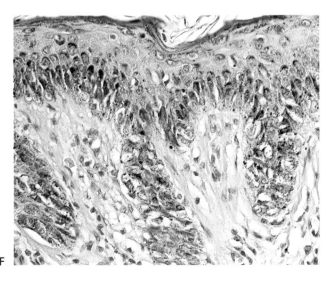

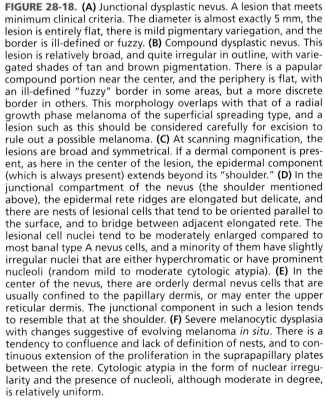

FIGURE 28-18. (A) Junctional dysplastic nevus. A lesion that meets minimum clinical criteria. The diameter is almost exactly 5 mm, the lesion is entirely flat, there is mild pigmentary variegation, and the border is ill-defined or fuzzy. **(B)** Compound dysplastic nevus. This lesion is relatively broad, and quite irregular in outline, with variegated shades of tan and brown pigmentation. There is a papular compound portion near the center, and the periphery is flat, with an ill-defined "fuzzy" border in some areas, but a more discrete border in others. This morphology overlaps with that of a radial growth phase melanoma of the superficial spreading type, and a lesion such as this should be considered carefully for excision to rule out a possible melanoma. **(C)** At scanning magnification, the lesions are broad and symmetrical. If a dermal component is present, as here in the center of the lesion, the epidermal component (which is always present) extends beyond its "shoulder." **(D)** In the junctional compartment of the nevus (the shoulder mentioned above), the epidermal rete ridges are elongated but delicate, and there are nests of lesional cells that tend to be oriented parallel to the surface, and to bridge between adjacent elongated rete. The lesional cell nuclei tend to be moderately enlarged compared to most banal type A nevus cells, and a minority of them have slightly irregular nuclei that are either hyperchromatic or have prominent nucleoli (random mild to moderate cytologic atypia). **(E)** In the center of the nevus, there are orderly dermal nevus cells that are usually confined to the papillary dermis, or may enter the upper reticular dermis. The junctional component in such a lesion tends to resemble that at the shoulder. **(F)** Severe melanocytic dysplasia with changes suggestive of evolving melanoma *in situ*. There is a tendency to confluence and lack of definition of nests, and to continuous extension of the proliferation in the suprapapillary plates between the rete. Cytologic atypia in the form of nuclear irregularity and the presence of nucleoli, although moderate in degree, is relatively uniform.

traepidermal component extends by definition beyond the lateral border of the dermal component, forming a "shoulder" to the lesion histologically, and a "target-like" or "fried-egg" pattern clinically. Extension of melanocytes into the epidermis is absent or slight and limited to the lowermost layers. An inflammatory infiltrate, usually only of a mild or moderate degree and intermingled with melanophages, is present in the dermis beneath areas of junctional activity. The papillary dermis is also characteristically fibrotic, and typically lamellae of collagen encircle affected rete (concentric fibroplasia) and/or form stacked layers within dermal papillae (lamellar fibroplasia). The nevus cells in the dermis are mature, usually of the lymphocyte-like "type B" variety (Fig. 28-18E). They are often combined to the papillary dermis, or in 5% of cases may enter the upper reticular dermis (compound dysplastic nevus with congenital features [304]). Most dysplastic nevi are clinically stable (305), so that they are not "active" in the sense of continuing growth.

Cytologic Features

Cytologically, in addition to the lentiginous melanocytic hyperplasia, melanocytic nuclear atypia is required for the diagnosis. This atypia is characterized by irregularly shaped, large, hyperchromatic nuclei in some melanocytes. Most atypical melanocytes lie singly or in small groups, and the atypia involves only a minority of the lesional cells ("random" cytologic atypia) (Fig. 28-18D). Focal extension of atypical-appearing melanocytes into the lower spinous layer may be seen, but if this is prominent, transformation into melanoma *in situ* may have occurred. A borderline lesion may be a dysplastic nevus or an early superficial spreading melanoma that is still *in situ* or microinvasive. Since such early melanomas are curable after simple excision (306), this distinction does not carry the implication

of increased mortality, so long as the lesion is entirely removed. For lesions with severe dysplasia where the differential diagnosis includes the possibility of early melanoma, conservative re-excision is recommended for lesions that have been minimally or incompletely excised.

Melanocytic dysplasia appears to be a quantitative trait, and several authors have produced guidelines for grading dysplasia. McNutt et al. recently published a detailed schema for grading lesions from nevi without atypia to melanoma. This schema has been correlated with biology in that patients with more atypia in their nevus biopsies are more likely to have had a primary melanoma. In Table 28-4, key grading features are presented in schematic form. The critically important criteria for distinguishing between nevi and melanoma are discussed in more detail in Table 28-5. The features of severe dysplasia in this study included nests predominating over single cells in the epidermis, only rare upward migration of cells in the center and not at the periphery of the lesion, and a dermal component that tended to be abundant with more crowding of the dermal nests. Cytologically, the nuclei are usually larger than those of keratinocytes, and there was often an admixture of cells that include large bizarre hyperchromatic nuclei. Confluent ("uniform") atypia was not observed. Nucleoli were often prominent. The grading for each lesion was based on a combination of these architectural and cytologic features (307). Similar criteria for grading of dysplastic nevi have been published and illustrated by others (304,308–310). In general, in our opinion, lesions that show significant overlap with criteria for melanoma such as those listed above should be graded as severe dysplasia, with an indication, if appropriate, that evolving melanoma *in situ* cannot be ruled out (Fig. 28-18F). Such lesions should be managed by complete excision with, at a minimum, a clear margin of normal skin around the scar and any residual lesion. If melanoma *in situ* cannot be ruled out, current

TABLE 28-4. CRITERIA FOR DYSPLASTIC NEVUS GRADING

Atypia	None	Mild	Moderate	Severe	Malignant Melanoma
Lateral circumscription	+++	++	+	+	+/−
Symmetry	+++	+++	+++	+/−	+/−
Junctional extension	+/−	+++	+++	+++	++++
Rete ridge distortion	+/−	+/−	++	+++	++++
Concentric fibrosis	+/−	+	++	++	+/−
Diffuse fibrosis	+/−	+/−	+/−	+/−	+++
Lymphocytes	+/−	+	++	+++	++++
Upward migration	+/−	+/−	+/−	+/−	++++
Suprapapillary plates	−	−	−	+/−	++++
Nuclear size	+	+	++	++	+++
Nucleoli	−	+/−	+/−	+++	++++
Chromatin clumping	−	−	+/−	++	++++
Dermal mitoses	−	−	−	−	+++

Based on Arumi-Uria M, McNutt NS, Finnerty B. Grading of atypia in nevi: correlation with melanoma risk. *Mod Pathol* 2003;16:764–771.

guidelines would recommend consideration of excision with a 5-mm margin.

The diagnosis of melanocytic dysplasia has been found to be reproducible by two international multi-disciplinary groups that used agreed-upon criteria (311,312). In another study, including participants whose published criteria differed in their requirements for atypia and for a size criterion, it was concluded that the participating pathologists used different diagnostic criteria, but that their usage was consistent (313). It has been suggested that histologic criteria may be more specific when applied to larger lesions, and that cytologic atypia may play a key role in the identification and significance of these lesions. Slight melanocytic atypia may be subtle and poorly reproducible, and also may be of modest clinical significance. On the other hand, the diagnosis of higher-grade dysplasia (severe dysplasia) is likely to be both more reproducible, and of substantially greater biological significance (314,315). In our practice, we tend to distinguish between "mild to moderate" and "severe" dysplasia. Severe dysplasia shares sufficient characteristics with melanoma (Table 28-4) to suggest that it should be managed with complete excision and clear margins.

Pathobiology. After the early descriptions of dysplastic nevi as markers of high risk for melanoma in hereditary melanoma kindreds, it was widely assumed that identification of individuals in the community at high risk for melanoma required biopsy of a nevus to "rule out dysplasia." Subsequent studies have shown that risk is best assessed by the clinical evaluation of the patients' entire cutaneous phenotype. The total number of nevi and the number of large nevi (316), light skin color, and high freckle density (317) are all risk factors for development of melanoma, but the strongest single risk factor is the presence and number of dysplastic nevi (62). Family history of melanoma is another significant risk factor (306,318), as is a personal history of prior melanoma (319). In members of hereditary melanoma kindreds, the lifetime risk for melanoma approaches 100% in members who have clinically dysplastic nevi, corresponding to approximately 100-fold relative risk compared to the general population (319–321). In people without a family history of melanoma, the relative risk as determined in multiple cohort and case-control studies from different geographic regions is of the order of three- to ten-fold, depending on the number of dysplastic (clinically atypical) nevi on their skin (62,316,322–343). These data are based on clinical evaluation of nevi. Formal case-control studies of the risk associated with *histologically* dysplastic nevi do not exist, because of the difficulty of obtaining biopsies in adequate numbers of cases and controls. Also, clinical atypia does not necessarily correlate well with histologic atypia (344). Even when a biopsy can be obtained, usually only one or two nevi are sampled, whereas clinical examination considers the whole phenotype.

Nevertheless, it is clear that histologic atypia in dysplastic nevi is associated with melanoma risk. In one study, histologically verified clinically dysplastic nevi were associated with a relative risk of 4.6 for melanoma (324). In a multiobserver study where biopsies had been taken from 24 melanoma cases and 21 random controls, four of six observers (who had each used different criteria) found an increased prevalence of histologic dysplasia ranging up to a 3.5-fold increase in cases compared to controls (313). In an interesting study, Sagebiel et al. found that the degree of dysplasia in a nevus biopsy correlated with increasing age of the patient, with frank melanomas occupying the oldest age category (304). More recently, as discussed above (Table 28-4), McNutt et al. (307) in a very large, single-institution study demonstrated a clear relationship between the degree of atypia in clinically atypical (dysplastic) nevi submitted for biopsy, and the chance that a patient has had a melanoma, demonstrating that the risk of melanoma is greater for persons who tend to make nevi with high-grade histologic atypia.

Although melanomas in patients with dysplastic nevi may arise within a preexisting dysplastic nevus, the majority arise *de novo*. Histologic changes indistinguishable from those in dysplastic nevi are seen at the periphery of melanomas in approximately 20% to 30% of cases (97,250, 345–348), supporting the view that at least some cutaneous melanomas take origin in a dysplastic nevus. Even so, most dysplastic nevi are clinically stable (305), and will never evolve into melanomas. This paradox is explained by the fact that dysplastic nevi are vastly more common than melanomas in the general population, and provides a rationale against indiscriminate excision of clinically stable dysplastic nevi for prophylaxis of melanoma.

In keeping with their role as potential precursors and as simulants of melanoma, dysplastic nevi tend to occupy an intermediate position between nevi and melanomas in laboratory studies. In cell cycle proliferation marker studies, the reactivity of dysplastic nevi is intermediate, though closer to that of common nevi than of melanoma (349, 350). Electron microscopic studies of dysplastic nevi have shown abnormal spherical and partially melanized melanosomes similar to those seen in superficial spreading melanomas (351,352). Although most *in situ* hybridization or immunohistochemical studies have shown reactivity similar to common nevi, dysplastic nevi have reacted in an intermediate manner with some markers (353), while the reactivity with others has been more akin to that of melanomas (354), or intermediate (355). Interesting studies have shown that the amount of red pheomelanin is greater in dysplastic nevi than in common nevi or normal skin (356). Since pheomelanin may be a generator of toxic free radicals after UV irradiation, this attribute may increase the risk of genetic mutations in these lesions that may contribute to continued tumor progression. Genetic changes in nevi and dysplastic nevi are beginning to be cataloged. For example, loss of heterozygosity at the 9p locus (which contains the CDKN2A gene) was recently discovered in 64% of dysplastic nevi and 50% of benign nevi, while homozygous deletion of p16 was found in 29% of dysplastic nevi but never in benign nevi (357). Recent studies have demonstrated aberrations in DNA repair pathways in dysplastic nevi (358), and microsatellite instability in melanomas and nevi including dysplastic nevi (359,360). These findings are consistent with DNA repair deficiency in patients with dysplastic nevi, and tend to correlate with patient groups ordered according to increasing melanoma risk (360).

Differential Diagnosis and Management

The major importance of biopsy in an individual with dysplastic nevi is to rule out the possibility of melanoma in a problematic lesion. Key features in making this distinction are reviewed in Table 28-5. Lesions in which some features of dysplasia are observed but not judged to be diagnostic may be reported as "lentiginous (junctional or compound) nevi," or "nevus with architectural disorder," with an interpretive note. Such a note may indicate that additional evaluation of the patient could be appropriate to assess melanoma risk, and that periodic surveillance could be appropriate, especially if there are other clinically atypical (dysplastic) nevi, or a family or personal history of melanoma (361).

In conclusion, in patients with dysplastic nevi, periodic surveillance of the patient, and evaluation of first-degree relatives, may be indicated for early diagnosis of melanoma. This is especially so if the clinically dysplastic lesions are numerous, and in individuals who have a personal or family history of melanoma. There is evidence that surveillance and/or education of individuals at increased risk for melanoma can result in the diagnosis of melanomas in their early, curable stages (362). The major role of biopsy and of histologic examination of nevi in such individuals is to rule out melanoma in a clinically suspicious or changing lesion. Atypia is heterogeneous in these lesions, so complete excision biopsy is recommended (which can include shave or punch excisions as long as the entire lesion is included in the specimen (363). Lesions whose biopsy show severe dysplasia or changes suggestive of evolving melanoma *in situ* (Table 28-5) should be considered for conservative re-excision if their margins are close or involved (361).

MALIGNANT MELANOMA

Most malignant melanomas arise in the epidermis and these may be *in situ* (entirely within the epidermis), or may be invasive (extending from the epidermis into the dermis). Occasional invasive melanomas are entirely dermal at presentation. Invasive melanoma may be tumorigenic ("vertical growth phase"), or nontumorigenic ("radial growth phase"). Melanoma *in situ* and nontumorigenic invasive melanoma can be divided into (a) lentigo maligna, (b) superficial spreading, (c) acral lentiginous, and (d) mucosal lentiginous types. Tumorigenic melanoma may arise in relation to a preexisting nontumorigenic component of any of the above types, in which case it is named accordingly. Alternatively, tumorigenic melanoma may arise "*de novo*,"

TABLE 28-5. DYSPLASTIC NEVUS VERSUS RADIAL GROWTH–PHASE MELANOMA

Dysplastic Nevus	Radial Growth–Phase Melanoma
Pattern Features	
May be <6 mm in diameter, not often >10 mm	Usually >6 mm, often much >10 mm
Somewhat symmetrical	Often highly asymmetrical
Often symmetrically arranged about "shoulders" of a mature dermal nevus	If dermal nevus is present, it is likely to be asymmetrically placed
Uniformly elongated narrow, delicate rete ridges	Irregularly thickened epidermis, often with effaced rete ridges
No alteration of stratum corneum	May be hyperkeratotic
Nests predominate over single cells in epidermis	Single cells predominate except in late lesions
Little or no pagetoid spread of lesional cells into epidermis	Usually obvious pagetoid spread into epidermis, extending to stratum corneum
Patchy lymphocytic infiltrate in papillary dermis	Brisk band-like infiltrate
No regression	Regression common
Last lesional cells at lateral border are often in a nest	Last cells are often single, and may be above basal zone
Cytologic Features	
Scattered atypical epithelioid cells with dusty melanin pigment, nucleoli, anisokaryosis ("random atypia")	Epithelioid cells with dusty pigment, nucleoli, anisokaryosis predominate ("uniform atypia")
Most cells are not atypical	Most cells are atypical
No mitoses in epidermis or dermis	Intraepidermal mitoses in about one-third of cases; no mitoses in dermis
Cells in dermis, if any, are smaller than those in epidermis	Cells in dermis are similar to those in epidermis

without evidence of an adjacent *in situ* or microinvasive component at the time of detection, in which case it is termed (5) "nodular melanoma." However, some if not all of these lesions probably arise initially via a nontumorigenic intraepidermal component that fails to develop or persist as the tumorigenic component evolves. Important variants of tumorigenic melanoma include (6) desmoplastic melanoma and (7) neurotropic melanoma. Other unusual forms of tumorigenic melanoma will be discussed below.

All major types of melanoma originate almost invariably from melanocytes at the epidermal–dermal junction. Although the lesions are commonly associated with a preexisting nevus, more than half of them arise either *de novo*, or have completely supplanted the precursor nevus at the time of presentation. The majority of melanomas are thought to be caused by sunlight exposure, either intermittent (sunburn episodes) in the more common superficial spreading melanomas, or chronic in the lentigo maligna melanomas.

Classification of Melanoma

There are two major categories of melanoma, which represent sequential stages or "phases" of stepwise tumor progression (364). In the nontumorigenic *radial* or *horizontal growth phase*, the neoplastic melanocytes (melanoma cells) are confined to the epidermis (melanoma *in situ*), or to the epidermis and papillary dermis without formation of an expansile tumor mass (microinvasive melanoma). This phase may be followed after varying lengths of time by the focal appearance of the tumorigenic *vertical growth phase*, or a phase of dermal invasion with expansile tumor formation. Thus, a fully evolved melanoma may have two major lesional "compartments": the nontumorigenic, *in situ* or microinvasive radial growth phase; and an adjacent contiguous tumorigenic vertical growth phase compartment. In addition, dermal and/or epidermal compartments of an associated nevus may be recognized in some melanomas. Variants of each of the major compartments have been described and are listed in Table 28-6 (364,370).

For other variants (nevoid/minimal deviation, "balloon cell," "amelanotic," "spindle cell," malignant blue nevus, melanoma in congenital nevus, clear cell sarcoma, malignant melanocytic schwannoma, etc.) of low frequency, no definitive frequency estimates exist.

About 5% to 10% of melanomas in different series fall into "unclassified" or "other" categories (367,368). The fact that categorization of an individual case is occasionally difficult does not mean that classification of melanoma, after accounting for tumor thickness and site, is unnecessary, as has been stated (371). Even though in the tumorigenic stage, the prognosis is similar for all four types of melanoma, depending largely on the depth of invasion, the duration of the *in situ* phase preceding lentigo maligna melanoma is, on the average, longer than that of superficial spreading melanoma (372). Furthermore, there are differences in the apparent etiology of the various forms of melanoma, and in their molecular biology (373,374). Finally, the separate description of the morphologic variants has nosologic and pedagogic value, facilitating accurate diagnosis by enabling the recognition of the variant patterns.

TABLE 28-6. MELANOMA CLASSIFICATION

Radial growth phase (RGP)
Nontumorigenic melanoma
In situ or microinvasive
   Superficial spreading melanoma (SSM) — 67% of all
     melanomas
   Lentigo maligna melanoma (LMM) — 9%
   Acral-lentiginous melanoma (ALM) — 4%
   Unclassified radial growth phase (URGP) — 5%
Vertical growth phase (VGP)
Tumorigenic melanoma
No RGP compartment
   Nodular melanoma (NM) — 10% of all melanomas
RGP compartment present (may be SSM, LMM, ALM, URGP) —
   90%
   Usual vertical growth phase — 96%
   Desmoplastic — 3%, most are also neurotropic
   Neurotropic, not desmoplastic — 1%

Based on 1996 World Health Organization classification. From Clark WH Jr, Elder DE, Van Horn M. The biologic forms of malignant melanoma. *Hum Pathol* 1986;5:443–450; Baer SC, Schultz D, Synnestvedt M, et al. Desmoplasia and neurotropism: prognostic variables in patients with stage I melanoma. *Cancer* 1995;76:2242–2247; and Heenan PJ, Elder DE, Sobin LH, Histological classification of skin tumors. In: Heenan PJ, Elder DE, Sobin LH, eds. *Histological typing of skin tumors*. New York: Springer, 1996:3–10.

Morphology of Tumorigenic and Nontumorigenic Melanoma

In their nontumorigenic stage, melanomas tend to expand more or less inexorably along the radii of an imperfect circle as viewed clinically. The clinically derived term "radial" growth has no intuitive histologic meaning, and the histologic term "horizontal growth phase" has been suggested as an alternative. The major clinical diagnostic criteria have been summarized as "ABCD criteria" (375). These include lesional *asymmetry* (half of a lesion does not match the other half in shape or in color distribution); lesional *border* irregularity (lesions tend to have an indented coastline like the map of a small island); lesional *color* variegation (the surface is multicolored and may include shades of tan, brown, blue-black, gray-white and other variations); and lesional *diameter* generally >6 mm (although some melanomas are smaller) (Fig. 28-19).

Histologically, most of the lesional cells in the nontumorigenic melanomas are located in the epidermis. Microinvasion is here defined as the presence of a few lesional cells in the papillary dermis, without "tumorigenic proliferation," which is defined below. Microinvasive lesions are

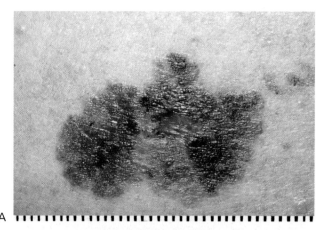

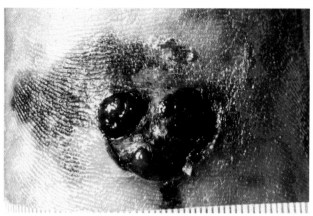

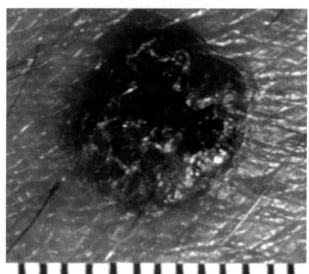

FIGURE 28-19. (A) Superficial spreading melanoma, nontumorigenic, radial growth phase only (microinvasive), with focal regression. The lesion is large, asymmetric, with irregular border, and variegated colors including reddish brown and focal areas of blue-black, as well as a focal grayish area of partial radial growth phase regression (near the middle of the lesion). This morphology could overlap with that of the severely dysplastic nevus in *(B)*. Each of these lesions is sufficiently atypical that it should be considered for excision for pathologic diagnosis. **(B)** Acral-lentiginous melanoma, tumorigenic, with extensive radial growth phase, partial regression of the radial growth phase, and a bulky, ulcerated, tumorigenic vertical growth–phase nodule. **(C)** Nodular melanoma. The tumorigenic vertical growth phase–nodule, lacking an adjacent radial growth phase by definition, is relatively small, symmetrical, and uniform in color. The focally ulcerated surface may lead to presenting symptoms of bleeding and oozing, which are signs of a relatively advanced melanoma.

not specifically distinguishable from *in situ* melanomas on clinical grounds. Whether microinvasive or *in situ*, nontumorigenic melanomas appear to lack competence for metastasis. In a database of 624 clinical stage I–invasive melanoma cases followed for more than 10 years, the 8-year survival rate from 161 microinvasive or *in situ* (pure radial growth phase) melanomas was 100 + 1%. In the same database, the patients with lesions having only radial growth phase were 4.3 years younger than those additionally having vertical growth phase, consistent with the hypothesis that the radial growth phase is antecedent, and relatively indolent (306,376).

Clinically, the tumorigenic vertical growth phase is qualitatively different from the plaque-like radial growth phase. The tumor appears as an expanding papule within a previously indolent plaque lesion, and grows in three dimensions in a balloon-like fashion to form a nodule (Fig. 28-19B). Typically, the ABCD criteria do not apply to the tumor nodule itself, which is commonly symmetrical, with smooth borders. The color is often quite uniform, and may

be pink rather than blue-black, and the diameter of the tumor nodule itself is often <6 mm, even in a quite high-risk lesion. For these reasons, clinical diagnosis of melanoma may be subtle in a nodular melanoma that lacks an adjacent nontumorigenic compartment (Fig. 28-19C).

The major histologic feature that distinguishes a tumorigenic melanoma is the capacity for proliferation of melanoma cells in the extracellular matrix of the dermis to form an expansile mass. In contrast, nontumorigenic melanoma cells may proliferate inexorably in the epidermal compartment, and may invade the dermis but do not proliferate there (Fig. 28-20). The lack of metastatic capacity in nontumorigenic melanomas may be explained by considering that cell proliferation in the extracellular matrix of a distant site is essential to the development of a metastasis. Thus, it is likely a tumor that cannot proliferate in the matrix at its local site of origin would not do so in a metastatic site either. Operational definitions for tumorigenic and nontumorigenic melanoma, and for radial and vertical growth phase follow (376,377).

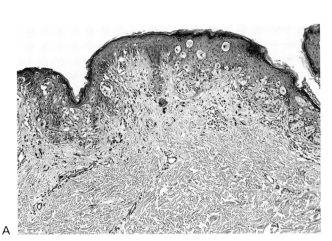

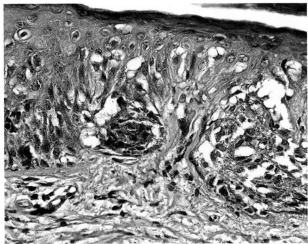

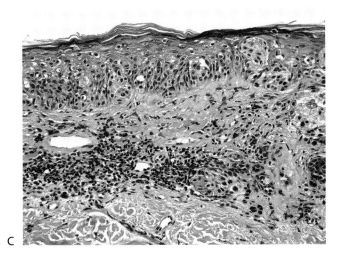

FIGURE 28-20. (A) Superficial spreading melanoma, microinvasive. At scanning magnification, a broad plaque that is asymmetrical in the distribution of the lesional cells, and in that of the responding lymphocytes and keratinocytes. **(B)** The lesional cells are uniformly atypical, and they tend to be arranged at least focally with single cells predominating and extending up into the epidermis in a pagetoid pattern. In this view, the basement membrane is intact (*in situ* radial growth phase). **(C)** In another portion of the lesion, scattered clusters of cells in the dermis are smaller than largest intraepidermal clusters, and there are no mitoses. These attributes define foci of microinvasive nontumorigenic melanoma (invasive radial growth phase).

Tumorigenic melanoma. A mass of melanoma cells is present in the dermis, defined as at least one cluster (nest) in the dermis that is larger than the largest intraepidermal cluster (indicative of a tumor with capacity for expansile growth in the dermis) (Fig. 28-21).

Nontumorigenic melanoma. No mass of melanoma cells is present in the dermis (there is no cluster larger than the largest intraepidermal cluster) (Fig. 28-20C).

Vertical growth phase (VGP). A lesion is classified as VGP if it is tumorigenic, or if there are any dermal mitoses. The presence of any mitoses in the dermal component of the melanoma is indicative of a tumor with capacity for expansile growth in the dermis and defines the concept of typical VGP even in the absence of a frank tumor mass (Fig. 28-21).

Radial growth phase (RGP). A lesion is classified as RGP only ("pure" RGP, or "radial growth phase confined") if it is nontumorigenic and there are no dermal mitoses. Alternatively, the RGP may be present as a "compartment" of a complex primary melanoma in which the above histologic criteria apply only to that portion of the melanoma adja-

cent to the VGP (Fig. 28-21). "Pure" RGP melanoma may be defined as "the absence of VGP in a primary melanoma" (Fig. 28-20).

In rare instances, a mass is formed in the dermal component of a melanoma by the "accretive" piling up of clusters of cells, in the absence of any single cluster of cells that is larger than the largest intraepidermal cluster (Fig. 28-22). These lesions have been described as "variant VGP" by Reed et al. (205). These lesions are nontumorigenic. However, if any mitoses were present in such a lesion, it would meet the criteria for VGP defined above. The prognostic significance of variant VGP is uncertain. Most examples are thin, with a good prognosis as judged by prognostic models. In our experience, rare instances of metastasis have been associated with the presence of variant VGP; the overall metastatic rate is exceedingly low, comparable with that associated with other nontumorigenic melanomas.

In a study conducted by the Pathology Panel of the Cancer Research Campaign in the United Kingdom, the level of agreement for recognition of VGP was "good" as

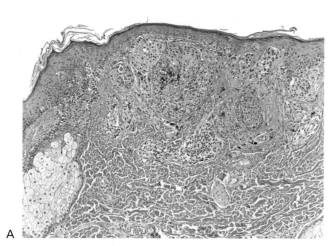

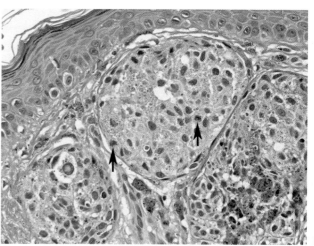

FIGURE 28-21. (A) Melanoma with early tumorigenic vertical growth phase. This lesion is Clark level II because the papillary dermis is expanded but not quite filled by the proliferation. The Breslow thickness is approximately 0.5 mm. Several of the clusters of cells in the dermis are slightly larger than the largest clusters in the epidermis, indicative of tumorigenic proliferation in the dermis. The cells in the epidermis are smaller than those in the dermis and they extend laterally as a predominantly *in situ* "radial growth phase compartment" in the primary melanoma. **(B)** At high magnification, there is uniform atypia, and there are scattered lesional cell mitoses in the early vertical growth phase. The melanin pigment is finely divided or "dusty."

judged by formal kappa analysis, and was improved after discussion of standardized criteria among members of the reviewing panel (378). Subsequently, two additional studies have confirmed this finding (379,380).

Molecular Pathology of Melanoma

Knowledge of the molecular pathology of melanoma has expanded dramatically since the discovery in 2001 of a high frequency of mutation of the oncogene BRAF in primary and metastatic melanomas (120). In a recent study, mutations resulting in the activating V599E amino-acid substitution were found in 68% of melanoma metastases, 80% of primary melanomas and, unexpectedly, in 82% of nevi (121). Activating mutations of the oncogene nRAS have also been described in melanomas and in tumor-associated and congenital nevi (122–124). Lesions that have mutated nRAS tend not to

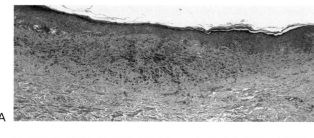

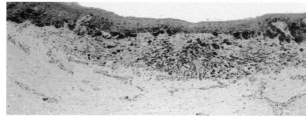

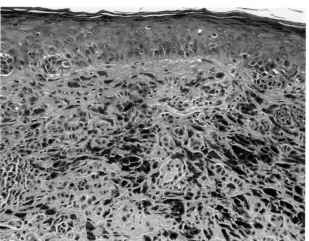

FIGURE 28-22. (A) Melanoma with variant vertical growth phase ("accretive VGP"). There is a region in the center of the lesion where the papillary dermis is expanded by a small mass. **(B)** The mass appears to have been formed by the accretive growth of numerous small nests, none of which are larger than the largest intraepidermal nests. **(C)** A Melan-A stain graphically demonstrates the smaller nests in the dermis, and the larger nests in the epidermis.

have mutated BRAF and vice versa (381). These data suggest that mutational activation of the RAS/RAF/MAPK mitogenic pathway in nevi is a critical step in the initiation of melanocytic neoplasia but alone is insufficient for melanoma tumorigenesis (121). The CDKN2A tumor suppressor gene product p16 is highly expressed in nevi (382,383), presumably restraining the proliferative pressure in these lesions despite the activating oncogene mutations. Loss of this suppressor in melanomas, in the context of activated mitogenic signaling pathways, may represent an important mechanism of progression (384).

NONTUMORIGENIC COMPARTMENT OF PRIMARY MALIGNANT MELANOMA (RADIAL GROWTH PHASE)

In the following sections, the morphology of the nontumorigenic compartments of the different forms of melanoma will be described. Next, the morphology of the tumorigenic VGP, which tends to be similar among the different forms, will be discussed. Typically, about 90% of all melanomas have a nontumorigenic compartment and about half of these also have a tumorigenic focus; and about 10% of melanomas, termed "nodular melanomas," have a tumorigenic but no *in situ* or invasive RGP compartment.

Two major patterns of nontumorigenic melanoma can be distinguished: pagetoid and lentiginous patterns. The lentiginous pattern recapitulates the pattern of focally contiguous proliferation of nevus cells in the simplest melanocytic neoplasm, the lentigo simplex. However, there is more uniform and complete contiguous basal replacement, and thus the proliferation is continuous, at least in part, between adjacent rete ridges. Pagetoid spread, graphically described as "buckshot scatter" of melanocytes within the epidermis, is the single best-known pattern of melanomas. However, many melanomas, including many of the lentiginous ones, are entirely or partly lacking in pagetoid proliferation. In many melanomas, as in nevi, nests of melanocytes are present at the dermal-dermal junction. These tend to differ from those in nevi in being more variable in size, shape, and orientation, and in their more irregular spacing along the junction (385).

Not all superficial melanocytic proliferations can reliably and reproducibly be distinguished as either a superficial melanoma or as a nevus. In such cases, we provide a descriptive designation, such as "superficial atypical melanocytic proliferation of uncertain significance" ("*SAMPUS*"), with a differential diagnosis. For example, a problematic lesion with dysplastic features and a small focus of pagetoid extension of slightly atypical melanocytes into the epidermis may be signed out as "junctional nevus with severe dysplasia and focal changes suggestive of evolving melanoma *in situ*." Because of the differential diagnosis in these

lesions of melanoma *in situ*, which could have locally persisting and recurring although not metastatic potential, we generally recommend a re-excision procedure for such lesions. The dimensions of such a procedure could follow guidelines for melanoma *in situ*, or at a minimum should be discussed with the patient and include a margin of normal tissue around the scar and any residual lesion.

Superficial Spreading Melanoma

Superficial spreading melanoma (SSM), also referred to as pagetoid melanoma (366) is the most frequent form of melanoma (about 70% of all cases), and may therefore be regarded as the "common" or "prototypic" form of melanoma. These lesions have been described in the past as "atypical melanocytic hyperplasia" (386) or as "precancerous melanosis," a term that dates back to one of the earliest descriptions of melanoma by Dubreuilh in 1912 (387). The lesions may occur on exposed skin but are rather more commonly found on intermittently exposed skin and are rare on unexposed skin. The most frequently involved sites are the upper back, especially in men, and the lower legs, especially in women. The lesions are slightly or definitely elevated, with a palpable border, and an irregular, partly arciform outline. There is often variation in color that includes not only tan, brown, and black, but also pink, blue, and gray. White areas may be seen at sites of spontaneous regression (Fig. 28-19A). Microinvasion may be clinically inapparent, but the onset of tumorigenic vertical growth is indicated by the development of a papule followed by nodularity and sometimes also ulceration, the latter usually a late feature. In rare instances the lesion has a verrucous surface in which case differentiation from a seborrheic keratosis may be difficult (388). In its early stage of development, superficial spreading melanoma may be indistinguishable clinically from a dysplastic nevus. Histologic examination is thus the "gold standard" and is necessary for accurate diagnosis.

Histopathology. Architectural pattern features of importance in the diagnosis include the large diameter of the lesions, poor circumscription (the last cells at the edge of the lesion tend to be small, single and scattered), and asymmetry (one half of the lesion does not mirror the other) (385). The epidermis is irregularly thickened and thinned (Fig. 28-20A). Rather uniformly rounded, large melanocytes are scattered in a pagetoid pattern throughout the epidermis. The large cells lie predominantly in nests in the lower epidermis and singly in the upper epidermis. The nests tend to vary a good deal in size and shape, and to become confluent. Dermal melanophages and a dermal infiltrate are regularly present. The lymphocytic infiltrate may be patchy and perivascular as in a dysplastic nevus, but is typically dense and band-like, especially in invasive lesions.

Cytologically, the lesional cells are rather uniform and have abundant cytoplasm containing varying amounts of melanin that often consists of small, "dusty" particles. They are almost entirely devoid of readily visible dendrites. The nuclei tend to be large and hyperchromatic, with irregular nuclear membranes and irregularly clumped chromatin (Fig. 28-20B). This "uniform cytologic atypia" is of considerable diagnostic importance and contrasts with the random atypia of dysplastic nevi.

When the lesion is *in situ*, the basement membrane is intact (as in the field seen in Fig. 28-20B) and there are no lesional cells in the dermis. In an invasive but nontumorigenic lesion (invasive RGP or "microinvasive" melanoma), cells similar to those in the epidermis are present in the dermis in the form of small nests, with no nests larger than those in the epidermis, and with no dermal mitoses (Fig. 28-20C). When tumorigenic VGP is present, there is at least one, or often more than one, cluster of cells in the dermis that is larger than the largest intraepidermal nest, and there may be lesional cell mitoses in the dermis as well (Figs. 28-21A and 21B).

Histogenesis. On electron microscopic examination, melanosomes are present in great numbers in the large pagetoid tumor cells. Their shape is largely spheroid, rather than ellipsoid as in normal melanocytes and in the tumor cells of lentigo maligna (389). They often also show other abnormalities, such as absence of cross linkages of the filaments within the melanosomes. Melanization within the melanosomes is variable but often incomplete (390). This accounts for the finely divided "dusty" character of the pigment in the cells of many melanomas.

Differential Diagnosis. A junctional nevus differs from superficial spreading melanoma in RGP by a lack of atypia in the tumor cells, particularly in their nuclei, by a lack of pagetoid upward extension of tumor cells, by the absence of a significant inflammatory infiltrate in the upper dermis, and by a sharper lateral demarcation. Salient features in the important distinction from junctional melanocytic dysplasia have been reviewed (Table 28-5), and include, at scanning magnification, larger size, asymmetry, an irregularly thickened and thinned epidermis, and a band-like lymphocytic infiltrate in superficial spreading melanoma. At higher power, indicators of melanoma include the presence of high-level and extensive pagetoid melanocytosis (large neoplastic cells scattered among benign keratinocytes), high-grade and/or uniform cytologic atypia, and lesional cell mitoses (the latter present in about one-third of cases). The differential diagnostic distinction from lentiginous melanomas is of less consequence, since the management is the same. In lentigo maligna, the epidermis is atrophic, and pagetoid melanocytosis is less prominent, and contiguous replacement of the basal cell layer by atypical melanocytes is the dominant pattern. Problematical cases can be reported as "malignant melanoma" (*in situ* or microinvasive, etc.) without designation as to type.

When tumorigenic VGP is present, it does not differ appreciably from that in any other form of melanoma, except for the adjacent RGP (Fig. 28-23). Classification of such "complex tumorigenic" primary melanomas is based on the morphology of the RGP.

Among the nonmelanocytic neoplasms that must be differentiated from a superficial spreading melanoma *in situ* are Paget's disease and pagetoid examples of Bowen's disease (squamous cell carcinoma *in situ*). Paget's disease (discussed in detail in Chapter 30) usually shows remnants of compressed basal cells beneath the tumor cells, while in superficial spreading melanoma the lesional cells extend to the basement membrane. In Paget's disease, the tumor cells

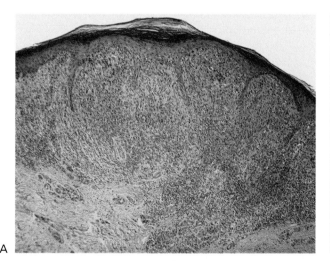
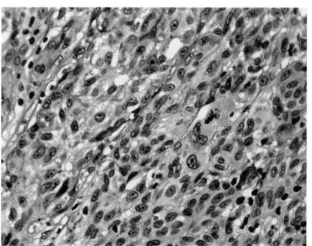

FIGURE 28-23. (A) Malignant melanoma, tumorigenic. At scanning magnification, there is a bulky ulcerated tumor nodule, which is eccentrically placed in contiguity with a broad plaque, the nontumorigenic, radial growth phase compartment (not shown, to the right of the image field). **(B)** The tumorigenic nodule is composed of uniformly atypical mitotically active fully malignant melanocytes (melanoma cells).

may stain positively for carcinoembryonic antigen and keratin, and are negative for HMB-45 and Melan-A. S-100 reactivity, though unusual, may be observed in Paget's disease Pagetoid Bowen's disease (discussed in Chapter 29) shows, as a rule, a well-preserved basal cell layer, except in areas in which dermal invasion has taken place, and immunohistochemically; it stains positively with antikeratin antibodies (e.g., AE1/AE3) (391). It does not stain with S-100 or with Melan-A or HMB-45. It should be noted that the cells of Paget's disease and of Bowen's disease may contain melanin pigment, because of transfer from reactive melanocytes in the adjacent skin.

Lentigo Maligna Melanoma

Lentigo maligna melanoma (LMM), previously referred to as melanosis circumscripta preblastomatosa of Dubreuilh and also as melanotic freckle of Hutchinson (of Hutchinson's melanotic freckle, HMF, a term used currently in Australia for this condition), accounts for about 10% of melanomas and typically occurs on the chronically exposed cutaneous surfaces of the elderly, most commonly on the face, and occasionally on the back, forearms or the lower legs (392). The term "lentigo maligna" may be regarded as synonymous with "lentigo maligna melanoma *in situ*" for most purposes. However, the term "lentigo maligna" is distinguished from melanoma *in situ* by some authors (see below) (393). In any case, these lesions, like other melanomas *in situ*, do not metastasize after complete excision, though they may persist and recur if not adequately excised. The lesion evolves slowly over many years, starting as an unevenly pigmented macule that gradually extends peripherally and may attain a diameter of several centimeters. It has an irregular border and, as long as it remains *in situ* or microinvasive, shows no induration. While extending in some areas, it may show spontaneous regression in others, resulting in irregular depigmented areas. The color varies from light brown to brown with minute dark brown or black flecks. Fine reticulated lines are usually also present and helpful in distinguishing the lesions from actinic lentigines. In contrast to SSM, the border is usually impalpable and indistinct. For this reason, the accurate clinical delineation of the border of a LMM can be problematical, and this not uncommonly results in unexpected positive or close margins in resection specimens. Occasionally, a lesion of lentigo maligna lacks melanin pigmentation (394–396). The clinical appearance then resembles that of a solar keratosis or Bowen's disease, or of an inflammatory patch, such as lupus. It is controversial whether lentigo maligna should be regarded as a form of melanoma *in situ* in all cases, or whether some cases should be regarded as precursor lesions (lentigo maligna) of *in situ* melanoma (melanoma *in situ*, lentigo maligna type) (393).

It has been suggested that the risk of progression from lentigo maligna to invasive lentigo maligna melanoma may

be about 5% (397), although some cases may progress rapidly (398). After adjustment for tumor thickness and other factors, lentigo maligna melanoma has the same prognosis as other forms of melanoma (399). However, its demographics and associations differ from those of the most common form of melanoma, superficial spreading melanoma. For example, patients with LMM have fewer nevi but more actinic keratoses than patients with SSM, consistent with a hypothesis of chronic sun exposure in the etiology of LMM (400).

Histopathology. Regarding architectural features, in its earliest stage, lentigo maligna may show at its periphery only hyperpigmentation with slight melanocytic proliferation, mainly in the basal cell layer. Toward the center of the lesion, there is a more pronounced increase in the concentration of basal melanocytes and some irregularity in their arrangement. Until there is contiguous proliferation of lesional melanocytes, these changes are not specific and may overlap with those of actinic lentigines. The epidermis is frequently flattened, in contrast to SSM, where it is irregularly thickened and thinned, or actinic lentigines where there is elongation of the rete. Although of diagnostic importance, this feature is less prominent than in superficial spreading melanoma (Fig. 28-24). Noteworthy is the tendency of the basal layer of follicular infundibula to also be involved by the lentiginous proliferation of atypical melanocytes in lentigo maligna.

Some nesting of melanocytes in the basal layer may be seen, but this is not usually pronounced until invasion of the dermis is developing (401). The atypical melanocytes within the nests usually retain their spindled shape, and they often "hang down" like rain droplets from the interface (367). Except in areas of nesting, the melanocytes tend to retain their dendritic processes. If the melanocytes are heavily melanized, some dendrites may be visible even in sections stained with hematoxylin-eosin; otherwise, staining with silver demonstrates the dendrites.

The upper dermis, which almost always shows severe elastotic solar degeneration, contains numerous melanophages and a rather pronounced, often band-like, inflammatory infiltrate. Invasion may be demonstrable in these areas of dermal inflammation. Since invasion in a lentigo maligna melanoma (as in other melanomas) is a focal process, one should ensure that the specimen is adequately grossed and sectioned in order not to miss such areas. The presence or absence of tumorigenic VGP is recognized using criteria already presented.

Cytologic Features

In fully evolved lesions of lentigo maligna, the lesional melanocytes in the epidermis show a marked increase in concentration, so that they come to lie in contiguity with one another, and their number in some areas exceeds that of the basal keratinocytes. Many of them are elongated and

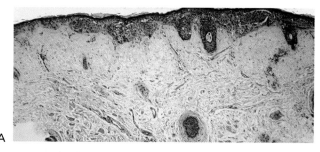

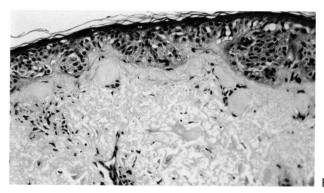

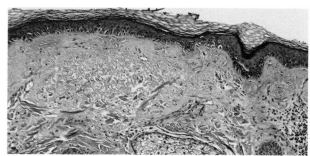

FIGURE 28-24. (A) Lentigo maligna melanoma, *in situ*. At low magnification, the lesions are broad and asymmetrical in the distribution of lesional and host responding cells. **(B)** The epidermis is atrophic, and there is usually severe actinic elastosis in the dermis. **(C)** As in superficial spreading melanoma, the lesional cells exhibit moderate to severe uniform cytologic atypia. There is usually some evidence of pagetoid proliferation in lentigo maligna melanoma, especially near areas of invasion. However, especially at the periphery of the lesion, this is much less prominent and the lesional cells are smaller than in superficial spreading melanoma.

spindle-shaped. Their nuclei appear atypical, being enlarged, hyperchromatic, and pleomorphic. However, the chromatin pattern is often not as open or "vesicular" as that seen in the more epithelioid cells of superficial spreading melanoma in its radial phase of growth. Frequently, atypical melanocytes extend along the basal cell layer of hair follicles, often for a considerable distance, frequently extending to the base of a shave biopsy specimen. Usually, the proliferating melanocytes contain moderate melanin, and melanin is present also in keratinocytes. There is usually some upward pagetoid extension of atypical melanocytes.

The question whether lentigo maligna should be regarded as a form of *in situ* melanoma in all instances is controversial. Flotte and Mihm have studied this issue and have identified two subsets of lesions (393). The first has atypical melanocytic hyperplasia, which they postulate to be correctly designated lentigo maligna. The second subset has the following features in addition to the melanocytic hyperplasia: individual and nests of cells at varying layers of the epidermis, confluence of the melanocytes replacing the basilar region, uniformity of the cytologic atypia, and nesting of uniformly atypical melanocytes. These lesions are designated as malignant melanoma *in situ*, lentigo maligna type. It is proposed that the lesions that have been termed lentigo maligna represent a spectrum of atypia and that the application of some of the traditional features for the diagnosis of melanoma may permit the segregation of more and less aggressive lesions (393). The properties of contiguous proliferation, and uniform cytologic atypia, in a broad, poorly circumscribed lesion are clearly of major importance in the diagnosis of *in situ* or microinvasive lentigo

maligna melanoma. These features are shared also with superficial spreading melanoma, while focal pagetoid melanocytosis, although often present, is less prominent. It should also be remembered that some individuals with chronic sun damage, may show diffuse, clinically covert, noncontiguous lentiginous proliferation of somewhat atypical melanocytes within the epidermal basal cell layer, and thus correlation with clinical appearance may be critical to determining the biological significance of low-grade atypical melanocytic hyperplasias. Mitotic figures are uncommonly present in the epidermal compartment of lentigo maligna melanoma; if present in the dermis, they are indicative of VGP. When tumorigenic vertical growth supervenes, it is often of the spindle cell type, including the desmoplastic and neurotropic variants.

Pathogenesis. As an explanation for the somewhat distinctive behavior of lentigo maligna, the theory has been offered that it is derived from spindle-shaped junctional melanocytes and thus represents a melanocyte-derived melanoma, in contrast to the superficial spreading melanoma that is derived from rounded junctional nevus cells and can be regarded as a nevus cell–derived melanoma (402). Electron microscopy provides some support for this concept. The melanocytes of lentigo maligna are large, synthetically active cells with many dendrites. The melanosomes are essentially normal, except that they appear somewhat more elongated than those present in normal melanocytes (389, 402). This is in contrast to superficial spreading melanomas, in which the melanosomes show considerable abnormalities. In a study of several immunohistochemical markers comparing lentigo maligna and superficial spreading melanomas, melanocytes of the latter showed greater proliferative activity, as reflected by PCNA staining, higher levels of bFGF, and more blood vessels. These results were considered to be in accordance with the biological behavior of superficial spreading and lentigo maligna melanomas, that is, the longer *in situ* phase of the latter (374). Although progression of lentigo maligna is often slow, some cases progress more rapidly, and complete excision of these lesions is recommended to prevent the development of a more dangerous melanoma (403).

Acral Lentiginous Melanoma

Acral melanoma occurs on the hairless skin of the palms and soles and in the ungual and periungual regions, the soles being the most common site (368,404). Acral melanoma is uncommon in all ethnic groups, but it is the predominant form of melanoma in individuals with darker skin. In groups such as Asians, Hispanics, Polynesians, and blacks where the overall incidence of melanoma is low, most melanomas are of the acral type. However, the absolute incidence of acral melanoma in these groups is similar to that in Caucasians who have a much higher inci-

dence of melanoma overall (405). These considerations suggest that different etiologic factors, likely not involving sunlight, are operative in acral than in other sites. Although the survival rate of patients with acral melanomas in most series is poor (406), this is likely due to their typically advanced microstage and/or stage at diagnosis.

Clinically, *in situ* or microinvasive acral lentiginous melanoma shows uneven pigmentation with an irregular, often indefinite border. The soles of the feet are most commonly involved. If the tumor is situated in the nail matrix, the nail and nail bed may show a longitudinal pigmented band, and the pigment may extend onto the nail fold (Hutchinson's sign). Tumorigenic vertical growth may be heralded by the onset of a nodule, with development of ulceration (Fig. 28-19B). However, some acral melanomas may be deeply invasive while remaining quite flat, because the thick stratum corneum acts as a barrier to exophytic growth.

Histopathology. The lesions are termed "lentiginous" because the majority of the lesional cells are single and located near the dermal–epidermal junction, especially at the periphery of the lesion (Fig. 28-25). However, usually some tumor cells can be found in the upper layers of the epidermis, especially near areas of invasion in the center of the

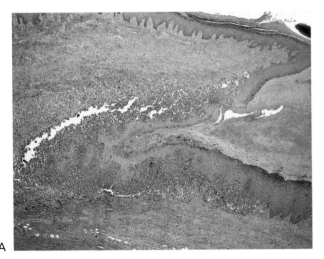

A

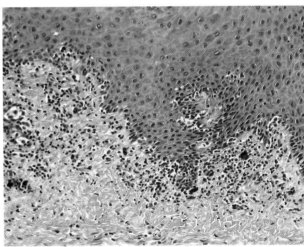

B

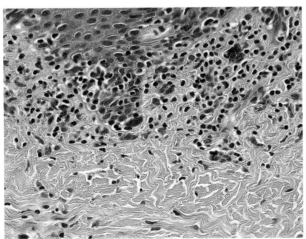

C

FIGURE 28-25. **(A)** Acral-lentiginous melanoma, subungual (radial growth phase). At low magnification, a lichenoid lymphocytic infiltrate along the dermal–epidermal junction is the clue to presence of the lesion. This feature may simulate an inflammatory condition. In this lesion, the process is seen to extend into the nail fold at the top of the image. **(B)** As in lentigo maligna and other lentiginous melanocytic proliferations, the lesional cells in acral-lentiginous melanoma tend to be arranged as single cells near the dermal–epidermal junction (lentiginous pattern), especially at the periphery of the lesion. **(C)** As in any melanoma, there is moderate to severe uniform cytologic atypia. Pagetoid melanocytosis may be present near the center of the lesion, but this is less prominent than in superficial spreading melanoma. When these features are less severe, the diagnosis may be subtle. Also, the neoplastic cells may be difficult to identify because of masking by the inflammatory infiltrate, as in this example.

lesions. The histologic picture differs from that of lentigo maligna, because of irregular acanthosis, the lack of elastosis in the dermis, and the frequently dendritic character of the lesional cells (407). Early *in situ* or microinvasive lesions may show, especially at the periphery, a deceptively subtle histologic picture consisting of an increase in basal melanocytes and hyperpigmentation with only focal atypia of the melanocytes. However, in the center of the lesions, there is usually readily evident uniform, severe cytologic atypia. There may be a lichenoid lymphocytic infiltrate that may largely obscure the dermal–epidermal junction, and in some cases this may be so dense as to simulate an inflammatory process. In most of the lesions, both spindle-shaped and round pagetoid tumor cells are seen, and, in many cases, pigmented dendritic cells are prominent. Pigmentation is often pronounced, resulting in the presence of melanophages in the upper dermis and of large aggregates of melanin in the broad stratum corneum. As in lentigo maligna, when tumorigenic VGP is present, it is often of the spindle cell type, and not uncommonly desmoplastic and/or neurotropic. In other instances, the invasive and tumorigenic cells in the dermis may be deceptively differentiated along nevoid lines.

Biology. Bastian et al. (373,408,409) have studied melanomas and nevi for copy number alterations by comparative genomic hybridization, and have shown that melanomas of the palms, soles, and subungual sites can be distinguished by the presence of multiple gene amplifications, about 50% of which are found at the cyclin D1 locus. Such amplifications are significantly less frequent in other cutaneous melanoma types and if present arise later in progression. Single basal melanocytes with similar gene amplifications have been identified in the histologically normal appearing skin immediately adjacent to a melanoma. These "field cells" appear to represent subtle melanoma *in situ* and may represent minimal residual disease that could lead to local recurrences if not excised. If the biological significance in terms of local recurrence of these cells can be confirmed, their identification may lead to recommendations for management of these lesions in the future.

Differential Diagnosis. The major consideration in the differential diagnosis of acral-lentiginous melanoma is the benign acral lentiginous nevus, discussed earlier (136,137). Features that distinguish this lesion from melanoma include smaller size, greater symmetry, lack of pagetoid lateral spread, absence of high-grade uniform atypia (not always present, however, in some melanomas), absence of mitotic activity in the dermal component, and evidence of dermal nevocytic differentiation (136,137).

Mucosal Lentiginous Melanoma

Next to the skin and eyes, melanoma is most apt to arise in the juxtacutaneous mucous membranes, such as the oral mucosa (410), nose and nasal sinuses (411), vagina (412), and anorectal mucosa (413). Mucosal melanomas are analogous to acral melanomas in histologic appearance and aggressiveness, which has led to the use of the histologic term "mucosal-lentiginous" melanoma (414).

TUMORIGENIC COMPARTMENT OF PRIMARY MALIGNANT MELANOMA (VERTICAL GROWTH PHASE)

The morphology of the variant forms of nontumorigenic melanoma has been discussed above. A tumorigenic VGP may develop in association with any of these to form a "complex" primary melanoma. In such cases, the histology shows a tumorigenic compartment adjacent to or within the confines of a nontumorigenic compartment. Nodular melanoma differs from these complex melanomas in that it is a tumorigenic melanoma with no clinically or histologically evident adjacent nontumorigenic compartment (367). The morphology of the "usual" or "common" forms of VGP is described in the next section.

Occasional melanomas exhibit variant patterns that may lead to diagnostic confusion because they may be more characteristically seen in nonmelanocytic tumors. Several variants of melanoma deserve a brief description in following sections: desmoplastic, neurotropic, polypoidal, verrucous, balloon cell, signet cell, myxoid, so-called "animal-type," nevoid, and minimal deviation melanoma. Other variants which will not be described here include small cell, adenoid/papillary, pleomorphic (fibrohistiocytic) (415), melanomas with rhabdoid cytoplasmic features (416,417), and the rare bone-forming or "osteogenic" melanoma (418).

Common Tumorigenic Melanoma Including Nodular Melanoma

Nodular melanoma by definition contains only tumorigenic vertical growth (sometimes associated with a precursor) and, because of this, has a poorer prognosis on the average than superficial spreading melanoma. However, when other risk factors such as thickness are controlled, the prognosis of nodular melanoma is not worse than that of other forms of melanoma (419). Nodular melanomas occur in slightly older patients than the common superficial spreading melanoma, and are relatively more frequent in men (367). A nodular melanoma starts as an elevated, variably pigmented papule that increases in size quite rapidly to become a nodule, and often undergoes ulceration. The ABCD criteria reviewed above do not apply to nodular melanomas, which often present clinically as quite small, symmetrical, and well-circumscribed papules or nodules (Fig. 28-19C). These may be conspicuously pigmented, oligomelanotic, or even amelanotic. The tumorigenic nodule that may develop in nodular melanoma does not differ clinically or histologically from that which may occur in relation to a preexisting nontumorigenic melanoma. Indeed, nodular melanomas may represent examples of "telescoped" tumor progression in which the antecedent radial phase has been so short-lived as to be inapparent (420).

Histopathology of Nodular Melanoma and Common Vertical Growth Phase (Tumorigenic Melanoma)

Architectural Features

In a typical tumorigenic melanoma, there is contiguous proliferation of neoplastic melanocytes in the dermis form-

ing a tumor mass that is larger (usually much larger) than the largest nest in the overlying epidermis. Asymmetry is often apparent at the cytologic level as variation in cell size, shape, and pigmentation, and in the distribution of the host response, such that one half of the lesion is not a mirror image of the other. However, the silhouette of the entire lesion may be quite symmetrical, especially in a nodular melanoma that lacks an adjacent nontumorigenic component (Fig. 28-26A). Conversely, if a nontumorigenic RGP compartment is present, asymmetry is likely to be more apparent, both at the clinical and histologic levels. The tumor mass is comprised of uniformly atypical cytologically fully malignant mitotically active cells usually

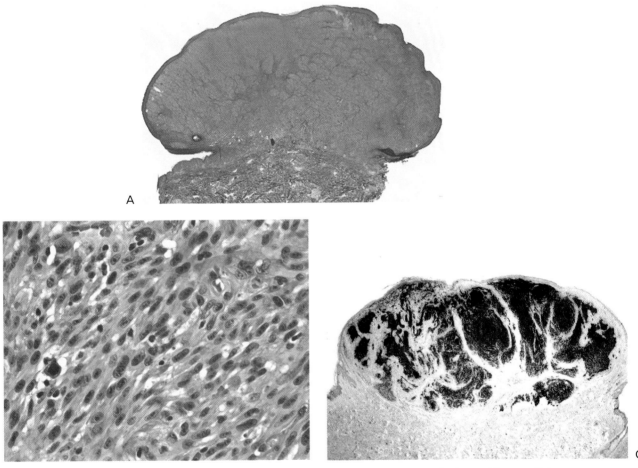

FIGURE 28-26. (A) Tumorigenic melanoma, nodular type (vertical growth phase without radial growth phase). The nodules of tumorigenic melanomas tend to be symmetrical at scanning magnification, though there may be an uneven distribution of pigment and of the lymphocytic response within many of the lesions. When there is no adjacent nontumorigenic radial growth phase component, as here, the lesion is termed "nodular melanoma." If a radial growth phase component is present, the melanoma is classified according to the type of compartment, such as "superficial spreading (or acral-lentiginous, etc.) melanoma with tumorigenic vertical growth phase." **(B)** The lesional cells of nodular melanoma exhibit severe uniform cytologic atypia, usually with readily evident mitoses. In any given high-power field such as this, appearances are indistinguishable from those of a vertical growth phase associated with a superficial spreading, lentigo maligna, or acral-lentiginous melanoma, or from those of a metastasis (compare Figs. 28-23B, 28-26B, 28-29C, 28-34, and 28-37B). **(C)** Nodular melanoma, S100 immunohistochemical stain. The brown reaction product in the lesional cells is striking, even at scanning magnification. Note the absence of S100-positive lesional cells in the adjacent skin.

growing in confluent nests or in sheets (Fig. 28-26B). Usually, the tumor mass fills and expands the papillary dermis (level III), or invades between coarse collagen fibers of the reticular dermis (level IV). Most level III melanomas and most melanomas >0.75 mm in thickness are tumorigenic while conversely, most level II or "thin" melanomas have no cluster in the dermis that is larger than the largest intraepidermal cluster, and are therefore nontumorigenic. The epidermis is frequently ulcerated, or there is an adherent scale-crust. It is often stretched and attenuated, or alternatively may be irregularly hyperplastic and even pseudoepitheliomatous.

Perhaps the best-known single criterion for melanoma is the upward "pagetoid" extension of tumor cells into the epidermis overlying the melanoma. However, this "pagetoid melanocytosis" or "pagetoid spread" is not specific for melanoma (138). While in nodular melanoma, permeation of the epidermis with tumor cells may be absent or may be limited to that portion overlying the dermal tumor, lateral extension of melanoma cells in the epidermis and papillary dermis beyond the confines of the dermal tumor is seen in the adjacent nontumorigenic compartment of complex primary melanomas (SSM, LMM, acral lentiginous melanoma [ALM]). This phenomenon greatly aids in histologic recognition of these tumors, and conversely, the recognition of nodular melanomas, which lack this adjacent component, may be difficult. For this reason, nodular melanoma may be difficult or impossible to distinguish from a metastatic melanoma in the skin, and when such a tumor is amelanotic, the distinction from other cutaneous neoplasms may be impossible without immunohistochemistry.

The amount of *inflammatory infiltrate* in tumorigenic melanomas varies. As a rule, early invasive malignant and many *in situ* melanomas show a band-like inflammatory infiltrate, often intermingled with melanophages, at the base of the tumor. In tumors that extend deep into the dermis, the inflammatory infiltrate is quite variable, but it is often only slight to moderate rather than pronounced. Lymphocytes extending among tumor cells are often associated with morphologic evidence of damage to individual tumor cells (apoptosis). These *tumor-infiltrating lymphocytes* (TILs) have been shown to have independent favorable prognostic significance (419). The lymphocytic infiltrate around melanomas is a T-cell response (421). TILs extracted from melanomas (mostly metastatic cases) may be cytotoxic and may be directed against immunogenic melanoma-associated antigens (422).

Cytologic Features

The tumor cells in the dermis show great variation in size and shape. Nevertheless, two major types of cells can be recognized—an epithelioid and a spindle-shaped cell type. Many tumors show both types of cells, but usually one type predominates. Generally, the "lentiginous" forms of melanoma (e.g., LMM and ALM) tend to show a predominance of spindle-shaped cells in their invasive dermal components, whereas superficial spreading and nodular melanomas tend to be composed largely of epithelioid cells (419). The epithelioid type of cell tends to lie in alveolar or nested formations, and the spindle-shaped type of cells in irregularly branching formations. The alveolar formations of the epithelioid cells are surrounded by thin fibers of collagen containing a few fibroblasts. Tumors in which spindle cells predominate may resemble sarcomas or other spindle cell tumors but in most cases differ from them by the presence of junctional melanocytic activity.

The uniformly atypical nuclei of the cells that constitute the tumor nodule are larger than those of melanocytes or nevus cells, with irregular nuclear membranes, hyperchromatic chromatin and, often, prominent nucleoli that tend to be irregular in size, shape, and number. The atypia is considered to be "uniform" if more than 50% of the cells have these characteristics, but more often than not, all or most of the cells are atypical. In addition to this uniform moderate or severe cytologic atypia, there is also a diagnostically important failure of the melanocytes in the deeper layers of the dermis to decrease in size (absence of "maturation") (Fig. 28-21). This must not be confused, however, with the presence of an intradermal nevus beneath a melanoma, a fairly common feature. Not uncommonly, melanoma cells will recapitulate nevic cell maturation, but in these instances the smaller cells at the base retain nuclear characteristics of malignant cells, and there will be cytologic "continuity" between these nevoid cells and the overlying more atypical lesional cells.

Mitotic figures are usually present in the lesional cells of the dermal and epidermal compartments of tumorigenic melanomas (they are present in the epidermal lesional cells in about one-third of nontumorigenic melanomas, and in the dermal compartment of 85% of tumorigenic melanomas) (419,423) (Fig. 28-23). Mitoses may also be seen in adjacent hyperplastic keratinocytes. The nuclei of these hyperplastic epidermal keratinocytes may be enlarged with prominent nucleoli, though they are not irregular or hyperchromatic. In contrast, mitotic figures are rarely seen in benign nevi other than Spitz nevi, and even in the latter lesions the rate is usually low or zero (160).

Differential Diagnosis. Great difficulty may be encountered in the differentiation of a melanoma from a junctional or compound nevus. The actual incidence of a wrong diagnosis is not inconsiderable, judging from the frequency with which pathologists disagree in their opinions. When there is doubt, the differential diagnosis should be clearly indicated, so that appropriate therapeutic intervention can be planned. Incisional biopsies are a common source of interpretive difficulty. The site of melanocytic lesions that have been partially removed by shave or punch biopsy should be excised to assure complete removal if there is any doubt at all about the diagnosis.

The most important attributes that differentiate the tumorigenic VGP of melanoma from nevi include *asymmetry*, *lack of maturation* of lesional cells with descent into the dermis, and *uniform cytologic atypia*.

Considerations in the important distinction between thin melanomas and dysplastic nevi are presented in Table 28-6. The most important differential diagnostic consideration for nodular melanoma is the Spitz nevus. The criteria for this distinction are presented in Table 28-3.

In some instances, it may be difficult to recognize a highly undifferentiated melanoma as such. The specific identification of a tumor as melanoma depends on the identification of melanin, or on appropriate immunohistochemical reactivity in an appropriate setting. The *amount of melanin* present varies greatly in melanomas. In some tumors, considerable melanin is found not only within the tumor cells but also within melanophages located in the stroma. In others, there may be no evidence of melanin in hematoxylin-eosin stains. However, a Fontana–Masson silver stain usually reveals at least a few cells containing melanin (424). Some melanomas are completely devoid of pigment (amelanotic melanoma). Although amelanotic melanomas tend to be aggressive lesions, the prognosis is not different from pigmented melanomas when other staging and microstaging attributes are taken into consideration (425). If appropriate tissue is available, the DOPA reaction may be positive in at least part of the tumor (426), and electron microscopy shows some melanosomes and premelanosomes in nearly all cases (415,424,427). However, in practice today, these methods have been largely supplanted by immunohistochemical techniques (415,424).

Immunohistochemistry. Most of the problems in distinguishing amelanotic or oligomelanotic tumorigenic melanomas from other tumors can be resolved by immunohistochemistry, using a panel of antibodies including S-100, HMB-45, keratin (low and intermediate molecular weight such as AE1/3), and LCA (40,428-431). On immunohistochemical testing, S-100 protein is nearly always positive in melanoma (431). A keratin stain should be done in addition to staining for S-100 protein, to rule out not uncommon S-100-positive carcinomas (432). A few studies have reported positive keratin reactivity in melanomas, but this is unusual when standard methods are used in paraffin sections (432–434). Reactivity of melanomas, mostly metastatic, has been described with polyclonal but not monoclonal CEA, and occasional melanomas react with the epithelial marker EMA (434). Melanomas, unlike most carcinomas, express vimentin, an intermediate filament that is usually associated with mesenchymal tissues (435). Lymphomas are usually positive with LCA, while S-100 and HMB-45 are negative. The anaplastic large-cell type of non-Hodgkin's lymphoma, which may present primarily in the skin, is quite likely to be confused with melanoma, and these tumors are usually positive for the CD30

(Ki-1) antigen, as well as LCA (CD45) (436). Occasional examples of histiocytic tumors such as epithelioid histiocytomas or juvenile xanthogranulomas may be confused with nodular melanomas, especially when foam cells or Touton giant cells are inconspicuous (198). It has been concluded that Melan-A and tyrosinase markers are sensitive and specific in making the diagnosis of a melanocytic lesion (200, 437).

Several more specific but less sensitive antigens, of which the antigen recognized by HMB-45 (gp100) is prototypic, are used in addition to S-100 in making the distinction between melanoma and nonmelanoma tumors. Like S-100, HMB-45 is positive in many benign melanocytic tumors and thus it is not specific for melanoma. Its sensitivity of about 70% overall is less than that of S-100 (close to 100% [432,433]), especially in desmoplastic and to a lesser extent other spindle cell melanomas where HMB-45 is usually negative (438). The specificity of the HMB-45 antigen depends on the context in which it is used. Benign melanocytic lesions that may react with HMB-45 include the junctional component of most nevi, and the dermal components of dysplastic nevi, blue nevi, cellular blue nevi, deep penetrating nevi, and Spitz nevi. Thus, HMB-45 cannot be used to distinguish benign from malignant melanocytic neoplasms. If on the other hand the diagnostic differential is between melanoma and carcinoma, lymphoma or sarcoma, the diagnostic specificity of a positive test is very high, albeit not 100%.

Use of HMB-45 has been augmented and in some institutions supplanted by other markers. Melan-A (MART-1), is an antigen initially recognized by T cells in melanoma patients, and like HMB-45 associated with the pigmentary apparatus. The sensitivity of this antigen is somewhat greater than HMB-45 and its specificity is about the same. The Melan-A antibody labels reactive cases strongly and clearly, but is less sensitive in spindle cell melanomas, and usually negative in the spindle cells of desmoplastic melanomas (430,439). Other markers that have been studied recently include the MAGE series of antigens (440), MITF (441–443), and others. In a recent study, Xu et al. evaluated reactivity for alternative markers in 14 HMB-45 negative, nondesmoplastic melanomas. Melanocyte-specific transcription factor was positive in 9, Melan-A in 9, tyrosinase in 6, and MAGE-1 in 11. In eight desmoplastic malignant melanomas, MAGE-1 was positive in three, and all other markers were negative. The five markers tested were negative in all but two schwannomas, one with focal melanocyte-specific transcription factor and the other with tyrosinase and weak MAGE-1 reactivity. It was concluded that MAGE-1, melanocyte-specific transcription factor, tyrosinase, and Melan-A are useful markers in the diagnosis of malignant melanocytic lesions when HMB-45 is negative (444).

In another recent study, a "pan-melanoma cocktail," composed of HMB 45, MART-1 and tyrosinase, labeled

98% of all melanomas but only 60% of desmoplastic melanoma, all of which were positive for S-100. The pan-melanoma cocktail is more specific than S-100 and might be considered as a complementary marker to polyclonal S-100 antibody, except for desmoplastic melanoma (445).

Desmoplastic and Neurotropic Melanoma

Desmoplastic melanomas present attributes of melanocytic, fibroblastic, and schwannian differentiation, often mixed within a single lesion (446). The lesions occur on chronically sun-damaged skin, usually in elderly patients. The lower lip is a relatively common site, sometimes in younger patients (447). Other cases occur, often in relation to lentiginous melanomas, in acral and mucosal sites (448–452). In a recent large series, the male-to-female ratio was 1.75:1 and the median patient age was 61 years. The median tumor thickness was 2.5 mm, and 44% of cases were amelanotic. Five-year survival was 75%. Significant predictors of overall survival were a high mitotic rate and tumor thickness. All the desmoplastic melanomas exceeded 1.5 mm in thickness and were Clark's level IV or V. There was a significant increase in local recurrence when neurotropism was present. The rate of local recurrence was not higher for desmoplastic melanoma than for other cutaneous melanomas (453).

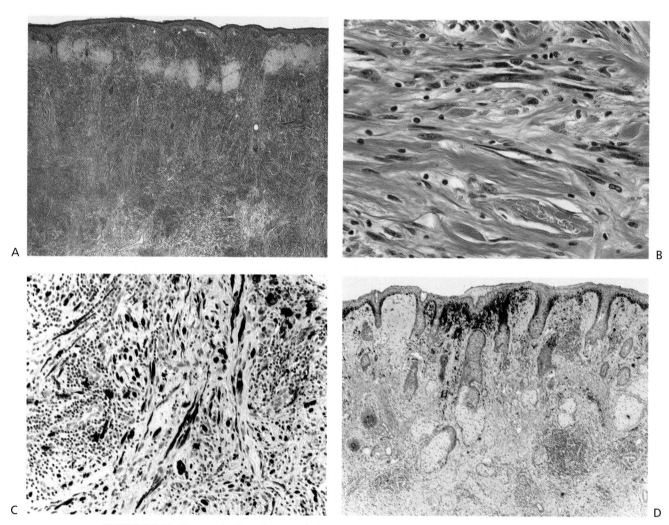

FIGURE 28-27. Desmoplastic melanoma. **(A)** At scanning magnification, the architecture of the reticular dermis is altered by a cellular infiltrate including nodule clusters of lymphocytes, appearances that can simulate an inflammatory infiltrate. **(B)** Atypical spindle cells arranged in loose fascicles extend into the deeper dermis and subcutis, beneath the epithelioid cell component. This subtle proliferation is easily overlooked, resulting in potential "undercalling" of the diagnosis and microstage. **(C)** Spindle cells are S100 positive. S100 stain is of great value in delineating the boundaries of desmoplastic melanomas, but should be interpreted cautiously as it is not specific for melanoma cells. **(D)** An immunohistochemical study for Melan-A focally stains the *in situ* and superficial dermal epithelioid cell component of the melanoma. The deeper spindle cells are uniformly negative.

Desmoplasia is most often seen in a spindle-cell VGP of lentigo maligna melanoma (454) or acral lentiginous melanoma (404,455). However, desmoplastic changes can be seen occasionally in tumors with rounded or undifferentiated melanoma cells. The collagen in desmoplastic melanomas is arranged as delicate fibrils that extend between the tumor cells and separate them from one another. The relationship between tumor cells and stroma is thus similar to that seen in sarcomas, in contrast to most melanomas, where an epithelial pattern of collagen fibers surrounding groups or clusters of tumor cells may be demonstrated, for example with a reticulin stain. Interestingly, neurotized nevi may also show the pattern of individual cells surrounded by collagen that characterizes desmoplastic melanomas, and the arrangement of the cells of desmoplastic melanomas in "wavy" fiber bundles comprised of "S-shaped" or "serpentine" cells may also recall the "schwannian" patterns of neurofibromas, neurotized nevi, and malignant schwannomas.

Histopathology. In desmoplastic melanoma, scanning magnification usually demonstrates an alteration of the architecture of the dermis, which may be subtle or more prominent. Frequently, this alteration extends throughout the full thickness of the reticular dermis into the fat. Typically, nodular clusters of lymphocytes and occasional plasma cells are present in the tumor or at its periphery, serving as a valuable scanning magnification clue (Fig. 28-27A). At higher magnification, the melanoma cells are usually elongated and amelanotic and are embedded in a markedly fibrotic stroma, so that it is often difficult to decide which are fibroblasts and which are melanoma cells. This problem is enhanced by the relative absence of nuclear atypia in many of the neoplastic spindle cells, although close scrutiny will usually reveal cells with nuclear hyperchromasia and contour irregularities not typical of resting or activated benign mesenchymal cells (Fig. 28-27B). Because of the frequent absence of melanin, differentiation from a fibrohistiocytic or a neural lesion may be difficult. Staining with S-100 protein antibody usually marks many of the spindle-shaped cells, indicating that they are not fibroblastic (456) (Fig. 28-27C), but nevi, neurofibromas, and neurogenic sarcomas are also typically S-100 positive. The HMB-45 or Melan-A antigens are usually not demonstrable in the spindle-cell compartment of desmoplastic melanomas, but they may be focally demonstrable in superficial dermal or *in situ* epithelioid melanocytes (Fig. 28-27D). Indeed, Melan-A reactivity in a spindle cell lesion (in the spindle cells themselves) may be taken as evidence against the diagnosis of a desmoplastic melanoma (22). The distinction from a neurogenic sarcoma may be very difficult or impossible in such cases where there is no pigment and there is no characteristic superficial RGP component (457). Some of these lesions might alternatively be regarded as superficial malignant epithelioid schwannomas. The prognostic implications are similar, whichever diagnostic term

is used. Desmoplastic melanomas have been shown to produce fibrogenic cytokines, neurotrophins, and neurotrophin receptors, which together can account for their desmoplastic and neurotropic propensities (458–460). Occasionally in desmoplastic malignant melanoma, the fibroplasia may be accompanied by cement production resulting in bone formation (461).

Although the reported survival rate for desmoplastic melanoma in the early literature was poor, this is likely because many of these cases had already recurred at the time the diagnosis was made. A report of a series of desmoplastic melanomas that had been prospectively diagnosed and definitively treated at their initial presentation showed that the survival was no different than for usual forms of melanoma, when thickness, mitotic rate, host response, and other risk factors were controlled. Indeed, the probability of survival is relatively good for prospectively diagnosed and definitively treated desmoplastic melanoma, because despite the considerable thickness of many of these lesions, the prognostically important mitotic rate and lymphocytic responses are often favorable (370).

Neurotropic melanoma is often a variant of desmoplastic melanoma (453,457,462–465). There are fascicles of desmoplastic melanoma that have invaded cutaneous nerves, usually in a spindle-cell vertical component with fibrosis (Fig. 28-28). However, some neurotropic melanomas lack these latter features of desmoplastic melanoma. Many of these are spindle-cell tumorigenic melanomas of acral-lentiginous or lentigo maligna type, but some are composed of epithelioid cells. Desmoplastic and spindle cell melanomas tend to express a high level of p75 neurotrophin receptor antigen, as well as other neurotrophins and their receptors, which may contribute to the high predisposition for per-

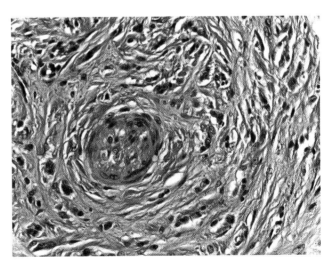

FIGURE 28-28. Neurotropism in a desmoplastic melanoma. A nerve in the center of the image contains atypical neoplastic spindle cells both in the nerve itself (endoneurial invasion) and in the perineurium (perineural invasion). The adjacent stroma contains neoplastic spindle cells separated by desmoplastic stroma.

ineural extension in the desmoplastic subset of spindled melanomas (459,460), and could be useful in diagnosis. Neurotropism in a primary melanoma is associated with increased risk for local recurrence, even after standard "definitive" therapy, and may also be associated with increased mortality (370).

Re-excision specimens. Evaluation of re-excision specimens for desmoplastic and neurotropic melanomas can present considerable difficulties. S-100 staining can be useful, but it has been demonstrated that S-100 positive cells may be present in benign scars (466–468). It is important that these procedures encompass a margin of normal tissue around the scar, both for completeness of excision, and because of the difficulty of excluding subtle melanoma involvement of the scar. In this regard, it is helpful to remember that residual melanoma is likely to present at the periphery of the scar, and to infiltrate normal tissue adjacent to it. The specimens should be carefully coated with India ink or colored dyes, and the inked margin should be carefully scrutinized for residual invasive melanoma, and for subtle neurotropic involvement of small nerves. A clue to the presence of melanoma, both in nerves and in the stroma, is the presence of clusters of lymphocytes, which sometimes may almost completely obscure the tumor cells themselves.

Immunohistochemistry. As previously discussed, desmoplastic and to a somewhat lesser extent other spindle cell melanomas tend to differ from the more common epithelioid cell melanomas in their immunohistochemical reactivity. Although S-100 is almost always positive, the more specific markers such as HMB-45, Melan-A are usually negative, except for occasional reactivity of a minor epithelioid cell component that is sometimes present in the epidermis or superficial dermal component of the neoplasm (Fig. 28-27D). In a recent study of 20 desmoplastic melanomas, all 20 were positive for S-100 protein, 7 were positive for MITF, 6 for HMB-45, and 11 for tyrosinase (443). In another study, only 4 of 13 spindle cell and desmoplastic melanomas (all positive with anti–S-100 and negative with HMB-45) were immunoreactive with A103 (two focally, two diffusely) (430). Thus, S-100 reactivity is of key importance in distinguishing these tumors from fibroblastic lesions. However, it is of no use in the distinction from neural tumors.

Differential Diagnosis. It is very important to differentiate desmoplastic melanoma from benign conditions, including benign melanocytic and neural tumors, fibrous and fibrohistiocytic tumors, and other spindle cell malignancies. Neurotized nevi and neurofibromas share serpentine spindle-cell and wavy fiber bundle patterns of schwannian differentiation with desmoplastic melanomas, but lack an *in situ* melanoma component, and lack atypia and mitotic activity as well as lymphocytic infiltrates in the dermal component. According to a study by Harris et al., similarities between desmoplastic nevi and desmoplastic melanomas included the presence of atypical cells and HMB-45 expression in the superficial portion of the lesions. The infrequent location on the head or neck, the absence of mitotic figures, a significantly lower number of Ki-67-reactive cells, and a decrease in HMB-45 expression in the deep area of the lesions helped distinguish desmoplastic nevi from desmoplastic melanoma (175). The diagnosis of desmoplastic melanoma should be made with great caution if the dermal spindle-cell component is positive for Melan-A (22). Fibrous tumors such as connective tissue nevi (469), or cellular dermatofibromas can be distinguished by immunohistochemical studies including negative S-100 staining. Other considerations include low-grade malignancies such as fibromatoses and dermatofibrosarcoma protuberans, and fully malignant lesions such as malignant schwannoma. The latter group of lesions may overlap biologically as well as morphologically, and their management is the same, namely complete excision and follow-up. Because spindle cell melanomas may be confused with other malignant spindle-cell neoplasms (e.g., malignant tumors of neural cells, smooth muscle, fibrohistiocytic cells, and spindle cell variants of squamous cell carcinoma), particularly when careful search fails to reveal evidence of *in situ* growth, immunohistochemical screening by the panel approach is recommended in such instances. Rarely, spindle cell melanomas may form vessel-like structures, and when such lesions occur on the scalp of elderly individuals, produce confusion with angiosarcoma. Immunohistochemical identification of S-100 protein and exclusion of CD31 endothelial reactivity may be helpful in such instances (470). Misdiagnosis of desmoplastic melanomas as one or another of the benign lesions listed above is not uncommon, because attributes of malignancy such as anaplasia or frequent mitoses are often not prominent features of these lesions. The large size and asymmetrical silhouette of many of these lesions differ from most benign lesions. An important sometimes subtle clue to the diagnosis at low power is the frequent presence of a lymphocytic infiltrate, distributed as nodular aggregates of infiltrating lymphocytes throughout the tumor, which are not seen in neurofibromas, nevi, or most fibrohistiocytic lesions. Lymphocytes may also be clustered about nerves involved by tumor cells in neurotropic melanomas. Other helpful diagnostic attributes, which may not be readily evident unless sought because of a high index of suspicion, include the presence of an atypical intraepidermal melanocytic component, which may be subtle and not always diagnostic of frank melanoma, and usually the presence of at least a few mitoses in the dermal component of the lesion.

Polypoid Melanoma

Also termed pedunculated melanoma, this term designates a melanoma that is confined, at least at first, to a nodule connected to the underlying skin by a pedicle or stalk

(471). The surface of the nodule often shows erosion or ulceration (472). Because these tumors are bulky, the prognosis is often poor, but probably not worse than predicted by other risk factors (473). By convention, polypoid melanomas, even when the greatly expanded papillary dermis is not filled, are considered to represent level III invasion unless tumor cells extend into the reticular dermis (level IV).

On histologic examination, the protruding nodule is filled with melanoma cells, while the underlying stalk or pedicle is free of tumor cells at first. Later, the tumor may infiltrate the pedicle and the dermis adjacent to the pedicle.

Verrucous Melanoma

These melanomas present as a markedly hyperkeratotic, tumorigenic nodule that may simulate a verruca or a verrucous carcinoma clinically (365,388,474–476). Histologically as well, the lesions are associated with marked keratosis and verrucous hyperplasia of keratinocytes that may assume pseudoepitheliomatous proportions and raise a question of squamous cell carcinoma unless the underlying neoplastic melanocytes are appreciated (477). Some other lesions are misdiagnosed histologically as benign nevi or seborrheic keratoses (475). "Verrucous" changes of adjacent keratinocytes are sometimes observed adjacent to acral and especially subungual melanomas, which are often mistaken clinically for warts upon initial presentation, if pigment is not prominent. In such instances, an inadequate biopsy that does not include the underlying neoplasm could appear to be consistent with a wart.

Balloon Cell Melanoma

Usually in addition to more characteristic melanoma cells of the epithelioid type, some melanomas contain aggregates of "balloon cells" (478). These balloon cells, characterized by their abundant, clear cytoplasm, may show relatively little nuclear atypia and thus may resemble those seen in a balloon cell nevus. The overall architecture of the lesion, and the presence of cytologic atypia, usually with mitotic activity, identify the tumor as a melanoma. Immunohistochemistry (Melan-A, HMB-45, and/or tyrosinase reactivity) may sometimes be required to distinguish the lesions from other clear cell tumors, such as renal cell carcinoma or xanthoma (479).

Transitions from the melanoma cells to balloon cells are usually seen. The metastases of a balloon cell melanoma may or may not be composed largely of balloon cells, and balloon cell metastases have been described from a melanoma that did not contain them in the primary tumor (480). Thus, this possibility should be considered in the differential diagnosis of metastatic clear cell tumors. The cells exhibit immunopathologic reactivity characteristic of melanoma.

Signet Cell Melanoma

Melanomas that contain prominent signet-ring cells may be confusing and must be distinguished from adenocarcinomas, tumors of vascular endothelium or adipose tissue, lymphomas, and epithelioid smooth muscle tumors (481–483). The signet cell morphology may be recognized in the primary tumors, or only in metastatic sites. Similar cells may be seen in benign nevi, and a somewhat similar change may also occur as a result of freezing artifact (482). Immunohistochemistry may be used to confirm the diagnosis of a melanocytic lesion and rule out competing possibilities. In evaluating these results, it should be recognized that expression of both CEA (only seen using polyclonal antibodies) (484,485) and keratin (434), have been described in melanomas.

Myxoid Melanomax

A histologic pattern of prominent myxoid stroma has been described in some primary and metastatic melanomas (486,487). The differential diagnosis may be very broad, including lipoblastic, myoblastic, fibroblastic, neurogenic or chondroblastic tumors with myxoid stroma (486). If the diagnosis is suspected, immunohistochemistry can be done to support the diagnosis. Fontana stain may reveal melanin pigment, and electron microscopy in a few cases has shown melanosomes.

Animal-Type Melanoma (Macrophagic Melanoma)

Rare tumors, comprised of nodules of heavily pigmented cells, mimic melanocytic neoplasms seen in horses and laboratory animals and thus have been termed animal type melanomas (488). The tumor cells are heavily stuffed with melanin granules, often obscuring the nucleus, and for this reason the tumors have been referred to as "melanophage-like" (489). Behavior of these lesions is unpredictable. In the only published series, of nine skin and one lymph node biopsy specimens from six patients the lesions were described as blue-black nodules with irregular borders from 1.0 to 4.0 cm in size, located on the scalp, lower extremities, back, and sacrum. Sections showed confluent dermal sheets of heavily melanized cells whose nuclei, where discernible, were large with irregularly thickened membranes, coarse chromatin, prominent, often spiculated nucleoli, and irregular parachromatinic clearing. Mitoses were infrequent. Four lesions had an epidermal component. One patient suffered metastases to regional lymph nodes, liver, and lungs with lethal effect, one experienced regional lymph node metastases but is still alive, one had local cutaneous metastases but was lost to follow-up (488). This rare dermal-based melanocytic neoplasm with prominent pigment synthesis, the animal type melanoma, has a biological behavior difficult to predict on morphologic grounds.

Pigmented Epithelioid Melanocytoma

A recently described melanocytic tumor that may resemble animal-type melanoma (as well as epithelioid blue nevi) as seen in Carney's complex and some cellular blue nevi is the pigmented epithelioid melanocytoma (PEM) (490). This lesion appears to represent a distinctive tumor that affects males and females equally and shows a median age of occurrence of 27 years (range 0.6 to 78 years). Multiple body sites may be affected, with extremities being the most common. Histologically there is a deep dermal nodule of heavily pigmented epithelioid and/or spindled melanocytes, and some lesions occur in association with combined nevi. Ulceration may be present in occasional lesions, a finding generally not present in epithelioid blue nevi. We have encountered one lesion that formed a bulky dermal nodule composed of typical heavily melanized cells identical to those of animal-type melanoma, less pigmented relatively bland epithelioid cells, and dendritic pigmented melanocytes resembling blue nevus cells. Although tumor cells may be deceptively bland and mitoses and necrosis inconspicuous or absent, regional lymph node involvement has been seen in 46% of cases studied. Nonetheless, extranodal spread is rare, and even with involvement of draining lymph nodes, the clinical course may be remarkably indolent.

Minimal Deviation Melanoma

Recognized by only some authors, this lesion is referred to as "borderline type" when it is limited to the papillary dermis and as "minimal deviation type" when it extends into the reticular dermis (205,491). These tumors are considered to exhibit less cytologic atypia than the common forms of melanoma, although the architectural characteristics of melanoma are usually present. The lesions in their vertical phase consist of uniformly expansile nodules, and the cells in the nodules tend to be arranged in uniform patterns. If the tumor cells are epithelioid in type, they may resemble cells of the ordinary acquired nevus. In the spindle cell variants, the tumor cells may resemble the cells of a Spitz nevus or, if pigmented or arranged in compact fascicles, a pigmented spindle-cell nevus. Because of the resemblance to nevus cells, the term nevoid melanoma has also been used. In a recent study, expression rates of the proliferation marker Ki-67 were intermediate between those seen in nevi and in superficial spreading melanomas (492). Even though recurrences, metastases, and death may occur, minimal deviation melanomas are thought to be biologically not as aggressive as common melanomas. However, in our opinion, prognosis is probably more accurately predicted by multivariable prognostic models.

Nevoid Melanoma

Although related to minimal deviation melanoma, this term has been used somewhat differently. Nevoid melanomas have been defined as lesions that, to a greater or lesser extent, mimic a benign nevus histologically, often with an emphasis on a nevoid architecture (in contrast to minimal deviation melanoma, where melanoma architecture tends to be preserved) (493,494). Usually, the resemblance is most apparent at scanning magnification, where lesions may appear symmetrical, nested, and devoid of radial growth, features which can lead to a missed diagnosis if sufficient attention is not paid to cytologic and subtle architectural features (495). In the study by Schmoeckel et al., useful discriminating attributes included cellular atypia, mitoses, infiltration of adnexa, infiltrative growth in the deeper dermis, and the absence of maturation. Tumor thickness was the most important prognostic criterion (494). Nevoid melanomas are generally considered to have the same biological potential as other melanomas with similar microstaging attributes (111,494). Key to the recognition of a nevoid melanoma is a high index of suspicion, and the identification of mitotic activity and cytologic atypia in the dermal component of the lesion (111,494,495). According to McNutt, reactivity of the intradermal component for HMB-45 antigen, without antigen retrieval, or for Ki-67 antigen can show that the dermal cells have an immature phenotype and, in combination with histologic criteria, can support a diagnosis of nevoid malignant melanoma (496).

EPIDEMIOLOGY, PROGNOSIS, AND MANAGEMENT OF MELANOMA

Risk Factors for Development of Melanomas

The major phenotypic risk factors for the development of melanoma have been discussed in previous sections. These include the pigmentation phenotype, freckles (43), the total number of banal nevi, the presence of large nevi, and, especially, the presence and number of dysplastic nevi (62). In addition, type I skin that burns easily and tans poorly is a risk factor, as are indicators of acute sun exposure, such as living in a sunny climate, a history of weekend and vacation sun exposure, and a history of sunburn episodes (497). Among these risk factors, melanocytic nevi and indicators of "acute, intermittent" sun exposure are more strongly related to superficial spreading and nodular melanoma (498,499), while skin type, ethnic background, and measures of total accumulated exposure to the sun ("chronic, continuous sun exposure") are more strongly related to lentigo maligna melanoma (500). Age is also a strong risk factor, operating in a continuously progressive fashion in lentigo maligna melanoma in contrast to a more complex pattern for superficial and nodular melanoma (405). The etiologic factors that may be related to acral and mucosal melanomas are unknown.

Preexisting Melanocytic Nevus

It is well known that melanomas can develop in congenital nevi and in dysplastic nevi. Histologically, remnants of a banal nevus are found in a substantial number of melanomas, of the order of about 10% to 35%, and evidence of associated melanocytic dysplasia may be seen in up to about 40% (97,250,345–348,501,502). Analysis has demonstrated that this relationship is likely to be nonrandom (503). Remnants of a dysplastic nevus adjacent to a RGP (usually of the superficial spreading type) can be distin-

guished from the latter using the criteria presented in Table 28-3. Remnants of a dermal component of a nevus deep to a melanoma can be distinguished from the melanoma cells by the following criteria (Fig. 28-29): (a) the dermal nevus cells are smaller; (b) they are arranged in nests that tend to be small and uniform in size and shape; (c) there may be evidence of maturation from superficial to deep within the nevus but not the melanoma cell population; (d) there is no evidence of continuous differentiation from a more obviously malignant superficial component to the nevoid cells at the base of the tumor; (e) there is no high-grade atypia and there are no mitoses in the dermal nevus cells; and (f) nevus cells tend to disperse as single cells if they enter the reticular dermis, while melanoma cells tend to infiltrate as sheets or clusters (Fig. 28-30). This paradoxically

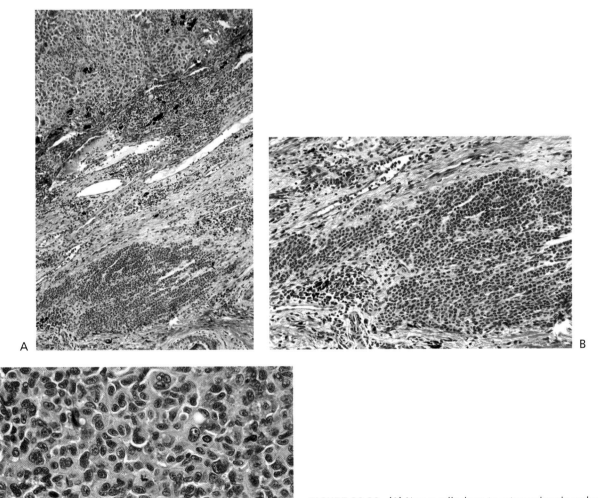

FIGURE 28-29. (A) Nevus cells deep to a tumorigenic melanoma. A collection of smaller cells is present at the interface of the papillary and reticular dermis deep to a tumor of vertical growth phase melanoma. **(B)** The nevus cells are smaller than the cells of the tumorigenic melanoma **(C)**. The tumorigenic melanoma cells have large, hyperchromatic nuclei with irregularly clumped nuclear chromatin, and with mitotic figures.

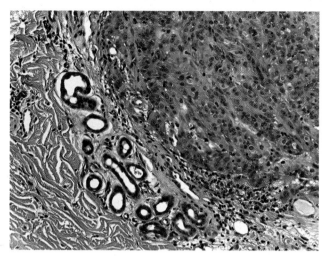

FIGURE 28-30. Infiltration of tumorigenic melanoma at base of lesion. The cells tend to be arranged in clusters or sheets. In benign nevi, the cells in the papillary dermis may be clustered but when they enter the reticular dermis they tend to disperse as single cells (compare with Fig. 28-10F).

less "invasive" pattern is related to the greater proliferative capacity of melanoma cells, invasion probably initially involves single cells which then proliferate to form the final pattern of sheets or fascicles in the reticular dermis. For the same reason, cutaneous metastases tend to be sharply demarcated, "expansive" lesions (104). Occasional examples of differentiated dermal melanoma cells may meet some of these criteria and thus present difficulties of interpretation (see Nevoid Melanoma section).

It has recently been demonstrated that in some cases, loss of heterozygosity at the 9p21 locus (the locus of the cell-cycle control gene CDKN2A) is detected simultaneously in a melanoma and its associated nevus (504). Recent studies have also demonstrated the same mutations in the oncogene nRAS in melanomas and in their associated nevi studied by microdissection (505). These results are consistent with a causal relationship for the development of melanoma within a preexistent associated nevus, and also support the hypothesis that these genetic alterations play an important role in early melanoma development, since they are found in histologically benign melanoma-associated nevi (504).

In addition to dysplastic nevi and banal dermal nevi, superficial and deep congenital pattern nevi are also commonly associated with melanomas (250). An exception to the general rule that melanoma arises at the epidermal–dermal border is observed occasionally in congenital nevi, in which a melanoma may arise deep in the dermis. However, these proliferations should be distinguished from benign cellular/proliferative nodules that may occur in congenital nevi (262). In very rare instances, a melanoma may develop within or beneath an intradermal nevus, resulting in a dermal nodule of atypical cells (506).

Multiple Primary Melanomas

People who have had a cutaneous melanoma are at risk of developing additional melanomas, with an incidence of approximately 5% in the first 10 years after diagnosis (507). The occurrence of multiple and familial melanomas has already been pointed out in relation to dysplastic nevi (508–512). A prior melanoma is a strong risk factor for subsequent melanoma, especially in young patients and in familial melanoma kindreds (319,321). It is important to differentiate an additional melanoma from a metastatic melanoma, especially from an epidermotropic metastasis (495,513), because the prognosis of an independent primary is likely to be much better than that of a metastasis. In a recent study, individuals with multiple primary melanomas were associated with a modest incidence of a family history of melanoma, dysplastic nevi and basal cell carcinoma and a small association with CDKN2A mutations (8%). Therefore, in addition to the multiple primary melanoma index case, other family members can benefit from screening and regular surveillance of their skin (514).

Malignant Melanoma in Infancy and Childhood

Malignant melanoma is a disease primarily of adults. The incidence of prepubertal melanoma is very low. In a few instances, it has occurred as multiple metastases resulting from transplacental transmission (515). Occasionally, a melanoma arises in infancy or childhood in a giant congenital nevus (225,229,230,234) (Fig. 28-12B). Outside of these situations, three patterns of primary melanoma have been described in children (516). In most instances, the melanoma shows a histologic picture similar to that in adults and the prognosis depends on thickness and other "microstaging" attributes. In other cases, the tumors are composed of small "blastic" malignant cells, and the course is usually aggressive, though sometimes unpredictably so, especially in tumors that arise in congenital nevi. In a few instances, the histologic picture is reminiscent of that seen in Spitz nevi (516–518). In some of these cases, metastases occur that are limited to the regional lymph nodes, and the child survives after adequate treatment (202,516). However, at least one example of a "Spitzean" melanoma with a fatal outcome in a child has been reported (516).

Biopsy of Melanoma

The question of whether an incisional biopsy is permissible in a lesion that is highly suspected of being a melanoma has been widely discussed. Several authors, especially from Europe, have opposed the performance of an incisional biopsy, because of a belief that it might cause metastatic spread (519). In other studies, no deleterious effect of a preceding biopsy was noted (520–523). It is difficult in studies of this sort to control for other risk factors, which might be expected to be more prevalent in the larger tumors for which an incisional biopsy might be contemplated.

Because a correct diagnosis and accurate prognostic staging are more likely to be accomplished when the entire tumor can be studied, an excisional biopsy is advisable whenever feasible, and only in occasional instances such as very large lesions is an incisional biopsy indicated (524). If a tumorigenic VGP is present, it should be entirely contained within the biopsy, if possible. A shave biopsy or curetting is not optimal, because it may result in inadequate material for diagnosis; it may also make impossible a determination of the depth of penetration of the tumor, which is very important for prognosis and for planning of the extent of surgical procedures (see next section). Shave or punch biopsies that completely encompass the lesion are, of course, acceptable.

Multivariable Prognostic Models

The "gold standard" for considering any putative prognostic marker to be clinically important is its inclusion as an independent variable in a multivariable analysis. So far, no such studies have been published for other than the traditional histopathologic and clinical variables reviewed above. Based on these multivariable analyses, prognostic models have been published, either requiring the use of a calculator to determine a regression function, or more simply, using published tables to provide a quantitative probability estimate (419,525–536). Although these models are useful in planning therapy, and especially in the development and execution of clinical trials, thickness and ulceration are the factors in predominant use for planning of therapy for stage I melanoma. Prognostic modeling may be considered as a form of staging of the primary tumor (so-called "microstaging").

Staging of Melanoma

The purpose of staging is to define subsets of cases with a similar prognosis for management and investigational purposes. The five-stage (0 to IV) clinicopathologic staging system of the American Joint Committee on Cancer (AJCC) primarily considers aspects of the tumor (T), the presence and size of nodal metastases (N) and the presence and sites of distant metastases (M) to determine a stage based on all three attributes (TNM). The 5-year survival for newly diagnosed localized primary melanoma cases (stages 0 to II) is about 80%, compared to 35% survival when lymph nodes are involved (stage III). Using prognostic models discussed below, subsets of cases with more or less favorable prognosis can be identified. When distant metastases are present, the survival at 5 years is of the order of 10% (534,537).

TNM Staging System for Melanoma

The tumor-node-metastasis (TNM) system of tumor staging considers factors related to the primary tumor, to regional lymph nodes (and other regional soft tissues), and to distant metastases to result in a classification that is associated with the probability of survival. The factors considered in the primary tumor (T) category include some of the microstaging attributes discussed above. Thus, the TNM classification combines staging and microstaging information in a single format. In the current system (which became official with the publishing of the sixth edition of the *AJCC Cancer Staging Manual* in 2002) (534,537,538), the T attributes are classified pathologically after excision of the melanoma (pT), as described below (537). The TNM model therefore considers pathologic attributes of the primaries, but staging for metastases is defined in part clinically. For example, lymph node metastases are defined in terms of the number of lymph nodes involved as well as volume, and are coded as "micrometastasis" if lymph node metastasis has been diagnosed at sentinel node biopsy or at elective lymphadenectomy, or as "macrometastasis" if clinically positive and pathologically confirmed by therapeutic lymphadenectomy (537). Among macrometastases, the size of nodes is no longer used in staging, based on evidence that the number of nodes but not their size is significant prognostically (539–544). In other prognostic models, it has been demonstrated that microstaging of the primary tumor retains prognostic significance in melanoma patients who are clinically negative but pathologically positive for metastases to regional nodes (545–547), and this is also reflected in the new AJCC staging system, where ulceration retains significance in some patients with nodal metastases. The new system was recently reviewed by Schuchter (548).

The recently published latest revision (2002) of the TNM categories is presented in Table 28-7, and the final stage groupings are in Table 28-8 (534,537,538). Clinical staging includes microstaging of the primary melanoma and clinical/radiologic evaluation for metastases. By convention, clinical staging should be used after complete excision of the primary melanoma, with clinical assessment for regional and distant metastases. Pathologic staging includes microstaging of the primary melanoma and pathologic information about the regional lymph nodes after partial or complete lymphadenectomy. Pathologic stage 0 or stage 1A patients do not require pathologic evaluation of their lymph nodes. There are no stage III subgroups for clinical staging. The definitions have been recommended by the AJCC Melanoma Staging Committee and approved by both the AJCC Executive Committee and the TNM Committee of the International Union Against Cancer (Union Internationale Contra Cancer, UICC). The revised melanoma staging system has been approved by the World Health Organization Melanoma Program as well as the Eu-

TABLE 28-7. MELANOMA TNM CLASSIFICATION

T Classification	Thickness	Ulceration/ Clark Level Status
	<1.0 mm	(a) Without ulceration and level II/III
		(b) With ulceration or level IV/V
T2	1.01–2.0 mm	(a) Without ulceration
		(b) With ulceration
T3	2.01–4.0 mm	(a) Without ulceration
		(b) With ulceration
T4	>4.0 mm	(a) Without ulceration
		(b) With ulceration

N Classification	No. of Metastatic Nodes	Nodal Metastatic Mass
N1	1 Node	(a) Micrometastasis[a]
		(b) Macrometastasis[b]
N2	2 to 3 Nodes	(a) Micrometastasis[a]
		(b) Macrometastasis[b]
		(c) In transit met(s)/ satellite(s) without metastatic nodes
N3	≥4 Metastatic nodes, or matted nodes, or in transit met(s)/satellite(s) with metastatic node(s)	

M Classification	Site	Serum Lactate Dehydrogenase
M1a	Distant skin, subcutaneous, or nodal metastases	Normal
M1b	Lung metastases	Normal
M1c	All other visceral metastases	Normal
	Any distant metastasis	Elevated

[a] Micrometastases are diagnosed after sentinel or elective lymphadenectomy.
[b] Macrometastases are defined as clinically detectable nodal metastases confirmed by therapeutic lymphadenectomy or when nodal metastasis exhibits gross extracapsular extension.
From Balch CM, Buzaid AC, Soong SJ, et al. Final version of the American Joint Committee on Cancer staging system for cutaneous melanoma. *J Clin Oncol* 2001;19:3635–3648; and Green FL, Page DL, Fleming ID, et al. Melanoma of the skin. In: *AJCC cancer staging manual, American Joint Committee on Cancer*, 6th ed. New York: Springer, 2002:209–217.

TABLE 28-8. STAGE GROUPINGS FOR CUTANEOUS MELANOMA

	Clinical Staging			Pathologic Staging		
	T	N	M	T	N	M
0	Tis	N0	M0	Tis	N0	M0
IA	T1a	N0	M0	T1a	N0	M0
IB	T1b	N0	M0	T1b	N0	M0
	T2a	N0	M0	T2a	N0	M0
IIA	T2b	N0	M0	T2b	N0	M0
	T3a	N0	M0	T3a	N0	M0
IIB	T3b	N0	M0	T3b	N0	M0
	T4a	N0	M0	T4a	N0	M0
IIC	T4b	N0	M0	T4b	N0	M0
III	Any T	N1	M0			
		N2				
		N3				
IIIA				T1–4a	N1a	M0
				T1–4a	N2a	M0
IIIB				T1–4b	N1a	M0
				T1–4b	N2a	M0
				T1–4a	N1b	M0
				T1–4a	N2b	M0
				T1–4a/b	N2c	M0
IIIC				T1–4b	N1b	M0
				T1–4b	N2b	M0
				Any T	N3	M0
IV	Any T	Any N	Any M1	Any T	Any N	Any M1

From Balch CM, Buzaid AC, Soong SJ, et al. Final version of the American Joint Committee on Cancer staging system for cutaneous melanoma. *J Clin Oncol* 2001;19:3635–3648; and Green FL, Page DL, Fleming ID, et al. Melanoma of the skin. In: *AJCC cancer staging manual, American Joint Committee on Cancer*, 6th ed. New York: Springer, 2002:209–217.

ropean Organization for Research and Treatment of Cancer Melanoma Group (549). These new definitions incorporate substantial revisions from previous (1983 and 1997) versions of the melanoma staging categories and classifications (538,550,551).

The TNM staging system differs from previously used, simple primarily clinical staging systems (localized, regional, and metastatic disease) in that pathologic attributes of the primary neoplasm ("microstaging attributes") are considered in the definition of the first three stages of the "stage groups." Tumors in stage groups I and II are non-

metastatic, and stage III may or not be associated with distant metastasis (Table 28-8). Stage IV is always metastatic. Since these stages are different from those defined in other staging systems, it is clear that the system in use (e.g., AJCC stage X) should be clearly specified when staging is used as a basis for therapy or prognosis.

The staging system is primarily based on survival studies done in several collaborating institutions. Survival rates for 17,600 patients categorized according to the AJCC staging system are shown in Table 28-9. Survival times were calculated from onset of primary melanoma diagnosis and are considered censored for patients who were alive at the last follow-up or who died without evidence of melanoma (534,537).

Pathology of Microstaging Attributes in Common Use

As discussed above, the 2002 AJCC staging system, which is currently used worldwide, incorporates several attributes of primary and metastatic melanomas, such as Breslow's thickness, Clark's levels of invasion, and the presence or absence of ulceration in the primary tumor. These and other

TABLE 28-9. SURVIVAL RATES FOR MELANOMA BY TNM AND STAGING CATEGORIES (537,538)

Path Stage	TNM	No. of Paths	1-Year Survival	2-Year Survival	5-Year Survival	10-Year Survival
IA	T1aN0M0	4,510	99.7±0.1	99.0±0.2	95.3±0.4	87.9±1.0
IB	T1b	1,380	99.8±0.1	98.7±0.3	90.9±1.0	83.1±1.5
	T2a	3,285	99.5±0.1	97.3±0.3	89.0±0.7	79.2±1.1
IIA	T2b	958	98.2±0.5	92.9±0.9	77.4±1.7	64.4±2.2
	T3a	1,717	98.7±0.3	94.3±0.6	78.7±1.2	63.8±1.7
IIB	T3b	1,523	95.1±0.6	84.8±1.0	63.0±1.5	50.8±1.7
	T4a	563	94.8±1.0	88.6±1.5	67.4±2.4	53.9±3.3
IIC	T4b	978	89.9±1.0	70.7±1.6	45.1±1.9	32.3±2.1
IIIA	N1a	252	95.9±1.3	88.0±2.3	69.5±3.7	63.0±4.4
	N2a	130	93.0±2.4	82.7±3.8	63.3±5.6	56.9±6.8
IIIB	N1a	217	93.3±1.8	75.0±3.2	52.8±4.1	37.8±4.8
	N2a	111	92.0±2.7	81.0±4.1	49.6±5.7	35.9±7.2
	N1b	122	88.5±2.9	78.5±3.7	59.0±4.8	47.7±5.8
	N2b	93	76.8±4.4	65.6±5.0	46.3±5.5	39.2±5.8
IIIC	N1b	98	77.9±4.3	54.2±5.2	29.0±5.1	24.4±5.3
	N2b	109	74.3±4.3	44.1±4.9	24.0±4.4	15.0±3.9
	N3	396	71.0±2.4	49.8±2.7	26.7±2.5	18.4±2.5
IV	M1a	179	59.3±3.7	36.7±3.6	18.8±3.0	15.7±2.9
	M1b	186	57.0±3.7	23.1±3.2	6.7±2.0	2.5±1.5
	M1c	793	40.6±1.8	23.6±1.5	9.5±1.1	6.0±0.9

TNM, aspects of tumor (T), presence and size of nodal metastases (N), and presence and sites of distant metastases (M).
From Balch CM, Buzaid AC, Soong SJ, et al. Final version of the American Joint Committee on Cancer staging system for cutaneous melanoma. *J Clin Oncol* 2001;19:3635–3648; and Green FL, Page DL, Fleming ID, et al. Melanoma of the skin. In: *AJCC cancer staging manual, American Joint Committee on Cancer*, 6th ed. New York: Springer, 2002:209–217.

attributes that may contribute to the assessment of prognosis are discussed in the following sections.

Vertical Growth Phase

The morphology of VGP has already been presented. Here we discuss its significance as a prognostic attribute in relatively thin melanomas with vertical growth, and in level II melanomas ostensibly without vertical growth. In one series, metastases occurred in 2% of melanomas <0.76 mm thick. The cases that metastasized all had tumorigenic VGP. The rate of metastasis for tumorigenic melanomas <0.76 mm in thickness was 15%, while in nontumorigenic (RGP) melanoma of any thickness (most are <1 mm), the metastatic rate was zero (306,376). In rare instances of metastasizing thin melanomas, VGP is absent; most if not all of these cases in our experience and in the literature have had extensive partial or complete regression (419, 552–555). As already mentioned, two reproducibility studies have been done for VGP in thin melanomas, and have concluded that this determination can be reliably made by practicing pathologists (380,556). A recent study investigated prognostic factors in metastasizing thin level II melanomas, and concluded that VGP was the only statistically significant factor. It was proposed that growth phase evaluation should be added to the recommendations for melanoma histologic reporting, at least for level II superfi-

cial spreading melanomas (379). Even though VGP is the most common "explanation" for metastasizing thin melanoma (306,379), not all such lesions contain this feature (557).

Levels of Invasion

Although tumor thickness is now considered to be the single most important prognostic attribute, the levels of invasion suggested by Clark (365,558) have prognostic value, at least in certain subsets of cases (559,560), or more broadly, depending on the databases studied (561). They also have descriptive value. The different levels appear to reflect the sequential acquisition of new properties by evolving tumors. They are as follows, with survival rates for prospectively diagnosed and definitively treated clinical stage I cases in parentheses (562).

In level I (100% 10-year disease-free survival), melanoma cells are confined to the epidermis and its appendages. These *in situ* melanomas (AJCC stage 0) presumably lack the capacity to invade through a basement membrane. In level II (96% survival), there is extension into the papillary dermis, with at most only a few melanoma cells extending to the interface between papillary and reticular dermis. These melanomas are "microinvasive," but lack the capacity to form tumors in all but a few cases. Almost all of the level II tumors that metastasize have a small tumorigenic papule (VGP), as previously defined. In level III (86% survival), there is extension of the tumor cells throughout the papillary dermis, filling it, and impinging upon the reticular dermis without, however, invading it. These melanomas are competent to form tumors in the papillary dermis, a loose mesenchyme that is specialized to support epithelium. Level IV (66% survival) tumors are not only invasive and tumorigenic, but also have the capacity to invade the dense, sparsely vascular mesenchyme of the reticular dermis. Level V (53% survival) tumors invade the subcutaneous fat. Observer agreement for Clark level has been found to be fair to good (563).

Thickness of Tumor

Tumor thickness is the single most important factor in predicting survival for stage I patients. Breslow, in 1970, first measured tumor thickness objectively with a micrometer (564,565). The depth of invasion is measured from the top of the granular layer to the deepest extension of the tumor; in ulcerated lesions, measurement is from the ulcer base overlying the deepest point of invasion. In the initial report, metastasis did not occur in lesions <0.76 mm in greatest thickness. Since then, there have been reports of metastases from "thin" melanomas, though this continues to be rare (566,567). Metastasis from "thin" melanomas, or from level II melanomas, appears usually to be explained by the presence of tumorigenic melanoma (VGP, see earlier section). In a computer simulation studying the biology of thickness development, tumor thickness was related not only to time

(the most important factor) but also to tumor cell motility, a decreased rate of tumor cell loss, and pronounced proliferation in the tumor cells, attributes that are also thought to correlate with aggressiveness of tumors (568).

In determining the depth of penetration, whether by level or by measurement, the following rules apply:

- Melanocytes in junctional nests are not considered invasive, even though they may "push" into the papillary dermis.
- If deep nests of melanoma cells arise from the epithelium of cutaneous appendages, they are not used in measurement from the surface.
- A column of melanocytes extending from the lower border of the lesion into the deep dermis at nearly a right angle is not measured, because it is likely that the column arises from an appendage; this supposition can usually be verified by serial sections or keratin stains (569) (Fig. 28-31). Observer agreement for Clark level has been found to be excellent (563).

Partial and Complete Regression of Melanoma

Partial regression is common in melanomas. Usually, it is observed in the nontumorigenic compartment ("RGP regression"). Regression is defined as a focal area in which there is delicate fibroplasia of the papillary dermis, often accompanied by proliferation of dilated blood vessels, and usually with a sprinkling of melanophages and lymphocytes, with melanoma present in the epidermis and/or papillary dermis to one or both sides, but not within the area of regression (Fig. 28-32). Paradoxically, partial regression of the RGP ("RGP regression") has been associated in some series with poorer prognosis (419,553–555,570), perhaps because a more significant dermal component had been present and had metastasized before it regressed. Interobserver agreement for regression as a prognostic attribute has been found to be poor in several studies (571,572), perhaps because of failure to agree upon criteria.

In contrast to the apparent negative correlation of RGP regression with prognosis, TILs within the VGP, which may be considered as a potentially different form of immunological regression ("VGP regression"), are associated with improved survival rates (419,573–575) (Fig. 28-33A). Regression of the VGP has not been well described. Occasionally, one sees an area of fibrosis and melanophages apparently partially replacing a portion of a tumor nodule, and very infrequently, this process may proceed to completion, resulting in a collection of melanophages in the dermis that could represent the residual evidence of a preexisting tumor nodule. This phenomenon has been aptly referred to as "tumoral melanosis" (576) (Fig. 28-33B). Not all of these cases are due to regression of a melanoma; pigmented basal cell carcinomas or other pigmented skin tumors may regress and produce similar findings (577).

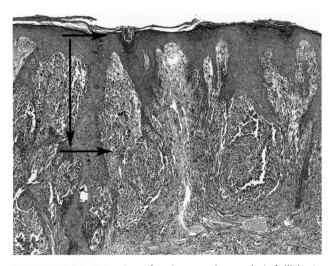

FIGURE 28-31. Extension of melanoma down a hair follicle. In a lentigo maligna melanoma (*right center*), a hair follicle is largely replaced by melanoma cells that are confined to the epidermis and adventitial dermis of the follicle. This melanoma is nontumorigenic. Invasive cells at the base of the follicle should not be used for thickness measurement. *Arrows* indicate where measurement should be taken perpendicularly from the top of the granular layer to the deepest invasive tumor cell.

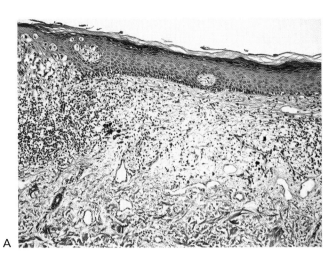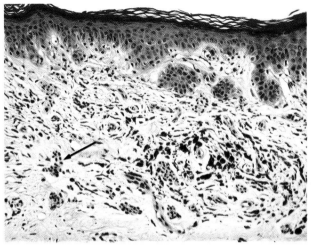

FIGURE 28-32. (A) Partial regression of radial growth phase. At *left*, there are melanoma cells in the epidermis and papillary dermis. To the *right*, there is fibrosis with lymphocytes and melanophages in the papillary dermis. **(B)** In another area of partial radial growth phase regression, the papillary dermis is widened by fibroblasts with lymphocytes and melanophages. Remnants of a nevus are seen in the regressive fibroplasia (*arrow*), apparently unaffected by the regression process.

In occasional cases of metastatic melanoma with no obvious primary tumor, clinical examination may reveal a hypopigmented or irregularly hyperpigmented atrophic patch in the skin of the nodal drainage region (578). Some other cases of apparently regressed primary melanoma may present as clinically pigmented, variegated lesions, clinically suspicious for melanoma. Some of these have presented with concomitant metastases, but some, in our experience, have not been associated with metastasis. Although the diagnosis of melanoma cannot be made with certainty in

these latter cases, we have seen at least one case in which metastatic melanoma developed after a period of follow-up. Histologic examination shows in the case of depigmented lesions telangiectasia and some pigmented macrophages in the papillary dermis, and in the case of still pigmented lesions an irregular band of melanophages and inflammatory cells in the upper part of the dermis. In some cases, serial sections may reveal a few melanoma cells in the dermis or in the subcutaneous tissue. It is presumed that in patients who present with metastatic melanoma without a

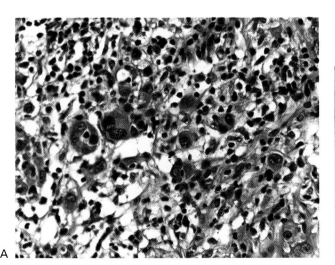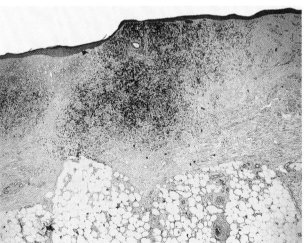

FIGURE 28-33. (A) Tumor-infiltrating lymphocytes at base of the vertical growth phase of a primary melanoma. Lymphocytes among the tumor cells, often associated with evidence of cell apoptosis, are a favorable prognostic attribute. **(B)** Tumoral melanosis. A localized collection of pigmented melanophages is present in the dermis, consistent with regression of a tumorigenic melanoma or other pigmented tumor.

clinically overt primary lesion, such completely regressed primary sites may be responsible, although they may evade detection. In such instances, it is important not to implicate other detectable melanocytic lesions (e.g., dysplastic nevi, melanoma *in situ*) as primary sources of metastasis by default.

Tumor-Infiltrating Lymphocytes

The presence of TILs that are actually among and in contact with the tumor cells of the VGP has been shown to have powerful independent prognostic significance (419, 573,579–582) (Fig. 28-33A). The prognosis is best for tumors with a "brisk" TIL response, defined as lymphocytes forming a continuous band beneath the tumor or diffusely throughout its substance. Tumors with "absent" TILs have the worst prognosis, and a "nonbrisk" response (discontinuous band) is associated with an intermediate prognosis. The presence of a noninfiltrative lymphocytic infiltrate around the tumor, usually at its base, is not associated with prognosis (583). The lymphocytic infiltrate tends to diminish with increasing thickness of the primary melanoma, and is usually scant in deeply invasive tumors. The histologic determination of the TIL response has been shown to be reproducible (584).

Mitotic Rate

Mitotic rate has been associated with prognosis in multiple studies (521,529,585–590). However, other well-conducted, large studies have not identified this relationship in multivariable models (533,588,589,591–594). The differences among these studies may have to do with differences in the determination of mitotic rate, or with interactions between mitotic rate and other variables such as ulceration; in some large studies, mitotic rate has not been systematically considered (534,537,595). When it is determined in the tumorigenic compartment of primary melanomas, the mitotic rate has been shown to have powerful independent significance (419). Areas where mitoses are counted should include those where they appear to be the highest (the "hot spot"). The prognosis is best when the mitotic rate is zero, and worst when the rate is greater than six mitoses per square millimeter (419). The presence of mitoses may also be useful in identifying thin melanomas with a propensity to metastasize (588,589,596) (Fig. 28-21B). Interobserver agreement for tumor mitotic rate has been found to be excellent (563).

Ulceration

Ulceration is defined by the loss of continuity of the epithelium over the surface of the tumor (Fig. 28-34). Evidence of a host reaction to the ulceration is also required, in order to exclude epithelial loss due to biopsy trauma

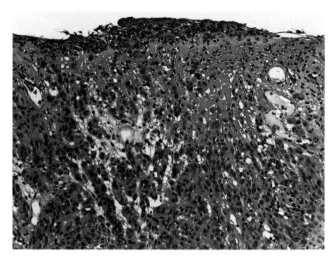

FIGURE 28-34. Ulcerated melanoma. An ulcer is defined as an area of loss of continuity of epithelium over the surface of the lesion, with evidence of a host reaction. The example here shows a neutrophilic and fibrinous exudate on the surface of the ulcer.

(597). Even with a host response, it may be difficult or impossible to determine whether ulceration is secondary to the tumor or a result of excoriation or environmental trauma. Nonetheless, this attribute has prognostic significance in most multivariable analyses (528,533,534,580, 594,598–606). Other studies, particularly those in which mitotic rate is an independent variable, have not identified ulceration as an independently significant prognostic attribute (419,529,585,586,607). In the AJCC staging data, ulceration in stage I reduces the 5-year survival rate from 88% to 83% (534). A potentially useful prognostic algorithm has been published in which ulceration is the primary stratifying variable (419,530). Ulceration is a key substratifying variable in the latest AJCC staging system for melanoma (see Tables 28-3 through 28-6) (534). Interobserver agreement for ulceration has been found to be excellent (563,597).

Vascular or Lymphatic Invasion

Although often correlated with survival as a single variable (419), the presence of vascular or lymphatic invasion has infrequently been found to correlate with survival in large series of cases studied by multivariable analysis (608). In a recent publication, two types of vascular invasion were studied: vascular invasion with tumor cells within blood or lymphatic vessels (Fig. 28-35); or "uncertain" vascular invasion, with melanoma cells present within the wall of the vessel, immediately adjacent to the endothelium. The presence of either type of vascular involvement significantly reduced the survival associated with melanoma. In a multivariate analysis, vascular involvement was the second most important factor (after tumor thickness) in the primary

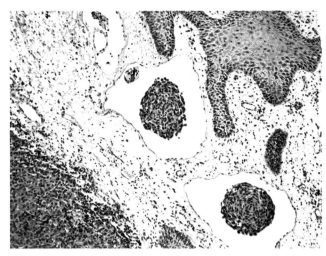

FIGURE 28-35. Lymphatic invasion. Although not often recognized, except in very thick tumors, lymphatic invasion is probably an adverse prognostic attribute.

tumor in predicting survival (609). Vascular invasion also appears to be a strong predictor of the development of in transit metastases in follow-up (610).

Tumor vascularity has also been correlated with survival in some but not all studies (611). In another matched-pair analysis, tumor vascularity was found not to correlate with survival rates (612). New markers are now available that distinguish between vascular and lymphatic channels in paraffin sections, which may make study of these variables more informative in the future.

Satellites

Satellites are defined as discontinuous foci of tumor (metastases) located within 5 cm of a primary melanoma, while in-transit metastases are beyond 5 cm but still regional. The presence of satellites is a significant staging attribute in the current AJCC staging system, defining a lesion as stage IV, with a poor prognosis (534,537,595). Microscopic satellites are independently associated with worse prognosis (613,614). These are defined as tumor nests, >0.05 mm in diameter, in the reticular dermis, panniculus, or vessels beneath the principal invasive tumor mass but separated from it by normal tissue on the section in which the Breslow measurement was taken (Fig. 28-36).

Other Clinicopathologic Prognostic Factors

Various factors in addition to thickness of the tumor have been cited as influencing the prognosis of clinical stage I melanoma but many of them are directly related to thickness. In different clinicopathologic databases, multivariate analyses have led to prognostic models that differ somewhat in the predictive variables that are shown to have independent significance. Several features, however, have appeared in two or more of the studies.

Lesional Location
Among the favorable clinical factors is location of the tumor on the hair-bearing portions of the limbs, in contrast to location on the trunk, neck and head, or palms and soles (533,580,601,615–618). In one of these studies, lower trunk, thigh, lower leg, foot, lower arms, hands, and face were identified as intermediate sites, with the remaining sites representing higher risk (615). In other studies, however, the palms and soles and the distal lower extremity have been included in the higher risk sites (419,618).

Gender
There is general agreement that women have a better prognosis than men, owing partly, but not entirely, to the

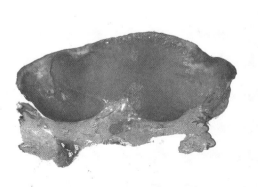

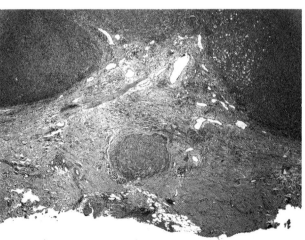

A   B

FIGURE 28-36. (A) Microscopic satellite present at the base of a bulky tumorigenic vertical growth phase melanoma. **(B)** The satellite is located in the superficial reticular dermis.

higher incidence in women of lesions on the extremities where the prognosis is favorable compared to the trunk (419,533,580,617,619–621). The age of the patient has an adverse prognostic effect in some series (533,535,580,617, 619,622).

Histogenetic Type

Among the histologic factors, the type of tumor, whether nodular or superficial spreading, does not, in most studies, independently affect the prognosis (399,419,623), despite a suggestion in some studies that the prognosis for lentigo maligna melanoma may be slightly better (624). Nodular melanomas, on average, are thicker than superficial spreading melanomas, and thus have a worse prognosis overall (625,626). However, the prognosis is the same for nodular and other types of melanoma of similar thickness, and in multivariable analyses, nodular type is not an independent predictor (419,529,580,624). The scarcity or absence of melanin in the tumor cells ("amelanotic melanoma"), indicative of poor differentiation, affect the prognosis adversely in some series, but does so most likely because of correlations with tumor thickness and other variables (419).

Biological Markers

Biological markers derived from the study of the primary tumors or of host attributes may be expected to add to the precision of present prognostic models. The most consistently useful marker studied to date appears to be the proliferation marker Mib-1 (Ki-67), which has been found to be significantly related to mortality risk in a number of studies (596,627–633). Other markers, in general, have not been studied in sufficiently large series of cases, or have not been reproduced in other data sets.

Local Excision

Formerly, the margin of resection of the primary tumor was regarded by most authors as optimal at about 5 cm beyond the perimeter of the lesion (634). However, a narrower margin is now acceptable. Margin width recommendations were reviewed by an NIH Consensus Conference in 1992 (635). A margin of 0.5 to 1.0 cm is recommended for excision of a melanoma *in situ*, with a margin of 1 cm for melanomas <1.0 mm thick, and a 2- to 3-cm skin margin for thicker lesions (636–638). A worldwide cooperative study showed that in patients with primary melanomas no thicker than 2 mm, excisions with margins of 1 cm gave results as good as excisions with margins of 3 cm (639). A critical review of the literature revealed no evidence of an adverse effect on outcome in terms of survival from melanoma with narrowing of margins to 1 cm. A slightly increased rate of local recurrence was observed in some studies, especially with thicker primary tumors. This analysis therefore did not support the use of resection margins

>1 cm for invasive melanoma of any thickness (640). Others have considered similar or lesser margins (641,642). This hypothesis may be worthy of testing in a future randomized trial (643).

In examining a resected specimen for melanoma, we generally serially embed the area of the biopsy scar, and sample the specimen margin with perpendicular sections. The specimen is first inked in order to identify the true margin surface. After taking the initial margin section, the specimen is bread-loafed macroscopically and any remaining lesions suspicious for possible satellites are also submitted for histologic examination. The margin widths discussed above are clinical margins, measured from the clinically visible periphery of the melanoma. Therefore, careful histologic examination of the excised tumor and its margins is mandatory, because margins may be involved in spite of a clinically normal appearance. It is not necessary, however, to measure the margin width histologically in the resection specimen, as long as the width is adequate. In our practice, we generally alert the clinician when the margin width is <0.1 cm (<1 mm) in a resection specimen. The dermis and subcutis should also be evaluated carefully (grossly and microscopically) for the presence of satellites, which may have prognostic significance, and which may occasionally be present at the margin. Satellites are rare in relation to thin tumors, but in one study, they were detected in 22% of the re-excision specimens from melanomas >2.25 mm in thickness (644). The presence of neurotropism should also be carefully sought and reported in melanoma resection specimens, especially of course if this neural invasion extends to the specimen margin.

Elective Lymph Node Dissection

A clinically positive lymph node in a patient with primary cutaneous melanoma should be biopsied, and if the node is histologically positive, a full regional node dissection should be done as a "therapeutic" procedure ("therapeutic regional lymph node dissection," TRLND) with curative intent and to gain local control (645). For clinically negative lymph nodes, the role of "elective regional lymph node dissection" (ERLND) is controversial. Theoretically, regional nodes could be regarded as necessary filters that must be bypassed by all melanomas that metastasize systematically. However, it is clear that many melanomas metastasize by the hematogenous route to distant organs without ever involving regional nodes. Thus, lymph node involvement in many cases may be simply a marker of a melanoma that has already metastasized.

The incidence of regional lymph node involvement increases with the thickness of the tumor. Involvement of the regional lymph nodes is extremely rare in melanomas with a thickness of <0.76 mm. It is therefore generally agreed that elective regional lymph node dissection is not indicated for these melanomas (most of which are nontumorigenic) (646–648). For tumors 0.76 mm thick or thicker, the data are conflicting (648–653), and recent therapeutic trials have not completely resolved the issues (604,654, 655). The next generation of trials of selective lymphadenectomy will likely be more conclusive.

Melanoma patients with palpable lymph nodes are at a high risk of having distant metastases. The number of involved lymph nodes and the depth of the tumor are important prognostic factors. Patients who have metastases in <20% of their resected regional lymph nodes and a tumor thickness of <3.5 mm have a 5-year disease-free survival rate of 80%, compared with 18% for patients who have a tumor thickness >3.5 mm or metastases in 20% or more of their resected lymph nodes (545). Curiously, the size of involved nodes is not related to survival (656). The presence of brisk TILs in a lymph node metastasis is a favorable prognostic attribute and was associated in one study with a survival rate of 83%, compared to 29% in patients whose metastases lacked TILs. Multivariate analysis confirmed the prognostic value of TILs in predicting disease-free survival in patients with regional node metastases (582).

Selective Lymphadenectomy (Sentinel Lymph Node Dissection)

Selective lymphadenectomy was developed by Morton et al. as a means of sampling regional lymph nodes while avoiding most of the complications of an elective dissection (657). The "sentinel" lymph node is identified by injections into the region of the melanoma of radioactive colloid and a vegetable dye ("blue dye"). The sentinel node is identified as the first in the regional lymph node basis to contain these markers ("hot and blue"). Studies have demonstrated that if the sentinel node is negative, the probability of metastases being found in the remainder of the lymph node basin is very low indeed. In early studies, the sentinel node was evaluated by frozen sections with rapid S-100 staining (658). Currently, the standard procedure is to examine the node with paraffin H&E sections, with S-100 as a sensitive marker, and with HMB-45 or, more recently, Melan-A, as a more specific although less sensitive marker (659). Use of a "cocktail" of antibodies to MART-1, Melan-A, and tyrosinase has also been proposed (660). In evaluating the S-100 stain, reactive dendritic cells, which are present in most sentinel nodes, must be distinguished from metastatic melanoma deposits. Capsular nevic rests must also be distinguished; these are located in capsular or sinusoidal collagen rather than in sinuses, lack significant cytologic atypia, and stain with S-100 and sometimes with HMB-45 or Melan-A, though usually less intensely than is seen in authentic melanoma deposits.

The Association of Directors of Anatomic and Surgical Pathology (ADASP) has recently published guidelines for the processing of lymph nodes including sentinel nodes submitted for evaluation of metastatic disease. It is recommended that small nodes be submitted in their entirety or that larger nodes be sections at 3- to 4-mm intervals and entirely submitted. Intraoperative examination should be limited to those cases where the procedure is likely to influence management (e.g., to confirm clinically and grossly positive nodes so that a complete node clearance can proceed). ADASP recommends that more than one section be performed on each sentinel node block. It is considered not currently to be clear how many sections and levels are optimal (661). Although the ADASP committee does not provide recommendations for immunostains, or even endorse this procedure unequivocally, in most centers it is currently the practice to perform S-100 (more sensitive, less specific), and either HMB-45 or Melan-A (more specific, less sensitive) staining on one profile from each submitted sentinel node.

MALIGNANT BLUE NEVUS

Malignant blue nevus is a rare tumor. It may arise in a blue or cellular blue nevus (662–664), a giant congenital nevus (258), or in a nevus of Ota (10), or it may be malignant from the start (665). Malignant blue nevi may involve the dermis and may be ulcerated, or may present as a deep-seated expansile mass (665). In some lesions classified as malignant blue nevus, metastases occur that are limited to the regional lymph nodes, and the patient survives after removal of the tumor and the involved lymph nodes (663). There may be overlap in these cases with the phenomenon of cellular blue nevi with regional metastases. In other cases, however, death occurs as the result of widespread metastases (41,662,665,666). Unfortunately, reliable distinction between these two groups of cases is not possible.

Histopathology. Recognition of the lesion as a malignant blue nevus rather than a common melanoma is based on the absence of junctional activity and the presence of at least some bipolar tumor cells with branching dendritic processes containing melanin granules (41,662, 665) (Fig. 28-37A through D). This may require silver staining, because melanin is often scant in malignant blue nevi arising from areas of cellular blue nevus. However, considerable amounts of melanin are seen in some malignant blue nevi (665).

In addition to showing the standard features of malignancy, such as invasiveness of the tumor, atypia with hyperchromatism, pleomorphism and irregularity of the nuclei, and presence of atypical mitoses, malignant blue nevi often show areas of necrosis as evidence of their malignant nature (663,665). The combination of uniform cytologic atypia, high-grade atypia, spontaneous tumor necrosis, and more than a few mitoses, may be considered diagnostic of malignant blue nevus in a lesion with a characteristic associated blue nevus pattern. Some lesions that do not meet all of these criteria, for example some lesions that have lacked

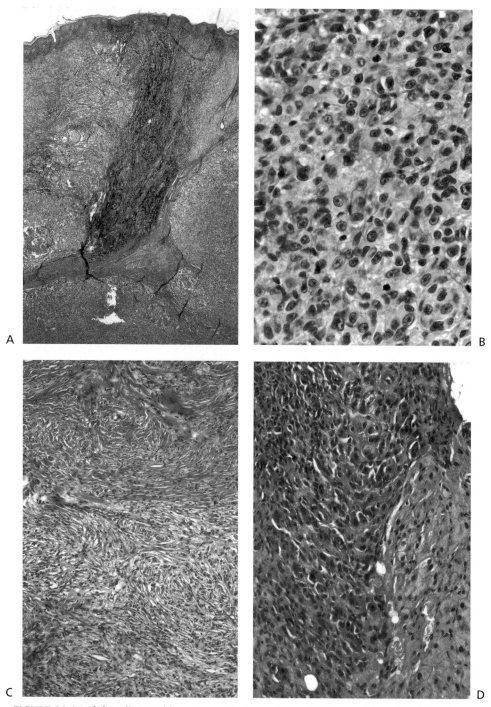

FIGURE 28-37. (A) Malignant blue nevus. A bulky melanocytic tumor with variegated patterns of architecture and pigmentation is present in the dermis, without an associated *in situ* component in the epidermis. **(B)** An area of solid growth showing severe uniform atypia and frequent mitoses. **(C)** An area of blue nevus-like pattern at the top, with a more cellular blue nevus-like pattern at the bottom. **(D)** Liver metastasis from a malignant blue nevus. Neoplastic melanocytes *(left)* in liver tissue *(right)* from a needle biopsy.

necrosis, have metastasized (664). Tumors with the overall appearance of cellular blue nevus that show only some of these features, especially if these are present in minor degree, may be signed out descriptively as "melanocytic tumor of uncertain potential" (MELTUMP) (see below).

Histogenesis. Although some authors have regarded the tumor cells as related to Schwann cells (663), electron microscopic studies have shown the presence of melanosomes in the cells and a lack of cytoplasmic enclosures of unmyelinated axons, which would be seen if the tumor cells were Schwann cells. Although the melanosomes in many cells are devoid of melanin (665), incubation with DOPA has shown that they are strongly DOPA-positive (41). Thus, it is evident that the tumor cells are melanocytes.

Differential Diagnosis. Malignant blue nevus differs from primary melanoma by the absence of junctional activity, and by the presence of associated common and/or cellular blue nevus. However, distinction of a malignant blue nevus from a metastatic melanoma can be difficult, because metastatic melanoma is occasionally found without a demonstrable primary melanoma. The primary melanoma may have involuted or may be located at an obscure internal site. The presence of dendritic cells indicative of an associated blue nevus or cellular blue nevus component is then the most reliable criterion favoring a diagnosis of malignant blue nevus instead of a metastatic melanoma. In doubtful cases, the differential diagnosis of metastatic melanoma should be expressed, and a workup for another primary should be considered clinically.

MELANOCYTIC TUMORS OF UNCERTAIN MALIGNANT POTENTIAL (MELTUMPS)

This is a descriptive term for a heterogeneous group of melanocytic tumors that exhibit some features indicative of possible malignancy, such as nuclear atypia, macronucleoli, mitotic activity, necrosis, or ulceration, but in number or degree insufficient to justify a malignant diagnosis (667). Accordingly, they reflect the biological reality that occasional melanocytic lesions that do not meet criteria for fully evolved melanoma cannot be predicted to be benign with 100% accuracy.

Histopathology. Tumors appropriately placed in this descriptive category may be quite bulky neoplasms of the order of several millimeters in diameter and thickness, composed of pigmented often spindle-shaped cells. The overall cellularity may be relatively low compared to fully malignant melanomas. There may be occasional mitoses, but not more than one or a few per section plane. Abnormal mitoses, if present, are usually indicative of frank malignancy. Focal areas of individual cell necrosis may be present, but if there are areas of confluent geographic necrosis, or if an ulcer is present, a frankly malignant diagnosis is appropriate. There may be a few enlarged melanocytes in the epidermis but, if there is an intraepidermal component that can be identified as a RGP of melanoma of any of the common types, a diagnosis of melanoma should be made.

Differential Diagnosis. This descriptive diagnosis is one of exclusion, and the differential diagnosis includes specific neoplasms described elsewhere in this chapter, including atypical and malignant Spitz nevi, minimal deviation melanomas, deep penetrating nevi, cellular neurothekeoma (discussed in Chapter 35), atypical cellular blue nevi, and melanoma.

Some lesions that may be placed in this descriptive category that have not been discussed elsewhere are composed of dendritic cells stuffed with abundant and coarsely divided pigment that obscures the nucleus (488). Sometimes these cells are difficult to distinguish from melanophages. They are also reminiscent of dermal melanophores seen in some vertebrates, which may occasionally in animals give rise to malignant tumor resembling malignant blue nevi. Some of these lesions may have prominent epidermal involvement, with pagetoid spread of the heavily pigmented lesional cells into the epidermis, and a dermal component that is broader in the papillary than in the reticular dermis. These lesions, despite their unusual cytology, have pattern features that are relatively characteristic of melanoma. Some related lesions, where criteria for malignancy are not deemed to have been fully met, may be placed in the descriptive category of "uncertain malignant potential." Yet other very rare lesions present as nodular clusters of authentic melanophages ("tumoral melanosis") (576). These lesions may be examples of complete regression of a pigmented VGP nodule, a very rare phenomenon that is quite differential from the partial regression frequently observed in the RGP compartment of common melanomas.

Management

The existence of these "difficult" or "uncertain" cases, where diagnostic agreement is not likely to be achieved even among experienced observers, suggests a need for a practical means of dealing with these cases in the best interests of the patients. In this regard, two principles apply. First, lesions should be managed by means sufficient to provide adequate therapy for the most clinically significant entity in the differential diagnosis of an uncertain neoplasm, and second, patients and their physicians deserve to know that their lesion cannot be diagnosed specifically with presently available means. A pathology report in such a case should not provide a false assurance of confidence in any given diagnosis. In these cases, we typically recommend management with the differential diagnosis of melanoma taken into consideration, and provide microstaging attributes sufficient at least for AJCC staging of the lesion as melanoma (668). The dimensions of a re-excision procedure could follow guidelines for the AJCC stage of the "melanoma," or at a minimum should be discussed with the patient and include a margin of normal tissue around the scar and any residual lesion.

In addition, a sentinel lymph node sampling procedure may be discussed with the patient. Sentinel lymph node sampling has been offered to patients with "atypical" or "uncertain" melanocytic tumors in a number of centers (669,670). Some of these cases have been found to be associated with lymph node metastases. In such circumstances, there may be a temptation to revise the diagnosis to "malignant melanoma." However, as previously discussed, there have been reports of lesions with characteristics of Spitz nevi that have metastasized to regional lymph nodes, sometimes followed by prolonged survival, perhaps indefinite survival (202,671,672). Similar situations have been reported in relation to cellular blue nevi (28). Therefore, in a situation where a "melanocytic tumor of uncertain malignant potential" is found to be associated with regional lymph node metastases, we report the metastasis as "metastatic melanocytic tumor of uncertain malignant potential." We indicate that the biological potential of this metastatic tumor remains uncertain. However, the prognosis is clearly more guarded than in the absence of such metastases, and in such circumstances, the possibility of adjuvant therapy including interferon may be taken into consideration (669).

METASTATIC MELANOMA

Metastatic spread, uncommon in thin melanomas, is quite common in tumors thicker than 2 mm. Lymph node metastases usually present earlier than hematogenous metastases. Although metastases tend to occur within 5 years after onset of the disease, their appearance may be delayed, especially in "thin" melanomas (673). Late metastases, beyond 10 years, do occur, but they are relatively rare (674,675).

The prognosis for patients with distant metastatic disease is very poor. In a recent study, the median survival overall was 7.5 months; patients with cutaneous, nodal, or gastrointestinal metastases had a median survival of 12.5 months, and an estimated 5-year survival rate of 14% (676). Resection of a solitary metastasis (e.g., to brain,

liver) may be associated with a remarkably good outcome, but such instances are exceedingly rare.

In about 4% to 10% of the patients who present initially with metastases of melanoma, no primary tumor can be found. The sex ratio, age incidence, family history, survival rates, and patterns of recurrence and further metastases in these patients with unknown primary tumors are consistent with an unnoticed cutaneous lesion as the site of origin for the metastatic disease (677). Although the primary tumor may in some instances be in an internal organ or perhaps secondary to malignant transformation of extracutaneous nevus cell rests (as in lymph node capsules), it can be assumed that it was in most instances located in the skin and regressed spontaneously. In a study of 40 patients with unknown primary melanoma, patients with lymph node metastasis survived significantly longer than patients diagnosed with lymph node metastasis concurrent with a known cutaneous primary melanoma. The prevalence of dysplastic nevi was intermediate between that reported among primary melanoma patients and that reported among population controls, suggesting the likelihood of a primary cutaneous origin for the metastatic melanoma (678). In some instances, there is a history of a spontaneously resolving pigmented lesion, and one may see at that site either a hypopigmented area or an irregular, flat, pigmented lesion, consistent with complete regression of a putative primary melanoma at that site (679).

Histopathology. The histologic appearance of melanoma *metastases in the skin* usually differs from that of a primary melanoma by the absence of an inflammatory infiltrate and of junctional activity (Fig. 28-38). However, primary melanomas may occasionally fail to involve the epidermis,

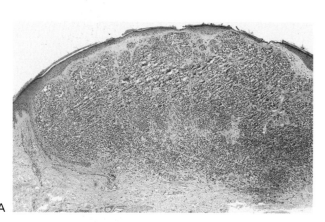

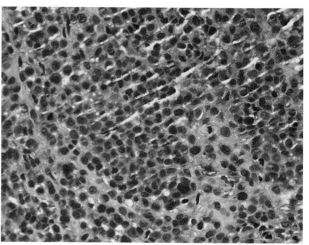

A   B

FIGURE 28-38. (A) Dermal metastatic melanoma. Metastatic melanoma often presents as a fairly symmetrical cellular nodule in the reticular dermis or subcutis. The lesions are often quite small at the time they are excised and presented for an initial diagnosis of metastatic spread. **(B)** Cytologically, the cells are uniformly atypical, as in tumorigenic primary melanomas (compare Figs. 28-23B, 28-26B, 28-29C, 28-34, and 28-37B with each other). Sometimes, especially in superficial or epidermotropic cutaneous metastases, atypia is deceptively minimal. The identification of mitotic activity, and of lymphatic invasion, may be very helpful in making the diagnosis.

and may also not show an inflammatory infiltrate, particularly when they are deeply invasive. Furthermore, in occasional instances, even metastases exhibit a prominent lymphocytic infiltrate (582), and can contact the overlying epidermis in a way that is suggestive of junctional activity, with nests of atypical melanocytes in the epidermis. Some metastatic melanomas may have a nevoid phenotype, and clinicopathologic correlation (e.g., follow-up) may be required to differentiate them from a primary nevoid melanoma or from a nevus (680).

Epidermotropic metastatic melanoma refers to a metastatic deposit that is initially localized to the papillary dermis and involves the overlying epidermis. Most of these lesions occur in an extremity regional to a distal primary melanoma. Epidermotropic metastasis is characterized by (a) thinning of the epidermis by aggregates of atypical melanocytes within the dermis; (b) inward turning of the rete ridges at the periphery of the lesion; and (c) usually no lateral extension of atypical melanocytes within the epidermis beyond the concentration of the metastasis in the dermis (681). However, this distinction can be very difficult at times, and cases have been reported in which there was lateral extension beyond the dermal component (513,682). In some other cases, the metastatic cells are small and nevoid, with few if any mitoses, and in these instances of *differentiated or nevoid epidermotropic metastatic melanoma* or "epidermotropic metastatic melanomas with maturation" the lesions can be mistaken for compound nevi (495).

Generalized Melanosis in Metastatic Melanoma

This is a rare phenomenon that may be associated with widespread melanoma metastases. It is characterized by diffuse slate blue discoloration of the entire skin, the conjunctivae, and the oral and pharyngeal mucous membranes, often with melanuria. Melanin granules have been observed also in blood smears within neutrophils and monocytes. Autopsy reveals a similar discoloration in the intima of the large arteries and of many visceral organs (683).

Histologically, numerous melanin granules are seen located within macrophages throughout the dermis, especially around capillaries. They stain with the Fontana–Masson stain and are dopapositive. In addition, some dermal vessels are focally plugged with dark, amorphous dopapositive material. In most instances, only melanophages have been found. It is assumed that the melanin is produced by distant melanoma cells, and then carried by the blood to the skin to be deposited within dermal melanophages (683,684). In a few cases, two types of pigmented cells have been identified in the dermis, particularly in semithin sections: melanophages and individually scattered melanoma cells appearing larger and less pigmented than the melanophages. On autopsy, melanin phagocytosis is seen in many organs, especially in the

Kupffer cells of the liver and the cells lining the sinusoids of the lymph nodes, spleen, and adrenal glands (684).

REFERENCES

1. Chan HH, Lam LK, Wong DS, et al. Nevus of Ota: a new classification based on the response to laser treatment. *Lasers Surg Med* 2001;28:267–272.
2. Kikuchi I, Inoue S. Natural history of the Mongolian spot. *J Dermatol* 1980;7:449–450.
3. Hidano A, Kajima H, Ikeda S, et al. Natural history of nevus of Ota. *Arch Dermatol* 1967;95:187.
4. Hidano A, Kajima H, Endo Y. Bilateral nevus Ota associated with nevus Ito. A case of pigmentation on the lips. *Arch Dermatol* 1965;91:357–359.
5. Burkhart CG, Gohara A. Dermal melanocyte hamartoma. A distinctive new form of dermal melanocytosis. *Arch Dermatol* 1981;117:102–104.
6. Dekio S, Koike S, Jidoi J. Nevus of ota with nevus of Ito—report of a case with cataract. *J Dermatol* 1989;16:164–166.
7. Bashiti HM, Blair JD, Triska RA, et al. Generalized dermal melanocytosis. *Arch Dermatol* 1981;117:791–793.
8. Mevorah B, Frenk E, Delacretaz J. Dermal melanocytosis. Report of an unusual case. *Dermatologica* 1977;154:107–114.
9. Hirayama T, Suzuki T. A new classification of Ota's nevus based on histopathological features. *Dermatologica* 1991;183:169–172.
10. Dorsey CS, Montgomery H. Blue nevus and its distinction from mongolian spot and the nevus of Ota. *J Invest Dermatol* 1954;22:225–236.
11. Patel BC, Egan CA, Lucius RW, et al. Cutaneous malignant melanoma and oculodermal melanocytosis (nevus of Ota): report of a case and review of the literature. *J Am Acad Dermatol* 1998;38:862–865.
12. Kopf AW, Bart RS. Malignant blue (Ota's?) nevus. *J Dermatol Surg Oncol* 1982;8:442–445.
13. Balmaceda CM, Fetell MR, O'Brien JL, et al. Nevus of Ota and leptomeningeal melanocytic lesions. *Neurology* 1993;43:381–386.
14. Arunkumar MJ, Ranjan A, Jacob M, et al. Neurocutaneous melanosis: a case of primary intracranial melanoma with metastasis. *Clin Oncol (R Coll Radiol)* 2001;13:52–54.
15. Piercecchi-Marti MD, Mohamed H, Liprandi A, et al. Intracranial meningeal melanocytoma associated with ipsilateral nevus of Ota. Case report. *J Neurosurg* 2002;96:619–623.
16. Rodriguez HA, Ackerman LV. Cellular blue nevus. *Cancer* 1968;21:393–405.
17. Harvell JD, White WL. Persistent and recurrent blue nevi. *Am J Dermatopathol* 1999;21:506–517.
18. Pittman JL, Fisher BK. Plaque-type blue nevus. *Arch Dermatol* 1976;112:1127–1128.
19. Gonzalez-Campora R, Galera-Davidson H, Vazquez-Ramirez FJ, et al. Blue nevus: classical types and new related entities. A differential diagnostic review. *Pathol Res Pract* 1994;190:627–635.
20. Misago N. The relationship between melanocytes and peripheral nerve sheath cells (Part II): blue nevus with peripheral nerve sheath differentiation. *Am J Dermatopathol* 2000;22:230–236.
21. Sun J, Morton TH Jr, Gown AM. Antibody HMB-45 identifies the cells of blue nevi. An immunohistochemical study on paraffin sections. *Am J Surg Pathol* 1990;14:748–751.
22. Kucher C, Zhang PJ, Pasha T, et al. Melan-A, Ki67 as useful markers to discriminate desmoplastic melanoma from sclerotic nevi. United States and Canadian Academy of Pathology Abstracts. 2004.

23. Michal M, Kerekes Z, Kinkor Z, et al. Desmoplastic cellular blue nevi. *Am J Dermatopathol* 1995;17:230–235.

24. Bhawan J, Cao SL. Amelanotic blue nevus: a variant of blue nevus. *Am J Dermatopathol* 1999;21:225–228.

25. Carr S, See J, Wilkinson B, et al. Hypopigmented common blue nevus. *J Cutan Pathol* 1997;24:494–498.

26. Ferrara G, Argenziano G, Zgavec B, et al. "Compound blue nevus": a reappraisal of "superficial blue nevus with prominent intraepidermal dendritic melanocytes" with emphasis on dermoscopic and histopathologic features. *J Am Acad Dermatol* 2002; 46:85–89.

27. Tran TA, Carlson JA, Basaca PC, et al. Cellular blue nevus with atypia (atypical cellular blue nevus): a clinicopathologic study of nine cases. *J Cutan Pathol* 1998;25:252–258.

28. Temple-Camp CR, Saxe N, King H. Benign and malignant cellular blue nevus. A clinicopathological study of 30 cases. *Am J Dermatopathol* 1988;10:289–296.

29. Rodriguez HA, Ackerman LV. Cellular blue nevus. Clinicopathologic study of forty-five cases. *Cancer* 1968;21:393–405.

30. Zembowicz A, Granter SR, McKee PH, et al. Amelanotic cellular blue nevus: a hypopigmented variant of the cellular blue nevus: clinicopathologic analysis of 20 cases. *Am J Surg Pathol* 2002;26:1493–1500.

31. Avidor I, Kessler E. "Atypical" blue nevus—a benign variant of cellular blue nevus. Presentation of three cases. *Dermatologica* 1977;154:39–44.

32. Marano SR, Brooks RA, Spetzler RF, et al. Giant congenital cellular blue nevus of the scalp of a newborn with an underlying skull defect and invasion of the dura mater. *Neurosurgery* 1986; 18:85–89.

33. Silverberg GD, Kadin ME, Dorfman RF, et al. Invasion of the brain by a cellular blue nevus of the scalp. A case report with light and electron microscopic studies. *Cancer* 1971;27:349–355.

34. Aloi F, Pich A, Pippione M. Malignant cellular blue nevus: a clinicopathological study of 6 cases. *Dermatology* 1996;192: 36–40.

35. Gonzalez-Campora R, Diaz-Cano S, Vazquez-Ramirez F, et al. Cellular blue nevus with massive regional lymph node metastases. *Dermatol Surg* 1996;22:83–87.

36. Bortolani A, Barisoni D, Scomazzoni G. Benign "metastatic" cellular blue nevus. *Ann Plast Surg* 1994;33:426–431.

37. Leopold JG, Richards DB. The inter-relationship of blue and common nevi. *J Pathol* 1968;95:37–43.

38. Pulitzer DR, Martin PC, Cohen AP, et al. Histologic classification of the combined nevus: analysis of the variable expression of melanocytic nevi. *Am J Surg Pathol* 1991;15:1111–1122.

39. Masson P. My conception of cellular nevi. *Cancer* 1951;4:19–38.

40. Skelton H, III, Smith KJ, Barrett TL, et al. HMB-45 staining in benign and malignant melanocytic lesions. A reflection of cellular activation. *Am J Dermatopathol* 1991;13:543–550.

41. Mishima Y. Cellular blue nevus. Melanogenic activity and malignant transformation. *Arch Dermatol* 1970;101:104–110.

42. Bastiaens M, ter Huurne J, Gruis N, et al. The melanocortin-1-receptor gene is the major freckle gene. *Hum Mol Genet* 2001; 10:1701–1708.

43. Bliss JM, Ford D, Swerdlow AJ, et al. Risk of cutaneous melanoma associated with pigmentation characteristics and freckling: systematic overview of 10 case-control studies. *Int J Cancer* 1995;62:367–376.

44. Rhodes AR, Albert LS, Barnhill RL, et al. Sun-induced freckles in children and young adults. A correlation of clinical and histopathologic features. *Cancer* 1991;67:1990–2001.

45. Breathnach AS, Wyllie LM. Electron microscopy of melanocytes and melanosomes in freckled human epidermis. *J Invest Dermatol* 42;389–394. 1964.

46. Benedict PH, Szabo G, Fitzpatrick TB, et al. Melanotic macules in Albright's syndrome and in neurofibromatosis. *JAMA* 1968; 205:618–626.

47. Barnhill RL, Albert LS, Shama SK, et al. Genital lentiginosis: a clinical and histopathologic study. *J Am Acad Dermatol* 1990;22: 453–460.

48. Maize JC. Mucosal melanosis. *Dermatol Clin* 1988;6:283–293.

49. Weathers DR, Corio RL, Crawford BE, et al. The labial melanotic macule. *Oral Surg Oral Med Oral Pathol* 1976;42:196–205.

50. Gupta G, Williams REA, MacKie RM. The labial melanotic macule: a review of 79 cases. *Br J Dermatol* 1997;136:772–775.

51. Sexton FM, Maize JC. Melanotic macules and melanoacanthomas of the lip. A comparative study with census of the basal melanocyte population. *Am J Dermatopathol* 1987;9:438–444.

52. Horlick HP, Walther RR, Zegarelli DJ, et al. Mucosal melanotic macule, reactive type: a simulation of melanoma. *J Am Acad Dermatol* 1988;19:786–791.

53. Becker SW. Concurrent melanosis and hypertrichosis in distribution of nevus unius lateris. *Arch Dermatol Syph* 60;155–160. 1949.

54. Fehr B, Panizzon RG, Schnyder UW. Becker's nevus and malignant melanoma. *Dermatologica* 1991;182:77–80.

55. Rower JM, Carr RD, Lowney ED. Progressive cribriform and zosteriform hyperpigmentation. *Arch Dermatol* 1978;114: 98–99.

56. Urbanek RW, Johnson WC. Smooth muscle hamartoma associated with Becker's nevus. *Arch Dermatol* 1978;114:104–106.

57. Tate PR, Hodge SJ, Owen LG. A quantitative study of melanocytes in Becker's nevus. *J Cutan Pathol* 1980;7:404–409.

58. Haneke E. The dermal component in melanosis naeviformis Becker. *J Cutan Pathol* 1979;6:53–58.

59. Happle R, Koopman RJ. Becker nevus syndrome. *Am J Med Genet* 1997;68:357–361.

60. Newman Dorland WA. *Dorland's illustrated medical dictionary*. Philadelphia: WB Saunders, 29:2000.

61. Mehregan AH. Lentigo senilis and its evolutions. *J Invest Dermatol* 1975;65:429–433.

62. Tucker MA, Halpern A, Holly EA, et al. Clinically recognized dysplastic nevi. A central risk factor for cutaneous melanoma. *JAMA* 1997;277:1439–1444.

63. McLean DI, Gallagher RP. "Sunburn" freckles, cafe-au-lait macules, and other pigmented lesions of schoolchildren: the Vancouver Mole Study. *J Am Acad Dermatol* 1995;32:565–570.

64. Elder DE, Murphy GF. Benign melanocytic tumors (nevi). In: Elder DE, Murphy GF, eds. *Melanocytic tumors of the skin*. Washington, DC: Armed Forces Institute of Pathology, 1991:5–81.

65. Bolognia JL. Reticulated black solar lentigo ("ink spot" lentigo). *Arch Dermatol* 1992;128:934–940.

66. Bastiaens MT, Westendorp RG, Vermeer BJ, et al. Ephelides are more related to pigmentary constitutional host factors than solar lentigines. *Pigment Cell Res* 1999;12:316–322.

67. Rhodes AR, Harrist TJ, Momtaz T. The PUVA-induced pigmented macule: a lentiginous proliferation of large, sometimes cytologically atypical, melanocytes. *J Am Acad Dermatol* 1983;9: 47–58.

68. Montagna W, Hu F, Carlisle K. A reinvestigation of solar lentigines. *Arch Dermatol* 1980;116:1151–1154.

69. Hodgson C. Lentigo senilis. *Arch Dermatol* 1963;87:197–207.

70. Andersen WK, Labadie RR, Bhawan J. Histopathology of solar lentigines of the face: a quantitative study. *J Am Acad Dermatol* 1997;36:444–447.

71. Abel EA, Reid H, Wood C, Hu CH. PUVA-induced melanocytic atypia: is it confined to PUVA lentigines? *J Am Acad Dermatol* 1985;13:761–768.

72. Mehregan DR, Hamzavi F, Brown K. Large cell acanthoma. *Int J Dermatol* 2003;42:36–39.

73. Gartmann H. The malignity of nevoid lentigo. A contribution to the early diagnosis and prevention of malignant melanoma and its preconditions. *Z Hautkr* 1978;53:91–100 (in German).
74. Ryu HJ, Jeong JT, Kye YC, et al. Generalized lentiginosis with strabismus. *Int J Dermatol* 2002;41:780–782.
75. Zahorcsek Z, Schneider I. Generalized lentiginosis manifesting through three generations. *Int J Dermatol* 1996;35:357–359.
76. Marchesi L, Naldi L, Di Landro A, et al. Segmental lentiginosis with "jentigo" histologic pattern. *Am J Dermatopathol* 1992;14:323–327.
77. Micali G, Nasca MR, Innocenzi D, et al. Agminated lentiginosis: case report and review of the literature. *Pediatr Dermatol* 1994;11:241–245.
78. Stewart DM, Altman J, Mehregan AH. Speckled lentiginous nevus. *Arch Dermatol* 1978;114:895–896.
79. Schaffer JV, Orlow SJ, Lazova R, et al. Speckled lentiginous nevus: within the spectrum of congenital melanocytic nevi. *Arch Dermatol* 2001;137:172–178.
80. Coppin BD, Temple IK. Multiple lentigines syndrome (LEOPARD syndrome or progressive cardiomyopathic lentiginosis). *J Med Genet* 1997;34:582–586.
81. Reed OM, Mellette JR Jr, Fitzpatrick JE. Cutaneous lentiginosis with atrial myxomas. *J Am Acad Dermatol* 1986;15:398–402.
82. Carney JA, Stratakis CA. Epithelioid blue nevus and psammomatous melanotic schwannoma: the unusual pigmented skin tumors of the Carney complex. *Semin Diagn Pathol* 1998;15:216–224.
83. Jeghers H, McKusick BA, Katz KH. Generalized intestinal polyposis and melanin spots of the oral mucosa, lips and digits. *N Engl J Med* 241;993–1005. 2003.
84. Cramer HJ. Nevus spilus. A histopathological study.Ger *Zentralbl Allg Pathol* 1977;121:122–128 (in German).
85. Choi HS, Park YJ, Park JG. Peutz–Jeghers syndrome: a new understanding. *J Korean Med Sci* 1999;14:2–7.
86. Boardman LA, Pittelkow MR, Couch FJ, et al. Association of Peutz–Jeghers-like mucocutaneous pigmentation with breast and gynecologic carcinomas in women. *Medicine (Baltimore)* 2000;79:293–298.
87. Selmanowitz VJ, Orentreich N, Felsenstein JM. Lentiginosis profusa syndrome (multiple lentigines syndrome). *Arch Dermatol* 1971;104:393–401.
88. Yamada K, Matsukawa A, Hori Y, et al. Ultrastructural studies on pigmented macules of Peutz–Jeghers syndrome. *J Dermatol* 1981;8:367–377.
89. Jimbow K, Horikoshi T. The nature and significance of macromelanosomes in pigmented skin lesions: their morphological characteristics, specificity for their occurrence, and possible mechanisms for their formation. *Am J Dermatopathol* 1982;4:413–420.
90. Konrad K, Wolff K, Honigsmann H. The giant melanosome: a model of deranged melanosome-morphogenesis. *J Ultrastruct Res* 1974;48:102–123.
91. Horikoshi T, Jimbow K, Sugiyama S. Comparison of macromelanosomes and autophagic giant melanosome complexes in nevocellular nevi, lentigo simplex and malignant melanoma. *J Cutan Pathol* 1982;9:329–339.
92. Shaffer, B. Pigmented nevi. *Arch Dermatol* 72;120–132. 1955.
93. Shoji T, Cockerell CJ, Koff AB, et al. Eruptive melanocytic nevi after Stevens–Johnson syndrome. *J Am Acad Dermatol* 1997;37:337–339.
94. Richert S, Bloom EJ, Flynn K, et al. Widespread eruptive dermal and atypical melanocytic nevi in association with chronic myelocytic leukemia: case report and review of the literature. *J Am Acad Dermatol* 1996;35:326–329.
95. Eady RAJ, Gilkes JJH, Wilson Jones E. Eruptive nevi: report of two cases with enzyme histochemical, light and electron microscopical findings. *Br J Dermatol* 1977;97:267–278.

96. Kanzler MH, Mraz-Gernhard S. Primary cutaneous malignant melanoma and its precursor lesions: diagnostic and therapeutic overview. *J Am Acad Dermatol* 2001;45:260–276.
97. Clark WH Jr, Elder DE, Guerry DIV, et al. A study of tumor progression: the precursor lesions of superficial spreading and nodular melanoma. *Hum Pathol* 1984;15:1147–1165.
98. Whimster IW. Recurrent pigment cell naevi and their significance in the problem of endogenous carcinogenesis. *Ann Ital Dermatol Clin Sper* 1965;19:168–191.
99. Kossard S, Wilkinson B. Small cell (naevoid) melanoma: a clinicopathologic study of 131 cases. *Australas J Dermatol* 1997; 38[Suppl 1]:S54–S58.
100. Eng AM. Solitary small active junctional nevi in juvenile patients. *Arch Dermatol* 1983;119:35–38.
101. Worret WI, Burgdorf WH. Which direction do nevus cells move? Abtropfung reexamined. *Am J Dermatopathol* 1998;20:135–139.
102. Miescher G, von Albertini A. Histologie de 100 cas de naevi pigmentaires d'apres les methodes de Masson. *Bull Soc Franc Dermatol Syph* 1935;42:1265–1273.
103. Goovaerts G, Buyssens N. Nevus cell maturation or atrophy. *Am J Dermatopathol* 1988;10:20–27.
104. Smolle J, Smolle-Juettner FM, Stettner H, et al. Relationship of tumor cell motility and morphologic patterns. Part 1. Melanocytic skin tumors. *Am J Dermatopathol* 1992;14:231–237.
105. Rhodes AR, Silverman RA, Harrist TJ, et al. A histologic comparison of congenital and acquired nevomelanocytic nevi. *Arch Dermatol* 1985;121:1266–1273.
106. Sagebiel RW. Histologic artifacts of benign pigmented nevi. *Arch Dermatol* 1972;106:691–693.
107. Fullen DR, Reed JA, Finnerty B, et al. S100A6 preferentially labels type C nevus cells and nevic corpuscles: additional support for Schwannian differentiation of intradermal nevi. *J Cutan Pathol* 2001;28:393–399.
108. Penneys NS, Mogollon R, Kowalczyk A, et al. A survey of cutaneous neural lesions for the presence of myelin basic protein. An immunohistochemical study. *Arch Dermatol* 1984;120:210–213.
109. Stegmaier OC. Natural regression of the melanocytic nevus. *J Invest Dermatol* 1959;32:[413]:419.
110. Foucar E, Bentley TJ, Laube DW, et al. A histopathologic evaluation of nevocellular nevi in pregnancy. *Arch Dermatol* 1985;121:350–354.
111. Zembowicz A, McCusker M, Chiarelli C, et al. Morphological analysis of nevoid melanoma: a study of 20 cases with a review of the literature. *Am J Dermatopathol* 2001;23:167–175.
112. Winkelmann RK. Cholinesterase in the cutaneous nevus. *Cancer* 1960;13:626–630.
113. Thorne EG, Mottaz JH, Zelickson AS. Tyrosinase activity in dermal nevus cells. *Arch Dermatol* 1971;104:619–624.
114. Niizuma K. Electron microscopic study of nevic corpuscle. *Acta Derm Venereol* 1975;55:283–289.
115. Lund HZ, Stobbe GD. The natural history of the pigmented nevus: factors of age and anatomic location. *Am J Pathol* 1949;6:1117–1147.
116. Maize JC, Foster G. Age-related changes in melanocytic naevi. *Clin Exp Dermatol* 1979;4:49–58.
117. Mishima Y. Macromolecular changes in pigmentary disorders. *Arch Dermatol* 1965;91:519–557.
118. Gilchrest BA, Treloar V, Grassi AM, et al. Characteristics of cultivated adult human nevocellular nevus cells. *J Invest Dermatol* 1986;87:102–107.
119. Gottlieb B, Brown AL Jr, Winkelmann RK. Fine structure of the nevus cell. *Arch Dermatol* 1965;92:81–87.
120. Davies H, Bignell GR, Cox C, et al. Mutations of the BRAF gene in human cancer. *Nature* 2002;417:949–954.

121. Pollock PM, Harper UL, Hansen KS, et al. High frequency of BRAF mutations in nevi. *Nat Genet* 2003;33:19–20.

122. Omholt K, Karsberg S, Platz A, et al. Screening of N-ras codon 61 mutations in paired primary and metastatic cutaneous melanomas: mutations occur early and persist throughout tumor progression. *Clin Cancer Res* 2002;8:3468–3474.

123. Demunter A, Stas M, Degreef H, et al. Analysis of N- and k-ras mutations in the distinctive tumor progression phases of melanoma. *J Invest Dermatol* 2001;117:1483–1489.

124. Jafari M, Papp T, Kirchner S, et al. Analysis of ras mutations in human melanocytic lesions: activation of the ras gene seems to be associated with the nodular type of human malignant melanoma. *J Cancer Res Clin Oncol* 1995;121:23–30.

125. Papp T, Pemsel H, Zimmermann R, et al. Mutational analysis of the N-ras, p53, p16INK4a, CDK4, and MC1R genes in human congenital melanocytic naevi. *J Med Genet* 1999;36:610–614.

126. Keller-Melchior R, Schmidt R, et al. Expression of the tumor suppressor gene product p16INK4 in benign and malignant melanocytic lesions. *J Invest Dermatol* 1998;110:932–938.

127. Sharpless E, Chin L. The INK4a/ARF locus and melanoma. *Oncogene* 2003;22:3092–3098.

128. Cachia AR, Indsto JO, McLaren KM, et al. CDKN2A mutation and deletion status in thin and thick primary melanoma. *Clin Cancer Res* 2000;6:3511–3515.

129. Goette DF, Doty RD. Balloon cell nevus. Summary of the clinical and histological characteristics. *Arch Dermatol* 1978;114:109–111.

130. Hashimoto K, Bale GF. An electron microscopic study of balloon nevus cells. *Cancer* 1972;30:530.

131. Okun MR, Donnellan B, Edelstein L. An ultrastructural study of balloon cell nevus. Relationship of mast cells to nevus cells. *Cancer* 1974;34:615–625.

132. MacLennan R, Kelly JW, Rivers JK, et al. The Eastern Australian Childhood Nevus Study: site differences in density and size of melanocytic nevi in relation to latitude and phenotype. *J Am Acad Dermatol* 2003;48:367–375.

133. Rongioletti F, Ball RA, Marcus R, et al. Histopathological features of flexural melanocytic nevi: a study of 40 cases. *J Cutan Pathol* 2000;27:215–217.

134. MacKie RM, English J, Aitchison TC, et al. The number and distribution of benign pigmented moles (melanocytic nevi) in a healthy British population. *Br J Dermatol* 1985;113:167–174.

135. Boyd AS, Rapini RP. Acral melanocytic neoplasms: a histologic analysis of 158 lesions. *J Am Acad Dermatol* 1994;31:740–745.

136. Clemente C, Zurrida S, Bartoli C, et al. Acral-lentiginous naevus of plantar skin. *Histopathology* 1995;27:549–555.

137. Han KH, Cho KH. Acral lentiginous nevus. *J Dermatol* 1998;25:23–27.

138. Haupt HM, Stern JB. Pagetoid melanocytosis: histologic features in benign and malignant lesions. *Am J Surg Pathol* 1995;19:792–797.

139. Baran R, Barriere H. Longitudinal melanonychia with spreading pigmentation in Laugier–Hunziker syndrome: a report of two cases. *Br J Dermatol* 1986;115:707–710.

140. Kouskoukis CE, Scher RK, Hatcher VA. Melanonychia striata longitudinalis. A case report. *J Dermatol Surg Oncol* 1982;8:284–286.

141. Baran R, Eichmann A. Longitudinal melanonychia associated with Bowen's disease: two new cases. *Dermatology* 1993;186:159–160.

142. Kemmett D, Ellis J, Spencer MJ, et al. The Laugier–Hunziker syndrome—a clinical review of six cases. *Clin Exp Dermatol* 1990;15:111–114.

143. Rich P. Nail biopsy. Indications and methods. *J Dermatol Surg Oncol* 1992;18:673–682.

144. Kopf AW, Albom M, Ackerman AB. Biopsy technique for longitudinal streaks of pigmentation in nails. A preliminary report. *Am J Dermatopathol* 1984;6:309–312.

145. Scher RK, Silvers DN. Longitudinal melanonychia striata. *J Am Acad Dermatol* 1991;24:1035–1036.

146. Molina D, Sanchez JL. Pigmented longitudinal bands of the nail. A clinicopathologic study. *Am J Dermatopathol* 1995;17:539–541.

147. Goettmann-Bonvallot S, Andre J, Belaich S. Longitudinal melanonychia in children: a clinical and histopathologic study of 40 cases. *J Am Acad Dermatol* 1999;41:17–22.

148. Takata M, Maruo K, Kageshita T, et al. Two cases of unusual acral melanocytic tumors: illustration of molecular cytogenetics as a diagnostic tool. *Hum Pathol* 2003;34:89–92.

149. Friedman RJ, Ackerman AB. Difficulties in the histologic diagnosis of melanocytic nevi on the vulvae of premenopausal women. In: Ackerman AB, ed., *Pathology of malignant melanoma.* New York: Masson, 1981:119–127.

150. Carlson JA, Mu XC, Slominski A, et al. Melanocytic proliferations associated with lichen sclerosus. *Arch Dermatol* 2002;138:77–87.

151. Clark WHJ, Hood AF, Tucker MA, et al. Atypical melanocytic nevi of the genital type with a discussion of reciprocal parenchymal-stromal interactions in the biology of neoplasia. *Hum Pathol* 1998;29[Suppl 1]:S1–S24.

152. Maize JC, Ackerman AB. *Pigmented lesions of the skin: clinicopathologic correlations.* Philadelphia: Lea & Febiger, 1987.

153. Christensen WN, Friedman KF, Woodruff JD, et al. Histologic characteristics of vulval nevocellular nevi. *J Cutan Pathol* 1987;14:87–91.

154. Rock B, Hood AF, Rock JA. Prospective study of vulvar nevi. *J Am Acad Dermatol* 1990;22:104–106.

155. Spitz S. Melanomas of childhood. *Am J Pathol* 1948;24:591–609.

156. Allen AC. Juvenile melanomas of children and adults and melanocarcinomas of children. *Arch Dermatol* 1960;82:325–335.

157. Paniago-Periera C, Maize JC, Ackerman AB. Nevus of large spindle and/or epithelioid cells (Spitz's nevus). *Arch Dermatol* 1978;114:1811–1823.

158. Harris MN, Hurwitz RM, Buckel LJ, et al. Congenital Spitz nevus. *Dermatol Surg* 2000;26:931–935.

159. Dal Pozzo V, Benelli C, Restano L, et al. Clinical review of 247 case records of Spitz nevus (epithelioid cell and/or spindle cell nevus). *Dermatology* 1997;194:20–25.

160. Weedon D, Little JH. Spindle and epithelioid cell nevi in children and adults. A review of 211 cases of the Spitz nevus. *Cancer* 1977;40:217–225.

161. Hulshof MM, Van Haeringen A, Gruis NA, et al. Multiple agminate Spitz naevi. *Melanoma Res* 1998;8:156–160.

162. Fass J, Grimwood RE, Kraus E, et al. Adult onset of eruptive widespread Spitz's nevi. *J Am Acad Dermatol* 2002;46:S142–S143.

163. McGovern VJ. Spitz nevus. In: McGovern VJ, ed. *Melanoma: histological diagnosis and prognosis.* New York: Raven Press, 1983:37–44.

164. Busam KJ, Barnhill RL. Pagetoid Spitz nevus. Intraepidermal Spitz tumor with prominent pagetoid spread. *Am J Surg Pathol* 1995;19:1061–1067.

165. Merot Y, Frenk E. Spitz nevus (large spindle cell and/or epithelioid cell nevus). Age-related involvement of the suprabasal epidermis. *Virchows Arch A Pathol Anat Histopathol* 1989;415:97–101.

166. Merot Y. Transepidermal elimination of nevus cells in spindle and epithelioid cell (Spitz) nevi [Letter]. *Arch Dermatol* 1988;124:1441–1442.

167. Kantor G, Wheeland RG. Transepidermal elimination of nevus cells. A possible mechanism of nevus involution. *Arch Dermatol* 1987;123:1371–1374.

168. Scott G, Chen KTK, Rosai J. Pseudoepitheliomatous hyperplasia in Spitz nevi: a possible source of confusion with squamous cell carcinoma. *Arch Pathol Lab Med* 1989;113:61–63.

169. Paniago-Pereira C, Maize JC, Ackerman AB. Nevus of large spindle and/or epithelioid cells (Spitz's nevus). *Arch Dermatol* 1978;114:1811–1823.

170. Smolle J, Taniguchi S, Kerl H. Relationship of tumor cell motility and morphologic patterns. Part 2. Analysis of tumor cell sublines with different motility in vitro. *Am J Dermatopathol* 1992;14:315–318.

171. Arbuckle S, Weedon D. Eosinophilic globules in the Spitz nevus. *J Am Acad Dermatol* 1982;7:324–327.

172. Kamino H, Flotte TJ, Misheloff E, et al. Eosinophilic globules in Spitz's nevi. New findings and a diagnostic sign. *Am J Dermatopathol* 1979;1:319–324.

173. Wesselmann U, Becker LR, Brocker EB, et al. Eosinophilic globules in Spitz nevi: no evidence for apoptosis. *Am J Dermatopathol* 1998;20:551–554.

174. Echevarria R, Ackerman LV. Spindle and epithelioid cell nevi in the adult. Clinicopathologic report of 26 cases. *Cancer* 1967;20: 175–189.

175. Harris GR, Shea CR, Horenstein MG, et al. Desmoplastic (sclerotic) nevus: an underrecognized entity that resembles dermatofibroma and desmoplastic melanoma. *Am J Surg Pathol* 1999;23:786–794.

176. MacKie RM, Doherty VR. The desmoplastic melanocytic naevus: a distinct histological entity. *Histopathology* 1992;20: 207–211.

177. Barr RJ, Morales RV, Graham JH. Desmoplastic nevus: a distinct histologic variant of mixed spindle cell and epithelioid cell nevus. *Cancer* 1980;46:557–564.

178. Lazzaro B, Rebers A, Herlyn M, et al. Immunophenotyping of compound and Spitz nevi and vertical growth phase melanomas using a panel of monoclonal antibodies reactive in paraffin sections. *J Invest Dermatol* 1993;313S–317S.

179. Bergman R, Azzam H, Sprecher E, et al. A comparative immunohistochemical study of MART-1 expression in Spitz nevi, ordinary melanocytic nevi, and malignant melanomas. *J Am Acad Dermatol* 2000;42:496–500.

180. Suster S. Hyalinizing spindle and epithelioid cell nevus. A study of five cases of a distinctive histologic variant of Spitz's nevus. *Am J Dermatopathol* 1994;16:593–598.

181. Diaz-Cascajo C, Borghi S, Weyers W. Angiomatoid Spitz nevus: a distinct variant of desmoplastic Spitz nevus with prominent vasculature. *Am J Dermatopathol* 2000;22:135–139.

182. Schreiner E, Wolff K. Die Ultrastruktur des benignen juvenilen Melanoms. *Arch Klin Exp Dermatol* 1970;237:749–768.

183. Evans MJ, Sanders DS, Grant JH, et al. Expression of Melan-A in Spitz, pigmented spindle cell nevi, and congenital nevi: comparative immunohistochemical study. *Pediatr Dev Pathol* 2000; 3:36–39.

184. Ribe A, McNutt NS. S100A6 Protein expression is different in Spitz nevi and melanomas. *Mod Pathol* 2003;16:505–511.

185. LeBoit PE, Van Fletcher H. A comparative study of Spitz nevus and nodular malignant melanoma using image analysis cytometry. *J Invest Dermatol* 1987;88:753–757.

186. Leitinger G, Cerroni L, Soyer HP, et al. Morphometric diagnosis of melanocytic skin tumors. *Am J Dermatopathol* 1990;12: 441–445.

187. Steiner A, Binder M, Mossbacher U, et al. Estimation of the volume-weighted mean nuclear volume discriminates Spitz's nevi from nodular malignant melanomas. *Lab Invest* 1994;70: 381–385.

188. Hofmann Wellenhof R, Rieger E, Smolle J, et al. Proliferative activity in Spitz's nevi compared with other melanocytic skin lesions. *Melanoma Research* 1993;3:313–317.

189. Penneys N, Seigfried E, Nahass G, et al. Expression of proliferating cell nuclear antigen in Spitz nevus. *J Am Acad Dermatol* 1995;32:964–967.

190. Tu P, Mitauchi S, Miki Y. Proliferative activities in Spitz nevus compared with melanocytic nevus and malignant melanoma using expression of PCNA/cyclin and mitotic rate. *Am J Dermatopathol* 1993;15:311–314.

191. Vogt T, Stolz W, Glassl A, et al. Multivariate DNA cytometry discriminates between Spitz nevi and malignant melanomas because large polymorphic nuclei in Spitz nevi are not aneuploid. *Am J Dermatopathol* 1996;18:142–150.

192. Winokur TS, Palazzo JP, Johnson WC, et al. Evaluation of DNA ploidy in dysplastic and Spitz nevi by flow cytometry. *J Cutan Pathol* 1990;17:342–347.

193. Bastian BC, Wesselmann U, Pinkel D, et al. Molecular cytogenetic analysis of Spitz nevi shows clear differences to melanoma. *J Invest Dermatol* 1999;113:1065–1069.

194. Matsuta M, Matsuta M, Kon S, et al. Interphase cytogenetics of melanocytic neoplasms: numerical aberrations of chromosomes can be detected in interphase nuclei using centromeric DNA probes. *J Cutan Pathol* 1994;21:1–6.

195. De Wit PEJ, Kerstens HMJ, Poddighe PJ, et al. DNA in situ hybridization as a diagnostic tool in the discrimination of melanoma and Spitz naevus. *J Pathol* 1994;173:227–233.

196. Skowronek J, Warchol JB, Karas Z, et al. Significance of DNA ploidy measurements in Spitz nevi. *Pol J Pathol* 2000;51:45–50.

197. Bastian BC, LeBoit PE, Pinkel D. Mutations and copy number increase of HRAS in Spitz nevi with distinctive histopathological features. *Am J Pathol* 2000;157:967–972.

198. Busam KJ, Rosai J, Iversen K, et al. Xanthogranulomas with inconspicuous foam cells and giant cells mimicking malignant melanoma: a clinical, histologic, and immunohistochemical study of three cases. *Am J Surg Pathol* 2000;24:864–869.

199. Gyorki DE, Busam K, Panageas K, et al. Sentinel lymph node biopsy for patients with cutaneous desmoplastic melanoma. *Ann Surg Oncol* 2003;10:403–407.

200. Busam KJ, Granter SR, Iversen K, et al. Immunohistochemical distinction of epithelioid histiocytic proliferations from epithelioid melanocytic nevi. *Am J Dermatopathol* 2000;22:237–241.

201. Crotty KA, Scolyer RA, Li L, et al. Spitz naevus versus Spitzoid melanoma: when and how can they be distinguished? *Pathology* 2002;34:6–12.

202. Smith KJ, Barett TL, Skelton HG, et al. Spindle cell and epithelioid cell nevi with atypia and metastasis (malignant Spitz tumor). *Am J Surg Pathol* 1989;13:931–939.

203. Casso EM, Grin-Jorgensen CM, Grant-Kels JM. Spitz nevi. *J Am Acad Dermatol* 1992;27:901–913.

204. Shapiro PE. Spitz nevi. *J Am Acad Dermatol* 1993;29:667–668.

205. Reed RJ, Ichinose H, Clark WH Jr, et al. Common and uncommon melanocytic nevi and borderline melanomas. *Semin Oncol* 1975;2:119–147.

206. Sau P, Graham JH, Helwig EB. Pigmented spindle cell nevus: a clinicopathologic analysis of ninety-five cases. *J Am Acad Dermatol* 1993;28:565–571.

207. Barnhill RL, Barnhill MA, Berwick M, et al. The histologic spectrum of pigmented spindle cell nevus: a review of 120 cases with emphasis on atypical variants. *Hum Pathol* 1991;22: 52–58.

208. Sagebiel RW, Chinn EK, Egbert BM. Pigmented spindle cell nevus. Clinical and histologic review of 90 cases. *Am J Surg Pathol* 1984;8:645–653.

209. Smith NP. The pigmented spindle cell tumor of Reed: an underdiagnosed lesion. *Semin Diagn Pathol* 1987;4:75–87.

210. Wistuba I, Gonzalez S. Eosinophilic globules in pigmented spindle cell nevus. *Am J Dermatopathol* 1990;12:268–271.

211. Walton RG, Jacobs AH, Cox AJ. Pigmented lesions in newborn infants. *Br J Dermatol* 1976;95:389–396.

212. Rivers JK, MacLennan R, Kelly JW, et al. The eastern Australian childhood nevus study: prevalence of atypical nevi, congenital nevus-like nevi, and other pigmented lesions. *J Am Acad Dermatol* 1995;32:957–963.

213. Mark GJ, Mihm MC Jr, Liteplo MG, et al. Congenital melanocytic nevi of the small and garment type. Clinical, histologic, and ultrastructural studies. *Hum Pathol* 1973;4:395–418.

214. Kopf AW, Bart RS, Hennessey P. Congenital nevocytic nevi and malignant melanomas. *J Am Acad Dermatol* 1979;1:123–130.

215. Rhodes AR. Melanocytic precursors of cutaneous melanoma. Estimated risks and guidelines for management. *Med Clin North Am* 1986;70:3–37.

216. Orkin M, Frichot BC III, Zelickson AS. Cerebriform intradermal nevus. A cause of cutis verticis gyrata. *Arch Dermatol* 1974;110:575–582.

217. Morishima T, Endo M, Imagawa I, et al. Clinical and histopathological studies on spotted grouped pigmented nevi with special reference to eccrine-centered nevus. *Acta Derm Venereol* 1976;56:345–352.

218. Botet MV, Caro FR, Sanchez JL. Congenital acral melanocytic nevi clinically stimulating acral lentiginous melanoma. *J Am Acad Dermatol* 1981;5:406–410.

219. Ruiz-Maldonado R, Orozco-Covarrubias L, Ridaura-Sanz C, et al. Desmoplastic hairless hypopigmented naevus: a variant of giant congenital melanocytic naevus. *Br J Dermatol* 2003;148:1253–1257.

220. Slaughter JC, Hardman JM, Kempe LG, et al. Neurocutaneous melanosis and leptomeningeal melanomatosis in children. *Arch Pathol* 1969;88:298–304.

221. Reed WB, Becker SW, Becker SW Jr, et al. Giant pigmented nevi, melanoma, and leptomeningeal melanosis. *Arch Dermatol* 1965;91:100–119.

222. Foster RD, Williams ML, Barkovich AJ, et al. Giant congenital melanocytic nevi: the significance of neurocutaneous melanosis in neurologically asymptomatic children. *Plast Reconstr Surg* 2001;107:933–941.

223. Rhodes AR, Sober AJ, Day CL, et al. The malignant potential of small congenital nevocellular nevi. An estimate of association based on a histologic study of 234 primary cutaneous melanomas. *J Am Acad Dermatol* 1982;6:230–241.

224. Rhodes AR, Melski JW. Small congenital nevocellular nevi and the risk of cutaneous melanoma. *J Pediatr* 1982;100:219–224.

225. Illig L. Small and giant congenital melanocytic nevi as precursors to melanoma in children and adults. *Pediatr Pol* 1986;61:475–483.

226. Swerdlow AJ, Green A. Melanocytic naevi and melanoma: an epidemiological perspective. *Br J Dermatol* 1987;117:137–146.

227. Ruiz-Maldonado R, Tamayo L, Laterza AM, et al. Giant pigmented nevi: clinical, histopathologic, and therapeutic considerations. *J Pediatr* 1992;120:906–911.

228. Shpall S, Frieden I, Chesney M, et al. Risk of malignant transformation of congenital melanocytic nevi in blacks. *Pediatr Dermatol* 1994;11:204–208.

229. Swerdlow AJ, English JS, Qiao Z. The risk of melanoma in patients with congenital nevi: a cohort study. *J Am Acad Dermatol* 1995;32:595–599.

230. Marghoob AA, Schoenbach SP, Kopf AW, et al. Large congenital melanocytic nevi and the risk for the development of malignant melanoma—a prospective study. *Arch Dermatol* 1996;132:170–175.

231. Naasan A, Al-Nafussi A, Quaba A. Cutaneous malignant melanoma in children and adolescents in Scotland, 1979–1991. *Plast Reconstr Surg* 1996;98:442–446.

232. DeDavid M, Orlow SJ, Provost N, et al. A study of large congenital melanocytic nevi and associated malignant melanomas: review of cases in the New York University Registry and the world literature. *J Am Acad Dermatol* 1997;36:409–416.

233. Scalzo DA, Hida CA, Toth G, et al. Childhood melanoma: a clinicopathological study of 22 cases. *Melanoma Res* 1997;7:63–68.

234. Egan CL, Oliveria SA, Elenitsas R, et al. Cutaneous melanoma risk and phenotypic changes in large congenital nevi: a follow-up study of 46 patients. *J Am Acad Dermatol* 1998;39:923–932.

235. Sahin S, Levin L, Kopf AW, et al. Risk of melanoma in medium-sized congenital melanocytic nevi: a follow-up study. *J Am Acad Dermatol* 1998;39:428-433.

236. Betti R, Inselvini E, Vergani R, et al. Small congenital nevi associated with melanoma: case reports and considerations. *J Dermatol* 2000;27:583–590.

237. Bittencourt FV, Marghoob AA, Kopf AW, et al. Large congenital melanocytic nevi and the risk for development of malignant melanoma and neurocutaneous melanocytosis. *Pediatrics* 2000;106:736–741.

238. Richardson SK, Tannous ZS, Mihm MC Jr. Congenital and infantile melanoma: review of the literature and report of an uncommon variant, pigment-synthesizing melanoma. *J Am Acad Dermatol* 2002;47:77–90.

239. Solomon LM. The management of congenital melanocytic nevi. *Arch Dermatol* 1980;116:1017.

240. Berg P, Lindelof B. Congenital nevocytic nevi: follow-up of a Swedish birth register sample regarding etiologic factors, discomfort, and removal rate. *Pediatr Dermatol* 2002;19:293–297.

241. Illig L, Weidner F, Hundeiker M, et al. Congenital nevi less than or equal to 10 cm as precursors to melanoma. 52 cases, a review, and a new conception. *Arch Dermatol* 1985;121:1274–1281.

242. Everett MA. Histopathology of congenital pigmented nevi. *Am J Dermatopathol* 1989;11:11–12.

243. Cribier BJ, Santinelli F, Grosshans E. Lack of clinical-pathological correlation in the diagnosis of congenital naevi. *Br J Dermatol* 1999;141:1004–1009.

244. Stenn KS, Arons M, Hurwitz S. Patterns of congenital nevocellular nevi. *J Am Acad Dermatol* 1983;9:388–393.

245. Kuehnl-Petzoldt C, Kunze J, Mueller R, et al. Histology of congenital nevi during the first year of life. A study by conventional and electron microscopy. *Am J Dermatopathol* 1984;6[Suppl]:81–88.

246. Barnhill RL, Fleischli M. Histologic features of congenital melanocytic nevi in infants 1 year of age or younger. *J Am Acad Dermatol* 1995;33:780–785.

247. Clemmensen OJ, Kroon S. The histology of "congenital features" in early acquired melanocytic nevi. *J Am Acad Dermatol* 1988;19:742–746.

248. Hurwitz RM, Buckel LJ. Superficial congenital compound melanocytic nevus. Another pitfall in the diagnosis of malignant melanoma. *Dermatol Surg* 1997;23:897–900.

249. Fontaine D, Parkhill W, Greer W, et al. Nevus cells in lymph nodes: an association with congenital cutaneous nevi. *Am J Dermatopathol* 2002;24:1–5.

250. Kaddu S, Smolle J, Zenahlik P, et al. Melanoma with benign melanocytic naevus components: reappraisal of clinicopathological features and prognosis. *Melanoma Res* 2002;12:271–278.

251. Rhodes AR, Wood WC, Sober AJ, et al. Nonepidermal origin of malignant melanoma associated with a giant congenital nevocellular nevus. *Plast Reconstr Surg* 1981;67:782–790.

252. Paull WH, Polley D, Fitzpatrick JE. Malignant melanoma arising intradermally in a small congenital nevus of an adult. *J Dermatol Surg Oncol* 1986;12:1176–1178.

253. Padilla RS, McConnell TS, Gribble JT, et al. Malignant melanoma arising in a giant congenital melanocytic nevus. A case report with cytogenetic and histopathologic analyses. *Cancer* 1988;62:2589–2594.

254. Sharpe RJ, Salasche SJ, Barnhill RL, et al. Nonepidermal origin of cutaneous melanoma in a small congenital nevus. *Arch Dermatol* 1990;126:1559–1561.

255. Weidner N, Flanders DJ, Jochimsen PR, et al. Neurosarcomatous malignant melanoma arising in a neuroid giant congenital melanocytic nevus. *Arch Dermatol* 1985;121:1302–1306.

256. Pack GT, Davis J. Nevus giganticus pigmentosus with malignant transformation. *Surgery* 1961;49;347–354.

257. Aroni K, Georgala S, Papachatzaki E, et al. Coexistence of plaque-type blue nevus and congenital melanocytic nevi. *J Dermatol* 1996;23:325–328.

258. Hendrickson MR, Ross JC. Neoplasms arising in congenital giant nevi: morphologic study of seven cases and a review of the literature. *Am J Surg Pathol* 1981;5:109–135.

259. Hoang MP, Sinkre P, Albores-Saavedra J. Rhabdomyosarcoma arising in a congenital melanocytic nevus. *Am J Dermatopathol* 2002;24:26–29.

260. Fromont HG, Fraitag S, Wolter M, et al. DNA content and cell proliferation in giant congenital melanocytic naevi (GCMN). An analysis by image cytometry. *J Cutan Pathol* 1998;25:401–406.

261. Lowes MA, Norris D, Whitfeld M. Benign melanocytic proliferative nodule within a congenital naevus. *Australas J Dermatol* 2000;41:109–111.

262. Xu X, Weber KS, Elenitsas R, et al. Clinical and histological cellular nodules in congenital nevi. *J Cutan Pathol* 2004;31:153–159.

263. Bastian BC, Xiong J, Frieden IJ, et al. Genetic changes in neoplasms arising in congenital melanocytic nevi: differences between nodular proliferations and melanomas. *Am J Pathol* 2002;161:1163–1169.

264. Williams HI. Primary malignant meningeal melanoma associated with benign hairy naevi. *J Pathol* 1969;99:171–172.

265. Chang CS, Hsieh PF, Chia LG, et al. Leptomeningeal malignant melanoma arising in neurocutaneous melanocytosis: a case report. *Zhonghua Yi Xue Za Zhi (Taipei)* 1997;60:316–320.

266. Mehregan DA, Mehregan AH. Deep penetrating nevus. *Arch Dermatol* 1993;129:328–331.

267. Seab JA Jr, Graham JH, Helwig EB. Deep penetrating nevus. *Am J Surg Pathol* 1989;13:39–44.

268. Cooper PH. Deep penetrating (plexiform spindle cell) nevus. A frequent participant in combined nevus. *J Cutan Pathol* 1992;19:172–180.

269. Barnhill RL, Mihm MC Jr, Magro CM. Plexiform spindle cell naevus: a distinctive variant of plexiform melanocytic naevus. *Histopathology* 1991;18:243–247.

270. Mehregan DR, Mehregan DA, Mehregan AH. Proliferating cell nuclear antigen staining in deep-penetrating nevi. *J Am Acad Dermatol* 1995;33:685–687.

271. Kopf AW, Morrill SD, Silberberg I. Broad spectrum of leukoderma acquisitum centrifugum. *Arch Dermatol* 1965;92:14–33.

272. Huynh PM, Lazova R, Bolognia JL. Unusual halo nevi—darkening rather than lightening of the central nevus. *Dermatology* 2001;202:324–327.

273. Berman A. Halo nevus with exceptional clinical features. Apparent arrest of nevus cell degeneration and return of pigment to halo. *Arch Dermatol* 1978;114:1081–1082.

274. Brownstein MH, Kazam BB, Hashimoto K. Halo congenital nevus. *Arch Dermatol* 1977;113:1572–1575.

275. Happle R, Echternacht K, Schotola I. Halonaevus ohne Halo. *Hautarzt* 1975;26;44–46.

276. Meyerson LB. A peculiar papulosquamous eruption involving pigmented nevi. *Arch Dermatol* 1971;103:510–512.

277. Pariser RJ. "Nevocentric" erythema multiforme. *J Am Acad Dermatol* 1994;31:491–492.

278. Elenitsas R, Halpern AC. Eczematous halo reaction in atypical nevi. *J Am Acad Dermatol* 1996;34:357–361.

279. Penneys NS, Mayoral F, Barnhill R, et al. Delineation of nevus cell nests in inflammatory infiltrates by immunohistochemical staining for the presence of S100 protein. *J Cutan Pathol* 1985;12:28–32.

280. Gauthier Y, Surleve-Bazeille JE, Gauthier O, et al. Ultrastructure of halo nevi. *J Cutan Pathol* 1975;2:71–81.

281. Swanson JL, Wayte DM, Helwig EB. Ultrastructure of halo nevi. *J Invest Dermatol* 1968;50:434–450.

282. Hashimoto K. A case of halo nevus with effete melanocytes. *Acta Derm Venereol* 1975;55:87–95.

283. Zeff RA, Freitag A, Grin CM, et al. The immune response in halo nevi. *J Am Acad Dermatol* 1997;37:620–624.

284. Musette P, Bachelez H, Flageul B, et al. Immune-mediated destruction of melanocytes in halo nevi is associated with the local expansion of a limited number of T cell clones. *J Immunol* 1999;162:1789–1794.

285. Kornberg R, Ackerman AB. Pseudomelanoma. Recurrent melanocytic nevus following partial surgical removal. *Arch Dermatol* 1975;111:1588–1590.

286. Duray PH, Livolsi VA. Recurrent dysplastic nevus following shave excision. *J Dermatol Surg Oncol* 1984;10:811–815.

287. Trau H, Orenstein A, Schewach-Miller M, et al. Pseudomelanoma following laser therapy for congenital nevus. *J Dermatol Surg Oncol* 1986;12:984–986.

288. Sexton M, Sexton CW. Recurrent pigmented melanocytic nevus: a benign lesion, not to be mistaken for malignant melanoma. *Arch Pathol Lab Med* 1991;115:122–126.

289. Park HK, Leonard DD, Arrington JH III, et al. Recurrent melanocytic nevi: clinical and histologic review of 175 cases. *J Am Acad Dermatol* 17;285–292. 1987.

290. Bong JL, Perkins W. Shave excision of benign facial melanocytic naevi: a patient's satisfaction survey. *Dermatol Surg* 2003;29:227–229.

291. Hoang MP, Prieto VG, Burchette JL, et al. Recurrent melanocytic nevus: a histologic and immunohistochemical evaluation. *J Cutan Pathol* 2001;28:400–406.

292. Alanko T, Rosenberg M, Saksela O. FGF expression allows nevus cells to survive in three-dimensional collagen gel under conditions that induce apoptosis in normal human melanocytes. *J Invest Dermatol* 1999;113:111–116.

293. Clark WH Jr, Reimer RR, Greene M, et al. Origin of familial malignant melanomas from heritable melanocytic lesions. "The B-K mole syndrome." *Arch Dermatol* 1978;114:732–738.

294. Lynch HT, Frichot BCI, Lynch JF. Familial atypical multiple mole-melanoma syndrome. *J Med Genet* 1978;15:352–356.

295. Elder DE, Goldman LI, Goldman SC, et al. Dysplastic nevus syndrome: a phenotypic association of sporadic cutaneous melanoma. *Cancer* 1980;46:1787–1794.

296. Rahbari H, Mehregan AH. Sporadic atypical mole syndrome. A report of five nonfamilial B-K mole syndrome-like cases and histopathologic findings. *Arch Dermatol* 1981;117:329–331.

297. Elder DE, Clark WH Jr, Elenitsas R, et al. The early and intermediate precursor lesions of tumor progression in the melanocytic system: common acquired nevi and atypical (dysplastic) nevi. *Semin Diagn Pathol* 1993;10:18–35.

298. National Institutes of Health: Consensus development conference. Precursors to malignant melanoma. *JAMA* 1984;251:1864–1866.

299. Kelly JW, Crutcher WA, Sagebiel RW. Clinical diagnosis of dysplastic melanocytic nevi. A clinicopathologic correlation. *J Am Acad Dermatol* 1986;14:1044–1052.

300. Ackerman AB, Mihara I. Dysplasia, dysplastic melanocytes, dysplastic nevi, the dysplastic nevus syndrome, and the relation between dysplastic nevi and malignant melanomas. *Hum Pathol* 1985;16:87–91.

301. Ackerman AB, Briggs PL, Bravo F. Dysplastic nevus, compound type vs. Clark's nevus, compound type. In: Ackerman AB, Briggs PL, Bravo F, eds. *Differential diagnosis in dermatopathology III.* Philadelphia: Lea & Febiger, 1993:158–161.

302. National Institutes of Health. National Institutes of Health Consensus Development Conference statement on diagnosis and treatment of early melanoma, January 27–29, 1992. *Am J Dermatopathol* 1993;15:34–43.

303. Shea CR, Vollmer RT, Prieto VG. Correlating architectural disorder and cytologic atypia in Clark (dysplastic) melanocytic nevi. *Hum Pathol* 1999;30:500–505.

304. Sagebiel RW, Banda PW, Schneider JS, et al. Age distribution and histologic patterns of dysplastic nevi. *J Am Acad Dermatol* 1985;13:975–982.

305. Halpern AC, Guerry DIV, Elder DE, et al. Natural history of dysplastic nevi. *J Am Acad Dermatol* 1993;29:51–57.

306. Guerry DIV, Synnestvedt M, Elder DE, et al. Lessons from tumor progression: the invasive radial growth phase of melanoma is common, incapable of metastasis, and indolent. *J Invest Dermatol* 1993;100:342S–345S.

307. Arumi-Uria M, McNutt NS, Finnerty B. Grading of atypia in nevi: correlation with melanoma risk. *Mod Pathol* 2003;16:764–771.

308. Rudolph PO. Atypical melanocyte hyperplasia. *Z Hautkr* 1986;61:724–726 (in German).

309. Bruijn JA, Berwick M, Mihm MC Jr, et al. Common acquired melanocytic nevi, dysplastic melanocytic nevi and malignant melanomas: an image analysis cytometric study. *J Cutan Pathol* 1993;20:121–125.

310. Duncan LM, Berwick M, Bruijn JA, et al. Histopathologic recognition and grading of dysplastic melanocytic nevi: an interobserver agreement study. *J Invest Dermatol* 1993;100:318S–321S.

311. Clemente C, Cochran A, Elder DE, et al. Histopathologic diagnosis of dysplastic nevi. Concordance among pathologists convened by the WHO melanoma programme. *Hum Pathol* 1991;22:313–319.

312. De Wit PEJ, Van't Hof-Grootenboer B, Ruiter DJ, et al. Validity of the histopathological criteria used for diagnosing dysplastic naevi. *Eur J Cancer [A]* 1993;29A. 831–839.

313. Piepkorn MW, Barnhill RL, Cannon-Albright LA, et al. A multiobserver, population-based analysis of histologic dysplasia in melanocytic nevi. *J Am Acad Dermatol* 1994;30:707–714.

314. Weinstock MA. Dysplastic nevi revisited. *J Am Acad Dermatol* 1994;30:807–810.

315. Kelly JW. Clinical diagnosis of dysplastic melanocytic nevi. A clinicopathologic correlation. 1986;14:1044–1052.

316. Holly EA, Kelly JW, Shpall SN, et al. Number of melanocytic nevi as a major risk factor for malignant melanoma. *J Am Acad Dermatol* 1987;17:459–468.

317. Evans RD, Kopf AW, Lew RA, et al. Risk factors for the development of malignant melanoma. I. Review of case-control studies. *J Dermatol Surg Oncol* 1988;14:393–408.

318. Ford D, Bliss JM, Swerdlow AJ, et al. Risk of cutaneous melanoma associated with a family history of the disease. The International Melanoma Analysis Group (IMAGE). *Int J Cancer* 1995;62:377–381.

319. Carey WP Jr, Thompson CJ, Synnestvedt M, et al. Dysplastic nevi as a melanoma risk factor in patients with familial melanoma. *Cancer* 1994;74:3118–3125.

320. Greene MH, Clark WH Jr, Tucker MA, et al. High risk of malignant melanoma in melanoma-prone families with dysplastic nevi. *Ann Intern Med* 1985;102:458–465.

321. Halpern AC, Guerry D, Elder DE, et al. A cohort study of melanoma in patients with dysplastic nevi. *J Invest Dermatol* 1993;100:346S–349S.

322. Albert LS, Rhodes AR, Sober AJ. Dysplastic melanocytic nevi and cutaneous melanoma: markers of increased melanoma risk for affected persons and blood relatives. *J Am Acad Dermatol* 1990;22:69–75.

323. Augustsson A. Melanocytic naevi, melanoma and sun exposure. *Acta Derm Venereol Suppl (Stockh)* 1991;166:1–34.

324. Augustsson A, Stierner U, Rosdahl I, et al. Common and dysplastic naevi as risk factors for cutaneous malignant melanoma in a Swedish population. *Acta Derm Venereol (Stockh)* 1991;71:518–524.

325. Baccarelli A, Landi MT. Risk factors of malignant skin melanoma in Italian population: review of results of a case-control study. *Epidemiol Prev* 2002;26:293–299 (in Italian).

326. Bakos L, Wagner M, Bakos RM, et al. Sunburn, sunscreens, and phenotypes: some risk factors for cutaneous melanoma in southern Brazil. *Int J Dermatol* 2002;41:557–562.

327. Bataille V, Bishop JAN, Sasieni P, et al. Risk of cutaneous melanoma in relation to the numbers, types and sites of naevi: a case-control study. *Br J Cancer* 1996;73:1605–1611.

328. Bauer J, Garbe C. Acquired melanocytic nevi as risk factor for melanoma development. A comprehensive review of epidemiological data. *Pigment Cell Res* 2003;16:297–306.

329. Bergman W, Voorst Vader PC, Ruiter DJ. Dysplastic nevi and the risk of melanoma: a guideline for patient care. Nederlandse Melanoom Werkgroep van de Vereniging voor Integrale Kankercentra. *Ned Tijdschr Geneeskd* 1997;141:2010–2014 (in German).

330. Byles JE, Hennrikus D, Sanson-Fisher R, et al. Reliability of naevus counts in identifying individuals at high risk of malignant melanoma. *Br J Dermatol* 1994;130:51–56.

331. Garbe C, Büttner P, Weiss J, Soyer HP, et al. Risk factors for developing cutaneous melanoma and criteria for identifying persons at risk: Multicenter case-control study of the Central Malignant Melanoma Registry of the German Dermatological Society. *J Invest Dermatol* 1994;102:695–699.

332. Grulich AE, Bataille V, Swerdlow AJ, et al. Naevi and pigmentary characteristics as risk factors for melanoma in a high-risk population: a case-control study in New South Wales, Australia. *Int J Cancer* 1996;67:485–491.

333. Halpern AC, Guerry DIV, Elder DE, et al. Dysplastic nevi as risk markers of sporadic (non-familial) melanoma: a case-control study. *Arch Dermatol* 1991;127:995–999.

334. Jackson A, Wilkinson C, Ranger M, et al. Can primary prevention or selective screening for melanoma be more precisely targeted through general practice? A prospective study to validate a self-administered risk score. *BMJ* 1998;316:34–38.

335. Kang S, Barnhill RL, Mihm MC Jr, et al. Melanoma risk in individuals with clinically atypical nevi. *Arch Dermatol* 1994;130:999–1001.

336. Kroon BB, Bergman W, Coebergh JW, et al. Consensus on the management of malignant melanoma of the skin in The Netherlands. Dutch Melanoma Working Party. *Melanoma Res* 1999;9:207–212.

337. Landi MT, Baccarelli A, Tarone RE, et al. DNA repair, dysplastic nevi, and sunlight sensitivity in the development of cutaneous malignant melanoma. *J Natl Cancer Inst* 2002;94:94–101.

338. MacKie RM. Incidence, risk factors and prevention of melanoma. *Eur J Cancer* 1998;34[Suppl 3]:S3–S6.

339. Nordlund JJ, Kirkwood J, Forget BM, et al. Demographic study of clinically atypical (dysplastic) nevi in patients with melanoma and comparison subjects. *Cancer Res* 1985;45:1855–1861.

340. Roush GC, Nordlund JJ, Forget B, et al. Independence of dysplastic nevi from total nevi in determining risk for nonfamilial melanoma. *Prev Med* 1988;17:273–279.

341. Schneider JS, Moore DH II, Sagebiel RW. Risk factors for melanoma incidence in prospective follow-up: the importance of atypical (dysplastic) nevi. *Arch Dermatol* 1994;130:1002–1007.

342. Slade J, Salopek TG, Marghoob AA, et al. Risk of developing cutaneous malignant melanoma in atypical-mole syndrome: New York University experience and literature review. *Recent Results Cancer Res* 1995;139:87–104.

343. Swerdlow AJ, English J, MacKie RM, et al. Benign melanocytic naevi as a risk factor for malignant melanoma. *BMJ* 1986;292:1555–1559.

344. Annessi G, Cattaruzza MS, Abeni D, et al. Correlation between clinical atypia and histologic dysplasia in acquired melanocytic nevi. *J Am Acad Dermatol* 2001;45:77–85.

345. Gruber SB, Barnhill RL, Stenn KS, et al. Nevomelanocytic proliferations in association with cutaneous malignant melanoma: a multivariate analysis. *J Am Acad Dermatol* 1989;21:773–780.

346. Sagebiel RW. Melanocytic nevi in histologic association with primary cutaneous melanoma of superficial spreading and nodular types: effect of tumor thickness. *J Invest Dermatol* 1993;100:322S–325S.

347. Skender-Kalnenas TM, English DR, Heenan PJ. Benign melanocytic lesions: risk markers or precursors of cutaneous melanoma? *J Am Acad Dermatol* 1995;33:1000–1007.

348. Rhodes AR, Harrist TJ, Day CL, et al. Dysplastic melanocytic nevi in histologic association with 234 primary cutaneous melanomas. *J Am Acad Dermatol* 1983;9:563–574.

349. Takahashi H, Strutton GM, Parsons PG. Determination of proliferating fractions in malignant melanomas by anti-PCNA/cyclin monoclonal antibody. *Histopathology* 1991;18:221–227.

350. Urso C, Bondi R, Balzi M, et al. Cell kinetics of melanocytes in common and dysplastic nevi and in primary and metastatic cutaneous melanoma. *Pathol Res Pract* 1992;323:329.

351. Jimbow K, Horikoshi T, Takahashi H, et al. Fine structural and immunohistochemical properties of dysplastic melanocytic nevi: comparison with malignant melanoma. *J Invest Dermatol* 1989;92:304S–309S.

352. Rhodes AR, Seki Y, Fitzpatrick TB, et al. Melanosomal alterations in dysplastic melanocytic nevi. A quantitative, ultrastructural investigation. *Cancer* 1988;61:358–369.

353. Elder DE, Rodeck U, Thurin J, et al. Antigenic profile of tumor progression stages in human melanocytic nevi and melanomas. *Cancer Res* 1989;49:5091–5096.

354. Smoller BR, McNutt NS, Hsu A. HMB-45 staining of dysplastic nevi. Support for a spectrum of progression toward melanoma. *Am J Surg Pathol* 1989;13:680–684.

355. Fogt F, Vortmeyer AO, Tahan SR. Nucleolar organizer regions (AgNOR) and Ki-67 immunoreactivity in cutaneous melanocytic lesions. *Am J Dermatopathol* 1995;17:12–17.

356. Yamada K, Salopek T, Jimbow K, et al. An extremely high content of pheomelanin in dysplastic nevi. *J Invest Dermatol* 1989;92:544a.

357. Tran TP, Titus-Ernstoff L, Perry AE, et al. Alteration of chromosome 9p21 and/or p16 in benign and dysplastic nevi suggests a role in early melanoma progression (United States). *Cancer Causes Control* 2002;13:675–682.

358. Korabiowska M, Brinck U, Kellner S, et al. Relation between two independent DNA-repair pathways in different groups of naevi. *In Vivo* 1999;13:243–245.

359. Hussein MR, Sun M, Tuthill RJ, et al. Comprehensive analysis of 112 melanocytic skin lesions demonstrates microsatellite instability in melanomas and dysplastic nevi, but not in benign nevi. *J Cutan Pathol* 2001;28:343–350.

360. Birindelli S, Tragni G, Bartoli C, et al. Detection of microsatellite alterations in the spectrum of melanocytic nevi in patients with or without individual or family history of melanoma. *Int J Cancer* 2000;86:255–261.

361. Tripp JM, Kopf AW, Marghoob AA, et al. Management of dysplastic nevi: a survey of fellows of the American Academy of Dermatology. *J Am Acad Dermatol* 2002;46:674–682.

362. Masri GD, Clark WH Jr, Guerry D, et al. Screening and surveillance of patients at high risk for malignant melanoma result in detection of earlier disease. *J Am Acad Dermatol* 1990;22:1042–1048.

363. Barr RJ, Linden KG, Rubinstein G, et al. Analysis of heterogeneity of atypia within melanocytic nevi. *Arch Dermatol* 2003;139:289–292.

364. Clark WH Jr, From L, Bernardino EA, et al. The histogenesis and biologic behavior of primary human malignant melanomas of the skin. *Cancer Res* 1969;29:705–727.

365. Clark WH Jr. A classification of malignant melanoma in man correlated with histogenesis and biologic behavior. In: Montagna W, Hu F, eds. *Advances in the biology of the skin*, vol. VIII. New York: Pergamon Press, 1967:621–647.

366. McGovern VJ. The classification of melanoma and its histologic reporting. *Pathology* 1970;2:85–98.

367. Clark WH Jr, Elder DE, Van Horn M. The biologic forms of malignant melanoma. *Hum Pathol* 1986;5:443–450.

368. McGovern VJ, Cochran AJ, Van der EEP, et al. The classification of malignant melanoma, its histological reporting and registration: a revision of the 1972 Sydney classification. *Pathology* 1986;18:12–21.

369. Heenan PJ, Elder DE, Sobin LH. Histological classification of skin tumors. In: Heenan PJ, Elder DE, Sobin LH, eds. *Histological typing of skin tumors*. New York: Springer, 1996:3–10.

370. Baer SC, Schultz D, Synnestvedt M, et al. Desmoplasia and neurotropism—prognostic variables in patients with stage I melanoma. *Cancer* 1995;76:2242–2247.

371. Ackerman AB. Malignant melanoma. A unifying concept. *Am J Dermatopathol* 1980;2:309–313.

372. Flotte TJ, Mihm MC Jr. Melanoma: the art versus the science of dermatopathology. *Hum Pathol* 1986;17:441–442.

373. Bastian BC. Understanding the progression of melanocytic neoplasia using genomic analysis: from fields to cancer. *Oncogene* 2003;22:3081–3086.

374. Auslender S, Barzilai A, Goldberg I, et al. Lentigo maligna and superficial spreading melanoma are different in their in situ phase: an immunohistochemical study. *Hum Pathol* 2002;33:1001–1005.

375. Rigel DS, Friedman RJ. The rationale of the ABCDs of early melanoma. *J Am Acad Dermatol* 1993;29:1060–1061.

376. Elder DE, Guerry DIV, Epstein MN, et al. Invasive malignant melanomas lacking competence for metastasis. *Am J Dermatopathol* 1984;6:55–62.

377. Elder DE, Murphy GF. *Melanocytic tumors of the skin*. Washington, DC: Armed Forces Institute of Pathology, 1991.

378. Cook MG, Clarke TJ, Humphreys S, et al. The evaluation of diagnostic and prognostic criteria and the terminology of thin cutaneous melanoma by the CRC Melanoma Pathology Panel. *Histopathology* 1996;28:497–512.

379. Lefevre M, Vergier B, Balme B, et al. Relevance of vertical growth pattern in thin level II cutaneous superficial spreading melanomas. *Am J Surg Pathol* 2003;27:717–724.

380. McDermott NC, Hayes DP, al-Sader MH, et al. Identification of vertical growth phase in malignant melanoma. A study of interobserver agreement. *Am J Clin Pathol* 1998;110:753–757.

381. Mercer KE, Pritchard CA. Raf proteins and cancer: B-Raf is identified as a mutational target. *Biochim Biophys Acta* 2003;1653:25–40.

382. Mihic-Probst D, Saremaslani P, Komminoth P, et al. Immunostaining for the tumour suppressor gene p16 product is a useful marker to differentiate melanoma metastasis from lymph-node nevus. *Virchows Arch* 2003;443:745–751.

383. Radhi JM. Malignant melanoma arising from nevi, p53, p16, and Bcl–2:expression in benign versus malignant components. *J Cutan Med Surg* 1999;3:293–297.

384. Keller-Melchior R, Schmidt R, Piepkorn M. Expression of the tumor suppressor gene product p16INK4 in benign and malignant melanocytic lesions. *J Invest Dermatol* 1998;110:932–938.

385. Price NM, Rywlin AM, Ackerman AB. Histologic criteria for the diagnosis of superficial spreading melanoma: formulated on the basis of proven metastatic lesions. *Cancer* 1976;38:2434–2441.

386. Sagebiel RW. Histopathology of borderline and early malignant melanomas. *Am J Surg Pathol* 1979;3:543–552.

387. Dubreuilh MW. De la melanose circonscrite precancereuse. *Ann Dermatol Syphiligr (Paris)* 1912;3:129.

388. Steiner A, Konrad K, Pehamberger H, et al. Verrucous malignant melanoma. *Arch Dermatol* 1988;124:1534–1537.

389. Mishima Y. Melanocytic and nevocytic malignant melanomas. Cellular and subcellular differentiation. *Cancer* 1967;20:632–649.

390. Clark WH Jr, Ainsworth AM, Bernardino EA, et al. The developmental biology of primary human malignant melanomas. *Semin Oncol* 1975;2:83–103.

391. Guldhammer B, Nrgaard T. The differential diagnosis of intraepidermal malignant lesions using immunohistochemistry. *Am J Dermatopathol* 1986;8:295–301.

392. Clark WH Jr, Mihm MC Jr. Lentigo maligna and lentigo-maligna melanoma. *Am J Pathol* 1969;55:39–67.

393. Flotte TJ, Mihm MCJ. Lentigo maligna and malignant melanoma in situ, lentigo maligna type. *Hum Pathol* 1999;30:533–536.

394. Rocamora V, Puig L, Romani J, et al. Amelanotic lentigo maligna melanoma: report of a case and review of the literature. *Cutis* 1999;64:53–56.

395. Rahbari H, Nabai H, Mehregan AH, et al. Amelanotic lentigo maligna melanoma: a diagnostic conundrum—presentation of four new cases. *Cancer* 1996;77:2052–2057.

396. Burket JM. Amelanotic lentigo maligna. *Arch Dermatol* 1979;115:496.

397. Weinstock MA, Sober AJ. The risk of progression of lentigo maligna to lentigo maligna melanoma. *Br J Dermatol* 1987;116:303–310.

398. Michalik EE, Fitzpatrick TB, Sober AJ. Rapid progression of lentigo maligna to deeply invasive lentigo maligna melanoma. Report of two cases. *Arch Dermatol* 1983;119:831–835.

399. Koh HK, Michalik E, Sober AJ, et al. Lentigo maligna melanoma has no better prognosis than other types of melanoma. *J Clin Oncol* 1984;2:994–1001.

400. Whiteman DC, Watt P, Purdie DM, et al. Melanocytic nevi, solar keratoses, and divergent pathways to cutaneous melanoma. *J Natl Cancer Inst* 2003;95:806–812.

401. Cramer SF, Kiehn CL. Sequential histologic study of evolving lentigo maligna melanoma. *Arch Pathol Lab Med* 1982;106:121–125.

402. Mishima Y, Matsunaka M. Pagetoid premalignant melanosis and melanoma: differentiation from Hutchinson's melanotic freckle. *J Invest Dermatol* 1975;65:434–440.

403. Kelly JW. Following lentigo maligna may not prevent the development of life- threatening melanoma. *Arch Dermatol* 1992;128:657–660.

404. Arrington JH 3d, Reed RJ, Ichinose H, et al. Plantar lentiginous melanoma: a distinctive variant of human cutaneous malignant melanoma. *Am J Surg Pathol* 1977;1:131–143.

405. Elder DE. Skin cancer: melanoma and other specific nonmelanoma skin cancers. *Cancer* 1995;75[Suppl: 245–256.

406. Coleman WP 3d, Loria PR, Reed RJ, et al. Acral lentiginous melanoma. *Arch Dermatol* 1980;116:773–776.

407. Paladugu RR, Winberg CD, Yonemoto RH. Acral lentiginous melanoma. A clinicopathologic study of 36 patients. *Cancer* 1983;52:161–168.

408. Sauter ER, Yeo UC, Von Stemm A, et al. Cyclin d1 is a candidate oncogene in cutaneous melanoma. *Cancer Res* 2002;62:3200–3206.

409. Bastian BC, Kashani-Sabet M, Hamm H, et al. Gene amplifications characterize acral melanoma and permit the detection of occult tumor cells in the surrounding skin. *Cancer Res* 2000;60:1968–1973.

410. Rapini RP, Golitz LE, Greer RO, et al. Primary malignant melanoma of the oral cavity. A review of 177 cases. *Cancer* 1985;55:1543–1551.

411. Mesara BW, Burton WD. Primary malignant melanoma of the upper respiratory tract. Clinicopathologic study. *Cancer* 1968;21:217–225.

412. Pandey M, Mathew A, Abraham EK, et al. Primary malignant melanoma of the mucous membranes. *Eur J Surg Oncol* 1998;24:303–307.

413. Wanebo HJ, Woodruff JM, Farr GH, et al. Anorectal melanoma. *Cancer* 1981;47:1891–1900.

414. Elder DE, Jucovy PM, Tuthill RJ, et al. The classification of malignant melanoma. *Am J Dermatopathol* 1980;2:315–320.

415. Nakhleh RE, Wick MR, Rocamora A, et al. Morphologic diversity in malignant melanomas. *Am J Clin Pathol* 1990;93:731–740.

416. Borek BT, McKee PH, Freeman JA, et al. Primary malignant melanoma with rhabdoid features: a histologic and immunocytochemical study of three cases. *Am J Dermatopathol* 1998;20:123–127.

417. Chang ES, Wick MR, Swanson PE, et al. Metastatic malignant melanoma with "rhabdoid" features. *Am J Clin Pathol* 1994;102:426–431.

418. Lucas DR, Tazelaar HD, Unni KK, et al. Osteogenic melanoma: a rare variant of malignant melanoma. *Am J Surg Pathol* 1993;17:400–409.

419. Clark WH Jr, Elder DE, Guerry DIV, et al. Model predicting survival in stage I melanoma based on tumor progression. *J Natl Cancer Inst* 1989;81:1893–1904.

420. Heenan PJ, Holman CD. Nodular malignant melanoma: a distinct entity or a common end stage? *Am J Dermatopathol* 1982; 4:477–478.

421. Kornstein MJ, Brooks JS, Elder DE. Immunoperoxidase localization of lymphocyte subsets in the host response to melanoma and nevi. *Cancer Res* 1983;43:2749–2753.

422. Spagnoli GC, Schaefer C, Willimann TE, et al. Peptide-specific CTL in tumor-infiltrating lymphocytes from metastatic melanomas expressing MART-I/Melan-A, gp100 and tyrosinase genes: a study in an unselected group of HLA-A2.1-positive patients. *Int J Cancer* 1995;64:309–315.

423. Stolz W, Schmoeckel C, Welkovich B, et al. Semiquantitative analysis of histologic criteria in thin malignant melanomas. *J Am Acad Dermatol* 1989;20:1115–1120.

424. Azar HA, Espinoza CG, Richman AV, et al. "Undifferentiated" large cell malignancies: an ultrastructural and immunocytochemical study. *Hum Pathol* 1982;13:323–333.

425. Koch SE, Lange JR. Amelanotic melanoma: the great masquerader. *J Am Acad Dermatol* 2000;42:731–734.

426. Morishima T, Tatsumi F, Fukada E, et al. Studies on amelanotic melanoma with the fluorescence method (Falck and Hillarp) and biochemical analysis of 5-S-cysteinyldopa in the tissues. *Arch Dermatol Res* 1983;275:329–333.

427. Clark WH Jr. Four types of cellular fine structure associated with human amelanotic melanoma. *Yale J Biol Med* 1973;46: 428.

428. DeLellis RA, Dayal Y. The role of immunohistochemistry in the diagnosis of poorly differentiated malignant neoplasms. *Semin Oncol* 1987;14:173–192.

429. Sheffield MV, Yee H, Dorvault CC, et al. Comparison of five antibodies as markers in the diagnosis of melanoma in cytologic preparations. *Am J Clin Pathol* 2002;118:930–936.

430. Busam KJ, Chen YT, Old LJ, et al. Expression of melan-A (MART1) in benign melanocytic nevi and primary cutaneous malignant melanoma. *Am J Surg Pathol* 1998;22:976–982.

431. Argenyi ZB, Cain C, Bromley C, et al. S–100 protein-negative malignant melanoma: fact or fiction? A light microscopic and immunohistochemical study. *Am J Dermatopathol* 1994;16: 233–240.

432. Drier JK, Swanson PE, Cherwitz DL, et al. S100 protein immunoreactivity in poorly differentiated carcinomas. Immunohistochemical comparison with malignant melanoma. *Arch Pathol Lab Med* 1987;111:447–452.

433. Zarbo RJ, Gown AM, Nagle RB, et al. Anomalous cytokeratin expression in malignant melamoma: one- and two-dimensional Western blot analysis and immunohistochemical survey of 100 melanomas. *Mod Pathol* 1990;3:494–501.

434. Ben-Izhak O, Stark P, Levy R, et al. Epithelial markers in malignant melanoma. A study of primary lesions and their metastases. *Am J Dermatopathol* 1994;16:241–246.

435. Puches R, Smolle J, Rieger E, et al. Expression of cytoskeletal components in melanocytic skin lesions. An immunohistochemical study. *Am J Dermatopathol* 1991;13:137–144.

436. Domagala W, Chosia M, Bedner E, et al. Immunocytochemical criteria in the differential diagnosis of malignant melanoma versus carcinoma, lymphoma and sarcoma in fine needle aspirates. *Pathol Pol* 1991;42:73–78.

437. Gyorki DE, Busam K, Panageas K, et al. Sentinel lymph node biopsy for patients with cutaneous desmoplastic melanoma. *Ann Surg Oncol* 2003;10:403–407.

438. Wick MR, Stanley SJ, Swanson PE. Immunohistochemical diagnosis of sinonasal melanoma, carcinoma and neuroblastoma with monoclonal antibodies HMB-45 and anti-synaptophysin. *Arch Pathol Lab Med* 1988;112:616–620.

439. Chen YT, Stockert E, Jungbluth A, et al. Serological analysis of Melan-A(MART–1), a melanocyte-specific protein homoge-

440. Busam KJ, Iversen K, Berwick M, et al. Immunoreactivity with the anti-MAGE antibody 57B in malignant melanoma: frequency of expression and correlation with prognostic parameters. *Mod Pathol* 2000;13:459–465.

441. King R, Weilbaecher KN, McGill G, et al. Microphthalmia transcription factor. A sensitive and specific melanocyte marker for melanoma diagnosis. *Am J Pathol* 1999;155:731–738.

442. Salti GI, Manougian T, Farolan M, et al. Micropthalmia transcription factor: a new prognostic marker in intermediate-thickness cutaneous malignant melanoma. *Cancer Res* 2000;60: 5012–5016.

443. Busam KJ, Iversen K, Coplan KC, et al. Analysis of microphthalmia transcription factor expression in normal tissues and tumors, and comparison of its expression with S-100 protein, gp100, and tyrosinase in desmoplastic malignant melanoma. *Am J Surg Pathol* 2001;25:197–204.

444. Xu X, Chu AY, Pasha TL, et al. Immunoprofile of MITF, tyrosinase, melan-A, MAGE–1 in HMB45-negative melanomas. *Am J Surg Pathol* 2002;26:82–87.

445. Orchard G. Evaluation of melanocytic neoplasms: application of a pan-melanoma antibody cocktail. *Br J Biomed Sci* 2002; 59:196–202.

446. Conley J, Lattes R, Orr W. Desmoplastic malignant melanoma (a rare variant of spindle cell melanoma). *Cancer* 1971;28: 914–935.

447. Hui JI, Linden KG, Barr RJ. Desmoplastic malignant melanoma of the lip: a report of 6 cases and review of the literature. *J Am Acad Dermatol* 2002;47:863–868.

448. Prasad ML, Jungbluth AA, Iversen K, et al. Expression of melanocytic differentiation markers in malignant melanomas of the oral and sinonasal mucosa. *Am J Surg Pathol* 2001;25: 782–787.

449. Mulvany NJ, Sykes P. Desmoplastic melanoma of the vulva. *Pathology* 1997;29:241–245.

450. Rogers RS III, Gibson LE. Mucosal, genital, and unusual clinical variants of melanoma. *Mayo Clin Proc* 1997;72:362–366.

451. Kilpatrick SE, White WL, Browne JD. Desmoplastic malignant melanoma of the oral mucosa—an underrecognized diagnostic pitfall. *Cancer* 1996;78:383–389.

452. Benda JA, Platz CE, Anderson B. Malignant melanoma of the vulva: a clinical-pathologic review of 16 cases. *Int J Gynecol Pathol* 1986;5:202–216.

453. Quinn MJ, Crotty KA, Thompson JF, et al. Desmoplastic and desmoplastic neurotropic melanoma: experience with 280 patients. *Cancer* 1998;83:1128–1135 (see also comments).

454. Labreque PG, Hu C–H, Winkelmann RK. On the nature of desmoplastic melanoma. *Cancer* 1976;38:1205–1213.

455. Kato T, Suetake T, Sugiyama Y, et al. Epidemiology and prognosis of subungual melanoma in 34 Japanese patients. *Br J Dermatol* 1996;134:383–387.

456. Reiman HM, Goellner JR, Woods JE, et al. Desmoplastic melanoma of the head and neck. *Cancer* 1987;60:2269–2274.

457. Jain S, Allen PW. Desmoplastic malignant melanoma and its variants. A study of 45 cases. *Am J Surg Pathol* 1989;13: 358–373.

458. Kubo M, Kikuchi K, Nashiro K, et al. Expression of fibrogenic cytokines in desmoplastic malignant melanoma. *Br J Dermatol* 1998;139:192–197.

459. Innominato PF, Libbrecht L, Van den Oord JJ. Expression of neurotrophins and their receptors in pigment cell lesions of the skin. *J Pathol* 2001;194:95–100.

460. Iwamoto S, Burrows RC, Agoff SN, et al. The p75 neurotrophin receptor, relative to other Schwann cell and mela-

noma markers, is abundantly expressed in spindled melanomas. *Am J Dermatopathol* 2001;23:288–294.

461. Moreno A, Lamarca J, Martinez R, et al. Osteoid and bone formation in desmoplastic malignant melanoma. *J Cutan Pathol* 1986;13:128–134.

462. Reed RJ, Leonard DD. Neurotropic melanoma. A variant of desmoplastic melanoma. *Am J Surg Pathol* 1979;3:301–311.

463. Carlson JA, Dickersin GR, Sober AJ, et al. Desmoplastic neurotropic melanoma: a clinicopathologic analysis of 28 cases. *Cancer* 1995;75:478–494.

464. Reed RJ, Martin P. Variants of melanoma. *Semin Cutan Med Surg* 1997;16:137–158.

465. Tsao H, Sober AJ, Barnhill RL. Desmoplastic neurotropic melanoma. *Semin Cutan Med Surg* 1997;16:131–136.

466. Chorny JA, Barr RJ. S100-positive spindle cells in scars: a diagnostic pitfall in the re-excision of desmoplastic melanoma. *Am J Dermatopathol* 2002;24:309–312.

467. Kamath NV, Ormsby A, Bergfeld WF, et al. A light microscopic and immunohistochemical evaluation of scars. *J Cutan Pathol* 2002;29:27–32.

468. Robson A, Allen P, Hollowood K. S100 expression in cutaneous scars: a potential diagnostic pitfall in the diagnosis of desmoplastic melanoma. *Histopathology* 2001;38:135–140.

469. Cesinaro AM, Morgan MB, Morgan MB. "Connective tissue nevus" and a serendipitous S-100 discovery. *Am J Dermatopathol* 2003;25:86–87.

470. Baron JA, Monzon F, Galaria N, et al. Angiomatoid melanoma: a novel pattern of differentiation in invasive periocular desmoplastic malignant melanoma. *Hum Pathol* 2000;31:1520–1522.

471. Kiene P, Petres-Dunsche C, Fölster-Holst R. Pigmented pedunculated malignant melanoma. A rare variant of nodular melanoma. *Br J Dermatol* 1995;133:300–302.

472. McGovern VJ, Shaw HM, Milton GW. Prognostic significance of a polypoid configuration in malignant melanoma. *Histopathology* 1983;7:663–672.

473. Plotnick H, Rachmaninoff N, VandenBerg HJ Jr. Polypoid melanoma: a virulent variant of nodular melanoma. Report of three cases and literature review. *J Am Acad Dermatol* 1990; 23:880–884.

474. Kuehnl-Petzoldt CH, Berger H, Wiebelt H. Verrucous-keratotic variants of malignant melanoma. A clinicopathologic study. *Am J Dermatopathol* 1982;4:403–410.

475. Blessing K, Evans AT, Al-Nafussi A. Verrucous naevoid and keratotic malignant melanoma: a clinico-pathological study of 20 cases. *Histopathology* 1993;23:453–458.

476. Hanly AJ, Jorda M, Elgart GW. Cutaneous malignant melanoma associated with extensive pseudoepitheliomatous hyperplasia. Report of a case and discussion of the origin of pseudoepitheliomatous hyperplasia. *J Cutan Pathol* 2000;27: 153–156.

477. Kamino H, Tam ST, Alvarez L. Malignant melanoma with pseudocarcinomatous hyperplasia—an entity that can simulate squamous cell carcinoma. A light-microscopic and immunohistochemical study of four cases. *Am J Dermatopathol* 1990;12: 446–451.

478. Kao GF, Helwig EB, Graham JH. Balloon cell malignant melanoma of the skin: a clinicopathologic study of 34 cases with histochemical, immunohistochemical, and ultrastructural observations. *Cancer* 1992;69:2942–2952.

479. Northcutt AD. Epidermotropic xanthoma mimicking balloon cell melanoma. *Am J Dermatopathol* 2000;22:176–178.

480. Mowat A, Reid R, MacKie R. Balloon cell metastatic melanoma: an important differential in the diagnosis of clear cell tumours. *Histopathology* 1994;24:469–472.

481. Sheibani K, Battifora H. Signet-ring cell melanoma. A rare morphologic variant of malignant melanoma. *Am J Surg Pathol* 1988;12:28–34.

482. Livolsi VA, Brooks JJ, Soslow R, et al. Signet cell melanocytic lesions. *Mod Pathol* 1992;5:515–520.

483. Bastian BC, Kutzner H, Yen T, et al. Signet-ring cell formation in cutaneous neoplasms. *J Am Acad Dermatol* 1999;41:606–613.

484. Sanders DSA, Evans AT, Allen CA, et al. Classification of CEA-related positivity in primary and metastatic malignant melanoma. *J Pathol* 1994;172:343–348.

485. Selby WL, Nance KV, Park HK. CEA immunoreactivity in metastatic malignant melanoma. *Mod Pathol* 1992;5:415–419.

486. Bhuta S, Mirra JM, Cochran AJ. Myxoid malignant melanoma. A previously undescribed histologic pattern noted in metastatic lesions and a report of four cases. *Am J Surg Pathol* 1986;10:203–211.

487. Hitchcock MG, McCalmont TH, White WL. Cutaneous melanoma with myxoid features: twelve cases with differential diagnosis. *Am J Surg Pathol* 1999;23:1506–1513.

488. Crowson AN, Magro CM, Mihm MCJ. Malignant melanoma with prominent pigment synthesis: "animal type" melanoma—a clinical and histological study of six cases with a consideration of other melanocytic neoplasms with prominent pigment synthesis. *Hum Pathol* 1999;30:543–550.

489. Elder DE, Murphy GF. Malignant tumors (melanomas and related lesions). In: Elder DE, Murphy GF, eds. *Melanocytic tumors of the skin*. Washington, DC: Armed Forces Institute of Pathology, 1991:103–206.

490. Zembowicz A, Carney JA, Mihm MC. Pigmented epithelioid melanocytoma: a low-grade melanocytic tumor with metastatic potential indistinguishable from animal-type melanoma and epithelioid blue nevus. *Am J Surg Pathol* 2004;28:31–40.

491. Muhlbauer JE, Margolis RJ, Mihm MC Jr, et al. Minimal deviation melanoma: a histologic variant of cutaneous malignant melanoma in its vertical growth phase. *J Invest Dermatol* 1983; 80:63S–65S.

492. Chorny JA, Barr RJ, Kyshtoobayeva A, et al. Ki-67 and p53 expression in minimal deviation melanomas as compared with other nevomelanocytic lesions. *Mod Pathol* 2003;16:525–529.

493. Levene A. On the histological diagnosis and prognosis of malignant melanoma. *J Clin Pathol* 1980;33:101–124.

494. Schmoeckel C, Castro CE, Braun-Falco O. Nevoid malignant melanoma. *Arch Dermatol Res* 1985;277:362–369.

495. Ruhoy SM, Prieto VG, Eliason SL, et al. Malignant melanoma with paradoxical maturation. *Am J Surg Pathol* 2000;24: 1600–1614.

496. McNutt NS. "Triggered trap": nevoid malignant melanoma. *Semin Diagn Pathol* 1998;15:203–209.

497. Armstrong BK, Kricker A. The epidemiology of UV induced skin cancer. *J Photochem Photobiol B* 2001;63:8–18.

498. Hemminki K, Zhang H, Czene K. Incidence trends and familial risks in invasive and in situ cutaneous melanoma by sun-exposed body sites. *Int J Cancer* 2003;104:764–771.

499. Nelemans PJ, Groenendal H, Kiemeney LA, et al. Effect of intermittent exposure to sunlight on melanoma risk among indoor workers and sun-sensitive individuals. *Environ Health Perspect* 1993;101:252–255.

500. Elwood JM, Gallagher RP, Worth AJ, et al. Etiological differences between subtypes of cutaneous malignant melanoma: Western Canada Melanoma Study. *J Natl Cancer Inst* 1987;78: 37–44.

501. Urso C, Giannotti V, Reali UM, et al. Spatial association of melanocytic naevus and melanoma. *Melanoma Res* 1991;1: 245–249.

502. Marks R, Dorevitch AP, Mason G. Do all melanomas come from "moles"? A study of the histological association between melanocytic naevi and melanoma. *Australas J Dermatol* 1990; 31:77–80.

503. Smolle J, Kaddu S, Kerl H. Non-random spatial association of melanoma and naevi—a morphometric analysis. *Melanoma Res* 1999;9:407–412.

504. Bogdan I, Smolle J, Kerl H, et al. Melanoma ex naevo: a study of the associated naevus. *Melanoma Res* 2003;13:213–217.

505. Eskandarpour M, Hashemi J, Kanter L, et al. Frequency of UV-inducible NRAS mutations in melanomas of patients with germline CDKN2A mutations. *J Natl Cancer Inst* 2003;95: 790–798.

506. Tajima Y, Nakajima T, Sugano I, et al. Malignant melanoma within an intradermal nevus. *Am J Dermatopathol* 1994;16: 301–306.

507. Slingluff CL Jr, Vollmer RT, Seigler HF. Multiple primary melanoma: incidence and risk factors in 283 patients. *Surgery* 1993;113:330–339.

508. Stam-Posthuma JJ, Duinen C, Scheffer E, et al. Multiple primary melanomas. *J Am Acad Dermatol* 2001;44:22–27.

509. Conrad N, Leis P, Orengo I, et al. Multiple primary melanoma. *Dermatol Surg* 1999;25:576–581.

510. Johnson TM, Hamilton T, Lowe L. Multiple primary melanomas. *J Am Acad Dermatol* 1998;39:422–427.

511. MacKie RM. Multiple melanoma and atypical melanocytic nevi—evidence of an activated and expanded melanocytic system. *Br J Dermatol* 1982;107:621–629.

512. Moseley HS, Giuliano AE, Storm FK 3d, et al. Multiple primary melanoma. *Cancer* 1979;43:939–944.

513. Abernethy JL, Soyer HP, Kerl H, et al. Epidermotropic metastatic malignant melanoma simulating melanoma in situ: a report of 10 examples from two patients. *Am J Surg Pathol* 1994;18:1140–1149.

514. Blackwood MA, Holmes R, Synnestvedt M, et al. Multiple primary melanoma revisited. *Cancer* 2002;94:2248–2255.

515. Skov-Jensen T, Hastrup J, Lambrethsen E. Malignant melanoma in children. *Cancer* 1966;19:620–626.

516. Barnhill RL, Flotte TJ, Fleischli M, et al. Cutaneous melanoma and atypical Spitz tumors in childhood. *Cancer* 1995;76: 1833–1845.

517. Crotty KA, McCarthy SW, Palmer AA, et al. Malignant melanoma in childhood: a clinicopathologic study of 13 cases and comparison with Spitz nevi. *World J Surg* 1992;16:179–185.

518. Wong TY, Duncan LM, Mihm MC Jr. Melanoma mimicking dermal and Spitz's nevus ("nevoid" melanoma). *Semin Surg Oncol* 1993;9:188–193.

519. Rampen FH, Van der Esch EP. Biopsy and survival of malignant melanoma. *J Am Acad Dermatol* 1985;12:385–388.

520. Lederman JS, Sober AJ. Does biopsy type influence survival in clinical stage I cutaneous melanoma? *J Am Acad Dermatol* 1985;13:983–987.

521. Sondergaard K, Schou G. Therapeutic and clinico-pathological factors in the survival of 1,469 patients with primary cutaneous malignant melanoma in clinical stage I. A multivariate regression analysis. *Virchows Arch [A]* 1985;408:249–258.

522. Landthaler M, Braun-Falco O, Leitl A, et al. Excisional biopsy as the first therapeutic procedure versus primary wide excision of malignant melanoma. *Cancer* 1989;64:1612–1616.

523. Bong JL, Herd RM, Hunter JA. Incisional biopsy and melanoma prognosis. *J Am Acad Dermatol* 2002;46:690–694.

524. Hauschild A, Rosien F, Lischner S. Surgical standards in the primary care of melanoma patients. *Onkologie* 2003;26:218–222.

525. Day CL Jr, Sober AJ, Kopf AW, et al. A prognostic model for clinical stage I melanoma of the upper extremity. The importance of anatomic subsites in predicting recurrent disease. *Ann Surg* 1981;193:436–440.

526. Day CL Jr, Sober AJ, Kopf AW, et al. A prognostic model for clinical stage I melanoma of the lower extremity. Location on

527. Day CL Jr, Sober AJ, Kopf AW, et al. A prognostic model for clinical stage I melanoma of the trunk Location near the midline is not an independent risk factor for recurrent disease. *Am J Surg* 1981;142:247–251.

528. MacKie RM, Aitchison T, Sirel JM, et al. Prognostic models for subgroups of melanoma patients from the Scottish Melanoma Group database 1979–86, and their subsequent validation. *Br J Cancer* 1995;71:173–176.

529. Barnhill RL, Fine JA, Roush GC, et al. Predicting five-year outcome for patients with cutaneous melanoma in a population-based study. *Cancer* 1996;78:427–432.

530. Mackie RM, Hole D, Hunter JA, et al. Cutaneous malignant melanoma in Scotland: incidence, survival, and mortality 1979–94. *Br Med J* 1997;315:1117–1121.

531. Schuchter L, Schultz DJ, Synnestvedt M, et al. A prognostic model for predicting 10-year survival in patients with primary melanoma. *Ann Intern Med* 1996;125:369–375.

532. Soong S-J, Weiss HL. Predicting outcome in patients with localized melanoma. In: Balch CM, Houghton AN, Sober AJ, et al., eds. *Cutaneous melanoma*. St. Louis: Quality Medical Publishing, 1998:51–64.

533. Cochran AJ, Elashoff D, Morton DL, Elashoff R. Individualized prognosis for melanoma patients. *Hum Pathol* 2000;31: 327–331.

534. Balch CM, Soong SJ, Gershenwald JE, et al. Prognostic factors analysis of 17,600 melanoma patients: validation of the american joint committee on cancer melanoma staging system. *J Clin Oncol* 2001;19:3622–3634.

535. Ferrone CR, Panageas KS, Busam K, et al. Multivariate prognostic model for patients with thick cutaneous melanoma: importance of sentinel lymph node status. *Ann Surg Oncol* 2002; 9:637–645.

536. Gimotty PA, Guerry D, Elder DE. Validation of prognostic models for melanoma. *Am J Clin Pathol* 2002;118:489–491.

537. Balch CM, Buzaid AC, Soong SJ, et al. Final version of the american joint committee on cancer staging system for cutaneous melanoma. *J Clin Oncol* 2001;19:3635–3648.

538. Green FL, Page DL, Fleming ID, et al. Melanoma of the skin. In: Green FL, et al., eds. *AJCC cancer staging manual/American Joint Committee on Cancer*. New York: Springer/Verlag, 2002: 209–217.

539. Kretschmer L, Neumann C, Preusser KP, et al. Superficial inguinal and radical ilioinguinal lymph node dissection in patients with palpable melanoma metastases to the groin—an analysis of survival and local recurrence. *Acta Oncol* 2001;40:72–78.

540. Hughes TM, A'Hern RP, Thomas JM. Prognosis and surgical management of patients with palpable inguinal lymph node metastases from melanoma. *Br J Surg* 2000;87:892–901.

541. Kretschmer L, Preusser KP, Marsch WC, et al. Prognostic factors of overall survival in patients with delayed lymph node dissection for cutaneous malignant melanoma. *Melanoma Res* 2000;10:483–489.

542. Messaris GE, Konstadoulakis MM, Ricaniadis N, et al. Prognostic variables for patients with stage III malignant melanoma. *Eur J Surg* 2000;166:233–239.

543. Mann GB, Coit DG. Does the extent of operation influence the prognosis in patients with melanoma metastatic to inguinal nodes? *Ann Surg Oncol* 1999;6:263–271 (see also comments).

544. Strobbe LJ, Jonk A, Hart AA, et al. Positive iliac and obturator nodes in melanoma: survival and prognostic factors. *Ann Surg Oncol* 1999;6:255–262 (see also comments).

545. Day CL Jr, Sober AJ, Lew RA, et al. Malignant melanoma patients with positive nodes and relatively good prognoses: microstaging retains prognostic significance in clinical stage I mel-

anoma patients with metastases to regional nodes. *Cancer* 1981;47:955–962.

546. Balch CM, Soong SJ, Murad TM, et al. A multifactorial analysis of melanoma. III. Prognostic factors in melanoma patients with lymph node metastases (stage II). *Ann Surg* 1981;193: 377–388.

547. Cochran AJ, Lana AMA, Wen D-R. Histomorphometry in the assessment of prognosis in stage II malignant melanoma. *Am J Surg Pathol* 1989;13:600–604.

548. Schuchter LM. Review of the 2001 AJCC staging system for cutaneous malignant melanoma. *Curr Oncol Rep* 2001;3: 332–337.

549. Ruiter DJ, Testori A, Eggermont AM, et al. The AJCC staging proposal for cutaneous melanoma: comments by the EORTC Melanoma Group. *Ann Oncol* 2001;12:9–11.

550. Beahrs OH, Myers MH. *Manual for staging of cancer*. Philadelphia: Lippincott, 1983:117–122.

551. Buzaid AC, Ross MI, Balch CM, et al. Critical analysis of the current American Joint Committee on Cancer staging system for cutaneous melanoma and proposal of a new staging system. *J Clin Oncol* 1997;15:1039–1051.

552. Abramova L, Slingluff L, Patterson JW. Problems in the interpretation of apparent "radial growth phase" malignant melanomas that metastasize. *J Cutan Pathol* 2002;29:407–414.

553. Sondergaard K, Hou Jensen K. Partial regression in thin primary cutaneous malignant melanomas clinical stage I. A study of 486 cases. *Virchows Arch [A]* 1985;408:241–247.

554. Ronan SG, Eng AM, Briele HA, et al. Thin malignant melanomas with regression and metastases. *Arch Dermatol* 1987;123:1326–1330.

555. Prehn RT. The paradoxical association of regression with a poor prognosis in melanoma contrasted with a good prognosis in keratoacanthoma. *Cancer Res* 1996;56:937–940.

556. Cook MG, Clarke TJ, Humphreys S, et al. A nationwide survey of observer variation in the diagnosis of thin cutaneous malignant melanoma including the MIN terminology. *J Clin Pathol* 1997;50:202–205.

557. Cook MG, Spatz A, Brocker EB, et al. Identification of histological features associated with metastatic potential in thin (<1.0 mm) cutaneous melanoma with metastases. A study on behalf of the EORTC Melanoma Group. *J Pathol* 2002;197: 188–193.

558. Mihm MC Jr, Clark WH Jr, From L. The clinical diagnosis, classification and histogenetic concepts of the early stages of cutaneous malignant melanomas. *N Engl J Med* 1971;284: 1078–1082.

559. Morton DL, Davtyan DG, Wanek LA, et al. Multivariate analysis of the relationship between survival and the microstage of primary melanoma by Clark level and Breslow thickness. *Cancer* 1993;71:3737–3743.

560. Kelly JW, Sagebiel RW, Clyman S, et al. Thin level IV malignant melanoma. A subset in which level is the major prognostic indicator. *Ann Surg* 1985;202:98–103.

561. Marghoob AA, Koenig K, Bittencourt FV, et al. Breslow thickness and clark level in melanoma: support for including level in pathology reports and in American Joint Committee on Cancer Staging. *Cancer* 2000;88:589–595 (see also comments).

562. Büttner P, Garbe C, Bertz J, et al. Primary cutaneous melanoma: optimized cutoff points of tumor thickness and importance of Clark's level for prognostic classification. *Cancer* 1995;75:2499–2506.

563. Scolyer RA, Shaw HM, Thompson JF, et al. Interobserver reproducibility of histopathologic prognostic variables in primary cutaneous melanomas. *Am J Surg Pathol* 2003;27:1571–1576.

564. Breslow A. Thickness, cross-sectional areas and depth of invasion in the prognosis of cutaneous melanoma. *Ann Surg* 1970; 172:902–908.

565. Breslow A. Tumor thickness, level of invasion and node dissection in stage I cutaneous melanoma. *Ann Surg* 1975;182: 572–575.

566. Oliveira Filho RS, Ferreira LM, Biasi LJ, et al. Vertical growth phase and positive sentinel node in thin melanoma. *Braz J Med Biol Res* 2003;36:347–350.

567. Bedrosian I, Faries MB, Guerry D, et al. Incidence of sentinel node metastasis in patients with thin primary melanoma (< or = 1 mm) with vertical growth phase. *Ann Surg Oncol* 2000; 7:262–267 (see also comments).

568. Smolle J. Biological significance of tumor thickness. Theoretical considerations based on computer simulation. *Am J Dermatopathol* 1995;17:281–286.

569. Breslow A. Prognostic factors in the treatment of cutaneous melanoma. *J Cutan Pathol* 1979;6:208–212.

570. Guitart J, Lowe L, Piepkorn M, et al. Histological characteristics of metastasizing thin melanomas: a case-control study of 43 cases. *Arch Dermatol* 2002;138:603–608.

571. Corona R, Mele A, Amini M, et al. Interobserver variability on the histopathologic diagnosis of cutaneous melanoma and other pigmented skin lesions. *J Clin Oncol* 1996;14:1218–1223.

572. Lock-Andersen J, Hou-Jensen K, Hansen JPH, et al. Observer variation in histological classification of cutaneous malignant melanoma. *Scand J Plast Reconstr Surg Hand Surg* 1995;29: 141–148.

573. Clemente CG, Mihm MG, Bufalino R, et al. Prognostic value of tumor infiltrating lymphocytes in the vertical growth phase of primary cutaneous melanoma. *Cancer* 1996; 77:1303–1310.

574. Håkansson A, Gustafsson B, Krysander L, et al. Tumour-infiltrating lymphocytes in metastatic malignant melanoma and response to interferon alpha treatment. *Br J Cancer* 1996;74: 670–676.

575. Massi D, Franchi A, Borgognoni L, et al. Thin cutaneous malignant melanomas (< or = 1.5 mm): identification of risk factors indicative of progression. *Cancer* 1999;85:1067–1076.

576. Barr RJ. The many faces of completely regressed malignant melanoma. In: LeBoit PE, ed. *Malignant melanoma and melanocytic neoplasms*. Philadelphia: Hanley & Belfus, 1994: 359–370.

577. Flax SH, Skelton HG, Smith KJ, et al. Nodular melanosis due to epithelial neoplasms: a finding not restricted to regressed melanomas. *Am J Dermatopathol* 1998;20:118–122.

578. Jonk A, Kroon BBR, Rümke P, et al. Lymph node metastasis from melanoma with an unknown primary site. *Br J Surg* 1990;77:665–668.

579. Tuthill RJ, Unger JM, Liu PY, et al. Risk assessment in localized primary cutaneous melanoma: a Southwest Oncology Group study evaluating nine factors and a test of the Clark logistic regression prediction model. *Am J Clin Pathol* 2002;118: 504–511.

580. Masback A, Olsson H, Westerdahl J, et al. Prognostic factors in invasive cutaneous malignant melanoma: a population-based study and review. *Melanoma Res* 2001;11:435–445.

581. Hernberg M, Turunen JP, Muhonen T, et al. Tumor-infiltrating lymphocytes in patients with metastatic melanoma receiving chemoimmunotherapy. *J Immunother* 1997;20:488–495.

582. Mihm MC Jr, Clemente CG, Cascinelli N. Tumor infiltrating lymphocytes in lymph node melanoma metastases: a histopathologic prognostic indicator and an expression of local immune response. *Lab Invest* 1996;74:43–47.

583. Clark WH Jr, Elder DE, Guerry D, et al. Model predicting survival in stage I melanoma based on tumor progression. *J Natl Cancer Inst* 1989;81:1893–1904.

584. Busam KJ, Antonescu CR, Marghoob AA, et al. Histologic classification of tumor-infiltrating lymphocytes in primary cutaneous malignant melanoma. A study of interobserver agreement. *Am J Clin Pathol* 2001;115:856–860.

585. Azzola MF, Shaw HM, Thompson JF, et al. Tumor mitotic rate is a more powerful prognostic indicator than ulceration in patients with primary cutaneous melanoma: an analysis of 3661 patients from a single center. *Cancer* 2003;97:1488–1498.

586. Ostmeier H, Fuchs B, Otto F, et al. Can immunohistochemical markers and mitotic rate improve prognostic precision in patients with primary melanoma? *Cancer* 1999;85:2391–2399.

587. Karjalainen JM, Eskelinen MJ, Nordling S, et al. Mitotic rate and S-phase fraction as prognostic factors in stage I cutaneous malignant melanoma. *Br J Cancer* 1998;77:1917–1925.

588. Schmoeckel C, Bockelbrink A, Bockelbrink H, et al. Low- and high-risk malignant melanoma. I. Evaluation of clinical and histological prognosticators in 585 cases. *Eur J Cancer Clin Oncol* 1983;19:227–235.

589. Schmoeckel C, Bockelbrink A, Bockelbrink H, et al. Low- and high-risk malignant melanoma. II. Multivariate analyses for a prognostic classification. *Eur J Cancer Clin Oncol* 1983;19:237–243.

590. Larsen TE, Grude TH. A retrospective histological study of 669 cases of primary cutaneous malignant melanoma in clinical stage I. 2. The relation of cell type, pigmentation, atypia and mitotic count to histological type and prognosis. *Acta Pathol Microbiol Scand [A]* 1978;86A:513–522.

591. Talve LA, Collan YU, Ekfors TO. Nuclear morphometry, immunohistochemical staining with Ki-67 antibody and mitotic index in the assessment of proliferative activity and prognosis of primary malignant melanomas of the skin. *J Cutan Pathol* 1996;23:335–343.

592. Bentzen JK, Hansen HS, Nielsen HW. The prognostic importance of volume-weighted mean nuclear volume, mitotic index, and other stereologically measured quantitative parameters in supraglottic laryngeal carcinoma. *Cancer* 1999;86:2222–2228.

593. Cherpelis BS, Haddad F, Messina J, et al. Sentinel lymph node micrometastasis and other histologic factors that predict outcome in patients with thicker melanomas. *J Am Acad Dermatol* 2001;44:762–766.

594. Zettersten E, Sagebiel RW, Miller JR III, et al. Prognostic factors in patients with thick cutaneous melanoma (> 4 mm). *Cancer* 2002;94:1049–1056.

595. Keilholz U, Martus P, Punt CJ, et al. Prognostic factors for survival and factors associated with long-term remission in patients with advanced melanoma receiving cytokine-based treatments. Second analysis of a randomised EORTC Melanoma Group trial comparing interferon-alpha2a (IFNalpha) and interleukin 2 (IL–2) with or without cisplatin. *Eur J Cancer* 2002;38:1501–1511.

596. Frahm SO, Schubert C, Parwaresch R, et al. High proliferative activity may predict early metastasis of thin melanomas. *Hum Pathol* 2001;32:1376–1381.

597. Spatz A, Cook MG, Elder DE, et al. Interobserver reproducibility of ulceration assessment in primary cutaneous melanomas. *Eur J Cancer* 2003;39:1861–1865.

598. Larsen TE, Grude TH. A retrospective histological study of 669 cases of primary cutaneous malignant melanoma in clinical stage I. 4. The relation of cross-sectional profile, level of invasion, ulceration and vascular invasion to tumour type and prognosis. *Acta Pathol Microbiol Scand [A]* 1979;87A:131–138.

599. Balch CM, Wilkerson JA, Murad TM, et al. The prognostic significance of ulceration of cutaneous melanoma. *Cancer* 1980;45:3012–3017.

600. Tan GJ, Baak JP. Evaluation of prognostic characteristics of stage I cutaneous malignant melanoma. *Anal Quant Cytol* 1984;6:147–154.

601. Sondergaard K, Schou G. Survival with primary cutaneous malignant melanoma, evaluated from 2012 cases. A multivariate regression analysis. *Virchows Arch A Pathol Anat Histopathol* 1985;406:179–195.

602. Mraz-Gernhard S, Sagebiel RW, Kashani-Sabet M, et al. Prediction of sentinel lymph node micrometastasis by histological features in primary cutaneous malignant melanoma. *Arch Dermatol* 1998;134:983–987.

603. Balch CM, Buzaid AC, Atkins MB, et al. A new American Joint Committee on *Cancer* staging system for cutaneous melanoma. *Cancer* 2000;88:1484–1491.

604. Balch CM, Soong S, Ross MI, et al. Long-term results of a multi-institutional randomized trial comparing prognostic factors and surgical results for intermediate thickness melanomas (1.0 to 4.0 mm). Intergroup Melanoma Surgical Trial. *Ann Surg Oncol* 2000;7:87–97 (see also comments).

605. Massi D, Borgognoni L, Franchi A, et al. Thick cutaneous malignant melanoma: a reappraisal of prognostic factors. *Melanoma Res* 2000;10:153–164.

606. Retsas S, Henry K, Mohammed MQ, et al. Prognostic factors of cutaneous melanoma and a new staging system proposed by the American Joint Committee on Cancer (AJCC). Validation in a cohort of 1284 patients. *Eur J Cancer* 2002;38:511–516.

607. Niezabitowski A, Czajecki K, Rys J, et al. Prognostic evaluation of cutaneous malignant melanoma: a clinicopathologic and immunohistochemical study. *J Surg Oncol* 1999;70:150–160.

608. Straume O, Akslen LA. Independent prognostic importance of vascular invasion in nodular melanomas. *Cancer* 1996;78:1211–1219.

609. Kashani-Sabet M, Sagebiel RW, Ferreira CM, et al. Vascular involvement in the prognosis of primary cutaneous melanoma. *Arch Dermatol* 2001;137:1169–1173.

610. Borgstein PJ, Meijer S, Van Diest PJ. Are locoregional cutaneous metastases in melanoma predictable? *Ann Surg Oncol* 1999;6:315–321.

611. Kashani-Sabet M, Sagebiel RW, Ferreira CM, et al. Tumor vascularity in the prognostic assessment of primary cutaneous melanoma. *J Clin Oncol* 2002;20:1826–1831.

612. Busam KJ, Berwick M, Blessing K, et al. Tumor vascularity is not a prognostic factor for malignant melanoma of the skin. *Am J Pathol* 1995;147:1049–1056.

613. Harrist TJ, Rigel DS, Day CL Jr, et al. "Microscopic satellites" are more highly associated with regional lymph node metastases than is primary melanoma thickness. *Cancer* 1984;53:2183–2187.

614. León P, Daly JM, Synnestvedt M, et al. The prognostic implications of microscopic satellites in patients with clinical stage I melanoma. *Arch Surg* 1991;126:1461–1468.

615. Garbe C, Büttner P, Bertz J, et al. Primary cutaneous melanoma: prognostic classification of anatomic location. *Cancer* 1995;75:2492–2498.

616. Huang X, Soong SJ, McCarthy WH, et al. Classification of localized melanoma by the exponential survival trees method. *Cancer* 1997;79:1122–1128.

617. Sahin S, Rao B, Kopf AW, et al. Predicting ten-year survival of patients with primary cutaneous melanoma—corroboration of a prognostic model. *Cancer* 1997;80:1426–1431.

618. Hsueh EC, Lucci A, Qi K, et al. Survival of patients with melanoma of the lower extremity decreases with distance from the trunk. *Cancer* 1999;85:383–388.

619. Averbook BJ, Fu P, Rao JS, et al. A long-term analysis of 1018 patients with melanoma by classic Cox regression and tree-structured survival analysis at a major referral center: implications on the future of cancer staging. *Surgery* 2002;132:589–604.
620. Måsbäck A, Westerdahl J, Ingvar C, et al. Cutaneous malignant melanoma in southern Sweden 1965, 1975, and 1985—prognostic factors and histologic correlations. *Cancer* 1997;79:275–283.
621. Stidham KR, Johnson JL, Seigler HF. Survival superiority of females with melanoma: a multivariate analysis of 6383 patients exploring the significance of gender in prognostic outcome. *Arch Surg* 1994;129:316–324.
622. Averbook BJ, Russo LJ, Mansour EG. A long-term analysis of 620 patients with malignant melanoma at a major referral center. *Surgery* 1998;124:746–755.
623. Langford FP, Fisher SR, Molter DW, et al. Lentigo maligna melanoma of the head and neck. *Laryngoscope* 1993;103:520–524.
624. O'Brien CJ, Coates AS, Petersen-Schaefer K, et al. Experience with 998 cutaneous melanomas of the head and neck over 30 years. *Am J Surg* 1991;162:310–314.
625. Larsen TE, Grude TH. A retrospective histological study of 669 cases of primary cutaneous malignant melanoma in clinical stage I. 3. The relation between the tumour-associated lymphocyte infiltration and age and sex, tumour cell type, pigmentation, cellular atypia, mitotic count, depth of invasion, ulceration, tumour type and prognosis. *Acta Pathol Microbiol Scand [A]* 1978;86A:523–530.
626. Larsen TE, Grude TH. A retrospective histological study of 669 cases of primary cutaneous malignant melanoma in clinical stage I. I. Histological classification, sex and age of the patients, localization of tumour and prognosis. *Acta Pathol Microbiol Scand [A]* 1978;86A:437–450.
627. Moretti S, Spallanzani A, Chiarugi A, et al. Correlation of Ki-67 expression in cutaneous primary melanoma with prognosis in a prospective study: different correlation according to thickness. *J Am Acad Dermatol* 2001;44:188–192.
628. Korabiowska M, Brinck U, Middel P, et al. Proliferative activity in the progression of pigmented skin lesions, diagnostic and prognostic significance. *Anticancer Res* 2000;20:1781–1785.
629. Straume O, Sviland L, Akslen LA. Loss of nuclear p16 protein expression correlates with increased tumor cell proliferation (Ki-67) and poor prognosis in patients with vertical growth phase melanoma. *Clin Cancer Res* 2000;6:1845–1853.
630. Vlaykova T, Talve L, Hahka-Kemppinen M, et al. MIB-1 immunoreactivity correlates with blood vessel density and survival in disseminated malignant melanoma. *Oncology* 1999;57:242–252.
631. Sparrow LE, English DR, Taran JM, et al. Prognostic significance of MIB-1 proliferative activity in thin melanomas and immunohistochemical analysis of MIB-1 proliferative activity in melanocytic tumors. *Am J Dermatopathol* 1998;20:12–16.
632. Böni R, Doguoglu A, Burg G, et al. MIB-1 immunoreactivity correlates with metastatic dissemination in primary thick cutaneous melanoma. *J Am Acad Dermatol* 1996;35:416–418.
633. Ramsay JA, From L, Iscoe NA, et al. MIB-1 proliferative activity is a significant prognostic factor in primary thick cutaneous melanomas. *J Invest Dermatol* 1995;105:22–26.
634. Ringborg U, Andersson R, Eldh J, et al. Resection margins of 2 versus 5 cm for cutaneous malignant melanoma with a tumor thickness of 0.8 to 2.0 mm—a randomized study by the Swedish melanoma study group. *Cancer* 1996;77:1809–1814.
635. National Institutes of Health. Consensus Development Conference. Diagnosis and treatment of early melanoma. *JAMA* 1992;268:1314–1319.
636. Lens MB, Dawes M, Goodacre T, et al. Excision margins in the treatment of primary cutaneous melanoma: a systematic review of randomized controlled trials comparing narrow vs wide excision. *Arch Surg* 2002;137:1101–1105.
637. Balch CM, Soong SJ, Smith T, et al. Long-term results of a prospective surgical trial comparing 2 cm vs. 4 cm excision margins for 740 patients with 1–4 mm melanomas. *Ann Surg Oncol* 2001;8:101–108.
638. Balch CM, Urist MM, Karakousis CP, et al. Efficacy of 2-cm surgical margins for intermediate-thickness melanomas (1 to 4 mm). Results of a multi-institutional randomized surgical trial. *Ann Surg* 1993;218:262–267.
639. Veronesi U, Cascinelli N, Adamus J, et al. Thin stage I primary cutaneous malignant melanoma. Comparison of excision with margins of 1 or 3 cm. *N Engl J Med* 1988;318:1159–1162.
640. Piepkorn M. Melanoma resection margin recommendations, unconventionally based on available facts. *Semin Diagn Pathol* 1998;15:230–234.
641. Heenan PJ. Melanoma: margins for error. *ANZ J Surg* 2002;72:300–303.
642. Ackerman AB, Scheiner AM. How wide and deep is wide and deep enough? A critique of surgical practice in excisions of primary cutaneous malignant melanoma. *Hum Pathol* 1983;14:743–744.
643. Balch CM. Surgical margins for melanoma: is 2 cm too much? *ANZ J Surg* 2002;72:251–252.
644. Elder DE, Guerry DIV, Heiberger RM, et al. Optimal resection margin for cutaneous malignant melanoma. *Plast Reconstr Surg* 1983;71:66–72.
645. Serpell JW, Carne PW, Bailey M. Radical lymph node dissection for melanoma. *ANZ J Surg* 2003;73:294–299.
646. Breslow A. Surgical pros and cons. The debate over immediate lymph node dissection in melanoma. *Surg Gynecol Obstet* 1979;149:731–732.
647. Balch CM, Soong SJ, Milton GW, et al. A comparison of prognostic factors and surgical results in 1,786 patients with localized (stage I) melanoma treated in Alabama, USA, New South Wales, Australia. *Ann Surg* 1982;196:677–684.
648. Milton GW, Shaw HM, McCarthy WH, et al. Prophylactic lymph node dissection in clinical stage I cutaneous malignant melanoma: results of surgical treatment in 1319 patients. *Br J Surg* 1982;69:108–111.
649. Veronesi U. Regional lymph node dissection in melanoma of the limbs. Stage I. A cooperative international trial (WHO Collaborating Centers for diagnosis and treatment of melanoma). *Recent Results Cancer Res* 1977;62:8.
650. Veronesi U, Adamus J, Bandiera DC, et al. Inefficacy of immediate node dissection in stage 1 melanoma of the limbs. *N Engl J Med* 1977;297:627–630.
651. Sim FH, Taylor WF, Ivins JC, et al. A prospective randomized study of the efficacy of routine elective lymphadenectomy in management of malignant melanoma. Preliminary results. *Cancer* 1978;41:948–956.
652. Balch CM, Soong SJ, Murad TM, et al. A multifactorial analysis of melanoma III. Prognostic factors in melanoma patients with lymph node metastases (stage II). *Ann Surg* 193:377–388.
653. Elder DE, Guerry DIV, VanHorn M, et al. The role of lymph node dissection for clinical stage I malignant melanoma of intermediate thickness (1.51–3.99 mm). *Cancer* 1985;56:413–418.
654. Essner R. Surgical treatment of malignant melanoma. *Surg Clin North Am* 2003;83:109–156.
655. Zimmermann T, Andresen S, Schmitt H, et al. Elective lymph node dissection. *Zentralbl Chir* 2001;126:279–282.

656. Buzaid AC, Tinoco LA, Jendiroba D, et al. Prognostic value of size of lymph node metastases in patients with cutaneous melanoma. *J Clin Oncol* 1995;13:2361–2368.

657. Morton DL, Thompson JF, Essner R, et al. Validation of the accuracy of intraoperative lymphatic mapping and sentinel lymphadenectomy for early-stage melanoma: a multicenter trial. Multicenter Selective Lymphadenectomy Trial Group. *Ann Surg* 1999;230:453–463.

658. Morton DL, Wen DR, Foshag LJ, et al. Intraoperative lymphatic mapping and selective cervical lymphadenectomy for early-stage melanomas of the head and neck. *J Clin Oncol* 1993;11:1751–1756.

659. Shidham VB, Qi DY, Acker S, et al. Evaluation of micrometastases in sentinel lymph nodes of cutaneous melanoma: higher diagnostic accuracy with Melan-a and Mart-1 compared with S-100 protein and Hmb-45. *Am J Surg Pathol* 2001;25:1039–1046.

660. Shidham VB, Qi D, Rao RN, et al. Improved immunohistochemical evaluation of micrometastases in sentinel lymph nodes of cutaneous melanoma with "MCW melanoma cocktail"—a mixture of monoclonal antibodies to MART-1, Melan-A, tyrosinase. *BMC Cancer* 2003;3:15.

661. Association of Directors of Anatomic and Surgical Pathology. ADASP recommendations for the processing and reporting of lymph node specimens submitted for evaluation of metastatic disease. *Mod Pathol* 2001;14:629–632.

662. Kwittken J, Negri L. Malignant blue nevus. Case report of a Negro woman. *Arch Dermatol* 1966;94:64–69.

663. Merkow LP, Burt RC, Hayeslip DW, et al. A cellular and malignant blue nevus: a light and electron microscopic study. *Cancer* 1969;24:888–896.

664. Granter SR, McKee PH, Calonje E, et al. Melanoma associated with blue nevus and melanoma mimicking cellular blue nevus: a clinicopathologic study of 10 cases on the spectrum of so-called "malignant blue nevus". *Am J Surg Pathol* 2001;25:316–323.

665. Hernandez FJ. Malignant blue nevus. A light and electron microscopic study. *Arch Dermatol* 1973;107:741–744.

666. Goldenhersh MA, Savin RC, Barnhill RL, et al. Malignant blue nevus. Case report and literature review. *J Am Acad Dermatol* 1988;19:712–722.

667. McGinnis KS, Lessin SR, Elder DE, et al. Pathology review of cases presenting to a multidisciplinary pigmented lesion clinic. *Arch Dermatol* 2002;138:617–621.

668. Balch CM, Buzaid AC, Soong SJ, et al. New TNM melanoma staging system: linking biology and natural history to clinical outcomes. *Semin Surg Oncol* 2003;21:43–52.

669. Su LD, Fullen DR, Sondak VK, et al. Sentinel lymph node biopsy for patients with problematic Spitzoid melanocytic lesions: a report on 18 patients. *Cancer* 2003;97:499–507.

670. Kelley SW, Cockerell CJ. Sentinel lymph node biopsy as an adjunct to management of histologically difficult to diagnose melanocytic lesions: a proposal. *J Am Acad Dermatol* 2000;42:527–530.

671. Mihic-Probst D, Zhao J, Saremaslani P, et al. Spitzoid malignant melanoma with lymph-node metastasis. Is a copy-number loss on chromosome 6q a marker of malignancy? *Virchows Arch* 2001;439:823–826.

672. Barnhill RL, Argenyi ZB, From L, et al. Atypical Spitz nevi/tumors: lack of consensus for diagnosis, discrimination from melanoma, and prediction of outcome. *Hum Pathol* 1999;30:513–520.

673. Rogers GS, Kopf AW, Rigel DS, et al. Hazard-rate analysis in stage I malignant melanoma. *Arch Dermatol* 1986;122:999–1002.

674. Steiner A, Wolf C, Pehamberger H, et al. Late metastases of cutaneous malignant melanoma. *Br J Dermatol* 1986;114:737–740.

675. Raderman D, Giler S, Rothem A, et al. Late metastases (beyond ten years) of cutaneous malignant melanoma. Literature review and case report. *J Am Acad Dermatol* 1986;15:374–378.

676. Barth A, Wanek LA, Morton DL. Prognostic factors in 1,521 melanoma patients with distant metastases. *J Am Coll Surg* 1995;181:A193-A201.

677. Baab GH, McBride CM. Malignant melanoma: the patient with an unknown site of primary origin. *Arch Surg* 1975;110:896–900.

678. Anbari KK, Schuchter LM, Bucky LP, et al. Melanoma of unknown primary site: presentation, treatment, and prognosis—a single institution study. University of Pennsylvania Pigmented Lesion Study Group. *Cancer* 1997;79:1816–1821.

679. Bottger D, Dowden RV, Kay PP. Complete spontaneous regression of cutaneous primary malignant melanoma. *Plast Reconstr Surg* 1992;89:548–553.

680. McNutt NS, Urmacher C, Hakimian J, et al. Nevoid malignant melanoma: morphologic patterns and immunohistochemical reactivity. *J Cutan Pathol* 1995;22:502–517.

681. Kornberg R, Harris M, Ackerman AB. Epidermotropically metastatic malignant melanoma. Differentiating malignant melanoma metastatic to the epidermis from malignant melanoma primary in the epidermis. *Arch Dermatol* 1978;114:67–69.

682. Heenan PJ, Clay CD. Epidermotropic metastatic melanoma simulating multiple primary melanomas. *Am J Dermatopathol* 1991;13:396–402.

683. Konrad K, Wolff K. Pathogenesis of diffuse melanosis secondary to malignant melanoma. *Br J Dermatol* 1974;91:635–655.

684. Adrian RM, Murphy GF, Sato S, et al. Diffuse melanosis secondary to metastatic malignant melanoma. Light and electron microscopic findings. *J Am Acad Dermatol* 1981;5:308–318.

TUMORS AND CYSTS
OF THE EPIDERMIS

NIGEL KIRKHAM

CLASSIFICATION OF TUMORS
OF THE EPIDERMIS

Epidermal tumors can be divided into tumors of the surface epidermis and tumors of the epidermal appendages. In each of the two classes, benign and malignant tumors occur.

Benign tumors in general are characterized by (a) a symmetrical architecture and a circumscribed profile, (b) a tendency to differentiate along organized tissue lines, (c) uniformity in the appearance of the tumor cell nuclei, (d) architectural order in the arrangement of the tumor cell nuclei, (e) restraint in the rate of growth, and (f) absence of metastases.

Malignant tumors, in contrast, are characterized by (a) a less symmetrical architecture and a poorly circumscribed profile; (b) a variable but often poorly differentiated phenotype; (c) atypicality in the appearance of the tumor cell nuclei, which show pleomorphism, that is, great variability in size and shape, and anaplasia, that is, hyperplasia and hyperchromasia; (d) architectural disorder in the arrangement of the tumor cell nuclei with loss of polarity; (e) rapid growth with the presence of mitoses, including atypical mitoses; and (f) potentiality to give rise to metastases.

Of the criteria of malignancy just cited, only the potentiality to give rise to metastases is decisive evidence for the malignancy of a tumor. For metastases to form, the tumor cells must possess a degree of autonomy that nonmalignant cells do not have. This autonomy enables malignant tumor cells to induce foreign tissue to furnish the necessary stroma in which they can multiply.

In addition to malignant tumors, one finds in the surface epidermis so-called premalignant tumors, better regarded as tumors located largely *in situ*. Although cytologically malignant, they are biologically still benign.

The tumors of the surface epidermis have been classified by the World Health Organization as shown in Table 29-1 (1).

LINEAR EPIDERMAL NEVUS

Linear epidermal nevi, or verrucous nevi, may be either localized or systematized. In the *localized type*, which is present usually but not invariably at birth, only one linear lesion is present. It consists of closely set, papillomatous, hyperkeratotic papules. It may be located anywhere—on the head, trunk, or extremities. Being located on only one side of the patient, it is often referred to as *nevus unius lateris*. In its configuration, the localized type of linear epidermal nevus resembles the inflammatory linear verrucous epidermal nevus (ILVEN), but the latter differs clinically by the presence of erythema and pruritus and histologically by the presence of inflammation and parakeratosis (1a,b) (see Chapter 7).

In the *systematized type*, papillomatous hyperkeratotic papules in a linear configuration are present not just as one linear lesion, as in the localized type, but as many linear lesions. These linear lesions often show a parallel arrangement, particularly on the trunk. They may be limited to one side of the patient or may have a bilateral, symmetric distribution. The term *ichthyosis hystrix* is occasionally used, perhaps unnecessarily, for instances of extensive bilateral lesions (2).

Localized and, more commonly, systematized linear epidermal nevi may be associated with skeletal deformities and central nervous system deficiencies, such as mental retardation, epilepsy, and neural deafness (3).

The presence of a basal cell epithelioma within a linear epidermal nevus has been observed occasionally, particularly on the head in cases in which the linear epidermal nevus has been associated with either a nevus sebaceus or a syringocystadenoma papilliferum (4) (see Chapter 30). In areas other than the head, it is very rare (5). Similarly, development of a squamous cell carcinoma has been described only rarely (6,7), but in one instance the squamous cell carcinoma had metastasized to a regional lymph node (8).

Histopathology. Nearly all cases of the localized type of linear epidermal nevus and some cases of the systematized

TABLE 29-1. CLASSIFICATION OF SURFACE EPIDERMIS TUMORS BY WORLD HEALTH ORGANIZATION

Epithelial Tumors
Benign
  Epidermal
    Epidermal nevus
    Seborrheic keratosis
      Irritated
      Adenoid
      Plane
      With an intraepidermal epithelioma pattern
      Melanoacanthoma
      Inverted follicular keratosis
      Benign squamous keratosis
    Clear cell acanthoma
      (Also nevus comedonicus, epidermolytic acanthoma,
        acantholytic acanthoma, oral white sponge nevus)
    Fibroepithelial polyp
    Warty dyskeratoma
    Actinic keratosis
      (Also precancerous leukoplakia, oral florid papillomato-
        sis, Bowen's disease, erythroplasia of Queyrat)
    Keratoacanthoma
      Giant keratoacanthoma
      Keratoacanthoma centrifugum marginatum
      Subungual keratoacanthoma
      Multiple keratoacanthomas
      Multiple eruptive keratoacanthomas
    Benign lichenoid keratosis
Malignant
  Squamous cell carcinoma
    Spindle cell
    Acantholytic
    Verrucous
    Horn forming
    Lymphoepithelial
  Basal cell carcinoma
    Multifocal superficial (superficial multicentric)
    Nodular (solid, adenoid cystic)
    Infiltrating
    Nonsclerosing
    Sclerosing (desmoplastic morpheic)
  Fibroepithelial
  Basal cell carcinoma with adnexal differentiation
    Follicular
    Eccrine
  Basosquamous carcinoma
  Keratotic basal cell carcinoma
  Pigmented basal cell carcinoma
  Basal cell carcinoma in basal cell nevus syndrome
  Micronodular basal cell carcinoma
This chapter also includes details on cysts that are classified as
  follows:
  Follicular cysts
    Infundibular cyst
    Trichilemmal cyst
    Steatocystoma multiplex
    Dermoid cyst
    Eruptive vellus hair cyst
  Milia
  Bronchogenic and thyroglossal duct cysts
  Cutaneous ciliated cyst
  Median raphe cyst of the penis

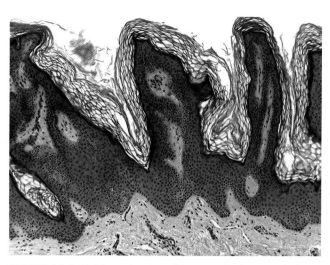

FIGURE 29-1. Epidermal nevus. This example shows orthokeratotic hypekeratosis, papillary projections with a flat surface.

type show the histologic picture of a benign papilloma (2,9). One observes considerable hyperkeratosis, papillomatosis, and acanthosis with elongation of the rete ridges resembling seborrheic keratosis (Fig. 29-1).

Occasionally in cases of the localized type, but quite frequently in cases of the systematized type, particularly those with a widespread distribution, one observes the rather striking histologic picture referred to either as *epidermolytic hyperkeratosis* (10), or as *granular degeneration of the epidermis* (11). It is the same process that was first recognized in all cases of bullous congenital ichthyosiform erythroderma, a disorder that is often referred to as *epidermolytic hyperkeratosis* (Chapter 6). It has since been found to occur in several other conditions as well (see Isolated and Disseminated Epidermolytic Acanthoma section).

The salient histologic features of epidermolytic hyperkeratosis are (a) perinuclear vacuolization of the cells in the stratum spinosum and in the stratum granulosum; (b) peripheral to the vacuolization, irregular cellular boundaries; (c) an increased number of irregularly shaped, large keratohyaline granules; and (d) compact hyperkeratosis in the stratum corneum (11,12).

In some instances, histologic examination of unilateral linear lesions reveals features of acantholytic dyskeratosis as seen in Darier's disease (see Chapter 6). In some patients, these linear lesions have been present since birth or infancy (13), but in most instances they have arisen in adult life (14). Because acantholytic dyskeratosis is not specific for Darier's disease, the proposal has been made to designate such cases not as Darier's disease but as acantholytic dyskeratotic epidermal nevus (14).

Differential Diagnosis. The histologic picture of a benign papilloma, as found in most cases of linear epidermal nevus, can also be seen in seborrheic keratosis, verruca vulgaris, and acanthosis nigricans. Even though these four conditions have in common hyperkeratosis and papillomatosis, they can be differentiated easily in typical cases; however, one is occasionally unable to make a diagnosis any more specific than benign papilloma. Thus, in the following three situations, clinical data are required for differentiation from linear epidermal nevus: (a) the hyperkeratotic type of seborrheic keratosis, which is characterized by the absence of basaloid cells and horn cysts and instead shows upward extension of epidermis-lined papillae; (b) old verrucae vulgaris, which no longer show vacuolization of epidermal cells or columns of parakeratosis (see Chapter 25); and (c) acanthosis nigricans showing more pronounced acanthosis and greater elongation of the rete ridges than usual (see Chapter 17).

NEVOID HYPERKERATOSIS OF NIPPLE AND AREOLA

Nevoid hyperkeratosis and papillomatosis of nipples and areola presents as sharply demarcated papules and plaques, often appearing at puberty or during pregnancy and persisting unchanged. There are no associated systemic or dermatologic conditions. The main differential diagnosis is seborrheic keratosis (14a).

Histopathology. There are papillomatous elongations of the epidermis with hyperkeratosis and areas of keratotic plugging (15). This condition represents a nevoid form of hyperkeratosis (16).

NEVUS COMEDONICUS

A nevus comedonicus consists of closely set, slightly elevated papules that have in their center a dark, firm hyperkeratotic plug resembling a comedo. Nevus comedonicus, like linear epidermal nevus, usually has a linear configuration and occurs as a single lesion. In some instances, however, there are multiple bilateral linear lesions (17) or lesions that are randomly distributed rather than linear (18). Lesions may be present on the palms or soles in addition to other areas (19,20). Such cases may represent a combination of nevus comedonicus with a porokeratotic eccrine duct nevus.

Histopathology. Each comedo is represented by a wide, deep invagination of the epidermis filled with keratin. These invaginations resemble dilated hair follicles; in fact, as evidence that they actually represent rudimentary hair follicles, one occasionally finds in the lower portion of an invagination one or even several hair shafts (17). One or two small sebaceous gland lobules may also be seen opening into the lower pole of invaginations (18).

In several instances, the keratinocytes composing the follicular epithelial wall have shown the typical changes of epidermolytic hyperkeratosis (see discussion below) (21),

indicative of a relationship of nevus comedonicus to systematized nevus verrucosus (see Chapter 30).

POROKERATOTIC ECCRINE OSTIAL AND DERMAL DUCT NEVUS

Porokeratotic eccrine ostial and dermal duct nevus may be limited to a palm (22) or to a sole (23), but may be present on both hands and feet and elsewhere (24,24a). It also may involve not only eccrine ducts but also hair follicles on the hairy parts of the body (25).

Histopathology. In the porokeratotic eccrine duct nevus, each invagination consists of a dilated eccrine duct containing a parakeratotic plug. The absence of the granular layer at the base of the plug together with the presence of keratinocytes showing vacuolization of their cytoplasm results in a histologic picture resembling that of porokeratosis (22–24) (see Chapter 6).

ISOLATED AND DISSEMINATED EPIDERMOLYTIC ACANTHOMA

Isolated epidermolytic acanthoma, histologically characterized by the presence of "epidermolytic hyperkeratosis," does not have a characteristic clinical appearance or location. Usually it occurs as a solitary papillomatous lesion less than 1 cm in diameter (26–28). Occasionally, several lesions are seen in a localized area (29,30). One case has been described, which was probably secondary to trauma (30a).

Disseminated epidermolytic acanthoma occurs as numerous discrete, flat, brownish papules 2 to 6 mm in diameter, resembling seborrheic keratoses. The upper trunk, especially the back, is the site of predilection (31,32).

Histopathology. In addition to hyperkeratosis and papillomatosis, pronounced epidermolytic hyperkeratosis is observed, also referred to as *granular degeneration*, throughout the stratum malpighii, sparing only the basal layer, just as seen in linear epidermal nevi with epidermolytic changes. One observes both intracellular and intercellular edema of the epidermal cells and keratohyaline granules that are coarser than normal and extend to a greater depth in the stratum malpighii (26).

Differential Diagnosis. Myrmecia warts, caused by human papilloma virus type 1 (HPV-1), also show perinuclear vacuolization and an abundance of keratohyaline granules, representing a type of "granular degeneration" similar to that seen in epidermolytic hyperkeratosis. However, in myrmecia warts, the keratohyaline granules are eosinophilic and coalesce in the upper layers of the epidermis to form large, homogeneous, eosinophilic "inclusion bodies." In verrucae vulgaris, usually caused by HPV-2, foci of vacuolated cells and clumped basophilic keratohyaline granules may be present, but these changes are limited to the upper layers of the epidermis. In addition, both myrmecia warts and verrucae vulgaris show focal parakeratosis, rather than orthokeratosis as seen in epidermolytic hyperkeratosis (see Chapter 25).

INCIDENTAL EPIDERMOLYTIC HYPERKERATOSIS

Epidermolytic hyperkeratosis is seen not only in isolated and disseminated epidermolytic hyperkeratosis (see previous discussion) but also as a *regular* finding in epidermolytic hyperkeratosis, or bullous congenital ichthyosiform erythroderma (Chapter 6), and in epidermolytic keratosis palmaris et plantaris and as an *occasional* finding in linear epidermal nevus and nevus comedonicus. In addition, epidermolytic hyperkeratosis may represent an *incidental* histologic finding in many different types of lesions, largely but not exclusively tumors. It has also been observed in normal oral mucosa adjacent to lesions of squamous cell carcinoma and basal cell epithelioma (33).

Histopathology. Epidermolytic hyperkeratosis may be seen throughout an entire lesion of solar keratosis (34) and in the entire lining of trichilemmal cyst (35). More commonly, however, the histologic features of epidermolytic hyperkeratosis are seen as a small focus, often limited to a single epidermal rete ridge, in such diverse lesions as sebaceous hyperplasia (36), intradermal nevus, hypertrophic scar (37), superficial basal cell epithelioma (38), seborrheic keratosis, the margin of a squamous cell carcinoma, lichenoid amyloidosis, and granuloma annulare (10). In some instances, the process is limited to one or two intraepidermal sweat duct units (37). It is more frequently seen in dysplastic nevi than in ordinary melanocytic nevi (37a).

ISOLATED AND DISSEMINATED ACANTHOLYTIC ACANTHOMA

This condition usually occurs as a solitary papule or small nodule (39), although there may be multiple lesions (40, 41). No characteristic clinical appearance or location exists, although multiple lesions have been seen largely in the genital region (23,42).

Histopathology. Acantholysis is the most prominent feature. The pattern may resemble that of pemphigus vulgaris, pemphigus vegetans, pemphigus foliaceus, or benign familial pemphigus (39). Acantholysis may be combined with dyskeratosis, in which case the histologic picture resembles that of Darier's disease as the result of the presence of corps ronds and grains (10,40,41). Because of this, the alternative name of *dyskeratotic acanthoma* has been suggested (41a).

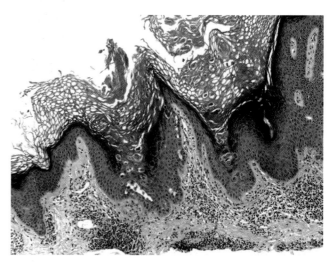

FIGURE 29-2. Incidental focal acantholytic dyskeratosis. Focally, within the biopsy, there is suprabasal cleft formation with overlying dyskeratotic cells.

INCIDENTAL FOCAL ACANTHOLYTIC DYSKERATOSIS

Analogous to epidermolytic hyperkeratosis, acantholytic dyskeratosis is seen as a *regular* histologic feature in Darier's disease (see Chapter 6), transient acantholytic dermatosis, and warty dyskeratoma. It also is an *occasional* finding in acantholytic dyskeratotic epidermal nevus, a variant of linear epidermal nevus. In addition, again like epidermolytic hyperkeratosis, focal acantholytic dyskeratosis is observed occasionally as an *incidental* histologic finding in a variety of lesions including vascular nevi (41b).

Histopathology. Focal suprabasal clefts with overlying acantholytic and dyskeratotic cells, some of which have the appearance of corps ronds, have been seen as a single focus in the epidermis overlying such diverse lesions as dermatofibroma, basal cell epithelioma, melanocytic nevus, and chondrodermatitis nodularis helicis (35), as well as in pityriasis rosea (43) and acral lentiginous malignant melanoma (44) (Fig. 29-2).

ORAL WHITE SPONGE NEVUS

First described in 1935 (45), oral white sponge nevus is a benign autosomal dominant disorder that affects noncornifying, stratified squamous epithelia. It may be present at birth or have its onset in infancy, childhood, or adolescence (46). Extensive areas of the oral mucosa and sometimes the entire oral mucosa have a thickened, folded, creamy white appearance. In some instances, the rectal mucosa (45), vagina (47), nasal mucosa (48), or esophagus (49) is also involved. This distribution of lesions suggests that mutations in the epithelial keratins K4 and/or K13 may be responsible: a three base-pair deletion in the helix initiation peptide of K4 has been reported in affected members of two families (50). Further studies of one large family suggested that a K13 gene was responsible (50a).

The oral lesions seen in pachyonychia congenita are both clinically and histologically indistinguishable from a white sponge nevus (Chapter 6) (48).

Histopathology. The oral epithelium shows hyperplasia with much more pronounced hydropic swelling of the epithelial cells than is normal for the oral mucosa. The swelling, although extensive, is focal (51). It extends into the rete ridges but spares the basal layer (52). The nuclei appear smaller than normal (46). The surface shows parakeratosis, as does the normal oral mucosa, and only rarely are there small accumulations of keratohyaline granules (47).

Pathogenesis. On electron microscopic examination, large cytoplasmic areas of the epithelial cells appear optically empty or contain only faint granular material. Tonofilaments are limited to the perinuclear and peripheral areas. The intercellular areas show irregular dilatation, and large, irregularly shaped vacuoles are present within the cytoplasm (53). A possibly fundamental disturbance is the presence of numerous intracellular Odland bodies or membrane-coating granules (Chapter 3), which are not extruded into the intercellular spaces (54).

Differential Diagnosis. The histologic picture of oral white sponge nevus is identical to that seen in pachyonychia congenita (see previous discussion), oral focal epithelial hyperplasia (53), and leukoedema of the oral mucosa (see text below).

LEUKOEDEMA OF ORAL MUCOSA

Leukoedema of the oral mucosa is a common condition that, when pronounced, shows a clinical and histologic resemblance to oral white sponge nevus. However, leukoedema differs from white sponge nevus by being patchy rather than diffuse, by having exacerbations and remissions and adult onset, and by not being inherited (55).

Histopathology. In leukoedema of the oral mucosa, as in oral white sponge nevus, the suprabasal epithelial cells show marked intracellular edema. The nuclei appear smaller than normal.

LINGUA GEOGRAPHICA

In *lingua geographica* (geographic tongue), also referred to as superficial migratory glossitis, the dorsum of the tongue shows irregularly shaped red patches surrounded by a whitish, raised border a few millimeters wide (56). It is usually asymptomatic, with local loss of filiform papillae

leading to the development of ulcer-like lesions that rapidly change color and size (56a).

Histopathology. Whereas the dorsum of the tongue normally shows a granular and a horny layer, these layers are absent in the red patches of lingua geographica. Along the whitish border, the epithelium shows irregular thickening and infiltration of neutrophils. In its upper portion, the epithelium shows collections of neutrophils within the interstices of a sponge-like network formed by degenerated and thinned epithelial cells (57,58). The histologic picture thus shows Kogoj's spongiform pustules, which are indistinguishable from those seen in pustular psoriasis.

Pathogenesis. The presence of spongiform pustules generally is regarded as diagnostic of pustular psoriasis and as almost specific for it (see Chapter 8), even though it rarely occurs in other pustules, such as those caused by *Candida albicans* (59). It has therefore been suggested that geographic tongue represents a localized form of pustular psoriasis (60). However, even though pustular psoriasis and lingua geographica may both show annular lesions on the tongue, pustular psoriasis of the mouth generally shows clinical evidence of pustules and is usually seen also in other areas of the mouth. It is therefore best to regard lingua geographica as a separate entity.

SEBORRHEIC KERATOSIS

Seborrheic keratoses are very common lesions: sometimes single but often multiple. They occur mainly on the trunk and face but also on the extremities, with the exception of the palms and soles. Seborrheic keratoses usually do not appear before middle age, but are present in about 20% of the elderly (61). They are sharply demarcated, brownish in color, and slightly raised, so that they often look as if they are stuck on the surface of the skin. Most of them have a verrucous surface, which has a soft, friable consistency. Some, however, have a smooth surface but characteristically show keratotic plugs. Although most lesions measure only a few millimeters in diameter, a lesion may occasionally reach a size of several centimeters. Crusting and an inflammatory base are found if the lesion has been subjected to trauma. Occasionally, small seborrheic keratoses are pedunculated, especially on the neck and upper chest, and then clinically resemble soft fibromas (see Chapter 32).

Histopathology. Seborrheic keratoses show a considerable variety of histologic appearances. Six types are generally recognized: irritated, adenoid or reticulated, plane, clonal, melanoacanthoma, inverted follicular keratosis, and benign squamous keratosis (Figs. 29-3 to 29-8). Often more than one type is found in the same lesion. In addition, two clinical variants of seborrheic keratosis will be described. They are dermatosis papulosa nigra and stucco keratosis.

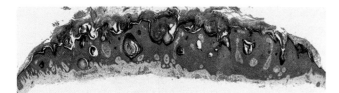

FIGURE 29-3. Seborrheic keratosis. Scanning magnification. The lesion is radially symmetrical with keratin on its surface and several horn cysts.

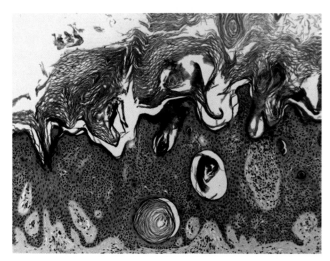

FIGURE 29-4. Seborrheic keratosis. Most of the cells have a basaloid appearance, with interspersed horn cysts filled with keratin.

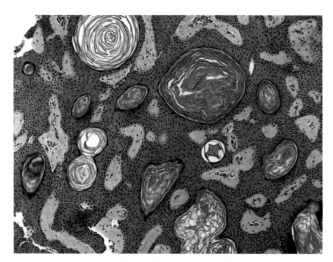

FIGURE 29-5. Seborrheic keratosis. Medium magnification. Keratin-filled horn cysts are surrounded by basaloid cells.

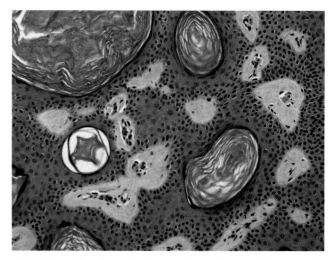

FIGURE 29-6. Seborrheic keratosis. High magnification. The cells have a basaloid appearance, with interspersed horn cysts filled with keratin.

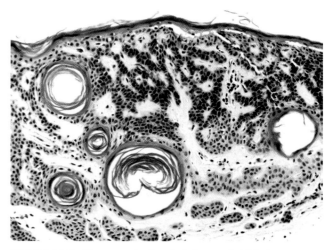

FIGURE 29-7. Pigmented seborrheic keratosis. Thin interwoven cords of basaloid cells show cytoplasmic melanin pigmentation. Horn cysts are also present.

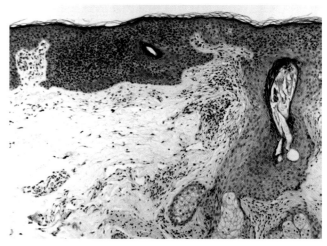

FIGURE 29-8. Seborrheic keratosis. Clonal type. Basaloid cells are surrounded by more eosinophilic squamous cells.

All types of seborrheic keratosis have in common hyperkeratosis, acanthosis, and papillomatosis. The acanthosis in most instances is due entirely to upward extension of the tumor. Thus, the lower border of the tumor is even and generally lies on a straight line that may be drawn from the normal epidermis at one end of the tumor to the normal epidermis at the other end (Fig. 29-2). Two types of cells are usually seen in the acanthotic epidermis: squamous cells and basaloid cells. The former have the appearance of squamous cells normally found in the epidermis; the basaloid cells are small and uniform in appearance and have a relatively large nucleus. In areas of slight intercellular edema, intercellular bridges can be easily recognized (61). Thus, they resemble the basal cells found normally in the basal layer of the epidermis.

Irritated Type and Inverted Follicular Keratosis

In the irritated, or activated, type of seborrheic keratosis, squamous cells outnumber basaloid cells. The characteristic feature is the presence of numerous whorls or eddies composed of eosinophilic flattened squamous cells arranged in an onion-peel fashion, resembling poorly differentiated horn pearls (Figs. 29-9 and 29-10). These "squamous eddies" are easily differentiated from the horn pearls of squamous cell carcinoma by their large number, small size, and circumscribed configuration. Irritated seborrheic keratoses, in addition, may show areas of downward proliferation breaking through the horizontal demarcation generally present in nonirritated seborrheic keratoses (62,63). Frequently, some of these proliferations are seen to originate from the walls of keratin-filled invaginations. Inflammation beneath irritated seborrheic keratoses usually is mild or absent, indicating that irritated seborrheic keratoses are different from inflamed seborrheic keratoses.

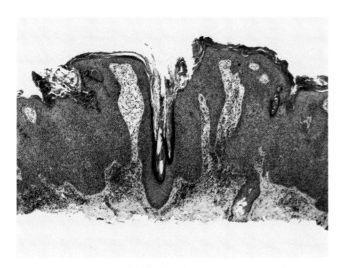

FIGURE 29-9. Inverted follicular keratosis. An endophytic proliferation of mature squamous epithelium.

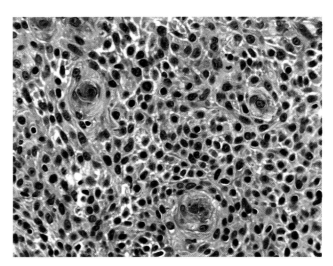

FIGURE 29-10. Inverted follicular keratosis. Squamous eddies are present, composed of whorls of squamous cells. There is no substantial cytologic atypia.

In a few instances, acantholysis has been observed within tumor nests composed of squamous cells (64). These acantholytic changes differ from those occurring in incidental focal acantholytic dyskeratosis by not showing suprabasal location or dyskeratotic cells resembling corps ronds (65).

Pathogenesis. The formation of numerous squamous eddies is the result of the "activation" of resting basaloid cells into squamous cells. This unique and highly diagnostic feature of irritated or activated seborrheic keratoses, as well as their downward proliferation, is the result of irritation. This has been proved experimentally by the excision of seborrheic keratoses either after a previous biopsy (66) or after irritation with croton oil (67).

The identical histologic picture as seen in irritated seborrheic keratosis has been described under the designations of *inverted follicular keratosis* (68,69) and *follicular poroma* (70,71). As these terms indicate, the authors regard the keratin-filled invaginations as follicular infundibula and the proliferations arising from them as composed of cells of the follicular infundibulum. The follicular infundibulum consists of cells with the same type of keratinization as the surface epidermis, and there is evidence that seborrheic keratoses incorporate cells of the infundibular portion of the hair follicle and are partially derived from these cells. Seborrheic keratoses, like inverted follicular keratoses, occur exclusively on hair-bearing skin. Some seborrheic keratoses even contain aggregates of vellus hairs within the keratinous invaginations, an occurrence analogous to trichostasis spinulosa (72) (see Chapter 18). Although some authors merely concede that irritated seborrheic keratoses and inverted follicular keratoses may be histologically indistinguishable (63,73,74) others regard the two disorders as identical (62,72,75). Because of their histologic similarity and particularly because of the highly specific appearance of the squamous eddies that occur in these two conditions, they are best regarded as identical.

Adenoid or Reticulated Type

In the adenoid or reticulated type of seborrheic keratosis, numerous thin tracts of epidermal cells extend from the epidermis and show branching and interweaving in the dermis. Many tracts are composed of only a double row of basaloid cells. Horn cysts and pseudo-horn cysts are absent in purely reticulated lesions; however, the reticulated type often also shows areas of the acanthotic type, and horn cysts and pseudo-horn cysts are commonly seen in these areas. The basaloid cells of the reticulated type of seborrheic keratosis usually show marked hyperpigmentation.

There is both clinical and histologic evidence of a close relationship between solar or senile lentigo senilis and the reticulated type of seborrheic keratosis. A lesion of solar lentigo may even become a reticulated seborrheic keratosis through exaggeration of the process of downward budding of pigmented basaloid cells (76) (see Chapter 28).

Acanthotic Type

In the acanthotic type, the most common type of seborrheic keratosis, hyperkeratosis and papillomatosis often are slight, but the epidermis is greatly thickened. Although only narrow papillae are included in the thickened epidermis in some cases, one can see in other lesions a retiform pattern composed of thick, interwoven tracts of epithelial cells surrounding islands of connective tissue. Horny invaginations that on cross sections appear as pseudo-horn cysts are numerous. In addition, there also are true horn cysts, which, like the pseudo-horn cysts, show sudden and complete keratinization with only a very thin granular layer.

The true horn cysts begin as foci of orthokeratosis within the substance of the lesion (77). In time, they enlarge and are carried by the current of epidermal cells toward the surface of the lesion, where they unite with the invaginations of surface keratin. In the greatly thickened epidermis, basaloid cells usually outnumber squamous cells.

The amount of melanin in seborrheic keratoses of the acanthotic type is often greater than normal. Excess amounts of melanin are seen in about one-third of the specimens stained with hematoxylin-eosin (78); staining with silver reveals excess amounts in about two-thirds of the cases (79). In dopa-stained sections, melanocytes are limited to the dermal–epidermal junctional layer present at the base of the tumor and at the interfaces between the tumor tracts and the islands of dermal stroma (67). The melanin, largely present in keratinocytes, is in most instances also limited to keratinocytes located at the dermal-epidermal junction. Only deeply pigmented lesions show melanin widely distributed throughout the tumor within basaloid cells (80).

A mononuclear inflammatory infiltrate is seen quite frequently in the dermis underlying a seborrheic keratosis. The inflammation may impinge on the tumor in a lichenoid or eczematous pattern. In the lichenoid pattern, a band-like infiltrate is seen hugging the basal cell layer of the tumor. In the eczematous pattern, there is exocytosis leading to spongiosis. Squamous eddies, typical of irritated seborrheic keratoses, are only rarely seen in inflamed seborrheic keratoses (81).

Formation of an *in situ* carcinoma within an acanthotic seborrheic keratosis, so-called Bowenoid transformation, is seen occasionally (82,83). It seems to occur predominantly in lesions located in sun-exposed areas of the skin, so that sun damage may be a factor (84). In one reported case, a metastasis in a regional lymph node was found (85). On rare occasions, a basal cell epithelioma may form within an acanthotic seborrheic keratosis and may extend from there into the underlying dermis (86,87).

Pathogenesis. Electron microscopic examination has confirmed the light microscopic impression that the small basaloid cells seen in the acanthotic type of seborrheic keratosis are related to cells of the epidermal basal cell layer rather than to the basaloma cells of basal cell epithelioma. They possess a fair number of desmosomes and a moderate number of tonofilaments that differ from those present in cells of the epidermal basal cell layer only by showing less orientation (88).

Hyperkeratotic Type

In the hyperkeratotic type, also referred to as the digitate or serrated type, hyperkeratosis and papillomatosis are pronounced, whereas acanthosis is not very conspicuous. The numerous digitate upward extensions of epidermis-lined papillae often resemble church spires. The histologic picture then resembles that seen in acrokeratosis verruciformis of Hopf (see Chapter 6). The epidermis consists largely of squamous cells, although small aggregates of basaloid cells may be seen here and there. As a rule, no excess amounts of melanin are found.

Clonal Type

In the clonal, or nesting, type of seborrheic keratosis, well-defined nests of cells are located within the epidermis. In some instances, the nests resemble foci of basal cell epithelioma, since the nuclei appear small and dark-staining, and intercellular bridges are seen in only a few areas (89) (Fig. 29-8). The histologic picture in such cases has been erroneously interpreted by some authors as representing an intraepidermal epithelioma of Borst–Jadassohn (90) (see Chapter 30). In other instances of clonal seborrheic keratosis, the nests are composed of fairly large cells showing distinct intercellular bridges, with the nests separated from one another by strands of cells exhibiting small dark nuclei.

Melanoacanthoma

This rather rare variant of pigmented seborrheic keratosis (80) differs from the usual type of pigmented seborrheic keratosis by showing a marked increase in the concentration of melanocytes. Rather than being confined to the basal layer of the tumor lobules, many melanocytes are scattered throughout the tumor lobules (80,91). In some instances, well-defined islands of basaloid cells intermingled with many melanocytes are distributed through the tumor (92). The melanocytes are large and richly dendritic and contain variable amounts of melanin. The block in transfer of melanin from melanocytes to keratinocytes often is only partial (91), although in some instances nearly all the melanin is retained in the melanocytes (93).

Pathogenesis. Melanoacanthoma is a benign mixed tumor of melanocytes and keratinocytes (80).

DERMATOSIS PAPULOSA NIGRA

Dermatosis papulosa nigra is found in about 35% of all adult blacks, often has its onset during adolescence (94), and has been described in a 3-year-old child (95). The lesions are located predominantly on the face, especially in the malar regions, but may also occur on the neck and upper trunk. They usually consist of small, smooth, pigmented papules, except on the neck and trunk, where some of them may be pedunculated.

Histopathology. The lesions have the histologic appearance of seborrheic keratoses but are smaller. Most lesions are of the acanthotic type and show thick interwoven tracts of epithelial cells. The cells are largely squamous in appearance, with only a few basaloid cells (94). Horn cysts are quite common. An occasional lesion shows a reticulated pattern, in which the tracts are composed of a double row of basaloid cells. Melanin pigmentation is pronounced in all lesions.

STUCCO KERATOSIS

Stucco keratoses are small, gray-white seborrheic keratoses 1 to 3 mm in diameter, located in symmetric arrangement on the distal portions of the extremities, especially the ankles. They can easily be scraped off without any resultant bleeding.

Histopathology. Stucco keratoses have the appearance of the hyperkeratotic type of seborrheic keratosis, showing the church-spire pattern of upward-extending papillae (96,97). Horn cysts and basaloid cells are usually absent (98).

LESER-TRÉLAT SIGN

The Leser-Trélat sign is characterized by the sudden appearance of numerous seborrheic keratoses in association with a malignant tumor. Although many reports have appeared in recent years concerning this sign and although its existence is accepted, it is not always easy to decide which cases should be included. In some instances, numerous seborrheic keratoses develop on inflamed skin, but this does not represent the Leser-Trélat sign (81). A review of 40 cases that were accepted as representing the Leser-Trélat sign (99) showed that 30% had "malignant" acanthosis nigricans (Chapter 17), either accompanying (100) or following the sign (101). Thus, the Leser-Trélat sign has been interpreted as "an incomplete form of acanthosis nigricans" (102), or as "potentially representing an early stage of acanthosis nigricans" (101).

Although the malignant tumor in 67% of the reported cases consisted of an abdominal adenocarcinoma (99,103) the remaining 33% included many different types of malignancies, including leukemia (104) or mycosis fungoides (105). More controversially a case-control study failed to demonstrate a specific association between eruptive seborrheic keratoses and internal cancer risk (106).

Histopathology. The seborrheic keratoses in the Leser-Trélat sign are the same as other seborrheic keratoses. The hyperkeratotic form is indistinguishable from malignant acanthosis nigricans (99,107).

LARGE CELL ACANTHOMA

Large cell acanthoma occurs as a slightly hyperkeratotic, sharply demarcated patch, usually on sun-exposed skin of the head or extremities. As a rule, it measures less than 1 cm in size. Generally, it is a solitary lesion: occasionally multiple lesions are observed (108–110).

Histopathology. Within a well-demarcated area of the epidermis, the scattered large keratinocytes are about twice the normal size and have proportionally large nuclei. There may be a disordered arrangement of the keratinocytes.

Pathogenesis. The lesion is aneuploid, with various stages of development, and is probably related to stucco keratosis (108,110).

CLEAR CELL ACANTHOMA

Clear cell acanthoma, a tumor that is clinically and histologically quite distinct, was first described in 1962 (111). It is not rare. Typically the lesions are solitary and occur on the legs. They are slowly growing, sharply delineated, red nodules or plaques 1 to 2 cm in diameter and usually covered with a thin crust and exuding some moisture. A collarette is often seen at the periphery. It has been said that the lesion appears stuck on, like a seborrheic keratosis, and is vascular, like a granuloma pyogenicum (112,113).

Histopathology. Within a sharply demarcated area of the epidermis, all epidermal cells, with the exception of cells of

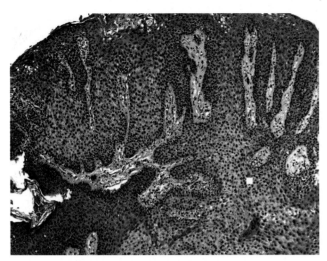

FIGURE 29-11. Clear cell acanthoma. The cells within the lesion appear pale by comparison with the adjacent normal epidermis.

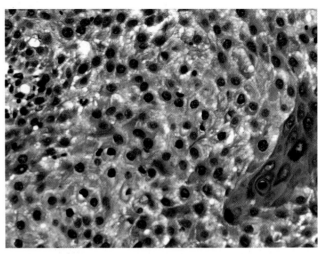

FIGURE 29-12. Clear cell acanthoma. High magnification. Neutrophils and nuclear dust are scattered through the clear cells of the lesion.

the basal cell layer, appear strikingly clear and slightly enlarged (Figs. 29-10 and 29-11). The nuclei of the clear epidermal cells appear normal. When staining is carried out with the periodic acid–Schiff (PAS) reaction, the presence of large amounts of glycogen is revealed within the cells (111,114).

Slight spongiosis is present between the clear cells. The rete ridges are elongated and may show intertwining (115). The surface shows parakeratosis with few or no granular cells. The acrosyringia and acrotrichia within the tumor retain their normal stainability (116). There is an absence of melanin within the tumor cells, but dendritic melanocytes containing melanin are occasionally seen interspersed between the clear cells (114,117).

A conspicuous feature in most lesions is the presence throughout the epidermis of numerous neutrophils, many of which show fragmentation of their nuclei (Fig. 29-12). The neutrophils often form microabscesses in the parakeratotic horny layer (118,119). Dilated capillaries are seen in the elongated papillae and often also in the dermis underlying the tumor (114). In addition, a mild to moderately severe cellular infiltrate composed largely of lymphoid cells is present in the dermis. Some clear cell acanthomas appear papillomatous, so that they have the configuration of a seborrheic keratosis (120).

Beneath the tumor, some cases have shown hyperplasia of sweat ducts (118) or syringoma-like proliferations (121).

Pathogenesis. On histochemical examination, phosphorylase is absent in clear cell acanthoma except for the basal cell layer. This enzyme normally is present in the epidermis and is necessary for the degradation of glycogen (122).

Electron microscopy reveals glycogen granules in the tumor cells, except in the cells of the basal cell layer. In the lower portion of the tumor, the glycogen granules are seen largely around the nuclei. In the upper portion, however, the amount of glycogen is increased, and the granules are seen to infiltrate between the tonofilaments (122).

Although the melanocytes, including their dendrites, contain melanosomes, hardly any melanosomes are present within the tumor cells, indicating a blockage in the transfer of melanosomes from the melanocytes to the tumor cells (123).

EPIDERMAL OR INFUNDIBULAR CYST

Epidermal cysts are slowly growing, elevated, round, firm, intradermal or subcutaneous tumors that cease growing after having reached 1 to 5 cm in diameter. They occur most commonly on the face, scalp, neck, and trunk. Although most epidermal cysts arise spontaneously in hair-bearing areas, occasionally they occur on the palms or soles (124,125) or form as the result of trauma (126). Usually a patient has only one or a few epidermal cysts, rarely many. In Gardner's syndrome, however, numerous epidermal cysts occur, especially on the scalp and face (Chapter 32).

Histopathology. Epidermal cysts have a wall composed of true epidermis, as seen on the skin surface and in the infundibulum of hair follicles, the infundibulum being the uppermost part of the hair follicle that extends down to the entry of the sebaceous duct. In young epidermal cysts, several layers of squamous and granular cells can usually be recognized (Fig. 29-13). In older epidermal cysts, the wall often is markedly atrophic, either in some areas or in the entire cyst, and may consist of only one or two rows of greatly flattened cells. The cyst is filled with horny material arranged in laminated layers. In sections stained with hematoxylin-eosin, melanocytes and melanin pigmentation of keratinocytes can be seen only rarely in epidermal

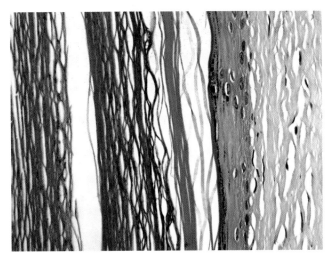

FIGURE 29-13. Epidermal cyst. The cyst is lined by stratified squamous epithelium with a granular layer. The cyst is filled with keratin flakes.

cysts of whites but frequently in epidermal cysts of blacks. Silver stains reveal that most of the melanin is located in the basal layer of the cyst lining, but some melanin is seen also in the contents of the cyst (127).

When an epidermal cyst ruptures and the contents of the cyst are released into the dermis, a considerable foreign-body reaction with numerous multinucleated giant cells results, forming a *keratin granuloma*. The foreign-body reaction usually causes disintegration of the cyst wall. However, it may lead to a pseudocarcinomatous proliferation in remnants of the cyst wall, simulating a squamous cell carcinoma (128). Melanocytes, melanin, and melanophages have been reported in the walls of epidermal cysts in some Indians (128a) and a Japanese patient (128b).

Development of a basal cell epithelioma (129), a lesion of Bowen's disease (130), or a squamous cell carcinoma (131) in epidermal cysts is a rare event. In cases of squamous cell carcinoma, the tumor is apt to be of low malignancy and does not metastasize. It is likely that some cases that were regarded in the past as malignant degeneration of epidermal cysts now are interpreted either as pseudocarcinomatous hyperplasia in a ruptured epidermal cyst (128) or as proliferating trichilemmal tumor (132) (Chapter 30).

Pathogenesis. It is widely assumed that most spontaneously arising epidermal cysts are related to the follicular infundibulum. The occurrence of hybrid cysts with partially epidermal and partially trichilemmal lining favors this assumption (133). Epidermal cysts in nonfollicular regions, such as the palms or soles, probably form as a result of the traumatic implantation of epidermis into the dermis or subcutis (124,125).

As seen by electron microscopy, the keratinization in epidermal cysts is identical to that in the surface epidermis and in the pilosebaceous infundibulum, since the keratin located within the keratinized cells consists of relatively electron-lucent tonofilaments embedded in an electron-dense interfilamentous substance derived from keratohyaline granules. The keratinized cells of the cyst content have a markedly flattened, elongated appearance and are surrounded by a thick marginal band rather than by a plasma membrane. Desmosomes are no longer present (134).

MILIA

Milia are multiple, superficially located, white, globoid, firm lesions, generally only 1 to 2 mm in diameter. A distinction is made between primary milia, which arise spontaneously on the face in predisposed individuals, and secondary milia, which occur either in diseases associated with subepidermal bullae, such as bullous pemphigoid, dystrophic epidermolysis bullosa (135,135a) and porphyria cutanea tarda, or after dermabrasion (136) and other trauma.

Histopathology. Primary milia of the face are derived from the lowest portion of the infundibulum of vellus hairs at about the level of the sebaceous duct. The milia often are still connected with the vellus hair follicle by an epithelial pedicle. Primary milia are small cysts differing from epidermal cysts only in size. They are lined by a stratified epithelium a few cell layers thick and contain concentric lamellae of keratin (136).

Secondary milia have the same histologic appearance as primary milia (136). They may develop from any epithelial structure and on serial sections may still show a connection to the parent structure, whether a hair follicle, sweat duct, sebaceous duct, or epidermis (137). Secondary milia that follow blistering arise in most instances from the eccrine sweat duct and very rarely from a hair follicle. In a certain percentage, however, no connection is found with any skin appendage, suggesting that the milia have developed from aberrant epidermis (138). In milia derived from eccrine sweat ducts, the sweat ducts are frequently seen to enter the cyst wall at the bottom of the milium (136,138).

Pathogenesis. Primary milia of the face represent a keratinizing type of benign tumor (136). In contrast, secondary milia represent retention cysts caused by proliferative tendencies of the epithelium after injury (139).

TRICHILEMMAL OR PILAR CYST

Trichilemmal or pilar cysts are clinically indistinguishable from epidermal cysts. They differ from epidermal cysts, however, in frequency and distribution. They are less common than epidermal cysts, constituting only about 25% of the combined material; about 90% of trichilemmal cysts occur on the scalp. Trichilemmal cysts often show an autosomal dominant inheritance pattern and are solitary in only 30% of the cases, with 10% of patients having more than ten cysts (140). Furthermore, in contrast to epidermal

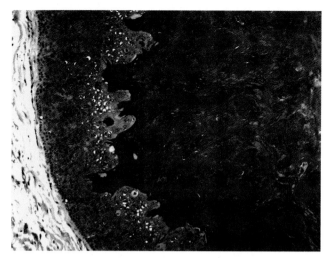

FIGURE 29-14. Trichilemmal cyst. The cyst is lined by a squamous epithelium with no granular layer and with swelling of the cells close to the cyst cavity that is filled with homogeneous horny material.

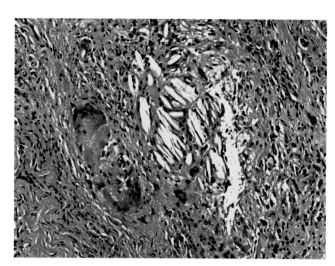

FIGURE 29-15. Keratin granuloma. At the edge of a partially ruptured cyst cholesterol clefts form part of a kertin granuloma.

cysts, trichilemmal cysts are easily enucleated and appear as firm, smooth, white-walled cysts (141).

Histopathology. The wall of trichilemmal cysts is composed of epithelial cells possessing no clearly visible intercellular bridges. The peripheral layer of cells shows a distinct palisade arrangement not seen in epidermal cysts. The epithelial cells close to the cystic cavity appear swollen and are filled with pale cytoplasm (Fig. 29-14). These swollen cells do not produce a granular layer but generally undergo abrupt keratinization, although nuclear remnants are occasionally retained in a few cells. The content of the cysts consists of homogeneous eosinophilic material (134).

Whereas focal calcification of the cyst content does not occur in epidermal cysts, foci of calcification are seen in approximately one-fourth of trichilemmal cysts (140). A considerable foreign-body reaction results when the wall of a trichilemmal cyst ruptures, and the cyst may then undergo partial or complete disintegration (Fig. 29-15).

Trichilemmal cysts frequently disclose small, acanthotic foci in their walls that are indistinguishable from solid areas, as seen in a proliferating trichilemmal cyst (142). The association of a trichilemmal cyst with tumor lobules of a proliferating trichilemmal cyst is also seen occasionally (Chapter 30) (140).

Pathogenesis. Trichilemmal cysts, also referred to as pilar cysts, originally were called sebaceous cysts. The name was changed when it became apparent that the keratinization in them is analogous to the keratinization that takes place in the outer root sheath of the hair, or trichilemma (143). The outer root sheath of the hair does not keratinize wherever it covers the inner root sheath. It keratinizes normally in two areas, the follicular isthmus of anagen hairs and the sac surrounding catagen and telogen hairs, because in these

two regions the inner root sheath has disappeared. The follicular isthmus of anagen hairs is the short, middle portion of the hair follicle, extending upward from the attachment of the arrector pili muscle to the entrance of the sebaceous duct. At the lower end of the follicular isthmus, the inner root sheath sloughs off, exposing the outer root sheath, which, in its exposed portion, undergoes a specific type of homogeneous keratinization without the interposition of a granular layer. This type of trichilemmal keratinization also takes place in the sac surrounding catagen and telogen hairs, because hairs in these stages have lost their inner root sheath. The differentiation toward hair keratin in trichilemmal cysts has been confirmed by immunohistochemical staining because they stain with antikeratin antibodies derived from human hair, in contrast to epidermal cysts, which stain with antikeratin antibodies obtained from human callus (144).

Electron microscopic examination of the epithelial lining of trichilemmal cysts shows that, on their way from the peripheral layer toward the center, the epithelial cells have an increasing number of filaments in their cytoplasm. The transition from nucleate to anucleate cells is abrupt and is associated with the loss of all cytoplasmic organelles. The junction between the keratinizing and keratinized cells shows interdigitations (145). The keratinized cells are filled with tonofilaments and, unlike those in epidermal cysts, retain their desmosomal connections (134).

Differential Diagnosis. Even though both the trichilemmal cyst and the proliferating trichilemmal cyst show trichilemmal types of keratinization and can occur together, one is essentially a cyst and the other essentially a solid, tumorlike proliferation. The latter is therefore discussed under Tumors with Differentiation Toward Hair Structures (see Chapter 30).

STEATOCYSTOMA MULTIPLEX

Steatocystoma multiplex is inherited in an autosomal dominant pattern. One observes numerous small, rounded, moderately firm, cystic nodules that are adherent to the overlying skin and usually measure 1 to 3 cm in diameter. When punctured, the cysts discharge an oily or creamy fluid and, in some instances, also small hairs (146, 146a,b,c). They are found most commonly in the axillae, in the sternal region, and on the arms. Steatocystoma also occurs occasionally as a solitary, noninherited tumor in adults, where it is referred to as *steatocystoma simplex* (147).

Histopathology. The cysts have walls that are intricately folded with several layers of epithelial cells, although in atrophic areas only two or three layers of flat cells may be present. Elsewhere is a basal layer in palisade arrangement, above which are two or three layers of swollen cells without recognizable intercellular bridges. Central to these cells there is a thick, homogeneous, eosinophilic horny layer that forms without an intervening granular layer. It protrudes irregularly into the lumen in a fashion simulating the decapitation secretion of apocrine glands (148) (Fig. 29-16).

A characteristic feature seen in most lesions of steatocystoma is the presence of flattened sebaceous gland lobules either within or close to the cyst wall (149). In some cysts, invaginations resembling hair follicles extend from the cyst wall into the surrounding stroma, and in rare instances true hair shafts are seen within them, indicating that the invaginations represent the outer root sheath of hairs. In a few cysts, the lumen contains clusters of hair, mainly of lanugo size but partially of intermediate character (150). When stained with the PAS reaction, the cells of the cyst wall are found to be rich in glycogen.

Pathogenesis. Electron microscopic examination has shown that the cyst wall consists of keratinizing cells. Nearest to the lumen, the cyst wall consists of several layers of flattened, very elongated horny cells interconnected by desmosomes.

It appears likely that differentiation in the cyst wall of steatocystoma multiplex is to a large extent in the direction of the sebaceous duct (151,152). The sebaceous duct and the outer root sheath are composed of similar cells, but undulation and thinning of the horny layer and the existence of sebaceous cells in the cyst wall are characteristic features of the sebaceous gland side of the sebaceous duct (152). Sebaceous duct cells, like outer root sheath cells, contain abundant glycogen and amylophosphorylase, keratinize without the interposition of keratohyaline granules, and on electron microscopic examination, after keratinization retain their desmosomes (148).

PIGMENTED FOLLICULAR CYST

This is an uncommon pigmented lesion resembling a nevus.

Histopathology. The cyst wall consists of infundibular epidermis. The cyst contains, in addition to laminated keratin, numerous large pigmented hair shafts. One or two growing hair follicles are seen in the wall of the cyst (153).

DERMOID CYST

Dermoid cysts are subcutaneous cysts that usually are present at birth. They occur most commonly on the head, mainly around the eyes, and occasionally on the neck. When located on the head, they often are adherent to the periosteum. Usually they measure between 1 and 4 cm in diameter.

Histopathology. Dermoid cysts, in contrast to epidermal cysts, are lined by an epidermis that possesses various epidermal appendages that are usually fully matured (Figs. 29-17

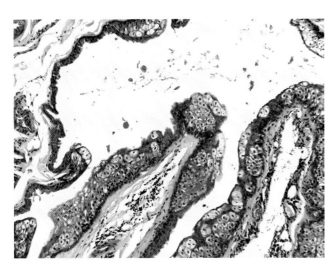

FIGURE 29-16. Steatocystoma multiplex. The cyst wall shows intricate folding. The lining stratified squamous epithelium has sebaceous gland lobules within and close to it.

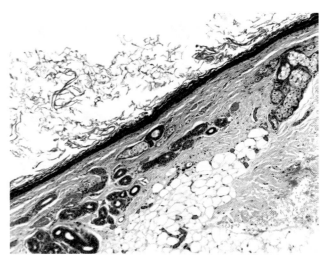

FIGURE 29-17. External angular dermoid cyst. The cyst is lined by stratified squamous epithelium, with adnexal structures in the wall.

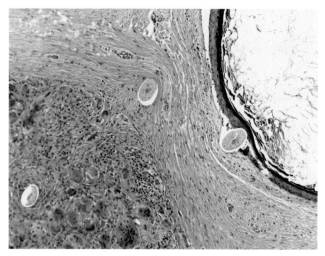

FIGURE 29-18. External angular dermoid cyst. In this example, the cyst has ruptured, producing an adjacent granuloma containing hair shafts derived from the cyst.

and 29-18). Hair follicles containing hairs that project into the lumen of the cyst are often present. In addition, the dermis of dermoid cysts usually contains sebaceous glands, often eccrine glands, and in about 20% of the cases, apocrine glands that have matured (154).

Pathogenesis. Dermoid cysts are a result of the sequestration of skin along lines of embryonic closure.

BRONCHOGENIC AND THYROGLOSSAL DUCT CYSTS

Bronchogenic cysts are rare. They are small, solitary lesions seen most commonly in the skin or subcutaneous tissue just above the sternal notch. Rarely, they are located on the ante-

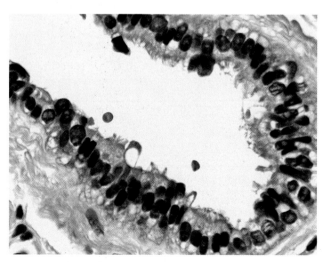

FIGURE 29-19. Bronchogenic cyst. High magnification. The lining epithelium is columnar with a ciliated surface.

rior aspect of the neck or on the chin. As a rule, they are discovered shortly after birth. They may show a draining sinus.

Thyroglossal duct cysts are clinically indistinguishable from bronchogenic cysts, except that they are usually located on the anterior aspect of the neck.

Histopathology. Bronchogenic cysts are lined by a mucosa consisting of ciliated pseudostratified columnar epithelium (Fig. 29-19). Goblet cells may be interspersed. The wall frequently contains smooth muscle and mucous glands but only rarely contains cartilage (153).

Thyroglossal duct cysts differ from bronchogenic cysts in that they do not contain smooth muscle and they frequently contain thyroid follicles (155).

Pathogenesis. On electron microscopy the cilia show two central microtubules surrounded by nine paired microtubules (156).

CUTANEOUS CILIATED CYST

Cutaneous ciliated cysts are found very rarely in females as a single lesion, largely on the lower extremities, and even more rarely in males and on the back (157–159,159a). They usually measure several centimeters in diameter. They are either unilocular or multilocular and are filled with clear or amber fluid. The finding of one on the perineum led the authors to suggest a primitive tailgut origin to this cyst, probably from the embryonic remnants of cloacal membrane (159b).

Histopathology. Cutaneous ciliated cysts show numerous papillary projections lined by a simple cuboidal or columnar ciliated epithelium. Mucin-secreting cells are absent (159).

Pathogenesis. The epithelial lining of the cysts resembles that seen in the fallopian tube. On electron microscopy, the cilia show two central filaments encircled by nine pairs of filaments (160).

MEDIAN RAPHE CYST OF THE PENIS

Median raphe cysts of the penis arise usually in young adults. They are located on the ventral aspect of the penis, most commonly on the glans. They are solitary and measure only a few millimeters in diameter (161). However, they may extend over several centimeters in a linear fashion (162). It seems that, in some instances, median raphe cysts have been erroneously reported as apocrine cystadenoma of the penis (163,164) (Fig. 29-20) (see also Chapter 31).

Histopathology. The cysts are lined by pseudostratified columnar epithelium varying from one to four cells in thickness, mimicking the transitional epithelium of the urethra. Some of the epithelial cells have clear cytoplasm, mucin-containing cells are uncommon, and a case lined by ciliated epithelium has been described (165).

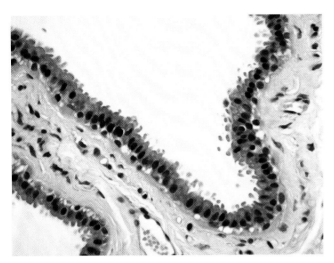

FIGURE 29-20. Apocrine cyst. In this small dermal cyst the lining epithelium forms a single layer with apocrine snouting secretion.

Pathogenesis. It is likely that median raphe cysts do not represent a defective closure of the median raphe, but rather the anomalous budding and separation of urethral columnar epithelium from the urethra (166).

ERUPTIVE VELLUS HAIR CYSTS

In eruptive vellus hair cysts, a condition first described in 1977 (167), asymptomatic follicular papules 1 to 2 mm in diameter occur, most commonly on the chest but in some instances elsewhere. Some of the papules have a crusted or umbilicated surface. The condition is usually seen in children and young adults but can develop at any age. Spontaneous clearing may take place in a few years. Autosomal dominant inheritance has been described (168,169). Cytokeratin studies have shown that epidermoid cysts expressed cytokeratin 10 and eruptive vellus hair cysts expressed cytokeratin 17, whereas trichilemmal cysts and steatocystoma multiplex showed expression of both cytokeratin 10 and cytokeratin 17, supporting the opinion that eruptive vellus hair cysts, which stained negative for cytokeratin 10, and steatocystoma multiplex are distinct entities and not variants of a single disorder (169a).

Histopathology. A cystic structure is usually seen in the mid-dermis lined by squamous epithelium. It contains laminated keratinous material and varying numbers of transversely and obliquely cut vellus hairs (167). In some cysts, vellus hairs are seen emerging from follicle-like invaginations of the cyst wall (170). In other cysts, a telogen hair follicle is seen extending from the lower surface toward the subcutis (167). Crusted or umbilicated lesions show either a cyst communicating with the surface and extruding its contents (169,171), or partial destruction of a cyst

by a granulomatous infiltrate and elimination of vellus hairs to the surface of the skin (172).

Pathogenesis. Eruptive vellus hair cysts represent a developmental abnormality of vellus hair follicles that predisposes them to occlusion at their infundibular level. This results in retention of hairs, cystic dilatation of the proximal part of the follicle, and secondary atrophy of the hair bulbs (167,171). There is a close relationship with steatocystoma multiplex (173). Both processes could be described as multiple pilosebaceous cysts (174).

WARTY DYSKERATOMA

Warty dyskeratoma, first described in 1957 (175) usually occurs as a solitary lesion, most commonly on the scalp, face, or neck, although a case with multiple lesions has been described (176). It has also been reported in non–sun-exposed skin including the oral mucosa, usually on the hard palate or an alveolar ridge (177,178). Although its clinical appearance is not always distinctive, it often occurs as a slightly elevated papule or nodule with a keratotic umbilicated center (179). The lesion, after having reached a certain size, persists indefinitely.

Histopathology. The center of the lesion is occupied by a large, cup-shaped invagination connected with the surface by a channel filled with keratinous material (Figs. 29-21, 29-22, and 29-23). The large invagination contains numerous acantholytic, dyskeratotic cells in its upper portion. The lower portion of the invagination is occupied by numerous villi, that is, markedly elongated dermal papillae that are often lined with only a single layer of basal cells and project upward from the base of the cup-shaped invagination (175,180–182) (Fig. 29-21). Typical corps ronds can usually be seen in the thickened granular layer

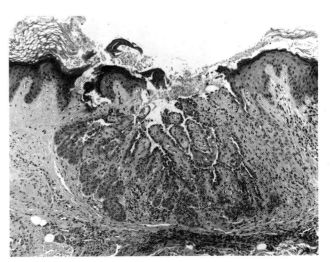

FIGURE 29-21. Warty dyskeratoma. Low magnification. A large invagination is connected to the by a channel.

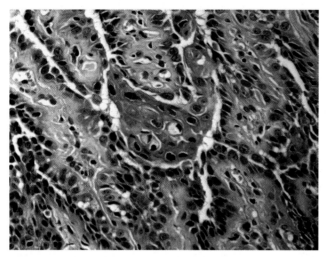

FIGURE 29-22. Warty dyskeratoma. The villi at the base of the invagination are covered with a single layer of cells. Acantholytic, dyskeratotic cells lie above the villi.

lining the channel at the entrance to the invagination (179,183) (Fig. 29-22).

Pathogenesis. The central cup-shaped invagination has been interpreted by several observers as a greatly dilated hair follicle, because in early lesions a hair follicle or sebaceous gland is often connected with the invagination (180). Occasionally, two or three adjoining follicles seem to be involved (179). The fact, however, that warty dyskeratoma can arise on the oral mucosa indicates that, as in Darier's disease, the dyskeratotic, acantholytic process is not always derived from a pilosebaceous structure.

Although attempts were made at first to correlate warty dyskeratoma with Darier's disease, it is now generally agreed that warty dyskeratoma represents an entity, "a be-

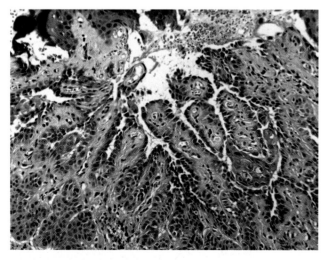

FIGURE 29-23. Warty dyskeratoma. High magnification. Acantholytic and dyskeratotic cells lie above the basal layer of epithelial cells.

nign cutaneous tumor that resembles Darier's disease microscopically" (175).

ACTINIC KERATOSIS

Solar keratoses are also known as actinic keratoses. The adjective *solar* is more specific, because it refers to the sun as the cause, whereas the adjective *actinic* refers to a variety of rays (184). Even among the sun rays, action spectrum evaluations indicate that the ultraviolet B (UVB) rays (290 to 320 nm) are the most damaging ("carcinogenic") rays, although UVA rays (320 to 400 nm) can augment the damaging effects of UVB rays (185).

Actinic keratoses are usually seen as multiple lesions in sun-exposed areas of the skin in middle-aged or older persons who have fair complexions. Excessive exposure to sunlight over many years and inadequate protection against it are the essential predisposing factors. Actinic keratoses are seen most commonly on the face and the dorsa of the hands and in the bald portions of the scalp in men (186).

Usually, the lesions measure less than 1 cm in diameter. They are erythematous, are often covered by adherent scales, and except in their hypertrophic form, show little or no infiltration. Some actinic keratoses are pigmented and show peripheral spreading, making clinical differentiation from lentigo maligna difficult (187). Occasionally, lesions show marked hyperkeratosis and then have the clinical aspect of cutaneous horns. A lesion analogous to actinic keratosis occurs on the vermilion border of the lower lip as *solar cheilitis* and may show areas of erosion and hyperkeratosis (188–190).

Actinic keratosis and solar cheilitis can develop into squamous cell carcinoma. However, the incidence of this transformation is difficult to determine, because the borderline between actinic keratosis and squamous cell carcinoma is not clear-cut (see Histopathology section). It has been estimated that in 20% of patients with actinic keratoses squamous cell carcinoma develops in one or more of the lesions (191). Usually, squamous cell carcinomas arising either in actinic keratoses or *de novo* in sun-damaged skin do not metastasize. The incidence of metastasis in different series varies from 0.5% (192) to 3% (193). In carcinoma of the vermilion border of the lip, however, metastases have been found in 11% of the cases (193).

Histopathology. Actinic keratoses are keratinocytic dysplasias or squamous cell carcinomas *in situ*. This definition is preferable to their designation as precancerous, because most of them never progress to cancers. Biologically, the lesions are still benign; invasion into the dermis, if present at all, is limited to the most superficial portion, the papillary dermis (see Differential Diagnosis section).

Five types of actinic keratosis can be recognized histologically: hypertrophic, atrophic, bowenoid, acantholytic, and pigmented (Figs. 29-24 to 29-33). Transitions and

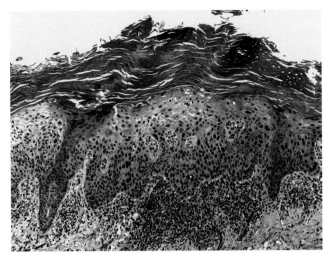

FIGURE 29-24. Actinic keratosis. Tall columns of parakeratotic keratin alternate with bands of orthokeratotic keratin with moderate atypia of the underlying keratinocytes.

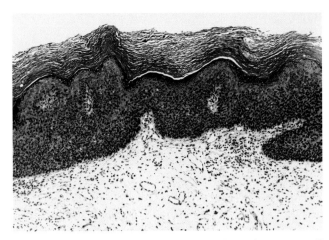

FIGURE 29-27. Actinic keratosis, Bowenoid type (squamous cell carcinoma *in situ*). Low magnification. Beneath a thick layer of parakeratotic keratin the epidermis shows cytologic atypia.

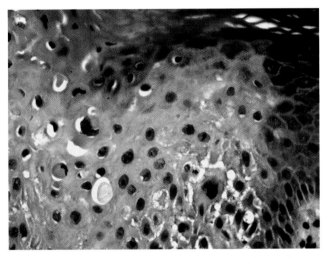

FIGURE 29-25. Actinic keratosis. Beneath a thick layer of parakeratotic keratin the epidermis shows cytologic atypia.

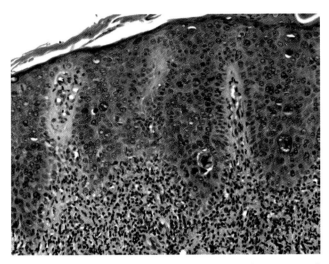

FIGURE 29-28. Actinic keratosis, Bowenoid type (squamous cell carcinoma *in situ*). Medium magnification. Marked cellular and nuclear pleomorphism are present together with frequent and atypical mitoses in a Bowenoid actinic keratosis (squamous cell carcinoma *in situ*).

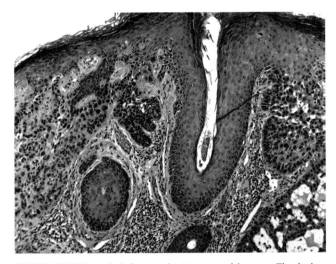

FIGURE 29-26. Actinic keratosis, Hypertrophic type. The lesion shows hyperkeratosis and papillomatosis with prominent cytologic atypia. There is a moderate lymphocytic infiltrate in the underlying papillary dermis.

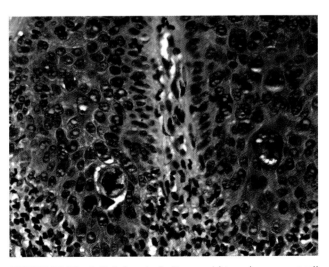

FIGURE 29-29. Actinic keratosis, Bowenoid type (squamous cell carcinoma *in situ*). High magnification. Large atypical mitoses are prominent in this Bowenoid actinic keratosis.

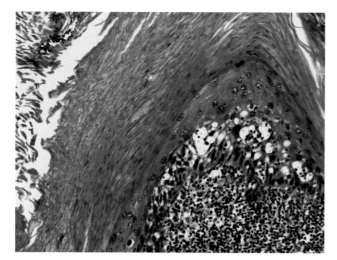

FIGURE 29-30. Actinic keratosis, acantholytic type. Low magnification. The epidermis is markedly hyperkeratotic. In the dermis, there is a dense lichenoid inflammatory infiltrate. The keratosis shows focal acantholytic change.

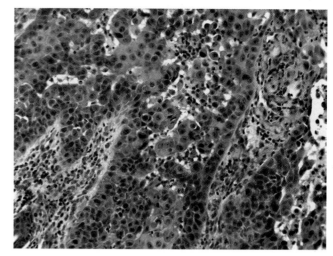

FIGURE 29-32. Actinic keratosis, acantholytic type. High magnification. Keratinocytes in the basal layer are crowded, with an increased nuclear-cytoplasmic ratio, and they tend to become separated from one another and to adopt a rounded configuration. This process of "secondary acantholysis" may in some instances result in the formation of pseudoglandular spaces that may mimic a glandular pattern of differentiation.

combinations among these five types occur. In addition, many cutaneous horns prove on histologic examination to be actinic keratoses.

In the *hypertrophic type* of actinic keratosis, hyperkeratosis is pronounced and is usually intermingled with areas of parakeratosis (194). This variety of keratosis, sometimes referred to as *florid keratosis*, may easily be overdiagnosed as invasive squamous cell carcinoma by the unwary. Mild or moderate papillomatosis may be present. The epidermis is thickened in most areas and shows irregular downward proliferation that is limited to the uppermost dermis and does not represent frank invasion (Fig. 29-26). A varying proportion of the keratinocytes in the stratum malpighii

show a loss of polarity and thus a disorderly arrangement. Some of these cells show pleomorphism and atypicality ("anaplasia") of their nuclei, which appear large, irregular, and hyperchromatic. Often the nuclei in the basal layer are closely crowded together. Some of the cells in the midportion of the epidermis show premature keratinization, resulting in dyskeratotic cells or apoptotic bodies characterized by homogeneous, eosinophilic cytoplasm with or without a nucleus. In contrast to the epidermal keratinocytes, the cells of the hair follicles and eccrine ducts that penetrate the epidermis within actinic keratoses retain

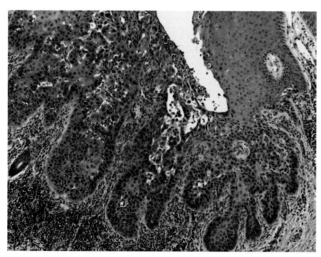

FIGURE 29-31. Actinic keratosis, acantholytic type. Medium magnification. In the dermis, there is a dense lichenoid inflammatory infiltrate. The keratosis shows focal acantholytic change.

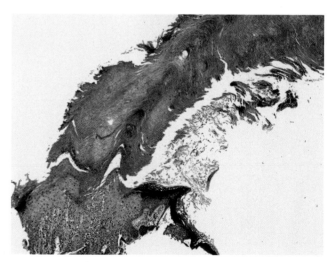

FIGURE 29-33. Cutaneous horn. The horn consists of a column of keratin arising in an actinic keratosis.

their normal appearance and keratinize normally (195, 196). Occasionally, cells of the normal adnexal epithelium extend over the atypical cells of the epidermis in an umbrella-like fashion. In some cases, abnormal keratinocytes extend downward on the outside of the follicular infundibulum to the level of the sebaceous duct and, less commonly, along the eccrine duct (196).

A variant of the hypertrophic type of actinic keratosis is the lichenoid actinic keratosis, which demonstrates nuclear atypia, irregular acanthosis and hyperkeratosis, the presence of basal cell liquefaction, degeneration of the basal cell layer, and a bandlike "lichenoid" infiltrate in close apposition to the epidermis (197). Fairly numerous eosinophilic, homogeneous apoptotic bodies are seen in the upper dermis as so-called Civatte bodies. Aside from the presence of nuclear atypicality, there is considerable resemblance to lichen planus and benign lichenoid keratosis (see Chapter 7).

In rare instances of actinic keratosis of the hypertrophic type, in addition to finding anaplastic nuclei in the lower epidermis, one finds areas of epidermolytic hyperkeratosis in the upper epidermis. These changes are like those seen in bullous congenital ichthyosiform erythroderma, in linear epidermal nevus, and as incidental epidermolytic hyperkeratosis in a variety of lesions. In areas of epidermolytic hyperkeratosis, one observes in the upper epidermis clear spaces around the nuclei and a thickened granular layer with large, irregularly shaped keratohyaline granules (34). Epidermolytic hyperkeratosis may occur also in lesions of solar cheilitis (198).

In the *atrophic type* of actinic keratosis, hyperkeratosis usually is slight. The epidermis is thinned and devoid of rete ridges. Atypicality of the cells is found predominantly in the basal cell layer, which consists of cells with large hyperchromatic nuclei that lie close together. The atypical basal layer may proliferate into the dermis as buds and duct-like structures. It may also surround as cell mantles the upper portion of pilosebaceous follicles and sweat ducts, the epithelium of which otherwise appears normal (196).

The *bowenoid type* of actinic keratosis is histologically indistinguishable from Bowen's disease, and may also be referred to as squamous cell carcinoma *in situ*. As in Bowen's disease, there is within the epidermis considerable disorder in the arrangement of the nuclei, as well as clumping of nuclei and dyskeratosis (Figs. 29-27, 29-28, and 29-29).

In the *acantholytic type* of actinic keratosis, immediately above the atypical cells composing the basal cell layer there are clefts or lacunae similar to those seen in Darier's disease (Chapter 6) (199). These clefts form as a result of anaplastic changes in the lowermost epidermis, resulting in dyskeratosis and loss of the intercellular bridges (Fig. 29-28). A few acantholytic cells may be present within the clefts (Figs. 29-30, 29-31, and 29-32). Because the acantholysis is preceded by cellular changes, it is referred to as secondary acantholysis, in contrast to the primary acantholysis seen in the "acantholytic" diseases, such as pem-

phigus vulgaris and Darier's disease. Above the acantholytic clefts, the epidermis shows varying degrees of atypicality but generally less atypicality than is seen in the basal cell layer. The anaplastic cells of the basal cell layer frequently show extensions into the upper dermis as buds or short, duct-like structures. Suprabasal acantholysis may be seen also around hair follicles and sweat ducts in the upper dermis. When atypia is full-thickness or high-grade, the term *acantholytic squamous cell carcinoma in situ* may be applied.

In the *pigmented type* of actinic keratosis, excessive amounts of melanin are present, especially in the basal cell layer. In some cases, the atypical keratinocytes are well melanized (200). In others, almost all the melanin is retained within the cell bodies and dendrites of the melanocytes, indicating some block in melanin transfer. Numerous melanophages are seen in most cases in the superficial dermis (187).

In all five types of actinic keratosis, the upper dermis usually shows a fairly dense, chronic inflammatory infiltrate composed predominantly of lymphoid cells but often also containing plasma cells. Solar cheilitis, more frequently than actinic keratosis of the skin, shows an inflammatory infiltrate in which plasma cells predominate (188). Although the upper dermis usually shows solar or basophilic degeneration, this may be absent in areas with a pronounced inflammatory reaction, probably because the inflammation has resulted in a regeneration of collagen.

In instances in which the histologic diagnosis is actinic keratosis but the clinical diagnosis is squamous cell carcinoma, it is advisable to section more deeply into the block of tissue, because progression into squamous cell carcinoma may have taken place in another area. Because no sharp line of demarcation exists between the two conditions, it is not always possible to decide whether a lesion can still be regarded as an actinic keratosis or should be classified as an early squamous cell carcinoma. Thus, some authors regard squamous cell carcinoma as a lesion in which irregular aggregates of atypical keratinocytes are found in the papillary dermis, not in continuity with the overlying epidermis (201); others call a lesion that does not extend downward to the level of the reticular dermis an actinic keratosis without qualification (202). This decision is rarely a vital one, because early squamous cell carcinoma arising in an actinic keratosis rarely causes metastases, although it may become deeply invasive and destructive through further growth. Because carcinomas arising in solar cheilitis have a significantly higher tendency to metastasize than carcinomas arising in actinic keratosis, and because invasion of the dermis in solar cheilitis may be focal, lesions of solar cheilitis require thorough examination by means of step sections (189).

Pathogenesis. On electron microscopic examination, only a difference in degree was found to exist between actinic keratosis and squamous cell carcinoma (203). In applying blood group antigens as indicators of malignancy to sections of actinic keratosis, areas of positive staining alternate with areas showing no staining, the lack of staining being indicative of anaplasia. Areas of irregular downward proliferation or early invasion are consistently negative (204).

Differential Diagnosis. In actinic keratoses showing relatively slight atypicality, or anaplasia, of the tumor cells, diagnosis may be difficult. Thus, a hypertrophic actinic keratosis with a lichenoid inflammatory infiltrate may show a close histologic resemblance to the lesion known as *benign lichenoid keratosis*. In fact, this lesion was at one time thought to be a variant of actinic keratosis (205). Benign lichenoid keratosis differs from actinic keratosis by showing dissolution rather than atypicality of the basal cell layer, analogous to lichen planus (206,207) (Chapter 7).

An atrophic actinic keratosis may closely resemble lupus erythematosus, because both types of lesions show flattening of the epidermis. Although lupus erythematosus shows vacuolization and actinic keratosis shows atypicality of the cells in the basal layer, these two changes are not always easily distinguished from one another. Therefore, other findings, such as follicular plugging and a patchy, periappendageal infiltrate in lupus erythematosus, are necessary for differentiation (Chapter 10).

A pigmented actinic keratosis may resemble lentigo maligna, particularly if the melanin is seen largely within the melanocytes (187). Usually, however, lentigo maligna shows more flattening of the epidermis than pigmented actinic keratosis and, more important, a great increase in the number of melanocytes, together with atypicality in the melanocytes but not in the basal keratinocytes (Chapter 28).

CUTANEOUS HORN

Cutaneous horn, or *cornu cutaneum*, is the clinical term for a circumscribed, conical, markedly hyperkeratotic lesion in which the height of the keratotic mass amounts to at least half of its largest diameter (208). The term refers to a reaction pattern and not to a specific lesion (209).

Histopathology. On histologic examination, different types of lesions can be seen at the base of the conical hyperkeratosis of a cornu cutaneum. Most commonly, an actinic keratosis is encountered (210) (Fig. 29-33). In some instances, a filiform verruca, a seborrheic keratosis, or a squamous cell carcinoma is found (208). On rare occasions, a trichilemmoma (209) or a basal cell epithelioma is seen (211). (For a description of trichilemmal horn, see Chapter 30.)

ORAL LEUKOPLAKIA

The term *leukoplakia* was used in the past by dermatologists and gynecologists (212) to designate white patches of the oral mucosa or the vulva that showed early, *in situ*, anaplastic changes; the term *leukokeratosis* was used for patches with a histologically benign appearance. However, leukoplakia has been redefined on the basis of the concept proposed by oral pathologists (213), and this concept has been accepted by the World Health Organization (214).

According to this concept, the term *leukoplakia* carries no histologic connotation and is used only as a clinical description. It is defined as a white patch or plaque that will not rub off and that cannot be characterized clinically or histologically as any specific disease (e.g., lichen planus, lupus erythematosus, candidiasis, white sponge nevus) (215). The reason for using the term leukoplakia as a purely clinical designation is that a distinction between benign leukoplakia and leukoplakia with dysplastic changes cannot be made on clinical grounds. It is therefore essential that all white plaques that either are idiopathic in origin or persist for 3 to 4 weeks after any existing irritation has been eliminated be examined histologically (216). In many cases of oral leukoplakia, either chemical irritation through tobacco or mechanical irritation through dental stumps or ill-fitting dentures plays a role. Although the leukoplakia clears in some instances after the irritation has been removed, it persists in others. However, the transformation of a benign leukoplakia into a malignant leukoplakia is regarded as rare (217). Still, any leukoplakia that is growing or altering its appearance requires a repeat biopsy (28).

Clinically, lesions of leukoplakia on the oral mucosa consist of one or several white patches that may not be raised and that appear ill defined. However, if they are slightly elevated, they appear sharply demarcated, with an irregular outline.

Erythroplakia of the oral mucosa consists of red, sharply delineated patches that vary greatly in size. Some of these lesions are sprinkled or intermingled with patches of leukoplakia and are then referred to as *speckled erythroplakia* (218).

On examination by histology, scraping, or culture, both leukoplakia and erythroplakia frequently show *C. albicans* as a secondary invader, a finding that may give rise to an incorrect diagnosis of candidiasis (219). However, infection with *C. albicans* may cause oral lesions that are clinically indistinguishable from leukoplakia (220).

The analysis of oral leukoplakias and oral invasive carcinomas for human papillomavirus-related DNA has shown a significant percentage of these lesions to be reactive with papillomavirus antibodies, allowing the conclusion that they are induced by papillomaviruses, especially by HPV-11 and HPV-16 (221,222) (Chapter 25).

Histopathology. The white color of leukoplakia is the result of hydration of a thickened horny layer. On histologic examination, about 80% of the lesions of oral leukoplakia are found to be benign (215,219). Such lesions show hyperkeratotic or parakeratotic thickening of the horny layer, acanthosis, and a chronic inflammatory infiltrate (Fig. 29-34). Of the remaining 20% of the cases, 17% show varying degrees of dysplasia or *in situ* carcinoma, and 3% show in-

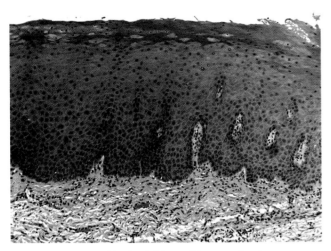

FIGURE 29-34. Oral leukoplakia. In this example, the squamous epithelium is hyperkeratotic and acanthotic but shows no evidence of dysplasia.

filtrating squamous cell carcinoma (215). Ultimate development of carcinoma has been observed in 7% to 13% of all cases of leukoplakia (214). Localization of the leukoplakia seems to play an important role in the presence of malignancy. Leukoplakias on the buccal mucosa were found to be benign in 96% of the cases; whereas on the floor of the mouth, only 32% of the leukoplakias were benign, 31% showed a carcinoma *in situ*, and 37% an invasive carcinoma (223).

In situ carcinoma, also referred to as precancerous leukoplakia, may have a similar histologic appearance to the hypertrophic type of actinic keratosis. Thus, the most important features observed within a moderately acanthotic epithelium are, first, pleomorphism and atypicality of the nuclei, which appear large, irregular, and hyperchromatic, and, second, loss of polarity, resulting in a disorderly arrangement of the cells. In some instances, one finds as additional features premature keratinization resulting in dyskeratotic cells in the midportion of the epithelium, crowding of nuclei in the basal cell layer, and irregular downward proliferations of the epithelium. There is considerable histologic, philosophical, and biological overlap among lesions categorized as high-grade dysplasia and carcinoma *in situ* in oral as in other mucous membranes.

Erythroplakia of the oral mucosa, in contrast to leukoplakia, invariably shows nuclear atypicality. One observes *in situ* carcinoma in half of the cases and invasive carcinoma in the other half (218). The red appearance is explained by the absence of the normal surface covering of orthokeratin or parakeratin.

Differential Diagnosis. A decision as to whether *in situ* carcinoma exists in a leukoplakia can be difficult, since some pleomorphism of nuclei and some loss of polarity of the cells can be seen occasionally also in various inflamma-

tory conditions, including benign leukoplakia (216). In doubtful cases, step sections throughout the biopsy specimen are required, as well as, possibly, examination of additional biopsy specimens. The decision as to whether a leukoplakia is benign or low grade or is a high-grade dysplasia or a carcinoma *in situ* is of great importance. In comparison with squamous cell carcinoma of the skin developing in an actinic keratosis, squamous cell carcinoma of the oral mucosa developing in a leukoplakia with *in situ* carcinoma has a much greater tendency to metastasize.

Also, differentiation of leukoplakia from oral lichen planus may cause difficulties both clinically and histologically. In lichen planus, no atypia is seen and there often is partial absence of basal cells. In addition, the prevalence of Langerhans cells in lesions of lichen planus may aid in the differentiation (224).

VERRUCOUS HYPERPLASIA, VERRUCOUS CARCINOMA OF ORAL MUCOSA

Verrucous hyperplasia of the oral mucosa consists of extensive verrucous, white patches that may arise as such or develop from lesions of leukoplakia. Verrucous hyperplasia and verrucous carcinoma are indistinguishable clinically. They may coexist, or verrucous carcinoma may develop from verrucous hyperplasia. In some instances, verrucous hyperplasia develops into frank squamous cell carcinoma rather than into verrucous carcinoma (225).

Verrucous carcinoma of the oral mucosa is also known as *oral florid papillomatosis*. Clinically, white, cauliflower-like lesions are observed that may involve large areas of the oral mucosa and that gradually extend and coalesce. Extensive local tissue destruction may occur. However, metastases are rare and, if they occur, remain limited to the regional lymph nodes (226–228).

Histopathology. Verrucous hyperplasia shows a hyperplastic epithelium with upward extension of verrucous projections located predominantly superficial to the adjacent epithelium (225).

Verrucous carcinoma (oral florid papillomatosis) differs in its early stage from verrucous hyperplasia by showing, in addition to the surface verrucous projections, extension of the lesion into the underlying connective tissue (225). The downward extensions of the epithelium are round and club-shaped and appear well demarcated from the surrounding stroma. Nuclear pleomorphism or hyperchromasia and formation of horn pearls are absent.

Some lesions of verrucous carcinoma persist in this stage for many years, although ultimately they show in the areas of deepest extension a moderate loss of polarity, increased cytoplasmic basophilia, nuclear hyperchromasia, and frequent mitotic figures. These features, however, do not suffice for a diagnosis of squamous cell carcinoma (229). Other lesions show sufficient nuclear atypicality and loss of polarity in the downward proliferations to indicate the presence of a well-differentiated squamous cell carcinoma (230). In about 10% of the cases of verrucous carcinoma, transformation into a classic squamous cell carcinoma takes place (227,228). (For a more detailed discussion of verrucous carcinoma, see page 836.)

NECROTIZING SIALOMETAPLASIA

One or occasionally two ulcers showing a rolled border and measuring 1 to 2 cm in diameter are found usually on the hard palate, but occasionally on the soft palate. If located on the hard palate, bone may be exposed at the base of the ulcer. Spontaneous healing takes place within 6 to 12 weeks. The importance of necrotizing sialometaplasia, a rare condition first reported in 1973 (231), lies in its clinical and histologic resemblance to carcinoma (186).

Histopathology. Histologic examination shows coagulative necrosis of salivary gland lobules and squamous metaplasia within adjacent viable lobules. The connective tissue framework of the necrotic glands remains intact, thereby preserving the lobular architecture of the salivary gland. Faintly basophilic material representing sialomucin is seen within the necrotic glands. This is both PAS positive and Alcian-blue positive. Adjacent to the necrotic glands, normal-appearing salivary gland acini may be seen. Other salivary gland structures show either partial squamous metaplasia, with a peripheral rim of squamous cells, or complete replacement by squamous epithelium. The squamous metaplasia also involves the salivary ducts (232,233).

Pathogenesis. The abrupt clinical onset and rapid spontaneous healing suggest that an acute vascular insult results in infarction and coagulation necrosis of the salivary acini (232).

Differential Diagnosis. To pathologists not familiar with this condition, the apparent irregular proliferation and deep extension of squamous epithelium may suggest a diagnosis of carcinoma. However, the confinement of cytologically benign squamous epithelium to the preexisting lobular pattern of salivary glands should permit the correct diagnosis (234).

EOSINOPHILIC ULCER OF THE TONGUE

One or two asymptomatic ulcers measuring 0.8 to 2.0 cm in diameter arise suddenly on the tongue. Spontaneous healing takes place within a few weeks.

Histopathology. A dense cellular infiltrate is present at the base of the ulcer, extending through the submucosa into the striated muscle bundles of the tongue. Most of the cells are eosinophils, but there are also lymphocytes and histiocytes (235,236). In one case, focal leukocytoclastic vasculitis was present (237).

Differential Diagnosis. This lesion differs from eosinophilic granuloma of histiocytosis X (see Chapter 26) clinically by its tendency to arise and heal rapidly, and histologically by the smaller number and smaller size of the histiocytes (235).

BOWEN'S DISEASE

Bowen's disease usually consists of a solitary lesion. It may occur on exposed or on unexposed skin. It may be caused on exposed skin by exposure to the sun and on unexposed skin by the ingestion of arsenic (see Pathogenesis section below and subsequent Arsenical Keratosis and Carcinoma section). Lesions of Bowen's disease can form in lesions of epidermodysplasia verruciformis caused by HPV-5 (see Chapter 25). Not infrequently the fingers, including the nail fold or nail bed, are involved (238).

Bowen's disease manifests itself as a slowly enlarging erythematous patch of sharp but irregular outline, showing little or no infiltration. Within the patch are generally areas of scaling and crusting. Although Bowen's disease may resemble a superficial basal cell epithelioma, it differs from it by the absence of a fine pearly border and lack of a tendency to heal with central atrophy. Bowen's disease lesions can occur on the glans penis, where they are referred to also as erythroplasia of Queyrat.

Bowenoid papulosis of the genitalia, because of its probable relationship to genital warts, is discussed in Chapter 25.

Histopathology. Bowen's disease is an intraepidermal squamous cell carcinoma referred to also as squamous cell carcinoma *in situ*. Thus, it represents biologically but not morphologically a *precancerous dermatosis,* under which designation it was described originally in 1912 (239).

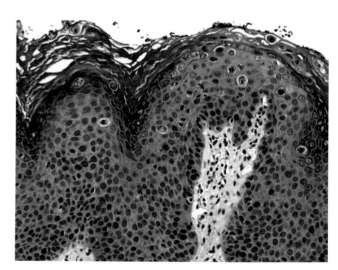

FIGURE 29-35. Bowen's disease. The epidermis is irregularly thickened. The normal maturation pattern is effaced.

The epidermis shows acanthosis with elongation and thickening of the rete ridges, often to such a degree that the papillae located between the rete ridges are reduced to thin strands (Fig. 29-35). Throughout the epidermis, the cells lie in complete disorder, resulting in a "windblown" appearance (Fig. 29-36). Many cells appear highly atypical, showing large, hyperchromatic nuclei. Multinucleated epidermal cells containing clusters of nuclei are often present. The horny layer usually is thickened and consists largely of parakeratotic cells with atypical, hyperchromatic nuclei (240).

A common and rather characteristic feature is the presence of cells showing atypical individual cell keratinization. Such dyskeratotic cells are large and round and have a homogeneous, strongly eosinophilic cytoplasm and a hyperchromatic nucleus. The infiltrate of atypical cells in Bowen's disease frequently extends into follicular infundibula and causes replacement of the follicular epithelium by atypical cells down to the entrance of the sebaceous duct (184).

Even though the marked atypicality of the epidermal cells includes the cells of the basal layer, the border between the epidermis and dermis everywhere appears sharp, and the basement membrane remains intact. The upper dermis usually shows a moderate amount of a chronic inflammatory infiltrate.

An occasional finding in Bowen's disease is vacuolization of the cells, especially in the upper portion of the epidermis (241). Also, in exceptional cases, multiple nests of atypical cells are scattered through a normal epidermis, sometimes with sparing of the basal cell layer. This results in a histologic picture that used to be interpreted as intraepidermal epithelioma of Borst–Jadassohn (184,242) (Chapter 31).

In a small percentage of cases of Bowen's disease, an invasive squamous cell carcinoma develops. The usual figure quoted is 3% to 5% (243). The highest incidence given is 11% (244). On the opposite end is a statement that, in the vast majority of cases, Bowen's disease remains a carcinoma *in situ* during the lives of those affected (245). If invasion happens, it usually takes place after many years' duration of the disease. The invasive tumor retains the cytologic characteristics of the intraepidermal tumor, and invasion may occur at first in only a limited area. To avoid missing such an area, it is advisable to examine representative sections throughout the entire tissue block. As soon as invasion has taken place, the prognosis changes. So long as Bowen's disease remains in its intraepidermal stage, metastases do not occur. However, once invasion of the dermis has occurred, there exists the possibility of regional and even visceral metastases (244).

Pathogenesis. No agreement exists about the frequency with which visceral carcinoma develops in patients with Bowen's disease. The first authors to point out an association between Bowen's disease and visceral cancer found that of 35 patients with Bowen's disease who were known to have died, 20 (57%) had an associated internal cancer (244). In a subsequent series, however, a significant increase in the incidence of associated internal cancer was observed only in patients in whom the lesions of Bowen's disease were located in areas not exposed to the sun (33%); in patients in whom the lesions were in exposed areas, the incidence of visceral cancer was low (5%) (246). Subsequent studies, with one exception (247), have not demonstrated in patients with Bowen's disease a significantly increased risk of internal malignancy (184,248–250).

Electron microscopic examination of lesions of Bowen's disease has demonstrated the presence of many dyskeratotic cells. The perinuclear aggregation and condensation of tonofilaments in these dyskeratotic cells are similar to but more pronounced than in the dyskeratotic cells of Darier's disease (251). Some of the markedly dyskeratotic cells in Bowen's disease disintegrate, and portions of such cells are phagocytized by other epidermal cells, which may contain, in addition to the phagocytized dyskeratotic material, phagocytized desmosomes in their cytoplasm (251, 252). In other instances, the intracellularly located desmosomes are not phagocytized but are drawn into the dyskeratotic cells of Bowen's disease together with aggregating tonofilaments (253). The phenomenon of intracytoplasmic desmosomes, however, is not specific for Bowen's disease, although it is found most commonly in this condition. Thus, intracytoplasmic desmosomes have been observed within dyskeratotic keratinocytes in Darier's disease (254), squamous cell carcinoma (255), and keratoacanthoma (256); within nondyskeratotic keratinocytes in extramammary Paget's disease (257) and malignant melanoma (258); and even within normal keratinocytes in both the epidermis (259) and the oral mucosa (260). It can be assumed that the occasional occurrence of invaginations of the plasma membrane is a normal event in keratinocytes

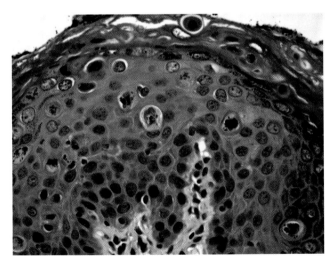

FIGURE 29-36. Bowen's disease. Throughout the epidermis, the cells lie in disarray, with frequent large atypical mitoses.

and that the invaginated plasma membrane can contain desmosomal structures. These structures are more resistant to enzymatic destruction than the plasma membrane and thus may be found free in the cytoplasm (260).

Two types of epidermal giant cells can be recognized in Bowen's disease. In one type, an entire dyskeratotic cell has been "cannibalized" by another keratinocyte and is located within the cytoplasm of the phagocytizing cell (261). In the second type, multiple nuclei lie in the center of the giant cell surrounded by dyskeratotic tonofilaments. It seems that, by becoming entangled with the spindles of the mitotic apparatus, the dyskeratotic tonofilaments interfere with the normal division of the cell so that nuclear division can take place, but cellular division cannot (251,252).

Differential Diagnosis. No histologic difference exists between bowenoid actinic keratosis and Bowen's disease. They may differ merely in size, the bowenoid actinic keratosis usually being smaller than Bowen's disease.

Paget's disease may share with Bowen's disease the presence of vacuolated cells, but, in contrast with Bowen's disease, it shows no dyskeratosis. In addition, the material contained in Paget cells is often PAS positive and diastase resistant, whereas the PAS-positive material that is sometimes present in the vacuolated cells of Bowen's disease is glycogen and therefore diastase labile (262).

ERYTHROPLASIA OF QUEYRAT (BOWEN'S DISEASE OF THE GLANS PENIS, CARCINOMA *IN SITU*)

Erythroplasia of Queyrat is the term often used for carcinoma *in situ* located on the glans penis. Clinically and histologically, it is identical to Bowen's disease, and this designation would seem preferable for simplicity's sake. The only reason for keeping the term erythroplasia of Queyrat alive is that it was introduced in 1911 (263), 1 year before the description of Bowen's disease (239).

Erythroplasia or Bowen's disease of the glans penis is seen almost exclusively in uncircumcised men. It manifests itself as an asymptomatic, sharply demarcated, bright red, shiny, very slightly infiltrated plaque on the glans penis, or less often, in the coronal sulcus or on the inner surface of the prepuce (264).

Histopathology. Erythroplasia of Queyrat of the glans penis has the same histologic appearance as Bowen's disease. Progression into an invasive squamous cell carcinoma has been observed in up to 30% of the patients (265), with metastases in about 20% of the patients with invasive erythroplasia (266). It thus has a greater tendency toward invasion and metastasis than Bowen's disease of the skin (265).

Differential Diagnosis. A clinical diagnosis of erythroplasia of Queyrat requires histologic examination of an adequate biopsy for confirmation, since differentiation from balanitis circumscripta plasmacellularis is not possible on a clinical basis.

BALANITIS CIRCUMSCRIPTA PLASMACELLULARIS

A disorder first described by Zoon in 1952 (267), balanitis circumscripta plasmacellularis has the same clinical appearance as erythroplasia of Queyrat or Bowen's disease of the glans penis. In some instances, erosions with a tendency to bleed are present (268). Like erythroplasia, this disorder is seen almost exclusively in uncircumcised males (269). On rare occasions, an analogous lesion referred to as *vulvitis circumscripta plasmacellularis* is observed on the vulva (270,271).

Histopathology. The epidermis appears thinned and often shows absence of its upper layers (272). It may be partially detached as a result of subepidermal cleavage or even absent (268,273). If present, the epidermis often has a rather distinctive appearance; in addition to being thinned and flattened, it is composed of diamond- or lozenge-shaped, flattened keratinocytes that are separated from each other by uniform intercellular edema (269). Erythrocytes may be seen permeating the epidermis. In some cases, the keratinocytes appear degenerated or necrotic (272).

The upper dermis shows a bandlike infiltrate in which numerous plasma cells are often seen (267,272). In some cases, however, their number is only moderate (269) or even small (273). In addition, the capillaries are dilated, and there may be extravasations of erythrocytes and deposits of hemosiderin (274).

Pathogenesis. It has been pointed out that plasma cells frequently predominate in the inflammatory response at mucocutaneous junctions in a variety of benign and malignant processes. Thus, the term *circumorificial plasmacytosis* was introduced for benign plasma cell infiltrates on the glans penis, vulva, and lips (275–277). However, the combination of histologic and clinical features seen in balanitis circumscripta plasmacellularis, and probably also in vulvitis circumscripta plasmacellularis, is unique and deserves recognition as an entity (269,270,272).

SQUAMOUS INTRAEPITHELIAL NEOPLASIA (DYSPLASIA) OF THE VULVA

The term leukoplakia of the vulva is purely a clinical designation requiring histologic examination for clarification of the diagnosis, especially to decide whether or not atypicality of the epithelial cells exists. The clinical aspect of leukoplakia of the vulva is more variable than that of oral leukoplakia because it does not always consist just of white patches as in the mouth but may have a papular or verrucous appearance. The reason is that on the vulva, human papilloma virus (HPV) infections can occur as flat papular condylomas (278), often in association with similar lesions on the cervix. Also the condition previously described as bowenoid papulosis, in the presence of multiple, coalescing papules, may result in a verrucous aspect of the leukoplakia (279) (Chapter 25). A clear-cut histologic decision often is not possible unless adequate clinical data are available.

The further investigation of dysplastic lesions in the vulva has shown that there are two types of vulvar intraepithelial neoplasia (VIN) (279a). The first of these is *undifferentiated VIN*, which is associated with human papillomavirus infection, occurs mainly in younger women, tends to be multicentric and is of the undifferentiated or bowenoid type. This is probably what has previously been called bowenoid papulosis. The second type is *differentiated VIN* which is not associated with human papillomavirus infection, typically occurs in older women and is often unifocal. It is commonly associated with lichen sclerosus or squamous hyperplasia and carries a substantial risk of progression to invasive squamous cell carcinoma.

Histopathology. Flat condylomas, which may be associated with VIN, show intracellular vacuolization that may result in a somewhat atypical appearance of the epithelium referred to as *koilocytotic atypia*. This may be difficult to differentiate from true atypia (278). In undifferentiated VIN the changes are those of undifferentiated basaloid or Bowenoid dysplasia. In differentiated VIN the epithelium is thickened and parakeratotic with elongated and anastomosing rete ridges. The characteristic feature is the presence of large basal or parabasal eosinophilic keratinocytes with abnormal vesicular nuclei and prominent intercellular bridges. Intraepithelial pearls may be present in the rete ridges. There is little or no atypia above the basal layer of the epidermis.

ARSENICAL KERATOSIS AND CARCINOMA

Inorganic arsenic was a frequently used oral medication for a number of dermatoses until evidence accumulated in the 1930s that, besides its long-known tendency to form arsenical keratoses on the palms and soles, inorganic arsenic quite frequently causes carcinoma of the skin (280). In the 1950s, it became apparent that inorganic arsenic could cause visceral carcinoma. The most common form in which inorganic arsenic has been administered was Fowler's solution containing 1% potassium arsenite.

Careless handling of industrial wastes can introduce arsenic into well water used for domestic consumption, resulting in "epidemic" occurrences of arsenical keratoses and cutaneous carcinomas (281,282).

Arsenical keratoses of the palms and soles, consisting of verrucous papules without surrounding inflammation, are a common manifestation of prolonged arsenic ingestion. Thus, in a follow-up study of 262 patients who had been

taking Fowler's solution for 6 to 26 years before this study, arsenical keratoses of the palms and soles were observed in 40%, and arsenic-induced carcinomas of the skin in 8% (283). In the study from Taiwan, 80% of the 428 patients with arsenical carcinomas of the skin had arsenical keratoses of the palms and soles (284). The minimal latent period between the beginning of arsenic intake and the onset of arsenical keratoses of the palms and soles has been found to be 2.5 years, and the average latent period 6 years (283).

Cutaneous carcinomas following arsenic ingestion are usually multiple, and about three-fourths of them are located on the trunk (284). They consist of erythematous, scaling, occasionally crusted patches that slowly increase in size. Carcinomas can also arise in arsenical keratoses of the palms and soles (283,284). The average latency between the beginning of arsenic intake and the onset of carcinoma has been 18 years, with a range from 3 to 40 years (285).

Visceral carcinoma can be caused by arsenic intake, but the actual incidence is difficult to determine because of the long latent period, which may vary from 13 to 50 years, with an average of 24 years (286). The most common locations appear to be bronchi and the genitourinary system (283,286). There are on record two incidences of prolonged arsenic intake in which lung cancer occurred in a high percentage of the patients: one report concerned vineyard workers exposed to an arsenic insecticide (287), and the other dealt with villagers exposed to arsenic-containing drinking water (288). In the latter series, the onset of pulmonary cancer started 30 years after the arsenic exposure.

Because Bowen's disease is the most common cutaneous carcinoma produced by arsenic, the possibility of a relationship between Bowen's disease and visceral carcinoma is of interest. This association, first pointed out in 1959 (244) appears to be greatest in those cases of Bowen's disease in which the lesions are located in unexposed areas and thus are not caused by sun exposure. In one report, an association with internal carcinoma was found in about one-third of the cases (246). It has been suggested that arsenic is the common denominator in such cases, causing both Bowen's disease and internal carcinoma. However, subsequent studies have shown no significant relationship between Bowen's disease in covered areas and internal malignancy (248); or, if such a relationship has been found to exist, no arsenic ingestion has been found in most of the patients (247).

Histopathology. In arsenical keratoses of the palms and soles, one may find, in some instances, only hyperkeratosis and acanthosis without evidence of nuclear atypicality (284). However, when one cuts deeper into the tissue block, atypicality may become apparent. Whereas some arsenical keratoses show only mild nuclear atypicality, the findings in others are those of a squamous cell carcinoma *in situ* and are analogous to Bowen's disease or an actinic keratosis. Disorder in the arrangement of the squamous cells and nuclear atypicalities is observed, such as hyperchromasia, clumping, or dyskeratosis (289). Atrophy of the epidermis and basophilic degeneration of the upper dermis, as seen in some actinic keratoses, are absent in arsenical keratoses. Evidence of development into an invasive squamous cell carcinoma may be seen in some arsenical keratoses (283,284,289).

The type of cutaneous carcinoma that follows arsenic ingestion can be either squamous cell carcinoma or basal cell carcinoma, usually as multiple lesions. Squamous cell carcinomas usually occur as *in situ* lesions analogous to Bowen's disease, and basal cell carcinomas occur most commonly as superficial basal cell carcinomas, although invasive squamous cell carcinomas and basal cell carcinomas occur occasionally. Invasive tumors may arise *de novo* or may develop within preexisting lesions of Bowen's disease or superficial basal cell carcinoma.

A matter of controversy has been whether arsenical carcinomas occur more commonly as lesions of Bowen's disease or as superficial basal cell carcinomas. For many years, it was accepted that lesions of Bowen's disease were the usual reaction (241). However, two more publications have stated that superficial basal cell carcinomas are far more prevalent than lesions of Bowen's disease (283,290); yet, in two other publications, Bowen's disease was found to be much more common (284,289). The most likely explanation for this discrepancy appears to be that, in many instances, lesions of Bowen's disease have been misinterpreted as superficial basal cell carcinoma (289). The distinction can indeed be difficult; one author who found mainly superficial basal cell carcinomas conceded that 25% of them showed "squamous metaplasia," (290), and another author has proposed the concept of "combined forms" consisting of a "mixture of superficial basal cell carcinoma and intraepidermal carcinoma" (284). It appears likely that lesions designated as superficial basal cell carcinoma with squamous metaplasia or as combined forms represent lesions of Bowen's disease. (For histologic descriptions of Bowen's disease and superficial basal cell carcinoma, see page 836.)

Pathogenesis. In vitro experiments concerning the effects of inorganic arsenic on human epidermal cells have shown that arsenic depresses premitotic DNA replication. Furthermore, incubation with inorganic arsenic and subsequent exposure of the cell cultures to ultraviolet light causes interruption of the enzymatic "dark repair mechanism" in the epidermal cells. Among other enzymes, arsenic seems to block predominantly DNA polymerase by attaching itself to sulfhydryl groups. The damaging effect of arsenic on DNA may explain its carcinogenic effect (291).

SQUAMOUS CELL CARCINOMA

Squamous cell carcinoma may occur anywhere on the skin and on mucous membranes with squamous epithelium. It rarely arises from normal-appearing skin. Most commonly, it arises in sun-damaged skin, either as such or from an actinic keratosis. Next to sun-damaged skin, squamous cell carcinomas arise most commonly in scars from burns and in stasis ulcers, termed *Marjolin's ulcers* (292). Regarding metastases, carcinomas arising in sun-damaged skin have a very low propensity to metastasize, the incidence amounting to only about 0.5% (192). This is in contrast to a metastatic rate of 2% to 3% for all patients with squamous cell carcinoma of the skin, with death resulting in about three-fourths of the patients with metastases (193,293). Carcinomas of the lower lip, even though in most cases also induced by exposure to the sun, have a much higher incidence of metastasis, about 16%, with death occurring in about half of these patients as the result of metastases (294). Also, the rate of metastases is higher in adenoid and mucin-producing squamous cell carcinomas of the skin than in the common type.

Cutaneous squamous cell carcinomas that arise secondary to inflammatory and degenerative processes have a much higher rate of metastasis than those developing in sun-damaged skin. Thus, the rate of metastasis was found to be 31% in squamous cell carcinomas arising in osteomyelitic sinuses (295), 20% in radiation-induced skin cancer (296), and 18% in carcinomas developing in burn scars (297). Furthermore, carcinomas arising from modified skin, such as the glans penis and the vulva, and from the oral mucosa have a rather high rate of metastasis unless recognized and adequately treated at an early stage.

The incidence of squamous cell carcinomas, like that of other malignant neoplasms, is significantly increased in immunosuppressed patients (298). The incidence of cutaneous squamous cell carcinoma has been found to be 18 times greater in patients with a renal transplant and immunosuppression than in the average population (299). Squamous cell carcinomas may also show greater aggressiveness in such patients (300).

Clinically, squamous cell carcinoma of the skin most commonly consists of a shallow ulcer surrounded by a wide, elevated, indurated border. Often the ulcer is covered by a crust that conceals a red, granular base. Occasionally, raised, fungoid, verrucous lesions without ulceration occur. Multiprofessional guidelines for the management of patients with squamous cell carcinoma have been published (300a).

Three variants of squamous cell carcinoma, *adenoid squamous cell carcinoma*, *mucin-producing squamous cell carcinoma*, and *verrucous carcinoma*, will be discussed later.

Histopathology. Squamous cell carcinoma of the skin is a true, invasive carcinoma of the surface epidermis. On histologic examination, one finds the tumor to consist of irregular masses of epidermal cells that proliferate downward into the dermis (Figs. 29-37 through 29-49). The invading tumor masses are composed in varying proportions of normal squamous cells and of atypical (anaplastic) squamous

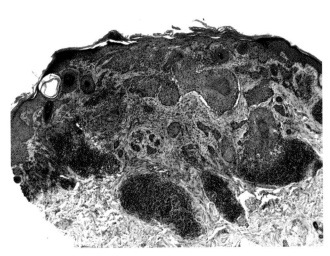

FIGURE 29-37. Squamous cell carcinoma arising in actinic keratosis. Low magnification. The epidermis shows features of an actinic keratosis. There is invasion of the dermis by epidermal masses. The dermis shows a marked inflammatory reaction.

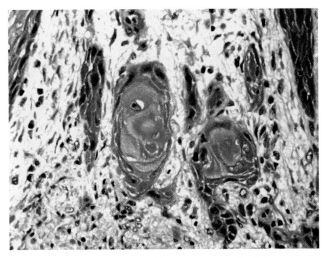

FIGURE 29-39. Squamous cell carcinoma, well differentiated. High magnification. There is invasion of the dermis by epidermal masses, the cells of which are predominantly mature squamous cells showing relatively slight atypicality. Occasional eosinophils are present in the dermis.

cells. The number of atypical squamous cells is higher in the more poorly differentiated tumors (Fig. 29-44). Atypicality of squamous cells expresses itself in such changes as great variation in the size and shape of the cells, hyperplasia and hyperchromasia of the nuclei, absence of intercellular bridges, keratinization of individual cells, and the presence of atypical mitotic figures (Fig. 29-45).

Differentiation in squamous cell carcinoma is in the direction of keratinization. Keratinization often takes place in the form of horn pearls, which are very characteristic structures composed of concentric layers of squamous cells showing gradually increasing keratinization toward the center. The center shows usually incomplete and only

rarely complete keratinization. Keratohyaline granules within the horn pearls are sparse or absent.

Marjolin's ulcer is a term applied to tumors that arise at the periphery of a chronic ulcer or a scar (292). The scar may be due to a remote burn or to radiation, or there may be a chronic inflammatory process such as a draining osteomyelitis sinus. The tumors often are well differentiated and may arise in a background of pseudoepitheliomatous hyperplasia, making diagnosis difficult (Fig. 29-50 and 29-51). The tumors may be highly invasive (Fig. 29-47).

Spindle cell squamous cell carcinoma in particular may show a great resemblance to atypical fibroxanthoma (301). In some instances, spindle-cell squamous cell carcinomas

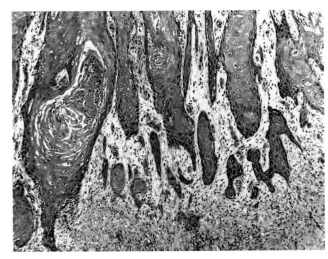

FIGURE 29-38. Squamous cell carcinoma, well differentiated. Low magnification. There is invasion of the dermis by epidermal masses.

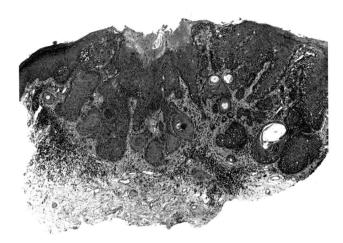

FIGURE 29-40. Squamous cell carcinoma, acantholytic type. Scanning magnification. Invasive cell masses extend into the reticular dermis. There is focal acantholysis superficially. (Same lesion as in Figs. 29-41 and 29-42.)

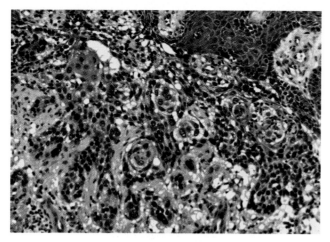

FIGURE 29-41. Squamous cell carcinoma, acantholytic type. There is focal acantholysis in the upper part of the lesion. (Same lesion as in Figs. 29-40 and 29-42.)

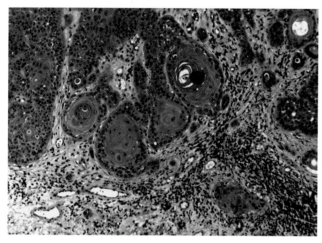

FIGURE 29-42. Squamous cell carcinoma, acantholytic type. In the deep part of the lesion the invasive cell masses show much less keratinization than in a well-differentiated tumor. (Same lesion as in Figs. 29-40 and 29-41.)

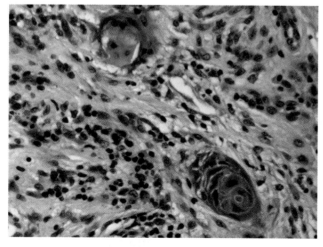

FIGURE 29-43. Squamous cell carcinoma. High magnification. Small groups of malignant squamous cells infiltrate the dermis surrounded by an inflammatory cell infiltrate in which eosinophils are present.

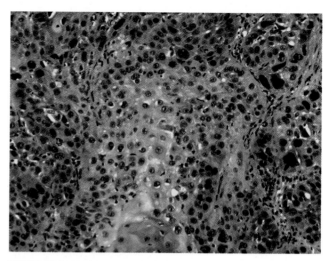

FIGURE 29-44. Squamous cell carcinoma, poor differentiation. High magnification. Pleomorphic, hyperchromatic malignant squamous cells infiltrate the dermis surrounded by an inflammatory cell infiltrate in which eosinophils are present.

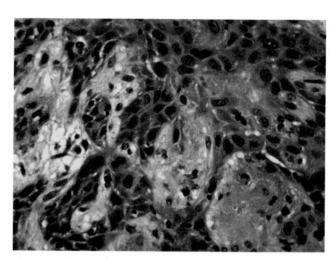

FIGURE 29-45. Squamous cell carcinoma, poor differentiation. High magnification. Pleomorphic, hyperchromatic malignant squamous cells infiltrate the dermis.

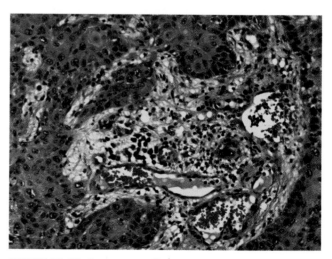

FIGURE 29-46. Squamous cell carcinoma, poor differentiation. High magnification. In this example, excised from the ear, single malignant cells invade the dermis adjacent to blood vessels.

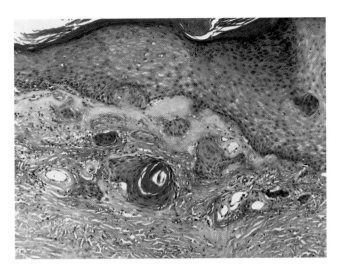

FIGURE 29-47. Postradiotherapy squamous cell carcinoma. This lesion, arising in an area treated many years previously with radiotherapy, shows a combination of invasive keratinizing squamous cell carcinoma and stromal damage secondary to radiotherapy.

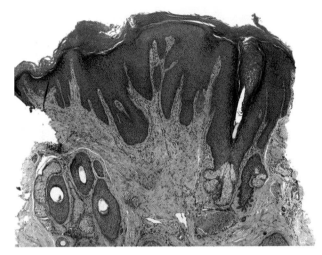

FIGURE 29-49. Lichen simplex chronicus with pseudocarcinomatous (pseudoepitheliomatous) hyperplasia. This punch biopsy specimen shows how epidermal hyperplasia can involve hair follicles and surface epidermis to produce a proliferative lesion mimicking an invasive process.

contain areas in which the cells either show intercellular bridges and beginning keratinization or show evidence of origin from the epidermis. In other cases, however, such areas cannot be detected. The spindle cells are intermingled with collagen and may be arranged in whorls (302). Not infrequently, pleomorphic giant cells are seen (301). In such instances, distinction from atypical fibroxanthoma may be difficult: differential diagnosis by immunohistochemical examination is required (see Pathogenesis section).

Raised, verrucous lesions of squamous cell carcinoma may show a considerable histologic resemblance to keratoacanthoma by having a central keratin-filled crater with

peripheral buttresses. In most instances, however, one finds less cellular maturation and evidence of nuclear atypicality.

Pathogenesis. Electron microscopy of squamous cell carcinoma, in comparison with normal epidermal squamous cells, shows a reduction in the number of desmosomes on the cell surface. In their place, microvilli extend into the widened intercellular spaces. Desmosomes can be seen within the cytoplasm of some of the tumor cells, either by themselves or attached to bundles of tonofilaments (255). Their intracytoplasmic location may be the result of either phagocytosis or invagination of the plasma membrane. However, it is not a specific finding for squamous cell car-

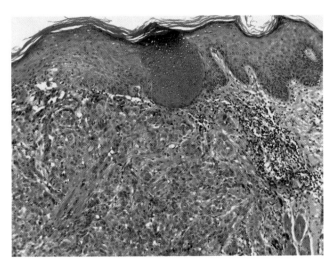

FIGURE 29-48. Metastatic squamous cell. A nodule of squamous cell carcinoma infiltrates the dermis beneath an epidermis devoid of dysplasia. The tumor was metastatic from a bronchial primary.

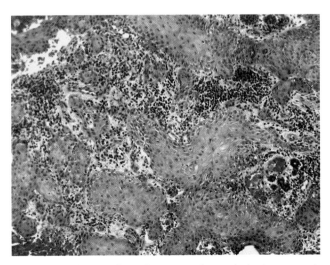

FIGURE 29-50. Pseudocarcinomatous hyperplasia. Low magnification. This curetting specimen shows a proliferative squamous lesion without substantial atypia and mimicking an invasive lesion.

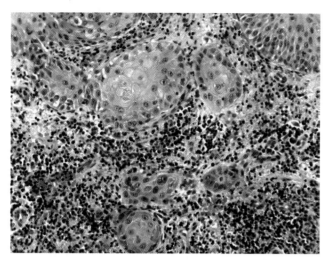

FIGURE 29-51. Pseudocarcinomatous hyperplasia. High magnification. At high magnification the proliferative squamous lesion, without substantial atypia and mimicking an invasive lesion, is seem more clearly. There may be overlap with well-differentiated squamous cell carcinoma, and a more generous excisional biopsy may be required in many if not most instances to differentiate between the two processes.

cinoma; intracytoplasmic desmosomes can be found also in keratoacanthoma and Bowen's disease, as well as in several unrelated epidermal proliferations and even in normal keratinocytes.

At the dermal-epidermal junction, the basement membrane shows sporadic discontinuities through which long cytoplasmic protrusions penetrate, indicating invasion of the dermis by epidermal keratinocytes (303).

In early squamous cell carcinoma, lymphocytes are often seen in close contact with tumor cells, some of which show degenerative changes such as disruption of the plasma membrane, as well as fragmentation and subsequent release of organelles into the intercellular spaces. This can be interpreted as the cellular expression of an immune reaction against tumor cells (304).

The epithelial nature of the sarcoma-like cells in *spindle-cell squamous cell carcinoma* is supported by electron microscopic findings, which have shown that these cells contain tonofilaments and occasional desmosome-like structures (302,305). Electron microscopy has also shown that structures diagnosed by light microscopy as atypical fibroxanthomas represent a heterogeneous group of neoplasms and that some are in actuality spindle-cell squamous cell carcinomas (301,306).

Immunohistochemical methods are of considerable value in the differentiation of squamous cell carcinoma from mesodermal tumors, such as atypical fibroxanthoma and malignant fibrous histiocytoma, and from malignant melanoma. For the identification of keratinocytes, primary antibodies directed against high-molecular-weight cytokeratins, such as cytokeratin 13, may be used. In contrast,

atypical fibroxanthoma and malignant fibrous histiocytomas react with vimentin (see Chapter 34) and malignant melanoma with S-100 protein (see Chapter 28). At times, even differentiation of a squamous cell carcinoma from a lymphoma may be difficult, in which case a positive reaction with monoclonal antileukocyte antibody (LCA) would favor lymphoma (307) (see Chapter 31). The immunohistochemistry may also be valuable in identifying tumor cells of a squamous cell carcinoma in the midst of an inflammatory infiltrate and can thus aid in deciding whether or not the margins of an excised specimen are free of tumor cells (308). The immunohistochemical differential diagnosis of spindle cell neoplasms in the skin is discussed also in Chapters 4, 28, and 34.

Differential Diagnosis. The diagnosis of squamous cell carcinoma, although easily made in typical cases, may sometimes be difficult.

The differences between squamous cell carcinoma *in situ* and actinic keratosis lie in the degree rather than the type of changes. In both conditions, one finds atypicality of cells, with dyskeratosis of individual cells and downward proliferation of the epidermis. However, only in frank squamous cell carcinoma is there invasion of the reticular dermis. No sharp line of demarcation exists between the two conditions, and not infrequently, on step sectioning for a lesion, the histologic appearance of actinic keratosis reveals one or several areas in which the changes have progressed to squamous cell carcinoma. Metastatic squamous cell carcinoma, for example from another skin primary or from a mucous membrane or visceral lesion, usually shows a greater degree of cytological atypia, may be located deeper in the dermis or subcutis, and lacks an overlying *in situ* component (Fig. 29-48).

For discussions of differentiation of squamous cell carcinoma from pseudocarcinomatous hyperplasia, see page 836; from keratoacanthoma, page 849; and from basal cell carcinoma, page 836.

ACANTHOLYTIC (ADENOID) SQUAMOUS CELL CARCINOMA

As a result of dyskeratosis and subsequent acantholysis, squamous cell carcinomas occasionally show what may appear to be tubular and alveolar formations on histologic examination. Such lesions have been termed *adenoid* or *pseudoglandular* squamous cell carcinomas, but they are better termed *acantholytic.* Clinically, they are found almost exclusively in sun-damaged skin of elderly patients, especially on the face and ears (309,310). They have also been seen on the vermilion border of the lower lip (311). Two instances of occurrence on the oral mucosa have been reported, but both were recurrences after radiation therapy (312).

On sun-exposed skin, acantholytic squamous cell carcinomas may arise as such or may develop from an actinic keratosis (310,313). In most instances, they do not differ in clinical appearance from the usual type of squamous cell carcinoma and thus commonly show a central ulceration surrounded by a raised, indurated border. Occasionally, they greatly resemble a keratoacanthoma in clinical appearance (314). The incidence of metastases varies. In one series it was only 2% (310), but in another series 14% of the patients had fatal metastases (315). Tumor size of greater than 1.5 cm correlates with the risk of an adverse outcome.

Histopathology. The adenoid changes may be seen in only a portion of a squamous cell carcinoma or throughout the lesion. Not infrequently, an actinic keratosis of the acantholytic type is seen overlying the lesion. There are tubular and alveolar lumina lined with one or several layers of epithelium (Figs. 29-40, 29-41, and 29-42). In areas in which the lumina are lined with a single layer of epithelium, the epithelial cells resemble glandular cells, but in areas with several layers of epithelium, squamous and partially keratinized cells usually form the inner layers. The lumina are filled with desquamated acantholytic cells, many of which are partially or fully keratinized (310,314,316). In some cases, the eccrine ducts at the periphery of these tumors show signs of dilatation and proliferation (309, 316). These ductal changes probably are induced by the surrounding inflammatory infiltrate.

Pathogenesis. These tumors represent squamous cell carcinomas of lobular growth in which there is considerable dyskeratosis with individual cell keratinization resulting in acantholysis in the center of the lobular formations. This process is analogous to the suprabasal clefts seen in some actinic keratoses (314). Acantholytic squamous cell carcinomas differ from sweat gland carcinomas (see Chapter 30), in which the single row of cuboidal cells lining the lumina consists of true glandular cells (317,318). These latter tumors may in some instances be highly malignant.

MUCIN-PRODUCING SQUAMOUS CELL CARCINOMA

This rare variant of squamous cell carcinoma is associated with a more aggressive clinical course than are most cutaneous squamous cell carcinomas (319). The 11 cases have been reported under different designations, such as mucoepidermoid carcinoma (320) and adenosquamous carcinoma of the skin (319). The latter designation may lead to confusion with adenoid squamous cell carcinoma.

Histopathology. Varying numbers of mucin-producing cells are found within tumors that have the appearance of a squamous cell carcinoma. These cells generally appear large and pale and stain positively with the PAS method and with mucicarmine (319,321). Treatment of sections with sialidase eliminates the mucicarmine staining material, whereas treatment with hyaluronidase fails to do so. Thus, the material is epithelial mucin (sialomucin) (319). Occa-

sionally, true glandular lumina are present (319,322). Some of the lumina resemble distorted eccrine ducts and stain positively for carcinoembryonic antigen (322).

VERRUCOUS CARCINOMA

Verrucous carcinoma is a low-grade squamous cell carcinoma first described in 1948 (323) as occurring in the oral cavity. The diagnosis of verrucous carcinoma requires evaluation of the clinical and microscopic appearance and biologic behavior of the neoplasm. It is a slowly growing, at first exophytic, verrucous, and fungating tumor that may ultimately penetrate deep into the tissue. However, it causes regional metastases only very late, if at all. Because of its high degree of histologic differentiation, it is often not recognized as a carcinoma for a long time. Three major forms of verrucous carcinoma are recognized, all of them occurring in areas of maceration.

Verrucous carcinoma of the oral cavity, also called oral florid papillomatosis, shows white, cauliflower-like lesions that may involve large areas of the oral mucosa.

Verrucous carcinoma of the genitoanal region, also called giant condylomata acuminatum of Buschke and Loewenstein, most commonly occurs on the glans penis and foreskin of uncircumcised males, where it consists of papillomatous proliferations. Ultimately, it may penetrate into the urethra. It may also occur on the vulva in females and in the anal region (Chapter 25).

Plantar verrucous carcinoma, also called epithelioma cuniculatum (324), at first shows a striking resemblance to an intractable plantar wart. As the exophytic mass grows, it shows a great tendency toward deep, penetrating growth, resulting in numerous deep crypts filled with horny material and pus. The crypts resemble the burrows of rabbits, hence the name *cuniculatum.* The tumor ultimately penetrates the plantar fascia (325) and may even destroy metatarsal bones and invade the skin of the dorsum of the foot (326).

The occurrence of verrucous carcinoma has been described occasionally in many other areas, such as the face (327) and back (328), as well as in preexisting lesions, such as chronic ulcers and draining sinuses of hidradenitis suppurativa (329).

Histopathology. For the diagnosis of verrucous carcinoma, a large, deep biopsy is essential. The superficial portions generally resemble a verruca by showing hyperkeratosis, parakeratosis, and acanthosis. The keratinocytes appear well differentiated, stain lightly with eosin, and possess a small nucleus. The tumor invades with broad strands that often contain keratin-filled cysts in their center. There are large, bulbous, downward proliferations that compress the collagen bundles and push them aside. Thus, the tumor has been said to invade by "bulldozing rather than stabbing" (330). Even in the deep portions of the tumor, nuclear atypia, individual cell keratinization, and horn pearls are absent (331).

However, in some instances, particularly in the oral cavity (227,230) but occasionally also in the genitoanal region (332) and on the plantar surface (333,334), verrucous carcinoma may ultimately show sufficient nuclear atypicality and loss of polarity to indicate the development of a true squamous cell carcinoma. In rare instances, the development of regional lymph node metastases has been observed in verrucous carcinoma of the mouth (228) the genitals (332) and the soles of the feet (334). Radiation therapy has led in some instances of oral verrucous carcinoma to anaplastic transformation and extensive metastases (335).

Pathogenesis. Although a viral cause of verrucous carcinoma has been suspected for a long time, demonstration of viral particles by electron microscopy has been possible in only a few instances of verrucous carcinoma. Virus-like particles were demonstrated in one case of plantar verrucous carcinoma presumed to be associated with a plantar wart (336) in the superficial epithelium of 5 of 13 cases of plantar verrucous carcinoma (337) and in one case of verrucous carcinoma of the vagina. The recently introduced, more sensitive, and more specific method of demonstrating various types of human papilloma viruses by means of DNA hybridization has succeeded in proving the presence of HPV-6, and less frequently of HPV-11, in Buschke–Loewenstein tumors of the external genitals in both sexes (338). Similarly, HPV-6 was found in a vulvar tumor of Buschke–Loewenstein through molecular hybridization (339).

PSEUDOCARCINOMATOUS HYPERPLASIA

Pseudocarcinomatous hyperplasia or *pseudoepitheliomatous hyperplasia*, as it is often called, represents a considerable downward proliferation of the epidermis into the dermis. Clinically and histologically, this downward proliferation may suggest a squamous cell carcinoma. It occurs occasionally (a) in chronic proliferative inflammatory processes, such as bromoderma, blastomycosis, blastomycosis-like pyoderma (pyoderma vegetans) (340), or hidradenitis suppurativa (341); and (b) at the edges of chronic ulcers, as seen in the following conditions: after burns or in stasis dermatitis (342), pyoderma gangrenosum, basal cell epithelioma (343), lupus vulgaris, osteomyelitis, scrofuloderma, gumma, and granuloma inguinale. In addition, granular cell tumor is known to evoke quite frequently a pseudocarcinomatous hyperplasia.

Histopathology. Histologically, pseudocarcinomatous hyperplasia shows an epithelial hyperplasia that often closely resembles moderately or well-differentiated squamous cell carcinoma. Although squamous cell carcinoma may develop at the edges of chronic ulcers, it is likely that some cases that are regarded as such actually represent pseudo-

carcinomatous hyperplasia. Nevertheless, a lesion starting out as pseudocarcinomatous hyperplasia at the edge of an ulcer may eventually develop into a squamous cell carcinoma and even metastasize (344,345).

The histologic picture of pseudocarcinomatous hyperplasia shows irregular invasion of the dermis by uneven, jagged, often sharply pointed epidermal cell masses and strands with horn-pearl formation and often numerous mitotic figures (Figs. 29-49, 29-50, and 29-51). These irregular proliferations of the epidermis may extend below the level of the sweat glands, where they appear in sections as isolated islands of epidermal tissue (341). However, the squamous cells usually are well differentiated, and atypicalities, such as individual cell keratinization and nuclear hyperplasia and hyperchromasia, are minimal or absent (Fig. 29-51). Furthermore, one often sees invasion of the epithelial proliferations by leukocytes and disintegration of some of the epidermal cells in pseudocarcinomatous hyperplasia, findings that usually are absent in squamous cell carcinoma (342). Nevertheless, even when all of these criteria are taken into account, it may still be difficult to differentiate squamous cell carcinoma from pseudocarcinomatous hyperplasia by the study of just one histologic section (341). Multiple biopsies and detailed clinical data may be necessary for differentiation.

In every section in which a diagnosis of squamous cell carcinoma is contemplated, it is worthwhile to study the inflammatory infiltrate for the possible presence of granulomas, as seen in tuberculosis and the deep mycoses, or of intraepidermal abscesses, as seen in bromoderma. If such evidence is found, one may be dealing with pseudocarcinomatous hyperplasia instead of squamous cell carcinoma.

Differential Diagnosis. Differentiation of pseudocarcinomatous hyperplasia from verrucous carcinoma rarely causes difficulties, because in verrucous carcinoma there is verrucous upward proliferation and downward proliferation. Also, verrucous carcinoma shows more pronounced keratinization in the downward extensions, which appear bulbous rather than sharply pointed.

BASAL CELL CARCINOMA

Basal cell carcinomas are seen almost exclusively on hair-bearing skin, especially on the face. Except in the nevoid basal cell carcinoma syndrome (see Chapter 30), they rarely occur on the palms (346,347) or on the soles (348,349). Their occurrence on the mucous membrane is doubted; instances of basal cell carcinoma of the oral mucosa reported in the literature (350) probably are ameloblastomas (351).

Basal cell carcinomas usually occur as single lesions, although the occurrence of several lesions, either simultaneously or subsequently, is not infrequent. About 40% of patients who have had a basal cell carcinoma will have one or more basal cell carcinomas within 10 years (352). Basal cell carcinomas generally occur in adults, although they may be seen in children (353–355). However, there are three rare forms of basal cell carcinoma with early onset. In the linear, unilateral basal cell nevus, all lesions are present at birth. In the nevoid basal cell syndrome and the Bazex syndrome, some patients manifest lesions before puberty.

Predisposing Factors. Although basal cell carcinomas may arise without apparent reason, there are several predisposing factors. The most common of them is a light skin color in association with prolonged exposure to strong sunlight (356). The predisposing effect of sun exposure is particularly evident in patients with xeroderma pigmentosum, in whom both basal cell carcinoma and squamous cell carcinoma are common (see Chapter 6). That prolonged sun exposure alone does not suffice to produce basal cell carcinomas is suggested by their great rarity on the dorsa of hands and fingers (357). Additional factors that predispose a person to develop both basal cell carcinoma and squamous cell carcinoma are large or numerous doses of roentgen rays (358,359) and, less commonly, burn scars (360,361) and other scars (362). In contrast, most carcinomas of the skin caused by the prolonged intake of inorganic arsenic are squamous cell carcinomas, which often, like Bowen's disease, are located *in situ* (241,289). Occasionally, however, basal cell carcinomas, particularly superficial basal cell carcinomas, can result (283,284) (see Arsenical Keratosis and Carcinoma section).

Occurrence of Metastases. As a rule, basal cell carcinomas do not metastasize. However, there are exceptions. The incidence of metastasis ranges from 0.01% in pathologic specimens (363), through 0.028% in dermatologic patients (364), to 0.1% in patients from surgical centers (365). A review published in 1984 described 175 cases with histologically proven metastases (366).

The typical case history of a metastatic basal cell carcinoma is that of a large, ulcerated, locally invasive, and destructive primary lesion that has recurred despite repeated surgical procedures or radiotherapy (367,a,b). However, massive size, ulceration, and history of multiple recurrences are not absolute prerequisites for metastasis (368). Most observers have found no specific histologic type of basal cell carcinoma that is more capable of metastasizing than others (369–371). Also, no evidence exists that the hosts' immunologic defenses are severely compromised (366). However, some authors assert that the metatypical or basosquamous type of basal cell carcinoma is the most likely to metastasize (372).

In contrast to metastatic squamous cell carcinoma of the skin, which shows lymphogenic metastases to lymph nodes in 80% to 90% of cases, in metastatic basal cell carcinoma, hematogenic and lymphogenic spread show about an even distribution (366). Although about 50% of the patients with metastatic basal cell carcinoma have metastases to lymph nodes as their first site of spread, lungs and bones also are frequently the first sites of involvement. Metastases to the liver, other viscera, and to the skin or subcutaneous tissues have occurred. However, these areas were usually involved only when at least one of the three major sites of metastasis was also affected (373). The average survival time after metastasis to the lungs, bones, or internal organs is about 10 months (374).

Clinical Appearance. Five clinical types of basal cell carcinoma occur: (a) noduloulcerative basal cell carcinoma, including rodent ulcer, by far the most common type; (b) pigmented basal cell carcinoma; (c) morphea-like or fibrosing basal cell carcinoma; (d) superficial basal cell carcinoma; and (e) fibroepithelioma. In addition, there are three clinical syndromes in which basal cell carcinomas play an important part. They are (a) the nevoid basal cell carcinoma syndrome; (b) the linear unilateral basal cell nevus; and (c) the Bazex syndrome, showing follicular atrophoderma with multiple basal cell carcinomas.

Noduloulcerative basal cell carcinoma begins as a small, waxy nodule that often shows a few small telangiectatic vessels on its surface. The nodule usually increases slowly in size and often undergoes central ulceration. A typical lesion then consists of a slowly enlarging ulcer surrounded by a pearly, rolled border. This represents the so-called rodent ulcer.

Most rodent ulcers possess a limited potential for growth; however, occasionally they can be infiltrative and aggressive and then can reach considerable size and invade deeply. On the face, they may destroy the eyes and nose (375), or they may penetrate the skull and invade the dura mater (376). Death may then ensue. (Such destructive basal cell carcinomas are seen occasionally also in the nevoid basal cell carcinoma syndrome; see discussion below.)

Pigmented basal cell carcinoma differs from the noduloulcerative type only by the brown pigmentation of the lesion.

Morphea-like or fibrosing basal cell carcinoma manifests itself as a solitary, flat or slightly depressed, indurated, yellowish plaque. The surface is smooth and shiny. The border is often ill defined. The overlying skin remains intact for a long time before ulceration finally occurs. The term arises from a clinical resemblance to localized scleroderma or morphea. The tumors, despite being deeply infiltrative, may be mistaken clinically for a lesion of morphea, or for a scar.

Superficial basal cell carcinoma consists of one or several erythematous, scaling, only slightly infiltrated patches that slowly increase in size by peripheral extension. The patches are often surrounded, at least in part, by a fine, threadlike, pearly border. The patches usually show small areas of superficial ulceration and crusting. In addition, their center may show smooth, atrophic scarring. In contrast to the first three types of basal cell carcinoma that are commonly situated on the face, superficial basal cell carcinoma occurs predominantly on the trunk.

Fibroepithelioma consists of usually only one but occasionally of several raised, moderately firm, slightly pedunculated nodules, covered by smooth, slightly reddened skin. Clinically, they resemble fibromas. The most common location is the back.

The *nevoid basal cell carcinoma syndrome* is an autosomal dominant disorder with low penetration. Small nodules appear between puberty and 35 years of age, and there may be hundreds or thousands of them (377). During the "nevoid" stage, the nodules slowly increase in number and size. They are haphazardly distributed over the face and body. During adulthood, many of the basal cell carcinomas undergo ulceration, and later in life, the disease sometimes enters a "neoplastic" stage, in which some of the basal cell carcinomas, especially of the face, become invasive, destructive, and mutilating. Occasionally, even death occurs as the result of invasion of an orbit and of the brain (378–380). There also may be metastases to the lung (378).

Half of adult patients with the nevoid basal cell carcinoma syndrome show numerous palmar and plantar pits 1 to 3 mm in diameter. These pits usually develop during the second decade of life and represent *formes frustes* of basal cell carcinoma (381) (see Histopathology section). Also, epidermal cysts are quite common (382).

Most patients show multiple skeletal and central nervous system anomalies (379) among which are odontogenic keratocysts of the jaws, anomalies of the ribs, scoliosis, mental retardation, and calcification of the falx cerebri. In several reported cases, there were also cerebellar medulloblastomas (383) or fibrosarcomas of a mandible or maxilla (384). In the jaw cysts, an ameloblastoma may arise (385).

The *linear unilateral basal cell nevus* is very rare. There is an extensive unilateral linear or zosteriform eruption, usually present since birth, consisting of closely set nodules of basal cell carcinoma (386). They may be interspersed with comedones (387,388) and striae-like areas of atrophy (389). The lesions do not increase in size with aging of the patient.

The *Bazex syndrome*, first described in 1966 (390), is dominantly inherited and shows as its main features (a) follicular atrophoderma characterized by widened follicular openings like "ice-pick marks" mainly on the extremities; and (b) multiple, small basal cell carcinomas on the face, usually arising first in adolescence or early adulthood (391), but occasionally in late childhood (392). In addition, there may be localized anhidrosis or generalized hypohidrosis, and congenital hypotrichosis on the scalp and elsewhere (392).

Histopathology. Basal cell carcinomas tend to share the common features of a predominant basal cell type, peripheral palisading of lesional cell nuclei, a specialized stroma, and clefting artifact between the epithelium and the stroma. In addition, there are variable degrees of cytologic atypia and mitotic activity; some degree of these latter changes is virtually always present (Figs. 29-52 through 29-76). In the

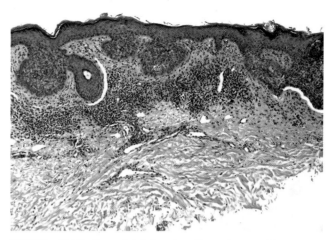

FIGURE 29-52. Superficial basal cell carcinoma. The tumor shows buds and irregular proliferations of tumor tissue attached to the undersurface of the epidermis. A cleft is also present at the interface with the dermis **(far right)**.

common solid type of basal cell carcinoma, nodular masses of basaloid cells are formed that extend into the dermis in relation to a delicate, specialized tumor stroma (Figs. 29-57 and 29-60). Cystic spaces may form as a result of tumor necrosis or cellular dyshesion (Fig. 29-56). The characteristic cells of basal cell carcinoma, referred to by some as basaloma cells, have a large, oval, or elongated nucleus and relatively little cytoplasm. Often, the cytoplasm of individual cells is poorly defined, so that it may appear as if their nuclei are embedded in a symplasmatic mass. The nuclei resemble those of basal cells of the epidermis, but basaloma cells differ from basal cells by having a larger ratio of nucleus to cy-

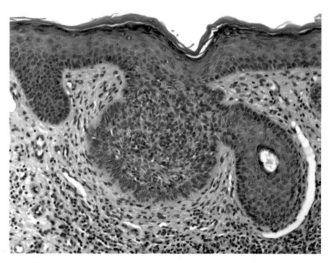

FIGURE 29-53. Superficial basal cell carcinoma. High magnification. The tumor shows a bud of cells in the bulge zone of a hair follicle similar to the primary epithelial germ buds in embryonal skin.

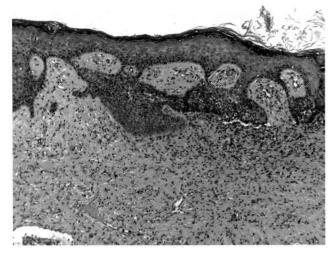

FIGURE 29-54. Dermatofibroma. There is a basal proliferation of basaloid cells mimicking the appearances of a superficial basal cell carcinoma. The lesion lacks the specialized basal cell stroma and there is little or no atypia. Clefting artifact is focally present, indicating that this finding is not specific for a basal cell carcinoma.

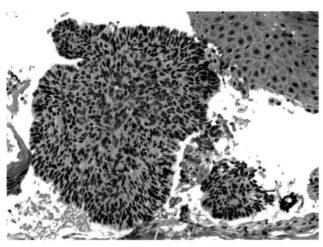

FIGURE 29-55. Basal cell carcinoma, solid type. In this curetting specimen nests of cells from a nodular basal cell carcinoma show peripheral palisading.

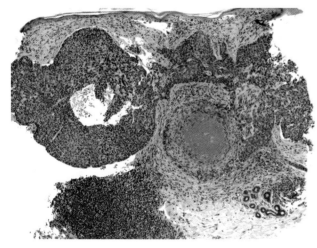

FIGURE 29-56. Basal cell carcinoma, solid type with cystic degeneration. In an originally solid basal cell carcinoma, cystic spaces have formed within the large cell masses as the result of tumor cell disintegration.

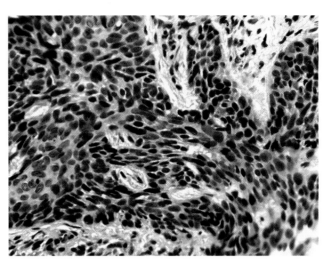

FIGURE 29-57. Basal cell carcinoma, solid type. High magnification. The basaloid tumor cells flow through the dermis with a variable degree of peripheral palisading.

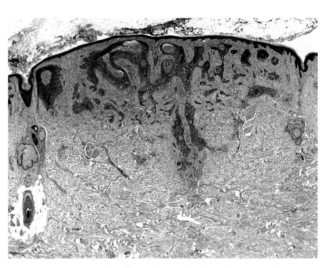

FIGURE 29-58. Basal cell carcinoma, infiltrative. Scanning magnification. Basaloid cells infiltrate the dermis in an excision specimen, but the infiltration is relatively limited in extent.

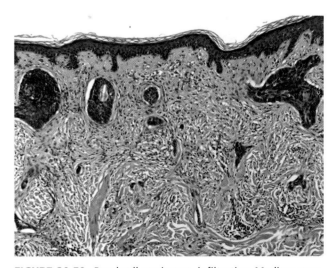

FIGURE 29-59. Basal cell carcinoma, infiltrative. Medium magnification. Basaloid cells infiltrate the dermis in an excision specimen. In the upper dermis, the cells form nests of variable size.

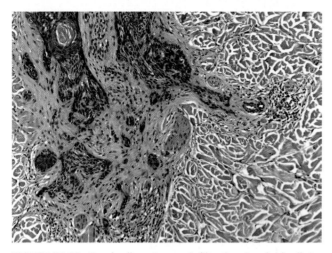

FIGURE 29-60. Basal cell carcinoma, infiltrative. Basaloid cells infiltrate the dermis in an excision specimen. In the deeper part of the lesion, tumor cells infiltrate within their specialized stroma.

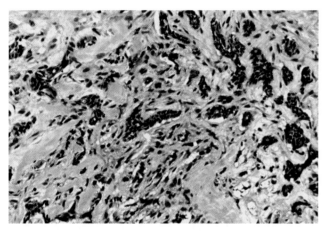

FIGURE 29-61. Basal cell carcinoma, infiltrative, morpheic. There is more atypia than in most basal cell carcinomas. The infiltrating cords of basaloid cells are slender and widely infiltrative, consistent with the so-called morpheic variant of basal cell carcinoma.

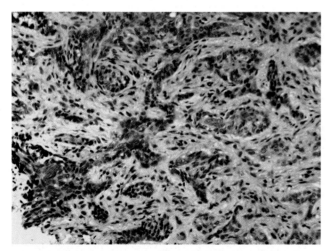

FIGURE 29-62. Basal cell carcinoma, infiltrative, metatypical. There is more atypia than in most basal cell carcinomas, and there is focal squamous differentiation within the infiltrating cords of basaloid cells, consistent with the so-called metatypical variant of basal cell carcinoma.

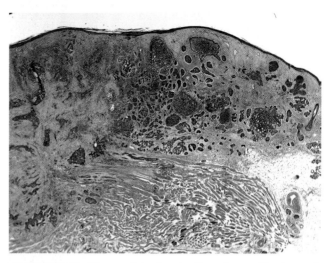

FIGURE 29-63. Micronodular basal cell carcinoma. The tumor is relatively symmetrical and circumscribed, but with a more infiltrative element at its base.

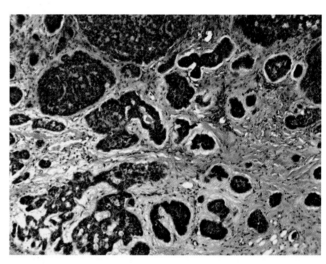

FIGURE 29-64. Micronodular basal cell carcinoma. High magnification. The infiltrative element at the base of the tumor contains small rounded nests of tumor cells.

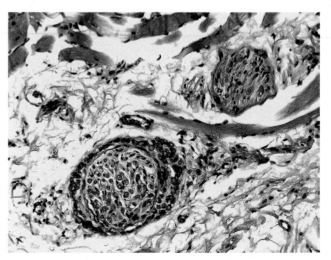

FIGURE 29-65. Micronodular basal cell carcinoma. High magnification. Tumor cells infiltrate around a dermal nerve close to the excision margin.

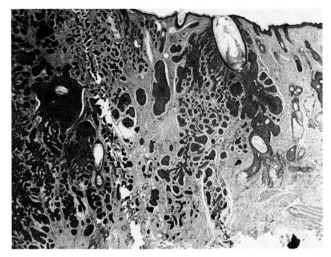

FIGURE 29-66. Micronodular basal cell carcinoma. The tumor shows larger nests of cells towards the surface but with widespread deeper infiltration by smaller, rounded cell nodules.

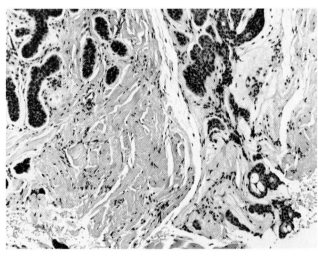

FIGURE 29-67. Micronodular basal cell carcinoma. Micronodules of tumor extend focally to the deep excision margin.

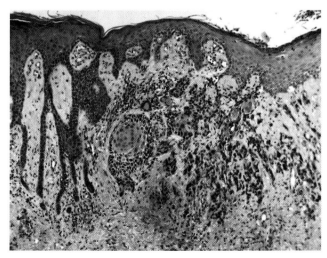

FIGURE 29-68. Basosquamous carcinoma. The tumor shows predominant architectural features of a basal cell carcinoma, but with a prominent element of squamous differentiation.

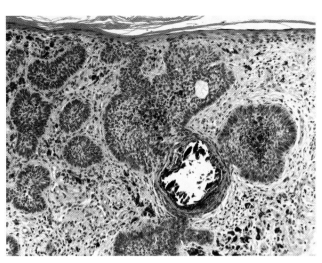

FIGURE 29-69. Pigmented basal cell carcinoma. Melanin pigment is present within solid islands of basal cell carcinoma and in macrophages between the islands of tumor cells.

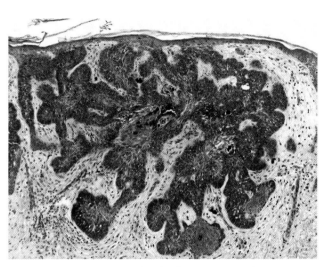

FIGURE 29-70. Pigmented basal cell carcinoma. Melanin pigment is present within solid islands of basal cell carcinoma and to a lesser extent in macrophages between the islands of tumor cells.

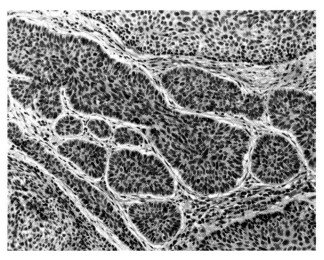

FIGURE 29-71. Nodular basal cell carcinoma. Medium magnification. The islands of tumor cells show peripheral palisading as well as mitotic and apoptotic figures.

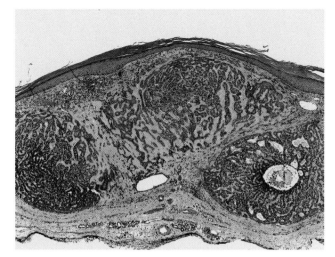

FIGURE 29-72. Adenoid basal cell carcinoma. Scanning magnification. The strands of epithelial cells form nodules with a lacelike pattern of cells within the nodules.

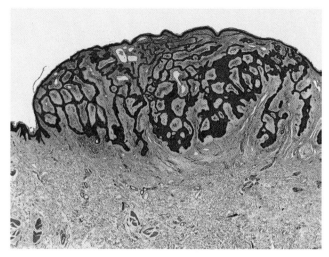

FIGURE 29-74. Fibroepithelioma of Pinkus (fibroepithelial basal cell carcinoma). The tumor has an elevated nodular appearance with, in this instance, a focus of superficial ulceration and hemorrhage.

toplasm (393), and by not showing intercellular bridges. The nuclei in basal cell carcinomas as a rule have a rather uniform, nonanaplastic appearance. They usually show no pronounced variation in size or intensity of staining and no abnormal mitoses, even in the rare instances of basal cell carcinoma with metastases. In the exceptional cases of basal cell carcinoma in which one finds, interspersed among the usual cells of basal cell carcinoma, cells with large hyperchromatic nuclei, multiple nuclei, and bizarre "star-burst" mitoses, the clinical course is not different from that of the usual basal cell carcinoma (394,395). Although most basal cell carcinomas appear well demarcated, some show an infiltrative growth. They are now widely recognized as a distinct histologic subtype.

The connective tissue stroma proliferates with the tumor and is arranged in parallel bundles around the tumor masses, so that a mutual relationship seems to exist between the parenchyma of the tumor and its stroma (396,397). The stroma adjacent to the tumor masses often shows numerous young fibroblasts; in addition, it may appear mucinous (398,399). Frequently there are areas of retraction of the stroma from tumor islands, resulting in peritumoral lacunae (Figs. 29-52 and 29-53). These lacunae once were regarded as a fixation artifact, but peritumoral lacunae can be observed also on cryostat sections. Immunostaining with antibodies to laminin, type IV collagen, and bullous pemphigoid has revealed the presence of laminin and type IV collagen on the stroma side of the lacunae, but bullous

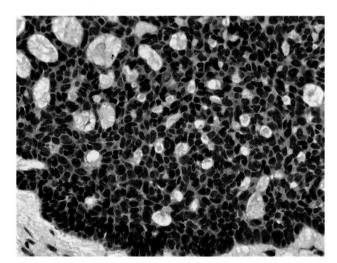

FIGURE 29-73. Adenoid basal cell carcinoma. The strands of epithelial cells present a lacelike pattern. The stroma has a mucoid appearance.

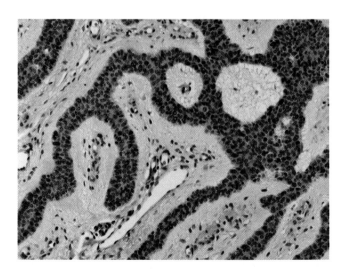

FIGURE 29-75. Fibroepithelioma of Pinkus (fibroepithelial basal cell carcinoma). Long, thin, branching, anastomosing strands of basal cell carcinoma are embedded in a fibrous stroma.

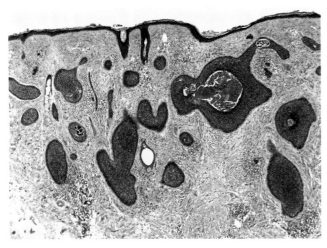

FIGURE 29-76. Basal cell carcinoma showing follicular differentiation. Epithelium and stroma form structures reminiscent of follicular germs, and there is formation of a horn cyst resembling a follicular structure.

pemphigoid antigen is absent at the site of lacunae (400). Even though bullous pemphigoid antigen is diminished in other areas of basal cell carcinoma (401), it is likely that loss of this antigen contributes to the formation of peritumoral lacunae (400). Because these lacunae are quite typical for some basal cell carcinomas, their presence aids in the differentiation of basal cell carcinoma from other tumors, such as squamous cell carcinoma. Also, stromal or intratumor deposits of amyloid are found quite frequently (402) (see Pathogenesis section). A mild inflammatory infiltrate is often seen in the stroma of nonulcerated basal cell carcinomas but may be entirely lacking. If ulceration occurs, there usually is a rather pronounced inflammatory reaction.

From a histologic point of view, basal cell carcinomas can be divided into two groups: undifferentiated and differentiated. Those of the latter group show a slight degree of differentiation toward the cutaneous appendages of hair, sebaceous glands, apocrine glands, or eccrine glands. A sharp dividing line between the two groups cannot be drawn, because many undifferentiated basal cell carcinomas show differentiation in some areas, and most differentiated basal cell carcinomas show areas lacking differentiation. By correlating the clinical classification with the histologic classification, it can be stated that the noduloulcerative type of basal cell carcinoma, as well as the lesions of the nevoid basal cell carcinoma syndrome, the linear unilateral basal cell nevus, and the Bazex syndrome, may show differentiation or no differentiation, but the other four types of basal cell carcinoma—pigmented basal cell carcinoma, fibrosing basal cell carcinoma, superficial basal cell carcinoma, and fibroepithelioma—usually show little or no differentiation.

From a clinical point of view it is probably more relevant to classify basal cell carcinomas into those with a low

risk of recurrence (nodular, nodulocystic, and fibroepithelioma of Pinkus) and those with a high risk of local recurrence (superficial, infiltrative, morpheic, metatypical, micronodular). Of these the *micronodular basal cell carcinoma* has received the least recognition, but probably carries as high a risk of local recurrence as the others in the high-risk group (Figs. 29-63 through 29-67). They vary between symmetrical, circumscribed examples and others that are asymmetrical and infiltrate between collagen bundles. The risk of local recurrence may be related to the presence of perineural invasion (which may occur in other types of basal cell carcinoma as well (Fig. 29-65), and to the focal nature in which the tumor may infiltrate deeply into the dermis to involve the excision margin (Fig. 29-67). There is an overlap of appearances between morpheic and micronodular basal cell carcinomas. In deciding on which subtype one is dealing with, the element representing more than 50% of the whole tumor should take precedence.

Basal cell carcinomas showing no differentiation are called *solid* basal cell carcinomas. They can be subdivided into *circumscribed* and *infiltrative*. Those with differentiation toward hair structures are called *keratotic*; toward sebaceous glands, *basal cell carcinomas with sebaceous differentiation*; and toward tubular glands, *adenoid* basal cell carcinomas. A *signet ring cell* variant has also been described (402a). In many differentiated basal cell carcinomas, differentiation is directed toward more than one of these cutaneous appendages. For example, areas of keratinization may be found in a tumor that also shows adenoid structures. No difference exists in the rate of growth between undifferentiated and differentiated basal cell carcinomas.

Solid basal cell carcinoma of the *circumscribed* type shows tumor masses of various sizes and shapes embedded in the dermis (Figs. 29-55 and 29-56). In more than 90% of basal cell carcinomas, a connection between tumor cell formations and the surface epidermis can be shown to exist (403). Occasionally, a tumor mass is found in contact with an outer root sheath. The peripheral cell layer of the tumor masses often shows a palisade arrangement, whereas the nuclei of the cells inside lie in a haphazard fashion. Solid basal cell carcinomas containing large aggregates of tumor cells occasionally show disintegration of their cells in the center of the tumor masses, resulting in cyst formation (404) (Fig. 29-56). Some solid basal cell carcinomas, although they show little or no structural differentiation toward any of the epidermal appendages, nevertheless show two types of cells: a large cell with an oval, pale nucleus, and a small cell with an elongated, dark nucleus (404) (Fig. 29-71).

Solid basal cell carcinomas of the *infiltrative* type, also referred to as *aggressive* basal cell carcinomas, show the basaloid cells predominantly arranged as elongated strands, only a few layers thick and with little or no palisading of the peripheral cells. Such strands can invade deeply. The demarcation of the tumor from the stroma is often poor (405). There are cell aggregates that display an irregular, spiky configuration (406). The cells and their nuclei show great variations in size and shape (407) (Figs. 29-57 and 29-61). There is little or no increase in the density of stroma collagen and no significant increase in the number of fibroblasts. There may be foci of squamous differentiation (Fig. 29-62). The number of inflammatory cells depends to some degree on the extent of ulceration. There often is perineural infiltration (405) and, on the face, there may be invasion of bone (376).

Keratotic basal cell carcinoma shows parakeratotic cells and horn cysts in addition to undifferentiated cells. The parakeratotic cells possess elongated nuclei and a slightly eosinophilic cytoplasm, in contrast to the deeply basophilic cytoplasm of undifferentiated cells. The parakeratotic cells may lie in strands, in concentric whorls, or around the horn cysts. It is likely that they are cells with initial keratinization somewhat similar to the nucleated cells in the keratogenic zone of normal hair shafts. The horn cysts, which are composed of fully keratinized cells, represent attempts at hair shaft formation (408). Just as in the keratinization of the hair shaft, the horn cysts form without the interposition of granular cells. Some keratotic basal cell carcinomas possess horn cysts of considerable size.

Keratotic basal cell carcinoma shares with trichoepithelioma the presence of horn cysts, and it is sometimes difficult to decide whether a lesion represents a keratotic basal cell carcinoma or a trichoepithelioma (see Chapter 30). Clinical data may be necessary for a decision to be reached. The horn cysts must not be confused with the horn pearls that occur in squamous cell carcinoma (see Differential Diagnosis section).

Basal cell carcinoma with sebaceous differentiation shows essentially a basal cell carcinoma in which there are interspersed aggregates of sebaceous cells and cells transitional from basaloma cells to sebaceous cells. The transitional cells have granules that stain positive with Sudan III and other lipid stains (388) (see Chapter 4). A clear-cut separation from sebaceoma (sebaceous epithelioma) is at times impossible because transitions exist. Most examples of lesions thought to represent basal cell carcinomas with sebaceous differentiation are probably actually sebaceomas (409).

Adenoid basal cell carcinoma shows formations suggesting tubular, gland-like structures. The cells are arranged in intertwining strands and radially around islands of connective tissue, resulting in a tumor with a lace-like pattern (Figs. 29-72 and 29-73). In rare instances, lumina may be surrounded by cells that have the appearance of secretory cells. The lumina may be filled with a colloidal substance or with an amorphous granular material, but definite evidence of secretory activity of the cells lining the lumina cannot be obtained, even with histochemical methods. Similarly, because of the low degree of differentiation of the cells, histochemical reactions that would indicate either apocrine or eccrine differentiation are negative (410). The tumor originally described as a basal cell tumor with ec-

crine differentiation (411) is now regarded as an eccrine carcinoma and referred to as *syringoid eccrine carcinoma* (see Chapter 30).

Four uncommon histologic variants of basal cell carcinoma have been described: an adamantinoid type, a granular type, a clear cell type, and a type with matricial differentiation. *Adamantinoid basal cell carcinoma* shows a great histologic resemblance to dental ameloblastoma or adamantinoma (412). One observes solid masses of basaloma cells with palisading at the periphery. Inside this layer, the cells show elongated nuclei and stellate cytoplasm stretched as thin, connecting bridges across empty spaces, as seen in adamantinoma. In *granular basal cell carcinoma*, some of the tumor cells have the usual appearance of basaloma cells, whereas others show a gradual transition to granular cells. The granular cells show in their cytoplasm numerous eosinophilic granules with a tendency to coalesce (413,414). The eosinophilic lysosome-like granules greatly resemble those seen in granular cell tumor (see Chapter 35). In the *clear cell basal cell carcinoma*, the clear cell pattern may occupy all or part of the tumor islands. The clear cells contain vacuoles of different sizes filled with glycogen (415). The vacuoles often cause peripheral displacement of the nucleus, giving the cells a signet-ring appearance (416). In *basal cell carcinoma with matricial differentiation*, islands of shadow cells, as seen in pilomatricoma, are located within a basal cell carcinoma (417).

Noduloulcerative basal cell carcinoma, clinically the most common type of basal cell carcinoma, may on histologic examination appear solid, keratotic, or adenoid. The histologic descriptions given previously for solid, keratotic, and adenoid basal cell carcinoma apply in general to the noduloulcerative type of basal cell carcinoma.

Although about 75% of basal cell carcinomas are found on staining with dopa to contain melanocytes, and melanin is present in about 25% of them (418), large amounts of melanin are encountered only rarely (Figs. 29-69 and 29-70). The melanin is produced by benign melanocytes that colonize the tumor. These tumors are called *pigmented basal cell carcinomas*.

Basal cell carcinomas with large amounts of melanin are shown on staining with silver to contain melanocytes interspersed between the tumor cells. These melanocytes have numerous melanin granules in their cytoplasm and dendrites (418). This contrasts with normal epidermal melanocytes of whites, in which there are only a few rather small melanin granules because most of the melanin is located within the keratinocytes (419). The tumor cells in some pigmented basal cell carcinomas may contain very little melanin, but there are many melanophages in the connective tissue stroma surrounding the tumor masses.

Connective tissue participation is much greater in the *morphea-like or fibrosing* variant than in the other types of basal cell carcinoma. Embedded in a dense fibrous stroma are innumerable groups of tumor cells arranged in elongated strands (420) (Fig. 29-61). Most of the strands are narrow, often only one cell thick, so that they resemble the narrow strands of tumor cells seen in the skin in metastatic scirrhous carcinoma of the breast. However, on searching, one usually finds at least a few larger aggregates of tumor cells and some strands of tumor cells showing branching. The strands of tumor cells often extend deep into the dermis.

Superficial basal cell carcinoma shows buds and irregular proliferations of tumor tissue attached to the undersurface of the epidermis (Figs. 29-52 and 29-53). The peripheral cell layer of the tumor formations often shows palisading. In most cases, there is little penetration into the dermis. The overlying epidermis usually shows atrophy. Fibroblasts, often in a fairly large number, are arranged around the tumor cell proliferations. In addition, a mild or moderate amount of a nonspecific chronic inflammatory infiltrate is present in the upper dermis.

Some superficial basal cell carcinomas, after having persisted as such for various lengths of time, become invasive basal cell carcinomas. Because this change may be limited at first to a few areas, representative sections throughout the entire block should be examined. (For a discussion of the evidence that superficial basal cell carcinoma is unicentric, see Pathogenesis section.)

In *fibroepithelioma*, first described in 1953 (396), long, thin, branching, anastomosing strands of basal cell carcinoma are embedded in a fibrous stroma (396,421) (Figs. 29-74 and 29-75). Many of the strands show connections with the surface epidermis. Here and there, small groups of dark-staining cells showing a palisade arrangement of the peripheral cell layer may be seen along the epithelial strands, like buds on a branch. Usually, the tumor is quite superficial and is well demarcated at its lower border. Fibroepithelioma combines features of the intracanalicular fibroadenoma of the breast, the reticulated type of seborrheic keratosis, and superficial basal cell carcinoma (396). Fibroepithelioma can change into an invasive and ulcerating basal cell carcinoma (422).

The multiple basal cell carcinomas seen in the *nevoid basal cell carcinoma syndrome* present no features that distinguish them from ordinary basal cell carcinoma, even while they are still in the early nevoid stage and have not yet become invasive and destructive, as they may be later in the neoplastic stage (423). All the diverse features of basal cell carcinoma, such as solid, adenoid, cystic, keratotic, superficial, and fibrosing formations, can be seen in the lesions of the nevoid basal cell carcinoma syndrome (424). Usually, a histologic distinction between the nevoid basal cell carcinoma syndrome and typical trichoepithelioma is easy, because keratotic cysts are more prominent in the latter. However, some lesions of trichoepithelioma show relatively few horn cysts. A histologic distinction in such cases may be impossible (425), and clinical data will be necessary (see Chapter 30).

The palmar and plantar pits are a result of the premature desquamation of most of the horny layer (426). On histologic examination, the epidermal rete ridges beneath the pits are found to be crowded with cells resembling those of basal cell carcinoma. Overlying these rete ridges, there is a markedly thinned granular layer topped by a very thin layer of loose keratin (381). In some patients, the pits actually show at their base the presence of small basal cell carcinomas (427). In rare instances, one or several clinically visible basal cell carcinomas arise on the palms or soles in patients with palmar and plantar pits (426,428,429).

The jaw cysts represent odontogenic keratocysts. They are lined by a festooned epithelium consisting of two to five layers of squamous cells that form keratin without the presence of a granular cell layer (430). Each jaw cyst may consist of either one large cyst or multiple microcysts (424). Some of the cutaneous cysts, instead of being epidermal cysts, have the appearance of the jaw cysts and are similar to those cysts seen in steatocystoma multiplex but without showing sebaceous lobules (430).

The basal cell carcinomas in *linear unilateral basal cell nevus* have a variable histologic appearance. The tumor formations may be solid, adenoid, keratotic, or cystic (387, 431). In addition, there may be areas resembling trichoepithelioma (386) or eccrine spiradenoma (432). The walls of the comedones show numerous buds of basal cell carcinoma extending into the surrounding dermis (387,389).

The basal cell carcinomas encountered in the *Bazex syndrome* have a variable histologic appearance. Some of them are indistinguishable from trichoepithelioma (391,392). The areas of follicular atrophoderma show a dilated follicular ostium leading into a distorted and underdeveloped pilosebaceous unit (392).

The tumor described in 1926 by Jadassohn and regarded by him as an intraepidermal epithelioma analogous to one previously reported by Borst has been referred to subsequently as *Borst–Jadassohn epithelioma*. For a long time this tumor and similar tumors subsequently described were thought to be intraepidermal basal cell carcinomas, because the cells composing the intraepidermal islands usually are small and have a deeply basophilic cytoplasm (433). However, on careful examination, it became evident that the cells composing the intraepidermal islands in the presumed intraepidermal basal cell carcinomas possess intercellular bridges and are seborrheic keratoses of the clonal type (66,434). The existence of an intraepidermal basal cell carcinoma is also unlikely because the close relationship that exists between tumor and stroma in basal cell carcinoma excludes the formation of intraepidermal nests, which would lack any contact with the stroma (435).

However, there are several types of tumors, some benign and some malignant, that on occasion show well-defined islands of cells within the epidermis that differ in their appearance from the surrounding epidermal cells (90). This is referred to as the *Jadassohn phenomenon*. Among the tumors that occasionally have an intraepidermal location are the following:

Clonal seborrheic keratosis. Some of these tumors show intraepidermal aggregates of basaloid cells suggestive of a basal cell carcinoma *in situ* (66) (Fig. 29-8), whereas others show intraepidermal islands of an irritated seborrheic keratosis simulating a squamous cell carcinoma *in situ.*

Bowen's disease. Occasionally, one observes clonal aggregates of Bowen's disease within the epidermis (436). At a later stage, there may be dermal invasion (437).

Intraepidermal poroma, also referred to as hidroacanthoma simplex (438,439) (Chapter 30).

Intraepidermal malignant eccrine poroma. In cases of intraepidermal metastases of malignant eccrine poroma, the tumor masses extend through the superficial lymphatics from the dermis into the epidermis (440,441) (see Chapter 31).

The concept of intraepidermal tumors has been extended also to include Paget's disease of the breast, extramammary Paget's disease (Chapter 30), intraepidermal junction nevus (see Chapter 28), and malignant melanoma *in situ* (90) (see Chapter 28).

Some authors still regard the intraepidermal epithelioma of Jadassohn as a distinct entity that may invade the dermis and occasionally cause metastases (442). It has been postulated that this tumor arises from acrosyringium keratinocytes or pluripotential adnexal cells and represents an adnexal carcinoma (442).

The existence of *basal cell carcinomas with features of squamous cell carcinoma* was first postulated in 1922 (443). Two types of basal squamous cell epitheliomas, referred to as *metatypical epitheliomas,* were recognized: a mixed and an intermediary type. The mixed type was described as showing focal keratinization consisting of pearls with a colloidal or parakeratotic center, and the intermediary type as showing within a network of narrow strands two kinds of cells, an outer row of dark-staining basal cells and an inner layer of cells appearing larger, lighter, and better defined than the basal cells and regarded as intermediate in character between basal and squamous cells (Fig. 29-68).

Several authors have accepted the existence of basal squamous cell epitheliomas or metatypical epitheliomas (372,444–446). They are considered by some to represent a transition from basal cell carcinoma to squamous cell carcinoma. It has been stated that a continuum extends from basal cell carcinoma at one extreme to squamous cell carcinoma at the other (446). The incidence of basal squamous cell carcinomas among basal cell carcinomas has been judged to be 3% (446) 8% (445) and even 12% (444). It has also been stated that basal squamous cell epitheliomas show a greater tendency to metastasize than basal cell carcinomas (372,444,446).

However, the existence of basal squamous cell epitheliomas is questioned by many (397,447–451). It would seem that the entirely different genesis of squamous cell carcinoma, a true anaplastic carcinoma of the epidermis, and basal cell carcinoma, a tumor composed of immature rather than anaplastic cells, makes the occurrence of transitional forms quite unlikely (see Pathogenesis section). It can be assumed that the so-called mixed type of basal squamous cell epithelioma represents a keratotic basal cell carcinoma (Fig. 29-68) and that the intermediate type represents a basal cell carcinoma with differentiation into two types of cells (basal cell carcinoma with squamous differentiation). This form of differentiation is often seen deep to an area of ulceration. Other putative examples of basosquamous differentiation are better interpreted as *basal cell carcinoma with follicular differentiation* (Fig. 29-76).

Mixed carcinoma shows a squamous cell carcinoma contiguous to a basal cell carcinoma as a so-called collision tumor. It is likely that, in most instances, the squamous cell carcinoma develops secondary to the basal cell carcinoma. Like other chronic ulcerative lesions, such as burns and stasis ulcers, basal cell carcinoma may stimulate the development of a squamous cell carcinoma. Before making a diagnosis of mixed carcinoma, however, one must rule out the possibility of pseudocarcinomatous hyperplasia occurring in a basal cell carcinoma.

Pathogenesis. Krompecher, who first described basal cell carcinoma, stated in 1903 that he regarded this tumor as a carcinoma of the basal cells of the epidermis and that those tumors that show a tendency toward gland formation are imitating the potential of the basal cells to form cutaneous glands (452). Krompecher's view is still supported by some (453–455). According to Geschickter and Koehler, only those basal cells with a potential to develop into glandular cells give rise to basal cell carcinoma. They suggested the designation *appendage cell carcinoma.* Mallory held the opinion that basal cell carcinomas are carcinomas of hair matrix cells. In 1947, Foot expressed the view that basal cell carcinomas are carcinomas that have developed from distorted primordia of dermal adnexa rather than from ordinary epidermal basal cells (408). He stated that the tumors imitate the embryonal development of one or all three types of adnexal primordia, that is, hair, sebaceous gland, and sweat gland.

The first author to express doubts that basal cell carcinomas are carcinomas was Adamson; in 1914, he stated that, in his opinion, basal cell carcinomas are nevoid tumors originating "from latent embryonic foci aroused from their dormant state at a later period in life" (456). He believed that the latent embryonic foci usually are embryonic pilosebaceous follicles but occasionally are embryonic sweat ducts. Several other authors have since reached similar conclusions, among them Wallace and Halpert, who stated in 1950 that they regarded basal cell carcinomas as benign tumors arising from cells destined to form hair follicles (457). They proposed the term *trichoma* for them.

In 1948, Lever expressed his belief that basal cell carcinomas are not carcinomas and are not derived from basal cells, but rather are nevoid tumors, or hamartomas, derived from primary epithelial germ cells. In other words, basal cell carcinomas originate from incompletely differentiated, immature cells and not from anaplastic cells. Although gamma-glutamyl transpeptidase activity is observed in the atypical cells in squamous cell carcinoma, Bowen's disease, and actinic keratoses, no gamma-glutamyl transpeptidase activity is expressed in the cells of basal cell carcinoma (458). In this view, basal cell carcinoma represents the least differentiated of the appendage tumors.

It was originally assumed, analogous to Adamson's view, that the primary epithelial germ cells giving rise to basal cell carcinoma are in all instances embryonic cells that lay dormant until the onset of neoplasia. Even though this view applies to the linear unilateral basal cell nevus, which is usually present from birth, it is likely that, as suggested by Pinkus, basal cell carcinomas occurring later in life arise not from dormant embryonic primary epithelial germ cells but from pluripotential cells that form continuously during life and, like embryonic primary epithelial germ cells, have the potential of forming hair, sebaceous glands, and apocrine glands (396). The fact that basal cell carcinomas may arise in sun-exposed areas and in areas of radiodermatitis supports this view. Their tendency to local invasion and tissue destruction, their capacity for local persistence and recurrence if not ablated, and their occasional capacity for metastasis support the concept that these lesions are carcinomas, albeit in most instances with little or no capacity for metastasis.

It is now widely accepted that disruption of the hedgehog-patched pathway is a key event in development of basal cell cancer. In addition to patched gene alterations, p53 gene mutations are also frequently present (396a,b,c,d,e,f,g,h,i,j). Lever's view that basal cell carcinomas are derived from primary epithelial germ cells has been developed in light of the recognition and characterization of epidermal stem cells.

Pilar Differentiation

Differentiation in basal cell carcinoma is predominantly toward pilar keratin. The presence of citrulline in keratinized structures indicates that the origin of the keratin is the hair matrix, because epidermal keratin contains no citrulline (449). Studies with monoclonal cytokeratin antibodies support the assumption of pilar differentiation in basal cell carcinoma. Thus, a cytokeratin antibody binding to the follicular epithelium but not to the interfollicular epidermis stains all cells of basal cell carcinoma (459). Also, a monoclonal antibody against basal cell carcinoma keratin stains, in addition to the cells of basal cell carcinoma, all follicular cells below the isthmus portion of normal anagen hair follicles (460). These findings contribute to the general view that basal cell carcinoma should be regarded as a hair follicle tumor rather than an epidermal tumor.

Stromal Factor

The importance of stroma in the development of basal cell carcinomas is borne out by the fact that autotransplants of basal cell carcinomas survive only when they include connective tissue stroma (461). Also, the rarity of basal cell carcinomas on the palms and soles and the fact that the palmar and plantar pits of the nevoid basal cell carcinoma syndrome very rarely show a full-fledged basal cell carcinoma suggest that the palms and soles do not possess the stromal factor necessary for the formation of basal cell carcinomas (462).

Lack of Autonomy

Basal cell carcinomas, when transplanted to the anterior chamber of the rabbit's eye together with their connective tissue stroma, fail to grow, in contrast to squamous cell carcinoma (463). Furthermore, basal cell carcinomas, in contrast to many human tumors, do not grow when transplanted subcutaneously to athymic nude mice (464). These observations suggest a lack of autonomy of the cells of at least some basal cell carcinomas. Because autonomy of the tumor cell is a prerequisite for the formation of metastases and represents a characteristic feature of malignant tumors (465), the absence of autonomy in basal cell carcinoma is consistent with its inability to metastasize in most instances.

Site of Origin

The usual site of origin of basal cell carcinoma appears to be the surface epidermis. Occasionally, however, the tumor may originate from the outer root sheath of a hair follicle (466,467).

Of particular interest is the manner of growth of *superficial basal cell carcinoma*. Routine sectioning carried out perpendicular to the skin surface shows seemingly independent nests of basal cell carcinoma suggestive at times of the growth of primary epithelial germs in the embryonic skin. Thus, it was at one time widely assumed that the peripheral extension seen in superficial basal cell carcinoma was based on a "multicentric" growth characterized by the formation of new buds of tumor tissue at the periphery. However, on the basis of findings in serial sections and in wax reconstructions of superficial basal cell carcinomas, Madsen has favored the theory of a "unicentric" origin (468,469). Madsen was able to show that the tumor strands are continuous but are attached to the undersurface of the epidermis only at intervals, like garlands. Madsen found not only in his wax reconstructions but also in sections cut parallel to the surface of the skin that individual tumor islands are interconnected. Oberste-Lehn (470), using a technique of separating the epidermis from the dermis by maceration, could not find such interconnections, but the possibility could not be excluded, as Madsen pointed out, that the interconnections had ruptured as a result of the maceration. It was subsequently shown when trypsin was used for the separation of the epidermis from the dermis that interconnections exist between tumor cell nests in superficial basal cell carcinoma. Similarly, three-dimensional reconstruction by means of serial, horizontal microscopic sections and a special computer confirmed a unicentric origin (471).

Electron Microscopy. The predominant cell in undifferentiated basal cell carcinoma is characterized by a large nucleus, poorly developed desmosomes, and rather sparse tonofilaments. Thus, the tumor cells differ from normal epidermal basal cells. They resemble the cells of the undifferentiated hair matrix (472) or the immature basal cells of the embryonic epidermis, particularly those of the primary epithelial germ (473,474). In addition to the prevalent large, light cells, a few cells that are smaller, darker, and more irregularly shaped can be found (404,473). The darkness of the latter cells is due to the abundance of ribonucleoprotein particles in their cytoplasm. A well-developed basement membrane separates the tumor from the dermis (472). Processes from the tumor cells do not usually penetrate the basement membrane in basal cell carcinoma, in contrast to squamous cell carcinoma, in which processes extend through a fragmented basement membrane into the stroma (475).

Keratinization is commonly observed by electron microscopy in basal cell carcinoma, especially in the keratotic type. In addition to well-developed desmosomes and many thick bundles of tonofilaments, dense clumps of homogeneous, dyskeratotic material are present in many keratinizing cells. A small number of keratohyaline granules are often seen. They probably represent trichohyalin granules, which occur in the process of keratinization of the inner root sheath and its cuticle (473).

Some basal cell carcinomas show areas of adenoid differentiation in which cells are grouped around gland-like lumina. Such cells may show pronounced infolding of the plasma membrane at their lateral borders as seen normally in eccrine ductal cells (404).

In pigmented basal cell carcinomas, most of the melanin is found within melanocytes of the tumor and in melanophages located in the connective tissue stroma. Although numerous melanosomes are present in the dendrites of the melanocytes, the tumor cells generally do not phagocytize the melanin-containing dendrites, resulting in a blockage of the transfer of melanin from melanocytes to the tumor cells (476,477). This is analogous to the blocked transfer from melanocytes to tumor cells in some pigmented seborrheic keratoses referred to as melanoacanthoma. Nevertheless, in occasional instances of pigmented basal cell carcinoma, some transfer of melanosomes to the tumor cells takes place. The tumor cells then contain melanosomes, which are located largely as melanosome complexes within lysosomes (473).

Presence of Amyloid

Cell proliferation in basal cell carcinoma is considerable. The experimentally determined cell-doubling time of 9 days, however, does not conform with the clinical observation that basal cell carcinoma, as a rule, is a very slowly growing tumor (478). This suggests that there must be cell death. In addition to phagocytosis by neighboring tumor cells and macrophages, apoptosis of tumor cells also often takes place, with transformation of the cells into colloid bodies and subsequently into amyloid (402,479). This conversion of epithelial cells into amyloid is analogous to that occurring in lichenoid and macular amyloidosis. Colloid bodies, demonstrable by direct immunofluorescence for immunoglobulin M (IgM), have been found in 89% of basal cell carcinomas (402). Amyloid has been observed in the stroma and inside the tumor islands both by histochemistry and by electron microscopy in as many as 65% of basal cell carcinomas (402,480). This amyloid shows positive staining with antikeratin antiserum, indicating that it is derived from tonofilaments (481). The fact that the amyloid is permanganate-resistant indicates that it is not secondary amyloid (482). The presence of amyloid may contribute to an apparent lack of sensitivity to radiotherapy (482a).

Differential Diagnosis. Differentiation of basal cell carcinoma from squamous cell carcinoma can sometimes be difficult, so difficult that some authors believe that intermediate forms (basal squamous cell epitheliomas) occur. However, as a rule, differentiation is fairly easy. One of the best points of differentiation is that most cells of basal cell carcinoma stain deeply basophilic, whereas most cells of squamous cell carcinoma, at least in low-grade lesions, have an eosinophilic tint due to partial keratinization. The cells in high-grade squamous cell carcinoma may appear basophilic because of the absence of keratinization. However, they differ from basal cell carcinoma by showing much greater atypicality of their nuclei and their mitotic figures. It is important to remember that keratinization is not a prerogative of squamous cell carcinoma; it occurs also in basal cell carcinoma with differentiation toward hair structures (see Keratotic Basal Cell Carcinoma section). Keratinization in basal cell carcinomas may be partial and then result in parakeratotic bands and whorls, or it may be complete and result in horn cysts. The keratinization seen in the horn cysts differs from that seen in the horn pearls of squamous cell carcinomas by being abrupt and complete rather than gradual and incomplete. The fairly common presence in basal cell carcinoma of areas of retraction of the tumor cell masses from the surrounding connective tissue also aids in the differentiation of this tumor from squamous cell carcinoma, in which such areas of retraction are rarely found.

The differential diagnosis of basal cell carcinoma from trichoepithelioma is discussed in Chapter 31. Of particular importance is the differentiation of fibrosing basal cell carcinoma from the only recently described desmoplastic trichoepithelioma. Both tumors have in common thin strands of small basaloid cells embedded in a dense, fibrous stroma, but desmoplastic trichoepithelioma also shows a considerable number of horn cysts. Many tumors originally diagnosed as basal cell carcinomas in children and teenagers could be reclassified as desmoplastic trichoepithelioma (483).

In making a biopsy diagnosis, it is important to have sections that adequately represent the lesion. It is curious that in punch biopsies the initial sections may not show the tumor. Further sections should always be examined if the clinical diagnosis is one of basal cell carcinoma (483b). There is also a limited evidence base to recommend the most effective and economical excision margins. It seems likely that a margin of 3 mm may be adequate in most cases, but in high-risk basal cell carcinoma this may be insufficient (483c,d,e,f).

EPIDERMAL TUMORS IN IMMUNOSUPPRESSED HOSTS

The widespread use of immunosuppressive therapy as part of organ transplantation and in the treatment of some immunologically mediated diseases has led to a new phenomenon of rapidly developing warts and epidermal tumors (483a). There is a spectrum of squamous atypia ranging from typical viral warts through dysplastic or atypical warts to squamous cell carcinomas, which are often very poorly differentiated (Fig. 29-77). The squamous cell carcinomas have been shown to have similar proliferative potential to similar lesions in hosts with normal immune function

(484), although they lack the host immune response that would normally be present (485). They also share the same early expression of keratin 17 seen in a number of epidermal hyperproliferative states (486). Mutations of p53 may play a part in the development of the tumors (487). Rapidly progressing multiple squamous cell carcinomas have also been reported in association with chronic myeloid leukemia (488). Basal cell carcinomas tend to show an infiltrative rather than a nodular growth pattern more frequently in the immunosuppressed (489). Kaposi's sarcoma can also present as a fulminant process following liver or kidney transplantation (490,491), and may recur with the introduction of cyclosporin A therapy (492). It has also been suggested that HIV-positive hosts have an increased risk of developing malignant melanoma (493).

KERATOACANTHOMA

Two types of keratoacanthoma exist: solitary and multiple.

Solitary Keratoacanthoma

Solitary keratoacanthoma was first described in 1889 by Hutchinson as a "crateriform ulcer of the face," and since 1950 has been recognized as an entity and differentiated from squamous cell carcinoma, which it often resembles clinically and histologically (493a,494,495). Solitary keratoacanthoma occurs in elderly persons usually as a single lesion; however, occasionally, there are several lesions, or new lesions develop. The lesion consists of a firm, dome-shaped nodule 1.0 to 2.5 cm in diameter with a horn-filled crater in its center. The sites of predilection are exposed areas, where about 95% of solitary keratoacanthomas occur, but they may occur on any hairy cutaneous site (496). They have not been reported on the palms, soles, or mucous surfaces, although, in rare instances, they occur subungually (see discussion below). Keratoacanthomas located on the vermilion border of the lip probably arise from hair follicles in the adjacent skin (497). Keratoacanthomas usually reach their full size within 6 to 8 weeks and involute spontaneously, generally in less than 6 months. Healing takes place with a slightly depressed scar. In some instances, a keratoacanthoma increases in size for more than 2 months and takes up to 1 year to involute (496).

An increased incidence of keratoacanthoma is observed in immunosuppressed patients (498). Also, keratoacanthomas commonly occur in the Muir–Torre syndrome of sebaceous neoplasms and keratoacanthomas associated with visceral carcinomas (Chapter 30). Keratoacanthomas may be the only type of cutaneous tumor present in this syndrome (499,500).

There are three rare clinical variants of solitary keratoacanthoma. In two forms, giant keratoacanthoma and keratoacanthoma centrifugum marginatum, the keratoacan-

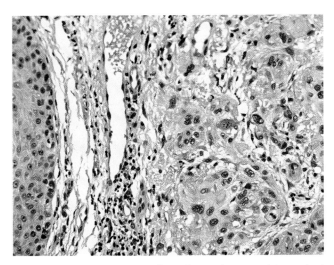

FIGURE 29-77. Squamous cell carcinoma in a renal transplant recipient. The dermis is infiltrated by a squamous cell carcinoma with very marked cellular pleomorphism.

thoma attains a large size. In *giant keratoacanthoma*, the growth rapidly reaches a size of 5 cm or more and may cause destruction of underlying tissues. Nevertheless, spontaneous involution takes place after several months, often accompanied by detachment of a large keratotic plaque. The most common sites are the nose (501,502) and the eyelids (498,503,504). In *keratoacanthoma centrifugum marginatum*, the lesion may reach 20 cm in diameter. There is no tendency toward spontaneous involution; instead, there is peripheral extension with a raised, rolled border and atrophy in the center of the lesion. The most common locations are the dorsa of the hands (505,506) and the legs (507,508). The third rare variant is *subungual keratoacanthoma*, which shows a destructive crateriform lesion with keratotic excrescences under the distal portion of a fingernail. It fails to regress spontaneously, is tender, and by roentgenogram shows damage to the terminal phalanx by pressure erosion (509–511).

Claims have been made that keratoacanthoma can undergo transformation into a squamous cell carcinoma either spontaneously (505,512), or as a result of immunosuppression (498,513). It appears more likely, however, that the squamous cell carcinoma existed from the beginning in such instances (496,514) (see Differential Diagnosis section).

Histopathology. The architecture of the lesion in a keratoacanthoma is as important to the diagnosis as the cellular characteristics. Therefore, if the lesion cannot be excised in its entirety, it is advisable that a fusiform specimen be excised for biopsy from the center of the lesion and that this specimen includes the edge at least of one side and preferably of both sides of the lesion (515). A shave biopsy is inadvisable, since the histologic changes at the base of the lesion are often of great importance in the differentiation from squamous cell carcinoma. Frequently a curettage specimen will be submitted, in which case clear distinction between keratoacanthoma and squamous cell carcinoma may be impossible to achieve with confidence.

In the early proliferative stage, one observes a horn-filled invagination of the epidermis from which strands of epidermis protrude into the dermis. These strands are poorly demarcated from the surrounding stroma in many areas, and may contain cells showing nuclear atypia (516) as well as many mitotic figures (517). Even atypical mitoses may be seen occasionally (518). Dyskeratotic cells, that is, cells showing individual cell keratinization, may also be seen in areas that otherwise do not show advanced keratinization. However, even at this early stage, some of the tumor areas show a fairly pronounced degree of keratinization, giving them an eosinophilic, glassy appearance. In the dermis, a rather pronounced inflammatory infiltrate is present (517). Perineural invasion is occasionally seen in the proliferative phase of keratoacanthoma and should not be misinterpreted as evidence of malignancy (519,520).

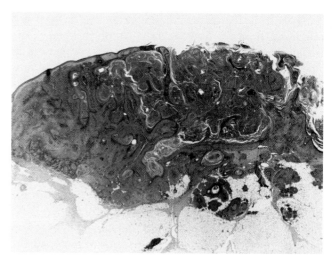

FIGURE 29-78. Keratoacanthoma. Low magnification. There is a large, central keratin-filled crater. Epidermis extends like a buttress over the side of the crater (**right**). Irregular epidermal proliferations extend downward from the base of the crater into the dermis.

A fully developed lesion shows in its center a large, irregularly shaped crater filled with keratin (Fig. 29-78). The epidermis extends like a lip or a buttress over the sides of the crater. At the base of the crater, irregular epidermal proliferations extend both upward into the crater and downward from the base of the crater. These proliferations may still appear somewhat atypical, but less so than in the initial stage; the keratinization is extensive and fairly advanced, with only a thin shell of one or two layers of basophilic, nonkeratinized cells at the periphery of the proliferations, whereas the cells within this shell appear eosinophilic and glassy as a result of keratinization (Fig. 29-79). There are many horn pearls, most of which show complete keratinization in their center. The base of a fully developed keratoacanthoma appears regular and well demarcated and usually does not extend below the level of the sweat glands. A rather dense inflammatory infiltrate is often present at the base of the lesion (496,521) (Fig. 29-80).

In the involuting stage, proliferation has ceased, and most cells at the base of the crater have undergone keratinization. There may be shrunken, eosinophilic cells analogous to colloid or Civatte bodies among the tumor cells located nearest to the stroma as well as in the stroma, suggesting that cell degeneration followed by apoptosis contributes to the involution of the keratoacanthoma (507). Gradually, the crater flattens and finally disappears during healing.

Pathogenesis. It is generally agreed that the lesion starts with hyperplasia of the infundibulum of one or several adjoining hair follicles and with squamous metaplasia of the attached sebaceous glands (522). The application of cutaneous carcinogens to the skin of animals frequently pro-

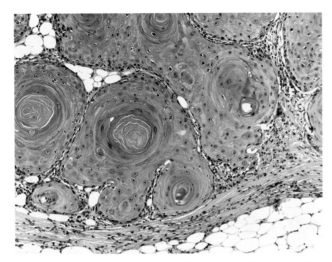

FIGURE 29-79. Keratoacanthoma. Higher magnification of the epidermal proliferations at the base of the crater shows their resemblance to squamous cell carcinoma. However, there is more keratinization than is usually seen in squamous cell carcinoma, giving the tumor islands a glassy appearance.

duces, among other tumors, lesions with the histologic appearance of keratoacanthomas, and these tumors also have their origin in the infundibulum of one or several hair follicles (523).

The cause of keratoacanthoma is not known. The theory of a viral genesis has not been confirmed. The electron microscopic findings are largely nonspecific. However, keratoacanthomas, like squamous cell carcinomas and lesions of Bowen's disease, often show the presence of fairly numerous intracytoplasmic desmosomes (524,525).

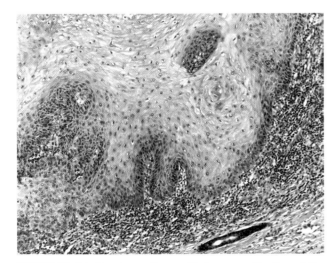

FIGURE 29-80. Keratoacanthoma. Higher magnification of the epidermal proliferations at the base of the crater shows their resemblance to squamous cell carcinoma. However, the basal layer is well defined with no evidence of any invasive element.

Differential Diagnosis. Differentiation of typical, mature lesions of keratoacanthoma from squamous cell carcinoma generally is not difficult. In favor of a diagnosis of keratoacanthoma are the architecture of a crater surrounded by buttresses and the high degree of keratinization, which is manifested by the eosinophilic, glassy appearance of many of the cells. Clinical data are also of great value: rapid development of an exophytic lesion showing a central, horn-filled crater speaks for keratoacanthoma rather than for squamous cell carcinoma.

The greatest difficulties in the differentiation of a keratoacanthoma from a squamous cell carcinoma are encountered in very early lesions, because a horn-filled invagination may be seen in squamous cell carcinoma and cells with an atypical appearance may occur in a keratoacanthoma. Occasionally, an early keratoacanthoma shows a greater degree of nuclear atypia than do some squamous cell carcinomas (526). Also, individual cell keratinization can occur in keratoacanthoma. On rare occasions, even adenoid formations caused by dyskeratosis and acantholysis can occur in keratoacanthoma (527). Thus, it was found on reclassification in one study that in only 81% of the cases of keratoacanthoma could a diagnosis of squamous cell carcinoma be fully excluded and that in only 86% of the cases of squamous cell carcinoma could keratoacanthoma be ruled out with certainty. These findings explain why, on rare occasions, lesions classified as keratoacanthoma cause metastases (514). Great caution is indicated in the diagnosis of giant keratoacanthomas. Several cases diagnosed as such turned out to be squamous cell carcinomas, either by metastasizing (528) or by deep invasion into muscle (529).

Because it is widely agreed that squamous cell carcinomas can masquerade as keratoacanthomas clinically and histologically (496,530), it is best to err on the safe side in a doubtful case and to proceed on the assumption that the lesion is a squamous cell carcinoma.

Attempts at differentiating between keratoacanthoma and squamous cell carcinoma by histochemical or immunohistochemical methods have shown distinct differences in typical cases but not necessarily in borderline cases.

There are two variants of *multiple keratoacanthoma*: the multiple self-healing epitheliomas of the skin, or Ferguson Smith type, and the eruptive keratoacanthomas, or Grzybowski type. Both variants are rare in comparison with solitary keratoacanthoma.

In *multiple self-healing epitheliomas* of the skin, lesions begin to appear in childhood or adolescence on any part of the skin, including the palms and soles, but especially on the face and the extremities. Subungual lesions have also been described (510). Generally, there are no more than a dozen lesions at any one time (531). The lesions may reach the same size as solitary keratoacanthomas and after a few months heal with a depressed scar (532,533). In some cases, however, the lesions do not heal (534). In some patients, the condition is inherited (534,535).

In *eruptive keratoacanthoma*, lesions do not appear until adult life. Many hundreds of follicular papules are present, measuring from 2 to 3 mm in diameter (536,537). The oral mucosa and larynx may be involved (538,539).

Histopathology. The histologic appearance of the lesions of multiple self-healing epitheliomas of the skin is similar to that of solitary keratoacanthoma (531,533). More frequently than in solitary keratoacanthoma, the cutaneous proliferations in multiple self-healing epitheliomas of the skin are seen to be continuous with the follicular epithelium (540). The cutaneous lesions in eruptive keratoacanthoma show less crater formation than those in solitary keratoacanthoma. The mucosal lesions lack a crater and can easily be misinterpreted as squamous cell carcinoma (538,539).

Pathogenesis. It appears likely that multiple keratoacanthoma basically represents the same condition as solitary keratoacanthoma and that predisposition or genetic factors are responsible for the greater number of lesions (541). In multiple as in solitary keratoacanthoma, lesions arising in hair-bearing parts of the skin have their onset in the upper portion of a hair follicle, whereas the site of origin of lesions arising on the palms, soles, and mucous membranes is not apparent (538).

PAGET'S DISEASE

Paget's disease of the breast occurs almost exclusively in women. Only a few instances of its occurrence in the male breast have been described (542). Of interest is its occurrence in the male breast after treatment of a carcinoma of the prostate with estrogen (543). The cutaneous lesion in Paget's disease of the breast begins either on the nipple or the areola of the breast and extends slowly to the surrounding skin. It is always unilateral and consists of a sharply defined, slightly infiltrated area of erythema showing scaling, oozing, and crusting. There may or may not be ulceration or retraction of the nipple.

The cutaneous lesion is nearly always associated with carcinoma of the breast, and in more than half of the patients, a mass can be felt on palpation of the breast. Metastases in the axillary lymph nodes were found by one group of investigators in about 67% of their patients with a palpable mass of the breast and in 33% of those without a palpable mass (544). This contrasts with the experience of others, who encountered no axillary metastases in the absence of a palpable mass of the breast (545).

A clinical picture indistinguishable from that of early Paget's disease of the nipple may be seen in erosive adenomatosis of the nipple, a benign neoplasm of the major nipple ducts (546) (see Chapter 30).

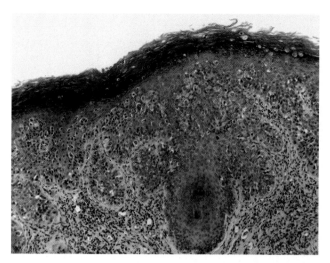

FIGURE 29-81. Paget's disease. The epidermis is permeated with numerous Paget cells lying singly and in groups. There is no invasion of the dermis by Paget cells.

Histopathology. In early lesions of Paget's disease of the breast, the epidermis usually shows only a few scattered Paget cells. They are large, rounded cells that are devoid of intercellular bridges and contain a large nucleus and ample cytoplasm. The cytoplasm of these cells stains much lighter than that of the adjacent squamous cells (Figs. 29-81 and 29-82). As the number of Paget cells increases, they compress the squamous cells to such an extent that the latter may merely form a network, the meshes of which are filled with Paget cells lying singly and in groups. In particular, one often observes flattened basal cells lying between Paget cells and the underlying dermis.

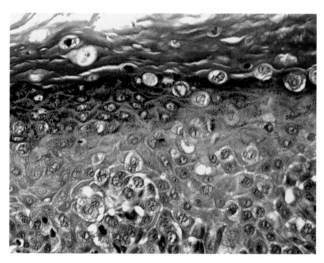

FIGURE 29-82. Paget's disease. High magnification. Paget cells are scattered through the epidermis. They are large rounded cells devoid of intercellular bridges, with ample pale-staining cytoplasm.

Histochemical staining of the Paget cells within the epidermis in Paget's disease of the breast has given inconsistent results. In contrast with extramammary Paget's disease in which the presence of sialomucin can be demonstrated in abundance in nearly all cases, the Paget cells in Paget's disease of the breast stain with the PAS reaction in only some of the cases (547), and if positive, the number of positively staining cells is rather small (548). The PAS-positive cells may be diastase-resistant, but often they are not (549). Similarly, the Alcian blue stain at pH 2.5 is only weakly positive in scattered Paget cells in some of the cases and negative in others (549). Occasionally, Paget cells contain some melanin (550); however, they are dopa negative (551).

The dermis in Paget's disease shows a moderately severe chronic inflammatory reaction. Although Paget cells do not invade the dermis from the epidermis, they may be seen extending from the epidermis into the epithelium of hair follicles (552).

Histologic examination of the mammary ducts and glands nearly always shows malignant changes in some of them. At first, the carcinoma is confined within the walls of the ducts and glands, but the tumor cells ultimately invade the connective tissue. From then on, lymphatic spread and metastases occur, just as in other types of mammary carcinoma. In mammary Paget's disease, the malignant changes have their onset in the lactiferous ducts and from there extend into the epidermis (547), but there are rare instances in which the malignant cells are confined to the epidermis of the nipple or involve only the most distal portion of one lactiferous duct (553).

Pathogenesis. As long as electron microscopic examination constituted the major factor in analyzing the derivation or the direction of differentiation of the cells in Paget's disease of the nipple, no clear decision could be reached whether the constituting cells were keratinocytes or glandular cells. The presence of desmosomes between neighboring Paget cells and between Paget cells and keratinocytes seemed to support a derivation from keratinocytes (554). On the other hand, scattered desmosomes are normally found connecting the cells of the lactiferous ducts (555), and wherever cytoplasmic processes of Paget cells lie in contact with the basal lamina, no hemidesmosomes are present, as they would be in the case of keratinocytes (549). Also, Paget cells can be found bordering small lumina in areas in which groups of Paget cells lie together (549,555,556).

Immunohistochemical studies in recent years have proved beyond any doubt the glandular derivation of the Paget cells of both mammary and extramammary Paget's disease. Thus, carcinoembryonic antigen is regularly found in Paget cells. Whereas intervening keratinocytes and melanocytes do not stain, carcinoembryogenic antigen is present in the cells of normal eccrine and apocrine glands (557). Furthermore, Paget cells express cytokeratins typical of glandular epithelia but do not react with antibodies to epidermal keratin (558). CAM 5.2 is a low-molecular-weight cytokeratin marker that stains Paget's cells in 70% to 90% of cases. The adjacent epidermis, which is rich in molecular weight cytokeratins, does not stain. Cytokeratin 7 is a more sensitive, but not specific, marker for Paget's disease. As well as staining Paget's cells it may also stain intraepidermal Merkel cells and Toker cells, so positive staining needs to be correlated with morphology when interpreting appearances in a section (559).

Enzyme histochemistry in Paget's disease of the breast has shown the presence of an apocrine enzymatic pattern in the intraepidermal Paget cells consisting of a strong reactivity for acid phosphatase and esterase and only a weakly positive reaction for aminopeptidase and succinic dehydrogenase (559). This finding suggests that the intraepidermal Paget cells in Paget's disease of the breast are derived from mammary gland cells, because the mammary gland represents a modified apocrine gland.

Differential Diagnosis. Paget's disease of the breast must be differentiated from Bowen's disease and the superficial spreading or "pagetoid" type of malignant melanoma *in situ*. Although vacuolated cells may occur in both Paget's disease and Bowen's disease, one observes clear-cut transitions between the vacuolated cells and epidermal cells only in Bowen's disease. Furthermore, one may observe in Bowen's disease, but not in Paget's disease, clumping of nuclei within multinucleated epidermal cells and individual cell keratinization. In addition, the cells in Bowen's disease do not contain carcinoembryonic antigen but react with prekeratin contained in rabbit antihuman prekeratin antiserum (560).

In the superficial spreading or pagetoid type of malignant melanoma *in situ*, as in the epidermis of Paget's disease of the breast, there are large, vacuolated cells scattered through the epidermis (548). The difficulty in distinguishing between the two types of cells may be increased by the fact that Paget cells occasionally also contain melanin (550). The most important points to remember in differentiating the two types of cells are as follows: (a) Paget cells are separated in many areas from the dermis by flattened basal cells, whereas melanoma cells border directly on the dermis; (b) Paget cells do not invade the dermis, whereas melanoma cells often do; (c) the tumor cells of malignant melanoma contain abundant cytoplasmic S-100 protein, but in tissues from Paget's disease, S-100 protein is usually absent in the tumor cells, although it may be seen in myoepithelial cells, Langerhans cells, and Schwann cells of cutaneous nerves (561); (d) Paget cells are dopa negative, unlike melanoma cells; and (e) melanoma cells, unlike Paget cells, may be positive for the HMB-45 antigen.

EXTRAMAMMARY PAGET'S DISEASE

Extramammary Paget's disease most commonly affects the vulva (279a), less commonly the male genital area (562), or the perianal area (551), and, in exceptional cases only, the axillae, the region of the ceruminal glands (563) or that of Moll's glands (564). In cases with involvement of the axillae, the genital area may also be affected (565). Thus, extramammary Paget's disease involves areas in which apocrine glands are normally encountered. Only very few cases of an association between mammary and vulvar Paget's disease have been described (566). In rare instances, extramammary Paget's disease is a secondary event caused by extension of an adenocarcinoma either of the rectum to the perianal region (551), of the cervix to the vulvar region (567), or of the urinary bladder to the urethra and glans penis (568) or to the groin (569). On the other hand, longstanding genital Paget's disease can extend inward to the cervix and urinary tract (570).

In extramammary Paget's disease, the clinical picture shows a slowly enlarging reddish patch with oozing and crusting. The patch resembles an eczematous lesion, but has a sharp, irregular border. In extramammary Paget's disease, in contrast to the mammary type, itching is common.

Histopathology. Extramammary Paget's disease shares with Paget's disease the presence of varying numbers of Paget cells within the epidermis. In some instances, the Paget cells are found to be limited to the epidermis. Frequently, Paget cells can also be identified within the epithelium of some hair follicles or eccrine sweat ducts (571). Such *in situ* malignancy associated with extramammary Paget's disease has the same favorable prognosis, as does extramammary Paget's disease limited to the epidermis. However, the prognosis is much more serious in cases in which the Paget cells have invaded the dermis from the epidermis (571,572), or from an underlying sweat gland carcinoma (573). In this respect, extramammary Paget's disease differs from mammary Paget's disease, in which invasion of the dermis from the overlying epidermis does not occur (552). Glandular clusters with a central lumen, absent in mammary Paget's disease, may be seen in the lower epidermis in extramammary Paget's disease (571,574).

On histochemical staining, the Paget cells seen in the epidermis and in the adnexa show a positive reaction for sialomucin in almost all cases of extramammary Paget's disease. Thus, the cytoplasm of the Paget cells is PAS-positive, diastase-resistant, stains with Alcian blue at pH 2.5 but not at pH 0.4, and is hyaluronidase-resistant (Chapter 4). It usually stains positive also with colloidal iron and mucicarmine (547). Nevertheless, these stains can be negative in cases of extramammary and of mammary Paget's disease (548).

Immunohistochemical staining typically shows that in primary Paget's disease the Paget cells stain positively for cytokeratin 7, whereas in secondary cases the cells may be cytokeratin 20 positive (548a).

In cases of "secondary" extramammary Paget's disease, the process extends either from a mucus-secreting adenocarcinoma of the rectum to the perianal skin (551,575, 576), from a mucus-secreting endocervical carcinoma to

the vulva (567), or from a transitional cell carcinoma of the urinary bladder with urethral extension (568,569). In such cases, the Paget cells in the perianal or vulvar skin are derived from the preexisting carcinoma and contain mucus that always is PAS positive and diastase resistant, and always shows a positive staining reaction with Alcian blue at pH 2.5 that is hyaluronidase resistant. The mucus represents sialomucin, a nonsulfated acid mucopolysaccharide (551). The prognosis in secondary extramammary Paget's disease is poor.

The prognosis of "primary" extramammary Paget's disease generally is better than that of mammary Paget's disease. In two large combined series of 123 patients with vulvar Paget's disease, only 26 patients (21%) showed an underlying invasive carcinoma in the dermis at the time of operation (571,572). In the other 79%, the Paget cells were present only within the epidermis and the epithelium of the cutaneous appendages, so that the process was still *in situ.* Thus, one author observed only two examples of invasive sweat gland carcinoma among more than 100 cases of extramammary Paget's disease (573) and another author reported none among 12 cases (558). However, the rate of local recurrence is high even after seemingly adequate excision. The reasons for this are that (a) the extent of histologically demonstrable disease is often far greater than that of the clinically visible lesion, and (b) extramammary Paget's disease, in contrast to mammary Paget's disease, can arise multifocally even in clinically normal-appearing areas of the skin (577).

Pathogenesis. At one time, the view was widely accepted that in primary extramammary Paget's disease the Paget cells in the epidermis are there as a result of an *in situ* upward extension of an *in situ* adenocarcinoma of sweat glands along eccrine or apocrine ducts (574,578). This view is analogous to the generally accepted views that secondary extramammary Paget's disease represents an extension of a rectal, cervical, or urinary bladder adenocarcinoma and that the development of mammary Paget's disease is an extension of an epidermotropic lactiferous duct carcinoma. The fact that an underlying *in situ* adenocarcinoma often could not be demonstrated was explained by the anatomic differences between the breast, which has only 20 large, conspicuous lactiferous ducts, and the genital skin, which has thousands of small apocrine and eccrine glands, making location of the particular small gland involved by carcinoma technically difficult (574). Staining with antikeratin monoclonal antibodies has indicated that upward extension of an *in situ* adenocarcinoma derived from malignant secretory cells present within sweat ducts can occur (579).

Even though in some cases extramammary Paget's disease is the result of extension of an underlying apocrine or eccrine sweat gland carcinoma to the overlying epidermis, in most instances it has its origin within the epidermis (572). Careful subserial total sectioning of excised lesions of vulvar Paget's disease has shown that the lesions within the epidermis and its appendages have a multifocal origin (577). Another pertinent argument in favor of the independence of the epidermal foci from any appendageal foci is the observation that in cases with extensive epidermal lesions, involvement of eccrine ducts and glands is often sparse and involvement of apocrine ducts and glands almost invariably absent, even though some Paget cells form apocrine glandular structures in the epidermis (571). Even if there is continuity between the epidermal and the ductal foci, there is no certain way of determining whether the extension is in an upward or downward direction. However, the clinching argument in favor of the autonomy of the epidermal foci in primary extramammary Paget's disease is the fact that, in contrast to mammary Paget's disease, dermal invasion generally originates from the epidermis, not ductal or glandular structures (571,572).

In cases in which the extramammary Paget's disease arises within the epidermis and extends from there at a later date into the adnexa and still later from the epidermis into the dermis, the question is: Which cell gives rise to the Paget cell? Two possibilities have been suggested, although proof for either is lacking. The first is that the Paget cell arises within the poral portion of an apocrine duct (580). The second is that, because the disease tends to occur in areas rich in apocrine glands and because there is in some cases unequivocal evidence of apocrine differentiation in the epidermis, intraepidermal Paget cells may be formed by pluripotential germinative cells within the epidermis that go awry trying to form apocrine structures (562,571).

Immunohistochemical studies indicate an apocrine genesis of extramammary Paget's disease. It is true that carcinoembryonic antigen merely indicates that the extramammary Paget cells are glandular rather than epidermal cells, and does not decide whether they are apocrine or eccrine (557,558). However, two immunoreactants for apocrine glands, gross cystic disease fluid protein (581), and apocrine epithelial antigen (558) have been shown to react with the Paget cells of extramammary Paget's disease, providing evidence for an apocrine derivation.

The majority of cases of mammary and extramammary Paget's disease are cytokeratin 7 positive. Those few cases that are negative have been reported to be more commonly associated with the presence of an underlying malignancy. In contrast, cytokeratin 20 is found more frequently in cases of extramammary Paget's disease with an underlying malignancy. The pattern of cytokeratin expression can therefore be used to predict the likelihood of the presence or absence of an associated internal malignancy (582).

Differential Diagnosis. Extramammary Paget's disease, like Paget's disease of the breast, must be differentiated from Bowen's disease and especially from superficial spreading or pagetoid malignant melanoma *in situ* (see Paget's Disease, Differential Diagnosis section).

REFERENCES

1. Heenan PJ, Elder DE, Sobin LH. *Histological typing of skin tumours.* Berlin: Springer-Verlag, 1996.
1a. Lee SH, Rogers M. Inflammatory linear verrucous naevi: a review of 23 cases. *Australas J Dermatol* 2001;42:252.
1b. Miteva LG, Dourmishev AL, Schwartz RA. Inflammatory linear verrucous epidermal nevus. *Cutis* 2001;68:327.
2. Basler RSW, Jacobs SI, Taylor WB. Ichthyosis hystrix. *Arch Dermatol* 1978;114:1059.
3. Solomon LM, Fretzin DF, Dewald RL. The epidermal nevus syndrome. *Arch Dermatol* 1968;97:273.
4. Winer LH, Levin GH. Pigmented basal-cell carcinoma in verrucous nevi. *Arch Dermatol* 1961;83:960.
5. Horn MS, Sausker WF, Pierson DL. Basal cell epithelioma arising in a linear epidermal nevus. *Arch Dermatol* 1981;117:247.
6. Dogliotti M, Frenkel A. Malignant change in a verrucous nevus. *Int J Dermatol* 1978;17:225.
7. Cramer SF, Mandel MA, Hauler R, et al. Squamous cell carcinoma arising in linear epidermal nevus. *Arch Dermatol* 1981;117:222.
8. Levin A, Amazon K, Rywlin AM. A squamous cell carcinoma that developed in an epidermal nevus. *Am J Dermatopathol* 1984;6:51.
9. Su WPD. Histopathologic varieties of epidermal nevus. *Am J Dermatopathol* 1982;4:161.
10. Ackerman AB. Histopathologic concept of epidermolytic hyperkeratosis. *Arch Dermatol* 1970;102:253.
11. Braun-Falco O, Petzoldt D, Christophers E, et al. Die granulöse degeneration bei naevus verrucosus bilateralis. *Arch Klin Exp Dermatol* 1969;235:115.
12. Zeligman I, Pomeranz J. Variations of congenital ichthyosiform erythroderma. *Arch Dermatol* 1965;91:120.
13. Demetree JW, Lang PG, St Clair JT. Unilateral linear zosteriform epidermal nevus with acantholytic dyskeratosis. *Arch Dermatol* 1979;115:875.
14. Starink TM, Woerdeman MJ. Unilateral systematized keratosis follicularis: a variant of Darier's disease or an epidermal nevus (acantholytic dyskeratotic epidermal naevus)? *Br J Dermatol* 1981;105:207.
14a. Baykal C, Buyukbabani N, Kavak A, et al. Nevoid hyperkeratosis of the nipple and areola: a distinct entity. *J Am Acad Dermatol* 2002;46:414.
15. Mehregan AH, Rahbari H. Hyperkeratosis of nipple and areola. *Arch Dermatol* 1977;113:1691.
16. Ortonne JP, El Baze P, Juhlin L. Nevoid hyperkeratosis of the nipple and areola mammae. *Acta Derm Venereol (Stockh)* 1986;66:175.
17. Fritsch P, Wittels W. Ein fall von bilateralem naevus comedonicus. *Hautarzt* 1971;22:409.
18. Paige TN, Mendelson CG. Bilateral nevus comedonicus. *Arch Dermatol* 1967;96:172.
19. Wood MG, Thew MA. Nevus comedonicus. *Arch Dermatol* 1968;98:111.
20. Harper KE, Spielvogel RL. Nevus comedonicus of the palm and wrist. *J Am Acad Dermatol* 1985;12:185.
21. Barsky S, Doyle JA, Winkelmann RK. Nevus comedonicus with epidermolytic hyperkeratosis. *Arch Dermatol* 1981;117:86.
22. Marsden RA, Fleming K, Dawber RPR. Comedo naevus of the palm: a sweat duct naevus? *Br J Dermatol* 1979;101:717.
23. Abell E, Read SI. Porokeratotic eccrine ostial and dermal duct nevus. *Br J Dermatol* 1980;103:435.
24. Aloi FG, Pippione M. Porokeratotic eccrine ostial and dermal duct nevus. *Arch Dermatol* 1986;122:892.

24a. Sassmannshausen J, Bogomilsky J, Chaffins M. Porokeratotic eccrine ostial and dermal duct nevus: a case report and review of the literature. *J Am Acad Dermatol*. 2000;43:364.

25. Coskey RJ, Mehregan AH, Hashimoto K. Porokeratotic eccrine duct and hair follicle nevus. *J Am Acad Dermatol* 1982; 6:940.

26. Shapiro L, Baraf CS. Isolated epidermolytic acanthoma. *Arch Dermatol* 1970;101:220.

27. Gebhart W, Kidd RL. Das solitäre epidermolytische akanthom. *Z Hautkr* 1972;47:1.

28. Niizuma K. Isolated epidermolytic acanthoma. *Dermatologica* 1979;159:30.

29. De Coninck A, Willemsen M, De Dobbeleer G, et al. Vulvar localization of epidermolytic acanthoma. *Dermatologica* 1986; 172:276.

30. Zina AM, Bundino S, Pippione MG. Acrosyringial epidermolytic papulosis neviformis. *Dermatologica* 1985;171:122.

30a. Sanchez-Carpintero I, Espana A, Idoate MA. Disseminated epidermolytic acanthoma probably related to trauma. *Br J Dermatol* 1999;141:728.

31. Hirone T, Fukushiro R. Disseminated epidermolytic acanthoma. *Acta Derm Venereol (Stockh)* 1973;53:393.

32. Miyamoto Y, Ueda K, Sato M, et al. Disseminated epidermolytic acanthoma. *J Cutan Pathol* 1979;6:272.

33. Goette DK, Lapins NA. Epidermolytic hyperkeratosis as an incidental finding in normal oral mucosa. *J Am Acad Dermatol* 1984;10:246.

34. Ackerman AB, Reed RJ. Epidermolytic variant of solar keratosis. *Arch Dermatol* 1973;107:104.

35. Ackerman AB. Focal acantholytic dyskeratosis. *Arch Dermatol* 1972;106:702.

36. Nagashima M, Matsuoka S. So-called granular degeneration as incidental histopathological finding. *Jpn J Dermatol (Series B)* 1971;81:494.

37. Mehregan A. Epidermolytic hyperkeratosis. *J Cutan Pathol* 1978;5:76.

37a. Conlin PA, Rapini RP. Epidermolytic hyperkeratosis associated with melanocytic nevi: a report of 53 cases. *Am J Dermatopathol* 2002;24:23.

38. González SB. Epidermolytic hyperkeratosis associated with superficial basal cell carcinoma. *Arch Dermatol* 1983;119:186.

39. Brownstein MH. Acantholytic acanthoma. *J Am Acad Dermatol* 1988;19:783.

40. Chorzelski TP, Kudejko J, Jablonska S. Is papular acantholytic dyskeratosis of the vulva a new entity? *Am J Dermatopathol* 1984;6:557.

41. Coppola G, Muscardin LM, Piazza P. Papular acantholytic dyskeratosis. *Am J Dermatopathol* 1986;8:364.

41a. Roten SV, Bhawan J. Isolated dyskeratotic acanthoma. A variant of isolated epidermolytic acanthoma. *Am J Dermatopathol* 1995;17:63.

41b. Gambichler T, Rapp S, Sauermann K, et al. Uncommon vascular naevi associated with focal acantholytic dyskeratosis. *Clin Exp Dermatol* 2002;27:195.

42. Megahed M, Scharffetter-Kochanek K. Acantholytic acanthoma. *Am J Dermatopathol* 1993;15:283.

43. Stern JK, Wolf JE Jr, Rosan T. Focal acantholytic dyskeratosis in pityriasis rosea. *Arch Dermatol* 1979;115:497.

44. Botet MV, Sánchez JL. Vesiculation of focal acantholytic dyskeratosis in acral lentiginous malignant melanoma. *J Dermatol Surg Oncol* 1979;5:798.

45. Cannon AB. White sponge nevus of the mucosa: Naevus spongiosus albus mucosae. *Arch Dermatol Syph* 1935;31:365.

46. Jorgenson RJ, Levin S. White sponge nevus. *Arch Dermatol* 1981;117:73.

47. Zegarelli EV, Everett FG, Kutscher AH, et al. Familial white folded dysplasia of the mucous membranes. *Arch Dermatol* 1959; 80:59.

48. Witkop CJ Jr, Gorlin RJ. Four hereditary mucosal syndromes. *Arch Dermatol* 1961;84:762.

49. Haye KR, Whitehead FIH. Hereditary leukokeratosis of the mucous membranes. *Br J Dermatol* 1968;80:529.

50. Rugg EL, McLean WH, Allison WE, et al. A mutation in the mucosal keratin K4 is associated with oral white sponge nevus. *Nat Genet* 1995;11:450.

50a. Terrinoni A, Rugg EL, Lane EB, et al. A novel mutation in the keratin 13 gene causing oral white sponge nevus. *J Dent Res* 2001;80:919.

51. Cooke BED, Morgan J. Oral epithelial nevi. *Br J Dermatol* 1959;71:134.

52. Stüttgen G, Berres HH, Will W. Leukoplakische epitheliale naevi der mundschleimhuat. *Arch Klin Exp Dermatol* 1965; 221:433.

53. Kuhlwein A, Nasemann T, Jänner M. Nachweis von papillomviren bei fokaler epithelialer hyperplasie heck und die differentialdiagnose zum weissen schleimhautnävus. *Hautarzt* 1981;32:617.

54. Metz J, Metz G. Der naevus spongiosus albus mucosae. *Z Hautkr* 1979;54:604.

55. Duncan SC, Su WPD. Leukoedema of the oral mucosa. *Arch Dermatol* 1980;116:906.

56. Sigal MJ, Mock D. Symptomatic benign migratory glossitis: report of two cases and literature review. *Pediatr Dent* 1992;14:392.

56a. Assimakopoulos D, Patrikakos G, Fotika C, et al. Benign migratory glossitis or geographic tongue: an enigmatic oral lesion. *Am J Med* 2002;113:751.

57. Dawson TAJ. Microscopic appearance of geographic tongue. *Br J Dermatol* 1969;81:827.

58. Marks R, Radden BG. Geographic tongue. *Australas J Dermatol* 1981;22:75.

59. Degos R, Garnier G, Civatte J. Pustulose par Candida albicans avec lésions psoriasiformes rappelant le psoriasis pustuleux. *Bull Soc Fr Dermatol Syphiligr* 1962;69:231.

60. O'Keefe E, Braverman IM, Cohen I. Annulus migrans: identical lesions in pustular psoriasis, Reiter's syndrome, and geographic tongue. *Arch Dermatol* 1973;107:240.

60a. Baer RL, Garcia RL, Partsalidou V, et al. Papillated squamous cell carcinoma in situ arising in a seborrheic keratosis. *J Am Acad Dermatol* 1981;5:561.

61. Andrade R, Steigleder GK. Contribution à l'étude histologique et histochimique de la verrue seborrhéique (papillome basocellulaire). *Ann Dermatol Syphiligr* 1959;86:495.

62. Sim-Davis D, Marks R, Wilson Jones E. The inverted follicular keratosis. *Acta Derm Venereol (Stockh)* 1976;56:337.

63. Indianer L. Controversies in dermatopathology. *J Dermatol Surg Oncol* 1979;5:321.

64. Uchiyama N, Shindo Y. An acantholytic variant of seborrheic keratosis. *J Dermatol* 1986;13:222.

65. Tagami H, Yamada M. Seborrheic keratosis: an acantholytic variant. *J Cutan Pathol* 1978;5:145.

66. Morales A, Hu F. Seborrheic verruca and intraepidermal basal cell epithelioma of Jadassohn. *Arch Dermatol* 1965;91:342.

67. Mevorah B, Mishima Y. Cellular response of seborrheic keratosis following croton oil irritation and surgical trauma. *Dermatologica* 1965;131:452.

68. Helwig EB. Inverted follicular keratosis. In: Proceedings of Seminar on the skin: neoplasms and dermatoses. 20th Seminar of the American Society of Clinical Pathologists, Washington, DC, 1954. Washington, DC: American Society of Clinical Pathologists, 1955:38.

69. Mehregan AH. Inverted follicular keratosis. *Arch Dermatol* 1964; 89:229.

70. Duperrat B, Mascaro JM. Une tumeur développée aux dépens de l'acrotrichium ou partie intraépidermique du follicule pilaire: porome folliculaire. *Dermatologica* 1963;126:291.

71. Grosshans E, Hanau D. L'adénome infundibulaire: un porome folliculaire à différenciation sebacée et apocrine. *Ann Dermatol Venereol* 1981;108:59.

72. Kossard S, Berman A, Winkelmann RK. Seborrheic keratoses and trichostasis spinulosa. *J Cutan Pathol* 1979;6:492.

73. Headington JT. Tumors of the hair follicle: a review. *Am J Pathol* 1976;85:480.

74. Brownstein MH, Shapiro L. The pilosebaceous tumors. *Int J Dermatol* 1977;16:340.

75. Lever WF. Inverted follicular keratosis is an irritated seborrheic keratosis. *Am J Dermatopathol* 1983;5:474.

76. Mehregan AH. Lentigo senilis and its evolutions. *J Invest Dermatol* 1975;65:429.

77. Sanderson KF. The structure of seborrheic keratoses. *Br J Dermatol* 1968;80:588.

78. Becker SW. Seborrheic keratosis and verruca with special reference to the melanotic variety. *Arch Dermatol Syphiligr* 1951;63:358.

79. Lennox B. Pigment patterns in epithelial tumors of the skin. *J Pathol Bacteriol* 1949;61:587.

80. Mishima Y, Pinkus H. Benign mixed tumor of melanocytes and malpighian cells. *Arch Dermatol* 1960;81:539.

81. Berman A, Winkelmann RK. Inflammatory seborrheic keratoses with mononuclear cell infiltration. *J Cutan Pathol* 1978; 5:353.

82. Rahbari H. Bowenoid transformation of seborrheic verrucae (keratoses). *Br J Dermatol* 1979;101:459.

83. Baer RL, Garcia RL, Partsalidou V, et al. Papillated squamous cell carcinoma in situ arising in a seborrheic keratosis. *J Am Acad Dermatol* 1981;5:561.

84. Booth JC. Atypical seborrheic keratosis. *Australas J Dermatol* 1977;18:10.

85. Christeler A, Delacrétaz J. Verrues séborrhéiques et transformation maligne. *Dermatologica* 1966;133:33.

86. Mikhail GR, Mehregan AH. Basal cell carcinoma in seborrheic keratosis. *J Am Acad Dermatol* 1982;6:500.

87. Goette DK. Basal cell carcinoma arising in seborrheic keratosis. *J Dermatol Surg Oncol* 1985;11:1014.

88. Braun-Falco O, Kint A, Vogell W. Zur histogenese der verruca seborrhoica. II. Mitteilung. Elektronenmikroskopische befunde. *Arch Klin Exp Dermatol* 1963;217:627.

89. Okun MF, Edelstein LM. Clonal seborrheic keratosis. In: Okun MF, Edelstein LM. *Gross and microscopic pathology of the skin*, vol 2. Boston: dermatopathology Foundation Press, 1976:576.

90. Mehregan AH, Pinkus H. Intraepidermal carcinoma: a critical study. *Cancer* 1964;17:609.

91. Schlappner OLA, Rowden G, Phillips TM, et al. Melanoacanthoma: ultrastructural and immunological studies. *J Cutan Pathol* 1978;5:127.

92. Prince C, Mehregan AH, Hashimoto K, et al. Large melanoacanthomas: a report of five cases. *J Cutan Pathol* 1984;11:309.

93. Delacrétaz J. Mélano-acanthome. *Dermatologica* 1975;151:236.

94. Hairston MA Jr, Reed RJ, Derbes VJ. Dermatosis papulosa nigra. *Arch Dermatol* 1964;89:655.

95. Babapour R, Leach J, Levy H. Dermatosis papulosa nigra in a young child. *Pediatr Dermatol* 1993;10:356.

96. Willoughby C, Soter NA. Stucco keratosis. *Arch Dermatol* 1972; 105:859.

97. Braun-Falco O, Weissmann I. Stukkokeratosen. *Hautarzt* 1978; 29:573.

98. Kocsard E, Carter JJ. The papillomatous keratoses: the nature and differential diagnosis of stucco keratosis. *Australas J Dermatol* 1971;12:80.

99. Stieler W, Plewig G. Acanthosis nigricans maligna und Leser-Trélat-Zeichen bei doppelmalignom von mamma und magen. *Z Hautkr* 1987;62:344.

100. Schwartz RA, Burgess GH. Florid cutaneous papillomatosis. *Arch Dermatol* 1978;114:1803.

101. Ronchese F. Keratoses, cancer and the sign of Leser-Trélat. *Cancer* 1965;18:1003.

102. Sneddon IB, Roberts JBM. An incomplete form of acanthosis nigricans. *Gut* 1962;3:269.

103. Liddell K, White JE, Caldwell JW. Seborrheic keratoses and carcinoma of the large bowel. *Br J Dermatol* 1975;92:449.

104. Kechijian P, Sadick NS, Mariglio J, et al. Cytarabine-induced inflammation in the seborrheic keratoses of Leser-Trélat. *Ann Intern Med* 1979;91:868.

105. Lambert D, Fort M, Legoux A, et al. Le signe de Leser-Trélat. *Ann Dermatol Venereol* 1980;107:1035.

106. Lindelof B, Sigurgeirsson B, Melander S. Seborrheic keratoses and cancer. *J Am Acad Dermatol* 1992;26:947.

107. Venencie PY, Perry HO. Sign of Leser-Trélat. *J Am Acad Dermatol* 1984;10:83.

108. Argenyi ZB, Huston BM, Argenyi EE, et al. Large-cell acanthoma of the skin: a study by image analysis cytometry and immunohistochemistry. *Am J Dermatopathol* 1994;16:140.

109. Rabinowitz AD, Inghirami G. Large-cell acanthoma: a distinctive keratosis. *Am J Dermatopathol* 1992;14:136.

110. Sanchez Yus E, Del Rio E, Requena L. Large-cell acanthoma is a distinctive condition. *Am J Dermatopathol* 1992;14:140.

111. Degos R, Civatte J. Clear-cell acanthoma: experience of 8 years. *Br J Dermatol* 1970;83:248.

112. Fine RM, Chernosky ME. Clinical recognition of clear-cell acanthoma (Degos). *Arch Dermatol* 1969;100:559.

113. Innocenzi D, Barduagni F, Cerio R, et al. Disseminated eruptive clear cell acanthoma: a case report with review of the literature. *Clin Exp Dermatol* 1994;19:249.

114. Wells GC, Wilson Jones E. Degos' acanthoma: acanthome à cellules claires. *Br J Dermatol* 1967;79:249.

115. Kerl H. Das klarzellenakanthom. *Hautarzt* 1977;28:456.

116. Zak FG, Girerd RJ. Das blasszellige akanthom (Degos). *Hautarzt* 1968;19:559.

117. Pierard GE. Mélanoacanthome à cellules claires. *Ann Dermatol Venereol* 1986;113:253.

118. Wilson Jones E, Wells GC. Degos' acanthoma: acanthome à cellules claires. *Arch Dermatol* 1966;94:286.

119. Trau H, Fisher BK, Schewach-Millet M. Multiple clear cell acanthomas. *Arch Dermatol* 1980;116:433.

120. Fukushiro S, Takei Y, Ackerman AB. Pale-cell acanthosis. *Am J Dermatopathol* 1985;7:515.

121. Cramer HJ. Klarzellenakanthom (Degos) mit syringomatösen und naevus-sebaceus-artigen anteilen. *Dermatologica* 1971;143: 265.

122. Desmons F, Breuillard F, Thomas P, et al. Multiple clear-cell acanthoma (Degos). *Int J Dermatol* 1977;16:203.

123. Hu F, Sisson JK. The ultrastructure of pale cell acanthoma. *J Invest Dermatol* 1969;52:185.

124. Leonforte JF. Palmoplantare epidermiszyste. *Hautarzt* 1978; 29:657.

125. Fisher BK, MacPherson M. Epidermoid cyst of the sole. *J Am Acad Dermatol* 1986;15:1127.

126. Onuigbo WIB. Vulval epidermoid cysts in the Igbos of Nigeria. *Arch Dermatol* 1976;112:1405.

127. Fieselman DW, Reed RJ, Ichinose H. Pigmented epidermal cyst. *J Cutan Pathol* 1974;1:256.

128. Raab W, Steigleder GK. Fehldiagnosen bei horncysten. *Arch Klin Exp Dermatol* 1961;212:606.

128a. Shet T, Desai S. Pigmented epidermal cysts. *Am J Dermatopathol* 2001;23:477.

128b. Akasaka T, Imamura Y, Kon S. Pigmented epidermal cyst. *J Dermatol* 1997;24:475.

129. Delacrétaz J. Keratotic basal-cell carcinoma arising from an epidermoid cyst. *J Dermatol Surg Oncol* 1977;3:310.

130. Shelley WB, Wood MG. Occult Bowen's disease in keratinous cysts. *Br J Dermatol* 1981;105:105.

131. McDonald LW. Carcinomatous change in cysts of skin. *Arch Dermatol* 1963;87:208.

132. Wilson Jones E. Proliferating epidermoid cysts. *Arch Dermatol* 1966;94:11.

133. Brownstein MH. Hybrid cyst: a combined epidermoid and trichilemmal cyst. *J Am Acad Dermatol* 1983;9:872.

134. McGavran MH, Binnington B. Keratinous cysts of the skin. *Arch Dermatol* 1966;94:499.

135. McGrath JA, Schofield OM, Eady RA. Epidermolysis bullosa pruriginosa: dystrophic epidermolysis bullosa with distinctive clinicopathological features. *Br J Dermatol* 1994;130:617.

135a. Wolfe SF, Gurevitch AW. Eruptive milia. *Cutis* 1997;60:183.

136. Epstein W, Kligman AM. The pathogenesis of milia and benign tumors of the skin. *J Invest Dermatol* 1956;26:1.

137. Leppard B, Sneddon IB. Milia occurring in lichen sclerosus et atrophicus. *Br J Dermatol* 1975;92:711.

138. Tsuji T, Sugai T, Suzuki S. The mode of growth of eccrine duct milia. *J Invest Dermatol* 1975;65:388.

139. Pinkus H. In discussion of Epstein W, Kligman AM. *J Invest Dermatol* 1956;26:10.

140. Leppard BJ, Sanderson KV. The natural history of trichilemmal cysts. *Br J Dermatol* 1976;94:379.

141. Leppard BJ, Sanderson KV, Wells RS. Hereditary trichilemmal cysts. *Clin Exp Dermatol* 1977;2:23.

142. Brownstein MH, Arluk DJ. Proliferating trichilemmal cyst: a simulant of squamous cell carcinoma. *Cancer* 1981;48:1207.

143. Pinkus H. "Sebaceous cysts" are trichilemmal cysts. *Arch Dermatol* 1969;99:544.

144. Cotton DWK, Kirkham N, Young BJJ. Immunoperoxidase anti-keratin staining of epidermal and pilar cysts. *Br J Dermatol* 1984;111:63.

145. Kimura S. Trichilemmal cysts. *Dermatologica* 1978;157:164.

146. Contreras MA, Costello MJ. Steatocystoma multiplex with embryonal hair formation. *Arch Dermatol* 1957;76:720.

146a. Cho S, Chang SE, Choi JH, et al. Clinical and histologic features of 64 cases of steatocystoma multiplex. *J Dermatol* 2002;29:152.

146b. Hohl D. Steatocystoma multiplex and oligosymptomatic pachyonychia congenita of the Jackson–Sertoli type. *Dermatology* 1997;195:86.

146c. Setoyama M, Mizoguchi S, Usuki K, et al. Steatocystoma multiplex: a case with unusual clinical and histological manifestation. *Am J Dermatopathol* 1997;19:89.

147. Brownstein MH. Steatocystoma simplex: a solitary steatocystoma. *Arch Dermatol* 1982;118:409.

148. Hashimoto K, Fisher BK, Lever WF. Steatocystoma multiplex. *Hautarzt* 1964;15:299.

149. Oyal H, Nikolowski W. Sebocystomatosen. *Arch Klin Exp Dermatol* 1957;204:361.

150. Kligman AM, Kirschbaum JD. Steatocystoma multiplex: a dermoid tumor. *J Invest Dermatol* 1964;42:383.

151. Plewig G, Wolff HH, Braun-Falco O. Steatocystoma multiplex: anatomic reevaluation, electron microscopy, and autoradiography. *Arch Dermatol Res* 1982;272:363.

152. Kimura S. An ultrastructural study of steatocystoma multiplex and the normal pilosebaceous apparatus. *J Dermatol* 1981;8:459.

153. Sandoval R, Urbina F. Pigmented follicular cyst. *Br J Dermatol* 1994;131:130.

154. Brownstein MH, Helwig EB. Subcutaneous dermoid cysts. *Arch Dermatol* 1973;107:237.

155. Ambiavagar PC, Rosen Y. Cutaneous ciliated cyst on the chin: probable bronchogenic cyst. *Arch Dermatol* 1979;115:895.

156. Van der Putte SCJ, Toonstra J. Cutaneous "bronchogenic" cyst. *J Cutan Pathol* 1985;12:404.

157. Ashton MA. Cutaneous ciliated cyst of the lower limb in a male. *Histopathology* 1995;26:467.

158. Sickel JZ. Cutaneous ciliated cyst of the scalp: a case report with immunohistochemical evidence for estrogen and progesterone receptors. *Am J Dermatopathol* 1994;16:76.

159. Tresser NJ, Dahms B, Berner JJ. Cutaneous bronchogenic cyst of the back: a case report and review of the literature. *Pediatr Pathol* 1994;14:207.

159a. Fontaine DG, Lau H, Murray SK, et al. Cutaneous ciliated cyst of the abdominal wall: a case report with a review of the literature and discussion of pathogenesis. *Am J Dermatopathol* 2002;24:63.

159b. Sidoni A, Bucciarelli E. Ciliated cyst of the perineal skin. *Am J Dermatopathol* 1997;19:93.

160. Clark JV. Ciliated epithelium in a cyst of the lower limb. *J Pathol* 1969;98:289.

161. Cole LA, Helwig EB. Mucoid cysts of the penile skin. *J Urol* 1976;115:397.

162. Dupré A, Lassère J, Christol B, et al. Canaux et kystes dysembryoplasiques du raphé génito-périnéal. *Ann Dermatol Venereol* 1982;109:81.

163. Ahmed A, Jones AW. Apocrine cystadenoma. *Br J Dermatol* 1969;81:899.

164. Powell RF, Palmer CH, Smith EB. Apocrine cystadenoma of the penile shaft. *Arch Dermatol* 1977;113:1250.

165. Romani J, Barnadas MA, Miralles J, et al. Median raphe cyst of the penis with ciliated cells. *J Cutan Pathol* 1995;22:378.

166. Paslin D. Urethroid cyst. *Arch Dermatol* 1983;119:89.

167. Esterly NB, Fretzin DF, Pinkus H. Eruptive vellus hair cysts. *Arch Dermatol* 1977;113:500.

168. Stiefler RE, Bergfeld WF. Eruptive vellus hair cysts: an inherited disorder. *J Am Acad Dermatol* 1980;3:425.

169. Piepkorn MW, Clark L, Lombardi DL. A kindred with congenital vellus hair cysts. *J Am Acad Dermatol* 1981;5:661.

169a. Tomkova H, Fujimoto W, Arata J. Expression of keratins (K10 and K17) in steatocystoma multiplex, eruptive vellus hair cysts, and epidermoid and trichilemmal cysts. *Am J Dermatopathol* 1997;19:250.

170. Lee S, Kim JG. Eruptive vellus hair cyst. *Arch Dermatol* 1979;115:744.

171. Burns DA, Calnan CD. Eruptive vellus hair cysts. *Clin Exp Dermatol* 1981;6:209.

172. Bovenmyer DA. Eruptive vellus hair cysts. *Arch Dermatol* 1979;115:338.

173. Redondo P, Vazquez-Doval J, Idoate M, et al. Multiple pilosebaceous cysts. *Clin Exp Dermatol* 1995;20:328.

174. Ohtake N, Kubota Y, Takayama O, et al. Relationship between steatocystoma multiplex and eruptive vellus hair cysts. *J Am Acad Dermatol* 1992;26:876.

175. Szymanski FJ. Warty dyskeratoma. *Arch Dermatol* 1957;75:567.

176. Azuma Y, Matsukawa A. Warty dyskeratoma with multiple lesions. *J Dermatol* 1993;20:374.

177. Gorlin RJ, Peterson WC Jr. Warty dyskeratoma: a note concerning its occurrence in the oral mucosa. *Arch Dermatol* 1967;95:292.

178. Harrist TJ, Murphy GF, Mihm MC Jr. Oral warty dyskeratoma. *Arch Dermatol* 1980;116:929.

179. Tanay A, Mehregan AH. Warty dyskeratoma (review). *Dermatologica* 1969;138:155.

180. Graham JH, Helwig EB. Isolated dyskeratosis follicularis. *Arch Dermatol* 1958;77:377.

181. Delacrétaz J. Dyskératomes verruqueux et kératoses séniles dyskératosiques. *Dermatologica* 1963;127:23.

182. Metz J, Schröpl F. Zur nosologie des dyskeratoma segregans: "Warty dyskeratoma." *Arch Klin Exp Dermatol* 1970; 238:21.

183. Furtado TA, Szymanski FJ. Ètude histologique du dyskératose verruqueux. *Ann Dermatol Syphiligr* 1961;88:633.

184. Brownstein MH, Rabinowitz AD. The precursors of cutaneous squamous cell carcinoma. *Int J Dermatol* 1979;18:1.

185. Epstein JH. Photocarcinogenesis, skin cancer, and aging. *J Am Acad Dermatol* 1983;9:487.

186. Sober AJ, Burstein JM. Precursors to skin cancer. *Cancer* 1995;75:645.

187. James MP, Wells GC, Whimster IW. Spreading pigmented actinic keratosis. *Br J Dermatol* 1978;98:373.

188. Koten JW, Verhagen ARHB, Frank GL. *Histopathology* of actinic cheilitis. *Dermatologica* 1967;135:465.

189. Cataldo E, Doku HC. Solar cheilitis. *J Dermatol Surg Oncol* 1981;7:989.

190. Piscascia DD, Robinson JK. Actinic cheilitis: a review of the etiology, differential diagnosis, and treatment. *J Am Acad Dermatol* 1987;17:255.

191. Montgomery H, Dörffel J. Verruca senilis und keratoma senile. *Arch Dermatol Syph* 1932;166:286.

192. Lund HZ. How often does squamous cell carcinoma of the skin metastasize? *Arch Dermatol* 1965;92:635.

193. Müller R, Reymann F, Hou-Jensen K. Metastases in dermatological patients with squamous cell carcinoma. *Arch Dermatol* 1979;115:703.

194. Billano RA, Little WP. Hypertrophic solar keratosis. *J Am Acad Dermatol* 1983;7:484.

195. Halter K. Uber ein wenig beachtetes histologisches kennzeichen des keratoma senile. *Hautarzt* 1952;3:215.

196. Pinkus H. Keratosis senilis. *Am J Clin Pathol* 1958;29:193.

197. Tan CY, Marks R. Lichenoid solar keratosis: prevalence and immunologic findings. *J Invest Dermatol* 1982;79:365.

198. Vakilzadeh F, Happle R. Epidermolytic leukoplakia. *J Cutan Pathol* 1982;9:267.

199. Carapeto FJ, García-Pérez A. Acantholytic keratosis. *Dermatologica* 1974;148:233.

200. Braun-Falco O, Schmoeckel C, Geyer C. Pigmentierte aktinische keratosen. *Hautarzt* 1986;37:676.

201. Kerl H. What is the boundary that separates a thick solar keratosis and a thin squamous cell carcinoma? *Am J Dermatopathol* 1984;6:305.

202. Ackerman AB. What is the boundary that separates a thick solar keratosis and a thin squamous cell carcinoma? *Am J Dermatopathol* 1984;6:306.

203. Mahrle G, Thiele B. Epidermal dysplasia in solar keratosis. *J Cutan Pathol* 1983;10:295(abst).

204. Schaumburg-Lever G, Alroy J, Gavris V, et al. Cell-surface carbohydrates in proliferative epidermal lesions. *Am J Dermatopathol* 1984;6:583.

205. Hirsch P, Marmelzat WL. Lichenoid actinic keratosis. *Dermatol Int* 1967;6:101.

206. Shapiro L, Ackerman AB. Solitary lichen planus-like keratosis. *Dermatologica* 1966;132:386.

207. Scott MA, Johnson WC. Lichenoid benign keratosis. *J Cutan Pathol* 1976;3:217.

208. Bart RS, Andrade R, Kopf AW. Cutaneous horn. *Acta Derm Venereol (Stockh)* 1968;48:507.

209. Brownstein MH, Shapiro EE. Trichilemmal horn: cutaneous horn overlying trichilemmoma. *Clin Exp Dermatol* 1979;4:59.

210. Cramer HJ, Kahlert G. Das cornu cutaneum: Selbständiges krankheitsbild oder klinisches symptom? *Dermatol Wochenschr* 1964;150:521.

211. Sandbank M. Basal cell carcinoma at the base of cutaneous horn: cornu cutaneum. *Arch Dermatol* 1971;104:97.

212. McAdams AJ Jr, Kistner RW. The relationship of chronic vulvar disease, leukoplakia, and carcinoma in situ to carcinoma of the vulva. *Cancer* 1958;11:740.

213. Shklar G. Oral leukoplakia: studies in enzyme histochemistry. *J Invest Dermatol* 1967;48:153.

214. Pindborg JJ. Pathology of oral leukoplakia. *Am J Dermatopathol* 1980;2:277.

215. Waldron CA, Shafer WG. Leukoplakia revisited: a clinicopathologic study of 3256 leukoplakias. *Cancer* 1975;36:1386.

216. Hornstein OP. Klinik, ätiologie und therapie der oralen leukoplakien. *Hautarzt* 1979;30:40.

217. Shklar G. Modern studies and concepts of leukoplakia in the mouth. *J Dermatol Surg Oncol* 1981;7:996.

218. Shafer WG, Waldron CA. Erythroplakia of the oral cavity. *Cancer* 1975;36:1021.

219. Grässel-Pietrusky R, Hornstein OP. Histologische untersuchungen zur häufigkeit des *Candidabefalls* präkanzeröser oraler leukoplakien. *Hautarzt* 1980;31:21.

220. Cawson RA, Lehner T. Chronic hyperplastic candidiasis: candidal leukoplakia. *Br J Dermatol* 1968;80:9.

221. Löning T, Ikenberg H, Becker J, et al. Analysis of oral papillomas, leukoplakias, and invasive carcinomas for human papillomavirus type related DNA. *J Invest Dermatol* 1985;84:417.

222. Gassenmaier A, Hornstein OP. Presence of papillomavirus DNA in benign and precancerous oral leukoplakias and squamous cell carcinomas. *Dermatologica* 1988;176:224.

223. Schell H, Schönberger A. Zur lokalisationshäufigkeit von benignen und präkanzerösen leukoplakien und von karzinomen in der mundhöhle. *Z Hautkr* 1987;62:798.

224. Rich AM, Reade PC. A quantitative assessment of Langerhans' cells in oral mucosal lichen planus and leukoplakia. *Br J Dermatol* 1989;120:223.

225. Shear M, Pindborg JJ. Verrucous hyperplasia of the oral mucosa. *Cancer* 1980;46:1855.

226. Kraus FT, Perez-Mesa C. Verrucous carcinoma. *Cancer* 1966; 19:26.

227. Samitz MH, Ackerman AB, Lantis LR. Squamous cell carcinoma arising at the site of oral florid papillomatosis. *Arch Dermatol* 1967;96:286.

228. Grinspan D, Abulafia J. Oral florid papillomatosis: verrucous carcinoma. *Int J Dermatol* 1979;18:608.

229. Wechsler HL, Fisher ER. Oral florid papillomatosis. *Arch Dermatol* 1962;86:480.

230. Kanee B. Oral florid papillomatosis complicated by verrucous squamous carcinoma. *Arch Dermatol* 1969;99:196.

231. Abrams AM, Melrose RJ, Howell FV. Necrotizing sialometaplasia: a disease simulating malignancy. *Cancer* 1973;32:130.

232. Raugi GJ, Kessler S. Necrotizing sialometaplasia: a condition simulating malignancy. *Arch Dermatol* 1979;115:329.

233. Piette F, Sauque E, Pellerin P, et al. Sialométaplasie nécrosante. *Ann Dermatol Venereol* 1980;107:821.

234. Fechner RE. Necrotizing sialometaplasia: a source of confusion with carcinoma of the palate. *Am J Clin Pathol* 1977;67: 315.

235. Shapiro L, Juhlin EA. Eosinophilic ulcer of the tongue. *Dermatologica* 1970;140:242.

236. Burgess GH, Mehregan AH, Drinnan AJ. Eosinophilic ulcer of the tongue. *Arch Dermatol* 1977;113:644.

237. Borroni G, Pericoli R, Gabba P, et al. Eosinophilic ulcers of the tongue. *J Cutan Pathol* 1984;11:322.

238. Baran RL, Gormley DE. Polydactylous Bowen's disease of the nail. *J Am Acad Dermatol* 1987;17:201.

239. Bowen JT. Precancerous dermatosis. *J Cutan Dis* 1912;30: 241.
240. Montgomery H. Precancerous dermatosis and epithelioma in situ. *Arch Dermatol Syph* 1939;39:387.
241. Montgomery H, Waisman M. Epithelioma attributable to arsenic. *J Invest Dermatol* 1941;4:365.
242. Strayer DS, Santa Cruz DJ. Carcinoma in situ of the skin: a review of histopathology. *J Cutan Pathol* 1980;7:244.
243. Kao GF. Editorial: carcinoma arising in Bowen's disease. *Arch Dermatol* 1986;122:1124.
244. Graham JH, Helwig EB. Bowen's disease and its relationship to systemic cancer. *Arch Dermatol* 1959;80:133.
245. Ackerman AB. Reply to Mascaro JM: Bowenoid papulosis. *J Am Acad Dermatol* 1981;4:608.
246. Peterka ES, Lynch FW, Goltz RW. An association between Bowen's disease and internal cancer. *Arch Dermatol* 1961;84: 623.
247. Callen JP, Headington J. Bowen's and non–Bowen's squamous intraepidermal neoplasia of the skin. *Arch Dermatol* 1980; 116:422.
248. Andersen SL, Nielsen H, Raymann F. Relationship between Bowen's disease and internal malignant tumors. *Arch Dermatol* 1973;108:367.
249. Reymann F, Ravnborg L, Schon G, et al. Bowen's disease and internal malignant disease. *Arch Dermatol* 1988;124:677.
250. Chuang TY, Reizner GT. Bowen's disease and internal malignancy. *J Am Acad Dermatol* 1988;19:47.
251. Seiji M, Mizuno F. Electron microscopic study of Bowen's disease. *Arch Dermatol* 1969;99:3.
252. Olson RL, Nordquist R, Everett MA. Dyskeratosis in Bowen's disease. *Br J Dermatol* 1969;81:676.
253. Sato A, Seiji M. Electron microscopic observations of malignant dyskeratosis in leukoplakia and Bowen's disease. *Acta Derm Venereol Suppl (Stockh)* 1973;53:101.
254. Arai H, Hori Y. An ultrastructural observation of intracytoplasmic desmosomes in Darier's disease. *J Dermatol* 1977;4:223.
255. Klingmüller G, Klehr HU, Ishibashi Y. Desmosomen im cytoplasma entdifferenzierter keratinocyten des plattenepithelcarcinoms. *Arch Klin Exp Dermatol* 1970;238:356.
256. Fisher ER, McCoy MM II, Wechsler HL. Analysis of histopathologic and electron microscopic determinants of keratoacanthoma and squamous cell carcinoma. *Cancer* 1972;29: 1387.
257. Ishibashi Y, Niimura M, Klingmüller G. Elektronenmikroskopischer beitrag zur morphologie von Paget–Zellen. *Arch Dermatol Forsch* 1972;245:402.
258. Klug H, Haustein UF. Vorkommen von intrazytoplasmatischen desmosomen in keratinozyten. *Dermatologica* 1974;148: 143.
259. Komura J, Watanabe S. Desmosome-like structures in the cytoplasm of normal human keratinocyte. *Arch Dermatol Res* 1975;253:145.
260. Schenk P. Desmosomale strukturen im cytoplasma normaler und pathologischer keratinocyten. *Arch Dermatol Res* 1975; 253:23.
261. Olson RL, Nordquist R, Everett MA. An electron microscopic study of Bowen's disease. *Cancer Res* 1968;28:2078.
262. Raiten K, Paniago-Pereira C, Ackerman AB. Pagetoid Bowen's disease vs. extramammary Paget's disease. *J Dermatol Surg Oncol* 1976;2:24.
263. Queyrat L. Erythroplasie du gland. *Bull Soc Fr Dermatol Syphiligr* 1911;22:378.
264. Goette DK. Erythroplasia of Queyrat. *Arch Dermatol* 1974; 110:271.
265. Mikhail GR. Cancers, precancers, and pseudocancers on the male genitalia. *J Dermatol Surg Oncol* 1980;6:1027.
266. Graham JH, Helwig EB. Erythroplasia of Queyrat. In: Graham JH, Johnson WC, Helwig EB, eds. *Dermal pathology.* Hagerstown, MD: Harper & Row, 1972:597.
267. Zoon JJ. Balanoposthite chronique circonscrite bénigne à plasmocytes. *Dermatologica* 1952;105:1.
268. Eberhartinger C, Bergmann M. Balanoposthitis chronica circumscripta plasmacellularis Zoon und Phimose. *Z Hautkr* 1971;46:251.
269. Souteyrand P, Wong E, MacDonald DM. Zoon's balanitis: balanitis circumscripta plasmacellularis. *Br J Dermatol* 1981; 105:195.
270. Mensing H, Jänner M. Vulvitis plasmacellularis Zoon. *Z Hautkr* 1981;56:728.
271. Davis J, Shapiro L, Baral J. Vulvitis circumscripta plasmacellularis. *J Am Acad Dermatol* 1983;8:413.
272. Brodin M. Balanitis circumscripta plasmacellularis. *J Am Acad Dermatol* 1980;2:33.
273. Jonquières EDL, De Lutzky FK. Balanites et vulvites pseudoérythroplasiques chroniques. *Ann Dermatol Venereol* 1980; 107:173.
274. Nödl F. Zur klinik und histologie der balanoposthitis chronica circumscripta benigna plasmacellularis. *Arch Dermatol Syph* 1954;198:557.
275. Schuermann H. Plasmocytosis circumorificialis. *Dtsch Zahnarztl Z* 1960;15:601.
276. Moldenhauer E. Die cheilitis plasmacellularis: ein beitrag zur plasmocytosis circumorificialis. *Dermatol Wochenschr* 1966; 152:636.
277. Baughman RD, Berger P, Pringle WM. Plasma cell cheilitis. *Arch Dermatol* 1974;110:725.
278. Crum CP, Liskow A, Petras P, et al. Vulvar intraepithelial neoplasia: severe atypia and carcinoma in situ. *Cancer* 1984;54:1429.
279. Ulbright TM, Stehman FB, Roth LM, et al. Bowenoid dysplasia of the vulva. *Cancer* 1982;50:2910.
279a. Fox H, Wells M. Recent advances in the pathology of the vulva. *Histopathology* 2003;42:209.
280. Montgomery H. Arsenic as an etiologic agent in certain types of epithelioma. *Arch Dermatol Syph* 1935;32:218.
281. Mazumder DN, Das Gupta J, Chakraborty AK, et al. Environmental pollution and chronic arsenicosis in south Calcutta. *Bull World Health Organ* 1992;70:481.
282. Das D, Chatterjee A, Mandal BK, et al. Arsenic in ground water in six districts of West Bengal, India: the biggest arsenic calamity in the world. Part 2. Arsenic concentration in drinking water, hair, nails, urine, skin-scale and liver tissue (biopsy) of the affected people. *Analyst* 1995;120:917.
283. Fierz U. Katamnestische untersuchungen über die nebenwirkungen der therapie mit anorganischem arsen bei hautkrankheiten. *Dermatologica* 1965;131:41.
284. Yeh S. Skin cancer in chronic arsenicism. *Hum Pathol* 1973; 4:469.
285. Neubauer O. Arsenical cancer. *Br J Cancer* 1947;1:192.
286. Sommers SC, McManus RG. Multiple arsenical cancers of skin and internal organs. *Cancer* 1953;6:347.
287. Roth F. Über die chronische arsenvergiftung der moselwinzer unter besonderer berücksichtigung des arsenkrebses. *Z Krebsforsch* 1956;61:287.
288. Miki Y, Kawatsu T, Matsuda K, et al. Cutaneous and pulmonary cancers associated with Bowen's disease. *J Am Acad Dermatol* 1982;6:26.
289. Hundeiker M, Petres J. Morphogenese und formenreichtum der arseninduzierten Präkanzerosen. *Arch Klin Exp Dermatol* 1968;231:355.
290. Ehlers G. Klinische und histologische untersuchungen zur frage arzneimittelbedingter arsen-tumoren. *Z Hautkr* 1968;43: 763.

291. Jung EG, Trachsel B. Molekularbiologische untersuchungen zur arsencarcinogenese. *Arch Klin Exp Dermatol* 1970;237: 819.

292. Barr LH, Menard JW. Marjolin's ulcer. *Cancer* 1983;52:173.

293. Epstein E, Epstein NN, Bragg K, et al. Metastases from squamous cell carcinomas of the skin. *Arch Dermatol* 1968;97: 245.

294. Frierson HF Jr, Cooper PH. Prognostic factors in squamous cell carcinoma of the lower lip. *Hum Pathol* 1986;17:346.

295. Sedlin ED, Fleming JL. Epidermal carcinoma arising in chronic osteomyelitic foci. *J Bone Joint Surg* 1963;45:827.

296. Martin H, Strong E, Spiro RH. Radiation-induced skin cancer of the head and neck. *Cancer* 1970;25:61.

297. Arons MS, Lynch JB, Lewis SR, et al. Scar tissue carcinoma. I. A clinical study with special reference to burn scar carcinoma. *Ann Surg* 1965;161:170.

298. Hoxtell EO, Mandel JS, Murray SS, et al. Incidence of skin carcinoma after renal transplantation. *Arch Dermatol* 1977; 113:436.

299. Gupta AK, Cardella CJ, Haberman HF. Cutaneous malignant neoplasms in patients with renal transplants. *Arch Dermatol* 1986;122:1288.

300. Turner JE, Callen JP. Aggressive behavior of squamous cell carcinoma in a patient with preceding lymphocytic lymphoma. *J Am Acad Dermatol* 1981;4:446.

300a. Motley R, Kersey P, Lawrence C, et al. Multiprofessional guidelines for the management of the patient with primary cutaneous squamous cell carcinoma. *Br J Dermatol* 2002;146: 18.

301. Evans HL, Smith JL. Spindle cell squamous carcinoma and sarcoma-like tumors of the skin. *Cancer* 1980;45:2687.

302. Manglani KS, Manaligod JR, Ray B. Spindle cell carcinoma of the glans penis. *Cancer* 1980;46:2266.

303. Kobayasi T. Dermo-epidermal junction in invasive squamous cell carcinoma. *Acta Derm Venereol (Stockh)* 1969;49:445.

304. Boncinelli U, Fornieri C, Muscatello U. Relationship between leukocytes and tumor cells in precancerous and cancerous lesions of the lip: a possible expression of immune reaction. *J Invest Dermatol* 1978;71:407.

305. Battifora H. Spindle cell carcinoma: ultrastructural evidence of squamous origin and collagen production by the tumor cells. *Cancer* 1976;37:2275.

306. Barr RJ, Wuerker RB, Graham JH. Ultrastructure of atypical fibroxanthoma. *Cancer* 1977;40:736.

307. Gatter KC, Alcock C, Heryet A. The differential diagnosis of routinely processed anaplastic tumors using monoclonal antibodies. *Am J Clin Pathol* 1984;82:33.

308. Robinson JK, Gottschalk R. Immunofluorescent and immunoperoxidase staining of antibodies to fibrous keratin. *Arch Dermatol* 1984;120:199.

309. Lever WF. Adenoacanthoma of sweat glands. *Arch Dermatol Syph* 1947;56:157.

310. Johnson WC, Helwig EB. Adenoid squamous cell carcinoma: adenoacanthoma. *Cancer* 1966;19:1639.

311. Borelli D. Aspetti pseudoglandolari nell'epithelioma discheratosico: "Adenoacanthoma of sweat glands" di Lever. *Dermatologica* 1948;97:193.

312. Takagi M, Sakota Y, Takayama S, et al. Adenoid squamous cell carcinoma of the oral mucosa: report of two autopsy cases. *Cancer* 1977;40:2250.

313. Chorzelski T. Ein fall von übergang einer keratosis senilis mit dyskeratose vom typ des morbus Darier in ein dyskeratotisches spinaliom. *Hautarzt* 1963;14:37.

314. Muller SA, Wilhelmj CM Jr, Harrison EG Jr, et al. Adenoid squamous cell carcinoma: adenoacanthoma of Lever. *Arch Dermatol* 1964;89:589.

315. Wick MR, Pettinato G, Nappi O. Adenoid (acantholytic) squamous carcinoma of the skin. *J Cutan Pathol* 1988;15: 351(abst).

316. Delacrétaz J, Madjedi AS, Loretan R. Epithelioma spinocellulare segregans: Über die sogenannten "adenoacanthome der schweissdrüsen" (Lever). *Hautarzt* 1957;8:512.

317. Lasser A, Cornog JL, Morris J MCL. Adenoid squamous cell carcinoma of the vulva. *Cancer* 1974;33:224.

318. Underwood JW, Adcock LL, Okagari T. Adenosquamous carcinoma of skin appendages (adenoid squamous cell carcinoma, pseudoglandular squamous cell carcinoma, adenoacanthoma of sweat glands of Lever) of the vulva. *Cancer* 1978; 42:1851.

319. Weidner N, Foucar E. Adenosquamous carcinoma of the skin: an aggressive mucin- and gland-forming carcinoma. *Arch Dermatol* 1985;121:775.

320. Gallager HS, Miller GV, Grampa G. Primary mucoepidermoid carcinoma of the skin. *Cancer* 1959;12:286.

321. Fulling KH, Strayer DS, Santa Cruz DJ. Adnexal metaplasia in carcinoma in situ of the skin. *J Cutan Pathol* 1981;8:79.

322. Friedman KJ. Low-grade primary cutaneous adenosquamous (mucoepidermoid) carcinoma. *Am J Dermatopathol* 1989;11: 43.

323. Ackerman LV. Verrucous carcinoma of the oral cavity. *Surgery* 1948;23:670.

324. Aird I, Johnson HD, Lennox B, et al. Epithelioma cuniculatum: a variety of squamous carcinoma peculiar to the foot. *Br J Surg* 1954;42:245.

325. Brown SM, Freeman RG. Epithelioma cuniculatum. *Arch Dermatol* 1976;112:1295.

326. Reingold IM, Smith BP, Graham JH. Epithelioma cuniculatum pedis: a variant of squamous cell carcinoma. *Am J Clin Pathol* 1978;69:561.

327. Nguyen KQ, McMarlin SL. Verrucous carcinoma of the face. *Arch Dermatol* 1984;120:383.

328. Sanchez-Yus E, Velasco E, Robledo A. Verrucous carcinoma of the back. *J Am Acad Dermatol* 1986;14:947.

329. Klima M, Kurtis B, Jordan PH Jr. Verrucous carcinoma of the skin. *J Cutan Pathol* 1980;7:88.

330. Mohs FE, Sahl WJ. Chemosurgery for verrucous carcinoma. *J Dermatol Surg Oncol* 1979;5:302.

331. Brodin MB, Mehregan AH. Verrucous carcinoma. *Arch Dermatol* 1980;116:987.

332. Dawson DF, Duckworth JK, Bernhardt H, et al. Giant condyloma and verrucous carcinoma of the genital area. *Arch Pathol* 1965;79:225.

333. Seehafer JR, Muller SA, Dicken CH, et al. Bilateral verrucous carcinoma of the feet. *Arch Dermatol* 1979;115:1222.

334. McKee PH, Wilkinson JD, Corbett MF, et al. Carcinoma cuniculatum: a case metastasizing to skin and lymph nodes. *Clin Exp Dermatol* 1981;6:613.

335. Perez CA, Kraus FT, Evans JC, et al. Anaplastic transformation in verrucous carcinoma of the oral cavity after radiation therapy. *Radiology* 1966;86:108.

336. Wilkinson JD, McKee PH, Black MM, et al. A case of carcinoma cuniculatum with coexistent viral plantar wart. *Clin Exp Dermatol* 1981;6:619.

337. McKee PH, Wilkinson JD, Black MM, et al. Carcinoma (epithelioma) cuniculatum. *Histopathology* 1981;5:425.

338. Gross G, Gissmann L. Urogenitale und anale papillomvirus-infektionen. *Hautarzt* 1986;37:587.

339. Mathieu A, Avril MF, Duvillard P, et al. Tumeurs de Buschke-Löwenstein: trois localisations vulvaires. Association à l'HPV6 dans un cas. *Ann Dermatol Venereol* 1985;112:745.

340. Su WPD, Duncan SC, Perry HO. Blastomycosis-like pyoderma. *Arch Dermatol* 1979;115:170.

341. Sommerville J. Pseudo-epitheliomatous hyperplasia. *Acta Derm Venereol (Stockh)* 1953;33:236.

342. Winer LH. Pseudoepitheliomatous hyperplasia. *Arch Dermatol Syph* 1940;42:856.

343. Freeman RG. On the pathogenesis of pseudoepitheliomatous hyperplasia. *J Cutan Pathol* 1974;1:231.

344. Ju DMC. Pseudoepitheliomatous hyperplasia of the skin. *Dermatol Int* 1967;6:82.

345. Wagner RF Jr, Grande DJ. Pseudoepitheliomatous hyperplasia vs. squamous cell carcinoma. *J Dermatol Surg Oncol* 1986; 12:632.

346. Johnson DE. Basal-cell epithelioma of the palm. *Arch Dermatol* 1960;82:253.

347. Hyman AB, Barsky AJ. Basal cell epithelioma of the palm. *Arch Dermatol* 1965;92:571.

348. Hyman AB, Michaelides P. Basal-cell epithelioma of the sole. *Arch Dermatol* 1963;87:481.

349. Lewis HM, Stensaas CO, Okun MR. Basal cell epithelioma of the sole. *Arch Dermatol* 1965;91:623.

350. Williamson JJ, Cohney BC, Henderson BM. Basal cell carcinoma of the mandibular gingiva. *Arch Dermatol* 1967; 95:76.

351. Urmacher C, Pearlman S. An uncommon neoplasm of the oral mucosa. *Am J Dermatopathol* 1983;5:601.

352. Schubert H, Wolfram G, Güldner G. Basaliomrezidive nach behandlung. *Dermatol Monatsschr* 1979;165:89.

353. Murray JE, Cannon B. Basal-cell cancer in children and young adults. *N Engl J Med* 1960;262:440.

354. Maron H. Basaliom bei kindern. *Dermatol Wochenschr* 1963; 147:545.

355. Milstone EB, Helwig EB. Basal cell carcinoma in children. *Arch Dermatol* 1973;108:523.

356. Gellin GA, Kopf AW, Garfinkel L. Basal cell epithelioma. *Arch Dermatol* 1965;91:38.

357. Schubert H. Häufigkeit und lokalisation von basaliomen im Kopf-Hals-Bereich. *Dermatol Monatsschr* 1984;170:453.

358. Anderson NP, Anderson HE. Development of basal cell epithelioma as a consequence of radiodermatitis. *Arch Dermatol Syph* 1951;63:586.

359. Schwartz RA, Burgess GH, Milgrom H. Breast carcinoma and basal cell epitheliomas after x-ray therapy for hirsutism. *Cancer* 1979;44:1601.

360. Gaughan LJ, Bergeron JR, Mullins JF. Giant basal cell epithelioma developing in acute burn site. *Arch Dermatol* 1969;99: 594.

361. Margolis MH. Superficial multicentric basal cell epithelioma arising in thermal burn scar. *Arch Dermatol* 1970;102:474.

362. Wechsler HL, Krugh FJ, Domonkos AN, et al. Polydysplastic epidermolysis bullosa and development of epidermal neoplasms. *Arch Dermatol* 1970;102:374.

363. Weedon D, Wall D. Metastatic basal cell carcinoma. *Med J Aust* 1975;2:177.

364. Paver K, Poyzen K, Burry N, et al. The incidence of basal cell carcinoma and their metastases in Australia and New Zealand. *Australas J Dermatol* 1973;14:53.

365. Cotran RS. Metastasizing basal cell carcinomas. *Cancer* 1961; 14:1036.

366. Von Domarus H, Stevens PJ. Metastatic basal cell carcinoma: report of five cases and review of 170 cases in the literature. *J Am Acad Dermatol* 1984;10:1043.

367. Amonette RA, Salasche SJ, Chesney T McC, et al. Metastatic basal cell carcinoma. *J Dermatol Surg* 1981;7:397.

367a. Jones VS, Chandra S, Smile SR, et al. A unique case of metastatic penile basal cell carcinoma. *Indian J Pathol Microbiol* 2000;43:465.

367b. Ribuffo D, Alfano C, Ferrazzoli PS, et al. Basal cell carcinoma of the penis and scrotum with cutaneous metastases. *Scand J Plast Reconstr Surg Hand Surg* 2002;36:180.

368. Dzubow LM. Metastatic basal cell carcinoma originating in the supra-parotid region. *J Dermatol Surg Oncol* 1986;12: 1306.

369. Assor D. Basal cell carcinoma with metastasis to bone. *Cancer* 1967;20:2125.

370. Wermuth BM, Fajardo LF. Metastatic basal cell carcinoma. *Arch Pathol* 1970;90:458.

371. Soffer D, Kaplan H, Weshler Z. Meningeal carcinomatosis due to basal cell carcinoma. *Hum Pathol* 1985;16:530.

372. Farmer ER, Helwig EB. Metastatic basal cell carcinoma: a clinicopathologic study of 17 cases. *Cancer* 1980;46:748.

373. Mikhail GR, Nims LP, Kelly AP Jr, et al. Metastatic basal cell carcinoma. (review) *Arch Dermatol* 1977;113:1261.

374. Safai B, Good RA. Basal cell carcinoma with metastasis. *Arch Pathol* 1977;101:327.

375. Dvoretzky I, Fisher BK, Haker O. Mutilating basal cell epithelioma. *Arch Dermatol* 1978;114:239.

376. Gormley DE, Hirsch P. Aggressive basal cell carcinoma of the scalp. *Arch Dermatol* 1978;114:782.

377. Gorlin RJ. Nevoid basal-cell carcinoma syndrome. *Medicine (Baltimore)* 1987;66:98.

378. Taylor WB, Anderson DE, Howell JB, et al. The nevoid basal cell carcinoma syndrome. *Arch Dermatol* 1968;98:612.

379. Southwick GJ, Schwartz RA. The basal cell nevus syndrome: disasters occurring among a series of 36 patients. *Cancer* 1979;44:2294.

380. Berendes U. Die klinische bedeutung der onkotischen phase des basalzellnaevus-syndroms. *Hautarzt* 1971;22:261.

381. Howell JB, Mehregan AH. Pursuit of the pits in the nevoid basal cell carcinoma syndrome. *Arch Dermatol* 1970;102: 586.

382. Leppard BJ. Skin cysts in the basal cell naevus syndrome. *Clin Exp Dermatol* 1983;8:603.

383. Hermans EH, Grosfeld JCM, Spaas JAJ. The fifth phakomatosis. *Dermatologica* 1965;130:446.

384. Reed JC. Nevoid basal cell carcinoma syndrome with associated fibrosarcoma of the maxilla. *Arch Dermatol* 1968;97:304.

385. Happle R. Naevobasaliom und ameloblastom. *Hautarzt* 1973; 24:290.

386. Anderson TE, Best PV. Linear basal cell nevus. *Br J Dermatol* 1962;74:20.

387. Carney RG. Linear unilateral basal cell nevus with comedones. *Arch Dermatol Syph* 1952;65:471.

388. Horio M, Egami K, Maejima K, et al. Electron microscopic study of sebaceous epithelioma. *J Dermatol* 1978;5:139.

389. Bleiberg J, Brodkin RH. Linear unilateral basal cell nevus with comedones. *Arch Dermatol* 1969;100:187.

390. Bazex A, Dupré A, Christol B. Atrophodermie folliculaire, proliférations basocellulaires et hypotrichose. *Ann Dermatol Syphil.igr (Paris)* 1966;93:241.

391. Viksnins P, Berlin A. Follicular atrophoderma and basal cell carcinomas. *Arch Dermatol* 1977;113:948.

392. Plosila M, Kiistala R, Niemi KM. The Bazex syndrome: follicular atrophoderma with multiple basal cell carcinoma, hypotrichosis and hypohidrosis. *Clin Exp Dermatol* 1981;6:31.

393. Rupec M, Kint A, Himmelmann GW, et al. Zur ultrastruktur des soliden basalioms. *Dermatologica* 1975;151:288.

394. Okun MR, Blumental G. Basal cell epithelioma with giant cells and nuclear atypicality. *Arch Dermatol* 1964;89:598.

395. Rupec M, Vakilzadeh F, Korb G. Über das vorkommen von mehrkernigen riesenzellen in basaliomen. *Arch Klin Exp Dermatol* 1969;235:198.

396. Pinkus H. Premalignant fibroepithelial tumors of the skin. *Arch Dermatol Syph* 1953;67:598.

396a. Bale AE, Yu KP. The hedgehog pathway and basal cell carcinomas. *Hum Mol Genet* 2001;10:757.

396b. Bonifas JM, Pennypacker S, Chuang PT, et al. Activation of expression of hedgehog target genes in basal cell carcinomas. *J Invest Dermatol* 2001;116:739.

396c. Ling G, Ahmadian A, Persson A, et al. PATCHED and p53 gene alterations in sporadic and hereditary basal cell cancer. *Oncogene* 22–11–2001;20:7770.

396d. Saldanha G, Shaw JA, Fletcher A. Evidence that superficial basal cell carcinoma is monoclonal from analysis of the Ptch1 gene locus. *Br J Dermatol* 2002;147:931.

396e. Saldanha G. The Hedgehog signalling pathway and cancer. *J Pathol* 2001;193:427.

396f. Toftgard R. Hedgehog signalling in cancer. *Cell Mol Life Sci* 2000;57:1720.

396g. Wicking C, McGlinn E. The role of hedgehog signalling in tumorigenesis. *Cancer Lett* 2001;173:1.

396h. Sardi I, Piazzini M, Palleschi G, et al. Molecular detection of microsatellite instability in basal cell carcinoma. *Oncol Rep* 2000;7:1119.

396i. Tojo M, Kiyosawa H, Iwatsuki K, et al. Expression of a sonic hedgehog signal transducer, hedgehog-interacting protein, by human basal cell carcinoma. *Br J Dermatol* 2002;146:69.

396j. Zedan W, Robinson PA, Markham AF, et al. Expression of the sonic hedgehog receptor "PATCHED" in basal cell carcinomas and odontogenic keratocysts. *J Pathol* 2001;194:473.

397. Pinkus H. Epithelial and fibroepithelial tumors. *Arch Dermatol* 1965;91:24.

398. Fanger H, Barker BE. Histochemical studies of some keratotic and proliferating skin lesions. *Arch Pathol* 1957;64:143.

399. Moore RD, Stevenson J, Schoenberg MD. The response of connective tissue associated with tumors of the skin. *Am J Clin Pathol* 1960;34:125.

400. Mérot Y, Faucher F, Didierjean L, et al. Loss of bullous pemphigoid antigen in peritumoral lacunae of basal cell epitheliomas. *Acta Derm Venereol (Stockh)* 1984;64:209.

401. Stanley JR, Beckwith JB, Fuller RP, et al. A specific antigenic defect of the basement membrane is found in basal cell carcinoma but not in other epidermal tumors. *Cancer* 1982;50:1486.

402. Weedon D, Shand E. Amyloid in basal cell carcinomas. *Br J Dermatol* 1979;101:141.

402a. Aroni K, Lazaris AC, Nikolaou I, et al. Signet ring basal cell carcinoma. A case study emphasizing the differential diagnosis of neoplasms with signet ring cell formation. *Pathol Res Pract* 2001;197:853.

403. Hundeiker M, Berger H. Zur morphogenese der basaliome. *Arch Klin Exp Dermatol* 1968;231:161.

404. Reidbord HE, Wechsler HL, Fisher ER. Ultrastructural study of basal cell carcinoma and its variants with comments on histogenesis. *Arch Dermatol* 1971;104:132.

405. Mehregan AH. Aggressive basal cell epithelioma on sunlight-protected skin. *Am J Dermatopathol* 1983;5:221.

406. Jacobs GH, Rippey JJ, Altini M. Prediction of aggressive behavior in basal cell carcinoma. *Cancer* 1982;49:533.

407. Lang PJ Jr, Maize JC. Histologic evaluation of recurrent basal cell carcinoma and treatment implications. *J Am Acad Dermatol* 1986;14:186.

408. Foot NC. Adnexal carcinoma of the skin. *Am J Pathol* 1947;23:1.

409. Troy JL, Ackerman AB. Sebaceoma: a distinctive benign neoplasm of adnexal epithelium differentiating toward sebaceous cells. *Am J Dermatopathol* 1984;6:7.

410. Wood MG, Pranich K, Beerman H. Investigation of possible apocrine gland component in basal-cell epithelioma. *J Invest Dermatol* 1958;30:273.

411. Freeman RG, Winkelmann RK. Basal cell tumor with eccrine differentiation. *Arch Dermatol* 1969;100:234.

412. Lerchin E, Rahbari H. Adamantinoid basal cell epithelioma. *Arch Dermatol* 1975;111:586.

413. Barr RJ, Graham JH. Granular cell basal cell carcinoma. *Arch Dermatol* 1979;115:1064.

414. Mrak RE, Baker GF. Granular basal cell carcinoma. *J Cutan Pathol* 1987;14:37.

415. Barnadas MA, Freeman RG. Clear cell basal cell epithelioma. *J Cutan Pathol* 1988;15:1.

416. Cohen RE, Zaim MT. Signet-ring clear-cell basal cell carcinoma. *J Cutan Pathol* 1988;15:183.

417. Aloi FG, Molinero A, Pippione M. Basal cell epithelioma with matricial differentiation. *Am J Dermatopathol* 1988;10:509.

418. Deppe R, Pullmann H, Steigleder GK. Dopa-positive cells and melanin in basal cell epithelioma. *Arch Dermatol Res* 1976;256:79.

419. Zelickson AS, Goltz RW, Hartmann JF. A histologic and electron microscopic study of a pigmenting basal cell epithelioma. *J Invest Dermatol* 1961;36:299.

420. Caro MR, Howell JB. Morphea-like epithelioma. *Arch Dermatol Syph* 1952;63:471.

421. Hornstein O. Über die Pinkussche varietät der basaliome. *Hautarzt* 1957;8:406.

422. Degos R, Hewitt J. Tumeurs fibro-épithéliales prémalignes de Pinkus et épithélioma baso-cellulaire. *Ann Dermatol Syphiligr (Paris)* 1955;82:124.

423. Howell JB, Caro MR. The basal-cell nevus. *Arch Dermatol* 1959;79:67.

424. Mason JK, Helwig EB, Graham JH. Pathology of the nevoid basal cell carcinoma syndrome. *Arch Pathol* 1965;79:401.

425. Jablonska S. Basaliome naevoider abkunft. *Hautarzt* 1961;12:147.

426. Howell JB, Freeman RG. Structure and significance of the pits with their tumors in the nevoid basal cell carcinoma syndrome. *J Am Acad Dermatol* 1980;2:224.

427. Holubar K, Matras H, Smalik AV. Multiple palmar basal cell epitheliomas in basal cell nevus syndrome. *Arch Dermatol* 1970;101:679.

428. Ward WH. Nevoid basal cell carcinoma associated with a dyskeratosis of the palms and soles. *Australas J Dermatol* 1960;5:204.

429. Taylor WB, Wilkins JW Jr. Nevoid basal cell carcinoma of the palm. *Arch Dermatol* 1970;102:654.

430. Barr RJ, Headley JL, Jensen JL, et al. Cutaneous keratocysts of nevoid basal cell carcinoma syndrome. *J Am Acad Dermatol* 1986;14:572.

431. Horio T, Komura J. Linear unilateral basal cell nevus with comedo-like lesions. *Arch Dermatol* 1978;114:95.

432. Blanchard L, Hodge SJ, Owen LG. Linear eccrine nevus with comedones. *Arch Dermatol* 1981;117:357.

433. Sims CF, Parker RL. Intraepidermal basal cell epithelioma. *Arch Dermatol Syph* 1949;59:45.

434. Steffen C, Ackerman AB. Intraepidermal epithelioma of Borst–Jadassohn. *Am J Dermatopathol* 1985;7:5.

435. Holubar K, Wolff K. Intraepidermal eccrine poroma. *Cancer* 1969;23:626.

436. Okun MR, Edelstein LM. *Gross and microscopic pathology of the skin*, vol. 2. Boston: Dermatopathology Foundation Press, 1976.

437. Berger P, Baughman R. Intra-epidermal epithelioma: report of a case with invasion after many years. *Br J Dermatol* 1974;90:343.

438. Smith JLS, Coburn JG. Hidroacanthoma simplex. *Br J Dermatol* 1956;68:400.

439. Mehregan AH, Levson DN. Hidroacanthoma simplex. *Arch Dermatol* 1969;100:303.

440. Bardach H. Hidroacanthoma simplex with in situ porocarcinoma. *J Cutan Pathol* 1978;5:236.

441. Pinkus H, Mehregan AH. Epidermotropic eccrine carcinoma. *Arch Dermatol* 1963;88:597.

442. Graham JH, Johnson WC, Helwig EB, eds. *Dermal pathology*. Hagerstown, MD: Harper & Row, 1972.

443. Darier J, Ferrand M. L'épithéliome pavimenteux mixte et intermédiaire. *Ann Dermatol Syphiligr (Paris)* 1955;82:124.

444. Montgomery H. Basal squamous cell epithelioma. *Arch Dermatol Syph* 1928;18:50.

445. Gertler W. Zur epithelverbundenheit der basaliome. *Dermatol Wochenschr* 1965;151:673.

446. Borel DM. Cutaneous basosquamous carcinoma: review of the literature and report of 35 cases. *Arch Pathol* 1973;95:293.

447. Welton DG, Elliott JA, Kimmelstiel P. Epithelioma. *Arch Dermatol Syph* 1949;60:277.

448. Lennox B, Wells AL. Differentiation in the rodent ulcer group of tumours. *Br J Cancer* 1951;5:195.

449. Holmes EJ, Bennington JL, Haber SL. Citrulline-containing basal cell carcinomas. *Cancer* 1968;22:663.

450. Smith OD, Swerdlow MA. Histogenesis of basal-cell epithelioma. *Arch Dermatol* 1956;74:286.

451. Freeman RG. Histopathologic considerations in the management of skin cancer. *J Dermatol Surg* 1976;2:215.

452. Krompecher E. *Der basalzellenkrebs*. Jena: Gustav Fischer, 1903.

453. Montgomery H. *Dermatopathology*. New York: Harper & Row, 1967;923.

454. Teloh HA, Wheelock MC. Histogenesis of basal cell carcinoma. *Arch Pathol* 1949;48:447.

455. Ten Seldam REJ, Helwig EB. *Histological typing of skin tumours*. Geneva: World Health Organization, 1974.

456. Adamson HG. On the nature of rodent ulcer: its relationship to epithelioma adenoides cysticum of Brooke and to other trichoepitheliomata of benign nevoid character;its distinction from malignant carcinoma. *Lancet* 1914;1:810.

457. Wallace SA, Halpert B. Trichoma: tumor of hair anlage. *Arch Pathol* 1950;50:199.

458. Chiba M, Jimbow K. Expression of gamma-glutamyl transpeptidase in normal and neoplastic epithelial cells of human skin. *Br J Dermatol* 1986;114:459.

459. Kariniemi AL, Holthöfer H, Vartto T, et al. Cellular differentiation of basal cell carcinoma studies with fluorescent lectins and cytokeratin antibodies. *J Cutan Pathol* 1984;11:541.

460. Shimizu N, Ito M, Tazawa T, et al. Anti-keratin monoclonal antibody against basal cell epithelioma keratin: BKN-1. *J Dermatol* 1987;14:359.

461. Van Scott EJ, Reinertson RP. The modulating influence of stromal environment on epithelial cells studied in human autotransplants. *J Invest Dermatol* 1961;36:109.

462. Covo JA. The pits in the nevoid basal cell carcinoma syndrome. *Arch Dermatol* 1971;103:568.

463. Gerstein W. Transplantation of basal cell epithelioma to the rabbit. *Arch Dermatol* 1963;88:834.

464. Grimwood RE, Johnson CA, Ferris CF, et al. Transplantation of human basal cell carcinoma to athymic mice. *Cancer* 1985;56:519.

465. Greene HSN. The heterologous transplantation of embryonic mammalian tissue. *Cancer Res* 1943;3:809.

466. Zackheim HS. Origin of the human basal cell epithelioma. *J Invest Dermatol* 1963;40:283.

467. Brown AC, Crounse RB, Winkelmann RK. Generalized hairfollicle hamartoma. *Arch Dermatol* 1969;99:478.

468. Madsen A. De l'épithélioma baso-cellulaire superficiel. *Acta Derm Venereol (Stockh)* 1941;22[Suppl]7:1.

469. Madsen A. Studies on basal-cell epithelioma of the skin. *Acta Pathol Microbiol* 1965;65[Suppl]177:7.

470. Oberste-Lehn H. Zur histogense des Basalioms. *Z Hautkr* 1954;16:334.

471. Lang PG Jr, McKelvey AC, Nicholson JH. Three dimensional reconstruction of the superficial multicentric basal cell carcinoma. *Am J Dermatopathol* 1987;9:198.

472. Zelickson AS. An electron microscope study of the basal cell epithelioma. *J Invest Dermatol* 1962;39:183.

473. Lever WF, Hashimoto K. Electron microscopic and histochemical findings in basal cell epithelioma, squamous cell carcinoma and some appendage tumors. XIII International Dermatology Congress, vol 1. Berlin: Springer-Verlag, 1968:3.

474. Kumakiri M, Hashimoto K. Ultrastructural resemblance of basal cell epithelioma to primary epithelial germ. *J Cutan Pathol* 1978;5:53.

475. Cutler B, Posalaky Z, Katz I. Cell processes in basal cell carcinoma. *J Cutan Pathol* 1980;7:310.

476. Zelickson AS. The pigmented basal cell epithelioma. *Arch Dermatol* 1967;96:524.

477. Bleehen SS. Pigmented basal cell epithelioma. *Br J Dermatol* 1975;93:361.

478. Weinstein GO, Frost P. Cell proliferation in human basal cell carcinoma. *Cancer Res* 1970;30:724.

479. Hashimoto K, Kobayashi H. Histogenesis of amyloid in the skin. *Am J Dermatopathol* 1980;2:165.

480. Hashimoto K, Brownstein MH. Localized amyloidosis in basal cell epithelioma. *Acta Derm Venereol (Stockh)* 1973;53:331.

481. Masu S, Hosokawa M, Seiji M. Amyloid in localized cutaneous amyloidosis: immunofluorescence studies with antikeratin antiserum especially concerning the difference between systemic and localized cutaneous amyloidosis. *Acta Derm Venereol (Stockh)* 1981;61:381.

482. Looi LM. Localized amyloidosis in basal cell carcinoma. *Cancer* 1983;52:1833.

482a. Cox NH, Nicoll JJ, Popple AW. Amyloid deposition in basal cell carcinoma: a cause of apparent lack of sensitivity to radiotherapy. *Clin Exp Dermatol* 2001;26:499.

483. Rahbari H, Mehregan AH. Basal cell epithelioma (carcinoma) in children and teenagers. *Cancer* 1982;49:350.

483a. Berg D, Otley CC. Skin cancer in organ transplant recipients: epidemiology, pathogenesis, and management. *J Am Acad Dermatol* 2002;47:1.

483b. Haupt HM, Stern JB, Dilaimy MS. Basal cell carcinoma: clues to its presence in histologic sections when the initial slide is nondiagnostic. *Am J Surg Pathol* 2000;24:1291.

483c. Bisson MA, Dunkin CS, Suvarna SK, et al. Do plastic surgeons resect basal cell carcinomas too widely? A prospective study comparing surgical and histological margins. *Br J Plast Surg* 2002;55:293.

483d. Dieu T, Macleod AM. Incomplete excision of basal cell carcinomas: a retrospective audit. *Aust N Z J Surg* 2002;72:219.

483e. Kumar P, Watson S, Brain AN, et al. Incomplete excision of basal cell carcinoma: a prospective multicentre audit. *Br J Plast Surg* 2002;55:616.

483f. Robinson JK, Fisher SG. Recurrent basal cell carcinoma after incomplete resection. *Arch Dermatol* 2000;136:1318.

484. Hoyo E, Kanitakis J, Euvrard S, et al. Proliferation characteristics of cutaneous squamous cell carcinomas developing in organ graft recipients: comparison with squamous cell carcinomas of nonimmunocompromised hosts by counting argyrophilic proteins associated with nucleolar organizer regions. *Arch Dermatol* 1993;129:324.

485. Viac J, Chardonnet Y, Euvrard S, et al. Langerhans' cells, inflammation markers and human papillomavirus infections in benign and malignant epithelial tumors from transplant recipients. *J Dermatol* 1992;19:67.

486. Proby CM, Churchill L, Purkis PE, et al. Keratin 17 expression as a marker for epithelial transformation in viral warts. *Am J Pathol* 1993;143:1667.

487. McGregor JM, Farthing A, Crook T, et al. Posttransplant skin cancer: a possible role for p53 gene mutation but not for oncogenic human papillomaviruses. *J Am Acad Dermatol* 1994;30:701.

488. Angeli-Besson C, Koeppel MC, Jacquet P, et al. Multiple squamous-cell carcinomas of the scalp and chronic myeloid leukemia. *Dermatology* 1995;191:321.

489. Oram Y, Orengo I, Griego RD, et al. Histologic patterns of basal cell carcinoma based upon patient immunostatus. *Dermatol Surg* 1995;21:611.

490. Hertzler G, Gordon SM, Piratzky J, et al. Case report: fulminant Kaposi's sarcoma after orthotopic liver transplantation. *Am J Med Sci* 1995;309:278.

491. Abouna GM, Kumar MS, Samhan M. Kaposi's sarcoma in renal transplant recipients: a case report. *Transpl Sci* 1994;4:20.

492. Al-Sulaiman MH, Mousa DH, Dhar JM, et al. Does regressed posttransplantation Kaposi's sarcoma recur following reintroduction of immunosuppression? *Am J Nephrol* 1992;12:384.

493. McGregor JM, Newell M, Ross J, et al. Cutaneous malignant melanoma and human immunodeficiency virus (HIV) infection: a report of three cases. *Br J Dermatol* 1992;126:516.

493a. Hutchinson J. The crateriform ulcer of the face: a form of epithelial cancer. *Trans Pathol Soc (London)* 1889;40:275.

494. Musso L, Gordon H. Spontaneous resolution of molluscum sebaceum. *Proc R Soc Med* 1950;43:838.

495. Rook A, Whimster IW. Le kératoacanthome. *Arch Belg Dermatol Syphiligr* 1950;6:137.

496. Ghadially FN. Keratoacanthoma. In: Fitzpatrick TB, Eisen AZ, Wolff K, et al., eds. *Dermatology in general medicine*, 2nd ed. New York: McGraw-Hill, 1979:383.

497. Silberberg I, Kopf A, Baer RL. Recurrent keratoacanthoma of the lip. *Arch Dermatol* 1962;86:44.

498. Sullivan JJ, Colditz GA. Keratoacanthoma in a subtropical climate. *Australas J Dermatol* 1979;20:34.

499. Muir EG, Bell AJY, Barlow KA. Multiple primary carcinomata of the colon, duodenum, and larynx associated with keratoacanthomata of the face. *Br J Surg* 1967;54:191.

500. Poleksic S. Keratoacanthoma and multiple carcinomas. *Br J Dermatol* 1974;91:461.

501. Rapaport J. Giant keratoacanthoma of the nose. *Arch Dermatol* 1975;111:73.

502. Bart RS, Popkin GL, Kopf AW, et al. Giant keratoacanthoma. *J Dermatol Surg* 1975;1:49.

503. Kallos A. Giant keratoacanthoma. *Arch Dermatol* 1958;78:207.

504. Obermayer ME. Das keratoakanthom: seine zur gewebsdestruktion führende wachstumskapazität. *Hautarzt* 1964;15:628.

505. Belisario JC. Brief review of keratoacanthoma and description of keratoacanthoma centrifugum marginatum. *Australas J Dermatol* 1965;8:65.

506. Miedzinski F, Kozakiewicz J. Das keratoakanthoma centrifugum: eine besondere varietät des keratoakanthoms. *Hautarzt* 1962;13:348.

507. Weedon D, Barnett L. Keratoacanthoma centrifugum marginatum. *Arch Dermatol* 1975;111:1024.

508. Heid E, Grosshans E, Lazrak B, et al. Keratoacanthoma centrifugum marginatum. *Ann Dermatol Venereol* 1979;106:367.

509. Macaulay WL. Subungual keratoacanthoma. *Arch Dermatol* 1976;112:1004.

510. Stoll DM, Ackerman AB. Subungual keratoacanthoma. *Am J Dermatopathol* 1980;2:265.

511. Keeney GL, Banks PM, Linscheid RL. Subungual keratoacanthoma. *Arch Dermatol* 1988;124:1074.

512. Rook A, Whimster I. Keratoacanthoma: a 29-year retrospect. *Br J Dermatol* 1979;100:41.

513. Poleksic S, Yeung KY. Rapid development of keratoacanthoma and accelerated transformation into squamous cell carcinoma of the skin. *Cancer* 1978;41:12.

514. Kern WH, McGray MK. The histopathologic differentiation of keratoacanthoma and squamous cell carcinoma of the skin. *J Cutan Pathol* 1980;7:318.

515. Popkin GL, Brodie SJ, Hyman AB, et al. A technique of biopsy recommended for keratoacanthoma. *Arch Dermatol* 1966;94:191.

516. Wade TR, Ackerman AB. The many faces of keratoacanthoma. *J Dermatol Surg Oncol* 1978;4:498.

517. De Moragas JM, Montgomery H, McDonald JR. Keratoacanthoma versus squamous-cell carcinoma. *Arch Dermatol* 1957;77:390.

518. Giltman LI. Tripolar mitosis in a keratoacanthoma. *Acta Derm Venereol (Stockh)* 1981;61:362.

519. Janecka IP, Wolff M, Crikelair GF, et al. Aggressive histological features of keratoacanthoma. *J Cutan Pathol* 1978;4:342.

520. Lapins NA, Helwig EB. Perineural invasion by keratoacanthoma. *Arch Dermatol* 1980;116:791.

521. Levy EJ, Cahn MM, Shaffer B, et al. Keratoacanthoma. *JAMA* 1954;155:562.

522. Calnan CD, Haber H. Molluscum sebaceum. *J Pathol Bacteriol* 1955;69:61.

523. Ghadially FN. The role of the hair follicle in the origin and evolution of some cutaneous neoplasms of man and experimental animals. *Cancer* 1961;14:801.

524. Takaki Y, Masutani M, Kawada A. Electron microscopic study of keratoacanthoma. *Acta Derm Venereol (Stockh)* 1971;51:21.

525. Von Bülow M, Klingmüller G. Elektronenmikroskopische untersuchungen des keratoakanthoms. *Arch Dermatol Forsch* 1971;241:292.

526. Chalet MD, Connors RC, Ackerman AB. Squamous cell carcinoma vs. keratoacanthoma: criteria for histologic differentiation. *J Dermatol Surg* 1975;1:16.

527. Stevanovic DV. Keratoacanthoma dyskeratoticum and segregans. *Arch Dermatol* 1965;92:666.

528. Piscioli F, Boi S, Zumiani G, et al. A gigantic, metastasizing keratoacanthoma. *Am J Dermatopathol* 1984;6:123.

529. Goldenhersh MA, Olsen TG. Invasive squamous cell carcinoma initially diagnosed as giant keratoacanthoma. *J Am Acad Dermatol* 1984;10:372.

530. Nikolowski W. Zur problematik des keratoakanthoms. *Dermatol Monatsschr* 1970;156:148.

531. Sullivan JJ, Donoghue MF, Kynaston B, et al. Multiple keratoacanthomas. *Australas J Dermatol* 1980;21:16.

532. Ferguson Smith J. A case of multiple primary squamous-celled carcinomata of the skin in a young man with spontaneous healing. *Br J Dermatol* 1934;46:267.

533. Tarnowski WM. Multiple keratoacanthomata. *Arch Dermatol* 1966;94:74.

534. Hilker O, Winterscheidt M. Familiäre multiple keratoakanthome. *Z Hautkr* 1987;62:280.

535. Sommerville J, Milne JA. Familial primary self-healing squamous epithelioma of the skin (Ferguson Smith type). *Br J Dermatol* 1950;62:485.

536. Grzybowski M. A case of peculiar generalized epithelial tumours of the skin. *Br J Dermatol* 1950;62:310.

537. Sterry W, Steigleder GK, Pullmann H, et al. Eruptive keratoakanthome. *Hautarzt* 1981;32:119.

538. Rossman RE, Freeman RG, Knox JM. Multiple keratoacanthomas. *Arch Dermatol* 1964;89:374.

539. Winkelmann RK, Brown J. Generalized eruptive keratoacanthoma. *Arch Dermatol* 1968;97:615.

540. Wright AL, Gawkrodger DJ, Branford WA, et al. Self-healing epitheliomata of Ferguson–Smith. *Dermatologica* 1988;176:22.

541. Rook A, Moffat JL. Multiple self-healing epithelioma of Ferguson Smith type. *Arch Dermatol* 1956;74:525.

542. Lancer HA, Moschella SL. Paget's disease of the male breast. *J Am Acad Dermatol* 1982;7:393.

543. Hadlich J, Göring HD, Linse R. Morbus Paget beim mann nach Östrogenbehandlung. *Dermatol Monatsschr* 1981;167:305.

544. Ashikari R, Park K, Huvos AG, et al. Paget's disease of the breast. *Cancer* 1970;26:680.

545. Paone JF, Baker RR. Pathogenesis and treatment of Paget's disease of the breast. *Cancer* 1981;48:825.

546. Lewis HM, Ovitz ML, Golitz LE. Erosive adenomatosis of the nipple. *Arch Dermatol* 1976;112:1427.

547. Sitakalin C, Ackerman AB. Mammary and extramammary Paget's disease. *Am J Dermatopathol* 1985;7:335.

548. Hopsu-Havu VK, Sonck CE. The problem of extramammary Paget's disease: report of four cases with "pagetoid" cells. *Z Hautkr* 1971;46:41.

548a. Lloyd J, Flanagan AM. Mammary and extramamary Paget's disease. *J Clin Pathol* 2000;53:742.

549. Ordoñez NG, Awalt H, MacKay B. Mammary and extramammary Paget's disease. *Cancer* 1987;59:1173.

550. Culberson JD, Horn RC Jr. Paget's disease of the nipple. *Arch Surg* 1956;72:224.

551. Helwig EB, Graham JH. Anogenital (extramammary) Paget's disease: a clinicopathologic study. *Cancer* 1963;16:387.

552. Orr JW, Parish DJ. The nature of the nipple changes in Paget's disease. *J Pathol Bacteriol* 1962;84:201.

553. Lagios MD, Westdahl PR, Rose MR, et al. Alternative management in cases without or with minimal extent of underlying breast carcinoma. *Cancer* 1984;54:545.

554. Sagebiel RW. Ultrastructural observations on epidermal cells in Paget's disease of the breast. *Am J Pathol* 1969;57:49.

555. Ebner H. Zur ultrastruktur des morbus Paget mamillae. *Z Hautkr* 1969;44:297.

556. Caputo R, Califano A. Ultrastructural features of extramammary Paget's disease. *Arch Klin Exp Dermatol* 1970;236:121.

557. Nadji M, Morales AR, Girtanner RE, et al. Paget's disease of the skin: a unifying concept of histogenesis. *Cancer* 1982;50:2203.

558. Kariniemi AL, Forsman L, Wahlström T, et al. Expression of differentiation antigen in mammary and extramammary Paget's disease. *Br J Dermatol* 1984;110:203.

559. Belcher RW. Extramammary Paget's disease: enzyme histochemical and electron microscopic study. *Arch Pathol* 1972;94:59.

560. Penneys NS, Nadji M, Morales A. Carcinoembryonic antigen in benign sweat gland tumors. *Arch Dermatol* 1982;118:225.

561. Glasgow BJ, Wen DR, Al-Jitawi S, et al. Antibody to S-100 protein aids the separation of pagetoid melanoma from mammary and extramammary Paget's disease. *J Cutan Pathol* 1987;14:223.

562. Murrell TW Jr, McMullan FH. Extramammary Paget's disease. *Arch Dermatol* 1962;85:600.

563. Fligiel Z, Kaneko M. Extramammary Paget's disease of the external ear canal in association with ceruminous gland carcinoma. *Cancer* 1975;36:1072.

564. Whorton CM, Patterson JB. Carcinoma of Moll's glands with extramammary Paget's disease of the eyelid. *Cancer* 1955;8:1009.

565. Duperrat B, Mascaro JM. Maladie de Paget abdomino-scrotale (3e présentation): apparition d'un épithéliome apocrine de l'aisselle et de lésions de maladie de Paget sur la peau axillaire sus-jacente. *Bull Soc Fr Dermatol Syphiligr* 1964;71:176.

566. Fetissoff F, Arbeille-Brassart B, Lansac J, et al. Association d'une maladie de Paget mammaire et vulvaire. *Ann Dermatol Venereol* 1981;109:43.

567. McKee PH, Hertogs KT. Endocervical adenocarcinoma and vulval Paget's disease: a significant association. *Br J Dermatol* 1980;103:443.

568. Metcalf JS, Lee RE, Maize JC. Epidermotropic urothelial carcinoma involving the glans penis. *Arch Dermatol* 1985;121:532.

569. Ojeda VJ, Heenan PJ, Watson SH. Paget's disease of the groin associated with adenocarcinoma of the urinary bladder. *J Cutan Pathol* 1987;14:227.

570. Powell FC, Bjornsson J, Doyle JA, et al. Genital Paget's disease and urinary tract malignancy. *J Am Acad Dermatol* 1985;13:84.

571. Jones RE Jr, Austin C, Ackerman AB. Extramammary Paget's disease. *Am J Dermatopathol* 1979;1:101.

572. Hart WR, Millman JB. Progression of intraepithelial Paget's disease of the vulva to invasive carcinoma. *Cancer* 1977;40:2333.

573. Wick MR, Goellner JR, Wolfe JT III, et al. Vulvar sweat gland carcinomas. *Arch Pathol* 1985;109:43.

574. Lee SC, Roth LM, Ehrlich C, et al. Extramammary Paget's disease of the vulva. *Cancer* 1977;39:2540.

575. Yoell JH, Price WG. Paget's disease of the perianal skin with associated adenocarcinoma. *Arch Dermatol* 1960;82:986.

576. Wood WS, Culling CFA. Perianal Paget disease. *Arch Pathol* 1975;99:442.

577. Gunn RA, Gallager HS. Vulvar Paget's disease. *Cancer* 1980;46:590.

578. Koss LG, Brockunier A Jr. Ultrastructural aspects of Paget's disease of the vulva. *Arch Pathol* 1969;87:592.

579. Tazawa T, Ito M, Fujiwara H, et al. Immunologic characteristics of keratin in extramammary Paget's disease. *Arch Dermatol* 1988;124:1063.

580. Pinkus H, Mehregan AH. *A guide to dermatopathology.* 3rd ed. New York: Appleton-Century-Crofts, 1981.

581. Mérot Y, Mazoujian G, Pinkus G, et al. Extramammary Paget's disease of perianal and perineal regions: evidence of apocrine derivation. *Arch Dermatol* 1985;121:750.

582. Lloyd J, Flanagan AM. Mammary and extramammary Paget's disease. *J Clin Pathol* 2000;53:742.

TUMORS OF THE EPIDERMAL APPENDAGES

WALTER KLEIN
EDWARD CHAN
JOHN T. SEYKORA

CLASSIFICATION OF APPENDAGEAL TUMORS

Historically, tumors of the epidermal appendages have been classified into four groups that exhibit histologic features analogous to hair follicles, sebaceous glands, apocrine glands, and eccrine glands. In general, this type of diagnostic nosology based on the microscopic attributes of appendageal structures has been practical for the classification of adnexal lesions.

However, in some cases, the diagnosis of adnexal neoplasms presents unique difficulties, in part, related to the wide variety of tumors, the substantial frequency of one lesion exhibiting histologic features of two or more adnexal lines and the complicated nomenclature (1–5). Histogenesis is a concept that implies that the histologic appearance of a tumor is similar to the histology of the organ/structure from which the tumor arose ("cell of origin"). These concepts of appendageal tumorigenesis are being modified by new information pertaining to mechanisms governing the proliferation and differentiation of pluripotent cells that may be situated within multiple compartments in the epidermis and associated adnexa.

In general, tumors are not derived directly from mature (differentiated, postmitotic) cells; rather, tumors originate from multipotential undifferentiated cells present within the epidermis or its appendageal structures (6). Such cells, when undergoing neoplastic transformation, may aberrantly express one or more lines of appendageal differentiation to varying degrees given that these cells are not a priori restricted to one line of differentiation. Taken together, these concepts predict that the histologic features of a tumor are related to the activation of molecular pathways responsible for forming the mature adnexal structure. The degree to which the eccrine, apocrine, sebaceous, and follicular differentiation pathways are activated and recapitulated gives a tumor its histologic features. These concepts predict that tumors, including adnexal tumors, may imprecisely resemble their mature counterparts and that multiple lines of differentiation may be seen simultaneously in the same tumor (6). Given that tumor cell physiology is somewhat abnormal, it is remarkable that a significant percentage of adnexal neoplasms manifest predominantly one line of differentiation (Table 30-1).

Benign adnexal tumors in which there is an admixture of follicular, eccrine, sebaceous, and/or apocrine adnexal differentiation, such as sebaceous units in combination with either eccrine and/or apocrine elements, are a source of diagnostic confusion that likely results from multidirectional differentiation involving pluripotential cells of the epidermis or of adnexal structures. Differentiation is probably influenced not only by genetic potential, but also by field effects such as regional vascularity and molecular microenvironmental attributes of the epidermis, dermis, or subcutis (6). In human skin, keratinocytes with markers of stem cells appear to reside in the "bulge," and cells with capability of proliferating and differentiating along appendageal lines (progenitor cells) appear to traffic from this site to the basilar epidermis, the sebaceous gland, and the hair follicle (7–9).

In addition to benign tumors, there are carcinomas of the epidermal appendages, which have the potential to metastasize. Three types of glandular carcinoma are recognized: carcinoma of sebaceous glands, of eccrine glands, and of apocrine glands. Other epithelial carcinomas exhibiting various types of follicular differentiation have been reported, such as pilomatrical carcinoma, malignant proliferating trichilemmal cyst, trichilemmal carcinoma, and trichoblastic carcinoma (Table 30-1).

As alluded to above, the histopathology of a tumor often can be interpreted by comparing it to the histology of skin appendages. For example, clear or pale cell change due to cytoplasmic glycogen may recapitulate the embryonic acrosyringium in a nodular hidradenoma or the glycogenated follicular outer root sheath in a trichilemmoma. Cytoplasmic fat vacuoles that indent the nucleus are typical of sebaceous differentiation that is seen in sebaceous glands,

TABLE 30-1. CLASSIFICATION OF TUMORS OF EPIDERMAL APPENDAGES

Lesion Type	Follicular Differentiation	Sebaceous Differentiation	Apocrine Differentiation	Eccrine Differentiation
Hyperplasias, hamartomas	Hair follicle nevus Dilated pore Generalized hair follicle hamartoma Basaloid follicular hamartoma	Nevus sebaceous Sebaceous hyperplasia	Apocrine nevus	Eccrine nevus
Benign neoplasms	Trichofolliculoma Pilar sheath acanthoma Fibrofolliculoma Trichodiscoma Trichoepithelioma Trichoblastoma Trichoadenoma Pilomatricoma Trichilemmoma Tumor of follicular infundibulum Trichilemmal horn Proliferating trichilemmal cyst	Sebaceous adenoma Sebaceoma	Aprocrine hidrocystoma Hidroadenoma papilliferum Syringocystadenoma papilliferum Tubular apocrine adenoma Erosive adenomatosis of the nipple Apocrine cylindroma	Eccrine hidrocystoma Syringoma Eccrine cylindroma Eccrine poroma Eccrine syringofibroadenoma Mucinous syringometaplasia Eccrine spiroadenom Papillary eccrine adenoma Nodular hidradenoma Chondroid syringoma
Malignant neoplasms	Pilomatrix carcinoma Malignant proliferating trichilemmal tumor Trichilemmal carcinoma Trichoblastic carcinoma	Sebaceous carcinoma	Malignant apocrine cylindroma	Porocarcinoma Malignant eccrine spiroadenoma Malignant nodular hidradenoma Malignant chrondroid syringoma Eccrine adenocarcinoma Microcystic adnexal carcinoma Aggressive digital papillary adenocarcinoma Adenoid cystic carcinoma Mucinous eccrine carcinoma Syringoid eccrine carcinoma Malignant eccrine cylindroma

sebaceous adenomas, and sebaceous carcinomas. Many adnexal tumors contain a distinctive, fibrotic, eosinophilic hyaline stroma that envelops the epithelial elements. This stroma assists in differentiating many basaloid adnexal neoplasms from basal cell carcinoma. Eccrine tumors commonly exhibit a nearly acellular hyalinized eosinophilic stroma with dilated thin-walled vessels (e.g., nodular hidradenoma, eccrine poroma). Tubule formation and focal keratinization occurring in eccrine tumors tend to differentiate them from renal cell or other metastatic clear cell carcinomas. Historically, immunohistochemistry has been of little value in definitively distinguishing among the phenotypic patterns of adnexal neoplasms (10). However, specific mutations in genes associated with appendageal neoplasms

such as CYLD1 in cylindromas may provide molecular signatures for lesions (11). Further research on these tumors using current technologies, especially DNA microarrays and proteomic studies, may yield additional molecular markers useful for classifying these lesions.

Lesional histology evolves with time and in response to local effects. For example, a trichilemmal cyst, possibly stimulated by inflammatory mediators, may, as it ages, transform into a proliferating trichilemmal cyst and ultimately into the solid pilar tumor of the scalp. It is almost certain that tumor progression, the "process whereby tumors go from bad to worse" also operates in adnexal tumors, as it does in most tumor types. From a clinical point of view, adnexal neoplasms should not be regarded as obligate precursors of malignancy.

Classification of the Benign Appendageal Tumors

The four groups of benign appendage tumors with differentiation toward hair, sebaceous glands, apocrine glands, and eccrine glands can be divided, according to a gradient of decreasing differentiation, into three major subgroups: hyperplasias, hamartomas, and cysts; benign tumors; and malignant tumors (Table 30-1). This classification is similar to the approach of the recent World Health Organization's *International Histological Classification of Tumours* monograph (12).

Of the three subgroups of benign appendageal lesions, the hyperplasias, hamartomas, and cysts are composed of mature or nearly mature structures. The benign neoplasms, in general, show less complete differentiation than the hyperplasias; nonetheless, well-developed, differentiated, or partially differentiated structures are present. The malignant neoplasms are a further step down with regard to degree of differentiation, and it may be difficult to recognize the type of structure that the tumor is attempting to form.

Although most of the benign appendage tumors fit well into one of the entities listed in Table 30-1, tumors in an intermediate stage of differentiation are occasionally encountered (13).

Ontogeny of Benign Appendageal Tumors

Three possibilities exist for the development of benign appendageal tumors: development from primary epithelial germs, from pluripotential cells, or from cells of preexisting structures. In 1948, the thesis was advanced that cutaneous tumors differentiating toward hair, sebaceous glands, or apocrine glands developed from primary epithelial germ cells and were primary epithelial germ tumors; further, that the hyperplasias, adenomas, and benign epitheliomas arose from primary epithelial germ cells that had attained a certain degree of differentiation before the onset of neoplasia (14).

Given that pluripotent stem cells give rise to cutaneous appendageal structures, and that stem cells are continually present in the skin, it is likely that the benign appendageal tumors arise from these cells that possess the potential of differentiating into tumors with hair, sebaceous gland, or apocrine structures (6). Appendageal tumors associated with genetic syndromes, such as multiple cylindromas, multiple trichoepitheliomas, and the nevoid basal cell carcinoma syndrome, are probably derived from abnormally regulated pluripotent cells that are directed to form abnormal appendageal structures rather than mature appendages. This scenario is likely to be true in sporadic occurrences of these same adnexal tumors. In some instances, pluripotent cells differentiate in more than one direction, as is seen most commonly on the scalp, where a syringocystadenoma may exhibit three different lines of appendageal differentiation.

Terminology

The terms *nevus*, *hamartoma*, and *carcinoma* used in the classification of the benign appendage tumors require definition.

The term *nevus* is used in the literature in two different ways, referring (a) to a tumor composed of nevus cells derived from melanocytes (nevocellular nevus, melanocytic nevus, pigmented nevus), or (b) to a lesion that is usually present at birth and is composed of mature or nearly mature structures, such as nevus sebaceus, eccrine nevus, nevus verrucosus, and nevus flammeus. To avoid confusion, it is advisable to use the term nevus with a qualifying adjective, and to assume that nevus without a qualifying adjective designates a tumor composed of melanocytic nevus cells.

The term *hamartoma* is appropriate for those nevi that have no melanocytic nevus cells and, like congenital hyperplasias, are composed of mature or nearly mature structures. Hamartoma, derived from the Greek word *hamartanein* (to fail, to err), was chosen as the designation for "tumor-like malformations showing a faulty mixture of the normal components of the organ in which they occur" (15).

Many authors have used the term *epithelioma* as a synonym for carcinoma. However, since the literal meaning of the word is "tumor of the epithelium," the term may be employed as a designation of benign as well as of malignant tumors of the epithelium, provided that a qualifying adjective is added (16). Because the term has been used for both benign and malignant neoplasms, it seems best to avoid its use except in a clearly defined historical context. The term *carcinoma* is used for malignant epithelial tumors, including those that are characterized by a tendency to inexorable growth with local invasion and tissue destruction as well as those that may in addition have capacity for distant metastasis. As in previous editions, we have selected terms that are widely understood and used, not necessarily those that are above all semantic scrutiny (17).

TUMORS WITH DIFFERENTIATION TOWARD HAIR STRUCTURES

Hair Follicle Nevus

This rare, small tumor presents as a small nodule on the face, often at birth. It has also been referred to as congenital vellus hamartoma (18). Recently, a few reported cases have raised the possibility of a novel neurocutaneous syndrome (19).

Histopathology. There are numerous, small, well-differentiated vellus hair follicles, occasionally accompanied by a few small sebaceous glands (20) (Figs. 30-1 and 30-2).

Differential Diagnosis. The small vellus hair follicles present in the central part of the face greatly resemble the hair follicles in a hair follicle nevus. Other entities to con-

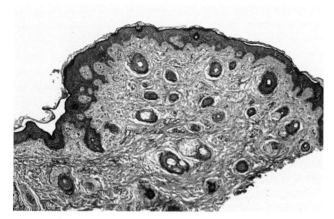

FIGURE 30-1. Hair Follicle Nevus. Increased numbers of small hairs are seen localized in the dermis.

sider in the differential diagnosis are accessory tragus and hair follicle hamartoma (21,22).

Trichofolliculoma

Trichofolliculoma occurs in adults as a solitary lesion, usually on the face but occasionally on the scalp or neck. It consists of a small, skin-colored, dome-shaped nodule. Frequently, there is a central pore. If such a central pore is present, a wool-like tuft of immature, usually white hairs may be seen emerging from it, a highly diagnostic clinical feature (23).

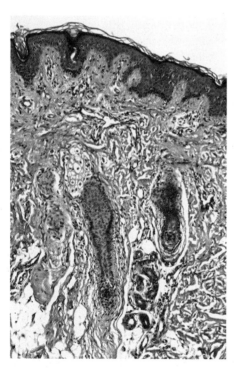

FIGURE 30-2. Hair Follicle Nevus. The small hairs mature normally and are associated with sebaceous glands.

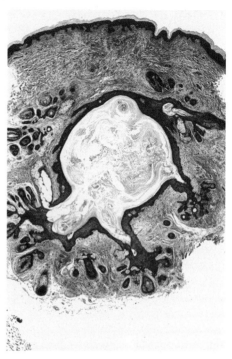

FIGURE 30-3. Trichofolliculoma. In the dermis, there is a keratin-filled cyst lined by squamous epithelium associated with follicular structures.

Histopathology. On histologic examination, the dermis contains a large cystic space that is lined by squamous epithelium and contains horny material and frequently fragments of birefringent hair shafts (24) (Fig. 30-3). In cases with a central pore, the large cystic space is continuous with the surface epidermis, an indication that it represents an enlarged, distorted hair follicle. In some cases, one or two additional cystic spaces are present in the dermis. Radiating from the wall of these "primary" hair follicles, one sees many small but usually fairly well-differentiated "secondary" hair follicles (Fig. 30-4). Well-developed secondary hair follicles often show a hair papilla (Fig. 30-4). Furthermore, they usually show an outer and an inner root sheath, the latter of which may contain eosinophilic trichohyalin granules and, located in the center, a fine hair (Fig. 30-4). These fine hairs are visualized best where the secondary hair follicles appear in cross sections. Small groups of sebaceous gland cells may be embedded in the walls of the secondary hair follicles (25) (Fig. 30-4). In some of the more rudimentary secondary follicles, one observes a central horn cyst in place of a hair, as seen also in trichoepithelioma (26). The stroma is rich in fibroblasts and is oriented in parallel bundles of fibers that encapsulate the epithelial proliferations in a manner resembling that of the normal fibrous root sheath (27). Glycogen can be demonstrated in the outer root sheath of the secondary hair follicles, just as it is seen in the outer root sheath of mature hair structures (24).

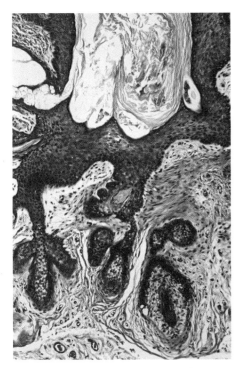

FIGURE 30-4. Trichofolliculoma. Emanating from the cyst wall are numerous small "secondary" hair follicles, some of which show, in addition to a hair and an outer root sheath, an inner root sheath with trichohyalin granules.

In all trichofolliculomas, epithelial strands interconnect the secondary hair follicles. Since these epithelial strands differentiate in the direction of the outer root sheath, the peripheral cell row is palisaded, and because of their glycogen content, the cells within the strands appear large and vacuolated (27).

Additional Studies. Recent evidence suggests that trichofolliculomas undergo morphologic changes corresponding to the normal hair follicle cycle (28). The folliculosebaceous cystic hamartoma (which is characterized by a folliculosebaceous proliferation with cyst-like infundibular dilatation and a stromal mesenchymal component with variable fibroplasia, vascular and neural proliferation and adipocyte metaplasia) may represent a late-stage trichofolliculoma in that it has more prominent sebaceous differentiation linked to the cystic infundibulum with more prominent surrounding stroma (29,30). Transgenic mice that overexpress a stabilized form of the beta-catenin protein develop trichofolliculomas (31); therefore, increased signaling through the β-catenin pathway may play a role in the development of trichofolliculomas in humans.

Sebaceous Trichofolliculoma

Sebaceous trichofolliculoma, a variant of trichofolliculoma, occurs in areas rich in sebaceous follicles, such as the nose. It is a centrally depressed lesion with a fistula-like opening from which terminal hairs and vellus hairs protrude (32).

Histopathology. There is a rather large, irregularly shaped, centrally located cavity lined by squamous epithelium. Many radially arranged pilosebaceous follicles connect to the cavity. These contain sebaceous ducts and numerous well-differentiated, large sebaceous lobules, as well as hair follicles containing partially terminal and partially vellus hairs (32).

Differential Diagnosis. Unlike folliculosebaceous cystic hamartoma which presents as a solitary papule or nodule, sebaceous trichofolliculoma clinically presents with a central pore-like opening that exhibits protruding hairs. Histopathologically, folliculosebaceous cystic hamartoma is additionally characterized by stromal mesenchymal abnormalities, a finding not seen in the previously reported cases of sebaceous trichofolliculoma (33).

Dilated Pore and Pilar Sheath Acanthoma

Dilated pore and pilar sheath acanthoma clinically share with trichofolliculoma and sebaceous trichofolliculoma the presence of a central pore and histologically the presence of a large cystic space that is continuous with the surface epidermis, lined by squamous epithelium, and filled with keratinous material.

The *dilated pore*, described in 1954 by Winer (34), occurs on the face, usually as a solitary lesion and predominantly in adult males. It has the appearance of a giant comedone and does not possess any palpable induration.

The *pilar sheath acanthoma*, described in 1978 (35), is usually found on the skin of the upper lip of adults. It is seen elsewhere on the face only rarely. It occurs as a solitary skin-colored nodule with a central pore-like opening.

Histopathology. The dilated pore differentiates toward the infundibulum both architecturally and cytologically (36). It shows a markedly dilated pilar infundibulum lined by an epidermis that is atrophic near the ostium but hypertrophic deeper in the cystic cavity, where it shows many rete ridges and irregular thin proliferations into the surrounding stroma (Figs. 30-5 and 30-6). The keratin-filled cystic cavity may extend into the subcutaneous fat. In the lower portion, small sebaceous gland lobules and vellus hair follicles may be attached to the lining epidermis (34).

The pilar sheath acanthoma differs from the dilated pore by showing a larger, irregularly branching cystic cavity. In place of thin proliferations, as seen in the dilated pore, numerous lobulated masses of cells radiate from the wall of the cystic cavity into the dermis and the subcutaneous tissue (35). The pilar sheath acanthoma can exhibit some features of the outer root sheath in that some areas may show peripheral palisading and contain varying amounts of glycogen (37). It has been suggested that pilar sheath acanthomas can differentiate toward all components of the folliculosebaceous unit (36,38).

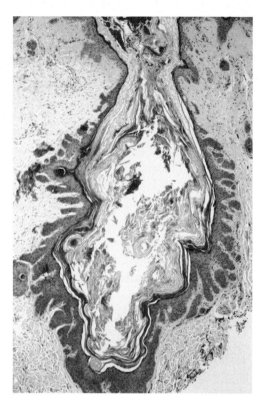

FIGURE 30-5. Dilated Pore of Winer. An irregular cystic cavity is present in the dermis.

Fibrofolliculoma and Trichodiscoma

Fibrofolliculomas and trichodiscomas consist of 2- to 4-mm large, yellow-white, smooth, dome-shaped lesions, often on the face. The lesions can be solitary or multiple. Multiple fibrofolliculomas have been described in association with trichodiscomas and acrochordons (39,40). This triad is now referred to as the Birt–Hogg–Dubé syndrome and is inherited in an autosomal dominant fashion (39).

In patients with the Birt–Hogg–Dubé syndrome the lesions are present in considerable number mainly on the face and neck. In such cases, the trichodiscomas are clinically indistinguishable from the fibrofolliculomas (41). In this syndrome, there is an increased risk for the development of renal tumors and colonic polyps (42,43). In a reported patient with a large connective tissue nevus, fibrofolliculomas were present in large numbers within as well as around the connective tissue nevus (41).

Besides occurring in association with multiple fibrofolliculomas, multiple trichodiscomas also occur without them, as small papules either widely disseminated or localized to one area (44,45).

Histopathology. Fibrofolliculomas show in their center a hair follicle that often appears distorted. It is surrounded by a thick mantle of basophilic, mucoid stroma (Fig. 30-7). Numerous thin, anastomosing bands of follicular epithelium extend into this stroma (39,41) (Fig. 30-8).

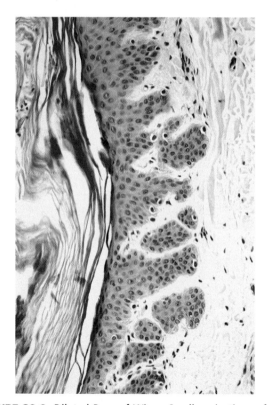

FIGURE 30-6. Dilated Pore of Winer. Small projections of epithelial cells extend from the wall of the cyst into the surrounding dermis.

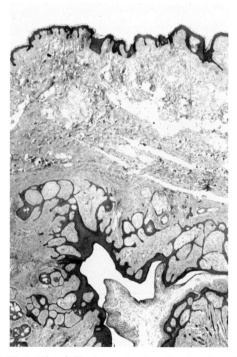

FIGURE 30-7. Fibrofolliculoma. In the dermis, there is a distorted cystic structure associated with epithelial cords and a fibrous stroma.

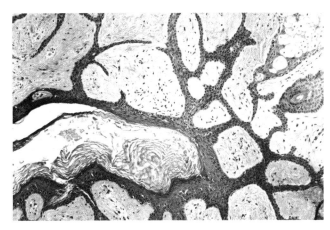

FIGURE 30-8. Fibrofolliculoma. Numerous thin, anastomosing bands of follicular epithelium extend into the bland fibrocellular stroma.

Trichodiscomas are seen in the dermis as an area of fine fibrillary connective tissue containing ectatic blood vessels (Figs. 30-9 and 30-10). Epithelial hyperplasia resembling that seen in fibrofolliculomas is often seen. A hair follicle is usually found at the margin of the lesion (39,41). Trichodiscomas have been regarded as hamartomas of the mesodermal component of hair disks (44).

The pedunculated acrochordons seen in association with multiple fibrofolliculomas may contain only dermal connective tissue. However, in some instances, they contain thin, anastomosing strands of epithelium; they are regarded as fibrofolliculomas displaying the configuration of an acrochordon (44).

Additional Studies. Steffen and Ackerman (46) consider that histopathologically, fibrofolliculoma and trichodiscoma are hamartomas of follicular epithelium, follicular mantles, and perifollicular connective tissue. The immunophenotypic characteristics of syndromic-associated and

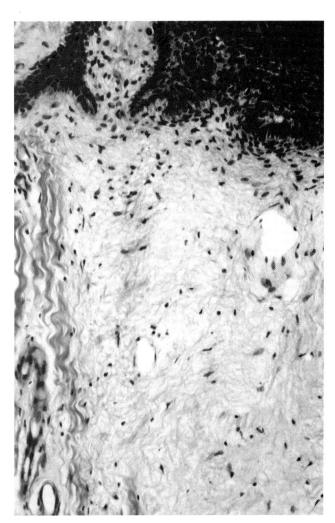

FIGURE 30-10. Trichodiscoma. The altered connective tissue exhibits ectatic vessels, a myxomatous appearance, and increased numbers of mature fibrocytic cells.

sporadic types are identical and consist of perifollicular spindle cells that are positive for vimentin and CD34, and negative for factor XIII. This suggests that these lesions originate from the hair follicle mantle (47).

Trichoepithelioma

Trichoepithelioma occurs either in multiple lesions or as a solitary lesion. The name *trichoepithelioma* is preferable to other designations, such as *epithelioma adenoides cysticum* and *multiple benign cystic epithelioma*, because it indicates that the differentiation of this tumor is directed toward hair structures.

Multiple trichoepitheliomas are transmitted as an autosomal dominant trait (48). In most instances, the first lesions appear in childhood and gradually increase in number (49). Numerous rounded, skin-colored, firm papules and nodules, usually between 2 and 8 mm in diameter located

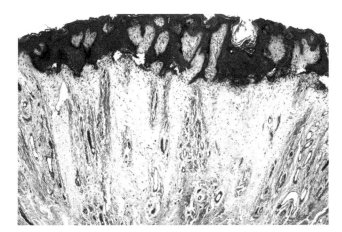

FIGURE 30-9. Trichodiscoma. Present in the dermis are areas of fine, fribrillar connective tissue.

mainly in the nasolabial folds, but also the nose, forehead, and upper lip are seen. Occasionally, lesions are seen also on the scalp, neck, and upper trunk. Ulceration of the lesions occurs rarely. Transformation of one or several lesions into basal cell carcinomas is a very rare event. Most of the cases reported as such in the past are now regarded as instances of nevoid basal cell carcinoma syndrome (18,50). Nevertheless, there have been a few cases of basal cell carcinoma arising in the setting of multiple trichoepitheliomas (51–53). The simultaneous presence of trichoepithelioma and cylindroma, the latter of which is also dominantly inherited, has been observed repeatedly (see Cylindroma section).

Solitary trichoepithelioma occurs more commonly than multiple trichoepitheliomas (49). It is not inherited and consists of a firm, elevated, flesh-colored nodule, usually less than 2 cm in diameter. Its onset usually is in childhood or early adult life (54). Most commonly, the lesion is seen on the face, but it may occur elsewhere. The presence within the same tumor of a solitary trichoepithelioma and an apocrine adenoma has been described (55).

Giant solitary trichoepithelioma, measuring several centimeters in diameter, is a distinct variant of trichoepithelioma (56). It arises in later life and occurs most commonly on a thigh and in the perianal region (56,57).

Histopathology. As a rule, multiple trichoepitheliomas are superficial dermal lesions. They appear well circumscribed, small, and symmetrical on histologic examination. Horn cysts are the most characteristic histologic feature, although they may be absent in some lesions. They consist of a fully keratinized center surrounded by basophilic cells that have the same appearance as the cells in the basal cell carcinoma ("basalioma cells"), except that they tend to lack high-grade atypia and mitoses, as are prominent in some but not all carcinomas (Figs. 30-11 and 30-12). The keratinization is abrupt and complete, in the manner of so-called "trichilemmal" keratinization, as opposed to the horn pearls of squamous cell carcinoma. Quite frequently,

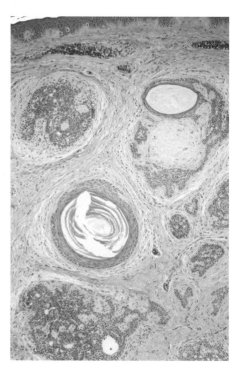

FIGURE 30-12. Trichoepithelioma. Fibroblasts encircle and are tightly associated with the basaloid epithelial islands, lacking the retraction artifact typical of basal cell carcinoma. The walls of the horn cysts are formed by a few layers of cells. Some of the basophilic islands resemble follicular papillae.

one observes one or a few layers of cells with eosinophilic cytoplasm and large, oval, pale, vesicular nuclei situated between the basophilic cells and the horn cysts (49).

Tumor islands composed of basophilic cells constitute a second major component of multiple trichoepitheliomas. They have the same appearance as epidermal or skin appendage basal cells that usually are arranged in a lace-like or adenoid network but occasionally also as solid aggregates (Fig. 30-12). These tumor islands show peripheral palisading of their cells and are surrounded by a stroma with a moderate number of fibroblasts. The fibroblasts encircle and are tightly associated with the basaloid islands, lacking the retraction artifact typical of basal cell carcinoma (Fig. 30-12). Both the adenoid and the solid aggregates show invaginations, which contain numerous fibroblasts and thus resemble follicular papillae (Fig. 30-12).

Additional findings, observed in some but not all multiple trichoepitheliomas, are the presence of a foreign-body giant cell reaction in the vicinity of ruptured horn cysts, calcium deposits either within the foci of the foreign-body reaction or within intact horn cysts, and amyloid (49,58).

Occasionally, some lesions in patients with multiple trichoepitheliomas show relatively little differentiation toward hair structures. They contain only a few horn cysts with many areas resembling basal cell carcinoma (49). Such lesions can be difficult to distinguish from those of a kera-

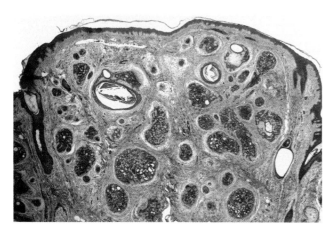

FIGURE 30-11. Trichoepithelioma. The two major components are horn cysts of varying sizes and basaloid epithelial formations.

totic basal cell carcinoma, which may also show horn cysts. Thus, on a histologic basis, it may be difficult to definitively distinguish between multiple trichoepitheliomas and basal cell carcinoma (see Differential Diagnosis).

Solitary trichoepithelioma often have a high degree of differentiation toward hair structures. Solitary lesions with relatively little differentiation toward hair structures are best classified as keratotic basal cell carcinoma. If a lesion is to qualify for the diagnosis of solitary trichoepithelioma, it should contain numerous horn cysts and abortive hair papillae and show only few areas with the appearance of basal cell carcinoma (54). Mitotic figures should be very rare or absent, and the lesion should not be unduly large, asymmetrical, or infiltrative.

Additional Studies. It is assumed that the basophilic cells surrounding horn cysts are similar to hair matrix cells and that the horn cysts represent attempts at hair shaft formation. The eosinophilic cells seen occasionally around horn cysts probably represent cells with initial keratinization and are similar to the nucleated cells seen in normal hair shafts at the keratogenous zone.

Histochemical staining with the Gomori stain for alkaline phosphatase has shown positive staining in many invaginations at the periphery of tumor islands and strands, indicative of a differentiation toward hair papillae (59). An immunohistochemical analysis using a panel of monoclonal antikeratin antibodies suggests that trichoepitheliomas differentiate toward the outer root sheath (60). The expression of cytokeratin 15 in trichoepitheliomas suggests that these tumors contain cells that are related to hair follicle stem cells in the follicular bulge (61). Electron microscopic study has confirmed that the horn cysts of trichoepithelioma represent immature hair structures, with abrupt development of the horn cells from hair matrix cells (62).

The putative gene for multiple familial trichoepitheliomas has been localized to chromosome 9p21 (63). Several known tumor suppressor genes, including *p15*, *p16*, and *p19* have been assigned to this region (64). However loss of heterozygosity on chromosome 9p21 has not been found in sporadic trichoepitheliomas (65). Conversely, in sporadic trichoepitheliomas loss of heterozygosity has been found on chromosome 9q23 (65). In addition, deletions causing overexpression of the human homologue of the Drosophila patched gene (*Ptch*) have been found in trichoepitheliomas as in basal cell carcinoma (66).

The close relationship between trichoepithelioma and basal cell carcinoma has been explained on the basis of the assumption that they have a common genesis from pluripotential cells, which, like primary epithelial germ cells, may develop toward hair structures (14). This hypothesis is supported by the fact that *patched* gene mutations are seen in both tumors (67). Because cells of various degrees of maturity may occur in the same lesion, trichoepithelioma may have areas consistent with the histologic picture of basal cell carcinoma and vice versa.

Differential Diagnosis. The difficulty of differentiating multiple trichoepitheliomas from keratotic basal cell carcinoma on histologic grounds has been pointed out, and the need for clinical data has been stressed. Diagnosis may be assisted, in a given case, by clinical data, such as the number and distribution of the lesions and the presence of hereditary transmission. In addition, certain histologic features as well as immunohistochemical stains can assist in differentiating between the two. The presence of well-formed horn cysts, papillary-mesenchymal bodies (distinct fibroblastic aggregations around the basaloid islands), and lack of high-grade atypia and mitoses favor the diagnosis of trichoepithelioma (68). Histologic features that favor basal cell carcinoma include the presence of myxoid stroma and stromal retraction or clefting around the basaloid islands (58). In trichoepitheliomas, focal positive CD34 staining of the fibroblastic stroma has been shown, whereas in basal cell carcinoma, this staining pattern was not seen (69). However, in a separate study similar CD34 staining was found in trichoepitheliomas, but also in many metatypical basal cell carcinomas (70). Staining of the outermost epithelial layer with *bcl-2* has been seen in several trichoepitheliomas. In contrast, basal cell carcinomas frequently stain diffusely (70,71).

The differentiation of multiple trichoepitheliomas from the nevoid basal cell carcinoma syndrome on histologic grounds can be just as difficult. This, too, often requires clinical information. Although both diseases are dominantly inherited and have multiple lesions, the lesions in multiple trichoepitheliomas present mainly in the nasolabial fold, remain small, and hardly ever ulcerate, whereas the lesions in the nevoid basal cell carcinoma syndrome are haphazardly distributed and, especially in the late "neoplastic" phase, can grow to considerable size, ulcerate deeply, and show severely destructive growth. In addition, patients with the nevoid basal cell carcinoma syndrome almost invariably show multiple skeletal and central nervous system anomalies and frequently show multiple palmar and plantar pits.

Desmoplastic Trichoepithelioma

Desmoplastic trichoepithelioma, a nonfamilial and usually solitary lesion, was formerly considered a solitary trichoepithelioma (49,54). However, it has sufficient clinical and histologic characteristics to be regarded as a distinct variant of trichoepithelioma. The term *desmoplastic* trichoepithelioma appears preferable to the designation *sclerosing epithelial hamartoma* because it stresses the relationship of the lesion to solitary trichoepithelioma (72,73).

Clinically, the tumor almost always is located on the face, measures from 3 to 8 mm in diameter, and is markedly indurated. In many instances, there is a raised, annular border and a depressed nonulcerated center, causing the lesion to resemble granuloma annulare (72). Most commonly, the lesion appears in early adulthood, but it quite frequently appears in the second decade of life (73). It is much more common in females than in males (72). Familial desmoplastic trichoepitheliomas have been reported infrequently (74,75).

Histopathology. The three characteristic histologic features are narrow strands of tumor cells, horn cysts, and a desmoplastic stroma (72) (Figs. 30-13 and 30-14). The tumor strands usually are from one to three cells thick and are composed of small basaloid cells with prominent oval nuclei and scant cytoplasm. Usually there are numerous horn cysts, which in some cases are large (76). Considerable amounts of densely collagenous and hypocellular stroma are present. Large aggregates of tumor cells are not seen. Foreign-body granulomas at the site of ruptured horn cysts and areas of calcification within some of the horn cysts are seen in many tumors.

Differential Diagnosis. The resemblance to microcystic adnexal (eccrine) carcinoma and syringoma may be considerable, especially if a superficial specimen is taken for biopsy. Like desmoplastic trichoepithelioma, microcystic adnexal carcinoma has horn cysts, strands of basaloid cells, and a dense desmoplastic stroma. It differs, however, by showing ductal structures, a deeply infiltrating growth, and often perineural invasion (77). The diagnosis of microcystic adnexal carcinoma should be considered in any tumor resembling a trichoepithelioma or a syringoma in which the lesional cells extend to the base of a superficial biopsy. Syringomas, which usually are periorbital, rarely have horn cysts, foreign-body granulomas, or calcification (72).

Desmoplastic trichoepithelioma may also resemble morphea-like (fibrosing) basal cell carcinoma. However, in morphea-like basal cell carcinoma, horn cysts are absent.

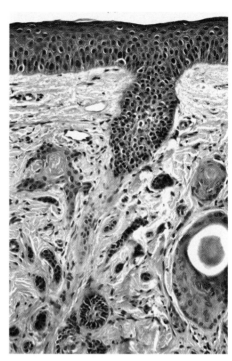

FIGURE 30-14. Desmoplastic Trichoepithelioma. The strands of tumor cells are comprised of small basaloid cells and are usually one to three cells thick.

Of value in ruling out basal cell carcinoma, especially the morphea-like form, are the absence of mitoses, individual cell necrosis, and mucinous stroma and the lack of foci of separation artifact of lesional epithelium and stroma (72). The immunostains for the CD34 and *bcl-2* molecules, discussed above, also may assist in discriminating between the two lesions (70,71,78). In addition, matrix metalloproteinase stromelysin-3 (ST-3) expression has been demonstrated in morphea-like basal carcinomas but not desmoplastic trichoepitheliomas (79). The presence of Merkel cells has been shown in desmoplastic trichoepitheliomas and not morphea-like basal cell carcinomas (80).

Occasional lesions of solitary or desmoplastic trichoepithelioma cannot reliably be distinguished from keratotic or morphea-like basal cell carcinomas, respectively. A descriptive report and a recommendation for complete excision are appropriate in such cases.

Trichoblastoma

Trichoblastomas are benign skin lesions that recapitulate in some form in the developing hair follicle. They differ from trichoepitheliomas in size, location, and lack of keratinizing cysts (81). Trichoblastomas are up to 1.0 cm in size and most commonly occur on the scalp (82). Multiple lesions

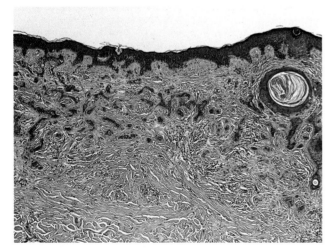

FIGURE 30-13. Desmoplastic Trichoepithelioma. Horn cysts and narrow strands of epithelial cells are embedded in a fibrous stroma.

have been described (83). As mentioned, these lesions are benign, and aggressive forms may represent a type of basal cell carcinoma (84,85).

Histopathology. Trichoblastomas consist of a proliferation of follicular germ cells manifested by a combination of various proportions of mesenchymal and epithelial cells. A spectrum of lesions is seen depending on the proportions of mesenchymal and epithelial components. At one end is the predominantly mesenchymal variant, termed the *trichogenic fibroma*, and at the other is classic trichoblastoma with predominantly basaloid epithelial cells (82). The classic large lesion comprised of islands of basaloid cells occupying the dermis (Fig. 30-15) with occasional extension into the subcutaneous fat. These basaloid islands demonstrate peripheral palisading and a fibrocellular stroma similar to that surrounding follicles (Fig. 30-16). There is no overlying epidermal connection (Fig. 30-15). Less common variants have been described including giant, clear cell, pigmented, rippled-pattern trichoblastomas, and cutaneous lymphadenoma (86–90).

Similar lesions that are infiltrative, exhibit cytologic atypia, and mitotic activity may be termed *trichoblastic carcinoma*, but these lesions may overlap with basal cell carcinoma (Figs. 30-17 and 30-18). Such problematic lesions may be signed out descriptively as *malignant adnexal neoplasm* with a description of the apparent differentiation. Criteria that may have value in distinguishing trichoblastomas and trichilemmomas from basal cell carcinomas include the following: the presence in the former of symmetry, of circumscription with smooth margins and "shelling out" of the normal tissue, of follicular and "racemiform" patterns of lesional cells, the lack of a clefting artifact between stroma and epithelium that is characteristic of basal cell carcinoma, the lack of stromal edema and lymphocytes, the formation of a delicate stroma reminiscent of that formed around immature hair follicles, and the lack of ulceration (91).

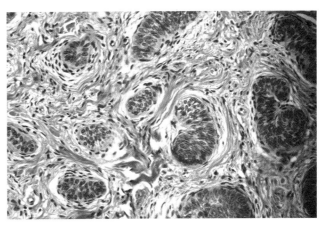

FIGURE 30-16. Trichoblastoma. Higher power showing epithelial structures embedded in a fibrotic stroma that are reminiscent of follicular germs.

Trichoadenoma

A rare, solitary tumor first described in 1958 (92), trichoadenoma usually occurs on the face or buttocks as a solitary nodular lesion and varies from 3 to 15 mm in diameter (93). It may arise anytime during adult life. It may clinically mimic basal cell carcinoma.

Histopathology. Numerous horn cysts are present throughout the dermis (Fig. 30-19). They are surrounded by eosinophilic cells, which greatly resemble the eosinophilic cells that

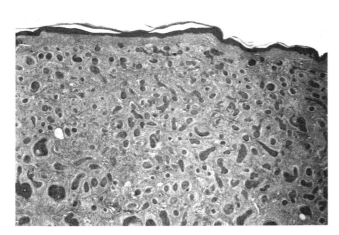

FIGURE 30-15. Trichoblastoma. This is a bulky tumor that spans the dermis and is comprised of islands of tumor cells.

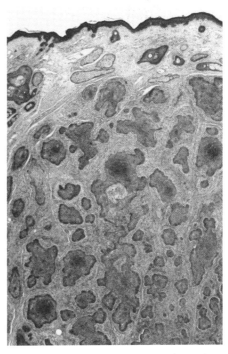

FIGURE 30-17. Trichoblastic Carcinoma. A large dermal tumor comprised of irregular epithelial islands.

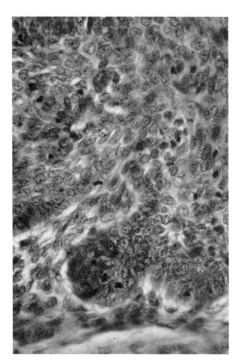

FIGURE 30-18. Trichoblastic Carcinoma. Higher power demonstrates cytologic atypia, numerous mitoses, and a fibrocellular stroma.

are often seen in trichoepithelioma located between the basophilic cells and the central horn cysts (Fig. 30-20). In some instances, a single layer of flattened granular cells is interpolated between the horn cysts and the surrounding eosinophilic cells (93–95). Some islands consist only of eosinophilic epithelial cells without central keratinization. Sparse intercellular bridges have been observed between the eosinophilic cells. Foci of foreign-body granuloma are present at the sites of ruptured horn cysts (92). A variant has been de-

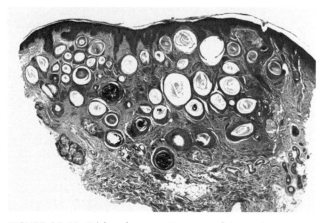

FIGURE 30-19. Trichoadenoma. Numerous horn cysts are present in the dermis.

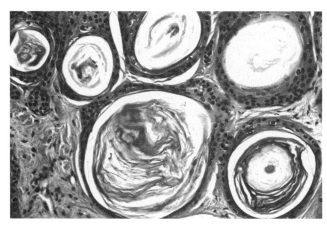

FIGURE 30-20. Trichoadenoma. The horn cysts are comprised of eosinophilic cells containing keratin.

scribed, termed verrucous trichoadenoma, which clinically resembles a seborrheic keratosis (96).

Additional Studies. In terms of morphologic differentiation, the trichoadenoma is situated between a trichofolliculoma and trichoepithelioma (97). The general architecture of trichoadenoma greatly resembles that of trichoepithelioma and thus suggests the development of immature hair structures. However, because the cyst wall consists of epidermoid cells and the keratinization may take place with formation of keratohyaline, it has been suggested that the tumor differentiates largely toward the infundibular portion of the pilosebaceous unit (93).

Generalized Hair Follicle Hamartoma and Basaloid Follicular Hamartoma

Only a few cases have been described of generalized hair follicle hamartoma, a distinctive condition characterized by progressive alopecia starting in adulthood, diffuse papules and plaques of the face, and an association with myasthenia gravis (98–101).

Basaloid follicular hamartoma was originally described as a localized patch of alopecia on the scalp (102). Solitary and multiple familial lesions have since been described (103,104). A few rare syndromes have been described which among their many manifestations have lesions reminiscent of basaloid follicular hamartomas (98,105). Recently, an autosomally dominant inherited form with multiple basaloid follicular hamartomas has been described and named *dominantly inherited, generalized basaloid follicular hamartoma syndrome.* These syndromes all may represent contiguous gene syndromes or different mutations in the same related genes (106,107).

Histopathology. In both hamartomas, the hair loss is the result of damage inflicted on each hair follicle by gradually growing "hair follicle hamartomas."

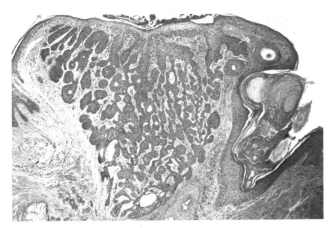

FIGURE 30-21. Basaloid Follicular Hamartoma. Present is a stable small, well-circumscribed lesion comprised of strands of epithelial cells with scattered cystic structures.

In the generalized hair follicle hamartoma, areas of alopecia without papules or plaques reveal more or less advanced replacement of the hair follicles by a lace-like network of basaloid cells with follicular differentiation resembling trichoepithelioma (98,100). The papules and plaques of the face show a complete lack of hair structures and extensive proliferations of basaloid cells embedded in a cellular stroma with formation of horn cysts in some areas. The histologic appearance is indistinguishable from that of trichoepithelioma (99).

The basaloid follicular hamartoma reveals strands and cords of small, basaloid cells emanating from the infundibular portion of the hair follicle (107,108) (Figs. 30-21 and 30-22). The tumor stroma is mildly fibrocellular. There is no significant clefting between tumor and stroma, and mitotic activity is rare (Fig. 30-22). These lesions may have a similar appearance to infundibulocystic basal cell

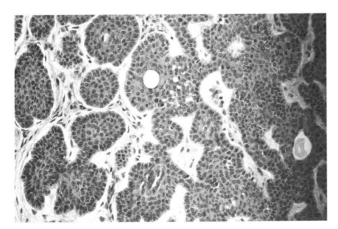

FIGURE 30-22. Basaloid Follicular Hamartoma. The lesion exhibits small basaloid cells lacking necrosis of mitotic activity. A mildly fibrocellular stroma is seen.

carcinoma, but usually can be distinguished on clinical and histologic grounds (107,109,110).

Differential Diagnosis. Linear unilateral basal cell nevus shows similar basaloid proliferations, some of which may resemble trichoepithelioma and basal cell carcinoma. However, the clinical picture is different because the lesion is congenital and unilateral (111).

Pilomatricoma

Pilomatricoma (pilomatrixoma), or calcifying epithelioma of Malherbe, is a tumor with differentiation toward hair cells, particularly hair cortex cells. Pilomatricoma occurs usually as a solitary lesion. The face and the upper extremities are the most common sites. Generally, the tumor varies in diameter from 0.5 to 3.0 cm, but it may be as large as 5 cm. The tumors may arise in persons of any age, but about 40% of them arise in children younger than 10, and about 60% in persons in the first two decades of life (112).

It frequently presents as a firm, deep-seated nodule that is covered by normal skin. Occasionally, however, the tumor is more superficially located, causing a blue-red discoloration of the overlying skin, and, rarely, it protrudes as a sharply demarcated, dark red nodule. Rapid enlargement of a pilomatricoma may occur as the result of formation of a hematoma (113). Perforation may take place with extrusion of parts of the contents (114). Although, as a rule, pilomatricoma is not hereditary, there are a few instances of familial occurrence, and in some of these cases the tumor is associated with myotonic dystrophy (115,116). Pilomatricoma-type changes can be seen in the epidermal cysts of Gardner's syndrome (117). Unusual clinical variants include large, extruding, or perforating examples, multiple eruptive cases, familial cases, and malignant examples termed *pilomatrix carcinoma* (118–122) (see below).

Histopathology. The tumor is sharply demarcated and often surrounded by a connective tissue capsule (Fig. 30-23). It is usually located in the lower dermis and extends into the subcutaneous fat. Embedded in a rather cellular stroma, irregularly shaped islands of epithelial cells are present. As a rule, two types of cells, *basophilic cells* and *shadow cells*, compose the islands (123) (Figs. 30-24 and 30-25). In some tumors, however, basophilic cells are absent. The basophilic cells possess round or elongated, deeply basophilic nuclei and scanty cytoplasm, so that the nuclei lie close together (Fig. 30-24). The cellular borders of the basophilic cells often are indistinct, so that it appears as if the nuclei were embedded in a symplasmic mass. The basophilic cells are arranged either on one side or along the periphery of the tumor islands. In some areas, the transition of basophilic cells into shadow cells is abrupt, whereas in others the transition is gradual. In

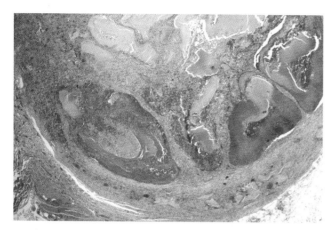

FIGURE 30-23. Pilomatricoma. The tumor is often well-circumscribed and composed of epithelial islands embedded in a rather cellular stroma. Two types of cells comprise the islands: basophilic cells and shadow cells. The basophilic cells resemble hair matrix cells. The shadow cells show a central unstained shadow at the site of the lost nucleus. In the center of the field, one can see transformation of the basophilic cells into shadow cells.

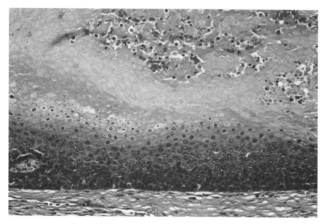

FIGURE 30-24. Pilomatricoma. The transformation of basaloid cells into shadow cells is associated with loss of nuclei.

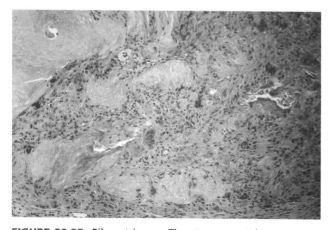

FIGURE 30-25. Pilomatricoma. The stroma contains numerous multinucleated giant cells reacting to tumoral keratin.

areas of gradual transition there are cells showing a gradual loss of nuclei and ultimately appearing as faintly eosinophilic, keratinized shadow cells. The shadow cells have a distinct border and possess a central unstained area as a shadow of the lost nucleus (Figs. 30-24 and 30-25). In tumors of recent origin, numerous areas of basophilic cells usually are present. As the lesion ages, the number of basophilic cells decreases because of development into shadow cells, and in tumors of long standing, few or no basophilic cells remain.

In many tumors, small, round, eosinophilic centers of keratinization are seen within areas of basophilic cells or within aggregates of shadow cells. The keratinization within these centers is abrupt and complete (124). In some tumors, melanin is present, as can be expected in tumors with differentiation toward hair bulbs. It is found most commonly in shadow cells or within melanophages of the stroma. A variant of pilomatricoma with numerous dendritic melanocytes located in the islands of basophilic cells has been described and termed melanocytic matricoma (125–127).

With the von Kossa stain, calcium deposits are found in approximately 75% of the tumors (128). Usually, the calcium is already apparent as deeply basophilic deposits in sections stained with hematoxylin-eosin. Most of the tumors containing calcium are composed largely of shadow cells. The calcium is seen either as fine basophilic granules within the cytoplasm of the shadow cells or as large sheets of amorphous, basophilic material replacing the shadow cells. Occasionally, foci of calcification are seen in the stroma of the tumors. Areas of ossification are seen in 15% to 20% of the cases (129). Ossification takes place in the stroma next to areas of shadow cells, probably through metaplasia of fibroblasts into osteoblasts. Bone morphogenic protein (BMP-2) has been shown in the cytoplasm of shadow cells but not in basophilic cells, indicating a possible role in bone formation (130). Calcium-rich shadow cells may act as inducing factors (131). The stroma of pilomatricomas often shows a considerable foreign-body reaction containing many giant cells adjacent to the shadow cells (Fig. 30-25).

Additional Studies. Pilomatricoma was originally described in 1880 as calcified epithelioma of sebaceous glands; however, it was recognized in 1942 that the cells of the tumor differentiate in the direction of hair cortex cells, a finding that was subsequently confirmed by electron microscopic studies (132,133). On this basis, the designation *pilomatricoma* was suggested (129).

Histochemical studies have revealed in most tumor cells a strongly positive reaction with the periodic acid–Schiff stain for sulfhydryl or disulfide groups. This reaction is indicative of keratinization (128,129,134). As further evidence of keratinization, the shadow cells show strong birefringence in polarized light (135). A very similar birefringence is seen in the keratogenous zone of hair (129).

Electron microscopic examination has revealed a few desmosomes and a moderate number of tonofilaments in the areas of basophilic cells (136). In cells that are in transition to shadow cells, numerous tonofilaments are seen aggregated into thick keratin fibrils. They form keratin without the appearance of keratohyaline granules. A striking resemblance exists between cells that are in transition to shadow cells and cells in the keratogenous zone of normal hair, because both types of cells show thick keratin fibrils concentrically arranged around a faintly visible nucleus. Fully developed shadow cells show numerous fused, electron-dense keratin fibrils surrounding the empty nuclear area (134,136,137).

Several more recent studies, using immunohistochemistry and in-situ hybridization with various cytokeratins and hair specific keratins, further support that pilomatrixomas differentiate toward cortical cells of the normal hair shaft during their maturation process (138–140).

Mutations in β-catenin (*CTNNB1*) have been described in pilomatricomas (141,142). The resulting mutation stabilizes the β-catenin protein, which translocates into the nucleus, where it activates gene transcription through members of the Lef/Tcf family of transcription factors (143).

Differential Diagnosis. The wall of trichilemmal cysts also contains basophilic cells, which as they keratinize gradually lose their nuclei and often undergo calcification. The peripheral layer of basophilic cells in trichilemmal cysts, however, shows a palisading pattern, whereas the basophilic cells of pilomatricoma do not. Furthermore, shadow cells characterized by a central unstained area at the site of the disintegrated nucleus are seen only in pilomatricomas and, exceptionally, in basal cell carcinomas with foci of matricial differentiation (144).

Pilomatrix Carcinoma

Pilomatrix carcinoma is the rare malignant counterpart of pilomatricoma. The lesions have a male predominance and

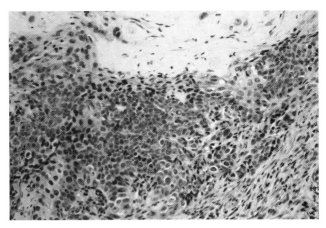

FIGURE 30-27. Pilomatrix Carcinoma. Hyperchromatic, anaplastic cells focally transition into shadow cells (top).

occur in older patients. Some pilomatricomas show apparent transformation into carcinomas (145,146). Other cases are malignant from the onset (147,148). Pilomatrix carcinomas are not necessarily larger than benign pilomatricomas. Pulmonary and bone metastases may occur (120,149,150). The lesions have a tendency to recur if not widely excised (119).

Histopathology. Pilomatrix carcinomas are asymmetrical, cellular, infiltrative neoplasms (Fig. 30-26). Many areas, especially at the periphery of the tumor, show proliferations of large, anaplastic, hyperchromatic basophilic cells with numerous mitoses (Figs. 30-27 and 30-28); however, this can be seen in pilomatricomas on occasion (146). Toward the center of the tumor, there may be transformation of basophilic cells into eosinophilic shadow cells of the type seen in benign pilomatricomas, or there may be large cystic centers containing necrotic debris (148,151). Features which are helpful in making the diagnosis include asymmetry and poor circumscription, presence of several markedly sized and variably shaped basaloid aggregations of tumor cells,

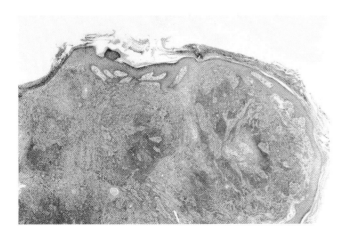

FIGURE 30-26. Pilomatrix Carcinoma. There is a cellular, asymmetrical tumor that infiltrates the dermis.

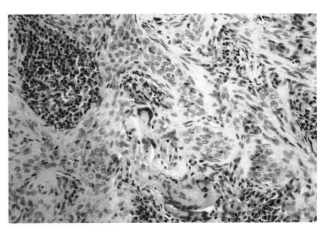

FIGURE 30-28. Pilomatrix Carcinoma. The lesion also focally demonstrates an infiltrative pattern.

continuity of basaloid cells with the epidermis, extensive areas of necrosis en masse, infiltrative growth pattern (Fig. 30-28), and presence of ulceration (152).

Proliferating Trichilemmal Cyst

The proliferating trichilemmal cyst, also referred to as proliferating trichilemmal tumor, is nearly always a single lesion; rarely, there are two proliferating trichilemmal cysts (153,154). Another common designation used for this lesion is proliferating pilar tumor. About 90% of the cases occur on the scalp, with the residual 10% occurring mainly on the back. More than 80% of the patients are women, most of them elderly (155).

Starting as a subcutaneous nodule suggestive of a wen, the tumor may grow into a large, elevated, lobulated mass that may undergo ulceration and thus greatly resemble a squamous cell carcinoma (155). The tumor may occur in association with one or even several trichilemmal cysts of the scalp (156,157) (see Chapter 30). There is evidence that a proliferating trichilemmal cyst may develop from an ordinary trichilemmal cyst (155,158). However, the tumor may also give rise to one or several trichilemmal cysts, which ultimately may separate from it (154). In several instances, rapid enlargement of nodular scalp lesions has indicated malignant transformation (159). In such cases, metastases may arise.

Histopathology. The proliferating trichilemmal cyst, or proliferating trichilemmal tumor, usually is well demarcated from the surrounding tissue (160). It is composed of multiple, variably sized lobules composed of squamous epithelium (Fig. 30-29). Some of the lobules are surrounded by a vitreous layer and show palisading of their peripheral cell layer (154). Characteristically, the epithelium in the center of the lobules abruptly changes into eosinophilic amorphous keratin (Fig. 30-30). This amorphous keratin is of the same type as that seen in the cavity of ordinary trichilemmal cysts (161). In addition to showing trichilemmal keratinization, some proliferating trichilemmal cysts exhibit changes resembling the keratinization of the follicular infundibulum. These changes consist of epidermoid keratinization resulting in horn pearls, some of which resemble "squamous eddies" (155).

The tumor cells in many areas show some degree of nuclear atypia, as well as individual cell keratinization, which at first glance suggests a squamous cell carcinoma (see Fig. 30-30) (156,162). The tumor differs from a squamous cell carcinoma by a rather sharp demarcation from the surrounding stroma as well as an abrupt mode of keratinization (160). Foci of calcification, although generally small, are often present in the areas of amorphous keratin (157,160). Some tumors show vacuolization or clear cell formation of some of the tumor cells as a result of glycogen storage (156,161).

Differential Diagnosis. In addition to its well-circumscribed nature, the presence of numerous sharply demarcated areas of amorphous eosinophilic keratin in the center

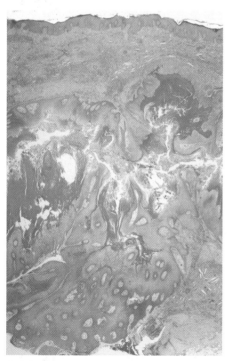

FIGURE 30-29. Proliferating trichilemmal cyst. The tumor is composed of irregularly shaped lobules of squamous epithelium undergoing an abrupt change into amorphous keratin. Central portions of the lobules demonstrate amorphous keratin.

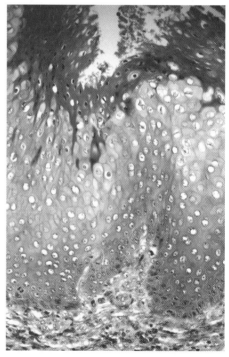

FIGURE 30-30. Proliferating trichilemmal cyst. Large, pale keratinocytes undergo abrupt keratinization without keratohyaline granules.

of the tumor strands and lobules, and the absence of extensive areas of severe atypia and of invasion of the surrounding tissue usually permit differentiation from squamous cell carcinoma.

Additional Studies. Keratinization in proliferating trichilemmal cysts is of the same type as in ordinary trichilemmal cysts. The "trichilemmal" keratinization in both is analogous to that of the outer root sheath as seen normally at the follicular isthmus above the zone of sloughing of the inner root sheath and in the sac surrounding the lower end of the telogen hair (156,163). Analogous to the outer root sheath, proliferating trichilemmal cysts show (a) an abrupt change of squamous epithelium into amorphous keratin; (b) vacuolated cells containing glycogen, like the cells of the outer root sheath; and (c) a prominent glassy layer of collagen surrounding some tumor formations (161). Focal calcification within the amorphous keratin is a feature that proliferating trichilemmal cysts and ordinary trichilemmal cysts have in common.

Malignant Proliferating Trichilemmal Tumor

In rare instances, malignant transformation of proliferating trichilemmal cysts takes place, indicated by rapid enlargement of the nodule (159). There have been several reported instances of metastases, most of them regional (156,164, 165). In one instance, however, the metastases were generalized and fatal (166). Penetration of the tumor into cerebral sinuses has occurred, causing death (167).

Histopathology. Malignant proliferating trichilemmal tumors show extensive areas of severe atypia and invasion of the surrounding tissue (159). Even though areas of trichilemmal keratinization are still evident, tissue invasion and the presence of nuclear atypia and giant nuclei indicate malignancy (166).

Additional Studies. Unlike proliferating trichilemmal cyst, there is loss of CD34 expression (168). DNA aneuploidy and a higher proliferation index have also been observed (168). There appears to be a spectrum of cases ranging from a proliferative trichilemmal cyst to a frankly malignant proliferating trichilemmal tumor (169). In addition, similar to squamous cell carcinomas, loss of heterozygosity at chromosome 17p and increased p53 immunoreactivity has been observed in proliferating trichilemmal cysts (170,171). It has been proposed by some that proliferating trichilemmal cysts may be low-grade carcinomas (172,173). Regardless, both lesions should be treated with wide local excision and adequate follow-up (169).

Trichilemmoma

Trichilemmoma is a fairly common solitary tumor. In addition, multiple facial trichilemmomas are specifically associated with Cowden's disease.

Solitary Trichilemmoma

Solitary trichilemmoma, first recognized as an entity in 1962, generally is a small tumor, 3 to 8 mm in diameter, occurring usually on the face (174,175). Occasionally, it measures several centimeters in diameter (176). It has no characteristic clinical appearance. In some instances, it is found at the base of a cutaneous horn (177).

Histopathology. One or several lobules are seen descending from the surface epidermis into the dermis. In some instances, the lobules are oriented about a central hair-containing follicle (174). A variable number of tumor cells have the appearance of clear cells because of their content of glycogen (Figs. 30-31 and 30-32). The periphery of the tumor lobules usually shows palisading of columnar cells and a distinct, often thickened basement membrane zone resembling the vitreous layer surrounding the lower portion of normal hair follicles (175) (Fig. 30-32). Paradoxically, trichilemmomas do not show the trichilemmal type of keratinization seen in trichilemmal cysts and proliferating trichilemmal cysts. Rather, at the surface, trichilemmomas display epidermoid keratinization, which is frequently pronounced and may even lead to the formation of an overlying cutaneous horn (178).

In *desmoplastic trichilemmoma* there are irregular extensions of cells of the outer root sheath type that project into sclerotic collagen bundles and mimic invasive carcinoma (179) (Figs. 30-33 and 30-34). Superficially, the lesion shows changes of a trichilemmoma, a finding which aids in the distinction from an invasive carcinoma. Additionally, unlike basal cell carcinomas, desmoplastic trichilemmomas stain with CD34 (180).

Differential Diagnosis. In instances with relatively few clear cells and marked hypergranulosis and hyperkeratosis, differentiation from a verruca vulgaris may be difficult. A PAS stain for the demonstration of glycogen may aid in differentiating these two lesions. However, old verrucae,

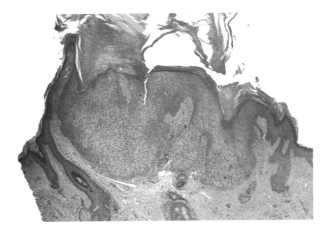

FIGURE 30-31. Trichilemmoma. The tumor shows verrucous hyperplasia with lobular formations extending into the superficial dermis. As a result of their differentiation toward outer root sheath cells, many cells appear clear.

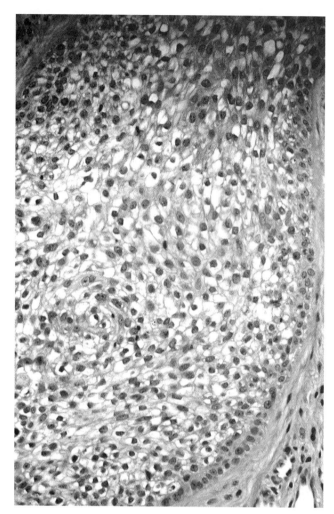

FIGURE 30-32. Trichilemmoma. Many cells demonstrate clear cytoplasm. The peripheral epithelial cells demonstrate palisading.

which often lack viral cytopathic changes, may acquire cytoplasmic glycogen and mimic many features of trichilemmoma. Trichilemmomas differ from ordinary verrucae by their lobulated rather than papillary (verrucous) configuration, by their localization about follicular infundibula, by the presence of basaloid palisading at the periphery of tumor lobules, and by the presence of a thickened, hyalinized basement membrane which can be highlighted by a PAS stain. Molecular studies have not supported the notion that all trichilemmomas result from human papillomavirus infection (181).

Multiple Trichilemmomas in Cowden's Disease

Cowden's disease, or multiple hamartoma syndrome, is an autosomal dominant genodermatosis with distinctive mucocutaneous and systemic findings (182). The syndrome is characterized by multiple hamartomas in several organ sys-

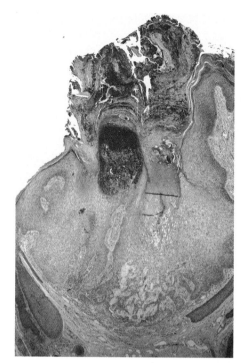

FIGURE 30-33. Desmoplastic trichilemmoma. The lesion exhibits features of a trichilemmoma with focal infiltrative growth in the dermis.

tems including the skin, breast, thyroid, gastrointestinal tract, endometrium, and brain. The mucocutaneous lesions are a near constant manifestation and include trichilemmomas, oral papillomatoses, and acral and palmoplantar keratoses. The most frequent systemic findings include fibrocystic breast disease, breast fibroadenomas, thyroid adenomas, goiter, and intestinal polyposis (183). Individuals are at highest risk for the development of breast cancer, but other visceral malignancies including thyroid and endometrial carcinomas may occur (184,185). An association with

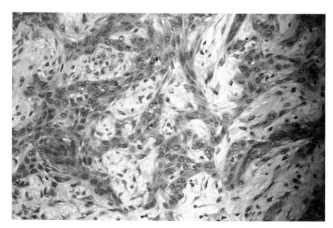

FIGURE 30-34. Desmoplastic trichilemmoma. Cords of bland epithelial cells infiltrate the dermis mimicking invasive carcinoma.

Lhermitte–Duclos disease (dysplastic cerebellar gangliocytoma) and Bannayan–Riley–Ruvalcaba syndrome (macrocephaly, lipomatosis, hemangiomatosis, and speckled penis) has been noted, suggesting that they are all overlapping syndromes characterized by germline phosphatase and tensin homologue (PTEN) mutations (186–189).

Multiple trichilemmomas are found in all patients with Cowden's disease (184). They are limited to the face, where they are found mainly about the mouth, nose, and ears. They consist of flesh-colored, pink or brown papules that may resemble verrucae vulgaris (190). Multiple trichilemmomas precede the development of breast cancer and thus can identify women with a high risk of developing this cancer (184). Thus, recognition of Cowden's disease is important because of the high incidence of breast cancer in women with this disease. In addition, there may be closely set oral papules, giving the lips, gingiva, and tongue a characteristic "cobblestone" appearance, as well as multiple small acral keratoses. Small hyperkeratotic papillomas are commonly found on the distal portions of the extremities (191).

The gene for Cowden's disease was localized to chromosome 10q22-23 and subsequently identified as *PTEN* (deleted on chromosome 10) (192,193). PTEN encodes a dual-specificity phosphatase and is the major 3-phosphatase in the phosphoinositol-3-kinase pathway that inactivates signals from (PI-3K)/AKT kinases, an antiapoptotic pathway; therefore, loss of PTEN function results in increased antiapoptotic signaling in the PI-3K/AKT pathway (194). Mutational analysis has revealed germline mutations in the gene in multiple members of afflicted families (195,196).

Histopathology. Multiple biopsy specimens may be needed to find the diagnostic histologic picture of trichilemmoma in the facial lesions. Thus, in one series, only 29 of 53 facial lesions showed findings diagnostic of trichilemmoma (178).

The oral lesions may show a fibromatous nodule composed of relatively acellular fibers patterned in whorls (sclerotic fibroma) or fibrovascular tissue with acanthosis (178, 191,197). The extrafascial cutaneous lesions may resemble verruca vulgaris or acrokeratosis verruciformis (see Chapters 6 and 26). Only few specimens show mild follicular hyperplasia as seen in trichilemmoma (191).

Differential Diagnosis. See Differential Diagnosis in Solitary Trichilemmoma section.

Tumor of the Follicular Infundibulum

The tumor of the follicular infundibulum was first described in 1961 (198). It usually occurs as a solitary, flat, keratotic papule on the face (198). Clinically, it may resemble a basal cell carcinoma. Rarely, multiple papules are present (199). Additionally, lesions may occur in Cowden's disease and nevus sebaceous (200).

Histopathology. There is a plate-like growth of epithelial cells in the upper dermis extending parallel to the epi-

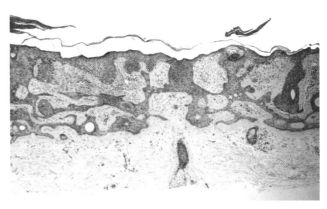

FIGURE 30-35. Tumor of the follicular infundibulum. A plate-like growth of anastamosing epithelial cords extends parallel to the epidermis in the upper dermis and shows multiple connections with the epidermis.

dermis and showing multiple connections with the lower margin of the epidermis (Fig. 30-35). The peripheral cell layer of the tumor plate shows palisading, and the centrally located cells show a pale-staining cytoplasm as a result of their glycogen content; small cysts resembling the follicular infundibulum are often seen (Fig. 30-36). Small hair follicles enter the tumor plate from below and lose their identity; they are then no longer recognizable (198). Along the lower margin of the plate, there may be invaginations that resemble hair papillae (199). Focal sebaceous differentiation and ductal proliferation have been seen (201,202).

Differential Diagnosis. The plate-like growth with multiple connections to the epidermis resembles superficial basal cell carcinoma, which may also show peripheral palisading. However, the cells of the tumor of the follicular infundibulum possess a greater amount of cytoplasm, in which, furthermore, PAS-positive material is present (203). Atypia, necrosis, and mitotic activity are generally lacking. Other

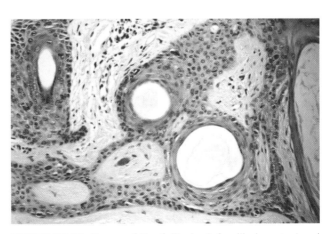

FIGURE 30-36. Tumor of the follicular infundibulum. Lesional cells demonstrate focal cytoplasmic clearing, horn cyst formation, and peripheral palisading.

entities to consider are trichilemmoma, inverted follicular keratosis, and a seborrheic keratosis (154). The key histologic finding in tumor of the follicular infundibulum, as mentioned above, is the presence of a plate-like growth of epithelium with multiple connections to the epidermis.

Trichilemmal Horn and Trichilemmoma Horn

Trichilemmal and trichilemmoma horns clinically have the appearance of a cutaneous horn, as seen in several other conditions. Both are solitary. The more common trichilemmal horn may be seen in many different areas; the trichilemmoma horn occurs on the face or scalp (177,204).

Histopathology. In a *trichilemmal horn*, trichilemmal keratinization occurs. At the base of the lesion, there is a prominent basement membrane zone, with palisading of the basal cell layer and a tendency of the viable epithelial cells to become large and pale staining. As trichilemmal cells, they keratinize without a granular layer (204,205). Some nuclear atypicality analogous to a carcinoma *in situ* has been observed (206). A seborrheic keratosis or verruca vulgaris with exuberant trichilemmal keratinization may mimic a trichilemmal horn (207). Immunohistochemical staining with CD34 has been shown confirming an outer root sheath origin (208).

In a trichilemmoma horn, a trichilemmoma is seen at the base of the lesion. At the surface, the trichilemmoma shows a cutaneous horn displaying epidermoid keratinization that is frequently pronounced, with a thick granular layer and massive hyperkeratosis (177) (Fig. 30-31).

Trichilemmal Carcinoma

Trichilemmal carcinoma occurs largely on the face or ears as a slow-growing epidermal papule, indurated plaque, or nodule that may ulcerate (209–213). Unlike trichilemmomas, trichilemmal carcinoma is an unusual finding in Cowden's disease (214). Recurrence and metastases are uncommon, and conservative surgical excision with clear margins is curative (209,211,215).

Histopathology. This tumor is histologically invasive and consists of cytologically atypical clear cells resembling those of the outer root sheath (18). The lesional cells have abundant glycogenated clear cytoplasm. The lesional cells form solid, lobular, or trabecular growth patterns with foci of pilar-type keratinization and with peripheral palisading of cells with subnuclear vacuolization. Cytologic atypia is prominent, and there may be pagetoid spread of lesional cells into the epidermis, mimicking melanoma. The cells have hyperchromatic, pleomorphic, very large nuclei (215). The cytoplasm contains glycogen, and this is PAS-positive and diastase sensitive (213). Areas of trichilemmal keratinization are frequently present (216).

Differential Diagnosis. A trichilemmal carcinoma may resemble a trichilemmoma by showing a lobular architecture or may resemble a "tumor of the follicular infundibulum" by replacing the surface epidermis (213,215). Differentiation from other carcinomas with clear cell features such as squamous cell carcinoma, basal cell carcinoma, and sebaceous carcinoma may be difficult. Typical features of these carcinomas are usually seen adjacent to the clear cell component.

Additional Studies. The pathogenesis of trichilemmal carcinomas is unclear. The distribution of lesions suggests that sunlight may play a role. A few cases have been reported in association with a burn scar, irradiation, and xeroderma pigmentosa (212,217,218). Loss of p53 has been shown in a trichilemmal carcinoma arising from a proliferating trichilemmal cyst (219).

TUMORS WITH SEBACEOUS DIFFERENTIATION

Nevus Sebaceus

Nevus sebaceus of Jadassohn is nearly always located on the scalp or the face as a single lesion and is present at birth. In childhood, it consists of a circumscribed, slightly raised, hairless plaque that is often linear in configuration but may be round or irregularly shaped. In puberty, the lesion becomes verrucous and nodular (220).

Less commonly, nevus sebaceus consists of multiple extensive lesions found on the face, neck, or trunk. Usually, at least some of the lesions have a linear configuration (221). In addition, some patients with extensive nevus sebaceus show as evidence of a "neurocutaneous syndrome," epilepsy and mental retardation, neurologic defects, or skeletal deformities (222–225). In some patients, the linear nevus is partially a linear nevus sebaceus and partially a linear epidermal nevus (223,224). Thus, the "neurocutaneous syndrome" that is associated with nevus sebaceus overlaps with the abnormalities associated with the epidermal nevus syndrome, in which skeletal deformities and central nervous system abnormalities may also occur (226). The involvement of the central nervous system that may be seen in extensive cases of both linear nevus sebaceus and linear epidermal nevus closely resembles that of tuberous sclerosis by computed tomography and x-ray studies (227) (see Chapter 33).

Histopathology. The sebaceous glands in nevus sebaceus follow the pattern of normal sebaceous glands during infancy, childhood, and adolescence. In the first few months of life, they are well developed (228). During childhood the sebaceous glands in nevus sebaceus are underdeveloped, and therefore, greatly reduced in size and number. Thus, the diagnosis of nevus sebaceus may be missed. However, the presence of incompletely differentiated hair structures is typical of nevus sebaceus. There often are cords of undifferentiated cells resembling the embryonic stage of hair follicles (220). Some hair structures consist of dilated, keratin-filled infundibula showing multiple buds of undifferentiated cells.

At puberty, the lesion assumes its diagnostic histologic appearance. Large numbers of mature or nearly mature sebaceous glands and overlying papillomatous hyperplasia of the epidermis are seen (Fig. 30-37). The hair structures remain small except for occasional dilated infundibula. There are often buds of undifferentiated cells that resemble foci of basal cell carcinoma and represent malformed hair germs (229) (Fig. 30-38). Ectopic apocrine glands develop in about two-thirds of the patients at puberty and sometimes at a younger age (220,229) (Fig. 30-37). These glands are located deep in the dermis beneath the masses of sebaceous gland lobules.

Quite commonly, in addition to the infantile and adolescent phases, there is a third stage in adulthood when various types of appendageal tumors develop secondarily within lesions of nevus sebaceus. A syringocystadenoma papilliferum has been found in 8% to 19% of the lesions of nevus sebaceus (220) (Figs. 30-37 and 30-39). In two recent large case series, the most commonly associated appendageal tumors were trichoblastoma and syringocystadenoma papilliferum (230,231). Less commonly found appendage tumors include nodular hidradenoma, syringoma, sebaceous epithelioma, chondroid syringoma, trichilemmoma, and proliferating trichilemmal cyst (220,232,233).

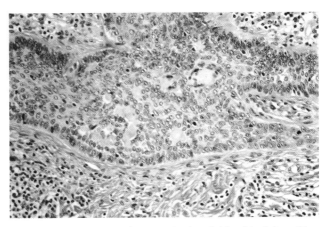

FIGURE 30-38. Nevus sebaceus. The basaloid epithelial proliferations often resemble basal cell carcinoma. However, these proliferations also demonstrate features of appendageal neoplasms as evidenced by the deposition of hyaline material within the lesion.

Basaloid epithelial proliferations resembling basal cell carcinoma are clinically evident in 5% to 7% of the cases of nevus sebaceus (Fig. 30-38) (229,234). In many instances, however, basal cell carcinomas are found that are small, clinically not apparent, and that show no aggressive growth pattern (229). It is not always possible to differentiate histologically between a basal cell carcinoma and "basaloid proliferations" that arise in malformed hair germs and that are seen in as many as half of all cases of nevus sebaceus (Fig. 30-38) (234). As original evidence that the basal cell carcinoma-like proliferations in many instances are not true basal cell carcinomas, some proliferations contain Sudan-positive granules as an indication of sebaceous differentiation or glycogen as an indication of pilar differentiation (235). Other proliferations show follicular differentiation with formation of hair papillae and hair bulbs. Furthermore in critical reviews, several groups have proposed that most reported basal cell carcinomas

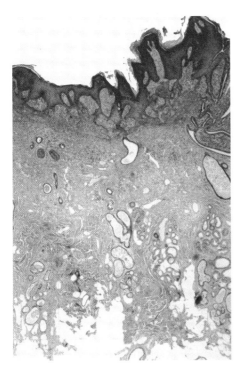

FIGURE 30-37. Nevus sebaceus. There is epidermal hyperplasia and papillomatosis. Superficially, a basaloid epithelial neoplasm is seen and dilated apocrine glands are present in the dermis. This scalp lesion lacks anagen follicles.

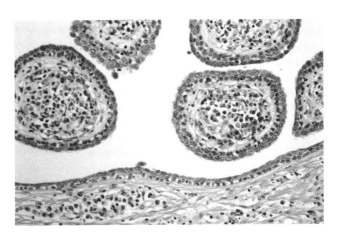

FIGURE 30-39. Nevus sebaceus. A syringocystadenoma papilleferum was also present in this lesion.

arising in nevus sebaceous are actually trichoblastomas (230,231,236).

In only rare instances does a squamous cell carcinoma develop within a nevus sebaceus. This may be associated either with regional lymph node metastasis or with generalized metastases (237). Apocrine carcinomas and, in one instance, a malignant eccrine poroma have developed in nevi sebaceae, and these lesions, too, may lead to regional or even generalized metastases (237,238).

Additional Studies. The frequent association of nevus sebaceus with other appendageal tumors and with apocrine glands suggests that nevus sebaceus is derived from the primary epithelial germ (229). Moreover as has been reported in basal cell carcinomas (239,240), loss of heterozygosity of the human homologue of the Drosophila patched gene (*Ptch*) has been demonstrated in nevus sebaceus (241). This could partly explain the association of basal cell carcinomas and other basaloid appendageal tumors with nevus sebaceus. However, a separate study of eleven lesions of nevus sebaceus found no demonstrable loss of heterozygosity (242). The reason for the discrepancy is uncertain; however, differences such as sampling during microdissection of other cell populations may account for the observed difference (242).

Sebaceous Hyperplasia

The lesions of sebaceous hyperplasia nearly always occur on the face, chiefly on the forehead and cheeks, in elderly persons. It has also been reported in the vulva, penis, and areola (243–246). The hyperplasia rarely occurs in early adult life (247). Apparent familial forms have also been reported (76,248). It clinically presents as one or, more commonly, several elevated, small, soft, yellow, slightly umbilicated papules. The usual size is 2 to 3 mm in diameter.

Histopathology. Most lesions consist of a single greatly enlarged sebaceous gland composed of numerous lobules grouped around a centrally located, wide sebaceous duct (Fig. 30-40). Its opening to the surface corresponds to the central umbilication of the lesion. Serial sections show that all sebaceous lobules grouped around the central duct are connected with that duct. Large lesions may consist of several enlarged sebaceous glands and contain several ducts, with sebaceous lobules grouped around each of them. Although some sebaceous gland lobules appear fully mature, others show more than one peripheral row of undifferentiated, generative cells in which there are few or no lipid droplets (249).

Additional Studies. Labeling with tritiated thymidine has shown that the migration of sebocytes from the basal cell area to the center of the sebaceous lobules and into the sebaceous duct is distinctly slower in cases of sebaceous hyperplasia than in normal sebaceous glands (249). Microsatellite instability has been detected in very few cases of sebaceous hyperplasia as compared to true sebaceous

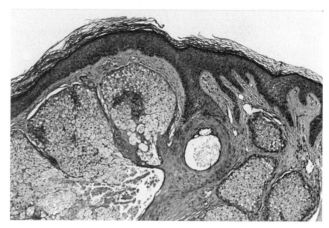

FIGURE 30-40. Sebaceous hyperplasia. The lesion consists of an enlarged sebaceous gland lying in close proximity to the epidermis.

neoplasms (250,251) (see Muir–Torre syndrome). Immunohistochemical staining for androgen receptors has been shown to be fairly specific for sebaceous lesions as compared to basal cell carcinomas, squamous cell carcinomas, and clear cell acanthomas (252).

Differential Diagnosis. In rhinophyma, which also shows large sebaceous glands and ducts, there is no grape-like grouping of the sebaceous lobules around the ducts, and the lesion is not sharply demarcated. In nevus sebaceus, ductal structures are less apparent than in sebaceous hyperplasia, and apocrine glands are often found beneath the sebaceous glands.

Fordyce's Spots and Montgomery's Tubercles

In Fordyce's spots, groups of minute, yellow, globoid lesions are observed on the vermilion border of the lips or on the oral mucosa. The incidence of the disorder increases with age, so that 70% to 80% of elderly persons show such lesions, which represents ectopic sebaceous glands (253). Montgomery's tubercles are ectopic mature sebaceous glands located on the areola of the breast (254).

Histopathology. Each lesion consists of a group of small but mature sebaceous lobules situated around a small sebaceous duct leading to the surface epithelium (253,255) (Fig. 30-41). Because of the small size of the sebaceous duct, serial sections may be required to demonstrate the duct.

Sebaceous Adenoma

Sebaceous adenoma presents as a yellow, circumscribed nodule located on either the face or scalp. Prior to 1968, sebaceous adenoma was regarded as a rare solitary tumor, and there were few publications about it (256–258). Since then, however, both solitary and multiple lesions have been

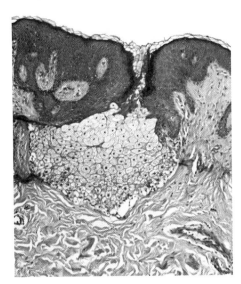

FIGURE 30-41. Montgomery's Tubercle. A mature sebaceous lobule in continuity with the epidermis is seen.

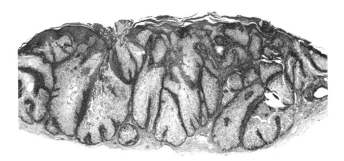

FIGURE 30-42. Sebaceous adenoma. The tumor is composed of enlarged sebaceous lobules of varying size and shape.

well documented in patients with Muir–Torre syndrome (see below).

Histopathology. On histologic examination, sebaceous adenoma is sharply demarcated from the surrounding tissue. It is composed of incompletely differentiated sebaceous lobules that are irregular in size and shape (Fig. 30-42). Two types of cells are present in the lobules. The cells of the first type are identical to the cells present at the periphery of normal sebaceous glands and represent undifferentiated basaloid cells (Fig. 30-43). The cells of the second type are mature sebaceous cells (Fig. 30-43). In addition, there often are some cells in a transitional stage between these two types (259). Distribution of the basaloid and sebaceous cells within the lobules varies. Some lobules contain mainly sebaceous cells and thereby resemble mature sebaceous lobules. Frequently, the proportion of mature sebaceous cells exceeds the surrounding basaloid cells (Fig. 30-43). However, at most the two types of cells occur in approximately equal proportions. Fat stains on properly preserved specimens reveal the presence of lipid material in the sebaceous and transitional cells. Some large lobules contain cystic spaces in their center formed by the disintegration of mature sebaceous cells. Also, there may be foci of squamous epithelium with keratinization. These foci probably represent areas with differentiation toward cells of the infundibulum. Cystic sebaceous adenomas seem to occur exclusively in patients with Muir–Torre syndrome (260).

Differential Diagnosis. In terms of differentiation, sebaceous adenoma stands between sebaceous hyperplasia, in which sebaceous lobules appear fully or nearly fully matured, and sebaceous epithelioma or sebaceoma (see below), in which the tumor is composed predominantly or irregularly shaped cell masses and the percentage of tumor cells with sebaceous differentiation is far less than 50%. Sebaceous adenoma and sebaceous epithelioma lack nuclear atypia and invasive, asymmetric growth patterns, which are hallmarks of sebaceous carcinoma. Considerable mitotic activity in the basaloid regions may be present in either, however.

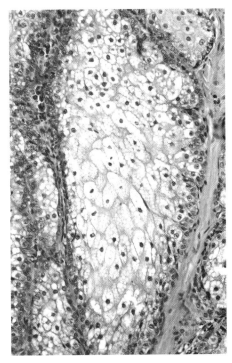

FIGURE 30-43. Sebaceous adenoma. In the lobules, two types of mature cells can be recognized: basaloid and sebaceous. However, sebaceous cells predominate. Cytologic atypia is not seen.

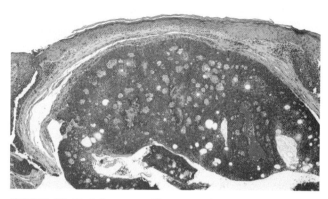

FIGURE 30-44. Sebaceoma. The tumor is a well-circumscribed nodule exhibiting focal cystic change and containing basaloid epithelial cells. Scattered areas of clearer (sebaceous) cells are seen.

Sebaceoma (Sebaceous Epithelioma)

Clinically, sebaceoma, or sebaceous epithelioma, varies from a circumscribed nodule to that of an ill-defined plaque. Some of the lesions are yellow (261). Most lesions are located on the face or scalp. In addition to occurring as a primary lesion, a sebaceous epithelioma occasionally arises within a nevus sebaceus (220,229). Sebaceous epitheliomas may also be found among the multiple sebaceous neoplasms that occur in association with multiple visceral carcinomas and are referred to as Muir–Torre syndrome (see below).

Histopathology. The histologic spectrum extends from that seen in sebaceous adenoma to lesions that may be difficult to distinguish from sebaceous carcinoma. Generally, a sebaceoma shows either a well-circumscribed nodule or irregularly shaped cell masses in which more than half of the cells are undifferentiated basaloid cells but in which there are significant aggregates of mature sebaceous cells and of transitional cells (262) (Figs. 30-44 and 30-45). Disintegra-

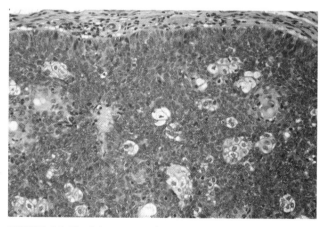

FIGURE 30-45. Sebaceoma. The majority of the lesion is composed of undifferentiated basaloid cells with islands of sebaceous cells.

tion of sebaceous cells is seen in some areas (261). Lesions verging on a sebaceous carcinoma show some degree of irregularity in the arrangement of the cell masses, and, although the majority of cells are basaloid cells, many cells show differentiation toward sebaceous cells (263). Recently a verruca/seborrheic keratosis type of sebaceoma has been described, in which the upper part of the lesion mimics a verruca or seborrheic keratosis (264).

Differential Diagnosis. Criteria that may be of assistance in differentiating sebaceous adenoma from sebaceoma include the often greater size and depth of the latter, and the lack of structures resembling normal sebaceous lobules. Nuclear atypia is "rare," and mitoses may be numerous in sebaceomas, in contrast to adenomas, in which they are few or absent (265).

Muir–Torre Syndrome

The Muir–Torre syndrome is defined by the combined occurrence of at least one sebaceous skin tumor and one internal malignancy in the same patient. Since 1967, when the first publication by Muir appeared concerning the coexistence of frequently multiple sebaceous tumors and usually multiple visceral carcinomas, scores of cases have been reported (266,267). Keratoacanthomas also have occurred in these patients, in some cases without sebaceous lesions, in association with visceral malignancies (268,269). The cutaneous lesions can often precede the first manifestation of internal malignancy (270).

Among the internal malignancies, carcinoma of the colon is the most common malignancy, although a wide tumor spectrum exists including carcinomas of the genitourinary tract (including bladder, renal pelvis, ovary, and uterus), breast, head and neck, small intestinal, and lymphoma (267, 270). Also common are adenomatous colonic polyps. Many of the malignant tumors are of relatively low malignancy, with only a slight tendency to metastasize (271).

Cutaneous lesions vary from just 1 to more than 100 lesions (272). Although the lesion in many instances is recognizable as a sebaceous tumor by its color or as a keratoacanthoma by its crater, histologic examination may be required to establish a diagnosis.

Histopathology. Sebaceous adenomas are the most distinctive cutaneous markers of the Muir–Torre syndrome. They may be solid, cystic, or keratoacanthoma-like (259). Cystic sebaceous adenomas seem to occur exclusively in patients with Muir–Torre syndrome (260,273). Although ordinary keratoacanthomas occur in the Muir–Torre syndrome, often they have an accompanying sebaceous proliferation (274). In addition to sebaceous adenomas, sebaceomas, and basal cell carcinomas with sebaceous differentiation, there are tumors with unusual appearance, so that a hard-to-classify sebaceous proliferation should be considered as a possible manifestation of the Muir–Torre syndrome (274). Also, sebaceous carcinomas occur, but no metastases have been reported (272,275).

Genetics. A genetic predisposition was described in some cases of the Muir–Torre syndrome, and the Muir–Torre syndrome has been found in association with the "cancer family syndrome," now known as hereditary nonpolyposis colorectal carcinoma (267,276). Muir–Torre syndrome shares several clinical and pathologic characteristics with hereditary nonpolyposis colorectal carcinoma syndrome (276). Microsatellite instability has been demonstrated in a subset of patients with Muir–Torre syndrome (277). Subsequently, germline mutations in the DNA mismatch repair genes *hMLH1* and *hMSH2* have been found (278–280). The presence of microsatellite instability in sebaceous neoplasms and even benign skin lesions is helpful in the detection of an underlying inherited DNA mismatch repair defect (250,281). Moreover, immunohistochemical staining for MSH2 or MLH1 protein expression in MTS-associated skin tumors can also be used as a diagnostic screening tool to identify patients with germline mutations (282,283).

Sebaceous Carcinoma

Sebaceous carcinomas have been traditionally classified into ocular and extraocular types. The ocular type most frequently occurs on the eyelids, where it originates from the meibomian glands and less commonly from the glands of Zeis. Extraocular sebaceous carcinoma has been reported most commonly on the head and neck, but also in the vulva, penis, and rarely other locations (284–286). On the eyelids, sebaceous carcinoma may be easily mistaken for chronic blepharoconjunctivitis or a chalazion (287). On extraocular sites, sebaceous carcinoma usually manifests itself as a nodule that may or may not be ulcerated (263,288).

Sebaceous carcinomas of the eyelids quite frequently cause regional metastases. Also, there may be orbital invasion, and in 22% of the cases reported in one study, death resulted from visceral metastases (289). Extraocular sebaceous carcinomas also may cause regional metastases (290–292). However, death resulting from visceral metastasis in extraocular sebaceous carcinomas originally was thought to be uncommon (288,293). Recently it has been suggested that extraocular sebaceous carcinoma can widely metastasize and cause death just as frequently as ocular types (294). The sebaceous carcinomas that may be found among the multiple sebaceous neoplasms occurring in association with multiple visceral carcinomas in the Muir–Torre syndrome do not metastasize, although the visceral malignant tumors may (295). In some instances, a sebaceous carcinoma represents the only cutaneous manifestation of the syndrome (296).

Histopathology. The irregular lobular formations show great variations in the size of the lobules (Fig. 30-46). Al-

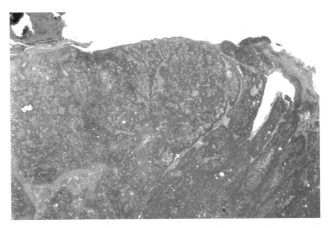

FIGURE 30-46. Sebaceous carcinoma. Irregular epithelial lobules are associated with epidermal ulceration and an infiltrative growth pattern in the dermis composed of sebaceous and undifferentiated cells showing considerable variation in the shape and size of their nuclei. The undifferentiated cells differ from the undifferentiated cells of sebaceous epithelioma by showing greater atypicality of their nuclei and an eosinophilic rather than a basophilic cytoplasm.

though many cells are undifferentiated, distinct sebaceous cells showing a foamy cytoplasm are present in the center of most lobules (288) (Figs 46 and 47). Many undifferentiated cells and sebaceous cells appear atypical, showing considerable nuclear and nucleolar pleomorphism (292) (Fig. 30-47). Also, many of the undifferentiated cells have an eosinophilic cytoplasm, and when fat stains are used on frozen sections, the cells are found to contain fine lipid globules (287). Some of the large lobules show areas composed of atypical keratinizing cells, as seen in squamous cell carcinoma (263).

Sebaceous carcinomas of the eyelids in nearly half of the cases examined show a pagetoid spread of malignant cells in the conjunctival epithelium or the epidermis of the skin of the lid or both (289). These changes are seen very rarely in

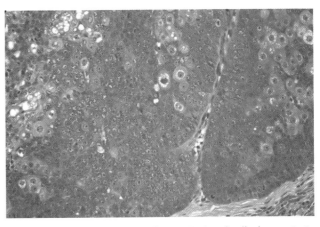

FIGURE 30-47. Sebaceous carcinoma. Lesional cells demonstrate marked cytologic atypia, mitotic activity, and focal sebaceous differentiation.

extraocular sebaceous carcinoma (293). The pagetoid cells contain no mucopolysaccharides but stain positively for fat with oil red O (289). Recognition of the pagetoid growth pattern in biopsy material can be essential to recognition of the existence of an underlying sebaceous carcinoma (297).

Additional Studies. Certain strains of human papilloma virus have been implicated in the pathogenesis of sebaceous carcinoma (298). Mutations in the p53 gene have been seen in invasive but not *in situ* sebaceous carcinoma, and p53 immunohistochemical staining for proliferating cell nuclear antigen seem to have some prognostic value (299,300).

Differential Diagnosis. The tumor cells in sebaceous carcinoma are often large and squamoid in appearance, or show basaloid differentiation with only inconspicuous lipidization. In the latter case, the tumor must be distinguished from basal cell carcinomas with sebaceous differentiation, and in the former case the differential diagnosis includes squamous cell carcinomas with hydropic changes (301,302). Other malignant neoplasms with clear cells must also be considered, including metastatic lesions (294).

Sebaceous carcinomas do not show the typical changes seen in basal cell carcinomas. Instead, the undifferentiated cells of sebaceous carcinoma show a more eosinophilic cytoplasm, greater cytologic atypia, and greater invasiveness (303). Clear-cell squamous cell carcinoma usually shows evidence of keratinization in the form of dyskeratotic cells and squamous parakeratotic whorls. Using an immunohistochemical battery, including epithelial membrane antigen (EMA), anti-BCA-255 (BRST-1), and CAM 5.2 can be helpful in distinguishing sebaceous carcinoma from basal cell carcinoma and squamous cell carcinoma (304).

The malignant neoplasms with clear cells do not show sebaceous differentiation. The cytoplasmic clearing is due to glycogen accumulation, which causes the nuclei to be positioned eccentrically. In contrast, neoplastic cells with sebaceous differentiation show scalloped centrally situated nuclei and microvacuolated cytoplasm secondary to lipid deposits. When sebaceous carcinoma is suspected or found at frozen section, additional sections should be saved for fat stains. Sebaceous ductal differentiation consists of ductal structures lined by an eosinophilic corrugated cuticle similar to that of the normal sebaceous duct. Finally, metastases to the skin from malignant neoplasms composed of clear cells, namely, renal, breast, bladder, and prostatic carcinoma or melanoma, may mimic also sebaceous carcinoma. Histochemical and immunohistochemical methods can be helpful in narrowing the differential diagnosis appropriately (304).

As in other malignant adnexal neoplasms, zones of necrosis, marked nuclear atypia, and abnormal mitotic figures are common in sebaceous carcinoma (Fig. 30-47). Pagetoid proliferation of tumor cells in the epidermis or conjunctiva may extend widely and confers a poorer prognosis. Other adverse prognostic attributes include multi-

centric involvement, poor differentiation (i.e., sparse lipid), necrosis, paucity of reactive lymphocytes, extensive local invasion, and vascular or bony invasion (300). Metastases first involve regional lymph nodes of the periauricular, submaxillary, and cervical chains. Visceral spread may occur and lead to death. Additional criteria that may be of assistance in differentiating sebaceous carcinoma and sebaceoma are that carcinomas are larger, asymmetric, and poorly circumscribed, whereas sebaceomas may extend into the subcutis but are circumscribed and symmetrical. Carcinomas may ulcerate the epidermis, and there may be extensive necrosis ("necrosis en masse"). The relative percentage of differentiated (vacuolated) to undifferentiated (nonvacuolated) sebocytes varies but tends to be higher in sebaceomas. Nuclear atypia is often striking, and mitotic figures are numerous and sometimes atypical in carcinomas. Sebaceomas in contrast lack striking nuclear atypia, but may have few or many mitoses (265).

TUMORS WITH APOCRINE DIFFERENTIATION

Apocrine Nevus

Large numbers of mature apocrine glands are frequently present in lesions of nevus sebaceus and syringocystadenoma papilliferum. However, the pure apocrine nevus is a rare tumor. Apocrine nevi have presented as papules, facial nodules, and, most frequently, as soft tissue masses of the axillae (305–309).

Histopathology. These lesions are comprised of increased numbers of apocrine glands, usually situated in the reticular dermis with occasional extension into subcutaneous tissue (305–313).

Immunohistochemistry. Studies demonstrate positive staining for carcinoembryonic antigen, gross cystic disease fluid protein, epithelial membrane antigen, and low-molecular-weight keratins (307,313,314). Lesions are typically negative for S-100 and high-molecular-weight keratins.

Apocrine Hidrocystoma

Apocrine hidrocystoma occurs usually as a solitary, translucent cystic nodule (315–317). The term "apocrine cystadenoma" has also been used to describe these lesions (315). Lesional diameter usually ranges from 1 to 15 mm; however, "giant" lesions measuring 20 mm have been described (318). Frequently, the lesions have a blue hue and can resemble a blue nevus. The usual location of apocrine hidrocystoma is on the face, but it is occasionally seen on the ears, scalp, chest, shoulders, or vulva (317,319–324). Multiple apocrine hidrocystomas are rarely encountered (325,326). Lesions described as occurring on the penis have been reclassified as median raphe cysts (327).

The blue color in some of the cysts is not fully explained. According to most authors, it is a Tyndall effect caused by the scattering of light in a colloidal system and the resultant reflection of blue light (319,325).

Histopathology. The dermis contains one or several large cystic spaces into which papillary projections often extend (Fig. 30-48). The inner surface of the cyst and the papillary projections are lined by a row of columnar secretory cells of variable height showing "decapitation" secretion indicative of apocrine secretion (Fig. 30-49). Peripheral to the layer of secretory cells are elongated myoepithelial cells, their long axes running parallel to the cyst wall (319). In some cases, one finds superficially located lumina lined by a double layer of ductal epithelium in addition to the cysts lined by secretory cells (315).

Additional Studies. The apocrine nature of the secretion of the luminal cells has been demonstrated by the presence of numerous large PAS-positive, diastase-resistant granules in the secretory cells, and by electron microscopy. Electron microscopic examination shows abundant secretory granules of moderate density and uniform internal structure in the secretory cells of apocrine hidrocystoma, particularly in their luminal portion, and evidence of apocrine secretion (328–330).

The apocrine hidrocystoma can be regarded as a cystic adenoma rather than as a retention cyst because the secretory cells do not appear flattened, as they would be in a retention cyst, and because papillary projections extend into the lumen of the cystic spaces (315).

Differential Diagnosis. Eccrine hidrocystomas, which are lined by ductal cells, differ from apocrine hidrocystomas by the absence of decapitation secretion, of PAS-positive granules, and of myoepithelial cells. However, those portions of an apocrine hidrocystoma in which the cystic spaces are lined by ductal epithelium have the same appearance as the cystic spaces in eccrine hidrocystomas, except that the lat-

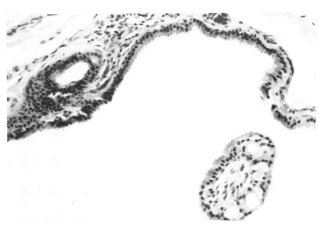

FIGURE 30-49. Apocrine hidrocystoma (cystadenoma). The cyst is lined by a single row of columnar cells showing *decapitation secretion*. Peripheral to the row of secretory cells are elongated myoepithelial cells.

ter usually are unilocular, and apocrine hidrocystomas are often multilocular. Median raphe cysts of the penis, which have been mistakenly reported as apocrine hidrocystomas, show a pseudostratified columnar cyst wall without evidence of decapitation secretion and without a row of myoepithelial cells (327).

Hidradenoma Papilliferum

Hidradenoma papilliferum usually occurs in women, usually on the labia majora or in the perineal or perianal region (331–334). In males, it has been reported as a perineal lesion or ectopically as an arm lesion (335,336). Occurrences on the upper eyelid and in the external ear canal have been reported (337,338). The tumor is covered by normal skin and measures only a few millimeters in diameter. Malignant changes have been reported in hidradenoma papilliform, as aggressive adenosquamous or squamous cell carcinomas (339,340).

Histopathology. The tumor represents an adenoma with apocrine differentiation (341). Located in the dermis, it is well circumscribed and surrounded by a fibrous capsule, and shows no connection with the overlying epidermis (Fig. 30-50). Some tumors have a peripheral epithelial wall showing areas of keratinization (197). Within the tumor, one observes tubular and cystic structures (Fig. 30-51). Papillary folds project into the cystic spaces. The lumina are lined occasionally with only a single row of columnar cells, which show an oval, pale-staining nucleus located near the base, a faintly eosinophilic cytoplasm, and active decapitation secretion as seen in the secretory cells of apocrine glands (341) (Fig. 30-52). Usually, the lumina are surrounded by a double layer of cells consisting of an inner layer of secretory cells and of an outer layer of small cuboidal cells with deeply basophilic nuclei, which are myoepithelial cells (342) (Fig. 30-52).

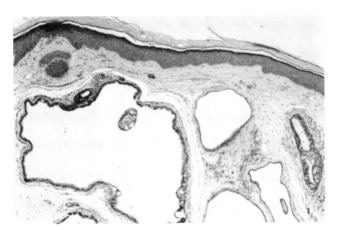

FIGURE 30-48. Apocrine hidrocystoma (cystadenoma). The dermis contains a multi-loculated cystic lesion lined by epithelial cells with occasional papillary projections.

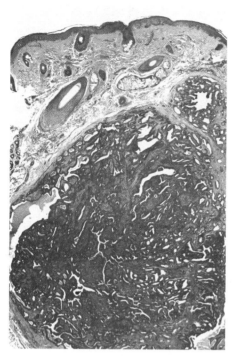

FIGURE 30-50. Hidradenoma papilliferum. The tumor consists of a well-circumscribed dermal nodule with scattered cystic and branching spaces.

Additional Studies. The apocrine nature of the secretion in hidradenoma papilliferum has been established by histochemical, enzyme histochemical, and electron microscopic examinations.

Histochemically, the luminal cells contain many large, PAS-positive, diastase-resistant granules as seen in the secretory cells of apocrine glands. In addition, the luminal cells are positive for nonspecific esterase and acid phosphatase, the so-called apocrine enzymes, and negative for phosphorylase, a typical eccrine enzyme. Furthermore, the

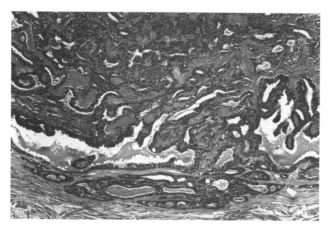

FIGURE 30-51. Hidradenoma papilliferum. Numerous papillary projections are seen within the lesion.

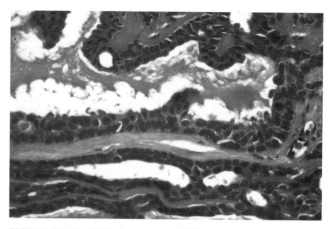

FIGURE 30-52. Hidradenoma papilliferum. The papillary folds are lined by one layer of high cylindric cells, which show evidence of active "decapitation" secretion like that seen in apocrine glands. A basal layer of small cuboidal cells is also present.

outer row of cells stains positive for alkaline phosphatase, as myoepithelial cells normally do (341).

Electron microscopic examination demonstrates two features of the luminal cells that are regarded as characteristic for apocrine secretory cells. First, numerous membrane-limited, secretory granules that are of varying size and density and that contain lipid droplets are present in the apical portion of these cells. Second, as evidence of decapitation secretion, portions of apical cytoplasm containing large secretory granules are released into the lumen (342). The peripheral layer of cells contains numerous myofilaments.

Syringocystadenoma Papilliferum

Syringocystadenoma papilliferum occurs most commonly on the scalp or the face; however, in about one-fourth of the cases, it is seen elsewhere (343–346). It is usually first noted at birth or in early childhood and presents as a papule or several papules in a linear arrangement, or as a plaque. The lesion increases in size at puberty, becoming papillomatous and often crusted (347). On the scalp, syringocystadenoma papilliferum frequently arises around puberty within a nevus sebaceus that has been present since birth.

Histopathology. The epidermis shows varying degrees of papillomatosis. One or several cystic invaginations extend downward from the epidermis (Fig. 30-53). The upper portion of the invaginations and, in some instances, large segments of the cystic invaginations are lined by squamous, keratinizing cells similar to those of the surface epidermis (348). In the lower portion of the cystic invaginations, numerous papillary projections extend into the lumina of the invaginations. The papillary projections and the lower portion of the invaginations are lined by glandular epithelium often consisting of two rows of cells (Fig. 30-54). The luminal row of cells consists of high columnar cells with oval nuclei and faintly eosinophilic cytoplasm. Occasion-

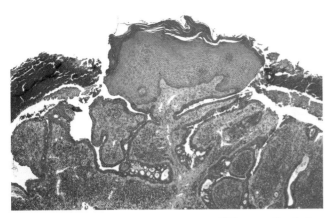

FIGURE 30-53. Syringocystadenoma papilliferum. The lesion exhibits a cystic invagination extends with numerous papillary projections.

ally, some of these cells show active decapitation secretion, and cellular debris is found in the lumina (14,349). The outer row of cells consists of small cuboidal cells with round nuclei and scanty cytoplasm. In some areas, the cells of the luminal layer are arranged in multiple layers and form a lace-like pattern resulting in multiple small, tubular lumina (344) (Fig. 30-53).

Beneath the cystic invaginations, deep in the dermis, one can find in many cases groups of tubular glands with large lumina. The cells lining the large lumina often show evidence of active decapitation secretion, indicating that they are apocrine glands (14,347) (Fig. 30-54). Connections of the apocrine glands deep in the dermis with the cystic invaginations in the upper dermis can be traced when step sections are carried out (14).

A highly diagnostic feature is the almost invariable presence of a fairly dense cellular infiltrate composed nearly

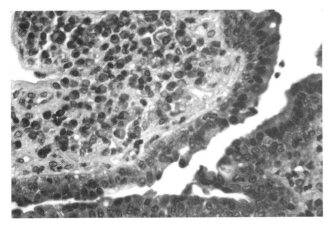

FIGURE 30-54. Syringocystadenoma papilliferum. The papillary projections are lined by two rows of cells. The luminal row of cells consists of columnar cells with evidence of active "decapitation" secretion. The outer row of cells consists of small cuboidal cells. Plasma cells are usually seen in the papillary core.

entirely of plasma cells in the stroma of this tumor, especially in the papillary projections (Fig. 30-54). These are predominantly of the IgG and IgA classes (350,351).

Frequently, there are malformed sebaceous glands and hair structures in the lesions of syringocystadenoma papilliferum (347). In about one-third of the cases, syringocystadenoma papilliferum is associated with a nevus sebaceus. In about 10% of the cases, a basaloid epithelial proliferation resembling basal cell carcinoma develops, but this is noted only in lesions that also exhibit a nevus sebaceus (344). A few instances of transition of a syringocystadenoma papilliferum into an adenocarcinoma with regional lymph node metastases have been reported (351a,351b).

Additional Studies. Syringocystadenoma papilliferum can exhibit both apocrine and of eccrine differentiation. For example, positive immunoreactivity for gross cystic disease fluid proteins 15 and 24 (GCDFP-15 and 24) and zinc alpha-2 glycoprotein demonstrates evidence of apocrine differentiation (314,352). On the other hand, immunohistochemical analysis of cytokeratins in syringocystadenoma papilliferum demonstrates similarities to eccrine poromas and the ductal component of eccrine glands (353). In addition, light and electron microscopic features of some lesions show evidence of eccrine differentiation (13). It is probable that syringocystadenoma papilliferum arises from undifferentiated cells with the potential to exhibit both apocrine and eccrine modes of epithelial secretion. Interestingly, the view expressed by Pinkus (347) probably is correct: most lesions of syringocystadenoma papilliferum exhibit apocrine differentiation; however, some demonstrate eccrine features. Studies have demonstrated loss of heterozygosity for patched and p16, a negative regulator of the cell cycle, in syringocystadenoma papilliferum, suggesting that these molecules may play a role in the pathogenesis of these lesions (354).

Tubular Apocrine Adenoma

First described in 1972 (355), additional cases of tubular apocrine adenoma have been reported (356–360). The tumor typically presents as a well-defined nodule that is located on the scalp. Most tumors are under 2 cm in diameter, although one reported lesion located on the scalp measured 7 by 4 cm (355).

Histopathology. This tumor manifests numerous irregularly shaped tubular structures that are usually lined by two layers of epithelial cells (Figs. 30-55 and 30-56). The peripheral layer consists of cuboidal or flattened cells, and the luminal layer is composed of columnar cells (355). Some of the tubules have a dilated lumen with papillary projections extending into it (Fig. 30-56). Decapitation secretion of the luminal cells is seen in many areas. In addition, cellular fragments and eosinophilic granular debris are seen in some lumina. In some cases, tubular apocrine adenomas can arise in association with syringocystadenoma

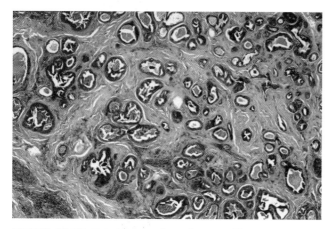

FIGURE 30-55. Tubular apocrine adenoma. There are numerous irregularly shaped tubular structures in the dermis.

papilliferum (SCAP); often the SCAP is situated in the superficial portion of the "combined" lesion (357,359,361).

Additional Studies. Electron microscopy has revealed secretory granules and evidence of apocrine-type decapitation secretion in the luminal cells (355,358). In contrast to hidradenoma papilliferum, the peripheral cell layer contains no myofilaments. Enzyme histochemistry is also consistent with apocrine differentiation (355).

Differential Diagnosis. In tubular apocrine adenomas with marked papillary proliferations, there may be some nuclear pleomorphism, which suggests sweat gland carcinoma or a metastatic adenocarcinoma. However, the presence of a peripheral layer of cuboidal or flattened cells is a feature favoring benignity (356).

Tubular apocrine adenomas resemble papillary eccrine adenoma, and at one time these two tumors were regarded as identical (359). Because of their differences in decapitation secretion, in enzyme histochemistry, and in electron

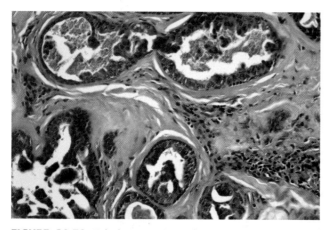

FIGURE 30-56. Tubular apocrine adenoma. The tubules are usually lined by two layers of epithelial cells, an indicator of benignancy. The peripheral layer consists of cuboidal or flattened cells, and the luminal layer is composed of columnar cells. Some of the tubules have a dilated lumen with papillary projections. Eosinophilic debris can be seen in the tubular lumens.

microscopy, the suggestion was made that they be referred to as *tubulopapillary hidradenoma*, with apocrine or eccrine differentiation as the case may be (362). (For a description of papillary eccrine adenomas, see below.) The term tubulopapillary hidradenoma may be considered to conceptualize a spectrum of lesions that includes tubular apocrine adenoma and papillary eccrine adenoma, and these are also closely related to syringocystadenoma papilliferum (363,364).

Apocrine Adenoma, Apocrine Fibroadenoma

Rare variants of apocrine adenomas can occur in apocrine areas, such as in the axilla (365), and in the perianal region (366,367).

Histopathology. Apocrine lumina are readily recognized by the presence of decapitation secretion. In addition, there may be cystically dilated spaces (365,366). A stromal component resembling that in fibroadenomas of the breast has been described (367).

Erosive Adenomatosis of the Nipple

Erosive adenomatosis (papillary adenoma, florid papillomatosis) of the nipple represents an adenoma of the major nipple ducts (368–371). In the early lesions, the nipple appears eroded and inflamed often with a serous discharge. During this early erosive phase, clinical differentiation from Paget's disease of the breast may be impossible. Later, the nipple shows nodular thickening; then, differentiation from Paget's disease is easier. Peak incidence for erosive adenomatosis is the fifth decade of life; cases in eight-year-old girls have been reported (372).

Histopathology. Extending downward from the epidermis are irregular, dilated tubular structures resembling those seen in tubular apocrine adenoma (368). These tubules are lined by a peripheral layer of cuboidal cells and a luminal layer of columnar cells that occasionally demonstrate secretory projections at their luminal border (368). Some of the tubules demonstrate papillary proliferations of columnar cells that extend into the lumen; these proliferations may be so pronounced as to nearly fill the entire lumen. In other areas, detached, partially necrotic cells may be seen in the tubular lumina. In some lesions, considerable acanthosis of the epidermis is seen, with extension of squamous epithelium into some of the superficial ductal structures.

Differential Diagnosis. Erosive adenomatosis of the nipple must be differentiated from intraductal carcinoma, which shows larger cuboidal cells and uniform atypicality of the nuclei, frequently with necrosis. Immunohistochemical studies have demonstrated myoepithelial cells within lesions of erosive adenomatosis, which would help differentiate these lesions from intraductal carcinoma (373). Hidradenoma papilliferum, in contrast to erosive adenomatosis of the nipple, shows no connections of the tubular structures with the surface epidermis (374).

Cylindroma

Cylindroma occurs more often as a solitary lesion than as multiple lesions (375). Cases with multiple lesions are dominantly inherited and show numerous dome-shaped, smooth nodules of various sizes on the scalp. Occasionally, scattered nodules are also present on the face and, in rare instances, on the trunk and the extremities (376). The lesions begin to appear in early adulthood and increase in number and size throughout life. They vary in size from a few millimeters to several centimeters. Nodules on the scalp may be present in such large numbers as to cover the entire scalp like a turban. For this reason, they are referred to occasionally as turban tumors.

The association of multiple lesions of cylindroma with multiple lesions of trichoepithelioma is quite common (375,377–380). In these cases, the lesions of the scalp are cylindromas, and those elsewhere are partially cylindromas and partially trichoepitheliomas. Brooke–Spiegler syndrome refers to a dominantly inherited disorder in which patients demonstrate multiple cylindromas, spiradenomas, and trichoepitheliomas (378,380–383). In several instances, multiple cylindromas have been found in association with eccrine spiradenoma (375,384,385).

Sporadic, solitary cylindromas are not inherited; they appear in adulthood and occur either on the scalp or the face. Their histologic appearance is the same as that of multiple cylindromas (375).

Histopathology. Cylindromas represent a tumor that may manifest both apocrine and eccrine differentiation; however, features of apocrine differentiation usually predominate (375). The tumors of cylindroma are composed of numerous islands of epithelial cells. Varying considerably in size and shape and lying close together, separated often only by their hyaline sheath and a narrow band of collagen, the islands of epithelial cells seem to fit together like pieces of a jigsaw puzzle (Figs. 30-57 and 30-58). The hyaline sheath surrounding the tumor islands, like a cylinder, is quite variable in thickness. In addition, droplets of hyalin are present in many islands, and some islands consist largely of hyalin and contain only a few cells. The hyalin is PAS-positive and diastase resistant (349).

Two types of cells constitute the islands: cells with small, dark-staining nuclei are present predominantly at the periphery of the islands, often in a palisade arrangement, and cells with large, light-staining nuclei lie in the center of the islands (Fig. 30-58). In addition, tubular lumina are often present. In some cases, they are quite numerous, whereas in others only a few are found after a thorough search. The lumina are lined by cells that usually have the appearance of ductal cells (386). Occasionally, however, the luminal cells show active secretion, like the secretory cells of apocrine glands (14). Often, amorphous material is found within

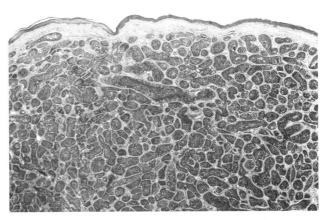

FIGURE 30-57. Cylindroma. The tumor is composed of irregularly shaped islands that fit together like pieces of a jigsaw puzzle. The islands are surrounded by a hyaline sheath.

the lumina; it contains both neutral and acid mucopolysaccharides, as demonstrated by positive staining with the PAS reaction and Alcian blue (349).

Additional Studies. The ultrastructural and immunohistochemical features best-fit differentiation toward the intradermal coiled duct region of eccrine sweat glands (387–389) with myoepithelial cell participation (390).

Electron microscopic examination, similar to examination by light microscopy, has revealed two major types of cells; undifferentiated basal cells with small, dark nuclei, and differentiating cells with large, pale nuclei. Most of the differentiating cells still appear immature as "indeterminate cells," but some show a certain degree of differentiation toward secretory or ductal cells and are in part arranged around lumina (386,391,392).

Interestingly, an early study of two large pedigrees led to the conclusion that cylindromas and trichoepitheliomas are different manifestations of the same disorder and not

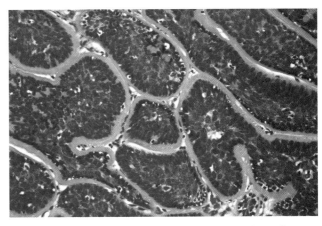

FIGURE 30-58. Cylindroma. Two types of epithelial cells comprise the islands: cells with small dark nuclei representing undifferentiated cells, and cells with large pale nuclei, representing cells with a certain degree of differentiation toward ductal or secretory cells. Droplets of hyaline material are seen in the island.

merely examples of genetic linkage (380). More recently, genetic studies have identified a single gene, CYLD1, on 16q12-q13 as being altered in familial cylindromatosis syndrome (Brooke–Spiegler) (11). Loss of heterozygosity at the 16q12-q13 locus has been demonstrated in familial cylindromatosis and sporadic cylindromas (11). The CYLD1 gene has been cloned; the molecule contains cytoskeletal binding domains and domains similar to ubiquitin hydrolases (393). Frameshift mutations in the CYLD1 gene have also been associated with familial cylindromatosis (394). The various tumors associated with familial cylindromatosis may arise from different types of mutations in the CYLD1 gene; however, this has not been definitively demonstrated (394).

The thick hyaline band surrounding the tumor islands of cylindroma is composed mainly of an amorphous substance identical to the subepidermal lamina densa. It is connected with the tumor cells by half-desmosomes. Enmeshed in it are aggregated anchoring fibrils and thin collagen fibrils (13). This thick hyaline membrane and also the particles of hyaline present between the cells of the tumor islands react positively to staining with antibodies against type IV collagen and laminin, analogous to the subepidermal lamina densa. This hyaline is synthesized by the tumor cells and is similar to the deposits of basement membrane protein demonstrated in hyalinosis cutis et mucosae (395).

Malignant Cylindroma

Cylindromas rarely undergo malignant degeneration; however, a number of cases have been reported (396–402). In most of these patients, there were multiple cylindromas of the scalp, but in several cases a single tumor was present (396–404). Usually only one tumor was malignant, but in some cases malignant progression had occurred in several tumors (405,406).

Death usually ensued through visceral metastases, but in a few patients it occurred as the result of invasion of the skull with ensuing hemorrhage or meningitis. Local excision of the tumors of the scalp may result in a cure.

Histopathology. Areas of malignant degeneration are characterized by islands of cells showing marked anaplasia and pleomorphism of the nuclei, many atypical mitotic figures, loss of the hyaline sheath, loss of palisading at the periphery, and invasion into the surrounding tissue.

TUMORS WITH ECCRINE DIFFERENTIATION

Eccrine Nevus

Eccrine nevi are very rare. They may show a circumscribed area of hyperhidrosis (407,408), a solitary sweat-discharging pore (409), or papular lesions in a linear arrangement (410).

In the so-called eccrine angiomatous hamartoma, there may be one or several nodules (411) or a solitary large plaque

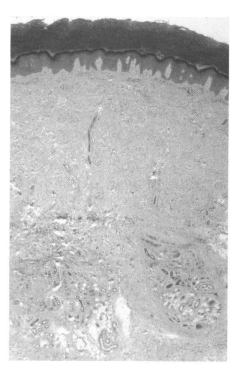

FIGURE 30-59. Eccrine angiomatous hamartoma. There is an increased number of eccrine structures with intermingled capillary channels in the deep dermis.

(412). The lesions are generally present on an extremity at birth. Hyperhidrosis and/or pain may be apparent (413).

Histopathology. Eccrine nevi show an increase in the size of the eccrine coil or in both the size and the number of coils. In other cases there is ductal hyperplasia consisting of thickening of the walls and dilatation of the lumina.

Eccrine angiomatous hamartomas usually lie in the deep dermis and contain increased numbers of eccrine structures and numerous capillary channels surrounding or intermingled with the eccrine structures (414) (Figs. 30-59 and 30-60). These hamartomas may also contain fatty tissue and pilar structures (415,416).

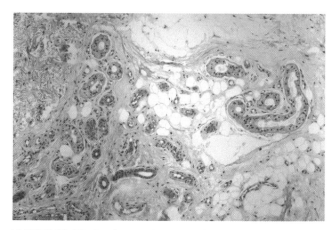

FIGURE 30-60. Eccrine angiomatous hamartoma. The eccrine coils and capillaries are associated with fatty tissue.

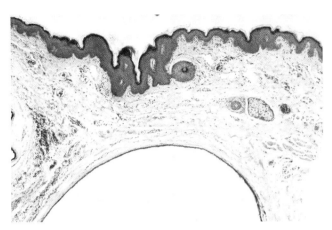

FIGURE 30-61. Eccrine hidrocystoma. A solitary cystic lesion is seen in the dermis.

Eccrine Hidrocystoma

In this condition, usually one lesion, but occasionally several, and rarely numerous lesions are present on the face (417). As in apocrine hidrocystoma, the lesion consists of a small, translucent, cystic nodule 1 to 3 mm in diameter that often has a bluish hue. In some patients with numerous lesions, the number of cysts increases in warm weather and decreases during winter (418).

Histopathology. Eccrine hidrocystoma shows a single cystic cavity located in the dermis (Fig. 30-61). The cyst wall usually shows two layers of small, cuboidal epithelial cells (417) (Fig. 30-62). In some areas, only a single layer of flattened epithelial cells can be seen, their flattened nuclei extending parallel to the cyst wall. Small papillary projections extending into the cavity of the cyst are observed only rarely (419). Eccrine secretory tubules and ducts are often located below the cyst and in close approximation to it, and, on serial sections, one may find an eccrine duct leading into the cyst from below (391). However, no connection can be found between the cyst and the epidermis.

Additional Studies. Electron microscopy of eccrine hidrocystoma has established that the cyst wall is composed of ductal cells, since the luminal cell membrane shows numerous microvilli and no secretory granules (420). Tonofilaments are seen in the luminal portion of the cells, and desmosomes connect the cells (421). Enzyme histochemistry in cases with numerous cysts has revealed phosphorylase and succinic dehydrogenase, which are eccrine enzymes, in the cyst walls (420,421).

It is likely that obstruction of eccrine ducts lead to either temporary or permanent retention of sweat (421).

Differential Diagnosis. For a discussion of differentiation of eccrine from apocrine hidrocystoma, see Apocrine hidrocystomer.

Syringoma

Based on histochemical and electron microscopic findings, syringoma represents an adenoma of intraepidermal eccrine ducts. It occurs predominantly in women at puberty or later in life. Although occasionally solitary, the lesions usually are multiple and may be present in great numbers. They are small, skin-colored or slightly yellow, soft papules, usually only 1 or 2 mm in diameter. In many patients, the lesions are limited to the lower eyelids. Other sites of predilection are the cheeks, thighs, axillae, abdomen, and vulva (265, 422–425). In so-called eruptive hidradenoma or syringoma, the lesions arise in large numbers in successive crops on the anterior trunk of young persons (426). Rarely, the lesions of syringoma show a unilateral, linear arrangement (427). In rare instances, occult syringomas of the scalp are associated with diffuse thinning of the hair (428) or with cicatricial alopecia. Inapparent syringoma has been found incidentally in close approximation to basal cell carcinoma (429).

Histopathology. Embedded in a fibrous stroma are numerous small ducts (Fig. 30-63), the walls of which are lined usually by two rows of epithelial cells (Fig. 30-64). In most instances, these cells are flat. Occasionally, the cells

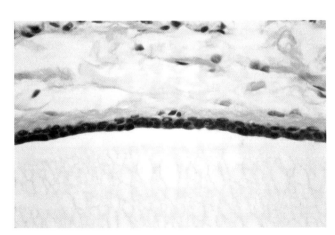

FIGURE 30-62. Eccrine hidrocystoma. The cyst is lined by a single layer of cuboidal epithelium.

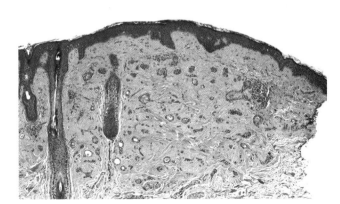

FIGURE 30-63. Syringoma. In the dermis, numerous tubular structures are embedded in a dense, collagenous stroma.

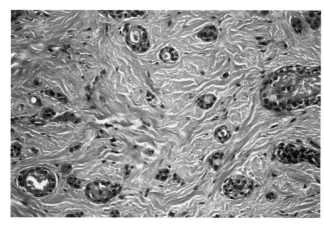

FIGURE 30-64. Syringoma. The walls of the ducts are predominantly lined by two rows of epithelial cells. Some ducts are lined by an eosinophilic cuticle, others have have comma-like tails. Granular eosinophilic material is seen in some ducts.

of the inner row appear vacuolated. The lumina of the ducts contain amorphous debris (Fig. 30-64). Some of the ducts possess small, comma-like tails of epithelial cells, giving them the appearance of tadpoles. In addition, there are solid strands of basophilic epithelial cells independent of the ducts.

Near the epidermis, there may be cystic ductal lumina filled with keratin and lined by cells containing keratohyaline granules (426). These keratin cysts resemble milia. Sometimes they rupture, producing a foreign-body reaction.

In rare instances, many of the tumor cells appear as clear cells secondary to glycogen accumulation (430). Typically, one observes only a few ductal structures and epithelial cords but predominantly cell islands that are irregular in shape and size. With the occasional exception of the peripheral cell layer, these islands are usually composed entirely of clear cells and have more cell layers than are generally seen in ordinary syringomas (431) (Fig. 30-65).

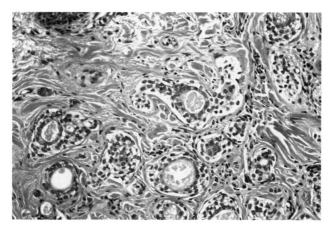

FIGURE 30-65. Syringoma. In this rare variant, the tumor islands consist largely of clear cells as a result of glycogen accumulation.

Additional Studies. Enzyme histochemical and electron microscopic studies have established syringoma as a tumor with differentiation toward intraepidermal eccrine sweat ducts (391,432). The enzyme pattern in the cells of syringoma shows a prevalence of eccrine enzymes such as succinic dehydrogenase, phosphorylase, and leucine aminopeptidase (433,434). In contrast to apocrine structures, syringomas react only weakly to lysosomal apocrine enzymes such as acid phosphatase and β-glucuronidase, except in a narrow, lysosome-rich periluminal zone (426).

Electron microscopic examination reveals that the lumina of the ducts are lined not by secretory but by ductal cells showing numerous short microvilli, interconnecting desmosomes, a periluminal band of tonofilaments, and many lysosomes. In some tumor cells, intracytoplasmic cavities are formed by lysosomal action. Coalescence of several such intracytoplasmic cavities to form an intercellular lumen is the mode by which the ductal lumina are formed in syringoma; this is identical with the mode of formation of the embryonic and the regenerating intraepidermal eccrine ducts (391,426).

The finding of cystic ductal lumina filled with keratin near the epidermis is compatible with the natural keratinizing propensity of the luminal cells of the intraepidermal eccrine sweat duct toward the upper strata of the epidermis (426).

Differential Diagnosis. The solid strands of basophilic epithelial cells embedded in a fibrous stroma seen in some cases of syringoma have an appearance similar to that of the strands seen in fibrosing basal cell carcinoma. However, fibrosing basal cell carcinoma lacks ductal structures containing amorphous material. The horn cysts near the epidermis in syringoma resemble those occurring in trichoepithelioma, and their presence in syringoma was formerly misinterpreted as the occurrence of both types of tumors within the same lesion (14). Although trichoepithelioma (including desmoplastic trichoepithelioma) shows solid strands of basophilic epithelial cells and horn cysts, it lacks ductal structures. Syringoma can be distinguished from microcystic adnexal carcinoma by its smaller size, greater symmetry, superficial dermal location, lack of prominent horn cyst formation, and infrequent single-file strand formation. Also, microcystic adnexal carcinoma, a much larger tumor than syringoma, extends into the subcutaneous tissue (77). The diagnosis of microcystic adnexal carcinoma should always be considered in any apparently syringomatous or trichoepitheliomatous neoplasm that extends to the base of a superficial biopsy.

Eccrine Poroma

Initially described in 1956, eccrine poroma is a fairly common solitary tumor (435). In about two-thirds of the cases, it is found on the sole or the sides of the foot, occurring next in frequency on the hands and fingers (436). Eccrine poroma has also been observed in many other areas of the skin, such as the neck, chest, nose, and eyelid (437–440). Eccrine poroma generally arises in middle-aged persons. The tumor has a rather firm consistency, is raised, is asymptomatic, often slightly pedunculated, and usually measures less than 2 cm in diameter.

An unusual clinical variant is *eccrine poromatosis* in which more than 100 papules are observed on the palms and soles (441); in one reported case, the papular poromas, in addition to involving the palms and soles, showed a widespread, diffuse distribution (442).

Histopathology. In its typical form, eccrine poroma arises within the lower portion of the epidermis, from where it emanates downward into the dermis as tumor masses that often consist of broad, anastomosing bands of epithelial cells (Fig. 30-66). The border between epidermis and tumor is readily apparent because of the distinctive appearance of the tumor cells: they are smaller than epidermal keratinocytes, have a uniform cuboidal appearance, a round, deeply basophilic nucleus, and are connected by intercellular bridges (Fig. 30-67). The lesional cells tend not to keratinize within the tumor, but they are able to keratinize on the surface of the tumor in instances in which the tumor has replaced the overlying epidermis. Although the border between tumor formations and the stroma is sharp, tumor cells located at the periphery show no palisading.

Characteristically, the tumor cells contain significant amounts of glycogen that is associated with cytoplasmic clearing, usually in an uneven distribution (443) (Fig. 30-67). Melanocytes and melanin often are absent, although they may be present in tumors from various racial backgrounds (444–446).

In a majority of eccrine poromas, narrow ductal lumina and occasionally cystic spaces are found within the tumor bands (443). They are lined by an eosinophilic, PAS-positive, diastase-resistant cuticle similar to that lining eccrine sweat ducts.

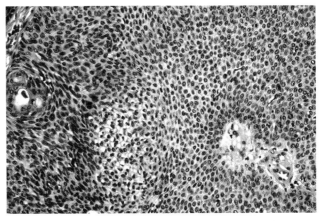

FIGURE 30-67. Eccrine poroma. The cells comprising the tumor have a uniformly small cuboidal appearance and are connected by intercellular bridges. A ductal lumen is present. The tumor vessels demonstrate a hyalinized stroma.

Poromas can be situated entirely within the epidermis, where the lesion appears as a number of distinct cellular aggregates. Such intraepidermal poromas were first described under the designation *hidroacanthoma simplex*, about the same time at which poroma was first described (447,448) (Fig. 30-68). These lesions represent one example of the so-called Borst–Jadassohn phenomenon of intraepithelial epitheliomas. A few ductal lumina lined by an eosinophilic cuticle can often be seen within the intraepidermal islands (449). Eccrine poromas may also be located largely or entirely within the dermis, where they consist of variously shaped tumor islands containing ductal lumina; these lesions are referred to as dermal duct tumors (450).

Syringoacanthoma of Rahbari represents a clonal variant of eccrine poroma in which variously sized nests of small, deeply basophilic, ovoid or cuboidal sweat duct-like cells are embedded within an acanthotic epidermis (451).

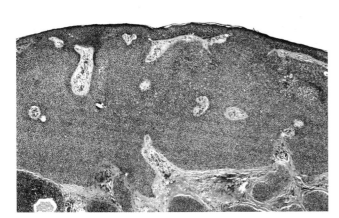

FIGURE 30-66. Eccrine poroma. The tumor consists of broad anastomosing bands emanating from the epidermis.

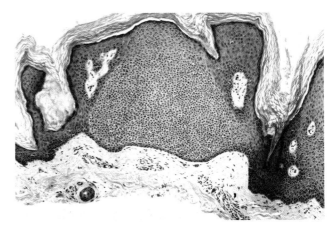

FIGURE 30-68. Hidroacanthoma simplex. There are discrete aggregates of small cells in the epidermis, constituting one example of the so-called Borsst-Jadassohn phenomenon of intraepithelial epitheliomas.

Additional Studies. Enzyme histochemical staining has shown the prevalence of eccrine enzymes in eccrine poromas, particularly phosphorylase and succinic dehydrogenase (450,452,453).

Electron microscopic examination reveals that the tumor cells, except for the luminal cells, contain a moderate number of tonofilaments, are connected with each other by desmosomes, and appear identical to the cells that compose the outer layer of the intraepidermal eccrine duct (poral epithelial cells) (452). The luminal cells show a periluminal filamentous zone and, extending into the lumen, numerous tortuous microvilli coated with amorphous material that forms the eosinophilic cuticle seen by light microscopy. Some of the tumor cells may also exhibit features considered indicative of dermal duct differentiation (391,454).

Differential Diagnosis. Eccrine poroma must be differentiated from basal cell carcinoma and seborrheic keratosis. In basal cell carcinoma, the cells have no visible intercellular bridges, are more variable in size, often show peripheral palisading, and contain little or no glycogen. The cells of eccrine poroma greatly resemble the small basaloid cells of seborrheic keratosis, especially because they possess clearly visible intercellular bridges. However, seborrheic keratoses have an even demarcation at their lower border; moreover, their cells have the potential to keratinize, and when they keratinize, they form horn cysts. Also, both basal cell carcinoma and seborrheic keratosis lack ductal lumina lined with an eosinophilic cuticle. Furthermore, these two types of tumors very rarely occur on the sole of the foot.

Malignant Eccrine Poroma (Porocarcinoma)

Malignant eccrine poroma, or porocarcinoma, may arise *de novo* (455,456); however, it usually develops in a long-standing eccrine poroma (446,457–459). The tumor favors extremities, particularly legs and feet, usually in adults of either sex. In some instances, the malignant eccrine poroma is localized, manifesting itself as a nodule, plaque, or ulcerated tumor (456,457,459,460). In other cases, there are multiple cutaneous metastases, which are usually associated with visceral metastases, resulting in death (446,458–460). The propensity to form multiple cutaneous metastases is an unusual feature of malignant eccrine poroma.

Histopathology. Malignant eccrine poroma may be seen associated with an eccrine poroma or a lesion of hidroacanthoma simplex (457,459). In such cases, one observes areas composed of eccrine poroma cells with a benign appearance adjacent to areas of anaplastic cells.

In the primary tumor, the malignant cells may be limited to the epidermis or may extend into the dermis (Fig. 30-69). Some islands of tumor cells may lie free in the dermis. The epidermis often shows considerable acanthosis as a result of the proliferation of numerous well-defined tumor cell nests

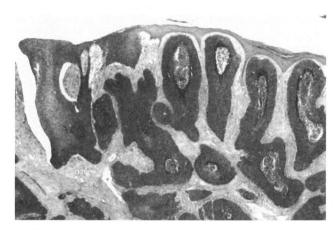

FIGURE 30-69. Porocarcinoma. Large islands of tumor cells are seen, many with central necrosis.

within it. Cystic lumina may be seen within the epidermal and dermal tumor nests (Fig. 30-69). The malignant cells have large, hyperchromatic, irregularly shaped nuclei and may be multinucleated (459) (Fig. 30-70). Lesional cells are rich in glycogen (455). The tumors are asymmetrical, with cords and lobules of polygonal tumor cells, typically with a cribriform pattern. Nuclear atypia is evident, with frequent mitoses and necrosis (Fig. 30-70). Useful clues to eccrine differentiation include spiraling ductular structures, ducts lined by cuticular material, zones of cytoplasmic glycogenation, and also intraepidermal cells in discrete aggregates, often centered on acrosyringeal pores. Foci of squamous differenti-

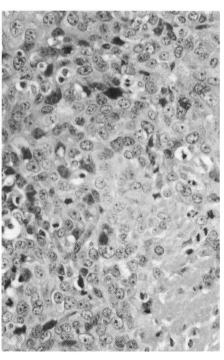

FIGURE 30-70. Porocarcinoma. Lesional cells demonstrate marked atypia, mitotic activity, and necrosis (upper right).

ation may resemble well-differentiated squamous cell carcinoma (461). The stroma may be fibrotic, hyalinized, highly myxoid, or frankly mucinous. The distinction from metastatic adenocarcinoma, especially of breast and lung origin, can be difficult, especially for less-differentiated tumors. Ductular differentiation with formation of a PAS-positive cuticle is strong evidence against a metastasis. An extracutaneous primary adenocarcinoma should be clinically ruled out.

The term ductal eccrine carcinoma has been used to refer to tumors that may appear in the dermis as an infiltrative poroma (porocarcinoma) or as a moderately differentiated adenocarcinoma (462). About one-third of ductal eccrine carcinomas are fatal, usually because of distant metastasis (463).

Malignant eccrine poroma, analogous to its benign variant, can show a clonal ("intraepithelial epithelioma") pattern of its anaplastic acrosyringeal cells. The intraepidermal clones of *such malignant syringoacanthomas* may remain *in situ* or become invasive (451).

In cutaneous metastases, numerous nests of tumor cells are present in both the epidermis and the dermis. In the epidermis, sharply defined small and large nests of tumor cells are seen surrounded by the squamous cells of the hyperplastic epidermis, resulting in a "pagetoid" pattern (446,455). Some of the tumor nests in the dermis are located within dilated lymphatic vessels, suggesting spread of the tumor in the lymphatics of the skin (455). From the lymphatics, the tumor cells invade the overlying epidermis because of the "epidermotropic" nature of the tumor cells.

Eccrine Syringofibroadenoma

First described in 1963, this usually is a solitary, hyperkeratotic, nodular plaque, several centimeters in diameter, on one extremity (464–466). Eccrine syringofibroadenoma and acrosyringeal nevi have many similarities, and some, but not all, consider them to be equivalent lesions (464–468). In one

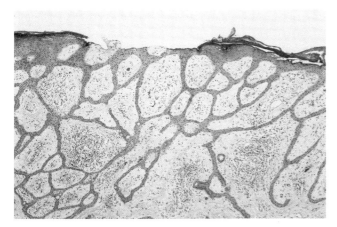

FIGURE 30-71. Eccrine syringofibroadenoma. The tumor is composed of anastomosing epithelial cords associated with a fibrous stroma.

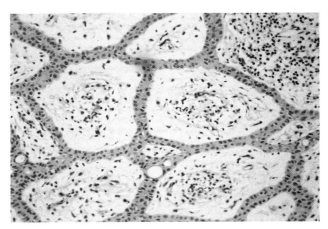

FIGURE 30-72. Eccrine syringofibroadenoma. The epithelial strands are comprised of mature acrosyringeal cells, which may form lumina and are embedded in a fibrovascular stroma.

instance, a linear lesion has been reported to extend along a lower extremity (469). Eccrine syringofibroadenomatosis has been associated with inherited palmar-plantar keratodermas including hidrotic ectodermal dysplasia and Schopf syndrome (470–472).

Histopathology. Slender, anastomosing epithelial cords of acrosyringeal cells, with or without formation of lumina, are embedded in a fibrovascular stroma (465) (Figs. 30-71 and 30-72). The net-like pattern of epithelial cells resembles that seen in fibroepithelioma (469). Lesions demonstrating prominent clear cell change have been described (473,474).

Additional Studies. Immunohistochemical studies and electron microscopy studies provide evidence for acrosyringeal differentiation in eccrine syringofibroadenomas (475–479).

Mucinous Syringometaplasia

A rare condition first described in 1974, mucinous syringometaplasia occurs as a solitary lesion in two different forms: as a verrucous lesion in an acral location on the sole of a foot or a finger and as a plaque resembling a basal cell carcinoma in a more central location (288,480,481). With pressure, serous fluid can often be expressed (288).

Histopathology. An invagination lined by squamous epithelium extends into the dermis. One or several eccrine ducts lead into the invagination. They are lined in part by mucin-laden goblet cells (288). In addition, there may be mucinous metaplasia in the underlying eccrine coils (481, 482). The epithelial mucin is PAS-positive and Alcian-blue-reactive, suggesting that it is sialomucin.

Eccrine Spiradenoma

Eccrine spiradenoma usually occurs as a solitary intradermal nodule measuring 1 to 2 cm in diameter. Occasionally, there are several lesions, and rarely, there are numerous small nodules in a zosteriform pattern or large nodules, up to 5 cm, in a linear arrangement (483–486). In most instances, eccrine spiradenoma arises in early adulthood. Lesions can arise in a variety of locations, and the nodules are often tender and occasionally painful.

Histopathology. The tumor may consist of one large, sharply demarcated lobule, but more commonly there are several lobules located in the dermis without connections to the epidermis (Fig. 30-73). The lobules are evenly and sharply demarcated and may display a fibrous capsule (487) (Fig. 30-73). On low magnification, the tumor lobules often appear deeply basophilic because of the dense packing of nuclei.

On higher magnification, the epithelial cells within the tumor lobules are found to be arranged in intertwining cords (488,489). These cords may enclose small, irregularly shaped islands of edematous connective tissue (490). Two types of epithelial cells are present in the cords, both of which possess only scant amounts of cytoplasm (Fig. 30-74). The cells of the first type possess small, dark nuclei; they are generally located at the periphery of the cellular aggregates. The cells of the second type have large, pale nuclei; they are located in the center of the aggregates and may be arranged partially around small lumina observed in about half of the tumors (Fig. 30-74) (487). The lumina frequently contain small amounts of a granular, eosinophilic material that is PAS-positive and diastase resistant (488). In the absence of lumina, the cells with pale nuclei may show a rosette arrangement. Glycogen is absent in the tumor cells or is present in insignificant amounts.

In some cases of eccrine spiradenoma, hyaline material is focally present in the stroma that surrounds the cords of tumor cells (Fig. 30-74). In addition, hyalin may be seen within some of the cords among the tumor cells as hyaline droplets (488). The stroma surrounding the tumor lobules occasionally shows lymphedema with dilated blood vessels or lymphatics (488). A heavy diffuse lymphocytic infil-

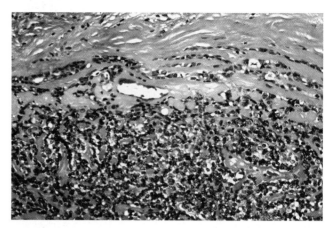

FIGURE 30-74. Eccrine spiradenoma. The epithelial cells are arranged in intertwining bands. Two types of cells can be seen. Cells with small dark nuclei lie at the periphery of the bands; they represent undifferentiated cells. Cells with large pale nuclei lie in the center of the bands and around small lumina. Collections of hyalinized material are seen.

trate, mainly of T cells, may be present (491). Malignant progression is rare.

Additional Studies. Enzyme histochemical staining has revealed a prevalence of eccrine enzymes in eccrine spiradenoma, but the reactions are not as strong as in syringoma or eccrine poroma (485,490,492).

Electron microscopic examination, similar to light microscopic examination, has shown two types of cells: undifferentiated basal cells with small, dark nuclei, and differentiating cells with large, pale nuclei. Most of the differentiating cells are immature ("indeterminate cells") and, in some tumors, may show no further differentiation (490). In most instances, however, there is some degree of differentiation toward intradermal eccrine ductal cells or toward eccrine secretory cells. Around the same lumen, some cells may show numerous microvilli and a well-developed periluminal zone of tonofilaments and thus resemble ductal cells, whereas other cells have only a few thin microvilli and thus resemble secretory cells (391,485). All secretory cells demonstrate features of serous cells (clear cells) (493). A few myoepithelial cells with typical myofilaments are present occasionally at the periphery of tubular structures (485).

Eccrine spiradenoma exhibits features of both the dermal duct and the secretory segment of the eccrine sweat gland. However, the weakness and inconsistency of the enzyme histochemical reactions, the presence largely of undifferentiated and indeterminate cells, and the absence of dark mucous cells indicate a rather low degree of differentiation. Immunohistochemical studies for cytokeratins demonstrate that the large, pale epithelial cells expressed keratins similar to those of luminal cells in the transitional portions, between the secretory portions and the coiled ducts (494). The small, dark cells expressed cytokeratins similar to the basal cells in the transitional portions of the eccrine gland.

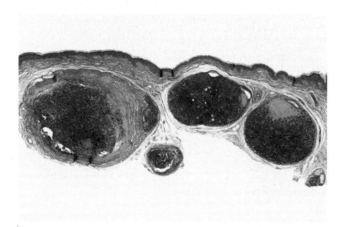

FIGURE 30-73. Eccrine spiradenoma. Well circumscribed aggregates of tumor cells are seen in the dermis.

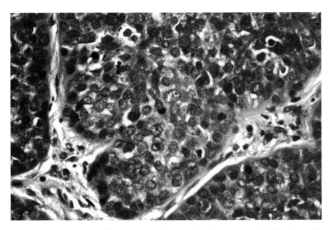

FIGURE 30-75. Malignant eccrine spiradenoma. Lesional cells demonstrate marked atypia with loss of the two cell types. Mitotic activity is also seen.

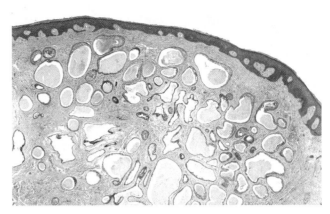

FIGURE 30-76. Papillary eccrine adenoma. The tumor is well circumscribed, symmetrical, and consists of dilated, occasionally branching tubular structures.

Malignant Eccrine Spiradenoma

Occasionally, malignant degeneration occurs in eccrine spiradenomas, usually the lesions have been present for years (404,495,496). However, malignant transformation of spiradenomas has been reported in lesions with a clinical history of seven months (497). Metastases can occur; fortunately, few patients die of generalized metastases (496–498). Regional lymph node metastasis has been reported (497,499). Notable clinical features may include a history of enlargement in a previously stable lesion.

Histopathology. In malignant lesions, two distinct components typically are seen: benign eccrine spiradenoma and carcinomatous regions associated with areas of transition (497,499). However, lesions consisting of well-demarcated zones of spiradenoma and spiradenocarcinoma have also been described (497). The carcinomatous lesion may display glandular formation, squamous differentiation, sarcomatous change, or no evidence of differentiation (497,499–503). Although mitoses may be seen in benign eccrine spiradenomas, malignant spiradenomas usually show a high mitotic rate (497,499) (Fig. 30-75). Other histologic features indicative of malignancy include the loss of two cell populations, increased nuclear to cytoplasmic ratio, and hyperchromasia (497) (Fig. 30-75). Because the malignant changes may be focal in a benign spiradenoma, the malignancy may be missed if the specimen is inadequately sampled (504).

Papillary Eccrine Adenoma

Papillary eccrine adenoma (PEA) is a benign tumor that exhibits prominent eccrine differentiation and architectural features similar to tubular apocrine adenoma. First described in 1977, it occurs most commonly on the distal portions of the extremities as a small, solitary nodule (505).

Histopathology. As in tubular apocrine adenoma, the tumor is comprised of a well-circumscribed, symmetrical collection of dilated, occasionally branching tubular struc-

tures, lined by two layers of epithelial cells (Figs. 30-76 and 30-77). Papillary projections extend into the lumina (505). The ducts may contain amorphous eosinophilic material (Fig. 30-77) (506). However, evidence of decapitation secretion is lacking (362). Small microcysts representing dilated ducts may be present (362,507–510). The low-power impression may suggest a benign breast lesion, such as intraductal hyperplasia, especially when, as is characteristic, the tumor is located within the superficial and deep dermis and is not continuous with the overlying epidermis. Amorphous and granular eosinophilic secretions are present in many of the duct lumens, and occasionally there are small, keratin-filled cysts. Adenomatous regions present variably spaced ducts and glands lined by one to several layers of cuboidal epithelium. The presence of a dense fibrovascular stromal tissue distinguishes this lesion from dermal endometriosis, which has a more cellular stroma. The tumor may recur locally but does not metastasize systemically.

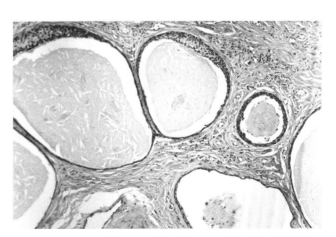

FIGURE 30-77. Papillary eccrine adenoma. The dilated tubular structures are lined by two layers of cells and contain amorphous eosinophilic material.

Additional Studies. The amylophosphorylase reaction indicating eccrine differentiation is prominent, but the reaction with acid phosphatase, an apocrine enzyme, shows practically no staining in the tumor (362). Immunoreactivity for S-100 protein, CEA, and EMA is typically present, consistent with differentiation toward the secretory epithelium of sweat glands (506,509,510).

Nodular Hidradenoma

Nodular hidradenoma is a fairly common cutaneous neoplasm that has been referred to as *clear cell myoepithelioma, clear cell hidradenoma, eccrine sweat gland adenoma of the clear cell type, solid cystic hidradenoma,* and *eccrine acrospiroma* (492,511–516). Nodular hidradenoma can arise in a variety of anatomic sites.

Nodular hidradenoma exhibits eccrine differentiation based on its enzyme histochemical and electron microscopic features (517). The tumor is usually solitary; however, on rare occasions, multiple lesions have been reported (517). The tumors present themselves as intradermal nodules and in most instances measure between 0.5 and 2.0 cm in diameter, although they may be larger. They are usually covered by intact skin, but some tumors show superficial ulceration and discharge serous material (515). Although clinically the tumor only rarely gives the impression of being cystic, gross examination of the specimen often reveals the presence of cysts (513,516).

Histopathology. The tumor is well circumscribed and may appear encapsulated. It is composed of epithelial lobules located in the dermis, which may extend into the subcutaneous fat. Within the lobulated masses, tubular lumina of various sizes are often present (Figs. 30-78 and 30-79). However, such lumina may be absent or few in number, so that step sectioning is needed to find them. The tubular lumina in some instances are branched. There are often cystic

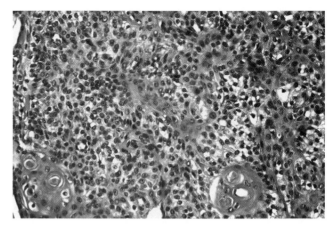

FIGURE 30-79. Nodular hidradenoma. The tumor is comprised of clear cell and polyhedral cells, some of which appear fusiform. Foci of squamous differentiation are seen as are small ductal lumina.

spaces, which may be of considerable size and contain a faintly eosinophilic, homogeneous material (515) (Fig. 30-78). The tubular lumina are lined by cuboidal ductal cells or by columnar secretory cells. Occasionally, the secretory cells show active secretion suggestive of decapitation secretion (513,517). The wide cystic spaces are only rarely lined by a single row of luminal cells; more frequently, they are bordered by tumor cells that show no particular orientation and occasionally show degenerative changes (513). This suggests that the cystic spaces may result from tumor cell degeneration.

In solid portions of the tumor, two types of cells can be recognized (513,515,518,519). The proportion of these two types of cells varies considerably from tumor to tumor. One cell type is polyhedral with a rounded nucleus and slightly basophilic cytoplasm. These cells may appear fusiform and show an elongated nucleus (Fig. 30-79). Another cell type is usually round and contains very clear cytoplasm, so that the cell membrane is distinctly visible; the cell nucleus appears small and dark (Fig. 30-79). There also are cells with features of both varieties; these cells usually show a rather light, eosinophilic cytoplasm. The clear cells contain considerable amounts of glycogen, but they may show, in addition, significant amounts of PAS-positive, diastase-resistant material along their periphery (518). In some tumors, squamoid differentiation is seen, with the cells appearing large and polyhedral and showing eosinophilic cytoplasm (520) (Fig. 30-79). There even may be keratinizing cells with formation of horn pearls (513,514) (Fig. 30-79). In other tumors, groups of squamous cells are arranged around small lumina that are lined with a well-defined eosinophilic cuticle and thus resemble the intraepidermal portion of the eccrine duct (516,518).

In most cases, no connections of the tumor lobules with the surface epidermis are noted; however, in some instances, the tumor replaces the epidermis centrally and

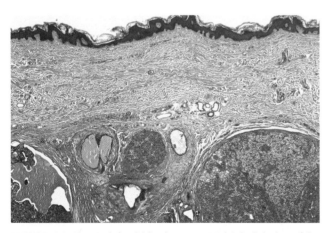

FIGURE 30-78. Nodular hidradenoma. Multiple lobules of lesional cells are present in the dermis. Focal cystic change is seen. The cystic spaces seem to form as a result of degeneration of tumor cells.

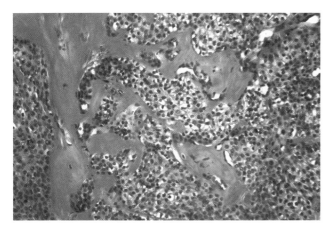

FIGURE 30-80. Nodular hidradenoma. The tumor contains small collections of a characteristic eosinophilic hyalinized stroma.

merges with the acanthotic epidermis at the periphery of the tumor (513,514,516). The tumor nodules are frequently associated with foci of a characteristic eosinophilic hyalinized stroma (Fig. 30-80).

Additional Studies. The polyhedral and fusiform cells, because of their location peripheral to the luminal cells and because of their shape, were originally regarded as cells exhibiting myoepithelial differentiation (513,517). However, the absence of alkaline phosphatase and, ultrastructurally, of myofilaments has disproved their relationship to myoepithelial cells.

Enzyme histochemical staining has established the presence in nodular hidradenoma of high concentrations of eccrine enzymes, particularly phosphorylase and respiratory enzymes, including succinic dehydrogenase and diphosphopyridine nucleotide (DPNH) diaphorase (492,519). Immunohistochemical reactivity for keratin, EMA, CEA, S-100 protein, and vimentin is characteristic (521).

Electron microscopy has demonstrated tonofilaments in the polyhedral and fusiform cells, and an abundance of glycogen in the clear cells. These tumor cell types resemble those of eccrine poroma and those that compose the outer layers of the intraepidermal eccrine duct (519). In addition, four types of luminal cells can be recognized: a secretory type, dermal-ductal and epidermal-ductal types, and an immature type (519). It can be concluded that nodular hidradenoma shows differentiation toward intraepidermal and intradermal eccrine structures ranging from the poral epithelium to the secretory segment (511, 519). Thus, ultrastructurally nodular hidradenoma seems to be intermediate between eccrine poroma, with its largely intraepidermal ductal differentiation, and eccrine spiradenoma, with its dermal-ductal and secretory differentiation. From this point of view, the clear cells represent immature poral epithelial cells, and the horn-pearl formation can be regarded as the keratinization of poral epithelial cells.

Differential Diagnosis. Nodular hidradenoma shares with trichilemmoma the presence of clear cells rich in glycogen. Foci of keratinization may also be found in both. However, only nodular hidradenoma usually shows the presence of large cystic spaces and of tubular lumina, and only trichilemmoma shows peripheral palisading of its tumor cells.

Although tumor nuclei may be hyperchromatic and there may be coarsely clumped chromatin, marked pleomorphism and frequent or atypical mitoses are not observed. If such changes are present, the tumor should be considered to have a potential for aggressive behavior. Zonal or diffuse patterns of necrosis also suggest malignancy, but the most important indicator of malignancy is an infiltrative, poorly circumscribed, and asymmetrical perimeter.

Nodular hidradenomas may occasionally reform after local excision. Associated distortion and fibrosis may impede the diagnostic interpretation when the histology of the primary lesion is unknown or unavailable. Lesions that have frequent mitoses or nuclear atypia but which lack clear evidence of asymmetric invasive growth may be termed atypical, and a re-excision to ensure that their complete removal may be contemplated.

Malignant Nodular Hidradenoma

Malignant nodular hidradenomas are rare, and usually malignant from their inception; however, malignant lesions may arise from benign nodular hidradenomas (522,523). Malignant nodular hidradenomas usually present as a solitary nodule on the head, trunk, or distal extremity. Most reported cases are in patients over 50 years of age, though they may occur at any age. These lesions tend to metastasize, and may cause death. Although there is insufficient evidence in the literature, the recurrence rate may be estimated at about 50%, and the metastasis rate is about 60%, including metastases to regional nodes, bone, viscera, and skin (523–527).

Histopathology. While nodular hidradenomas are typically well demarcated, malignant nodular hidradenomas are usually larger, asymmetrical, and show invasion into the surrounding tissue. In addition, there may be angiolymphatic invasion (528). Mitoses are usually easily detected, and some may be atypical. Tumor necrosis, areas of high cellularity, and focal or diffuse areas of marked cytologic atypia in which differentiated elements are unrecognizable are present in some examples. In these, the diagnosis of malignancy may be evident, but the recognition of adnexal origin and the precise subclassification may be problematical. In some cases of malignant nodular hidradenomas, nuclear anaplasia may be only slight to moderate or even absent in both the primary tumor and the metastases (529). Nuclear anaplasia, if present, may be limited to the clear cells or affect both the polyhedral and clear cells.

Chondroid Syringoma (Mixed Tumor of the Skin)

The term chondroid syringoma, introduced in 1961, is also known as the mixed tumor of the skin because the tumor is epithelial with associated mesenchymal changes (530,531). Chondroid syringomas are firm intradermal or subcutaneous nodules. Although the overlying skin may be attached to the tumor, it otherwise appears normal. Mixed tumors occur most commonly on the head and neck (530, 531). Their usual size is between 0.5 and 3.0 cm.

Histopathology. Histologically, two types of chondroid syringomas can be recognized: one with tubular, cystic, partially branching lumina, and the other with small, tubular lumina (531). The former type is much more common than the latter.

Chondroid syringoma with tubular, branching lumina shows marked variation in the size and shape of the tubular lumina; it also shows cystic dilatation and branching (Figs. 30-81 and 30-82). Embedded in an abundant stroma, the tubular lumina are lined by two layers of epithelial cells: a luminal layer of cuboidal cells, and a peripheral layer of flattened cells (Fig. 30-82). Furthermore, there are large and small aggregates of epithelial cells without lumina as well as single epithelial cells widely scattered through the stroma. It appears that cells from the peripheral cell layer of the tubular structures and from the solid aggregates proliferate into the stroma (530). In most instances, the tubular lumina contain small amounts of amorphous, eosinophilic

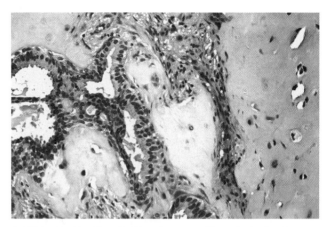

FIGURE 30-82. Chondroid syringoma. The tubular lumina are lined by two layers of cells: a luminal layer of cuboidal cells and a peripheral layer of flattened cells. Cells in the mucoid stroma have the appearance of chondrocytes.

material that is PAS-positive and resistant to digestion with diastase. In general, the tubular structures are suggestive of eccrine differentiation (530). Occasionally, the luminal cells show an apocrine type of decapitation secretion, at least in some areas (Fig. 30-82) (531–535).

The abundant stroma in many areas has a mucoid, faintly basophilic appearance. As a result of shrinkage of the mucoid substance, the fibroblasts and epithelial cells that are scattered through it are surrounded by a halo, so that they resemble the cells of cartilage (Fig. 30-82). The mucoid stroma stains with Alcian blue, mucicarmine, and aldehyde-fuchsin. The Alcian blue material is not appreciably decreased by predigestion with hyaluronidase (530). Furthermore, on staining with toluidine blue or the Giemsa stain, there is distinct metachromasia (532). Therefore, it can be concluded that the mucin consists largely of sulfated acid mucopolysaccharides, or chondroitin sulfate. The stroma is histochemically similar to normal cartilage (530). In a few areas, the stroma may appear homogeneous and eosinophilic, like hyalin, and is then PAS-positive and diastase resistant (530,534).

Chondroid syringoma with small, tubular lumina shows numerous small ducts as well as small groups of epithelial cells and solitary epithelial cells scattered through a mucoid stroma. The tubular lumina are lined by only a single layer of flat epithelial cells, from which small, comma-like proliferations often extend into the stroma, resembling a syringoma (531). The mucoid stroma contains acid mucopolysaccharides that stain metachromatically with toluidine blue.

Additional Studies. By immunohistochemistry, the inner layer cells express cytokeratin, CEA, and EMA. The outer cell layer is positive for vimentin, S-100 protein, NSE, and, occasionally, glial fibrillary acidic protein (536–539). The tumor can show either eccrine or apocrine differentiation. In three cases examined by electron microscopy, eccrine differentiation was noted (534,540). On the other hand, immunohistochemical examination with gross cystic dis-

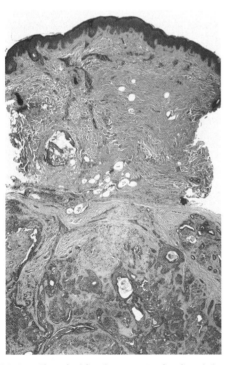

FIGURE 30-81. Chondroid syringoma. In the dermis is a nodular tumor comprised of tubular epithelial element embedded in an abundant stroma.

ease fluid protein has indicated apocrine differentiation in both cases tested (352). The stroma appears to evolve over time. Initially, delicate stellate fibroblast-like cells possibly related to ductal myoepithelial cells are suspended in the Alcian blue–positive, hyaluronidase-resistant myxoid stroma. Stromal cells may acquire cytoplasmic lipid, resulting in a scattering of mature signet ring fat cells within the myxoid background. In some lesions, there is complete synthesis and secretion of solid hyaline cartilage populated by cells in lacunae showing ultrastructural features of true chondrocytes and S-100 positivity.

Electron microscopy demonstrates that both ductal and secretory lumina are present, with the secretory lumina lined by clear and dark cells as in eccrine secretory lumina (540). The cells of the outer layer of the tubuloalveolar and ductal structures, like myoepithelial cells, contain numerous filaments and extend into the chondroid matrix, which they apparently produce (534). No chondrocytes were seen in the chondroid matrix in one study (534). In another study, the stroma showed epithelial cells and fibroblasts embedded in a fibrocollagenous matrix and islands of cartilaginous tissue containing chondrocytes with ultrastructural features similar to mature cartilage (540). In this particular case, foci of ossification were also observed, indicating that metaplasia into cartilage and bone had taken place.

Differential Diagnosis. Although most mixed tumors do not recur after surgical excision, seeding and regrowth of stromal and epithelial elements may occur, especially after an incomplete curettage. Lack of symmetry and an infiltrative pattern of growth are important features in distinguishing between benign mixed tumors and the rarely encountered malignant variant (see below) (541).

Malignant Chondroid Syringoma

In most cases of malignant chondroid syringoma, anaplastic changes are present from the beginning (542). Rarely, a chondroid syringoma of many years' duration suddenly

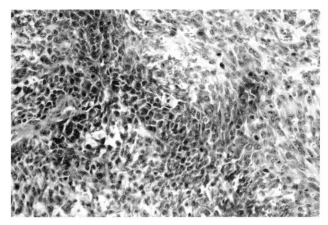
FIGURE 30-84. Malignant chondroid syringoma. Sheets of anaplastic cells are present.

undergoes malignant changes with widespread metastases (543,544). The degree of aggressive behavior varies with malignant chondroid syringomas. For example, there may be only a local recurrence, but some cases have shown regional lymph node metastases or an osseous metastasis (542,545,546). In several cases, fatal visceral metastases have occurred (543,547–549). When this tumor metastasizes, it generally does so as an adenocarcinoma, often losing the tendency to form chondroid stroma.

Histopathology. Histologically, malignant chondroid syringoma is composed of epithelial structures with glandular differentiation and carcinomatous features, embedded in a mucinous stroma with spindle mesenchymal cells and areas of chondroid differentiation (Figs. 30-83, 30-84, and 30-85). Sheets of atypical cells with increased mitotic activity can also be seen (Fig. 30-84). Unlike biphasic synovial sarcoma, in which both components express cytokeratins, only the epithelial structures of malignant chondroid syringoma are cytokeratin-positive. The malignant tumor and its metastases are recognizable as chondroid syringoma

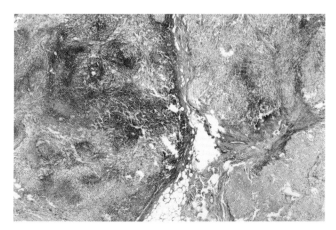
FIGURE 30-83. Malignant chondroid syringoma. An asymmetrical cellular tumor is seen in the dermis.

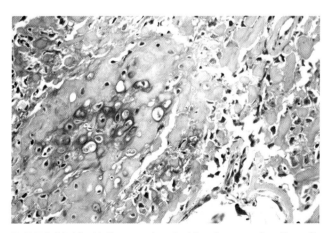
FIGURE 30-85. Malignant chondroid syringoma. Focally, cells embedded in a mucoid stroma reminiscent of chondroid syringoma are seen.

through their chondroid stroma and tubular structures (Fig. 30-85). However, tubular differentiation is much less evident than in benign lesions (547). Most of the epithelial cells in the malignant tumor are arranged in irregular cords or sheets (545) (Fig. 30-84). The tumor cells appear atypical and hyperchromatic (546). In addition, an increased mitotic rate, vascular invasion, infiltration into the surrounding tissue, and necrosis have been noted (542).

CARCINOMAS OF APOCRINE AND ECCRINE GLANDS

Carcinomas exhibiting apocrine and eccrine differentiation can be classified in several different ways. One logical classification scheme distinguishes lesions based on whether the carcinoma may frequently evolve from a benign lesion. In reality, this group of tumors may derive either from a benign precursor through tumor progression or *de novo* as a malignant lesion. In this group are malignant cylindroma, malignant eccrine poroma, malignant eccrine spiradenoma, malignant nodular hidradenoma, and malignant chondroid syringoma, lesions that have already been discussed. The second group comprises apocrine and eccrine carcinomas that appear to have no benign precursor. In this group are carcinoma of apocrine glands, eccrine adenocarcinoma, syringoid eccrine carcinoma, microcystic adnexal carcinoma, mucinous (adenocystic) carcinoma, adenoid cystic carcinoma, and aggressive digital papillary adenocarcinoma.

CARCINOMA OF APOCRINE GLANDS

Carcinomas of apocrine glands are rare tumors (365,550–554). These lesions occur primarily in the axillae and in other anatomic regions endowed with apocrine glands, including the anogenital region (365,551). Lesions can occur elsewhere on the skin (550,552). Apocrine carcinomas can also occur in the external auditory meatus, where ceruminous glands, which represent modified apocrine glands, are located (555,556). These tumors may extend to the ear and preauricular skin (557).

Some cases of carcinoma of apocrine glands exhibit only local invasiveness, but other lesions metastasize to regional lymph nodes (365,551,552). In fact, some patients have died from widespread metastases (550,552).

Histopathology. The histologic picture is that of an adenocarcinoma that may be well, moderately, or poorly differentiated (365).

In well-differentiated apocrine gland carcinomas, nuclear atypicality and invasiveness are limited. Well-developed glandular lumina are present; these lumina may be cystic and show branching (365). The cytoplasm of the tumor cells is strongly eosinophilic. Evidence of decapitation secretion, typical of apocrine glands, is present, at least in some areas. In addition, the cytoplasm of the tumor cells contains PAS-positive, diastase-resistant granules, and often contains iron-positive granules (365). Myoepithelial cells are seen rarely (552).

In moderately or poorly differentiated apocrine gland carcinomas, recognition of apocrine histopathologic features may be difficult to assess, although even poorly differentiated tumors often demonstrate regions with prominent apocrine differentiation (365).

Additional Studies. Enzyme histochemical determinations are of value in establishing an apocrine genesis. Apocrine gland carcinomas show strong activity for apocrine enzymes, such as acid phosphatase, β-glucuronidase, and indoxyl acetate esterase, and low activity or absence of eccrine enzymes, such as phosphorylase and succinic dehydrogenase (550,552).

Differential Diagnosis. Apocrine gland carcinoma of the axilla must be differentiated from a carcinoma arising in ectopic breast tissue. Features that favor the diagnosis of a carcinoma of apocrine glands are the presence of neoplastic glands high in the dermis, apocrine glands near the tumor, and intracytoplasmic granules of iron (365).

Classic Type of Eccrine Adenocarcinoma

Only a few lesions of primary eccrine carcinoma possess a clinical appearance suggesting eccrine malignancy. Although they may arise on the palms or on the soles, they more commonly arise elsewhere, particularly in the head and neck region (13,558–560).

The classic type of eccrine gland adenocarcinoma has a high incidence of metastases. Of 68 patients followed for 5 years or more, 29 had regional lymph node metastases, and visceral metastases were present in 26 (561).

Histopathology. The histologic configuration in the classic type of eccrine gland adenocarcinoma varies from areas of fairly well-differentiated tubular structures to anaplastic cells in other areas, not recognizable by themselves as eccrine sweat gland structures (559). The tubular structures usually show only small lumina that are lined by either a single layer or a double layer of cells (559). In some areas, the lumina are lined by secretory cells, which appear large and vacuolated because of the presence of glycogen and which often contain also PAS-positive, diastase-resistant granules (13,562).

Additional Studies. Immunohistochemical techniques have been of little help in characterizing these lesions (558). So-called eccrine enzymes, such as amylophosphorylase and succinic dehydrogenase, may be present in moderate amounts, but their role in identifying the tumors as eccrine rather than as metastatic has not been well defined (13,563).

Differential Diagnosis. It is often difficult to differentiate the classic type of eccrine sweat gland carcinoma from a metastatic adenocarcinoma. Therefore, the diagnosis of metastatic adenocarcinoma should always be given serious consideration before a diagnosis of eccrine sweat gland carcinoma is decided upon.

Syringoid Eccrine Carcinoma

This tumor was originally referred to in 1969 as *basal cell tumor with eccrine differentiation* (564), and subsequently as *eccrine epithelioma* (565); the term *syringoid eccrine carcinoma* is preferable because the tumor differs from basal cell carcinoma in its cytologic and enzymatic patterns. It represents a relatively well-differentiated form of eccrine carcinoma (566). Although first reported as a deeply invasive and destructive tumor of the scalp (564), it also occurs in other locations, and metastases rarely occur (566).

Histopathology. Syringoid eccrine carcinoma resembles syringoma by showing ductal, cystic, and comma-like epithelial components and by containing eccrine enzymes such as phosphorylase and succinic dehydrogenase (564). It differs from syringoma by its cellularity, anaplasia, and deep invasiveness. This uncommonly diagnosed tumor is probably related to the microcystic adnexal carcinoma. A clear cell variant of syringoid eccrine carcinoma has been described (567,568).

Additional Studies. Immunohistochemical analysis revealed that most tumor cells expressed simple epithelial cytokeratins (CKs 7, 8, 18, 19) consistent with sweat gland secretory differentiation (569).

Microcystic Adnexal Carcinoma

Microcystic adnexal carcinoma, or sclerosing sweat duct carcinoma, may best be considered as a sclerosing variant of ductal eccrine carcinoma (570,571). This tumor is most commonly seen on the skin of the upper lip, but occasion-

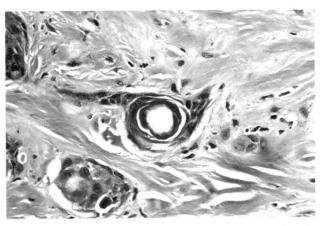

FIGURE 30-87. Microcystic adnexal carcinoma. Superficially, keratin-filled cystic glands are present and may be mistaken for the cysts of a trichoepithelioma, but the lesion invades deeply into the dermis.

ally also on the chin, nasolabial fold, or cheek (571,572). Microcystic adnexal carcinoma is an aggressive neoplasm that invades deeply. Local recurrence is common; however, metastases have not been reported.

Histopathology. Microcystic adnexal carcinoma is a poorly circumscribed dermal tumor that may extend into the subcutis and skeletal muscle (Fig. 30-86). Continuity with the epidermis or follicular epithelium may be seen. Two components within a desmoplastic stroma may be evident. In some areas, basaloid keratinocytes are seen, some of which contain horn cysts and abortive hair follicles; in other areas, ducts and gland-like structures lined by a two-cell layer predominate (572) (Figs. 30-87 and 30-88). The tumor islands typically reduce in size as the tumor extends deeper into the dermis. *Cells* with clear cytoplasm may be present, and sebaceous differentiation has been reported (573). Cytologically, the cells are bland without significant atypia; mitoses are rare or absent. Perineural invasion may be seen, a feature that may account for the high recurrence rate.

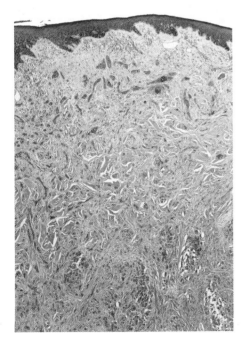

FIGURE 30-86. Microcystic adnexal carcinoma. There is a large, poorly circumscribed tumor comprised of epithelial cords that invades deeply into the dermis.

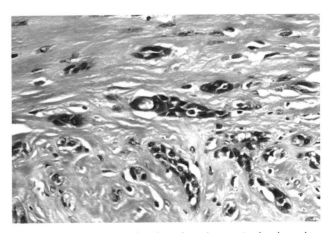

FIGURE 30-88. Microcystic adnexal carcinoma. In the deep dermis, cords of bland epithelial cells demonstrate focal ductal differentiation. A marked desmoplastic response is noted.

Additional Studies. Immunoperoxidase staining for carcinoembryonic antigen stains the glandular structures but not the pilar structures (571). The presence of both pilar and eccrine structures allows differentiation from desmoplastic trichoepithelioma and syringoma. Lack of circumscription, deep dermal involvement, and perineural involvement all aid in diagnosis, since the cytology mimics benign adnexal neoplasms. This diagnosis should always be considered and complete excision contemplated when a syringomatous or trichoepithelioma-like proliferation extends to the base of a biopsy, especially in an elderly patient.

Mucinous Eccrine Carcinoma

First described in 1971, mucinous eccrine carcinoma is a rather uncommon tumor that metastasizes to regional lymph node metastases occasionally (574,575). Widespread metastases have been described very rarely (576).

Histopathology. The histologic appearance of mucinous eccrine carcinoma is highly characteristic (577). The tumor is divided into numerous compartments by strands of fibrous tissue. In each compartment, abundant amounts of pale-staining mucin surround nests or cords of moderately anaplastic epithelial cells, some of which show a tubular lumen (574,578) (Figs. 30-89 and 30-90). The mucin shows strongly positive reactions with both PAS and colloidal iron. The mucinous material is resistant to diastase and hyaluronidase but is sensitive to digestion with siali-

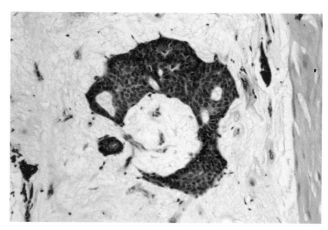

FIGURE 30-90. Mucinous eccrine adenocarcinoma. The islands of tumor cells show mild cytologic atypia and focal duct formation.

dase. The reaction with Alcian blue is positive at pH 2.5 but negative at pH 1.0 and pH 0.4, which indicates that the mucin is nonsulfated (579). It can be concluded that the mucin represents sialomucin, an epithelial mucin (574,578).

Additional Studies. Enzyme histochemical studies have revealed a prevalence of eccrine enzymes in these tumors (578). Electron microscopy has revealed two types of secretory cells in the tumor, dark and light, analogous to the two types normally encountered in eccrine coils. The sialomucin is secreted by the dark cells (580). Immunohistochemical results also suggest differentiation toward eccrine secretory coil (581).

It is important to differentiate this tumor from a metastatic mucinous adenocarcinoma, in which the primary lesion most commonly is located in the large intestines (574). In both primary and metastatic mucinous adenocarcinoma, islands of tumor cells appear to be floating in lakes of mucin, but the tumor cells are more atypical in the metastatic type and the atypical cells invade between collagen bundles at the margin of the nodule (582). Exclusion of primary visceral carcinomas is often impossible by histology alone.

Mucoepidermoid (Low-Grade Adenosquamous) Carcinoma

This tumor, which combines well-differentiated squamous and glandular epithelium, is histologically identical to that of salivary glands, and may occur as a primary cutaneous malignancy (583–585).

Adenoid Cystic Carcinoma

One of the rarest types of eccrine carcinomas is the adenoid cystic carcinoma, first described in 1975 (586). Metastases have been reported but are uncommon (587). This indolent tumor, like its more aggressive counterpart in salivary

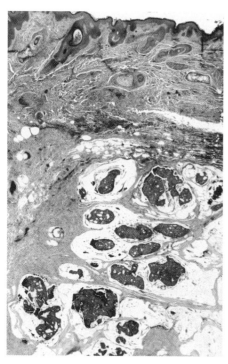

FIGURE 30-89. Mucinous eccrine adenocarcinoma. The tumor is divided into numerous compartments. In each compartment, abundant amounts of mucin surround small islets of tumor cells.

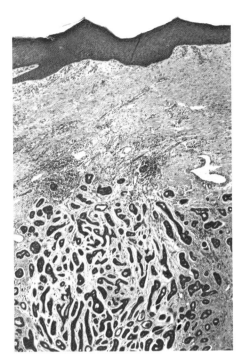

FIGURE 30-91. Adenoid cystic carcinoma of eccrine glands. A large cell mass shows an adenoid or cribriform pattern. In addition, many small, solid epithelial islands are present.

glands, spreads in perineural spaces. Therefore, it recurs in 20% of cases (587,588).

Histopathology. Microscopic examination reveals lesions exhibiting an adenoid or cribriform pattern comprised of many small, epithelial islands (Fig. 30-91). Round spaces formed by malignant epithelial cells and containing amphophilic basement membrane-like material occur in the cribriform type and tubular variants (589) (Fig. 30-92). Through the accumulation of mucin, the adenoid spaces may be transformed into multiple cystic spaces lined by a flattened cuboidal epithelium. The adenoid and cystic

spaces contain pale-staining mucin that in some cases is hyaluronidase sensitive, but in others was resistant to hyaluronidase digestion and reacted with the Alcian blue stain at pH 2.5 and at pH 0.5 (590,591). In several instances, there has been extension along perineural spaces.

Additional Studies. Adenoid cystic carcinoma is immunoreactive for carcinoembryonic antigen, amylase, and S-100 protein (591).

Adenoid cystic carcinoma of eccrine glands must be distinguished from the adenoid type of basal cell carcinoma, from which it differs by lack of continuity with the epidermis or hair sheath and by the absence of peripheral palisading (590). In addition, the adenoid type of basal cell carcinoma shows negative reactions to carcinoembryonic antigen, amylase, and S-100 protein (591). Cutaneous extension from a parotid tumor or scar recurrence should be ruled out in adjacent body sites.

Aggressive Digital Papillary Adenocarcinoma

These tumors, originally described in 1987, occur on the fingers, toes, and adjacent skin of the palms and soles, especially in adult males, as a single, often cystic mass that rarely ulcerates but often invades soft tissue (592).

Histopathology. Aggressive digital papillary adenocarcinoma shares some histologic features with papillary eccrine adenoma. These tumors are usually cellular, dermal nodules with cystic cavities (Fig. 30-93). Characteristic histologic findings of this lesion include tubuloalveolar and ductal structures associated with papillary projections protruding into cystically dilated lumina (Figs. 30-94 and 30-95). Macropapillae lined by atypical epithelial cells project into microcysts. These areas may merge with more cellular regions of moderately differentiated adenocarcinoma. Mitotic activity and cytologic atypia are often

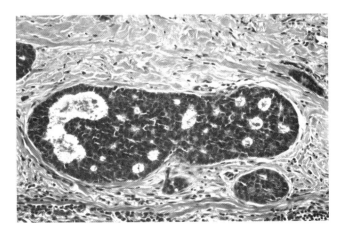

FIGURE 30-92. Adenoid cystic carcinoma of eccrine glands. Some epithelial islands demonstrate a cribiform pattern.

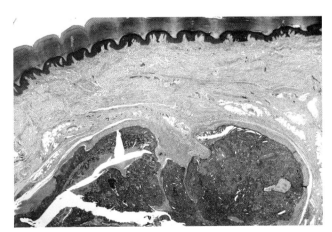

FIGURE 30-93. Aggressive digital papillary adenocarcinoma. A large lobulated dermal tumor with focal cystic change is seen in the dermis of acral skin.

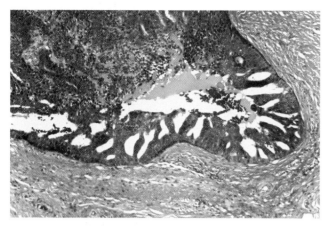

FIGURE 30-94. Aggressive digital papillary adenocarcinoma. Micropapillary structures are seen.

present (Fig. 30-95). Metastatic papillary carcinoma from breast, lung, thyroid, and ovary are in the histologic differential. Initially, a low-grade variant, "aggressive digital papillary adenoma," was described that differed from adenocarcinoma based on degree of pleomorphism, mitotic rate, and necrosis (592). However, recent studies suggest that histologic features alone cannot reliably predict clinical behavior, and therefore, all lesions should be considered aggressive digital papillary adenocarcino-

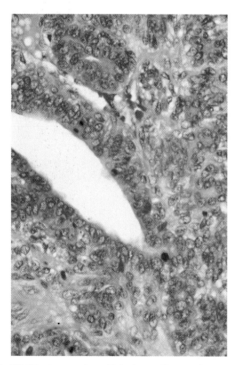

FIGURE 30-95. Aggressive digital papillary adenocarcinoma. Gland formation with cytologic atypia and mitotic activity are present.

mas (593,594). When metastases develop, they often involve the lung.

REFERENCES

1. Wong TY, Suster S, Cheek RF, et al. Benign cutaneous adnexal tumors with combined folliculosebaceous, apocrine, and eccrine differentiation. Clinicopathologic and immunohistochemical study of eight cases [Comment]. *Am J Dermatopathol* 1996;18:124–136.
2. Buchi ER, Peng Y, Eng AM, et al. Eccrine acrospiroma of the eyelid with oncocytic, apocrine and sebaceous differentiation. Further evidence for pluripotentiality of the adnexal epithelia. *Eur J Ophthalmol* 1991;1:187–193.
3. Sanchez Yus E, Requena L, Simon P, et al. Complex adnexal tumor of the primary epithelial germ with distinct patterns of superficial epithelioma with sebaceous differentiation, immature trichoepithelioma, and apocrine adenocarcinoma. *Am J Dermatopathol* 1992;14:245–252.
4. Weyers W, Nilles M, Eckert F, et al. Spiradenomas in Brooke–Spiegler syndrome. *Am J Dermatopathol* 1993;15:156–161.
5. Massa MC, Medenica M. Cutaneous adnexal tumors and cysts: a review. Part I. Tumors with hair follicular and sebaceous glandular differentiation and cysts related to different parts of the hair follicle. *Pathol Annu* 1985;20:189–233.
6. Perez-Losada J, Balmain A. Stem-cell hierarchy in skin cancer. Nature reviews. *Cancer* 2003;3:434–443.
7. Oshima H, Rochat A, Kedzia C, et al. Morphogenesis and renewal of hair follicles from adult multipotent stem cells. *Cell* 2001;104:233–245.
8. Lyle S, Christofidou-Solomidou M, Liu Y, et al. Human hair follicle bulge cells are biochemically distinct and possess an epithelial stem cell phenotype. *J Invest Dermatol Symp Proc* 1999;4:296–301.
9. Taylor G, Lehrer MS, Jensen PJ, et al. Involvement of follicular stem cells in forming not only the follicle but also the epidermis. *Cell* 2000;102:451–461.
10. Penneys NS. Immunohistochemistry of adnexal neoplasms. *J Cutan Pathol* 1984;11:357–364.
11. Biggs PJ, Chapman P, Lakhani SR, et al. The cylindromatosis gene (cyld1) on chromosome 16q may be the only tumour suppressor gene involved in the development of cylindromas. *Oncogene* 1996;12:1375–1377.
12. Heenan P, Elder DE, Sobin LH. Histological typing of skin tumours. Vol 3. Berlin Heidelberg: Springer, 1996.
13. Hashimoto K, Lever W. *Appendage Tumors of the Skin.* Vol. 47. Springfield, IL: Charles C. Thomas, 1968.
14. Lever WF. Pathogenesis of benign tumors of cutaneous appendages and of basal cell epithelioma. *Arch Dermatol Syph* 1948;57:679.
15. Albrecht E. Uber hamartome. *Verh Dtsch Ges Pathol* 1904;7:153.
16. Jadassohn J. Die benignen epitheliome. *Arch Dermatol Syph* 1914;117:705, 833.
17. Murphy G, Elder DE. *Nomenclature, Classification and Staging.* Vol 1. Washington, DC: Armed Forces Institute of Pathology, 1990.
18. Headington JT. Tumors of the hair follicle. A review. *Am J Pathol* 1976;85:479–514.
19. Ikeda S, Kawada J, Yaguchi H, et al. A case of unilateral, systematized linear hair follicle nevi associated with epidermal nevus-like lesions. *Dermatology* 2003;206:172–174.
20. Pippione M, Aloi F, Depaoli MA. Hair-follicle nevus. *Am J Dermatopathol* 1984;6:245–247.

21. Ban M, Kamiya H, Yamada T, et al. Hair follicle nevi and accessory tragi: variable quantity of adipose tissue in connective tissue framework. *Pediatr Dermatol* 1997;14:433–436.
22. Germain M, Smith KJ. Hair follicle nevus in a distribution following Blaskho's lines. *J Am Acad Dermatol* 2002;46[Suppl 1]: S125–127.
23. Pinkus H, Sutton RLJ. Trichofolliculoma. *Arch Dermatol* 1965; 91:46.
24. Gray HR, Helwig EB. Trichofolliculoma. *Arch Dermatol* 1962; 86:619.
25. Hyman AB, Clayman SJ. Hair follicle nevus. *Arch Dermatol* 1957;75:678.
26. Sanderson KV. Hair follicle nevus. *Trans St Johns Hosp Dermatol Soc* 1961;47:154.
27. Kligman AM, Pinkus H. The histogenesis of nevoid tumors of the skin. *Arch Dermatol* 1960;81:922.
28. Schulz T, Hartschuh W. The trichofolliculoma undergoes changes corresponding to the regressing normal hair follicle in its cycle. *J Cutan Pathol* 1998;25:341–353.
29. Kimura T, Miyazawa H, Aoyagi T, et al. Folliculosebaceous cystic hamartoma. A distinctive malformation of the skin. *Am J Dermatopathol* 1991;13:213–220.
30. Schulz T, Hartschuh W. Folliculo-sebaceous cystic hamartoma is a trichofolliculoma at its very late stage. *J Cutan Pathol* 1998; 25:354–364.
31. Gat U, DasGupta R, Degenstein L, et al. De novo hair follicle morphogenesis and hair tumors in mice expressing a truncated beta-catenin in skin. *Cell* 1998;95:605–614.
32. Plewig G. Sebaceous trichofolliculoma. *J Cutan Pathol* 1980;7: 394–403.
33. El-Darouty MA, Marzouk SA, Abdel-Halim MR, et al. Folliculosebaceous cystic hamartoma. *Int J Dermatol* 2001;40:454–457.
34. Winer L. The dilated pore, a trichoepithelioma. *J Invest Dermatol* 1954;23:181.
35. Mehregan AH, Brownstein MH. Pilar sheath acanthoma. *Arch Dermatol* 1978;114:1495–1497.
36. Steffen C. Winer's dilated pore: the infundibuloma. *Am J Dermatopathol* 2001;23:246–253.
37. Bhawan J. Pilar sheath acanthoma. A new benign follicular tumor. *J Cutan Pathol* 1979;6:438–440.
38. Lee JY, Hirsch E. Pilar sheath acanthoma. *Arch Dermatol* 1987; 123:569–570.
39. Birt AR, Hogg GR, Dube WJ. Hereditary multiple fibrofolliculomas with trichodiscomas and acrochordons. *Arch Dermatol* 1977;113:1674–1677.
40. Fujita WH, Barr RJ, Headley JL. Multiple fibrofolliculomas with trichodiscomas and acrochordons. *Arch Dermatol* 1981; 117:32–35.
41. Weintraub R, Pinkus H. Multiple fibrofolliculomas (Birt–Hogg–Dube) associated with a large connective tissue nevus. *J Cutan Pathol* 1977;4:289–299.
42. Schulz T, Hartschuh W. Birt–Hogg–Dube syndrome and Hornstein-Knickenberg syndrome are the same. Different sectioning technique as the cause of different histology. *J Cutan Pathol* 1999;26:55–61.
43. Pavlovich CP, Walther MM, Eyler RA, et al. Renal tumors in the Birt–Hogg–Dube syndrome. *Am J Surg Pathol* 2002;26: 1542–1552.
44. Pinkus H, Coskey R, Burgess GH. Trichodiscoma. A benign tumor related to haarscheibe (hair disk). *J Invest Dermatol* 1974; 63:212–218.
45. Grosshans E, Dungler T, Hanau D. Pinkus' trichodiscoma [author's translation]. *Ann Dermatol Venereol* 1981;108:837–846.
46. Steffen C, Ackerman AB. Fibrofolliculoma, trichodiscoma, and Birt–Hogg–Dubé syndrome. In: Ackerman AB, ed. *Neoplasms with Sebaceous Differentiation*. Philadelphia: Lea & Febiger, 1994:205.
47. Collins GL, Somach S, Morgan MB. Histomorphologic and immunophenotypic analysis of fibrofolliculomas and trichodiscomas in Birt–Hogg–Dube syndrome and sporadic disease. *J Cutan Pathol* 2002;29:529–533.
48. Gaul LE. Heredity of multiple benign cystic epithelioma. *Arch Dermatol Syph* 1953;68:517.
49. Gray HR, Helwig EB. Epithelioma adenoides cysticum and solitary trichoepithelioma. *Arch Dermatol* 1963;87:102.
50. Howell JB, Anderson DE. Transformation of epithelioma adenoides cysticum into multiple rodent ulcers: fact or fallacy. A historical vignette. *Br J Dermatol* 1976;95:233–241.
51. Pariser RJ. Multiple hereditary trichoepitheliomas and basal cell carcinomas. *J Cutan Pathol* 1986;13:111–117.
52. Johnson SC, Bennett RG. Occurrence of basal cell carcinoma among multiple trichoepitheliomas. *J Am Acad Dermatol* 1993; 28:322–326.
53. Wallace ML, Smoller BR. Trichoepithelioma with an adjacent basal cell carcinoma, transformation or collision? *J Am Acad Dermatol* 1997;37:343–345.
54. Zeligman I. Solitary trichoepithelioma. *Arch Dermatol* 1960; 82:35.
55. Müller-Hess S, Delacretaz J. Trichoepitheliom mit strukturen eines apokrinen adenoms. *Dermatologica* 1973;146:170–176.
56. Tatnall FM, Jones EW. Giant solitary trichoepitheliomas located in the perianal area: a report of three cases. *Br J Dermatol* 1986; 115:91–99.
57. Filho GB, Toppa NH, Miranda D, et al. Giant solitary trichoepithelioma. *Arch Dermatol* 1984;120:797–798.
58. Bettencourt MS, Prieto VG, Shea CR. Trichoepithelioma: a 19-year clinicopathologic re-evaluation. *J Cutan Pathol* 1999;26: 398–404.
59. Kopf AW. The distribution of alkaline phosphatase in normal and pathologic human skin. *Arch Dermatol* 1957;75:1.
60. Ohnishi T, Watanabe S. Immunohistochemical analysis of cytokeratin expression in various trichogenic tumors. *Am J Dermatopathol* 1999;21:337–343.
61. Jih DM, Lyle S, Elenitsas R, et al. Cytokeratin 15 expression in trichoepitheliomas and a subset of basal cell carcinomas suggests they originate from hair follicle stem cells. *J Cutan Pathol* 1999; 26:113–118.
62. Kyllönen AP, Stenbäck F, Väänänen R. Trichoepitheliomatous tumors: morphology and ultrastucture. *J Cutan Pathol* 1981;8: 167(abst).
63. Harada H, Hashimoto K, Ko MS. The gene for multiple familial trichoepithelioma maps to chromosome 9p21. *J Invest Dermatol* 1996;107:41–43.
64. Hussussian CJ, Struewing JP, Goldstein AM, et al. Germline p16 mutations in familial melanoma. *Nat Genet* 1994;8:15–21.
65. Matt D, Xin H, Vortmeyer AO, et al. Sporadic trichoepithelioma demonstrates deletions at 9q22.3. *Arch Dermatol* 2000; 136:657–660.
66. Vorechovsky I, Unden AB, Sandstedt B, et al. Trichoepitheliomas contain somatic mutations in the overexpressed PTCH gene: support for a gatekeeper mechanism in skin tumorigenesis. *Cancer Res* 1997;57:4677–4681.
67. Vorechovsky I, Unden AB, Sandstedt B, et al. Trichoepitheliomas contain somatic mutations in the overexpressed PTCH gene: support for a gatekeeper mechanism in skin tumorigenesis. *Cancer Res* 1 1997;57:4677–4681.
68. Brooke JD, Fitzpatrick JE, Golitz LE. Papillary mesenchymal bodies: a histologic finding useful in differentiating trichoepitheliomas from basal cell carcinomas. *J Am Acad Dermatol* 1989; 21:523–528.

69. Kirchmann TT, Prieto VG, Smoller BR. CD34 staining pattern distinguishes basal cell carcinoma from trichoepithelioma. *Arch Dermatol* 1994;130:589–592.

70. Swanson PE, Fitzpatrick MM, Ritter JH, et al. Immunohistologic differential diagnosis of basal cell carcinoma, squamous cell carcinoma, and trichoepithelioma in small cutaneous biopsy specimens. *J Cutan Pathol* 1998;25:153–159.

71. Poniecka AW, Alexis JB. An immunohistochemical study of basal cell carcinoma and trichoepithelioma. *Am J Dermatopathol* 1999;21:332–336.

72. Brownstein MH, Shapiro L. Desmoplastic trichoepithelioma. *Cancer* 1977;40:2979–2986.

73. Macdonald DM, Jones EW, Marks R. Sclerosing epithelial hamartoma. *Clin Exp Dermatol* 1977;2:153–160.

74. Dervan PA, O'Hegarty M, O'Loughlin S, et al. Solitary familial desmoplastic trichoepithelioma. A study by conventional and electron microscopy. *Am J Dermatopathol* 1985;7:277–282.

75. Shapiro PE, Kopf AW. Familial multiple desmoplastic trichoepitheliomas. *Arch Dermatol* 1991;127:83–87.

76. Dupré A, Bonafé JL, Lassére J. Hamartome épithélial sclérosant: forme clinique du trichoépithéliome. *Ann Dermatol Venereol* 1980;107:649–654.

77. Goldstein DB, RJ, Santa Cruz DJ. Microcystic adnexal carcinoma: a distinct clinicopathologic entity. *Cancer* 1982;50:566.

78. Kirchmann TT, Prieto VG, Smoller BR. Use of CD34 in assessing the relationship between stroma and tumor in desmoplastic keratinocytic neoplasms. *J Cutan Pathol* 1995;22:422–426.

79. Thewes M, Worret WI, Engst R, et al. Stromelysin-3: a potent marker for histopathologic differentiation between desmoplastic trichoepithelioma and morphealike basal cell carcinoma. *Am J Dermatopathol* 1998;20:140–142.

80. Hartschuh W, Schulz T. Merkel cells are integral constituents of desmoplastic trichoepithelioma: an immunohistochemical and electron microscopic study. *J Cutan Pathol* 1995;22:413–421.

81. Gilks CB, Clement PB, Wood WS. Trichoblastic fibroma. *Am J Dermatopathol* 1989;11:397.

82. Headington JT, French AJ. Primary neoplasms of the hair follicle. Histogenesis and classification. *Arch Dermatol* 1962;86:430.

83. Cohen C, Davis TS. Multiple trichogenic adnexal tumors. *Am J Dermatopathol* 1986;8:241.

84. Cowen EW, Helm KF, Billingsley EM. An unusually aggressive trichoblastoma. *J Am Acad Dermatol* 2000;42:374–377.

85. Helm KF, Cowen EW, Billingsley EM, et al. Trichoblastoma or trichoblastic carcinoma? *J Am Acad Dermatol* 2001;44:547.

86. Diaz-Cascajo C, Borghi S, Rey-Lopez A, et al. Cutaneous lymphadenoma. A peculiar variant of nodular trichoblastoma. *Am J Dermatopathol* 1996;18:186.

87. Kanitakis J, Brutzkus A, Butnaru AC, et al. Melanotrichoblastoma: immunohistochemical study of a variant of pigmented trichoblastoma. *Am J Dermatopathol* 2002;24:498–501.

88. Yamamoto O, Hisaoka M, Yasuda H, et al. A rippled-pattern trichoblastoma: an immunohistochemical study. *J Cutan Pathol* 2000;27:460.

89. Tronnier M. Clear cell trichoblastoma in association with a nevus sebaceous. *Am J Dermatopathol* 2001;23:143.

90. Requena L, Barat A. Giant trichoblastoma on the scalp. *Am J Dermatopathol* 1993;15:497.

91. Ackerman AB, de Viragh PA, Chonchitnant N. Trichoblastoma: trichoepithelioma. In: *Tumors with Follicular Differentiation*. Philadelphia: Lea & Febiger, 1993:359.

92. Nikolowski W. Tricho-adenom. *Arch Klin Exp Dermatol* 1958; 207:34.

93. Rahbari H, Mehregan A, Pinkus H. Trichoadenoma of Nikolowski. *J Cutan Pathol* 1977;4:90–98.

94. Undeutsch W, Rassner G. [Trichoadenoma (Nikolowski). A clinical and histologic case report]. *Hautarzt* 1984;35:650–652.

95. Nikolowski W. Trichoadenom. *Z Hautkr* 1977;53:87.

96. Jaqueti G, Requena L, Sanchez Yus E. Verrucous trichoadenoma. *J Cutan Pathol* 1989;16:145–148.

97. Reibold R, Undeutsch W, Fleiner J. Trichoadenoma of Nikolowski—review of four decades and seven new cases [German]. *Hautarzt* 1998;49:925–928.

98. Brown AC, Crounse RG, Winkelmann RK. Generalized hairfollicle hamartoma, associated with alopecia, aminoacidura, and myasthenia gravis. *Arch Dermatol* 1969;99:478–493.

99. Ridley CM, Smith N. Generalized hair follicle hamartoma associated with alopecia and myasthenia gravis: report of a second case. *Clin Exp Dermatol* 1981;6:283–289.

100. Starink TM, Lane EB, Meijer CJ. Generalized trichoepitheliomas with alopecia and myasthenia gravis: clinicopathologic and immunohistochemical study and comparison with classic and desmoplastic trichoepithelioma. *J Am Acad Dermatol* 1986; 15:1104–1112.

101. Weltfriend S, David M, Ginzburg A, et al. Generalized hair follicle hamartoma: the third case report in association with myasthenia gravis. *Am J Dermatopathol* 1987;9:428–432.

102. Mehregan AH, Baker S. Basaloid follicular hamartoma: three cases with localized and systematized unilateral lesions. *J Cutan Pathol* 1985;12:55–65.

103. Brownstein MH. Basaloid follicular hamartoma: solitary and multiple types. *J Am Acad Dermatol* 1992;27:237–240.

104. Girardi M, Federman GL, McNiff JM. Familial multiple basaloid follicular hamartomas: a report of two affected sisters. *Pediatr Dermatol* 1999;16:281–284.

105. Goeteyn M, Geerts ML, Kint A, et al. The Bazex–Dupre–Christol syndrome. *Arch Dermatol* 1994;130:337–342.

106. Metry D, Guill C. Generalized basaloid follicular hamartoma syndrome. *J Am Acad Dermatol* 2001;45:644–646.

107. Jih DM, Shapiro M, James WD, et al. Familial basaloid follicular hamartoma: lesional characterization and review of the literature. *Am J Dermatopathol* 2003;25:130–137.

108. Brownstein MH. Basaloid follicular hamartoma: solitary and multiple types. *J Am Acad Dermatol* 1992;27:237–240.

109. Walsh N, Ackerman AB. Basaloid follicular hamartoma: solitary and multiple types. *J Am Acad Dermatol* 1993;29:125–129.

110. Walsh N, Ackerman AB. Infundibulocystic basal cell carcinoma: a newly described variant. *Mod Pathol* 1990;3:599–608.

111. Mehregan AH, Baker S. Basaloid follicular hamartoma: three cases with localized and systematized unilateral lesions. *J Cutan Pathol* 1985;12:55–65.

112. Moehlenbeck FW. Pilomatrixoma (calcifying epithelioma). A statistical study. *Arch Dermatol* 1973;108:532–534.

113. Swerlick RA, Cooper PH, Mackel SE. Rapid enlargement of pilomatricoma. *J Am Acad Dermatol* 1982;7:54–56.

114. Uchiyama N, Shindo Y, Saida T. Perforating pilomatricoma. *J Cutan Pathol* 1986;13:312–318.

115. Chiaramonti A, Gilgor RS. Pilomatricomas associated with myotonic dystrophy. *Arch Dermatol* 1978;114:1363–1365.

116. Demircan M, Balik E. Pilomatricoma in children: a prospective study. *Pediatr Dermatol* Nov-1997;14:430–432.

117. Cooper PH, Fechner RE. Pilomatricoma-like changes in the epidermal cysts of Gardner's syndrome. *J Am Acad Dermatol* 1983;8:639–644.

118. Panico L, Manivel JC, Pettinato G, et al. Pilomatrix carcinoma. A case report with immunohistochemical findings, flow cytometric comparison with benign pilomatrixoma and review of the literature. *Tumori* 1994;80:309–314.

119. Sau P, Lupton GP, Graham JH. Pilomatrix carcinoma. *Cancer* 1993;71:2491–2498.

120. Gould E, Kurzon R, Kowalczyk AP, et al. Pilomatrix carcinoma with pulmonary metastasis. Report of a case. *Cancer* 1984;54: 370–372.

121. Hanly MG, Allsbrook WC, Pantazis CG, et al. Pilomatrical carcinosarcoma of the cheek with subsequent pulmonary metastases. A case report. *Am J Dermatopathol* 1994;16:196–200.

122. Kawakami M, Akiyama M, Kimoto M, et al. Extraordinarily large calcifying epithelioma without aggressive behavior. *Dermatology* 2001;202:74–75.

123. Solanki P, Ramzy I, Durr N, et al. Pilomatrixoma. Cytologic features with differential diagnostic considerations. *Arch Pathol Lab Med* 1987;111:294–297.

124. Lever WF, Griesemer RD. Calcifying epithelioma of Malherbe. *Arch Dermatol Syph* 1949;59:506.

125. Cazers JS, Okun MR, Pearson SH. Pigmented calcifying epithelioma. Review and presentation of a case with unusual features. *Arch Dermatol* 1974;110:773–774.

126. Carlson JA, Healy K, Slominski A, et al. Melanocytic matricoma: a report of two cases of a new entity. *Am J Dermatopathol* 1999;21:344–349.

127. Resnik KS. Is melanocytic matricoma a bona fide entity or is it just one type of matricoma? *Am J Dermatopathol* 2003;25:166.

128. Peterson WCJ, Hult AM. Calcifying epithelioma of Malherbe. *Arch Dermatol* 1964;90:404.

129. Forbis RJ, Helwig EB. Pilomatrixoma: calcifying epithelioma. *Arch Dermatol* 1961;83:606.

130. Kurokawa I, Kusumoto K, Bessho K, et al. Immunohistochemical expression of bone morphogenetic protein-2 in pilomatricoma. *Br J Dermatol* 2000;143:754–758.

131. Wiedersberg H. Das epithelioma calcificans Malherbe. *Dermatol Monatsschr* 1971;157:867.

132. Turhan B, Krainer L. Bemerkungen über die sogenannten verkalkenden epitheliome der haut und ihre genese. *Dermatologica* 1942;85:73.

133. Malherbe A, Chenantais J. Note sur l'épithéliome calcifié des glandes sébacées. *Prog Med* 1880;8:826.

134. Hashimoto K, Nelson RG, Lever WF. Calcifying epithelioma of Malherbe. Histochemical and electron microscopic studies. *J Invest Dermatol* 1966;46:391–408.

135. Lever WF, Hashimoto K. Die Histogenese einiger Hautanhangstumoren im Lichte histochemischer und elektronenmikroskopischer Befunde (Ekkrines Porom, ckkrines Spiradenom, Syringom, Cylindrom und verkalkendes Epitheliom). *Hautarzt* 1966;17:161–173.

136. McGavran MH. Ultrastructure of pilomatrixoma (calcifying epithelioma). *Cancer* 1965;18:1445–1456.

137. Hashimoto K, Lever WF. Histogenesis of skin appendage tumors. *Arch Dermatol* 1969;100:356–369.

138. Cribier B, Asch PH, Regnier C, et al. Expression of human hair keratin basic 1 in pilomatrixoma. A study of 128 cases. *Br J Dermatol* 1999;140:600–604.

139. Cribier B, Peltre B, Langbein L, et al. Expression of type I hair keratins in follicular tumours. *Br J Dermatol* 2001;144:977–982.

140. Watanabe S, Wagatsuma K, Takahashi H. Immunohistochemical localization of cytokeratins and involucrin in calcifying epithelioma: comparative studies with normal skin. *Br J Dermatol* 1994;131:506–513.

141. Chan EF, Gat U, McNiff JM, et al. A common human skin tumour is caused by activating mutations in beta-catenin. *Nat Genet* 1999;21:410–413.

142. Moreno-Bueno G, Gamallo C, Perez-Gallego L, et al. Beta-catenin expression in pilomatrixomas. Relationship with beta-catenin gene mutations and comparison with beta-catenin expression in normal hair follicles. *Br J Dermatol* 2001;145:576–581.

143. Behrens J, von Kries JP, Kuhl M, et al. Functional interaction of beta-catenin with the transcription factor LEF-1. *Nature* 1996;382:638–642.

144. Aloi FG, Molinero A, Pippione M. Basal cell carcinoma with matrical differentiation. Matrical carcinoma. *Am J Dermatopathol* 1988;10:509–513.

145. van der Walt JD, Rohlova B. Carcinomatous transformation in a pilomatrixoma. *Am J Dermatopathol* 1984;6:63–69.

146. Lopansri S, Mihm MC Jr. Pilomatrix carcinoma or calcifying epitheliocarcinoma of Malherbe: a case report and review of literature. *Cancer* 1980;45:2368–2373.

147. Wood MG, Parhizgar B, Beerman H. Malignant pilomatricoma. *Arch Dermatol* 1984;120:770–773.

148. Green DE, Sanusi ID, Fowler MR. Pilomatrix carcinoma. *J Am Acad Dermatol* 1987;17:264–270.

149. O'Donovan DG, Freemont AJ, Adams JE, et al. Malignant pilomatrixoma with bone metastasis. *Histopathology*. 1993;23:385–386.

150. Mir R, Cortes E, Papantoniou PA, et al. Metastatic trichomatricial carcinoma. *Arch Pathol Lab Med* 1986;110:660–663.

151. Weedon D, Bell J, Mayze J. Matrical carcinoma of the skin. *J Cutan Pathol* 1980;7:39–42.

152. Hardisson D, Linares MD, Cuevas-Santos J, et al. Pilomatrix carcinoma: a clinicopathologic study of six cases and review of the literature. *Am J Dermatopathol* 2001;23:394–401.

153. Poiares Baptista A, Garcia ESL, Born MC. Proliferating trichilemmal cyst. *J Cutan Pathol* 1983;10:178–187.

154. Hanau D, Grosshans E. Trichilemmal tumor undergoing specific keratinization: "keratinizing trichilemmoma." *J Cutan Pathol* 1979;6:463–475.

155. Brownstein MH, Arluk DJ. Proliferating trichilemmal cyst: a simulant of squamous cell carcinoma. *Cancer* 1 1981;48:1207–1214.

156. Holmes EJ. Tumors of lower hair sheath. Common histogenesis of certain so-called "sebaceous cysts," acanthomas and "sebaceous carcinomas." *Cancer* 1968;21:234–248.

157. Korting GW, Hoede N. Zum sogenannten "pilar tumor of the scalp." *Arch Klin Exp Dermatol* 1969;234:409–419.

158. Leppard BJ, Sanderson KV. The natural history of trichilemmal cysts. *Br J Dermatol* 1976;94:379–390.

159. Mehregan AH, Lee KC. Malignant proliferating trichilemmal tumors—report of three cases. *J Dermatol Surg Oncol* 1987;13:1339–1342.

160. Wilson Jones E. Proliferating epidermoid cysts. *Arch Dermatol* 1966;94:11.

161. Reed RJ, Lamar LM. Invasive hair matrix tumors of the scalp. Invasive pilomatrixoma. *Arch Dermatol* 1966;94:310–316.

162. Dabska M. Giant hair matrix tumor. *Cancer* 1971;28:701–706.

163. Pinkus H. "Sebaceous cysts" are trichilemmal cysts. *Arch Dermatol* 1969;99:544–555.

164. Saida T, Oohara K, Hori Y, et al. Development of a malignant proliferating trichilemmal cyst in a patient with multiple trichilemmal cysts. *Dermatologica* 1983;166:203–208.

165. Park BS, Yang SG, Cho KH. Malignant proliferating trichilemmal tumor showing distant metastases. *Am J Dermatopathol* 1997;19:536–539.

166. Amaral AL, Nascimento AG, Goellner JR. Proliferating pilar (trichilemmal) cyst. Report of two cases, one with carcinomatous transformation and one with distant metastases. *Arch Pathol Lab Med* 1984;108:808–810.

167. Hödl S, Smolle J, Scharnagl E. Zur dignität der proliferierenden trichilemmalzyste. *Hautarzt* 1984;35:640–644.

168. Herrero J, Monteagudo C, Ruiz A, et al. Malignant proliferating trichilemmal tumours: an histopathological and immunohistochemical study of three cases with DNA ploidy and morphometric evaluation. *Histopathology* 1998;33:542–546.

169. Sau P, Graham JH, Helwig EB. Proliferating epithelial cysts. Clinicopathological analysis of 96 cases. *J Cutan Pathol* 1995;22:394–406.

170. Takata M, Quinn AG, Hashimoto K, et al. Low frequency of loss of heterozygosity at the nevoid basal cell carcinoma locus and other selected loci in appendageal tumors. *J Invest Dermatol* 1996;106:1141–1144.

171. Fernandez-Figueras MT, Casalots A, Puig L, et al. Proliferating trichilemmal tumour: p53 immunoreactivity in association with p27Kip1 over-expression indicates a low-grade carcinoma profile. *Histopathology* 2001;38:454–457.

172. Lopez-Rios F, Rodriguez-Peralto JL, Aguilar A, et al. Proliferating trichilemmal cyst with focal invasion: report of a case and a review of the literature. *Am J Dermatopathol* 2000;22:183–187.

173. Noto G. "Benign" proliferating trichilemmal tumour: does it really exist? *Histopathology* 1999;35:386–387.

174. Headington JT, French AJ. Primary neoplasms of the hair follicle. *Arch Dermatol* 1962;107:866.

175. Brownstein MH, Shapiro L. Trichilemmoma. Analysis of 40 new cases. *Arch Dermatol* 1973;107:866–869.

176. Mehregan AH, Medenica M, Whitney D, et al. A clear cell pilar sheath tumor of scalp: case report. *J Cutan Pathol* 1988;15:380–384.

177. Brownstein MH, Shapiro EE. Trichilemmomal horn: cutaneous horn overlying trichilemmoma. *Clin Exp Dermatol* 1979;4:59–63.

178. Brownstein MH, Mehregan AH, Bikowski JB, et al. The dermatopathology of Cowden's syndrome. *Br J Dermatol* 1979;100:667–673.

179. Crowson AN, Magro CM. Basal cell carcinoma arising in association with desmoplastic trichilemmoma. *Am J Dermatopathol* 1966;18:43.

180. Illueca C, Monteagudo C, Revert A, et al. Diagnostic value of CD34 immunostaining in desmoplastic trichilemmoma. *J Cutan Pathol* 1998;25:435–439.

181. Leonardi CL, Zhu WY, Kinsey WH, et al. Trichilemmomas are not associated with human papillomavirus DNA. *J Cutan Pathol* 1991;18:193–197.

182. Lloyd KM, Denis M. Cowden's disease: a possible new symptom complex with multiple system involvement. *Ann Intern Med* 1963;58:136–142.

183. Allen BS, Fitch MH, Smith JG Jr. Multiple hamartoma syndrome. A report of a new case with associated carcinoma of the uterine cervix and angioid streaks of the eyes. *J Am Acad Dermatol* 1980;2:303–308.

184. Brownstein MH, Wolf M, Bikowski JB. Cowden's disease: a cutaneous marker of breast cancer. *Cancer* 1978;41:2393–2398.

185. Starink TM, van der Veen JP, Arwert F, et al. The Cowden syndrome: a clinical and genetic study in 21 patients. Clin Genet. 1986;29:222–233.

186. Albrecht S, Haber RM, Goodman JC, et al. Cowden syndrome and Lhermitte–Duclos disease. *Cancer* 1992;70:869–876.

187. Padberg GW, Schot JD, Vielvoye GJ, et al. Lhermitte–Duclos disease and Cowden disease: a single phakomatosis. *Ann Neurol* 1991;29:517–523.

188. Gorlin RJ, Cohen MM Jr, Condon LM, et al. Bannayan–Riley-Ruvalcaba syndrome. *Am J Med Genet* 1 1992;44:307–314.

189. Marsh DJ, Kum JB, Lunetta KL, et al. PTEN mutation spectrum and genotype-phenotype correlations in Bannayan–Riley–Ruvalcaba syndrome suggest a single entity with Cowden syndrome. *Hum Mol Genet* 1999;8:1461–1472.

190. Thyresson HN, Doyle JA. Cowden's disease (multiple hamartoma syndrome). *Mayo Clin Proc* 1981;56:179–184.

191. Starink TM, Hausman R. The cutaneous pathology of facial lesions in Cowden's disease. *J Cutan Pathol* 1984;11:331–337.

192. Nelen MR, Padberg GW, Peeters EA, et al. Localization of the gene for Cowden disease to chromosome 10q22–23. *Nat Genet* 1996;13:114–116.

193. Li J, Yen C, Liaw D, et al. PTEN, a putative protein tyrosine phosphatase gene mutated in human brain, breast, and prostate cancer. *Science* 28 1997;275:1943–1947.

194. Waite KA, Eng C. Protean PTEN: form and function. *Am J Hum Genet* 2002;70:829–844.

195. Liaw D, Marsh DJ, Li J, et al. Germline mutations of the PTEN gene in Cowden disease, an inherited breast and thyroid cancer syndrome. *Nat Genet* 1997;16:64–67.

196. Nelen MR, van Staveren WC, Peeters EA, et al. Germline mutations in the PTEN/MMAC1 gene in patients with Cowden disease. *Hum Mol Genet* 1997;6:1383–1387.

197. Weary PE, Gorlin RJ, Gentry WC Jr, et al. Multiple hamartoma syndrome (Cowden's disease). *Arch Dermatol* 1972;106:682–690.

198. Mehregan AH, Buttler JD. A tumor of follicular infundibulum. *Arch Dermatol* 1961;83:294.

199. Johnson WC, Hookerman BJ. Basal cell hamartoma with follicular differentiation. *Arch Dermatol* 1972;105:105–106.

200. Cribier B, Grosshans E. Tumor of the follicular infundibulum: a clinicopathologic study. *J Am Acad Dermatol* 1995;33:979–984.

201. Mahalingam M, Bhawan J, Finn R, et al. Tumor of the follicular infundibulum with sebaceous differentiation. *J Cutan Pathol* 2001;28:314–317.

202. Horn TD, Vennos EM, Bernstein BD, et al. Multiple tumors of follicular infundibulum with sweat duct differentiation. *J Cutan Pathol* 1995;22:281–287.

203. Chan P, White SW, Pierson DL, et al. Trichilemmoma. *J Dermatol Surg Oncol* 1979;5:58–59.

204. Brownstein MH. Trichilemmal horn: cutaneous horn showing trichilemmal keratinization. *Br J Dermatol* 1979;100:303–309.

205. Nakamura K. Two cases of trichilemmal-like horn. *Arch Dermatol* 1984;120:386–387.

206. Grouls V. Tricholemmale keratose und tricholemmales karzinom. *Hautarzt* 1987;38:335–341.

207. DiMaio DJ, Cohen PR. Trichilemmal horn: case presentation and literature review. *J Am Acad Dermatol* 1998;39:368–371.

208. Poblet E, Jimenez-Reyes J, Gonzalez-Herrada C, et al. Trichilemmal keratosis. A clinicopathologic and immunohistochemical study of two cases. *Am J Dermatopathol* 1996;18:543–547.

209. Wong TY, Suster S. Tricholemmal carcinoma. A clinicopathologic study of 13 cases. *Am J Dermatopathol* 1994;16:463–473.

210. Hunt SJ, Abell E. Malignant hair matrix tumor ("malignant trichoepithelioma") arising in the setting of multiple hereditary trichoepithelioma. *Am J Dermatopathol* 1991;13:275–281.

211. Boscaino A, Terracciano LM, Donofrio V, et al. Tricholemmal carcinoma: a study of seven cases. *J Cutan Pathol* 1992;19:94–99.

212. Reis JP, Tellechea O, Cunha MF, et al. Trichilemmal carcinoma: review of 8 cases. *J Cutan Pathol* 1993;20:44–49.

213. ten Seldam RE. Tricholemmocarcinoma. Australas *J Dermatol* 1977;18:62–72.

214. O'Hare AM, Cooper PH, Parlette HL 3rd. Trichilemmomal carcinoma in a patient with Cowden's disease (multiple hamartoma syndrome). *J Am Acad Dermatol* 1997;36:1021–1023.

215. Schell H, Haneke E. Tricholemmales karzinom: Berich über 11 fälle. *Hautarzt* 1986;37:384–387.

216. Swanson PE, Cherwitz DL, Wick MR. Trichilemmal carcinoma: a clinicopathologic study of 6 cases. *J Cutan Pathol* 1988;14:374(abst).

217. Ko T, Tada H, Hatoko M, et al. Trichilemmal carcinoma developing in a burn scar: a report of two cases. *J Dermatol* 1996;23:463–468.

218. Chan KO, Lim IJ, Baladas HG, et al. Multiple tumour presentation of trichilemmal carcinoma. *Br J Plast Surg* 1999;52:665–667.

219. Takata M, Rehman I, Rees JL. A trichilemmal carcinoma arising from a proliferating trichilemmal cyst: the loss of the

wild-type p53 is a critical event in malignant transformation. *Hum Pathol* 1998;29:193–195.

220. Mehregan A, Pinkus H. Life history of organoid nevi. *Arch Dermatol* 1965;91:574.

221. Lentz C, Altman J, Mopper C. Nevus sebaceus of Jadassohn. *Arch Dermatol* 1968;97:294.

222. Marden P, Venters HD. A new neurocutaneous syndrome. *Am J Dis Child* 1966;112:79.

223. Wauschkuhn J, Rohde B. Systematisierte talgdrüsen-, pigment-, und epitheliale naevi mit neurologischer symptomatik: Feuerstein–Mimssches neuroektodermales syndrom. *Hautarzt* 1971;22:10.

224. Hornstein O, Knickenberg M. Zur kenntnis des Schimmelpenning–Feuerstein–Mims–syndroms. *Arch Dermatol Forsch* 1974; 250:33.

225. Feuerstein R, Mims L. Linear nevus sebaceus with convulsions and mental retardation. *Am J Dis Child* 1962;104:675.

226. Solomon LW, Fretzin DF, Dewald RL. The epidermal nevus syndrome. *Arch Dermatol* 1968;97:273.

227. Kuokkanen K, Koivikko M, Alavaikko M. Organoid nevus phakomatosis. *Acta Derm Venereol (Stockh)* 1980;60:534.

228. Lantis S, Leyden J, Thew M, et al. Nevus sebaceus of Jadassohn: part of a new neurocutaneous syndrome. *Arch Dermatol* 1968; 98:117.

229. Wilson Jones E, Heyl T. Naevus sebaceus. *Br J Dermatol* 1970; 82:99.

230. Cribier B, Scrivener Y, Grosshans E. Tumors arising in nevus sebaceus: a study of 596 cases. *J Am Acad Dermatol* 2000;42: 263–268.

231. Jaqueti G, Requena L, Sanchez Yus E. Trichoblastoma is the most common neoplasm developed in nevus sebaceus of Jadassohn: a clinicopathologic study of a series of 155 cases. *Am J Dermatopathol* 2000;22:108–118.

232. Rahbari H, Mehregan A. Development of proliferating trichilemmal cyst in organoid nevus. *J Am Acad Dermatol* 1986; 14:123.

233. Bonvalet D, Barrandon V, Foix C, et al. Tumeurs annexielles bénignes de survenue tardive sur naevus verrucosébacé (Jadassohn). *Ann Dermatol Venereol* 1983;110:337.

234. Brownstein M, Shapiro L. The pilosebaceous tumors. *Int J Dermatol* 1977;16:340.

235. Morioka S. The natural history of nevus sebaceus. *J Cutan Pathol* 1985;12:200.

236. Steffen CH, Ackerman AB. *Neoplasms with Sebaceous Differentiation*. Philadelphia: Lea & Febiger, 1996:89.

237. Domingo J, Helwig EB. Malignant neoplasms associated with nevus sebaceus of Jadassohn. *J Am Acad Dermatol* 1979;1:545–556.

238. Tarkhan, II, Domingo J. Metastasizing eccrine porocarcinoma developing in a sebaceous nevus of Jadassohn. Report of a case. *Arch Dermatol* 1985;121:413–415.

239. Gailani MR, Stahle-Backdahl M, Leffell DJ, et al. The role of the human homologue of Drosophila patched in sporadic basal cell carcinoma. *Nat Genet* 1996;14:78–81.

240. Shen T, Park WS, Boni R, et al. Detection of loss of heterozygosity on chromosome 9q22.3 in microdissected sporadic basal cell carcinoma. *Hum Pathol* 1999;30:284.

241. Xin H, Matt D, Qin JZ, et al. The sebaceous nevus: a nevus with deletions of the PTCH gene. *Cancer Res* 1999;59:1834–1836.

242. Takata M, Tojo M, Hatta N, et al. No evidence of deregulated patched-hedgehog signaling pathway in trichoblastomas and other tumors arising within nevus sebaceous. *J Invest Dermatol* 2001;117:1666–1670.

243. Ortiz-Rey JA, Martin-Jimenez A, Alvarez C, et al. Sebaceous gland hyperplasia of the vulva. *Obstet Gynecol* 2002;99:919–921.

244. Rocamora A, Santonja C, Vives R, et al. Sebaceous gland hyperplasia of the vulva: a case report. *Obstet Gynecol* 1986;68 [Suppl 3]:63S–65S.

245. Carson HJ, Massa M, Reddy V. Sebaceous gland hyperplasia of the penis. *J Urol* 1996;156:1441.

246. Belinchon I, Aguilar A, Tardio J, et al. Areolar sebaceous hyperplasia: a case report. *Cutis* 1996;58:63–64.

247. De Villez RL, Roberts LC. Premature sebaceous gland hyperplasia. *J Am Acad Dermatol* 1982;6:933–935.

248. Boonchai W, Leenutaphong V. Familial presenile sebaceous gland hyperplasia. *J Am Acad Dermatol* 1997;36:120–122.

249. Luderschmidt C, Plewig G. Circumscribed sebaceous gland hyperplasia: autoradiographic and histoplanimetric studies. *J Invest Dermatol* 1978;70:207–209.

250. Kruse R, Rutten A, Schweiger N, et al. Frequency of microsatellite instability in unselected sebaceous gland neoplasias and hyperplasias. *J Invest Dermatol* 2003;120:858–864.

251. Popnikolov NK, Gatalica Z, Colome-Grimmer MI, et al. Loss of mismatch repair proteins in sebaceous gland tumors. *J Cutan Pathol* 2003;30:178–184.

252. Bayer-Garner IB, Givens V, Smoller B. Immunohistochemical staining for androgen receptors: a sensitive marker of sebaceous differentiation. *Am J Dermatopathol* 1999;21:426–431.

253. Miles A. Sebaceous glands in the lip and cheek mucosa of man. *Br Dent J* 1958;105:235.

254. Smith DM Jr, Peters TG, Donegan WL. Montgomery's areolar tubercle. A light microscopic study. *Arch Pathol Lab Med* 1982; 106:60–63.

255. Chambers SO. The structure of Fordyce's disease as demonstrated by wax reconstruction. *Arch Dermatol Syph* 1928;18:666.

256. Woolhandler HW, Becker WS. Adenoma of sebaceous glands: adenoma sebaceum. *Arch Dermatol Syph* 1942;45:734.

257. Lever WF. Sebaceous adenoma: review of the literature and report of a case. *Arch Dermatol Syph* 1948;57:102.

258. Essenhigh DM, Jones D, Rack JH. A sebaceous adenoma. *Br J Dermatol* 1964;76:330.

259. Banse-Kupin L, Morales A, Barlow M. Torre's syndrome. *J Am Acad Dermatol* 1984;10:803.

260. Rutten A, Burgdorf W, Hugel H, et al. Cystic sebaceous tumors as marker lesions for the Muir–Torre syndrome: a histopathologic and molecular genetic study. *Am J Dermatopathol* 1999; 21:405–413.

261. Troy JL, Ackerman AB. Sebaceoma. A distinctive benign neoplasm of adnexal epithelium differentiating toward sebaceous cells. *Am J Dermatopathol* 1984;6:7–13.

262. Hori M, Egami K, Maejima K, et al. Electron microscopic study of sebaceous epithelioma. *J Dermatol* 1978;5:139.

263. Urban FH, Winkelmann RK. Sebaceous malignancy. *Arch Dermatol* 1961;84:63.

264. Misago N, Mihara I, Ansai S, et al. Sebaceoma and related neoplasms with sebaceous differentiation: a clinicopathologic study of 30 cases. *Am J Dermatopathol* 2002;24:294–304.

265. Steffen C, Ackerman AB. Sebaceoma. In: Steffen C, Ackerman AB. *Neoplasms with Sebaceous Differentiation*. Philadelphia: Lea & Febiger, 1994:385.

266. Muir EG, Bell AJ, Barlow KA. Multiple primary carcinomata of the colon, duodenum, and larynx associated with keratoacanthomata of the face. *Br J Surg* 1967;54:191–195.

267. Finan MC, Connolly SM. Sebaceous gland tumors and systemic disease: a clinicopathologic analysis. *Medicine (Baltimore)* 1984; 63:232.

268. Poleksic S. Keratoacanthoma and multiple carcinomas. *Br J Dermatol* 1974;91:461–463.

269. Fathizadeh A, Medenica MM, Soltani K, et al. Aggressive keratoacanthoma and internal malignant neoplasm. *Arch Dermatol* 1982;118:112–114.

270. Schwartz RA, Torre DP. The Muir–Torre syndrome: a 25-year retrospect. *J Am Acad Dermatol* 1995;33:90–104.

271. Rulon DB, Helwig EB. Multiple sebaceous neoplasms of the skin: an association with multiple visceral carcinomas, especially of the colon. *Am J Clin Pathol* 1973;60:745–752.

272. Torre D. Multiple sebaceous tumors. *Arch Dermatol* 1968;98:549–551.

273. Abbott JJ, Hernandez-Rios P, Amirkhan RH, et al. Cystic sebaceous neoplasms in Muir–Torre syndrome. *Arch Pathol Lab Med* 2003;127:614–617.

274. Burgdorf WH, Pitha J, Fahmy A. Muir–Torre syndrome. Histologic spectrum of sebaceous proliferations. *Am J Dermatopathol* 1986;8:202–208.

275. Worret WI, Burgdorf WH, Fahmy A, et al. Torre–Muir syndrome. Sebaceous gland neoplasms, keratoacanthomas, multiple internal cancers and heredity [German]. *Hautarzt* 1981;32:519–524.

276. Lynch HT, Lynch PM, Pester J, et al. The cancer family syndrome. Rare cutaneous phenotypic linkage of Torre's syndrome. *Arch Intern Med* 1981;141:607–611.

277. Honchel R, Halling KC, Schaid DJ, et al. Microsatellite instability in Muir–Torre syndrome. *Cancer Res* 1994;54:1159–1163.

278. Kolodner RD, Hall NR, Lipford J, et al. Structure of the human MSH2 locus and analysis of two Muir–Torre kindreds for msh2 mutations. *Genomics* 1994;24:516–526.

279. Kruse R, Rutten A, Lamberti C, et al. Muir–Torre phenotype has a frequency of DNA mismatch-repair-gene mutations similar to that in hereditary nonpolyposis colorectal cancer families defined by the Amsterdam criteria. *Am J Hum Genet* 1998;63:63–70.

280. Kruse R, Lamberti C, Wang Y, et al. Is the mismatch repair deficient type of Muir–Torre syndrome confined to mutations in the hMSH2 gene? *Hum Genet* 1996;98:747–750.

281. Swale VJ, Quinn AG, Wheeler JM, et al. Microsatellite instability in benign skin lesions in hereditary non-polyposis colorectal cancer syndrome. *J Invest Dermatol* 1999;113:901–905.

282. Machin P, Catasus L, Pons C, et al. Microsatellite instability and immunostaining for MSH-2 and MLH-1 in cutaneous and internal tumors from patients with the Muir–Torre syndrome. *J Cutan Pathol* 2002;29:415–420.

283. Mathiak M, Rutten A, Mangold E, et al. Loss of DNA mismatch repair proteins in skin tumors from patients with Muir–Torre syndrome and MSH2 or MLH1 germline mutations: establishment of immunohistochemical analysis as a screening test. *Am J Surg Pathol* 2002;26:338–343.

284. Carlson JW, McGlennen RC, Gomez R, et al. Sebaceous carcinoma of the vulva: a case report and review of the literature. *Gynecol Oncol* 1996;60:489–491.

285. Escalonilla P, Grilli R, Canamero M, et al. Sebaceous carcinoma of the vulva. *Am J Dermatopathol* 1999;21:468–472.

286. Oppenheim AR. Sebaceous carcinoma of the penis. *Arch Dermatol* 1981;117:306–307.

287. Dixon RS, Mikhail GR, Slater HC. Sebaceous carcinoma of the eyelid. *J Am Acad Dermatol* 1980;3:241–243.

288. King DT, Barr RJ. Syringometaplasia: mucinous and squamous variants. *J Cutan Pathol* 1979;6:284–291.

289. Rao NA, Hidayat AA, McLean IW, et al. Sebaceous carcinomas of the ocular adnexa: a clinicopathologic study of 104 cases, with five-year follow-up data. *Hum Pathol* 1982;13:113–122.

290. Hernández-Pérez E, Baños E. Sebaceous carcinoma: report of two cases with metastasis. *Dermatologica* 1978;156:184.

291. Mellette JR, Amonette RA, Gardner JH, et al. Carcinoma of sebaceous glands on the head and neck. *J Dermatol Surg Oncol* 1981;7:404.

292. Rulon DB, Helwig EB. Cutaneous sebaceous neoplasms. *Cancer* 1974;33:82–102.

293. Wick MR, Goellner JR, Wolfe JT 3rd, et al. Adnexal carcinomas of the skin. II. Extraocular sebaceous carcinomas. *Cancer* 1985;56:1163–1172.

294. Moreno C, Jacyk WK, Judd MJ, et al. Highly aggressive extraocular sebaceous carcinoma. *Am J Dermatopathol* 2001;23:450–455.

295. Leonard DD, Deaton WR Jr. Multiple sebaceous gland tumors and visceral carcinomas. *Arch Dermatol* 1974;110:917–920.

296. Graham R, McKee P, McGibbon D, et al. Torre–Muir syndrome. An association with isolated sebaceous carcinoma. *Cancer* 1985;55:2868–2873.

297. Russell WG, Page DL, Hough AJ, et al. Sebaceous carcinoma of meibomian gland origin. The diagnostic importance of pagetoid spread of neoplastic cells. *Am J Clin Pathol* 1980;73:504–511.

298. Hayashi N, Furihata M, Ohtsuki Y, et al. Search for accumulation of p53 protein and detection of human papillomavirus genomes in sebaceous gland carcinoma of the eyelid. *Virchows Arch* 1994;424:503–509.

299. Gonzalez-Fernandez F, Kaltreider SA, Patnaik BD, et al. Sebaceous carcinoma. Tumor progression through mutational inactivation of p53. *Ophthalmology* 1998;105:497–506.

300. Hasebe T, Mukai K, Yamaguchi N, et al. Prognostic value of immunohistochemical staining for proliferating cell nuclear antigen, p53, and c-erbB-2 in sebaceous gland carcinoma and sweat gland carcinoma: comparison with histopathological parameter. *Mod Pathol* 1994;7:37–43.

301. Friedman KJ, Boudreau S, Farmer ER. Superficial epithelioma with sebaceous differentiation. *J Cutan Pathol* 1987;14:193–197.

302. Kuo T. Clear cell carcinoma of the skin. A variant of the squamous cell carcinoma that simulates sebaceous carcinoma. *Am J Surg Pathol* 1980;4:573–583.

303. Prioleau PG, Santa Cruz DJ. Sebaceous gland neoplasia. *J Cutan Pathol* 1984;11:396–414.

304. Sinard JH. Immunohistochemical distinction of ocular sebaceous carcinoma from basal cell and squamous cell carcinoma. *Arch Ophthalmol* 1999;117:776–783.

305. Perez-Oliva N, del Pozo Hernando LJ, Tejerina JA, et al. Nevus apocrino. *Med Cut Ibero Lat Am* 1990;18:67–69.

306. Rabens SF, Naness JI, Gottlieb BF. Apocrine gland organic hamartoma (apocrine nevus). *Arch Dermatol* 1976;112:520–522.

307. Schwartz RA, Rojas-Corona R, Lambert WC. The polymorphic apocrine nevus: a study of a unique tumor including carcinoembryonic antigen staining. *J Surg Oncol* 1984;26:183–186.

308. Ando K, Hashikawa Y, Nakashima M, et al. Pure apocrine nevus. A study of light-microscopic and immunohistochemical features of a rare tumor. *Am J Dermatopathol* 1991;13:71–76.

309. Civatte J, Tsoitis G, Preaux J. Le naevus apocrine. Etude de 2 cas. *Ann Dermatol Syph* 1974;101:251–261.

310. Burden PA, Gentry RH, Fitzpatrick JE. Piloleiomyoma arising in an organoid nevus: a case report and review of the literature. *J Dermatol Surg Oncol* 1987;13:1213–1218.

311. Kim JH, Hur H, Lee CW, et al. Apocrine nevus. *J Am Acad Dermatol* 1988;18:579–581.

312. Mori O, Hachisuka H, Sasai Y. Apocrine nevus. *Int J Dermatol* 1993;32:448–449.

313. Neill JS, Park HK. Apocrine nevus: light microscopic, immunohistochemical and ultrastructural studies of a case. *J Cutan Pathol* 1993;20:79–83.

314. Mazoujian G. Immunohistochemistry of GCDFP-24 and zinc alpha2 glycoprotein in benign sweat gland tumors. *Am J Dermatopathol* 1990;12:452–457.

315. Mehregan AH. Apocrine cystadenoma. *Arch Dermatol* 1964;90:274.

316. Mehregan AH, Rahbari H. Benign epithelial tumors of the skin. IV: Benign apocrine gland tumors. *Cutis* 1978;21:53–56.

317. Benisch B, Peison B. Apocrine hidrocystoma of the shoulder. *Arch Dermatol* 1977;113:71–72.
318. Schewach-Millet M, Trau H. Congenital papillated apocrine cystadenoma: a mixed form of hidrocystoma, hidradenoma papilliferum, and syringocystadenoma papilliferum. *J Am Acad Dermatol* 1984;11:374–376.
319. Smith JD, Chernosky ME. Apocrine hidrocystoma (cystadenoma). *Arch Dermatol* 1974;109:700–702.
320. Ter Poorten HJ. Apocrine hidrocystoma of the right scapula. *Arch Dermatol* 1977;113:1730.
321. Shields JA, Eagle RC Jr, Shields CL, et al. Apocrine hidrocystoma of the eyelid. *Arch Ophthalmol* 1993;111:866–867.
322. Adeloye A, Aghadiuno PU, Adesina MA, et al. A large apocrine hidrocystoma located over the thoracic spine in a Nigerian. *Central African J Med* 1987;33:74–76.
323. De Fontaine S, Van Geertruyden J, Vandeweyer E. Apocrine hidrocystoma of the finger. *J Hand Surg [Br]* 1998;23:281–282.
324. Glusac EJ, Hendrickson MS, Smoller BR. Apocrine cystadenoma of the vulva. *J Am Acad Dermatol* 1994;31:498–499.
325. Kruse TV, Khan MA, Hassan MO. Multiple apocrine cystadenomas. *Br J Dermatol* 1979;100:675–681.
326. Alessi E, Gianotti R, Coggi A. Multiple apocrine hidrocystomas of the eyelids. *Br J Dermatol* 1997;137:642–645.
327. Asarch RG, Golitz LE, Sausker WF, et al. Median raphe cysts of the penis. *Arch Dermatol* 1979;115:1084–1086.
328. Hassan MO, Khan MA, Kruse TV. Apocrine cystadenoma. An ultrastructural study. *Arch Dermatol* 1979;115:194–200.
329. Gross BG. The fine structure of apocrine hidrocystoma. *Arch Dermatol* 1965;92:706–712.
330. Schaumburg-Lever G, Lever WF. Secretion from human apocrine glands: an electron microscopic study. *J Invest Dermatol* 1975;64:38–41.
331. Virgili A, Marzola A, Corazza M. Vulvar hidradenoma papilliferum. A review of 10.5 years' experience. *J Reprod Med* 2000;45:616–618.
332. Vortel V, Kraus Z, Andrys J. Hidroadenoma papilliferum vulvae. *Ceskoslovenska Gynekologie* 1972;37:58–59.
333. Ioannides G. Hidradenoma papilliferum. *Am J Obstet Gynecol* 1966;94:849–853.
334. Goette DK. Hidradenoma papilliferum. *J Am Acad Dermatol* 1988;19:133–135.
335. Loane J, Kealy WF, Mulcahy G. Perianatal hidradenoma papilliferum occurring in a male: a case report. *Irish J Med Sci* 1998;167:26–27.
336. Vang R, Cohen PR. Ectopic hidradenoma papilliferum: a case report and review of the literature. *J Am Acad Dermatol* 1999;41:115–118.
337. Santa Cruz DJ, Prioleau PG, Smith ME. Hidradenoma papilliferum of the eyelid. *Arch Dermatol* 1981;117:55–56.
338. Nissim F, Czernobilsky B, Ostfeld E. Hidradenoma papilliferum of the external auditory canal. *J Laryngol Otol* 1981;95:843–848.
339. Shenoy Y. Malignant perianal papillary hidradenoma. *Arch Dermatol* 1961;83:965.
340. Bannatyne P, Elliott P, Russell P. Vulvar adenosquamous carcinoma arising in a hidradenoma papilliferum, with rapidly fatal outcome: case report. *Gynecol Oncol* 1989;35:395–398.
341. Meeker JN, RD, Helwig EG. Hidradenoma papilliferum. *Am J Clin Pathol* 1962;37:182–195.
342. Hashimoto K. Hidradenoma papilliferum. An electron microscopic study. *Acta Derm Venereol* 1973;53:22–30.
343. Rostan SE, Waller JD. Syringocystadenoma papilliferum in an unusual location. Report of a case. *Arch Dermatol* 1976;112:835–836.
344. Helwig EH, VC. Syringocystadenoma papilliferum. *Arch Dermatol* 1955;71:361.
345. Goldberg NS, Esterly NB. Linear papules on the neck of a child. Syringocystadenoma papilliferum. *Arch Dermatol* 2001;121:1198.
346. de Bliek JP, Starink TM. Multiple linear syringocystadenoma papilliferum. *J Eur Acad Dermatol Venereol* 1999;12:74–76.
347. Pinkus H. Life history of naevus syringoadenomatosus papilliferus. *Arch Dermatol Syph* 1954;69:305.
348. Hashimoto K. Syringocystadenoma papilliferum. An electron microscopic study. *Archiv fur Dermatologische Forschung* 1972;245:353–369.
349. Fusaro RG, RW. Histochemically demonstrable carbohydrates of appendageal tumors of the skin: II. Benign apocrine gland tumors. *J Invest Dermatol* 1962;38:137.
350. Mambo N. Immunohistochemical study of the immunoglobulin classes of the plasma cells in papillary syringadenoma. *Virchows Archiv* 1982;397:1.
351. Vanatta PR, Bangert JL, Freeman RG. Syringocystadenoma papilliferum. A plasmacytotropic tumor. *Am J Surg Pathol* 1985;9:678–683.
351a. Seco Navado MA, Fresno Forcelledo M, Orduna Domingo A, et al. Syringocystadenoma papillifere à évolution maligne. *Ann Dermatol Venereol* 1982;109:685.
351b. Numata M, Hosoe S, Itoh N, et al. Syringadenocarcinoma papilliferum. *J Cutan Pathol* 1985;12:13.
352. Mazoujian G, Margolis R. Immunohistochemistry of gross cystic disease fluid protein (GCDFP-15) in 65 benign sweat gland tumors of the skin. *Am J Dermatopathol* 1988;10:28–35.
353. Noda Y, Kumasa S, Higashiyama H, et al. Immunolocalization of keratin proteins in sweat gland tumours by the use of monoclonal antibody. *Pathol Res Pract* 1988;183:284–291.
354. Boni R, Xin H, Hohl D, et al. Syringocystadenoma papilliferum: a study of potential tumor suppressor genes. *Am J Dermatopathol* 2001;23:87–89.
355. Landry M, Winkelmann RK. An unusual tubular apocrine adenoma. *Arch Dermatol* 1972;105:869–879.
356. Okun MR, Finn R, Blumental G. Apocrine adenoma versus pocrine carcinoma. Report of two cases. *J Am Acad Dermatol* 1980;2:322–326.
357. Toribio J, Zulaica A, Peteiro C. Tubular apocrine adenoma. *J Cutan Pathol* 1987;14:114–117.
358. Umbert P, Winkelmann RK. Tubular apocrine adenoma. *J Cutan Pathol* 1976;3:75–87.
359. Civatte J, Belaich S, Lauret P. Adenome tubulaire apocrine (quatre cas). *Ann Dermatol Venereol* 1979;106:665–669.
360. Burket JM, Zelickson AS. Tubular apocrine adenoma with perineural invasion. *J Am Acad Dermatol* 1984;11:639–642.
361. Ansai S, Watanabe S, Aso K. A case of tubular apocrine adenoma with syringocystadenoma papilliferum. *J Cutan Pathol* 1989;16:230–236.
362. Falck VG, Jordaan HF. Papillary eccrine adenoma. A tubulopapillary hidradenoma with eccrine differentiation. *Am J Dermatopathol* 1986;8:64–72.
363. Ishiko A, Shimizu H, Inamoto N, et al. Is tubular apocrine adenoma a distinct clinical entity? *Am J Dermatopathol* 1993;15:482–487.
364. Fox SB, Cotton DW. Tubular apocrine adenoma and papillary eccrine adenoma. Entities or unity? *Am J Dermatopathol* 1992;14:149–154.
365. Warkel RL, Helwig EB. Apocrine gland adenoma and adenocarcinoma of the axilla. *Arch Dermatol* 1978;114:198–203.
366. Weigand DA, Burgdorf WH. Perianal apocrine gland adenoma. *Arch Dermatol* 1980;116:1051–1053.
367. Assor D, Davis JB. Multiple apocrine fibroadenomas of the anal skin. *Am J Clin Pathol* 1977;68:397–399.
368. Smith NP, Jones EW. Erosive adenomatosis of the nipple. *Clin Exp Dermatol* 1977;2:79–84.

369. Smith EJ, Kron SD, Gross PR. Erosive adenomatosis of the nipple. *Arch Dermatol* 1970;102:330–332.
370. Pratt-Thomas HR. Erosive adenomatosis of the nipple. *J South Carolina Med Assoc* 1968;64:37–40.
371. Lewis HM, Ovitz ML, Golitz LE. Erosive adenomatosis of the nipple. *Arch Dermatol* 1976;112:1427–1428.
372. Albers SE, Barnard M, Thorner P, et al. Erosive adenomatosis of the nipple in an eight-year-old girl. *J Am Acad Dermatol* 1999;40:834–837.
373. Diaz NM, Palmer JO, Wick MR. Erosive adenomatosis of the nipple: histology, immunohistology, and differential diagnosis. *Mod Pathol* 1992;5:179–184.
374. Brownstein MH, Phelps RG, Magnin PH. Papillary adenoma of the nipple: analysis of fifteen new cases. *J Am Acad Dermatol* 1985;12:707–715.
375. Crain RCH, Helwig EB. Dermal cylindroma: dermal eccrine cylindroma. *Am J Clin Pathol* 1961;35:504.
376. Baden H. Cylindromatosis simulating neurofibromatosis. *N Engl J Med* 1962;267:296.
377. Lausecker H. Beitrag zu den naevo-epitheliomen. *Arch Dermatol Syph* 1952;194:639.
378. Gottschalk HR. Proceedings: dermal eccrine cylindroma, epithelioma adenoides cysticum of Brooke, and eccrine spiradenoma. *Arch Dermatol* 1974;110:473–474.
379. Headington JT, Batsakis JG, Beals TF, et al. Membranous basal cell adenoma of parotid gland, dermal cylindromas, and trichoepitheliomas. Comparative histochemistry and ultrastructure. *Cancer* 1977;39:2460–2469.
380. Welch JP, Wells RS, Kerr CB. Ancell-Spiegler cylindromas (turban tumours) and Brooke–Fordyce trichoepitheliomas: evidence for a single genetic entity. *J Med Genet* 1968;5:29–35.
381. Berberian BJ, Sulica VI, Kao GF. Familial multiple eccrine spiradenomas with cylindromatous features associated with epithelioma adenoides cysticum of Brooke. *Cutis* 1990;46:46–50.
382. Burrows NP, Jones RR, Smith NP. The clinicopathological features of familial cylindromas and trichoepitheliomas (Brooke–Spiegler syndrome): a report of two families. *Clin Exp Dermatol* 1992;17:332–336.
383. Delfino M, D'Anna F, Ianniello S, et al. Multiple hereditary trichoepithelioma and cylindroma (Brooke–Spiegler syndrome). *Dermatologica* 1991;183:150–153.
384. Goette DK, McConnell MA, Fowler VR. Cylindroma and eccrine spiradenoma coexistent in the same lesion. *Arch Dermatol* 1982;118:274–274.
385. Ferrandiz C, Campo E, Baumann E. Dermal cylindromas (turban tumour) and eccrine spiradenomas in a patient with membranous basal cell adenoma of the parotid gland. *J Cutan Pathol* 1985;12:72–79.
386. Urbach FG, Graham JH. Dermal eccrine cylindroma. *Arch Dermatol* 1963;88:880.
387. Kallioinen M. Immunoelectron microscope demonstration of the basement membrane components laminin and type IV collagen in the dermal cylindroma. *J Pathol* 1985;147:97–102.
388. Penneys NS, Kaiser M. Cylindroma expresses immunohistochemical markers linking it to eccrine coil. *J Cutan Pathol* 1993;20:40–43.
389. Cotton DW, Braye SG. Dermal cylindromas originate from the eccrine sweat gland. *Br J Dermatol* 1984;111:53–61.
390. Tellechea O, Reis JP, Ilheu O, et al. Dermal cylindroma. An immunohistochemical study of thirteen cases. *Am J Dermatopathol* 1995;17:260–265.
391. Hashimoto K, Lever WF. Histogenesis of skin appendage tumors. *Arch Dermatol* 1969;100:356.
392. Munger BL, GJ, Helwig EB. Ultrastructure and histochemical characteristics of dermal eccrine cylindroma: turban tumor. *J Invest Dermatol* 1962;39:577.
393. Bignell GR, Warren W, Seal S, et al. Identification of the familial cylindromatosis tumour-suppressor gene. *Nat Genet* 2000;25:160–165.
394. Gutierrez PP, Eggermann T, Holler D, et al. Phenotype diversity in familial cylindromatosis: a frameshift mutation in the tumor suppressor gene CYLD underlies different tumors of skin appendages. *J Invest Dermatol* 2002;119:527–531.
395. Weber L, Wick G, Gebhart W, et al. Basement membrane components outline the tumour islands in cylindroma. *Br J Dermatol* 1984;111:45–51.
396. Lin PY, Fatteh SM, Lloyd KM. Malignant transformation in a solitary dermal cylindroma. *Arch Pathol Lab Med* 1987;111:765–767.
397. Gerretsen AL, van der Putte SC, Deenstra W, et al. Cutaneous cylindroma with malignant transformation. *Cancer* 1993;72:1618–1623.
398. Bondeson L. Malignant dermal eccrine cylindroma. *Acta Derm Venereol* 1979;59:92–94.
399. Durani BK, Kurzen H, Jaeckel A, et al. Malignant transformation of multiple dermal cylindromas. *Br J Dermatol* 2001;145:653–656.
400. Hammond DC, Grant KF, Simpson WD. Malignant degeneration of dermal cylindroma. *Ann Plast Surg* 1990;24:176–178.
401. Lotem M, Trattner A, Kahanovich S, et al. Multiple dermal cylindroma undergoing a malignant transformation. *Int J Dermatol* 1992;31:642–644.
402. Ma A, Goldberg R, Medenica M, et al. Malignant cylindroma of the scalp. *J Am Acad Dermatol* 1991;25:960–964.
403. Urbanski SJ, From L, Abramowicz A, et al. Metamorphosis of dermal cylindroma: possible relation to malignant transformation. Case report of cutaneous cylindroma with direct intracranial invasion. *J Am Acad Dermatol* 1985;12:188–195.
404. Galadari E, Mehregan AH, Lee KC. Malignant transformation of eccrine tumors. *J Cutan Pathol* 1987;14:15–22.
405. Beideck MKA. Maligne entartung bei kutanen zylindromen. *Z Hautkr* 1985;60:73.
406. Luger A. Das cylindrom der haut und seine maligne degeneration. *Arch Dermatol Syph* 1949;188:155.
407. Goldstein N. Ephidrosis (local hyperhidrosis): Nevus sudoriferus. *Arch Dermatol* 1967;96:67.
408. Arnold H. Nevus seborrheicus et sudoriferus. *Arch Dermatol* 1945;51:370.
409. Herzberg J. Ekkrines syringocystadenom. *Arch Klin Exp Dermatol* 1962;214:600.
410. Imai S, Nitto H. Eccrine nevus with epidermal changes. *Dermatologica* 1983;166:84–88.
411. Hyman AB, Harris H, Brownstein MH. Eccrine angiomatous hamartoma. *New York St J Med* 1968;68:2803–2806.
412. Zeller DJ, Goldman RL. Eccrine-pilar angiomatous hamartoma. Report of a unique case. *Dermatologica* 1971;143:100–104.
413. Challa VR, Jona J. Eccrine angiomatous hamartoma: a rare skin lesion with diverse histological features. *Dermatologica* 1977;155:206–209.
414. Sanmartin O, Botella R, Alegre V, et al. Congenital eccrine angiomatous hamartoma. *Am J Dermatopathol* 1992;14:161–164.
415. Velasco JA, Almeida V. Eccrine-pilar angiomatous nevus. *Dermatologica* 1988;177:317–322.
416. Donati P, Amantea A, Balus L. Eccrine angiomatous hamartoma: a lipomatous variant. *J Cutan Pathol* 1989;16:227–229.
417. Smith JD, Chernosky ME. Hidrocystomas. *Arch Dermatol* 1973;108:676–679.
418. Cordero A, Montes LF. Eccrine hidrocystoma. *J Cutan Pathol* 1976;3:292.
419. Hassan MO, Khan MA. Ultrastructure of eccrine cystadenoma. A case report. *Arch Dermatol* 1979;115:1217–1221.

420. Sperling LS, Sakas EL. Eccrine hidrocystomas. *J Am Acad Dermatol* 1982;7:763.

421. Ebner JE, Erlach E. Ekkrine hidrozystome. *Dermatol Monatsschr* 1975; 161:739.

422. Brown SM, Freeman RG. Syringoma limited to the vulva. *Arch Dermatol* 1971;104:331.

423. Goyal S, Martins CR. Multiple syringomas on the abdomen, thighs, and groin. *Cutis* 2000;66:259–262.

424. Lo JS, Dijkstra JW, Bergfeld WF. Syringomas on the penis. *Int J Dermatol* 1990;29:309–310.

425. Thomas J, Majmudar B, Gorelkin L. Syringoma localized to the vulva. *Arch Dermatol* 1979;115:95–96.

426. Hashimoto K, DiBella RJ, Borsuk GM, et al. Eruptive hidradenoma and syringoma. Histological, histochemical, and electron microscopic studies. *Arch Dermatol* 1967;96:500–519.

427. Yung CW, Soltani K, Bernstein JE, et al. Unilateral linear nevoidal syringoma. *J Am Acad Dermatol* 1981;4:412–416.

428. Shelley WB, Wood MG. Occult syringomas of scalp associated with progressive hair loss. *Arch Dermatol* 1980;116:843–844.

429. Spitz DF, Stadecker MJ, Grande DJ. Subclinical syringoma coexisting with basal cell carcinoma. *J Dermatol Surg Oncol* 1987;13:793–795.

430. Headington JT, Koski J, Murphy PJ. Clear cell glycogenosis in multiple syringomas. Description and enzyme histochemistry. *Arch Dermatol* 1972;106:353–356.

431. Feibelman CE, Maize JC. Clear-cell syringoma. A study by conventional and electron microscopy. *Am J Dermatopathol* 1984;6:139–150.

432. Asai Y, Ishii M, Hamada T. Acral syringoma: electron microscopic studies on its origin. *Acta Derm Venereol* 1982;62:64–68.

433. Winkelmann R, Muller SA. Sweat gland tumors. *Arch Dermatol* 1964;89:827.

434. Mustakallio K. Succinic dehydrogenase activity of syringomas. *Acta Dermatol* 1964;89:827.

435. Pinkus HR, Rogin JR, Goldman P. Eccrine poroma. *Arch Dermatol* 1956, 74:511.

436. Hyman AB, Brownstein MH. Eccrine poroma. An analysis of forty-five new cases. *Dermatologica* 1969;138:29–38.

437. Moore TO, Orman HL, Orman SK, et al. Poromas of the head and neck. *J Am Acad Dermatol* 2001;44:48–52.

438. Vu PP, Whitehead KJ, Sullivan TJ. Eccrine poroma of the eyelid. *Clin Exp Ophthalmol* 2001;29:253–255.

439. Okun MA, Ansell HB. Eccrine poroma. *Arch Dermatol* 1963; 88:561.

440. Penneys NS, Ackerman AB, Indgin SN, et al. Eccrine poroma: two unusual variants. *Br J Dermatol* 1970;82:613–615.

441. Goldner R. Eccrine poromatosis. *Arch Dermatol* 1970;101:606–608.

442. Wilkinson RD, Schopflocher P, Rozenfeld M. Hidrotic ectodermal dysplasia with diffuse eccrine poromatosis. *Arch Dermatol* 1977;113:472–476.

443. Freeman RK, Knox JM, Spiller WF. Eccrine poroma. *Am J Clin Pathol* 1961;36:444.

444. Yasuda TK, Kawadg A, Yoshida K. Eccrine poroma. *Arch Dermatol* 1964;90:428.

445. Knox JS, Spiller WF. Eccrine poroma. *Arch Dermatol* 1958;77:726.

446. Krinitz K. Malignes itraepidermales ekkrines Porom. *Zeitschrift fur Haut- und Geschlechtskrankheiten* 1972;47:9–17.

447. Pinkus HR, Rogin JR, Goldman P. Eccrine poroma. *Arch Dermatol* 1956;74:511.

448. Smith JC, Coburn JG. Hidroacanthoma simplex. *Br J Dermatol* 1956;68:400.

449. Mehregan AL, Levson DN. Hidroacanthoma simplex. *Arch Dermatol* 1969;100:303.

450. Winkelmann RM, McLeod WA. The dermal duct tumor. *Arch Dermatol* 1966;94:50.

451. Rahbari H. Syringoacanthoma. Acanthotic lesion of the acrosyringium. *Arch Dermatol* 1984;120:751–756.

452. Hashimoto KL, Lever WF. Eccrine poroma: histochemical and electron microscopic studies. *J Invest Dermatol* 1964;43:237.

453. Sanderson KR, Ryan EA. The histochemistry of eccrine poroma. *Br J Dermatol* 1963;75:86.

454. Hu CM, Manques AS, Winkelmann RK. Dermal duct tumor. *Arch Dermatol* 1978;114:1659.

455. Pinkus HM, Mehregan AH. Epidermotropic eccrine carcinoma. *Arch Dermatol* 1963;88:597.

456. Mishima Y, Morioka S. Oncogenic differentiation of the intraepidermal eccrine sweat duct: eccrine poroma, poroepithelioma and porocarcinoma. *Dermatologica* 1969;138:238–250.

457. Bardach H. Hidroacanthoma simplex with in situ porocarcinoma. A case suggesting malignant transformation. *J Cutan Pathol* 1978;5:236–248.

458. Gschnait F, Horn F, Lindlbauer R, et al. Eccrine porocarcinoma. *J Cutan Pathol* 1980;7:349–353.

459. Mohri S, Chika K, Saito I, et al. A case of porocarcinoma. *J Dermatology* 1980;7:431–434.

460. Ishikawa K. Malignant hidroacanthoma simplex. *Arch Dermatol* 1971;104:529.

461. Pena J, Suster S. Squamous differentiation in malignant eccrine poroma. *Am J Dermatopathol* 1993;15:492–496.

462. Urso CP, Paglierani M, Bondi R. Histologic spectrum of carcinomas with eccrine ductal differentiation: Sweat-gland ductal carcinomas. *Am J Dermatopathol* 1993;15:435.

463. Kolde G, Macher E, Grundmann E. Metastasizing eccrine porocarcinoma. Report of two cases with fatal outcome. *Pathol Res Pract* 1991;187:477–481.

464. Weedon DL, Lewis J. Acrosyringeal nevus. *J Cutan Pathol* 1977; 4:166.

465. Mehregan AH, Marufi M, Medenica M. Eccrine syringofibroadenoma (Mascaro). Report of two cases. *J Am Acad Dermatol* 1985;13:433–436.

466. Mascaro J. Considérations sur les tumeurs fibroépithéliales: le syringofibroadénome eccrine. *Ann Dermatol Syphilgr* 1963;90:143.

467. Weedon D. Eccrine syringofibroadenoma versus acrosyringeal nevus. *J Am Acad Dermatol* 1987;16:622–623.

468. Hurt MA, Igra-Serfaty H, Stevens CS. Eccrine syringofibroadenoma (Mascaro). An acrosyringeal hamartoma. *Arch Dermatol* 1990;126:945–949.

469. Ogino A. Linear eccrine poroma. *Arch Dermatol* 1976;112:841.

470. Gkolfinopoulos T, Ingen-Housz-Oro S, Cavelier-Balloy B, et al. Syndrome de Schopf–Schulz–Passarge: 2 observations. *Dermatology* 1997;195:309–310.

471. Simpson EL, Styles AR, Cockerell CJ. Eccrine syringofibroadenomatosis associated with hidrotic ectodermal dysplasia. *Br J Dermatol* 1998;138:879–884.

472. Starink TM. Eccrine syringofibroadenoma: multiple lesions representing a new cutaneous marker of the Schopf syndrome, and solitary nonhereditary tumors. *J Am Acad Dermatol* 1997; 36:569–576.

473. Fretzin DF, Sloan JB, Beer K, et al. Eccrine syringofibroadenoma. A clear-cell variant. *Am J Dermatopathol* 1995;17:591–593.

474. Fouilloux B, Perrin C, Dutoit M, et al. Clear cell syringofibroadenoma (of Mascaro) of the nail. *Br J Dermatol* 2001;144:625–627.

475. Kanitakis J, Zambruno G, Euvrard S, et al. Eccrine syringofibroadenoma. Immunohistological study of a new case. *Am J Dermatopathol* 1987;9:37–40.

476. Ishida-Yamamoto A, Iizuka H, Eady RA. Filaggrin immunoreactive composite keratohyalin granules specific to acrosyringia and related tumours. *Acta Derm Venereol* 1994;74:37–42.

477. Ohnishi T, Suzuki T, Watanabe S. Eccrine syringofibroadenoma. Report of a case and immunohistochemical study of keratin expression. *Br J Dermatol* 1995;133:449–454.

478. Ishida-Yamamoto A, Iizuka H. Eccrine syringofibroadenoma (Mascaro). An ultrastructural and immunohistochemical study. *Am J Dermatopathol* 1996;18:207–211.

479. Sueki H, Miller SJ, Dzubow LM, et al. Eccrine syringofibroadenoma (Mascaro): an ultrastructural study. *J Cutan Pathol* 1992;19:232–239.

480. Kwittken J. Muciparous epidermal tumors. *Arch Dermatol* 1974;109:554.

481. Scully K, Assaad D. Mucinous syringometaplasia. *J Am Acad Dermatol* 1984;11:503–508.

482. Mehregan AH. Mucinous syringometaplasia. *Arch Dermatol* 1980;116:988–989.

483. Shelley W, Wood MG. A zosteriform network of spiradenoma. *J Am Acad Dermatol* 1980;2:59.

484. Munger BB, Berghorn BM, Helwig EB. A light and electron-microscopic study of a case of multiple eccrine spiradenoma. *J Invest Dermatol* 1962;38:289.

485. Hashimoto K, Gross BG, Nelson RG, et al. Eccrine spiradenoma. Histochemical and electron microscopic studies. *J Invest Dermatol* 1966;46:347–365.

486. Tsur H, Lipskier E, Fisher BK. Multiple linear spiradenomas. Plastic & Reconstructive Surgery 1981;68:100–102.

487. Mambo NC. Eccrine spiradenoma: clinical and pathologic study of 49 tumors. *J Cutan Pathol* 1983;10:312–320.

488. Kersting D, Helwig EB. Eccrine spiradenoma. *Arch Dermatol Syph* 1956;73:199.

489. Lever W. Myoepithelial sweat gland tumor: myoepithelioma. *Arch Dermatol Syph* 1948;57:332.

490. Castro C, Winkelmann, RK. Spiradenoma: histochemical and electron microscopic study. *Arch Dermatol* 1974;109:40.

491. van den Oord JJ. Perivascular spaces in eccrine spiradenoma: a clue to its histological diagnosis [Comment]. *Am J Dermatopath* 1995;17:266.

492. Winkelmann RK, Wolff K. Histochemistry of hidradenoma and eccrine spiradenoma. *J Invest Dermatol* 1967;49:173–180.

493. Hashimoto K, Kanzaki T. Appendage tumors of the skin: histogenesis and ultrastructure. *J Cutan Pathol* 1984;11:365–381.

494. Watanabe S, Hirose M, Sato S, et al. Immunohistochemical analysis of cytokeratin expression in eccrine spiradenoma: similarities to the transitional portions between secretory segments and coiled ducts of eccrine glands. *Br J Dermatol* 1994;131:799–807.

495. Cooper PH, Frierson HF Jr, Morrison AG. Malignant transformation of eccrine spiradenoma. *Arch Dermatol* 1985;121:1445–1448.

496. Wick MR, Swanson PE, Kaye VN, et al. Sweat gland carcinoma ex eccrine spiradenoma. *Am J Dermatopathol* 1987;9:90–98.

497. Granter SR, Seeger K, Calonje E et al. Malignant eccrine spiradenoma (spiradenocarcinoma): a clinicopathologic study of 12 cases. *Am J Dermatopathol* 2000;22:97–103.

498. Dabska M. Malignant transformation of eccrine spiradenoma. *Pol Med J* 1972;11:388–396.

499. Evans HL, Su D, Smith JL, et al. Carcinoma arising in eccrine spiradenoma. *Cancer* 1979;43:1881–1884.

500. Herzberg A, Elenitsas R, Strohmeyer CR. Unusual case of early malignant transformation of spiradenoma. *Dermatol Surg Oncol* 1995;21:1.

501. McKee PH, Fletcher CD, Stavrinos P, et al. Carcinosarcoma arising in eccrine spiradenoma. A clinicopathologic and immunohistochemical study of two cases. *Am J Dermatopathol* 1990;12:335–343.

502. Saboorian MH, Kenny M, Ashfaq R, et al. Carcinosarcoma arising in eccrine spiradenoma of the breast. Report of a case and review of the literature. *Arch Pathol Lab Med* 1996;120:501–504.

503. Itoh T, Yamamoto N, Tokunaga M. Malignant eccrine spiradenoma with smooth muscle cell differentiation: histological and immunohistochemical study. *Pathol Int* 1996;46:887–893.

504. Argenyi ZB, Nguyen AV, Balogh K, et al. Malignant eccrine spiradenoma. A clinicopathologic study. *Am J Dermatopathol* 1992;14:381–390.

505. Rulon DB, Helwig EB. Papillary eccrine adenoma. *Arch Dermatol* 1977;113:596–598.

506. Urmacher C, Lieberman PH. Papillary eccrine adenoma. Light-microscopic, histochemical, and immunohistochemical studies. *Am J Dermatopathol* 1987;9:243–249.

507. Nova M, Kress Y, Jennings TA, et al. Papillary eccrine adenoma and low-grade eccrine carcinoma: a comparative histologic, ultrastructural, and immunohistochemical study. *Surg Pathol* 1990;3:179.

508. Sexton M, Maize JC. Papillary eccrine adenoma. A light microscopic and immunohistochemical study. *J Am Acad Dermatol* 1988;18:1114–1120.

509. Megahed M, Holzle E. Papillary eccrine adenoma. A case report with immunohistochemical examination. *Am J Dermatopathol* 1993;15:150–155.

510. Aloi F, Pich A. Papillary eccrine adenoma. A histopathological and immunohistochemical study. *Dermatologica* 1991;182:47–51.

511. O'Hara J, Bensch KG. Fine structure of eccrine sweat gland adenoma, clear cell type. *J Invest Dermatol* 1967, 49:261.

512. Lund H. Tumors of the skin. In: *Atlas of Tumor Pathology*. Sec. I, Fasc. 2. Washington, DC: Armed Forces Institute of Pathology, 1957.

513. Lever W, Castleman, B. Clear cell myoepithelioma of the skin. *Am J Pathol* 1952;28:691.

514. O'Hara J, Bensch K, Ioannides G, et al. Eccrine sweat gland adenoma, clear cell type. *Cancer* 1966;19:1438.

515. Winkelmann RK, Wolff K. Solid-cystic hidradenoma of the skin. Clinical and histopathologic study. *Arch Dermatol* 1968;97:651–661.

516. Johnson BL Jr, Helwig EB. Eccrine acrospiroma. A clinicopathologic study. *Cancer* 1969;23:641–657.

517. Efskind J, Eker R. Myo-epitheliomas of the skin. *Acta Derm Venereol (Stockh)* 1954;34:279.

518. Kersting D. Clear cell hidradenoma and hidradenocarcinoma. *Arch Dermatol* 1963;87:323.

519. Hashimoto K, DiBella RJ, Lever WF. Clear cell hidradenoma. Histological, histochemical, and electron microscopic studies. *Arch Dermatol* 1967;96:18–38.

520. Stanley RJ, Sanchez NP, Massa MC, et al. Epidermoid hidradenoma. A clinicopathologic study. *J Cutan Pathol* 1982;9:293–302.

521. Haupt HM, Stern JB, Berlin SJ. Immunohistochemistry in the differential diagnosis of nodular hidradenoma and glomus tumor. *Am J Dermatopathol* 1992;14:310–314.

522. Biddlestone LR, McLaren KM, Tidman MJ. Malignant hidradenoma—a case report demonstrating insidious histological and clinical progression. *Clin Exp Dermatol* 1991;16:474–477.

523. Mambo NC. The significance of atypical nuclear changes in benign eccrine acrospiromas: a clinical and pathological study of 18 cases. *J Cutan Pathol* 1984;11:35–44.

524. Mehregan A, Hashimoto K, Rahbari H. Eccrine adenocarcinoma: a clinicopathologic study of 35 cases. *Arch Dermatol* 1983;119:104.

525. Keasbey L, Hadley GC. Clear-cell hidradenoma: report of three cases with widespread metastases. *Cancer* 1954;7:934.

526. Santler R, Everhartinger C. Malignes klarzellen-myoepitheliom. *Dermatologica* 1965;130:340.

527. Hernandez-Perez E, Cestoni-Parducci R. Nodular hidradenoma and hidradenocarcinoma. A 10-year review. *J Am Acad Dermatol* 1985;12:15–20.

528. Headington JT, Niederhuber JE, Beals TF. Malignant clear cell acrospiroma. *Cancer* 1978;41:641–647.

529. Stromberg BV, Thorne S, Dimino-Emme L, et al. Malignant clear cell hidradenoma: a case report and literature review. *Nebraska Med J* 1991;76:166–170.

530. Hirsch P, Helwig EB. Chondroid syringoma. *Arch Dermatol* 1961;84:835.

531. Headington J. Mixed tumors of the skin: eccrine and apocrine types. *Arch Dermatol* 1961;84:989.

532. Gartmann H, Pullmann H. Chondroides Syringom. *Zeitschrift fur Hautkrankheiten* 1979;54:908–913.

533. Tsoitis G, Brisou B, Destombes P. Mummified cutaneous mixed tumor. *Arch Dermatol* 1975;111:194–196.

534. Varela-Duran J, Diaz-Flores L, Varela-Nunez R. Ultrastructure of chondroid syringoma: role of the myoepithelial cell in the development of the mixed tumor of the skin and soft tissues. *Cancer* 1979;44:148–156.

535. Welke S, Goos M. Das chondroide Syringom. *Hautarzt* 1982;33:15–17.

536. Iglesias F, Forcelledo FF, Sanchez TS, et al. Chondroid syringoma: a histological and immunohistochemical study of 15 cases. *Histopathology* 1990;17:311.

537. Banerjee SS, Harris M, Eyden BP, et al. Chondroid syringoma with hyaline cell change. *Histopathology* 1993;22:235–245.

538. Hassab-el-Naby HM, Tam S, White WL, et al. Mixed tumors of the skin. A histological and immunohistochemical study. *Am J Dermatopathol* 1989;11:413–428. [Erratum: *Am J Dermatopathol* 1990;12:108.]

539. Kanitakis J, Zambruno G, Viac J, et al. Expression of neural-tissue markers (S-100 protein and Leu-7 antigen) by sweat gland tumors of the skin. An immunohistochemical study. *J Am Acad Dermatol* 1987;17:187–191.

540. Hernandez F. Mixed tumors of the skin of the salivary gland type: a light and electron microscopic study. *J Invest Dermatol* 1976;66:49.

541. Trown K, Heenan PJ. Malignant mixed tumor of the skin (malignant chondroid syringoma). *Pathology* 1994;26:237–243.

542. Harrist TA, Aretz TH, Mihm MC Jr, et al. Malignant chondroid syringoma. *Arch Dermatol* 1981;117:719.

543. Shvili D, Rothem A. Fulminant metastasizing chondroid syringoma of the skin. *Am J Dermatopathol* 1986;8:321–325.

544. Metzler G, Schaumburg-Lever G, Hornstein O, et al. Malignant chondroid syringoma: immunohistopathology. *Am J Dermatopathol* 1996;18:83–89.

545. Botha JB, Kahn LB. Aggressive chondroid syringoma. Report of a case in an unusual location and with local recurrence. *Arch Dermatol* 1978;114:954–955.

546. Hilton JM, Blackwell JB. Metastasising chondroid syringoma. *J Pathol* 1973;109:167–170.

547. Matz LR, McCully DJ, Stokes BA. Metastasizing chondroid syringoma: case report. *Pathology* 1969;1:77–81.

548. Redono C, Rocamora A, Villoria F, et al. Malignant mixed tumor of the skin: malignant chondroid syringoma. *Cancer* 1982;49:1690–1696.

549. Ishimura E, Iwamoto H, Kobashi Y, et al. Malignant chondroid syringoma. Report of a case with widespread metastasis and review of pertinent literature. *Cancer* 1983;52:1966–1973.

550. Baes H, Suurmond D. Apocrine sweat gland carcinoma. Report of a case. *Br J Dermatol* 1970;83:483–486.

551. Futrell JW, Krueger GR, Chretien PB, et al. Multiple primary sweat gland carcinomas. *Cancer* 1971;28:686–691.

552. Sakamoto F, Ito M, Sato S, et al. Basal cell tumor with apocrine differentiation: apocrine epithelioma. *J Am Acad Dermatol* 1985;13:355–363.

553. Paties C, Taccagni GL, Papotti M, et al. Apocrine carcinoma of the skin. A clinicopathologic, immunocytochemical, and ultrastructural study. *Cancer* 1993;71:375–381.

554. Nishikawa Y, Tokusashi Y, Saito Y, et al. A case of apocrine adenocarcinoma associated with hamartomatous apocrine gland hyperplasia of both axillae. *Am J Surg Pathol* 1994;18:832–836.

555. Neldner KH. Ceruminoma. *Arch Dermatol* 1968;98:344–348.

556. Michel RG, Woodard BH, Shelburne JD, et al. Ceruminous gland adenocarcinoma: a light and electron microscopic study. *Cancer* 1978;41:545–553.

557. Lynde CW, McLean DI, Wood WS. Tumors of ceruminous glands. *J Am Acad Dermatol* 1984;11:841–847.

558. Swanson PE, Cherwitz DL, Neumann MP, et al. Eccrine sweat gland carcinoma: an histologic and immunohistochemical study of 32 cases. *J Cutan Pathol* 1987;14:65–86.

559. Teloh H, Balkin RB, Grier JP. Metastasizing sweat gland carcinoma. *Arch Dermatol* 1957;76:80.

560. Grant R. Sweat gland carcinoma with metastases. *JAMA* 1960;173:490.

561. el-Domeiri AA, Brasfield RD, Huvos AG, et al. Sweat gland carcinoma: a clinico-pathologic study of 83 patients. *Ann Surg* 1971;173:270–274.

562. Dave VK. Eccrine sweat gland carcinoma with metastases. *Br J Dermatol* 1972;86:95–97.

563. Orbaneja J, Yus ES, Diaz-Flores L, et al. Adenocarcinom der ekkrinen schweissdrüsen. *Hautarzt* 1973;24:197.

564. Freeman R, Winkelmann RK. Basal cell tumor with eccrine differentiation. *Arch Dermatol* 1969;100:234.

565. Sanchez N, Winkelmann RK. Basal cell tumor with eccrine differentiation: eccrine epithelioma. *J Am Acad Dermatol* 1982;6:514.

566. Mehregan AH, Hashimoto K, Rahbari H. Eccrine adenocarcinoma. A clinicopathologic study of 35 cases. *Arch Dermatol* 1983;119:104–114.

567. Sanchez Yus E, Requena Caballero L, Garcia Salazar I, et al. Clear cell syringoid eccrine carcinoma. *Am J Dermatopathol* 1987;9:225–231.

568. Ramos D, Monteagudo C, Carda C, et al. Clear cell syringoid carcinoma: an ultrastructural and immunohistochemical study. *Am J Dermatopathol* 2000;22:60–64.

569. Ohnishi T, Kaneko S, Egi M, et al. Syringoid eccrine carcinoma: report of a case with immunohistochemical analysis of cytokeratin expression. *Am J Dermatopathol* 2002;24:409–413.

570. Cooper PH. Sclerosing carcinomas of sweat ducts (microcystic adnexal carcinoma). *Arch Dermatol* 1986;122:261–264.

571. Nickoloff BJ, Fleischmann HE, Carmel J, et al. Microcystic adnexal carcinoma. Immunohistologic observations suggesting dual (pilar and eccrine) differentiation. *Arch Dermatol* 1986;122:290–294.

572. Goldstein DJ, Barr RJ, Santa Cruz DJ. Microcystic adnexal carcinoma: a distinct clinicopathologic entity. *Cancer* 1982;50:566–572.

573. Nelson BR, Lowe L, Baker S, et al. Microcystic adnexal carcinoma of the skin. A reappraisal of the differentiation and differential diagnosis of an underrecognized neoplasm. *J Am Acad Dermatol* 1993;29:840–845.

574. Mendoza S, Helwig EB. Mucinous (adenocystic) carcinoma of the skin. *Arch Dermatol* 1971;103:68–78.

575. Santa-Cruz DJ, Meyers JH, Gnepp DR, et al. Primary mucinous carcinoma of the skin. *Br J Dermatol* 1978;98:645–653.

576. Yeung KY, Stinson JC. Mucinous (adenocystic) carcinoma of sweat glands with widespread metastasis. Case report with ultrastructural study. *Cancer* 1977;39:2556–2562.

577. Snow SN, Reizner GT. Mucinous eccrine carcinoma of the eyelid. *Cancer* 1992;70:2099–2104.

578. Headington JT. Primary mucinous carcinoma of skin: histochemistry and electron microscopy. *Cancer* 1977;39:1055–1063.

579. Baandrup U, Leftarr, Gaard H. Mucinous (adenocystic) carcinoma of the skin. *Dermatologica* 1982;164:338.

580. Wright J, Font RL. Mucinous sweat gland adenocarcinoma of the eyelid. *Cancer* 1979;44:1757.

581. Hein R, Kuhn A, Landthaler M, et al. Cytokeratin expression in mucinous sweat gland carcinomas: an immunohistochemical analysis of four cases. *Br J Dermatol* 1994;130:432–437.

582. Schmid U, Hardmeier T, Altmannsberger M, et al. Mucinous carcinoma. *Histopathology* 1992;21:161–165.

583. Landman G, Farmer ER. Primary cutaneous mucoepidermoid carcinoma: report of a case. *J Cutan Pathol* 1991;18:56–59.

584. Wenig BL, Sciubba JJ, Goodman RS, et al. Primary cutaneous mucoepidermoid carcinoma of the anterior neck. *Laryngoscope* 1983;93:464–467.

585. Friedman KJ. Low-grade primary cutaneous adenosquamous (mucoepidermoid) carcinoma. Report of a case and review of the literature. *Am J Dermatopathol* 1989;11:43–50.

586. Boggio R. Letter: adenoid cystic carcinoma of scalp. *Arch Dermatol* 1975;111:793–794.

587. Seab JA, Graham JH. Primary cutaneous adenoid cystic carcinoma. *J Am Acad Dermatol* 1987;17:113–118.

588. Cooper PH, Adelson GL, Holthaus WH. Primary cutaneous adenoid cystic carcinoma. *Arch Dermatol* 1984;120:774–777.

589. Fukai K, Ishii M, Kobayashi H, et al. Primary cutaneous adenoid cystic carcinoma: ultrastructural study and immunolocalization of types I, III, IV, V collagens and laminin. *J Cutan Pathol* 1990;17:374–380.

590. Headington JT, Teears R, Niederhuber JE, et al. Primary adenoid cystic carcinoma of skin. *Arch Dermatol* 1978;114:421–424.

591. Wick MR, Swanson PE. Primary adenoid cystic carcinoma of the skin. A clinical, histological, and immunocytochemical comparison with adenoid cystic carcinoma of salivary glands and adenoid basal cell carcinoma. *Am J Dermatopathol* 1986;8:2–13.

592. Kao GF, Helwig EB, Graham JH. Aggressive digital papillary adenoma and adenocarcinoma. A clinicopathological study of 57 patients, with histochemical, immunopathological, and ultrastructural observations. *J Cutan Pathol* 1987;14:129–146.

593. Duke WH, Sherrod TT, Lupton GP. Aggressive digital papillary adenocarcinoma (aggressive digital papillary adenoma and adenocarcinoma revisited). *Am J Surg Pathol* 2000;24:775–784.

594. Jih DM, Elenitsas R, Vittorio CC, et al. Aggressive digital papillary adenocarcinoma: a case report and review of the literature. *Am J Dermatopathol* 2001;23:154–157.

31

CUTANEOUS LYMPHOMAS AND LEUKEMIAS

GEORGE F. MURPHY
ROLAND SCHWARTING

OVERVIEW

The subject of cutaneous lymphoma and leukemia has long been one of conceptual confusion and diagnostic challenge. Aside from the inherent difficulties in differentiating hyperplastic from neoplastic hematopoietic cells in skin, the recent evolution in classification schemas for lymphoma and leukemia have contributed significantly to this dilemma. Moreover, some traditional didactic treatments of this issue too often provide information so abundant as to confound the overview necessary for a practical, confident, and accurate diagnostic approach to potential lymphoproliferative disorders of skin.

The classification system adapted to skin and used in this chapter is that of the World Health Organization (WHO) Classification of Tumours of the Haematopoietic and Lymphoid Tissues (1). This recent and seminal contribution represents a classification based on the "Revised European-American Classification of Lymphoid Neoplasms" (REAL classification) (2), and serves to offer pathologists, oncologists, and geneticists a universal system for lymphoma/leukemia classification that is based primarily on histopathologic and genetic features. In addition to myeloid neoplasms, the WHO classification recognizes three principal categories of lymphoid neoplasia: those of T and of NK cells, B cells, and Hodgkin lymphoma. The artificial separation between leukemia and lymphoma is de-emphasized in view of the fact that both solid (lymphomatous) and circulating (leukemic) phases are present in many lymphoid neoplasms (e.g., as with B-cell small lymphocytic lymphoma and B-cell chronic lymphocytic leukemia). Because neoplasms within this category tend to recapitulate either early or late stages of lymphoid differentiation, the respective modifiers "precursor" and "peripheral/mature" are often applied to these tumors. Importantly, the system pays special attention to recognizing only those diseases that represent distinct clinicopathologic entities. In this regard, a synthesis of morphology, immunophenotype, genetic features, and clinical features are often required to define distinct disease entities.

The treatment of lymphoproliferative disorders detailed below is in no small part indebted to the outstanding foundations that have been developed in previous editions of this text. In particular, the classification, images, and related commentary provided by LeBoit and McCalmont (3) were invaluable to the development of the present material and represent a major advance in the textural treatment of this difficult and rapidly evolving topic.

Lymphoproliferative disorders of the skin fall into two major categories: primary cutaneous neoplasms (those where skin involvement often precedes or coexists with detectable extracutaneous disease), and extracutaneous neoplasms that may secondarily involve the skin. The specific diseases that follow will thus be grouped according to the following schema in order to include the vast majority of conditions recognized by the current WHO classification that have specific relevance to the skin (Table 31-1).

CUTANEOUS HEMATOPOIETIC INFILTRATES: OVERVIEW AND GENERAL CONCEPTS

T- and B-Cell Infiltration Patterns

While numerous exceptions exist, there are fundamental and often reproducible trends in the patterns produced when lymphocytes infiltrate the skin (4). This is based in part on differences in adhesive ligands between B and T cells, resulting in differential affinity for various compartments within the skin. Moreover, chemokinetic and chemotactic signals may influence the migration of various classes of lymphoid cells in different ways. The best example of this is the tendency for both benign and malignant T cells, but not B cells, to migrate into epithelial structures, including the epidermis and its adnexae. This results in the phenomena of "epidermotropism" and "folliculotropism," accounting for the tendency to identify T cells within the epidermal layer and often as a band of cells within the

TABLE 31-1. CLASSIFICATION OF PRIMARY AND SECONDARY LYMPHOMAS/LEUKEMIAS OF SKIN

Primary cutaneous B-cell lymphoproliferative disorders
B-cell lymphomatoid hyperplasia
B-cell neoplasms
  Cutaneous follicle center cell lymphoma
  Extraosseous plasmacytoma
  Extranodal marginal B-cell lymphoma (MALT lymphoma)
  Diffuse large B-cell lymphoma, extranodal type
  Lymphomatoid granulomatosis initially presenting in skin
Secondary B-cell lymphoproliferative disorders affecting skin
B-cell neoplasms
  Precursor B-lymphoblastic leukemia/lymphoma
  Chronic lymphocytic leukemia/small lymphocytic lymphoma
  Follicular lymphoma
  Mantle cell lymphoma
  Diffuse B-cell lymphoma, nodal type
  Intravascular large B-cell lymphoma
  Lymphomatoid granulomatosis
Hodgkin lymphoma
Primary cutaneous T-cell lymphoproliferative disorders
T-cell lymphomatoid hyperplasias
T-cell and NK-cell neoplasms
  Mycosis fungoides
  Sezary syndrome
  Primary cutaneous CD30-positive T-cell lymphoproliferative disorders
  Subcutaneous panniculitis-like T-cell lymphoma
Secondary T/NK-cell lymphoproliferative disorders affecting skin
Nodal
  Peripheral T-cell lymphoma
  Anaplastic large-cell lymphoma
Extranodal
  Extranodal NK/T-cell lymphoma, nasal type
Leukemic/disseminated
  Adult T-cell leukemia/lymphoma
  Precursor T-lymphoblastic leukemia/lymphoblastic lymphoma
  T-cell prolymphocytic leukemia
Uncertain lineage/differentiation
  Blastic NK-cell lymphoma
Primary cutaneous myeloid hyperplasia and neoplasia
  Extramedullary hematopoiesis
  Myeloid sarcoma
Secondary myeloid neoplasms affecting skin
  Acute and chronic myeloid leukemia

underlying papillary dermis (Fig. 31-1A). Occasionally, as is the case in epidermotropic phases of mycosis fungoides, T cells may align along the basement membrane zone of the dermal–epidermal junction, a finding that may have a basis in expression by these cells of integrin receptors for the specific membrane components (5). This "T-cell pattern" of infiltration is not invariable among T-cell malignancies, however, and epidermotropism may be blunted as tumors evolve and progress to more aggressive and poorly differentiated states. B cells, on the other hand, do not demonstrate the same affinity for the epidermis and adnexae, and seldom are these cells detected in significant numbers within the epidermis or papillary dermis. The sparing of the latter produces the characteristic "grenz zone" seen in B-cell pattern infiltrates of the skin. Moreover, perhaps because of the innate proclivity of B cells to aggregate into follicular structures, B-cell infiltrates in the skin often (but not invariably) show a nodular architecture (Fig. 31-1B).

T- and B-cell patterns are potentially helpful in presumptive assignment of cell lineage, but they are not invariable, cannot be used as a reliable surrogate for immunohistochemical detection of lineage-related antigens, and do not permit separation of reactive from dysplastic and malignant. Although this latter distinction frequently depends on cytology, immunophenotype, and genotype, the architecture or "trafficking patterns" of hematopoietic cells in the skin may also provide insight into biological potential for aggressive behavior.

Abnormal Trafficking: Distinction from Inflammation

Skin is a lymphoid organ, and both the epidermal and dermal layers represent interactive immune systems that contribute to and partially regulate inflammatory cell trafficking (6,7). In both T- and B-cell responses in skin, circulating lymphocytes initially adhere to activated endothelium lining of dermal postcapillary venules. Migration across the vessel wall results in perivascular or angiocentric dermati-

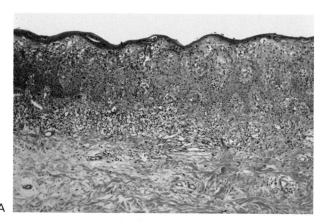
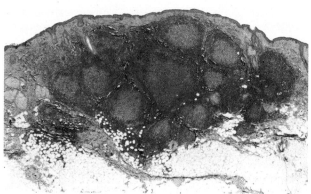

A   B

FIGURE 31-1. Patterns of T and B-cell infiltration. **(A)** T-cell pattern. **(B)** B-cell pattern with grenz zone and germinal center formation.

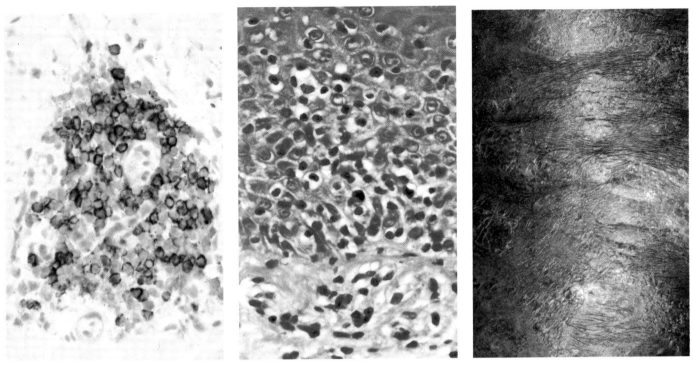

FIGURE 31-2. Normal and abnormal trafficking patterns. **(A)** T-cell immunohistochemistry of angiocentric pattern. **(B)** Abnormal epidermotropism into a "passive" epidermis. **(C)** Scaling patches and plaques as a consequence of altered epidermal maturation associated with T-cell epidermotropism (mycosis fungoides).

tis (Fig. 31-2A). If further migration is stunted, this exclusive angiocentric localization may produce a pattern that may lead to a specified number of differential diagnostic considerations based on correlation with clinical parameters (e.g., as in erythema chronicum migrans). Migration away from the vessel wall is presumably swift enough that in the case of T cells, papillary dermal accumulation and epidermotropism, in addition to a persistent angiocentric pattern, may result. However, activated T cells on an immunologic mission, as in the case of contact hypersensitivity, psoriasis, or cytotoxic dermatitis, generally alter the epidermis as they enter it by way of the cytokines and growth factors that they produce. Thus, reactive T-cell epidermotropism is often accompanied by epithelial spongiosis, acanthosis, or apoptosis. In the case of malignant T-cell infiltration, in contrast, the epidermis tends to be "passive," with T-cell infiltration resulting in permissive aggregation of variably atypical lymphocytes within the epidermis (Fig. 31-2B) and sometimes also or exclusively in adnexal epithelium. This infiltration is not generally associated with reactive epithelial alteration in the form of spongiosis or apoptosis, but rather may be associated with epithelial injury in the form of localized mucinous degeneration, a potential contributing factor to the development of Pautrier microabscesses and follicular mucinosis that may accompany mycosis fungoides (8). Moreover, as the epidermis becomes more extensively infiltrated, impaired maturation often manifests as clinical abnormalities in scale production. Hence, many T-cell lymphoproliferative disorders

will show surface hyperkeratosis that in early stages may mimic dermatitis clinically (Fig. 31-2C).

Infiltration of the skin by reactive B cells often results in a perivascular accumulation of cells usually without significant epidermotropism or papillary dermal/interstitial involvement (i.e., producing a grenz zone of papillary dermal sparing). With persistence of antigenic stimulus, as may occur in the setting of some insect bite reactions, nodular aggregates of B cells may form in order to variably recapitulate the formation of germinal centers within the dermis (Fig. 31-3A). These patterns of infiltration contrast sharply with those of malignant B cells. Although malignant B cells may also form nodules vaguely reminiscent of germinal centers, or even induce the formation of associated reactive B-cell infiltrates, the former tends to show a destructive relationship to preexisting structures (Fig. 31-3B). Accordingly, malignant B cells will frequently infiltrate in an interstitial pattern (versus perivascular), resulting in splaying apart of collagen bundles and mesenchymal cells (e.g., smooth muscle cells forming arrector pili muscles) within the reticular dermis. Moreover, nodular aggregation of malignant B cells tends to displace adnexal epithelium, resulting in their distortion and occasionally in their ischemic destruction in the process.

Circulating leukemic cells, like inflammatory cells, may show a perivascular pattern of infiltration upon initial infiltration of skin. However, unlike reactive and malignant T cells, they will avoid epithelial infiltration, and like other malignant cells, they will soon infiltrate in an interstitial

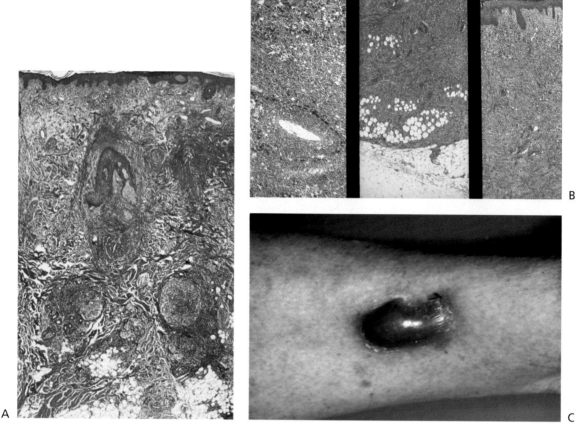

FIGURE 31-3. Normal and abnormal trafficking patterns. **(A)** B-cell pattern showing nondestructive infiltration of superficial and deep dermis. **(B)** B-cell lymphomas showing vascular invasion (*left*), replacement of subcutis (*middle*), and diffuse interstitial pattern (*right*). **(C)** Plum-colored nodule covered by thinned, glistening epidermis due to B-cell dermal infiltration.

pattern within the dermis. This interstitial architecture, albeit suggestive of abnormal trafficking inherent to malignancy, does not invariably correlate with a malignant phenotype. In this regard, it should be recalled that histiocytes in the setting of certain evolutionary stages of palisaded granulomatous dermatitis, lymphocytes in early inflammatory lesions of morphea, and immature myeloid cells, in the setting of extramedullary hematopoiesis may also show similar interstitial patterns.

The tendency for progressive dermal infiltration with relative sparing of the epidermal layer in both B-cell and many leukemic malignancies results in clinical lesions that are red to plum-colored and covered by thin, shiny (nonkeratotic) epidermal surfaces (Fig. 31-3C).

Hematopoietic Cell Lineage and Differentiation: Relevance to Leukemia/Lymphoma

Most hematologic malignancies affecting the skin have lineage relationships to normal evolutionary stages of cellular maturation. Malignant T cells and myeloid cells thus tend to recapitulate morphologic and antigenic features of cells

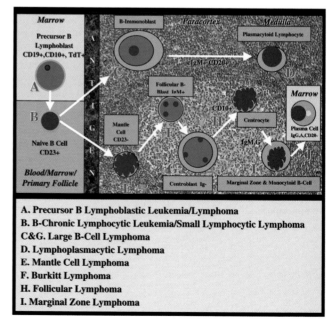

A. Precursor B Lymphoblastic Leukemia/Lymphoma
B. B-Chronic Lymphocytic Leukemia/Small Lymphocytic Lymphoma
C&G. Large B-Cell Lymphoma
D. Lymphoplasmacytic Lymphoma
E. Mantle Cell Lymphoma
F. Burkitt Lymphoma
H. Follicular Lymphoma
I. Marginal Zone Lymphoma

FIGURE 31-4. Schematic diagram of B-cell differentiation in relationship to sites of nodal maturation, relevant markers, and corresponding lymphomas that may develop.

undergoing intrathymic/post-thymic and intraosseous maturation, respectively. Malignant B cells also have definite developmental relationships to normal B-cell ontogeny within bone marrow and lymphoid organs. Because B-cell malignancies compose a clinically and morphologically diverse group of diseases, it is helpful conceptually to relate specific disorders to developmental stages of normal B-cell maturation. Figure 31-4 is an adaptation from the current WHO classification schema (2) that attempts to achieve this end.

PRIMARY CUTANEOUS B-CELL LYMPHOPROLIFERATIVE DISORDERS

B-Cell Lymphomatoid Hyperplasia

Critical to consideration of B-cell malignancies of the skin is understanding the patterns and compositions inherent to forms of cutaneous lymphoid hyperplasia where B cells predominate. Because such lesions have been confused with true lymphomatous infiltrates, the unfortunate term "pseudolymphoma" has been coined, and its use is discouraged for obvious semantic reasons.

Clinical Features. Typically, B-cell cutaneous lymphomatoid hyperplasia develops as one or several clustered nodular lesions without evidence of epidermal involvement (e.g., scaling). The head, neck, and trunk are most frequently involved in our experience, although any site is potentially vulnerable. The color is often red to purple, and thus the clinical appearance may overlap with that of true B-cell lymphoma (Fig. 31-5A). Lesions may persist for many months before resolution occurs, and on occasion, evolution to lymphoma has been documented.

Histopathology. Infiltrates may show a nodular or diffuse architecture, and though many lesions will be most concentrated in the more superficial dermal layers, equal or preferential involvement of the deeper dermis and subcutis

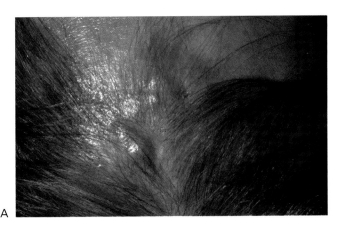

A

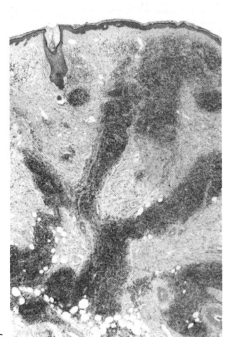
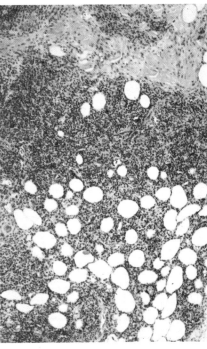

B, C

FIGURE 31-5. Clinical and histological features of B-cell lymphomatoid hyperplasia. **(A)** Clinical lesions. **(B)** Scanning magnification of dermal infiltrate. **(C)** Involvement of deep dermis and subcutis.

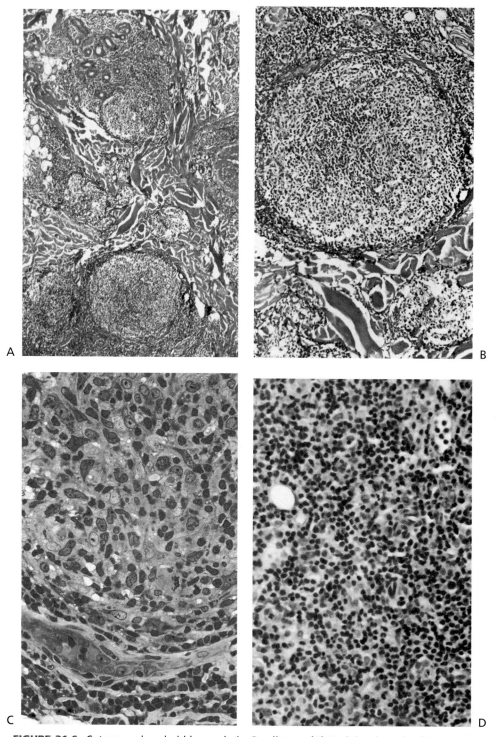

FIGURE 31-6. Cutaneous lymphoid hyperplasia, B-cell type. **(A)** Nodular dermal infiltration by lymphoid cells with formation of germinal centers. **(B)** Higher magnification of germinal center. **(C)** One-micron toluidine blue-stained section of germinal center composed of admixture of lymphocytes in various stages of maturation. **(D)** Reactive germinal center characterized by mitotically active follicular center lymphocytes.

may be seen (Fig. 31-5B and C). This "bottom-heavy" pattern of infiltration, which by convention has been associated with B-cell malignancies, does not reliably permit exclusion of B-cell cutaneous lymphoid hyperplasia. Unlike true B-cell lymphoma, however, hyperplastic B-cell infiltrates generally do not exhibit a pattern of infiltration that destroys preexisting structures (e.g., vessels, adnexae). While hair follicles may be distorted and hyperplastic in certain cases where primary follicular pathology presumably incites the B-cell proliferative response (so-called pseudolymphomatous folliculitis), this is distinct from secondary follicular injury that may be seen in the setting of true lymphoma.

The hallmark of B-cell cutaneous lymphoid hyperplasia is the formation of true lymphoid follicles (Fig. 31-6A). These follicles contain a cytologic continuum of B-cell maturation, and this exhibits lymphocytes with small and large and cleaved and uncleaved nuclear contours (Fig. 31-6B and C), immunoblasts, and tingible body macrophages (macrophages containing particulate basophilic debris within their cytoplasm). Mitotic figures and apoptotic cells may be numerous in follicles showing florid evidence of immune activation (Fig. 31-6D). Reactive follicles may show expanded mantle zones, whereas follicle-like structures formed in certain B-cell lymphomas tend to show thinned or absent mantle zones. Because reactive follicles are generally polyclonal, both kappa and lambda light chains are expressed by immunohistochemistry. Moreover, immunoglobulin gene rearrangements are usually not present, although clonal proliferation within B-cell cutaneous lymphoid hyperplasia has been described (9), and this feature alone should not be used to separate reactive from malignant infiltrates of B cells.

Histogenesis. The cause is often unknown, although persistent localized immune responses to injected or extruded antigens, as may occur with arthropod bite assaults or even in the context of follicular cyst rupture, have been implicated. Certain drugs may also result in B-cell, as well as T-cell–pattern cutaneous infiltrates that may mimic lymphoma both clinically and histologically (10,11).

Differential Diagnosis. B-cell cutaneous lymphoid hyperplasia must be differentiated from follicular lymphoma, a lesion that generally shows a follicular pattern of dermal infiltration. Immunohistochemical and molecular analyses generally permit differentiation in difficult cases where cytologic features that separate reactive from neoplastic lymphoid follicles are not present (see below). It is noteworthy that establishing the presence of reactive germinal centers in a skin infiltrate does not definitively exclude lymphoma, because some forms of B-cell lymphoma are typically associated with admixed reactive follicles (e.g., extranodal marginal cell lymphoma). Moreover, as has been mentioned, patients with established B-cell cutaneous lymphoid hyperplasia must be monitored over time in recognition of the fact that on occasion, this presentation will be a harbinger of eventual development of a clonal B-cell malignancy. Numerous eosinophils may be observed in association with some forms of B-cell cutaneous lymphoid hyperplasia, including lesions of angiolymphoid hyperplasia with eosinophilia and its localized variants.

Table 31-2 summarizes distinguishing characteristics that may be useful in differential diagnosis of the B-cell lymphoproliferative disorders in the skin.

Cutaneous Follicle Center-Cell Lymphoma

Cutaneous follicular lymphoma, one of the most common types of primary B-cell lymphoma of the skin (12), is a neoplasm derived from follicular center B cells (centrocytes/cleaved follicular center cells) and centroblasts/noncleaved follicular center cells. Many of the histopathologic and antigenic features of this lymphoma are identical to follicular lymphoma occurring primarily in lymph nodes, and accordingly, many of these details also are presented for this

TABLE 31-2. SALIENT DIFFERENTIAL FEATURES OF SOME CUTANEOUS B-CELL PROLIFERATIONS

Condition	Follicle Composition	Follicle Architecture	Interfollicular Region
MCL with mantle zone pattern	Benign, polymorphous, polyclonal	Small, round circumscribed	Neoplastic B-cells, CD23⁻, cyclin D1⁺ CD5⁺
Follicular Lymphoma	Neoplastic, monomorphous, clonal	Variable size and circumscription	Residual or compressed normal tissue BCL2⁺ sometimes
B-cutaneous lymphoid hyperplasia	Benign, polymorphous, polyclonal	Variable size and circumscription	Non-neoplastic T-cells, see below
B-small lymphocytic lymphoma	Proliferation centers, pro-lymphocytes and paraimmunoblasts	Uniform pale zones, evenly dispersed	Neoplastic B-cells, CD23⁺, cyclin D1⁻
Extranodal marginal zone lymphoma	Benign, polymorphous, polyclonal	Variable, irregular (when colonized by neoplastic cells)	Small lymphocytes, plasma cells, immunoblasts, eosinophils, histiocytes CD35⁺. CD5⁻, CD10⁻,CD23⁻
Common to most B-cell proliferations	Tendency to form follicles	Tend to loss of zonation	CD19⁺, CD20⁺,CD79a⁺ CD22⁺, CD3⁻

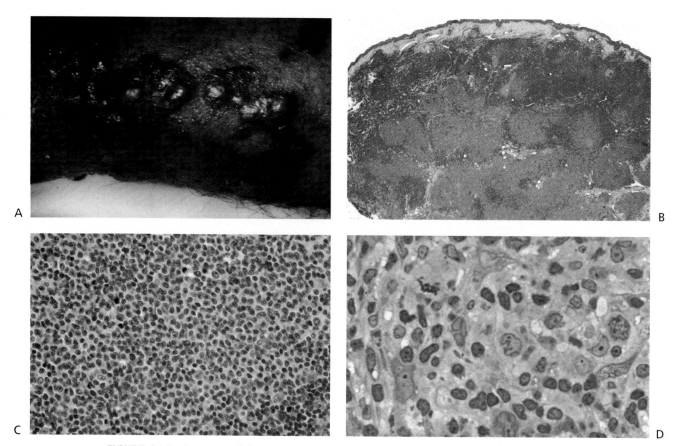

FIGURE 31-7. Cutaneous follicle center cell lymphoma. **(A)** Clustered plum-colored nodules covered by thinned, glistening epidermal layer. **(B)** Scanning magnification showing coalescent nodules forming follicle-like architecture. **(C)** Higher magnification of malignant centrocytes and centroblasts. **(D)** One-micron, toluidine blue-stained section showing cytologic features of centrocytes and centroblasts.

topic under secondary B-cell lymphoproliferative disorders (below).

Clinical Features. Cutaneous follicular lymphoma occurs primarily as one to several red to plum-colored nodules (Fig. 31-7A) often on the head and trunk, and unlike overt nodal follicular lymphoma, tends to remain localized in the skin where local therapy may be effective (13). Lesions with exclusive skin involvement tend to show a more favorable prognosis than is the case when skin is infiltrated secondary to nodal disease (14,15).

Histopathology. Primary skin involvement (16,17) presents as nodular dermal infiltrates that may initially resemble germinal centers (18). Lesions may also show overlap to mucosal lymphoma (MALToma) and marginal zone lymphoma of spleen. The dermal nodules initially may resemble germinal centers but are composed of neoplastic cells devoid of mantle zones (16). These follicular regions are devoid of polarization and do not show a prominent "starry-sky" pattern, and other regions may be characterized by a more diffuse pattern with associated sclerosis. Based on these architectural features (Fig. 31-

7B), lesions may be classified as follicular (greater than 75% follicular architecture), follicular and diffuse (25% to 75% follicular architecture), and minimally follicular (less than 25% follicular). Rarely, exclusively diffuse follicle center cell lymphomas may also be seen, where the diagnosis must be based on cellular composition. Cytologically, two types of neoplastic lymphocytes are observed in follicular lymphoma (Fig. 31-7C and D). The predominant cell is the centrocyte, or cleaved FCC, a small- to medium-sized lymphocyte with scant cytoplasm and with angulated, infolded, or twisted nuclear contours and inconspicuous nucleoli. Similar but often smaller centrocytes may also be present in the interfollicular regions. Centroblasts, or noncleaved FCC, are larger transformed lymphocytes with round to oval nuclei with vesicular chromatin and several visible nucleoli. On occasion, an even admixture of centrocytes and centroblasts, or even a predominance of centroblasts may be encountered. These ratios provide the basis for a grading system based on proportional numbers of centroblasts in ten neoplastic follicles, with Grade 1 = average count of 0 to 5/high power field (HPF), Grade 2 = 6 to 15/HPF, and Grade 3 = more than 15/HPF (19–21).

Although recurrences are often observed, the overall prognosis is good, with spread beyond the skin being exceedingly rare.

Histogenesis. Germinal center B cells are believed to represent the cell of origin of follicular lymphoma. Tumor cells tend to express surface immunoglobulins (IgM, IgD, IgG, and rarely IgA), BCL2, CD10, and the B-cell–associated markers CD20, CD19, CD22, and CD79a. Most cases are negative for CD5 (in contrast to CLL/SLL) and CD4 (3). Although BCL2 expression is useful in differentiating neoplastic follicles in extracutaneous sites from normally negative hyperplastic germinal centers, it should be noted that in primary cutaneous follicular lymphoma, BCL2 is frequently negative. Rearrangement of immunoglobulin heavy- and light-chain genes is the rule (Fig. 31-8), and cytogenetic abnormalities are almost always present (22), with the t(14;18)(q32;q21) rearrangement of the BCL2 gene the most common.

Differential Diagnosis. Cutaneous follicular lymphoma must be differentiated from cutaneous lymphoid hyperplasia of the B-cell type (B-CLH) (23,24) and other conditions associated with the formation of reactive follicles (e.g., marginal and mantle zone lymphoma). B-CLH often is clinically manifested by one or more erythematous to plum-colored plaques and nodules. Any site may be affected, but there is a predilection for skin of the face and scalp. The underlying cause is often unknown, although speculated etiologies include reactions to topical agents or to injected antigens, as may occur in insect bites or localized infection with the spirochete *Borrelia burgdorferi* (25–27). Histologically, there may be a nodular to diffuse interstitial infiltrate that often involves the deep dermis and occasionally the subcutis. Germinal center formation may be variably pronounced, but occasionally these structures are indistinguishable from those encountered in reactive lymph nodes. Specifically, in addition to smaller lymphocytes with cleaved nuclei (centrocytes) and larger lymphocytes with noncleaved nuclei (centroblasts), they will contain an admixture of immunoblasts, antigen-presenting follicular dendritic cells, and macrophages containing phagocytized cellular debris (tingible body macrophages). Moreover, there tends to be aggregation of centroblasts and tingible body macrophages at one pole of the hyperplastic follicle, and of centrocytes at the opposite pole, producing darker- and lighter-staining regions, respectively. Immunohistochemistry will reveal both kappa and lambda Ig light-chain expression in B-CLH, as opposed to monotypic expression in follicular lymphoma. Genotypic analysis may also be of assistance when in establishing a diagnosis of B-CLH when it fails to reveal clonal immunoglobulin gene rearrangements. However, it must be noted that on occasion, cases of B-CLH appear to evolve over time into more aggressive clonal processes, or may harbor a malignant clone in the midst of otherwise reactive histologic and immunophenotypic changes (28).

Extraosseous Plasmacytoma

Extraosseous plasmacytoma is a neoplasm of plasma cells that occurs at primary sites other than bone marrow and, as such, represents only a small percentage of all plasma cell neoplasms (29).

Clinical Features. The majority of affected individuals are middle-aged adult males (male/female ratio is 2:1). Although lesions may present in skin, most such tumors occur in tissues of the oropharynx, nasopharynx and nasal sinuses, and larynx (30). Approximately 15% to 20% of patients will have a monoclonal gammopathy, but neoplastic cells, by definition, spare the bone marrow and peripheral blood. Prognosis seems to be related primarily to the presence of solitary versus multiple lesions, with the former responding well to either surgical excision or radiotherapy, and the latter associated with a significant rate of mortality.

Histopathology. There is diffuse to nodular dermal infiltration by mature and occasionally less differentiated (plasmablastic) plasma cells (Fig. 31-9A). Occasional cells may have polylobated nuclear contours, nucleoli, and/or binucleation (Fig. 31-9B). It is of note that nuclear immaturity

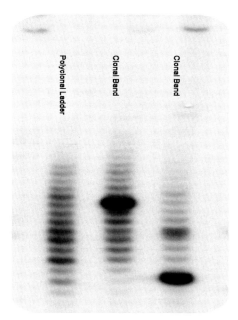

FIGURE 31-8. Polymerase chain reaction analysis for clonal IgH gene rearrangements. The left lane shows a polyclonal ladder with no evidence of gene rearrangement, whereas the middle and right lanes show dominant bands in a background polyclonal ladder, indicating clonal IgH gene rearrangement in two cases of B-cell lymphoma.

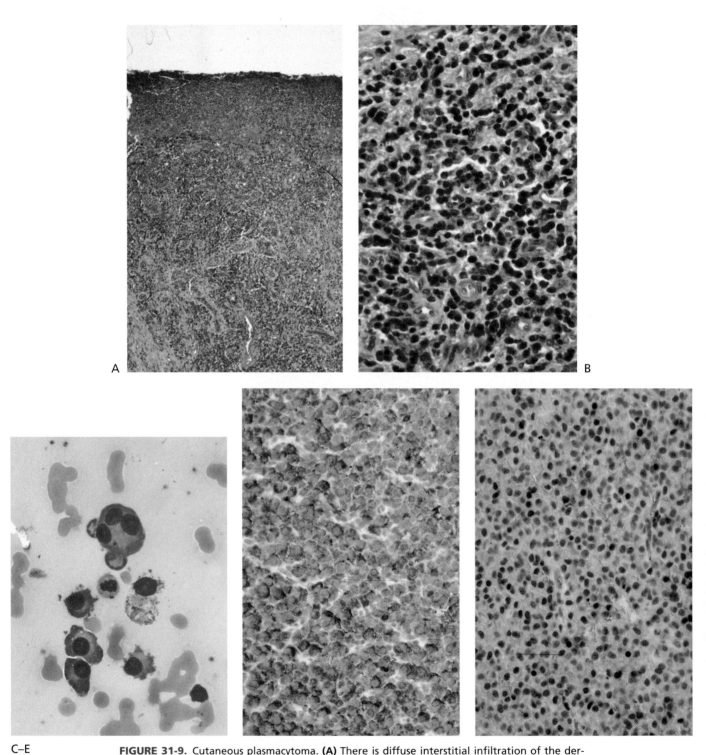

FIGURE 31-9. Cutaneous plasmacytoma. **(A)** There is diffuse interstitial infiltration of the dermis associated with surface erosion. **(B)** Higher magnification, showing cellular infiltrate composed of plasmacytoid cells, some with binucleation. **(C)** Atypical plasma cells in bone marrow aspirate from patient with multiple myeloma. **(D)** Paraffin immunohistochemistry of cutaneous plasmacytoma for lambda light chains. **(E)** Paraffin immunohistochemistry of cutaneous plasmacytoma for kappa light chains.

and pleomorphism tend not to occur in the setting of reactive plasma cell infiltrates. The cytoplasm of the neoplastic plasma cells may contain a variety of inclusions usually related to abnormal accumulation of immunoglobulin, including round eosinophilic (Russell) bodies. Such cytoplasmic changes are not, however, specific for neoplastic plasma cells. In cases where systemic dissemination occurs or when primary myeloma involves skin secondarily, abnormal plasma cells may be detected in bone marrow aspirates (Fig. 31-9C).

Histogenesis. Clonal transformation of a peripheral plasma cell is the most likely cell of origin. A key feature therefore is the expression of monotypic cytoplasmic immunoglobulin and light-chain restriction that, unlike cell surface–associated monotypic immunoglobulin in B-cell lymphomas, is generally demonstrable in formalin-fixed, paraffin-embedded material (Fig. 31-9D and E). CD38 and CD79a are usually expressed, although most but not all plasma cells lack pan–B-cell antigens, CD19 and CD20. Molecular studies generally reveal rearrangement of immunoglobulin genes.

Differential Diagnosis. The differential diagnosis includes extranodal, marginal zone B-cell lymphoma (MALT type; see below) with marked plasmacytic differentiation, and reactive, plasma cell-rich, immune responses.

Extranodal Marginal B-Cell Lymphoma (MALT Lymphoma)

MALT lymphoma is an indolent, radiosensitive extranodal neoplasm composed of heterogeneous populations of small B cells, including marginal zone (centrocyte-like) cells, monocytoid cells, immunoblasts, and small lymphocytes. The term MALT refers to mucosal-associated lymphoid tissue, in which these neoplasms were first recognized (31,32).

Clinical Features. MALT lymphoma is responsible for less than 10% of all B-cell lymphomas, and the gastrointestinal tract is the primary site of involvement in 50% of cases (31,32). Other sites may be affected, with skin infiltration noted in 11% of cases (33). Males and females are affected in a 1:1.2 ratio, and the median age of occurrence is 61 (31). Chronic lymphoid hyperplasia caused by antigenic stimulation may be a predisposing feature, with *Helicobacter pylori*–associated chronic gastritis (34,35), Hashimoto thyroiditis (36–38), and autoimmune sialadenitis (39,40) representing important examples. Other examples of MALT lymphoma being associated with an infectious agent are orbital lymphoma (*Chlamydia psittaci*) and cutaneous MALT lymphoma (*B. burgdorferi*) (41–44). Patients with hepatitis C have a higher incidence of splenic marginal zone lymphoma (45). Conceptually, MALT lymphomas are divided into a "native" type that arises in extranodal anatomic compartments where lymphoid tissue is normally present and into an "acquired"

type that emanates from tissue that normally lacks lymphoid tissue. In general, MALT lymphoma is an indolent form of lymphoma that responds well to a variety of therapeutic modalities, including eradication of chronic antigenic stimulus in cases where infectious agents are implicated.

Histopathology. A characteristic feature of MALT lymphoma is the tendency of the neoplastic cells to infiltrate around reactive B-cell follicles. This infiltration is in a marginal zone distribution (external to the mantle zone), and expansion of these areas may result in confluent zones that displace and separate the reactive follicles (46,47). Marginal zone B cells have small- to medium-sized nuclei with slightly irregular contours and inconspicuous nuclei, and thus resemble centrocytes (Fig. 31-10). The cytoplasm is variably visible and pale, with cells showing less cytoplasm resembling small lymphocytes and those with more ample cytoplasm acquiring a monocytoid appearance. Variable plasmacytic differentiation may also be present. A minority population of centroblasts and immunoblasts may also be observed. Colonization of the reactive germinal centers by neoplastic cells may occasionally produce a picture that initially resembles follicular lymphoma. Transformation to diffuse, large B-cell lymphoma (see below) has been described.

Histogenesis. The cell of origin is speculated to be a post–germinal center, marginal zone B-cell. Tumor cells express immunoglobulins (most often IgM) and show light-chain restriction. Typical immunophenotypes are CD20$^+$, CD79$^+$, CD21$^+$, CD35$^+$, CD5$^-$, CD10$^-$, and CD23$^-$, although a marker entirely specific for MALT lymphoma does not presently exist. Immunoglobulin genes are rearranged. More recently, we have been able to further our understanding of the underlying genetic abnormalities in MALT lymphoma (48–51). The most common recurrent structural abnormality in MALT lymphoma is t(11;18)

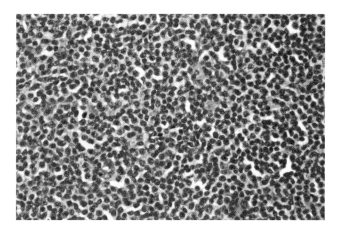

FIGURE 31-10. Extranodal marginal B-cell lymphoma (MALT lymphoma). The interfollicular confluent infiltrate is composed of B cells that resemble centrocytes.

(q21;q21), in which the apoptosis inhibitor gene API2 on chromosome 11 partners with the MALT1 gene on chromosome 18. t(11;18) is present in approximately 25% of MALT lymphomas irrespective of anatomic site. A much less common translocation is t(1;14)(p22;q32), which involves the gene encoding the nuclear protein BCL-10 in tumor cells with this translocation. BCL-10 regulates cell survival. It is expressed in the *nucleus* of MALT lymphoma cells in both t(11;18) and t(1;14) positive cases, while negative cases show *cytoplasmic* expression for BCL-10 protein. While the abovementioned translocations are seemingly unrelated, they both engage in activation of NF6B, which is a transcription factor with a pivotal role in activating genes involved in immunity, inflammation, and apoptosis. It is proposed that enhanced NF6B activity is critical in tumor progression.

Differential Diagnosis. The differential diagnosis includes other small B-cell lymphomas as well as cutaneous lymphoid hyperplasia. Absence of CD5 and cyclin D1 are useful in separating MALT lymphoma from mantle cell lymphoma, absence of CD5 alone in excluding small lymphocytic lymphoma, and absence of CD10 in ruling out follicular lymphoma. Presence of expanded interfollicular zones by B cells with cytologic and immunophenotypic features of MALT lymphoma should distinguish this entity from most cases of cutaneous lymphoid hyperplasia where interfollicular regions, if expanded, should contain a predominant population of T cells. See also Table 31-2.

Diffuse Large B-Cell Lymphoma, Extranodal Type

Diffuse large B-cell lymphoma (DLBCL) is a high-grade neoplasm composed of large B cells. It may present as a rapidly enlarging, often symptomatic tumor involving a single lymph node or an extranodal site, although staging often discloses disease dissemination. The discussion for primary cutaneous DLBCL is essentially the same as for its primary nodal counterpart with secondary dissemination of skin, and therefore this topic is discussed in detail below under the topic of secondary B-cell lymphoproliferative disorders.

Lymphomatoid Granulomatosis Initially Presenting in Skin

Lymphomatoid granulomatosis (LYG) is a form of angiocentric and angiodestructive B-cell lymphoproliferative disease. While it generally presents in the lung, skin may occasionally be the initial site of involvement. The salient features of LYG in the skin are identical for both primary and secondary lesions, and thus this disorder is discussed

in detail below under its more common occurrence as a secondary B-cell lymphoproliferative disorder affecting the skin.

SECONDARY B-CELL LYMPHOPROLIFERATIVE DISORDERS AFFECTING SKIN

Precursor B-Lymphoblastic Lymphoma

Precursor B-lymphoblastic lymphoma (B-LBL) is a relatively rare neoplasm of B-lymphoblasts with a tendency for skin, lymph node, and bone marrow involvement. It may also present primarily in a leukemic phase, where it is known as precursor B-cell acute lymphoblastic leukemia (B-ALL). Lymphoblastic lymphomas may be of either T- or B-cell lineage (see separate discussion of precursor T-lymphoblastic leukemia/lymphoma under secondary T/NK lymphoproliferative disorders below). Although the majority of systemic lymphoblastic lymphomas are of T-cell lineage, those with a tendency for cutaneous involvement have shown a curious tendency toward B-cell lineage (52).

Clinical Features. B-LBL generally tends to affect children and young adults aged less than 35 years. Bone marrow involvement is generally extensive at time of presentation, with associated anemia and thrombocytopenia and symptoms related to bone or joint pain. Patients may show lymphadenopathy as well as hepatic and splenic enlargement upon physical examination. Skin lesions, which may occasionally occur without blood or marrow involvement (53,54), may take the form of multiple papules and nodules that often involve the head and neck. The outlook is favorable if skin is exclusively involved at the time of diagnosis, as compared to an unfavorable prognosis if the disease is disseminated (55). There tends to be a high rate of remission, with median survival of approximately 5 years (53).

Histopathology. Skin involvement may be nodular or diffuse within the dermis, consisting of homogeneous infiltration by mitotically active lymphoblasts with variably convoluted nuclei containing finely stippled chromatin and inconspicuous nucleoli (Fig. 31-11A). Cytoplasm is sparse, and may be difficult to detect in routinely prepared tissue. The epidermis is spared, often separated from the region of dermal involvement by a thin subepidermal mantle of unaffected dermis (Grenz zone). Further classification, including differentiation between T- and B-cell lymphoblastic differentiation, requires immunohistochemical analysis.

Histogenesis. The neoplastic cells of B-LBL lack surface immunoglobulin expression and may harbor cytoplasmic μ chain (pre–B-cell leukemia) or no immunoglobulin (progenitor B-cell leukemia), and thus are generally considered to be precursor B cells. The characteristic cytochemical/

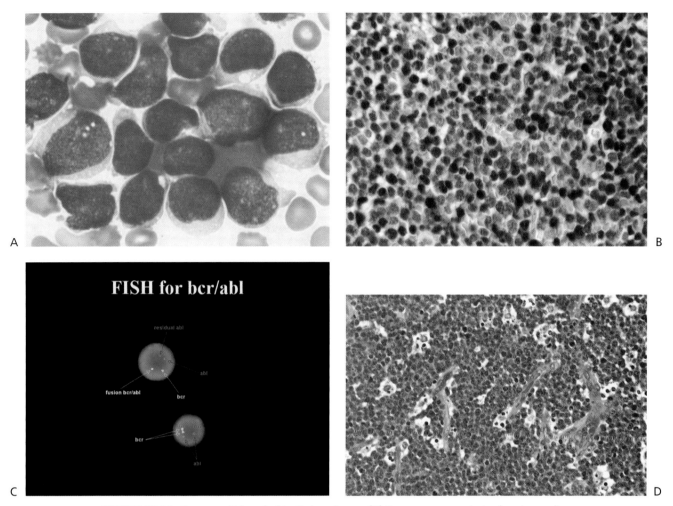

FIGURE 31-11. Precursor B-lymphoblastic lymphoma. **(A)** Bone marrow aspirate showing malignant lymphoblasts. **(B)** Nuclear reactivity for terminal deoxynucleotidyl transferase (TdT). **(C)** FISH in a patient with acute lymphoblastic leukemia positive for the Philadelphia chromosome. (Upper cell: green dot is BCR gene on chromosome 22; red dot to lower right is normal ABL gene on chromosome 9; yellow dot is fusion BCR/ABL; red dot to upper left is residual ABL gene adjacent to breakpoint. Lower cell is normal gene pattern for comparison.) **(D)** "Starry sky" pattern of Burkitt lymphoma that must be distinguished from mitotically active lesions of precursor B-lymphoblastic lymphoma.

immunohistochemical profile consists of positive terminal deoxynucleotidyl transferase (TdT) (Fig. 31-11B), as well as CD19, cytoplasmic CD79a, CD10 (also known as CALLA, or common acute lymphocytic leukemia antigen), and CD24+, and variable reactivity for CD22 and CD20. Stains for surface immunoglobulin and myeloperoxidase are characteristically negative. Cytogenetic abnormalities are numerous and frequently correlate with prognosis and treatment protocols, particularly in pediatric patients (56–58). The arsenal of tests assessing molecular abnormalities includes conventional cytogenetics, polymerase chain reaction, and fluorescence *in situ* hybridization (FISH). Hyperdiploid karyotypes with more than 50 chromosomes ordinarily convey favorable prognosis, while hypodiploidy predicts unfavorable outcome. t(9;22)

(Philadelphia chromosome), t(4;11) involving the mixed lineage leukemia (MLL) gene locus, and t(1;19) are examples of LBL with adverse clinical outcomes. Along with chronic myelogenous leukemia, some lymphoblastic leukemias/lymphomas express the chimeric bcr-abl gene that encodes for a tyrosine kinase that is constitutively activated, thus playing a key role in leukemogenesis (Fig. 31-11C).

Differential Diagnosis. Lesions may be differentiated from morphologically similar infiltrates of malignant T-cell lymphoblasts and myeloblasts by cytochemistry/immunohistochemistry. Occasionally, mitotically active lesions in children may resemble the starry-sky pattern of Burkitt lymphoma (Fig. 31-11D), and lesions in adults may mimic mantle cell lymphoma; TdT determination is of value in establishing a diagnosis of B-LBL in such cases (59,60).

Chronic Lymphocytic Leukemia/Small Lymphocytic Lymphoma

Chronic lymphocytic leukemia/small lymphocytic lymphoma (CLL/SLL) is an indolent disseminated or solid neoplastic proliferation of a monotonous population of small lymphocytes of B-cell lineage.

Clinical Features. CLL/SLL is relatively common, generally affects older adults, and shows a 2:1 male/female ratio. Patients diagnosed with CLL have bone marrow and peripheral blood involvement, and lymph nodes, liver, and spleen are also typically infiltrated. Other sites of occasional infiltration by leukemic cells are the skin, breast, and ocular adnexae. When tissue infiltration occurs without evidence of bone marrow involvement, a diagnosis of SLL can be made histologically. Although not usually curable, the disease tends to run an indolent course, unless transformation to a high-grade, large B-cell lymphoma supervenes. This phenomenon, known as Richter syndrome, occurs in approximately 3.5% of cases. When cases with plasmacytoid differentiation (previously termed immunocytoma or

plasmacytoid lymphoma) affect skin primarily, there is often a single nodule on the trunk or extremity, and less frequently on the head and neck. Lesions tend to be multiple with secondary cutaneous involvement and may be associated with immunoglobulin production, resulting in autoimmune sequelae, or in the case of secretion of IgM, a Waldenstrom macroglobulinemia picture.

Cutaneous involvement may produce papules and nodules, or occasionally more diffuse skin infiltration that results in irregular thickening and furrowing (61). Occasionally leukemic cells may infiltrate sites of preexisting dermatitis where adhesive interactions with inflamed vessels are presumably augmented.

Histopathology. Involved tissues are infiltrated by uniform populations of small lymphocytes containing rounded hyperchromatic nuclei and a variably inconspicuous nucleolus (62,63) (Fig. 31-12). In lymph nodes and occasionally in other sites, pseudofollicles (alternatively termed proliferation or growth centers) that contain a continuum small to large lymphocytes, including prolymphocytes and paraimmunoblasts, will produce a nodular pattern of regularly distributed pale-staining areas at scanning magnification. Cases with plasmacytoid differentiation may preferentially affect the superficial dermis or show a vertically oriented

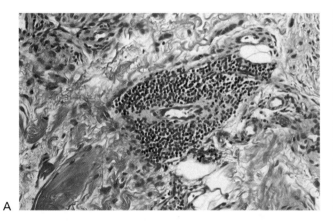

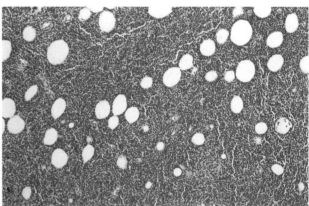

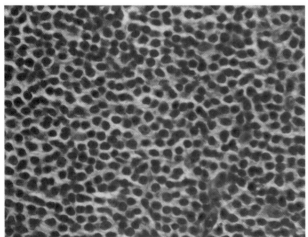

FIGURE 31-12. Chronic lymphocytic leukemia/small lymphocytic lymphoma. **(A)** Early angiocentric infiltration within the dermis by small uniform lymphoid cells. **(B)** Advanced replacement of the subcutis by similar cells. **(C)** Diffuse, cellular infiltrate composed of uniform populations of small lymphocytes containing rounded, hyperchromatic nuclei with inconspicuous nucleoli.

perifollicular distribution and be composed of heterogeneous populations of cells, including, in addition to plasmacytoid lymphocytes, immunoblasts, plasma cells, histiocytes, eosinophils, and reactive lymphoid follicles (16,64).

Skin involvement may take the form of an angiocentric pattern within the superficial and deep dermis and subcutis (Fig. 31-12A), and interstitial pattern where small lymphocytes are present among collagen bundles and adipocytes (Fig. 31-12B) as well as around vessels, and a mixed diffuse/nodular pattern (65). In the latter, proliferation centers similar to those typical of nodal involvement may occasionally be encountered. As with B-cell pattern infiltrates, the epidermis and follicular epithelium is spared, and the papillary dermis is usually uninvolved, producing a typical grenz zone. Cytologically, the infiltrating cells are identical to those that involve lymph nodes and other extranodal sites (Fig. 31-12C).

Histogenesis. The typical immunophenotype of the tumor cells consists of positivity for CD5, CD19, CD79a, CD23, and CD43. They generally only weakly express surface IgM or IgM and IgD, CD20, CD22, and CD11c, and are negative for CD10 and cyclin D1. It should be recalled that light-chain restriction is confined to surface immunoglobulin in CLL/SLL, and thus unlike plasma cells that contain cytoplasmic immunoglobulin, immunoglobulin restriction can only be demonstrated in fresh, frozen (unfixed) sections. Heavy- and light-chain immunoglobulin genes are rearranged, and this can be demonstrated by molecular analysis using polymerase chain reaction (PCR). At the molecular level, two groups of CLL can be distinguished, one without somatic mutations in the immunoglobulin VH regions being the equivalent of recirculating CD5+, CD23+, IgM+, and IgD+ naive B cells that are normally detected in blood and in primary follicles and mantle zones (66,67), and one with somatic mutations in the variable genes corresponding to post–germinal center B cells. The majority of CLL exhibit chromosomal abnormalities. Unmutated types of CLL are more commonly associated with trisomy 12, while the mutated forms may present with deletions at 13q14. Previous cases with reported clonal bcl-1 gene rearrangement may have been misdiagnosed cases of mantle cell lymphoma. Distinguishing between the two ontogenetic types of CLL carries prognostic significance: the prospect of CLL with germline VH genes is significantly less favorable than those with hypermutated VH genes. Flow cytometric detection of CD38 (68,69) and, more recently, of zeta-associated protein 70 (ZAP-70) (70–75) that appears to enhance signal transduction, have been utilized as surrogate markers to detect germline VH gene types of CLL with predictable poor outcome.

Differential Diagnosis. In certain cases, the small lymphocytes of CLL/SLL may show moderate irregularity of nuclear contour, raising suspicion for mantle cell lymphoma. The presence of pseudofollicles or prolymphocytes and paraimmunoblasts will permit a diagnosis of CLL/SLL in such instances (76,77). It should also be noted that in occasional cases there may be plasmacytoid differentiation by the neoplastic lymphocytes, corresponding to so-called plasmacytoid immunocytoma of previous classification systems (78) and resulting in potential diagnostic confusion with marginal zone and MALT lymphoma (14).

The perivascular pattern in CLL/SLL may result in confusion with forms of dermatitis characterized by a predominant or exclusive angiocentric architecture of inflammatory cell infiltration. This differential would therefore include polymorphous light eruption (Chapter 12), dermal forms of lupus erythematosus (Chapter 10), certain dermal delayed hypersensitivity responses to drug or injected antigen (Chapter 11), and the family of gyrate erythemas (e.g., erythema annulare centrifugum and erythema chronicum migrans) (Chapter 7). Although all of these conditions contain small lymphocytes, the cells of CLL/SLL tend to be more homogeneous at high magnification. Moreover, most forms of dermatitis are predominated by T cells, not B cells, and the B cells of CLL/SLL will also characteristically aberrantly express CD5.

Follicular Lymphoma

Follicular lymphoma is a relatively common, often low-grade neoplasm of B-lymphocytes differentiating toward follicle center cells (centrocytes or cleaved follicle center cells; FCC) and centroblasts (noncleaved FCC). These tumors at least focally show a nodular/follicular architecture upon tissue infiltration. This section will include some descriptive overlap with cutaneous follicle center-cell lymphoma, discussed previously.

Clinical Features. This type of lymphoma affects primarily older adults, with a median age of 59 and a male/female ratio of 1:1 (79). When children are affected, lesions tend to be localized to the head and neck, and approximately half of tumors are of the large-cell type (see below). In addition to lymph node involvement, bone marrow, spleen, blood, Waldeyer ring, gastrointestinal tract, and skin and soft tissues may be affected. Primary follicular lymphoma of the skin ("cutaneous follicle center cell lymphoma") is one of the most common types of B-cell lymphomas affecting the skin (12). This variant occurs primarily as one to several red to plum-colored nodules on the head and trunk, and unlike overt nodal follicular lymphoma, tends to remain localized in the skin where local therapy may be effective (13). However, most patients have widespread disease at time of presentation (31), although symptoms and signs tend to be restricted to lymph node enlargement. Of all cases of nodal follicular lymphoma, approximately 4% will show evidence of secondary skin involvement. Follicular lymphoma is generally incurable, showing an indolent waxing and waning course. The overall median survival is 7 to 9 years regardless of whether therapy is aggressive or symptomatic.

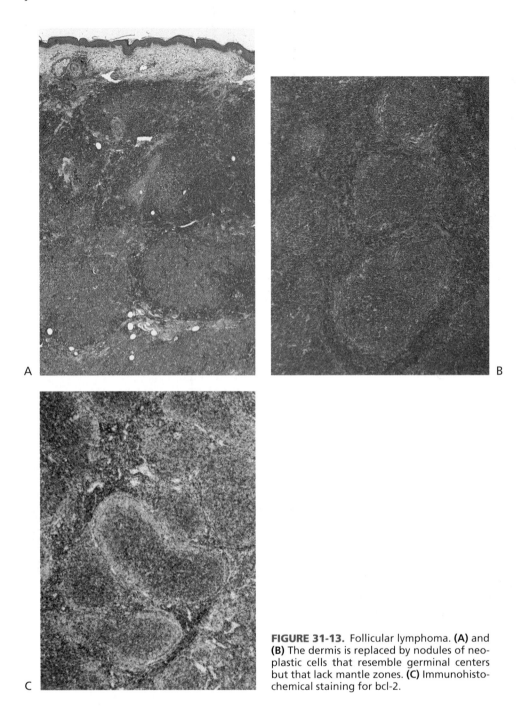

FIGURE 31-13. Follicular lymphoma. **(A)** and **(B)** The dermis is replaced by nodules of neoplastic cells that resemble germinal centers but that lack mantle zones. **(C)** Immunohistochemical staining for bcl-2.

Histopathology. The characteristic architecture consists of multiple closely packed nodules that initially may resemble germinal centers but that are composed of neoplastic cells devoid of mantle zones (16) (Fig. 31-13A and B). These follicular regions are devoid of polarization and do not show a prominent starry-sky pattern, and other regions may be characterized by a more diffuse pattern with associated sclerosis. Based on these architectural features, lesions may be classified as follicular (greater than 75% follicular architecture), follicular and diffuse (25% to 75% follicular architecture), and minimally follicular (less than 25% fol-

licular). Rarely, exclusively diffuse follicle center cell lymphomas may also be seen, where the diagnosis must be based on cellular composition. Cytologically, two types of neoplastic lymphocytes are observed in follicular lymphoma. The predominant cell is the centrocyte, or cleaved FCC, a small- to medium-sized lymphocyte with scant cytoplasm and with angulated, infolded, or twisted nuclear contours and inconspicuous nucleoli. Similar but often smaller centrocytes may also be present in the interfollicular regions. Centroblasts, or noncleaved FCC, are larger transformed lymphocytes with round to oval nuclei with vesicular chromatin and several visible nucleoli (Fig. 31-7). On occasion, an even admixture of centrocytes and centroblasts, or even a predominance of centroblasts may be encountered. These ratios provide the basis for a grading system based on proportional numbers of centroblasts in ten neoplastic follicles, with Grade 1 = average count of 0 to 5/HPF, Grade 2 = 6 to 15/HPF, and Grade 3 = more than 15/HPF (19–21).

Skin involvement, either secondary (with established nodal disease) or primary (16,17), presents as nodular dermal infiltrates that may initially resemble germinal centers (18). Whereas secondary cutaneous involvement tends to have significant morphologic overlap with features seen in lymph nodes, primary cutaneous follicular lymphoma may also show overlap to mucosal lymphoma (MALToma) and marginal zone lymphoma of spleen. Moreover, lesions with exclusive skin involvement tend to share with these entities a more favorable prognosis (15,16).

Histogenesis. Germinal-center B cells are believed to represent the cell of origin of follicular lymphoma. Tumor cells tend to express surface immunoglobulins (IgM, IgD, IgG, and rarely IgA, BCL2, CD10), and the B-cell–associated markers CD20, CD19, CD22, and CD79a. Most cases are negative for CD5 (in contrast to CLL/SLL) and CD43. Although BCL2 expression is useful in differentiating neoplastic follicles (Fig. 31-13C) from normally negative hyperplastic germinal centers, it should be noted that in cases where skin is exclusively involved at the time of presentation ("cutaneous follicular center cell lymphoma"), BCL2 is frequently negative. Rearrangement of immunoglobulin heavy- and light-chain genes is the rule, and cytogenetic abnormalities are almost always present (22), with the t(14;18)(q32;q21) rearrangement of the BCL2 gene the most common. The BCL-2 protein is situated on mitochondrial membranes, and serves as an inhibitor of programmed cell death. Consequently, BCL-2 expression in nodal follicular lymphoma appears to lend the tumor cells a distinct survival advantage when compared to their benign germinal center counterparts that undergo apoptosis.

Differential Diagnosis. Cutaneous involvement by follicular lymphoma must be differentiated from cutaneous lymphoid hyperplasia of the B-cell type (B-CLH) (23,24) and other conditions associated with the formation of reactive follicles (e.g., marginal and mantle zone lymphoma). B-CLH often is clinically manifested by one or more erythematous to plum-colored plaques and nodules. Any site may be affected, but there is a predilection for skin of the face and scalp. The underlying cause is often unknown, although a reaction to injected, as may occur in insect bites or localized infection with the spirochete *B. burgdorferi* (25–27). Histologically, there may be a nodular to diffuse interstitial infiltrate that often involves the deep dermis and occasionally the subcutis. Germinal center formation may be variably pronounced, but occasionally these structures are indistinguishable from those

encountered in reactive lymph nodes. Specifically, in addition to smaller lymphocytes with cleaved nuclei (centrocytes) and larger lymphocytes with noncleaved nuclei (centroblasts), they will contain an admixture of immunoblasts, antigen-presenting follicular dendritic cells, and macrophages containing phagocytized cellular debris (tingible body macrophages). Moreover, there tends to be aggregation of centroblasts and tingible body macrophages at one pole of the hyperplastic follicle, and of centrocytes at the opposite pole, producing darker and lighter-staining regions, respectively. Immunohistochemistry will reveal both kappa and lambda Ig light-chain expression in B-CLH, as opposed to monotypic expression in follicular lymphoma. Genotypic analysis may also be of assistance when in establishing a diagnosis of B-CLH when it fails to reveal clonal immunoglobulin gene rearrangements. However, it must be noted that on occasion, cases of B-CLH appear to evolve over time into more aggressive clonal processes, or may harbor a malignant clone in the midst of otherwise reactive histologic and immunophenotypic changes (28). Some of these differences are summarized in Table 31-2.

Mantle Cell Lymphoma

Mantle cell lymphoma (MCL) is a B-cell neoplasm that is composed of uniform populations of small- to medium-sized lymphocytes that resemble follicular center cells, or centrocytes, but that tend to have somewhat less irregular nuclear contours (80–85). The normal cellular counterpart thus resides in the mantles that surround secondary lymphoid follicles in lymph nodes. Unlike follicular lymphoma, which accounts for approximately one-third of all non-Hodgkin lymphomas in the United States, MCL is considerably less common, accounting for only 3% to 10% (31). Unlike B-SLL, proliferation centers are absent. Because it rarely involves skin, it is discussed here briefly.

Clinical Features. This disease affects middle-aged and older individuals with a 2:1 male/female ratio (31,82,83, 86–88). Disease is usually advanced at time of detection (stage III or IV) and generally affects lymph nodes, spleen, and bone marrow with or without peripheral blood involvement, and gastrointestinal tract involvement may also be observed (82,88–90). When multiple sites of polypoid gastrointestinal involvement by lymphoma are encountered, the diagnosis is generally MCL (91–93). Occurrence in skin is rare but potentially underreported. Presentation in skin is generally followed by development of overt extracutaneous involvement, consistent with the notion that primary skin MCL is a more aggressive process than primary cutaneous follicular lymphoma or plasmacytoid B-CLL variants (18,94). Median survival is 3 to 5 years, and cure is unusual (87–90,95,96).

Histopathology. The majority of cases shows a vaguely nodular to diffuse pattern of growth composed of small- to

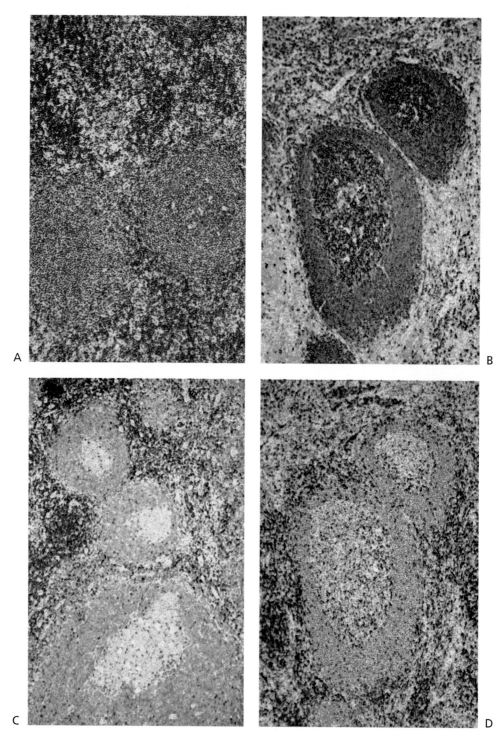

FIGURE 31-14. Mantle cell lymphoma. **(A)** There is a vaguely nodular to diffuse infiltrate composed of small to medium-sized lymphocytes. **(B)** Immunophenotypically, the cells are characterized by strong reactivity for the B-cell marker CD20. **(C)** Reactivity for CD5, which is compared here to T cells (*upper left*), forms a mantle zone pattern about compressed lymphoid follicles. **(D)** Negativity for the T-cell marker CD3.

medium-sized lymphocytes with variably irregular nuclear contours (Fig. 31-14A). The chromatin pattern is dispersed and nucleoli are inconspicuous. These cells most closely resemble centrocytes. Smaller cells resembling those of B-CLL may also be present. Transformed tumor cells (e.g., those resembling centroblasts, immunoblasts, or paraimmunoblasts) and pseudofollicles are not seen. Other cells that are sometimes admixed include occasional plasma cells, histiocytes dispersed in a pattern that may resemble the starry sky of Burkitt lymphoma, and endothelial cells forming hyalinized vascular profiles. A characteristic feature of some lesions of MCL is the tendency of neoplastic lymphocytes to surround and compress nonneoplastic lymphoid follicles (so-called mantle zone pattern). Skin infiltration may be nodular to diffuse, and occasional lesions will show preferential infiltration of the more superficial dermal layers. Rarely, recurrent lesions will show more nuclear atypia and numerous mitoses, qualifying for the designation of "blastoid MCL."

Histogenesis. The tumor is believed to arise from a peripheral B-cell of the inner mantle zone of the lymphoid follicle. Accordingly, the tumor is characterized by a clonal proliferation of CD20+ B cells (Fig. 31-14B) that express surface IgM with or without associated IgD (81,82,85,95). They also tend to express CD5 (Fig. 31-14C), CD43, and BCL-2 protein, and are negative for CD10 and CD23 (82,95,97–102) (Fig. 31-14D). CD5 negativity does occasionally occur, and may be associated with more indolent biological behavior (103). Interestingly, gastrointestinal lesions are associated with expression of the gut homing receptor, alpha4 beta7 (104). The clonal nature of the process may be demonstrated via rearrangements of immunoglobulin heavy- and light-chain genes, and virtually all cases have cytogenetic abnormalities using FISH (105, 106). Most cases of mantle cell lymphoma have undergone clonal heavy- and light-chain gene rearrangement with germline configuration in the VH gene region, which is consistent with pre-germinal center origin. t(11;14)(q13;q32), with participation of the cyclin-D1 gene and the immunoglobulin heavy-chain locus, is the cytogenetic hallmark of MCL (95,107–111). Cyclin D1 (Prad-1, bcl-1) is an important cell-cycle regulatory protein involved in restriction point control between G1 and S phase. The genetic abnormality is detectable by conventional cytogenetics, FISH analysis, or PCR; overexpression of the gene product can be readily assessed by immunohistochemical stains with antibodies directed against the nuclear cyclin D1 protein. More recently, pathogenesis of MCL has been linked to alterations of the ataxia-telangiectasia mutated (ATM) gene which encodes a protein critically involved in the cellular response to DNA damage (112–114). It has been known for a long time that patients with hereditary ataxia telangiectasia are predisposed to develop malignant lymphomas. Of all malignant lymphomas, MCL is most commonly associated with mutations of the

ATM gene, most of which are nonsense mutations resulting in truncated proteins followed by missense mutations. The underlying molecular mechanism leading to ATM mutations in MCL is unknown.

Differential Diagnosis. The most common differential diagnostic problem is differentiation of MCL from other process where lymphoid follicles or their mimics are present. Table 31-2 summarizes the salient differential features for MCL compared to other cutaneous B-cell lymphomas.

Diffuse Large B-Cell Lymphoma, Nodal Type

Diffuse large B-cell lymphoma (DLBCL) is a relatively common type of non-Hodgkin lymphoma that affects primarily adults and frequently presents with involvement of extranodal sites, including skin. It is an aggressive lymphoma characterized by diffuse tissue infiltration by monotonous populations of large, "histiocytoid" malignant lymphocytes.

Clinical Features. Although elderly individuals are most often affected, with the median age in the seventh decade, the disease may affect a wide age range, and children are occasionally affected (31,86). Patients often present with signs or symptoms of a rapidly enlarging tumor at either a nodal or extranodal site, the latter of which commonly involve skin, soft tissue, and numerous viscera (2). Upon more thorough staging, disease is often found to be advanced and thus disseminated (31,86), although this aggressive lymphoma is potentially curable with aggressive chemotherapy. Lesions generally arise *de novo*, although some lesions represent transformation within preexisting more indolent lymphomas (e.g., SLL, follicular lymphoma, lymphomatoid granulomatosis, or marginal zone lymphoma). One important predisposing factor is immunodeficiency, particularly in the presence of seropositivity for Epstein–Barr virus (EBV).

In the skin, DLBCL form red to purpuric papules, nodules, and infiltrated plaques. Occasionally, only skin is found to be involved after careful staging work-up, and such cases may be considered to be primary in the skin, including skin of the back (115). Such lesions confined exclusively to the skin have proven to be more amenable to treatment (e.g., localized irradiation), although those involving the lower extremities have been noted to be more aggressive (116).

Histopathology. Tissue infiltration in DLBCL generally results in local destruction and effacement of preexisting structures (Fig. 31-15A), occasionally associated with zones of fibrosis. The dermal infiltrates may be diffuse or nodular, and frequently deep dermis is preferentially affected, producing a so-called "bottom-heavy" pattern. Cytologically, there is a uniform, monomorphous population of large transformed lymphoid cells resembling centroblasts (Fig. 31-15B). These cells have scant cytoplasm, large nuclei with vesicular nuclear chromatin patterns, and often prominent nucleoli. Immunoblastic, T-cell/histiocyte–rich, and anaplastic variants have been described, but significant

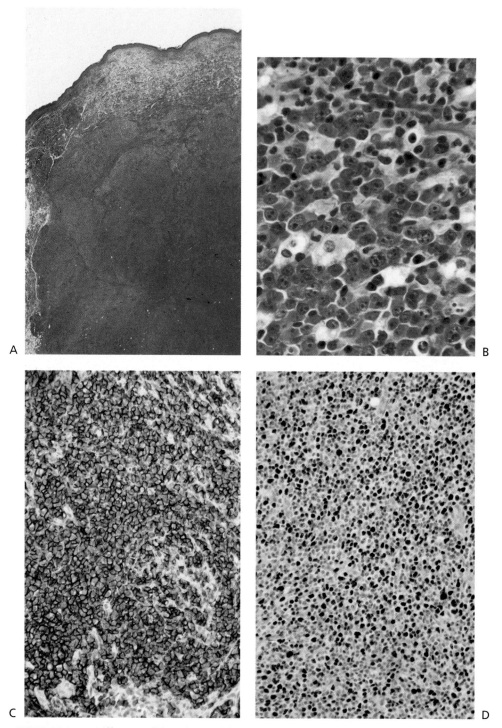

FIGURE 31-15. Diffuse B-cell lymphoma. **(A)** The dermis is diffusely effaced by a destructive infiltrate. **(B)** High magnification showing infiltrate composed of large neoplastic lymphocytes. **(C)** Immunohistochemistry shows the malignant cells to express CD20. **(D)** Evidence of a high proliferative rate based on Ki-67 reactivity.

problems exist in terms of interobserver variability in subclassifying lesions according to variant forms (2).

Histogenesis. The presumed cell of origin is a peripheral germinal center or post-germinal center B-cell. Accordingly, one or more pan–B-cell markers (e.g., CD19, CD20, CD22, CD79a) are expressed (Fig. 31-15C). Surface or cytoplasmic immunoglobulin is demonstrable in the majority of cases, the latter tending to correlate with plasmacytoid features of the large malignant B cells (117,118), and immunoglobulin gene rearrangements are regularly encountered. Anaplastic variants tend to express CD30 more consistently than their nonanaplastic counterparts (119). CD5 and BCL2 expressions are also variably encountered in DLBCL (120). Twenty-five percent of DLBCL demonstrate alterations of the BCL-6 (LAZ-3) gene at 3q27, which encodes a zinc finger protein with homology to several *Drosophila* transcription factors (121–128). BCL-6 protein is readily recognizable by immunohistochemistry and expressed in normal germinal center lymphocytes. It should be emphasized that DLBC lymphoma represents a heterogeneous group of malignancies reflected in variable immunophenotypical and genetic expression. Gene expression data obtained from microarrays suggest two distinct groups of DLBCL, one of which resembles the genetic makeup of germinal center cells (GCC), while the other one corresponds to the genetic makeup of nongerminal center B cells. DLBCL derived from GCC consistently express BCL-6, and have a significantly better prognosis than DLBCL derived from non-GCC (129). High proliferative rates may be attested to upon Ki-67 staining (Fig. 31-15D).

Differential Diagnosis. Occasional lesions may be dominated by medium-sized lymphoid cells, resulting in confusion with leukemia cutis or Burkitt lymphoma, and immunohistochemistry is required for definitive classification. Unlike blastoid variants of MCL, cells of DLBCL are negative for cyclin D1 expression. Anaplastic lesions may raise the differential diagnosis of dermal involvement by anaplastic carcinoma and amelanotic melanoma, and in such cases, immunohistochemical screening for lineage-related markers (e.g., CD45, cytokeratins, Melan A) is a useful initial point of departure for diagnostic evaluation.

Intravascular Large B-Cell Lymphoma

Considered a rare subtype of DLBCL, intravascular (angiotropic) B-cell lymphoma (formerly and mistakenly termed "malignant angioendotheliomatosis") is an aggressive process that prototypically demonstrates intralumenal aggregation of large malignant B cells within vessels of involved tissues (130–136).

Clinical Features. Intravascular large B-cell lymphoma is a disease of adults. It presents as widely disseminated involvement of extranodal tissues, including skin, lung, central nervous system, kidney, and adrenal glands. Because signs and symptoms relate primarily to vascular occlusion,

clinical presentation tends to be highly variable. Skin lesions tend to be red plaques and nodules. Telangiectasia and epidermal changes due to ischemia, including scaling and ulceration, also may be observed.

Histopathology. Involved vessels are either entirely or partially occluded by populations of large, malignant-appearing lymphoid cells (Fig. 31-16A). In the case of the latter, these cells may adhere to inconspicuous and attenuated underlying endothelium, producing the false impression of endothelial atypia or malignancy (Fig. 31-16B). Cytologically, tumor cells contain large nuclei with vesicular chromatin patterns and prominent nucleoli.

Histogenesis. The malignant B cells of peripheral germinal center or post-germinal center origin are believed to express defective homing receptors (e.g., CD11a/CD18), resulting in their tendency for intravascular accumulation due to impaired ability for diapedesis (137,138). Confirmation of B-cell origin may be accomplished by immunohistochemistry for CD20 (Fig. 31-16C). There is variable expression of CD5 (139–146). Diffuse large B-cell lymphoma with hemophagocytic syndrome (BCL-HS) has been reported mainly in Asia and is regarded as a distinct variant of intravascular lymphoma. Rare cases or intravascular lymphoma with a T-cell phenotype have been documented (147,148).

Differential Diagnosis. Because lesions so typically show malignant cells to be exclusively confined to vascular lumens, the primary differential diagnosis involves differentiation of these cells from malignant endothelium (e.g., angiosarcoma). In this regard, it should be remembered that both endothelial cells and many cells of hematopoietic origin express the C34 marker. Differentiation from other intravascular malignant deposits (e.g., inflammatory carcinoma of the breast) may be confirmed using lineage-related immunohistochemical markers.

Lymphomatoid Granulomatosis

Lymphomatoid granulomatosis (LYG) is a rare and variably aggressive lymphoproliferative disorder characterized by angiocentric and angiodestructive infiltration of extranodal tissues, including skin, by EBV-transformed B cells and reactive T cells (149–151).

Clinical Features. Adult males are generally affected by LYG (2:1 male/female ratio), although immunosuppressed children may also present with this disease. Although multiple organs may be involved, the lung is the most common and, if not infiltrated at time of presentation, tends to be affected at some point during the natural evolution of disease. Skin involvement is quite common, being demonstrable in 25% to 50% of all cases. Nodal tissue and spleen are rarely affected (152–155).

Histopathology. Unlike most non-Hodgkin lymphomas, LYG shows an angiocentric and angiodestructive architecture and a polymorphous cytology (152,154) (Fig. 31-17). The infiltrating mononuclear cells show permeation and

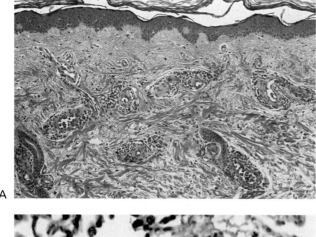

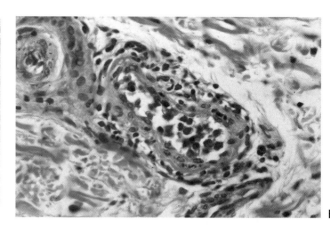

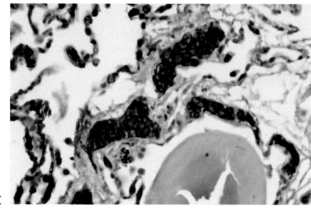

FIGURE 31-16. Intravascular large B-cell lymphoma. **(A)** Superficial dermal vessels are partially occluded by hyperchromatic malignant cells. **(B)** Higher magnification discloses malignant-appearing lymphocytes partially adherent to the endothelial surface of involved vessels. **(C)** CD20 reactivity for malignant B cells within pulmonary vessels from a patient with diffuse extracutaneous involvement.

focal destruction and fibrinoid necrosis of vessel walls (156), and adjacent zones of ischemic necrosis may result. The cellular composition includes variably atypical lymphocytes with cleaved and elongated nuclear contours, immunoblasts, plasma cells, and histiocytes (157,158). Although mycosis fungoides may rarely produce angiodestructive lesions (159), the lymphoid cells in LYG tend not to have true cerebriform contours. Scattered immunoblasts and histiocytoid cells with some morphologic overlap with Reed–Sternberg

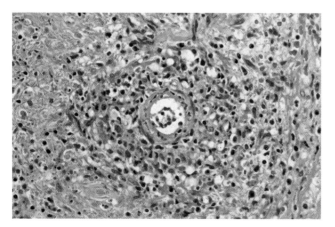

FIGURE 31-17. Lymphomatoid granulomatosis. Atypical lymphocytes have infiltrated and partially destroyed the involved vessel walls.

variants may express B-cell markers as well as EBV protein. Occasional foci of epidermotropism may be observed in some lesions. Grading of lesions (I to III) based on proportion of EBV⁺ cells, extent of atypia, and necrosis may correlate with biological behavior for some lesions (160).

Histogenesis. The underlying cause of LYG appears to be related to EBV-driven abnormal B-cell proliferation in the setting of immunodeficiency (161,162). Large EBV⁺ cells are also reactive for CD20, variably positive for CD30, and negative for CD15. The background lymphocytes are CD3⁺, with CD4 greater than CD8. Higher-grade lesions tend to show clonality of immunoglobulin genes (155,163).

Differential Diagnosis. LYG must be differentiated from hematopoietic malignancies that also may show an angiodestructive growth pattern, such as extranodal NK/T-cell lymphoma of the nasal type (163), and rare instances of mycosis fungoides with a vasculitic component (159). Identification of EBV⁺ cells that express CD20 is helpful in separating LYG from these entities. There should not be diagnostic confusion with intravascular large B-cell lymphoma, which fails to show true primary vascular destruction.

Hodgkin Lymphoma

Hodgkin lymphoma (HL) constitutes a group of a relatively common type of lymphoproliferative conditions that share the common features of frequent origin in cer-

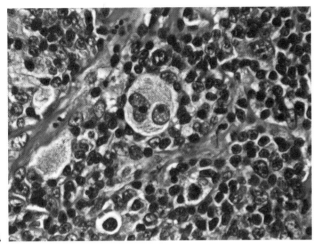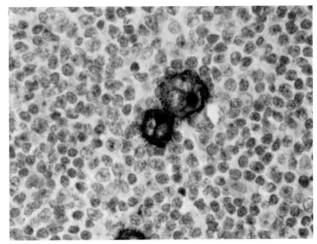

FIGURE 31-18. Hodgkin lymphoma. **(A)** Classic Hodgkin lymphoma showing pleomorphic infiltrate and characteristic Reed–Sternberg cell that **(B)** is reactive for the CD30 antigen.

vical lymph nodes, tendency toward occurrence in young adults, presence of Reed–Sternberg cells and their variants, and instances of rosette-like rimming of these cells by T-lymphocytes. Although skin is rarely involved, HL is discussed here briefly because it may be considered in the differential diagnosis of other cutaneous lymphoproliferative disorders (164–169).

Clinical Features. There are two major variants of HL; the common classic Hodgkin lymphoma (CHL) and the far less frequently encountered nodular lymphocyte predominant Hodgkin lymphoma (NLPHL). The former consists of four histologic subtypes (see below). CHL tends to affect adolescents and young adults and typically presents as peripheral lymphadenopathy localized to one or several node groups. NLPHL affects young to middle-aged patients with a male predominance. Slightly less than half of these patients will also have systemic signs of disease (fever, sweats, weight loss).

Histopathology. All forms of HL result in a polymorphous hematopoietic infiltrate that may efface nodal architecture and preexisting tissue structure. The histologic variant forms of CHL are lymphocyte rich (LRCHL), nodular

sclerosis (NSHL), mixed cellularity (MCHL), and lymphocyte depleted (LDHL). CLH contains variable numbers of neoplastic Reed–Sternberg (HRS) cells with abundant cytoplasm and at least two nuclear lobes, each containing prominent eosinophilic nucleoli and C30 expression by immunohistochemistry (Fig. 31-18A and B). By contrast, NLPHL is characterized by cytologically and immunophenotypically distinct neoplastic cells known as L&H cells (lymphocytic and/or histiocytic Reed–Sternberg cell variants). These cells have infolded and multilobed nuclei that may resemble "popcorn" that contain often multiple, small, basophilic nucleoli. The key features of each type of HL are summarized in Table 31-3.

Skin involvement by HL generally resembles nodal disease. Architecturally, dermal infiltration is nodular or diffuse with an absence of epidermotropism.

Histogenesis. The majority of cases of classic type HL are believed to be derived from mature germinal center B cells (170,171) that are rich in somatic mutations in the VH immunoglobulin genes. NLPHL is uniformly positive for B-cell markers (CD19, CD20, CD22, etc.), while classic types of HD express CD30 (172) in most instances. It

TABLE 31-3. KEY FEATURES OF EACH TYPE OF HODGKIN LYMPHOMA

	NLPHL	LRCLH	NSHL	MCHL	LDHL
Architecture	Nodular or nodular & diffuse	Usually nodular, rarely diffuse	Nodular, with collagen bands	Diffuse, no collagen bands	Highly variable
Cytology	Polymorphous, with L&H cells	Small lymphocytes, admixed with HRS cells	Polymorphous, HRS cells often in lacunar spaces	Polymorphous, HRS cells, granulomas	Variable, high ratio of HRS to lymphocytes
Immunophenotype	L&H cells CD20⁺, CD30⁻, CD15EMA⁺/⁻	HRS cells variably CD20⁺, CD30⁺, CD15⁺ EMA⁻	HRS cells variably CD20⁺, CD30⁺, CD15⁺ EMA⁻	HRS cells variably CD20⁺, CD30⁺, CD15⁺ EMA⁻	HRS cells variably CD20⁺, CD30⁺, CD15⁺ EMA⁻
EBV status	Negative	Many positive	Many positive	Many positive	

appears that Hodgkin lymphoma, in spite of morphologic similarities, represents a spectrum of disease entities rather than a single malady. NLPHL shows invariable expression of nuclear transcription factor oct-2 that regulates the immunoglobulin promoter gene together with its cofactor BOB-1 (173–176). Classical types of HD tend to be positive for PAX-5 encoded B-cell–specific activator protein (BSAP) (175,177–180), and show variable expression for EBV in the tumor cells (181–184), either decorated by antibodies against latent membrane protein (LMP-1 and EBNA-1), or visualized by *in situ* hybridization to the RNA of EBV (EBER-1). A plethora of cytokines (interleukins, colony stimulating factors, TGF-β, etc.) contributes to the variegated histologic appearance of HD (185–188).

Differential Diagnosis. HL only rarely involves skin, and such events are almost always secondary to nodal disease. HL involving skin may be confused, however, with T-cell–rich large B-cell lymphoma, diffuse large B-cell lymphoma, anaplastic T-cell lymphoma, and reactive lymphoid hyperplasia. Careful correlation of clinical, histologic, and immunophenotypic features will generally assist in definitively excluding HL from these differential diagnostic considerations.

CD30⁺ cells may occur in a variety of settings in addition to HL, including anaplastic T-cell lymphoma, mycosis fungoides, and lymphomatoid papulosis, and these conditions occasionally may develop in the same patient, resulting in speculation that they may be biologically interrelated (189). Careful evaluation and correlation of coexisting clinical parameters, immunohistochemical, and molecular studies may be necessary for accurate classification of atypical cutaneous infiltrates containing more than occasional CD30⁺ large lymphoid cells. Fortunately, skin involvement by HL in the absence of overt nodal disease is so rare as to make its inclusion in this differential an academic one.

PRIMARY CUTANEOUS T-CELL LYMPHOPROLIFERATIVE DISORDERS

T-Cell Lymphomatoid Hyperplasias

T-cell lymphomatoid hyperplasia refers to the occurrence of epidermotropic cutaneous immune responses composed of activated/proliferative T cells that produce a pattern that may mimic mycosis fungoides and its variants. It is arbitrarily divided into several clinicopathologic variants here in order to better illustrate the patterns most likely to result in potential diagnostic confusion with T-cell malignancy.

Clinical Features. Because these conditions all share the feature of epitheliotropism, they, like various forms of mycosis fungoides, may be associated with the formation of scaling erythematous and variably indurated patches and plaques, and occasionally with foci of alopecia. On occasion, subacute to chronic spongiotic or lichenoid dermatitis may be associated with lymphoid epidermotropism in the

relative absence of intercellular edema or apoptosis, thus bringing to mind consideration of possible T-cell dyscrasia. Certain immune responses may also show a T-cell pattern in the setting of drug-induced immune dysregulation, and therefore mimic T-cell dyscrasia or lymphoma.

Histopathology. Dermatitis with epidermotropism in the relative absence of associated spongiosis or evidence of cytotoxic injury will generally show more typical findings upon evaluation of deeper sections. Multiple biopsies may occasionally be required to better assess the sequential evolution of lesions and to identify stages where more characteristic inflammatory changes predominate. The finding of Langerhans cell microgranulomas (190) favors a reactive process, although care must be taken not to confuse these structures with true Pautrier microabscesses (Fig. 31-19A; see below). Importantly, many examples of T-cell–pattern lymphomatoid dermatitis will lack the uniform cytologic atypia within the epidermotropic component more characteristically seen in mycosis fungoides. Exceptions to this, however, are T-cell–pattern reactive infiltrates occurring in patients with altered immune function, as may be seen in certain lymphomatoid drug eruptions (Fig. 31-19B), as described by Brady et al. (191). In these settings, cytologically atypical epidermotropic infiltrates may closely mimic mycosis fungoides, and even may show immunophenotypic (e.g., diminished CD7 expression) or genotypic (e.g., T-cell receptor gene rearrangements) abnormalities that are reversible upon drug cessation (192).

Histogenesis. The histogenesis of T-cell–pattern drug-induced lymphoid dyscrasia seems to relate to the concurrence of cutaneous hypersensitivity reactions caused by drugs that themselves are capable of inciting some level of immune dysregulation. These drugs include anticonvulsants, antidepressants, phenothiazines, calcium channel blockers, and angiotensin-converting enzyme inhibitors.

Differential Diagnosis. The primary differential diagnosis is the T-cell–pattern immune response in the setting of immune dysregulation. Careful consideration of clinical factors, including duration of lesions, response to previous therapy, and potential relationship to drugs that influence lymphocyte function should be undertaken before definitively excluding a lymphomatoid drug eruption in the differential diagnosis of epidermotropic T-cell malignancies.

T-Cell and NK-Cell Neoplasms

Mycosis Fungoides

Mycosis fungoides is a cutaneous T-cell lymphoma that typically begins as slowly progressive dermatitis-like patches and plaques, and when untreated evolves to nodules and eventual systemic dissemination. The patch/plaque stage of the disease is the result of intraepidermal and superficial dermal infiltration by small- to medium-sized malignant T cells with characteristically cerebriform nuclear contours, while the more advanced stages develop as a consequence

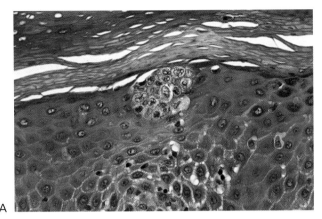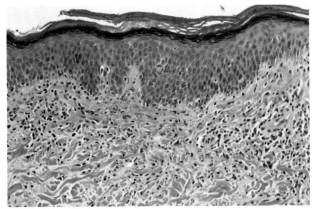

A   B

FIGURE 31-19. T-cell lymphomatoid hyperplasia. **(A)** Langerhans cell microgranuloma associated with T-cell immune response may mimic Pautrier microabscess. **(B)** Lymphomatoid drug eruption, with papillary dermal interstitial and focally epidermotropic infiltrate of variably activated lymphocytes in a characteristic T-cell pattern.

of exclusively dermal involvement by nonepidermotropic, often cytologically more atypical malignant T cells.

Clinical Features. Mycosis fungoides is relatively rare, accounting for less than 1% of non-Hodgkin lymphomas. However, of lymphomas that arise primarily in skin, it is the most common (12). It is a disease predominantly of adult males (2:1 male/female ratio), although children are occasionally affected. Lesions initially present as erythematous scaling patches and plaques that typically are resistant to antiinflammatory therapy (Fig. 31-20A). Lesions are generally large (many centimeters in diameter), and may show arcuate or polycyclic configurations. Zones of alopecia may occur due to infiltration and mucinous degeneration of hair follicles (alopecia mucinosa). Occasional lesions may show epidermal atrophy, prominently dilated superficial dermal blood vessels, and patchy hyper- and hypo-pigmentation (poikiloderma vasculare atrophicans variant), while others may show excessive epidermal thickening and scaling (psoriasiform variant). In one rare form

of the disease, lesions are generally solitary, involve acral skin, and clinically resemble squamous neoplasia as a result of epidermal thickening and scale formation (pagetoid reticulosis variant). The dermal component is occasionally associated with granulomatous inflammation that compromises the integrity of elastic fibers (granulomatous slack skin variant).

The natural history of mycosis fungoides is one of slow progression, with the patches and plaques giving rise over time to nodules that may eventually ulcerate (Fig. 31-20B). Rarely nodules are documented from the outset (d'emblee variant), although this rare presentation is not well characterized, and some of these patients may have other forms of T-cell malignancy (e.g., adult T-cell leukemia/lymphoma). Diffuse erythroderma may be associated with systemic dissemination, and may represent either a manifestation of late evolution of localized disease (193) or blood involvement from the outset (Sézary syndrome). When extracutaneous spread eventuates, lymph nodes, spleen, liver, and

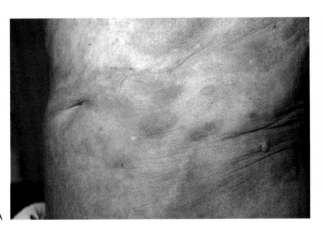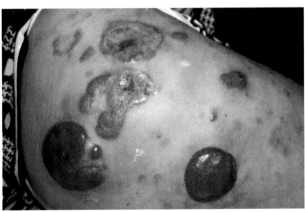

A   B

FIGURE 31-20. Mycosis fungoides: clinical features. **(A)** Erythematous scaling patches and plaques of early disease. **(B)** Plaques and nodules of advanced disease.

lungs are often involved, in addition to the peripheral blood. Lymph node enlargement at such advanced stages must be differentiated from nodal hyperplasia resulting from chronic drainage of involved sites (dermatopathic lymphadenopathy).

Clinical staging of mycosis fungoides involves four categories: stage I indicates disease confined to skin as localized (Ia) or disseminated (Ib) patches/plaques, or as tumors (Ic); stage II signifies nodal enlargement without histologic evidence of nodal lymphoma (generally dermatopathic changes only); stage III implies lymphomatous involvement of lymph nodes; and stage IV connotes visceral dissemination. Prognosis is directly related to extent of disease progression, with stage I and II lesions having an excellent outcome (12,193,194), and more advanced presentations (nodules and extracutaneous dissemination) showing aggressive courses.

Histopathology. Early lesions of mycosis fungoides show a diffuse lymphocytic infiltrate within the papillary dermis, often associated with coarse fibrosis (Fig. 31-21A and B). The lymphocytic component may be, in part, reactive, with an admixture of eosinophils, plasma cells, and monocytes, and in this mixture of cells the characteristic cytology of mycosis fungoides cells may be difficult to document. Care must be taken to identify foci of epidermotropism or folliculotropism that generally involve the malignant T-cell clone. These foci may consist of a lentiginous pattern (linear accumulation associated with the basement membrane zone) (Fig. 31-22A and B), or a pagetoid pattern

with either single-cell infiltration (Fig. 31-22C) or clustered exocytosis of atypical lymphocytes, also known as Pautrier microabscesses, into a "passive" epidermal layer (Fig. 31-22D). Lymphoid epidermotropism in mycosis fungoides, unlike its counterparts in dermatitis, is generally unassociated with significant epidermal or follicular spongiosis or evidence of cytotoxicity (basal cell layer vacuolization or apoptosis). Rather, the epithelium may appear passive, resulting in seemingly permissive accumulation of atypical lymphocytes within lacunar spaces that separate seemingly indifferent keratinocytes. These spaces appear by sequential analyses to result from minute regions of epithelial mucinosis. When hair follicles are infiltrated by malignant T cells, accumulation of mucin may produce widened intercellular spaces between epithelial cells and ultimately result in inability of follicles so affected to support existing or recycle new hair shafts (follicular mucinosis).

Cytologically, the malignant T cells in mycosis fungoides are small- to medium-sized lymphocytes that characteristically contain nuclei with dense heterochromatin and elaborately indented (cerebriform) nuclear contours (Fig. 31-23A and B). Occasionally, these cells may be difficult to differentiate from cytokine-activated T cells. However, one helpful feature is the tendency for epidermotropic malignant T cells to predominantly or exclusively show cerebriform nuclear features. Intraepithelial aggregates of malignant T cells in mycosis fungoides must be differentiated, however, from similar aggregates of larger mononuclear cells also with irregular, frequently indented, nuclear

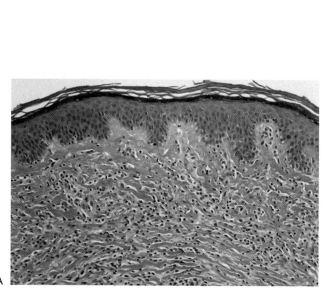

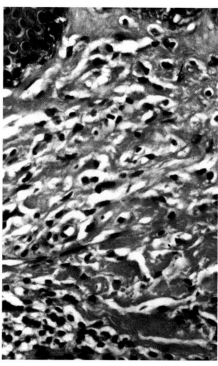

FIGURE 31-21. Mycosis fungoides: histologic features of early disease. **(A)** and **(B)** Papillary dermal interstitial lymphoid infiltration associated with coarse fibrosis.

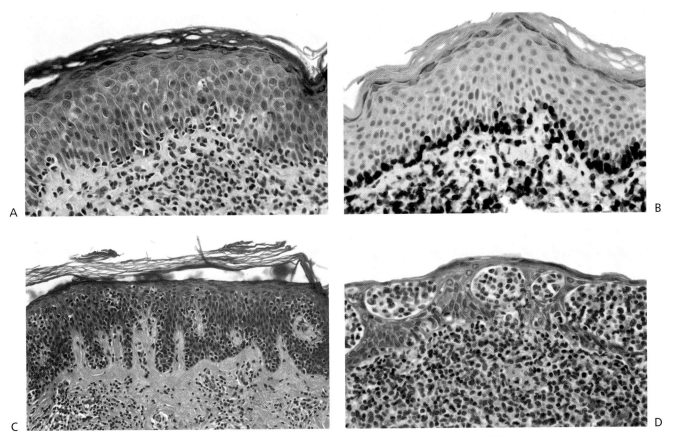

FIGURE 31-22. Mycosis fungoides: architectural patterns of epidermotropism. **(A)** Papillary dermal interstitial infiltrate associated with linear aggregation of neoplastic lymphocytes along the dermal–epidermal junction. **(B)** Adjacent section stained for CD4 emphasizing this linear pattern of early epidermotropism. **(C)** Early plaque-stage disease with single-cell epidermotropism by atypical lymphocytes into a "passive" epidermal layer. **(D)** Plaque-stage disease characterized by prominent clusters of atypical lymphocytes within the epidermis (Pautrier microabscesses).

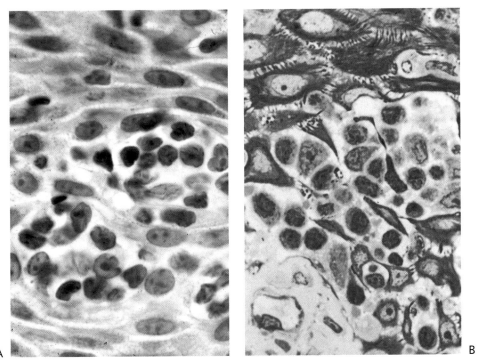

FIGURE 31-23. Mycosis fungoides: cytology. **(A)** Oil immersion conventional microscopy of atypical lymphocytes within the epidermal layer. **(B)** One-micron, toluidine blue-stained section of epidermotropic malignant lymphocytes showing characteristically infolded nuclear contours.

profiles (so-called Langerhans cell microgranulomas [7]; also see differential diagnosis section). Malignant T cells with cerebriform nuclei also may be detected within the dermal component of lesions. However, their frequent admixture with reactive lymphocytes, and mononuclear cells may make their reliable identification more difficult, especially in early lesions. With advanced disease when lesions become nodular, and there is often loss of epidermotropism, the dermal infiltrate is composed of nodular to diffuse interstitial populations of more uniform atypical T cells (Fig. 31-24A and B). Transformation to large, highly atypical lymphocytes in the dermal component is associated with development of an aggressive biological course (195,196).

There are a number of clinicopathologic variants of mycosis fungoides, which include *adnexotropic mycosis fungoides* (197). This form of the disease may occur anywhere, although skin of the face and scalp as well as sun-exposed extremities is often involved. Epidermotropism may be minimal to absent, and diagnosis may be overlooked when biopsies are too superficial. Infiltration of hair follicles by characteristically atypical T cells (198) may result in Pautrier microabscesses and be associated with follicular mucinosis where keratinocytes forming affected follicles produce intracellular mucin and eventually degenerate, culminating in alopecia (Fig. 31-25A, B, and C). Eccrine involvement may also be observed, with or without follicular lesions. Infiltration of the eccrine coil may be associated with syringometaplasia, but not mucinosis (Fig. 31-25D). Prognosis is generally favorable, although potentially less so than in early evolutionary stages of classical epidermotropic patch/plaque disease (12).

Pagetoid Reticulosis. This rare and peculiar form of mycosis fungoides is associated with exclusively epidermal infiltration by malignant T cells, often in the form of a solitary acral lesion where associated epidermal proliferation and hyperkeratosis results in the clinical impression of a squamous neoplasm (so-called Woringer–Kolopp disease).

Immunophenotypic studies have disclosed the malignant T-cell to be CD4+, CD8+, or double negative for both epitopes, and T-cell receptor gene rearrangements may be demonstrated (199). The prognosis is excellent.

Granulomatous Slack Skin. This variant indicates the presence of elastolytic granulomas that develop in association with the dermal lymphomatous component. As such, it may not be exclusive to mycosis fungoides, but rather a granulomatous reaction pattern that may occasionally accompany other types of lymphoma involving the skin. Clinically, zones of skin with increased folding and decreased elasticity slowly develop, with preferential involvement of intertriginous sites. Histologically, atypical T-cell infiltrates, often associated with epidermotropism or folliculotropism, are intimately associated with noncaseating dermal granulomas formed by histiocytes that may contain ingested elastic fibers (200).

Poikiloderma vasculare atrophicans. This is a reaction pattern that may occur in lesions of mycosis fungoides, although it is not synonymous with T-cell lymphoma and may be seen in other settings. Early lesions may involve either large plaques or small papules arranged in a net-like configuration. Lesions show erythema, mild scaling, epidermal thinning, mottled hypo- and hyperpigmentation, and telangiectasia, and the clinical picture may resemble changes of radiodermatitis. Histopathology discloses epidermal atrophy, epidermal infiltration by atypical lymphocytes, a variable band of lymphocytes, histiocytes, and melanophages in the papillary dermis, and ectasia of superficial dermal vessels. The finding of atypical lymphocytes, potentially supported by a characteristic immunophenotypic and molecular profile for mycosis fungoides, should assist in separating this rare variant from other causes of acquired poikiloderma, including dermatomyositis and lupus erythematosus.

Psoriasiform Mycosis Fungoides. This form of the disease may overlap with what has been described as pagetoid reticulosis with multiple lesions (so-called Ketron–Goodman

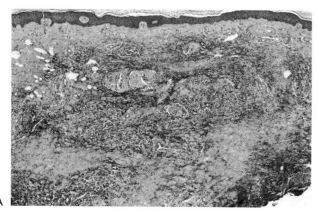
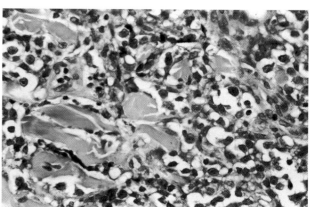

FIGURE 31-24. Mycosis fungoides: nonepidermotropic. **(A)** There is a nodular to diffuse dermal infiltrate with relative sparing of the superficial dermis and epidermis. **(B)** Cytologically, atypical lymphocytes produce an interstitial pattern of dermal infiltration.

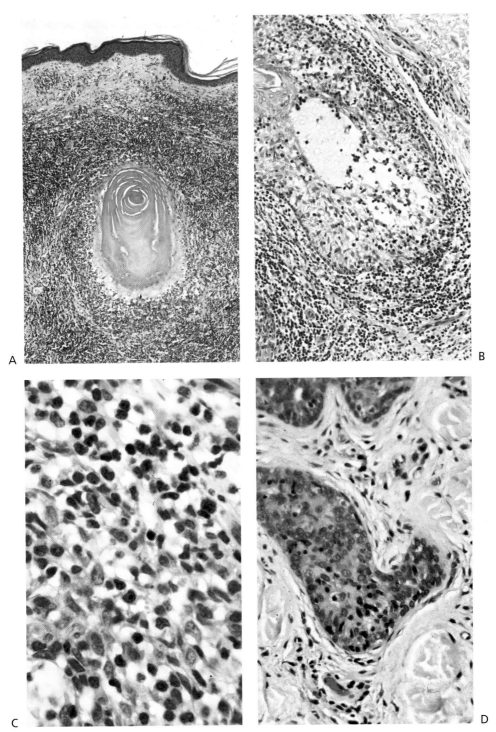

FIGURE 31-25. Adnexotropic mycosis fungoides. **(A)** Infiltration is associated with architectural distortion and destruction of follicular structures. **(B)** Follicular mucinosis characterized by pools of pale blue-staining mucin. **(C)** Atypical T cells in a mucinous background. **(D)** Eccrine involvement by atypical lymphocytes, associated with syringosquamous metaplasia.

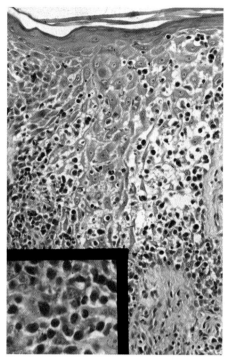

FIGURE 31-26. Psoriasiform mycosis fungoides. There is epidermal hyperplasia associated with pronounced epidermotropism by atypical lymphocytes (*inset*).

disease). In our experience this variant is rare, and may in some instances be the consequence of superimposed lichen simplex chronicus. Epidermotropism is present, consisting of accumulation of single and clustered, atypical small- to intermediate-sized lymphocytes within the epidermal layer (Fig. 31-26). However, there is marked acanthosis frequently in association with coarse papillary dermal fibrosis. In one study of 222 biopsies where mycosis fungoides produced patterns that mimicked various forms of dermatitis, including psoriasiform dermatitis, diagnostic clues included epitheliotropism in the relative absence of spongiosis, alignment of atypical lymphocytes in association with the basal cell layer, lymphoid atypia, and broad areas of compact hyperkeratosis with subtly interspersed parakeratosis (201).

Histogenesis. The cell of origin in mycosis fungoides is believed to be a peripheral epidermotropic T cell. The immunophenotype is CD2+, CD3+, CD4+, CD5+, and CD8− (Fig. 31-27A through E), although rare cases have been described that are CD8+ (202,203). Lesions often show absence of CD7, even at early evolutionary stages of the disease, although this finding in itself does not reliably permit differentiation of mycosis fungoides cells from reactive T cells (202). The skin-homing antigen, HECA, is expressed in most cases, consistent with association of the malignant clone with a peripheral epidermotropic T cell. In advanced disease, cytotoxic granule-associated proteins also may be demonstrated (204). Although occasional CD30+ cells may be identified in

the dermal infiltrates, this epitope is not expressed by most cells comprising the malignant clone. T-cell receptor genes are clonally rearranged, and this may be a helpful, albeit not entirely specific, diagnostic adjunct in early disease.

It is possible that very early evolutionary stages of mycosis fungoides involve a dysplastic phase in tumor progression. Such lesions may fulfill some but not all of the features required for a diagnosis of patch-stage disease. We generally refer to such lesions as being compatible with possible evolving T-cell dyscrasia, and recommend close follow-up and interval biopsy sampling to assess disease evolution. Some such lesions may be referred to by a variety of potentially confusing clinical descriptors, including as "large-plaque parapsoriasis." The notion that small-plaque parapsoriasis is an indolent form of mycosis fungoides is questionable in view of the accepted requirement for most malignant cells to exhibit features of tumor progression over time.

Differential Diagnosis. The practical differential diagnosis of epidermotropic mycosis fungoides involves primarily reactive T-cell infiltrates with epidermotropism or an abnormal papillary dermal homing pattern. True dermatitis may show lymphoid epidermotropism and development of Langerhans cell microgranulomas that superficially may resemble Pautrier microabscesses. However, the former is generally associated with spongiosis or evidence of cytotoxic epidermal injury, and the latter with large cells containing ample cytoplasm, pale-staining infolded nuclei, and CD1a positivity by immunohistochemistry (190). Adnexotropic lesions must be separated from forms of dermatitis primarily centered about hair follicles and sweat glands. Again, the finding of uniformly atypical epitheliotropic lymphocytes and their tendency to be predominantly CD4+ by immunohistochemistry should assist in this differential. While occasional cases of dermatitis show T-cell receptor gene rearrangements, most do not, and accordingly PCR analysis is also an important adjunct in differentiating mycosis fungoides from inflammatory imitators. As discussed above, careful clinical history is required to access relationship of onset of atypical T-cell–pattern epidermotropic infiltrates to drugs that may produce immune dysregulation and eruptions that are morphologically, immunophenotypically, and even genotypically difficult to differentiate from mycosis fungoides. Late-stage disease, where epithelial involvement is minimal to absent and cytologic features may be higher grade, must be distinguished from B-cell lymphomas involving the skin. Although rare variants of mycosis fungoides may result in expansive differential diagnostic categories, most cases will include these histologic presentations.

Sézary Syndrome

Sézary syndrome refers to a potentially aggressive form of systemic T-cell leukemia/lymphoma characterized by generalized redness and scaling of the skin (erythroderma), lymphadenopathy, and presence of malignant T cells in the

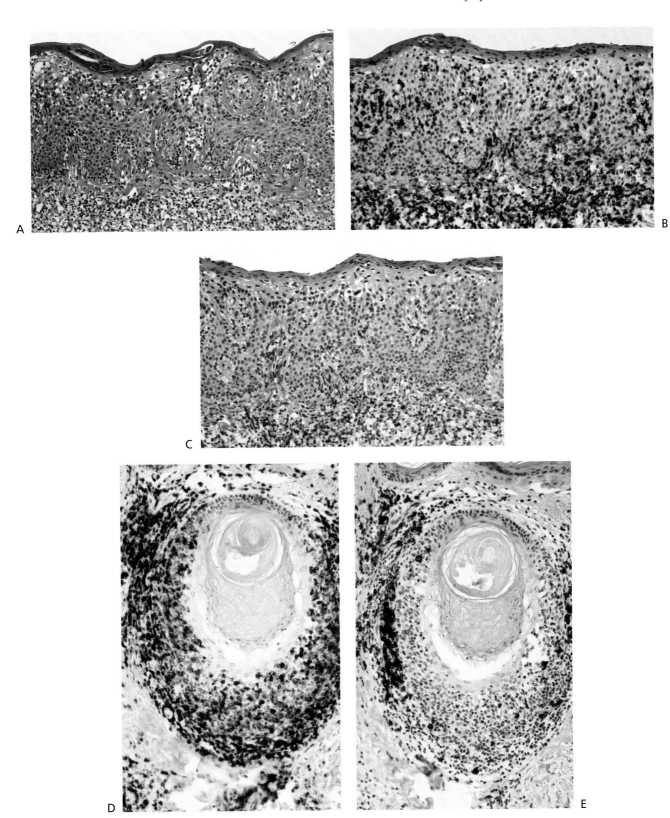

FIGURE 31-27. Immunophenotypic features of mycosis fungoides. Serial sections through a plaque-stage lesion with marked epidermotropism **(A)** reveal that most of the epidermotropic cells express CD4 **(B)**, but not CD8 **(C)**. Similar findings are observed for folliculotropic T cells: **(D)** = CD4, **(E)** = CD8.

skin and peripheral blood. Because these malignant T cells have phenotypic and antigenic overlap with those of mycosis fungoides, Sézary syndrome is sometimes regarded as a mycosis fungoides variant. However, important clinical and histopathologic differences exist between classical mycosis fungoides and Sézary syndrome.

Clinical Features. Patients generally present with diffuse skin erythema and lymphadenopathy. There may also be itching, hair loss, nail dystrophy, and hyperkeratosis affecting the skin of palms and soles (12). In addition to lymph node, skin, and blood involvement, malignant T cells may also infiltrate viscera in late stages, although bone marrow is often spared (12,193).

Histopathology. Affected skin may show changes similar to those of patch and plaque–stage mycosis fungoides, although the infiltrate is often sparse and multiple sections may be required in some cases to identify convincing epidermotropism by atypical lymphocytes (Fig. 31-28A). Involved lymph nodes are characterized by effacement of their architecture by infiltrates of atypical cells. The peripheral blood contains atypical lymphocytes with cerebriform nuclear contours, with smaller versions referred to as Lutzner cells, and larger ones as classical Sézary cells (Fig. 31-28B). Diagnosis of Sézary syndrome requires at least 1,000 such cells per square millimeter in most series (12,193). Flow cytometry will generally indicate elevation in CD4:CD8 ratio and increased numbers of cells with a CD4+CD7− phenotype. Molecular analysis will show clonal rearrangement of the T-cell receptor gene in most cases (12,205).

Histogenesis. The neoplastic peripheral epidermotropic T cells are CD2+, CD3+, CD4+, CD5+, and CD7+/−. Aberrant T-cell phenotypes are common; rare CD8+ variants have been described (12).

Differential Diagnosis. Sézary syndrome must be differentiated from other dermatitic causes of erythroderma (e.g., atopic dermatitis, seborrheic dermatitis, pityriasis rubra pilaris, psoriasis). Because the histopathology of skin involvement in Sézary syndrome may be subtle, it is often critical

also to examine routine buffy-coat preparations as well as flow cytometry of peripheral blood in establishing a diagnosis of Sézary syndrome. Immunohistochemistry to identify epidermotropism by predominantly to exclusively CD4+ T cells, loss of CD7, and molecular analysis for T-cell receptor gene rearrangements are also important adjuncts to correct diagnosis. Although patients with advanced mycosis fungoides also may develop leukemic dissemination by malignant cerebriform T cells, the clinical course and presence of advanced plaques and nodules should separate these individuals from patients with true Sézary syndrome. Patients with adult T-cell leukemia/ lymphoma have circulating atypical T cells. However, these tend to be polylobated rather than cerebriform, and cutaneous lesions are generally multiple nodules rather than diffuse erythroderma.

Primary Cutaneous CD30+ T-Cell Lymphoproliferative Disorders

This category refers to a spectrum of related, relatively low-grade disorders that primarily affect skin and develop from an activated or transformed large T cell that expresses the CD30 antigen (125,206–208). Although these conditions may occur together in a given patient and show clinical, histologic, and antigenic overlap, the clinicopathologic features are sufficiently distinctive for considering them in the context of the following categories: (a) primary cutaneous anaplastic large-cell lymphoma (C-ALCL); (b) lymphomatoid papulosis (LYP); and (c) borderline lesions.

Clinical Features. Skin lesions of C-ALCL consist of one or more localized nodules or occasionally papules (12,208). Lesions must be differentiated by careful staging from systemic ALCL with secondary skin involvement and from high-grade large-cell lymphomas that may also express CD30, since these latter conditions have a considerably worse prognosis. Partial or complete regression of individual lesions may occur, although relapse is common (208). Eventual extracutaneous dissemination

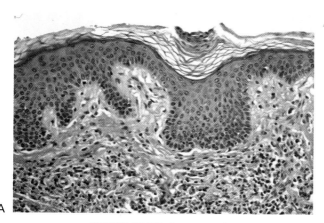
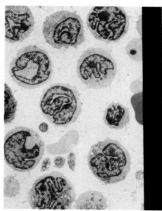
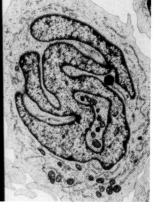

FIGURE 31-28. Sezary syndrome. **(A)** There is a band-like papillary dermal lymphoid infiltrate with minimal epidermotropism. **(B)** Ultrastructural examination of peripheral blood buffy coat reveals numerous Sezary cells.

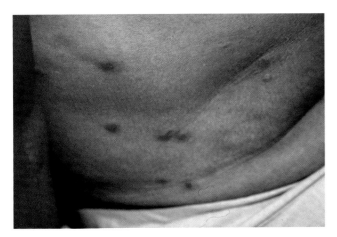

FIGURE 31-29. Primary CD30⁺ lymphoproliferative disorders: lymphomatoid papulosis. Lesions clinically present as multiple "juicy" red papules and nodules.

to lymph nodes occurs in about 10% of patients with primary skin involvement, particularly in individuals who have multiple primary lesions (206,208). LYP typically develops as multiple diffusely distributed "juicy" red papules and nodules that usually regress within one to several months (208) (Fig. 31-29). Lesions are generally less than 2.5 cm in diameter, and extracutaneous dissemination only occurs in a minority of cases that progress to overt lymphoma.

Histopathology. Nodules are formed by infiltrates that typically involve the superficial and deep dermis, and occasionally the subcutis, in a diffuse, interstitial pattern (12) (Fig. 31-30A). Cytologically, biopsies of C-ALCL may closely resemble those of systemic ALCL with secondary skin involvement (Fig. 31-30B), although Reed–Sternberg cells and highly pleomorphic, multinucleated giant cells may be more numerous in the former. The large atypical cells should account for the majority of cells composing the

infiltrate, although a background of secondary inflammatory elements may be observed. Marked epidermal hyperplasia, sometimes with keratoacanthoma-like features, invasion by atypical cells, and ulceration, is often present.

By contrast, the architecture of LYP tends to be more restricted, forming a wedge-shaped infiltrate extending from the superficial into the mid and deep dermis (Fig. 31-31A). This is composed of an admixture of various cell types, including variably activated lymphocytes, histiocytes, neutrophils, and eosinophils. An admixed minority population composed of atypical large lymphocytes, however, is required for the diagnosis, and these may either resemble Reed–Sternberg cells (type A LYP) or the cerebriform cells of mycosis fungoides (type B LYP). In the latter, epidermotropism similar to that seen in patch/plaque stage mycosis fungoides may be present. Occasional biopsies will show hybrid features between these two types of LYP. There is an angiocentric deposition of infiltrating atypical cells (Fig. 31-31B), often accompanied by vascular injury. Epidermal changes include hyperkeratosis, parakeratosis, and occasional foci of neutrophil infiltration and central erosion/shallow ulceration (Fig. 31-31C). In rare instances, clinical features of LYP may be present in the setting of histologic characteristics of C-ALCL (predominance of large atypical cells), and these lesions are referred to as borderline or type C LYP. Rarely, a solitary tumor more in keeping with C-ALCL will show histopathology more like LYP (atypical cells in the minority), and such lesions have been termed anaplastic lymphoma, LYP-like (208).

Histogenesis. All forms of primary cutaneous CD30⁺ T-cell lymphoproliferative disease are believed to be derived from an activated skin-homing T cell. In C-ALCL, in addition to CD30-positivity by more than 75% of the cells forming the infiltrate (12,209), there is CD4 expression as well as frequent expression of cytotoxic granule proteins (granzyme B, perforin, TIA-1) (209,210). Aberrant T-cell phenotypes, with loss of CD2, CD3, and/or CD5

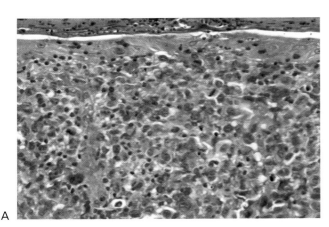

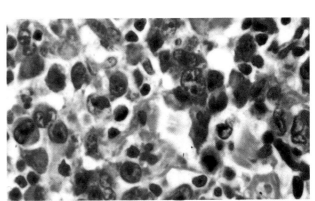

A   B

FIGURE 31-30. Histology of primary cutaneous anaplastic large cell lymphoma. **(A)** Skin infiltrate composed of tumoral infiltrate large atypical lymphocytes with associated incipient epidermal erosion. **(B)** High magnification of the large anaplastic lymphocytes forming an infiltrate in primary cutaneous anaplastic large-cell lymphoma.

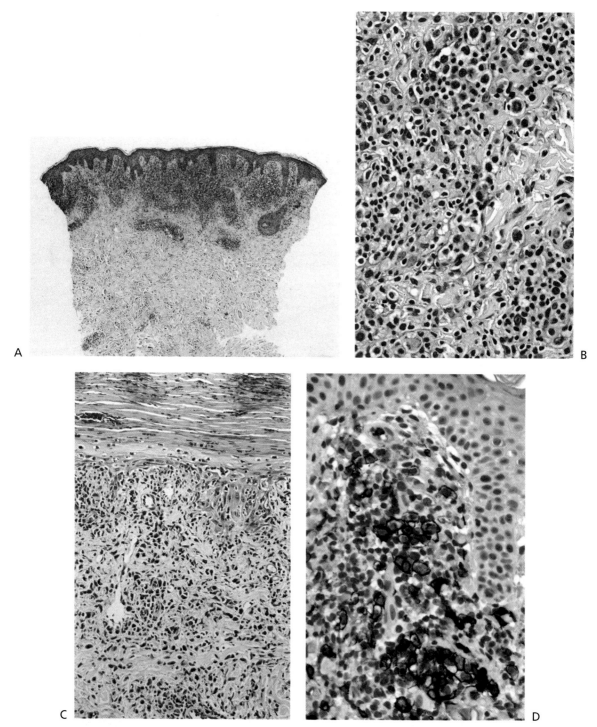

FIGURE 31-31. Histology of lymphomatoid papulosis. **(A)** Low power of localized infiltrate in superficial and mid-dermis, forming what will become a wedge-shaped angiocentric architecture. **(B)** Variably atypical lymphoid cells in the dermis. **(C)** Epidermal infiltration with associated scale abnormalities and neutrophil infiltration. **(D)** CD30+ cells are numerous within the superficial dermal component of the infiltrate.

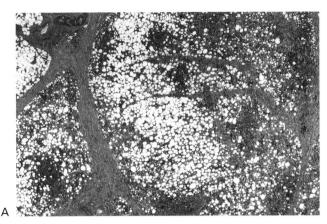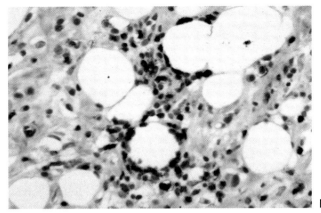

FIGURE 31-32. Subcutaneous panniculitis-like T-cell lymphoma. **(A)** Lobular and septal pattern of subcutaneous infiltration. **(B)** TIA-1 immunohistochemistry showing characteristic rimming about individual adipocytes.

may be observed. Importantly, unlike many cases of systemic CD30+ lymphomas, most primary cutaneous lesions are negative for epithelial membrane antigen (EMA) (12). A similar immunophenotype is expressed by the minority population of large atypical cells in type A LYP (Fig. 31-31D), although CD30 expression may not be detected in type B lesions in which Reed–Sternberg cells are infrequent to absent. Most cases of C-ALCL and about half of cases of LYP (predominantly the type A variant) show clonal rearrangements of the T-cell receptor.

Differential Diagnosis. The single most important consideration in the diagnosis of primary cutaneous CD30+ T-cell lymphoproliferative disorders is their differentiation from primary systemic lymphomas that may express CD30 and show a considerably worse prognosis. This may generally be accomplished by careful assessment of correlative clinical and histologic parameters, as well as by meticulous clinical staging. Distinction of C-ALCL from LYP is similarly possible by evaluation of clinical parameters and assessment of lesion architecture and relative percentages of large atypical CD30+ cells within the cutaneous infiltrates.

Subcutaneous Panniculitis-like T-cell Lymphoma

Subcutaneous panniculitis-like T-cell lymphoma (SPTCL) is defined as a rare lymphoma that (a) primarily infiltrates subcutaneous tissue; (b) shows high-grade cytologic features; and (c) is composed of T cells with a cytotoxic phenotype.

Clinical Features. While the majority of cases occur in young adults, a broad age range has been reported, and the disease tends to show an equal gender distribution (211). Affected individuals generally present with symptoms related to formation of deeply seated and variably sized cutaneous nodules often involving the extremities and/or trunk. Systemic symptoms and signs, when present, may relate to hemophagocytic syndrome with pancytopenia, fever, and

hepatosplenomegaly usually in the absence of lymphadenopathy (212). Immunosuppression appears to be a predisposing factor in some patients (213,214). Despite an aggressive natural history, particularly when complicated by the hemophagocytic syndrome, patients often respond favorably to initial rounds of chemotherapy (212,215,216).

Histopathology. There is a diffuse, variably cellular infiltrate involving both septae and lobules within the subcutis (Fig. 31-32A), with relative sparing of the overlying dermis. The infiltrate is composed of smaller lymphocytes with visible cytoplasm admixed with larger transformed cells with hyperchromatic nuclei. The initial biopsy in which the more atypical elements are not well represented may appear to be deceptively banal. Cells characteristically show peripheral alignment (rimming) about individual adipocytes (Fig. 31-32B). Fat necrosis and associated infiltration of reactive histiocytes may also be noted. Necrosis, nuclear fragmentation, and vascular injury may all be observed.

Histogenesis. The malignant cells express a mature CD8+ T-cell phenotype. In keeping with their presumed derivation from a cytotoxic T-cell, they also are reactive for the following proteins: granzyme, perforin, and T-cell intracellular antigen (TIA-1). About 75% of cases are derived from αβ T cells, and the remainder from γδ T cells, the latter often exhibiting both CD4 and CD8 negativity, but reactivity for CD56 (217). TCR genes are rearranged, and EBV sequences cannot be demonstrated.

SECONDARY T/NK-CELL LYMPHOPROLIFERATIVE DISORDERS AFFECTING SKIN

Peripheral T-Cell Lymphoma

This category corresponds to a relatively large group of predominantly nodal T-cell lymphomas that occur in Western countries and that frequently also show involvement of bone marrow, liver, spleen, peripheral blood, and skin (12,218–220). The WHO classification provides the modifier "unspecified" to emphasize that most cases are clinicopathologically heterogeneous, and thus do not fit well into better-defined entities of T-cell neoplasia. In skin, these lesions are separate from mycosis fungoides and Sézary syndrome, possessing distinctive histologic, antigenic, and genotypic attributes.

Clinical Features. The majority of cases involve adults without gender predilection, although reports of children being affected exist. Clinical presentation generally involves constitutional symptoms and lymphadenopathy. The lymphoepithelioid cell variant (see below) is a low-grade variant of peripheral T-cell lymphoma where systemic signs may include enlargement of cervical lymph nodes, hepatosplenomegaly, fever, and skin involvement in less than 10% of cases (221). Skin lesions may take the form of eczematous plaques or erythematous tumors; pruritus, peripheral eosinophilia, and hemophagocytic syndromes have also been described (218).

Histopathology. There are two variant forms of this entity: the *lymphoepithelioid cell variant* (previously referred to as Lennert lymphoma), and the T-zone variant. The lymphoepithelioid variant is characterized by small lymphocytes with variable, often minimal, irregularities in nuclear contour, admixed with clusters of epithelioid histiocytes, eosinophils, plasma cells, and occasional Reed Sternberg (RS)-like cells (222). These cells may infiltrate the dermis in a nodular or diffuse pattern, and the papillary dermis and epidermis may also be involved (223). The *T-zone variant* derives its name from its pattern of nodal involvement that primarily involves the interfollicular zones, with preservation of lymphoid follicles. Tumor cells are small- to intermediate in size and often lack significant pleomorphism (Fig. 31-33). As with the lympho-

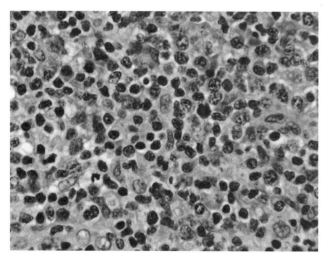

FIGURE 31-33. Peripheral T-cell lymphoma. Note relatively monomorphic lymphoid cells of intermediate size.

epithelioid variant, reactive cells, including plasma cells, epithelioid histiocyte, eosinophils, and RS-like cells may also be noted. It is likely that definitive separation of these two variants will require evaluation of lymph node, rather than skin involvement.

Histogenesis. The tumor is a malignancy of T cells, and the most common nodal immunophenotype is CD4+, CD30+, and CD8−, with frequently aberrant T-cell antigenic profiles (e.g., loss of pan–T-cell differentiation markers) (224,225). Moreover, there tend to be clonal rearrangements of TCR genes (226), as documented by PCR analysis. While there is no consistent trend in karyotypic abnormalities, an association between trisomy 3 and the lymphoepithelioid variant (Lennert's lymphoma) has been reported (227).

Differential Diagnosis. The lymphoepithelioid variant may occasionally mimic the granulomatous variant of mycosis fungoides, although the latter is characterized by clinical lesional evolution that involves initial formation of inconspicuous patches. Because lesions may be CD30+, they should not be confused with anaplastic large-cell lymphomas that differ cytologically. Whereas nodal cases also differ in that anaplastic large-cell lymphomas often express cytotoxic granule associated proteins (217,228–232), it must be noted that extranodal involvement by peripheral T-cell lymphoma may also have a cytotoxic T-cell phenotype, including CD56 expression (233). EBV is generally absent on tumor cells, but may be noted in the reactive components of lesions, in particular the RS-like cells (234). Because these cells may be noted, along with a polymorphous reactive component, care must be taken not to mistake lesions as the rare event of cutaneous involvement by Hodgkin lymphoma.

Anaplastic Large-Cell Lymphoma

Anaplastic large-cell lymphoma (ALCL) is a nodal T-cell malignancy that is characterized by homogeneous proliferation of large atypical lymphocytes that express the CD30 (Ki-1) antigen. It must be differentiated from primary cutaneous ALCL, a lesion with a considerably better prognosis.

Clinical Features. Of non-Hodgkin lymphomas, approximately 3% of adult lymphomas and 10–30% of lymphomas in children are accounted for by ALCL (235). Lesions may be further divided according to expression of anaplastic large-cell lymphoma kinase (ALK), with most positive cases affecting males in the second to third decades, and most negative cases occurring in older individuals with relatively equal distribution according to gender. Of extranodal sites, skin is involved in more than 20% of cases, followed by bone, soft tissue, lung, and liver (235,236). Fever and adenopathy are common, with presentation in advanced stages of disease the rule.

Histopathology. Although a wide morphologic spectrum has been described (2,237–242), most cases share the presence of large anaplastic mononuclear cells containing abundant cytoplasm and an eccentric, reniform nucleus (241) (Fig. 31-34A and B). Occasional intranuclear cytoplasmic inclusions ("doughnut" cells) and multinucleated forms may be observed (242). The chromatin pattern is generally finely aggregated, and nucleoli are variably prominent and usually multiple. In addition to lesions where these cells predominate (the common variant), others may show these cells to be admixed with large numbers of histiocytes (lymphohistiocytic variant) or with cytologically similar, albeit smaller atypical lymphocytes (small-cell variant). In general, however, the hallmark large anaplastic lymphocytes are recognizable cytologically and as a result of their tendency to aggregate about blood vessels. The dermal infiltrates tend to have a nodular architecture. The presence of epidermal hyperplasia tends to correlate with primary cutaneous ALCL rather than systemic ALCL.

Histogenesis. The presumed cell of origin for ALCL is a mature cytotoxic T cell. The majority of cases express T-cell antigens, and even those without T-cell antigen expression ("null cell" phenotype) have evidence of T-cell lineage at a genomic level (231). Pan–T-cell maturation markers (e.g., CD3, CD5, and CD7) are frequently negative, consistent with an aberrant T-cell phenotype. The majority of cases show strong CD30 reactivity on the cell membrane and in association with the Golgi zone (Fig. 31-34C). This reactivity is especially prominent on the hallmark large

anaplastic cells, and less pronounced on the smaller variant forms (241). ALK expression (see below) is present in 60% to 80% of cases, and the majority of these are also positive for epithelial membrane antigen (EMA) (237,241). In addition, most cases show positivity for cytotoxic-associated markers, including TIA-1, granzyme B, and/or perforin (230,231). Tumor cells are consistently negative for EBV, although they may show perinuclear staining for lysosomal enzymes as well as reactivity with some probes that identify CD68, and accordingly, caution must be exercised in not assuming histiocytic lineage in such instances (243). The majority of cases demonstrate clonal rearrangements in the TCR irrespective of expression of T-cell markers.

Overexpression of the ALK protein is caused by alterations of the ALK gene at chromosome 2. Most commonly, t(2;5)(p23;35) is seen with the participation of the ALK gene on chromosome 2 and nucleophosmin (NPM) gene on chromosome 5. However, breakpoints on chromosomes other than 5 can partner with the ALK gene. Classic t(2;5) leads to ALK protein overexpression resulting in both cytoplasmic and nuclear stain with antibodies directed against this molecule. The ALK protein functions as a tyrosine kinase receptor, and its gene belongs to the insulin receptor superfamily. ALCL are invariably negative for EBV genomes separating them from EBV⁺ classic types of Hodgkin lymphoma.

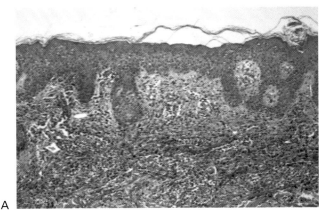

A

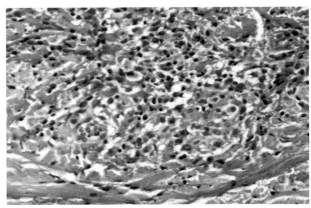

B

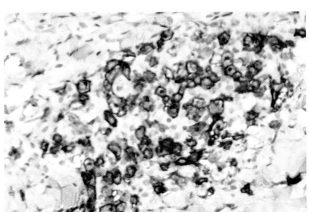

C

FIGURE 31-34. Anaplastic large cell lymphoma. Low **(A)** and higher magnification **(B)** showing dermal infiltrate by large anaplastic lymphoid cells. **(C)** Immunohistochemistry for CD30.

Differential Diagnosis. The primary differential diagnostic considerations include Hodgkin lymphoma, particularly when RS-like cells are present. However, the immunophenotypic profile of ALCL is sufficiently distinctive to permit distinction of ALCL from the rare occurrence of Hodgkin lymphoma with skin involvement. System ALCL (discussed here) presents in the skin in advanced stages, and therefore may be further differentiated from primary cutaneous ALCL and its regressing variants (e.g., lymphomatoid papulosis) based on clinical parameters (discussed in greater detail later).

Extranodal NK/T-Cell Lymphoma, Nasal Type

The nasal type of extranodal NK/T-cell lymphoma is characterized by angiocentric and angiodestructive infiltrates of malignant cells with NK or cytotoxic T-cell phenotype that often but not invariably involve tissues of the nasal cavity (244–247). It has been known by numerous appellations, including pleomorphic reticulosis and lethal midline granuloma.

Clinical Features. Extranodal NK/T-cell lymphoma tends to more often affect adult males, with a geographic distribution showing concentration in Asia, Mexico, Central America, and South America. Sites most often affected include the nasal cavity and nasopharynx, skin and soft tissues, gastrointestinal tract, and testis; secondary lymph node involvement is also common (233, 248–255). Nasopharyngeal involvement is often associated with extensive destruction of soft tissue and bone, and rapid and widespread dissemination may occur. Skin may be either a site of secondary spread or a primary manifestation of the disease. Cutaneous nodules, often with ulceration, are most often encountered. Advanced disease is the rule at the time of presentation, and an associated hemophagocytic syndrome may also be noted (251,256). Fever, cachexia, and other systemic symptoms are frequently documented (233,249,250,257). In those advanced cases where marrow and peripheral blood involvement are encountered, there is overlap with aggressive NK-cell leukemia. Prognosis is variable, although most cases occurring at sites other than the nasal cavity have a poor outcome.

Histopathology. The characteristic histopathology involves a diffuse, focally angiocentric and angiodestructive infiltrate of variably sized, mitotically active lymphoid cells with moderate quantities of pale cytoplasm and nuclei with irregular and occasionally elongated profiles. Chromatin tends to be coarsely granular, and nucleoli are inconspicuous. Some cases will show an admixture of reactive inflammatory cells, including activated lymphocytes, plasma cells, and eosinophils. Infiltration and fibrinoid necrosis of affected vessel walls and zones of necrosis and

apoptosis are characteristic findings (156). The epidermis or squamous epithelial mucosa may be ulcerated, or in some instances may show florid pseudoepitheliomatous hyperplasia.

Histogenesis. In most instances, the cell of origin is believed to be an NK cell or a cytotoxic T cell. The typical immunophenotype is CD2$^+$, CD56$^+$, and surface CD3$^-$ (163,248,258–260). Cytotoxic granule associated proteins (TIA-1, granzyme B, perforin) are usually detected, and CD4, CD5, and CD8 are generally negative. Interestingly, TCR and immunoglobulin genes are in the germline configuration in most cases of extranodal NK/T-cell lymphoma, although a variety of cytogenetic abnormalities have been recorded. There is a strong association with EBV, suggesting a possible causal role for this agent (261–266).

Differential Diagnosis. The differential diagnosis includes other neoplastic lymphocytic infiltrates that are angiocentric and angiodestructive. Lymphomatoid granulomatosis had historically been considered in the context of extranodal NK/T-cell lymphoma, although the former is now recognized to represent a form of EBV$^+$ B-cell lymphoproliferative disorder that may contain numerous reactive T cells (260). Vasculitic variants of mycosis fungoides have been described, although these can be distinguished by the absence of cytotoxic markers that characterize most cases of extranodal NK/T-cell lymphoma.

Adult T-Cell Leukemia/Lymphoma

Adult T-cell leukemia/lymphoma (ATLL) is a peripheral high-grade lymphoid neoplasm caused by the human retrovirus, human T-cell leukemia virus type 1 (HTLV-1).

Clinical Features. ATLL occurs most often as an endemic disorder, primarily in Japan, the Caribbean Basin, and Central Africa, with the disease distribution mirrored by the prevalence of HTLV-1 infection (267). The disease is also detected in populations in certain parts of the southeastern United States where HTLV-1 seropositivity is high. The virus may be transmitted by blood and body fluids, including breast milk, and the disease is believed to have a long latency period before becoming overt. The median age is 55, with men slightly more affected than women (268). Widespread lymphadenopathy and peripheral blood involvement are present from the outset. The skin is the most common extralymphatic site of involvement, with lesions documented in more than half of the cases. *H*ypercalcemia, *o*steolytic bone lesions, *T*-cell leukemia, and *s*kin lesions (HOTS) represents a clinical syndrome that, along with lymphadenopathy, represents a prototypic presentation for ATLL. Skin lesions generally take the form of multiple papules, plaques, and nodules that may be explosive in onset (Fig. 31-35A). Clinical course is variable, and acute (leukemia, rash, hypercalcemia), lymphomatous (lymphadenopathy without leuke-

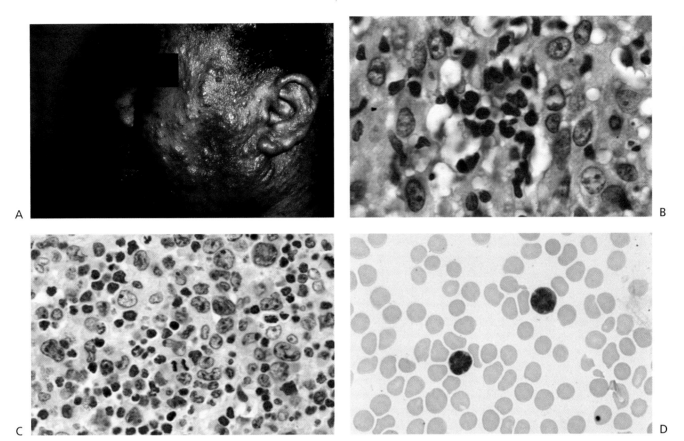

FIGURE 31-35. Adult T-cell leukemia/lymphoma. **(A)** Clinical appearance, where multiple nodules explosively developed within several weeks in this patient with hypercalcemia. **(B)** Epidermotropic atypical lymphocytes are indistinguishable by conventional paraffin histology from mycosis fungoides. **(C)** Tissue infiltration by tumor cells with variably hyperchromatic and convoluted nuclear contours. **(D)** Peripheral blood showing enlarged lymphoid cells with characteristically hyperlobated nuclear contours.

mia or hypercalcemia), and chronic/smoldering (skin lesions without leukemia or hypercalcemia) variants have been described. In general, individuals afflicted with the acute and lymphomatous types have a significantly worse prognosis (269).

Histopathology. Skin lesions may show nodular to diffuse infiltrates of atypical lymphocytes, with or without papillary dermal involvement or epidermotropism. Lesions thus are generally indistinguishable from mycosis fungoides in plaque to nodular stages of evolution (Fig. 31-35B). Cytologically, the neoplastic lymphocytes contain enlarged hyperchromatic nuclei with irregular, often convoluted nuclear profiles (Fig. 31-35C). Anaplastic cells with clumped nuclear chromatin and prominent nucleoli may also be observed (267,270). The peripheral blood contains atypical cells with characteristically hyperlobated nuclear profiles ("flower cells"), a feature that may serve to distinguish ATLL cells from those of Sézary syndrome and systemically disseminated forms of mycosis fungoides (Fig. 31-35D).

Histogenesis. Tumor cells are CD4+ T cells that also express T-cell associated antigens CD2, CD3, and CD5, but generally lack CD7 and CD8. As in all cases of T-cell lymphoma, rare cases that express CD8 but not CD4, or double negative (CD4−/CD8−) cases may occur. Tumor cells may also express CD30, but unlike anaplastic large-cell lymphoma, lack ALK, TIA-1, and granzyme B (271, 272). TCR gene rearrangements are present (273). Interestingly, the CD3+/CD4+ neoplastic cells of ATLL may demonstrate suppressor, rather than helper/inducer, function *in vitro*. Clonally integrated HTLV-1 is present. The HTLV-1 transactivator, Tax, has been implicated as the viral oncoprotein (274).

Differential Diagnosis. The differential diagnosis includes primarily mycosis fungoides and Sézary syndrome. The presence of patch-stage disease, both clinically and/or histologically, is of assistance in differentiating mycosis fungoides from ATLL. However, in more advanced lesions, distinction by histology alone may be impossible. Because most ATLL patients are not erythrodermic, this clinical feature may assist in differentiating this condition from Sézary syndrome. It should also be noted that the cytology of peripheral blood involvement in ATLL is distinctive, showing cells with hyperlobated, "flower-like" nuclear contours, rather than the cerebriform nuclei of Sézary cells. In suspected cases of ATLL, HTLV-1 serology should be performed (275), although definitive diagnosis ultimately will depend on demonstration of HTLV-1 gene integration within the malignant cells in skin or blood by Southern blot analysis (276).

Precursor T-Lymphoblastic Leukemia/Lymphoblastic Lymphoma

Precursor T-lymphoblastic leukemia (T-ALL)/lymphoblastic lymphoma (T-LBL) is a high-risk neoplasm that is derived from pre- and intra-thymic T-lymphocytes. The distinction between the designation of leukemia and lymphoma is somewhat arbitrary, with the former preferred when there is extensive marrow and blood involvement, and the latter when there is a mass lesion at presentation and less than 25% lymphoblasts in the marrow and minimal peripheral blood involvement (277).

Clinical Features. The most typical presentation is that of a mediastinal mass in children and young adults. Involvement of bone marrow and peripheral blood is frequent. Lymph nodes, liver, spleen, Waldeyer ring, central nervous system, gonads, and skin all may be involved. In-filtration of the skin results in erythematous to hemorrhagic papules and nodules, with skin of the head and neck region preferentially involved (55). Whereas the leukemic counterpart tends to affect children, the lymphomatous phase is more often encountered in adult males (37).

Histopathology. As with other poorly differentiated T-cell infiltrates of skin, the dermis is preferentially involved by a diffuse interstitial infiltrate, with little or no epidermotropism. Cytologically, the tumor cells are uniformly atypical, with scant cytoplasm and nuclei characterized by slightly irregular, sometimes grooved contours and moderately condensed to evenly dispersed chromatin patterns with inconspicuous nucleoli (55,278) (Fig. 31-36A). Occasionally eosinophils will be present within the dermal infiltrate.

Histogenesis. The cell of origin is believed to be a precursor T-lymphoblast. The tumor cells are TdT⁺ and may express CD1a, CD2, CD3, CD4, CD5, CD7, and/or CD8 to variable degree. Of these, reactivity for CD3 and CD7 are the most common (Fig. 31-36B and C). Lineage ambiguity of these primitive cells may occur, however, as evidenced by occasional expression of the B-cell marker CD79a or myeloid markers CD13 and/or CD33. Clonal rearrangements of the T-cell receptor are also commonly observed.

Differential Diagnosis. Skin involvement by T-ALL/ T-LBL must be differentiated from B-cell lymphoblastic

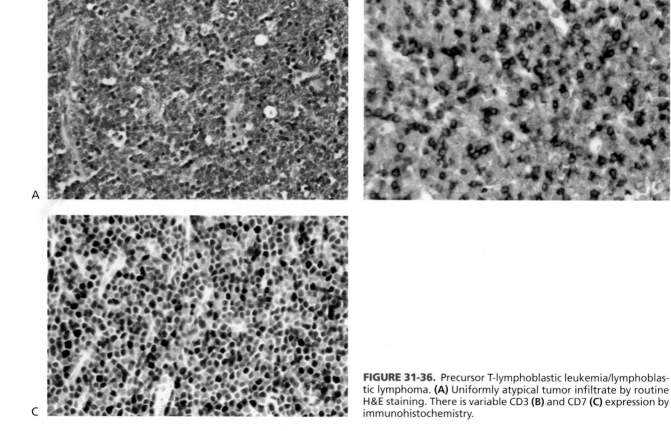

FIGURE 31-36. Precursor T-lymphoblastic leukemia/lymphoblastic lymphoma. **(A)** Uniformly atypical tumor infiltrate by routine H&E staining. There is variable CD3 **(B)** and CD7 **(C)** expression by immunohistochemistry.

leukemia/lymphoma and acute myeloid leukemia, and this requires immunohistochemistry and/or histochemistry for lineage-associated antigens and enzymes. In children, extranodal involvement by Burkitt lymphoma, and in adults, extranodal involvement by the blastoid variant of MCL, may enter into the differential diagnostic algorithm. Because lymphoblastic lymphoma is the only lymphoma that shows nuclear TdT positivity, these possibilities may be readily eliminated. Primary neuroendocrine carcinoma of the skin may occasionally be confused with T-ALL/T-LBL, especially when the former shows a diffuse interstitial pattern of dermal involvement. Again, immunohistochemistry will establish the hematopoietic and lineage characteristics of T-ALL/T-LBL in this setting.

T-Cell Prolymphocytic Leukemia

T-cell prolymphocytic leukemia (T-PLL) is a relatively rare, aggressive form of T-cell leukemia composed of cells of mature, post-thymic phenotype, that tend to involve lymph nodes, liver, spleen, and skin (20% of cases), in addition to blood and bone marrow (279).

Clinical Features. The vast majority of afflicted individuals are adults who present with generalized lymphadenopathy and enlargement of the spleen and liver. Anemia, thrombocytopenia, and atypical lymphocytosis are present; HTVL-1 serology is negative. Unlike Sézary syndrome, skin lesions are not erythrodermic, but rather infiltrative. The leukemic infiltrates tend to form plaques and nodules that are variably erythematous to hemorrhagic in appearance.

Histopathology. Skin involvement takes the form of dense dermal infiltrates with a focal tendency for periadnexal localization. Epidermotropism, however, is not present (280). Peripheral blood in most cases contains numerous (often more than $100 \times 10^3/l$) of small- to intermediate-sized lymphoid cells characterized by basophilic cytoplasm and nuclei with irregular contours and detectable nucleoli. Occasional cases will show such prominent irregularities in nuclear contour that the cells may resemble Sézary cells (281), while others will show a predominance of small lymphocytes with inconspicuous nucleoli (small-cell variant). Important common features, however, are the presence of cytoplasmic blebs from the plasma membranes and Golgi-region staining for alpha-naphthyl acetate esterase (282). Bone marrow will contain these cells as well, although the characteristic diagnostic features may be more difficult to establish in this tissue.

Histogenesis. Cases show various combinations of CD4 and CD8 reactivity, with most expressing CD4 and showing clonal rearrangements of TCR γ and β chains. Strong CD7 staining and coexpression of CD4 and CD8 in 25% of patients along with weak reactivity for CD3 suggest that T-PLL may be differentiating toward a stage intermediate between a cortical thymocyte and a mature peripheral blood T cell. Eighty percent of patients show inversion of chromosome 14 with breakpoints involving the long arm at q11 and q32 (283,284).

Differential Diagnosis. T-PLL must be differentiated from other forms of T-cell lymphoma showing skin involvement and a leukemic phase. The clinical features at presentation, absence of epidermotropism, absence of HTLV-1 positivity, characteristic cytoplasmic blebbing in peripheral blood smears, and cases where CD4 and CD8 are coexpressed (a feature virtually unique to T-PLL) should all assist in differential diagnostic exclusion of this rare yet aggressive condition.

Blastic NK-Cell Lymphoma

Blastic NK-cell lymphoma is an aggressive neoplasm of lymphoblast-like cells with features of commitment to NK lineage and a marked predilection for cutaneous involvement. A proportion of cases overlap with so-called precursor NK-cell lymphoblastic lymphoma/leukemia (285,286) and with primary cutaneous CD4+ CD56+ hematolymphoid neoplasm (287–293).

Clinical Features. This lymphoma tends to affect middle-aged and elderly individuals, who at time of presentation demonstrate skin lesions, often with soft tissue, lymph node, bone marrow, and/or peripheral blood involvement (294). Skin lesions may take the form of localized plum-colored tumors covered by a glistening, attenuated epidermal layer.

Histopathology. The dermis is diffusely infiltrated by a monotonous population of intermediate-sized lymphoid cells with a chromatin pattern that may suggest lymphoblastic or myeloblastic leukemia (Fig. 31-37; also see below). There is an absence of zonal necrosis or angiocentric infiltration, as may occur with extranodal NK/T-cell lymphoma of the nasal type. On rare occasion, tumor cells may aggregate to form rosette-like structures resembling Homer–Wright

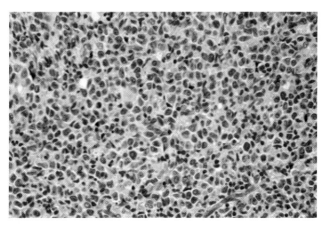

FIGURE 31-37. Blastic NK-cell lymphoma. The dermis is replaced by a monotonous infiltrate of intermediate-sized mononuclear cells with some morphologic overlap with myeloblasts.

rosettes (295). Azurophilic cytoplasmic granules are variably detected upon Giemsa staining (296).

Histogenesis. Although the precise lineage remains to be defined, a precursor NK-cell origin has been postulated. The neoplastic cells tend to be CD3⁻, CD4⁺, and CD56⁺. This disease entity is immunophenotypically somewhat ill defined, and the diagnosis should be made only in the absence of myeloid and T-lineage markers other than CD4, in particular in light of the fact that both AML and T-ALL can express CD56. The future will tell whether blastic NK-cell lymphoma will continue to be treated as a distinct disease category. Distinct from other NK-cell malignancies, EBV is invariably absent.

Differential Diagnosis. Because of potential confusion with myeloblastic and precursor T-lymphoblastic lymphoma/leukemia, the diagnosis of blastic NK-cell lymphoma is best made when neoplastic cells are negative for CD3, myeloperoxidase, and CD33, and preferable also when they fail to demonstrate TCR gene rearrangements.

PRIMARY CUTANEOUS MYELOID HYPERPLASIA/NEOPLASIA

Extramedullary Hematopoiesis

Extramedullary hematopoiesis refers to abnormal trilineage maturation of hematopoietic elements in tissues other than bone marrow. In skin, the process has been referred to as *dermal hematopoiesis.* Occasionally, extramedullary hematopoiesis is restricted to cells of erythroid lineage, a phenomenon termed *dermal erythropoiesis* that may occur in neonates in association with the stress of various viral infections, or in adults with myelofibrosis.

Clinical Features. Lesions typically present as macules, papules, and occasionally nodules that have a dull blue-red hue. Dermal hematopoiesis in neonates tends to affect the head and neck (so-called "blueberry muffin baby"). In adults, cutaneous extramedullary hematopoiesis frequently involves the trunk and occasionally in surgical scars after splenectomy, a procedure that in itself appears to augment the phenomenon.

Histopathology. Poorly formed micronodules of pleomorphic cells are present in the dermis, and the pattern may initially mimic leukemia cutis of an unusual dermal inflammatory reaction. Maturing erythrocytes can be identified as clustered "colonies" of cells containing round basophilic nuclei rimmed by eosinophilic cytoplasm. Admixed myeloblasts, metamyelocytes, and characteristically large megakaryocytes containing prominently multilobated nuclei are often also present. These latter cells are reactive for CD61, a helpful marker in further confirming their lineage identity.

Histogenesis. Although normal hematopoiesis occurs in bone marrow, the occurrence of extramedullary hemato-

poiesis in skin and other tissues underscores the fact that under certain conditions, extramedullary tissues contain the appropriate precursor cells and growth factors to serve as surrogates for the marrow microenvironment.

Differential Diagnosis. Extramedullary hematopoiesis in the skin must be distinguished from reactive and dysplastic polymorphous infiltrates that may contain large atypical cells (e.g., lymphomatoid papulosis containing large Reed–Sternberg cells) and from forms of leukemia cutis that harbor cells with primitive myeloid features. Clinical information may be helpful in determining whether patients have predisposing factors for this phenomenon. The morphologic identification of erythropoiesis and the presence of megakaryocytes, and further confirmation of the latter via immunohistochemistry for CD61, should assist in those rare circumstances when true extramedullary hematopoiesis is detected in the skin.

Myeloid Sarcoma

Myeloid sarcoma refers to a tumor formed by myeloblasts or immature myeloid cells that affects an extramedullary site, such as skin. The mass, also referred to as an extramedullary myeloid tumor, granulocytic sarcoma or chloroma, may precede or present simultaneously with a systemic myeloproliferative disorder, including acute and chronic myeloid leukemias (see below) and myelodysplastic syndromes, or represent a relapse of disease previously in remission. Acute monoblastic leukemia giving rise to extramedullary myeloid tumor is referred to as monoblastic sarcoma.

Clinical Features. Lesions may be solitary or multiple, and may show clinical features indistinguishable from secondary cutaneous involvement by acute and chronic myeloid leukemia (see below).

Histopathology. Most commonly, myeloid sarcoma is composed of an admixture of myeloblasts, neutrophil precursors, and mature neutrophils (granulocytic sarcoma). Less differentiated (blastic) variants are formed primarily by myeloblasts, whereas the immature and differentiated variants are composed primarily of myeloblasts and promyelocytes, or of promyelocytes and more mature forms, respectively. Rarely, myeloid sarcomas may be composed principally of monoblasts. In situations involving transformation of chronic myeloproliferative disease, trilineage hematopoiesis may also be observed.

Histogenesis. The postulated cell of origin is a myeloid hematopoietic cell. Tumor cells stain positively for myeloperoxidase, lysozyme, and chloroacetate esterase. The myeloblastic components may express CD13, CD33, and CD117, as also would be anticipated in acute myelogenous leukemia. Tumors with monoblastic differentiation may express CD14, CD116, and CD11c, as well as lysozyme and CD68. CD43 also is expressed by the majority of myeloid sarcomas.

Differential Diagnosis. Tumors containing primarily blastic and immature elements must be differentiated from various non-Hodgkin lymphomas, including lymphoblastic, Burkitt, and large-cell types. In general, in any poorly differentiated malignant skin infiltrate of confirmed hematopoietic lineage, myeloid differentiation should be considered and excluded by appropriate immunohistochemical panels.

SECONDARY MYELOID NEOPLASMS AFFECTING SKIN

Acute and Chronic Myeloid Leukemia

Leukemia cutis is an important differential consideration in the assessment of atypical hematopoietic/lymphoproliferative infiltrates of the skin. Some lymphomas may occur along a continuum with leukemic phases, and thus certain forms of leukemia have already been discussed under T- and B-cell lymphoid neoplasms. Because circulating leukemic cells may always potentially deposit in the skin, there are a wide range of disorders that come into consideration in this section. The WHO classification, for example, considers acute myeloid leukemias according to categories that relate to presence of recurrent genetic abnormalities, association with multilineage dysplasia and therapies, and those that are of ambiguous lineage or not otherwise categorized. Chronic myeloproliferative conditions are also classed into multiple groups, as is exemplified by chronic myelogenous, neutrophilic, and eosinophilic leukemias, and polycythemia vera, to name a few. Because the nuances of these classification schemes rely heavily on morphologic, immunophenotypic, and genotypic findings in the bone marrow, a detailed discussion is beyond the scope of this section that will focus on common features of neoplastic myeloid infiltrates of skin, and how to recognize them.

Clinical Features. Clinical symptoms and signs are often related to marrow replacement by malignant cells, and thus tend to relate to anemia, thrombocytopenia, and alteration in normal leukocyte function (infection). Peripheral blood generally shows leukocytosis as a result of involvement by malignant cells, although occasionally these may not be detectable in spite of massive marrow involvement. In such situations, involvement of solid tissues, such as skin, may be the initial presenting feature of leukemia in evolution. Chronic leukemias are more indolent neoplasms that are composed of more mature myeloid cells that slowly replace the marrow compartment and seed the blood. Acute leukemias are more aggressive neoplasms that are composed on less mature myeloid cells and that more rapidly and completely replace normal hematopoietic marrow and seed the blood. Cutaneous infiltrates may present as red to purpuric patches, plaques, papules, or nodules, with or without ulceration (297) (Fig. 31-38). Mucosae may also be affected. There exist, in addition, numerous paraneoplastic findings that may be associated with leukemia, including gingival hyperplasia, vasculitis, Sweet and pyo-

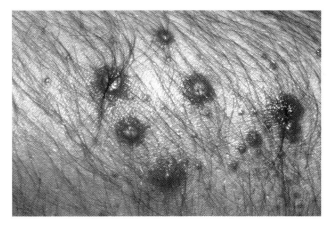

FIGURE 31-38. Acute myeloid leukemia. Multiple erythematous to hemorrhagic plaques and nodules are observed.

derma neutrophilic dermatitis, urticaria, erythema multiforme, and erythema nodosum, to name a few.

Histopathology. Myeloid leukemias may recapitulate various forms of myeloid lineage, and accordingly these neoplasms may be described as showing myeloid, myelomonocytic, monocytic, and megakaryocytic differentiation. Acute myeloid leukemia may be divided into M0 to M7 subtypes according to differentiation patterns described in Table 31-4.

TABLE 31-4. WORLD HEALTH ORGANIZATION CLASSIFICATION OF ACUTE MYELOID LEUKEMIAS

Acute myeloid leukemia with recurrent genetic abnormalities
 Acute myeloid leukemia with t(8;21)(q22;q22);(AML1/ETO)
 Acute myeloid leukemia with abnormal bone marrow eosinophils inv(16)(P13q22) or t(16;16)(p13;q22);(CBFβ/MYH11)
 Acute promyelocytic leukemia (AML with t(15;17)(q22;q12) (PML/RARα) and variants (M3)
 Acute myeloid leukemia with 11q23 (MLL) abnormalities
Acute myeloid leukemia with multilineage dysplasia
 Following a myelodysplastic syndrome or myelodysplastic syndrome/myeloproliferative disorder
 Without antecedent myelodysplastic syndrome
Acute myeloid leukemia and myelodysplastic syndromes, therapy-related
 Alkylating agent-related
 Topoisomerase type II inhibitor-related (some may be lymphoid)
 Other types
Acute myeloid leukemia not otherwise categorized
 Acute myeloid leukemia minimally differentiated (M0)
 Acute myeloid leukemia without maturation (M1)
 Acute myeloid leukemia with maturation (M2)
 Acute myelomonocytic leukemia (M4)
 Acute monoblastic and monocytic leukemia (M5)
 Acute erythroid leukemia (M6)
 Acute megakaryoblastic leukemia (M7)
 Acute basophilic leukemia
 Acute panmyelosis with myelofibrosis
Myeloid sarcoma

Architecturally, early acute myelogenous leukemia cutis may produce an angiocentric infiltrate, although interstitial permeation among collagen bundles within the reticular dermis soon supervenes (Fig. 31-39A). Vague nodules may form as the dermis becomes progressively expanded by malignant cells, which express myeloperoxidase (Fig. 31-39B). Malignant myeloid cells forming the dominant cell type of acute myeloid leukemia cutis tend to appear monotonous and homogeneous cytologically (Fig. 31-39C). Nuclei are round to oval, chromatin may be evenly dis-

persed, and nucleoli are multiple but potentially inconspicuous. On rare occasion, immature eosinophils containing typical cytoplasmic granules in the absence of bilobed nuclear contours may be helpful in assigning a presumptive diagnosis (Fig. 31-39D). However, histochemistry and immunohistochemistry are generally required for confirmation, as well as examination of peripheral blood and bone marrow (Fig. 31-39E).

It is noteworthy that myeloid leukemia cutis may mimic an angiocentric inflammatory infiltrate architecturally, and

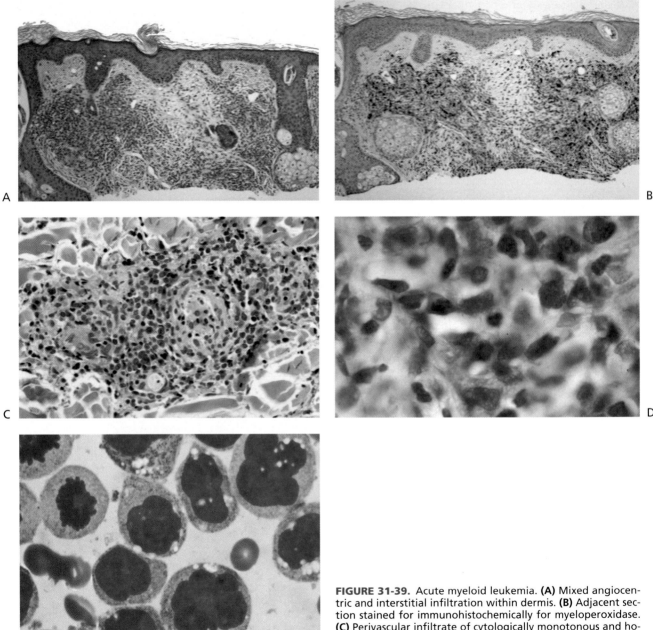

FIGURE 31-39. Acute myeloid leukemia. **(A)** Mixed angiocentric and interstitial infiltration within dermis. **(B)** Adjacent section stained for immunohistochemically for myeloperoxidase. **(C)** Perivascular infiltrate of cytologically monotonous and homogeneous myeloblasts. **(D)** Higher magnification revealing occasional eosinophilic myeloblasts. **(E)** Bone marrow aspirate in M5 acute myelogenous leukemia.

cytologically immature myeloid cells, although homogeneous, may not appear overtly anaplastic. Accordingly, it is appropriate to consider the differential possibility of acute myeloid leukemia cutis in the initial histologic evaluation of any atypical or malignant nonepidermotropic lymphoid infiltrate of presumed lymphoid origin (Fig. 31-39E). In cutaneous infiltrates with similar architectural features but containing mature myeloid elements, in addition to myeloblasts, the less common possibility of chronic myeloid leukemia cutis should be considered.

Histogenesis. Both acute and chronic forms of myeloid leukemia are derived from myeloid progenitors in the bone marrow. Accordingly, cells are histochemically positive for myeloperoxidase (Fig. 31-39B), Sudan black B, chloroacetate esterase, and Leder stains. Myeloid cells do not express B-lineage (CD19, CD20, CD22, CD19a) or T-lineage (CD2, CD3, CD5, CD7) markers, but may show immunohistochemical staining for the myeloid markers CD13, CD33, CD15, CD117, or megakaryoblastic antigens C41 and CD61.

Differential Diagnosis. In addition to possible confusion with T- and B-cell leukemia/lymphoma cutis, acute myeloid leukemia cutis must be differentiated from other interstitial dermal infiltrates dominated by monotonous populations of mononuclear cells. Mastocytosis may produce an interstitial pattern, and mast cells may react positively with the Leder stain, but not with more specific markers for myeloid differentiation (e.g., myeloperoxidase). Myeloblasts, along with more mature myeloid elements may occur in skin involved by chronic myelogenous leukemia as well as by extramedullary hematopoiesis. However, in the latter, maturing cells of erythrocyte and megakaryocytic differentiation are generally detectable.

REFERENCES

1. Jaffe ES, Harris NL, Stein H, et al., eds. *Tumours of hematopoietic and lymphoid tissues: World Health Organization classification of tumours.* Lyon: IARC Press, 2001.
2. Harris NL, Jaffe ES, Stein H, et al. A revised European-American classification of lymphoid neoplasms: a proposal from the International Lymphoma Study Group. *Blood* 1994;84: 1361–1392.
3. LeBoit PE, McCalmont TH. Cutaneous lymphomas and leukemias. In: Elder DE, et al., eds. *Lever's histopathology of the skin,* 8th ed. Philadelphia: Lippincott-Raven Publishers, 1995: 805–846.
4. Murphy GF, Mihm MC Jr. Benign, dysplastic, and malignant lymphoid infiltrates of the skin: an approach based on pattern analysis. In: Murphy GF, Mihm Jr MC, eds., *Lymphoproliferative disorders of the skin.* Boston: Butterworths, 1986:123–138.
5. Wayner EA, Gil SG, Murphy GF, et al. Epiligrin, a component of epithelial basement membranes, is an adhesive ligand for alpha 3 beta 1 positive T lymphocytes. *J Cell Biol* 1993;121: 1141–1152.
6. Murphy GF, Liu V. The dermal immune system. In: Bos JD, ed. *The skin immune system (SIS): cutaneous immunology and clinical immunodermatology,* 2nd ed. Boca Raton, FL: CRC Press, 1997: 347–364.
7. Murphy GF. The secret of "NIN": a novel neural immunological network potentially integral to immunologic function in human skin. In: Nickoloff, BJ, ed. *Dermal immune system.* Boca Raton, FL: CRC Press, 1993:227–244.
8. Nickoloff BJ. Epidermal mucinosis in mycosis fungoides. *J Am Acad Dermatol* 1986;15:83–86.
9. Nihal M, Mikkola D, Horvath N, et al. Cutaneous lymphoid hyperplasia: a lymphoproliferative continuum with lymphomatous potential. *Hum Pathol* 2003;34:617–622.
10. Mutasim DF. Lymphomatoid drug eruption mimicking digitate dermatosis: cross reactivity between two drugs that suppress angiotensin II function. *Am J Dermatopathol* 2003;25:331–334.
11. Ploysangam T, Breneman DL, Mutasim DF. Cutaneous pseudolymphomas [Review]. *J Am Acad Dermatol* 1998;38:877–895.
12. Willemze R, Kerl H, Sterry W, et al. EORTC classification for primary cutaneous lymphomas: a proposal from the Cutaneous Lymphoma Study Group of the European Organization for Research and Treatment of Cancer [Review]. *Blood* 1997;90:354–371.
13. Rijlaarsdam JU, Toonstra J, Meijer OW, et al. Treatment of primary cutaneous B-cell lymphomas of follicle center cell origin: a clinical follow-up study of 55 patients treated with radiotherapy or polychemotherapy. *J Clin Oncol* 1996;14:549–555.
14. Isaacson PG. Gastrointestinal lymphoma. *Hum Pathol* 1994;25: 1020–1029.
15. Giannotti B, Santucci M. Skin-associated lymphoid tissue (SALT)–related B-cell lymphoma (primary cutaneous B-cell lymphoma): a concept and a clinicopathologic entity. *Arch Dermatol* 1993;129:353–355.
16. Dabski K, Banks PM, Winkelmann RK. Clinicopathologic spectrum of cutaneous manifestations in systemic follicular lymphoma. A study of 11 patients. *Cancer* 1989;64:1480–1485.
17. Garcia CF, Weiss LM, Warnke RA, et al. Cutaneous follicular lymphoma. *Am J Surg Pathol* 1986;10:454–463.
18. Bertero M, Novelli M, Fierro MT, et al. Mantle zone lymphoma: an immunohistologic study of skin lesions. *J Am Acad Dermatol* 1994;30:23–30.
19. Mann RB, Berard CW. Criteria for the cytologic subclassification of follicular lymphomas: a proposed alternative method. *Hematol Oncol* 1983;1:187–192.
20. Metter GE, Nathwani BN, Burke JS, et al. Morphological subclassification of follicular lymphoma: variability of diagnoses among hematopathologists, a collaborative study between the Repository Center and Pathology Panel for Lymphoma Clinical Studies. *J Clin Oncol* 1985;3:25–38.
21. Nathwani BN, Metter GE, Miller TP, et al. What should be the morphologic criteria for the subdivision of follicular lymphomas? *Blood* 1986;68:837–845.
22. Tilly H, Rossi A, Stamatoullas A, et al. Prognostic value of chromosomal abnormalities in follicular lymphoma. *Blood* 1994;84: 1043–1049.
23. Smolle J, Torne R, Soyer HP, et al. Immunohistochemical classification of cutaneous pseudolymphomas: delineation of distinct patterns. *J Cutan Pathol* 1990;17:149–159.
24. Torne R, Roura M, Umbert P. Generalized cutaneous B-cell pseudolymphoma. Report of a case studied by immunohistochemistry. *Am J Dermatopathol* 1989;11:544–548.
25. Iwatsuki K, Yamada M, Takigawa M, et al. Benign lymphoplasia of the earlobes induced by gold earrings: immunohistologic study on the cellular infiltrates. *J Am Acad Dermatol* 1987; 16:83–88.
26. Hovmark A, Asbrink E, Olsson I. The spirochetal etiology of lymphadenosis benigna cutis solitaria. *Acta Derm Venereol* 1986; 66:479–484.

27. Blumental G, Okun MR, Ponitch JA. Pseudolymphomatous reaction to tattoos. Report of three cases. *J Am Acad Dermatol* 1982;6:485–488.

28. Wood GS, Ngan BY, Tung R, et al. Clonal rearrangements of immunoglobulin genes and progression to B cell lymphoma in cutaneous lymphoid hyperplasia. *Am J Pathol* 1989;135:13–19.

29. Alexiou C, Kau RJ, Dietzfelbinger H, et al. Extramedullary plasmacytoma: tumor occurrence and therapeutic concepts [Comment]. *Cancer* 1999;85:2305–2314.

30. Salmon SE, Cassady JR. Plasma cell neoplasms. In: DeVita VT, Hellman S, Rosenberg S, eds. *Cancer Updates*. Philadelphia: J.B. Lippincott, 1989.

31. A clinical evaluation of the International Lymphoma Study Group classification of non-Hodgkin's lymphoma. The Non-Hodgkin's Lymphoma Classification Project. *Blood* 1997;89:3909–3918.

32. Radaszkiewicz T, Dragosics B, Bauer P. Gastrointestinal malignant lymphomas of the mucosa-associated lymphoid tissue: factors relevant to prognosis. *Gastroenterology* 1992;102:1628–1638.

33. Thieblemont C, Bastion Y, Berger F, et al. Mucosa-associated lymphoid tissue gastrointestinal and nongastrointestinal lymphoma behavior: analysis of 108 patients. *J Clin Oncol* 1997;15:1624–1630.

34. Wotherspoon AC, Ortiz-Hidalgo C, Falzon MR, et al. Helicobacter pylori-associated gastritis and primary B-cell gastric lymphoma. *Lancet* 1991;338:1175–1176.

35. Isaacson PG, Spencer J. Is gastric lymphoma an infectious disease? *Hum Pathol* 1993;24:569–570.

36. Anscombe AM, Wright DH. Primary malignant lymphoma of the thyroid—a tumour of mucosa-associated lymphoid tissue: review of seventy-six cases. *Histopathology* 1985;9:81–97.

37. Pedersen RK, Pedersen NT. Primary non-Hodgkin's lymphoma of the thyroid gland: a population based study. *Histopathology* 1996;28:25–32.

38. Shumate MJ. MALTomas of the thyroid. *Arch Intern Med* 1997;157:1765.

39. Takahashi H, Cheng J, Fujita S, et al. Primary malignant lymphoma of the salivary gland: a tumor of mucosa-associated lymphoid tissue. *J Oral Pathol Med* 1992;21:318–325.

40. Harris NL. Lymphoid proliferations of the salivary glands. *Am J Clin Pathol* 1999;111:S94–103.

41. Garbe C, Stein H, Dienemann D, et al. Borrelia burgdorferi-associated cutaneous B cell lymphoma: clinical and immunohistologic characterization of four cases. *J Am Acad Dermatol* 1991;24:584–590.

42. Cerroni L, Zochling N, Putz B, et al. Infection by Borrelia burgdorferi and cutaneous B-cell lymphoma. *J Cutan Pathol* 1997;24:457–461.

43. Goodlad JR, Davidson MM, Hollowood K, et al. Borrelia burgdorferi–associated cutaneous marginal zone lymphoma: a clinicopathological study of two cases illustrating the temporal progression of B. burgdorferi–associated B-cell proliferation in the skin. *Histopathology* 2000;37:501–508.

44. Slater DN. Borrelia burgdorferi–associated primary cutaneous B-cell lymphoma. *Histopathology* 2001;38:73–77.

45. Weng WK, Levy S. Hepatitis C virus (HCV) and lymphomagenesis. *Leuk Lymphoma* 2003;44:1113–1120.

46. Isaacson PG, Spencer J. Malignant lymphoma of mucosa-associated lymphoid tissue. *Histopathology* 1987;11:445–462.

47. Isaacson PG, Wotherspoon AC, Diss T, et al. Follicular colonization in B-cell lymphoma of mucosa-associated lymphoid tissue. *Am J Surg Pathol* 1991;15:819–828.

48. Garbe C, Stein H, Dienemann D, et al. Borrelia burgdorferi-associated cutaneous B cell lymphoma: clinical and immunohistologic characterization of four cases. *J Am Acad Dermatol* 1991;24:584–590.

49. Cerroni L, Zochling N, Putz B, et al. Infection by Borrelia burgdorferi and cutaneous B-cell lymphoma. *J Cutan Pathol* 1997;24:457–461.

50. Goodlad JR, Davidson MM, Hollowood K, et al. Borrelia burgdorferi–associated cutaneous marginal zone lymphoma: a clinicopathological study of two cases illustrating the temporal progression of B. burgdorferi–associated B-cell proliferation in the skin. *Histopathology* 2000;37:501–508.

51. Slater DN. Borrelia burgdorferi-associated primary cutaneous B-cell lymphoma. *Histopathology* 2001;38:73–77.

52. Bernard A, Murphy SB, Melvin S, et al. Non-T, non-B lymphomas are rare in childhood and associated with cutaneous tumor. *Blood* 1982;59:549–554.

53. Lin P, Jones D, Dorfman DM, et al. Precursor B-cell lymphoblastic lymphoma: a predominantly extranodal tumor with low propensity for leukemic involvement. *Am J Surg Pathol* 2000;24:1480–1490.

54. Warnke RA, Weiss LM, Chan JKC, et al. *Atlas of tumor pathology: tumors of the lymph nodes and spleen*. Washington, DC: Armed Forces Institute of Pathology, 1995.

55. Sander CA, Medeiros LJ, Abruzzo LV, et al. Lymphoblastic lymphoma presenting in cutaneous sites. A clinicopathologic analysis of six cases. *J Am Acad Dermatol* 1991;25:1023–1031.

56. Okuda T, Fisher R, Downing JR. Molecular diagnostics in pediatric acute lymphoblastic leukemia. *Mol Diagn* 1996;1:139–151.

57. Pui CH, Campana D, Crist WM. Toward a clinically useful classification of the acute leukemias. *Leukemia* 1995;9:2154–2157.

58. Raimondi SC. Current status of cytogenetic research in childhood acute lymphoblastic leukemia [Review]. *Blood* 1993;81:2237–2251.

59. Coleman MS, Greenwood MF, Hutton JJ, et al. Adenosine deaminase, terminal deoxynucleotidyl transferase (TdT), and cell surface markers in childhood acute leukemia. *Blood* 1978;52:1125–1131.

60. Drexler HG, Menon M, Minowada J. Incidence of TdT positivity in cases of leukemia and lymphoma. *Acta Haematol* 1986;75:12–17.

61. Burg G, Braun-Falco O. *Cutaneous lymphomas, pseudolymphomas and related disorders*. New York: Springer-Verlag, 1983.

62. Ben Ezra J, Burke JS, Swartz WG, et al. Small lymphocytic lymphoma: a clinicopathologic analysis of 268 cases. *Blood* 1989;73:579–587.

63. Lennert K. *Malignant lymphomas other than Hodgkin's disease*. New York: Springer-Verlag, 1978.

64. Van Der Putte SC, Toonstra J, Schuurman HJ, et al. Immunocytoma of the skin simulating lymphadenosis benigna cutis. *Arch Dermatol Res* 1985;277:36–43.

65. Cerroni L, Zenahlik P, Hofler G, et al. Specific cutaneous infiltrates of B-cell chronic lymphocytic leukemia: a clinicopathologic and prognostic study of 42 patients. *Am J Surg Pathol* 1996;20:1000–1010.

66. MacLennan IC, Liu YJ, Oldfield S, et al. The evolution of B-cell clones [Review]. *Curr Top Microbiol Immunol* 1990;159:37–63.

67. Inghirami G, Foitl DR, Sabichi A, et al. Autoantibody-associated cross-reactive idiotype-bearing human B lymphocytes: distribution and characterization, including Ig VH gene and CD5 antigen expression. *Blood* 1991;78:1503–1515.

68. Damle RN, Wasil T, Fais F, et al. Ig V gene mutation status and CD38 expression as novel prognostic indicators in chronic lymphocytic leukemia. *Blood* 94;1999:1840–1847.

69. Hamblin TJ, Orchard JA, Gardiner A, et al. Immunoglobulin V genes and CD38 expression in CLL. *Blood* 2000;95:2455–2457.

70. Chen L, Widhopf G, Huynh L, et al. Expression of ZAP-70 is associated with increased B-cell receptor signaling in chronic lymphocytic leukemia. *Blood* 2002;100:4609–4614.

71. Wiestner A, Rosenwald A, Barry TS, et al. ZAP-70 expression identifies a chronic lymphocytic leukemia subtype with unmutated immunoglobulin genes, inferior clinical outcome, and distinct gene expression profile. *Blood* 2003;101:4944–4951.

72. Crespo M, Bosch F, Villamor N, et al. ZAP-70 expression as a surrogate for immunoglobulin-variable-region mutations in chronic lymphocytic leukemia. *N Engl J Med* 2003;348:1764–1775.

73. Murashige N, Kami M, Takaue Y. ZAP-70 in chronic lymphocytic leukemia. *N Engl J Med* 2003;349:506–507.

74. Durig J, Nuckel H, Cremer M, et al. ZAP-70 expression is a prognostic factor in chronic lymphocytic leukemia. *Leukemia* 2003;17:2426–2434.

75. Wiestner A, Staudt LM. Towards molecular diagnosis and targeted therapy of lymphoid malignancies. *Semin Hematol* 2003;40:296–307.

76. Perry DA, Bast MA, Armitage JO, et al. Diffuse intermediate lymphocytic lymphoma. A clinicopathologic study and comparison with small lymphocytic lymphoma and diffuse small cleaved cell lymphoma. *Cancer* 1990;66:1995–2000.

77. Bonato M, Pittaluga S, Tierens A, et al. Lymph node histology in typical and atypical chronic lymphocytic leukemia. *Am J Surg Pathol* 1998;22:49–56.

78. Andriko JA, Swerdlow SH, Aguilera NI, Abbondanzo SL. Is lymphoplasmacytic lymphoma/immunocytoma a distinct entity? A clinicopathologic study of 20 cases. *Am J Surg Pathol* 2001;25:742–751.

79. Glass AG, Karnell LH, Menck HR. The National Cancer Data Base report on non-Hodgkin's lymphoma. *Cancer* 1997;80:2311–2320.

80. Lennert K, Stein H, Kaiserling E. Cytological and functional criteria for the classification of malignant lymphomata. *Br J Cancer* 1975;31 suppl 2:29–43.

81. Tolksdorf G, Stein H, Lennert K. Morphological and immunological definition of a malignant lymphoma derived from germinal-centre cells with cleaved nuclei (centrocytes). *Br J Cancer* 1980;41:168–182.

82. Swerdlow SH, Habeshaw JA, Murray LJ, et al. Centrocytic lymphoma: a distinct clinicopathologic and immunologic entity. A multiparameter study of 18 cases at diagnosis and relapse. *Am J Pathol* 1983;113:181–197.

83. Lardelli P, Bookman MA, Sundeen J, et al. Lymphocytic lymphoma of intermediate differentiation. Morphologic and immunophenotypic spectrum and clinical correlations. *Am J Surg Pathol* 1990;14:752–763.

84. Banks PM, Chan J, Cleary ML, et al. Mantle cell lymphoma. A proposal for unification of morphologic, immunologic, and molecular data [Comment]. *Am J Surg Pathol* 1992;16:637–640.

85. Campo E, Raffeld M, Jaffe ES. Mantle-cell lymphoma [Review]. *Semin Hematol* 1999;36:115–127.

86. Armitage JO, Weisenburger DD. New approach to classifying non–Hodgkin's lymphomas: clinical features of the major histologic subtypes. Non–Hodgkin's Lymphoma Classification Project. *J Clin Oncol* 1998;16:2780–2795.

87. Velders GA, Kluin-Nelemans JC, de Boer CJ, et al. Mantle-cell lymphoma: a population-based clinical study. *J Clin Oncol* 1996;14:1269–1274.

88. Bosch F, Lopez-Guillermo A, Campo E, et al. Mantle cell lymphoma: presenting features, response to therapy, and prognostic factors. *Cancer* 1998;82:567–575.

89. Argatoff LH, Connors JM, Klasa RJ, et al. Mantle cell lymphoma: a clinicopathologic study of 80 cases. *Blood* 1997;89:2067–2078.

90. Norton AJ, Matthews J, Pappa V, et al. Mantle cell lymphoma: natural history defined in a serially biopsied population over a 20-year period. *Ann Oncol* 1995;6:249–256.

91. Ruskone-Fourmestraux A, Delmer A, Lavergne A, et al. Multiple lymphomatous polyposis of the gastrointestinal tract: prospective clinicopathologic study of 31 cases. Groupe D'etude des Lymphomes Digestifs. *Gastroenterology* 1997;112:7–16.

92. Kumar S, Krenacs L, Otsuki T, et al. bc1–1 rearrangement and cyclin D1 protein expression in multiple lymphomatous polyposis. *Am J Clin Pathol* 1996;105:737–743.

93. O'Briain DS, Kennedy MJ, Daly PA, et al. Multiple lymphomatous polyposis of the gastrointestinal tract. A clinicopathologically distinctive form of non-Hodgkin's lymphoma of B-cell centrocytic type41. *Am J Surg Pathol* 1989;13:691–699.

94. Geerts ML, Busschots AM. Mantle-cell lymphomas of the skin. *Dermatol Clin* 1994;12:409–417.

95. Zucca E, Stein H, Coiffier B. European Lymphoma Task Force (ELTF): report of the workshop on mantle cell lymphoma (MCL). *Ann Oncol* 1994;5:507–511.

96. Fisher RI, Dahlberg S, Nathwani BN, et al. A clinical analysis of two indolent lymphoma entities: mantle cell lymphoma and marginal zone lymphoma (including the mucosa-associated lymphoid tissue and monocytoid B-cell subcategories): a Southwest Oncology Group study. *Blood* 1995;85:1075–1082.

97. Zoldan MC, Inghirami G, Masuda Y, et al. Large-cell variants of mantle cell lymphoma: cytologic characteristics and p53 anomalies may predict poor outcome. *Br J Haematol* 1996;93:475–486.

98. Zukerberg LR, Medeiros LJ, Ferry JA, et al. Diffuse low-grade B-cell lymphomas. Four clinically distinct subtypes defined by a combination of morphologic and immunophenotypic features [Comment]. *Am J Clin Pathol* 1993;100:373–385.

99. Harris NL, Nadler LM, Bhan AK. Immunohistologic characterization of two malignant lymphomas of germinal center type (centroblastic/centrocytic and centrocytic) with monoclonal antibodies. Follicular and diffuse lymphomas of small-cleaved-cell type are related but distinct entities. *Am J Pathol* 1984;117:262–272.

100. Dorfman DM, Pinkus GS. Distinction between small lymphocytic and mantle cell lymphoma by immunoreactivity for CD23. *Mod Pathol* 1994;7:326–331.

101. Kumar S, Green GA, Teruya-Feldstein J, et al. Use of CD23 (BU38) on paraffin sections in the diagnosis of small lymphocytic lymphoma and mantle cell lymphoma. *Mod Pathol* 1996;9:925–929.

102. Utz GL, Swerdlow SH. Distinction of follicular hyperplasia from follicular lymphoma in B5–fixed tissues: comparison of MT2 and bcl-2 antibodies. *Hum Pathol* 1993;24:1155–1158.

103. Kaptain S, Zukerberg LR, Ferry JA, et al. BCL-1 cyclin D1+ CD5− mantle cell lymphoma. *Mod Pathol* 1998;11:133a-

104. Geissmann F, Ruskone-Fourmestraux A, Hermine O, et al. Homing receptor alpha4beta7 integrin expression predicts digestive tract involvement in mantle cell lymphoma. *Am J Pathol* 1998;153:1701–1705.

105. Li JY, Gaillard F, Moreau A, et al. Detection of translocation t(11;14)(q13;q32) in mantle cell lymphoma by fluorescence in situ hybridization. *Am J Pathol* 1999;154:1449–1452.

106. Vaandrager JW, Schuuring E, Zwikstra E, et al. Direct visualization of dispersed 11q13 chromosomal translocations in mantle cell lymphoma by multicolor DNA fiber fluorescence in situ hybridization. *Blood* 1996;88:1177–1182.

107. Luthra R, Hai S, Pugh WC. Polymerase chain reaction detection of the t(11;14) translocation involving the bcl-1 major translocation cluster in mantle cell lymphoma. *Diagn Mol Pathol* 1995;4:4–7.

108. Oka K, Ohno T, Kita K, et al. PRAD1 gene over-expression in mantle-cell lymphoma but not in other low-grade B-cell lymphomas, including extranodal lymphoma. *Br J Haematol* 1994;86:786–791.

109. Nakamura S, Seto M, Banno S, et al. Immunohistochemical analysis of cyclin D1 protein in hematopoietic neoplasms with special reference to mantle cell lymphoma. *Jpn J Cancer Res* 1994;85:1270–1279.

110. Bosch F, Jares P, Campo E, et al. PRAD-1/cyclin D1 gene over-expression in chronic lymphoproliferative disorders: a highly specific marker of mantle cell lymphoma. *Blood* 1994;84:2726–2732.

111. Williams ME, Swerdlow SH, Meeker TC. Chromosome t(11;14)(q13;q32) breakpoints in centrocytic lymphoma are highly localized at the bcl-1 major translocation cluster. *Leukemia* 1993;7:1437–1440.

112. Schaffner C, Idler I, Stilgenbauer S, et al. Mantle cell lymphoma is characterized by inactivation of the ATM gene. *Proc Natl Acad Sci U S A* 2000;97:2773–2778.

113. Camacho E, Hernandez L, Hernandez S, et al. ATM gene inactivation in mantle cell lymphoma mainly occurs by truncating mutations and missense mutations involving the phosphatidyl-inositol-3 kinase domain and is associated with increasing numbers of chromosomal imbalances. *Blood* 2002;99:238–244.

114. Fang NY, Greiner TC, Weisenburger DD, et al. Oligonucleotide microarrays demonstrate the highest frequency of ATM mutations in the mantle cell subtype of lymphoma. *Proc Natl Acad Sci U S A* 2003;100:5372–5377.

115. Pimpinelli N, Santucci M, Bosi A, et al. Primary cutaneous follicular centre-cell lymphoma—a lymphoproliferative disease with favourable prognosis. *Clin Exp Dermatol* 1989;14:12–19.

116. Willemze R, Meijer CJ, Sentis HJ, et al. Primary cutaneous large cell lymphomas of follicular center cell origin. A clinical follow-up study of nineteen patients. *J Am Acad Dermatol* 1987;16:518–526.

117. Stein H, Lennert K, Feller AC, et al. Immunohistological analysis of human lymphoma: correlation of histological and immunological categories [Review]. *Adv Cancer Res* 1984;42:67–147.

118. Doggett RS, Wood GS, Horning S, et al. The immunologic characterization of 95 nodal and extranodal diffuse large cell lymphomas in 89 patients. *Am J Pathol* 1984;115:245–252.

119. Piris M, Brown DC, Gatter KC, et al. CD30 expression in non-Hodgkin's lymphoma. *Histopathology* 1990;17:211–218.

120. Matolcsy A, Chadburn A, Knowles DM. De novo CD5-positive and Richter's syndrome–associated diffuse large B cell lymphomas are genotypically distinct. *Am J Pathol* 1995;147:207–216.

121. Hans CP, Weisenburger DD, Greiner TC, et al. Confirmation of the molecular classification of diffuse large B-cell lymphoma by immunohistochemistry using a tissue microarray. *Blood* 2004;103:275–282.

122. Liang R, Chan WP, Kwong YL, et al. Bcl-6 gene hypermutations in diffuse large B-cell lymphoma of primary gastric origin. *Br J Haematol* 1997;99:668–670.

123. Pescarmona E, Lo CF, Pacchiarotti A, et al. Analysis of the BCL-6 gene configuration in diffuse B-cell non-Hodgkin's lymphomas and Hodgkin's disease. *J Pathol* 1995;177:21–25.

124. Flenghi L, Ye BH, Fizzotti M, et al. A specific monoclonal antibody (PG-B6) detects expression of the BCL-6 protein in germinal center B cells. *Am J Pathol* 1995;147:405–411.

125. Cattoretti G, Chang CC, Cechova K, et al. BCL-6 protein is expressed in germinal-center B cells. *Blood* 1995;86:45–53.

126. Onizuka T, Moriyama M, Yamochi T, et al. BCL-6 gene product, a 92- to 98-kD nuclear phosphoprotein, is highly expressed in germinal center B cells and their neoplastic counterparts. *Blood* 1995;86:28–37.

127. Otsuki T, Yano T, Clark HM, et al. Analysis of LAZ3 (BCL-6) status in B-cell non–Hodgkin's lymphomas: results of rearrangement and gene expression studies and a mutational analysis of coding region sequences. *Blood* 1995;85:2877–2884.

128. Ye BH, Rao PH, Chaganti RS, et al. Cloning of bcl-6:the locus involved in chromosome translocations affecting band 3q27 in B-cell lymphoma. *Cancer Res* 1993;53:2732–2735.

129. Alizadeh AA, Eisen MB, Davis RE, et al. Distinct types of diffuse large B-cell lymphoma identified by gene expression profiling. *Nature* 2000;403:503–511.

130. Dedic K, Belada D, Zak P, et al. Intravascular large B-cell lymphoma presenting as cutaneous panniculitis. *Acta Medica (Hradec Kralove)* 2003;46:121–123.

131. Asagoe K, Fujimoto W, Yoshino T, et al. Intravascular lymphomatosis of the skin as a manifestation of recurrent B-cell lymphoma. *J Am Acad Dermatol* 2003;48:S1–S4.

132. Eros N, Karolyi Z, Kovacs A, et al. Intravascular B-cell lymphoma. *J Am Acad Dermatol* 2002;47:S260–S262.

133. Yegappan S, Coupland R, Arber DA, et al. Angiotropic lymphoma: an immunophenotypically and clinically heterogeneous lymphoma. *Mod Pathol* 2001;14:1147–1156.

134. Kamath NV, Gilliam AC, Nihal M, et al. Primary cutaneous large B-cell lymphoma of the leg relapsing as cutaneous intravascular large B-cell lymphoma. *Arch Dermatol* 2001;137:1657–1658.

135. Murase T, Nakamura S. An Asian variant of intravascular lymphomatosis: an updated review of malignant histiocytosis-like B-cell lymphoma. *Leuk Lymphoma* 1999;33:459–473.

136. Chang A, Zic JA, Boyd AS. Intravascular large cell lymphoma: a patient with asymptomatic purpuric patches and a chronic clinical course. *J Am Acad Dermatol* 1998;39:318–321.

137. Ferry JA, Harris NL, Picker LJ, et al. Intravascular lymphomatosis (malignant angioendotheliomatosis): a B-cell neoplasm expressing surface homing receptors. *Mod Pathol* 1988;1:444–452.

138. Ponzoni M, Arrigoni G, Gould VE, et al. Lack of CD 29 (beta1 integrin) and CD 54 (ICAM-1) adhesion molecules in intravascular lymphomatosis. *Hum Pathol* 2000;31:220–226.

139. Murase T, Nakamura S, Tashiro K, et al. Malignant histiocytosis-like B-cell lymphoma, a distinct pathologic variant of intravascular lymphomatosis: a report of five cases and review of the literature. *Br J Haematol* 1997;99:656–664.

140. Khalidi HS, Brynes RK, Browne P, et al. Intravascular large B-cell lymphoma: the CD5 antigen is expressed by a subset of cases. *Mod Pathol* 1998;11:983–988.

141. Shimazaki C, Inaba T, Nakagawa M. B-cell lymphoma-associated hemophagocytic syndrome. *Leuk Lymphoma* 2000;38:121–130.

142. Murase T, Nakamura S, Kawauchi K, et al. An Asian variant of intravascular large B-cell lymphoma: clinical, pathological and cytogenetic approaches to diffuse large B-cell lymphoma associated with haemophagocytic syndrome. *Br J Haematol* 2000;111:826–834.

143. Shimazaki C, Inaba T, Okano A, et al. Clinical characteristics of B-cell lymphoma-associated hemophagocytic syndrome (B-LAHS): comparison of CD5+ with CD5− B-LAHS. *Intern Med* 2001;40:878–882.

144. Tokura T, Murase T, Toriyama T, et al. Asian variant of CD5+ intravascular large B-cell lymphoma with splenic infarction. *Intern Med* 2003;42:105–109.

145. Ito M, Kim Y, Choi JW, et al. Prevalence of intravascular large B-cell lymphoma with bone marrow involvement at initial presentation. *Int J Hematol* 2003;77:159–163.

146. Khoury H, Dalal BI, Nantel SH. Intravascular lymphoma presenting with bone marrow involvement and leukemic phase. *Leuk Lymphoma* 2003;44:1043–1047.

147. Theaker JM, Gatter KC, Esiri MM, et al. Neoplastic angioendotheliosis—further evidence supporting a lymphoid origin. *Histopathology* 1986;10:1261–1270.

148. Sepp N, Schuler G, Romani N, et al. "Intravascular lymphomatosis" (angioendotheliomatosis): evidence for a T-cell origin in two cases. *Hum Pathol* 1990;21:1051–1058.

149. Culhaci N, Levi E, Sen S, et al. Pulmonary lymphomatoid granulomatosis evolving to large cell lymphoma in the skin. *Pathol Oncol Res* 2002;8:280–282.

150. Beaty MW, Toro J, Sorbara L, et al. Cutaneous lymphomatoid granulomatosis: correlation of clinical and biologic features. *Am J Surg Pathol* 2001;25:1111–1120.

151. Minars N, Kay S, Escobar MR. Lymphomatoid granulomatosis of the skin. A new clinocopathologic entity. *Arch Dermatol* 1975;111:493–496.

152. Katzenstein AL, Carrington CB, Liebow AA. Lymphomatoid granulomatosis: a clinicopathologic study of 152 cases. *Cancer* 1979;43:360–373.

153. Jaffe ES, Wilson WH. Lymphomatoid granulomatosis: pathogenesis, pathology and clinical implications [Review]. *Cancer Surv* 1997;30:233–248.

154. Koss MN, Hochholzer L, Langloss JM, et al. Lymphomatoid granulomatosis: a clinicopathologic study of 42 patients. *Pathology* 1986;18:283–288.

155. McNiff JM, Cooper D, Howe G, et al. Lymphomatoid granulomatosis of the skin and lung. An angiocentric T-cell–rich B-cell lymphoproliferative disorder. *Arch Dermatol* 1996;132:1464–1470.

156. Teruya-Feldstein J, Jaffe ES, Burd PR, et al. The role of Mig, the monokine induced by interferon-gamma, and IP-10, the interferon-gamma-inducible protein-10, in tissue necrosis and vascular damage associated with Epstein–Barr virus–positive lymphoproliferative disease. *Blood* 1997;90:4099–4105.

157. Jambrosic J, From L, Assaad DA, et al. Lymphomatoid granulomatosis. *J Am Acad Dermatol* 1987;17:621–631.

158. Chan JK, Ng CS, Ngan KC, et al. Angiocentric T-cell lymphoma of the skin. An aggressive lymphoma distinct from mycosis fungoides. *Am J Surg Pathol* 1988;12:861–876.

159. Fujiwara Y, Abe Y, Kuyama M, et al. CD8+ cutaneous T-cell lymphoma with pagetoid epidermotropism and angiocentric and angiodestructive infiltration. *Arch Dermatol* 1990;126:801–804.

160. Guinee DG Jr, Perkins SL, Travis WD, et al. Proliferation and cellular phenotype in lymphomatoid granulomatosis: implications of a higher proliferation index in B cells. *Am J Surg Pathol* 1998;22:1093–1100.

161. Wilson WH, Kingma DW, Raffeld M, et al. Association of lymphomatoid granulomatosis with Epstein–Barr viral infection of B lymphocytes and response to interferon-alpha 2b. *Blood* 1996;87:4531–4537.

162. Sordillo PP, Epremian B, Koziner B, et al. Lymphomatoid granulomatosis: an analysis of clinical and immunologic characteristics. *Cancer* 1982;49:2070–2076.

163. Jaffe ES, Chan JK, Su IJ, et al. Report of the Workshop on Nasal and Related Extranodal Angiocentric T/Natural Killer Cell Lymphomas. Definitions, differential diagnosis, and epidemiology. *Am J Surg Pathol* 1996;20:103–111.

164. Pagliaro JA, White SI. Specific skin lesions occurring in a patient with Hodgkin's lymphoma. *Australas J Dermatol* 1999;40:41–43.

165. Miazga-Janusz R, Kluz Z, Szczepaniak AM, et al. Nonspecific skin changes as early manifestation of Hodgkin's disease. *Wiad Lek* 1993;46:514–517.

166. Hayes TG, Rabin VR, Rosen T, et al. Hodgkin's disease presenting in the skin: case report and review of the literature. *J Am Acad Dermatol* 1990;22:944–947.

167. O'Bryan-Tear CG, Burke M, Coulson IH, et al. Hodgkin's disease presenting in the skin. *Clin Exp Dermatol* 1987;12:69–71.

168. Smith JL Jr, Butler JJ. Skin involvement in Hodgkin's disease. *Cancer* 1980;45:354–361.

169. Jones WC. Primary (extranodal) Hodgkin's disease of the skin. *Br J Clin Pract* 1974;28:209–211.

170. Kanzler H, Kuppers R, Hansmann ML, et al. Hodgkin and Reed–Sternberg cells in Hodgkin's disease represent the outgrowth of a dominant tumor clone derived from (crippled) germinal center B cells. *J Exp Med* 1996;184:1495–1505.

171. Marafioti T, Hummel M, Foss HD, et al. Hodgkin and reed-sternberg cells represent an expansion of a single clone originating from a germinal center B-cell with functional immunoglobulin gene rearrangements but defective immunoglobulin transcription. *Blood* 2000;95:1443–1450.

172. Schwarting R, Gerdes J, Durkop H, et al. BER-H2: a new anti-Ki-1 (CD30) monoclonal antibody directed at a formol-resistant epitope. *Blood* 1989;74:1678–1689.

173. Stein H, Marafioti T, Foss HD, et al. Down-regulation of BOB.1/OBF.1 and Oct2 in classical Hodgkin disease but not in lymphocyte predominant Hodgkin disease correlates with immunoglobulin transcription. *Blood* 2001;97:496–501.

174. Re D, Muschen M, Ahmadi T, et al. Oct-2 and Bob-1 deficiency in Hodgkin and Reed Sternberg cells. *Cancer Res* 2001;61:2080–2084.

175. Steimle-Grauer SA, Tinguely M, Seada L, et al. Expression patterns of transcription factors in progressively transformed germinal centers and Hodgkin lymphoma. *Virchows Arch* 2003;442:284–293.

176. Browne P, Petrosyan K, Hernandez A, et al. The B-cell transcription factors BSAP, Oct-2, and BOB.1 and the pan-B-cell markers CD20, CD22, and CD79a are useful in the differential diagnosis of classic Hodgkin lymphoma. *Am J Clin Pathol* 2003;120:767–777.

177. Krenacs L, Himmelmann AW, Quintanilla-Martinez L, et al. Transcription factor B-cell-specific activator protein (BSAP) is differentially expressed in B cells and in subsets of B-cell lymphomas. *Blood* 1998;92:1308–1316.

178. Foss HD, Reusch R, Demel G, et al. Frequent expression of the B-cell–specific activator protein in Reed–Sternberg cells of classical Hodgkin's disease provides further evidence for its B-cell origin. *Blood* 1999;94:3108–3113.

179. Torlakovic E, Torlakovic G, Nguyen PL, et al. The value of anti-pax-5 immunostaining in routinely fixed and paraffin-embedded sections: a novel pan pre-B and B-cell marker. *Am J Surg Pathol* 2002;26:1343–1350.

180. Schwering I, Brauninger A, Klein U, et al. Loss of the B-lineage–specific gene expression program in Hodgkin and Reed–Sternberg cells of Hodgkin lymphoma. *Blood* 2003;101:1505–1512.

181. Hummel M, Anagnostopoulos I, Dallenbach F, et al. EBV infection patterns in Hodgkin's disease and normal lymphoid tissue: expression and cellular localization of EBV gene products. *Br J Haematol* 1992;82:689–694.

182. Stein H, Herbst H, Anagnostopoulos I, et al. The nature of Hodgkin and Reed–Sternberg cells, their association with EBV, and their relationship to anaplastic large-cell lymphoma. *Ann Oncol* 1991;2 Suppl 2:33–38.

183. Wu TC, Mann RB, Charache P, et al. Detection of EBV gene expression in Reed–Sternberg cells of Hodgkin's disease. *Int J Cancer* 1990;46:801–804.

184. Anagnostopoulos I, Herbst H, Niedobitek G, et al. Demonstration of monoclonal EBV genomes in Hodgkin's disease and Ki-1–positive anaplastic large cell lymphoma by combined Southern blot and in situ hybridization. *Blood* 1989;74:810–816.

185. Hsu SM, Waldron JW Jr, Hsu PL, et al. Cytokines in malignant lymphomas: review and prospective evaluation. *Hum Pathol* 1993;24:1040–1057.

186. Tesch H, Feller AC, Jucker M, et al. Activation of cytokines in Hodgkin's disease. *Ann Oncol* 1992;3 Suppl 4:13–16.

187. Muller H, Takeshita M, Krause J, et al. Immunohistochemical in situ demonstration of cytokines in Hodgkin and non-Hodgkin lymphoma. *Verh Dtsch Ges Pathol* 1992;76:164–168.

188. Klein S, Jucker M, Diehl V, et al. Production of multiple cytokines by Hodgkin's disease derived cell lines. *Hematol Oncol* 1992;10:319–329.

189. LeBoit PE. Lymphomatoid papulosis and cutaneous CD30+ lymphoma. *Am J Dermatopathol* 1996;18:221–235.

190. Burkert KL, Huhn K, Menezes DW, et al. Langerhans cell microgranulomas (pseudo-pautrier abscesses): morphologic diversity, diagnostic implications and pathogenetic mechanisms. *J Cutan Pathol* 2002;29:511–516.

191. Brady SP, Magro CM, Diaz-Cano SJ, et al. Analysis of clonality of atypical cutaneous lymphoid infiltrates associated with drug therapy by PCR/DGGE. *Hum Pathol* 1999;30:130–136.

192. Magro CM, Crowson AN, Kovatich AJ, et al. Drug-induced reversible lymphoid dyscrasia: a clonal lymphomatoid dermatitis of memory and activated T cells. *Hum Pathol* 2003;34:119–129.

193. Kim YH, Hoppe RT. Mycosis fungoides and the Sézary syndrome. *Semin Oncol* 1999;26:276–289.

194. van Doorn R, Van Haselen CW, Voorst Vader PC, et al. Mycosis fungoides: disease evolution and prognosis of 309 Dutch patients. *Arch Dermatol* 2000;136:504–510.

195. Vergier B, De Muret A, Beylot-Barry M, et al. Transformation of mycosis fungoides: clinicopathological and prognostic features of 45 cases. French Study Group of Cutaneous Lymphomas. *Blood* 2000;95:2212–2218.

196. Diamandidou E, Colome-Grimmer M, Fayad L, et al. Transformation of mycosis fungoides/Sézary syndrome: clinical characteristics and prognosis. *Blood* 1998;92:1150–1159.

197. Jacobs MA, Kocher W, Murphy GF Combined folliculotropic/syringotropic cutaneous T-cell lymphoma without epidermal involvement: report of 2 cases and pathogenic implications. *Hum Pathol* 2003;34:1216–1220.

198. Gibson LE, Muller SA, Leiferman KM, et al. Follicular mucinosis: clinical and histopathologic study. *J Am Acad Dermatol* 1989;20:441–446.

199. Haghighi B, Smoller BR, LeBoit PE, et al. Pagetoid reticulosis (Woringer–Kolopp disease): an immunophenotypic, molecular, and clinicopathologic study. *Mod Pathol* 2000;13:502–510.

200. LeBoit PE. Granulomatous slack skin. *Dermatol Clin* 1994;12:375–389.

201. Shapiro PE, Pinto FJ. The histologic spectrum of mycosis fungoides/Sézary syndrome (cutaneous T-cell lymphoma). A review of 222 biopsies, including newly described patterns and the earliest pathologic changes. *Am J Surg Pathol* 1994;18:645–667.

202. Ralfkiaer E. Immunohistological markers for the diagnosis of cutaneous lymphomas. *Semin Diagn Pathol* 1991;8:62–72.

203. Munn SE, McGregor JM, Jones A, et al. Clinical and pathological heterogeneity in cutaneous gamma-delta T-cell lymphoma: a report of three cases and a review of the literature. *Br J Dermatol* 1996;135:976–981.

204. Vermeer MH, Geelen FA, Kummer JA, et al. Expression of cytotoxic proteins by neoplastic T cells in mycosis fungoides increases with progression from plaque stage to tumor stage disease. *Am J Pathol* 1999;154:1203–1210.

205. Russell-Jones R, Whittaker S. T-cell receptor gene analysis in the diagnosis of Sézary syndrome. *J Am Acad Dermatol* 1999;41:254–259.

206. McCarty MJ, Vukelja SJ, Sausville EA, et al. Lymphomatoid papulosis associated with Ki-1–positive anaplastic large cell lymphoma. A report of two cases and a review of the literature [Review]. 23 *Cancer* 1994;74:3051–3058.

207. Chott A, Vonderheid EC, Olbricht S, et al. The dominant T cell clone is present in multiple regressing skin lesions and associated T cell lymphomas of patients with lymphomatoid papulosis. *J Invest Dermatol* 1996;106:696–700.

208. Bekkenk MW, Geelen FA, Voorst Vader PC, et al. Primary and secondary cutaneous CD30(+) lymphoproliferative disorders: a report from the Dutch Cutaneous Lymphoma Group on the long-term follow-up data of 219 patients and guidelines for diagnosis and treatment. *Blood* 2000;95:3653–3661.

209. Kummer JA, Vermeer MH, Dukers D, et al. Most primary cutaneous CD30-positive lymphoproliferative disorders have a CD4-positive cytotoxic T-cell phenotype. *J Invest Dermatol* 1997;109:636–640.

210. Boulland ML, Wechsler J, Bagot M, et al. Primary CD30-positive cutaneous T-cell lymphomas and lymphomatoid papulosis frequently express cytotoxic proteins. *Histopathology* 2000;36:136–144.

211. Kumar S, Krenacs L, Medeiros J, et al. Subcutaneous panniculitic T-cell lymphoma is a tumor of cytotoxic T lymphocytes. *Hum Pathol* 1998;29:397–403.

212. Gonzalez CL, Medeiros LJ, Braziel RM, et al. T-cell lymphoma involving subcutaneous tissue. A clinicopathologic entity commonly associated with hemophagocytic syndrome. *Am J Surg Pathol* 1991;15:17–27.

213. Arnulf B, Copie-Bergman C, Delfau-Larue MH, et al. Nonhepatosplenic gammadelta T-cell lymphoma: a subset of cytotoxic lymphomas with mucosal or skin localization. *Blood* 1998;91:1723–1731.

214. Kaplan MA, Jacobson JO, Ferry JA, et al. T-cell lymphoma of the vulva in a renal allograft recipient with associated hemophagocytosis. *Am J Surg Pathol* 1993;17:842–849.

215. Salhany KE, Macon WR, Choi JK, et al. Subcutaneous panniculitis-like T-cell lymphoma: clinicopathologic, immunophenotypic, and genotypic analysis of alpha/beta and gamma/delta subtypes. *Am J Surg Pathol* 1998;22:881–893.

216. Koizumi K, Sawada K, Nishio M, et al. Effective high-dose chemotherapy followed by autologous peripheral blood stem cell transplantation in a patient with the aggressive form of cytophagic histiocytic panniculitis. *Bone Marrow Transplant* 1997;20:171–173.

217. Jaffe ES, Krenacs L, Kumar S, et al. Extranodal peripheral T-cell and NK-cell neoplasms [Review]. 82 *Am J Clin Pathol* 1999;111:S46–S55.

218. Ascani S, Zinzani PL, Gherlinzoni F, et al. Peripheral T-cell lymphomas. Clinico-pathologic study of 168 cases diagnosed according to the R.E.A.L. Classification. *Ann Oncol* 1997;8:583–592.

219. Gisselbrecht C, Gaulard P, Lepage E, et al. Prognostic significance of T-cell phenotype in aggressive non-Hodgkin's lymphomas. Groupe d'Etudes des Lymphomes de l'Adulte (GELA). *Blood* 1998;92:76–82.

220. Lopez-Guillermo A, Cid J, Salar A, et al. Peripheral T-cell lymphomas: initial features, natural history, and prognostic factors in a series of 174 patients diagnosed according to the R.E.A.L. Classification. *Ann Oncol* 1998;9:849–855.

221. Roundtree JM, Burgdorf W, Harkey MR. Cutaneous involvement in Lennert's lymphoma. *Arch Dermatol* 1980;116:1291–1294.

222. Suchi T, Lennert K, Tu LY, et al. Histopathology and immunohistochemistry of peripheral T cell lymphomas: a proposal for their classification [Review]. *J Clin Pathol* 1987;40:995–1015.

223. Braverman IM. Cutaneous T-cell lymphoma. *Curr Prob Dermatol* 1991;3–184.

224. Hastrup N, Ralfkiaer E, Pallesen G. Aberrant phenotypes in peripheral T cell lymphomas. *J Clin Pathol* 1989;42:398–402.

225. Pinkus GS, O'Hara CJ, Said JW. Peripheral/post-thymic T-cell lymphomas: a spectrum of disease. Clinical, pathologic,

and immunologic features of 78 cases. *Cancer* 1990;65:971–998.

226. Greiner TC, Raffeld M, Lutz C, et al. Analysis of T cell receptor-gamma gene rearrangements by denaturing gradient gel electrophoresis of GC-clamped polymerase chain reaction products. Correlation with tumor-specific sequences. *Am J Pathol* 1995;146:46–55.

227. Schlegelberger B, Himmler A, Godde E, et al. Cytogenetic findings in peripheral T-cell lymphomas as a basis for distinguishing low-grade and high-grade lymphomas. *Blood* 1994;83:505–511.

228. Boulland ML, Kanavaros P, Wechsler J, et al. Cytotoxic protein expression in natural killer cell lymphomas and in alpha beta and gamma delta peripheral T-cell lymphomas. *J Pathol* 1997;183:432–439.

229. Chan AC, Ho JW, Chiang AK, et al. Phenotypic and cytotoxic characteristics of peripheral T-cell and NK-cell lymphomas in relation to Epstein–Barr virus association. *Histopathology* 1999;34:16–24.

230. Krenacs L, Wellmann A, Sorbara L, et al. Cytotoxic cell antigen expression in anaplastic large cell lymphomas of T- and null-cell type and Hodgkin's disease: evidence for distinct cellular origin. *Blood* 1997;89:980–989.

231. Foss HD, Anagnostopoulos I, Araujo I, et al. Anaplastic large-cell lymphomas of T-cell and null-cell phenotype express cytotoxic molecules. *Blood* 1996;88:4005–4011.

232. Felgar RE, Macon WR, Kinney MC, et al. TIA-1 expression in lymphoid neoplasms. Identification of subsets with cytotoxic T lymphocyte or natural killer cell differentiation. *Am J Pathol* 1997;150:1893–1900.

233. Kern WF, Spier CM, Hanneman EH, et al. Neural cell adhesion molecule-positive peripheral T-cell lymphoma: a rare variant with a propensity for unusual sites of involvement. *Blood* 1992;79:2432–2437.

234. Quintanilla-Martinez L, Fend F, Moguel LR, et al. Peripheral T-cell lymphoma with Reed–Sternberg-like cells of B-cell phenotype and genotype associated with Epstein–Barr virus infection. *Am J Surg Pathol* 1999;23:1233–1240.

235. Stein H, Mason DY, Gerdes J, et al. The expression of the Hodgkin's disease associated antigen Ki-1 in reactive and neoplastic lymphoid tissue: evidence that Reed–Sternberg cells and histiocytic malignancies are derived from activated lymphoid cells. *Blood* 1985;66:848–858.

236. Brugieres L, Deley MC, Pacquement H, et al. CD30(+) anaplastic large-cell lymphoma in children: analysis of 82 patients enrolled in two consecutive studies of the French Society of Pediatric Oncology. *Blood* 1998;92:3591–3598.

237. Delsol G, al Saati T, Gatter KC, et al. Coexpression of epithelial membrane antigen (EMA), Ki-1, and interleukin-2 receptor by anaplastic large cell lymphomas. Diagnostic value in so-called malignant histiocytosis. *Am J Pathol* 1988;130:59–70.

238. Chan JK, Buchanan R, Fletcher CD. Sarcomatoid variant of anaplastic large-cell Ki-1 lymphoma [Comment]. *Am J Surg Pathol* 1990;14:983–988.

239. Kinney MC, Collins RD, Greer JP, et al. A small-cell-predominant variant of primary Ki-1 (CD30)+ T-cell lymphoma. *Am J Surg Pathol* 1993;17:859–868.

240. Pileri SA, Pulford K, Mori S, et al. Frequent expression of the NPM-ALK chimeric fusion protein in anaplastic large-cell lymphoma, lympho-histiocytic type. *Am J Pathol* 1997;150:1207–1211.

241. Benharroch D, Meguerian-Bedoyan Z, Lamant L, et al. ALK-positive lymphoma: a single disease with a broad spectrum of morphology. *Blood* 1998;91:2076–2084.

242. Jaffe ES. Post-thymic T-cell lymphomas. In: Jaffe ES, ed. *Surgical pathology of the lymph nodes and related organs*, 2nd ed. Philadelphia: WB Saunders, 1995:360.

243. Jaffe ES. Malignant histiocytosis and true histiocytic lymphomas. In: *Surgical pathology of lymph nodes and related organs*, 2nd ed. Philadelphia: WB Saunders, 1995:560–593.

244. Chan JK, Ng CS, Ngan KC, et al. Angiocentric T-cell lymphoma of the skin. An aggressive lymphoma distinct from mycosis fungoides. *Am J Surg Pathol* 1988;12:861–876.

245. Tsai TF, Su IJ, Lu YC, et al. Cutaneous angiocentric T-cell lymphoma associated with Epstein–Barr virus. *J Am Acad Dermatol* 1992;26:31–38.

246. Kanavaros P, Lescs MC, Briere J, et al. Nasal T-cell lymphoma: a clinicopathologic entity associated with peculiar phenotype and with Epstein–Barr virus. *Blood* 1993;81:2688–2695.

247. Santucci M, Pimpinelli N, Massi D, et al. Cytotoxic/natural killer cell cutaneous lymphomas. Report of EORTC Cutaneous Lymphoma Task Force Workshop. *Cancer* 2003;97:610–627.

248. Chan JK. Natural killer cell neoplasms [Review]. *Anat Pathol* 1998;3:77–145.

249. Nakamura S, Suchi T, Koshikawa T, et al. Clinicopathologic study of CD56 (NCAM)-positive angiocentric lymphoma occurring in sites other than the upper and lower respiratory tract [Comment]. *Am J Surg Pathol* 1995;19:284–296.

250. Chan JK, Sin VC, Wong KF, et al. Nonnasal lymphoma expressing the natural killer cell marker CD56: a clinicopathologic study of 49 cases of an uncommon aggressive neoplasm. *Blood* 1997;89:4501–4513.

251. Kwong YL, Chan AC, Liang R, et al. CD56+ NK lymphomas: clinicopathological features and prognosis. *Br J Haematol* 1997;97:821–829.

252. Suzumiya J, Takeshita M, Kimura N, et al. Sinonasal malignant lymphoma of natural killer cell phenotype associated with diffuse pancreatic involvement. *Leuk Lymphoma* 1993;10:231–236.

253. Tomita Y, Ohsawa M, Qiu K, et al. Epstein–Barr virus in lymphoproliferative diseases in the sino-nasal region: close association with CD56+ immunophenotype and polymorphic-reticulosis morphology. *Int J Cancer* 1997;70:9–13.

254. Petrella T, Delfau-Larue MH, Caillot D, et al. Nasopharyngeal lymphomas: further evidence for a natural killer cell origin. *Hum Pathol* 1996;27:827–833.

255. Chan JK, Ng CS, Lau WH, et al. Most nasal/nasopharyngeal lymphomas are peripheral T-cell neoplasms. *Am J Surg Pathol* 1987;11:418–429; erratum, *Am J Surg Pathol* 1987;11:742.

256. Cheung MM, Chan JK, Lau WH, et al. Primary non-Hodgkin's lymphoma of the nose and nasopharynx: clinical features, tumor immunophenotype, and treatment outcome in 113 patients. *J Clin Oncol* 1998;16:70–77.

257. Wong KF, Chan JK, Ng CS, et al. CD56 (NKH1)-positive hematolymphoid malignancies: an aggressive neoplasm featuring frequent cutaneous/mucosal involvement, cytoplasmic azurophilic granules, and angiocentricity. *Hum Pathol* 1992;23:798–804.

258. Agnello V, Chung RT, Kaplan LM. A role for hepatitis C virus infection in type II cryoglobulinemia. *N Engl J Med* 1992;327:1490–1495.

259. Chan JK, Tsang WY, Ng CS. Clarification of CD3 immunoreactivity in nasal T/natural killer cell lymphomas: the neoplastic cells are often CD3 epsilon+. *Blood* 1996;87:839–841.

260. Jaffe ES. Nasal and nasal-type T/NK cell lymphoma: a unique form of lymphoma associated with the Epstein–Barr virus [Comment]. *Histopathology* 1995;27:581–583.

261. Chan JK, Yip TT, Tsang WY, et al. Detection of Epstein–Barr viral RNA in malignant lymphomas of the upper aerodigestive tract [Review]. *Am J Surg Pathol* 1994;18:938–946; erratum, *Am J Surg Pathol* 1994;18:1274.

262. Arber DA, Weiss LM, Albujar PF, et al. Nasal lymphomas in Peru. High incidence of T-cell immunophenotype and Epstein–Barr virus infection [Comment]. *Am J Surg Pathol* 1993;17:392–399.

263. Elenitoba-Johnson KS, Zarate-Osorno A, Meneses A, et al. Cytotoxic granular protein expression, Epstein–Barr virus strain type, and latent membrane protein-1 oncogene deletions in nasal T-lymphocyte/natural killer cell lymphomas from Mexico. *Mod Pathol* 1998;11:754–761.

264. van Gorp J, Weiping L, Jacobse K, et al. Epstein–Barr virus in nasal T-cell lymphomas (polymorphic reticulosis/midline malignant reticulosis) in western China. *J Pathol* 1994;173:81–87.

265. Kanavaros P, Lescs MC, Briere J, et al. Nasal T-cell lymphoma: a clinicopathologic entity associated with peculiar phenotype and with Epstein–Barr virus. *Blood* 1993;81:2688–2695.

266. Quintanilla-Martinez L, Franklin JL, Guerrero I, et al. Histological and immunophenotypic profile of nasal NK/T cell lymphomas from Peru: high prevalence of p53 overexpression. *Hum Pathol* 1999;30:849–855.

267. Broder S, Bunn PA Jr, Jaffe ES, et al. NIH conference: T-cell lymphoproliferative syndrome associated with human T-cell leukemia/lymphoma virus [Review]. *Ann Intern Med* 1984;100: 543–557.

268. Yamaguchi K. Human T-lymphotropic virus type I in Japan. *Lancet* 1994;343:213–216.

269. Yamamura M, Yamada Y, Momita S, et al. Circulating interleukin-6 levels are elevated in adult T-cell leukaemia/lymphoma patients and correlate with adverse clinical features and survival. *Br J Haematol* 1998;100:129–134.

270. Manabe T, Hirokawa M, Sugihara K, et al. Angiocentric and angiodestructive infiltration of adult T-cell leukemia/lymphoma (ATLL) in the skin. Report of two cases. *Am J Dermatopathol* 1988;10:487–496.

271. Takeshita M, Akamatsu M, Ohshima K, et al. CD30 (Ki-1) expression in adult T-cell leukaemia/lymphoma is associated with distinctive immunohistological and clinical characteristics. *Histopathology* 1995;26:539–546.

272. Ohshima K, Suzumiya J, Sato K, et al. Nodal T-cell lymphoma in an HTLV-I-endemic area: proviral HTLV-I DNA, histological classification and clinical evaluation. *Br J Haematol* 1998; 101:703–711.

273. Ohshima K, Mukai Y, Shiraki H, et al. Clonal integration and expression of human T-cell lymphotropic virus type I in carriers detected by polymerase chain reaction and inverse PCR. *Am J Hematol* 1997;54:306–312.

274. Liu B, Liang MH, Kuo YL, et al. Human T-lymphotropic virus type 1 oncoprotein tax promotes unscheduled degradation of Pds1p/securin and Clb2p/cyclin B1 and causes chromosomal instability. *Mol Cell Biol* 2003;23:5269–5281.

275. Wieselthier JS, Koh HK. Sézary syndrome: diagnosis, prognosis, and critical review of treatment options. *J Am Acad Dermatol* 1990;22:381–401.

276. Gessain A, Moulonguet I, Flageul B, et al. Cutaneous type of adult T cell leukemia/lymphoma in a French West Indian woman. Clonal rearrangement of T-cell receptor beta and gamma genes and monoclonal integration of HTLV-I proviral DNA in the skin infiltrate. *J Am Acad Dermatol* 1990;23: 994–1000.

277. Murphy SB. Childhood non-Hodgkin's lymphoma. *N Engl J Med* 1978;299:1446–1448.

278. Quintanilla-Martinez L, Zukerberg LR, Harris NL. Prethymic adult lymphoblastic lymphoma. A clinicopathologic and immunohistochemical analysis. *Am J Surg Pathol* 1992;16:1075–1084.

279. Matutes E, Brito-Babapulle V, Swansbury J, et al. Clinical and laboratory features of 78 cases of T-prolymphocytic leukemia. *Blood* 1991;78:3269–3274.

280. Matutes E, Crockard AD, O'Brien M, et al. Ultrastructural cytochemistry of chronic T-cell leukaemias. A study with four acid hydrolases. *Histochem J* 1983;15:895–909.

281. Pawson R, Matutes E, Brito-Babapulle V, et al. Sézary cell leukaemia: a distinct T cell disorder or a variant form of T prolymphocytic leukemia? *Leukemia* 1997;11:1009–1013.

282. Matutes E, Crockard AD, O'Brien M, et al. Ultrastructural cytochemistry of chronic T-cell leukaemias. A study with four acid hydrolases. *Histochem J* 1983;15:895–909.

283. Brito-Babapulle V, Catovsky D. Inversions and tandem translocations involving chromosome 14q11 and 14q32 in T-prolymphocytic leukemia and T-cell leukemias in patients with ataxia telangiectasia. *Cancer Genet Cytogenet* 1991;55: 1–9.

284. Maljaei SH, Brito-Babapulle V, Hiorns LR, et al. Abnormalities of chromosomes 8:11:14, and X in T-prolymphocytic leukemia studied by fluorescence in situ hybridization. *Cancer Genet Cytogenet* 1998;103:110–116.

285. Koita H, Suzumiya J, Ohshima K, et al. Lymphoblastic lymphoma expressing natural killer cell phenotype with involvement of the mediastinum and nasal cavity. *Am J Surg Pathol* 1997;21:242–248.

286. Tamura H, Ogata K, Mori S, et al. Lymphoblastic lymphoma of natural killer cell origin, presenting as pancreatic tumour. *Histopathology* 1998;32:508–511.

287. Petrella T, Dalac S, Maynadie M, et al. CD4+ CD56+ cutaneous neoplasms: a distinct hematological entity? Groupe Francais d'Etude des Lymphomes Cutanes (GFELC). *Am J Surg Pathol* 1999;23:137–146.

288. Petrella T, Comeau MR, Maynadie M, et al. "Agranular CD4+ CD56+ hematodermic neoplasm" (blastic NK-cell lymphoma) originates from a population of CD56+ precursor cells related to plasmacytoid monocytes. *Am J Surg Pathol* 2002;26:852–862.

289. Kazakov DV, Mentzel T, Burg G, et al. Blastic natural killer-cell lymphoma of the skin associated with myelodysplastic syndrome or myelogenous leukaemia: a coincidence or more? *Br J Dermatol* 2003;149:869–876.

290. Falcao RP, Garcia AB, Marques MG, et al. Blastic CD4 NK cell leukemia/lymphoma: a distinct clinical entity. *Leuk Res* 2002; 26:803–807.

291. Bayerl MG, Rakozy CK, Mohamed AN, et al. Blastic natural killer cell lymphoma/leukemia: a report of seven cases. *Am J Clin Pathol* 2002;117:41–50.

292. Alvarez-Larran A, Villamor N, Hernandez-Boluda JC, et al. Blastic natural killer cell leukemia/lymphoma presenting as overt leukemia. *Clin Lymphoma* 2001;2:178–182.

293. DiGiuseppe JA, Louie DC, Williams JE, et al. Blastic natural killer cell leukemia/lymphoma: a clinicopathologic study. *Am J Surg Pathol* 1997;21:1223–1230.

294. Brody JP, Allen S, Schulman P, et al. Acute agranular CD4–positive natural killer cell leukemia. Comprehensive clinicopathologic studies including virologic and in vitro culture with inducing agents. *Cancer* 1995;75:2474–2483.

295. Ko YH, Kim SH, Ree HJ. Blastic NK-cell lymphoma expressing terminal deoxynucleotidyl transferase with Homer–Wright type pseudorosettes formation. *Histopathology* 1998;33:547–553.

296. Matano S, Nakamura S, Nakamura S, et al. Monomorphic agranular natural killer cell lymphoma/leukemia with no Epstein–Barr virus association. *Acta Haematol* 1999;101:206–208.

297. Su WP, Buechner SA, Li CY. Clinicopathologic correlations in leukemia cutis. *J Am Acad Dermatol* 1984;11:121–128.

TUMORS OF FIBROUS TISSUE INVOLVING THE SKIN

PETER J. HEENAN

BENIGN FIBROUS HISTIOCYTOMA (DERMATOFIBROMA)

Benign fibrous histiocytoma (BFH) has also been known as dermatofibroma, histiocytoma, and sclerosing hemangioma. These common tumors occur usually on the extremities of young adults, although they may arise elsewhere as firm, indolent single nodules; they are seen only rarely on the palms and soles (1). The occurrence of multiple tumors has been reported in patients receiving immunosuppressive therapy (2), in pregnancy (3), in patients with HIV infection (4), and after antiretroviral therapy (5). Although they are usually only a few millimeters in diameter, they occasionally measure 2 to 3 cm; most lesions are red, but they may be reddish-brown because of hyperpigmentation of the overlying skin or, rarely, blue-black due to large amounts of hemosiderin within the tumor. In the latter case, the clinical appearance may resemble malignant melanoma. The cut surface of the lesions varies in color from white to yellowish brown, depending on the proportions of fibrous tissue, lipid, and hemosiderin present (Fig. 32-1A). BFH usually persists indefinitely, although spontaneous involution has been observed (6).

Histopathology. The epidermis is usually hyperplastic, with hyperpigmentation of the basal layer and elongation of the rete ridges, separated by a clear (Grenz) zone from the tumor in the dermis (Fig. 32-1B), which is composed of fibroblast-like spindle cells, histiocytes, and blood vessels in varying proportions (Fig. 32-1C). Foamy histiocytes and multinucleate giant cells containing lipid or hemosiderin may be present, sometimes in large numbers, forming xanthomatous aggregates. Capillaries may be plentiful in the stroma, giving the lesion an angiomatous component; when associated with a sclerotic stroma, such lesions have been referred to as "sclerosing hemangioma." In some small lesions the spindle cells are distributed singly between the collagen bundles, forming a zone of subtly increased cellularity, whereas in larger tumors there is much denser cellularity and the spindle cells are arranged in sheets or interlocking strands in storiform pattern. The

dermal tumor is poorly demarcated on both sides, so that the fibroblasts and the young basophilic collagen extend between the mature, eosinophilic collagen bundles of the dermis and surround them, thus trapping normal collagen bundles at the periphery of the tumor nodule.

Pronounced hyperplasia of the overlying epidermis occurs in more than 80% of BFH (7), and is helpful in making the diagnosis and in distinguishing the atypical variant from atypical fibroxanthoma (8). Most commonly the hyperplasia consists of regular elongation of the rete ridges, which may be associated with hyperpigmentation of the basal layer. In some cases, the epidermal hyperplasia is reminiscent of seborrheic keratosis through the interlacing of thickened rete ridges. Occasionally, downgrowths are present that imitate the hair matrix to the point of having a connective tissue papilla (9). In 2% to 5% of the lesions, the downgrowths are indistinguishable from those of superficial basal cell carcinoma (10). Although the proliferations in most of these cases are regarded as similar to basal cell carcinoma, in rare instances a truly invasive basal cell carcinoma associated with ulceration develops (11,12).

VARIANTS OF BENIGN FIBROUS HISTIOCYTOMA

Cellular Benign Fibrous Histiocytoma

This is a very densely cellular tumor with fascicular and storiform growth patterns and frequent extension into the subcutis (Fig. 32-2A and B), sharing some features, therefore, with dermatofibrosarcoma protuberans (DFSP), which is discussed further below (13,14). Immunohistochemical features that may be helpful in making this distinction are listed in Table 32-1.

Aneurysmal Benign Fibrous Histiocytoma

In these tumors, collections of capillaries, foci of hemorrhage, siderophages, and foamy macrophages surround

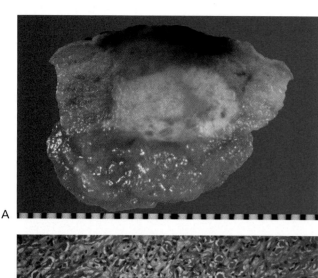

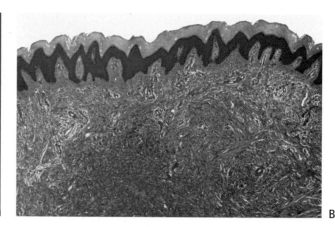

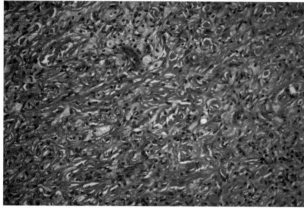

FIGURE 32-1. Benign fibrous histiocytoma (dermatofibroma). **A:** Gross specimen. A circumscribed nodular lesion with a yellow cut surface is present in the dermis. The epidermis shows brownish pigmentation and is separated from the underlying tumor by a clear zone. **B:** The epidermis is hyperplastic and separated by a narrow clear zone from a moderately cellular spindle cell tumor extending into the deep dermis. **C:** The tumor is composed of plump spindle cells with pale eosinophilic cytoplasm in a collagenous stroma, as well as groups of histiocytes with pale cytoplasm.

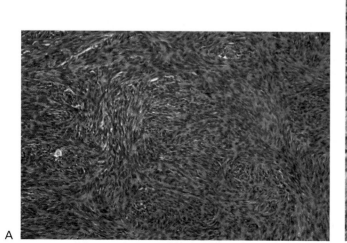

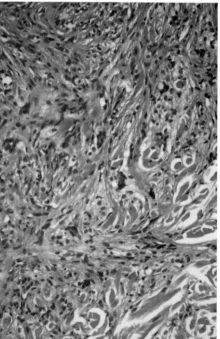

FIGURE 32-2. Cellular benign fibrous histiocytoma (dermatofibroma). **A:** The tumor consists of spindle cells arranged in densely cellular fascicular and storiform patterns. **B:** At the border of the lesion, the spindle cells surround individual collagen bundles.

TABLE 32-1. SUGGESTED IMMUNOHISTOCHEMICAL REACTIONS AS AN AID TO DIFFERENTIAL DIAGNOSIS OF CUTANEOUS SPINDLE CELL TUMORS

	Epithelioid Sarcoma	Atypical Fibroxanthoma	Dermatofibrosarcoma Protuberans	Cellular Benign Fibrous Histiocytoma	Spindle Cell Squamous Carcinoma	Desmoplastic Melanoma	Leiomyosarcoma
Cytokeratin	+	−	−	−	+	−	V
Vimentin	+	+	+	+	R	+	+
S100	−	−	−	−	−	+	R
Desmin	R	R	−	−	−	−	+
CD34	V	V	+	V	−	−	−
Factor XIIIa	−	V	V	+	−	−	−
Epithelial membrane antigen	+	−	−	−	−	−	−
Smooth muscle actin	V	V	V	V	−	V	+

This table is limited to reagents in common use. It is emphasized that the immunohistochemical reactions should be regarded as adjuncts to routine histologic methods.
V, variable; R, rare; U, unknown.

cleft-like and cavernous blood-filled spaces in the center of the tumor, simulating a vascular neoplasm but otherwise showing typical features of benign fibrous histiocytoma (15,16) (Fig. 32-3A and B).

Atypical Benign Fibrous Histiocytoma

Atypical cells are occasionally present in BFH and may lead to misdiagnosis as atypical fibroxanthoma, which may represent a dermal variant of malignant fibrous histiocytoma. Such lesions have been referred to as "atypical cutaneous fibrous histiocytoma" (8,17). They usually are less than 1.2 cm in diameter but occasionally are as large as 2.5 cm (18). The pseudomalignant changes may consist of scattered, strikingly atypical cells with an extremely large nucleus, referred to as monster cells (18,19), or there

may be marked focal cellular atypia with only a few normal mitoses. The atypical cells may also consist of multinucleate giant cells that possess bizarre, large, hyperchromatic nuclei with little cytoplasm or irregular, vesicular nuclei with abundant foamy cytoplasm (8) (Fig. 32-4A and B).

A recent study of atypical fibrous histiocytoma emphasized the presence of atypical cells with bizarre pleomorphic nuclei against a background of typical BFH (20). Some cases were larger (>2 cm in diameter), extended into the superficial subcutis, and contained zones of necrosis. Variable staining for smooth muscle actin and CD34 was present but no cases expressed factor XIIIa. Similar to cellular and aneurysmal BFH, atypical fibrous histiocytoma showed a higher tendency than common BFH to local recurrence and, in rare instances, metastasized (20).

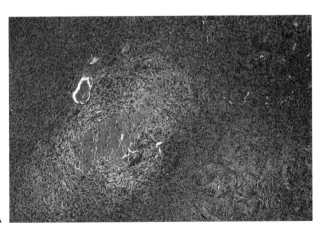

A

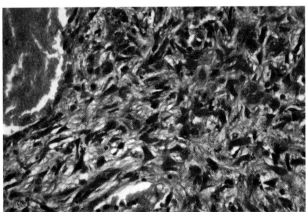

B

FIGURE 32-3. Aneurysmal benign fibrous histiocytoma (dermatofibroma). **A:** Central congested, dilated blood vessels and hemorrhage are surrounded by plump spindle cells. **B:** Spindle cells and siderophages are adjacent to blood-filled spaces.

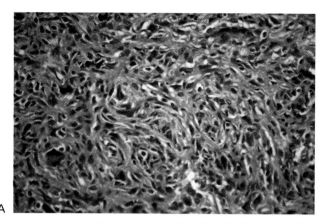
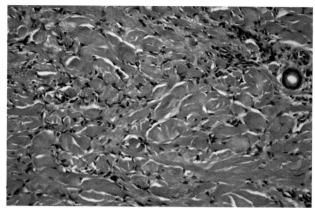

FIGURE 32-4. Atypical benign fibrous histiocytoma (dermatofibroma). **A:** This variant includes spindle cells, epithelioid cells, and giant cells with large, pleomorphic nuclei. **B:** At the border of this tumor, the cells are arranged around individual collagen bundles in the pattern typical of benign fibrous histiocytoma.

Epithelioid Benign Fibrous Histiocytoma

This distinctive variant, originally described as epithelioid cell histiocytoma (21), is composed of epithelioid cells with abundant eosinophilic cytoplasm, giant cells, foamy macrophages, and spindle cells forming an exophytic nodule or polypoid tumor with an epidermal collarette resembling pyogenic granuloma and intradermal Spitz nevus (22,23) (Fig. 32-5A and B).

Deep Benign Fibrous Histiocytoma

This is a rare form that develops entirely within subcutaneous tissue, deep soft tissue or in parenchymal organs (24). Unlike the cutaneous BFH, deep BFH tend to be well circumscribed with a pseudocapsule and foci of hemorrhage, and consist of monomorphic spindle cells resembling the cellular variant (25). Other less common variants that have been described include clear cell (26), granular

cell (27), lipidized (28), myxoid (29), myofibroblastic (30), osteoclastic (31), keloidal (32), atrophic (33), and palisading forms (34).

Neoplasm versus Reactive Process

The view has been expressed that BFH are not true neoplasms but reactive fibroblastic proliferation subsequent to trauma, including arthropod bites. These tumors have been referred to as "nodular subepidermal fibrosis" (35), and are regarded by some authorities as fibrosing inflammatory lesions, even in the presence of "monster cells" (18,36). The demonstration of clonality in some cases of dermatofibroma (37,38) and reports of metastasizing cellular dermatofibroma (39,40) suggest a neoplastic nature.

An analysis of HUMARA (androgen receptor gene) in BFH concluded that this lesion is a heterogeneous process in which the histiocytoid cells express a monoclonal genotype, whereas the fibroblastic cells may represent either re-

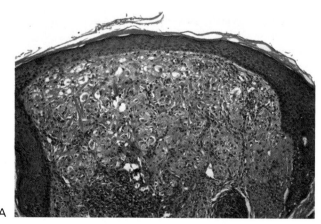
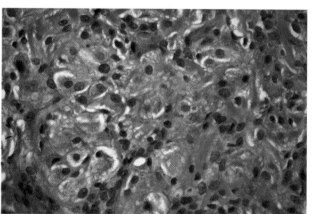

FIGURE 32-5. Epithelioid benign fibrous histiocytoma (dermatofibroma). **A:** The lesion is a small sharply circumscribed nodule with an epidermal collarette. **B:** Sheets of epithelioid histiocytes with eosinophilic cytoplasm.

active proliferation or a true neoplasm whose neoplastic cell type has been obscured by a prominent reactive fibroblastic component (41).

Hyperplasia of Epidermis

The hyperplasia of the epidermis overlying BFH has been attributed to stimulation by young collagen and abundant ground substance in the subepidermal dermis in a fashion similar to that of embryonic mesenchyme, causing the formation of immature hair structures (9) and even of primary epithelial germs (42) resembling basal cell carcinoma (10).

More recently, it has been proposed that mediators produced by BFH, including epidermal growth factor, may induce hair follicle formation and epidermal hyperplasia (43–45). The theory of induction of epidermal proliferation by the dermal fibrohistiocytic process has been further reinforced by a study that interpreted the varied expression of epidermal growth factor receptor, metallothionein, Ki-67 and keratins 1, 6, and 14 in simple hyperplasia of the epidermis as suggesting that the dermal process may trigger the induction of simple hyperplastic epidermis and then mediate both the abnormal keratinocyte differentiation and the transformation of simple hyperplastic epidermis to basaloid hyperplastic epidermis through the evolution of the dermal lesions (45).

Histogenesis. Dermatofibroma was originally described as fibroma simplex by Unna in 1894 (46), but subsequent studies showing that some dermatofibromas contain macrophages led to the introduction of the term *histiocytoma* (47,48). It became common practice, however, to refer to those tumors composed predominantly of collagen fibers and fibroblast-like spindle cells as *dermatofibromas*, and to tumors containing a larger component of histiocyte-like cells as *histiocytomas*.

More recent enzyme histochemical, electron microscopic, and immunohistochemical studies have indicated variously that these tumors demonstrate histiocytic, myofibroblastic, and fibroblastic differentiation and are probably of primitive mesenchymal origin (49). The term *benign fibrous histiocytoma* is now used as a general designation for this varied group of spindle cell neoplasms (49).

The alternative term *dermal dendrocytoma* has also been suggested for BFH on the basis of immunohistochemical studies using antibodies to factor XIIIa and MAC387 (50). Most cells in these tumors were found to react with factor XIIIa, whereas only a few were MAC387 positive. Factor XIIIa labels the normal dermal population of fixed connective tissue cells, or fibroblasts, also termed "dermal dendrocytes" because of their characteristic dendritic processes (51). MAC387, on the other hand, is expressed by monocyte-derived macrophages. Other investigators, however, believe that the factor XIIIa–positive cells seen in BFH represent reactive stromal cells rather than the true tumor cells (49,52), which often express vimentin and smooth muscle actin (52).

Electron Microscopy. Reports of electron microscopic studies have variously described the cells of benign fibrous histiocytoma as fibroblasts (53), histiocytes (54), and myofibroblasts (55).

Enzyme Histochemistry. The results of enzymic studies on BFH have also yielded varied results. Positive staining for lysozyme and α_1-antitrypsin have been interpreted as indicating histiocytic differentiation (56,57), whereas negative results for these enzymes have led to the speculation that both the fibroblastic and histiocyte-like cells in these tumors arise from primitive mesenchymal cells (58). The presence of HLA-DR antigens in the majority of cells in BFH has also been regarded as evidence in favor of histiocytic origin (59).

Differential Diagnosis. The cellular variant of BFH, frequently showing a storiform growth pattern and extending into the subcutis, shares these features with dermatofibrosarcoma protuberans (DFSP), from which it is distinguished by the overlying epidermal hyperplasia, polymorphism of the tumor cells and extension of tumor cells at the edge of the lesion to surround individual hyalinized collagen bundles (60). Cellular BFH also extends into the cutis along the interlobular septa or in a bulging, expansile pattern, rather than in the characteristic infiltrating honeycomb-like pattern of DFSP (14). DFSP is usually a much larger lesion at the time of diagnosis, often consisting of multiple nodules. Cellular BFH may also be confused with leiomyosarcoma which has plumper spindle cells with eosinophilic cytoplasm and nuclei with rounded ends, and shows positive staining for desmin and alpha smooth muscle actin (49) (Table 32-1).

Although previously CD34 expression was thought to offer strong support for the diagnosis of DFSP as against cellular BFH, it has recently been shown that some dermatofibromas express CD34 and some DFSP express factor XIIIa (61), suggesting a biologic spectrum between BFH and DFSP with coexistence of two different cell populations in these indeterminate lesions (62). Tenascin (an extracellular matrix glycoprotein) expression has been demonstrated immunohistochemically at the dermo–epidermal junction overlying BFH, but not DFSP, thus providing a new aid in the distinction between BFH and DFSP, perhaps compensating to some extent for the overlap in expression of CD34 and factor XIIIa (63,64).

Aneurysmal BFH may be confused with neoplasms of vascular origin and angiomatoid malignant fibrous histiocytoma. Benign and malignant angiomatous tumors are characterized by the formation of vascular structures lined by endothelial cells that stain positively for factor VIII, CD31, and CD34. Nodular Kaposi sarcoma, in particular, demonstrates slit-like spaces containing erythrocytes and a monomorphic CD34 positive spindle cell population (49). Aneurysmal BFH is distinguished from angiomatoid malignant fibrous histiocytoma by the presence in the latter tumor of eosinophilic histiocytoid cells, a prominent lymphocytic infiltrate and a thick pseudocapsule (65), and its presentation in a younger age group, occasionally with systemic symptoms, usually in a subcutaneous location (66).

The histologic features of epithelioid BFH resemble those of Spitz nevus and pyogenic granuloma. Epithelioid BFH differs from pyogenic granuloma in its greater density of epithelioid cells between blood vessels that are not arranged in lobules, with a less prominent inflammatory component and lack of protuberant endothelial cells (24). Intradermal Spitz nevus has a nested pattern in its superficial layers, spindle cells as well as epithelioid cells, intranuclear cytoplasmic invaginations, desmoplastic stroma, maturation in the deeper layers, and Kamino bodies are frequently present in the epidermis. Immunostaining of Spitz nevi is usually positive for S-100 protein and Melan A/MART 1, but negative for factor XIIIa.

Atypical fibroxanthoma differs from atypical BFH in its location on the sun-exposed skin of elderly patients, usually the head and neck, frequent ulceration, severe cellular pleomorphism and frequent mitoses, including bizarre forms, and the lack of a background of more typical BFH.

DERMATOFIBROSARCOMA PROTUBERANS

Dermatofibrosarcoma protuberans (DFSP) is a slowly growing dermal spindle cell neoplasm of intermediate malignancy that usually forms an indurated plaque on which multiple reddish purple, firm nodules subsequently arise, sometimes with ulceration (Fig. 32-6A). The tumors occur most frequently on the trunk or the proximal extremities of young adults and only rarely in the head and neck (67,68). A small proportion of cases have been reported in childhood and, rarely, as congenital lesions (69–71). Local recurrence is common but metastasis is rare (72,73).

Histopathology. DFSP is composed of densely packed, monomorphous, plump spindle cells arranged in a storiform (mat-like) pattern in the central areas of tumor nodules, whereas at the periphery there is diffuse infiltration of the dermal stroma, frequently extending into the subcutis and producing a characteristic honeycomb pattern (14) (Fig. 32-6B, C, and D). Infiltration into the underlying fascia and muscle is a late event (73). Lateral extension of irregular strands of spindle cells into the dermal stroma is

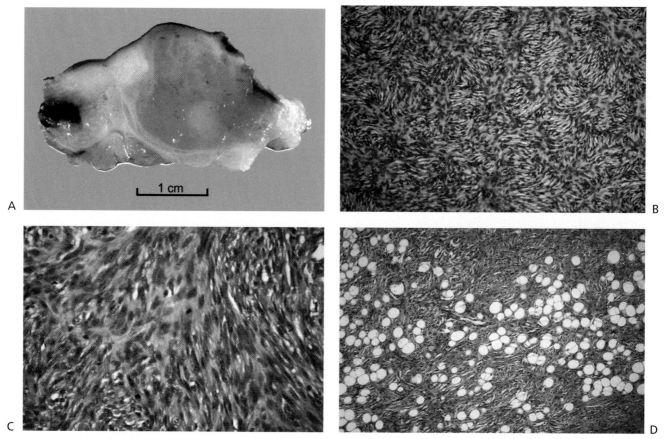

FIGURE 32-6. Dermatofibrosarcoma protuberans. **A:** Gross specimen of a myxoid variant of dermatofibrosarcoma protuberans forming a central nodule extending into the subcutis, with lateral extension in the dermis of a component of firmer white tissue. **B:** Densely packed spindle cells arranged in a storiform pattern. **C:** Uniform, plump spindle cells with scattered mitoses. **D:** Diffuse infiltration of the subcutis producing a honeycomb-like pattern.

often pronounced, where the peripheral elements of the tumor may have a deceptively bland appearance, approaching that of normal collagen. This can cause difficulty in determining the true extent of the tumor and may result in recurrence after presumed adequate resection.

Myxoid areas, sometimes resembling liposarcoma, include a characteristic vascular component of slit-like anastomosing thin-walled blood vessels presenting a crow's foot or chicken wire appearance (74) (Fig. 32-7A and B). Melanin-containing cells may be present in a small proportion of tumors, so-called Bednar tumor (pigmented DFSP, storiform neurofibroma) (75–77).

Fibrosarcomatous areas are seen in a small proportion of DFSP, characterized by a fascicular or herringbone growth pattern (78–80). This variant does not appear to have any greater propensity for local recurrence, which is related to the adequacy of primary surgical excision (80).

Giant cells are seen in a small proportion of otherwise typical DFSP. The histologic resemblance between giant cell fibroblastoma and DFSP, and recurrences of DFSP showing features of giant cell fibroblastoma, and vice versa, suggests that giant cell fibroblastoma is a juvenile variant of DFSP (81–86).

Histogenesis. On the basis of electron microscopic findings, the tumor cells have been regarded as fibroblasts, because they show active synthesis of collagen in a well-developed endoplasmic reticulum (87,88). In some tumors the presence of interrupted basement membrane–like material along the cell membrane has indicated that the cells are modified fibroblasts possessing features of perineural and endoneural cells (89). Immunohistochemical studies have suggested fibroblastic (90) or myofibroblastic (91) differentiation, but the expression of CD34 (human progenitor cell antigen) by DFSP has also been interpreted as supporting the view that these neoplasms are variants of nerve sheath tumors (92). Although DFSP is commonly regarded as a fibrohistiocytic tumor, the immunohistochemical and ultrastructural evidence suggests that fibroblastic origin is most likely (74,93) (Table 32-1).

Differential Diagnosis. DFSP shares common features with other dermal spindle cell neoplasms, but it is characterized by the uniformity of the spindle cells and a more prominent storiform pattern than is associated with benign or malignant fibrous histiocytoma. Superficial biopsies contribute to the difficulty in distinguishing between DFSP, benign fibrous histiocytoma (BFH), and diffuse neurofibroma. In contrast with cellular BFH, the epidermis overlying DFSP is usually attenuated or ulcerated rather than hyperplastic, and a clear zone between the epidermis and tumor may not be present (Fig. 32-8). DFSP is more densely cellular and monomorphic, with a more prominent storiform pattern, and the extension into the subcutis presents either the classic honeycomb-like pattern or a multilayered pattern, in contrast with the well-demarcated bulging deep margin of

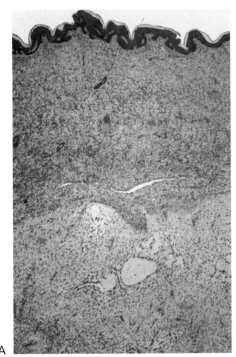
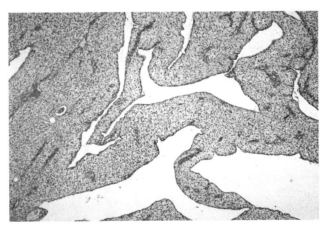

A

B

FIGURE 32-7. Myxoid dermatofibrosarcoma protuberans. **A:** This example of dermatofibrosarcoma protuberans has a myxoid component in the deeper dermis. **B:** Blood vessels in myxoid dermatofibrosarcoma protuberans producing a characteristic "crow's foot" or "chicken-wire" pattern.

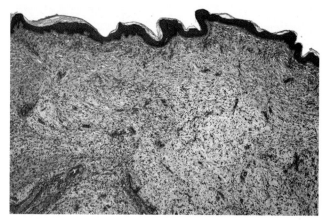

FIGURE 32-8. Dermatofibrosarcoma protuberans. The epidermis is not hyperplastic, and there is no Grenz zone between the epidermis and the underlying dermatofibrosarcoma protuberans.

cellular BFH, which may also extend into the subcutis, predominantly along the septa (14,60). Although immunostaining for CD34 is usually positive in DFSP and negative in most cellular BFH (92,94,95) (Fig. 32-9, Table 32-1), there is some overlap of expression of CD34 in BFH and DFSP (62). The expression of tenascin at the dermo–epidermal junction overlying BFH but not DFSP may help in the distinction between these tumors (63,64). The use of other immunohistochemical markers such as CD44 and hyaluronate (HA) may also prove useful in the distinction between BFH and DFSP according to a recent study which showed that BFH expressed CD44 strongly with only faint stromal HA, whereas in DFSP there was significantly reduced or absent CD44 and strong stromal HA deposition (96). Neurofibroma expresses S-100 protein, which is absent in DFSP, and it also has other histologic features of neural differentiation, without the dense, uniform cellularity of DFSP.

GIANT CELL FIBROBLASTOMA

Giant cell fibroblastoma (GCF), first described by Shmookler and Enzinger in 1982 (97), is a rare benign tumor occurring almost exclusively in children as a solitary dermal or subcutaneous nodule, most often on the back, thigh, or chest wall. Local recurrence following incomplete excision is common (98) but no metastases have been reported (99).

Histopathology. The dermal and subcutaneous nodules are composed of poorly circumscribed, loosely structured collections of pleomorphic spindle cells in a collagenous or myxoid stroma (Fig. 32-10A). Distinctive multinucleated giant cells line cleft-like, angiectid spaces (Fig. 32-10B). The apparently multiple nuclei of the giant cells have been shown by electron microscopy to represent multiple sausage-like lobations of a single nucleus (81). In the more solid, spindle-cell areas of the tumor, appearances resemble DFSP.

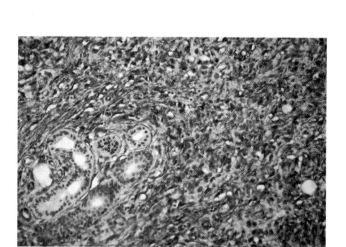

FIGURE 32-9. Dermatofibrosarcoma protuberans. Positive immunostaining for CD34.

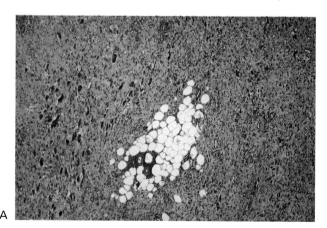

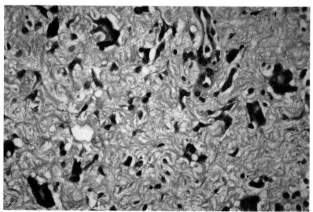

FIGURE 32-10. Giant cell fibroblastoma. **A:** The growth pattern resembles that of dermatofibrosarcoma protuberans with infiltration of subcutaneous fat by uniform spindle cells, with the additional feature of scattered giant cells. (Courtesy of Dr. Inara Strungs, Adelaide Children's Hospital, and Dr. P. W. Allen.) **B:** Spindle cells and numerous giant cells with mainly single, pleomorphic, multilobated nuclei.

Histogenesis. Ultrastructurally, the cells resemble fibroblasts. Immunohistochemical studies have shown that the tumors express vimentin but not S-100 protein or vascular markers, and positive immunostaining for CD34 has been demonstrated (100). The histologic similarity to DFSP, emphasized by reports of tumors sharing common features of both types and recorded cases in which recurrence of either DFSP or GCF has presented features of the other tumor, all suggest that GCF may be the juvenile counterpart of DFSP (81–86). Recent studies demonstrating GCF-like areas in further cases of DFSP, the expression of CD34 and the demonstration of the gene fusion transcripts COL 1A1-PDGFB from the T (17;22) (Q22; Q13) translocation in both tumors, have provided further evidence for a close relationship between these tumors (101,102). GCF with a Bednar tumor (pigmented dermatofibrosarcoma protuberans) component has also been reported (103,104).

DESMOID-TYPE FIBROMATOSIS (AGGRESSIVE FIBROMATOSIS, DESMOID TUMOR, AND MUSCULOAPONEUROTIC FIBROMATOSIS)

Desmoid-type fibromatoses are benign clonal fibroblastic proliferations that arise as firm nontender masses from muscular aponeuroses and tend to invade the muscle; this infiltrative growth pattern predisposes to local recurrence, but the lesions do not metastasize. Their rate of growth is slow, but the lesions may attain considerable size, as large as 25 cm in diameter (105). Although usually solitary, they may be multiple (106). Desmoid fibromatoses may occur in children but they are seen mainly in young adults, particularly in women, the most common type arising from the rectus abdominis muscle following pregnancy. The lesions also occur as extra-abdominal masses in older adults in equal gender distribution (107).

In addition, desmoid fibromatoses occur in Gardner syndrome, mainly as mesenteric masses. Inactivation of the APC (adenomatous polyposis coli) gene occurs in desmoid-type fibromatosis in patients with familial polyposis and less commonly in sporadic lesions (108). Trisomies for chromosomes 8 and/or 20 have been demonstrated in some cell subpopulations (109,110).

Histopathology. Desmoid fibromatoses are composed of poorly circumscribed bundles of uniform spindle cells surrounded by abundant collagen that may include keloid-like areas, hyalinization, and myxoid change (Fig. 32-11A). The nuclei are small, regular, and pale staining with a variable mitotic rate. The lesions frequently infiltrate adjacent striated muscle, entrapping degenerate muscle fibers (105) (Fig. 32-11B and C).

Histogenesis. Ultrastructurally, the spindle cells of desmoid fibromatosis show the features of fibroblasts or myo-

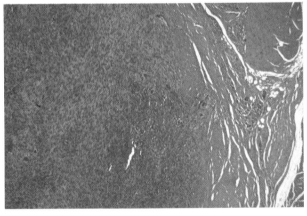

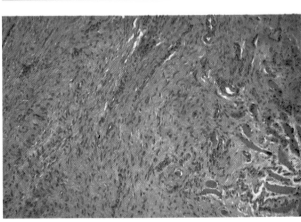

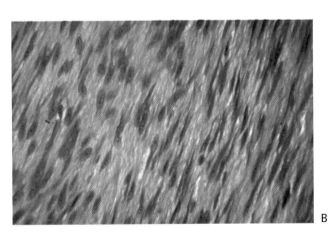

FIGURE 32-11. Desmoid type fibromatosis (desmoid tumor). **A:** A mass composed of dense bundles of eosinophilic spindle cells is present within striated muscle. **B:** The tumor cells are monomorphous, with regular nuclei and pale cytoplasm; there are no mitoses or giant cells. **C:** In this area, the spindle cells are more dispersed and infiltrate the striated muscle, isolating degenerate segments of muscle fibers.

fibroblasts (106,111,112). Immunostaining is strongly positive for vimentin, and variable for smooth muscle actin and muscle-specific actin (113).

PLEXIFORM FIBROHISTIOCYTIC TUMOR

Plexiform fibrohistiocytic tumor is a rare multinodular neoplasm of the dermis and subcutis, composed of histiocyte-like cells, fibroblasts, and, usually, multinucleate giant cells in a plexiform pattern (114). This distinctive lesion occurs as a slowly growing mass, usually involving the upper extremity of children and young adults, more often in females. Local recurrence is common; small numbers of regional lymph node and visceral metastases have also been recorded (115).

Histopathology. Nodules of histiocytes and osteoclast-like giant cells are surrounded by fascicles of spindle cells intersecting the stroma in a plexiform pattern (Fig. 32-12). Cases without osteoclast-like giant cells or with only few of these cells have also been described (116–118).

Histogenesis. Ultrastructural and immunocytochemical studies have indicated histiocytic and myofibroblastic differentiation (115,119).

Differential Diagnosis. Cellular benign fibrous histiocytoma and dermatomyofibroma do not have the distinctive nodules of histiocytic-like cells of plexiform fibrohistiocytic tumor, whereas fibromatosis and nodular fasciitis are usually more deeply situated and lack the characteristic plexiform growth pattern. Fibrous hamartoma of infancy has no histiocytic nodules or giant cells (116).

DERMATOMYOFIBROMA

Dermatomyofibroma (120)—also called plaque-like dermal fibromatosis (121)—is a benign, dermal plaque-like proliferation of fibroblasts and myofibroblasts, occurring mainly in young adults, more commonly in the shoulder region of females, but also in children, especially on the posterior neck of prepubescent males (122).

Histopathology. Uniform spindle cells in elongated and intersecting fascicles arranged mainly parallel to the epidermal surface form a well-circumscribed plaque in the reticular dermis and may extend into the upper subcutis (120, 123) (Fig. 32-13A and B).

Histogenesis. Immunohistochemical reactivity for vimentin and nonspecific muscle actin and the ultrastructural features suggest myofibroblastic differentiation (120,123–125).

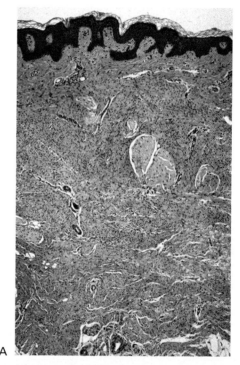

A

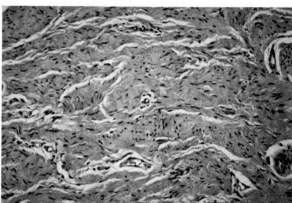

B

FIGURE 32-13. Dermatomyofibroma. **A:** The epidermis shows elongation of the rete ridges, which overlie a plaque of increased cellularity extending into the reticular dermis, surrounding but not replacing appendages. **B:** The plaque is composed of uniform spindle cells with eosinophilic cytoplasm arranged parallel to the epidermal surface.

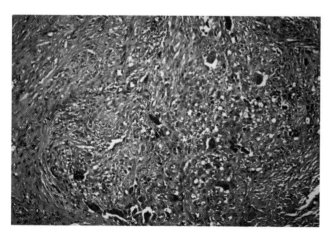

FIGURE 32-12. Plexiform fibrohistiocytic tumor. Epithelioid and osteoclast-like giant cells are surrounded by fascicles of spindle cells in a plexiform pattern.

Differential Diagnosis. The orientation parallel to the epidermis of monomorphic spindle cells and their location in the reticular dermis and upper subcutis are points of distinction from benign fibrous histiocytoma, and dermatomyofibroma does not express factor XIIIa or CD34 (123,124).

MALIGNANT FIBROUS HISTIOCYTOMA

Malignant fibrous histiocytoma (MFH) is a pleomorphic sarcoma that is the most common soft tissue sarcoma of middle and late adulthood (126); rare cases have also been reported in childhood (127,128). The most common sites of origin are the proximal extremities, particularly the thigh and buttock (126,129). The tumors are multilobular fleshy masses, often apparently circumscribed on gross examination, although the microscopic growth pattern is frequently infiltrative along fascial planes and between muscle fibers, accounting for the high rate of local recurrence. Involvement of the dermis, occasionally with ulceration, is rare (130); most tumors occur in striated muscle, less than 10% being confined to the subcutis. The risk of metastasis is related to tumor size, depth, and grade (126). The rates of local recurrence and metastasis have improved in the more recent studies, probably because of more effective primary surgical therapy. An overall survival rate of 50%, local recurrence rate of 25%, and a metastatic rate of 34% have been reported (131).

Histopathology. MFH is a highly cellular, pleomorphic tumor composed of fibroblast-like spindle cells, histiocyte-like cells, foam cells, and giant cells. Mitotic figures, including atypical forms, are plentiful (132,133). Four subtypes are recognized:

Storiform-pleomorphic (126,134)
Myxoid (myxofibrosarcoma) (135,136)
Giant cell (malignant giant cell tumor of soft parts) (137)
Inflammatory (xanthosarcoma, malignant xanthogranuloma) (138)

Angiomatoid fibrous histiocytoma, formerly regarded as another subtype of malignant fibrous histiocytoma (139), has been reclassified as a fibrohistiocytic tumor of intermediate grade (140) on the basis of its excellent prognosis (66,141).

The most common variant is the storiform-pleomorphic type, composed of spindle cells, plump histiocyte-like cells, and pleomorphic multinucleate giant cells. The spindle cells are arranged in whorled or storiform pattern, with a delicate collagenous stroma. Tumors containing a high proportion of relatively uniform spindle cells in a storiform pattern may resemble DFSP, whereas other tumors are anaplastic. The myxoid variant shows marked myxoid change in the stroma and more cellular foci of pleomorphic type. The giant cell variant contains osteoclast-like giant cells with abundant cytoplasm and numerous vesicular nuclei of uniform size (142). The inflammatory variant is characterized by a dense infiltrate of neutrophils and numerous xanthoma cells, as seen in fibroxanthosarcoma (138).

Histogenesis. It was originally assumed that MFH was composed of malignant histiocytes capable of acting as facultative fibroblasts (143). Electron microscopic studies indicated that the progenitor cell in MFH is a mesenchymal cell capable of both histiocytic and fibroblastic differentiation (132,144). Some tumors demonstrating the light microscopic criteria for malignant MFH, however, also express intermediate filaments including keratin (145–147). It has also been suggested that pleomorphic MFH may not be a distinct entity, but rather a collection of mesenchymal and nonmesenchymal tumors in which a large proportion could be reclassified more specifically on the basis of careful examination of extensively sampled material, immunohistochemistry, and electron microscopy (148,149). The diagnosis of pleomorphic MFH, therefore, is now reserved for a small group of undifferentiated pleomorphic sarcomas showing no definable line of differentiation (150). Immunohistochemistry has demonstrated that many high-grade pleomorphic sarcomas that might previously have been diagnosed as MFH are, in fact, leiomyosarcoma, liposarcoma, rhabdomyosarcoma, or myxofibrosarcoma (149). Cytogenetic aberrations have been detected in many cases but are difficult to evaluate because of the changing diagnostic criteria over time (151).

Atypical fibroxanthoma is histologically indistinguishable from pleomorphic MFH, its almost invariably benign course being attributed to its superficial location in the dermis (152). Lesions reported as metastasizing atypical fibroxanthoma are regarded by other authorities as MFH on the basis of their deep invasion, necrosis, or vascular invasion (152).

ANGIOMATOID FIBROUS HISTIOCYTOMA

This tumor was previously termed *angiomatoid malignant fibrous histiocytoma* (139). In recognition of the relatively good prognosis of this distinctive neoplasm of children and young adults (66), however, the term *malignant* has been deleted from the title (140). The tumor occurs most often on the extremities as a slowly growing nodular or cystic mass of the dermis or subcutis, sometimes associated with systemic symptoms, including anemia, pyrexia, and weight loss, and less often with local pain and tenderness.

Histopathology. The tumors characteristically include hemorrhagic cystic pseudoangiomatous structures, multinodular proliferation of eosinophilic histiocytoid or myoid cells, and an infiltrate of lymphocytes and plasma cells (141). The lymphoid tissue may include follicles with germinal centers and a thick pseudocapsule, thus resembling lymph node architecture. The hemorrhagic cystic structures are lined by flattened tumor cells rather than endothelium.

Histogenesis. Immunohistochemical studies have produced conflicting results with regard to histiocytic differentiation (65,153). The expression of desmin in some cases has been interpreted as evidence of myoid or myofibroblastic differentiation (65,141).

ATYPICAL FIBROXANTHOMA (PSEUDOSARCOMA AND PARADOXICAL FIBROSARCOMA)

Atypical fibroxanthoma (AFX) is a pleomorphic spindle cell neoplasm of the dermis that, despite apparently malignant histologic features, usually follows an indolent or locally aggressive course. It is a fairly common tumor, first described in 1963 (154), and interpreted as a benign reactive lesion (155,156). Because a small number of metastases have been reported, AFX has become regarded as a neoplasm of low-grade malignancy related to malignant fibrous histiocytoma, from which it is indistinguishable histologically (157,158). According to this view, the more favorable prognosis of AFX is related to its small size and superficial location (158,159). The specificity of pleomorphic malignant fibrous histiocytoma as an entity, its relationship with AFX, and the precise nature of cases of AFX reported to have metastasized (160,161) have been questioned (49,149,162,163). AFX usually presents as a solitary nodule less than 2 cm in diameter on the exposed skin of the head and neck or dorsum of the hand of elderly patients, often with a short history of rapid growth. The lesions are usually associated with severe actinic damage, and a few have arisen in areas treated by radiation. Several cases described on the trunk and extremities of younger persons

(164,165) may have represented cases of atypical benign fibrous histiocytoma (166).

Histopathology. AFX is an exophytic, densely cellular neoplasm, unencapsulated but with only limited infiltration of the stroma, frequently bounded by an epidermal collarette (Fig. 32-14A). The tumor may extend to the dermoepidermal junction, but there is no direct continuity with the squamous epithelium, although ulceration is often present. Severe solar elastosis is present in the adjacent dermis. The classical tumor is composed of pleomorphic histiocyte-like cells and atypical giant cells, often with bizarre nuclei and numerous mitotic figures, including abnormal forms (156,158,164) (Fig. 32-14B); the cells are arranged in compact, although disorderly pattern, surrounding but not destroying adnexal structures. Fibroblast-like spindle cells in variable numbers and cells of morphology intermediate between these spindle cells and histiocyte-like cells are also present (157,167). Scattered inflammatory cells and numerous small blood vessels are present, commonly with focal hemorrhage.

The spindle cell variant of AFX consists of eosinophilic spindle cells with vesicular nuclei and eosinophilic nucleoli arranged in fascicular pattern (168). Clear cell AFX is a rare variant composed of sheets of large cells with foamy cytoplasm and hyperchromatic, pleomorphic nuclei with frequent atypical mitoses (169,170) (Fig. 32-15A and B). Rare pigmented AFX, due to deposition of hemosiderin (171), and a granular cell variant have been reported (172).

Histogenesis. Electron microscopic (157,173) and immunohistochemical (91,174) studies indicate that, as for malignant fibrous histiocytoma, the progenitor cell is an undifferentiated mesenchymal cell, capable of showing histiocytic, fibroblastic, and myofibroblastic differentiation. The concept that AFX is a form of pleomorphic malignant fibrous histiocytoma has received further support from a

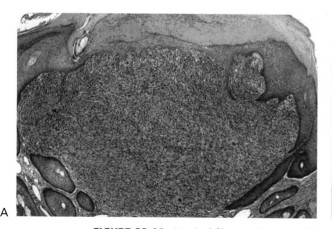
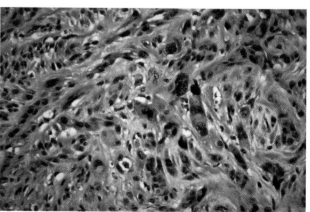

FIGURE 32-14. Atypical fibroxanthoma. **A:** The tumor is an exophytic densely cellular nodule, with a collarette of epidermis. **B:** The cytologic characteristics are very similar to those of malignant fibrous histiocytoma, with pleomorphic spindle cells, giant cells, and scattered mitoses, including atypical forms.

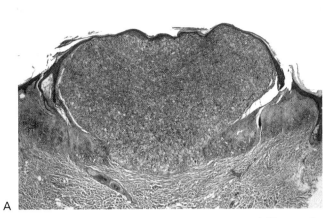
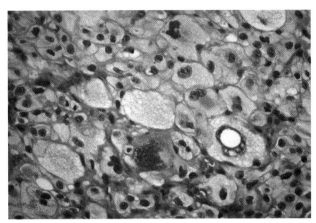

A   B

FIGURE 32-15. Clear-cell atypical fibroxanthoma. **A:** A well-defined, exophytic nodule with an epidermal collarette. **B:** Sheets of large cells with abundant clear or foamy cytoplasm and pleomorphic, hyperchromatic nuclei.

study in which no significant difference between AFX and malignant fibrous histiocytoma in their apoptotic behavior, proliferation indices, P53 protein expression or presence of bcl2 product was demonstrated (159).

Differential Diagnosis. The histologic features of most cases of AFX are diagnostic. In some cases, especially the less pleomorphic tumors, immunohistochemical staining is helpful in distinguishing AFX from other spindle cell and pleomorphic neoplasms. AFX expresses vimentin and, in many cases, actin and CD68, and is nonreactive for cytokeratin, carcino-embryonic antigen (CEA), S-100 protein, Melan-A, and usually desmin, thereby excluding most other neoplasms which share some of the histologic features of AFX (91,170,174) (Table 32-1).

EPITHELIOID SARCOMA

Epithelioid sarcoma, thus designated by Enzinger (175) in 1970, is a distinctive rare, highly malignant soft tissue neoplasm of uncertain origin, occurring most commonly in the distal extremities of young adult males as a slowly growing nodule or plaque (176) (Fig. 32-16), but also in a wide range of anatomic sites, including the head, neck, and pelvis in children (177–179), and the penis (180,181) and vulva (182). This aggressive neoplasm is characterized by multiple recurrences and a high rate of metastasis (176). The most important prognostic factors are sex of the patient and size of the tumor (183,184). The more favorable prognosis for females was emphasized by a study in which the 5-year survival rate was 80% for females, as against 40% for males (183).

Proximal type epithelioid sarcoma is an aggressive variant that occurs predominantly in the pelvis, perineum, and genital tract in older adults than in the usual distal type and frequently shows rhabdoid microscopic features simulating malignant extrarenal rhabdoid tumor (185,186).

Histopathology. The tumors are composed of irregular nodules of atypical epithelioid cells with eosinophilic cytoplasm of variable amount and pleomorphic nuclei, merging with spindle cells. These aggregates are embedded in collagenous fibrous tissue in which there may be focal hemorrhage, hemosiderin, and mucin deposition with a patchy lymphocytic infiltrate. Mitoses are present in varied frequency, vascular invasion is a common feature, and foci of necrosis are present in the centers of tumor nodules presenting a pseudogranulomatous appearance. Foci of pseudo-angiosarcomatous pattern, calcification and ossification may be present. Ulceration follows epidermal involvement by the larger tumor nodules, and invasion extends diffusely into the subcutis and deeper soft tissues (Fig. 32-17A through F).

A *spindle cell variant of epithelioid sarcoma* also occurs, in which the spindle cell pattern predominates without the characteristic epithelioid cells and nodularity (187,188) (Fig. 32-18).

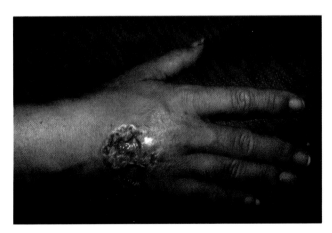

FIGURE 32-16. Epithelioid sarcoma (clinical photograph). Ulcerated nodules on the dorsum of the hand of a 32-year-old woman. The patient died from systemic metastases 18 months later.

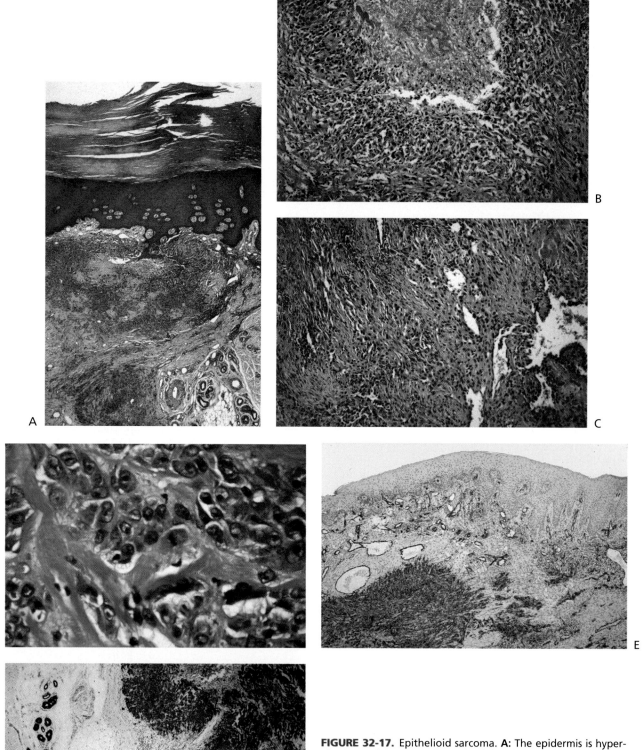

FIGURE 32-17. Epithelioid sarcoma. **A:** The epidermis is hyperplastic overlying several poorly defined nodules in the dermis with central foci of necrosis. **B:** Epithelioid cells with eosinophilic cytoplasm and pleomorphic nuclei surround a central zone of necrosis. **C:** Atypical epithelioid cells line irregular spaces, in angiosarcoma-like pattern, with spindle cells in the intervening stroma. **D:** Irregular groups of atypical epithelioid cells with pale eosinophilic cytoplasm, pleomorphic nuclei, prominent nucleoli and frequent mitoses, embedded in collagenous stroma. **E:** Positive staining for CD34. **F:** Intensely positive immunostaining for cytokeratins AE1 and AE3.

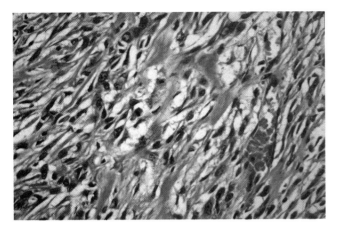

FIGURE 32-18. Epithelioid sarcoma: spindle cell variant. Predominant population of plump, atypical spindle cells.

Histogenesis. The histogenesis of epithelioid sarcoma is still uncertain, but the ultrastructural features of desmosome-like intercellular junctions, numerous microvilli and whorled arrangements of intermediate filaments (177,189, 190) and immunoreactivity for epithelial membrane antigen, cytokeratin, vimentin and, in many cases, CD34 and actin, suggest an origin from primitive mesenchymal cells with the capacity for epithelial differentiation (191). Cytogenetic studies have shown various chromosomal deletions and gains, none of which is specific for epithelioid sarcoma (192).

Differential Diagnosis. At low power, the neoplasm may suggest a granulomatous process such as granuloma annulare, necrobiosis lipoidica, or rheumatoid nodule. The cellular atypia, diffuse stromal invasion, and foci of necrosis involving tumor cells and not only stroma, as in the necrobiotic granulomatous processes (189), identify the process as malignant, and the diagnosis is supported by positive immunostaining for cytokeratin, vimentin, epithelial membrane antigen and, frequently, CD34 (191) (Table 32-1). Epithelioid sarcoma may also be confused with other neoplasms, including malignant fibrous histiocytoma, synovial sarcoma, fibrosarcoma, angiosarcoma, desmoid fibromatosis, hemangioendothelioma, malignant extrarenal rhabdoid tumor, and amelanotic melanoma. The characteristic clinical, morphologic, and immunocytochemical features usually permit distinction from these tumors, although the diagnosis may be difficult. Although epithelioid sarcoma, like synovial sarcoma, shows both mesenchymal and epithelial differentiation, it lacks the characteristic biphasic pattern of synovial sarcoma (190), which usually does not express CD34 (193). The lack of reactivity for cytokeratins 5/6 in most cases of epithelioid sarcoma may be a helpful feature in distinguishing superficial epithelioid sarcoma from squamous cell carcinoma, which consistently expresses that antigen (194) (Table 32-1).

SYNOVIAL SARCOMA

Synovial sarcoma most commonly occurs on the extremities, particularly the thigh, of young and middle-aged adults. Superficial lesions adjacent to the joints of the hand, foot or knee, sometimes present with dermal involvement (195, 196). A specific chromosomal translocation, t(X,18) (p11; q11), has been described in the majority of cases of synovial sarcoma (197).

Histopathology The tumor typically presents a biphasic pattern including an epithelioid cell component forming pseudoglandular spaces, and a uniform small spindle cell component resembling fibrosarcoma. Monophasic synovial sarcoma is composed usually only of spindle cells. Purely glandular monophasic synovial sarcoma theoretically exists but without cytogenetic analysis would be indistinguishable from adenocarcinoma (193). Most tumors express low and high molecular weight cytokeratins including cytokeratins 7 and 19, which are not found in malignant peripheral nerve, sheath tumor or Ewing's sarcoma (193).

Histogenesis Immunohistochemical and ultrastructural differences between normal synovial cells and the cells of synovial sarcoma indicate that the tumor is not derived from synovium, leading to suggestions of alternative terms including connective tissue carcinosarcoma and soft tissue carcinoma (198,199). An immunohistochemical study of the distribution of collagens, fibronectin, laminin, and tenascin in synovial sarcoma has produced results suggesting similarities between synovial sarcoma and the embryonic development of epithelia from mesenchymal cells, supporting the concept that synovial sarcoma is a soft tissue carcinosarcoma (200).

INFANTILE DIGITAL FIBROMATOSIS (RECURRING DIGITAL FIBROUS TUMOR OF CHILDHOOD AND INCLUSION BODY FIBROMATOSIS)

Infantile digital fibromatosis occurs as single or multiple nodules on the fingers or toes, excluding the great toe and the thumb. They may be present at birth, but they usually appear during the first year of life or, less commonly, later in childhood. The nodules rarely exceed 2 cm in diameter and involute spontaneously. In about 75% of the cases, recurrences are observed during early childhood (201).

Histopathology. The dermis is infiltrated by uniform spindle cells and collagen bundles arranged in interlacing fascicles, extending from just below the epidermis into the subcutis (Fig. 32-19A). A characteristic diagnostic feature is the presence of eosinophilic cytoplasmic inclusion bodies, 3 to 10 μm in diameter, often indenting the nucleus (202) (Fig. 32-19B). In hematoxylin-eosin sections, they resemble erythrocytes. These inclusions stain deep red with Masson trichome and purple with phosphotungstic acid–hematoxylin, and express vimentin and actin (203,204).

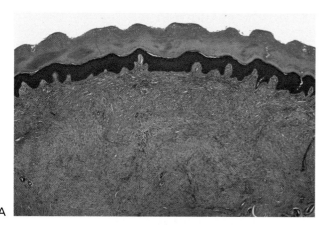
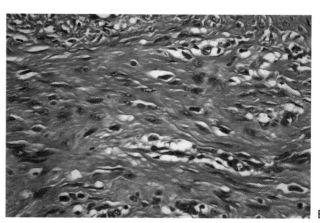

FIGURE 32-19. Infantile digital fibromatosis. **A:** Interlacing fascicles extend from the papillary dermis into the subcutis. **B:** Fascicles of spindle cells, some of which contain small, round, eosinophilic, cytoplasmic inclusions.

Histogenesis. Ultrastructurally, the spindle cells show the features of myofibroblasts and contain actin filaments that extend into and are continuous with the granular inclusions (206,207).

ACQUIRED DIGITAL FIBROKERATOMA (ACRAL FIBROKERATOMA)

Acquired digital fibrokeratoma presents as a solitary rounded, firm, more or less hyperkeratotic projection most commonly on a finger or toe, and occasionally on the palms or soles (207). Some appear to originate from the proximal nail fold (208). The outgrowth is either elongated or dome-shaped and slightly pedunculated, protruding from a collarette of slightly raised skin. In contrast to infantile digital fibromatosis, acquired fibrokeratoma occurs in adults. Rare cases of familial multiple acral mucinous fibrokeratoma and multiple acral fibromas associated with familial retinoblastoma have recently been reported, possibly examples of cutaneous markers of tumor suppressor gene germline mutation (209,210).

Histopathology. The epidermis is hyperkeratotic and acanthotic with thickened, often branching rete ridges. The core of the lesion is formed by thick, interwoven bundles of collagen, predominantly vertically oriented (211) (Fig. 32-20). Elastic fibers are usually present but are apt to be thin and sparse (212). Many tumors are highly vascular (207).

Differential Diagnosis. Although acquired digital fibrokeratoma may resemble a rudimentary supernumerary digit in its clinical and histologic appearance, rudimentary polydactyly almost always occurs at the base of the fifth finger, is present from birth, and is often bilateral. Histologically, rudimentary polydactyly differs from digital fibrokeratoma by the presence of numerous nerve bundles, especially at the base of the lesion (211).

TRICHODISCOMA AND FIBROFOLLICULOMA

Fibrofolliculoma and trichodiscoma are distinct, rare, benign dermal tumors, probably hamartomas, that originate from the mantle of the hair follicle and occur sporadically or in association with the Birt–Hogg–Dube syndrome (213,214). Their clinical features are similar; they occur as small flat or dome-shaped lesions, usually multiple, on the face, trunk, and extremities (215–220).

Histopathology. Trichodiscoma is a sharply defined fibrovascular lesion of the superficial dermis, associated with an adjacent hair follicle. The overlying epidermis is flattened, and the fibrillar collagen of the elliptical parafollicular lesion contains abundant connective tissue mucin. Fibrofolliculoma consists of a circumscribed proliferation of compact collagen and fibroblasts surrounding one or more distorted keratin-plugged hair follicles from which interlocking strands of basaloid cells protrude into the surrounding stroma.

FIGURE 32-20. Digital fibrokeratoma. A polypoid lesion with acanthotic epidermis overlying collagen bundles oriented mainly in the vertical plane.

Histogenesis. A recent study of trichodiscoma and fibro-folliculoma including sporadic cases and cases associated with Birt–Hogg–Dube syndrome demonstrated contiguous histologic features in those tumors associated with Birt–Hogg–Dube syndrome in contrast with the discrete epithelial and stromal patterns seen in the sporadic cases. The spindle cells within and surrounding the fibromyxoid component of the lesions expressed CD34 consistent with origin from the hair follicle mantle and were negative for factor XIIIa and smooth muscle actin (214).

FIBROUS PAPULE OF THE FACE

Fibrous papule of the face, a common lesion, occurs in mature persons nearly always as a solitary lesion on the lower portion of the nose or on the adjacent skin of the face. It is usually dome-shaped, firm, and small, not exceeding 5 mm in diameter. In most cases, it is skin colored, but it may be red or slightly pigmented. Originally described as an involuting melanocytic nevus (221,222), subsequent reports suggest that this lesion is an angiofibroma (223,224) and is synonymous with perifollicular fibroma (224).

Histopathology. The epidermis is raised, overlying a localized area of fibroplasia and vascular proliferation in the upper dermis. In nearly all cases, there are scattered, large triangular and stellate cells, some of which may be multinucleated (224,225). In some cases, an increased number of melanocytes is seen at the dermoepidermal junction (Fig. 32-21). In the perifollicular fibroma form a central hair follicle is surrounded by compact fibrous tissue (Fig. 32-22).

Histogenesis. The prevalence of melanocytes at the dermoepidermal junction and the resemblance of the large triangular and stellate cells in the dermis to nevus cells explain why authors in the past have regarded fibrous papules of the face as involuting melanocytic nevi. However, electron microscopic studies have identified the triangular or stellate

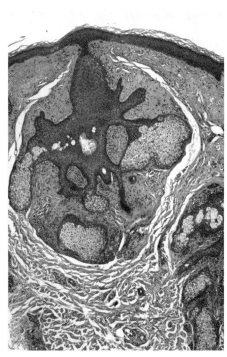

FIGURE 32-22. Fibrous papule; perifollicular fibroma type. A circumscribed zone of compact fibrous tissue surrounds a central hair follicle.

cells as fibroblasts rather than melanocytes (226,227). Several studies have shown that the spindle and stellate cells of fibrous papule express factor XIIIa but not S-100 protein, indicating that the tumors are composed of dermal dendritic cells or dermal fibroblasts rather than melanocytic nevus cells (228–232).

Differential Diagnosis. Because the facial lesions of tuberous sclerosis also show angiofibrosis and may contain stellate cells, differentiation from fibrous papule of the face may require clinical data (233).

PEARLY PENILE PAPULES

These small lesions (1 to 3 mm in diameter) are persistent pearly white papules that occur mainly on the coronal margin and sulcus of the penis and rarely on the glans in groups or rows in about 10% of young adult males.

Histopathology The features are those of an angiofibroma similar to fibrous papule of the face but lacking hair follicles (234).

TUBEROUS SCLEROSIS

Tuberous sclerosis, a dominantly inherited disorder, is characterized by the triad of mental deficiency, epilepsy, and angiofibromas of the face. The triad is not necessarily complete. The angiofibromas consist of numerous small, red,

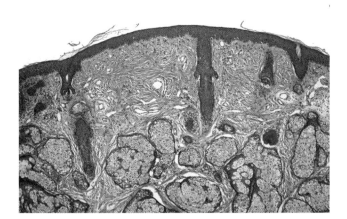

FIGURE 32-21. Fibrous papule of the face. The epidermis is slightly raised and overlies a zone of vascular fibroplasia in the superficial dermis, with scattered spindle and stellate cells in the upper layers.

smooth papules in symmetric distribution in the nasolabial folds, on the cheeks, and on the chin. Other organs are frequently involved (235).

Additional cutaneous manifestations may include asymmetrically arranged, large, raised, soft, brown fibromas on the face and the scalp, subungual and periungual fibromas, and so-called shagreen patches, usually found in the lumbosacral region and consisting of slightly raised and thickened areas of the skin. Scattered hypopigmented, leaf-shaped areas are present in more than half of the patients with tuberous sclerosis. Their diagnostic significance lies in the fact that they are present at birth or appear very early in life, and thus are the earliest cutaneous sign of tuberous sclerosis (236).

Genetic linkage studies show linkage to chromosome 9q34 (TSC 1) or to chromosome 16p31 (TSC 2) (237–239) in families with tuberous sclerosis. Two-thirds of cases are sporadic and are assumed to result from new mutations, many of which are in TSC 2 (239).

Systemic Lesions. Multiple tumors are commonly found in the brain (gliomas, often calcified) (240); retina (gliomas) (241); heart (rhabdomyomas) (242); and kidneys (angiomyolipomas) (243).

Histopathology. In the past, the symmetrically distributed, small, red angiofibromas of the face were mistakenly called adenoma sebaceum. However, the sebaceous glands are generally atrophic, and the main findings are dermal proliferation of spindle, stellate or multinucleate giant cells, and dilatation of capillaries. Occasionally, multinucleate giant cells are also present. In some cases, one observes vascular proliferation and perivascular proliferation of fibroblasts in addition to vascular dilatation (233). In old lesions, there may be perifollicular proliferation of collagen, leading to the compression of atrophic hair follicles by concentric layers of collagen. Elastic tissue is absent in the angiofibromas (Fig. 32-23A and B).

The larger, asymmetric fibromas on the face and scalp show markedly sclerotic collagen arranged in thick, concentric layers around atrophic pilosebaceous follicles. In contrast to the smaller lesions, dilated capillaries usually are absent. Giant angiofibroma (244) and a cluster growth of large nodules (245) have also been reported.

The ungual fibromas show fibrosis, occasionally with capillary dilatation. The shagreen patches have the histologic features of connective tissue nevi, with either a dense, sclerotic mass of very broad collagenous bundles in the lower dermis, mimicking morphea, or normal collagen bundles throughout the dermis in an interwoven pattern. The elastic tissue in some instances shows fragmentation and clumping (233), but generally is reduced in amount (246).

The hypopigmented, leaf-shaped areas show a normal number of melanocytes with decreased pigmentation. On electron microscopy, the melanosomes within the melanocytes and keratinocytes are smaller and show less melanization than normal melanosomes (236,246).

Differential Diagnosis. The angiofibromas of tuberous sclerosis are histologically indistinguishable from the solitary angiofibroma or fibrous papule of the face or nose. The shagreen patches of tuberous sclerosis differ from other connective tissue nevi by the regular absence of any increase in elastic tissue.

SOFT FIBROMA

Soft fibromas, also called "fibroepithelial polyps," "acrochordons," or "cutaneous tags," occur as three types: (a) multiple small, furrowed papules, especially on the neck and in the axillae, generally only 1 to 2 mm long; (b) single or multiple filiform, smooth growths in varying locations, about 2 mm wide and 5 mm long; and (c) solitary bag-like,

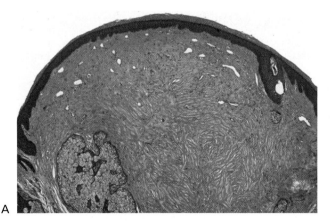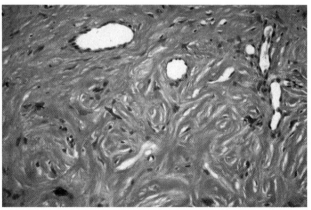

FIGURE 32-23. Angiofibroma of tuberous sclerosis. **A:** The epidermis is raised in a dome-shaped pattern overlying a zone of compact fibroplasia with prominent blood vessels in the upper half. **B:** Sclerotic, hyalinized collagenous stroma, with scattered spindle and stellate cells and telangiectatic blood vessels.

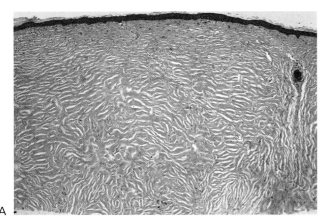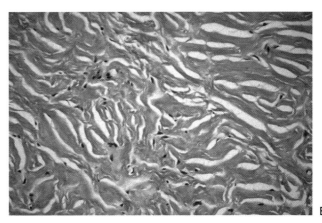

FIGURE 32-24. Sclerotic fibroma. **A:** The epidermis is flattened overlying a pale eosinophilic nodule extending into the deep dermis. **B:** Amorphous, eosinophilic collagen bundles in a laminated pattern.

pedunculated growths, usually about 1 cm in diameter but occasionally much larger, seen most commonly on the lower trunk (247–249).

Several reports have suggested an association between the presence of soft fibroma and colonic polyps (249–252); diabetes (253–255); and acromegaly (256). The association with colonic polyps, however, has not been confirmed by subsequent reports (257–261).

Histopathology. The multiple small furrowed papules usually show papillomatosis, hyperkeratosis, and regular acanthosis and occasionally also horn cysts within their acanthotic epidermis. Thus, there is often considerable resemblance to a pedunculated seborrheic keratosis.

The epidermis of the filiform, smooth growths shows slight to moderate acanthosis and occasionally mild papillomatosis. The connective tissue stalk is composed of loose collagen fibers and often contains numerous dilated capillaries filled with erythrocytes (247). Nevus cells are found in as many as 30% of the filiform growths, indicating that some of them represent involuting melanocytic nevi (262).

The bag-like, soft fibromas generally show a flattened epidermis overlying loosely arranged collagen fibers and mature fat cells in the center (258). In some instances, the dermis is quite thin, so that the fat cells compose a significant portion of the tumor, which may then be regarded as a lipofibroma (263).

SCLEROTIC FIBROMA

This is an uncommon neoplasm that occurs as solitary papules or nodules up to 3 cm in diameter (264) or as multiple papules in patients with Cowden disease (265).

Histopathology. The lesions are circumscribed nodules composed of interwoven fascicles of eosinophilic collagen bundles in laminated, storiform pattern with prominent

clefting (Fig. 32-24A and B). Immunostaining is positive for vimentin and factor XIIIa with focal positivity for CD34 (268,267).

Histogenesis. On the basis of similar fibrotic changes seen in dermatofibroma and in inflammatory lesions, it has been suggested that sclerotic fibromas may have diverse origins (268,269). The demonstration of type 1 collagen synthesis, however, has suggested that the lesion is a fibroblastic neoplasm (266).

PLEOMORPHIC FIBROMA

Pleomorphic fibroma typically presents as an exophytic nodule indistinguishable from a fibroepithelial polyp.

Histopathology. The epidermis is flattened overlying a circumscribed nodule composed of plump mononucleate and multinucleate cells with atypical nuclei and occasional mitoses, distributed sparsely in a fibrous stroma (Fig. 32-25A and B).

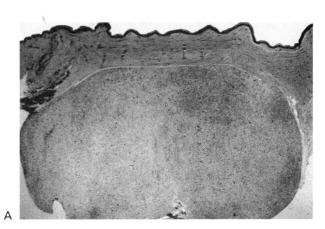

FIGURE 32-25. Pleomorphic fibroma. **A:** A sharply circumscribed nodule in the dermis and subcutis. *(continued)*

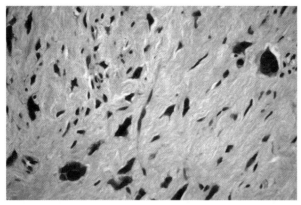

FIGURE 32-25. *(continued)* B: Spindle cells and giant cells with marked nuclear pleomorphism and hyperchromatism in a pale hyalinised stroma. (Courtesy of Dr. B. Dutta, Duttapath, Sydney, Australia.)

Histogenesis. In contrast to dermatofibroma with monster cells, pleomorphic fibroma expresses CD34, but is negative for Ki-M1p (270). Immunohistochemical studies have suggested either myofibroblastic or dendritic origin (270,271).

ANGIOFIBROBLASTOMA OF THE SKIN

Angiofibroblastoma of the skin is a recently described benign neoplasm that occurs as small solitary dermal nodules on the extremities of adults (272,273).

Histopathology. The lesions are composed of stellate and spindle fibroblasts embedded in a fibromyxoid and fibrous matrix with numerous capillaries. The spindle cells show reactivity for vimentin and focal positivity for muscle specific actin; factor XIIIa is present only in associated dendritic cells.

Differential Diagnosis. Angiofibroblastoma is more cellular than sclerotic fibroma and does not express CD34 (273).

COLLAGENOUS FIBROMA (DESMOPLASTIC FIBROBLASTOMA)

Collagenous fibroma is a recently described, rare benign tumor affecting mainly adult males, involving the subcutis or muscle, with rare involvement of the dermis (274–276). The tumors are usually small (1 to 4 cm in diameter), but examples up to 20 cm in diameter have been reported (277,278).

Histopathology. The lesions form circumscribed ovoid, elongated or disc-shaped masses that may be lobulated, composed of dense collagenous tissue, and scattered spindle or stellate fibroblasts and myofibroblasts. Focal myxoid change may be present and blood vessels are usually inconspicuous (278). The tumor cells express vimentin and, variably, alpha smooth muscle actin, and keratins AE1/AE3; the cells are negative for desmin, EMA, S-100 protein, and CD34 (278).

SOLITARY FIBROUS TUMOR

Solitary fibrous tumor is a rare mesenchymal neoplasm that most commonly involves the pleura, but has also been reported in extrapleural locations including the skin (279–281), as a circumscribed nodule, mainly on the head and neck (282). Rare metastases from pleural solitary fibrous tumors have been reported, but all documented cutaneous tumors of this type appear to have been benign (279).

Histopathology. The tumors are circumscribed nodules composed of spindle cells and prominent blood vessels, involving the dermis, subcutis, and fascia. The superficial layers of the tumor consist of bland spindle cells in a storiform pattern similar to dermatofibrosarcoma protuberans, whereas in the deeper layers there is a varied growth pattern including a vascular component of ectatic vessels and slit-like staghorn vessels presenting a hemangiopericytoma-like appearance, alternating with hypercellular fascicles of spindle cells with vesicular nuclei and eosinophilic cytoplasm (Fig. 32-26A and B).

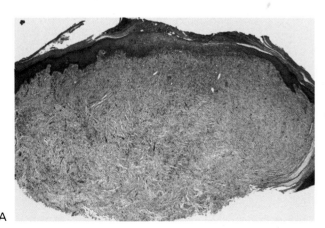
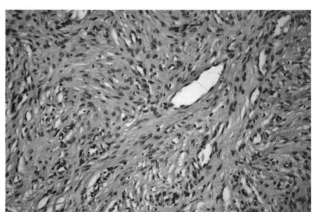

FIGURE 32-26. Solitary fibrous tumor. **A:** A circumscribed dermal nodule. **B:** Prominent vascularity including ectatic and slit-like vessels presenting a hemangiopericytoma-like pattern.

The cells express vimentin, CD34, CD99, and, focally, factor XIIIa, but they are negative for smooth muscle, neural, and epithelial markers (281).

GIANT CELL TUMOR OF TENDON SHEATH

Giant cell tumor of the tendon sheath occurs most commonly in young and middle-aged adults on the dorsum of the fingers, hands, and wrists, where it is attached to a tendon sheath. It is firm in consistency with a yellowish tan cut surface, measuring from 1 to 3 cm in diameter. There is no tendency towards spontaneous involution. The tumor may extend to the synovium of an adjacent joint space and, on rare occasions, may even extend into the overlying skin (283). Although it has been suggested that this tumor is an inflammatory proliferation (284), other reports indicate that the lesion is neoplastic (285).

Histopathology. The tumor consists of lobules of varied cellularity surrounded by dense collagen (Fig. 32-27A). In cellular areas, most cells are histiocyte-like cells with vesicular nuclei, foamy macrophages and siderophages. Less cellular areas consist of spindle cells within a fibrous or hyalinized stroma (283,286). The characteristic giant cells, resembling osteoclasts (287), are scattered through both the cellular and fibrous areas; their cytoplasm is deeply eosinophilic and they contain a variable number of haphazardly distributed nuclei (Fig. 32-27B). Although mitotic figures are seen in a large proportion of cases and may be frequent (288), there is no evidence that mitotic activity is related to metastasis, which is an extremely rare event in these tumors (289).

Histogenesis. Ultrastructural (287–290), enzymatic (286), and immunohistochemical studies (286,291–293) have indicated variously that the cells of this tumor may be related to synovial cells, monocytes, and osteoclasts.

FIBROMA OF TENDON SHEATH

Fibroma of the tendon sheath was first described in 1979 (294) as a distinct clinicopathologic entity. Its clinical characteristics resemble those of giant cell tumor of the tendon sheath (295). A clonal chromosomal abnormality, t(2;11) (q31–32; q12), has been demonstrated in one case (296); the identical translocation in collagenous fibroma suggests a genetic link (297).

Histopathology. The lesion is largely composed of interlacing bundles of hyalinized, hypocellular fibrous tissue with occasionally more cellular areas (298). A characteristic feature is the presence of slit-like vascular channels (295). No foam cells are seen, and multinucleated giant cells are very rare (298).

Histogenesis. The cells of fibroma of tendon sheath show myofibroblastic differentiation (299).

NODULAR FASCIITIS

Nodular fasciitis is a relatively common, benign soft tissue lesion that usually presents as a solitary, rapidly developing, sometimes tender subcutaneous nodule that reaches its ultimate size of 1 cm to 5 cm within a few weeks. The lesion is self-limited, and thus, even if it is incompletely excised, regresses, usually within a few months (300). Although the arm is the most common site, the lesion may occur in any subcutaneous area. The lesions occur in all age groups but more often in young adults, with an equal sex distribution.

The cause is unknown. Although trauma does not seem to play a role, the general view is that nodular fasciitis represents a reactive fibroblastic and vascular proliferation.

Histopathology. Nodular fasciitis occurs usually in the subcutis, less often in muscle and rarely in the dermis. A prominent feature is the infiltrative growth pattern along

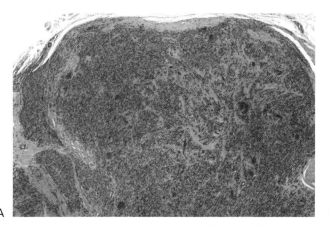
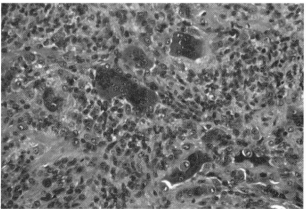

FIGURE 32-27. Giant-cell tumor of tendon sheath. **A:** The tumor is composed of sharply circumscribed, densely cellular lobules surrounded by fibrofatty tissue. **B:** Giant cells with multiple nuclei, resembling osteoclasts, are scattered among plump epithelioid and spindle cells.

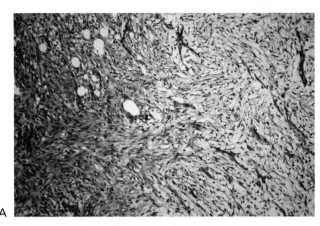
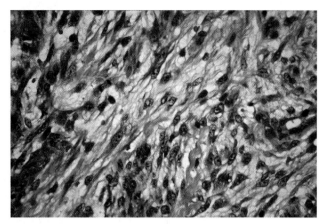

A   B

FIGURE 32-28. Nodular fasciitis. **A:** Plump spindle cells are arranged in varied cellularity in a loosely structured, vascular stroma. **B:** Plump spindle cells with ovoid, vesicular nuclei and scattered mitoses are embedded in a loosely structured stroma with capillaries, slit-like spaces, and scattered erythrocytes.

fibrous septa of the subcutis, resulting in poor demarcation. The nodule consists of plump fibroblasts growing haphazardly in a vascular, myxoid stroma presenting a tissue culture–like pattern (Fig. 32-28A and B). The vascular component includes well-formed capillaries and slit-like spaces with extravasation of red cells. The fibroblasts may show numerous mitoses, which are not atypical. Multinucleate, osteoclast-like giant cells are frequently present. In some instances degenerate muscle fibers simulate multinucleate giant cells (301). A lymphocytic infiltrate is often present, mainly at the periphery of the nodule (302). In older lesions, the fibroblasts appear more mature, showing a more compact arrangement of spindle cells with increased production of collagen (303).

Dermal fasciitis is a rare variant arising within the dermis (304–306). Postoperative/post-traumatic spindle cell nodule has also been described as the dermal analog of nodular fasciitis (307). Another variant, intravascular fasciitis (308), occurs in intimate association with blood vessels, forming small nodules of myofibroblasts, apparently originating from the vessel walls and protruding into the lumen. Proliferative fasciitis appears to be related to nodular fasciitis, but it includes giant cells resembling ganglion cells, similar to those of proliferative myositis and showing an abundant, irregularly outlined, basophilic cytoplasm with one or two large vesicular nuclei (309,310).

Histogenesis. The spindle cells in lesions of nodular fasciitis have the ultrastructural features of myofibroblasts (311). As in other myofibroblastic lesions, the cells are immunoreactant for vimentin, smooth muscle actin, and muscle-specific actin, but not for desmin (312).

Differential Diagnosis. The presence of numerous large, pleomorphic fibroblasts and the infiltrative type of growth may be suggestive of fibrosarcoma. In addition to rapid

growth and tenderness, however, the combination of fibroblastic and vascular proliferation is the most helpful diagnostic feature of nodular fasciitis. Other findings suggesting the diagnosis of nodular fasciitis are the presence of a mucoid ground substance and an inflammatory infiltrate, especially near the margin of the lesion. Because nodular fasciitis as a reactive lesion does not recur, the recurrence of a lesion originally diagnosed as such should spur a careful reappraisal of the histologic findings (309).

CRANIAL FASCIITIS OF CHILDHOOD

Cranial fasciitis of childhood is an unusual variant of nodular fasciitis that occurs in infants and children as a rapidly growing mass in the subcutaneous tissue of the scalp that extends into the underlying cranium. No recurrence has been reported after excision of the mass with resection or curettage of the underlying bone (313).

Histopathology. The histologic features closely resemble those of nodular fasciitis. An origin in one of the deep fascial layers of the scalp appears likely (313).

Histogenesis. The lesion contains fibroblasts and myofibroblasts (314).

MYOFIBROMA/MYOFIBROMATOSIS

Myofibroma and myofibromatosis are solitary or multiple benign neoplasms, occurring mainly in children, usually as congenital lesions although additional nodules may subsequently appear. The majority of lesions in both adults and children are solitary. The nodules are most commonly confined to the dermis, subcutis, and skeletal muscle of the head, neck, and trunk, but any site may be affected. In patients with myofibromatosis, multiple tumors may also involve bones and viscera, causing death in rare cases, especially those with pulmonary involvement (315–317). In adults the tumors are solitary and superficial (solitary cutaneous myofibroma) (318). In infants with visceral involvement, death may occur in the first few months of life, but in survivors and in those with superficial myofibromatosis, spontaneous involution of the lesions takes place, often within the first year of life, possibly mediated by apoptosis (319).

Histopathology. The cutaneous lesions consist of nodular dermal aggregates of plump spindle cells resembling smooth muscle cells arranged in short fascicles, sometimes with areas of central hyalinization (320) (Fig. 32-29A). Most tumors present a characteristic biphasic growth pattern. A peripheral component of leiomyoma-like fascicles of plump spindle cells surrounds a central hemangiopericytoma-like component where more rounded cells are arranged around the blood vessels (Fig. 32-29B). Collagen is present, but it is not abundant, and in less cellular areas the stroma may appear mucoid (321). A monophasic cellular variant has also been described recently; in these lesions the more characteristic biphasic pattern developed during the course of the disease (322).

Histogenesis. Ultrastructural evidence and immunoreactivity for vimentin and actin, with negative staining for desmin (318,323,324), have indicated that the spindle cells are myofibroblasts, but it has also been suggested that the spindle cells show true smooth muscle differentiation (325). The similarities between infantile myofibromas and infantile hemangiopericytoma indicate that they belong in the same spectrum (326) and that myofibromas are of pericytic origin (327).

FIBROUS HAMARTOMA OF INFANCY

Fibrous hamartoma of infancy occurs usually as one or, rarely, two subcutaneous nodules that may be present at birth or develop during the first 2 years of life (328–330). After an initial period of growth, there is no further increase in the size of the nodule. In a study of 40 cases, 29 patients were males and 11 were females, and the lesions were distributed in a wide range of anatomic sites (331).

Histopathology. The nodule consists of three different tissue components: cell-poor fibrous trabeculae, whorls of immature appearing spindle cells in a mucoid matrix, and mature adipose tissue (328,329) (Fig. 32-30A, B, and C). The fibrous component may vary in cellularity, pattern, and amount, resembling granulation tissue, deep fibrous histiocytoma, or fibromatosis in some areas (331).

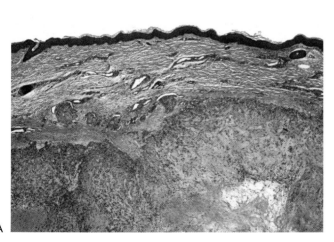
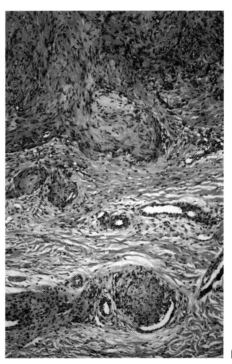

FIGURE 32-29. Infantile myofibromatosis. **A:** Circumscribed dermal nodules of varied size, with hyalinization in the center of the largest nodule. **B:** The nodules consist of fascicles of plump spindle cells with pale eosinophilic cytoplasm, some of which indent the walls of blood vessels.

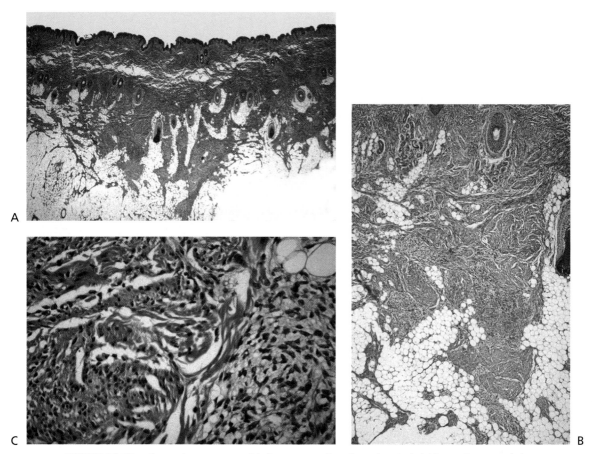

FIGURE 32-30. Fibrous hamartoma of infancy. **A:** Trabeculae of varied thickness intersect lobules of fat in the subcutis. **B:** The trabeculae are composed of spindle cells arranged in loosely structured myxoid areas and more densely collagenous foci. **C:** Whorls of immature spindle cells (*right*) and collagenous fibrous tissue (*left*).

JUVENILE HYALINE FIBROMATOSIS

A rare, recessively inherited disorder, juvenile hyaline fibromatosis starts in early infancy with flexural contractures, innumerable skin nodules that gradually increase in size, and a hypertrophic gingiva. The largest nodules are usually seen on the scalp (332). Juvenile hyaline fibromatosis has been reported in association with skull and encephalic abnormalities (333) and in the hand of an adult (334). The uncommon occurrence of widespread visceral involvement is known as infantile systemic hyalinosis (335).

Histopathology. The nodules are composed to varying degrees of fibroblasts and eosinophilic ground substance. Small, newly developed tumors are more cellular, whereas larger tumors contain much more ground substance (336,337). In paraffin-embedded, formalin-fixed material, empty spaces are seen around the fibroblasts as a shrinkage artifact, giving these cells a chondroid appearance (338).

Histogenesis. The spindle cells have the ultrastructural features of fibroblasts (339).

EWING'S SARCOMA AND PRIMITIVE NEUROECTODERMAL TUMOR

Ewing's sarcoma and primitive neuroectodermal tumor (PNET) are round cell sarcomas that show varying degrees of neuroectodermal differentiation. The term Ewing's sarcoma is used for those tumors that lack evidence of neuroectodermal differentiation whereas the term PNET is employed for tumors that demonstrate neuroectodermal features (340). Cutaneous extraskeletal Ewing's sarcoma is a highly malignant primary soft tissue neoplasm that rarely involves the skin (341), as distinct from extension of Ewing's sarcoma of bone into adjacent tissue.

Histopathology. Multiple tumor lobules in the subcutis may infiltrate the dermis. The nodules are composed of masses of uniform, round, or oval cells with round or ovoid nuclei, fine chromatin, and scanty clear or eosinophilic cytoplasm containing glycogen. Tumors with the histologic features of atypical Ewing's sarcoma or PNET show neural differentiation in the form of Homer–Wright rosettes and pseudorosettes, composed of more pleomorphic cells with a larger amount of eosinophilic cytoplasm and frequent mitoses (340).

Histogenesis. The overlapping light microscopic features, immunohistochemical features, and common genetic abnormalities among the tumors classified as Ewing's sarcoma of bone, peripheral primitive neuroectodermal tumor, extraskeletal Ewing's sarcoma, Askin tumor, and soft tissue PNET suggest that they are variants of a single entity. The tumor cells express the MIC2 gene recognized by CD99, and demonstrate several novel reciprocal chromosomal translocations and fusion gene transcripts (342–344).

CUTANEOUS MYXOMA

Cutaneous myxomas are sharply demarcated nodules of the dermis or subcutis, occurring as multiple lesions in association with cardiac and mammary myxomas, spotty pigmentation, and endocrine overactivity in Carney complex (345) or as solitary lesions, usually on the digits (346,347).

Histopathology. Cutaneous myxomas are sharply circumscribed lesions composed of stellate and spindle-shaped fibroblasts in a vascular, myxoid matrix (Fig. 32-31). An epithelial component is sometimes present, taking the form of strands of epithelium with trichoblastic features or small keratinous cysts (345,348). *Fibromyxoma* has been described as a lesion containing histiocytes and more fibroblasts than cutaneous myxoma in addition to the mucinous matrix. These lesions may occur as multiple tumors, clinically resembling dermatofibroma (349). For those lesions with more prominent vascularity the term *superficial angiomyxoma* is used (348,350).

Differential Diagnosis. Cutaneous myxoma is more sharply circumscribed and more vascular than cutaneous focal mucinosis (351). The tumors express vimentin, with variable positivity for CD34 and actin. The cells are usually

negative for S-100 protein, which is helpful in the distinction from neuroid tumors such as neurothekeoma (352).

DIGITAL MUCOUS CYST

It has been suggested that two types of digital mucous cysts exist (353,354). One type is analogous to focal mucinosis. It differs from focal mucinosis only by its location near the proximal nail fold and by its greater tendency to fluctuation. The other type is located on the dorsum of a finger near the distal interphalangeal joint and is due to a herniation of the joint lining, thus representing a ganglion (353). Another view is that digital mucous cyst and digital myxoma are identical, and that there is no anatomic connection with the interphalangeal joint (352).

Histopathology. According to the first concept, digital mucous cyst in its early stage has the same histologic appearance as that seen in focal mucinosis, namely, an ill-defined area of mucinous material. Subsequently, multiple clefts form and then coalesce into one large cystic space containing mucin composed largely of hyaluronic acid, which stains with Alcian blue and colloidal iron (355). The cystic space in early lesions is separated from the epidermis by mucinous stroma but in older lesions is found in a subepidermal location with thinning of the overlying epidermis. The collagen at the periphery of the cyst appears compressed. No lining of the cyst wall is apparent (355, 356) (Fig. 32-32).

Histogenesis. The type of digital mucous cyst that is analogous to focal mucinosis results from an overproduction of hyaluronic acid by fibroblasts (355). In the ganglion type of digital mucous cyst, the hyaluronic acid is derived from the joint fluid of the distal interphalangeal joint. The origin of the mucous material from the joint fluid is supported by the observation that, after the injection of methylene blue into the volar aspect of the distal

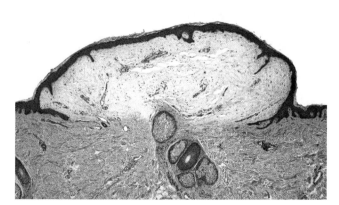

FIGURE 32-31. Cutaneous myxoma. The lesion is a sharply circumscribed nodule composed of a vascular mucinous matrix in which are scattered spindle cells.

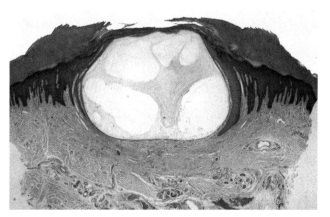

FIGURE 32-32. Digital mucous cyst. The epidermis is raised and attenuated and overlies a circumscribed mucinous cystic nodule, with an epidermal collarette.

interphalangeal joint space, the cyst regularly contains the dye (356,357).

MUCOUS CYST OF ORAL MUCOSA

Mucous cysts of the oral mucosa, also known as mucoceles, occur as solitary asymptomatic lesions, usually on the mucous surface of the lower lip and only rarely elsewhere on the oral mucosa (358). The cysts usually measure less than 1 cm in diameter, appear dome-shaped, are translucent, and contain a clear, viscous fluid. Mucous cysts of the oral mucosa usually are the result of minor trauma causing rupture of a mucous duct and release of sialomucin into the tissue. Although most patients with an oral mucous cyst have no preexisting abnormality, mucous cysts of the lower lip may occur in patients with *cheilitis glandularis*, a condition in which the labial mucous glands and ducts are hyperplastic (359).

Histopathology. Early lesions consist of multiple small spaces filled with sialomucin surrounded by or intermixed with granulation tissue in the submucosa. Older lesions show either a solitary large cystic space or several large spaces lined by a thick layer of granulation tissue composed of neutrophils, lymphocytes, fibroblasts, muciphages, and capillaries (358). The wall of some cysts shows a ruptured salivary duct opening into the cavity

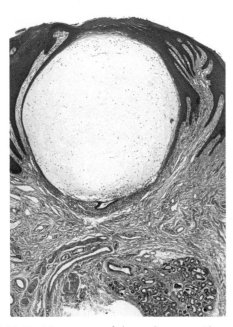

FIGURE 32-33. Mucous cyst of the oral mucosa. The squamous epithelium is raised with a collarette formation and overlies a circumscribed mucinous nodule. A segment of salivary gland duct opens into the base of the cyst.

(Fig. 32-33). The sialomucin within the cysts appears as amorphous, slightly eosinophilic material that is periodic acid–Schiff positive and diastase-resistant, and also stains with Alcian blue and colloidal iron. Superficial mucoceles are small, subepithelial, vesicular lesions. Minor salivary gland ducts in the underlying stroma provide a clue to the diagnosis (360).

HYPERTROPHIC SCAR AND KELOID

Hypertrophic scars and keloids represent the results of abnormal healing processes. Both lesions initially present the same clinical features of erythematous, shiny skin overlying firm scars. Keloids become much more prominent than hypertrophic scars and extend beyond the original site of injury, with a high rate of recurrence following surgical treatment (361). Keloids occur mainly on the head and neck, especially on the ear, upper chest and arms; they are very uncommon in the periocular region, and on the palms, soles, penis and scrotum (362,363). They affect all age groups, most commonly children older than 10 years and young adults.

Keloids usually follow an injury but some cases, especially presternal keloids, appear to occur spontaneously. Familial cases have been recorded (363) and keloids are much more common in black people (364). In the rare Rubinstein–Taybi syndrome, keloids may develop spontaneously in adolescence or early adulthood (365).

Histopathology. In hypertrophic scars and keloids, the formation of new collagen following the inflammatory stage wound healing is slower than in normally healing wounds, and in the early period of the fibroblastic stage of healing, the collagen fibers in the granulation tissue are arranged in a whorled or nodular pattern (366). In keloids the lesions include characteristic nodules of varied size composed of hypocellular fibrous tissue containing greatly thickened, compact, glassy, eosinophilic collagen bundles, in contrast to the more cellular nodules in hypertrophic scars lacking the more grossly abnormal collagen component (Fig. 32-34A and B).

Histogenesis. The pathophysiology of keloid formation has been summarized in a recent review of factors including abnormal fibroblast activity, increased hyaluronic acid production, and increased levels of transforming growth factor beta (TGFβ) and other cytokines (367). Among the mechanisms proposed as being of possible importance in this abnormal healing process, it has been suggested that decreased apoptosis may play a role, allowing the keloidal fibroblasts to proliferate and produce more collagen (367). The observation of decreased vascular density in keloid compared with hypertrophic scars and normal scars also suggests that hypoxia related to

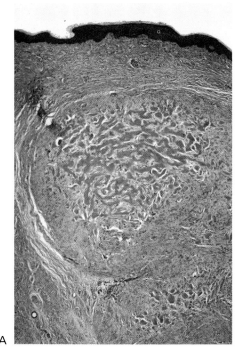
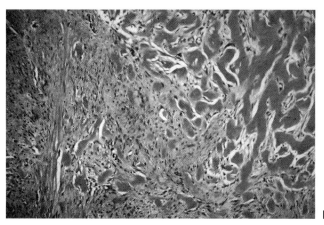

FIGURE 32-34. Keloid. **A:** Large nodules of cellular collagenous tissue extend into the deep dermis, with central collections of broad hyalinized collagen bundles. **B:** Irregular broad segments of hypereosinophilic, hyalinized collagen and adjacent strands of cellular collagen with plump fibroblasts.

their reduced level of vascularization may play an important role (363).

REFERENCES

1. Bedi TR, Pandhi RK, Bhutani LK. Multiple palmoplantar histiocytomas. *Arch Dermatol* 1976;112:1001–1003.
2. Bargman HB, Fefferman I. Multiple dermatofibromas in a patient with myasthenia gravis treated with prednisone and cyclophosphamide. *J Am Acad Dermatol* 1986;14:351–352.
3. Stainforth J, Goodfield MJD. Multiple dermatofibromata developing during pregnancy. *Clin Exp Dermatol* 1994;19:59–60.
4. Kanitakis J, Carbonnel E, Delmonte S, et al. Multiple eruptive dermatofibromas in a patient with HIV infection: case report and literature review. *J Cutan Pathol* 2000;27:54–56.
5. Bachmeyer C, Cordier F, Blum L, et al. Multiple eruptive dermatofibromas after highly active antiretroviral therapy. *Br J Dermatol* 2000;143:1336–1337.
6. Niemi KM. The benign fibrohistiocytic tumours of the skin [Review]. *Acta Derm Venereol (Stockh)* 1970;50:1–66.
7. Schoenfeld RJ. Epidermal proliferations overlying histiocytomas. *Arch Dermatol* 1964;90:266–270.
8. Leyva WH, Santa Cruz DJ. Atypical cutaneous fibrous histiocytoma. *Am J Dermatopathol* 1986;8:467–471.
9. Dalziel K, Marks R. Hair follicle-like changes over histiocytomas. *Am J Dermatopathol* 1986;8:462–466.
10. Bryant J. Basal cell carcinoma overlying longstanding dermatofibromas. *Arch Dermatol* 1977;113:1445–1446.
11. Goette DK, Helwig EB. Basal cell carcinomas and basal cell carcinoma-like changes overlying dermatofibroma. *Arch Dermatol* 1975;111:589–591.
12. Buselmeier TJ, Uecker JH. Invasive basal cell carcinoma with metaplastic bone formation associated with a long-standing dermatofibroma. *J Cutan Pathol* 1979;6:496–500.
13. Calonje E, Mentzel T, Fletcher CDM. Cellular benign fibrous histiocytoma: clinicopathologic analysis of 74 cases of a distinctive variant of cutaneous fibrous histiocytoma with frequent recurrence. *Am J Surg Pathol* 1994;18:668–676.
14. Kamino H, Jacobson M. Dermatofibroma extending into the subcutaneous tissue: differential diagnosis from dermatofibrosarcoma protuberans. *Am J Surg Pathol* 1990;14:1156–1164.
15. Santa Cruz DJ, Kyriakos M. Aneurysmal ("angiomatoid") fibrous histiocytoma of the skin. *Cancer* 1981;47:2053–2061.
16. Calonje E, Fletcher CDM. Aneurysmal benign fibrous histiocytoma: a clinicopathological analysis of 40 cases of a tumour frequently misdiagnosed as a vascular neoplasm. *Histopathology* 1995;26:323–331.
17. Fukamizu H, Oku T, Inoue K, et al. Atypical ("pseudocarcinomatous") cutaneous histiocytoma. *J Cutan Pathol* 1983;10:327–333.
18. Tamada S, Ackerman AB. Dermatofibroma with monster cells. *Am J Dermatopathol* 1987;9:380–387.
19. Setoyama M, Fukumaru S, Kanzaki T. Case of dermatofibroma with monster cells: a review and an immunohistochemical study. *Am J Dermatopathol* 1997;19:312–315.
20. Kaddu S, McMenamin ME, Fletcher CDM. Atypical fibrous histiocytoma of the skin: clinicopathologic analysis of 59 cases with evidence of infrequent metastasis. *Am J Surg Pathol* 2002;26:35–46.
21. Wilson Jones E, Cerio R, Smith NP. Epithelioid cell histiocytoma: a new entity. *Br J Dermatol* 1989;120:185–195.

22. Singh Gomez C, Calonje E, Fletcher CDM. Epithelioid benign fibrous histiocytoma of skin: clinico-pathological analysis of 20 cases of a poorly known variant. *Histopathology* 1994;24:123–129.

23. Glusac EJ, McNiff JM. Epithelioid cell histiocytoma: a simulant of vascular and melanocytic neoplasms. *Am J Dermatopathol* 1999;21:1–7.

24. Fletcher CD. Benign fibrous histiocytoma of subcutaneous and deep soft tissue. A clinicopathological analysis of 21 cases. *Am J Surg Pathol* 1990;14:801–809.

25. Coindre JM. Deep benign fibrous histiocytoma. In: Fletcher CDM, Unnik K, Mertens F, eds. *World Health Organisation Classification of Tumours. Pathology and Genetics of Tumours of Soft Tissue and Bone.* Lyon: International Agency for Research on Cancer Press, 2002:114–115.

26. Wambacher-Gasser B, Zelger B, Zelger BG, et al. Clear cell dermatofibroma. *Histopathology* 1997;30:64–69.

27. Zelger BG, Steiner H, Kutzner H, et al. Granular cell dermatofibroma. *Histopathology* 1997;31:258–262.

28. Iwata J, Fletcher CDM. Lipidized fibrous histiocytoma. Clinicopathologic analysis of 22 cases. *Am J Dermatopathol* 2000;22:126–134.

29. Zelger BG, Calonje E, Zelger B. Myxoid dermatofibroma. *Histopathology* 1999;34:357–364.

30. Usmani A, Lal P, Li H, et al. Myofibroblastic differentiation in dermatofibromas. *J Cutan Pathol* 2000;27:576(abst).

31. Kutchemeshgi M, Barr RJ, Henderson CD. Dermatofibroma with osteoclast-like giant cells. *Am J Dermatopathol* 1992;14:397–401.

32. Kuo T-t, Hu S, Chan H-L. Keloidal dermatofibroma. *Am J Surg Pathol* 1998;22:564–568.

33. Kiyohara T, Kumakiri M, Kobayashi H, et al. Atrophic dermatofibroma. Elastophagocytosis by the tumor cells. *J Cutan Pathol* 2000;27:312–315.

34. Schwob VS, Santa Cruz DJ. Palisading cutaneous fibrous histiocytoma. *J Cutan Pathol* 1986;13:403–407.

35. Klaus SN, Winkelman RK. The enzyme histochemistry of nodular subepidermal fibrosis. *Br J Dermatol* 1966;78:398–402.

36. Zelger BG, Zelger B. Dermatofibroma (fibrous histiocytoma): an inflammatory or neoplastic disorder? *Histopathology* 2001;38:379–381.

37. Calonje E. Is cutaneous benign fibrous histiocytoma (dermatofibroma) a reactive inflammatory process or a neoplasm? *Histopathology* 2000;37:278–280.

38. Chen T-C, Kuo T-t, Chan H-L. Dermatofibroma is a clonal proliferative disease. *J Cutan Pathol* 2000;27:36–39.

39. Colome-Grimmer MI, Evans HL. Metastasizing cellular dermatofibroma. A report of two cases. *Am J Surg Pathol* 1996;20:1361–1367.

40. Colby TV. Metastasizing dermatofibroma. *Am J Surg Pathol* 1997;21:976.

41. Hui P, Glusac EJ, Sinard JH, et al. Clonal analysis of cutaneous fibrous histiocytoma (dermatofibroma). *J Cutan Pathol* 2002;29:385–389.

42. Pinkus H. Pathobiology of the pilary complex. *Jpn J Dermatol [B]* 1967;77:304–330.

43. Cheng L, Amini SB, Zaim MT. Follicular basal cell hyperplasia overlying dermatofibroma. *Am J Surg Pathol* 1997;21:711–718.

44. Morgan MB, Howard HG, Everett MA. Epithelial induction in dermatofibroma: a role for the epidermal growth factor (EGF) receptor. *Am J Dermatopathol* 1997;19:35–40.

45. Han K-H, Huh C-H, Cho K-H. Proliferation and differentiation of the keratinocytes in hyperplastic epidermis overlying dermatofibroma. Immunohistochemical characterization. *Am J Dermatopathol* 2001;23:90–98.

46. Unna PG. Histopathologie der hautkrankheiten. Berlin: August Hirschwald, 1894;839–842.

47. Woringer F, Kviatkowski S. L'histiocytome de la peau. *Ann Dermatol Syph* 1932;3:998–1010.

48. Senear FE, Caro MR. Histiocytoma cutis. *Arch Dermatol Syph* 1936;33:209–226.

49. Calonje E, Fletcher CDM. Cutaneous fibrohistiocytic tumors: an update. *Adv Anat Pathol* 1994;1:2–15.

50. Cerio R, Spaull J, Wilson Jones E. Histiocytoma cutis: a tumor of dermal dendrocytes (dermal dendrocytoma). *Br J Dermatol* 1989;120:197–206.

51. Headington JT. The dermal dendrocyte. *Adv Dermatol* 1986;1:159–171.

52. Prieto VG, Reed JA, Shea CR. Immunohistochemistry of dermatofibroma and benign fibrous histiocytomas. *J Cutan Pathol* 1995;22:336–341.

53. Mihatsch-Konz B, Schaumburg-Lever G, Lever WF. Ultrastructure of dermatofibroma. *Arch Dermatol Forsch* 1973;246:181–192.

54. Aubock L. Zur Ultrastruktur fibroser und histiocytarer Hauttumoren. *Virchows Arch [A]* 1975;368:253–274.

55. Katenkamp D, Stiller D. Cellular composition of the so-called dermatofibroma (histiocytoma cutis). *Virchows Arch* 1975;367:325–336.

56. Kindblom LG, Jacobsen GK, Jacobsen M. Immunohistochemical investigations of tumors of supposed fibroblastic-histiocytic origin. *Hum Pathol* 1982;13:834–840.

57. Kerdel FA, Morgan EW, Holden CA. Demonstration of alpha-1–anti-trypsin and alpha-1–antichymotrypsin in cutaneous histiocytic infiltrates. *J Am Acad Dermatol* 1982;7:177–182.

58. Burgdorf W, Moreland A, Wasik R. Negative immunoperoxidase staining for lysozyme in nodular subepidermal fibrosis. *Arch Dermatol* 1982;118:241–243.

59. Kanitakis J, Schmitt D, Thivolet J. Immunohistologic study of cellular populations of histiocytofibromas ("dermatofibromas"). *J Cutan Pathol* 1984;11:88–94.

60. Zelger B, Sidoroff A, Stanzl U, et al. Deep penetrating dermatofibroma versus dermatofibrosarcoma protuberans. *Am J Surg Pathol* 1994;18:677–686.

61. Goldblum JR, Tuthill RJ. CD34 and factor XIIIa immunoreactivity in dermatofibrosarcoma protuberans and dermatofibroma. *Am J Dermatopathol* 1997;19:147–153.

62. Horenstein MG, Prieto VG, Nuckols JD, et al. Indeterminate fibrohistiocytic lesions of the skin. Is there a spectrum between dermatofibroma and dermatofibrosarcoma protuberans? *Am J Surg Pathol* 2000;24:996–1003

63. Franchi A, Santucci M. Tenascin expression in cutaneous fibrohistiocytic tumors. Immunohistochemical investigation of 24 cases. *Am J Dermatopathol* 1996;18:454–459.

64. Kahn HJ, Fekete E, From L. Tenascin differentiates dermatofibromas from dermatofibrosarcoma protuberans: comparison with CD34 and factor XIIIa. *Hum Pathol* 2001;32:50–56.

65. Fletcher CDM. Angiomatoid "malignant fibrous histiocytoma": an immunohistochemical study indicative of myoid differentiation. *Hum Pathol* 1991;22:563–568.

66. Costa MJ, Weiss SW. Angiomatoid malignant fibrous histiocytoma: a follow-up study of 108 cases with evaluation of possible histologic predictors of outcome. *Am J Surg Pathol* 1990;14:1126–1132.

67. Peters CW, Hanke CW, Pasarell HA, et al. Dermatofibrosarcoma protuberans of the face. *J Dermatol Surg Oncol* 1982;8:823–826.

68. Gutierrez G, Ospina JE, De Baez NE, et al. Dermatofibrosarcoma protuberans. *Int J Dermatol* 1984;23:396–401.

69. McKee PH, Fletcher CDM. Dermatofibrosarcoma protuberans presenting in infancy and childhood. *J Cutan Pathol* 1991;18:241–246.

70. Martin L, Combemale P, Dupin M, et al. The atrophic variant of dermatofibrosarcoma protuberans in childhood: a report of six cases. *Br J Dermatol* 1998;139:719–725.

71. Checketts SR, Hamilton TK, Baughman RD. Congenital and childhood dermatofibrosarcoma protuberans: a case report and review of the literature. *J Am Acad Dermatol* 2000;42:907–913.

72. Kahn LB, Saxe N, Gordon W. Dermatofibrosarcoma protuberans with lymph node and pulmonary metastases. *Arch Dermatol* 1978;114:599–601.

73. Taylor HB, Helwig EB. Dermatofibrosarcoma protuberans. *Cancer* 1961;15:717–725.

74. Fletcher CDM, Evans BJ, MacArtney JC, et al. Dermatofibrosarcoma protuberans: a clinicopathological and immunohistochemical study with a review of the literature. *Histopathology* 1985;9:921–938.

75. Bednar F. Storiform neurofibromas of the skin, pigmented and non-pigmented. *Cancer* 1957;10:368–376.

76. Dupree WB, Langloss JM, Weiss SW. Pigmented dermatofibrosarcoma protuberans (Bednar tumor). A pathologic, ultrastructural, and immunohistochemical study. *Am J Surg Pathol* 1985;9:630–639.

77. Fletcher CDM, Theaker JM, Flanagan A, et al. Pigmented dermatofibrosarcoma protuberans (Bednar tumour): melanocytic colonization or neuroectodermal differentiation? A clinicopathological and immunohistochemical study. *Histopathology* 1988;13:631–643.

78. Connelly JH, Evans HL. Dermatofibrosarcoma protuberans: a clinicopathologic review with emphasis on fibrosarcomatous areas. *Am J Surg Pathol* 1992;16:921–925.

79. Diaz-Cascajo C, Weyers W, Borrego L, et al. Dermatofibrosarcoma protuberans with fibrosarcomatous areas: a clinicopathologic and immunohistochemic study in four cases. *Am J Dermatopathol* 1997;19:562–567.

80. Goldblum JR, Reith JD, Weiss SW. Sarcomas arising in dermatofibrosarcoma protuberans. A reappraisal of biologic behavior in eighteen cases treated by wide local excision with extended clinical follow up. *Am J Surg Pathol* 2000;24:1125–1130.

81. Shmookler BM, Enzinger FM, Weiss SW. Giant cell fibroblastoma: a juvenile form of dermatofibrosarcoma protuberans. *Cancer* 1989;64:2154–2161.

82. Beham A, Fletcher DC. Dermatofibrosarcoma protuberans with areas resembling giant cell fibroblastoma: report of two cases. *Histopathology* 1990;17:165–167.

83. Alguacil-Garcia A. Giant cell fibroblastoma recurring as dermatofibrosarcoma protuberans. *Am J Surg Pathol* 1991;15:798–801.

84. Allen PW, Zwi J. Giant cell fibroblastoma transforming into dermatofibrosarcoma protuberans [Letter]. *Am J Surg Pathol* 1992;15:1127–1128.

85. Coyne J, Kaftan SM, Craig RD. Dermatofibrosarcoma protuberans recurring as a giant cell fibroblastoma. *Histopathology* 1992;21:184–187.

86. Michael M, Zamecnik M. Giant cell fibroblastoma with a dermatofibrosarcoma protuberans component. *Am J Dermatopathol* 1992;14:549–552.

87. Alguacil-Garcia A, Unni KH, Goellner JR. Histogenesis of dermatofibrosarcoma protuberans: an ultrastructural study. *Am J Clin Pathol* 1978;69:427–434.

88. Zina AM, Bundino S. Dermatofibrosarcoma protuberans: an ultrastructural study of five cases. *J Cutan Pathol* 1979;6:265–271.

89. Hashimoto K, Brownstein MH, Jacobiec FA. Dermatofibrosarcoma protuberans. *Arch Dermatol* 1974;110:874–885.

90. Lautier R, Wolff HH, Jones RE. An immunohistochemical study of dermatofibrosarcoma protuberans supports its fibroblastic character and contradicts neuroectodermal or histiocytic components. *Am J Dermatopathol* 1990;2:25–30.

91. Ma CK, Zarbo RJ, Gown AM. Immunohistochemical characterization of atypical fibroxanthoma and dermatofibrosarcoma protuberans. *Am J Clin Pathol* 1992;97:478–483.

92. Weiss SW, Nickoloff BJ. CD-34 is expressed by a distinctive cell population in peripheral nerve, nerve sheath tumors, and related lesions. *Am J Surg Pathol* 1993;17:1039–1045.

93. Calonje E, Fletcher CDM. Myoid differentiation in dermatofibrosarcoma protuberans and its fibrosarcomatous variant: clinicopathologic analysis of 5 cases. *J Cutan Pathol* 1996;23:30–36.

94. Aiba S, Tabata N. Ishil H, et al. Dermatofibrosarcoma protuberans is a unique fibrohistiocytic tumor expressing CD34. *Br J Dermatol* 1992;127:79–84.

95. Altman DA, Nickoloff BJ, Fivenson DP. Differential expression of factor XIIIa and CD34 in cutaneous mesenchymal tumors. *J Cutan Pathol* 1993;20:154–158.

96. Calikoglu E, Augsburger E, Chavaz P, et al. CD44 and hyaluronate in the differential diagnosis of dermatofibroma and dermatofibroma protuberans. *J Cutan Pathol* 2003;30:185–189.

97. Shmookler BM, Enzinger FM. Giant cell fibroblastoma: a peculiar childhood tumor. *Lab Invest* 1982;46:76A(abst).

98. Dymock RB, Allen PW, Stirling JW, et al. Giant cell fibroblastoma: a distinctive, recurrent tumor of childhood. *Am J Surg Pathol* 1987;11:263–272.

99. Weiss SW, Goldblum JR. Giant cell fibroblastoma. In: *Enzinger and Weiss's Soft Tissue Tumors*, 4th ed. Philadelphia: Mosby-Harcourt, 2001:507–516.

100. Harvell JD, Kilpatrick SE, White WL. Histogenetic relations between giant cell fibroblastoma and dermatofibrosarcoma protuberans. CD34 staining showing the spectrum and a simulator. *Am J Dermatopathol* 1998;20:339–345.

101. Dal Cin P, Sciot R, De Wever J, et al. Cytogenetic and immunohistochemical evidence that giant cell fibroblastoma is related to dermatofibrosarcoma protuberans. *Genes Chrom Cancer* 1996;15:73–75.

102. Terrier-Lacombe M-J, Guillou L, Maire G, et al. Dermatofibrosarcoma protuberans, giant cell fibroblastoma, and hybrid lesions in children: clinicopathological comparative analysis 28 cases with molecular data. *Am J Surg Pathol* 2003;27:27–39.

103. De Chadarevian JP, Coppola D, Billmure DF. Bednar tumor pattern in recurring giant cell fibroblastoma. *Am J Clin Pathol* 1993;100:164–166.

104. Zamecnik M, Michael M. Giant cell fibroblastoma with pigmented dermatofibrosarcoma protuberans component. *Am J Surg Pathol* 1994;18:736–740.

105. Gonatas K. Extra-abdominal desmoid tumors: report of six cases. *Arch Pathol* 1961;71:214–221.

106. Goellner JR, Soule EH. Desmoid tumors: an ultrastructural study of eight cases. *Hum Pathol* 1980;11:43–50.

107. Hayry P, Retamao JJ, Totterman S, et al. The desmoid tumor. II. Analysis of factors possibly contributing to the etiology and growth behavior. *Am J Clin Pathol* 1982;77:674–680.

108. Giarola M, Wells D, Mondini P, et al. Mutations of adenomatous polyposis cell (APC) gene are uncommon in sporadic desmoid tumours. *Br J Cancer* 1998;78:582–587.

109. Bridge JA, Swarts SJ, Buresh C, et al. Trisomies 8 and 20 characterize a subgroup of benign fibrous lesions arising in both soft tissue and bone. *Am J Pathol* 1999;154:729–733.

110. de Wever J, Dal Cin P, Fletcher CD, et al. Cytogenetic, clinical and morphologic correlations in 78 cases of fibromatosis: a report from the CHAMP Study Group. Chromosomes and morphology. *Mod Pathol* 2000;13:1080–1085.

111. Stiller D, Katenkamp D. Cellular features in desmoid fibromatosis and well differentiated fibrosarcomas: an electron microscopic study. *Virchows Arch [A]* 1975;369:155–164.

112. Hasegawa T, Hirose T, Kudo E, et al. Cytoskeletal characteristics of myofibroblasts in benign neoplastic and reactive fibroblastic lesions. *Virchows Arch [A]* 1990;416:375–382.

113. Goldblum J, Fletcher JA. Desmoid-type fibromatoses. In: Fletcher CDM, Unnik K, Mertens F, eds. *World Health Organisation Classification of Tumours. Pathology and Genetics of Tumours of Soft Tissue and Bone.* Lyon: International Agency for Research on Cancer Press, 2002:83–84.

114. Enzinger FM, Zhang R. Plexiform fibrohistiocytic tumor presenting in children and young adults. An analysis of 65 cases. *Am J Surg Pathol* 1988;12:818–826.

115. Remstein ED, Arndt CAS, Nascimento AG. Plexiform fibrohistiocytic tumor: clinicopathologic analysis of 22 cases. *Am J Surg Pathol* 1999;23:662–670.

116. Salamanca J, Rodríguez-Peralto JL, García de la Torre JP, et al. Plexiform fibrohistiocytic tumor without multinucleated giant cells. *Am J Dermatopathol* 2002;24:399–401.

117. Fisher C. Atypical plexiform fibrohistiocytic tumor. *Histopathology* 1997;30:271–273

118. Zelger B, Weinlich G, Steiner H, et al. Dermal and subcutaneous variants of plexiform fibrohistiocytic tumor. *Am J Surg Pathol* 1997;21:235–241.

119. Hollowood K, Holley MP, Fletcher CDM. Plexiform fibrohistiocytic tumor: clinicopathological, immunohistochemical and ultrastructural analysis in favour of a myofibroblastic lesion. *Histopathology* 1991;19:503–513.

120. Kamino H, Reddy VB, Guo M, et al. Dermatomyofibroma. *J Cutan Pathol* 1992;19:85–93.

121. Hugel H. Plaque-like dermal fibromatosis/dermatomyofibroma. *J Cutan Pathol* 1993;20:94.

122. Mortimore RJ, Whitehead KJ. Dermatomyofibroma: a report of two cases, one occurring in a child. *Australas J Dermatol* 2001;42:22–25.

123. Colome MI, Sanchez RL. Dermatomyofibroma: report of two cases. *J Cutan Pathol* 1994;21:371–376.

124. Mentzel T., Calonje E, Fletcher CDM. Dermatomyofibroma: additional observations on a distinctive cutaneous myofibroblastic tumour with emphases on differential diagnosis. *Br J Dermatol* 1993;129:69–73.

125. Ng WK, Cheung MF, Ma L. Dermatomyofibroma: further support of its myofibroblastic nature by electron microscopy. *Histopathology* 1996;29:181–183.

126. Weiss SW, Enzinger FM. Malignant fibrous histiocytoma: an analysis of 200 cases. *Cancer* 1978;41:2250–2266.

127. Lim S-C, Kim D-C, Jeong Y-K, et al. Malignant fibrous histiocytoma in a child's hand. *Histopathology* 1998;33:191–192.

128. Rothman AE, Lowitt MH, Pfau RG. Pediatric cutaneous malignant fibrous histiocytoma. *J Am Acad Dermatol* 2000;42:371–373.

129. Salo JC, Lewis JJ, Woodruff JM, et al. Malignant fibrous histiocytoma of the extremity. *Cancer* 1999;85:1765–1772.

130. Kempson RL, Kyriakos M. Fibroxanthosarcoma of the soft tissues: a type of malignant fibrous histiocytoma. *Cancer* 1972;29:961–976.

131. Pezzi CM, Rawlings MS Jr, Esgro JJ, et al. Prognostic factors in 227 patients with malignant fibrous histiocytoma. *Cancer* 1992;69:2098–2103.

132. Fu Y-S, Gabbiani G, Kaye GI, et al. Malignant soft tissue tumors of probable histiocytic origin (malignant fibrous histiocytomas): general considerations and electron microscopy and tissue culture studies. *Cancer* 1975;35:176–198.

133. Hardy TJ, An T, Brown PW, et al. Postirradiation sarcoma (malignant fibrous histiocytoma) of axilla. *Cancer* 1978;42:118–124.

134. Weiss SW. Malignant fibrous histiocytoma. *Am J Surg Pathol* 1982;6:773–784.

135. Weiss SW, Enzinger FM. Myxoid variant of malignant fibrous histiocytoma. *Cancer* 1977;39:1672–1685.

136. Lillemoe T, Steeper T, Manivel JC, et al. Myxoid malignant fibrous histiocytoma (MMFH) of the skin. *J Cutan Pathol* 1988; 15:324(abst).

137. Guccion JG, Enzinger FM. Malignant giant cell tumor of soft parts: an analysis of 32 cases. *Cancer* 1972;29:1518–1529.

138. Kyriakos M, Kempson RL. Inflammatory fibrous histiocytoma. *Cancer* 1976;37:1584–1606.

139. Enzinger FM. Angiomatoid malignant fibrous histiocytoma: a distinct fibrohistiocytic tumor of children and young adults simulating a vascular neoplasm. *Cancer* 1979;44:2147–2157.

140. Weiss SW. Histological Typing of Soft Tissue Tumours. *World Health Organization, Geneva International Histological Classification of Tumours*, No. 3, 2nd ed. Berlin and New York: Springer-Verlag, 1994:21..

141. Fanburg-Smith JC, Miettinen M. Angiomatoid "malignant" fibrous histiocytoma: a clinicopathologic study of 158 cases and further exploration of the myoid phenotype. *Hum Pathol* 1999;30:1336–1343.

142. Angervall L, Hagmar B, Kindblom LG, et al. Malignant giant cell tumor of soft tissue. *Cancer* 1981;47:736–747.

143. Soule EH, Enriquez P. Atypical fibrous histiocytoma, malignant fibrous histiocytoma, malignant histiocytoma, and epithelioid sarcoma: a comparative study of 65 tumors. *Cancer* 1974; 30:128–143.

144. Taxy JB, Battifora H. Malignant fibrous histiocytoma. *Cancer* 1977;40:254–267.

145. Roholl PJ, Prinsen I, Rademakers LP, et al. Two cell lines with epithelial cell-like characteristics established from malignant fibrous histiocytomas. *Cancer* 1991;68:1963–1972.

146. Litzky LA, Brooks JJ. Cytokeratin immunoreactivity in malignant fibrous histiocytoma and spindle cell tumors: comparison between frozen and paraffin-embedded tissues. *Mod Pathol* 1992;5:30–34.

147. Rosenberg AE, O'Connell JX, Dickerson GR, et al. Expression of epithelial markers in malignant fibrous histiocytoma of the musculoskeletal system: an immunohistochemical and electron microscopic study. *Hum Pathol* 1993;24:284–293.

148. Fletcher CDM. Pleomorphic malignant fibrous histiocytoma: fact or fiction? A critical reappraisal based on 159 tumors diagnosed as pleomorphic sarcoma. *Am J Surg Pathol* 1992;16: 213–228.

149. Hollowood K, Fletcher CDM. Malignant fibrous histiocytoma: morphologic pattern or pathologic entity? *Semin Diagn Pathol* 1995;12:210–220.

150. Weiss SW, Goldblum JR. Malignant fibrous histiocytoma. In: *Enzinger and Weiss's Soft Tissue Tumors*, 4th ed. Philadelphia: Mosby-Harcourt, 2001:539–569.

151. Fletcher CDM, van den Berg E, Molenaar WM. Pleomorphic malignant fibrous histiocytoma/undifferentiated high grade pleomorphic sarcoma. In: Fletcher CDM, Unnik K, Mertens F, eds. *World Health Organisation Classification of Tumours. Pathology and Genetics of Tumours of Soft Tissue and Bone.* Lyon: International Agency for Research on Cancer Press, 2002:120–122.

152. Weiss SW, Goldblum JR. Atypical fibroxanthoma. In: *Enzinger and Weiss's Soft Tissue Tumors*, 4th ed. Philadelphia: Mosby-Harcourt, 2001:536–539.

153. Smith ME, Costa MJ, Weiss SW. Evaluation of CD68 and other histiocytic antigens in angiomatoid malignant fibrous histiocytoma. *Am J Surg Pathol* 1991;15:757–763.

154. Helwig EB. Atypical fibroxanthoma. *Tex State J Med* 1963;59: 664–667.

155. Fretzin DFJ, Helwig EB. Atypical fibroxanthoma of the skin. *Cancer* 1973;31:1541–1552.

156. Kroe OJ, Pitcock JA. Atypical fibroxanthoma of the skin. *Am J Clin Pathol* 1969;51:487–492.

157. Barr RJ, Wuerker RB, Graham JH. Ultrastructure of atypical fibroxanthoma. *Cancer* 1977;40:736–743.

158. Enzinger FM. Atypical fibroxanthoma and malignant fibrous histiocytoma. *Am J Dermatopathol* 1979;1:185.

159. Westermann FN, Langlois NEI, Simpson JG. Apoptosis in atypical fibroxanthoma and pleomorphic malignant fibrous histiocytoma. *Am J Dermatopathol* 1997;19:228–231.

160. Jacobs DS, Edwards WD, Ye RC. Metastatic atypical fibroxanthoma of the skin. *Cancer* 1975;35:457–463.

161. Helwig EB, May D. Atypical fibroxanthoma of the skin with metastasis. *Cancer* 1986;57:368–376.

162. Zelger B, Soyer HP. Between Scylla and Charybdis: mythology in dermatology. *Dermatopathol Pract Conceptual* 2000;6:348–355.

163. Zelger BG, Soyer HP, Zelger B. Giant cell atypical fibroxanthoma: does it really exist? *Am J Dermatopathol* 1999;21:108–109.

164. Vargas-Cortes F, Winkelmann RK, Soule EH. Atypical fibroxanthoma of the skin. *Mayo Clin Proc* 1973;48:211–218.

165. Dahl I. Atypical fibroxanthoma of the skin. *Acta Pathol Microbiol Immunol Scand [A]* 1976;84:183–197.

166. Beham A, Fletcher CDM. Atypical "pseudosarcomatous" variant of cutaneous benign fibrous histiocytoma: a report of eight cases. *Histopathology* 1990;17:165–182.

167. Kemp JD, Stenn KS, Arons M, et al. Metastasizing atypical fibroxanthoma. *Arch Dermatol* 1978;14:1533–1535.

168. Calonje E, Wadden C, Wilson Jones E, Fletcher CDM. Spindle-cell non-pleomorphic atypical fibroxanthoma: analysis of a series and delineation of a distinctive variant. *Histopathology* 1992;22:247–254.

169. Requena L, Sangueza OP, Sinchez Yus E, et al. Clear-cell atypical fibroxanthoma: an uncommon histopathologic variant of atypical fibroxanthoma. *J Cutan Pathol* 1997;24:176–182.

170. Crowson AN, Carlson-Sweet K, MacInnis C, et al. Clear cell atypical fibroxanthoma: a clinicopathologic study. *J Cutan Pathol* 2002;29:374–381.

171. Diaz-Cascajo C, Borghi S, Bonczkowitz M. Pigmented atypical fibroxanthoma. *Histopathology* 1998;33:537–541.

172. Orosz Z. Atypical fibroxanthoma with granular cells. *Histopathology* 1998;33:88–89.

173. Alguacil-Garcia A, Unni KK, Goellner JR, et al. Atypical fibroxanthoma of the skin: an ultrastructural study of two cases. *Cancer* 1977;40:1471–1480.

174. Longacre TA, Smoller BR, Rouse RU. Atypical fibroxanthoma: multiple immunohistologic profiles. *Am J Surg Pathol* 1993;17:1199–1209.

175. Enzinger FM. Epithelioid sarcoma: a sarcoma simulating a granuloma or a carcinoma. *Cancer* 1970;26:1029–1041.

176. Chase DR, Enzinger FM. Epithelioid sarcoma: diagnosis, prognostic indicators and treatment. *Am J Surg Pathol* 1985;9:241–263.

177. Kodet R, Smelhais V, Newton WA, et al. Epithelioid sarcoma in childhood. *Pediatr Pathol* 1994;14:433.

178. Schmidt D, Harms D. Epithelioid sarcoma in children and adolescents: an immunohistochemical study. *Virchows Arch [A] Pathol Anat* 1987;410:423.

179. Billings SD, Hood AF. Epithelioid sarcoma arising on the nose of a child: a case report and review of the literature. *J Cutan Pathol* 2000;27:186–190.

180. Moore SW, Wheeler JE, Hefter LG. Epithelioid sarcoma masquerading as Peyronie's disease. *Cancer* 1975;35:1706–1710.

181. Huang DJ, Stanisic TH, Hansen KK. Epithelioid sarcoma of the penis. *J Urol* 1992;147:1370–1372.

182. Weismann D, Amenta PS, Kantor GR. Vulvar epithelioid sarcoma metastatic to scalp: a case report and review of the literature. *Am J Dermatopathol* 1990;12:462–468.

183. Bos GD, Pritchard DJ, Reiman HM, et al. Epithelioid sarcoma: an analysis of fifty-one cases. *J Bone Joint Surg Am* 1988;70:862–870.

184. Evans HL, Baer SC. Epithelioid sarcoma: a clinicopathologic and prognostic study of 26 cases. *Semin Diagn Pathol* 1993;10:286–291.

185. Guillou L, Wadden C, Coindre J-M, et al. "Proximal-type" epithelioid sarcoma, a distinctive aggressive neoplasm showing rhabdoid features. *Am J Surg Pathol* 1997;21:130–146.

186. Hasegawa T, Matsuno Y, Shimoda T, et al. Proximal-type epithelioid sarcoma: a clinicopathologic study of 20 cases. *Mod Pathol* 2001;14:655–663.

187. Mirra JM, Kessler S, Bhuta S, et al. The fibroma-like variant of epithelioid sarcoma: a fibrohistiocytic/myoid cell lesion often confused with benign and malignant spindle cell tumors. *Cancer* 1992;15:1382–1395.

188. Tan SH, Ong BH. Spindle cell variant of epithelioid sarcoma: an easily misdiagnosed tumor. *Australas J Dermatol* 2001;42:139–141.

189. Heenan PJ, Quirk CJ, Papadimitriou JM. Epithelioid sarcoma: a diagnostic problem. *Am J Dermatopathol* 1986;8:95–104.

190. Fisher C. Epithelioid sarcoma. *Hum Pathol* 1988;19:265–275.

191. Miettinen M, Fanburg-Smith JC, Virolainen M, et al. Epithelioid sarcoma: an immunohistochemical analysis of 112 classical and variant cases and a discussion of the differential diagnosis. *Hum Pathol* 1999;30:934–942.

192. Guillou L, Kaneko Y. Epithelioid sarcoma. In: Fletcher CDM, Unnik K, Mertens F, eds. *World Health Organisation Classification of Tumours. Pathology and Genetics of Tumours of Soft Tissue and Bone.* Lyon: International Agency for Research on Cancer Press, 2002:205–207.

193. Fisher C, de Bruijn DRH, Geurts van Kessel A. Synovial sarcoma. In: Fletcher CDM, Unnik K, Mertens F, eds. *World Health Organisation Classification of Tumours. Pathology and Genetics of Tumours of Soft Tissue and Bone.* Lyon: International Agency for Research on Cancer Press, 2002:203–204.

194. Lin L, Skacel M, Sigel JE, et al. Epithelioid sarcoma: an immunohistochemical analysis evaluating the utility of cytokeratin 5/6 in distinguishing superficial epithelioid sarcoma from spindled squamous cell carcinoma. *J Cutan Pathol* 2003;30:114–116.

195. Fletcher CDM, McKee PH. Sarcomas: III. Synovial sarcoma. *Clin Exp Dermatol* 1985;10:332–349.

196. Flieder DB, Moran CA. Primary cutaneous synovial sarcoma. A case report. *Am J Dermatopathol* 1998;20:509–512.

197. van de Rijn M, Barr FG, Collins MH, et al Absence of SYT-SSX fusion products in soft tissue tumors other than synovial sarcoma. *Am J Clin Pathol* 1999;112:43–49.

198. Miettinen M, Virtanen I. Synovial sarcoma: a misnomer. *Am J Pathol* 1984;117:18–25.

199. Ghadially FN. Is synovial sarcoma a carcinosarcoma of connective tissue? *Ultrastruct Pathol* 1987;11:147–151.

200. Guarino M, Christensen L. Immunohistochemical analysis of extracellular matrix components in synovial sarcoma. *J Pathol* 1994;172:279–286.

201. Santa Cruz DJ, Reiner CB. Recurrent digital fibroma of childhood. *J Cutan Pathol* 1978;5:339–346.

202. Shapiro L. Infantile digital fibromatosis and aponeurotic fibroma. *Arch Dermatol* 1969;99:37–42.

203. Choi KC, Hashimoto K, Setoyama M, et al. Infantile digital fibromatosis: Immunohistochemical and immunoelectron microscopic studies. *J Cutan Pathol* 1990;17:225–232.

204. Mukai M, Torikata C, Iri H, et al. Immunohistochemical identification of aggregated actin filaments in formalin-fixed, paraffin-embedded sections. *Am J Surg Pathol* 1992;16:110–115.

205. Bhawan J, Bacchetta C, Joris I. A myofibroblastic tumor: infantile digital fibroma. *Am J Pathol* 1979;94:19–36.

206. Hayashi T, Tsuda N, Chowbury PR, et al. Infantile digital fibromatosis: a study of the development and regression of cytoplasmic inclusion bodies. *Mod Pathol* 1995;8:548–552.

207. Verallo VVM. Acquired digital fibrokeratomas. *Br J Dermatol* 1968;80:730–736.

208. Kint A, Baran R. Histopathologic study of Koenen tumors: are they different from acquired digital fibrokeratoma? *J Am Acad Dermatol* 1988;18:369–372.

209. Dereure O, Savoy D, Doz F, et al Multiple acral fibromas in a patient with familial retinoblastoma: a cutaneous marker of tumour-suppressor gene germline mutation? *Br J Dermatol* 2000;143:856–859.

210. Moulin G, Balme B, Thomas L. Familial multiple acral mucinous fibrokeratomas. *J Am Acad Dermatol* 1998;38:999–1001.

211. Bart RS, Andrade R, Kopf AW, et al. Acquired digital fibrokeratomas. *Arch Dermatol* 1968;97:120–129.

212. Hare PJ, Smith PAJ. Acquired (digital) keratoma. *Br J Dermatol* 1969;81:667–670.

213. Ackerman AB, de Viragh PA, Chongchitnant N. Fibrofolliculoma and trichodiscoma. In: Ackerman AB, de Viragh PA, Chongchitnant N, eds. *Neoplasms with Follicular Differentiation*. Philadelphia/London: Lea & Febiger, 1993:244.

214. Collins GL, Somach S, Morgan MB. Histomorphologic and immunophenotypic analysis of fibrofolliculomas and trichodiscomas in Birt–Hogg–Dube syndrome and sporadic disease. *J Cutan Pathol* 2002;29:529–533.

215. Pinkus H, Coskey R, Burgess GH. Trichodiscoma: a benign tumor related to Haarscheibe (hair disk). *J Invest Dermatol* 1974;63:212–218.

216. Birt AR, Hogg GR, Dube WJ. Hereditary multiple fibrofolliculomas with trichodiscomas and acrochordons. *Arch Dermatol* 1977;113:1674–1677.

217. Fujita WH, Barr RJ, Headley JL. Multiple fibrofolliculomas with trichodiscomas and acrochordons. *Arch Dermatol* 1981; 117:32–35.

218. Foucar K, Rosen T, Foucar E, et al. Fibrofolliculoma: a clinicopathologic study. *Cutis* 1981;28:429–432.

219. Hornstein OP, Knickenberg M. Perifollicular fibromatosis cutis with polyps of the colon: a cutaneointestinal syndrome sui generis. *Arch Dermatol Res* 1975;253:161–175.

220. Starink TM, Kisch LS, Meijer CJLM. Familial multiple trichodiscomas: a clinicopathologic study. *Arch Dermatol* 1985; 121:888–891.

221. Graham JH, Saunders JB, Johnson WC, et al. Fibrous papule of the nose: a clinicopathological study. *J Invest Dermatol* 1965; 45:194–203.

222. Saylan T, Marks R, Wilson Jones E. Fibrous papule of the nose. *Br J Dermatol* 1971;85:111–118.

223. Reed RJ, Hairston MA, Palomeque FE. The histologic identity of adenoma sebaceum and solitary melanocytic angiofibroma. *Dermatol Int* 1966;5:3–11.

224. Meigel WN, Ackerman AB. Fibrous papule of the face. *Am J Dermatopathol* 1979;1:329–340.

225. McGibbon DH, Wilson Jones E. Fibrous papule of the nose. *Am J Dermatopathol* 1979;1:345–348.

226. Ragaz A, Berezowsky V. Fibrous papule of the face: a study of five cases by electron microscopy. *Am J Dermatopathol* 1979;1: 353–355.

227. Kimura S, Yamasaki Y. Ultrastructure of fibrous papule of the nose. *J Dermatol* 1983;10:571–578.

228. Spiegel J, Nadji M, Penneys NS. Fibrous papule: an immunohistochemical study with antibody to S100 protein. *J Am Acad Dermatol* 1983;9:360–362.

229. Nemeth AJ, Penneys NS, Bernstein HB. Fibrous papule: a tumor of fibrohistiocytic cells that contain factor XIIIa. *J Am Acad Dermatol* 1988;19:1102–1106.

230. Cerio R, Rao BK, Spaull J, et al. An immunohistochemical study of fibrous papule of the nose: 25 cases. *J Cutan Pathol* 1989;16:194–198.

231. Nemeth AJ, Penneys NS. Factor XIIIa is expressed by fibroblasts in fibrovascular tumors. *J Cutan Pathol* 1989;16:266–271.

232. Cerio R, Wilson Jones E. Factor XIIIa positivity in fibrous papule. *J Am Acad Dermatol* 1990;20:138–139.

233. Nickel WR, Reed WB. Tuberous sclerosis: special reference to the microscopic alterations in the cutaneous hamartomas. *Arch Dermatol* 1962;85:209–226.

234. Ackerman AB, Kornberg R. Pearly penile papules. Acral angiofibromas. *Arch Dermatol* 1973;108:673–675.

235. Sanchez NP, Wick MR, Perry HO. Adenoma sebaceum of Pringle: a clinicopathologic review, with a discussion of related pathologic entities. *J Cutan Pathol* 1981;8:395–403.

236. Fitzpatrick TB, Szabo G, Hori Y, et al. White leaf-shaped macules. *Arch Dermatol* 1968;98:1–6.

237. Kwiatkowski DJ, Short MP. Tuberous sclerosis. *Arch Dermatol* 1994;130:348–354.

238. Wienecke R, Maize JC Jr, Lowry DR, et al. The tuberous sclerosis gene TSC2 is a tumor suppressor gene whose protein product co-localizes with its putative substrate RAP1 in the *cis*/medial golgi. *J Invest Dermatol* 1996;106:811(abst).

239. Yamashita Y, Ono J, Okada S, et al Analysis of all exons of TSC1 and TSC2 genes for germline mutations in Japanese patients with tuberous sclerosis: report of 10 mutations. Am J Med Genet 2000;90:123–126.

240. Reed WB, Nickel WR, Campion G. Internal manifestations of tuberous sclerosis [Review]. *Arch Dermatol* 1963;87:715–728.

241. Scheig RL, Bornstein P. Tuberous sclerosis in the adult. *Arch Intern Med* 1961;108:789–795.

242. Morales JB. Congenital rhabdomyoma, tuberous sclerosis, and splenic histiocytosis. *Arch Pathol* 1961;71:485–493.

243. Price EB Jr, Mostofi FK. Symptomatic angiomyolipoma of the kidney. *Cancer* 1965;18:761–767.

244. Willis WF, Garcia RL. Giant angiofibroma in tuberous sclerosis. *Arch Dermatol* 1978;114:1843–1844.

245. Park YK, Hann SK. Cluster growths in adenoma sebaceum associated with tuberous sclerosis. *J Am Acad Dermatol* 1989; 20:918–920.

246. Kobayasi RT, Wolf-Jurgensen P, Danielsen L. Ultrastructure of shagreen patch. *Acta Derm Venereol (Stockh)* 1973;53:275–278.

247. Flegel H, Tessmann K. Gibt es ein weiches fibrom der haut? *Hautarzt* 1967;18:251–256.

248. Field LM. A giant pendulous fibrolipoma. *J Dermatol Surg Oncol* 1982;8:54–55.

249. Chobanian SJ, Van Ness MM, Winters C, Cattau EL. Skin tags as a marker for adenomatous polyps of the colon. *Ann Intern Med* 1985;103:892–893.

250. Beitler M, Eng A, Kilgour M, et al. Association between acrochordons and colonic polyps. *J Am Acad Dermatol* 1986;14: 1042–1049.

251. Chobanian SJ, Van Ness MM, Winters C. Skin tags as a screening marker for colonic neoplasia. *Gastrointest Endosc* 1986;32: 162.

252. Chobanian SJ. Skin tags and colonic polyps: a gastroenterologist's perspective. *J Am Acad Dermatol* 1987;16:407–409.

253. Margolis J, Margolis LS. Skin tags: a frequent sign of diabetes mellitus. *N Engl J Med* 1976;294:1184.

254. Kahana M, Grossman E, Feinstein A, et al. Skin tags: a cutaneous marker for diabetes mellitus. *Acta Derm Venereol (Stockh)* 1987;67:175–177.

255. Agarwal JK, Nigam PK. Acrochordon: a cutaneous sign of carbohydrate intolerance. *Australas J Dermatol* 1987;28:132–133.

256. Lawrence JH, Tobias CA, Linfoot JA, et al. Successful treatment of acromegaly: metabolic and clinical studies in 145 patients. *J Clin Endocrinol Metab* 1970;31:180–198.

257. Dalton AD, Coghill SB. No association between skin tags and colorectal adenomas. *Lancet* 1985;1:1332–1333.

258. Luk GD. Colonic polyps and acrochordons (skin tags) do not correlate in familial colonic polyposis kindreds. *Ann Intern Med* 1986;104:209–210.

259. Graffeo M, Cesari P, Buffoli F, et al. Skin tags: markers for colonic polyps? *J Am Acad Dermatol* 1989;21:1029–1030.

260. Da La Torre C, Ocampo C, Doval I, et al. Acrochordons are not a component of Birt–Hogg–Dube syndrome. Does this syndrome exist? Case reports and review of the literature. *Am J Dermatopathol* 1999;21:369–374.

261. Schulz T, Ebschner U, Hartschuh W. Localised Birt–Hogg–Dube syndrome with localised perivascular fibromas. *Am J Dermatopathol* 2001;23:149–153.

262. Stegmaier OC. Natural regression of the melanocytic nevus. *J Invest Dermatol* 1959;32:413–419.

263. Huntley AC. Eruptive lipofibromata. *Arch Dermatol* 1983;119:612–614.

264. Rapini RP, Golitz LE. Sclerotic fibromas of the skin. *J Am Acad Dermatol* 1989;20:266–271.

265. Starink TM, Meijer CJLM, Brownstein MH. The cutaneous pathology of Cowden's disease: new findings. *J Cutan Pathol* 1985;12:83–93.

266. Shitaba PK, Crouch EC, Fitzgibbon JF, et al. Cutaneous sclerotic fibroma. Immunohistochemical evidence of a fibroblastic neoplasm with ongoing type 1 collagen synthesis. *Am J Dermatopathol* 1995;17:339–343.

267. Hanft VN, Shea CR, McNutt NS, et al. Expression of CD34 in sclerotic ("plywood") fibromas. *Am J Dermatopathol* 2000;22:17–21.

268. Pujol RM, de Castro F, Schroeter AL, et al. Solitary sclerotic fibroma of the skin: a sclerotic dermatofibroma? *Am J Dermatopathol* 1996;18:620–624.

269. Chang S-N, Chun SI, Moon TK, et al. Solitary sclerotic fibroma of the skin. Degenerated sclerotic change of inflammatory conditions, especially folliculitis. *Am J Dermatopathol* 2000;22:22–25.

270. Rudolph P, Schubert C, Zelger BG, et al. Differential expression of CD34 and Ki-Mlp in pleomorphic fibroma and dermatofibroma with monster cells. *Am J Dermatopathol* 1999;21:414–419.

271. Kamino H, Lee JY-Y, Berke A. Pleomorphic fibroma of the skin; a benign neoplasm with cytologic atypia: a clinicopathologic study of eight cases. *Am J Surg Pathol* 1989;13:107–113.

272. Diaz-Cascajo C, Metze D. Angiofibroblastoma of the skin: a histological immunohistochemical, and ultrastructural report of two cases of an undescribed fibrous tumour. *Histopathology* 1999;35:109–113.

273. Diaz-Cascajo C, Schaefer D, Borghi S. Angiofibroblastoma of the skin: a report of seven cases in support of a distinctive entity. *J Cutan Pathol* 2002;29:534–539.

274. Jang J-G, Jung H-H, Suh K-S, et al. Desmoplastic fibroblastoma (collagenous fibroma). *Am J Dermatopathol* 1999;21:256–258.

275. Rudolph P, Schubert C, Harms D, et al. Giant cell collagenoma. A benign dermal tumor with distinctive multinucleate cells. *Am J Surg Pathol* 1998;22:557–563.

276. Junkins-Hopkins JM, Johnson WC. Desmoplastic fibroblastoma. *J Cutan Pathol* 1998;25:450–454.

277. Wesche WA, Cutlan RT. Collagenous fibroma: case report of a recently described benign soft tissue tumor. *J Cutan Pathol* 2000;27:576(abst).

278. Miettinen M, Fetsch JF. Collagenous fibroma (desmoplastic fibroblastoma): a clinicopathologic analysis of 63 cases of a distinctive soft tissue lesion with stellate-shaped fibroblasts. *Hum Pathol* 1998;29:676–682.

279. Chan JKC. Solitary fibrous tumour—everywhere, and a diagnosis in vogue. *Histopathology* 1997;31:568–576.

280. Okamura JM, Barr RJ, Battifora H. Solitary fibrous tumor of the skin. *Am J Dermatopathol* 1997;19:515–518.

281. Cowper SE, Kilpatrick T, Proper S, et al. Solitary fibrous tumor of the skin. *Am J Dermatopathol* 1999;21:213–219.

282. Morgan MB, Smoller BR. Solitary fibrous tumors are immunophenotypically distinct from mesothelioma(s). *J Cutan Pathol* 2000;27:451–454.

283. King DT, Millman AJ, Gurevitch AW. Giant cell tumor of the tendon sheath involving the skin. *Arch Dermatol* 1978;114:944–946.

284. Vogrincic GS, O'Connell JX, Gilks CB. Giant cell tumor of tendon sheath is a polyclonal cellular proliferation. *Hum Pathol* 1997;28:815–819.

285. de St. Aubain Somerhaussen N, Dal Cin P. Giant cell tumour of tendon sheath. In: Fletcher CDM, Unnik K, Mertens F, eds. *World Health Organisation Classification of Tumours. Pathology and Genetics of Tumours of Soft Tissue and Bone.* Lyon: International Agency for Research on Cancer Press, 2002:110–111.

286. Ushijima M, Hashimoto H, Tsuneyoshi M. Giant cell tumor of the tendon sheath (nodular tenosynovitis). *Cancer* 1986;57:875–884.

287. Carstens P. Giant cell tumors of tendon sheath. *Arch Pathol* 1978;102:99–103.

288. Rao AS, Vigorita VJ. Pigmented villonodular synovitis (giant cell tumor of the tendon sheath and synovial membrane): a review of 81 cases. *J Bone Joint Surg* 1984;66a:76.

289. Enzinger FM, Weiss SW. *Soft Tissue Tumors*, 3rd ed. St Louis: Mosby, 1995.

290. Alguacil-Garcia A, Unni KK, Goellner JR. Giant cell tumor of tendon sheath and pigmented villonodular synovitis: an ultrastructural study. *Am J Clin Pathol* 1978;69:6–17.

291. Wood GS, Beckstead JH, Medeiros LJ, et al. The cells of giant cell tumor of tendon sheath resemble osteoclasts. *Am J Surg Pathol* 1988;12:444–452.

292. Medeiros LJ, Beckstead JH, Rosenberg AE, et al. Giant cells and mononuclear cells of giant cell tumor of bone resemble histiocytes. *Appl Immunohistochem* 1993;1:115–122.

293. O'Connell JX, Fanburg JC, Rosenberg AE. Giant cell tumor of tendon sheath and pigmented villonodular synovitis: immunophenotype suggests a synovial cell origin. *Hum Pathol* 1995;26:771–775.

294. Chung EB, Enzinger FM. Fibroma of tendon sheath. *Cancer* 1979;44:1945–1954.

295. Cooper PH. Fibroma of tendon sheath. *J Am Acad Dermatol* 1984;11:625–628.

296. Dal Cin P, Sciot R, De Smet L, van den Berghe H. Translocation 2;11 in a fibroma of tendon sheath. *Histopathology* 1998;32:433–435.

297. Sciot R, Samson I, van den Berghe H, Van Damme B, et al. Collagenous fibroma (desmoplastic fibroblastoma): genetic link with fibroma of tendon sheath? *Mod Pathol* 1999;12:565–568.

298. Humphreys S, McKee PH, Fletcher CDM. Fibroma of tendon sheath. *J Cutan Pathol* 1986;13:331–338.

299. Hashimoto H, Tsuneyoshi M, Daimaru Y, et al. Fibroma of tendon sheath: a tumor of myofibroblasts. A clinicopathologic study of 18 cases. *Acta Pathol Jpn* 1985;35:1099–1107.

300. Hutter RVP, Stewart FW, Foote FW Jr. Fasciitis. *Cancer* 1962; 15:992–1003.

301. Bernstein KE, Lattes R. Nodular (pseudosarcomatous) fasciitis: a nonrecurrent lesion. *Cancer* 1982;49:1668–1678.

302. Mehregan AH. Nodular fasciitis. *Arch Dermatol* 1966;93:204–210.

303. Soule EH. Proliferative (nodular) fasciitis. *Arch Pathol* 1962;73:437–444.

304. Lai FM-M, Lam WY. Nodular fasciitis of the dermis. *J Cutan Pathol* 1993;20:66–69.

305. Goodlad JR, Fletcher CDM. Intradermal variant of nodular "fasciitis." *Histopathology* 1990;17:569–571.

306. Price S, Kahn LB, Saxe N. Dermal and intravascular fasciitis: unusual variants of nodular fasciitis. *Am J Dermatopathol* 1993; 15:539–543.

307. Wick MR, Mills SE, Ritter JH, et al. Postoperative/posttraumatic spindle cell nodule of the skin. The dermal analogue of nodular fasciitis. *Am J Dermatopathol* 1999;21:220–224.

308. Patchefsky AS, Enzinger FM. Intravascular fasciitis: a report of 17 cases. *Am J Surg Pathol* 1981;5:29–36.

309. Chung EB, Enzinger FM. Proliferative fasciitis. *Cancer* 1975; 36:1450–1458.

310. Diaz-Flores L, Martin Herrera AI, Garcia Montelongo R, et al. Proliferative fasciitis: ultrastructure and histogenesis. *J Cutan Pathol* 1989;16:85–92.

311. Wirman JA. Nodular fasciitis: a lesion of myofibroblasts. *Cancer* 1976;38:2378–2389.

312. Montgomery EA, Meis JM. Nodular fasciitis: its morphologic spectrum and immunohistochemical profile. *Am J Surg Pathol* 1991;15:942–948.

313. Lauer DH, Enzinger FM. Cranial fasciitis of childhood. *Cancer* 1980;45:401–406.

314. Patterson JW, Moran SL, Konerding H. Cranial fasciitis. *Arch Dermatol* 1989;125:674–678.

315. Venencie PV, Bigel P, Desgruelles C, et al. Infantile myofibromatosis. *Br J Dermatol* 1987;117:255–259.

316. Spraker MK, Stack C, Esterly NB. Congenital generalized fibromatosis. *J Am Acad Dermatol* 1984;10:365–371.

317. Stanford D, Rogers M. Dermatological presentations of infantile myofibromatosis: a review of 27 cases. *Australas J Dermatol* 2000;41:156–161.

318. Guitart J, Ritter JH, Wick MR. Solitary cutaneous myofibromas in adults: report of six cases and discussion of differential diagnosis. *J Cutan Pathol* 1996;23:437–444.

319. Fukasawa Y, Ishikura H, Takada A, et al. Massive apoptosis in infantile myofibromatosis: a putative mechanism of tumor regression. *Am J Pathol* 1994;144:480–485.

320. Chung EB, Enzinger FM. Infantile myofibromatosis. *Cancer* 1981;48:1807–1818.

321. Benjamin SP, Mercer RD, Hawk WA. Myofibroblastic contraction in spontaneous regression of multiple congenital mesenchymal hamartoma. *Cancer* 1977;40:2343–2352.

322. Zelger BWH, Calonje E, Sepp N, et al. Monophasic cellular variant of infantile myofibromatosis: an unusual histopathologic pattern in two siblings. *Am J Dermatopathol* 1995;17:131–138.

323. Smith KJ, Skelton HG, Barrett TL, et al. Cutaneous myofibroma. *Mod Pathol* 1989;2:603–609.

324. Daimaru Y, Hashimoto H, Enjoji M. Myofibromatosis in adults: adult counterpart of infantile myofibromatosis. *Am J Surg Pathol* 1989;13:859–865.

325. Fletcher CDM, Achu P, Van Noorden S, et al. Infantile myofibromatosis: a light microscopic, histochemical and immunohistochemical study suggesting true smooth muscle differentiation. *Histopathology* 1987;11:245–258.

326. Mentzel T, Calonje E, Nascimento AG, et al. Infantile hemangiopericytoma versus infantile myofibromatosis. Study of a series suggesting a continuous spectrum of infantile myofibroblastic lesions. *Am J Surg Pathol* 18:922–930.

327. Granter SR, Badizadegan K, Fletcher CDM. Myofibromatosis in adults, glomangiopericytoma and myopericytoma. A spectrum of tumors showing perivascular myoid differentiation. *Am J Surg Pathol* 1998;22:513–525.

328. Enzinger FM. Fibrous hamartoma of infancy. *Cancer* 1965;18:241–248.

329. Cooper PH. Fibrous proliferations of infancy and childhood. *J Cutan Pathol* 1992;19:257–267.

330. Scott DM, Peña JR, Omura EF. Fibrous hamartoma of infancy. *J Am Acad Dermatol* 1999;41:857–859.

331. Sotelo-Avila C, Bale PM. Subdermal fibrous hamartoma of infancy: pathology of 40 cases and differential diagnosis. *Pediatr Pathol* 1994;14:39–52.

332. Kitano Y. Juvenile hyalin fibromatosis. *Arch Dermatol* 1976; 112:86–88.

333. Gilaberte Y, Gonzalez Mediero I, Lopez Barrantes V, et al. Juvenile hyaline fibromatosis with skull-encephalic anomalies: a case report and review of the literature. *Dermatology* 1993; 187:144–148.

334. Hallock GG. Juvenile hyaline fibromatosis of the hand in an adult. *J Hand Surg [Am]* 1993;18:614–617.

335. Kan AE, Rogers M. Juvenile hyaline fibromatosis: an expanded clinicopathologic spectrum. *Pediatr Dermatol* 1989;6:68–75.

336. Kitano Y, Horiki M, Aoki T, et al. Two cases of juvenile hyalin fibromatosis. *Arch Dermatol* 1972;106:877–883.

337. Mayer-Da-Silva A, Polares-Baptista A, Rodrigo FG, et al. Juvenile hyalin fibromatosis. *Arch Pathol* 1988;112:928–931.

338. Remberger K, Krieg T, Kunze D, et al. Fibromatosis hyalinica multiplex (juvenile hyalin fibromatosis). *Cancer* 1985;56:614–624.

339. Winik BC, Boente MC, Asial R. Juvenile hyaline fibromatosis: ultrastructural study. *Am J Dermatopathol* 1998;20:373–378.

340. Ushigome S, Machinami R, Sorensen PH. Ewing sarcoma/primitive neuroectodermal tumour (PNET). In: Fletcher CDM, Unnik K, Mertens F, eds. *World Health Organisation Classification of Tumours. Pathology and Genetics of Tumours of Soft Tissue and Bone.* Lyon: International Agency for Research on Cancer Press, 2002:298–300.

341. Patterson JW, Maygarden SJ. Extraskeletal Ewing's sarcoma with cutaneous involvement. *J Cutan Pathol* 1986;13:46–58.

342. Ambros IM, Ambros PF, Strehl S, et al. MIC2 is a specific marker for Ewing's sarcoma and peripheral primitive neuroectodermal tumors. Evidence for a common histogenesis of Ewing's sarcoma and peripheral primitive neuroectodermal tumors from MIC2 expression and specific chromosome aberration. *Cancer* 1991;67:1886–1893.

343. Turc-Carel C, Aurias M, Mugneret F, et al. Chromosomes in Ewing's sarcoma. I. An evaluation of 85 cases and remarkable consistency of t(11;22)(q24;q12). *Cancer Genet Cytogenet* 1988;32:229–138.

344. Kempson RL, Fletcher CDM, Evans HL, et al. Cartilagenous and osseous tumors. In *Atlas of Tumor Pathology. Tumors of the Soft Tissues*, 3rd series, fasc. 30. Washington, DC: Armed Forces Institute of Pathology, 2001: 444–452.

345. Carney JA, Headington JT, Su WPD. Cutaneous myxomas: a major component of the complex of myxomas, spotty pigmentation, and endocrine overactivity. *Arch Dermatol* 1986;122:790–798.

346. Sanusi ID. Subungual myxoma. *Arch Dermatol* 1982;118:612–614.

347. Hill TL, Jones BE, Park KH. Myxoma of the skin of a finger. *J Am Acad Dermatol* 1990;22:343–345.

348. Allen PW, Dymock RB, MacCormac LB. Superficial angiomyxomas with and without epithelial components. *Am J Surg Pathol* 1988;12:519–530.

349. Zina AM, Bundino S. Multiple cutaneous fibromyxomas: a light and electron microscopic study. *J Cutan Pathol* 1980;7:335–341.

350. Guerin D, Calonje E, McCormick D, et al. Superficial angiomyxoma. Clinicopathologic analysis of a series of distinctive but poorly recognized cutaneous tumors with tendency for recurrence. *Am J Surg Pathol* 1999;23:910–917.

351. Wilk M, Schmoekel C. Cutaneous focal mucinosis: a histopathological and immunohistochemical analysis of 11 cases. *J Cutan Pathol* 1994;21:446–452.

352. Kempson RL, Fletcher CDM, Evans HL, et al. Digital Myxoma. In *Atlas of Tumor Pathology. Tumors of the Soft Tissues*, 3rd series, fasc. 30. Washington, DC: Armed Forces Institute of Pathology, 2001: 425–426.

353. Armijo M. Mucoid cysts of the fingers. *J Dermatol Surg Oncol* 1981;7:317–322.

354. Salasche SJ. Myxoid cysts of the proximal nail fold. *J Dermatol Surg Oncol* 1984;10:35–39.

355. Johnson WC, Graham JH, Helwig EB. Cutaneous myxoid cyst. *JAMA* 1965;191:15–20.

356. Goldman JA, Goldman L, Jaffe MS, et al. Digital mucinous pseudocysts. *Arthritis Rheum* 1977;20:997–1002.

357. Newmeyer WL, Kilgore ES Jr, Graham WP. Mucous cysts: the dorsal distal interphalangeal joint ganglion. *Plast Reconstr Surg* 1974;53:313–315.

358. Lattanand A, Johnson WC, Graham JH. Mucous cyst (mucocele). *Arch Dermatol* 1970;101:673–678.

359. Weir TW, Johnson WC. Cheilitis glandularis. *Arch Dermatol* 1971;103:433–437.

360. Jensen JL. Superficial mucoceles of the oral mucosa. *Am J Dermatopathol* 1990;12:88–92.

361. Ketchum LD, Cohen IK, Masters FW. Hypertrophic scars and keloids: a collective review. *Plast Reconstr Surg* 1974;53:140.

362. Murray JC, Pollack SV, Pinnel SR. Keloids: a review. *J Am Acad Dermatol* 1981;4:461–470.

363. Beer TW, Baldwin HC, Goddard JR, et al. Angiogenesis in pathological surgical scars. *Hum Pathol* 1998;29:1273–1278.

364. Onwukwe MF. Classification of keloids. *J Dermatol Surg Oncol* 1978;4:534–536.

365. Kurwa AR. Rubinstein-Taybi syndrome and spontaneous keloid. *Clin Exp Dermatol* 1978;4:251–254.

366. Linares HA, Larson DL. Early differential diagnosis between hypertrophic and nonhypertrophic healing. *J Invest Dermatol* 1974;62:514–516.

367. Shaffer JJ, Taylor SC, Cook-Boldin F. Keloidal scars: a review with a critical look at therapeutic options. *J Am Acad Dermatol* 2002;46:S63–S97.

VASCULAR TUMORS: TUMORS AND TUMOR-LIKE CONDITIONS OF BLOOD VESSELS AND LYMPHATICS

EDUARDO CALONJE
EDWARD WILSON-JONES

The classification of vascular lesions and in particular benign vascular tumors is far from satisfactory. The division between developmental, reactive, benign (neoplastic), and occasionally malignant vascular tumors is often blurred, and many conditions cannot be neatly classified into a specific category. This often reflects either limited knowledge about the pathogenesis or the presence of overlapping features among different entities. While advances in knowledge and research have undoubtedly led to the improvement of this situation, the classification of many vascular tumors still remains controversial. A few examples include pyogenic granuloma and angiolymphoid hyperplasia with eosinophilia (reactive vs neoplastic), and more importantly Kaposi's sarcoma (neoplastic vs infectious). The classification of vascular tumors proposed in this chapter and in Table 33-1 intends only to provide a framework to define and present different vascular tumors in a coherent manner based on recent developments. It does not intend to be definitive because future changes in our understanding of vascular tumors will give way to further modifications.

REACTIVE CONDITIONS

Intravascular Papillary Endothelial Hyperplasia (Masson's Hemangioendotheliome Vegetant Intravasculaire)

This condition that is not uncommon probably represents an unusual endothelial proliferation in an organizing thrombus that can be misdiagnosed as angiosarcoma (1). Intravascular papillary endothelial hyperplasia arises primarily within a venous channel or secondarily within a preceding angioma or some type of vascular anomaly, including hemorrhoids, as in Masson's original description (2). An exceptional case of an extravascular location in association with a hematoma has been reported (3). The lesions are almost always solitary, arising in the skin, subcutaneous tissue, or even muscle in the head and neck region, and the upper extremities. The fingers especially, are the most common sites. A rare instance of multiple lesions of the lower extremities simulating Kaposi's sarcoma has also been described (4). All ages can be affected, although there is a slight female predominance (5). Primary lesions are usually tender nodules less than 2 cm in size, whereas secondary lesions occur because some preceding vascular abnormality increases in size.

Histopathology. Often, low-power examination allows recognition of the intravascular nature of the process in a single thin-walled vein (Fig. 33-1) or as part of a preceding angiomatous condition. Extravascular lesions fail to reveal a blood vessel wall despite serial sectioning. The main lesion consists of a mass of anastomosing vascular channels with a variable degree of intraluminal papillary projections (Fig. 33-2). The stroma consists of hyalinized eosinophilic material that may merge with uncanalized thrombus remnants. The infiltrating vascular channels show enlarged and prominent endothelial cells that may be "heaped up" to give rise to intraluminal prominences, but atypia and mitotic activity are slight. Factor VIII–related antigen positivity of endothelial cells in the lesion may be related to vessel maturity (6).

Differential Diagnosis. The occurrence of areas of somewhat atypical endothelial-lined channels apparently showing a "dissection of collagen" appearance can closely simulate a well-differentiated angiosarcoma. However, the stroma is not collagen and thus is not refractile on polarization and the changes are localized and occur within a preceding vessel or a vascular anomaly. Usually angiosarcoma shows a much greater degree of nuclear atypia, multilayering, and mitotic activity.

Angioendotheliomatosis

Until the 1980s, two distinctive forms of angioendotheliomatosis were recognized: an aggressive variant with systemic involvement and poor prognosis, and a reactive self-limited form with a benign course usually restricted to

TABLE 33-1. CLASSIFICATION OF VASCULAR TUMORS

Reactive conditions
Intravascular papillary endothelial hyperplasia
Reactive angioendotheliomatosis
Glomeruloid hemangioma
Epithelioid hemangioma (angiolymphoid hyperplasia with eosinophilia)
Pyogenic granuloma (lobular capillary hemangioma)
Bacillary angiomatosis
Verruca peruana (not discussed)

Developmental abnormalities
Nevus flammeus (salmon patch, port-wine stain)
Angiokeratoma
Generalized essential telangiectasia
Unilateral nevoid telangiectasia
Angioma serpiginosum
Hereditary hemorrhagic telangiectasia (Osler–Rendu–Weber disease)
Nevus araneus (spider nevus)
Venous lake

Benign tumors
Capillary hemangioma
  Strawberry nevus
  Cherry angioma (Campbell de Morgan spot, senile angioma)
  Tufted angioma (angioblastoma)
Cavernous hemangioma
  Sinusoidal hemangioma
Verrucous hemangioma
Microvenular hemangioma
Hobnail hemangioma (targetoid hemosiderotic hemangioma)
Arteriovenous (venous) hemangioma (cirsoid aneurysm)
Angiomatosis
Spindle cell hemangioma

Low-grade malignant vascular tumors
Kaposi's sarcoma
Retiform hemangioendothelioma
Malignant endovascular papillary angioendothelioma
  (Dabska's tumor)
Kaposiform infantile hemangioendothelioma

Malignant vascular tumors
Epithelioid hemangioendothelioma
Angiosarcoma
  Idiopathic (head and neck)
  Associated with lymphoedema
  Postradiotherapy
  Epithelioid

Lymph vessel tumors
Lymphangioma circumscriptum
Cystic hygroma/cavernous lymphangioma
Progressive lymphangioma (benign lymphangioendothe-
  lioma)
Atypical vascular proliferation after radiotherapy

Tumors of perithelial and glomus cells
Glomus tumor
  Solid
  Glomangioma
  Glomangiomyoma
  Infiltrating glomus tumor
  Glomangiosarcoma
  Myopericytoma

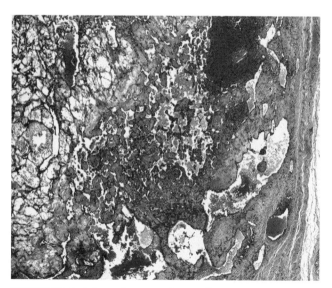

FIGURE 33-1. Primary intravascular papillary endothelial hyperplasia. Part of a markedly dilated vascular channel with prominent papillary structures intermixed with red blood cells and fibrin.

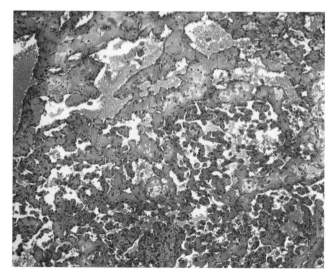

FIGURE 33-2. Intravascular papillary endothelial hyperplasia. Typical hyaline papillary projections lined by endothelial cells focally mimicking a dissection of collagen pattern.

the skin. However, with the advent of immunohistochemistry, many studies in recent years have demonstrated that malignant angioendotheliomatosis shows no endothelial differentiation but represents a form of angiotropic lymphoma that has been renamed *intravascular lymphomatosis* (see Chapter 32).

Reactive Angioendotheliomatosis

This is an uncommon condition that almost exclusively affects the skin and presents in patients of either gender with a wide anatomic distribution. Clinical presentation varies from erythematous or brown macules to papules and/or plaques that can be associated with purpura. A livedo-like pattern is sometimes present. In many cases, an association with systemic disease has been documented, including cryoglobulinemia (7), paraproteinemia, renal disease, amyloidosis (8), antiphospholipid syndrome (9), rheumatoid arthritis (10), cirrhosis (10), polymyalgia rheumatica (10), and systemic infections, especially bacterial endocarditis (11). Localized forms of the disease are less frequent and include a variant associated with peripheral vascular atherosclerotic disease described as diffuse dermal angiomatosis (12–14). The later presentation has also been described in association with iatrogenic arteriovenous fistulas (15).

Histopathology. Lesions are predominantly dermal and composed of closely packed, variably dilated vascular spaces (mainly capillaries) (Fig. 33-3) lined by bland but plump endothelial cells surrounded by pericytes. A minority of cases displays endothelial cells with focal epithelioid change (10). Small lumina might be apparent, but some are obliterated by endothelial cells or fibrin thrombi. Often the capillaries appear to proliferate in the lumina of dilated preexisting blood vessels. Hyaline refractile eosinophilic thrombi representing immunoglobulins are present in cases associated with cryoglobulinemia (7) (Fig. 33-4). In diffuse dermal angiomatosis, the proliferating endothelial cells are not

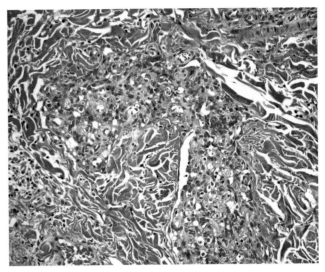

FIGURE 33-4. Reactive angioendotheliomatosis. Plump endothelial cells and intraluminal eosinophilic globules in a case associated with cryoglobulinemia.

present within vascular channels but can be found between dermal collagen fibers. Rare cases of patients presenting with a clinical and histologic picture similar to that of reactive angioendotheliomatosis but showing intravascular cells with a histiocytic immunophenotype have been described. It is not clear whether this represents the early stages of reactive angioendotheliomatosis or a distinctive entity (16).

Histogenesis. Reactive angioendotheliomatosis, in contrast to malignant angioendotheliomatosis, displays universal reactivity for endothelial markers and negativity for leukocyte common antigen, proving that the proliferating cells are endothelial cells (11). It has been proposed that the endothelial cell proliferation is induced by a circulating angiogenic factor or alternatively, especially in cases associated with cryoglobulinemia or atherosclerotic vascular disease, by occlusion of vascular spaces (7).

Differential Diagnosis. The histologic distinction from tufted angioma may be difficult but the clinical presentation of both entities is different and tufted angioma shows clusters of capillaries in a typical cannonball distribution throughout the dermis with crescent-like dilated spaces probably lymphatic in nature in the periphery of many of the vascular tufts.

Glomeruloid Hemangioma

This is a highly distinctive, rare, recently described reactive vascular proliferation that presents in patients with POEMS syndrome (polyneuropathy, organomegaly, endocrinopathy, M-protein, and skin changes), usually but not always in association with multicentric Castleman's disease (17–20). The skin changes in POEMS syndrome include hypertrichosis, hyperpigmentation, hyperhidrosis, sclerodermoid features, and multiple small vascular papules on the trunk and limbs.

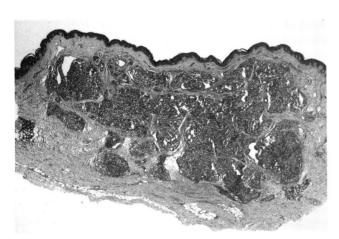

FIGURE 33-3. Reactive angioendotheliomatosis. Numerous closely packed capillaries within preexisting dilated blood vessels are seen throughout the dermis.

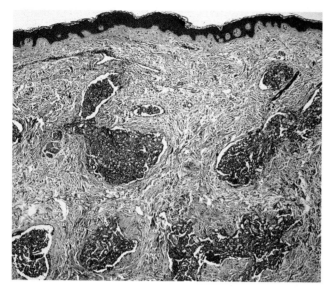

FIGURE 33-5. Glomeruloid hemangioma. Widely dilated pre-existing vascular channels filled with smaller blood vessels. Note the low-power resemblance to reactive angioendotheliomatosis.

Histopathology. Most vascular lesions in POEMS syndrome show the features of cherry angiomas, and only a small number of lesions have the appearance of a glomeruloid hemangioma. Other lesions may display histologic features that do not fit exactly into a definitive diagnostic category. In glomeruloid hemangioma, there are numerous ectatic vascular spaces throughout the dermis that contain in their lumina clusters of small congested capillaries surrounded by pericytes bearing a striking resemblance to renal glomeruli (Fig. 33-5 and 33-6). Although the endothelial cells are flat, a few scattered cells appear vacuolated and can show PAS-positive hyaline globules that correspond to deposition of immunoglobulins (18). Staining for human herpesvirus 8 is negative.

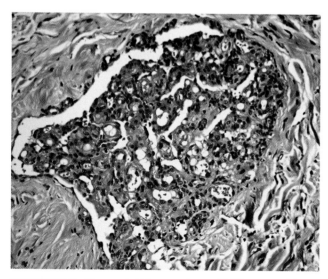

FIGURE 33-6. Glomeruloid hemangioma. Striking resemblance to a renal glomerulus.

Histogenesis. Glomeruloid hemangioma probably represents a variant of reactive angioendotheliomatosis. It has not been established what causes the vascular proliferation in POEMS syndrome, but it may be induced by an angiogenic factor, possibly the abnormal immunoglobulin in the vascular spaces.

Epithelioid Hemangioma (Angiolymphoid Hyperplasia with Eosinophilia)

The two terms of the title of this section highlight the controversy about whether this entity represents a vascular neoplasm or a reactive process consequent to trauma or some other stimulus. Previously, lesions included within this group were referred to as histiocytoid hemangiomas but this name has been abandoned because as originally proposed it included other entities that do not qualify as epithelioid hemangioma (21–24). It is not clear whether this entity represents a reactive proliferation secondary to diverse stimuli including trauma (25), or a neoplastic process but the later is favored. Therefore, the term *epithelioid hemangioma* is generally preferred to encompass vascular lesions at the benign end of the spectrum of conditions characterized by endothelial cells that have an epithelioid morphology (21–24).

Clinical Features. Most lesions arise either superficially in the dermis, or in the subcutaneous tissue or deeper tissues, although occasionally both superficial and deep tissues are affected together (26–29). Blood eosinophilia has been reported in up to 15% of patients (24,26).

Superficial Lesions. Young to middle-aged women are mainly affected with the development of pruritic papules and plaques at or around the external ear. The lesions can be numerous but are limited to one side. Typically the clinical course is chronic over several years despite excision and other treatment modalities. Such superficial lesions were originally referred to as pseudopyogenic granuloma (30). Occlusion of the external auditory canal can bring patients to the attention of ear, nose and throat specialists (31). Sometimes other areas in the head and neck region, especially the occipital region and the vicinity of the temporal artery, are affected.

Lesions of Subcutaneous and Deeper Tissues. Adults are mainly affected, and there is no gender predilection. The typical lesion is a solitary, slowly growing, firm, subcutaneous swelling 2 to 10 cm in size in the head and neck region with some predilection for the pre- or post-auricular sites. Sometimes more than one lesion arises. Most lesions are asymptomatic except for occasional pruritus. Lymphadenopathy is usually not seen. Occasionally other body sites are affected, such as the arm, hands, axillae, or inguinal region (25,26,32,33). Rare cases have been documented in association with a traumatically induced arteriovenous fistula involving the popliteal artery (34). Origin from the radial artery has also been documented (35). The condition can persist for years, but serious complications do not occur.

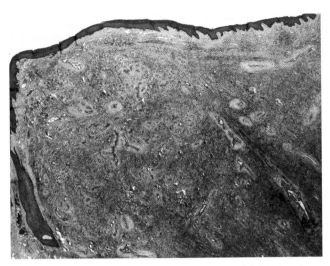

FIGURE 33-7. Epithelioid hemangioma. Superficial lesion from the ear showing typical lobular architecture and a prominent inflammatory cell infiltrate.

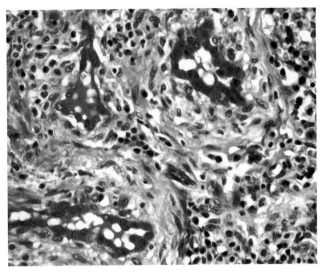

FIGURE 33-9. Epithelioid hemangioma. Prominent endothelial cells with abundant eosinophilic cytoplasm and numerous eosinophils in the surrounding stroma. Note perivascular fibrosis and numerous eosinophils.

Epithelioid hemangioma may also rarely occur in the oral cavity (36), tongue (37), lymph node (38), bone (39), and testis (40). A case has also been reported in an ovarian teratoma (41). Epithelioid hemangiomas occurring at sites different from the skin often lack the inflammatory component.

Histopathology. The main components of the pathology are as follows:

Proliferation of small to medium-sized blood vessels often showing a lobular architecture (Fig. 33-7). Many of these vascular channels are lined by greatly enlarged (epithelioid) endothelial cells (Figs. 33-8 and 33-9).

A perivascular inflammatory cell infiltrate composed mainly of lymphocytes and eosinophils.

Nodular areas of a lymphocytic infiltrate with rare follicle formation.

Frequent origin from a small artery or a vein. Rarely, the whole lesion is intravascular (Fig. 33-10). The condition described as intravenous atypical vascular proliferation represents a variant of intravascular epithelioid hemangioma (42).

In superficial lesions there is variable degree of vascular hyperplasia that can include areas in which the proliferation is almost angiomatous. A distinctive feature is the "cobblestone" appearance of enlarged endothelial cells that project into the lumina of some vessels. The nucleus of these cells is ovoid and orthochromatic without atypia

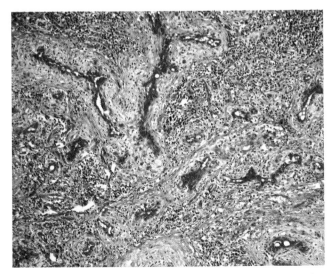

FIGURE 33-8. Epithelioid hemangioma. Numerous vascular channels lined by prominent large pink epithelioid endothelial cells and surrounded by inflammation.

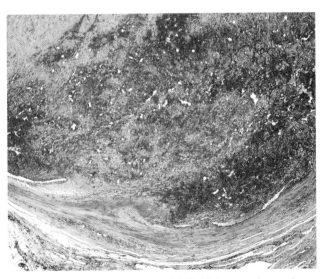

FIGURE 33-10. Intravascular epithelioid hemangioma. Some cases of epithelioid hemangioma are entirely intravascular.

or evidence of mitotic activity. Affected vessels often show endothelial cells with intracytoplasmic vacuoles, a prominent feature of some diagnostic value (30) (Fig. 33-9). The most abnormal blood vessels are usually surrounded by stellate and spindle-shaped cells in a mucoid stroma. The associated perivascular inflammatory cell infiltrate is usually loosely scattered around the affected vessel, but in places it may be almost completely absent. Generally, eosinophils make up 5% to 15% of the cells. Lesions with few inflammatory cells are rarely seen. Inflammatory cells also decrease markedly in late stages when a prominent fibrotic component is often present.

The epidermis above the lesions may show acanthosis or erosions due to superficial trauma. The skin appendages are usually unaffected except for the occasional finding of follicular mucinosis (43).

In subcutaneous lesions the inflammatory cell infiltrate is usually more massive, with a central, poorly circumscribed nodule that replaces the fat. The nodule is composed of confluent sheets of small lymphocytes and eosinophils in which a network of poorly canalized thick-walled capillaries is embedded. Satellite smaller islands of lymphoid cells with lymphoid follicles usually surround the central nodule. Eosinophils can form up to 50% of the cell population.

In about 50% of cases, evidence of involvement of medium- to large-sized arteries can be found (26). A variable degree of blood vessel damage occurs, with infiltration of the vessel wall by inflammatory cells and occlusion of the lumen. Partial loss of the internal elastic lamina is often seen.

Histogenesis. The etiology and pathogenesis of angiolymphoid hyperplasia is at present uncertain. Occasionally trauma (25) or external otitis can precede the onset of the disease. Ultrastructural studies have not confirmed that the enlarged endothelial cells are developing histiocytic properties, as has been suggested (22,23,30).

Differential Diagnosis. The proliferation of endothelial-lined channels with large irregular cells can be misinterpreted as angiosarcoma. The latter can be accompanied by a lymphocytic infiltrate, but eosinophils are rarely present. The main distinguishing feature is the presence of nuclear atypia with hyperchromatism, mitotic activity, and dissection of collagen pattern in angiosarcoma, but not in epithelioid hemangioma. Distinction from the recently described retiform hemangioendothelioma is easy: angiolymphoid hyperplasia lacks a retiform growth pattern and does not show tall, narrow endothelial cells with a typical hobnail appearance, as is the case in retiform hemangioendothelioma.

Angiolymphoid hyperplasia can be distinguished from most benign angiomas or ectasias by the absence of an intrinsic inflammatory cell infiltrate in the latter. Greatly enlarged endothelial cells with an eosinophilic cytoplasm are rarely seen in benign angiomas, although they can be seen focally in lobular capillary hemangioma (pyogenic granuloma).

Persistent insect bite reactions can show overlapping histologic features with angiolymphoid hyperplasia, but

the vascular proliferation is rarely as exuberant. A somewhat similar pathology can also arise as a reaction to injected vaccines (44–46). The histology is characterized by a deep lymphoid infiltrate with lymphoid follicles, tissue eosinophilia, and fibrosis. Vascular hyperplasia is, however, less marked than in angiolymphoid hyperplasia, and epithelioid endothelial cells are not a feature. A diagnostic feature is the presence of aluminium-containing histiocytes as demonstrated by solochrome-azurin when aluminium-adsorbed vaccines have been used (44). The presence of aluminium may also be demonstrated by energy-dispersive x-ray microanalysis.

When angiolymphoid hyperplasia with eosinophilia was first described in Western Europe, similarities to *Kimura's disease* as reported in Asia were noted. Indeed, many authors thought that both conditions might be part of one disease spectrum (26). However, more recently most authorities emphasize differences between the two entities (21,24,32,33,47–49). Subcutaneous angiolymphoid hyperplasia and Kimura's disease occur most commonly in the head and neck region in adults and both share the histologic features of extensive lymphoid proliferation, tissue eosinophilia, and evidence of vascular hyperplasia. Kimura's disease, however, demonstrates a wider age span with a male predominance and a tendency for more extensive lesions to occur, often with involvement of salivary tissue and lymph nodes and at sites distant from the head and neck region (50). Authors from Asia have stressed the histologic differences, the most important of which are the lesser degree of exuberant vascular hyperplasia, lacking prominent eosinophilic endothelial cells and the absence of uncanalized blood vessels in Kimura's disease. Other points of difference are eosinophilic abscesses and marked fibrosis around the lesions in Kimura's disease and the absence of lesions centered on damaged arteries. There is an important association between Kimura's disease and renal disease, particularly nephrotic syndrome (51).

Pyogenic Granuloma (Lobular Capillary Hemangioma)

Pyogenic granuloma is a common proliferative lesion that often occurs shortly after a minor injury or infection of the skin. Typically the lesion grows rapidly for a few weeks before stabilizing as an elevated, bright red papule, usually not more than 1 to 2 cm in size; it may then persist indefinitely unless destroyed. Recurrence after surgery or cautery is not rare. Pyogenic granuloma most often affects children or young adults of either gender, but the age range is wide; the hands, fingers, and face, especially the lips and gums, are the most common sites (52–54). Pyogenic granuloma of the gingiva in pregnancy (epulis of pregnancy) is a special subgroup.

A rare and alarming event is the development of multiple satellite angiomatous lesions at and around the site of a previously destroyed pyogenic granuloma (55,56). This usually occurs following lesions on the shoulder or upper trunk in children. Histologically, lesions that are similar to pyogenic granuloma can occur in the deep dermis, the subcutaneous tissue (57), and even within dilated venous channels (58,59). Widely scattered angiomatous lesions resembling pyogenic granulomas have also been described (60–63), sometimes in association with visceral disease.

Histopathology. The typical lesion presents as a polypoid mass of angiomatous tissue protruding above the surrounding skin. It is often constricted at its base by a collarette of acanthotic epidermis (Fig. 33-11). An intact flattened epidermis may cover the entire lesion, but surface erosions are common. In ulcerated lesions a superficial inflammatory cell reaction can give rise to an appearance suggestive of granulation tissue, but inflammation does not appear to be an intrinsic feature. Inflammation is usually slight in the deeper part of the lesion and may be absent when the epidermis is intact. The angiomatous tissue tends to occur in discrete masses or lobules, resembling a capillary hemangioma, hence the preference by Mills et al. (52) for the term "lobular capillary hemangioma" to describe this condition (Fig. 33-12). The angiomatous tissue is surrounded by myxoid stroma containing scattered spindle- and stellate-shaped connective tissue cells and occasional mast cells. The angiomatous tissue is composed of a variably dilated network of blood-filled capillary vessels and groups of poorly canalized vascular tufts. Mitotic activity varies and can be prominent. Feeding vessels often extend into the adjacent dermis and rare lesions show a deep component in the reticular dermis. Occasionally, foci of intravascular papillary endothelial hyperplasia occur within the larger deep vessels. Focal epithelioid endothelial cells can sometimes be seen.

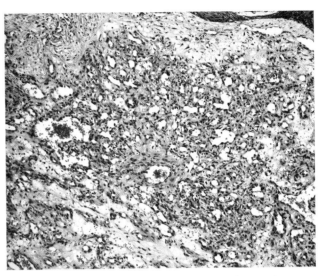

FIGURE 33-12. Lobular capillary hemangioma (Pyogenic granuloma). Distinctive lobules of dilated and congested capillaries in an edematous stroma.

Focal cytologic atypia may be present particularly in lesions arising in mucosal surfaces, such as the mouth (64). The histology of recurrent or satellite lesions is similar, but the angiomatous proliferation can extend more deeply into the dermis. Pyogenic granulomas of the subcutaneous tissue or in veins show similar histologic features but lack an inflammatory component. Intravascular lesions can so distend the veins that the surrounding muscle coat can be thinned and difficult to detect (Fig. 33-13).

Pathogenesis. It was once assumed that granuloma pyogenicum was caused by pyogenic infection. However, the histologic picture of early lesions suggests a capillary hemangioma, and even in eroded lesions that show inflamma-

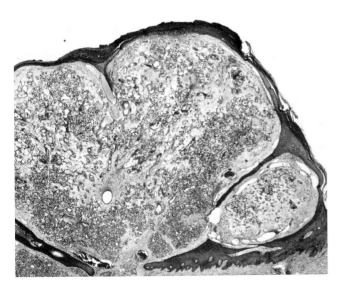

FIGURE 33-11. Lobular capillary hemangioma (Pyogenic granuloma). Early, nonulcerated lesion with the typical epithelial collarette.

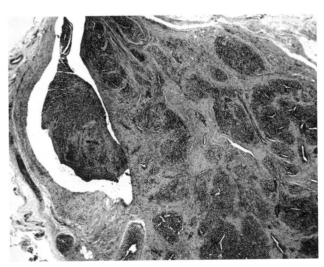

FIGURE 33-13. Intravascular lobular capillary hemangioma (pyogenic granuloma). Some cases occur entirely in an intravenous location.

tion, the appearance mimics that of a capillary hemangioma in its deeper portions. Therefore, terms like eruptive hemangioma (65) and lobular capillary hemangioma (52) have been suggested.

Immunohistochemical studies have demonstrated positive labeling of endothelial cells for factor VIII–related antigen, CD31, and also of perithelial cells for muscle-specific actin and type IV collagen. Antibodies to estrogen and progesterone-receptor proteins were negative (66). These studies tend to support a reactive rather than neoplastic etiology of pyogenic granuloma.

Differential Diagnosis. Both Kaposi's sarcoma and angiosarcoma should be considered as part of the differential diagnosis, especially when multiple lesions are present. Elevated polypoid lesions are rare in Kaposi's sarcoma; most show obvious spindle cells woven between delicate vascular spaces, unlike in pyogenic granuloma. A much greater degree of cell atypia with intraluminal spreading of malignant cells characterizes well-differentiated angiosarcomas. Focal areas of intravascular papillary endothelial hyperplasia within a pyogenic granuloma occasionally can simulate angiosarcoma, but, even so, nuclear atypia is slight.

In recent years, a further differential diagnosis of pyogenic granuloma is with bacillary angiomatosis, a recently described, infectious, vascular proliferation, common in HIV-infected patients, and caused by *Rochalimaea henselae*, a small, gram-negative rod belonging to the family Bartonellaceae (67,68) (see Chapter 21). Clinically, and especially histologically, lesions of bacillary angiomatosis can look remarkably similar to a pyogenic granuloma. The low-power architecture in superficial lesions may be almost identical to that seen in pyogenic granuloma (Fig. 33-14).

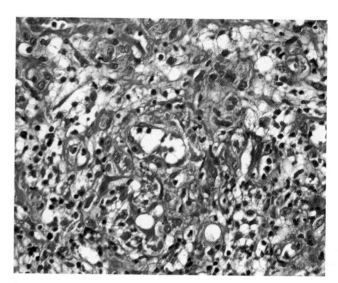

FIGURE 33-15. Bacillary angiomatosis. The vascular channels are lined by pale epithelioid endothelial cells. Often, neutrophils with nuclear dust are seen in the surrounding stroma.

In bacillary angiomatosis, however, the endothelial cells often have abundant pale cytoplasm (Fig. 33-15), and aggregates of neutrophils are present throughout the lesion, often in relation to clumps of granular basophilic material. This basophilic material shows bacilli when stained with Warthin–Starry (Fig. 33-16) or Giemsa stains.

Vascular granulomatous lesions mimicking pyogenic granulomas occasionally arise as a complication of retinoid therapy, but the histology is that of nonspecific vascular granulation tissue lacking a lobular architecture (69,70).

Distinction from a nodular lesion of orf or milker's nodule may be difficult, as the low-power architecture may resemble a lobular capillary hemangioma. However, in the former there is often prominent hyperplasia of the epider-

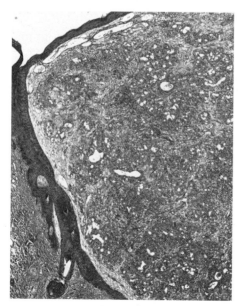

FIGURE 33-14. Bacillary angiomatosis. Similar low-power architecture to lobular capillary hemangioma but there is more prominent inflammation in the background.

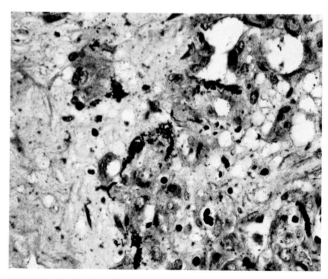

FIGURE 33-16. Bacillary angiomatosis. Warthin–Starry stain showing numerous clumps of bacilli.

mis and the infundibular portion of the hair follicles. The prominent vascular component represents granulation tissue with only a focal lobular architecture and the keratinocytes often show typical viral inclusions.

DEVELOPMENTAL ABNORMALITIES

Nevus Flammeus

The term nevus flammeus is often used to refer to two different lesions: the *salmon patch* and the *port-wine stain.* Although both lesions are congenital, the former tends to involute in the first years of life and usually has no association with other types of anomalies, while the latter tends to be persistent and is often related to other malformations. The salmon patch is present in up to 50% of newborns of either gender as an ill-defined, red to pale pink macule mainly in the nape of the neck, glabella, or eyelids (71,72). The port-wine stain occurs in about 0.3% of newborns as a macular, usually unilateral, red-pink lesion with a predilection for the face (72). Later in life the lesion becomes darker and raised.

Sturge–Weber syndrome (encephalotrigeminal angiomatosis) is characterized by the presence of a facial port-wine stain, often in the distribution of the trigeminal nerve associated with an ipsilateral leptomeningeal venous malformation, atrophy and calcification of the underlying cerebral cortex, epilepsy, mental retardation, ocular vascular malformations, glaucoma, and contralateral hemiparesis.

In *Klippel–Trenaunay syndrome* (osteohypertrophic nevus flammeus), one observes hypertrophy of the soft tissues and bones of one or several extremities affected with a nevus flammeus. Associated with this are varicosities or arteriovenous fistulas or both and less commonly, spindle-cell hemangioendotheliomas. Cases presenting with arteriovenous fistulas are sometimes known as Parkes–Weber syndrome. Complications of note are cutaneous ulcers and high-output cardiac failure.

Histopathology. In the *salmon patch,* dilated capillaries are seen in the papillary dermis. In the *port-wine stain,* no telangiectases are apparent histologically until the patient has reached about 10 years of age (73). The capillary ectasias thereafter gradually increase with age. Ultimately, when the lesion is raised or nodular, not only the superficial capillaries but also some of the blood vessels in the deeper layers of the dermis and in the subcutaneous layer are dilated. Many ectatic vessels are filled with red blood cells. Lesions with a deep component can be associated with a cavernous hemangioma or an arteriovenous malformation (73).

Histogenesis. Because no histologic abnormalities are present early in life with a port-wine stain, it appears likely that this malformation is the result of a congenital weakness of the capillary walls (73). Thus, the port-wine stain

represents a progressive telangiectasia. Antibodies directed against components of the blood vessel wall, collagenous basement–membrane protein (type IV collagen), fibronectin, and factor VIII–related antigen have an equivalent distribution and intensity in normal skin and nevus flammeus. Although this does not rule out a structural abnormality of these components, it has been suggested that the alteration may be related to the supporting dermal elements rather than to an intrinsic abnormality in the vessel wall (74). An abnormality in neuromodulation has been proposed as an alternate theory (75).

Angiokeratoma

Four types of angiokeratoma have been described that represent true ectasias of blood vessels of the superficial dermis (76):

Angiokeratoma corporis diffusum. Patients present with numerous clusters of tiny red papules in a symmetrical distribution usually in the "bathing-trunk" area. Although often considered synonymous with Fabry's disease, which is an X-linked genetic disorder associated with deficiency of the lysosomal enzyme A-galactosidase, identical clinical appearances have been described in patients with other enzymatic deficiencies including B-galactosidase, neuraminidase, and L-fucosidase (77,78). An exceptional case was reported in an individual with no detectable biochemical abnormalities (79).

Angiokeratoma of Mibelli. Several dark red papules with a slightly verrucous surface are seen on the dorsa of the fingers and toes. Usually the lesions appear during childhood or adolescence and measure 3 to 5 mm in diameter (80).

Angiokeratoma of Fordyce. Multiple vascular papules 2 to 4 mm in diameter are seen on the scrotum. Similar lesions have been described on the vulva (81). They arise in middle or later life. Early lesions are red, soft, and compressible; later, they become blue, keratotic, and noncompressible (82).

Solitary or multiple angiokeratomas. Usually one and occasionally several papular lesions arise in young adults, most commonly on the lower extremities. The lesions range from 2 to 10 mm in diameter. Early lesions appear bright red and soft, but they later become blue to black, firm, and hyperkeratotic (76). Thrombosed lesions are not uncommonly misdiagnosed clinically as malignant melanomas.

Histopathology. The histologic findings are essentially the same in all four above-mentioned types of angiokeratoma and consist of numerous, dilated, thin-walled, congested capillaries mainly in the papillary dermis underlying an epidermis that shows variable degrees of acanthosis with elongation of the rete ridges and hyperkeratosis (76) (Fig. 33-17). In cutaneous lesions of Fabry's disease, cytoplasmic

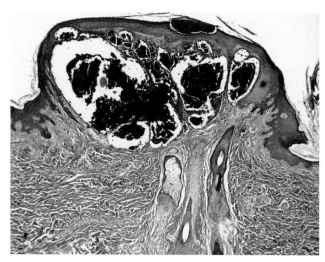

FIGURE 33-17. Angiokeratoma. Note ectatic blood vessels in the papillary dermis with overlying epidermal hyperplasia.

vacuoles representing lipids can sometimes be detected in endothelial cells, fibroblasts, and pericytes (83).

Generalized Essential Telangiectasia

Widespread linear telangiectases, mainly on the extremities, may gradually develop in adults, predominantly in women (84).

Histopathology. Dilated, often congested, vessels are seen in the papillary dermis. The walls of the vessels are composed only of endothelium. The absence of alkaline phosphatase activity suggests that it is the venous portion of the capillary loop that participates in the disease process (84).

Unilateral Nevoid Telangiectasia

Although unilateral nevoid telangiectasia may be congenital, in most instances its onset is related to high estrogen levels associated with pregnancy, puberty, and chronic hepatic disease associated with alcoholism (85). The telangiectases, which are largely punctate and stellate rather than linear, follow a dermatomal distribution, particularly those associated with the trigeminal nerve and cranial nerves III and IV. Rare cases are associated with gastric involvement (86).

Histopathology. Numerous dilated vessels are seen in the upper and middle dermis and, to a lesser extent, in the deeper part of the dermis.

Histogenesis. It has been proposed that the changes seen in this condition are induced by an increase in estrogen receptors in a dermatomal distribution (87).

Angioma Serpiginosum

Angioma serpiginosum is a rare acquired vascular lesion that usually presents in the first two decades of life with a predilection for females (88). Anatomic distribution is wide, but lesions often present on the lower extremities. The disorder is asymptomatic, and slow progression occurs over the years. Focal spontaneous regression rarely occurs. Most cases are sporadic but inherited cases have been reported (89). A typical lesion is characterized by deeply red nonpalpable puncta that are grouped closely together in a macular or netlike pattern. Irregular extension at the periphery of the macules may cause them to have serpiginous borders. The deeply red puncta represent dilated capillaries.

Histopathology. Dilated, thin-walled capillaries are seen in some of the dermal papillae and the superficial reticular dermis. Epidermal changes and extravasation of red blood cells does not occur.

Histogenesis. On electron microscopic examination, it is apparent that the thickening of the capillary walls is caused by a heavy precipitate of basement membrane–like material mixed with thin collagen fibers and an increased number of concentrically arranged pericytes (90). In addition, some of the dilated capillaries show slit-like protrusions of their lumina and endothelial lining into the surrounding thickened vessel walls. These findings indicate that angioma serpiginosum is not just a simple telangiectasia but represents a vascular malformation (90).

Hereditary Hemorrhagic Telangiectasia (Osler–Weber–Rendu Disease)

Osler–Weber–Rendu disease is inherited as an autosomal dominant trait. Although epistaxis may already begin in childhood, the characteristic telangiectases on the mucous membranes do not begin to appear until adolescence, and the cutaneous lesions often appear much later in life, involving particularly the upper part of the body. Typical lesions are small bright red nonpulsating papules.

Concomitant involvement of other organs including the gastrointestinal tract, liver, brain, lungs, spleen, kidneys, and adrenal glands is common. Associated vascular malformations are often a feature (91). Morbidity and mortality are mainly related to bleeding from internal organs.

Histopathology. Irregularly dilated capillaries and venules lined by flat endothelial cells are seen in the papillary and subpapillary dermis.

Histogenesis. On electron microscopy, the dilated vessels in the skin and oral mucosa are seen to be small postcapillary venules that normally do not possess pericytes. A defect in the perivascular supportive tissue has been found responsible for the breakdown of the junctions between endothelial cells and the resultant hemorrhage (92). The presence of a mild perivascular lymphocytic infiltrate has been regarded as important in inducing the pathologic changes (93).

Nevus Araneus (Spider Nevus)

Nevus araneus, or spider nevus, considered the most common form of telangiectasia, presents at any age, especially in children, with a predilection for the face and upper limbs (91,94). It is characterized by a central, slightly elevated, red punctum from which blood vessels radiate. Occasionally pulsation can be observed. Although spider nevi often arise spontaneously, pregnancy, the use of oral contraceptives, and liver disease are factors predisposing to their appearance (91). Spontaneous regression is common as children grow older and after pregnancy.

Histopathology. In the center of the lesion is an ascending artery that branches and communicates with multiple dilated capillaries.

Venous Lake

Venous lakes are small, dark blue, slightly raised, soft lesions occurring on the exposed skin of elderly persons. They can usually be emptied of most of their blood using sustained pressure. Usually several lesions are present. The face, ears, and lips are the most common sites.

Histopathology. Venous lakes represent telangiectasias. In the upper dermis, close to the epidermis, they show either one greatly dilated space or several interconnected dilated spaces filled with erythrocytes and lined by a single layer of flattened endothelial cells and a thin wall of fibrous tissue (95). In some instances, in place of fibrous tissue, there is a thin irregular noncontinuous smooth muscle layer (96).

BENIGN TUMORS

Capillary Hemangioma Variants

Strawberry Nevus (Juvenile Hemangioendothelioma, Juvenile Hemangioma)

Capillary hemangioma, mostly represented by strawberry nevus, constitutes the most common vascular tumor of infancy, affecting as many as one in every 100 live births. Overall, it comprises between 32% and 42% of all vascular tumors (97,98). Lesions usually first appear between the third and fifth week of life, increase in size for several months to 1 year, and then start to regress. A typical lesion consists of one or several bright red, soft, lobulated tumors that vary greatly in size, and have a wide anatomic distribution with a predilection for the head and neck area. Females are slightly more affected than males. On occasion lesions can involve deeper soft tissues or even internal organs and can be associated with high morbidity, especially if located near vital structures. Complete spontaneous resolution is common, occurring in about 70% of capillary hemangiomas by the time the patient has reached the age of 7 years.

Kasabach–Merritt syndrome consists of large capillary hemangiomas in infants associated with thrombocytopenia and purpura. However, this syndrome is seen occasionally in adults with numerous or very large cavernous hemangiomas and also in children with Kaposi-like infantile hemangioendothelioma (see below). The purpura is not just a result of thrombocytopenia, as first assumed, but represents a consumption coagulopathy within the hemangioma (99).

Histopathology. All tumors have a lobular architecture (Fig. 33-18), but microscopic features change as the lesion evolves. During their period of growth in early infancy, capillary hemangiomas show considerable proliferation of their endothelial cells. The endothelial cells are large, mitotically active, and aggregated predominantly in solid strands and masses in which there are only a few small capillary lumina. Not uncommonly crystalline intracytoplasmic inclusions can be seen in the endothelial cells. The lumina can be highlighted with the use of a reticulin stain. In maturing lesions, the capillary lumina are wider and the lining endothelial cells then appear flatter (Fig. 33-19). In mature lesions, some of the lumina may be greatly dilated, focally resembling a cavernous hemangioma. In the involuting phase, there is progressive fibrosis with disappearance of the blood vessels. The vascular nature of the tumor may be then difficult to establish. However, the lobular pattern is often preserved. A worrying but entirely benign feature seen in a number of capillary hemangiomas is the presence of perineural invasion (100,101).

Pathogenesis. Ultrastructural and immunohistochemical studies of capillary hemangiomas have demonstrated that tumors show remarkable cellular heterogeneity. A large proportion of the cells in a given tumor are endothelial cells and pericytes, but fibroblasts, mast cells, and a population of as yet unidentified factor XIIIa–positive cells have been described (102–104). A complex interaction among these cell populations may modulate the progression and

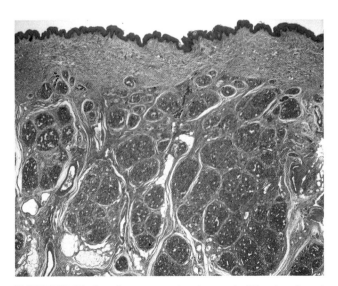

FIGURE 33-18. Stawberry nevus. Involvement of the dermis and subcutis by multiple lobules composed of capillaries.

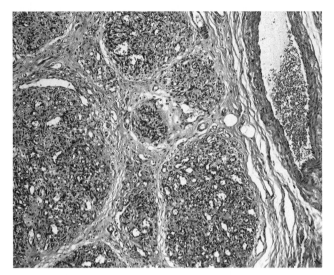

FIGURE 33-19. Strawberry nevus. Mature lesion with well-formed canalized capillaries and a neighboring feeding vessel.

later evolution of capillary hemangiomas (103). It has recently been described that juvenile hemangiomas share the same unique phenotype with human placenta (105).

Differential Diagnosis. Distinction from a vascular malformation is sometimes difficult as the later may have a prominent component composed of capillaries. Separating a strawberry nevus from a vascular malformation is important because the former involute spontaneously while the latter tend to persist. Immunohistochemical staining for GLUT-1, the human erythrocyte glucose transporter is useful to distinguish between both processes as juvenile hemangiomas are diffusely positive for this marker and vascular malformations are negative (106).

Cherry Hemangioma (Senile Angioma/Campbell de Morgan Spot)

Cherry hemangiomas are bright red lesions varying in size from a hardly visible punctum to a soft, raised, dome-shaped lesion measuring several millimeters in diameter. These very common lesions, often present in large numbers, may start appearing in early adulthood and the number of lesions increases with age. Cherry hemangiomas may occur anywhere on the skin, but the trunk and the upper limbs are the most common sites.

Histopathology. In the early stage of development, cherry hemangiomas have the appearance of true capillary hemangiomas, being composed of numerous newly formed capillaries with narrow lumina and prominent endothelial cells arranged in a lobular fashion in the subpapillary region (107). As the lesion ages the capillaries become dilated. In a fully mature cherry hemangioma, one observes numerous moderately dilated capillaries lined by flattened endothelial

cells. The intercapillary stroma shows edema and homogenization of the collagen. The epidermis is thinned and often surrounds most of the angioma as a collarette (108).

Differential Diagnosis. In its early stage, cherry hemangioma, like granuloma pyogenicum, shows capillary proliferation; however, endothelial proliferation is much less pronounced than in granuloma pyogenicum, so that solid aggregates of endothelial cells are not seen.

Tufted Angioma (Angioblastoma)

This benign angiomatous condition can be regarded as identical to the angioblastoma reported by Japanese authors (109,110). The angiomas affect the genders equally, usually arising between the age of 1 to 5 years (111); occasionally the lesions are present at birth, but they may develop in adults or even in old age (112). There are exceptional instances of angiomas arising in pregnancy with regression after parturition (113), the occurrence in several members of a family (114), and the development of lesions after liver transplantation (115). The most common sites for the angiomatous papules and plaques are the upper trunk, neck, and the proximal part of the limbs. The lesions usually slowly progress for several years and can come to cover wide segments of the body; some are tender on palpation and rare lesions regress (116).

Histopathology. Circumscribed foci of closely set capillaries are found scattered through the dermis and occasionally reach the subcutis. At lower magnification, these discrete, ovoid angiomatous lobules or tufts have been alluded to as giving rise to a "cannonball" appearance (111) (Fig. 33-20). The vascular nature of the tufts may not be immediately apparent as vascular lumina are compressed by enlarged endothelial cells and contain few red blood cells.

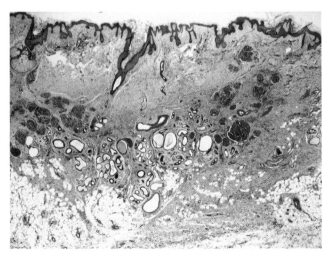

FIGURE 33-20. Tufted angioma. Scattered round or ovoid dermal lobules in a typical "cannonball" distribution.

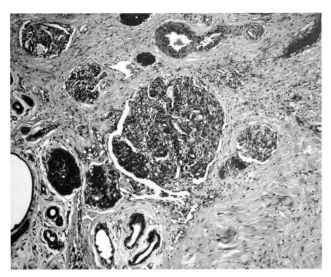

FIGURE 33-21. Tufted angioma. Lobule composed of blood-less capillaries surrounded by dilated crescent-shaped vascular channels.

Some of the vascular tufts appear to indent lymphatic-like channels (Figs. 33-21 and 33-22). Mitotic activity and cell atypia are insignificant.

Positivity for von Willebrand factor is usually limited to a few vessels (111,117). The presence of strong labeling for actin has been interpreted as indicating a prominent perithelial component among the tumor capillaries (117).

The main importance of this uncommon angioma, especially if it develops in adults, is the differential diagnosis from *Kaposi's sarcoma* or possibly a low-grade *angiosarcoma*. Endothelial cells in tufted angioma may show slight spindling but not the elongated spindle cells of Kaposi's sarcoma. The discrete focal arrangement of vascular tufts hav-

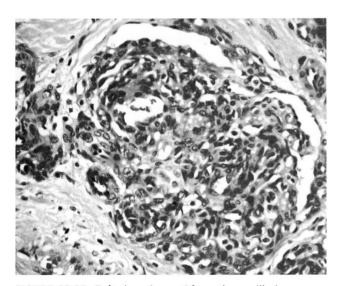

FIGURE 33-22. Tufted angioma. Often, the capillaries appear poorly canalized and pericytes are prominent.

ing few red blood cells also differs greatly from the mature lesions of Kaposi's sarcoma. The absence of cell atypia is the main distinguishing feature from angiosarcoma.

The hypertrophic cellular appearance of the tufts is similar to the angiomatous tissue in strawberry nevi, but the angiomatous aggregates are far more massive in the latter, where they tend to replace wide segments of the dermis and fat. It seems likely that tufted angioma is a variant of capillary hemangioma; this is supported by the finding of characteristic cytoplasmic crystalline lamellae in both disorders (118).

Cavernous Hemangioma

Sharing with strawberry nevus the same age, gender, and anatomic distribution, cavernous hemangioma is still less common and tends to be larger, deeper and less well-defined than the former and shows no tendency for spontaneous regression (97,98). Rare cavernous hemangiomas may be associated with an overlying capillary hemangioma. There are two rare conditions in which numerous cavernous hemangiomas occur: Maffucci's syndrome and the blue rubber bleb nevus.

Maffucci's Syndrome

The outstanding features of Maffucci's syndrome are dyschondroplasia resulting in defects in ossification; fragility of the bones, causing severe deformities, and osteochondromas, which may develop into chondrosarcomas (72). In addition, large, compressible subcutaneous cavernous hemangiomas may be present at birth or appear in childhood or early adulthood.

Blue Rubber Bleb Nevus

In the blue rubber bleb nevus, cavernous hemangiomas are present at birth, but may subsequently increase in size and number. The hemangiomas have a distinct appearance, and most of them are protuberant, dark blue, soft, and compressible, and some are pedunculated. They vary from a few millimeters to 3 cm in diameter. In addition, subcutaneous hemangiomas are felt on palpation. There are also hemangiomas in the oral mucosa, the gastrointestinal tract, and less commonly in other organs (72). Some blue rubber bleb nevi are probably telangiectatic glomangiomas in which the glomus cells are sparse.

Histopathology. Cavernous hemangiomas appear in the lower dermis and the subcutaneous tissue with large, irregular spaces containing red blood cells and fibrinous material (Fig. 33-23). The spaces are lined by a single layer of thin endothelial cells. Not uncommonly, a capillary

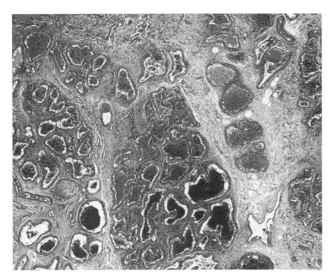

FIGURE 33-23. Cavernous hemangioma. Markedly dilated and congested vascular spaces.

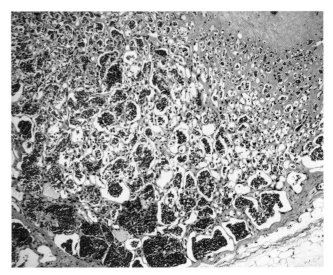

FIGURE 33-25. Sinusoidal hemangioma. Higher magnification reveals a typical sinusoidal appearance.

component is present, especially in the superficial portion of a tumor. Dystrophic calcification is often present.

Variant of Cavernous Hemangioma: Sinusoidal Hemangioma

Sinusoidal hemangioma is a relatively rare, recently described variant of cavernous hemangioma (119). The lesion presents as a bluish subcutaneous mass, especially in middle-aged adults, and has a predilection for females. Although the anatomic distribution is wide, tumors often present in the breast and in this setting angiosarcoma is considered in the differential diagnosis.

Histopathology. Sinusoidal hemangioma is lobular and focally ill-defined with partial or total replacement of sub-

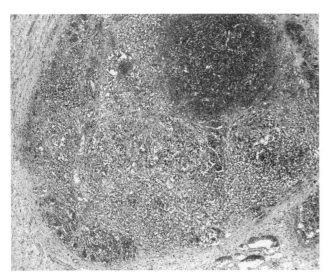

FIGURE 33-24. Sinusoidal hemangioma. Congested anastomosing vascular channels with a sieve-like appearance.

cutaneous fat lobules. The typical feature is the presence of gaping, markedly dilated and congested, thin walled, back-to-back vascular spaces in a sieve-like or sinusoidal arrangement (Fig. 33-24). Pseudopapillary structures due to cross-sectioning of these spaces focally resemble intravascular papillary endothelial hyperplasia (Fig. 33-25). The blood vessels are lined by bland, flat endothelial cells, which can be focally prominent and mildly pleomorphic. Thrombosis, hyalinization, dystrophic calcification, and even areas of infarction can be seen in older lesions. Distinction from a well-differentiated angiosarcoma is based on the presence in the latter of an infiltrative growth pattern, cytologic atypia, and multilayering. In breast lesions, it is worth remembering that mammary angiosarcomas are always intraparenchymal.

Verrucous Hemangioma

Verrucous hemangioma is a rare form of vascular malformation that is usually congenital and only rarely presents later in life. Most cases present as wart-like, dark blue papules or nodules with special predilection for the distal lower limbs. Although the majority of cases are solitary, an exceptional case with multiple lesions on different parts of the body has been reported (120). Often cases are confused clinically and histologically with angiokeratomas, but verrucous hemangiomas always have a deep component and recurrence after incomplete excision occurs in up to one third of cases (121,122).

In *Cobb syndrome*, a lesion identical to a verrucous hemangioma presents on the trunk with a dermatomal distribution and in association with an underlying meningospinal hemangioma (123).

Histopathology. The superficial portion of a verrucous hemangioma is indistinguishable from an angiokeratoma.

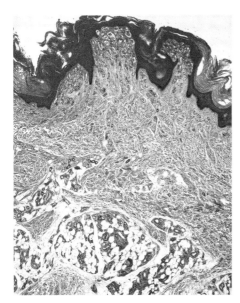

FIGURE 33-26. Verrucous hemangioma. Note the superficial component similar to angiokeratoma but with a deep component extending to the subcutaneous tissue.

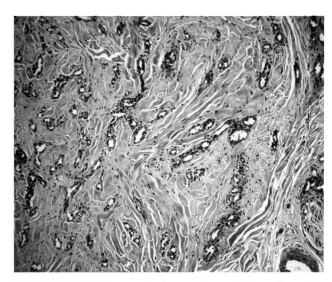

FIGURE 33-28. Microvenular hemangioma. Note small venules surrounded by somewhat hyalinized collagen bundles.

However, a combination of congested capillaries and cavern-like vascular spaces is seen extending into the deep dermis and subcutaneous tissue (Fig. 33-26). These vascular spaces are lined by flattened endothelial cells and are usually surrounded by a layer of pericytes. A lobular growth pattern is often apparent in the deep component.

Microvenular Hemangioma

This is a recently described uncommon acquired vascular lesion that usually arises as a small reddish lesion in young to middle-aged individuals of either gender (124,125). The arms, trunk, and legs are favored sites. The development of lesions in relationship to pregnancy or a change in the use of oral contraception may suggest a hormonal influence on the disease in women (126).

Histopathology. Histologically thin branching capillaries and small venules with narrow or slightly dilated lumina are found widely throughout the dermis (Fig. 33-27). There is no obvious endothelial cell atypia or accompanying inflammation, but slight dermal sclerosis is often present (Fig. 33-28). The collagen bundles around the vascular channels appear somewhat sclerotic. A fairly constant feature in many cases is the prominent infiltration of arrector pili muscles by the proliferating vascular channels (Fig. 33-29). The cells lining the vessels are strongly positive for

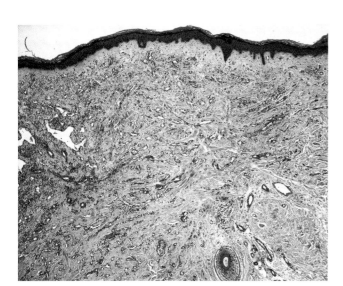

FIGURE 33-27. Microvenular hemangioma. Irregular, branching, thin-walled venules throughout the dermis.

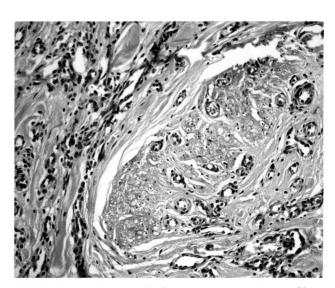

FIGURE 33-29. Microvenular hemangioma. Prominent infiltration of the arrector pili muscle.

von Willebrand factor and CD34. In two cases, angiomatous tufts in the deeper part of the lesion suggested a possible relationship with tufted angioma (125).

Differential Diagnosis. The importance of microvenular hemangioma as an acquired vascular anomaly in young persons lies in the differential diagnosis from an early or macular lesion of Kaposi's sarcoma. The lymphangioma-like channels of Kaposi's sarcoma are more delicate, do not contain erythrocytes, show angulated outlines, and tend to wrap around collagen bundles. Furthermore, plasma cells and other inflammatory cells are common in Kaposi's sarcoma but not in microvenular hemangioma.

Hobnail Hemangioma (Targetoid Hemosiderotic Hemangioma)

This is a relatively uncommon, vascular tumor that usually presents in the trunk or extremities of young or middle-aged adults with a male predominance (127–130). Rare cases occur in the oral mucosa. The descriptive name initially given to this tumor reflects a typical clinical appearance characterized by a small solitary lesion consisting of a brown to violaceous papule, 2 to 3 mm in diameter, surrounded by a thin, pale area and a peripheral ecchymotic ring. However, these features are only present in 20% of cases (129), and most often the clinical appearance is that of a red-blue or brown papule. The alternative name of *hobnail hemangioma*, which emphasizes a more constant special histologic feature, has therefore been proposed (see subsequent text) (129).

Histopathology. In the superficial reticular dermis there are a number of thin-walled, dilated, and irregular vascular spaces (Fig. 33-30) often lined by bland endothelial cells with scanty cytoplasm and rounded nuclei that protrude

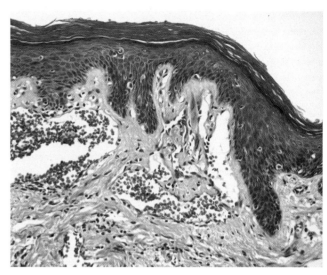

FIGURE 33-31. Hobnail hemangioma. Irregular congested vascular channels some of which are lined by hobnail endothelial cells.

into the lumina and closely resemble hobnails (Figs. 33-31 and 33-32). Focally, epithelioid cells are rarely present. Intraluminal papillary projections and fibrin thrombi can be seen in the superficial blood vessels (Fig. 33-32). The vascular channels in the deeper dermis become much less conspicuous and eventually disappear completely. These deeper channels are irregular and angulated, lined by flattened endothelial cells, and dissect between collagen bundles. Extensive red blood cell extravasation, inflammatory aggregates predominantly of lymphocytes, and, in a later stage, extensive stromal hemosiderin deposition are commonly seen.

Pathogenesis. Because there is a family of vascular tumors characterized by epithelioid endothelial cells, it has been

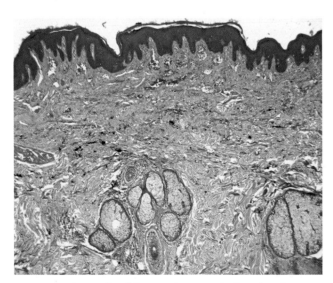

FIGURE 33-30. Hobnail hemangioma. Typical wedge-shape architecture with a prominent superficial component. Note prominent hemosiderin deposition.

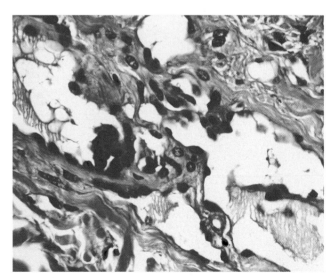

FIGURE 33-32. Hobnail hemangioma. Hobnail endothelial cells and small papillary projections.

proposed that this tumor represents the benign end of the spectrum of a group of vascular tumors characterized by hobnail endothelial cells that includes *Dabska's tumor* and *retiform hemangioendothelioma* (131). Based on the positivity of the endothelial cells for vascular endothelial growth factor receptor 3 (VEGFR-3), it has been proposed that these tumors display lymphatic differentiation (130). However, it has become apparent that VEGFR-3 is not a specific marker of lymphatic differentiation (132).

Differential Diagnosis. This includes patch-stage Kaposi's sarcoma, retiform hemangioendothelioma, and benign lymphangioendothelioma (see below).

Arteriovenous (Venous) Hemangioma (Cirsoid Aneurysm)

Arteriovenous (venous) hemangioma, or cirsoid aneurysm, usually occurs as a solitary dark-red papule or nodule on the face (especially the lip) or, less commonly, on the extremities of adults, with equal gender incidence (133,134). Rare cases present in the oral cavity (135). Most of the lesions measure less than 1 cm in diameter.

Histopathology. Within a circumscribed area, usually restricted to the dermis (Fig. 33-33), one observes densely aggregated, thick-walled and thin-walled vessels lined by a single layer of endothelial cells (Fig. 33-34). The walls of the thick-walled vessels consist mainly of fibrous tissue but in most instances also contain some smooth muscle. Internal elastic lamina is found in very few vessels, indicating that most of the blood vessels are veins. Many vessels contain red blood cells, and thrombi are occasionally seen (135). Lesions with similar histologic appearances can be seen in the deeper soft tissues of younger patients

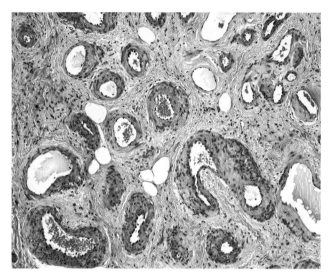

FIGURE 33-34. Cirsoid aneurysm. A combination of small veins and arteries.

and can be associated with hemodynamic complications due to shunting.

Histogenesis. It seems likely that many of these lesions represent pure venous hemangiomas, some of which have arterialized veins (135).

Angiomatosis

Angiomatosis is an uncommon condition that presents exclusively in children and adolescents and is defined as a diffuse proliferation of blood vessels affecting a large contiguous area of the body (136–138). Anatomic distribution is wide, but there is a preference for limb involvement. A typical case presents with involvement of the skin, underlying soft tissues, and even bones. Associated limb hypertrophy is common. Involvement of parenchymal organs and the central nervous system can be present. Due to extensive involvement, surgical treatment is difficult and recurrences are common.

Histopathology. Most tumors are composed of abundant mature fat intermixed with blood vessels in two histologic patterns (137). The most common pattern is a mixture of veins with irregular walls, cavernous vascular spaces, and capillaries. The veins often show an incomplete muscular layer, and smaller blood vessels can be seen in the walls of larger vessels. The second pattern is composed mainly of capillaries with a focal lobular architecture. Perineural invasion can be a feature in both patterns.

Spindle-Cell Hemangioma

This tumor was first described in 1986 (139) as a form of low-grade angiosarcoma, although mounting evidence in recent years widely favors a non-neoplastic process most

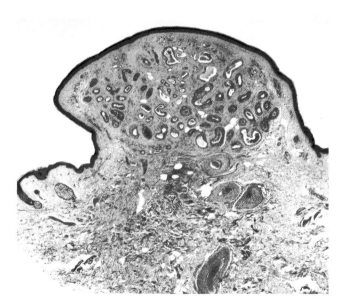

FIGURE 33-33. Cirsoid aneurysm. Polypoid superficial lesion composed of dilated thick-walled vascular channels.

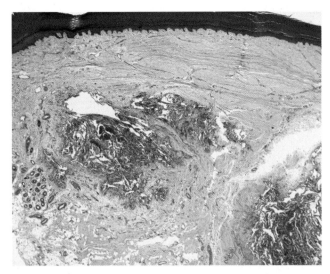

FIGURE 33-35. Spindle-cell hemangioma. Multifocal lesions combining dilated and congested vascular spaces and more cellular areas.

likely related to a vascular malformation (see Pathogenesis). Gender incidence is equal, and most lesions arise in the second or third decade of life. It presents as multiple red-blue nodules in the dermis and subcutaneous tissue, most commonly involving the distal aspects of the extremities with a predilection for the hands. Visceral lesions do not occur, and involvement of deeper soft tissues is rare (140). The clinical course is indolent with multiple new lesions appearing over the years. Spontaneous regression is exceptional. In approximately 10% of cases, associated anomalies include lymphoedema, Maffucci's syndrome, Klippel–Trenaunay syndrome, and early-onset varicose veins (139,141,142).

Histopathology. Tumors tend to be poorly circumscribed and may present totally or partially in an intravascular location especially involving medium-sized veins. A typical lesion is composed of two elements (Fig. 33-35): irregularly dilated, thin-walled, congested cavernous spaces often with organizing thrombi and phleboliths intermixed with more solid areas composed of spindle-shaped cells (Fig. 33-36) generally bland in appearance, although rare cases may show focal degenerative cytologic atypia. Mitotic figures are rare. Commonly in the solid areas focal aggregates of epithelioid cells with eosinophilic cytoplasm and bundles of smooth muscle are seen. The epithelioid cells may show vacuolation or intracytoplasmic lumina (Fig. 33-37). Slit-like vascular spaces are common in the solid areas and are accompanied by scattered extravasated red blood cells and hemosiderin-laden macrophages. Focal areas with changes resembling Masson's tumor can be a feature. Irregular, thick-walled vascular spaces reminiscent of those seen in vascular malformations are often seen in the periphery of many lesions. Occasionally, cases show combined features of epithelioid and spindle-cell hemangioendothelioma (143,144).

Pathogenesis. Original classification of this tumor as a form of low-grade angiosarcoma was based on the development of lymph node metastasis in one of the patients reported (139). However, the patient had been treated with radiotherapy, and it is very likely that the metastasis was from a radiation-induced sarcoma. Further case series in recent years have provided evidence favoring the theory that spindle-cell hemangioendothelioma represents a reactive condition or a form of vascular malformation (141,145–147).

By immunohistochemistry, the endothelial cells lining the vascular spaces and the epithelioid cells in the solid

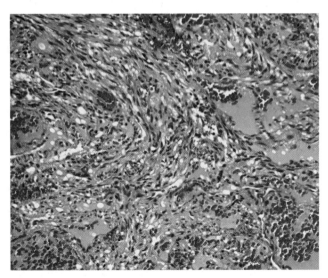

FIGURE 33-36. Spindle-cell hemangioma. Thin-walled dilated vascular spaces and bland spindle-shaped cells.

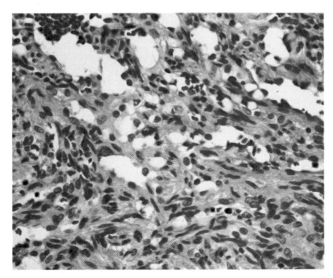

FIGURE 33-37. Spindle cell hemangioma. Spindle-shaped cells and focal epithelioid pale pink vacuolated cells.

areas stain variably with endothelial markers. The spindle cells stain focally with actin and less commonly with desmin.

Differential Diagnosis. The main differential diagnosis is with nodular-stage Kaposi's sarcoma, as discussed below.

LOW-GRADE MALIGNANT TUMORS

Malignant tumors of endothelial cell origin can be broadly divided into those of low- or high-grade malignancy (Table 31-1). Strictly used, the term low-grade malignant refers to a tumor that has an aggressive local behavior with a tendency for local recurrence but low or negligible potential for metastatic spread. There is a tendency to designate malignant vascular tumors with true potential for metastatic spread as angiosarcomas and low-grade tumors as hemangioendotheliomas. However, some authors use the terms interchangeably and progress in our understanding of some of these tumors has led to certain neoplasms being either up-graded as fully malignant (e.g., epithelioid hemangioendothelioma) or down graded as benign (e.g., spindle cell hemangioma). It must also be remembered that the term hemangioendothelioma was used in the past to refer to some benign vascular tumors, especially strawberry nevus in children. The category of low-grade malignant tumors also includes lesions like Kaposi's sarcoma a generally indolent process in which a truly neoplastic origin has not clearly been demonstrated.

Kaposi's Sarcoma

Until the late 1960s, Kaposi's sarcoma was described as an uncommon, slowly progressive, multifocal tumor arising mostly in elderly male patients of Eastern and Southern European descent, a clinical pattern now referred to as the "classic" form of the disease. The current intense interest in the disease stems from the recognition that Kaposi's sarcoma is an extremely common tumor in tropical Africa and that it is also a prime marker of acquired immunodeficiency syndrome (AIDS). In addition, Kaposi's sarcoma can arise in association with other causes of immunodeficiency, especially when drug induced. There remain many unusual facets about the disease; the genetic and epidemiologic aspects, the clinical course, the histopathologic features, the transmission, and the pathogenesis that as yet defy adequate scientific explanation. It is still controversial whether Kaposi's sarcoma is a multifocal reactive process or a neoplastic condition and the issue has still not been settled. Recently, all forms of Kaposi's sarcoma have been associated with a new type of herpesvirus named human herpesvirus 8 (see Histogenesis below).

Clinical Features. Nearly all cases of Kaposi's sarcoma can be classified into four groups (148–151):

Classic Kaposi's sarcoma. This arises 10 to 15 times more commonly in men than women, affecting mainly patients of Eastern European, Jewish, and Mediterranean origin. Studies of clusters of cases in the Peloponnese suggested a role for an infectious agent in the etiology of the disease (152). The disease mainly arises in patients over age 50 with the slow development of angiomatous nodules and plaques on the lower extremities. Affected patients may survive 10 to 20 years; even at late stages with widespread skin nodules, visceral disease is unusual, although asymptomatic involvement of lymph nodes, lungs, or gastrointestinal tract can often be found at necropsy (150). Occasionally before the advent of AIDS, an aggressive type of Kaposi's sarcoma occurred in young adults or children with early lymph node involvement (149). Various types of lymphoma have been reported to occur in the classic type of Kaposi's sarcoma with an incidence of 10% or more.

African Kaposi's sarcoma. In the 1960s, it was realized that Kaposi's sarcoma was very common among native blacks in Central Africa, representing the most common tumor in pathology departments in Uganda and parts of Zaire. In South Africa, it has been estimated that Kaposi's sarcoma is ten times more common in blacks than whites. In Africans, the disease can run a similar indolent course as in classic Kaposi's sarcoma, but a higher proportion of young people are affected, with a more aggressive disease manifested by widespread tumors, deep infiltrative or elevated fungating lesions, and bone involvement. A distinctive childhood type of Kaposi's sarcoma occurs with massive lymph node involvement and early death. Mucocutaneous lesions are usually a late or minor clinical feature in this lymphadenopathic form (149). The male-to-female ratio in these children is approximately 3:1.

AIDS-associated Kaposi's sarcoma. In the early 1980s, reports of groups of young homosexual males in New York and California who were developing Kaposi's sarcoma (153) were one of the keys in establishing the existence of AIDS. Originally about 40% of patients with AIDS had concomitant Kaposi's sarcoma, but this high percentage has gradually fallen to around 20% in the United States (148,151, 154) and Europe (155). Data from the Centers for Disease Control and Prevention in the United States suggested that Kaposi's sarcoma was at least 201,000 times more common with AIDS than in the general population (148). The risk of Kaposi's sarcoma occurring with AIDS is much greater in active homosexuals than in heterosexual males or females, such as hemophiliacs who receive contaminated blood products or drug abusers who share needles. These epidemiologic peculiarities call into question whether the human immunodeficiency virus (HIV) is the sole or main transmissible agent causing Kaposi's sarcoma.

The clinical features of AIDS-related Kaposi's sarcoma differ from the classic disease in the rapid evolution of the lesions, their atypical distribution affecting the trunk, and the mucosal involvement (150). Visceral involvement is very common at autopsy (156–159), but such internal lesions are often not apparent clinically during life. Visceral involvement may be present without any skin lesions. Most patients die as a result of infections due to immunodeficiency rather than from the direct effect of the sarcoma.

Kaposi's sarcoma and iatrogenic immunosuppression. Drug-induced immunosuppression to prevent rejection of transplanted organs greatly increases the risk of developing lymphomas and other tumors, including Kaposi's sarcoma. In one study, 13 cases of Kaposi's sarcoma arose in 820 kidney transplant recipients (160). A peculiarity of this type of Kaposi's sarcoma is the frequent regression or apparent cure on discontinuation of immunosuppressive therapy. The male-dominant gender ratio is much smaller in this group.

Histopathology. The histopathology of fully developed nodules of Kaposi's sarcoma in all types of the disease is distinctive and should rarely cause problems for pathologists. The diagnostic pitfalls lie mainly in the early macular lesions where misinterpretation as banal inflammation or some form of minor angiomatous or lymphatic anomaly is easy to make (161). A further difficulty is that in some late lesions, cytologic atypia increases and the vascular component of the nodules becomes effaced, giving rise to the differential diagnosis of other spindle-cell sarcomas.

For descriptive convenience, the histologic spectrum can be divided into stages roughly corresponding to the clinical type of lesion: early and late macules, plaques, nodules, and aggressive late lesions. In reality there is overlap between stages, and multiple biopsies taken at the same time or even a single biopsy may show features of different histologic stages. There are no differences in the pathology of the disease in the different risk groups.

Macular (patch stage). In early macules, there is usually a patchy, sparse, dermal perivascular infiltrate consisting of lymphocytes and plasma cells. Narrow cords of cells, insinuated between collagen bundles, may at first suggest histiocytes or connective tissue cells, but close inspection should reveal evidence of luminal differentiation or connection with discernible small vessels (Fig. 33-38). Usually a few dilated irregular or angulated lymphatic-like spaces lined by delicate endothelial cells are also present. Vessels with "jagged" outlines tending to separate collagen bundles are especially characteristic (153,162) (Fig. 33-39). Normal adnexal structures and preexisting blood vessels often protrude into newly formed blood vessels (Fig. 33-40). This finding known as the "promontory sign," is commonly present but is not specific to Kaposi's sarcoma. In late macular lesions, there is a more extensive infiltrate of vessels in the dermis: "jagged" vessels and cords of thicker-walled vessels similar to those in granulation tissue. Some of these vessels may in part be reactive rather than an intrinsic part of the tumor. At this stage, red blood cell extravasation and the presence of siderophages may be encountered. In some lesions, ramifying variably dilated bloodless lymphatic-like spaces dissect out collagen to give an appearance that suggests a well-differentiated angiosarcoma or progressive lymphangioma (163). This exaggerated lymphangioma-like appearance has led some authors to designate this as a special variant of the disease (162) (Fig. 33-41). Occasional fascicles of spindle-shaped cells may occur independent of blood vessels.

Plaque stage. In this stage a diffuse infiltrate of small blood vessels extends through most parts of the dermis and tends to displace collagen (Fig. 33-42). The vessels show variable morphology, some occurring as poorly canalized cords, some as blood-containing ovoid vessels, and some showing lymphatic-like features. Loosely distributed spindle

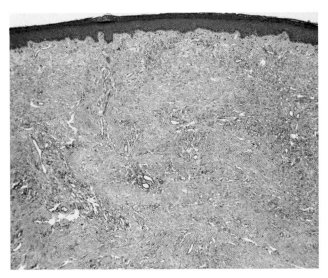

FIGURE 33-38. Patch-stage Kaposi's sarcoma. Numerous slit-like spaces throughout the dermis in the background of hemorrhage.

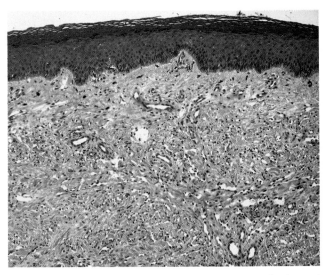

FIGURE 33-39. Patch-stage Kaposi's sarcoma. Irregular jagged thin-walled small vascular channels in association with hemosiderin deposition and focal inflammation.

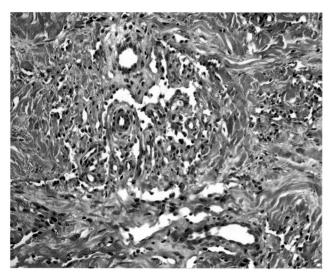

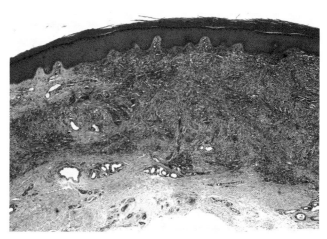

FIGURE 33-42. Plaque-stage Kaposi's sarcoma. A more cellular dermis with extensive hemorrhage.

FIGURE 33-40. Patch-stage Kaposi's sarcoma. A normal blood vessels protruding into newly formed blood vessels ("promontory sign") lined by bland endothelial cells.

cells, arranged in short fascicles, are also encountered (Fig. 33-43). Intracytoplasmic hyaline globules (164,165) may be found in areas with a denser infiltrate. These hyaline globules are seen more often in lesions from patients with AIDS.

Nodular stage. In the tumor stage, well-defined nodules composed of vascular spaces and spindle cells replace dermal collagen (Fig. 33-44). These tumor nodules tend to be compartmentalized by dense bands of fibrocollagenous tissue. Dilated lymphatic spaces can also be seen between tumor aggregates. The characteristic feature is a honeycomb-like network of blood-filled spaces or slits, closely associated with interweaving spindle cells (Fig. 33-45). Although generally vascular spaces and fascicles of

spindle cells are present, either element can focally predominate. The vascular lumina in the angiomatous tissue are so closely set that they lie next to each other in a "back-to-back" arrangement. Delicate flattened endothelial cells lining the vascular clefts are hardly discernible with routine stains but are easily seen with the immunocytochemical markers CD31 and CD34 (166). The vascular slits in the nodules appear to be in direct contact with spindle cells, leading to the suggestion that they are pseudovascular spaces (165). The presence of a closely set honeycomb-like pattern of vascular spaces is perhaps the single most important diagnostic feature of Kaposi's sarcoma. In the vascular spaces of pyogenic granuloma and most angiomas, the endothelial cells of the capillary walls are more prominent and the vessels are set farther apart by intervening stroma.

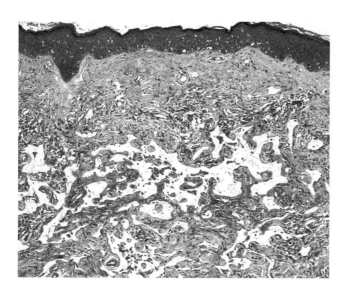

FIGURE 33-41. Lymphangiomatous Kaposi's sarcoma. Numerous irregular, dilated, bloodless vascular channels with a striking lymphangioma-like appearance.

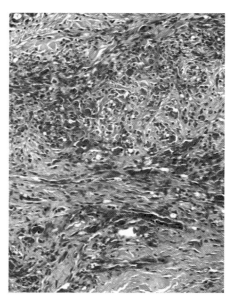

FIGURE 33-43. Plaque-stage Kaposi's sarcoma. Bland spindle-shaped cells with focal formation of cleft-like spaces containing red blood cells.

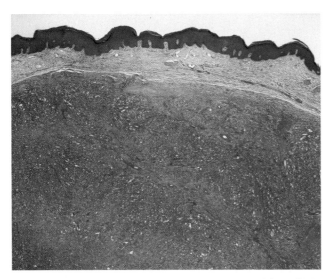

FIGURE 33-44. Nodular-stage Kaposi's sarcoma. Fairly well circumscribed dermal nodule.

Around the nodules, varying numbers of thicker-walled vessels are encountered that may represent reactive or "feeder" vessels and are not a basic component of the tumor. Blood pigment–containing macrophages are nearly always prominent adjacent to the nodules, especially in lesions at dependent sites.

The spindle cells in the nodules are elongated and fusiform with a well-defined cytoplasm. The nuclei are ovoid and somewhat flattened with finely granular chromatin in the long axis of the cells. The nucleoli are generally inconspicuous and nuclear atypia is absent or slight. Mitosis is infrequent. Prominent and consistent positivity for CD34 is seen in the spindle cell population.

Intra- and extra-cellular hyaline globules occur more frequently than in plaque-stage lesions. They present in groups as faintly eosinophilic spheres 1 to 7 μm in size and are PAS positive and diastase resistant (162). The globules probably represent partially digested erythrocytes (165). Although characteristic and of some diagnostic significance, hyaline globules are not entirely specific for Kaposi's sarcoma because they can be found occasionally in other connective tissue conditions with interstitial hemorrhage. Usually the epidermis and skin appendages remain intact.

Aggressive late-stage lesions. Mostly in Africans, but sometimes with other types of Kaposi's sarcoma, "infiltrating" lesions show a more obviously sarcomatous character with reduction or loss of the vascular component. The spindle cells demonstrate a greater degree of cytologic atypia with regard to size, shape, and nuclear features, with mitosis becoming frequent. In such lesions, phagocytosed erythrocytes and the presence of hyaline globules may provide clues about the tumor's origin. Very rarely angiosarcoma is mimicked by the development of vascular spaces lined by grossly atypical endothelial cells.

Tumor cells in all stages of Kaposi's disease regardless of the clinical category stain positive for human herpesvirus 8 antibody (see below) (Fig. 33-46).

It has been questioned whether the histologic features of Kaposi's sarcoma can be used as a guide to the prognosis. It seems reasonable to suggest that as the disease progresses from the macular to plaque and nodular stages, the presence of histologic characteristics of the polar macular and nodular stages may be a guide to the clinical evolution. Surprisingly this does not seem to be the case as a recent study (167) has indicated that lesions histologically indicative of nodular Kaposi's sarcoma carry a better prognosis than that of macular lesions.

A useful diagnostic tool is the demonstration of human herpesvirus 8 in cutaneous samples from patients with all

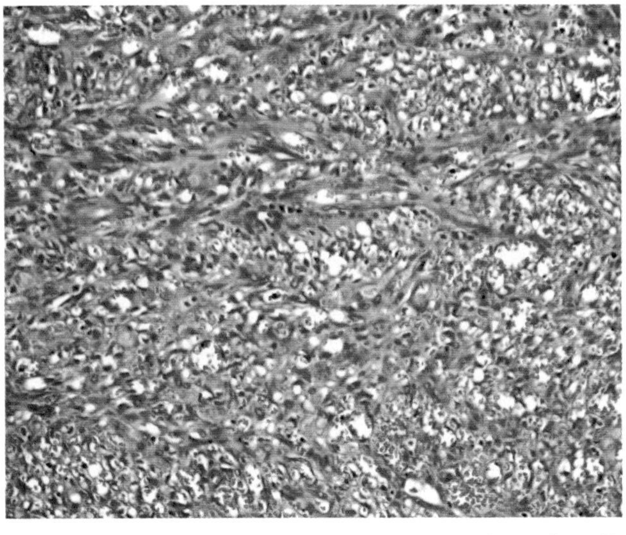

FIGURE 33-45. Nodular Kaposi's sarcoma. Bland spindle cells forming slit-like spaces occupied by red blood cells.

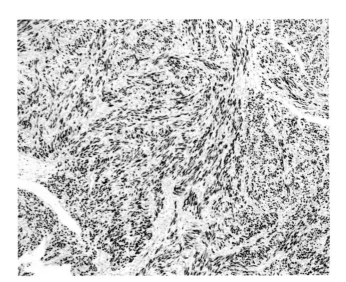

FIGURE 33-46. Nodular Kaposi's sarcoma. Diffuse staining of the nuclei of spindle-shaped cells with an antibody against human herpes virus 8 using the ABC method.

clinical subsets of Kaposi's sarcoma. Until recently, demonstration of the virus was only possible by *in situ* hybridization. This has been simplified by the development of a commercially available monoclonal antibody against the virus that can be used in routine practice.

Pathogenesis. The multifocal development, slow evolution of the classic form of the disease, occasional regression, and histology of inflammation that lacks cytologic atypia, has led many to suggest that at least initially Kaposi's sarcoma is a reactive condition and not a neoplastic process (149,152,168,169). Recent demonstration of clonality tends to favor the later but the issue remains far from settled (170). The morphogenesis of the differing tumor elements—in particular, the derivation of the spindle-cell component of plaque and nodular lesions—used to be controversial. Ultrastructural studies tend to indicate that the spindle cells represent transformed endothelial cells and have received strong support from recent immunohistochemical studies. The spindle cells label with endothelial cell markers CD31 and CD34 (166,171–173). CD34 is a less-specific label for endothelial cells than CD31 since labeling of other mesenchymal cells also occurs. The possibility of deriving spindle cells from dermal dendrocytes has not been supported by studies using markers against factor XIIIa, although reactive hyperplasia of dendrocytes occurs around Kaposi nodules (174). Nevertheless, Nickoloff suggests that activated dendrocytes may have an important role in the initiation of Kaposi lesions (171). Earlier cell-marker studies also provide evidence suggesting that the spindle cells of Kaposi's sarcoma are endothelial-cell derived (164, 175–178).

Dorfmann's (149) earlier morphologic observations led him to suggest that Kaposi's sarcoma may originate from lymphatic rather than vascular endothelial cells. This would account for lymphangioma-like instances of Kaposi's sarcoma (163). This suggestion has been supported by cell markers used by some authors (175,176) but not others (177). The positivity of endothelial cells in Kaposi's sarcoma to markers such as vascular endothelial growth factor receptor 3 has been advocated to support a lymphatic line of differentiation for Kaposi's sarcoma (179). However, the lack of specificity of this and other markers of lymphatic differentiation makes it impossible to confirm this theory (132). Dictor and Anderson (180) suggest, that because of the close association between veins and lymphatics, endothelium with hybrid characteristics could give rise to the lymphatic and blood-vascular aspects of the pathology. The role of growth-promoting factors causing angiogenesis and recruitment of other cells in Kaposi's sarcoma has also been studied using molecular biologic techniques (151,154).

The peculiar epidemiologic aspects of Kaposi's sarcoma have stimulated research for many years on whether viruses other than HIV or some other transmissible agent help to induce the disease. Initial studies of the fine structure of tumor cells in Kaposi's sarcoma revealed tuboreticular structures and cylindrical-confronting cisternae, suggestive of a cellular reaction to a viral infection. This was followed by an exceptional report of an association between cytomegalic virus and Kaposi's sarcoma and the identification of retrovirus-like structures (152,169). Recently, the riddle of the association between Kaposi's sarcoma and a virus has been resolved. Chang et al. (181) described a new human herpesvirus associated with Kaposi's sarcoma. This is a gamma herpesvirus closely associated to Epstein–Barr virus and has been named *human herpesvirus 8* (182,183). DNA sequences of this virus have been detected consistently in all variants of the disease including AIDS-related Kaposi's sarcoma (184), African endemic (184), Kaposi's sarcoma induced by iatrogenic immunosuppression, and Mediterranean (185) Kaposi's sarcoma. The virus can be found in the blood of patients before lesions of Kaposi's sarcoma develop (186).

Differential Diagnosis. The differential diagnosis is wide (161), with the most difficulties encountered with either early macular or late aggressive lesions. Vascular proliferations in stasis and multinucleate-cell angiohistiocytoma are discussed here in more detail because they are not described elsewhere in this chapter.

In *early macular lesions*, an inflammatory condition or a cell-poor (atrophic) histiocytoma may be suspected since the vascular nature of vessels with collapsed lumina may not be apparent. Appropriate cell markers may clarify the vascular nature of the underlying lesion. The cryptic vessels are universally positive with CD31 and CD34, but negative with factor XIIIa. Von Willebrand factor is negative in lymphangioma-like channels of Kaposi's sarcoma with positive labeling limited to thicker-walled vessels. In late macular lesions, the differential diagnosis includes a well-differentiated angiosarcoma, progressive lymphangioma, targetoid hemosiderotic hemangioma, and microvenular hemangioma. Angiosarcoma shows not only a "dissection" of collagen infiltrative pattern, but endothelial cell atypia with hyperchromatism and intraluminal shedding of malignant cells. Histologically, progressive lymphangioma is almost indistinguishable from Kaposi's sarcoma with prominent lymphangioma-like features, but inflammatory cells, especially plasma cells, tend to be absent in the former. When the clinical features are taken into account, distinction is not difficult. In targetoid hemosiderotic hemangioma, lymphangioma-like channels are mainly confined to the upper dermis; in places plump "hobnail" endothelial cells invaginate vascular spaces, inflammatory cells are rare, and hemosiderin deposition is prominent, unlike early Kaposi's sarcoma. Microvenular hemangioma differs by showing blood-containing vessels, many of which are surrounded by pericytes or smooth-muscle cells (positive for smooth-muscle actin) suggestive of venular differentiation.

Spindle-cell hemangioma, the rare, recently described kaposiform hemangioendothelioma of childhood, and moderately differentiated angiosarcomas with spindle-cell differentiation, are the most important histologic simulants of *nodular Kaposi's lesions.*

Spindle cell hemangioma differs by showing cavernous or widely dilated vascular spaces and collections of epithelioid cells with or without intracytoplasmic lumina.

Kaposiform hemangioendothelioma is mainly a disease of children that usually affects deep soft tissues although the skin can be affected (187–189). Histologically, the tumor shows intermediate features of capillary hemangioma and Kaposi's sarcoma and has a lobular growth pattern that is absent in Kaposi's sarcoma.

Sometimes spindle-cell differentiation is prominent in angiosarcoma, but usually markedly atypical cells are present, allowing differentiation from Kaposi's sarcoma.

Other acquired vascular conditions that can cause problems from the clinical and histologic point of view are bacillary angiomatosis, and pyogenic granuloma, especially if complicated by satellite lesions and tufted angioma. Spindle-cell fascicles with a bland cytologic appearance do not feature as a prominent component of any of these entities.

Aneurysmal benign fibrous histiocytoma is a nonvascular, highly cellular spindle-cell lesion with pseudovascular spaces and hemosiderin deposition that can be confused with nodular Kaposi's sarcoma (190). The variability of pathology, the presence of peripheral areas similar to common dermal fibrous histiocytoma, and immunohistochemistry should prevent error in diagnosis.

In *aggressive late-stage lesions,* many malignant spindle cell tumors can come into the differential diagnosis especially if clinical details are unavailable. The most important differential diagnoses are fibrosarcoma, leiomyosarcoma, monophasic synovial sarcoma, malignant cellular blue nevus with sparse melanin deposition, and desmoplastic malignant melanoma. Accurate diagnosis may be impossible unless reliable immunohistochemistry is available. CD31 and CD34 are particularly helpful in suggesting a vascular derivation even in poorly differentiated Kaposi's lesions.

Hypostasis and high venous pressure gives rise to vascular proliferation (pseudo-Kaposi's sarcoma/acroangiodermatitis). Angiomatous papules and plaques near the ankles that are secondary to high venous pressure result from incompetent veins and are common causes of Kaposi-like lesions (161,162). Less commonly, high venous pressure can arise due to congenital or acquired arteriovenous anomalies (191,192). Histologically, there is expansion of the whole capillary bed throughout the dermis. In the papillary dermis there is reduplication and corkscrewing of thick-walled capillaries, which increase in size and become angiomatous in appearance. Similarly, venules and deeper, vertically small veins become hypertrophied and tortuous. Erythrocyte extravasation, fibrosis with horizontally oriented spindle cells, and numerous siderophages are additional features. The angiomatous capillaries appear separated from each other by an edematous matrix, and they do *not* lie "back to back" as in Kaposi's sarcoma. To complicate matters, hypostatic vascular proliferation can coexist with Kaposi's sarcoma. A key difference between Kaposi's sarcoma and pseudo-Kaposi's sarcoma is that in the latter vascular hyperplasia results from hyperplasia of the preexisting vasculature, whereas in the former the vascular proliferation is mainly independent.

Multinucleate-cell angiohistiocytoma, a recently described reactive vascular condition, arises as slowly developing grouped vascular papules usually on the legs (193), but also at other sites including the face and hands (194). Most patients are older women. Histologically, an increased number of capillaries and venules with few inflammatory cells are found throughout the dermis, but the extent of the proliferation does achieve angiomatous proportions. Increased numbers of histiocytes and scattered multinucleate cells are usually found but not in every biopsy. Blood-pigment deposition is generally insignificant.

Immunohistochemical demonstration of human herpesvirus 8 is of great help in the histologic differential diagnosis of Kaposi's sarcoma as all the vascular and nonvascular entities previously discussed are usually not associated with this virus.

Retiform Hemangioendothelioma

Retiform hemangioendothelioma is a rare, recently described variant of low-grade angiosarcoma characterized by indolent clinical behavior (131,195,196). There is a predilection for young adults, and it presents as a slowly growing nondistinct tumor with equal gender incidence and a predilection for the extremities, especially the distal lower limbs. Rare cases can be associated with radiotherapy or chronic lymphedema. A single case with multiple primary tumors has been documented (197). Multiple recurrences are common, but metastasis has so far been reported in only two cases. One case metastasized to a regional lymph node and a second case presented with a soft tissue metastasis close to the primary tumor (198). Retiform hemangioendothelioma is part of the spectrum of a family of vascular tumors that are characterized by endothelial cells with a distinctive hobnail appearance. This includes a benign tumor originally described as targetoid hemosiderotic hemangioma (hobnail hemangioma) and another low-grade malignant lesion, Dabska's tumor.

Histopathology. Tumors are ill-defined and involve the reticular dermis with frequent extension into the subcutis. In most cases, there is a striking low-power resemblance to the normal rete testis conferred by the presence of elongated, arborizing blood vessels (Fig. 33-47) lined by monomorphic bland endothelial cells with prominent apical nuclei and scanty cytoplasm. These cells have been described as having a "matchstick" or hobnail appearance (Fig. 33-48). A lymphocytic inflammatory cell infiltrate is

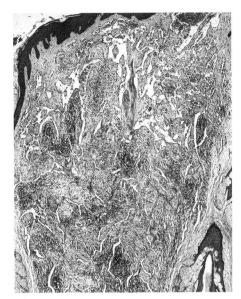

FIGURE 33-47. Retiform hemangioendothelioma. Branching blood vessels and a prominent lymphocytic inflammatory cell infiltrate.

frequently seen not only in the stroma but also in the vascular lumina (though not invariably present). The intravascular lymphocytes commonly appear in close contact with the hobnail endothelial cells. Occasional intravascular papillae with hyaline cores can be seen (Fig. 33-48). In most tumors, there are solid areas composed of bland spindle cells or epithelioid cells that stain for endothelial markers. Some lesions present a mini-retiform pattern that may be more difficult to recognize on low-power examination. A sclerotic stroma is seen in some cases.

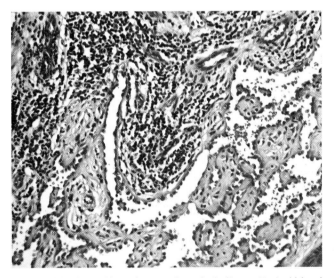

FIGURE 33-48. Retiform hemangioendothelioma. Typical bland hobnail endothelial cells and focal papillary projections.

Differential Diagnosis. Retiform hemangioendothelioma shares clinical and histologic features with Dabska's tumor. However, in Dabska's tumor, cavernous vascular spaces resembling lymphatics predominate, there is no retiform architecture, and intravascular papillae with collagenous cores are a striking feature. Hobnail hemangioma (targetoid hemosiderotic hemangioma) is more superficial, lacks a retiform architecture, and has hobnail endothelial cells that are mainly seen in vessels near the surface. Angiosarcoma often presents in a different clinical setting and shows cytologic atypia, mitoses, and absence of hobnail endothelial cells.

Papillary Intralymphatic Angioendothelioma (Malignant Endothelial Papillary Angioendothelioma, Dabska's Tumor)

Papillary intralymphatic angioendothelioma (PILA) is a very rare tumor that was first described in 1969 as malignant endolymphatic angioendothelioma (199). Until recently, only very few additional cases had been reported in the literature, and there seemed to be a lack of consensus regarding its specific histologic features. However, a recent series has delineated the histologic features of this tumor more accurately and the alternative name of PILA has been proposed (200). Tumors present mainly in infants and children but around 25% of patients are adults. Males and females are equally affected and most cases involve the limbs. Clinical presentation is that of a slowly growing, solitary, asymptomatic nodule or plaque. This tumor is classified amongst tumors with low-grade malignant potential based on reports of local recurrence and rare regional lymph node metastasis in the original series (199). However, follow-up in 8 of the 12 cases recently reported, showed no evidence of either local recurrence or distant spread (200). It is therefore likely that these tumors are benign, although confirmation of these findings is required in larger series with longer follow-up. Until this happens, complete excision of these tumors is advised.

Histopathology. Low-power examination reveals a dermal and often subcutaneous tumor composed of markedly dilated, thin-walled vascular channels resembling a cavernous lymphangioma (Fig. 33-49). These vascular channels are lined by bland hobnail endothelial cells with protruding nuclei and very scanty cytoplasm. A prominent intra- and extra-vascular lymphocytic inflammatory cell infiltrate is often present, and intravascular papillae with collagenous cores are a frequent finding (Fig. 33-50). Commonly, the lymphocytes appear to be in close apposition to the endothelial cells. Tumor cells stain for vascular markers including CD31, CD34, and von Willebrand factor.

Pathogenesis. Based on the close interaction between lymphocytes and endothelial cells in Dabska's tumor, it has been

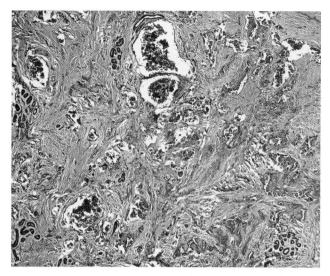

FIGURE 33-49. Papillary intralymphatic angioendothelioma. Cavernous lymphangioma-like vascular spaces and intravascular papillae.

proposed that the hobnail endothelial cells differentiate toward high endothelial cells, which are normally responsible for the selective homing of lymphocytes in lymphoid organs (201). A similar theory can be proposed for retiform hemangioendothelioma, which shares some histologic features with Dabska's tumor. The strong expression of vascular endothelial growth factor receptor 3 (VEGFR-3) by tumor cells has led to suggestions that these tumors display lymphatic differentiation (200). The specificity of this marker as an indicator of lymphatic differentiation is, however, doubtful.

Differential Diagnosis. See Differential Diagnosis for retiform hemangioendothelioma.

Composite Hemangioendothelioma

Composite hemangioendothelioma is a recently described low-grade malignant vascular tumor with a tendency for local recurrence but very low metastatic potential. It is defined as a neoplasm containing a mixture of histologic patterns including benign, intermediate, and/or malignant (202). It is a very rare tumor presenting mainly in adults and only exceptionally in children (202,203). There is no sex predilection and most tumors occur in the extremities with a predilection for the hands and feet. In a quarter of the patients, tumors arise in association with lymphoedema and lesions present as long-standing red/blue nodules or plaques. The rate of local recurrence is around 50% and this may occur years after excision of the primary tumor. Only a single case originating in the tongue has been reported to metastasize to a regional lymph node and to the soft tissues of the thigh.

Histopathology. Composite hemangioendothelioma is poorly circumscribed, with an infiltrative growth pattern and involvement of the dermis and subcutaneous tissue. The different components vary from tumor to tumor and may include retiform hemangioendothelioma (Fig. 33-51), epithelioid hemangioendothelioma, spindle cell hemangioma, conventional angiosarcoma (low and even high grade), lymphangioma circumscriptum and areas simulating an arteriovenous malformation. The prognosis is likely to be dictated by the component with the highest histologic grade but this should be estimated in larger series of cases with adequate follow-up. Immunohistochemistry displays positive staining for vascular markers including CD31, CD34, and von Willebrand factor.

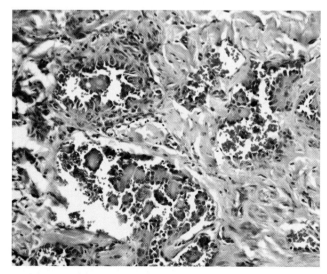

FIGURE 33-50. Papillary intralymphatic angioendothelioma. Bland hobnail endothelial cells and formation of numerous papillary projections with collagenous cores.

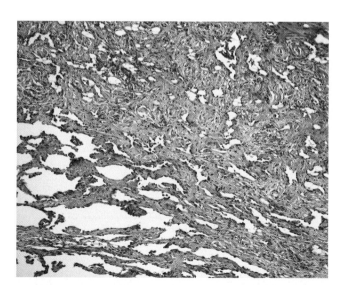

FIGURE 33-51. Composite hemangioendothelioma. Areas of retiform hemangioendothelioma and well-differentiated angiosarcoma. Elsewhere, the tumor contained areas resembling an epitheliod hemangioendothelioma.

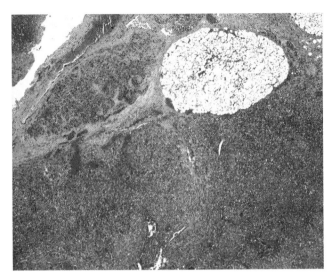

FIGURE 33-52. Kaposiform hemangioendothelioma. Typical lobular and infiltrative growth pattern with replacement of the subcutaneous tissue.

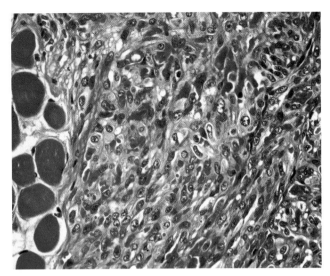

FIGURE 33-54. Kaposiform hemangioendothelioma. Note infiltration of skeletal muscle and frequent microthrombi within the capillaries.

Kaposiform Infantile Hemangioendothelioma

Although this tumor has only been described recently, individual cases of the same condition were reported in the past under different names (187–189,204,205). It is a rare vascular tumor that usually presents in the retroperitoneum or deep soft tissues of infants. A number of cases are associated with Kasabach–Merritt syndrome or lymphangiomatosis (168). It is classified as a low-grade, malignant vascular tumor because of its locally aggressive growth, yet metastases have not been reported. Cutaneous and superficial soft tissue tumors are relatively rare (169). Lesions with a superficial location tend to behave in

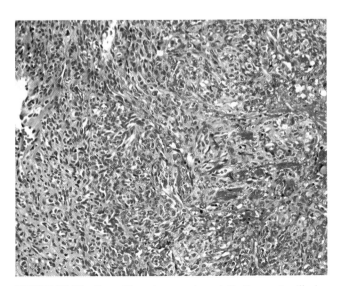

FIGURE 33-53. Kaposiform hemangioendothelioma. Capillaries intermixed with bland spindle-shaped cells.

a benign fashion except when associated with Kasabach–Merritt syndrome.

Histopathology. Low-power examination shows a tumor with a lobular and focally infiltrative growth pattern (Fig. 33-52). Bands of collagen separate tumor lobules. These lobules are composed of a mixture of congested capillaries surrounded by fascicles of bland spindle-shaped endothelial cells and pericytes (Fig. 33-53). Slit-like vascular spaces are often a feature. Focal areas with epithelioid cells containing abundant pale pink cytoplasm are often seen. In many areas, the tumor resembles a capillary hemangioma. Toward the periphery of the tumor lobules, small vascular channels frequently show intraluminal thrombi (Fig. 33-54). Hemosiderin deposition, hemorrhage, and very rare hyaline globules are additional findings. Distinction from Kaposi's sarcoma is discussed on page 000.

MALIGNANT TUMORS

Epithelioid Hemangioendothelioma

This neoplasm was initially described in 1982 as a low-grade tumor of vascular endothelial origin (206). Epithelioid hemangioendothelioma, however, is associated with high morbidity and mortality (see below) and should therefore be regarded as a neoplasm with full malignant potential (207). It mainly arises in the superficial and deep soft tissue and muscle of the extremities (208). The tumor can also arise at internal sites and in the viscera (especially the liver, lungs, and bone). Many of such tumors were described previously by different names (24,206,208). Middle-aged patients, with an equal gender distribution, are mainly affected, but the tumor has a wide age distribution. In about half the cases, the tumor apparently arises from a medium-sized vein or,

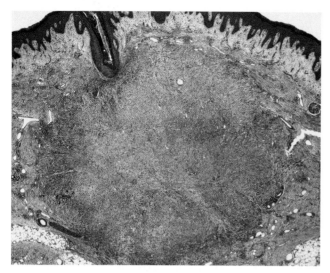

FIGURE 33-55. Epithelioid hemangioendothelioma. Purely cutaneous tumors often present as a fairly circumscribed nodule with hyalinization or myxoid change.

less often, an artery (206,207,209). Multicentricity is common in visceral lesions, particularly those affecting the lungs, liver, and bones. Skin involvement is uncommon and usually associated with an underlying soft tissue or bone lesion or with multicentric disease (208,210,211). Rare cases present with pure cutaneous involvement (212,213). Metastases develop in about 30% of cases involving superficial soft tissues with a mortality rate of 17% (207). The prognosis is worse for internal sites (208).

Histopathology. Typically, epithelioid hemangioendothelioma shows an infiltrative growth pattern. However, purely cutaneous tumors often consist of a fairly circum-

scribed dermal tumor (Fig. 33-55). Tumor cells are ovoid, cuboidal, or short and spindle-shaped with prominent eosinophilic cytoplasm. The nucleus is vesicular showing variable or no atypia, and the nucleolus lacks prominence (Fig. 33-56). Cells tend to be arranged in short fascicles, small nests, or in an "indian-file" pattern, often set in a distinctive hyalinized or mucoid stroma rich in sulphated acid mucopolysaccharides. There is often a chondroid appearance. Obvious vascular channels are generally lacking, but intracytoplasmic vacuoles, sometimes containing erythrocytes, are usually present (Fig. 33-56). Infiltration through large-vessel walls and evidence of endothelial origin may be found. A subset of the tumor with a more aggressive clinical course shows prominent cytologic atypia and a high mitotic rate, overlapping histologically with epithelioid angiosarcoma (207) (Fig. 33-57). Some cases are associated with a prominent osteoclast-like giant cell reaction (214,215). Although lesions with cytologic atypia and mitoses are associated with a poorer prognosis, the behavior of tumors with bland morphology is difficult to predict.

Tumor cells often stain for endothelial markers including CD31, CD34, and FVIII-RA. Positivity for pankeratin can be focally found in up to 20% to 30% of cases (207,216,217). Staining for epithelial membrane antigen is negative.

Cytogenetic analysis in two cases revealed a t(1;3) (p36.3;q25) (218). Analysis of a further case showed a complex translocation 7;22 (219).

Differential Diagnosis. The differential diagnosis includes epithelioid hemangioma (angiolymphoid hyperplasia with eosinophilia), which often has a lobular architecture, prominent inflammation, and numerous well-formed

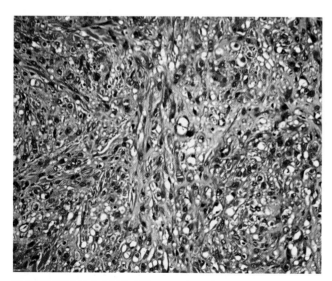

FIGURE 33-56. Epithelioid hemangioendothelioma. Epithelioid cells with variable atypia organized in short strands or individual units. Note formation of intracytoplasmic lumina.

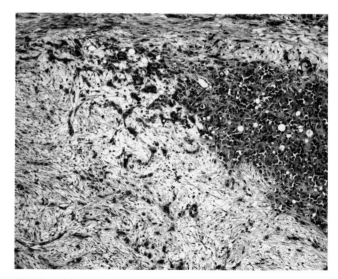

FIGURE 33-57. Epithelioid hemangioendothelioma. Transition between classic epithelioid hemangioendothelioma and solid, more pleomorphic areas with features of an epithelioid angiosarcoma.

blood vessels; metastatic adenocarcinoma, which is negative for endothelial markers and positive for mucin stains; myxoid chondrosarcoma, which has a lobular growth pattern, S-100 positive cells, and absence of intracytoplasmic lumina; and myoepithelioma, which usually lacks intracytoplasmic lumina and has cells that are variably positive for keratin, smooth-muscle actin, epithelial membrane antigen, and S-100.

Angiosarcoma

Most angiosarcomas of the skin arise in the following clinical settings: (a) angiosarcoma of the face and scalp in the elderly; (b) angiosarcoma (lymphangiosarcoma) secondary to chronic lymphoedema; and (c) angiosarcoma as a complication of chronic radiodermatitis or arising from the effects of severe skin trauma or ulceration (220).

Recently an aggressive variant known as epithelioid angiosarcoma (221) has been described, which is difficult to diagnose histologically without the help of immunohistochemistry because of undifferentiated cytomorphology (see below).

Apart from these circumstances, cutaneous angiosarcomas are extremely rare. Exceptional case reports include angiosarcoma arising in preceding benign vascular tumors or hamartomas (222–224), in a large blood vessel (225), in association with a plexiform neurofibroma in neurofibromatosis (226,227), in a schwannoma (228), in a malignant peripheral nerve sheath tumor (229,230), in xeroderma pigmentosum (231), and in vinyl chloride exposure (232). Angiosarcoma in children is exceptional (233,234). With the exception of epithelioid angiosarcoma, the histopathology of angiosarcomas is similar regardless of the clinical setting.

Angiosarcoma of the scalp and face of the elderly. This is almost invariably a fatal tumor that usually arises innocuously as erythematous or bruise-like lesions on the scalp or middle and upper face with a predilection for men (235–238). Subsequent plaques, nodules, or ulcerations develop; metastasis to nodes or internal organs usually arises as a late complication with many patients dying as a result of extensive local disease. This sarcoma has only rarely been reported in black patients; the disease mainly affects whites and sometimes Asians (239). Only a very small percentage of patients, with lesions less than 10 cm in diameter at presentation, can be successfully treated with radical widefield radiotherapy and surgery (235,240). The 5-year survival rate is very low and has been reported to be between 12% and 33%. A recent series combining idiopathic angiosarcoma of the face and scalp and angiosarcomas occurring in internal organs reports a 5-year survival rate of 24% (241).

Angiosarcoma following lymphedema (postmastectomy lymphangiosarcoma or the Stewart–Treves syndrome). Typi-

cally, the tumor presents in women who have had severe long-standing lymphedema of the arm following breast surgery (240,242,243). In most cases, lymphedema is present for about 10 years before the tumor arises, usually in the inner portion of the upper arm. Radiotherapy can usually be excluded as an etiologic factor because the sarcoma nearly always develops beyond the areas of chronic radiodermatitis. Lymphedema-induced angiosarcoma has also been described in men (244) and in a lower extremity (245) from causes other than cancer surgery, including congenital lymphedema (246) and tropical lymphedema due to filaria (247). The prognosis despite radical surgery is extremely poor (242). Exceptionally, a low-grade angiosarcoma with lesions simulating lymphangioma circumscriptum has been described as complicating chronic lymphedema after surgery (248).

Post-irradiation angiosarcoma. There are many reports of angiosarcoma arising in the skin after radiotherapy for internal cancer. The most common sites are the breast or chest wall (249–251) and the lower abdomen (252,253) after therapy for breast or gynecologic cancer. There are also rare reports of previous radiotherapy being a factor in the etiology of angiosarcoma of the head and neck region (235).

Histopathology. Usually the tumor extends well beyond the limits of the apparent clinical lesion (239). As a rule, the tumor shows varied differentiation in different biopsies, even within different fields in a single biopsy (Fig. 33-58). In well-differentiated areas, irregular anastomosing vascular channels lined by a single layer of somewhat enlarged endothelial cells permeate between collagen bundles (Figs. 33-59 and 33-60). Isolation and enclosure of collagen bundles, figuratively referred to as "dissection of collagen" by Rosai et al. (254), is a characteristic feature

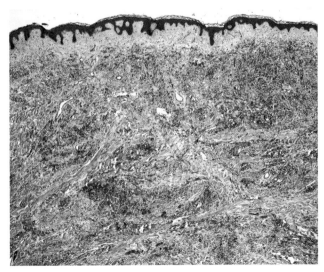

FIGURE 33-58. Well-differentiated angiosarcoma. Low-power view mimicking plaque stage of Kaposi's sarcoma.

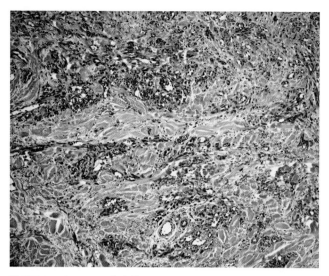

FIGURE 33-59. Well-differentiated angiosarcoma. Irregular and congested vascular channels infiltrating between collagen bundles.

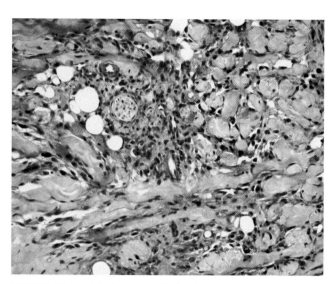

FIGURE 33-61. Moderately differentiated angiosarcoma. More cellular tumor with less-evident vascular differentiation and more cytologic atypia.

(Fig. 33-60). Nuclear atypia is always present and may be slight to moderate, but occasional large hyperchromatic cells may be encountered. At this stage the vascular lumens are generally bloodless, but they may contain free-lying shed malignant cells. Mitotic figures are invariably present and it has been suggested that a high mitotic rate correlate with a poor prognosis (255).

In less well-differentiated areas endothelial cells increase in size and number (Fig. 33-61), forming intraluminal papillary projections where there is enhanced mitotic activity. In poorly differentiated areas, solid sheets of large pleo-

morphic cells with little or no evidence of luminal differentiation can resemble metastatic carcinoma or melanoma (256). Focally, areas showing epithelioid cells are not uncommon. Other areas may simulate a poorly differentiated spindle cell sarcoma (Fig. 33-62). Interstitial hemorrhage and widely dilated blood-filled spaces may sometimes develop. Rare cases are composed of granular cells (257,258).

The histopathology of angiosarcomas secondary to lymphedema and radiotherapy shows a similar range of well-differentiated to poorly differentiated neoplasms as idiopathic angiosarcoma of the face and scalp. There are

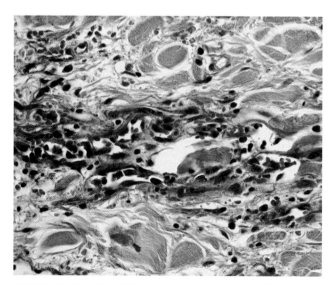

FIGURE 33-60. Well-differentiated angiosarcoma. Dissection of collagen pattern. Marked cytologic atypia and multilayering.

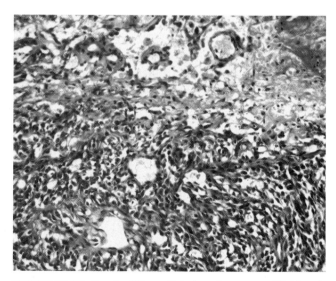

FIGURE 33-62. Poorly differentiated angiosarcoma. Highly cellular tumor composed of pleomorphic spindle-shaped cells and only focal suggestion of vascular differentiation.

no reliable histologic differentiating features, although sometimes evidence of chronic lymphedema or chronic radiation dermatitis may be apparent in the tissue adjacent to the sarcoma.

Histogenesis. It is doubtful whether sarcomas of probable lymphatic origin can be distinguished histologically from those of presumptive vascular endothelial origin; hence there is a tendency to disregard the term lymphangiosarcoma in favor of angiosarcoma. In fact, there is some evidence to suggest that not only angiosarcoma but also Kaposi's sarcoma could be of lymphatic endothelial cell origin.

Von Willebrand factor is the most specific but less sensitive vascular marker, and it is generally negative even in well-differentiated tumors (235). However, patchy, weak, diffuse staining may be found focally in less well-differentiated tumors that require caution in interpretation. CD34 and especially the more specific CD31 are much more reliable as sensitive markers of tumors of endothelial cell origin for use in routine biopsies (166) (Fig. 33-44). On electron microscopic examination, well-differentiated tumors may show the ovoid laminated organelle-like Weibel–Palade bodies characteristic of vascular endothelial cells, but they are absent in most tumors (254). The absence of von-Willebrand labeling and the paucity of Weibel–Palade bodies can be said to favor a lymphatic endothelial origin of this type of angiosarcoma (235).

Cytogenetics studies of soft tissue and cutaneous angiosarcoma are limited to a few case reports. Most analyzed cases have shown complex cytogenetic aberrations (259–261). In a single case of an angiosarcoma arising within a cavernous hemangioma, trisomy 5, and loss of the Y chromosome was the only abnormality demonstrated (262).

Differential Diagnosis. Well-differentiated angiosarcomas, if cell atypia is slight, may closely resemble early macular lesions of Kaposi's sarcoma and benign lymphangioendothelioma because all these conditions can demonstrate to a greater or lesser extent a "dissection of collagen" pattern. The major differences in clinical presentation of the disorders and absence of mitosis and the bland appearances of the endothelial cells in macular lesions of Kaposi's sarcoma and benign lymphangioendothelioma should prevent any difficulties. Focal dissection of collagen pattern is also mimicked in intravascular papillary endothelial hyperplasia by new vessels invading thrombotic material. In poorly differentiated angiosarcomas, it is usually possible to find evidence of channel formation in peripheral areas that allows diagnosis. However, the recent use of endothelial markers, especially CD31, is an important aid in diagnosis. Finally, occasionally adenoid squamous carcinomas or sarcomatoid squamous cell carcinoma, with or without intratumor hemorrhage, can simulate angiosarcoma (263–265). Immunohistochemistry is useful in these cases since only angiosarcomas with epithelioid morphology are positive for cytokeratin (221,266), but these also show staining for CD31 and CD34. Angiosarcomas are consistently negative for HHV-8 (267).

Epithelioid Angiosarcoma

This is a rare form of angiosarcoma that usually arises in deep soft tissues (221), but may also occur in the skin and internal organs, including the thyroid and adrenal gland (266,268). Personal experience indicates that cutaneous lesions are more common than previously thought, and it is likely that such lesions were diagnosed in the past as epithelial or melanocytic neoplasms. There is wide anatomic distribution, and cases present in adults with a slight predilection for males. Rare examples have been associated with radiation therapy (221), an arteriovenous fistula (269), and a foreign body (270). The outlook is extremely poor, although a slow course has been described for some skin tumors (268). However, the later is based on a small number of cases with short follow-up.

Histopathology. Tumors are composed of sheets of pleomorphic large cells with prominent eosinophilic cytoplasm, a large nucleus, and an eosinophilic nucleolus, usually with little evidence of vascular differentiation other than the occasional presence of intracytoplasmic vacuoles sometimes containing red blood cells (Fig. 33-63). This angiosarcoma can easily be mistaken for a carcinoma deposit or even malignant melanoma (Fig. 33-64). Usually the tumor cells demonstrate consistent positivity for von Willebrand factor and CD31. However, cytokeratin positivity is present in up to 50% of cases, and rare cases are focally positive for EMA; this might be a source of confusion with metastatic carcinoma and epithelioid sarcoma, which are negative for endothelial markers.

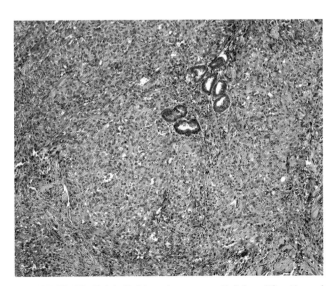

FIGURE 33-63. Epithelioid angiosarcoma. Solid proliferation of atypical epithelioid cells replacing the dermis.

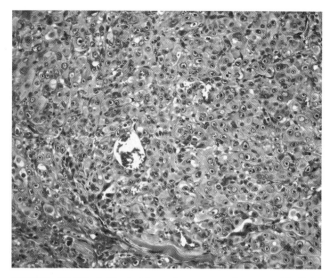

FIGURE 33-64. Epithelioid angiosarcoma. Large epithelioid cells with abundant pink cytoplasm, vesicular nuclei and a single prominent eosinophilic nucleolus. Note the resemblance to melanoma cells and the hemorrhage in the background.

TUMORS OF LYMPHATIC VESSELS

Lymphangiomas constitute only about 4% of all vascular tumors (271) and about 26% of benign vascular tumors in children (98). They can be classified into four types: (a) cavernous lymphangioma, (b) cystic hygroma, (c) lymphangioma circumscriptum (272), and (d) acquired progressive lymphangioma or benign lymphangioendothelioma (273–275). In addition, lesions of lymphangiectasia, which are indistinguishable from classic lymphangioma circumscriptum, may occur, though rarely, in association with congenital or acquired lymphedema (276). Although traditionally cavernous lymphangioma and cystic hygroma have been considered independent entities, it is likely that the latter is an ectatic variant of the former, which arises in areas of loose connective tissue; therefore, they will be discussed under the same heading (277). The existence of capillary lymphangioma is doubtful, and will not be considered further.

Histogenesis. The great majority of tumors of lymphatic vessels are benign, and most of them appear to represent developmental abnormalities rather than true neoplasms. Although in hemangiomas the endothelial cells stain positively for factor VIII–related antigen, the endothelial cells in lymphangiomas are for the most part negative for this marker (278). The presence of fragmented basal lamina and anchoring filaments in hemangiomas is a more reliable ultrastructural feature to use to distinguish lymphatics and blood vessels. However, distinction between angiomas and lymphangiomas is not always clear even when light microscopy is combined with immunohistochemistry and electron microscopy (279).

Cavernous Lymphangioma and Cystic Hygroma

Cavernous lymphangioma usually presents at birth or during the first 2 years of life with an equal gender incidence (280–282). The most common locations are the head and neck area (particularly the oral cavity) and, less often, the extremities. It presents as a large, diffuse, subcutaneous, often fluctuant soft mass. Recurrences are common after limited excision.

Cystic hygroma has a similar age and gender distribution, and lesions tend to affect the neck, axillae, and groin (281). Tumors tend to be better circumscribed than cavernous lymphangiomas, but there is also a tendency for local recurrence unless a wide excision is performed. Cystic hygroma of the neck is commonly associated with Turner's syndrome (281,283).

Histopathology. Cavernous lymphangioma shows large, irregularly shaped spaces in the dermis and subcutaneous tissue lined by a single layer of bland endothelial cells (Fig. 33-65). The surrounding stroma can be loose or fibrotic and shows a lymphocytic inflammatory cell infiltrate with scattered lymphoid follicles. An incomplete layer of smooth muscle can be seen in the walls of some vessels. The vascular lumina show pink proteinaceous fluid with lymphocytes, but erythrocytes can also be seen. Large cavernous lymphangiomas, particularly in areas of the lip or tongue, may extend between the muscle bundles, separating them from one another (272).

In cystic hygroma, microscopic features are similar to those of cavernous lymphangioma except for the pres-

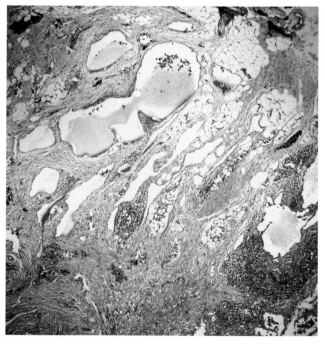

FIGURE 33-65. Cavernous lymphangioma. Dilated lymphatic channels and aggregates of lymphocytes in the stroma.

ence of numerous cystically dilated thin-walled lymphatic spaces.

Differential Diagnosis. Distinction from cavernous hemangioma can be impossible since the vascular channels in both conditions can show red blood cells in their lumina. The presence of lymphoid aggregates in the stroma tends to favor the diagnosis of lymphangioma.

Lymphangioma Circumscriptum

Lymphangioma circumscriptum is predominantly a developmental malformation of infancy with an equal gender incidence, but it may arise at any age (272,284). Similar acquired lesions arising in adults in relation to chronic lymphedema or radiotherapy are best regarded as *lymphangiectasia* (276). The anatomic distribution is wide, but the proximal portions of the limbs and limb girdle are most frequently affected. Association with cavernous lymphangioma, cystic hygroma, and even lymphangiomatosis is common. A typical lesion consists of collections of numerous vesicles containing clear fluid and less commonly, blood. Due to the presence of a deep component (see below), lesions arising in infancy tend to recur after simple excision.

Histopathology. Lymphangioma circumscriptum is composed of numerous dilated lymphatics in the superficial and papillary dermis (Fig. 33-66). There is clear fluid and, less frequently, red blood cells in their lumina. In the overlying epidermis there is some degree of acanthosis and hyperkeratosis. The surrounding stroma shows scattered lymphocytes. Lesions developing in infancy often show a large-caliber, muscular lymphatic space in the subcutaneous tissue, which has to be ligated at the time of excision to avoid recurrence (Fig. 33-67).

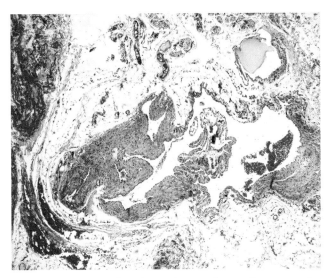

FIGURE 33-67. Lymphangioma circumscriptum. Deep muscular lymphatic. If this vessel is not ligated, the lesion will recur.

Progressive Lymphangioma (Benign Lymphangioendothelioma)

Progressive lymphangioma (benign lymphangioendothelioma) is a benign rare tumor that has a tendency to present in middle-aged to elderly adults and to evolve slowly over years. Males and females are equally affected, and although the anatomic distribution is wide, there is preferential involvement of the limbs (273–275,285). Clinically, a typical lesion is a solitary well-circumscribed erythematous macule or plaque. Recurrence after simple excision is exceptional, and occasional lesions can show focal or complete spontaneous regression (286).

Histopathology. Most lesions predominantly involve the superficial dermis but extension into the dermis and subcutis can be present (273,275). Irregular, horizontal, thin-walled vascular channels lined by a single layer of bland endothelial cells are seen dissecting collagen bundles (273,285) (Fig. 33-68). Endothelial cell atypia and mitotic figures are absent. The vascular channels appear empty or have scanty proteinaceous material and/or a few red blood cells.

Differential Diagnosis. The main differential diagnosis is with well-differentiated angiosarcoma and patch-stage Kaposi's sarcoma. Although sharing with angiosarcoma the presence of extensive dissection of collagen bundles, the latter conditions occur in completely different settings and in angiosarcoma there is usually, at least focally, cytologic atypia and mitotic figures. Patch-stage Kaposi's sarcoma often presents clinically with multiple lesions, and histologically the abnormal blood vessels tend to cluster around normal preexisting blood vessels. There is hemosiderin deposition with an inflammatory cell infiltrate with lymphocytes and plasma cells.

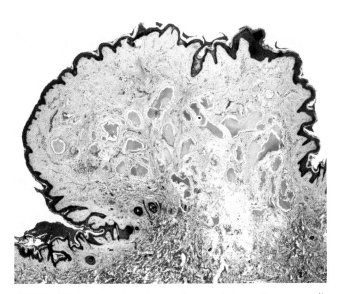

FIGURE 33-66. Lymphangioma circumscriptum. Numerous dilated lymphatic channels expand the papillary dermis.

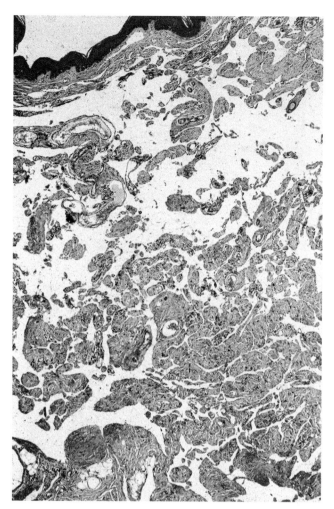

FIGURE 33-68. Progressive lymphangioma. Extensive dissection of collagen bundles by irregular vascular channels lined by bland flat endothelial cells.

Lymphangiomatosis

Lymphangiomatosis is a rare developmental abnormality that affects children with an equal gender incidence. Although most cases appear to be congenital the disease is often not diagnosed until childhood. The majority of cases involve soft tissues, skin, bone, and parenchymal organs. When vital organs are affected, the prognosis is very poor (287,288). Cases with involvement limited to skin and soft tissues of a limb (with or without bone involvement) have been described and are associated with a better prognosis (288). Rare cases can present in association with kaposiform hemangioendothelioma of infancy and childhood (168). Lymphangiomatosis is the lymphatic counterpart of angiomatosis. In some instances distinction between them can be difficult, although lymphangiographic studies can be very helpful in establishing the difference.

Histopathology. The appearance of lymphangiomatosis is very similar to that of progressive lymphangioma, but the changes in lymphangiomatosis are more extensive and diffuse with involvement of deeper soft tissues, fibrosis in long-standing cases, and stromal hemosiderin deposition.

Atypical Vascular Proliferation after Radiotherapy

These lesions usually develop a few months or years after radiotherapy for breast cancer (289–291). The clinical presentation is not distinctive and varies from skin-colored to red macules and papules. Occasional cases may mimic lymphangioma circumscriptum. The behavior appears to be entirely benign. A number of vascular lesions arising in the setting of radiotherapy have a completely innocent histologic appearance (291). The lesions described herein are those with atypical histologic features that may raise the possibility of malignancy.

Histopathology. Irregular lymphatic-like vascular channels lined by a single layer of endothelial cells are present focally in the superficial and/or deep dermis. An infiltrative growth pattern is lacking and lesions are usually fairly circumscribed (Fig. 33-69). The cells lining the channels often have a hobnail appearance and papillary projections may occasionally be seen. There is no cytologic atypia, multilayering, or mitotic figures (Fig. 33-70).

Differential Diagnosis. The differential diagnosis includes a well-differentiated angiosarcoma, hobnail hemangioma and Kaposi's sarcoma. As opposed to hobnail hemangioma, the lesion is not symmetrical, and the vascular channels do not have a predominant superficial dermal location. The clinical setting, the absence of inflammation and the presence of hobnail endothelial cells with focal papillary projections

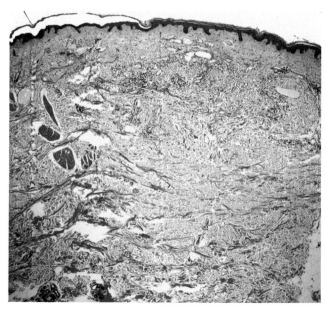

FIGURE 33-69. Atypical vascular proliferation after radiotherapy. Fairly localized superficial dermal vascular proliferation.

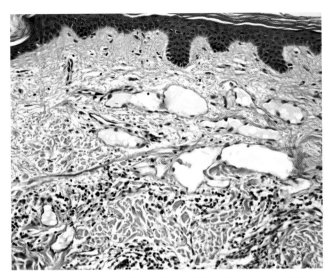

FIGURE 33-70. Atypical vascular proliferation after radiotherapy. Irregular vascular channels lined by slightly hyperchromatic endothelial cells, some of which have a hobnail appearance.

should allow distinction from Kaposi's sarcoma. Careful examination of multiple sections is recommended to make sure that there are no mitotic figures and cytologic atypia to distinguish it from a well-differentiated angiosarcoma. This distinction can be very difficult, especially in small biopsies.

TUMORS OF PERIVASCULAR CELLS

Glomus Tumor

Glomus tumors are relatively rare lesions that usually present in young adults between the third and fourth decade of life with no gender predilection except for subungual tumors that have a marked female predilection (292). The hand (particularly subungual region and palm) is the most commonly affected site, followed by the foot and forearm. Lesions, however, can occur with a wide anatomic distribution not only the skin, but also, rarely, in mucosae and internal organs. The later include the stomach (293), lung (294), trachea (295), bone (296), small bowel (297), pterygoid fossa (298), and mediastinum (299). Most tumors classically present as solitary, small (<1 cm), blue-red nodules that are characteristically associated with paroxysmal pain often elicited by changes in temperature (especially cold) or pressure. Subungual glomus tumors have been associated with neurofibromatosis type I (300–302).

A very small proportion of glomus tumors are multiple (in up to 10% of patients). As opposed to solitary glomus tumors, the latter usually arise in children, tend to be asymptomatic, are rarely subungual, and are thought to be inherited in an autosomal dominant fashion (303). The gene for multiple inherited glomus tumors has been linked to chromosome 1p21-22 (304,305). Clinically, multiple glomus tumors can

be confused with those of the blue rubber bleb nevus syndrome, and it is likely that cases of this condition reported in the past represented examples of multiple glomangiomas or glomangiomyomas. Histologically, multiple glomus tumors are predominantly glomangiomas (see below).

The glomus coccygeum is a prominent glomus body measuring up to several millimeters and located near the tip of the coccyx. Awareness of its existence is important because when found incidentally in biopsies, it may be confused with a neoplasm (306).

Local recurrence is very uncommon, and when seen, is usually in deep-seated tumors with an infiltrative growth pattern (so-called infiltrating glomus tumor) (307) (see below). Exceptionally, glomus tumors originate within a blood vessel (308,309) or nerve (310). Malignant glomus tumor or glomangiosarcoma is very rare and usually arises in deep soft tissues. It comprises around 1% of all glomus tumors (311). Glomangiosarcoma appears to be an aggressive tumor with a rate of metastasis of 40% (311).

Histopathology. Glomus tumors show varying proportions of glomus cells, blood vessels, and smooth muscle and are classified accordingly into *solid glomus tumor* (25% of cases), *glomangioma* (60% of cases), and *glomangiomyoma* (15% of cases). Most cases of glomus tumor are well circumscribed, and a classic solid lesion (Fig. 33-71) is composed of sheets of uniform cells with pale or eosinophilic cytoplasm, well-defined cell margins (highlighted distinctively by a PAS stain), and round or ovoid punched-out central nuclei (Fig. 33-72). Small blood vessels are uniformly distributed in the tumor but may not be apparent without the use of special stains. The stroma is often edematous, and extensive myxoid change may be present. Normal mitotic figures may be conspicuous in some cases, but cytologic atypia is

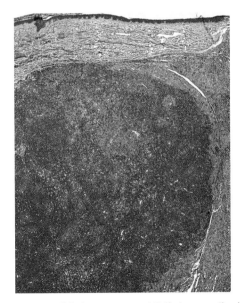

FIGURE 33-71. Solid glomus tumor. Well-circumscribed dermal nodule with only tiny vascular channels in the background.

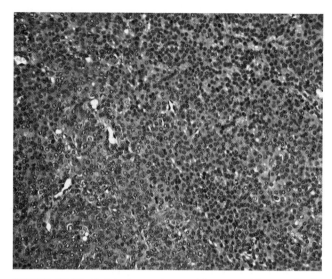

FIGURE 33-72. Solid glomus tumor. Monomorphic round cells with eosinophilic cytoplasm and central punched-out nuclei.

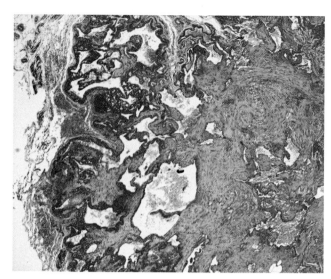

FIGURE 33-74. Glomangiomyoma. Spindle-shaped cells with pink cytoplasm combined with glomus cells.

usually absent. Numerous stromal nerve fibers may be highlighted with special stains. Exceptional cases show extensive oncocytic change (312). Tumor cells with epithelioid morphology have also been described (313). In glomangioma, there are numerous dilated, cavernous-like, thin-walled vascular spaces surrounded by one or a few layers of glomus cells (Fig. 33-73). In glomangiomyoma, there is an important number of spindle-shaped smooth-muscle cells, which tend to be distributed near the vascular spaces and blend with the adjacent collections of glomus cells (Fig. 33-74).

Infiltrating glomus tumor is a very rare variant that occurs in deep soft tissues and is characterized by solid nests of glomus cells with an infiltrative growth pattern (307). It is associated with a high recurrence rate.

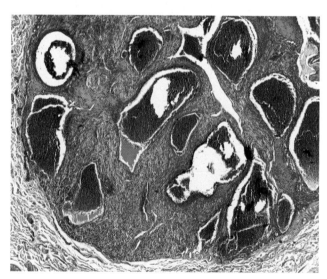

FIGURE 33-73. Glomangioma. Cavernous vascular spaces surrounded by layers of glomus cells.

The histologic diagnosis of glomangiosarcoma is difficult because of the sparsity of cases reported in the literature (307,314). Only recently, criteria for the histologic diagnosis of glomangiosarcoma have been delineated and include the following (311): (a) size greater than 2 cm and subfascial or visceral location, (b) atypical mitotic figures, or (c) marked nuclear atypia and any level of mitotic activity. A preexistent benign component is common but not invariably present. Tumors arising de novo have architectural features resembling a glomus but consist of cells with prominent atypia. In such cases, the diagnosis should be confirmed by positive immunohistochemical stain for smooth muscle actin and for collagen type IV (in a pericellular distribution) (311). Tumors with focal cytologic atypia but no evidence of other features suggestive of malignancy are classified as symplastic glomus tumors.

Histogenesis. Glomus tumors closely resemble the modified smooth muscle cells of a segment of a specialized arteriovenous anastomoses (Sucquet–Hoyer canal) that is involved in the regulation of temperature, the *glomus body*. Glomus bodies are usually found in acral skin, particularly on the hands. However, many glomus tumors arise from sites where glomus bodies are not known to exist. In view of this it is likely that some glomus tumors arise from differentiation of pluripotential mesenchymal cells or ordinary smooth-muscle cells. On immunohistochemical examination, glomus tumor cells stain for smooth-muscle actin, H-caldesmon, muscle-specific actin, and myosin (315,316). Staining for collagen type IV shows prominent pericellular positivity. Staining for desmin is only occasionally focally positive.

Differential Diagnosis. Solid glomus tumor can be distinguished from eccrine spiradenoma by the presence in the latter of two populations of cells, focal ductal differentiation, and positivity for epithelial markers. Occasionally intradermal nevus with pseudovascular spaces resembles a glomus tumor, but in the former there is always evidence of nesting, maturation, and positivity of lesional cells for S-100 (317).

Multiple glomus tumors differ from lesions of the blue rubber bleb nevus by the presence of glomus cells in nearly all tumors. It is likely that some if not all previously reported cases of blue rubber bleb nevus actually represented examples of multiple glomangiomas.

Myopericytoma

Traditionally, tumors thought to differentiate toward perivascular myoid cells or pericytes have been divided into two main categories: infantile hemangiopericytoma and adult hemangiopericytoma (318,319). Both variants, however, appear to have very little in common except for the histologic presence of a pericytomatous vascular pattern. Moreover, with the combination of immunohistochemistry and electron microscopy, most tumors classified as adult hemangiopericytoma on light microscopy show other lines of differentiation (320). These include synovial sarcoma, mesenchymal chondrosarcoma, solitary fibrous tumor, and deep benign fibrous histiocytoma. The few cases for which the line of differentiation remains obscure are the "true" adult hemangiopericytomas, but it is likely that they arise from an undifferentiated mesenchymal cell. These rare examples of "true" adult hemangiopericytomas do not usually occur in the skin and will not be discussed further in this chapter.

In recent years the concept of myopericytoma has been introduced to describe a spectrum of tumors composed of short oval to spindle-shaped cells with a myoid appearance and a distinctive concentric perivascular growth (321). These tumors tend to occur mainly in the deep dermis and subcutaneous tissue and include lesions classified in the past as glomangiopericytoma, myopericytoma, myofibroma, and myofibromatosis in adults. Infantile hemangiopericytoma and infantile myofibromatosis also represent part of the spectrum of tumors with true pericytic differentiation.

Infantile hemangiopericytoma usually presents at birth or in the first years of life as single or multiple dermal or subcutaneous nodules. Local recurrence is common, and distant spread has been described, but it is likely that spread represents multicentricity rather than true metastasis. Clinical and histologic features are almost identical to those of infantile myofibromatosis (see Chapter 33), and it has been proposed that both entities represent different maturation stages of the same condition (322,323).

Myopericytoma most commonly occurs in middle-aged adults with a predilection for the limbs especially, the distal lower limb. Lesions are small (<2 cm in diameter), long-standing, and usually asymptomatic, and may be single or less frequently, multiple. Rarely tumors are painful. In the setting of multiple myopericytomas, these often

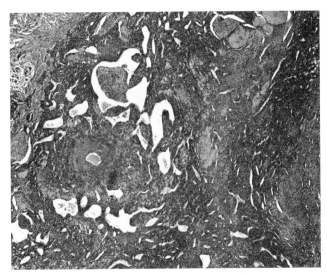

FIGURE 33-75. Infantile hemangiopericytoma. Biphasic tumor with numerous branching blood vessels.

develop simultaneously with a predilection for a single anatomic site. Recurrence is rare and frequently represents either persistence or the development of a new tumor. Very rare malignant examples of myopericytoma have been described (324).

Histopathology. Infantile hemangiopericytomas are multinodular and, show at least focally a biphasic growth pattern (Fig. 33-75). Hemangiopericytomatous areas composed of small, round hyperchromatic cells blend with areas composed of bundles and nodules of more mature spindle-shaped cells with eosinophilic cytoplasm resembling myofibroblasts (Fig. 33-76). This zoning phenomenon is identical to, although less pronounced than, that

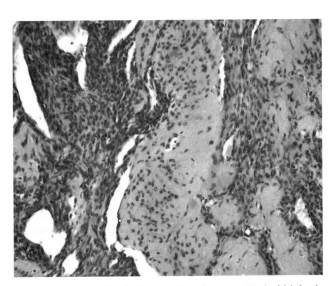

FIGURE 33-76. Infantile hemangiopericytoma. Typical biphasic pattern showing immature round cells with scanty cytoplasm (*left*) alternating with bundles of spindle cells with a myofibroblastic appearance (*right*).

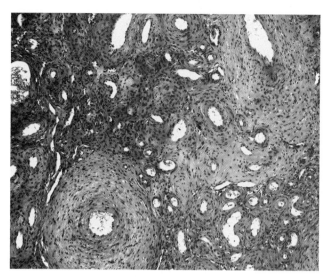

FIGURE 33-77. Myopericytoma. Biphasic pattern and prominent whirling of tumor cells around blood vessels.

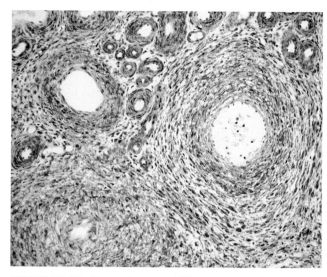

FIGURE 33-79. Myopericytoma. Diffuse staining of tumor cells with alpha-smooth muscle actin by the ABC method.

seen in infantile myofibromatosis (see Chapter 33). Mitosis, necrosis, and vascular invasion are common features.

In infantile hemangiopericytoma the darker, less mature cells in the pericytomatous areas usually do not stain for any markers whereas the more mature spindle-shaped cells resembling myofibroblasts stain for alpha-smooth muscle actin. Identical features are seen in infantile myofibromatosis, and it is believed that the two entities are part of the same spectrum (322,323).

The histologic spectrum of myopericytoma is very wide and varies from lesions that are very similar to myofibromatosis to tumors that closely resemble glomus tumors and even an angioleiomyoma. Tumors are well circumscribed and composed of a mixture of solid cellular areas intermixed

with variable numbers of vascular channels (Fig. 33-77). The later are often elongated and display prominent branching resulting in a stag-horn appearance (hemangiopericytoma-like). The cells in the solid areas are round or short and spindle-shaped with eosinophilic or amphophilic cytoplasm and vesicular nuclei. Cytologic atypia is not usually a feature and mitotic figures are very rare. A common and striking feature is the presence of concentric layers of tumor cells around vascular channels resulting in a typical onion ring appearance (Fig. 33-78). Myxoid change may be focally prominent. Occasional findings include hyalinization, cystic degeneration, and bone formation. Nodules of tumor cells may protrude into the lumina of vascular channels. Rare examples are entirely intravascular (324). In some cases, tumor cells closely resemble glomus cells and are characterized by round punched-out central nuclei and pale eosinophilic cytoplasm. These cases are referred to as glomangiopericytomas.

Glomangiopericytoma cells stain diffusely for smooth-muscle actin (Fig. 33-79) and are only very rarely, focally positive for desmin. Focal staining for CD34 may also be seen.

Differential Diagnosis. Some authors regard angioleiomyoma as part of the spectrum of myopericytoma. Angioleiomyoma however, is composed of uniform smooth-muscle cells, which stain diffusely for both smooth-muscle actin and desmin. Furthermore, concentric arrangement of tumor cells around vascular channels is not present.

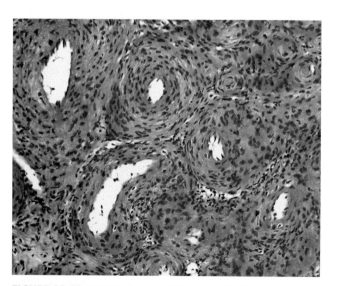

FIGURE 33-78. Myopericytoma. Bland spindle-shaped pericytes arranged in a concentric manner.

REFERENCES

1. Clearkin KP, Enzinger FM. Intravascular papillary endothelial hyperplasia. *Arch Pathol Lab Med* 1976;100:441.

2. Hashimoto H, Daimaru Y, Enjoji M. Intravascular papillary endothelial hyperplasia. A clinicopathologic study of 91 cases. *Am J Dermatopathol* 1983;5:539.

3. Pins MR, Rosenthal DI, Springfield DS, et al. Florid extravascular papillary endothelial hyperplasia (Masson's pseudosarcoma) presenting as a soft tissue sarcoma. *Arch Pathol Lab Med* 1993; 117:259.

4. Reed CN, Cooper PH, Swerlick RA. Intravascular papillary endothelial hyperplasia: multiple lesions simulating Kaposi's sarcoma. *J Am Acad Dermatol* 1984;10:110.

5. Miyamoto H, Nagatami T, Mohri S, et al. Intravascular papillary endothelial hyperplasia. *Clin Exp Dermatol* 1988;13:411.

6. Albretch S, Khan HJ. Immunohistochemistry of intravascular papillary endothelial hyperplasia. *J Cutan Pathol* 1990;17:16.

7. LeBoit PE, Solomon AR, Santa Cruz DJ, et al. Angiomatosis with luminal cryoprotein deposition. *J Am Acad Dermatol* 1992; 27:969.

8. Ortonne N, Vignon-Pennamen MD, Majdalani G, et al. Reactive angioendotheliomatosis secondary to dermal amyloid angiopathy. *Am J Dermatopathol* 2001;23:315.

9. Creamer D, Black MM, Calonje E. Reactive angioendotheliomatosis in association with the antiphospholipid syndrome. *J Am Acad Dermatol* 2000;45:903.

10. McMenamin ME, Fletcher CD. Reactive angioendotheliomatosis: a study of 15 cases demonstrating a wide clinicopathologic spectrum. *Am J Surg Pathol* 2002;26:685.

11. Wick MR, Rocamora A. Reactive and malignant "angioendotheliomatosis": a discriminant clinicopathological study. *J Cutan Pathol* 1988;15:260.

12. Krell JM, Sánchez RL, Solomon AR. Diffuse dermal angiomatosis: a variant of reactive cutaneous angioendotheliomatosis. *J Cutan Pathol* 1994;21:363.

13. Kim S, Elenitsas R, James WD. Diffuse dermal angiomatosis: a variant of reactive angioendotheliomatosis associated with peripheral vascular atherosclerosis. *Arch Dermatol* 2002;138:456.

14. Kimyai-Asadi A, Nousari HC, Ketabchi N, et al. Diffuse dermal angiomatosis: a variant of reactive angioendotheliomatosis associated with atherosclerosis. *J Am Acad Dermatol* 1999;40: 257.

15. Requena L, Farina MC, Renedo G, et al. Intravascular and diffuse dermal reactive angioendotheliomatosis secondary to iatrogenic arteriovenous fistulas. *J Cutan Pathol* 1999;26:159–164.

16. Rieger E, Soyer HP, LeBoit PE, et al. Reactive angioendotheliomatosis or intravascular histiocytosis? An immunohistochemical and ultrastructural study in two cases of intravascular histiocytic cell proliferation. *Br J Dermatol* 1999;140:497–504.

17. Chan JKC, Fletcher CDM, Hicklin GA, et al. Glomeruloid hemangioma: a distinctive cutaneous lesion of multicentric Castleman's disease associated with POEMS syndrome. *Am J Surg Pathol* 1990;14:1036.

18. Rongioletti F, Gambini C, Lerza R. Glomeruloid hemangioma: a cutaneous marker of POEMS syndrome. *Am J Dermatopathol* 1994;16:175.

19. Scheers C, Kolivras A, Corbisier A, et al. POEMS syndrome revealed by multiple glomeruloid angiomas. *Dermatology* 2002; 204:311–314.

20. Tsai CY, Lai CH, Chan HL, et al. Glomeruloid hemangioma—a specific cutaneous marker of POEMS syndrome. *Int J Dermatol* 2001;40:403–406.

21. Allen PW, Ramakrishna B, MacCormac LB. The histiocytoid hemangiomas and other controversies. *Pathol Ann* 1992;27:51.

22. Rosai J. Angiolymphoid hyperplasia with eosinophilia of the skin: its nosological position in the spectrum of histiocytoid hemangioma. *Am J Dermatopathol* 1982;4:175.

23. Rosai J, Gold J, Landy R. The histiocytoid hemangiomas: a unifying concept embracing several previously described entities of

skin, soft tissue, large vessels, bone and heart. *Hum Pathol* 1979; 10:707.

24. Tsang WYW, Chan JKC. The family of epithelioid vascular tumors. *Histol Histopathol* 1993;8:187.

25. Fetsch JF, Weiss SW. Observations concerning the pathogenesis of epithelioid hemangioma (angiolymphoid hyperplasia). *Mod Pathol* 1991;4:449.

26. Olsen TG, Helwig EB. Angiolymphoid hyperplasia with eosinophilia: a clinicopathologic study of 116 patients. *J Am Acad Dermatol* 1985;12:781.

27. Mehregan AH, Shapiro L. Angiolymphoid hyperplasia with eosinophilia. *Arch Dermatol* 1971;103:50.

28. Castro C, Winkelmann RK. Angiolymphoid hyperplasia with eosinophilia in the skin. *Cancer* 1974;34:1696.

29. Reed RJ, Terazakis N. Subcutaneous angiolymphoid hyperplasia with eosinophilia (Kimura's disease). *Cancer* 1972;29:489.

30. Eady RAJ, Wilson-Jones E. Pseudopyogenic granuloma: enzyme, histochemical and ultrastructural study. *Hum Pathol* 1977;8:653.

31. DelGaudio JM, Myers MW, Telian SA. Angiolymphoid hyperplasia with eosinophilia involving the external auditory canal. *Otolaryngol Head Neck Surg* 1994;111:669.

32. Chan JKC, Hui PK, Ng CS, et al. Epithelioid hemangioma (angiolymphoid hyperplasia with eosinophilia) and Kimura's disease in Chinese. *Histopathology* 1989;15:557.

33. Kuo TT, Shih LY, Chan HL. Kimura's disease: involvement of regional lymph nodes and distinction from angiolymphoid hyperplasia with eosinophilia. *Am J Surg Pathol* 1988;12:843.

34. Moesner J, Pallesen R, Sorensen B. Angiolymphoid hyperplasia with eosinophilia (Kimura's disease): a case with dermal lesions in the knee region and a popliteal arteriovenous fistula. *Arch Dermatol* 1981;117:650.

35. Morton K, Robertson SAJ, Hadden W. Angiolymphoid hyperplasia with eosinophilia: report of a case arising from the radial artery. *Histopathology* 1987;11:963.

36. Bartralot R, Garcia Patos V, Hueto J, et al. Angiolymphoid hyperplasia with eosinophils affecting the oral mucosa. *Br J Dermatol* 1996;134:744.

37. Razquin S, Mayayo E, Citores MA, et al. Angiolymphoid hyperplasia with eosinophilia of the tongue: report of a case and review of the literature. *Hum Pathol* 1991;22:837.

38. Suster S. Nodal angiolymphoid hyperplasia with eosinophilia. *Am J Clin Pathol* 1987;88:236–239.

39. O'Connell JX, Kattapuram SV, Mankin HJ, et al. Epithelioid hemangioma of bone. A tumor often mistaken for low-grade angiosarcoma or malignant hemangioendothelioma. *Am J Surg Pathol* 1993;17:610.

40. Banks ER, Mills SE. Histiocytoid (epithelioid) hemangioma of the testis. The so-called vascular variant of "adenomatoid tumor." *Am J Surg Pathol* 1990;14:584.

41. Madison JF, Cooper PH. A histiocytoid (epithelioid) vascular tumor of the ovary: occurrence within a benign cystic teratoma. *Mod Pathol* 1989;2:55.

42. Rosai J, Ackerman LR. Intravenous atypical vascular proliferation. A cutaneous lesion simulating a malignant blood vessel tumor. *Arch Dermatol* 1974;109:714.

43. Wolff HH, Kinney J, Ackerman AB. Angiolymphoid hyperplasia with follicular mucinosis. *Arch Dermatol* 1978;114:229.

44. Fawcett HA, Smith NP. Injection site granuloma due to aluminium. *Arch Dermatol* 1984;120:1318.

45. Hallam LA, Mackinlay GA, Wright AMA. Angiolymphoid hyperplasia with eosinophilia: Possible aetiological role for immunisation. *J Clin Pathol* 1989;42:944.

46. Miliauskas JR, Mukherjee T, Dixon B. Postimmunization (vaccination) injection-site reactions: a report of four cases and review of the literature. *Am J Surg Pathol* 1993;17:516.

47. Googe PB, Harris NL, Mihm MC Jr. Kimura's disease and angiolymphoid hyperplasia with eosinophilia: two distinct histopathological entities. *J Cutan Pathol* 1987;14:263.

48. Kung IT, Gibson JB, Bannatyne PM. Kimura's disease: a clinicopathological study of 21 cases and its distinction from angiolymphoid hyperplasia with eosinophilia. *Pathology* 1984;16:39.

49. Urabe A, Tsuneyoshi M, Enjoji M. Epithelioid hemangioma versus Kimura's disease: a comparative clinicopathologic study. *Am J Surg Pathol* 1987;10:758.

50. Kawada A. Morbus Kimura: Darstellung der erkrankung und ihre differential diagnose. *Hautarzt* 1976;27:309.

51. Yamada A, Mitsuhashi K, Miyakawa Y. Membranous glomerulonephritis associated with eosinophilic lymphfolliculosis of the skin (Kimura's disease): report of a case and review of the literature. *Clin Nephrol* 1982;18:211.

52. Mills SE, Cooper PH, Fechner RE. Lobular capillary hemangioma: the underlying lesion of pyogenic granuloma. A study of 73 cases from the oral and nasal mucous membranes. *Am J Surg Pathol* 1980;4:471.

53. Patrice SJ, Wiss K, Mulliken JB. Pyogenic granuloma (lobular capillary hemangioma): a clinicopathologic study of 178 cases. *Pediatr Dermatol* 1994;8:267.

54. Bhaskar SM, Jacoway JR. Pyogenic granuloma. Clinical features, incidence, histology and result of treatment: report of 242 cases. *J Oral Surg* 1961;24:391.

55. Blickenstaff RD, Roeningk RK, Peters MS, et al. Recurrent pyogenic granuloma with satellitosis. *J Am Acad Dermatol* 1989;21:1241.

56. Vicente MA, Estrach T, Zamora E, et al. Granuloma piogenico recidivante con lesiones satelites multiples: presentacion de dos casos. *Med Cutan Ibero Lat Am* 1990;18:331.

57. Cooper PH, Mills SE. Subcutaneous granuloma pyogenicum: lobular capillary hemangioma. *Arch Dermatol* 1982;118:30.

58. Saad RW, Sau P, Mulvaney MP, et al. Intravenous pyogenic granuloma. *Int J Dermatol* 1993;32:130.

59. Cooper PH, McAllister HA, Helwig EB. Intravenous pyogenic granuloma. A study of 18 cases. *Am J Surg Pathol* 1979;3:221.

60. Wilson BB, Greer KE, Cooper PH. Eruptive disseminated lobular capillary hemangioma (pyogenic granuloma). *J Am Acad Dermatol* 1989;21:391.

61. Nappi O, Wick MR. Disseminated lobular capillary hemangioma (pyogenic granuloma). *Am J Dermatopathol* 1986;8:379.

62. Torres JE, Sanchez JL. Disseminated pyogenic granuloma after an exfoliative dermatitis. *J Am Acad Dermatol* 1995;32:280.

63. Wilson BB, Greer KE, Cooper PH. Eruptive disseminated lobular capillary hemangioma (pyogenic granuloma). *J Am Acad Dermatol* 1989;21:391.

64. Renshaw AA, Rosai J. Benign atypical vascular lesions of the lip. A study of 12 cases. *Am J Surg Pathol* 1993;17:557.

65. Marsch WC. The ultrastructure of eruptive hemangioma ("pyogenic granuloma"). *J Cutan Pathol* 1981;8:144(abst).

66. Nichols GE, Gaffey MJ, Mills SE, et al. Lobular capillary hemangioma: an immunohistochemical study including steroid hormone status. *Am J Clin Pathol* 1992;97:770.

67. Cockerell CJ. Bacillary angiomatosis and related diseases caused by *Rochalimaea*. *J Am Acad Dermatol* 1995;32:783.

68. LeBoit PE, Berger TG, Egbert BM, et al. Bacillary angiomatosis. The histopathology and differential diagnosis of a pseudoneoplastic infection in patients with human immunodeficiency virus disease. *Am J Surg Pathol* 1989;13:909.

69. Exner JH, Dahod S, Pochi PE. Pyogenic granuloma-like acne lesions during isotretinoin therapy. *Arch Dermatol* 1983;119:808.

70. Valentic JP, Barr RJ, Weinstein GD. Inflammatory neovascular nodules associated with oral isotretinoin treatment of severe acne. *Arch Dermatol* 1983;119:871.

71. Leung AKC, Telmesani AMA. Salmon patches in Caucasian children. *Pediatr Dermatol* 1989;6:185.

72. Esterly NB. Cutaneous hemangiomas, vascular stains and malformations, and associated syndromes. *Curr Probl Dermatol* 1995;7:67.

73. Finley JL, Noe JM, Arndt KA, et al. Port-wine stains: morphologic variations and developmental lesions. *Arch Dermatol* 1984;120:1453.

74. Finley JL, Clark RAF, Colvin RB, et al. Immunofluorescent staining with antibodies to factor VIII, fibronectin, and collagenous basement membrane in normal human skin and port wine stains. *Arch Dermatol* 1982;118:971.

75. Smoller BP, Rosen S. Port-wine stains: a decrease of altered neural modulation of blood vessels? *Arch Dermatol* 1986;122:177.

76. Imperial R, Helwig EB. Angiokeratoma. *Arch Dermatol* 1967;95:166.

77. Epinette WW, Norins AL, Drew AL, et al. Angiokeratoma corporis diffusum with a L-fucosidase deficiency. *Arch Dermatol* 1973;107:754.

78. Ishibashi A, Tsuboi R, Shinmei M. B-galactosidase and neuraminidase deficiency associated with angiokeratoma corporis diffusum. *Arch Dermatol* 1984;120:1344.

79. Holmes RC, Fensom AH, McKee P, et al. Angiokeratoma corporis diffusum in a patient with normal enzyme activities. *J Am Acad Dermatol* 1984;10:384.

80. Hayes KR, Rebello DJA. Angiokeratoma of Mibelli. *Acta Derm Venereol (Stockh)* 1961;41:56.

81. Imperial R, Helwig EB. Angiokeratoma of the vulva. *Obstet Gynecol* 1967;29:307.

82. Agger P, Osmundsen PE. Angiokeratoma of the scrotum (Fordyce). *Acta Derm Venereol (Stockh)* 1970;50:221.

83. Tarnowski WM, Hashimoto K. New light microscopic findings in Fabry's disease. *Acta Derm Venereol (Stockh)* 1969;49:386.

84. McGrae JD Jr, Winkelmann RK. Generalized essential telangiectasia. *JAMA* 1963;185:909.

85. Wilken JK. Unilateral dermatomal superficial telangiectasia. *Arch Dermatol* 1984;120:579.

86. Anderson RL, Smith JG Jr. Unilateral nevoid telangiectasia with gastric involvement. *Arch Dermatol* 1975;111:617.

87. Uhlin SR, McCarty KS Jr. Unilateral nevoid telangiectatic syndrome: the role of estrogen and progesterone receptors. *Arch Dermatol* 1983;119:226.

88. Hunt SJ, Santa Cruz DJ. Acquired benign and "borderline" vascular lesions. *Dermatol Clin* 1992;10:97.

89. Marriott PJ, Munro O, Ryan T. Angioma serpiginosum: familial incidence. *Br J Dermatol* 1975;93:701.

90. Chavaz P, Laugier P. Angiome serpigineux de Hutchinson. *Ann Dermatol Venereol* 1981;108:429.

91. Abahamian LM, Rothe MJ, Grant-Kels JM. Primary telangiectasia of childhood. *Int J Dermatol* 1992;31:307.

92. Hashimoto K, Pritzker MS. Hereditary hemorrhagic telangiectasia: an electron microscopic study. *Oral Surg* 1972;34:751.

93. Braverman IM. Ultrastructure and organization of the cutaneous microvasculature in normal and pathological states. *J Invest Dermatol* 1989;93[2 Suppl]:2S.

94. Johnson WC. Pathology of cutaneous vascular tumors. *Int J Dermatol* 1976;15:239.

95. Bean WB, Walsh JR. Venous lakes. *Arch Dermatol* 1956;74:459.

96. Alcalay J, Sandbank M. The ultrastructure of cutaneous venous lakes. *Int J Dermatol* 1987;26:645).

97. Edgerton MT, Hiebert JM. Vascular and lymphatic tumors in infancy, childhood and adulthood: Challenge of diagnosis and treatment. *Curr Probl Cancer* 1978;2:4.

98. Coffin CM, Dehner LP. Vascular tumors in children and adolescents: a clinicopathologic study of 228 tumors in 222 patients. *Pathol Annu* 1993;28:97.

99. Esterly NB. Kasabach–Merritt syndrome in infants. *J Am Acad Dermatol* 1983;8:504.

100. Perrone T. Vessel-nerve intermingling in benign infantile hemangioendothelioma. *Hum Pathol* 1985;16:198.

101. Calonje E, Mentzel T, Fletcher CDM. Pseudosarcomatous neural invasion in capillary hemangiomas. *Histopathology* 1995; 26:159.

102. Taxy JB, Gray SR. Cellular angiomas of infancy: an ultrastructural study of two cases. *Cancer* 1979;43:2322.

103. Gonzales-Crussi F, Reyes-Mugica M. Cellular hemangiomas ("hemangioendotheliomas") in infants: light microscopic, immunohistochemical and ultrastructural observations. *Am J Surg Pathol* 1991;15:769.

104. Smoller BR, Apfelberg DB. Infantile (juvenile) capillary hemangioma: a tumor of heterogeneous cellular elements. *J Cutan Pathol* 1993;20:330.

105. North PE, Waner M, Mizeracki A, et al. A unique microvascular phenotype shared by juveniles hemangiomas and human placenta. *Arch Dermatol* 2001;137:559–570.

106. North PE, Waner M, Mizeracki A, et al. GLUT1 a newly discovered immunohistochemical marker for junvenile hemangiomas. *Hum Pathol* 2000;31:11–22.

107. Schnyder UW, Keller R. Zur klinik und histologie der angiome: iII. Mitteilung. Zur histologie und pathogenese der senilen angiome. *Arch Dermatol Syph (Berlin)* 1954;198:333.

108. Salamon T, Lazovic O, Milicecic M. Uber einige histologische befunde bei dem sogenannten angioma senile. *Dermatol Monatsschr* 1973;159:1021.

109. Cho KH, Kim SH, Park KC, et al. Angioblastoma (Nakagawa): is it the same as tufted angioma? *Clin Exp Dermatol* 1991;16: 110.

110. Kimura S. Ultrastructure of so-called angioblastoma of the skin before and after soft x-ray therapy. *J Dermatol* 1981;8:235.

111. Wilson Jones E, Orkin M. Tufted angioma (angioblastoma): a benign progressive angioma, not to be confused with Kaposi's sarcoma or low-grade angiosarcoma. *J Am Acad Dermatol* 1989; 20:214.

112. Alessi E, Bertoni E, Sala F. Acquired tufted angioma. *Am J Dermatopathol* 1986;8:426.

113. Kim YK, Kim HJ, Lee KG. Acquired tufted angioma associated with pregnancy. *Clin Exp Dermatol* 1992;17:458.

114. Heagerty AHM, Rubin A, Robinson TWE. Familial tufted angioma. *Clin Exp Dermatol* 1992;17:344.

115. Chu P, LeBoit PE. An eruptive vascular proliferation resembling acquired tufted angioma in the recipient of a liver transplant. *J Am Acad Dermatol* 1992;26:322.

116. Lam WY, Lai Mac-Moune F, Look CN, et al. Tufted angioma with complete regression. *J Cutan Pathol* 1994;21:461.

117. Padilla RS, Orkin M, Rosai J. Acquired "tufted" angioma (progressive capillary hemangioma). *Am J Dermatopathol* 1987;9: 292.

118. Kumakiri M, Muramoto F, Tsukniaga I. Crystalline lamellae in the endothelial cells of a type of hemangioma characterized by the proliferation of immature endothelial cells and pericytes: angioblastoma (Nakagawa). *J Am Acad Dermatol* 1983;8:68.

119. Calonje E, Fletcher CDM. Sinusoidal hemangioma: a distinctive benign vascular neoplasm within the group of cavernous hemangiomas. *Am J Surg Pathol* 1991;15:1130.

120. Cruces MJ, De La Torre C. Multiple eruptive verrucous hemangiomas: a variant of multiple hemangiomatosis. *Dermatologica* 1985;171:106.

121. Imperial R, Helwig EB. Verrucous hemangioma. *Arch Dermatol* 1967;96:247.

122. Chan JKC, Tsang WYW, Calonje E, et al. Verrucous hemangioma: a distinct but neglected variant of cutaneous hemangioma. *Int J Surg Pathol* 1995;2:171.

123. Jessen RT, Thompson S, Smith EB. Cobb syndrome. *Arch Dermatol* 1977;113:1587.

124. Hunt SJ, Santa Cruz DJ, Barr RJ. Microvenular hemangioma. *J Cutan Pathol* 1991;18:235.

125. Aloi F, Tomasini C, Pippione M. Microvenular hemangioma. *Am J Dermatopathol* 1993;15:534.

126. Satge D, Grande-Goburdhun J, Grosshans E. Hemangiome microcapillaire. *Ann Dermatol Venereol* 1993;120:297.

127. Santa Cruz DJ, Aronberg J. Targetoid hemosiderotic hemangioma. *J Am Acad Dermatol* 1988;19:550.

128. Rapini RP, Golitz LE. Targetoid hemosiderotic hemangioma. *J Cutan Pathol* 1990;17:233.

129. Ho C, McCalmont TH. Targetoid hemosiderotic hemangioma: report of 24 cases, with emphasis on unusual features and comparison to early Kaposi's sarcoma. *J Cutan Pathol* 1995;22: 67(abst).

130. Mentzel T, Partanen TA, Kutzner H. Hobnail hemangioma ("targetoid hemosiderotic hemangioma"): clinicopathologic and immunohistochemical analysis of 62 cases. *J Cutan Pathol* 1999;26:279.

131. Calonje E, Fletcher CDM, Wilson Jones E, et al. Retiform hemangioendothelioma: a distinctive form of low-grade angiosarcoma delineated in a series of 15 cases. *Am J Surg Pathol* 1994;18:115.

132. Partanen TA, Alitalo K, Miettinen M. Lack of lymphatic vascular specificity of vascular endothelial growth factor receptor 3 in 185 vascular tumors. *Cancer* 1999;86:2406.

133. Connelly MG, Winkelmann RK. Acral arteriovenous tumor: a clinicopathologic review. *Am J Surg Pathol* 1985;9:15.

134. Girard C, Graham JH, Johnson WC. Arteriovenous hemangioma (arteriovenous shunt). *J Cutan Pathol* 1974;1:73.

135. Koutlas IG, Jessurun J. Arteriovenous hemangioma: a clinicopathological and immunohistochemical study. *J Cutan Pathol* 1994;21:343.

136. Howat AJ, Campbell PE. Angiomatosis: a vascular malformation of infancy and childhood. Report of 17 cases. *Pathology* 1987;19:377.

137. Rao VK, Weiss SW. Angiomatosis of soft tissue: an analysis of the histologic features and clinical outcome in 51 cases. *Am J Surg Pathol* 1992;16:764.

138. Devaney K, Vinh TN, Sweet DE. Skeletal-extraskeletal angiomatosis. A clinicopathological study of fourteen patients and nosologic considerations. *J Bone Joint Surg Am* 1994;76:878.

139. Weiss SW, Enzinger FM. Spindle cell hemangioendothelioma: a low-grade angiosarcoma resembling cavernous hemangioma and Kaposi's sarcoma. *Am J Surg Pathol* 1986;10:521.

140. Ono CM, Mitsunaga MM, Lockett LJ. Intragluteal spindle cell hemangioendothelioma: an unusual presentation of a recently described vascular neoplasm. *Clin Orthop* 1992;281:224.

141. Fletcher CDM, Beham A, Schmid C. Spindle cell haemangioendothelioma: a clinicopathological and immunohistochemical study indicative of a non-neoplastic lesion. *Histopathology* 1991;18:291.

142. Scott GA, Rosai J. Spindle cell hemangioendothelioma: report of seven additional cases of a recently described vascular neoplasm. *Am J Dermatopathol* 1988;10:281.

143. Zoltie N, Roberts PF. Spindle cell haemangioendothelioma in association with epithelioid haemangioendothelioma. *Histopathology* 1989;15:544.

144. Azadeh B, Attallah MF, Ejeckam GC. Spindle cell hemangioendothelioma in association with epithelioid hemangioendothelioma. *Cutis* 1994;53:134.

145. Ding J, Hashimoto H, Imayama S, et al. Spindle cell hemangioendothelioma: probably a benign vascular lesion not a low-grade angiosarcoma. A clinicopathological, ultrastructural and immunohistochemical study. *Virchows Arch A* 1992;420:77.

146. Perkins P, Weiss SW. Spindle cell hemangioendothelioma: a clinicopathologic study of 78 cases. *Mod Pathol* 1994;7:9A.

147. Imayama S, Murakamai Y, Hashimoto H, et al. Spindle cell hemangioendothelioma exhibits the ultrastructural features of reactive vascular proliferation rather than of angiosarcoma. *Am J Clin Pathol* 1992;97:279.

148. Beral V, Peterman TA, Berkelman R, et al. Kaposi's sarcoma among persons with AIDS: a sexually transmitted infection. *Lancet* 1990;335:123.

149. Dorfmann RF. Kaposi's sarcoma with special reference to its manifestations in infants and children and to the concepts of Arthur Purdy Stout. *Am J Surg Pathol* 1986;10[Suppl]:68.

150. Friedman-Kien AE, Saltzman BR. Clinical manifestations of classical, endemic African, and epidemic AIDS-associated Kaposi's sarcoma. *J Am Acad Dermatol* 1990;22:1237.

151. Tappero JW, Conant MA, Wolfe SF, et al. Kaposi's sarcoma: epidemiology, pathogenesis, histology, clinical spectrum, staging criteria and therapy. *J Am Acad Dermatol* 1993;28:371.

152. Wolff K. The enigma of Kaposi's sarcoma: an answer at last? *Clin Exp Dermatol* 1992;17:146.

153. Gottlieb GJ, Ackerman AB. Kaposi's sarcoma: an extensively disseminated form in young homosexual men. *Hum Pathol* 1982;13:882.

154. Roth WK. HIV-associated Kaposi's sarcoma: New developments in epidemiology and molecular pathology. *J Cancer Res Clin Oncol* 1991;117:186.

155. Casabona J, Melbye M, Biggar RJ, et al. Kaposi's sarcoma and non-Hodgkin's lymphoma in European AIDS cases: no excess risk of Kaposi's sarcoma in Mediterranean countries. *Int J Cancer* 1991;47:49.

156. Lee WA, Hutckins GM. Cluster analysis of the metastatic patterns of human immunodeficiency virus-associated Kaposi's sarcoma. *Hum Pathol* 1992;23:306.

157. Lemlich G, Scham L, Lebwokl M. Kaposi's sarcoma and acquired immunodeficiency syndrome: postmortem findings in twenty-four cases. *J Am Acad Dermatol* 1987;16:319.

158. McKenzie R, Travis WD, Dolan SA, et al. The causes of death in patients with human immunodeficiency virus infection: a clinical and pathologic study with emphasis on the role of pulmonary diseases. *Medicine (Baltimore)* 1991;70:326.

159. Moskowitz LB, Hensley GT, Gould EW. Frequency and anatomic distribution of lymphadenopathic Kaposi's sarcoma in the acquired immunodeficiency syndrome: an autopsy series. *Hum Pathol* 1985;16:447.

160. Montagnimo G, Bencini PL, Tarantino A, et al. Clinical features and course of Kaposi's sarcoma in kidney transplant patients: report of 13 cases. *Am J Nephrol* 1994;14:121.

161. Blumenfield W, Egbert BM, Sagebiel RW. Differential diagnosis of Kaposi's sarcoma. *Arch Pathol Lab Med* 1985;109:123.

162. Chor PJ, Santa Cruz DJ. Kaposi's sarcoma: a clinicopathologic review and differential diagnosis. *J Cutan Pathol* 1992;19:6.

163. Gange RW, Wilson Jones E. Lymphangioma-like Kaposi's sarcoma: a report of three cases. *Br J Dermatol* 1979;100:327.

164. Facchetti F, Lucini L, Gavazzoni R, et al. Immunomorphological analysis of the role of blood vessel endothelium in the morphogenesis of cutaneous Kaposi's sarcoma: a study of 57 cases. *Histopathology* 1988;12:581.

165. Kao GF, Johnson FB, Sulica VI. The nature of hyaline (eosinophilic) globules and vascular slits of Kaposi's sarcoma. *Am J Dermatopathol* 1990;12:256.

166. Orchard GE, Wilson Jones E, Russell Jones R. Immunocytochemistry in the diagnosis of Kaposi's sarcoma and angiosarcoma. *Br J Biomed Sci* 1995;52:35.

167. Niedt GW, Myskowski PL, Urmacher C. Histologic predictors of survival in acquired immunodeficiency syndrome-associated Kaposi's sarcoma. *Hum Pathol* 1992;23:1419.

168. Brooks JJ. Kaposi's sarcoma: a reversible hyperplasia. *Lancet* 1986;2:1309.

169. Ioachim HL, Dorsett B, Melamed J, et al. Cytomegalovirus, angiomatosis, and Kaposi's sarcoma: new observations of a debated relationship. *Mod Pathol* 1992;5:169.

170. Rabkin CS, Janz S, Lash A, et al. Monoclonal origin of multicentric Kaposi's sarcoma lesions. *N Engl J Med* 1997;336:988–93.

171. Nickoloff BJ. PECAM–1(CD31) is expressed on proliferating endothelial cells, stromal-shaped cells, and dermal dendrocytes in Kaposi's sarcoma. *Arch Dermatol* 1993;129:250.

172. Nickoloff BJ. The human progenitor cell antigen (CD34) is localized on endothelial cells, dermal dendritic cells, and perifollicular cells in formalin-fixed normal skin, and on proliferating endothelial cells and stromal spindle-shaped cells in Kaposi's sarcoma. *Arch Dermatol* 1991;127:523.

173. Regezi JA, MacPhail LA, Daniels TE, et al. Human immunodeficiency virus-associated oral Kaposi's sarcoma: a heterogeneous cell population dominated by spindle-shaped endothelial cells. *Am J Pathol* 1993;143:240.

174. Gray MH, Trimble CL, Zirn J. Relationship of Factor XIIIa-positive dermal dendrocytes to Kaposi's sarcoma. *Arch Pathol Lab Med* 1991;115:791.

175. Beckstead JH, Wood GS, Fletcher V. Evidence for the origin of Kaposi's sarcoma from lymphatic endothelium. *Am J Pathol* 1985;119:294.

176. Russel Jones R, Spaull J, Wilson Jones E. Histogenesis of Kaposi's sarcoma in patients with and without acquired immune deficiency syndrome (AIDS). *J Clin Pathol* 1986;39:742.

177. Rutgers JL, Wieczoreck R, Bonetti F, et al. The expression of endothelial cell surface antigens by AIDS-associated Kaposi's sarcoma. *Am J Pathol* 1986;122:493.

178. Scully PA, Steinman HK, Kennedy C, et al. AIDS-related Kaposi's sarcoma displays differential expression of endothelial surface antigens. *Am J Pathol* 1988;130:244.

179. Lymboussaki A, Partanen TA, Olofsson B, et al. Expression of the vascular endothelial growth factor C receptor VEGFR–3 on lymphatic endothelium of the skin and on vascular tumors. *Am J Pathol* 1998;153:395.

180. Dictor M, Anderson C. Lymphaticovenous differentiation in Kaposi's sarcoma: Cellular phenotypes by stage. *Am J Pathol* 1988;130:411.

181. Chang Y, Cesarman E, Pessin MS. Identification of herpesvirus-like DNA sequences in AIDS-associated Kaposi's sarcoma. *Science* 1994;266:1865.

182. Levy JA. A new human herpesvirus KSHV or HHV8? *Lancet* 1995;346:786.

183. Geraminejad, P, Memar O, Aronson I., et al. Kaposi's sarcoma and other manifestations of human herpesvirus 8. *J Am Acad Dermatol* 2002;47:641.

184. Huang YQ, Li JJ, Kaplan MH, et al. Human herpesvirus-like nucleic acid in various forms of Kaposi's sarcoma. *Lancet* 1995;345:759.

185. Dupin N, Grandadam M, Calvez V, et al. Herpesvirus-like DNA sequences in patients with Mediterranean Kaposi's sarcoma. *Lancet* 1995;345:761.

186. Gao SJ, Kinsgley L, Hoover DR, et al. Seroconversion to antibodies against Kaposi's sarcoma-associated herpesvirus-related latent nuclear antigens before the development of Kaposi's sarcoma. *N Engl J Med* 1996;335:233.

187. Zukerberg LR, Nickoloff BJ, Weiss SW. Kaposiform hemangioendothelioma of infancy and childhood: an aggressive neoplasm associated with Kasabach–Merritt syndrome and lymphangiomatosis. *Am J Surg Pathol* 1993;17:321.

188. Lam WY, Lai FMM, To KF, et al. Cutaneous lesions of kaposiform hemangioendothelioma: report of two cases. *Int J Surg Pathol* 1995;2[Suppl]:521.

189. Lai FMM, Choi PCL, Leung PC, et al. Kaposiform hemangioendothelioma: five patients with cutaneous lesion and long follow-up. *Mod Pathol* 2001;14:1087.

190. Calonje E, Fletcher CDM. Aneurysmal benign fibrous histiocytoma: clinicopathological analysis of 40 cases of a tumour frequently misdiagnosed as a vascular neoplasm. *Histopathology* 1995;26:323.

191. Del-Rio E, Aguilar A, Ambrojo P, et al. Pseudo-Kaposi's sarcoma induced by minor trauma in a patient with Klippel–Trenaunay–Weber syndrome. *Clin Exp Dermatol* 1993;18:151.

192. Strutton G, Weedon D. Acro-angiodermatitis: a simulant of Kaposi's sarcoma. *Am J Dermatopathol* 1987;9:85.

193. Wilson Jones E, Cerio R, Smith NP. Multinucleate cell angiohistiocytoma: an acquired vascular anomaly to be distinguished from Kaposi's sarcoma. *Br J Dermatol* 1990;122:651.

194. Smolle J, Auboeck L, Gogg-Retzer I, et al. Multinucleate cell angiohistiocytoma: a clinicopathological, immunohistochemical and ultrastructural study. *Br J Dermatol* 1989;121:113.

195. Dufau JP, Pierre C, De SaintMaur PP, et al. Hemangioendothelioma retiforme. *Ann Pathol* 1997;17:47.

196. Fukunaga M, Endo Y, Masui F, et al. Retiform haemangioendothelioma. *Virchows Arch* 1996;428:301.

197. Duke D, Dvorak AM, Harrist TJ, et al. Multiple retiform hemangioendotheliomas. A low grade angiosarcoma. *Am J Dermatopathol* 1996;18:606.

198. Mentzel T, Stengel B, Katenkamp D. Retiform hemangioendothelioma. Clinico-pathologic case report and discussion of the group of low grade malignancy vascular tumors. *Pathologe* 1997;18:390.

199. Dabska M. Malignant endovascular papillary angioendothelioma of the skin in childhood: Clinicopathologic study of 6 cases. *Cancer* 1969;24:503.

200. Fanburg-Smith JC, Michal M, et al. Papillary intralymphatic angioendothelioma (PILA): a report of twelve cases of a distinctive vascular tumor with phenotypic features of lymphatic vessels. *Am J Surg Pathol* 1999;23:1004.

201. Manivel JC, Wick MR, Swanson PE, et al. Endovascular papillary angioendothelioma of childhood: a vascular lesion possibly characterized by "high" endothelial cell diferentiation. *Hum Pathol* 1986;17:1240.

202. Nayler SJ, Rubin BP, Calonje E, et al. Composite hemangioendothelioma: a complex, low-grade vascular lesion mimicking angiosarcoma. *Am J Surg Pathol* 2000;24:352.

203. Reis-Filho JS, Paiva ME, Lopes JM. Congenital composite hemangioendothelioma: case report and reappraisal of the hemangioendothelioma spectrum. *J Cutan Pathol* 2002;29:226.

204. Tsang WYW, Chan JCK. Kaposi-like infantile hemangioendothelioma: a distinctive vascular neoplasm of the retroperitoneum. *Am J Surg Pathol* 1991;15:982.

205. Tsang WYW, Chan JCK, Fletcher CDM. Recently characterized vascular tumors of skin and soft tissues. *Histopathology* 1991;19:489.

206. Weiss SW, Enzinger FM. Epithelioid hemangioendothelioma: a vascular lesion often mistaken for a carcinoma. *Cancer* 1982;50:970.

207. Mentzel T, Beham A, Calonje E, et al. Epithelioid hemangioendothelioma of skin and soft tissues: clinicopathologic and immunohistochemical study of 30 cases. *Am J Surg Pathol* 1997;21:363.

208. Weiss SW, Ishak KG, Dail DH, et al. Epithelioid hemangioendothelioma and related lesions. *Semin Diagn Pathol* 1986;3:259.

209. Angervall L, Kindblom L-G, Karlsson K, et al. Atypical hemangioendothelioma of venous origin. A clinicopathologic, angiographic, immunohistochemical and ultrastructural study of two endothelial tumors within the concept of histiocytoid hemangioma. *Am J Surg Pathol* 1985;9:504.

210. Tyring S, Guest P, Lee P, et al. Epithelioid hemangioendothelioma of the skin and femur. *J Am Acad Dermatol* 1989;20:362.

211. Malane SL, Sau P, Benson PM. Epithelioid hemangioendothelioma associated with reflex sympathetic dystrophy. *J Am Acad Dermatol* 1992;26:325.

212. Resnik KS, Kantor GR, Spielvogel RL, et al. Cutaneous epithelioid hemangioendothelioma without systemic involvement. *Am J Dermatopathol* 1993;15:272.

213. Quante M, Patel NK, Hill S, et al. Epithelioid hemangioendothelioma presenting in the skin. A clinicopathologic study of eight cases. *Am J Dermatopathol* 1998;20:541–546.

214. Suster S, Moran CA, Koss MN. Epithelioid hemangioendothelioma of the anterior mediastinum: clinicopathologic, immunohistochemical, and ultrastructural analysis of 12 cases. *Am J Surg Pathol* 1994;18:871.

215. Williams SB, Bulter CB, Gilkey GW, et al. Epithelioid hemangioendothelioma with osteoclast-like giant cells. *Arch Pathol Lab Med* 1993;117:315.

216. Gray MF, Rosenberg AE, Dickersin GR, et al. Cytokeratin expression in epithelioid vascular neoplasms. *Hum Pathol* 1990;21:211.

217. Van Haelst UJGM, Pruszczynski M, Ten Cate LN, et al. Ultrastructural and immunohistochemical study of epithelioid hemangioendothelioma of bone: coexpression of epithelial and endothelial markers. *Ultrastruct Pathol* 1990;14:141.

218. Mendlick MR, Nelson M, Pickering D, et al. Translocation t(1;3)(p36.3;q25) is a nonrandom aberration in epithelioid hemangioendothelioma. *Am J Surg Pathol* 2001;25:684.

219. Boudousquie AC, Lawce HJ, Sherman R, et al. Complex translocation (7;22) identified in an epithelioid hemangioendothelioma. *Cancer Genet Cytogenet* 1996;92:116.

220. Calixto MMP, Pacheco FA. Angiosarcoma of the leg in a patient with chronic osteomyelitis. *Skin Cancer* 1986;1:77.

221. Fletcher CDM, Beham A, Bekir S, et al. Epithelioid angiosarcoma of deep soft tissue: a distinctive tumor readily mistaken for an epithelial neoplasm. *Am J Surg Pathol* 1991;15:915.

222. Gloor M, Adler D, Bersch A, et al. Hamangiosarkom in einem naevus telangiectaticus lateralis. *Hautarzt* 1983;34:182.

223. Nagata M, Semba I, Ooya K, et al. Malignant endothelial neoplasm arising in the area of lymphangioma: immunohistochemical and ultrastructural observation. *J Oral Pathol* 1984;13:560.

224. Rossi S, Fletcher CD. Angiosarcoma arising in hemangioma/vascular malformation: report of four cases and review of the literature. *Am J Surg Pathol* 2002;26:1319.

225. Abratt RP, Williams M, Raff M, et al. Angiosarcoma of the superior vena cava. *Cancer* 1983;52:740.

226. Chadhuri B, Ronan SG, Manahgod JR. Angiosarcoma arising in a plexiform neurofibroma. *Cancer* 1980;46:605.

227. Brown RW, Tornos C, Evans HL. Angiosarcoma arising from malignant Schwannoma in a patient with neurofibromatosis. *Cancer* 1992;70:1141.

228. Trassard M, Le Doussal V, Bui BN, et al. Angiosarcoma arising in a solitary schwannoma (neurilemoma) of the sciatic nerve. *Am J Surg Pathol* 1996;20:1412.

229. Mentzel T, Katencamp D. Intraneural angiosarcoma and angiosarcoma arising in benign and malignant peripheral nerve sheath tumours: clinicopathological and immunohistochemical analysis of four cases. *Histopathology* 1999;35:114.

230. Morphopoulos GD, Banerjee SS, Ali HH, et al. Malignant peripheral nerve sheath tumour with vascular differentiation: a report of four cases. *Histopathology* 1996;28:401.

231. Leake J, Sheehan MP, Rampling D, et al. Angiosarcoma complicating xeroderma pigmentosum. *Histopathology* 1992;21:179.

232. Ghandur-Mnaymneh L, Gonzales MS. Angiosarcoma of the penis with hepatic angiomas in a patient with low vinyl chloride exposure. *Cancer* 1981;47:1318.

233. Kauffman SL, Stout AP. Malignant hemangioendothelioma in infants and children. *Cancer* 1961;14:1186.

234. Lezana-del Valle P, Gerald WL, Tsai J, et al. Malignant vascular tumors in young patients. *Cancer* 1998;83:1634.

235. Holden CA, Spittle MF, Wilson Jones E. Angiosarcoma of the face and scalp: prognosis and treatment. *Cancer* 1987;59:1046.

236. Mark RJ, Tron LM, Sercarz J, et al. Angiosarcoma of the head and neck: the UCLA experience 1955 through 1990. *Arch Otolaryngol Head Neck Surg* 1993;119:973.

237. Wilson Jones E. Malignant vascular tumours. *Clin Exp Dermatol* 1976;1:287.

238. Haustein U-F. Angiosarcoma of the face and scalp. *Int J Dermatol* 1991;30:851.

239. Matsumoto K, Inoue K, Fukamizu H, et al. Prognosis of cutaneous angiosarcoma in Japan: a statistical study of sixty-nine cases. *Chir Plastica* 1986;8:151.

240. Maddox JC, Evans HL. Angiosarcoma of the skin and soft tissue: a study of forty-four cases. *Cancer* 1981;48:1907.

241. Mark RJ, Pown JC, Tran LM, Fu YS, Juillard GF. Angiosarcoma. A report of 67 patients and a review of the literature. *Cancer* 1996;77:2400.

242. Woodward AH, Ivins JC, Soule EH Jr. Lymphangiosarcoma arising in chronic lymphedematous extremities. *Cancer* 1972;20:562.

243. Alessi E, Sala F, Berti E. Angiosarcomas in lymphedematous limbs. *Am J Dermatopathol* 1986;8:371.

244. Chen KTK, Bauer V, Flam MS. Angiosarcoma in postsurgical lymphedema: an unusual occurrence in a man. *Am J Dermatopathol* 1991;13:488.

245. Hultberg BM. Angiosarcomas in chronically lymphedematous extremities: two cases of Stewart–Treves syndrome. *Am J Dermatopathol* 1987;9:406.

246. Offori TW, Platt CC, Stephens M, et al. Angiosarcoma in congenital hereditary lymphedema (Milroy's disease): diagnostic beacons and a review of the literature. *Clin Exp Dermatol* 1993;18:174.

247. Muller R, Hajdu SI, Brennan MF. Lymphangiosarcoma associated with chronically lymphedematous extremities: two cases of Stewart–Treves syndrome. *Cancer* 1987;59:179.

248. Drachman D, Rosen L, Sharaf D, et al. Postmastectomy low-grade angiosarcoma: an unusual case resembling a lymphangioma circumscriptum. *Am J Dermatopathol* 1988;10:247.

249. Davies JD, Rees GJG, Mera SL. Angiosarcoma in irradiated post-mastectomy chest wall. *Histopathology* 1983;7:947.

250. Edeiken S, Russo DP, Knecht J, et al. Angiosarcoma after tylectomy and radiation therapy for carcinoma of the breast. *Cancer* 1992;70:644.

251. Moskaluk CA, Merino MJ, Danforth DN, et al. Low-grade angiosarcoma of the skin of the breast: a complication of lumpectomy and radiation therapy for breast carcinoma. *Hum Pathol* 1992;23:710.

252. Goette DK, Detlefs RL. Postirradiation angiosarcoma. *J Am Acad Dermatol* 1985;12:922.

253. Laaff H, Vibrans U. Cutaneous angiosarcoma after telecobalt irradiation. *Hautarzt* 1992;43:654.

254. Rosai J, Summer HW, Major MC, et al. Angiosarcoma of the skin: a clinicopathologic and fine structural study. *Hum Pathol* 1976;7:83.

255. Naka N, Ohsawa M, Tomita Y, et al. Prognostic factors in angiosarcoma: a multivariate analysis of 55 cases. *J Surg Oncol* 1996;61:170.

256. Matejka M, Konrad K. Cutaneous angiosarcoma of the face and scalp. *Clin Exp Dermatol* 1984;9:232.

257. McWilliam LJ, Harris M. Granular cell angiosarcoma of the skin: histology, electron microscopy and immunohistochem-

istry of a newly recognised tumor. *Histopathology* 1985;9:1205.

258. Hitchcock MG, Hurt MA, Santa Cruz DJ. Cutaneous granular cell angiosarcoma. *J Cutan Pathol* 1994;21:256.

259. Schuborg C, Mertens F, Rydholm A, et al. Cytogenetic analysis of four angiosarcomas from deep and superficial soft tissue. *Cancer Genet Cytogenet* 1998;100:52.

260. Molina A, Bangs CD, Donlon T. Angiosarcoma of the scalp with complex hypotetraploid karyotype. *Cancer Genet Cytogenet* 1989;41:268.

261. Kindblom LG, Stenman G, Angervall L. Morphological and cytogenetic studies of angiosarcoma in Stewart–Treves syndrome. *Vrichows Arch A Pathol Anat Histopathol* 1991;419:439.

262. Mandahl N, Jin YS, Heim S, et al. Trisomy 5 and loss of the Y chromosome as the sole cytogenetic anomalies in a cevernous hemangioma/angiosarcoma. *Genes Chrom Cancer* 1990;1:315.

263. Banerjee SS, Eyden BP, Wells S, et al. Pseudoakngiosarcomatous carcinoma: a clinicopathological study of seven cases. *Histopathology* 1992;21:13.

264. Nappi O, Wick MR, Pettinato G, et al. Pseudovascular adenoid squamous cell carcinoma of the skin: a neoplasm that may be mistaken for angiosarcoma. *Am J Surg Pathol* 1992;16:429.

265. McGrath JA, Schofield OM, Mayou BJ, et al. Metastatic squamous cell carcinoma resembling angiosarcoma complicating dystrophic epidermolysis bullosa. *Dermatologica* 1991;182:235.

266. Prescott RJ, Banerjee SS, Eyden BP, et al. Cutaneous epithelioid angiosarcoma: a clinicopathological study of four cases. *Histopathology* 1994;25:421.

267. Lasota J, Miettinen M. Absence of Kaposi's sarcoma-associated virus (human herpesvirus-8) sequences in angiosarcoma. *Virchows Arch* 1999;434:51–56.

268. Marrogi AJ, Hunt SJ, Santa Cruz DJ. Cutaneous epithelioid angiosarcoma. *Am J Dermatopathol* 1990;12:350.

269. Byers RJ, McMahon RFT, Freemont AJ, et al. Epithelioid angiosarcoma arising in an arteriovenous fistula. *Histopathology* 1992;21:87.

270. Jennings TA, Peterson L, Axiotis CA, et al. Angiosarcoma associated with foreign body material. *Cancer* 1988;62:2436.

271. Watson WL, McCarthy WB. Blood and lymph vessel tumors: a report of 1056 cases. *Surg Gynecol Obstet* 1940;71:569.

272. Peachey RDG, Lim CC, Whimster IW. Lymphangioma of the skin. *Br J Dermatol* 1970;83:519.

273. Wilson Jones E, Winkelmann RK, Zacharay CB, et al. Benign lymphangioendothelioma. *J Am Acad Dermatol* 1990;23:229.

274. Watanawe M, Kishiyama K, Ohkawara A. Acquired progressive lymphangioma. *J Am Acad Dermatol* 1993;8:663–667.

275. Guillou L, Flecher CDM. Benign lymphangioendothelioma (acquired progressive lymphangioma): a lesion not to be confused with well-differentiated angiosarcoma and patch stage Kaposi's sarcoma: clinicopathologic analysis of a series. *Am J Surg Pathol* 2000;24:1047–1057.

276. Prioleau PG, Santa Cruz DJ. Lymphangioma circumscription following radical mastectomy and radiation therapy. *Cancer* 1978;42:1989.

277. Zadvinskis DP, Benson MT, Kerr HH, et al. Congenital malformations of the cervicothoracic lymphatic system: embriology and pathogenesis. *Radiographics* 1992;12:1175.

278. Burgdorf WHC, Mukai K, Rosai J. Immunohistochemical identification of factor VIII-related antigen in endothelial cells of cutaneous lesions of alleged vascular nature. *Am J Clin Pathol* 1981;75:167.

279. Pearson JM, McWilliam LJ. A light microscopical, immunohistochemical, and ultrastructural comparison of hemangiomata and lymphangiomata. *Ultrastruct Pathol* 1990;14:497.

280. Harkins GA, Sabiston DC. Lymphangioma in infancy and childhood. *Surgery* 1960;47:811.

281. Chervenak FA, Isaacson G, Blakemore KJ, et al. Fetal cystic hygroma: cause and natural history. *N Engl J Med* 1983;309:822.

282. Alqahtani A, Nguyen LT, Flageole H, et al. 25 years experience with lymphangiomas in children. *J Pediatr Surg* 1999;34:1164.

283. Byrne J, Blanc WA, Warburton D, et al. The significance of cystic hygroma in fetuses. *Hum Pathol* 1984;15:61–67.

284. Flanagan BP, Helwig EB. Cutaneous lymphangioma. *Arch Dermatol* 1977;113:24.

285. Herron GS, Rouse RV, Kosek JC, et al. Benign lymphangioendothelioma. *J Am Acad Dermatol* 1994;31:362.

286. Mehregan DR, Mehregan AH, Mehregan DA. Benign lymphangioendothelioma: report of 2 cases. *J Cutan Pathol* 1992;19:502.

287. Ramani P, Shah A. Lymphangiomatosis: histologic and immunohistochemical analysis of four cases. *Am J Surg Pathol* 1993;17:329.

288. Singh Gomez C, Calonje E, Ferrar DW, et al. Lymphangiomatosis of the limbs: clinicopathologic analysis of a series. *Am J Surg Pathol* 1995;19:125.

289. Fineberg S, Rosen PP. Cutaneous angiosarcoma and atypical vascular lesion of the skin and breast after radiation therapy for breast carcinoma. *Am J Clin Pathol* 1994;102:757–763.

290. Diaz-Cascajo C, Borghi S, Weyers W, et al. Benign lymphangiomatous papules of the skin after radiotherapy: a report of five new cases and review of the literature. *Histopathology* 1999;35:319–327.

291. Requena L, Kutzner H, Mentzel T, et al. Benign vascular proliferations in irradiated skin. *Am J Surg Pathol* 2002;26:328–337.

292. Tsuneyoshi M, Enjoji M. Glomus tumor: a clinicopathologic and electron microscopic study. *Cancer* 1982;50:1601.

293. Haque S, Modlin IM, West AB. Multiple glomus tumors of the stomach with intravascular spread. *Am J Surg Pathol* 1992;16:291.

294. Gaertner EM, Steinberg DM, Huber M, et al. Pulmonary and mediastinal glomus tumors—report of five cases including a pulmonary glomangiosarcoma: a clinicopathologic study with literature review. *Am J Surg Pathol* 2000;24:1105.

295. Kim YI, Kim JH, Suh J, et al. Glomus tumor of the trachea. Report of a case with ultrastructural observations. *Cancer* 1989;64:881.

296. Sunderraj S, Al-Khalifa AA, Pal AK, et al. Primary intra-osseous glomus tumour. *Histopathology* 1989;14:532.

297. Geraghty JM, Everitt NJ, Blundell JW. Glomus tumor of the small bowel. *Histopathology* 1991;19:287–289.

298. Harvey JA, Walker F. Solid glomus tumor of the pterygoid fossa: a lesion mimicking an epithelial neoplasm of low grade malignancy. *Hum Pathol* 1987;18:965–966.

299. Hirose T, Hasegawa T, Seki K, et al. Atypical glomus tumor in the mediastinum: a case report with immunohistochemical and ultrastructural studies. *Ultrastruct Pathol* 1996;20:451.

300. Sawada S, Honda M, Kamide R, et al. Three cases of subungual glomus tumors with von Recklinghausen neurofibromatosis. *J Am Acad Dermatol* 1995;32:277–278.

301. Okada O, Demitsu T, Manabe M, et al. A case of multiple subungual glomus tumors associated with neurofibromatosis type 1. *J Dermatol* 1999;26:535.

302. Kim YC. An additional case of solitary subungual glomus tumor associated with neurofibromatosis 1. *J Dermatol* 2000;27:418.

303. Tran LP, Velanovich V, Kaufmann CR. Familial multiple glomus tumors: report of a pedigree and literature review. *Ann Plast Surg* 1994;32:89.

304. Boon LM, Brouillard P, Irrthum A, et al. A gene for inherited cutaneous venous anomalies ("glomangiomas") localizes to chromosome 1p21–22. *Am J Hum Genet* 1999;65:125.

305. Calvert JT, Burns S, Riney TJ, et al. Additional glomangioma family link to chromosome 1p: no evidence for genetic heterogeneity. *Hum Hered* 2001;51:180.

306. Albrecht S, Zbieranowski J. Incidental glomus coccygeum. When a normal structure looks like a tumor. *Am J Surg Pathol* 1990;14:922.

307. Gould EW, Manivel JC, Albores-Saavedra J, et al. Locally infiltrative glomus tumors and glomangiosarcoma: a clinical, ultrastructural and immunohistochemical study. *Cancer* 1990;65:310.

308. Beham A, Fletcher CDM. Intravascular glomus tumor: a previously undescribed phenomenon. *Virchows Arch [A]* 1991;418:175.

309. Googe PB, Griffin WC. Intravenous glomus tumor of the forearm. *J Cutan Pathol* 1993;20:359.

310. Calonje E, Fletcher CDM. Cutaneous intraneural glomus tumor: report of a case. *Am J Dermatopathol* 1995;15:395.

311. Folpe AL, Fanburg-Smith JC, Miettinen M, et al. Atypical and malignant glomus tumors: analysis of 52 cases, with a proposal for reclassification of glomus tumors. *Am J Surg Pathol* 2001;25:1–12.

312. Slater DN, Cotton DWK, Azzopardi JG. Oncocytic glomus tumor: a new variant. *Histopathology* 1987;11:523.

313. Pulitzer DR, Martin PC, Reed RJ. Epithelioid glomus tumor. *Hum Pathol* 1995;26:1022.

314. Aiba M, Hirayama A, Kuramochi S. Glomangiosarcoma in a glomus tumor. *Cancer* 1988;61:1467.

315. Dervan PA, Tobbin IN, Casey M, et al. Glomus tumour: an immunohistochemical profile of 11 cases. *Histopathology* 1989;14:483.

316. Porter PL, Bigler SA, McNutt M, et al. The immunophenotype of hemangiopericytomas and glomus tumors with special reference to muscle protein expression: an immunohistochemical study and review of the literature. *Mod Pathol* 1991;4:46.

317. Kaye VM, Dehner LP. Cutaneous glomus tumor: a comparative immunohistochemical study with pseudoangiomatous intradermal melanocytic nevi. *Am J Dermatopathol* 1991;13:2.

318. Enzinger FM, Smith BH. Hemangiopericytoma: an analysis of 106 cases. *Hum Pathol* 1976;7:61.

319. McMaster MJ, Soule EH, Ivins JC. Hemangiopericytoma: a clinicopathologic study and long-term follow-up of 60 patients. *Cancer* 1975;36:2232.

320. Fletcher CDM. Haemangiopericytoma: a dying breed? Reappraisal of an entity and its variants. *Curr Diagn Pathol* 1994;1:19.

321. Granter SR, Badizadegan K, Fletcher CD. Myofibromatosis in adults, glomangiopericytoma, and myopericytoma: a spectrum of tumors showing perivascular myoid differentiation. *Am J Surg Pathol* 1998;22:513.

322. Coffin CM, Dehner LP. Fibroblastic-myofibroblastic tumors in children and adolescents: a clinicopathologic study of 108 examples in 103 patients. *Pediatr Pathol* 1991;11:569.

323. Mentzel T, Calonje E, Nasciemento AG, et al. Infantile hemangiopericytoma versus infantile myofibromatosis: a study of a series suggesting a spectrum of infantile myofibroblastic lesions. *Am J Surg Pathol* 1994;18:922.

324. McMenamin ME, Fletcher CDM. Malignant myopericytoma: expanding the spectrum of tumors with myopericytic differentiation. *Histopathology* 2002;41:450.

TUMORS WITH FATTY, MUSCULAR, OSSEOUS, AND CARTILAGENOUS DIFFERENTIATION

BRUCE D. RAGSDALE

THE BASIC SCIENCE OF FAT RELEVANT TO TUMORS

Adipose tissue can be divided into two types, brown and white. In adults, most fat is the white, univesicular variety. White fat serves as the depot for stored lipid, which is an efficient energy reserve, and protects against external trauma. With hematoxylin and eosin staining, only the cell membrane and possibly an eccentric nucleus with or without vacuoles or pseudoinclusions of cytoplasmic fat (*lochkern*, German for "hole in the nucleus") are seen. The red-brown to tan color of brown adipose tissue results from cytochrome pigment in the numerous mitochondria of its finely vacuolated cells. Brown fat has been considered an immature or fetal stage in the development of white fat, but most evidence now substantiates the unique identity of brown fat and its role in basal metabolism and nonshivering thermogesis. In humans, brown fat is more prevalent in the newborn period than later in life, but it persists throughout adulthood in the neck, axilla, and mediastinum, as well as elsewhere, embedded within the common white fat (1), which, over time, tends to replace it.

Most investigators agree that perivascular cells resembling pericytes and fibroblasts play an important transition role in the development of benign and malignant lipoblasts. Both white and brown fat cells modulate (Fig. 34-1A) from these primitive fat organ precursors through multivesicular stages easily mistaken for histiocytes, to preadipocytes in which lipid inclusions coalesce and glycogen decreases, and finally to univacuolar adipocytes (Fig. 34-1B) (2) that are variably S-100 positive. The multivacuolar stage is observed in various tumors and is likely to reappear with involution following fat injury. In these settings, the cells with foamy cytoplasm are commonly mistaken for histiocytes—for example, the CD68-negative foam cells in subcutis following biopsy. This is the source of much nosologic confusion, particularly with regard to some of the lesions termed "histiocytomas" (3).

Normal fat has scattered CD 34 positive dendritic cells and small factor XIIIa positive dendritic cells, more numer-

ous near vessels and within fibrovascular septae. Subsets of them proliferate together in mesenchymal areas of spindle cell lipomas, pleomorphic lipomas, myxoid lipomas, and atypical lipoma/well-differentiated liposarcomas (4).

Fatty tumors of dermatologic interest are common and are generally situated in subcutaneous position (5).

Purely cutaneous lipogenic tumors are exceptionally rare and have different specific clinicopathologic features in comparison with more deeply located tumors (6). This fact, as with many other subsets of soft tissue tumors, makes correlation of histopathologic opinions with history and radiologic studies the surest route to accurate diagnoses.

NEVUS LIPOMATOSUS SUPERFICIALIS

Nevus lipomatosus superficialis is a fairly uncommon lesion showing groups of soft, flattened papules or nodules that have smooth or wrinkled surfaces and are skin-colored or pale yellow. Characteristically, the lesions are linearly distributed on one hip or buttock (nevus lipomatosus superficialis of Hoffman and Zurhelle) (7) (Fig. 34-2), from where they may overlap onto the adjacent skin of the back or the upper thigh (8). Other areas, such as the thorax or the abdomen, are only rarely affected. The lesions may be present at birth or may begin in infancy (nevus angiolipomatosus of Howell) (9) in which case the replacement of hypoplastic dermis may cause pseudotumorous yellow protrusions and be associated with skeletal and other malformations, but they develop most commonly during the first two decades of life and occasionally later. Multiple lesions may coalesce.

Solitary lesions that may not appear until after the fifth decade predilect the trunk and have been diagnosed as nevus lipomatosus superficialis (8), but it seems preferable to regard them instead as solitary, bag-like, soft fibromas (7) (Chapter 33), polypoid fibrolipomas or pedunculated lipofibromas (10).

Histopathology. Groups and strands of fat cells are found embedded among the collagen bundles of the dermis, often

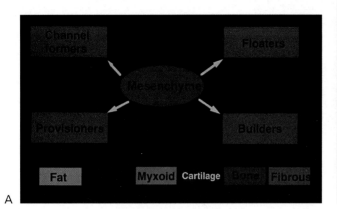

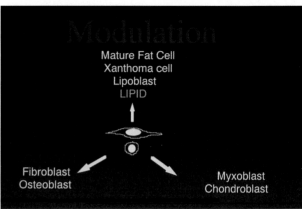

A   B

FIGURE 34-1. Mesenchymal modulation diagrams. **A:** Uncommitted mesenchyme is the product of *differentiation*, distinct from ectoderm and endoderm. Further adoption of specific function and corresponding cell structure (phenotype) is *modulation*, resulting in components of the circulatory system ("channel formers"); lympho-hematopoietic cells ("floaters"); structural connective tissue ("builders"); and fat-storing cells ("provisioners"). This normal panoply has its frequent neoplastic parallel in the multiple tissue types that can be found in mesenchymal tumors. **B:** Extracellular matrix products can be collagen-dominant (fibrous or osseous) or mucopolysaccharide-dominant (chondroid or myxoid). A signet-ring fat cell represents the end result of internal product storage rather than export, that is, accumulation of cytoplasmic fat, a process that begins as multiple small vacuoles. The structure and function of some fully modulated mesenchymal cells can change with altered systemic or local influences in the realms of metabolic, mechanical (e.g., trauma, friction, etc.), and/or circulatory (increased arterial flow vs. venous congestion) factors. Initially in this process, regression leads to spindle or round cells that can be easily mistaken for fibroblasts or lymphocytes. This is followed by cytoplasmic reorganization and acquisition, making possible new functions. Also, more than one modulational potential may be seen in mesenchymal tumors as they grow (e.g., Figs. 34-8 and 34-9).

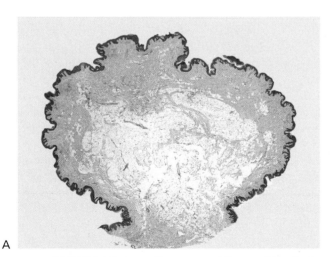

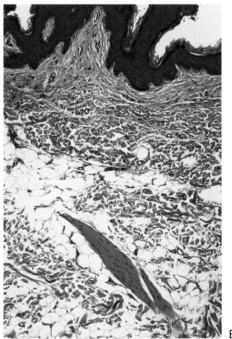

A   B

FIGURE 34-2. Nevus lipomatosus (45-year-old male, 2-cm lesion from buttock). **A:** A polypoidal projection of crenated epidermis has a fatty core. **B:** Mature signet-ring fat cells displace dermal collagen. A pilar muscle is surrounded by lesional fat.

as high as the papillary dermis (Fig. 34-2B). The proportion of fatty tissue varies greatly, from more than 50% of the dermis to less than 10%. In cases with only small deposits, the fat cells are apt to be situated in small foci around the subpapillary vessels. In instances with relatively large amounts of fat, the fat lobules are irregularly distributed throughout the dermis, and the boundary between the dermis and the hypoderm is ill-defined or lost. The fat cells may all be mature, but in some instances an occasional small, incompletely lipidized cell may be observed (8).

Aside from the presence of fat cells, the dermis may be entirely normal, but in some instances the density of the collagen bundles, the number of fibroblasts, and the vascularity are greater than in normal skin (7).

Pathogenesis. It is generally agreed that nevus lipomatosus represents, as the name implies, a nevoid anomaly. The ectopic fat cells in the dermis are derived from the perivascular mesenchymal tissue (8). This view has found support in electron microscopic studies of nevus lipomatosus superficialis, which in some instances showed, in the vicinity of capillaries, immature lipocytes containing numerous small lipid droplets and a centrally located nucleus (11,12).

Differential Diagnosis. In focal dermal hypoplasia, fat cells are also present in the dermis, often in close proximity to the epidermis but have concomitant extreme attenuation of collagen (Chapter 6). The rather common presence of fat cells within long-standing intradermal melanocytic nevi represents an involutionary phenomenon rather than an association of a nevus lipomatosus with a melanocytic nevus (Chapter 28) (13).

FOLDED SKIN WITH LIPOMATOUS NEVUS

Newborns, phenotypically likened to the "Michelin tire man" (14,15,16), have prominent skin folds due to excessive symmetric, circumferential folds of skin with underlying nevus lipomatosus affecting neck, forearms, and lower legs, and resolves spontaneously in childhood (16,17). Smooth muscle hamartoma (18) and multiple anomalies may coexist (19).

Histopathology. In some areas, fat lobules extend close to the epidermis, as in nevus lipomatosus superficialis, and surround adnexal structures. In other areas, the dermis is of normal thickness, but excessive amounts of adipose tissue are beneath the dermis and around adnexal structures. Several bands of fibrous tissue penetrate the subcutaneous fat (14).

Differential Diagnosis. Folded skin has also been reported overlying smooth muscle hamartoma (14).

PIEZOGENIC PAPULES

Fat pad thickness and septal integrity are both important to the mechanical characteristics of the heel fat pad (20).

In various diseases (e.g., rheumatoid arthritis and diabetes) and aging, the load-carrying ability of the heel pad is impaired (20). Septal wall fragmentation and increased width is noted in atrophic heel fat pads from patients with peripheral neuropathies (21). Non-neoplastic piezogenic papules due to the herniation of fat into the dermis present as multiple small papulonodules on the heels (22) or wrist (23) with or without pain. They tend to retract when unburdened and can be seen in the Ehlers–Danlos syndrome, possibly due to structural defects in the connective tissue with resultant poor compartmentalization of the fat (24).

Histopathology. The normally small fat compartments in lower dermis and subcutis coalesce due to loss of thin fibrous septations (23,25).

Differential Diagnosis. In bilateral congenital adipose plantar nodules (or congenital fibrolipomatous hamartoma) (26), well-defined lobules of mature fat occur in mid and deep dermis, mostly around adnexa (27).

LIPOMAS

Common lipomas consist of mature fat cells throughout (Fig. 34-3) and are the most common neoplasms of mesenchyme. Most lipomas (98%) occur as single or multiple subcutaneous growths that are soft, rounded or lobulated, and movable against the overlying skin. They often grow insidiously, displaying an initial growth phase followed by a period of quiescence. They come to clinical attention only if they reach inordinate size (Fig. 34-3A) or are perceived as blemishes in need of cosmetic removal. Approximately 6% of all cases are multifocal. The patient commonly presents with an asymptomatic, slow-growing round mass having a gelatinous or cystic consistency. Well-circumscribed lipomas are easily "shelled out" and only rarely regrow, generally when initially incompletely encapsulated or infiltrative. Deep-seated variants of ordinary lipomas tend to be less well circumscribed than their superficial counterparts, often sending out pseudopod-like processes within fascial planes, engulfing aponeuroses, and potentially compressing local structures. Large and even giant (28) size, rapid growth, deep location, fixation, pain, and thigh or retroperitoneal location are features that suggest the wisdom of preoperative radiographic characterization and a cautious surgical approach to exclude a more significant lesion.

Some lipomas are characterized by specific clinical presentation and location. A deep variant on the forehead (29) (Fig. 34-3B) is a rather common dermatologic specimen. *Perineural lipoma* involves the median nerve in nine of ten cases, and may be associated with macrodactyly. *Lumbosacral lipomas* frequently occur in conjunction with spina bifida and intraspinal lipoma. *Lipomas of tendon sheath and joint synovium* are centered on the named structures. *Diffuse articular lipomatosis (lipoma arborescens)* is a papillomatous synovial tumor with a tendency for repeated regrowth.

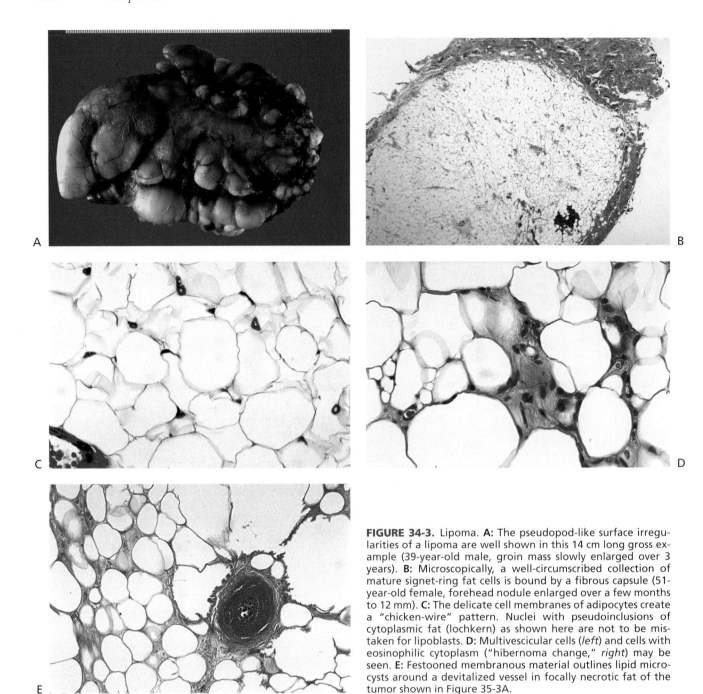

FIGURE 34-3. Lipoma. **A:** The pseudopod-like surface irregularities of a lipoma are well shown in this 14 cm long gross example (39-year-old male, groin mass slowly enlarged over 3 years). **B:** Microscopically, a well-circumscribed collection of mature signet-ring fat cells is bound by a fibrous capsule (51-year-old female, forehead nodule enlarged over a few months to 12 mm). **C:** The delicate cell membranes of adipocytes create a "chicken-wire" pattern. Nuclei with pseudoinclusions of cytoplasmic fat (lochkern) as shown here are not to be mistaken for lipoblasts. **D:** Multivescicular cells (*left*) and cells with eosinophilic cytoplasm ("hibernoma change," *right*) may be seen. **E:** Festooned membranous material outlines lipid microcysts around a devitalized vessel in focally necrotic fat of the tumor shown in Figure 35-3A.

Inter- and intra-muscular lipomas infiltrate muscle and tend to recur unless completely excised (30). *Myolipomas of soft tissue* are rarely subcutaneous (31). *Angiomyolipomas* are best known in the kidney. *Cutaneous angiomyolipoma* is rare, occurs in mainly middle-aged men (mean age, 53 years), and presents as a single, painless, subcutaneous nodule on an extremity (32). Here they are independent of tuberous sclerosis and of pulmonary lymphangiomyomatosis that can accompany the renal lesion. The *adenolipoma* is a dermal or subcutaneous variant of the common lipoma that does not deviate appreciably in presentation or gross appearance but microscopically has inclusions of sweat gland apparatus (33). Instances of malignant transformation of ordinary lipomas are anecdotal at best. *Atypical lipoma* is discussed in the section on liposarcoma.

In two rare conditions, multiple lipomas composed of mature fat cells arise in adult life. These conditions are *adiposis dolorosa* (Dercum's disease), in which there are tender, circumscribed or diffuse fatty deposits (34) with a predilection for the lower legs, abdomen, and buttocks (35, 36). In *multiple or benign symmetric lipomatosis (Madelung's disease)*, lipomas are present especially in the back, upper trunk, and neck in a "horse-collar" distribution (37–40). *Familial multiple lipomatosis* has hundreds of slow-growing subcutaneous (forearm, trunk and thigh) masses and deep or visceral lipomas that appear in the third decade (41,42). This and Dercum's disease can be inherited as an autosomal dominant trait. The *Bannayan–Zonana syndrome* is the congenital combination of multiple lipomas, including lipomas in body cavities in some instances, hemangiomas, and macrocephaly. *Diffuse lipomatosis* features infiltrating masses of mature adipose tissue in part of an extremity or trunk before age 2 years, possibly with concurrent tuberous sclerosis (43). *Nevus psiloliparus* (44) is the cutaneous component of subcutaneous scalp lipomas with overlying alopecia in *encephalocraniocutaneous lipomatosis* (45). Similarly hamartomatous, *infiltrating lipoma of the face* (46) is another variant of it. A thickened and soft scalp that may present as alopecia, *lipedematous scalp*, is a thickening of the subcutaneous fat of the scalp (47). Multiple lipomas and hemangiomas occur in *Cowden's syndrome. Fröhlich's syndrome* exhibits multiple lipomas, obesity, and sexual infantilism. The *Proteus syndrome* features multiple lipomatous lesions, including pelvic lipomatosis and fibroplasia of the feet and hands, skeletal hypertrophy, exostoses and scoliosis, and pigmented skin lesions. Use of protease inhibitors for HIV-1 can be associated with fat abnormalities including subcutaneous lipomas (48), angiolipomas (49), peripheral lipodystrophy, and benign symmetrical lipomatosis (50).

Histopathology. By definition, lipomas contain mature adipocytes as a principal component. They tend to be surrounded by a thin connective tissue capsule and are composed, often entirely, of normal fat cells that are indistinguishable from the fat cells in the subcutaneous tissue (Fig. 34-3C). Occasional "hibernoma-like" cells or multivesicular cells (Fig. 34-3D) around foci of necrosis should not be misinterpreted as lipoblasts, which differ in having coarse vacuoles and irregular nuclei. Membranous fat necrosis is a rare occurrence in lipomas of larger size (Fig. 34-3E) and has the typical staining reactions of ceroid pigment. Traumatic or ischemic causation is postulated (51).

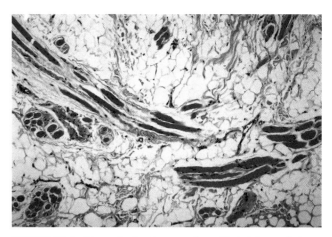

FIGURE 34-5. Normal subcutaneum, face. Skeletal muscle bundles are normally surrounded by mature fat on the face, and this is not to be mistaken for neoplasm.

Intramuscular (infiltrating) lipomas consist of mature fat cells that infiltrate muscle and splay fibers, but show no nuclear atypia (Fig. 34-4). A word of caution: mature fat is normally admixed with facial muscles of expression (Fig. 34-5). In some lipomas, one finds more or less of a connective tissue framework than in the normal subcutaneous fat. Those containing considerable proportions of fibrous connective tissue are called *fibrolipomas* (Fig. 34-6), or *sclerotic lipoma* if a prominent sclerotic stroma is in a storiform arrangement (52). Substantial basophilic mucopolysaccharide may fill regions of the tumor and recommends the term *myxolipoma* (Fig. 34-7). Focal chondroid (Fig. 34-8) and/or osteoid production (Fig. 34-9) have no significance other than underscoring the modulation potential of functional mesenchymal cells.

Myolipomas are comprised of variable amounts of benign smooth muscle and mature adipose tissue. The smooth muscle component of a cutaneous *angiomyolipoma*

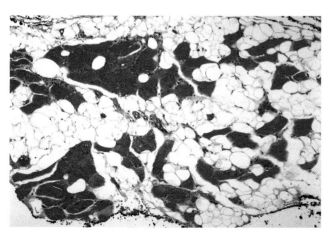

FIGURE 34-4. Intramuscular (infiltrating) lipoma (28-year-old female; 11-month history of a 1.5-cm shin nodule). Mature fat cells splay individual skeletal muscle fibers.

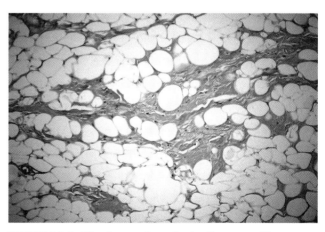

FIGURE 34-6. Fibrolipoma. Strands of collagenous, fibrous connective tissue can be seen within a tumor composed of mature adipocytes. In other cases, the nodule may be predominantly fibrous with little fat.

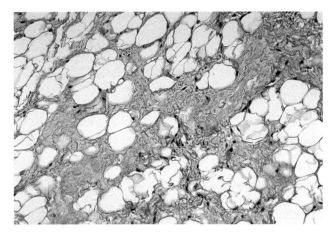

FIGURE 34-7. Myxolipoma (65-year-old female; small dorsal hand mass for 7 years, enlarging in the last several months to 2.8 cm). Basophilic myxoid substance between mature adipocytes is sparsely populated by nonatypical stellate and spindle shaped cells.

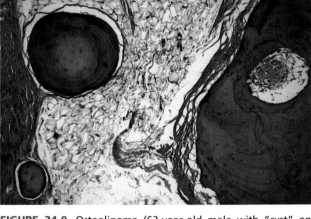

FIGURE 34-9. Osteolipoma (63-year-old male with "cyst" on forehead for many years). Rounded islands of bone are visible within a fibrofatty background in this mass. The largest ossicle (*right*) is undergoing haversianization.

comprised of mature adipose tissue, smooth muscle fascicles, and medium-sized blood vessels (Fig. 34-10) may show pronounced cellular and nuclear pleomorphism and hyperchromatism, as is common in the renal tumor of the same name (53). The distinctive feature of an *adenolipoma* (Fig. 34-11) is an admixture of displaced and distorted sweat glands within the fatty background (33). In *adiposis dolorosa* (Dercum's disease), most authors have found the lipomas to be indistinguishable histologically from ordinary lipomas. In some cases, the histologic appearance is that of an angiolipoma, a tumor that is often painful (see following text). In other cases, granulomas of the foreign-

body type have been noted within the fatty tissue (34). In *benign symmetric lipomatosis* (Madelung's disease), the lipomas have the histologic appearance characteristic of ordinary lipomas (38).

Efforts to distinguish true adipocyte neoplasms from lipomatous hamartomas and localized overgrowth of fat have been limited by the lack of reproducible markers for adipose neoplasms. Identification of a (12:16) (q13p11) translocation in myxoid liposarcomas, and of a similar translocation in lipomas with breakpoints at 12q14 (54), makes future prospects of resolving these issues of pathogenesis seem bright. For the present, lipomatous tumors are still classified morphologically (Table 34-1).

Differential Diagnosis. Growth pattern and size may suggest well-differentiated liposarcoma, but superficial (dermal or subcutaneous) liposarcomas are extremely rare. Lipomas do not contain diagnostic lipoblasts. This fact and the absence of the characteristic delicate capillary network distinguish lipomas with focal or substantial basophilic mucopolysaccharide from myxoid liposarcomas. Intramuscular (infiltrating) lipoma lacks the lipoblasts of well-differentiated (lipoma-like) liposarcoma, and the lobulation and multiple muscle involvement of the pediatric lipoblastoma. Deeply situated myolipomas can be confused with well-differentiated liposarcomas (31).

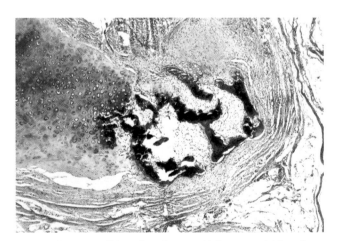

FIGURE 34-8. Ossifying chondromyxoid lipoma. Within a fatty and myxoid background are areas of chondrification (*left*) and ossification (*center*). The contact between the bone and cartilage to the left of center suggests that part of the bone was formed through the enchondral mechanism, analogous to longitudinal bone growth at the growth plate. A portion of the bone has formed directly from the fibrous background (intramembranous ossification). Including fat, this lesion manifests all three directions of modulation outlined in Figure 34-1B.

ANGIOLIPOMA

Angiolipomas usually occur as encapsulated subcutaneous lesions. As a rule, they arise in young adults. The forearm is the single most common location for this tumor, which accounts for 10% of tumors of fat (55,56). Clinically, angiolipomas resemble lipomas, although they have a greater tendency to be multiple. The size of these

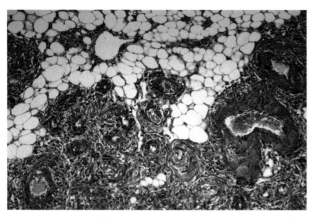
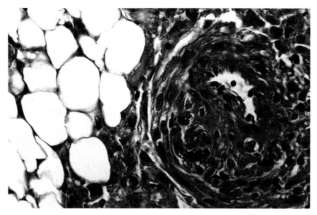

A   B

FIGURE 34-10. Angiomyolipoma. **A:** The basic components of this tumor are mature adipose tissue and thick-walled, medium-sized vascular channels from which sheets of plump, smooth muscle cells appear to be derived. **B:** Plump cells with features of smooth muscle appear to derive from the wall of a vessel within a fatty background. Moderate pleomorphism of the fatty and smooth muscle components is expected and does not connote malignancy.

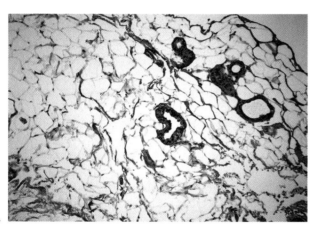
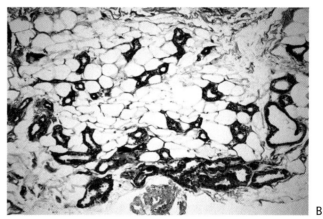

A   B

FIGURE 34-11. Adenolipoma. **A:** Excess mature fat in this medium-magnification view surrounds sweat gland coils and tubules (52-year-old male; 2-cm left neck nodule). **B:** Apocrine glandular elements (*bottom*) can be seen with sweat gland elements in a background of mature fat (62-year-old female; small axillary mass).

TABLE 34-1. BENIGN LIPOMATOUS TUMORS OF SKIN AND SOFT TISSUE

Hamartomas	Adiposis dolorosa (Dercum's disease)
Nevus lipomatosus cutaneous superficialis	Benign symmetric lipomatosis
Folded skin with lipomatous nevus	Familial multiple lipomatosis
Congenital lipomatosis	Pseudosarcomatous benign adipose tumors:
Proteus syndrome	Spindle cell lipoma
Benign neoplasms of white fat	Pleomorphic lipoma
Homogeneous:	Chondroid lipoma
Mature lipoma	Lipoblastoma and lipoblastomatosis
With heterogeneous mesenchymal elements:	Inter- and intra-muscular lipoma
Fibrolipoma	Cervical symmetrical lipomatosis
Myxolipoma	Pelvic lipomatosis
Ossifying lipoma	Diffuse lipomatosis
Angiolipoma	Benign neoplasm of brown fat
Myolipoma	Hibernoma
Angiomyolipoma	
With specific clinicopathogenic settings:	
Perineural lipoma	
Lipoma of tendon sheath and synovium	
Multiple lipoma syndromes	

yellow to yellow-red, circumscribed lesions is from 0.5 to 4.0 cm. They are often tender or painful when pressured or moved (57).

Histopathology. Inapparent at the gross level, angiolipomas microscopically show sharp encapsulation, numerous small-caliber vascular channels containing characteristic microthrombi, and variable amounts of mature adipose tissue (Fig. 34-12). These thrombi are well demonstrated by phosphotungstic acid–hematoxylin staining (58), and are likely artifacts of removal because they show no organization. The degree of vascularity is quite variable, ranging from only a few small angiomatous foci to lesions with a predominance of dense vascular and stromal tissue (57). The angiomatous foci are composed in part of well-formed, dilated capillaries engorged with erythrocytes. Other capillaries appear tortuous and have poorly formed lumina and prominent proliferation of pericytes. Perivascular fibrosis may be prominent. Fat cells are sparse and small vessels predominate in the cellular variant (59). With myxoid stroma, *angiomyxolipoma* (60) can be used. Scattered mast cells are expected. A normal karyotype implies hamartomatous pathogenesis.

Differential Diagnosis. Lesions with prominent perithelial fibrocytes may bring to mind spindle cell lipoma, which, however, lacks the conspicuous capillary channels with fibrin thrombi. Nearly all angiolipomas contain fibrin thrombi within their capillaries, often to a considerable degree. Cellular angiolipomas composed almost entirely of vascular channels and prominent spindle cells are sometimes confused with Kaposi's sarcoma or angiosarcoma. Subcutaneous position, encapsulation, septation, small size, diminutive nonatypical endothelial cells, microthrombi, and clinical presentation in healthy individuals help to exclude a malignant diagnosis (61). The term *infiltrating angiolipoma*, as used by Dionne and Seemayer (62) and by Puig et al. (63) is synonymous with *intramuscular angioma* (64), a vascular tumor with copious mature fat that is not

acknowledged in its name. Its vessels are larger, and this lesion has a significant recurrence rate. *Nodular-cystic fat necrosis*, also called mobile encapsulated lipoma (65), encapsulated angiolipoma, and encapsulated necrosis, can be shifted laterally perhaps several inches and cause pain. They are most often in the elbow or hip subcutis. They have no permanent attachment to a blood supply. Histologically, the fully developed lesions are thinly encapsulated, rounded nodules with well-preserved outlines of nonnucleated adipocytes devoid of inflammation or saponification but may calcify. This entity should be distinguished histologically from lipoma, angiolipoma, panniculitis associated with alpha 1–antitrypsin deficiency, membranous fat necrosis, and pancreatic fat necrosis (66).

SPINDLE CELL LIPOMA

A generally solitary, slow-growing subcutaneous tumor, spindle cell lipoma exhibits a predilection for the posterior neck and shoulder girdle region in men in their fifth to seventh decades. Clinically, the tumor is a slow-growing, painless nodule centered in the dermis or subcutis and measuring from 1 to 13 cm. This tumor does not recur or metastasize. Cytogenetics finds monosomy 16 or partial loss of 16q, a difference from liposarcoma (67). Abnormalities of chromosome 13 are reported (68).

Histopathology. Although the lesion is well circumscribed, it is seldom encapsulated. It is comprised of mature fat cells and uniform, slender spindle cells within a mucinous matrix (69). Spindle cell lipoma is polymorphous as a result of variations in cellularity, collagen content, and the ratio of spindle cells to mature adipocytes. In some areas, the neoplasm consists of a pure spindle cell population, often arranged in thick bundles, without fat cells. In other areas, the spindle cells are intermingled with scattered groups of mature fat cells (70) (Fig. 34-13).

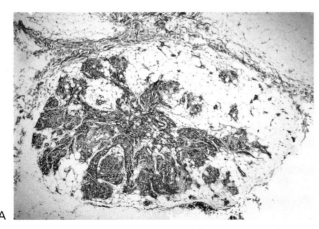
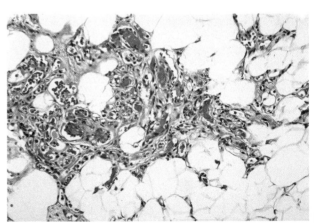

FIGURE 34-12. Angiolipoma. **A:** Prominent vessels radiate through a fibrous background into mature fat (incidental finding in a melanoma resection specimen). Prominent vascularity can impersonate a primary vascular neoplasm. **B:** At higher magnification, fibrin thrombi without organization occur in capillary lumina.

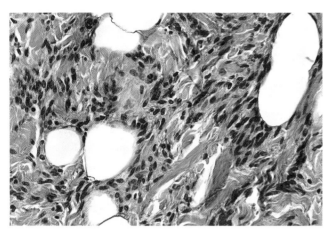

FIGURE 34-13. Spindle cell lipoma (62-year-old male; small back nodule). Uniform collagen-forming spindle cells expand the space between mature fat cells.

The spindle cells, functioning as fibroblasts, produce varying amounts of collagen. If abundant, the diagnosis is fibrous spindle cell lipoma (71). Numerous mast cells are scattered throughout the tumor (70). Some tumors also show a prominent admixture of blood vessels ranging from capillaries to thick-walled vessels containing smooth muscle bundles (72) to prominent sinusoidal channels that divide the tumor into irregular lobules. Irregular branching spaces between villiform, vascularized tumor projections constitute the *pseudoangiomatous* variant (73). Osseous or cartilaginous metaplasia is rare. The spindle cells are positive for CD34 and vimentin but not S-100. Some factor XIIIa–positive stromal cells are present. Ultrastructurally, they have abundant rough endoplasmic reticulum similar to fibroblasts and nonmembrane-bound lipid vacuoles (74). The cytogenetics parallels pleomorphic lipoma with loss of 16q material and less frequently 13q (75).

Differential Diagnosis. Nuclear palisading may be reminiscent of a neural tumor. Myxoid change and hypocellularity may bring myxoma to mind. A prominent hemangiopericytoma-like vascular pattern may be seen or a plexiform vascular pattern that may resemble myxoid liposarcoma. The diagnosis of liposarcoma or fibrosarcoma can usually be excluded without difficulty because of the uniformity of the proliferated spindle cells and the absence of multivacuolated lipoblasts, nuclear atypia or atypical mitotic figures in spindle cell lipoma (69). Larger unvacuolated cells with some atypia, with or without floret giant cells, constitute transitional features to pleomorphic lipoma.

PLEOMORPHIC LIPOMA

Like spindle cell lipomas, the great majority of pleomorphic (giant cell) lipomas are solitary tumors of the shoulder girdle and neck in men in the fifth to seventh decade. The

rare cutaneous spindle lipomas and pleomorphic lipomas, in contrast to subcutaneous forms, are more common in females and have a wider anatomic distribution (6). The lesion presents as a slow-growing, well-circumscribed dermal or subcutaneous mass averaging 5 cm, grossly resembling an ordinary lipoma (76) save for possible gelatinous gray areas on the cut surface. Like spindle cell lipoma, there is loss of chromosome 16q material (67). Despite occasional lipoblast-like cells and atypical mitotic figures, local excision should be curative.

Histopathology. This well-circumscribed tumor displays a wide morphologic spectrum. Although areas of mature fat cells are present, some of them show enlarged, hyperchromatic nuclei (77). In addition, most fat cells show marked variation in size. About half of the tumors contain occasional multivacuolated cells that have the appearance of lipoblasts (76). The mature and immature fat cells are situated singly and in groups in a mucinous stroma traversed by dense collagen bundles. Pseudopapillary structures as in the pseudoangiomatous spindle cell lipoma may be seen (78). A very helpful feature in the diagnosis of pleomorphic lipoma is the presence of characteristic multinucleated giant cells, which are found in most but not all cases (77). These giant cells exhibit, within an eosinophilic cytoplasm, multiple, marginally placed, and often overlapping hyperchromatic nuclei. This peculiar arrangement is not unlike that of the petals of a small flower, and these giant cells are therefore referred to as *floret-type giant cells* (76,79) (Fig. 34-14). Rarely, pleomorphic lipoma histology comprises a sharply demarcated nodule within an otherwise ordinary lipoma. Also, small foci of spindle cell lipoma may be encountered in some pleomorphic lipomas (76). Some pleomorphic lipomas have inflammatory cells, including lymphocytes, plasma cells, mast cells, and occasional histiocytes in a perivascular or diffuse stromal distribution. Mitoses are rare.

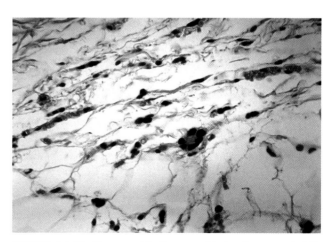

FIGURE 34-14. Pleomorphic lipoma with local regrowth (59-year-old male; interscapular local regrowth that had regained its original size of 9 cm, 8 years after initial surgery). A characteristic floret-type giant cell with multiple peripherally placed nuclei and deeply eosinophilic cytoplasm is near center.

Differential Diagnosis. No single feature confirms the diagnosis of pleomorphic lipoma and excludes liposarcoma. Only a multivariate analysis leads to the correct diagnosis, and such an analysis should consider the age and sex of the patient, anatomic location, size, epicenter of growth (deep or superficial), degree of local invasion, and histologic appearance. Liposarcomas differ from pleomorphic lipomas by their infiltrative growth, greater cellularity, more nuclear atypicality including atypical mitoses, more numerous multivacuolated lipoblasts, prominent necrosis, and absence of thick collagen bundles. Floret-type giant cells are rarely seen in liposarcomas, and then only in small numbers (76).

CHONDROID LIPOMA

Chondroid lipoma is an uncommon firm, yellow tumor, averaging 3 to 5 cm, generally encountered in adults, comprised of vacuolated fat cells similar to brown fat in a chondro-mucinous stroma. Based on 20 cases (80), the age range is 14 to 70 years with a 4:1 female predominance and predilection for the limbs and limb girdles. These nonpainful masses of weeks or years duration range from 1.5 to 11 cm in diameter, with a median of 4 cm. Perhaps half of these well-demarcated, encapsulated, yellow-to-white or gray-tan masses are in the subcutis or involve the superficial fascia of the skeletal muscle (Figs. 34-15A and B). The remaining masses are more deeply situated, possibly within muscles. The lower extremity is the most common location. This lesion, almost invariably mistaken for a sarcoma, especially myxoid liposarcoma or myxoid chondrosarcoma (80), is nonaggressive, and has a benign clinical course without local regrowth or metastases in the original 12 cases with follow-up (80). A three-way translocation between chromosomes 1, 2, and 5, together with an 11;16 translocation with a breakpoint in 11q13, are reported (81).

Histopathology. In chondroid lipoma, a variable background of mature adipose tissue is associated with a predominant, partially fibrinous to hyalinized myxoid matrix (Fig. 34-15C). Within this matrix are nests, strands, and sheets of eosinophilic and vacuolated cells, which contain glycogen and fat droplets, resembling brown fat cells, lipoblasts, and chondroblasts. The eosinophilic cells frequently contain one or several clear lipid vacuoles and an appearance similar or indistinguishable from lipoblasts. Vacuolated cell forms (hibernoma-like cells) simulate lipoblasts or chondroblasts. These cells lack pleomorphism and mitoses and adopt a lacunar appearance when surrounded by the prominent myxoid or hyalin matrix (Fig. 34-15D). The characteristic reaction panel is positivity for S100 protein, CD68, and KP1. Chondroid lipoma can be diagnosed by fine-needle aspiration biopsy (82), but more confidently in cell-block sections where immunochemistry and special stains can be brought to bear (83). The sulfated stroma is strongly metachromatic with toluidine blue at pH 4.0, Alcian blue-positive, hyaluronidase resistant, and aldehyde fuchsin-positive at pH 1.7.

Differential Diagnosis. The differential diagnosis includes primarily extraskeletal myxoid chondrosarcoma (where myxoid matrix obscures the mature fatty component), soft tissue chondroma (mainly hands and feet), myxoid liposarcoma, hyaline variant of chondroid syringoma and occasionally, myoepithelial tumors. The plexiform, capillary-like vasculature and myxoid matrix allow recognition of myxoid liposarcoma (80).

Pathogenesis. Electron microscopy reveals that the tumor cells have abundant intracytoplasmic lipid and glycogen, and also numerous pinocytotic vesicles characteristic of adipocytes rather than chondroblasts. This favors the view

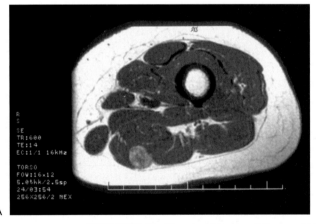
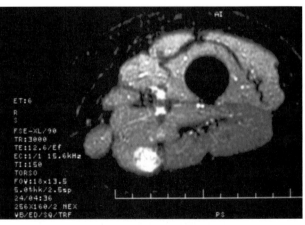

FIGURE 34-15. Chondroid lipoma (60-year-old female; 6-month history of posterior leg nodule). **A:** A T1-weighted MRI image of proximal thigh reveals a well-demarcated intramuscular mass with areas of high and low to intermediate signal consistent with fat. **B:** In a STIR image, the foci of high T1 signal suppression indicates fat. Much of it has high signal consistent with increased water content (myxoid) and cartilage. *(continued)*

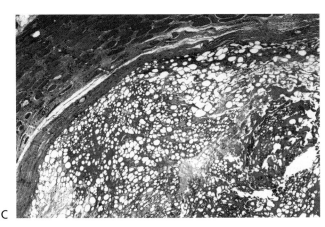

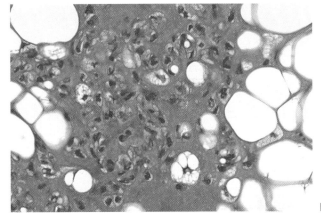

C   D

FIGURE 34-15. (continued) C: Chondroid lipoma is a lobular, well-circumscribed tumor comprised of strands and nests of rounded or polygonal eosinophilic cells in a stroma of mature fat, myxoid and chondroid material, and partly hyalinized fibrous tissue. **D:** The eosinophilic tumor cells have lipid vacuoles and grossly simulate lipoblasts. They contain neutral fat and glycogen and stain positively with oil red O and PAS stains. They are positive for vimentin and S-100 protein.

that chondroid lipoma is a tumor of pure white adipocytes with a hyalinized extracellular matrix that resembles cartilage under light microscopy (84). Another view is that the cells have features of embryonal fat and embryonal cartilage (85). Female predominance raises the possibility of hormonal factors in pathogenesis (80).

HIBERNOMA

Hibernoma (86) is a rare, benign soft tissue tumor. As of 1998, approximately 110 cases of hibernomas were in the world's literature (87). Hibernomas may appear in childhood and slowly increase in size (42), but occur chiefly in adults, with a peak incidence during the third decade of life, on average considerably younger than those with ordinary (mature) lipoma. This rare tumor arises most frequently at the few sites in which brown fat is encountered in adults, such as in the subcutis of the shoulder girdle, posterior neck, axilla (88), and mediastinum (89). Vestigial remnants of brown adipose tissue are the proposed origin (87). But some hibernomas occur at more unusual sites, such as abdomen (90), retroperitoneum (91), thigh (92,93), popliteal fossa, neck (94), chest wall, inguinal area, larynx (95), parotid region (96), mammary (97), and intradural extramedullary spinal (87). The tumor is rarely described in the dermatologic literature because locations where a dermatologist would likely be consulted, such as scalp (98) or forehead (99), are of virtually unique incidence. Clinically, hibernomas are indistinguishable from common lipomas. They are slow growing and painless, typically occurring in subcutis or rarely in muscle, and often noted several years before excision. Although usually asymptomatic, they are occasionally tender (99). Overlying skin may have increased warmth (100). This benign, moderately firm, solitary, subcutaneous,

tan or red-brown tumor is generally from 5 to 10 cm diameter, although examples up to 20 cm have been reported. The CT and MRI findings are "almost the same as those of other lipomatous tumors" (87) (Fig. 34-16A), and the MRI may "resemble liposarcoma" (93). On gross cross-section, the well-circumscribed, somewhat lobulated mass varies from tan to a deep red-brown. The distinct brown color of the gross cut surface (Fig. 34-16B) is due to prominent vascularity and a profusion of mitochondria in the granular tumor cells. Adequate treatment consists of complete excision (98, 101,102), sparing vital structures "with meticulous hemostasis" (93). Like lipomas, hibernomas have little tendency to recur locally after excision, although continued enlargement has been reported after 70% removal of an 11-cm infraclavicular tumor (103). A malignant counterpart of hibernoma (104) remains speculative.

Histopathology. Histologic examination reveals that the tumor is divided into numerous lobules by well-vascularized connective tissue (Fig. 34-16C). In contrast to ordinary lipoma of white fat, the highly vascular nature of the tumor is readily apparent in most sections. Constituent cells resemble those of brown fat tissue, which is present in the human fetus and newborn infants, but gradually diminishes in quantity throughout adult life (91). The tumor cells are round or polygonal and are closely apposed to one another within the lobules (Fig. 34-16D). Three principal types of cells (105) in varying proportions can be recognized: (a) a small cell (average, 37 microns) with granular, eosinophilic cytoplasm and with or without rare, multiple small oil-red O-positive lipid droplets and centrally placed nuclei and distinct cellular membranes; (b) a larger, multivacuolated fat cell (average, 54 microns) with scanty granular, eosinophilic cytoplasm, referred to as a mulberry cell; and (c) a still larger, univacuolated fat cell (average, 64 microns) with peripherally placed nucleus, variably present, and perhaps

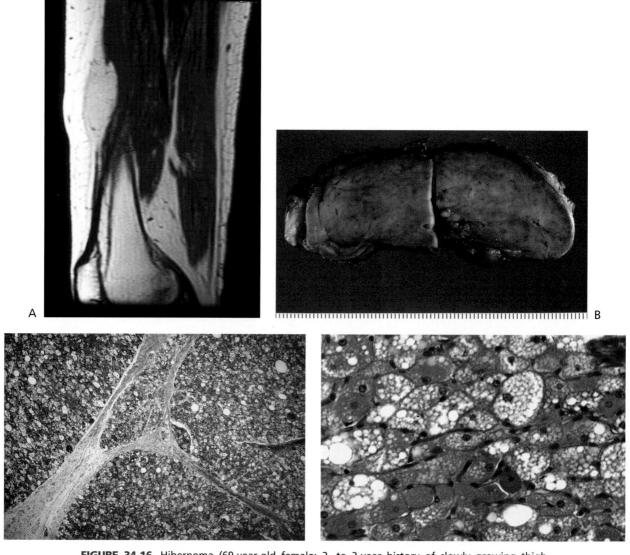

FIGURE 34-16. Hibernoma (69-year-old female; 2- to 3-year history of slowly growing thigh mass). **A:** A longitudinal MRI of the thigh discloses a fusiform tumor between subcutaneous fat and muscle with less T1 signal than mature fat. **B:** The characteristic brown color of this hibernoma contrasts with the pale yellow color of attached pericapsular white fat on each end of it. It results from the prominent vascularity and many mitochondria in tumor cells. **C:** A low-magnification view displays the distinct lobular pattern characteristic of hibernoma. **D:** At higher magnification, hibernoma cells show varying degrees of complete modulation to signet-ring fat cells. These cells range from uniform round to oval granular eosinophilic cells to multivacuolated cells with multiple small oil-red, O-positive lipid droplets and centrally placed nuclei, to intermixed univacuolar cells with one or more large lipid droplets and peripherally placed nuclei (lipocytes).

predominating, making distinction from ordinary lipoma difficult. The nuclei of the granular and multivacuolated cells are usually centrally located; and the nuclei of the univacuolated fat cells are peripheral. Cells of the three principal types, with transitional forms, usually are dispersed randomly throughout the lobules. In most tumors, multivacuolated "mulberry cells" predominate. Some tumors, however, contain a few lobules, particularly at their peripheries, that are composed entirely of univacuolated cells (90). The vacuoles in both the multivacuolated and univacuolated cells stain positively with Sudan black (106). Nuclear pleomor-

phism or hyperchromatism and lobate nuclei are rarely seen (104) and mitoses are absent.

Ultrastructure: Each tumor cell is invested by a basal lamina. There is an inverse relationship between lipid droplet size and the number of mitochondria per unit of cytoplasm that conspicuously lacks membrane systems. Pleomorphic mitochondria have dense matrices and transverse lamellar cristae, micropinocytotic vesicles, and periodic short plasmalemmal densities (105).

Pathogenesis. The term *hibernoma* reflects the fact that these tumors are composed of cells that resemble the brown fat of hibernating animals. The incomplete modulation of the mulberry cells may be attributable to underdevelopment of enzyme systems (106). Like many other benign lipomatous tumors, hibernoma has a characteristic cytogenetic abnormality, specifically, abnormalities of the long arm of chromosome 11 (11q13–21) (107) and 10q22 (108).

Differential Diagnosis. Hibernomas are to be distinguished from granular cell tumors that have no lipid vacuoles, and also from certain forms of round cell liposarcoma that usually contain diagnostic multivacuolar lipoblasts. The larger, univacuolated fat cell may predominate, making distinction from ordinary lipoma difficult.

LIPOFIBROMATOSIS

Lipofibromatosis is a rare pediatric neoplasm that has been variously interpreted as a type of infantile or juvenile fibromatosis, a variant of fibrous hamartoma of infancy, and a fibrosing lipoblastoma. Although it is likely that this tumor comprises part of the spectrum of what has been referred to in the literature as infantile/juvenile fibromatosis, its clinicopathologic features and, in particular, its distinctive tendency to contain fat as an integral component, warrant separate classification as a "lipofibromatosis." Males predominate two to one. The patients present with a soft tissue mass from 1 to 7 cm involving the hand, arm, leg, foot, trunk, or head that may be evident at birth. Histologically, adipose tissue has a spindled fibroblastic element with focal fascicular growth that typically has limited mitotic activity and chiefly involves the septa of fat and skeletal muscle, generally without extensive architectural effacement of fat as is common with conventional fibromatoses. The primitive nodular fibromyxoid component of fibrous hamartoma of infancy is absent. The fibroblastic element exhibits cytologic atypia and occasional mitoses. Small collections of univacuolated cells are often present at the interface between some of the fibroblastic fascicles and the mature adipocytes. The tumor entraps vessels, nerves, skin adnexa, and skeletal muscle. Focal immunoreactivity is present in some tumors for CD99, CD34, alpha-smooth muscle actin, BCL-2, and less frequently, S-100 protein, muscle actin (HUC 1-1), and EMA. However, no reactivity is detected for desmin (D33 and D-ER-1 clones), keratins, or CD57. Follow-up data for 25 individuals (median follow-up period, 6 years, 7 months) found regrowth of the tumor or persistent disease documented in 17 (72%), correlating with congenital onset, male sex, hand and foot location, incomplete excision, and mitotic activity in the fibroblastic element (109).

BENIGN LIPOBLASTOMA

Lipoblastoma and lipoblastomatosis (110) are rare benign neoplasms of fetal white fat that occur almost exclusively in infants and children (111), and typically as a stable or slowly to rapidly enlarging, asymptomatic soft lobular masses in the superficial or deep layers of soft tissue on the trunk or extremities, especially lower (112). Other sites of occurrence include the head, neck, and retroperitoneum, trunk, back, extremities, heel (113), buttock, inguinal canal, scrotum, retroperitoneum, peritoneal cavity, and lung (114). In a child under 3 months of age, images showing a predominantly fatty but inhomogeneous soft-tissue mass are suggestive of lipoblastoma (115). Two basic forms of benign lipoblastoma occur. One, which is a variant called lipoblastomatosis, is deeply situated and poorly circumscribed and tends to grow into the surrounding tissue spaces and musculature (106). The other is relatively superficial and encapsulated (111). Each form commonly presents as a painless nodule or mass, affecting boys twice as frequently as girls. They may cause dysfunction of other organ systems due to mass effect. Lipoblastomas occurring on the back can have intraspinal extension (116). Circumscribed lipoblastoma is more common than diffuse infiltrative lipoblastomatosis. Sizes range from 1 to over 20 cm in greatest dimension.

Complete surgical excision is recommended. Patients with focal lipoblastoma are unlikely to require further surgery after initial resection. Patients with diffuse lipoblastoma (lipoblastomatosis) are likely to have recurrent disease (usually within 2 years) and should undergo close follow-up (117). Cellular maturation has been reported in serial biopsies over time. A "wait-and-see" approach may be justified at least in infants with huge invasive lesions requiring a mutilating excision since complete spontaneous resolution of a diffuse lipoblastoma in the thigh was shown in a 2-day-old male at 1 year by magnetic resonance imaging (118).

Histopathology. Peripheral immature lipoblasts with fat vacuoles of various sizes and central mature fat cells containing single, large, fat vacuoles are characteristic (Fig. 34-17) whether the tumor is deeply or superficially situated. The lipoblasts vary in size. Most of them contain single vac-

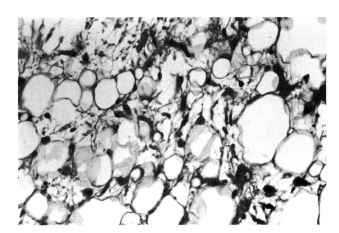

FIGURE 34-17. Lipoblastomatosis. The tumor is comprised of partly differentiated lipoblasts and has a prominent capillary vascular pattern with areas of mucoid matrix. Cells with large hyperchromatic nuclei are absent.

uoles that are variable in size but smaller than those found in mature fat cells. These vacuoles displace the nuclei against the cytoplasmic membrane (106). A few small lipoblasts contain two, three, or occasionally more vacuoles. Some benign lipoblastomas also show lipoblasts with finely vacuolar cytoplasm and centrally placed nuclei resembling hibernoma cells (119). Nonvacuolated cells that are spindle shaped or stellate are observed in the mucinous stroma with a fine vascular network striking similar to myxoid liposarcoma, and from which it may be indistinguishable. Fibrous septa partition lobules in the circumscribed form.

Differential Diagnosis. Only the age of the patient, the abundance of lipoblasts, the absence of atypical mitoses (119), and a sometimes subtle lobularity distinguish it from liposarcoma—especially the myxoid type (120). Although liposarcomas occur very rarely in infants and young children, the distinction may be impossible by light microscopy alone. Therefore, when performing a biopsy of a childhood adipose tumor with unusual features, such as progressive or invasive growth, fresh tissue should be submitted for cell culture. The tumor karyotype will, in most cases, aid in differentiating lipoblastoma from myxoid liposarcoma (121). Rearrangements of the chromosome 8 q11-q13 region are a discriminative marker that distinguishes lipoblastoma and lipoblastomatosis from myxoid liposarcoma (122). FISH can serve as a decisive tool in the differential diagnosis of lipoblastoma and lipoma-like liposarcoma apart from its role in the distinction between lipoblastoma and myxoid/round cell liposarcoma (123). Confusion with typical lipoma may occur. In fact, its early occurrence, ability to mature into a simple lipoma, cellular composition of mainly mature adipocytes, and benign course, suggest that it may more accurately be termed an "infantile lipoma" (124).

LIPOSARCOMA

Liposarcomas, constituting 15% to 20% of all soft tissue sarcomas, are generally deep-seated tumors most likely in the retroperitoneum or the deep soft tissues in or below the buttocks (125). Most commonly, they originate in the intermuscular fascial planes, with a special predilection for the thighs (126). From a fascial plane, they can extend to subcutaneous tissue. Liposarcoma can occur in subcutaneous location and rarely in dermis. As with most other dermal sarcomas, local recurrence is a more frequent problem than distant metastases (127).

Liposarcomas arise as such and for practical purposes do not develop from lipomas. The average age of onset is 50 years. Occasionally, liposarcomas arise in children from 10 to 15 years of age, comprising 4% of childhood soft tissue sarcomas (128), but are exceedingly rare, if not nonexistent, in children younger than 10 years (129). Liposarcomas are slightly more prevalent in males and tend to occur on the right side of the body more commonly than on the left. Infrequently, liposarcomas may be multicentric.

Four major types of liposarcomas are generally recognized and have epidemiologic and prognostic differences: (a) well differentiated, (b) myxoid, (c) round cell, and (d) pleomorphic (126,130). In some tumors, more than one type can be recognized. Myxoid variants are more common in the young, whereas well-differentiated and pleomorphic subtypes are more often encountered in older patients. The well-differentiated and myxoid types have better prognoses than the round cell and pleomorphic types (131).

Well-differentiated liposarcomas are further divided into three closely related subtypes: (a) "lipoma-like," (b) inflammatory, and (c) sclerosing. Well-differentiated liposarcomas are low grade and may regrow locally but do not metastasize. The clinical outcome of well-differentiated lipoma-like liposarcoma is best predicted by anatomic location (132). In the subcutis they are usually cured by local excision, rarely regrow, and do not metastasize. Therefore, the term atypical lipoma has been introduced for the subcutaneous form of well-differentiated liposarcoma (133). This is the form of liposarcoma most likely to be biopsied by the dermatologist. Because of this benign course, Evans (134) has suggested an even less committal designation for this neoplasm: atypical lipomatous tumor. It has been recommended that this term be restricted to subcutaneous tumors, especially those of small size with minimal atypical changes, and the term "well-differentiated liposarcoma" for the same histology at other sites (135).

For the more aggressive liposarcomas, circumscription of the lesion may offer false hope of eradication by simply shelling out the tumor. In reality, liposarcomas extend microscopic pseudopod-like extensions that commonly insinuate between fascial planes. Occasionally, small satellite nodules become separated from the lobulated sarcomatous mass, leading to an erroneous impression of multicentricity. Biopsy and resection should be carefully planned, guided by MRI and radiographic findings in a manner that eliminates prior biopsy tracts and any plane potentially contaminated by surgical exposure or spreading hematoma. The depth of atypical and malignant neoplasms showing lipomatous differentiation correlates with the tendency for local recurrence, which is particularly unlikely in subcutaneous locations (132).

Metastases are common, especially in round cell and pleomorphic liposarcomas where increased numbers of mitoses, in either the primary tumor or a local recurrence, predict metastases (132). Lungs and liver are the most common sites. Myxoid and round cell liposarcoma sarcoma have marked propensity to involve intra-abdominal sites, as well as other soft tissue areas (especially the neck) and bone. Therefore, abdominal CT and bone scan are recommended in the initial evaluation and follow-up of high-risk patients with larger, locally recurrent or high-grade tumors of any size (125). Myxoid liposarcoma metastasizes preferentially to serosal surfaces, such as the pleura, pericardium, and pelvic sidewall. If found in a trunk biopsy, an occult primary tumor in an extremity should be sought (136).

Histopathology. Liposarcoma is diagnosed only when there is convincing evidence of synthesis and storage of fat by the tumor cells (125), the hallmark of which is the lipoblast. For a cell to be designated as a lipoblast, it must show the ability to synthesize and accumulate non–membrane-bound lipid in the cytoplasmic matrix. Acceptable malignant lipoblasts are quite variable because they may recapitulate any stage in the normal maturation sequence. Their common morphologic denominator is well-demarcated cytoplasmic lipid that displaces or indents one or more irregular hyperchromatic nuclei. The nucleus conforms to the contours of the lipid droplet, creating an apparent delicate scalloping of the nuclear membrane. Hyperchromaticity and variability from lipoblast to lipoblast support a malignant diagnosis. Despite these criteria, the distinction between malignant lipoblast and "atypical lipocyte" is at times subjective, especially in the more well-differentiated, lipoma-like variants of liposarcoma. A "true" lipoblast is defined not only by a multivacuolated or univacuolated fat cell with indented or scalloped nucleus, but also by its histologic context (80). Benign fat necrosis, myxoid changes in structural fat, lipogranulomas, lymphomas with signet-ring changes, and carcinomas can contain vacuolated cells that mimic lipoblasts. Lesions such as pleomorphic lipomas and lipoblastomas illustrate that even unequivocal lipoblasts do not always signal malignancy.

The cells of liposarcoma bear a close resemblance to different stages in the development of fat and are found in variable proportions as a function of histologic subtype, but show a much greater individual variability.

In *well-differentiated lipoma-like liposarcoma,* the tumor is composed predominantly of univacuolated fat cells of various sizes. The nuclei of the fat cells are slightly pleomorphic, and some of them are hyperchromatic. *Atypical lipoma* histologically features distended fat cells that vary slightly in size and shape, with occasional interspersed lipoblasts. Broad, fibrous septa-containing cells with enlarged hyperchromatic atypical nuclei are a characteristic feature (Fig. 34-18). Foci of well-differentiated smooth muscle may be found but do not influence the behavior (137). The emergence of a high-grade sarcoma pattern within a well-differentiated liposarcoma or in recurrence is known by the biologically imprecise term "dedifferentiation" and is limited for practical purposes to these tumors when they are located in body spaces, especially retroperitoneum (138).

Myxoid liposarcoma (Fig. 34-19) is the most common type of liposarcoma and display various quantities of four elements: (a) proliferating lipoblasts, (b) delicate plexiform capillaries, (c) myxoid matrix, and (d) acid mucopolysaccharide lakes (Fig. 34-19A). Mitotic figures are conspicuously absent. These tumors have been subdivided into a well-differentiated type with little tendency to metastasize and a poorly differentiated type that commonly metastasizes (126). A well-differentiated myxoid liposarcoma contains, in addition to lipoblasts with spindle-shaped nuclei and several lipid vacuoles, more highly differentiated fat cells, such as so-called *signet-ring* cells (Fig. 34-19B), which have single large vacuoles occupying a major portion of the cytoplasm, and even mature fat cells. The tumor cells are arranged loosely in a myxoid stroma. In a poorly differentiated myxoid liposarcoma, the spindle-shaped lipoblasts have large, atypical nuclei and usually only small numbers of lipid droplets. Depending

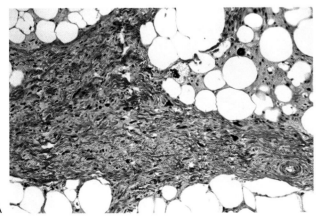

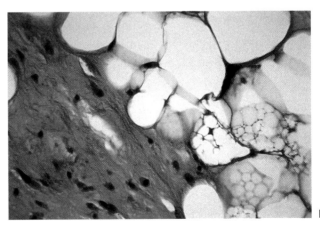

FIGURE 34-18. Well-differentiated lipoma-like liposarcoma (atypical lipoma). **A:** A broad, fibrous septum containing cells with atypical hyperchromatic nuclei partitions a tumor of fat-filled rounded cells, some of which are lipoblasts. (Courtesy of Andrew E. Rosenberg.) **B:** A higher magnification shows hyperchromatic nuclei in the fibrous septum and a dark-staining triangular lipoblast nucleus in adjacent fat (compare to Figure 34-3C and D). Prolonged searching may be required to find enlarged, irregular, hyperchromatic nuclei, some indented by clear lipid vacuoles, in atypical lipoma.

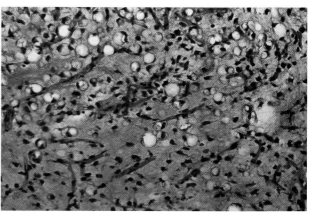

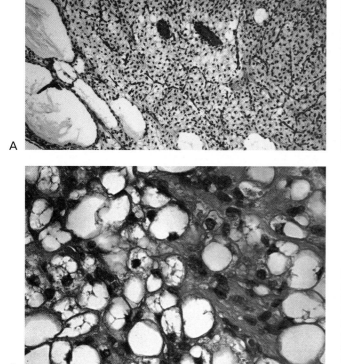

FIGURE 34-19. Myxoid liposarcoma. **A:** Angular hyperchromatic nuclei of densely packed lipoblasts might be mistaken for stellate cells of a myxoma. Pooling of myxoid material may result in a cribriform or lacelike pattern (*lower left*). **B:** Variously lipidized tumor cells occur in an abundant myxoid background and are served by a plexiform capillary network of vessels with thinner walls than in a myxofibrosarcoma (myxoid malignant fibrous histiocytoma). **C:** Lipoblasts are in varying stages of cytoplasmic lipid accumulation.

on the amount of myxoid stroma, there is considerable resemblance to either a myxosarcoma or an undifferentiated fibrosarcoma, because the latter may also have a certain amount of myxoid stroma.

Because of the more aggressive behavior of *round cell liposarcoma*, accurate diagnosis is important. As indicated by its name, round cell liposarcoma is characterized by an excessive proliferation of uniform, closely packed, rounded or oval cells, some of which contain no lipid. Others contain only small cytoplasmic vacuoles or a thin rim of clear cytoplasm (Fig. 34-20). These cells are vaguely reminiscent of Ewing's sarcoma (and, similarly, may contain glycogen), malignant lymphoma, or small-cell anaplastic carcinoma. Their association with other patterns of liposarcoma points to their liposarcomatous nature. Multivacuolated lipoblasts are few in number. Most tumor cells have hyperchromatic and atypical nuclei, with frequent mitoses. This tumor can be thought of as a less differentiated modification of liposarcoma in which the cells are largely incapable of lipid accumulation. At least focal transition toward the myxoid variant, or, less frequently, a well-differentiated or pleomorphic subtype, is always present. As previously indicated, these transitions are central to the correct diagnosis of round cell liposarcoma.

Myxoid and round cell liposarcoma account for about 30% to 35% of all liposarcomas and, even if still classified by the World Health Organization as two distinct subtypes, share both clinical and morphologic features. Lesions combining both patterns are frequent and wide agreement exists in considering round cell liposarcoma as the high-grade counterpart of myxoid liposarcoma. Furthermore, myxoid and round cell liposarcoma share the same characteristic

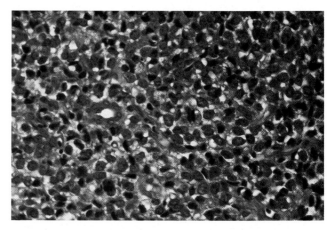

FIGURE 34-20. Round cell liposarcoma. Small, dark-staining tumor cells have little or no lipid accumulation. Because glycogen is involved in lipogenesis, these cells are PAS-positive, and this should not be taken as evidence for Ewing's sarcoma.

chromosome change represented most frequently by a reciprocal translocation t(12;16)(q13;p11) that fuses the chop gene with the TLS gene (139). Clinically, myxoid and round cell liposarcoma tend to occur in the limbs with a peak incidence ranging between the third and the fifth decade. In general, when more than 25% of the cellular elements are round cells, the diagnosis of round cell liposarcoma should be made. However, a >5% round cell component in a myxoid liposarcoma portends a higher risk of metastasis or death from disease (140). A peculiar tendency to metastasize to the soft tissue is observed that should not be interpreted as multicentricity (139).

Pleomorphic liposarcoma, an unlikely prebiopsy diagnosis (141), is characterized by a disorderly growth pattern, an extreme degree of cellular pleomorphism and bizarre giant cells. Two histologic variants of pleomorphic liposarcoma have been described. The majority of pleomorphic liposarcomas display limited numbers of lipoblasts admixed with smaller, polygonal, round or spindle-shaped cells with eosinophilic cytoplasm. Mitotic figures are usually rare. In any given microscopic field lacking a lipoblast, the separation of this entity from the pleomorphic storiform variant of malignant fibrous histiocytoma is difficult if not impossible. A less common variant contains giant lipoblasts. These extremely large cells have numerous cytoplasmic lipid droplets of variable size (Fig. 34-21). Multinucleation and amphophilia of the cytoplasm causes these cells to have the appearance of atypical mulberry cells, so that the tumor is suggestive of a malignant hibernoma. No myogenic (skeletal or smooth) ultrastructural features and vimentin positivity but nonreactivity for desmin or alpha-smooth muscle actin are expected (142).

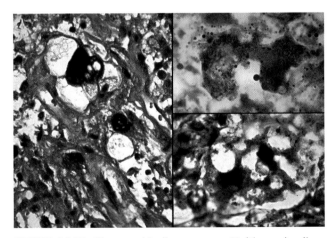

FIGURE 34-21. Pleomorphic liposarcoma. Multivacuolar lipoblasts have large, irregular hyperchromatic nuclei (*left panel*). The cytoplasmic lipid content of lipoblasts (lost in routine processing) can be demonstrated by frozen sections on fresh (*top right*) or formalin-fixed (*bottom right*) tissues stained with oil red O.

A subtype of pleomorphic liposarcoma is known by the pathobiologically imprecise designation, "dedifferentiated" liposarcoma. A peculiar biology is displayed that at least in most cases show neither "anaplasia" nor "dedifferentiation," but "transdifferentiation" of part of the neoplastic cells to a cellular phenotype of a different mesenchymal differentiation lineage (143). A well-differentiated (lipoma-like) or myxoid liposarcoma (144) component has superimposed nonlipogenic areas resembling high-grade fibrosarcoma or malignant fibrous histiocytoma with the full range of potential patterns from storiform pleomorphic and myxoid to the less common giant cell and inflammatory forms. Less common are undifferentiated large round cells resembling carcinoma or melanoma, meningothelial-like whorls (145, 146) or myofibroblastic, rhabdomyosarcomatous, leiomyosarcomatous, even osteoblastic differentiation. The interface between the two zones is usually abrupt.

The histologic subgroups of pleomorphic liposarcoma have not been shown to have prognostic value, perhaps because of the limited number of cases available for study. Its karyotype is complex (147). DNA flow analysis shows benign and low-grade liposarcomas to be diploid, and high-grade tumors to be generally aneuploid, regardless of histologic subtype (148).

Differential Diagnosis. A poorly differentiated myxoid liposarcoma may contain very little lipid material. A lipid stain then often aids in the diagnosis. The demonstration of neutral lipid in cells with special stains (e.g., Sudan black, oil red O) on frozen sections of tumor tissue is insufficient for a diagnosis of liposarcoma unless lipoblasts are also found. Many other mesenchymal tumors and some carcinomas (e.g., of kidney and adrenal) routinely contain fat, as do tumors injured by ischemia or radiation. The differential diagnosis of myxoid liposarcoma includes benign lesions, such as myxoid spindle cell lipoma, intramuscular myxoma and lipoblastoma, and malignant ones such as low-grade myxofibrosarcoma (a.k.a. myxoid malignant fibrous histiocytoma) and extraskeletal myxoid chondrosarcoma.

The main utility of immunohistochemistry in the diagnosis of liposarcoma is one of exclusion, because no specific or useful immunohistochemical marker has been found for malignant fatty tumors. Immunohistochemistry can be quite helpful in revealing the true identities of various sarcomas that may contain vacuolated bizarre cells, such as malignant schwannoma (S-100 protein), rhabdomyosarcoma (myoglobin), and leiomyosarcoma (desmin). But smooth muscle and even rhabdomyosarcomatous differentiation (149) can be found in primary liposarcoma. Alpha-1-antitrypsin and alpha-1-antichymotrypsin can be demonstrated in malignant fibrous histiocytoma (MFH) regardless of subtype, and are constant and diagnostically useful characteristics. However, these markers may also be present in other spindle-cell malignant tumors. By electron microscopy, cytoplasmic lipid is not membrane bound in liposarcoma, unlike in MFH (125).

TUMORS OF SMOOTH MUSCLE

Smooth muscle in the skin serves as the substrate for tumors, and consists of arrector pili muscles, mural muscle of blood vessels, and specialized muscle in genital sites, that is, scrotum (dartos), vulva, and nipple (areolar).

SMOOTH MUSCLE HAMARTOMA

Smooth muscle hamartoma usually presents as a single patch several centimeters in diameter, on extremities or trunk, most commonly in the lumbar region and rarely scrotal (150). It may be present at birth or may arise in childhood or early adulthood (151). Typically, there are small, follicular papules throughout the patch, although the entire lesion may be slightly elevated and/or linear (152). Transient elevation (pseudo-Darier sign) can often be elicited on rubbing (153,154). Associated vermiform movements are rarely seen, suggesting that the lesion is acting as an innervated functional (although abnormal) unit (151). The patch shows hyperpigmentation and hypertrichosis in some patients (155,156), but not in others (157). If hyperpigmentation and hypertrichosis are present, an association with Becker's melanosis (Chapter 28) exists (158). These two entities represent different poles of the same developmental spectrum of hamartomatous change (156). There is no known associated systemic involvement beyond being a potential component of the "Michelin tire syndrome" (see above) or malignant transformation (151). Induration, hyperpigmentation, and localized hypertrichosis diminish with time (159).

Histopathology. Numerous thick, long, straight, well-defined bundles of smooth muscle fibers are scattered throughout the dermis and extend in various directions (Fig. 34-22) without the circumscription of a cutaneous leiomyoma. Smooth muscle bundles can be readily distinguished from collagen bundles by the Masson trichrome stain, which stains smooth muscle red, and collagen green or blue. The overlying basal layer is often pigmented and above that, hyperkeratosis and papillomatosis (151). Hypertrichosis, if present, is due to increased hair shaft diameter and length, not increased hair density (151); some of the smooth muscle bundles show connections with large hair follicles (155,158).

Differential Diagnosis. The arrangement of the smooth muscle bundles in the dermis differs from that observed in piloleiomyoma, in which the smooth muscle bundles form a large aggregate.

Pathogenesis. In fetal life, hair muscles originate in a diffuse metachromatic zone of the mesoderm, near but not part of the fibroepithelial hair germ. Overproduction in these pilar fields may lead to stable hamartomatous overgrowths or progressive neoplasms (160). Intermediate lesions support the hypothesis that congenital smooth mus-

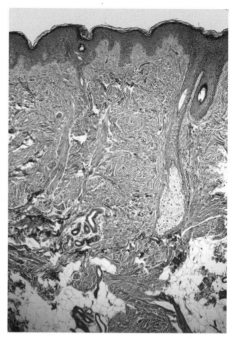

FIGURE 34-22. Smooth muscle hamartoma. Numerous thick, long, straight, well-defined bundles of smooth muscle fibers extend in various directions throughout the dermis.

cle hamartoma is one end of a spectrum of dermal smooth muscle proliferative disorders with Becker melanosis at the other end. However, the former is present at birth and the latter acquired beginning in the first or second decade with hyperpigmentation preceding hypertrichosis (151).

LEIOMYOMA

Five types of leiomyomas of the skin include (a) multiple piloleiomyomas and (b) solitary piloleiomyomas, both arising from arrectores pilorum muscles; (c) solitary genital leiomyomas, arising from the dartoic, vulvar, or mammillary muscles; (d) solitary angioleiomyomas, arising from the muscles of veins; and (e) leiomyomas with additional mesenchymal elements.

Multiple piloleiomyomas, by far are the most common type of leiomyoma, are small, firm, red or brown intradermal nodules arranged in a group or in a linear pattern, primarily affecting the trunk and extremities, but may occur on the face and neck and rarely in the mouth (161). Lesions may run into the hundreds, or cluster to form plaques, zosteriform groups, or in symmetrical distribution (162,163) (nevus leiomyomatosus systematicus) (164). Often, two or more areas are affected. Usually, but not always, the lesions are tender and give rise to occasional painful paroxysms (160). Pain can be spontaneous or triggered by exposure to cold, pressure, trauma, or emotion (161). Uterine leiomyomas (165–167) or erythropoietic activity (161) are rare associations. When multiple, excision of larger lesions and analgesics for pain, even oral nitroglycerin, phenoxybenzamine, nifedipine, and calcium channel-blocking drugs can be tried, either alone or in combination (161).

Solitary piloleiomyomas (168,169) are intradermal nodules that are usually larger than those of multiple piloleiomyomas, measuring up to 2 cm in diameter. Females predominate. Congenital occurrence is rare (166). Most of them are tender and also occasionally painful (170). Simple excision may suffice for one or a few lesions (161). Genital leiomyomas originate from the dartoic, vulvar, or mammary smooth muscle (171,172).

Solitary genital leiomyomas are located on the scrotum, the labia majora (173,174) or, rarely, nipples (173). Supernumerary breasts (polymastia) and supernumerary nipples (polythelia areolaris) are not uncommon along the course of the embryologic milk line. This extends from the anterior axillary fold to the inner thigh on either side of the midline. Supernumerary breast tissue (173) or aberrant areolae (172) located outside the milk line are extraordinary. Genital leiomyomas are intradermal and, in contrast to the other leiomyomas, most are asymptomatic (170).

Solitary angioleiomyomas are usually subcutaneous and only rarely intracutaneous in location. As a rule, they do not exceed 4 cm in diameter. The lower extremities are the most common sites. Pain and tenderness are evoked by most, but not all, angioleiomyomas (160).

The rare *cutaneous angiolipoleiomyoma* is an acquired asymptomatic tumor, always acral. The lesion has a strong male rather than female predilection (175). Unlike the renal counterpart, there is no association with tuberosclerosis. Recurrence after surgery is not anticipated.

Histopathology. Piloleiomyomas, whether multiple or solitary, and genital leiomyomas are similar in histologic appearance (170). They are poorly demarcated and are composed of interlacing bundles of smooth muscle fibers with which varying amounts of collagen bundles are intermingled (Fig. 34-23). The muscle fibers composing the smooth muscle bundles are generally straight, with little or no waviness; they contain centrally located, thin, very long, blunt-edged, "eel-like" nuclei. Hair follicles may persist in the lesion (176). Rare variants show granular (177) or clear cell (178) change. Pleomorphic multinucleated tumor giant cells can occur in cutaneous "symplastic" leiomyomas

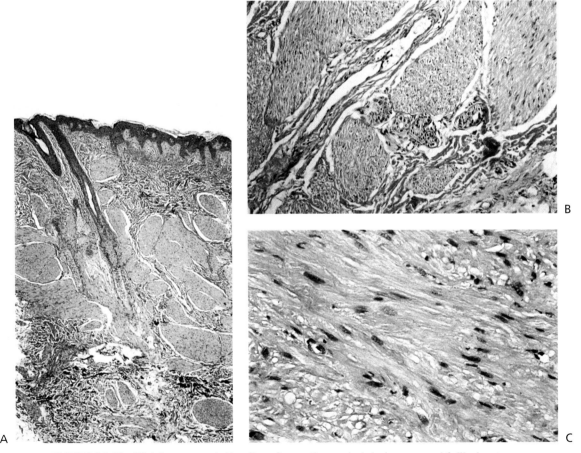

FIGURE 34-23. Piloleiomyoma. **A:** Bundles of smooth muscle interlace around follicular structures in the dermis. **B:** Well-defined smooth muscle bundles resembling pilar muscles surround sweat gland coils. **C:** Benign smooth muscle cells have some variation in nuclear size and chromaticity, blunt nuclear ends, and no conspicuous mitotic activity.

and pleomorphic angioleiomyoma, but more commonly in the uterus (179,180). Vulval leiomyomas express estrogen and progesterone receptors, unlike pilar tumors (181).

Angioleiomyomas differ from the other types of leiomyomas in that they are encapsulated and contain numerous vessels (Fig. 34-24). As a rule, they contain only small amounts of collagen. The numerous veins that are present vary in size and have muscular walls of varying thickness. On this basis, angioleiomyomas have been subdivided into a capillary or solid type, a cavernous type, and a venous type (182). In the capillary type, the vascular channels are numerous but small. Tumors of the cavernous type are composed of dilated vascular channels with small amounts of smooth muscle. Tumors of the venous type exhibit veins with thick muscular walls. In venous tumors, smooth muscle cells extend tangentially from the peripheries of the veins and merge with the intervascular tumor substance (Fig. 34-24B). The veins usually have a rounded or slit-like lumen, but some, because of contraction of their muscular tissue, have a stellate lumen. The veins have no elastic lamina. Areas of mucinous alteration are often present, especially in large angioleiomyomas. The smooth muscle may exhibit pleomorphism (182). An intravascular variant is rare (183).

Lipoleiomyomas comprise long, intersecting bundles of bland, smooth muscle mixed with the additional mesenchymal element of nests of mature fat cells (184).

Cutaneous angiolipoleiomyoma (Fig. 34-25) could arguably be considered an angioleiomyoma with fat cell modulation. However, elastic laminae completely or par-tially rim the vascular channels. These subcutaneous, well-circumscribed tumors are composed of benign smooth muscle, vascular spaces, connective tissue, and mature fat that may predominate. Masson trichrome will separate the muscular from fibrous components that are invariably present. The smooth muscle cells have a more mature fascicular arrangement than in the renal analog. Blood vessels in these subcutaneous well-circumscribed tumors intermittently have an elastic lamina (Fig. 34-25C) (175). Cutaneous angiolipoleiomyomas are unreactive for HMB-45, in contrast to renal and extrarenal angiomyolipoma (175, 177,185) yet have been reported under the term angiomyolipoma (185,186).

The muscle bundles of various leiomyoma variants stain pink with hematoxylin-eosin, just as collagen does, but can be distinguished from collagen bundles by the following differences in appearance. The nuclei of the fibroblasts located in the collagen are shorter than the nuclei located in the smooth muscle fibers and show tapering at their ends whereas smooth muscle nuclei tend to have blunt ends; the cytoplasm of the smooth muscle cell is more conspicuous than in quiescent fibroblasts. In contrast to collagen bundles, smooth muscle bundles usually show slight vacuolization, especially in cross-sections, as a result of a perinuclear clear zone. Reliable differentiation between muscle and collagen bundles is possible with the aid of one of the collagen stains, such as the aniline blue stain or the trichrome stain. With the aniline blue stain, muscle stains red and collagen blue; with the trichrome

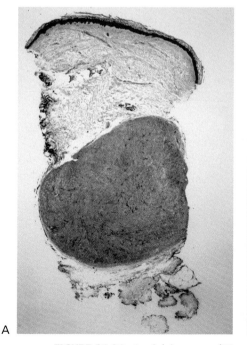
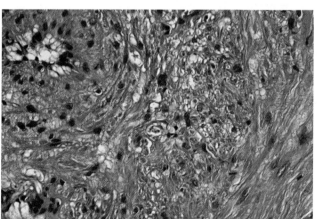

FIGURE 34-24. Angioleiomyoma (44-year-old female; firm, tender, 4-mm leg nodule). **A:** A low-magnification view shows the well-circumscribed border of a nodule at the dermal-subcutaneous boundary. **B:** At high magnification, the blood vessel walls are continuous with the benign smooth muscle cells comprising the tumor substance.

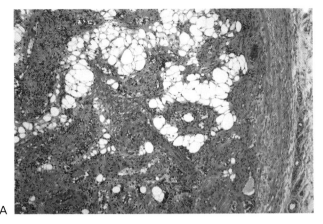

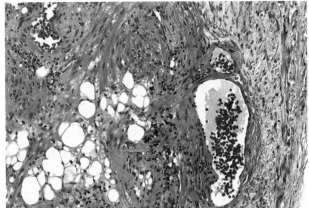

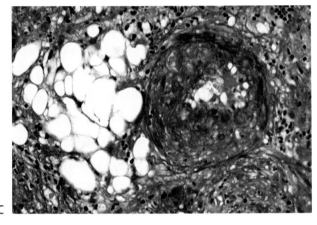

FIGURE 34-25. Angiolipoleiomyoma (51-year-old male; non-painful 1.5-cm knee "cyst" present 10 years but enlarging). **A:** A well-circumscribed subcutaneous nodule has prominent vascular spaces, redundant smooth muscle and much mature fat. **B:** The smooth muscle cells have a fascicular arrangement. **C:** Elastic lamina partly rim a representative vascular channel (elastic tissue stain).

stain, muscle stains dark red and collagen green or blue. The Masson technique is superior to Gomori's. Longitudinal intracytoplasmic myofibrils often can be visualized as striations in H&E sections and can be more easily resolved if stained with phosphotungstic acid–hematoxylin, where they appear as purple threads.

Differential Diagnosis. The discrete bundles set in dermal collagen of smooth muscle hamartoma are unlike the circumscription of most cutaneous leiomyomas and the scant intralesional collagen common in the multiple papular variant of pilar leiomyoma (187). The differential diagnosis of angiolipoleiomyoma includes angiolipoma with fibrosis (lacks muscle on Masson trichrome), angioleiomyoma (usually lacks elastic laminae and has female predominance), arteriovenous hemangioma (but it is uncircumscribed and without a fibrous pseudocapsule, fascicles of smooth muscle and intermixed lipocytes), and even cavernous hemangioma (but with larger vascular spaces having thinner walls and no surrounding fascicles of smooth muscle or fibrous pseudocapsule) (175). The histologic differential diagnosis of lesions with an intravascular growth pattern includes intravascular angioleiomyoma, intravascular pyogenic granuloma, papillary endothelial hyperplasia, reactive angioendotheliomatosis, intravascular nodular fasciitis, hemangiopericytoma, and intravascular glomus tumor (183). *Palisaded angioleiomyoma,* a histopathologic variant

of angioleiomyoma with prominent Verocay body formation, should be added to the ever-expanding list of tumors that demonstrate nuclear palisades along with neurilemoma, but immunohistochemistry gives positive reactions for actin and desmin and is negative for S-100 (188).

Pathogenesis. Arrectores pilorum gives rise to smooth muscle tumors. Electron microscopic examination has shown that piloleiomyomas are composed of normal-appearing smooth muscle cells. Each of these cells has a central nucleus surrounded by an area containing endoplasmic reticulum and mitochondria and, peripheral to this area, numerous myofilaments arranged in bundles. Both cytoplasmic and marginal dense bodies are present. The cause of the frequent pain or tenderness has not been satisfactorily determined. Some authors have observed, by electron microscopy, ultrastructural damage to nerve fibers through distortion and disruption of the myelin sheath (189) and only scanty unmyelinated nerve fibers (190) are postulated factors. It is probable, therefore, that the pain is a result of muscular contractions. Familial cases of multiple piloleiomyomas have been reported in autosomal dominant–incomplete penetrance mode (161). Since cutaneous leiomyomas show no positive staining for er-1d5 or pgr-1a6 antibodies, the tumorigenesis of cutaneous leiomyomas does not appear to be related to estrogen or progesterone receptor–mediated effects (181).

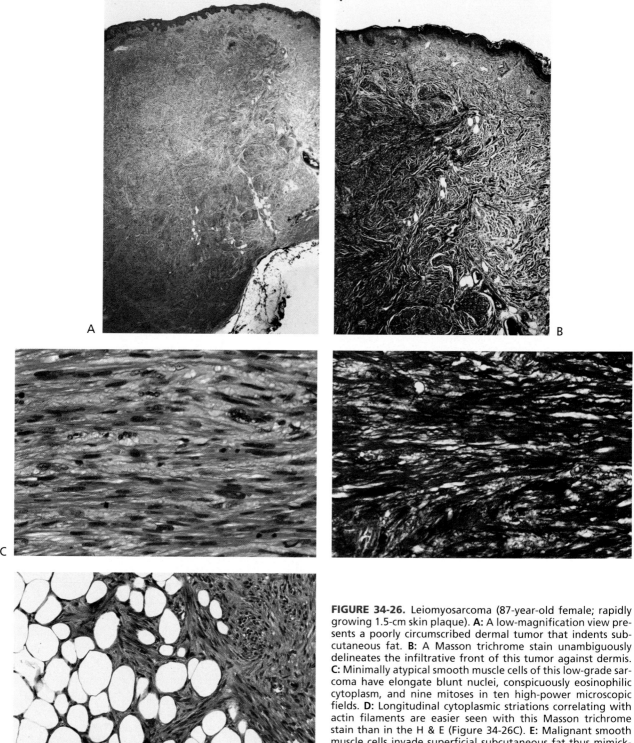

FIGURE 34-26. Leiomyosarcoma (87-year-old female; rapidly growing 1.5-cm skin plaque). **A:** A low-magnification view presents a poorly circumscribed dermal tumor that indents subcutaneous fat. **B:** A Masson trichrome stain unambiguously delineates the infiltrative front of this tumor against dermis. **C:** Minimally atypical smooth muscle cells of this low-grade sarcoma have elongate blunt nuclei, conspicuously eosinophilic cytoplasm, and nine mitoses in ten high-power microscopic fields. **D:** Longitudinal cytoplasmic striations correlating with actin filaments are easier seen with this Masson trichrome stain than in the H & E (Figure 34-26C). **E:** Malignant smooth muscle cells invade superficial subcutaneous fat thus mimicking dermatofibrosarcoma protuberans, but have elliptical rather than discoidal nuclei and bipolar eosinophilic cytoplasmic extensions.

LEIOMYOSARCOMA

Leiomyosarcomas, malignant nonepithelial tumors with smooth muscle differentiation, are generally deemed derived from mural smooth muscle cells of vessels or in viscera such as uterus or stomach, the urogenital system or in the retroperitoneal space. Leiomyosarcomas of the dermis and subcutaneous tissues are rare, accounting for less than 5% of all soft tissue sarcomas in adults. In 1992, fewer than 125 cases of cutaneous and subcutaneous leiomyosarcoma could be found in the English-language literature (191). Superficial leiomyosarcomas are most common in the fifth and sixth decades; reports differ as to whether there is (192) or is not (193) male predominance.

Cutaneous leiomyosarcomas (Fig. 34-26) exhibit a predilection for proximal extremity extensor surface location (194), which coincide with the areas of greatest hair distribution. They are believed to derive from the erector pili muscles, smooth muscle that surrounds sweat glands in the nearby adipose tissue or from vessel walls (193). Clinically, a solitary red-pink nodule may be painful or tender (160), but only rarely ulcerates. In some cases, several nodules are present (195), but this should arouse suspicion of metastases, for example, from a retroperitoneal, uterine, or alimentary tract primary (196), which favor the scalp and back. Leiomyosarcoma has been reported in an ectopic areola (197). Radiation dermatitis, trauma, lupus vulgaris (198), and origin in an angioleiomyoma (199) are other associations for leiomyosarcoma.

Subcutaneous leiomyosarcomas (200) are deemed to be vascular in origin and analogous to angioleiomyomas. Radiation dermatitis may be a substrate (198). They are subcutaneous nodules or diffuse swellings over which the nondiscolored skin usually is freely movable. They cause pain of a local or radiating nature in only a few patients. Wide surgical excision of leiomyosarcoma with close follow-up is recommended (193) since local recurrence is common (40% to 60%), with inadequate excision as the presumed risk factor (191). They are relatively radioresistant, according to a small number of treated cases (192,201).

The division of superficial leiomyosarcoma into two distinctly different histogenetic and prognostic categories (cutaneous and subcutaneous) (202) is more significant in predicting metastatic potential than is mitotic activity (192). Cutaneous leiomyosarcomas have a good prognosis. When confined to the dermis, the sarcoma may recur in up to half of all cases. Metastases to regional lymph nodes may occur, but they are not usually fatal (191). In at least one reported instance, however, distant metastases ultimately led to the death of the patient (196). Subcutaneous leiomyosarcomas are more aggressive, exhibiting higher growth rate, greater recurrence (40% to 60%), metastatic potential (30% to 60%), and ultimately fatal outcome (30% to 40%) than their cutaneous counterparts (191). Subcutaneous leiomyosarcoma may cause hematogenous metastases, usually to the lungs (192), but only rarely to lymph nodes (203,204) and lead to death in about one-third of the patients (192). Aneuploid tumors are more prone to metastasize than diploid tumors (205).

Purely subcutaneous leiomyosarcomas must be differentiated from leiomyosarcomas involving skeletal muscle or fascia that can present as a skin or subcutaneous tumor (Fig. 34-27) and are often fatal (206,207). In assessing depth, remember that subcutaneous leiomyosarcoma may invade the dermis and that cutaneous leiomyosarcoma generally is contained within the dermis, although larger lesions may extend into the adjacent subcutis and epidermis (191). MRI may be helpful in the distinction (Fig. 34-27A).

Vulvar and scrotal leiomyosarcomas tend to be larger and better circumscribed than those in skin or subcutaneous locations. Their traditional inclusion under the general heading of cutaneous leiomyosarcoma has been challenged (202,206).

Histopathology. Cutaneous leiomyosarcomas (Fig. 34-26) vary from moderately well to poorly delimited, nodular or diffuse (208) intradermal tumors that may extend into the subcutaneous tissue. In the center, the tumor shows nodular aggregates and densely packed, interlacing bundles of smooth muscle cells. At the margin of the tumor, strands of smooth muscle cells extend between collagen bundles. Cutaneous leiomyosarcomas, with their fascicular, infiltrative, peripheral growth pattern, presumably are derived from arrectores pilorum muscles (192). Minimal criteria for malignancy in a well-differentiated lesion include crowded cellularity, some plump and hyperchromatic nuclei constituting cellular atypia, irregular extension into dermis, and a few mitoses (Fig. 34-25C). Areas of lesser differentiation are present in all tumors, although to varying degrees. They show numerous irregularly shaped, anaplastic nuclei and usually also atypical giant cells with bizarre nuclei (Fig. 34-27B) (192). Still, the nature of the sarcoma usually can be established even in rather anaplastic tumors, because in some areas there are bundles of fairly well-differentiated smooth muscle cells in which delicate myofibrils can be revealed by staining with phosphotungstic acid–hematoxylin (78) or trichrome. Epithelioid leiomyosarcoma, mainly occurring in the uterus, can rarely occur in extremity soft tissue, skin, in superficial veins and venules of skin and in subcutis (209). Granular cell (210) inflammatory (211) and desmoplastic (212) leiomyosarcoma are other rare variants.

The number of mitoses may be high in anaplastic areas even when there will be no metastases (207). A given leiomyosarcoma may have "mitotic hot spots" that might not be represented in single samples (207). Percentage of S-phase cells correlates with mitotic count but, like absence of desmin reactivity, is not predictive of patient survival (205). Although notable mitotic rate remains the main criterion for leiomyosarcoma (e.g., three or more per ten high-power fields) (213), other histopathologic features of the tumor are important, as with uterine leiomyosarcoma

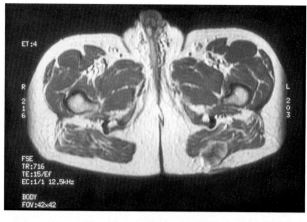

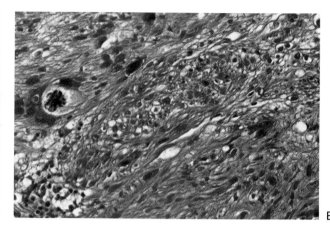

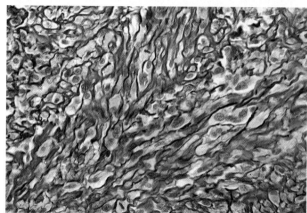

FIGURE 34-27. Intramuscular leiomyosarcoma (45-year-old male; nodule on left buttocks noted upon sitting. No evidence of disease 4 months after removal and local irradiation.) **A:** Two-thirds of an oval 4-cm × 5-cm buttock mass is within skeletal muscle (lower right) favoring its origin there, with secondary extension to subcutaneous fat where a biopsy might be mistaken for a superficial tumor. **B:** Substantial atypia and bizarre mitoses characterize this high grade leiomyosarcoma which manifests brightly eosinophilic cytoplasm. **C:** A delicate reticulin network envelopes each tumor cell (reticulin stain).

(214) including atypical smooth-muscle cells with peripheral extension into the surrounding tissue (195), pleomorphism, giant cells, and necrosis (192). Antidesmin positivity is found in 47% to 85% of superficial leiomyosarcomas, and is less common in higher-grade tumors. For those rare tumors in which routine histology and immunohistochemistry fail to provide a classification, electron microscopy offers another means for diagnosis (205).

Subcutaneous leiomyosarcomas may be well circumscribed and partially surrounded by a compressed rim of connective tissue. Irregular aggregates of more or less atypical smooth muscle cells can be seen intertwining haphazardly without the fascicular pattern characteristic of cutaneous leiomyosarcomas. Subcutaneous leiomyosarcomas show endothelium-lined, thin-walled blood vessels with variously shaped but often large lumina surrounded by smooth muscle cells (192). Vascular invasion is an adverse finding (215). Mitoses should be easily found (207). Osteoclast-like giant cells (216) or myxoid change (217) should not deter diagnosis. No correlation seems to exist between the degree of histologic malignancy of the tumor and metastases, which occur in up to 40% of the cases (206). DNA content, as determined by flow cytometry, was a strong predictor of metastatic potential in one study (205). Involvement of underlying muscular fasciae or skeletal muscle is a likely harbinger of metastases (206).

Pathogenesis. Immunohistochemical staining of deparaffinized sections shows expression of desmin in all cutaneous leiomyosarcomas and of muscle-specific actin in the great majority (196). Only about half of the subcutaneous leiomyosarcomas show significant numbers of tumor cells that are positive for desmin and actin (206). These smooth muscle markers may be demonstrated in "myofibroblastic" lesions and therefore are not absolute diagnostic criteria. Some hold that ultrastructural study is a more reliable means for definite identification. Positivity for cytokeratin may be found and is attributed to "phenotypic shift" in terms of vimentin and cytokeratin expression (218). Losses in the 13q4-21 region are the most frequent abnormality (219).

Electron microscopic examination has shown that the tumor cells have the characteristics of smooth muscle cells even when there is marked nuclear atypicality (207). Thus, the tumor cells show skeins of intermediate filaments punctuated by dense bodies, subplasmalemmal plaques, pinocytotic vesicles, and external pericellular lamina (194, 207). However, in some instances the basal lamina is discontinuous (196).

Differential Diagnosis. The presence of bizarre giant cells in cutaneous leiomyosarcomas may cause a resemblance to malignant fibrous histiocytoma (207) and atypical fibroxanthoma. However, at least in some areas, there are greatly elongated, thin, blunt-ended nuclei characteristic of smooth muscle cells. Also, demonstration of the enhancement of longitudinal striation due to myofibrils by staining with trichrome or phosphotungstic acid–hematoxylin will aid in the distinction. The same holds true for subcutaneous leiomyosarcomas, in which the presence of endothelial-lined vessels may suggest a hemangiopericytoma. The more extended histologic differential diagnosis includes fibrosarcoma, rhabdomyosarcoma, dermatofibroma, dermatofibrosarcoma protuberans, malignant schwannoma, nodular fasciitis, and synovial sarcoma.

RHABDOMYOMATOUS MESENCHYMAL HAMARTOMA OF SKIN (STRIATED MUSCLE HAMARTOMA)

This rare lesion principally occurs in the face and neck of newborns. The typical presentation is as a small, solitary dome-shaped papule or a polypoid pedunculated lesion, from a few millimeters to 1 to 2 cm. There is a strong male predominance.

Histopathology: Single or small groups of mature-appearing skeletal muscle fibers lie in dermis and subcutaneous tissue below normal epidermis. Mature fat, nerves,

and adnexal structures may be admixed and central calcification or ossification may be noted (220).

Differential Diagnosis. Nevus lipomatosus superficialis and fibrous hamartoma of infancy will have fat, but not skeletal muscle fibers. A benign Triton tumor (neuromuscular choristoma), a rare subcutaneous, peripheral nerve-associated lesion, is composed of mature skeletal muscle and neural tissue. A cutaneous embryonal rhabdomyosarcoma will show much less differentiation.

RHABDOMYOMA

Rhabdomyomas are extremely rare benign tumors of striated muscle that are divided into cardiac and extracardiac types, and then further subtyped on the basis of clinical and morphologic differences. *Adult-type rhabdomyomas* are slow-growing lesions that nearly always occur in the head and neck areas of elderly persons (Fig. 34-28). *Fetal-type rhabdomyomas* occur in the head and neck areas of children and adults. *Genital-type rhabdomyomas* are polypoidal tumor masses in the vagina and vulva of middle-aged women.

Histopathology. Adult rhabdomyomas contain cells with cytoplasmic vacuoles due to glycogen content but without easily observable cross-striations on H&E staining (Fig.

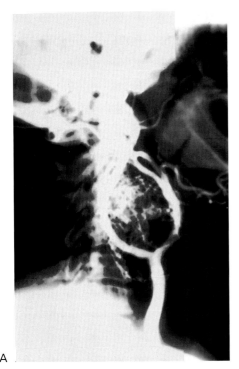
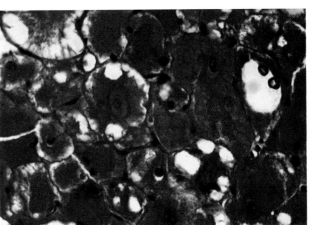

FIGURE 34-28. Adult-type rhabdomyoma (55-year-old male with 4-cm lateral neck mass). **A:** A hypervascular mass splays the carotid bifurcation in this carotid angiogram. **B:** Variably sized, deeply eosinophilic polygonal cells comprising this tumor have peripherally situated nuclei. Cytoplasmic cross-striations may be seen. Tissue processing removes intracellular glycogen and results in the pronounced vacuolated appearance of many of the cells. This lesion should not be mistaken for a granular cell tumor.

34-28B). Residual strands of cytoplasm between the vacuoles define "spider web cells" (221). The *fetal type* consists of immature skeletal muscle fibers. *Genital rhabdomyomas* contain interlacing fascicles or bundles of polymorphous cells, many with cross-striations, bland nuclei, and no mitoses. Immunohistochemical reactions identify positivity for desmin, myoglobin, actin and myosin (222) and possibly weak S-100 staining (223). The tumor cells are surrounded by basement membrane laminin and type IV collagen (224).

Differential Diagnosis. Exclude a supernumerary (225) accessory, or hypertrophic (226) muscle presenting as a tumor-like mass.

RHABDOMYOSARCOMA

Although rare in adults, rhabdomyosarcomas (RMS) are the most common soft tissue sarcomas in children. Most of these tumors are located in intramuscular locations or the genitourinary tract, usually deep to the introitus, most often in the vagina and less so in the vulva and perineum (227). Involvement of the skin is rare (228) and since skele-

tal muscle in skin occurs only in the face, that site is common (229). Only a few RMS present as dermal nodules (230–232). Subcutaneous indurations, congenital rashes (233), or multiple cutaneous metastases have been reported.

Histopathology. RMS often exhibit a low degree of differentiation so that their identification requires immunohistochemical studies (Fig. 34-29B). Only some of these tumors contain cells recognizable as rhabdomyoblasts by virtue of their cytoplasm exhibiting cross-striation that is best revealed by phosphotungstic acid–hematoxylin staining (230). Round cells of the embryonal variant, unlike those of lymphoma, neuroblastoma, trabecular carcinoma, and Ewing's sarcoma, tend to have cytoplasmic rims that are stained red by trichrome (Fig. 34-29C). The botryoid type, a gross, morphologic description meaning grapelike, is a variant of the embryonal type found mainly in mucosa-lined hollow organs, but a few may be encountered in skin-covered surfaces such as the eyelid or the anal region (228). Some tumors show alveolar spaces lined with small, round, dyshesive neoplastic cells, with tumor giant cells floating within these spaces (alveolar RMS) (230,234) (Fig. 34-30A). A mixed form such as embryonal RMS with focal alveolar features is not uncommon, and for staging and prognostic purposes, are classi-

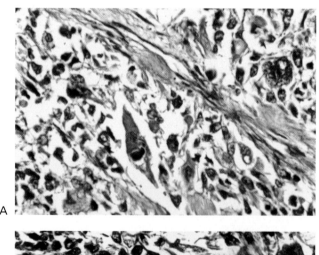

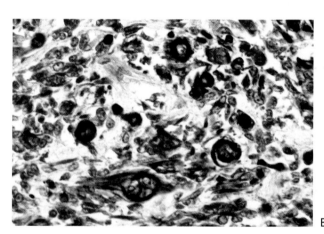

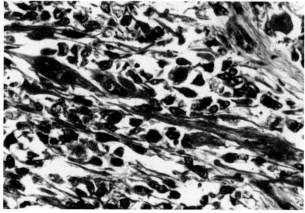

FIGURE 34-29. Embryonal rhabdomyosarcoma (14-year-old male; 3-month history of a mass, ultimately 11-cm × 7-cm, partly cystic and hemorrhagic, mass along the spermatic cord. The patient is disease free three years after removal of the tumor and ipsilateral iliac nodal metastases, plus radiation and chemotherapy.) **A:** Cytologically malignant round and elongate tumor cells occur together. **B:** The tumor cells are reactive for actin (but were negative for desmin) by immunoperoxidase technique. **C:** Myoplasm stains bright red in this Masson trichrome preparation.

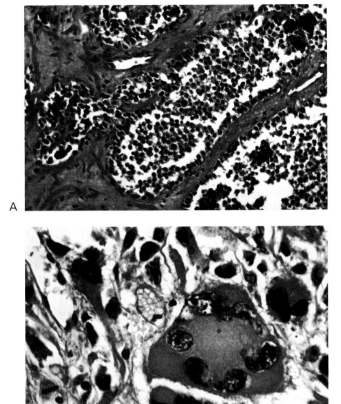

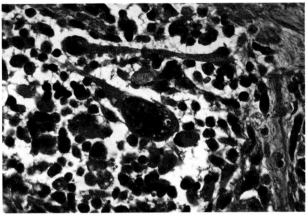

FIGURE 34-30. Other rhabdomyosarcoma variants. **A:** Alveolar rhabdomyosarcoma is comprised of rounded cells with eosinophilic cytoplasmic rims, lining spaces that contain similar or larger tumor cells. **B:** Round, "tadpole," and strap-shaped rhabdomyoblasts occur with atypical mitoses in alveolar rhabdomyosarcoma. **C:** Bizarre tumor giant cells accompany strap cells in pleomorphic rhabdomyosarcoma. The differential diagnosis would include liposarcoma and malignant fibrous histiocytoma.

fied as the alveolar type (228), which has a more aggressive clinical course. Pleomorphic cytologic features may be encountered in pediatric tumors still properly classified as embryonal or alveolar. Cells with elongated eosinophilic cytoplasm, so-called "strap cells," are suggestive but not diagnostic of RMS (234) (Fig. 34-30B), and may be found in the pleomorphic type (Fig. 34-30C). A sclerosing variant has cords of small, round malignant cells embedded in a densely hyalinized matrix having both a chondroid and osteoid-like appearance (235).

Histogenesis. Immunohistochemical studies of deparaffinized tissue may show undifferentiated cells to be positive only for vimentin, indicating a mesenchymal phenotype. More differentiated cells may be positive for desmin and myoglobin, which is indicative of muscular differentiation (230,234).

Differential Diagnosis. In younger patients, poorly differentiated round and spindle cell sarcomas should be excluded. Immunoreactions for muscle markers lack complete specificity. Rhabdomyosarcomatous differentiation can be seen in other sarcomas, such as "dedifferentiated" chondrosarcoma and malignant peripheral nerve sheath (malignant Triton) tumor, and in less expected settings such as Merkel cell (primary neuroendocrine) carcinoma (236). Benign reactive lesions such as proliferative

myositis and skeletal muscle regenerative giant cells in scars must be excluded.

MALIGNANT EXTRARENAL RHABDOID TUMOR

Rhabdoid sarcoma (malignant rhabdoid sarcoma), 2% of renal tumors, is a phenotype characterized histopathology by the presence of eosinophilic cytoplasmic inclusions corresponding to masses of intermediate filaments on electron microscopy, and can arise in subcutaneous sites (237) congenitally or in adults (238). Metastatic skin disease has been reported only in infants (239). The PASD and vimentin positive eosinophilic round cytoplasmic inclusions are negative for muscle-specific antigens. Prognosis is poor (240).

Differential Diagnosis. Carcinomas of various types including Merkel cell carcinoma (241), as well as melanoma (242) and lymphoma (243), may have rhabdoid features.

Pathogenesis. It is arguable whether the rhabdoid phenotype may represent a "final common pathway" that many tumors take in escalating grade and aggressivity (244) or a clinicopathologic entity in its own right. Deletions and/

or translocations of chromosomes 11p15 and 22q11 are found (245).

CUTANEOUS CHONDRO-OSSEOUS LESIONS

Extraskeletal osseous and cartilaginous tumors and tumor-like conditions of the extremities can often be differentiated radiologically; for those that cannot, knowledge of the spectrum of lesions will allow a suitably ordered differential diagnosis. Of the osseous lesions (myositis ossificans, fibro-osseous pseudotumor, fibrodysplasia ossificans progressiva, soft tissue osteoma, and extraskeletal osteosarcoma), all but myositis ossificans are relatively rare. The differential diagnosis for these extraskeletal osseous and cartilaginous lesions includes soft tissue sarcoma, calcified tophi in gout, melorheostosis, pilomatricoma, and tumoral calcinosis (246).

CUTANEOUS OSSIFICATION

Cutaneous bone formation may be primary or secondary. If it is primary, there is no preceding cutaneous lesion; if it is secondary, bone forms through metaplasia within a preexisting lesion. Primary cutaneous ossification can occur in Albright's hereditary osteodystrophy and as osteoma cutis.

Albright's Hereditary Osteodystrophy

In Albright's hereditary osteodystrophy (AHO), first described in 1952 (247), multiple areas of subcutaneous or intracutaneous ossification are often encountered (Fig. 34-31). These areas may be present at birth or may arise later in life. No definite area of predilection seems to exist; areas of ossification have been described on the trunk (248), extremities (249), and scalp. The areas of ossification may be so small as to be hardly perceptible or as large as 5 cm in diameter (250). Those located in the skin may cause ulceration, and bony spicules may be extruded through the ulcer (249). In addition to cutaneous and subcutaneous osteomas, bone formation may be observed in some cases along fascial planes (250).

AHO includes the syndromes of pseudohypoparathyroidism and pseudopseudohypoparathyroidism. Patients with the former condition have hypocalcemia with a failure to respond to parathyroid hormone, whereas patients with the latter syndrome fail to respond to parathyroid hormone but have normal serum calcium values (250). Patients with AHO have short stature, round facies, and multiple skeletal abnormalities, such as curvature of the radius and shortening of some of the metacarpal bones (250). As a result of this shortening, some knuckles are

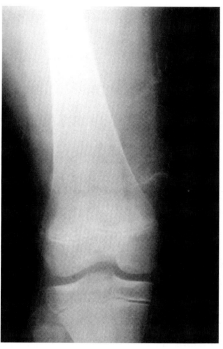

FIGURE 34-31. Heterotopic ossification in pseudohypoparathyroidism. A plain film of a juvenile's thigh features irregular branching spicules and cords of bone in dermis and subcutaneous tissue medial to the femur.

absent when the fists are clenched, and depressions or dimples are apparent there instead (the Albright dimpling sign). Additional manifestations include basal ganglia calcification and mental retardation.

Pathogenesis. An autosomal dominant condition, AHO results from heterozygous inactivation of G(s)alpha, encoded by the GNAS1 locus on the distal long arm of chromosome 20. Small insertions and deletions or point mutations of GNAS1 are found in approximately 80% of patients with AHO. The remainder may be accounted for by larger genomic rearrangements (251).

Histopathology. Spicules of bone of various sizes may be found within the dermis (252) or in the subcutaneous tissue (250). The bone contains fairly numerous osteocytes as well as cement lines that are best revealed with a strong (e.g., Harris) hematoxylin or in polarized light. In addition, osteoblasts with elongated nuclei can usually be seen along the margins of the bone where new bone is being laid down. The osteoblasts that form bone in all forms of primary cutaneous ossification originate in preexisting fibrous connective tissue, and thus their product is termed *intramembranous* rather than *enchondral* bone. Osteoclasts, if present, are cells with multiple large nuclei resembling multinucleated foreign-body giant cells but are distinguished by their attachment to a bone surface. They excavate surface pits called Howship's lacunae into the bone substance as the initial step in remodeling. Osteons with haversian canals containing blood vessels and connective tissue are produced through internal remodeling and indicate the passage of significant time. The spicules of bone may enclose, either partially or completely, areas of mature fat cells (250) that represent the maturation of the lesion with establishment of a medullary cavity. Hematopoietic elements, however, are observed only rarely among the fat cells.

The incidence of cutaneous ossification in AHO is fairly high, estimated at 42% of patients with pseudohypoparathyroidism and in 27% of those with pseudohypoparathyroidism (253). However, the reason for the bone formation is not clear. Because the association of AHO with cutaneous ossification was not recognized until 1965 (254), the question arises as to how many cases of primary cutaneous ossification reported before then occurred in association with AHO. In a review examining this question (252), several cases originally reported as primary osteoma of the skin were recognized as showing evidence of AHO (249). Although the conclusion that most cases of primary osteoma cutis are associated with AHO seems somewhat exaggerated, it is nevertheless apparent that patients with extensive foci of ossification usually have AHO.

Differential Diagnosis. Progressive osseous heteroplasia (POH) is a genetic disorder of mesenchymal differentiation in females characterized by dermal ossification during infancy and progressive heterotopic ossification of cutaneous, subcutaneous, and deep connective tissues during childhood (255). It is clinically distinguishable from AHO and fibrodysplasia (myositis) ossificans progressiva (FOP), which can present as fibrous scalp nodules (256). The initial skin involvement tends to be plaquelike or papulovesicular rash or reddened in duration, with dermal ossification. The disorder can be distinguished from FOP by the presence of cutaneous ossification, the absence of congenital malformations of the skeleton, the absence of inflammatory tumorlike swellings, the asymmetric mosaic distribution of lesions, the absence of predictable regional patterns of heterotopic ossification. Also, in FOP, cartilage production precedes ossification of deeper tissues (enchondral ossification), whereas the predominant pathway of bone formation in POH and AHO is intramembranous. POH can be distinguished from AHO by the progression of heterotopic ossification from skin and subcutaneous tissue into skeletal muscle, the presence of normal endocrine function, and the absence of a distinctive habitus associated with AHO. The genetic basis of POH is unknown; it may lie at one end of a clinical spectrum of ossification disorders mediated by abnormalities in GNAS1 expression and impaired activation of adenylyl cyclase (255).

Osteoma Cutis

The term *osteoma cutis* is applied to cases of primary cutaneous ossification in which there is no evidence of AHO in either the patients or their families. Congenital osteomas occur in Gardner's syndrome and AHO, or in patients presenting with numerous, spontaneous osteoma cutis lesions without systemic manifestations, or disease (257). Multiple miliary osteoma cutis, a disfiguring disorder, can occur unassociated with Albright's heredity osteodystrophy (258). Most commonly, this entity occurs in the face of a young woman with a long history of acne vulgaris. Less noticeable facial osteoma cutis is likely more common than reported since in a series of randomly selected patients with histories of long-term acne vulgaris, three of seven had x-ray evidence of multiple cutaneous opaque deposits on the face (259).

The four groups of patients with osteoma cutis have osteomas limited in extent in all but the first group: (a) patients with widespread osteomas since birth or early life but without evidence of Albright's hereditary osteodystrophy (260); (b) patients with single, large plaquelike osteomas present since birth either in the skin of the scalp (261,262) or in the skin or subcutaneous tissue of an extremity (263); (c) patients with single small osteomas arising in later life in various locations (263); and (d) patients with multiple miliary osteomas of the face. In some instances of the latter, all of them women, the osteomas do not appear until late in life (264). In others, they are observed in young women in association with long-standing acne vulgaris (265,266) and in these, the miliary osteomas have been interpreted as metaplastic ossification within acne scars. However, the absence of acne vulgaris among the patients in the older age group and the presence in one case of miliary osteomas also in the scalp where acne does not occur (264) raise the possibility that the acne vulgaris is coincidental. Large facial lesions can have an oral mucosal manifestation (267).

Histopathology. The histologic findings in osteoma cutis are the same as in primary cutaneous ossification occurring in conjunction with Albright's hereditary osteodystrophy. These small foci of ossification are within the dermis, sometimes demonstrably around extravasated keratin debris (Fig. 34-32A) or hair shafts (Fig. 34-32B), or in the stroma of another lesion such as a melanocytic nevus (Fig. 34-32C and D). They are formed by the activities of flattened osteoblasts that appear to be derived through modulation from dermal fibroblasts (Fig. 34-32E). A minority of the formative cells persists in the osseous product as resident osteocytes. Osteomas undergo a high rate of remodeling (258), enlarging by continued bone application at the surface with eventual central remodeling beginning with osteoclastic erosion (Fig. 34-32F). A circular outline is commonly achieved, with central hollowing that creates a space for fatty marrow, at which time they are at risk for all disorders of genuine skeletal members. In cases with transepidermal elimination, some patients show fragments of bone within channels lined by epidermis and leading to the surface (Figs. 34-32 G and H), and others show such fragments within

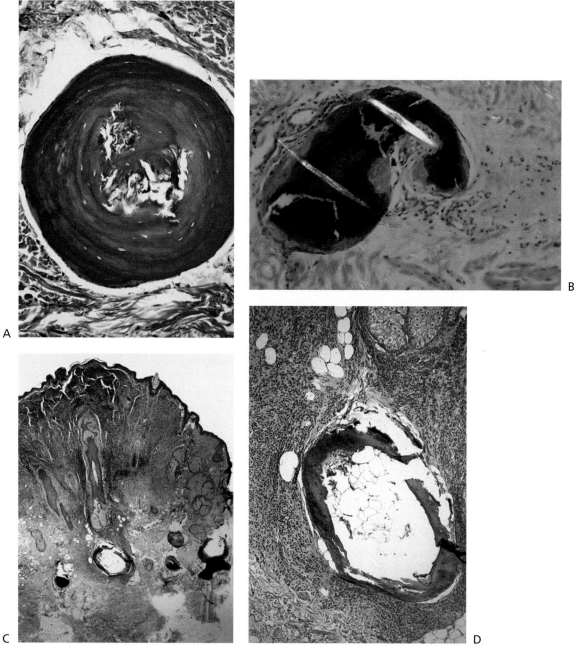

FIGURE 34-32. Osteoma cutis. **A:** A spherical osteoma cutis has resident osteocytes in oval lacunae of its laminations about a central nidus of mature squames (keratin flakes) that were likely extruded from a follicle or cyst (80-year-old female; shoulder). **B:** A polarized light view highlights two hair shafts crossing an irregular osteoma cutis (70-year-old male; mid-back). **C:** Five rounded ossifications are in the base of this compound nevus (44-year-old female; cheek). **D:** Fat is in the central chamber of one of the osteomas shown in Figure 34-32C. *(continued)*

breaks in the epidermis. A sinus tract draining an osteomyelitis or septic joint should enter the differential.

Pathogenesis. Postulation of "embryonal cell nests" or "primitive mesenchymal cells" as the source for the osteoblasts (268) is unnecessary, since in the genesis of osteoma cutis, dermal fibroblasts have the ability to differentiate into osteoblasts. They actively deposit type I collagen, as in mature bone, also constitutes 80% to 85% of collagen in the skin. *In situ* hybridization techniques further indicate that, given appropriate stimulation, indigenous fibroblasts have the ability to modulate into osteoblastic cells (see Fig. 34-1B) that have the same properties as those of

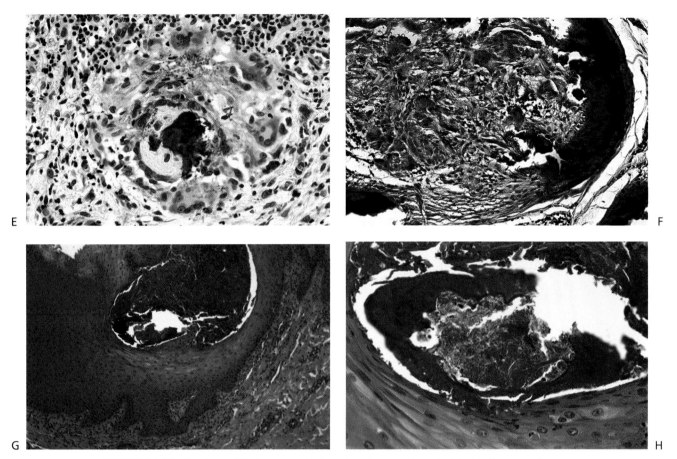

FIGURE 34-32. *(continued)* **E:** A very early stage in osteogenesis is depicted as it occurred upon mineralized debris near ruptured folliculitis (43-year-old male; back). **F:** Exuberant osteoclasia is hollowing out this osteoma that occurred in a nevus (36-year-old female; face). **G:** An epidermal-lined channel is evacuating a small osteoma, no longer in dermis (74-year-old male; toe). **H:** A high-power view of the osteoma from Figure 34-32G depicts osteoclastic erosions (Howship's lacunae) and autolysis of associated inflammatory exudate (osteomyelitis in osteoma cutis).

osteoblasts, such as high-alkaline phosphatase activity and a high expression of osteonectin (269). In multiple miliary osteoma cutis, a dynamic bone study using a tetracycline double-labeling technique demonstrated a high rate of internal remodeling (270).

Metaplastic or Secondary Ossification

This occurs within a preexisting lesion. It may be observed in association with cutaneous tumors, scars, or inflammatory processes. A simple prerequisite seems to be some antecedent relatively rigid substrate.

Histopathology. The tumor that most commonly shows metaplastic ossification is pilomatricoma (calcifying epithelioma of Malherbe) (Chapter 30), in 14% to 20% (263). Calcification of shadow cells attracts osteoclastic giant cells. Osteoclastic erosion of mineralized epithelium is followed by ("coupled to") osteoblastic deposition of osteoid against

remnants of the shadow cell islands. The process is therefore similar to enchondral ossification wherein mineralized cartilage is the inducing factor and can lead to a fat-filled cancellous network with thin cortex resembling a normal rib cross-section. Ossification is also rarely found in basal cell carcinoma, where it takes place usually in the stroma, but sometimes around mineralizing keratin microcysts. Some basal cell carcinomas with ossification are in the nevoid basal cell carcinoma syndrome (271). In intradermal nevi, ossification usually follows folliculitis. In desmoplastic malignant melanoma, fibroplasia may be accompanied by bone formation (272,273). Rare melanomas in which there is osteoid synthesis by S-100–positive tumor cells have been termed "osteogenic melanomas" (274). Ossification may also occur in chondroid syringomas or mixed tumors of the skin by means of the enchondral mechanism. In contrast to metaplastic ossification in association with tumors, metaplastic ossification in scars and in inflammatory processes of

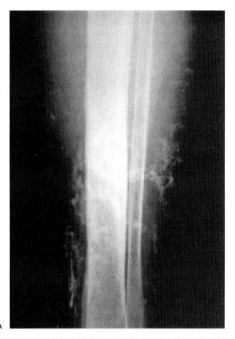

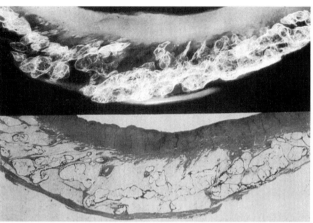

A   B

FIGURE 34-33. Heterotopic subcutaneous ossification associated with chronic venous stasis (60-year-old female with chronic venous stasis of lower legs). **A:** In this plain film radiograph, irregular bony deposits unrelated to veins can be seen in the absence of fat necrosis or abnormal serum calcium or phosphorus. **B:** A specimen radiograph (*top*) correlates well with the large format histologic section (*bottom*) in showing the distribution of irregular lobulated ossific plates in and around subcutaneous fat. The ossification has taken place in interlobular septa. In the histologic view, fibrosis markedly thickens dermis. Thick-walled veins are present in subcutaneous fat (e.g., *left of center*).

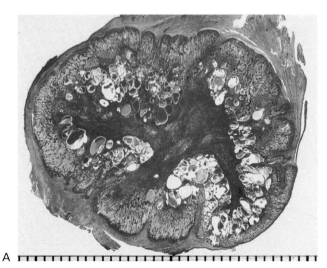

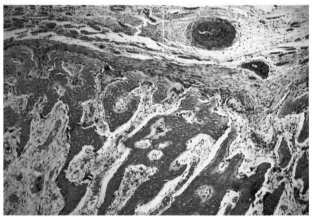

A   B

FIGURE 34-34. Myositis ossificans. **A:** A rounded 3-cm mass has central cellular bands without ossification and cancellous bone forming in the periphery. **B:** Involuting skeletal muscle fibers in what could be called a periosteum around the mass leave no doubt that interstitial connective tissue cells in injured muscle are the modulating osteogenic cells condensing to form the bone.

the skin, such as morphea, systemic scleroderma, and dermatomyositis (275) or venous stasis (Fig. 34-33), is rare.

Postinjury Ossification

Myositis ossificans (Fig. 34-34) results from a postinjury modulation of osteoblasts and can occur in a sufficiently superficial location to come to the attention of dermatologists (276). The characteristic radiologic appearance is that of a mass with a peripheral rim of radiodensity correlating with the most advanced and mature bony parts of the lesion, and relatively lucent, maximally injured, and somewhat ischemic central area. Other non-neoplastic soft tissue processes with bone formation such as *pseudomalignant osseous tumor of soft tissues* (Fig. 34-35), *florid reactive periostitis*, and *bizarre parosteal osteochondromatous proliferation* occur more commonly in acral location than myositis ossificans. A differential diagnosis of these lesions includes periosteal and parosteal osteosarcoma, periosteal chondroma, and osteomyelitis.

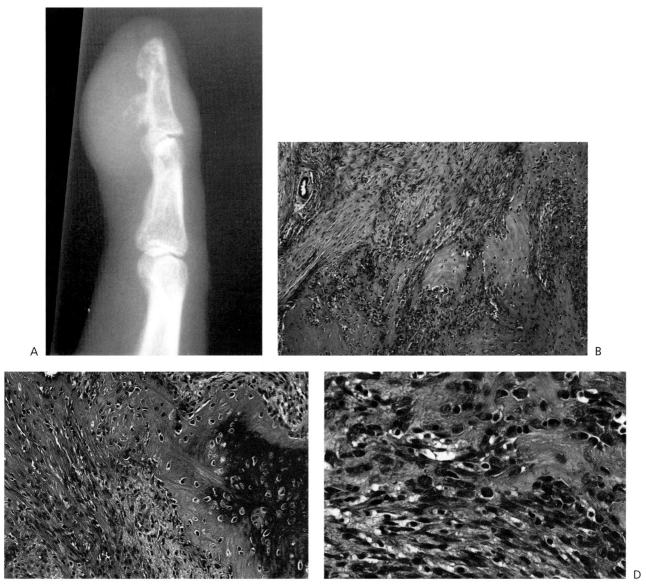

FIGURE 34-35. Fibro-osseous pseudotumor of digit (42-year-old male; rapidly enlarging finger tip with no recalled history of trauma). **A:** The terminal phalange of the fifth finger in this plain film radiograph has undergone bulbous enlargement and has some internal ossific density that may partly extend from the periosteal surface. **B:** A chaotic pattern of osteoid is emerging in an active spindle cell background. A sweat gland duct is at upper left. **C:** A medium-power view of this highly cellular reactive lesion shows basophilic mineralization of part of the osteoid product (*right*). **D:** The cellularity lacks the pleomorphism and abnormal mitoses of osteosarcoma.

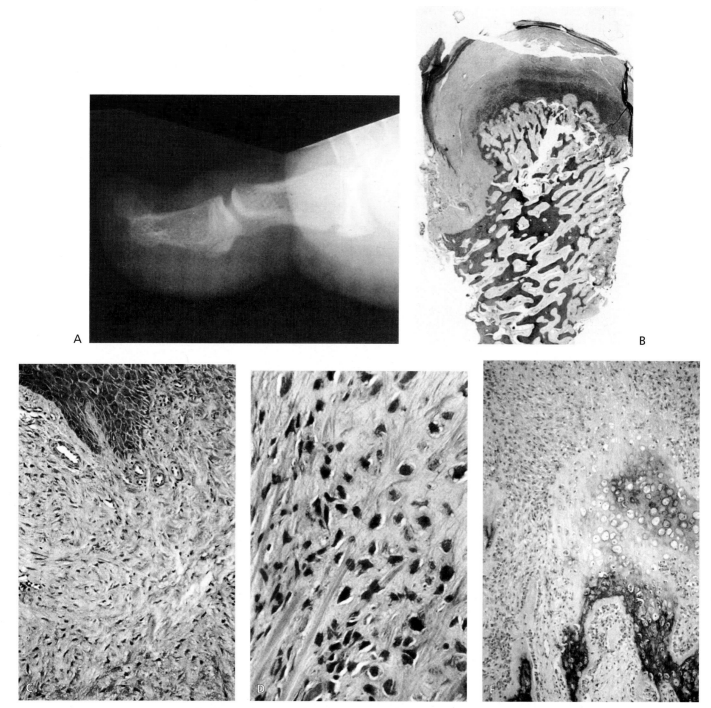

FIGURE 34-36. Subungual exostosis (14-year-old female; 4 months previously, a horse stepped on her great toe). **A:** A polypoid bony projection extends from the tuft of terminal phalanx beneath the nail. An osteocartilaginous exostosis (osteochondroma) would be expected to be attached to the metaphyseal (more proximal) region of the phalanx, not to the tip. **B:** The excised exostosis consists of a cartilaginous cap (*top*) emerging from dermis beneath stretched epidermis and nail bed epithelium. This cartilage overlies a cancellous bony stalk built largely through the process of enchondral ossification. **C:** The earliest stage in the progressive enlargement of a subungual exostosis is the elaboration of myxoid material between dermal fibroblasts (*bottom*). **D:** With time, the myxoid material assumes the solidity of hyaline cartilage and the intervening cells occupy lacunae within it. Deletion by osteoclastic erosion and substitution of bone tends to follow. **E:** Exuberant and reactive/reparative chondro-osseous tissue, as illustrated from another case, can be histologically disconcerting.

Subungual extososis (Fig. 34-36), first described by Dupuytren (277), is a fairly common benign bony projection that occurs on a distal phalanx beneath or beside the nail, often leading to nail deformity (278). It has also been reported as subungual osteochondroma (279) a term correctly applied only to the common anomalous tumor of epiphyseal cartilage generally seen in the growth years (280). The great toe is the most common site but other toes and fingers can be affected. Although the nodule usually measures only a few millimeters in diameter, it can be larger and cause swelling of the entire distal phalanx, possibly with ulceration that is treated for a time as an ingrown nail with infection. There is frequently an association with trauma (281), and these anecdotes argue persuasively for traumatic induction. Radiographs reveal a bony projection from the edge of the terminal phalangeal tuft (Fig. 34-36A) and are indispensable in avoiding assigning an incorrect alternative diagnosis (282). The length and radiologic density are proportional to duration. The treatment is surgical.

Histopathology. Myositis ossificans and its subcutaneous counterpart, *panniculitis ossificans*, in early postinjury stages can mimic a cellular, mitotically active spindle cell sarcoma in its early posttrauma growth, but lacks the abnormal mitoses and extreme pleomorphism of malignancy and manifests uniform nuclear chromaticity. Later, greater density and maturity of the bony product in the periphery around the disturbingly cellular central zones is less of a diagnostic challenge since it is the reverse of the architecture of soft tissue osteosarcoma and would not be seen in nodular fasciitis.

The earliest change in an *exostosis* (Fig. 34-36B) is mucopolysaccharide and osteoid elaboration by periosteum and modulated fibroblasts in the closely approximated contiguous dermis (Fig. 34-35C), eventuating in a gradational continuum of chondroid and osteoid that can be alarmingly cellular (Fig. 34-36E). As the cartilage achieves solid hyalin qualities, it becomes focally eroded along its deep surface by osteoclastic giant cells, followed immediately by enchondral bone deposition on any chondral remnant. In this way, a cancellous bony stalk is built out from original cortex at the expense of cartilage. The process continues, aggravated perhaps from ongoing irritation by footwear and as long as dermal fibroblasts continue to modulate into matrix-producing cells (282).

Extraskeletal Osteosarcoma

This aggressive tumor characterized by atypical mesenchymal cells synthesizing osteoid (Fig. 34-37), is extremely rare, especially in the skin (283). Primary cutaneous osteosarcoma is extremely rare but can occur in the skin with no associated predisposing conditions (284) or in an old burn scar (285). There should be no connection to deeper structures, and no demonstrable primary bone lesion (286). Other extraskeletal sites for primary osteosarcoma that may come to the attention of dermatologists include the penis (287) and tongue (288). Origin in antecedent myositis ossificans is possible (289). When osteosarcoma is concurrent with a distinct carcinoma pattern, such as basal cell

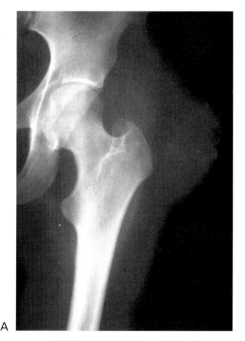
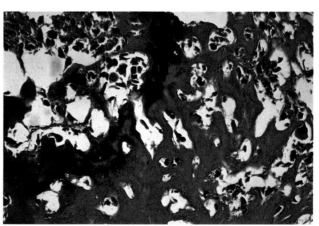

FIGURE 34-37. Extraskeletal osteosarcoma. **A:** In this plain film, an oval mass lateral to the hip joint has irregular central bony density, unlike the peripheral ossification of myositis ossificans. **B:** Cytologically malignant cells are forming osteoid. (Compare to Figure 34-35D)

carcinoma (284), the term carcinosarcoma can be used. Alkaline phosphatase staining compared with immunohistochemistry has proved to be superior in the differentiation from other pleomorphic sarcomas (290).

Differential Diagnosis. Metaplastic and reactive ossification may occur in and around various tumors with specific identity such as the ossifying fibromyxoid tumor of soft tissue (291). Sarcomatoid malignant melanoma, "fibrohistiocytic" tumors such as atypical fibroxanthoma and malignant fibrous histiocytoma, peripheral nerve sheath tumors (e.g., malignant Triton tumor), and Merkel cell carcinoma (292) may demonstrate "divergent" differentiation into bone, cartilage, or myogenous tissue. Electron microscopy can assist in detecting these tumors with differing biologic behaviors (293).

Fibro-osseous pseudotumor typically occurs in the digits of the hand and is characterized histopathologically by a fibroblastic proliferation with foci of osseous differentiation lacking the well-defined zonal pattern of myositis ossificans (246) (Fig. 34-35B). Because of its rapid growth and aggressive histopathologic appearance, this lesion can be mistaken for extraskeletal or parosteal osteosarcoma (294). A 1996 review of cutaneous metastasis from skeletal osteosarcoma found only three cases and added one (295).

BENIGN CARTILAGINOUS TUMORS OF SKIN AND SOFT TISSUE

Soft Tissue Chondromas

The hallmark of all differentiated chondrogenic tumors is the presence of neoplastic chondrocytic cells responsible for the formation of the characteristic cartilaginous tumor matrix (143). Benign cartilage nodules and masses independent of bone, including cutaneous cartilage tumors, are variously regarded as neoplastic, metaplastic, or anomalous. Generically referred to as soft part or *extraskeletal chondromas* (Fig. 34-38), most of these nodules are located in the hands and feet, especially in the fingers of middle-aged adults, but other sites (e.g., back) (296) and ages, including infants (297), are not immune. Most are solitary and may attach to tendons, tendon sheaths, or joint capsules (298,299) (Fig. 34-38A). These slowly enlarging nodules are seldom painful or tender and rarely exceed 3 cm in diameter. Soft tissue chondroma may present as a painful finger (300), an acute inflammatory episode (301), trigger finger (302), or compression neuropathy (303). Few recur locally. True *cutaneous chondromas*, primarily located in the dermis, are rarely described in the dermatologic literature (304), but can be familial (305).

Synovial chondroma (intracapsular and periarticular) and multiple purely cartilaginous (chondromatosis) or chondro-osseous (osteochondromatosis) nodules in tenosynovium or joint synovium are metaplastic changes of subsynovial fibrous tissue that may create a mass around a joint or along a tendon. When near a joint, intracapsular and para-articular chondromas are to be differentiated from synovial chondromatosis (306) (Fig. 34-39). Extraskeletal osteochondromas are painless, slow-growing masses of mature hyaline cartilage, with extensive enchondral ossification (307). Tenosynovial osteochondroma can cause carpal tunnel syndrome (308). Because of location, these tumors come to the attention of the dermatopathologist only rarely. Primary synovial chondrosarcoma is anecdotally rare (309).

Enchondromas are benign intraosseous hyaline cartilage tumors whose location in the distal phalanx is rare, but may be responsible for nail dystrophy (310).

Histopathology. Soft tissue chondromas appear to develop and grow at their periphery by the metaplastic enlargement of fibroblasts into plump cells that inflate the preexisting structural fibrous tissue with mucopolysaccharides, creating hyalin cartilage (Fig. 34-38C). The plump chondrocytes frequently have distinctive reniform and elongated nuclei rather than the expected round shape in most cartilage (Fig. 34-38D). A minority exhibits central or peripheral (311) secondary stippled or heavy deposits of calcium pyrophosphate dihydrate (312) and hydroxyapatite crystals. The well-circumscribed, solid-appearing cartilage may exhibit focal fibrosis, enchondral ossification (soft tissue osteochondroma), myxoid change (myxochondroma), cystification, and/or hemorrhage. Hyaline globules, spherical intracytoplasmic eosinophilic droplets deemed secretory products of probable glycoprotein nature, are in a minority of soft tissue chondromas. Ultrastructurally these are spherical, non-membrane-bound bodies having complex architectural features associated with profiles of rough endoplasmic reticulum with electron probe x-ray microanalytic peaks of sulfur and calcium (313). Hypercellular soft-tissue chondromas composed of enlarged chondrocytes within a variable amount of chondroid matrix that often demonstrates delicate calcifications and contain numerous osteoclast-like multinucleated giant cells, closely resemble chondroblastoma of bone (314,315). There may be a granulomatous reaction (315) ("chondrogranuloma") with multinucleated giant cells along the margins and interlobular vascular channels (Fig. 34-38E). Interpretation should ignore substantial atypia in what is radiologically or clinically a small lesion to avoid unnecessary disfiguring surgery. Plump, immature-appearing chondrocytes that are bi- or multi-nucleated are not uncommon and, as in bone lesions, do not necessarily connote malignancy (Fig. 34-38D); lesions associated with them behave no differently from the well-differentiated forms. Aspiration cytology of soft tissue chondroma presents myxofibrillary material and pleomorphic cells; the clinical, radiologic and cytologic triad are critical for the correct cytologic diagnosis of soft tissue chondroma despite worrisome cell atypia (316). Immunohistochemically, most of the tumor cells except for multinucleated giant cells are positive for vimentin. Cells positive for S-100 protein will be scattered throughout the tumor. Ultrastructurally, the chondroblastic cells have a characteristic microvillous cell border (315).

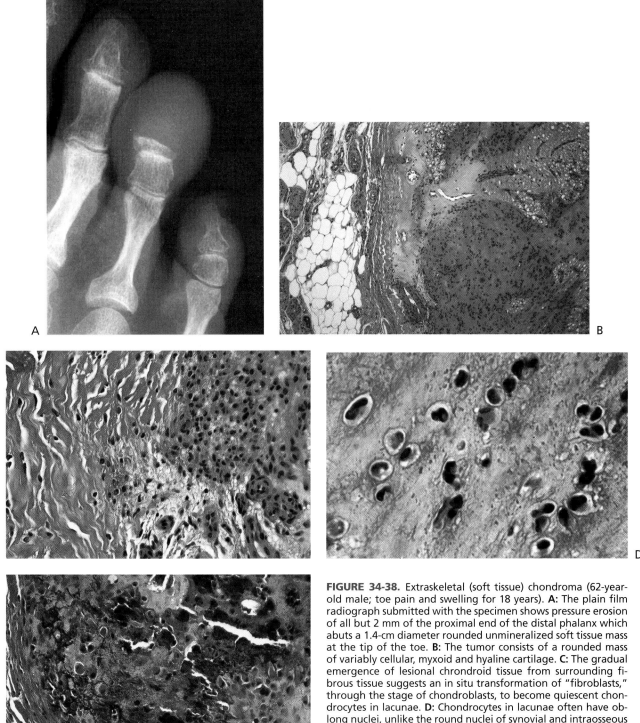

FIGURE 34-38. Extraskeletal (soft tissue) chondroma (62-year-old male; toe pain and swelling for 18 years). **A:** The plain film radiograph submitted with the specimen shows pressure erosion of all but 2 mm of the proximal end of the distal phalanx which abuts a 1.4-cm diameter rounded unmineralized soft tissue mass at the tip of the toe. **B:** The tumor consists of a rounded mass of variably cellular, myxoid and hyaline cartilage. **C:** The gradual emergence of lesional chrondroid tissue from surrounding fibrous tissue suggests an in situ transformation of "fibroblasts," through the stage of chondroblasts, to become quiescent chondrocytes in lacunae. **D:** Chondrocytes in lacunae often have oblong nuclei, unlike the round nuclei of synovial and intraosseous chondromas. Nuclear size variation and binucleate cells are commonplace in this benign lesion. **E:** Particulate mineralizations and lacy basophilic mineral deposits around tumor cells in the matrix correlate with the speckled radiographic densities from another case that are seen in one-third of these tumors.

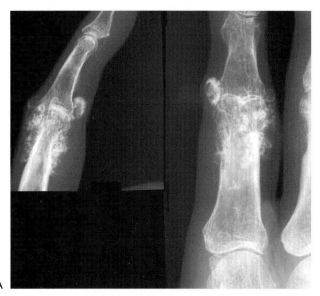
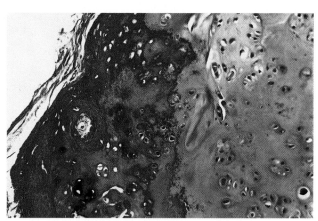

A   B

FIGURE 34-39. Synovial osteochondromatosis (71-year-old male; 5-year history of postinjury finger enlargement). **A:** Multiple lobules of the lesion around a proximal interphalangeal joint have radio-dense rims correlating with rims of enchondral bone. **B:** Between radiolucent, moderately cellular, solid-appearing hyaline cartilage (*right*) and the eosinophilic bone that rims it (*left*) is a basophilic zone of mineralized cartilage. (Courtesy of Newton Sampaio.)

Differential Diagnosis. Chondromas of soft tissue are defined by asymptomatic and harmless clinical course, lack of connection between the tumor and the underlying bone, slow tumor development, absence of age and sex predominance, and characteristic tumor histologic picture (317). Extraskeletal chondromas are to be distinguished from developmental cartilaginous rests of branchial origin (usually in the lateral neck in children or infants). Several soft tissue processes may contain histologically disconcerting cartilage, including mixed tumors (apocrine or eccrine), juvenile aponeurotic fibroma, giant cell tumor of tendon sheath, fibromatosis, metaplastic cartilage in occasional lipoma varieties, (teno)synovial (osteo)chondromatosis, cartilage produced in myositis ossificans and fracture callus, metaplastic cartilage in and around tophaceous pseudogout, and soft tissue recurrence of a bone tumor such as chondromyxoid fibroma (318). Heavily calcified chondromas show granular areas with giant cell reaction resembling tumoral calcinosis or tenosynovial giant-cell tumors. Radiographs can distinguish tumors extending from bone, such as osteochondroma or subungual exostosis (319). Extraskeletal chondromas with mineralization of the chondroid matrix will show on plain film radiographs (320), and the remainder can be imaged by MRI (321) or sonography (322).

Pathogenesis. Cytogenetic analyses of soft tissue chondroma report aberrations of chromosomes 6, 11, and 12q13-q15 (323).

Calcifying Aponeurotic Fibroma

This rare soft tissue tumor primarily occurs in children and adolescents and has a strong predilection for the distal por-

tion of the extremities—especially the hands and feet—but can occur in uncommon extra-acral sites such as the lumbosacral (324) area, back, knee region, thigh, forearm, elbow, and arm (325). Typically, a painless mass is present from 2 weeks to years before resection. Often adherent to dense fibrous connective tissue (e.g., tendon, fascia, or periosteum), this tumor is 1.0 to 5.0 cm in maximum dimension, lobulated, and poorly circumscribed, and has a dense fibrous consistency. Minute calcific foci may be evident grossly. Microscopically, spindled fibroblasts with a fascicular growth pattern and scattered epithelioid fibroblastic cells and multinucleated cells border chondroid foci with or without mineralization. It has been diagnosed by FNA where cytologic examination reveals benign-appearing spindled cells, chondroid cells, multinucleated giant cells, and calcific debris (326). Immunoreactivity always finds vimentin positivity, and possibly also reactivity for muscle-specific actin, smooth muscle actin, CD99, CD34, EMA, S-100 protein, and CD68. Approximately 50% develop one or more recurrences.

Differential Diagnosis. Familiarity with this entity should help to avoid confusion with other processes, including infantile and extra-abdominal fibromatoses, chondroma of soft parts, and fibrous hamartoma of infancy (325).

CHONDROSARCOMA

Extraskeletal Myxoid Chondrosarcoma

This type of chondrosarcoma is uncommon, and is known also as chordoid sarcoma because of the resemblance to chordoma (327). It usually affects adult males (328–330) with a median age at the time of diagnosis in the fifth decade of life (328,330). Only a small minority has been reported in children (328,331,332). The tumor frequently arises in the deep soft tissues, especially of the lower extremities (328). A gradually enlarging mass may or may not be associated with pain (328). Radiographically, the neoplasm is a nodular, radiolucent mass rich in water. Most extraskeletal myxoid chondrosarcomas are large, ovoid, pseudoencapsulated, well-circumscribed tumors with a lobular architecture. The cut surface is tan, gelatinous, and frequently hemorrhagic (Fig. 34-39A).

Histopathology. Extraskeletal myxoid chondrosarcoma is characterized by a proliferation of ovoid and bipolar cells that are enmeshed in a prominent myxoid matrix that is rich in chondroitin and keratin sulfate (328,333,334) (Fig. 34-40B). It has a repetitive lobular pattern and chains of neoplastic cells that seem to progress from the periphery toward the center of lobules. Hemorrhage and hemosiderin in the fibrous tissue surrounding the nodules is characteristic. The tumor cells have small to moderate amounts of eosinophilic cytoplasm and the nuclei are uniform and not pleomorphic. Occasionally, individual tumor cells are surrounded by lacunar spaces; however, the formation of well-developed hyaline cartilage is uncommon. Mitoses are not numerous and multinucleated giant cells are absent. There may be marked collagenization, spindling of tumor cells, and matrix poor regions in which the tumor cells grow in solid sheets. Ultrastructurally, the tumor cells of myxoid chondrosarcoma resemble chondroblasts. They are round to elongate and frequently have microvilli. The cytoplasm contains abundant dilated rough endoplasmic reticulum (RER), glycogen, free ribosomes, well-developed Golgi complexes and mitochondria (335–338). Aggregates of microtubules within the RER are a distinguishing feature (336,339). The cells may connect by desmosome-like intercellular junctions or those of the macula adherens type (327,338). The extracellular matrix is rich in amorphous material, small electron-dense particles, and scattered collagen fibers (335–338). The

neoplastic cells usually stain with antibodies to vimentin and S-100 protein (327,333,339,340). Some studies have shown that they also may be positive for Leu-7 and EMA. Uniformly, they have been negative for keratin.

Differential Diagnosis. Myxoid tumors of soft tissue encompass a heterogeneous group of lesions characterized by a marked abundance of extracellular mucoid (myxoid) matrix, with marked differences in biologic potential that generates diagnostic challenges for the clinician and pathologist alike (341). The differential diagnosis of extraskeletal myxoid chondrosarcoma is broad and includes many reactive processes and epithelial and mesenchymal neoplasms, chief among them, intramuscular myxoma, juxta-articular myxomas, neural neoplasms, cutaneous and soft tissue myoepitheliomas (342), benign polymorphous mesenchymal tumor of soft parts (343), myxoid liposarcoma, myxofibrosarcoma (myxoid malignant fibrous histiocytoma), metastatic carcinoma, metastatic melanoma with myxoid stroma, and chordoma. Myxoid chondrosarcoma does not have the vascular pattern typical of myxoid liposarcoma and lacks lipoblasts. Immunohistochemistry will help sort it out.

Pathogenesis. Cytogenetic studies are few but so far have shown reciprocal translocations involving chromosomes 9 and 22 (344) and translocations between chromosomes 2 and 13. Behavior resembles a low-grade sarcoma.

Mesenchymal Chondrosarcoma

Mesenchymal chondrosarcoma represents the prototypic neoplasm of prechondrogenic cells undergoing multifocal chondrocytic differentiation (143) and can involve the skin (345).

Chondroid-type calcifications and foci of low signal intensity within enhancing lobules reflect its dual histopathologic morphologic characteristics of differentiated cartilage islands interspersed within highly cellular undifferentiated mesenchyme (346) (Fig. 34-41). The

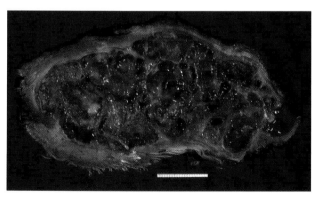
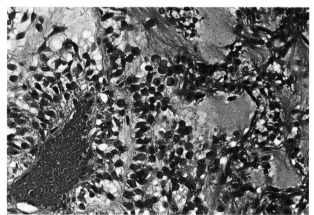

FIGURE 34-40. Extraskeletal myxoid chondrosarcoma (63-year-old male; 17 × 8 × 8 cm anterior thigh mass; death unrelated to tumor 28 months post-op). **A:** The tumor has a glistening myxoid and hemorrhagic cut surface. **B:** Ovoid and stellate tumor cells form perivascular arrays and cords in a basophilic myxoid background.

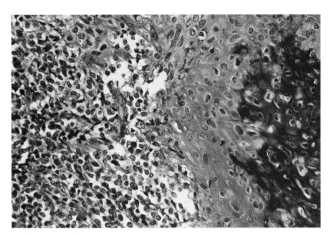

FIGURE 34-41. Mesenchymal chondrosarcoma. Small, round, undifferentiated cells (*left*) might easily be mistaken for Ewing sarcoma or lymphoma were it not for the sporadic island of cartilaginous product (*right*).

cartilaginous areas are S-100 positive and show strong CD99 reactivity in more than 50% of the small round blue cells with a distinct membrane pattern of staining (347). The expression of p30/32 (MIC2) is typically restricted to the small cell component. Positivity of small cells for desmin and/or smooth muscle actin may be seen, and in rare cases, more diffuse rhabdomyoblastic differentiation indicating mesenchymal chondrosarcoma is another primitive neoplasm with polyphenotypic differentiation and features that overlap those of other small cell malignancies of bone and soft tissue (348).

Differential Diagnosis. The cellular areas of mesenchymal chondrosarcoma can mimic fibrosarcoma, Ewing sarcoma, malignant hemangiopericytoma, peripheral neuroectodermal tumor, and synovial sarcoma.

Pathogenesis: An identical Robertsonian translocation involving chromosomes 13 and 21 [der(13;21)(q10;q10)] was detected in two cases of mesenchymal chondrosarcoma, possibly representing a characteristic rearrangement for this histopathologic entity (349).

CHONDROID LESIONS, RARER STILL

The appearance of cutaneous lesions in a patient with a prior history of chondrosarcoma should alert the clinician to the rare possibility of a *metastatic chondrosarcoma* (350). Such metastases preceding the diagnosis of primary chondrosarcoma are anecdotal. These metastases can be either single or multiple with a slight predilection for the head and neck region (351).

Metaplastic carcinoma (carcinosarcoma, sarcomatoid carcinoma, malignant mixed tumor) is a biphasic tumor comprising malignant epithelial and heterologous mesenchymal elements. Primary cutaneous cases are rare, with only seven documented in the English-language literature

by 1997. A review adding four further cases (352) included three that developed in association with squamous cell carcinoma and one in an eccrine porocarcinoma. Malignant heterologous malignant mesenchymal elements included osteosarcoma, chondrosarcoma, leiomyosarcoma, and rhabdomyosarcoma. In contrast to metaplastic carcinomas arising in visceral sites, those primarily arising in the skin do not appear to behave in a very aggressive manner.

Breast carcinoma is the most common origin of cutaneous metastasis in women, but is usually ductal or lobular histologic type. *Sarcomatoid (metaplastic) carcinoma of the breast,* although a well-established aggressive neoplasm, is very uncommon. Its metaplastic elements, derived from carcinomatous elements, span all types of mesenchymal differentiation. Skin metastasis from such lesions is extremely rare but can be chondrosarcomatous (353). *Malignant mesenchymoma,* defined as a sarcoma with three or more lines of differentiation, can occur in skin, such as a tumor in an abdominal incision scar composed of leiomyosarcoma, chondrosarcoma, and osteosarcoma (354).

Malignant melanomas showing foci of osteocartilaginous differentiation are extremely rare with only 18 cases reported as of 1998 (355) in a review that added two primary mucosal malignant melanomas (vagina and oral cavity). Chondroid change in the absence of osseous differentiation is extremely rare in malignant melanoma, but melanoma should be considered in the differential diagnosis of primary cutaneous neoplasms exhibiting cartilaginous differentiation (356). Oral mucosal melanomas with osteocartilaginous differentiation are to be distinguished from malignant change in a pleomorphic adenoma, sarcomatoid carcinoma, osteogenic sarcoma and mesenchymal chondrosarcoma. Primary vaginal melanoma with cartilaginous differentiation must be distinguished from primary malignant mixed Müllerian tumor (355).

Atypical fibroxanthoma can contain areas of chondroid differentiation that resemble chondrosarcoma and have S-100 positivity (357).

REFERENCES

1. Seemayer TA, Knaack J, Wang N, et al. On the ultrastructure of hibernoma. *Cancer* 1975;36:1785.
2. Napolitano L. The differentiation of white adipose cells: an electron microscope study. *Anat Rec* 1963;147:273.
3. Headington JT. The histiocyte in memoriam. *Arch Dermatol* 1986;122:532.
4. Silverman JS, Tamsen A. Fibrohistiocytic differentiation in subcutaneous fatty tumors. *J Cutan Pathol* 1997;24:484–493.
5. Ragsdale BD, Dupree WB. Fatty neoplasms. In: Bogumill GP, Fleegler EJ, eds. *Tumors of the Hand and Upper Limb.* Edinburgh: Churchill Livingstone, 1993:254.
6. Mentzel T. Cutaneous lipomatous neoplasms. *Semin Diagn Pathol* 2001;18:250–257.
7. Mehregan AH, Tavafoghi V, Ghandchi A. Nevus lipomatosus cutaneus superficialis (Hoffmann–Zurhelle). *J Cutan Pathol* 1975; 2:307.

8. Wilson-Jones E, Marks R, Pongsehirun D. Naevus superficialis lipomatosus. *Br J Dermatol* 1975;93:121.
9. Howell JB. Nevus lipomatosus vs focal dermal hypoplasia. *Arch Dermatol* 1965;92:238.
10. Nogita T, Wong T-Y, Hidano A, et al. Pedunculated lipofbroma. *Am Acad Dermatol* 1994;31:235–240.
11. Reymond JL, Stoebner P, Amblard P. Nevus lipomatosus cutaneus superficialis: an electron microscopic study of four cases. *J Cutan Pathol* 1980;7:295.
12. Dotz W, Prioleau PG. Nevus lipomatosus cutaneus superficialis: a light and electron microscopic study. *Arch Dermatol* 1984;120: 376.
13. Maize JC, Foster G. Age-related changes in melanocytic nevi. *Clin Exp Dermatol* 1979;4:49.
14. Gardner EW, Miller HM, Lowney ED. Folded skin associated with underlying nevus lipomatosus. *Arch Dermatol* 1979;115:978.
15. Burgdorf WHC, Doran CK, Worret WI. Folded skin with scarring: Michelin tire baby syndrome? *J Am Acad Dermatol* 1982; 7:90.
16. Ross CM. Generalized folded skin with underlying lipomatosus nevus: the Michelin tire baby [Letter]. *Arch Dermatol* 1972;106: 766.
17. Ciatti S, Del Monaco M, Hyde P, et al. Encephalocraniocutaneous lipomatosis: a rare neurocucaneous syndrome. *J Am Acad Dermatol* 1998;38:102–104.
18. Oku T, Iwasaki K, Fujita H. Folded skin with an underlying cutaneous smooth muscle hamartoma. *Br J Dermatol* 1993;129:606.
19. Schnur RE, Herzberg AJ, Spinner N, et al. Variability in the Michelin tire syndrome. *J Am Acad Dermatol* 1993;28:364–370.
20. Jahss MH, Kummer F, Michelson JD. Investigations into the fat pads of the sole of the foot: heel pressure studies. *Foot Ankle* 1992;13:227–232.
21. Buschmann WR, Jahss MH, Kummer F, et al. Histology and histomorphometric analysis of the normal and atrophic heel fat pad. *Foot Ankle Int* 1995;16:254–258.
22. Boni R, Dummer R. Compression therapy in painful piezogenic pedal papules. *Arch Dermatol* 1996;132:127–128.
23. Laing VB, Fleischer AB Jr. Piezogenic wrist papules: a common an asymptomatic finding. *Am Acad Dermatol* 1991;24:415–417.
24. Kahana M, Feinstein A, Tabachnic E, et al. Painful piezogenic pedal papules in patients with Ehlers–Danlos syndrome. *J Am Acad Dermatol* 1987;17:205–209.
25. Schlappner OLA, Wood MG, Gerstein W, et al. Painful and non-painful piezogenic pedal papules. *Arch Dermatol* 1972;106:729–733.
26. Ortega-Monzo C, Molina-Gallardo I, Monceagudo-Castro C, et al. Precalcaneal congenital fibrolipomatous hamartoma: a report of four cases. *Pediatr Dermatol* 2000;17:429–431.
27. Espana A, Pujol RM, Ideate MA, et al. Bilateral congenital adipose plantar nodules. *Br J Dermatol* 2000;142:1262–1264.
28. Sanchez MR, Golomb FM, Moy JA, et al. Giant lipoma: case report and review of the literature. *J Am Acad Dermatol* 1993;28: 266–268.
29. Salasche SJ, McCollough ML, Angeloni VL, et al. Frontalis-associated lipoma of the forehead. *J Am Acad Dermatol* 1989; 20:462–468.
30. Kashima M, Saito K. A case of atypical inter-muscular lipoma (Evans). *J Dermatol* 1991;18:532.
31. Meis JM, Enzinger FM. Myolipoma of soft tissue. *Am J Surg Pathol* 1991;15:121.
32. Mehregan DA, Mehregan DR, Mehregan AH. Angiomyolipoma. *J Am Acad Dermatol* 1992;27:331.
33. Hitchcock MG, Hurt MA, Santa Cruz DJ. Adenolipoma of the skin. A report of nine cases. *J Am Acad Dermatol* 1993;29:82.
34. Blomstrand R, Juhlin L, Nordenstam H, et al. Adiposis dolorosa associated with defects of lipid metabolism. *Acta Derm Venereol (Stockh)* 1971;51:243.
35. Blomstrand R, Juhlin L, Nordenstam H, et al. Adiposis dolorosa associated with defects of lipid metabolism. *Acta Derm Venereol* 1971;51:243–250.
36. Held JL, Andrew JA, Kohn SR. Surgical amelioration of Dercum's disease: a report and review. *J Dermatol Surg Oncol* 1989; 15:1294–1296.
37. Enzi G. Multiple symmetric lipomatosis:an updated clinical report. *Medicine (Baltimore)* 1984;63:56–64.
38. Ruzicka T, Vieluf D, Landchaler M, Braun-Falco O. Benign symmetric lipomatosis Launois-Bensaude. Report of ten cases and review of the literature. *Am Acad Dermatol* 1987;17:663–674.
39. Carlin MC, Ratz JL. Multiple symmetric lipomatosis: treatment with liposuction. *Am Acad Dermatol* 1988:18:359–362.
40. Ross M, Goodman MM. Multiple symmetric lipomatosis (Launois–Bensaude syndrome). *Int J Dermatol* 1992;31:80–82.
41. Leffell DJ, Braverman IM. Familial multiple lipomatosis. Report of a case and a review of the literature. *J Am Acad Dermatol* 1986;15:275–279.
42. Tsao H, Sober AJ. Multiple lipomatosis in a patient with familial atypical mole syndrome. *Br Dermatol* 1998;139:1118–1119.
43. Klein JA, Barr RJ. Diffuse lipomatosis and tuberous sclerosis. *Arch Dermatol* 1986;122:1298–1302.
44. Happle R, Kuster W. Nevus psiloliparus: a distinct fatty tissue nevus. *Dermatology* 1998;197:6–10.
45. Grimalt R, Ermacora E, Mistura L, et al. Encephalocraniocutaneous lipomatosis: case report and review of the literature. *Pediatr Dermatol* 1993;10:164–168.
46. Slavin SA, Baker DC, McCarthy JG, et al. Congenital infiltrating lipomatosis of the face: linicopathologic evaluation and treatment. *Plant Reconstr Surg* 1983;72:158–164.
47. Lee JH, Sung YH, Yoon JS, Park JK. Lipedematous scalp. *Arch Dermatol* 1994;130:802–803.
48. Bornhovd E, Sakrauski AK, Brdhl H, et al. Multiple circumscribed subcutaneous lipomas associated with use of human immunodeficiency virus protease inhibitors? *Br J Dermatol* 2000; 143:1113–1114.
49. Dank JP, Colven R. Protease-inhibitor associated angiolipomatosis. *J Am Acad Dermatol* 2000;42:129–131. 20:285–289.
50. Chen D, Misra A, Garg A. Clinical review 153: Lipodystrophy in human immunodeficiency virus-infected patients. *J Clin Endocrinol Metab.* 2002;87:4845–4856.
51. Ramdial PK, Madaree A, Singh B. Membranous fat necrosis in lipomas. *Am J Surg Pathol* 1997;21:841–846.
52. Zelger BG, Zelger B, Steiner H, et al. Sclerotic lipoma: lipomas simulating sclerotic fibroma. *Histopathology* 1997;31:174–181.
53. Rodriguez-Fernández A, Caro-Manilla A. Cutaneous angiomyolipoma with pleomorphic changes. *J Am Acad Dermatol* 1993; 29:115.
54. Mrozek K, Karakousis CP, Bloomfield CD. Chromosome 12 breakpoints are cytogenetically different in benign and malignant lipogenic tumors. Localization of breakpoints in lipoma to 12q15 and in myxoid liposarcoma to 12q13.3. *Cancer Res* 1993; 53:1670.
55. Dixon AY, McGregor DH, Lee SH. Angiolipomas: an ultrastructural and clinicopathological study. *Hum Pathol* 1981;12:739–747.
56. Goodfield MJD, Rowell NR. The clinical presentation of cutaneous angiolipomata and the response to 3-blockade. *Clin Exp Dermatol* 1988;13:190–192.
57. Howard WR, Helwig EB. Angiolipoma. *Arch Dermatol* 1960; 82:924.
58. Dixon AY, McGregor DH, Lee SH. Angiolipomas: an ultrastructural and clinicopathological study. *Hum Pathol* 1981;12:737.
59. Kanik AB, Oh CH, Bhawan J. Cellular angiolipoma. *Am J Dermatopathol* 1995;17:312–315.
60. Zamecnik M. Vascular myxolipoma (angiomyxolipoma) of subcutaneous tissue. *Histopathology* 1999;34:180–181.

61. Hunt SJ, Santa Cruz DJ, Barr RJ. Cellular angiolipoma. *Am J Surg Pathol* 1990;14:75.
62. Dionne GP, Seemayer TA. Infiltrating lipomas and angiolipomas revisited. *Cancer* 1974;33:732.
63. Puig L, Moreno S, DeMoragas JM. Infiltrating angiolipoma. *J Dermatol Surg Oncol* 1986;12:617.
64. Allen PW, Enzinger FM. Hemangiomas of skeletal muscle: an analysis of 89 cases. *Cancer* 1972;29:8.
65. Sahl WJ Jr. Mobile encapsulated lipomas. Formerly called encapsulated angiolipomas. *Arch Dermatol* 1978;114:1684–1686.
66. Hurt MA, Santa Cruz DJ. Nodular-cystic fat necrosis. A reevaluation of the so-called mobile encapsulated lipoma. *J Am Acad Dermatol* 1989;21:493–498.
67. Rubin BP, Fletcher CDM. The cytogenetics of lipomatous tumours. *Histopathology* 1997;30:507–511.
68. Dal Cin P, Sciot R, Polito P, et al. Lesions of I3q may occur independently of deletion of 16q in spindle cell/pleomorphic lipomas. *Histopathology* 1997;31:222–225.
69. Enzinger FM, Harvey DA. Spindle cell lipoma. *Cancer* 1975;36:1852.
70. Brody HJ, Meltzer HD, Someren A. Spindle cell lipoma. *Arch Dermatol* 1978;114:1065.
71. Diaz-Cascajo C, Borghi S, Weyers W. Fibrous spindle cell lipoma. Report of a new variant. *Am J Dermatopathol* 2001;23:112–115.
72. Warkel RL, Rehme CG, Thompson WH. Vascular spindle cell lipoma. *J Cutan Pathol* 1982;9:113.
73. Richmond I, Banerjee SS. Spindle cell lipoma—a pseudoangiomatous variant. *Histopathology* 1995;27:201.
74. Pitt MA, Roberts IS, Curry A. Spindle cell and pleomorphic lipoma: an ultrastructural study. *Ultrastruct Pathol* 1995;19:475–480.
75. Dal Cin P, Sciot R, Polito P, et al. Lesions of 13q may occur independently of deletion of 16q in spindle cell/pleomorphic lipomas. *Histopathology* 1997;31:222–225.
76. Shmookler BM, Enzinger FM. Pleomorphic lipoma. A benign tumor simulating liposarcoma. *Cancer* 1981;47:126.
77. Evans HL, Soule EH, Inkelmann RK. Atypical lipoma, atypical intramuscular lipoma, and well differentiated retroperitoneal liposarcoma. *Cancer* 1979;43:574.
78. Miettinen M, Lehto VP, Virtanen I. Antibodies to intermediate filament proteins. The differential diagnosis of cutaneous tumors. *Arch Dermatol* 1985;121:736–741.
79. Bryant J. A pleomorphic lipoma in the scalp. *J Dermatol Surg Oncol* 1981;7:323.
80. Meis JM, Enzinger FM. Chondroid lipoma: a unique tumor simulating liposarcoma and myxoid chondrosarcoma. *Am J Surg Pathol* 1993;17:1103.
81. Gisselsson D, Domanski HA, Hoglund M, et al. Unique cytological features and chromosome aberrations in chondroid lipoma. *Am J Surg Pathol* 1999;23:1300–1304.
82. Yang YJ, Damron TA, Ambrose JL. Diagnosis of chondroid lipoma by fine-needle aspiration biopsy. *Arch Pathol Lab Med* 2001;125:1224–1226.
83. Yang, JT. Diagnosis of chondroid lipoma by fine-needle aspiration biopsy [Reply to letter]. *Arch Pathol Lab Med* 2002;126:773–774.
84. Nielsen GP, O'Connell JX, Dickersin GR, et al. Chondroid lipoma, a tumor of white fat cells: a brief report of two cases with ultrastructural analysis. *Am J Surg Pathol* 1995;19:1272.
85. Kindblom L-G, Meis-Kindblom JM. Chondroid lipoma: an ultrastructural and immunohistochemical analysis with further observations regarding its differentiation. *Hum Pathol* 1995;26:706–715.
86. Rigor VU, Goldstone SE, Jones J, et al. Hibernoma: a case report and a discussion of a rare tumor. *Cancer* 1986;57:2207.
87. Chitoku S, Kawai S, Watabe Y, et al. Intradural spinal hibernoma: case report. *Surg Neurol* 1998;49:509–513.
88. Lay K, Velasco C, Akin H, et al. Axillary hibernoma: an unusual soft tissue tumor. *Am Surg* 2000;66:787–788.
89. Santambrogio L, Cioffi U, De Simone M, et al. Cervicomediastinal hibernoma. *Ann Thorac Surg* 1997;64:1160–1162.
90. Dardick I. Hibernoma: a possible model of brown fat histogenesis. *Hum Pathol* 1978;9:321.
91. Cabello Rodriguez M, Somaza de Saint-Palais M, Fernandez Lobato R, et al. Retroperitoneal hibernoma [Spanish]. *Rev Esp Enferm Dig* 1993;84:207–210.
92. Alvine G, Rosenthal H, Murphey M, et al. Hibernoma. *Skeletal Radiol* 1996;25:493–496.
93. Lewandowski PJ, Weiner SD. Hibernoma of the medial thigh. Case report and literature review. *Clin Orthop* 1996;330:198–201.
94. Florio G, Cicia S, Del Papa M, et al. Neck hibernoma: case report and literature review. *G Chir* 2000;21:339–341.
95. Sellari Franceschini S, Segnini G, Berrettini S, et al. Hibernoma of the larynx. Review of the literature and a new case. *Acta Otorhinolaryngol Belg* 1993;47:51–53.
96. Vinayak BC, Reddy KT. Hibernoma in the parotid region. *J Laryngol Otol* 1993;107:257–258.
97. Gardner-Thorpe D, Hirschowitz L, Maddox PR. Mammary hibernoma. *Eur J Surg Oncol* 2000;26:430.
98. Muszynski CA, Robertson DP, Goodman JC, et al. Scalp hibernoma: case report and literature review. *Surg Neurol* 1994;42:343–345.
99. Wilhelm KP, Eisenbeiss W, Wolff HH. Hibernoma of the forehead. A rare tumor of brown fatty tissue in an unusual site [German]. *Hautarzt* 1993;44:735–737.
100. Brines OA, Johnson MH. Hibernoma, a special fatty tumor. Report of a case. *Am J Pathol* 1949;25:467–479.
101. Chen DY, Wang CM, Chan HL. Hibernoma. Case report and literature review. *Dermatol Surg* 1998;24:393–5.
102. Abemayor E, McClean PH, Cobb CJ, et al. Hibernomas of the head and neck. *Head Neck Surg* 1987;9:362–7.
103. Lele SM, Chundru S, Chaljub G, et al. Hibernoma: a report of 2 unusual cases with a review of the literature. *Arch Pathol Lab Med* 2002;126:975–978.
104. Hashimoto H, Enjoji M. Liposarcoma: a clinicopathologic subtyping of 52 cases. *Acta Pathol Jpn* 1982;32:933–948.
105. Gaffney EF, Hargreaves HK, Semple E, et al. Hibernoma: Distinctive light and electron microscopic features and relationship to brown adipose tissue. *Hum Pathol* 1983;14:677.
106. Vellios F, Baez J, Shumacker HB. Lipoblastomatosis: a tumor of fetal fat different from hibernoma. *Am J Pathol* 1958;34:1149.
107. Mertens F, Rydholm A, Brosjo O, et al. Hibernomas are characterized by rearrangements of chromosome bands 11q13–21. *Int J Cancer* 199415;58:503–5.
108. Meloni AM, Spanier SS, Bush CH, et al. Involvement of 10q22 and 11q13 in hibernoma. *Cancer Genet Cytogenet* 1994;72:59–64.
109. Fetsch JF, Miettinen M, Laskin WB, et al. A clinicopathologic study of 45 pediatric soft tissue tumors with an admixture of adipose tissue and fibroblastic elements, and a proposal for classification as lipofibromatosis. *Am J Surg Pathol* 2000;24:1491–500.
110. Mentzel T, Calonje E, Fletcher CDM. Lipoblastoma and lipoblastomatosis: a clinicopathological study of 14 cases. *Histopathology* 1993;23:527–533.
111. Chung EB, Enzinger FM. Benign lipoblastomatosis: an analysis of 35 cases. *Cancer* 1973;32:483.
112. Coffin CM, Williams RA. Congenital lipoblastoma of the hand. *Pediatr Pathol* 1992;12:857.

113. Young RJ 3rd, Warschaw KE, Elston DM, et al. Acral lipoblastoma. *Cutis* 2000;65:243–245.

114. Hicks J, Dilley A, Patel D, et al. Lipoblastoma and lipoblastomatosis in infancy and childhood: histopathologic, ultrastructural, and cytogenetic features. *Ultrastruct Pathol* 2001;25:321–333.

115. Reiseter T, Nordshus T, Borthne A, et al. Lipoblastoma: MRI appearances of a rare paediatric soft tissue tumour. *Pediatr Radiol* 1999;29:542–545.

116. Chun YS, Kim WK, Park KW, et al. Lipoblastoma. *J Pediatr Surg* 2001;36:905–907.

117. Dilley AV, Patel DL, Hicks MJ, et al. Lipoblastoma: pathophysiology and surgical management. *J Pediatr Surg* 2001;36:229–231.

118. Mognato G, Cecchetto G, Carli M, et al. Is surgical treatment of lipoblastoma always necessary? *J Pediatr Surg* 2000;35:1511–1513.

119. Chaudhuri B, Ronan SG, Ghosh L. Benign lipoblastoma. *Cancer* 1980;46:611.

120. Mentzel T, Calonje E, Fletcher CD. Lipoblastoma and lipoblastomatosis: a clinicopathological study of 14 cases. *Histopathology* 1993;23:527.

121. Miller GG, Yanchar NL, Magee JF, et al. Tumor karyotype differentiates lipoblastoma from liposarcoma. *J Pediatr Surg* 1997;32:1771–1772.

122. Harrer J, Hammon G, Wagner T, et al. Lipoblastoma and lipoblastomatosis: a report of two cases and review of the literature. *Eur J Pediatr Surg* 2001;11:342–349.

123. Kuhnen C, Mentzel T, Fisseler-Eckhoff A, et al. Atypical lipomatous tumor in a 14-year-old patient: distinction from lipoblastoma using FISH analysis. *Virchows Arch* 2002;441:299–302.

124. O'Donnell KA, Caty MG, Allen JE, et al. Lipoblastoma: better termed infantile lipoma? *Pediatr Surg Int* 2000;16:458–461.

125. Spanier SS, Floyd J. A clinicopathologic comparison of malignant fibrous histiocytoma and liposarcoma. *Instr Course Lect* 1989;38:407–417. This does not appear to be published source. Please provide details on provider/publisher of course notes

126. Enterline HT, Culberson JD, Rochlin DB, et al. Liposarcoma. *Cancer* 1960;13:932.

127. Dei Tos AP, Mentzel T, Fletcher CD. Primary liposarcomas of the skin; a rare neoplasm with unusual high grade features. *Am J Dermatopathol* 1998;20:332–338.

128. Miser JS, Pizzo PA. Soft tissue sarcomas in childhood. *Pediatr Clin North Am* 1985;32:779.

129. Shmookler BM, Enzinger FM. Liposarcoma occurring in children: an analysis of 17 cases and review of the literature. *Cancer* 1983;52:567.

130. Enzinger FM, Winslow DJ. Liposarcoma: a study of 103 cases. *Virchows Arch Pathol* Anat 1962;335:367.

131. Reitan JB, Kaalhus O, Brennhovd IO, et al. Prognostic factors in liposarcoma. *Cancer* 1985;55:2482.

132. Azumi N, Curtis J, Kempson RL, et al. Atypical and malignant neoplasms showing lipomatous differentiation: a study of 111 cases. *Am J Surg Pathol* 1987;11:161.

133. Evans HL, Soule EH, Winkelman RK. Atypical lipoma, atypical intramuscular lipoma, well-differentiated retroperitoneal liposarcoma. *Cancer* 1979;43:574.

134. Evans HL. Liposarcomas and atypical lipomatous tumors. A study of 66 cases followed for a minimum of 10 years. *Surg Pathol* 1988;1:41.

135. Weiss S, Goldblum JR, eds. Liposarcoma. In *Enzinger and Weiss's Soft Tissue Tumors*, 4th ed. St. Louis: Mosby, 2001:662.

136. Pearlstone DB, Pisters PW, Bold RJ, et al. Patterns of recurrence in extremity liposarcoma: implications for staging and follow-up. *Cancer* 1999;85:85–92.

137. Evans HL. Smooth muscle in atypical lipomatous tumors. *Ann J Surg Pathol* 1990;14:714.

138. Kransdorf MJ, Meis JM, Jelinek JS. Dedifferentiated liposarcoma of the extremities. Imaging and findings in four patients. *Am J Radiol* 1993;161:127.

139. Orvieto E, Furlanetto A, Laurino L, et al. Myxoid and round cell liposarcoma: a spectrum of myxoid adipocytic neoplasia. *Semin Diagn Pathol* 2001;18:267–73.

140. Smith TA, Easley KA, Goldblum JR. Myxoid/round cell liposarcoma of the extremities: a clinicopathologic study of 29 cases with particular attention to extent of round cell liposarcoma. *Am J Surg Pathol* 1996;20:171.

141. Geltinger S, Thewes M, Abeck D, et al. A pleomorphic liposarcoma imitated a subcutaneous cyst [Letter]. *Acta Derm Venereol* 1997. 77:482–483.

142. Sührch W, Bégin LR, Seemayer TA, et al. Pleomorphic soft tissue myogenic sarcomas of adulthood: a reappraisal in the mid–1990's. *Am J Surg Pathol* 1996;20:131.

143. Aigner T. Towards a new understanding and classification of chondrogenic neoplasias of the skeleton—biochemistry and cell biology of chondrosarcoma and its variants. *Virchows Arch* 2002;441:219–30.

144. Mentzel T, Fletcher CDM. Dedifferentiated myxoid liposarcoma: a clinicopathological study suggesting a closer relationship between myxoid and well-differentiated liposarcoma. *Histopathology* 1997;30:457–463.

145. Fanburg-Smith JC, Miettinen M. Liposarcoma with meningothelial-like whorls: a study of 17 cases of a distinctive histological pattern associated with dedifferentiated liposarcoma. *Histopathology* 1998;33:414–424.

146. Nascimento AG, Kurtin PJ, Guillou L, et al. Dedifferentiated liposarcoma. A report of nine cases with a peculiar neurallike whorling pattern associated with metaplastic bone formation. *Am J Surg Pathol* 1998;22:945–955.

147. Dei Tos AP. Lipomatous tumours. *Curr Diagn Pathol* 2001;7:8–16.

148. Kreichbergs A, Tribukait B, Willems J, et al. DNA flow analysis of soft tissue tumors. *Cancer* 1987;59:128.

149. Shanks JH, Banerjee SS, Eyden BP, Focal rhabdomyosarcomatous differentiation in primary liposarcoma. *J Clin Pathol* 1996. 49:770–772.

150. Quinn TR, Young RH. Smooth-muscle hamartoma of the tunica dartos of the scrotum: report of a case. *Cutan Pathol* 1997;24:322–326.

151. Gagne, EJ, Su WPD. Congenital smooth muscle hamartoma of the skin. *Pediatr Dermatol* 1993;10:142.

152. Jang H-S, Kim MB, Oh C-K, et al. Linear congenital smooth muscle hamartoma with follicular spotted appearance. *Br J Dermatol* 2000;142:138–142.

153. Berberian BJ, Burnett JW Congenital smooth muscle hamartoma: a case report. *Br J Dermatol* 1986;115:711–714.

154. Gagne EJ, Su WPD. Congenital smooth muscle hamartoma of the skin. *Pediatr Dermatol* 1993;10:142–145.

155. Bronson DM, Fretzin DF, Farrell LN. Congenital pilar and smooth muscle nevus. *J Am Acad Dermatol* 1983;8:111.

156. Slifman NR, Harrist TJ, Rhodes AR. Congenital arrector pili hamartoma. *Arch Dermatol* 1985;121:1034.

157. Darling TN, Kamino H, Murray JC. Acquired cutaneous smooth muscle hamartoma. *J Am Acad Dermatol* 1993;28:844.

158. Urbanek RW, Johnson WC. Smooth muscle hamartoma associated with Becker's nevus. *Arch Dermatol* 1978;114:104.

159. Zvulunov A, Rotem A, Merlob P, et al. Congenital smooth muscle hamartoma. Prevalence, clinical findings, and follow-up in 15 patients. *Am J Dis Child* 1990;144:782–4.

160. Montgomery H, Winkelmann RK. Smooth-muscle tumors of the skin. *Arch Dermatol* 1959;79:32.

161. Straka BF, Wilson BB. Multiple papules on the leg. *Arch Dermatol* 1991;127:1717–1722.

162. Smith CG, Glaser DA, Leonardi C. Zosteriform multiple leiomyomas. *Am Acad Dermatol* 1998;38:272–273.

163. Agarwalla A, Thakur A, Jacob M, et al. Zosteriform and disseminated lesions in cutaneous leiomyoma. *Acta Derm Venereol* 2000;80:446.

164. Peters CW, Hanke CW, Reed JC. Nevus leiomyomatosus systematicus. *Cutis* 1981;27:484–486.

165. Jolliffe DS. Multiple cutaneous leiomyomata. *Clin Exp Dermatol* 1978;3:89–92.

166. Venencie PY, Puissant A, Boffa GA, et al. Multiple cutaneous leiomyomata and erythrocytosis with demonstration of erythropoietic activity in the cutaneous leiomyomata. *Br J Dermatol* 1982;107:483–486.

167. Engelke H, Christophers E. Leiomyomatosis cutis et uteri. *Acta Derm Venereol Suppl (Stockh)* 1979;59:51–54.

168. Orellana-Diaz 0, Hernandez-Perez E. Leiomyoma cutis and leiomyosarcoma: a 10-year study and a short review. *J Dermatol Surg Oncol* 1983;9:283–287.

169. Stout AP Solitary cutaneous and subcutaneous leiomyoma. *Am Cancer* 1937;29.435–469.

170. Fisher WC, Helwig EB. Leiomyomas of the skin. *Arch Dermatol* 1963;88:510.

171. De Cholnoky T. Acessory breast tissue in the axilla. *N Y State J Med* 1951;51;2245–2248.

172. Shewmake SW, Izuno GT. Supernummary areolae. *Arch Dermatol* 1977;113:823–825.

173. Newman PL, Fletcher CDM. Smooth muscle tumours of the external genitalia: clinicopathological analysis of a series. *Histopathology* 1991;18:523–529.

174. Jansen LH. Leiomyoma cutis. *Acta Derm Venereol* 1952;32: 40–50.

175. Fitzpatrick JE, Mellette JR, Hwang RJ, et al. Cutaneous angiolipoleiomyoma. *J Am Acad Dermatol* 1990;23:1093.

176. Fisher WC, Helwig ES. leiomyomas of the skin. *Arch Dermatol* 1963;88:510–520.

177. Mentzel T, Wadden C, Fletcher CDM. Granular cell change in smooth muscle tumours of skin and soft tissue. *Histopathology* 1994;24:223–231.

178. Dobashi Y, Iwabuchi K, Nakahata J, et al. Combined clear and granular cell leiomyoma of soft tissue: evidence of transformation to a histiocytic phenotype. *Histopathology* 1999;34:526–531.

177. De Rosa G, Bosciano A, Giordano G, et al. Symplastic leiomyoma of the scrotum. A case report. *Pathologica* 1996;88:55–57.

180. Kawagishi N, Kashiwagi T, The M, et al. Pleomorphic angioleiomyoma. Report of two cases with immunohistochemical studies. *Am J Dermatopathol* 2000;22:268–271.

181. McGinley KM, Bryant S, Kattine AA, et al. Cutaneous leiomyomas lack estrogen and progesterone receptor immunoreactivity. *J Cutan Pathol* 1997;24:241–245.

182. Hachisuga T, Hashimoto H, Enjoji M. Angioleiomyoma: a clinicopathologic reappraisal of 562 cases. *Cancer* 1984;54: 126.

183. Sajben FP Barnette DJ, Barrett TL. Intravascular angioleiomyoma. *J Cutan Pathol* 1999;26:165–167.

184. Scurry JP, Carey MP, Targett CS, et al. Soft tissue lipoleiomyoma. *Pathology* 1991;23:360.

185. Buyukbabani N, Tetikkurt S, Ozturk AS. Cutaneous angiomyolipoma: report of two cases with emphasis on HMB 45 utility. *J Eur Acad Dermatol Venereol* 1998. 11:151–154.

186. Rodriguez-Fernandez A, Caro-Mancilla A. Cutaneous angiomyolipoma with pleomorphic changes. *J Am Acad Dermatol* 1993;29:115–116.

187. Lun KR, Spelman LJ. Multiple piloleiomyomas. *Australas J Dermatol* 2000;41:185–186.

188. Baugh W, Quigley MM, Barrett TL. Palisaded angioleiomyoma. *J Cutan Pathol* 2000;27:526–8.

189. Mann PR. Leiomyoma cutis: an electron microscope study. *Br J Dermatol* 1970;82:463.

190. Seifert HW. Ultrastructural investigation on cutaneous angioleiomyoma. *Arch Dermatol Res* 1981;271:91.

191. Wascher RA, Lee MY. Recurrent cutaneous leiomyosarcoma. *Cancer* 1992;70:490.

192. Fields JP, Helwig EB. Leiomyosarcoma of the skin and subcutaneous tissue. *Cancer* 1981;47:156.

193. Schadendorf D, Haas N, Ostmeir H, et al. Primary leiomyosarcoma of the skin. A histological and immunolistachemical analysis. *Acta Derm Venereol (Stockh)* 1993;73:143–145.

194. Manivel JC, Wick MR, Dehner LP. Non-vascular sarcomas of the skin. In: Wick MR, ed. *Pathology of Unusual Malignant Cutaneous Tumors.* New York: Marcel Dekker, 1985:211.

195. Jegasothy BV, Gilgor RS, Hull DM. Leiomyosarcoma of the skin and subcutaneous tissue. *Arch Dermatol* 1981;117:478.

196. Swanson PE, Stanley MW, Scheithauer BW, et al. Primary cutaneous leiomyosarcoma. *J Cutan Pathol* 1988;15:129.

197. Alessi E, Sala F. Leiomyosarcoma in ectopic areola. *Am J Dermatopathol* 1992;14:165.

198. Yamamura T, Takada A, Higashiyama M, et al. Subcutaneous leiomyosarcoma developing in radiation dermatitis. *Dermatologica* 1991;183:154.

199. White IR, MacDonald DM. Cutaneous leiomyosarcoma with coexistent superficial angioleiomyoma. *Clin Exp Dermatol* 1981;6:333–337.

200. Yamamura T, Takada A, Higashiyama M, et al. Subcutaneous leiomyosarcoma. *Br J Dermatol* 1991;124:252.

201. Phelan JT, Sherer W, Mesa P. Malignant smooth muscle tumors (leiomyosarcoma) of soft tissue origin. *N Engl J Med* 1962; 266:1027.

202. Newman PL, Fletcher CD. Smooth muscle tumors of the external genitalia: Clinicopathologic analysis of a series. *Histopathology* 1991;18:523.

203. Levack J, Dick A. Cutaneous leiomyosarcoma with lymphatic spread: a report of two cases. *Glasgow Med J* 1955;36:337–342.

204. Haim S, Gellei B. Leiomyosarcoma of the skin. Report of two cases. *Dermatologica* 1970;140:30–55.

205. Oliver GF, Reiman HM, Gonchoroff NJ, et al. Cutaneous and subcutaneous leiomysarcoma. *Br J Dermatol* 1991;124:252.

206. Hashimoto H, Daimaru Y, Tsuneyoshi M, et al. Leiomyosarcoma of the external soft tissue. *Cancer* 1986;57:2077.

207. Headington JT, Beals TF, Niederhuber JE. Primary leiomyosarcoma of skin: a report and critical appraisal. *J Cutan Pathol* 1977;4:308.

208. Kaddu S, Beham A, Cerroni L, et al. Cutaneous leiomyosarcoma. *Am J Surg Pathol* 1997;21:979–987.

209. Yamamoto T, Minami R, Ohbayashi C, et al. Epithelioid leiomyosarcoma of the external deep soft tissue. *Arch Pathol Lab Med* 2002;126:468–470.

210. Sironi M, Assi A, Pasquinelli G, Cenacchi G. Not all granular cell tumors show Schwann cell differentiation: a granular cell leiomyosarcoma of the thumb, a case report. *Am J Dermatopathol* 1999;21:307–309.

211. Aubain Somerhausen N de S, Fletcher CD. Leiomyosarcoma of soft tissue in children. Clinicopathologic analysis of 20 cases. *Am J Surg Pathol* 1999;23:755–763.

212. Diaz-Cascajo C, Borghi S, Weyers W. Desmoplastic leiomyosarcoma of the skin. *Am J Dermatopathol* 2000:22:251–255.

213. Chen KTK, Tseng-Tong K, Hoffman KD. Leiomyosarcoma of the breast. *Cancer* 1981;47:1883–1886.

214. Perrone T, Dehner LP. Prognostically favorable "mitotically active" smooth-muscle tumors of the uterus. A clinicopathologic study of ten cases. *Am J Surg Pathol* 1988;12:1–8.

215. Gustafson PWillen H, Baldetorp B, et al. Soft tissue leiomyosarcoma. *Cancer* 1992;70:114–119.

216. Mentzel T Calonje E, Fletcher CDM. Leiomyosarcoma with prominent osteoclast-like giant cells. *Am J Surg Pathol* 1994;18:258–265.

217. Rubin BP, Fletcher CDM. Myxoid leiomyosarcoma of soft tissue, an underrecognized variant. *Am J Surg Pathol* 2000:24:927–936.

218. Lundgren L, Kindblom LG, Seidal T, et al. Intermediate and fine cytofilaments in cutaneous and subcutaneous leiomyosarcomas. *APMIS* 1991;99:820.

219. Derre J, Lagace R, Nicolas A, et al. Leiomyosarcomas and most malignant fibrous histiocytomas share very similar comparative genomic hybridization imbalances: an analysis of a series of 27 leiomyosarcomas. *Lab Invest* 2001;81:211–215.

220. Sahn EE, Garen PD, Pai GS, et al. Multiple rhabdomyomatous mesenchymal hamartomas of skin. *Am J Dermatopathol* 1990;12:485–91.

221. Verdolini R, Goteri G, Brancorsini D, et al. Adult rhabdomyoma: report of two cases of rhabdomyoma of the lip and of the eyelid. *Am J Dermatopathol* 2000;22:264–267.

222. Willis J, Abdul-Karim FW, di Sant' Agnese PA. Extracardiac rhabdomyomas. *Semin Diagn Pathol* 1994;11:15–25.

223. Cronin CT, Keel SB, Grabbe J, et al. Adult rhabdomyoma of the extremity: a case report and review of the literature. *Hum Pathol* 2000;31:1074–1080.

224. Lin GY, Sun X, Badve S. Pathologic quiz case. Vaginal wall mass in a 47-year-old woman. *Arch Pathol Lab Med* 2002;126:1241–1242.

225. Weiss S, Goldblum JR, eds. Rhabdomyoma. In *Enzinger and Weiss's Soft Tissue Tumors*, 4th ed. St. Louis: Mosby, 2001:781.

226. Wade WM Jr, Roy EW. Idiopathic masseter muscle hypertrophy: report of case. *J Oral Surg* 1971;29:196–200.

227. Bond SJ, Seibel N, Kapur S, Newman KD. Rhabdomyosarcoma of the clitoris. *Cancer* 1994;1984–1986.

228. Gong Y, Chao J, Bauer B, Sun X, et al. Primary cutaneous alveolar rhabdomyosarcoma of the perineum. *Arch Pathol Lab Med* 2002;126:982–984.

229. Schmidt D, Fletcher CD, Harms D. Rhabdomyosarcomas with primary presentation in the skin. *Pathol Res Pract* 1993;189:422–427.

230. Wiss K, Solomon AR, Raimer SS. Rhabdomyosarcoma presenting as a cutaneous nodule. *Arch Dermatol* 1988;124:1687.

231. Chang Y, Dehner LP, Egbert B. Primary cutaneous rhabdomyosarcoma. *Am J Surg Pathol* 1990;14:977–982.

232. Wong T-Y, Suster S. Primary cutaneous sarcomas showing rhabdomyoblastic differentiation. *Histopathology* 1995;26:25–32.

233. Godambe SV, Rawal J. Blueberry muffin rash as a presentation of alveolar cell rhabdomyosarcoma in a neonate. *Acta Paediatr* 2000;89:115–117.

234. Agamanolis DP, Dasu S, Krill CE Jr. Tumors of skeletal muscle. *Hum Pathol* 1986;17:778.

235. Folpe AL, McKenney JK, Bridge JA, et al. Sclerosing rhabdomyosarcoma in adults: report of four cases of a hyalinizing, matrix-rich variant of rhabdomyosarcoma that may be confused with osteosarcoma, chondrosarcoma, or angiosarcoma. *Am J Surg Pathol* 2002;26:1175–1183.

236. Fernandez-Figueras MT, Puig L, Gilaberte M, et al. Merkel cell (primary neuroendocrine) carcinoma of the skin with nodal metastasis showing rhabdomyosarcomatous differentiation. *J Cutan Pathol* 2002;29:619–622.

237. Dabbs DJ, Parks HK. Malignant rhabdoid skin tumor: an uncommon primary skin neoplasm. Ultrastructural and immunohistochemical analysis. *J Cutan Pathol* 1988;15:109–115.

238. Weeks DA, Beckwith JB, Mieran GW. Rhabdoid tumor: an entity or a phenotype? *Arch Pathol Lab Med* 1989;113:113–114.

239. Daniney A, Paller AS, Gonzolez-Crussi F. Congenital rhabdoid sarcoma with cutaneous metastases. *J Am Acad Dermatol* 1990;22:969–974.

240. Berry PJ, Vujanic GM. Malignant rhabdoid tumor. *Histopathology* 1992;20:189–193.

241. Leong FJ, Leong AS. Malignant rhabdoid tumor in adults—heterogenous tumors with a unique morphological phenotype. *Pathol Res Pract* 1996;192:796–807.

242. Borek BT, McKee PH, Freeman JA, et al. Primary malignant melanoma with rhabdoid features: a histologic and immunocytochemical study of three cases. *Am J Dermatopathol* 1998;20:123–127.

243. Weiss S, Goldblum JR, eds. Malignant soft tissue tumors of uncertain type. In *Enzinger and Weiss's Soft Tissue Tumors*, 4th ed. St. Louis: Mosby, 2001:1545.

244. Wick MR, Ritter JH, Dehner LP. Malignant rhabdoid tumors: a clinicopathologic review and conceptual discussion. *Semin Diagn Pathol* 1995;12:233–248.

245. White FV, Dehner LP, Belchis DA, et al. Congenital disseminated malignant rhabdoid tumor. A distinct clinicopathologic entity demonstrating abnormalities of chromosome 22gl I. *Am J Surg Pathol* 1999;23:249–256.

246. Kransdorf MJ, Meis JM. From the archives of the AFIP. Extraskeletal osseous and cartilaginous tumors of the extremities. *Radiographics* 1993;13:853–84.

247. Albright F, Forbes AP, Henneman PH. Pseudohypoparathyroidism. *Trans Assoc Am Physicians* 1952;65:337.

248. Peterson WC Jr, Mandel SL. Primary osteomas of skin. *Arch Dermatol* 1963;87:626.

249. Donaldson EM, Summerly R. Primary osteoma cutis and diaphyseal aclasis. *Arch Dermatol* 1962;85:261.

250. Eyre WG, Reed WB. Albright's hereditary osteodystrophy with cutaneous bone formation. *Arch Dermatol* 1971;104:636.

251. Aldred MA, Aftimos S, Hall C, et al. Constitutional deletion of chromosome 20q in two patients affected with albright hereditary osteodystrophy. *Am J Med Genet* 2002;113:167–72.

252. Goeteyn V, De Potter CR, Naeyaert JM. Osteoma cutis in pseudohypoparathyroidism. *Dermatology.* 1999;198:209–211.

253. Spranger J. Skeletal dysplasia: albright's hereditary osteodystrophy. In: Bergsma D, ed. *The First Conference on the Clinical Delineation of Birth Defects.* New York: National Foundation March of Dimes, 1968;122.

254. Piesowicz AT. Pseudohypoparathyroidism with osteoma cutis. *Proc R Soc Med* 1965;58:126.

255. Kaplan FS, Shore EM. Progressive osseous heteroplasia. *J Bone Miner Res* 2000;15:2084–2094.

256. McFarland GS, Robinowitz B, Say B. Fibrodysplasia ossificans progressiva presenting as fibrous scalp nodules. *Cleve Clin Q* 1984;51:549–552.

257. Oikarinen A, Tuomi M-L, Kallionen M, et al. A study of bone formation in osteoma cutis emplying biochemical, histochemical and in situ hybridization techniques. *Acta Derm Venereol (Stockh)* 1992;72:172–174.

258. Goldminz D, Greenberg RD. Multiple military osteoma cutis. *J Am Acad Dermatol* 1991;24:878–881.

259. Baslèr RSW, Taylor WB, Peacor DP. Postacne osteoma cutis. X-ray diffraction analysis. *Arch Dermatol* 1974;110:113–114.

260. O'Donnell TF Jr, Geller SA. Primary osteoma cutis. *Arch Dermatol* 1971;104:325.

261. Sanmartin O, Alegre V, Martinez-Aparicio A, et al. Congenital platelike osteoma cutis. Case report and review literature. *Pediatr Dermatol* 1993;10:182.

262. Monroe AB, Burgdorf WHC, Sheward S. Platelike cutaneous osteoma. *J Am Acad Dermatol* 1987;16:481.

263. Burgdorf W, Nasemann T. Cutaneous osteomas. A clinical and histopathologic review. *Arch Dermatol Res* 1977;260:121.

264. Helm F, De La Pava S, Klein E. Multiple miliary osteomas of the skin. *Arch Dermatol* 1967;96:681.

265. Basler RSW, Taylor WB, Peacor DR. Postacne osteoma cutis. *Arch Dermatol* 1974;110:113.

266. Moritz DL, Elewski B. Pigmented post acne osteoma cutis in a patient treated with minocycline: report and review of the literature. *J Am Acad Dermatol* 1991;24:851.

267. Farhood VW, Steed DL, Krolls SO. Osteoma cutis: cutaneous ossification with oral manifestations. *Oral Surg Oral Med Oral Pathol* 1978;45:98–103.

268. Takato T, Yanai A, Tanaka H, et al. Primary osteoma cutis of the back. *Plast Reconstr Surg* 1986;77:309–311.

269. Oikarinen A, Tuomi M-L, Kallionen M, et al. A study of bone formation in osteoma cutis employing biochemical, histochemical and in situ hybridization techniques. *Acta Derm Venereol (Stockh)* 1992;72:172.

270. Goldminz D, Greenberg RD. Multiple miliary osteoma cutis. *J Am Acad Dermatol* 1991;24:878.

271. Mason JK, Helwig EB, Graham JH. Pathology of the nevoid basal cell carcinoma syndrome. *Arch Pathol* 1965;79:401.

272. Urmacher C. Unusual stromal pattern in truly recurrent and satellite metastatic lesions of malignant melanoma. *Am J Dermatopathol* 1984;1[Suppl]:331.

273. Moreno A, Lamarca J, Martinez R, et al. Osteoid and bone formation in desmoplastic malignant melanoma. *J Cutan Pathol* 1986;13:128.

274. Lucas DR, Tazelaar HD, Unni KK, et al. Osteogenic melanoma: a rare varient of malignant melanoma. *Am J Surg Pathol* 1993;17:400.

275. Roth SI, Stowell RE, Helwig EB. Cutaneous ossification. *Arch Pathol* 1963;76:44.

276. De Maeseneer M, Jaovisidha S, Lenchik L, et al. Myositis ossificans of the foot. *J Foot Ankle* Surg 1997;36:290–293.

277. Dupuytren G. On the injuries and disease of the toes. In: Clark F, ed. *Publications of the Sydenham Society, London.* London: Sydenham Society, 1847;20:408–410.

278. Cohen PR, Scher RK. Geriatric nail disorders: diagnosis and treatment. *J Am Acad Dermatol* 1992;26:521–531.

279. Dumontier CA, Abimelec P. Nail unit enchondromas and osteochondromas: a surgical approach. *Dermatol Surg* 2001;27:274–279.

280. Kim SW, Moon SE, Kim JA. A case of subungual osteochondroma. *J Dermatol* 1998;25:60–62.

281. Davis DA, Cohen PR. Subungual exostosis: case report and review of the literature. *Pediatr Dermatol* 1996;13:212–218.

282. Ragsdale, BD. Morphologic analysis of skeletal lesions: correlation of imaging studies and pathologic findings. In: Reynaldo A, Weinstein RS, eds. *Advances in Pathology and Laboratory Medicine.* St. Louis: Mosby Year Book, 1993;445.

283. Pillay P, Simango S, Govender D. Extraskeletal osteosarcoma of the scalp. *Pathology* 2000;32:154–157.

284. Kuo TT. Primary cutaneous osteosarcoma. *Am J Dermatopathol* 1996;18:109.

285. Drut R, Barletta L. Osteogenic sarcoma arising in an old burn scar. *J Cutan Pathol* 1975;2:302–306.

286. Kobos JW, Yu GH, Varadarajan S, et al. Primary cutaneous osteosarcoma. *Am J Dermatopathol* 1995;17:53–57.

287. Bacetic D, Knezevic M, Stojsic Z, et al. Primary extraskeletal osteosarcoma of the penis with amalignant fibrous histiocytoma-like component. *Histopathology* 1998;33:185–186.

288. Dubey SP, Murthy DP, Cooke RA, et al. Primary osteogenic sarcoma of the tongue. *J Laryngol Otol* 1999;113:376–379.

289. Konishi E, Kusuzaki K, Murata H, et al. Extraskeletal osteosarcoma arising in myositis ossificans. *Skeletal Radiol* 2001;30:39–43.

290. Lidang Jensen M, Schumacher B, Myhre Jensen O, et al. Extraskeletal osteosarcomas: a clinicopathologic study of 25 cases. *Am J Surg Pathol* 1998;22:588–594.

292. Velasco-Pastor AM, Martinez-Escribano J, del Pino Gil-Mateo M, et al. Ossifying fibromyxoid tumor of soft parts. *J Cutan Pathol* 1996;23:381–384.

292. Fernandez-Figueras MT, Puig L, Gilaberte M, et al. Merkel cell (primary neuroendocrine) carcinoma of the skin with nodal metastasis showing rhabdomyosarcomatous differentiation. *Cutan Pathol* 2002;29:619–622.

293. Wick MR, Fitzgibbon J, Swanson PE. Cutaneous sarcomas and sarcomatoid neoplasms of the skin. *Semin Diagn Pathol* 1993;10:148–518.

294. Nishio J, Iwasaki H, Soejima O, et al. Rapidly growing fibroosseous pseudotumor of the digits mimicking extraskeletal osteosarcoma. *J Orthop Sci* 2002;7:410–3.

295. Setoyama M, Kanda A, Kanzaki T. Cutaneous metastasis of an osteosarcoma. A case report. *Am J Dermatopathol* 1996;18:629–632.

296. Pollock L, Malone M, Shaw DG. Childhood soft tissue chondroma: a case report. *Pediatr Pathol Lab Med* 1995;15:437–441.

297. Gangopadhyay AN, Khurana SK, Rastogi BL, et al. Soft tissue chondroma in an infant. *J Indian Med Assoc* 1991;89:315.

298. Chung EB, Enzinger FM. Chondroma of soft parts. *Cancer* 1978;41:1414.

299. DelSignore JL, Torre BA, Miller RJ. Extraskeletal chondroma of the hand: Case report and review of the literature. *Clin Orthop* 1990;254:147.

300. Wong L, Dellon AL. Soft tissue chondroma presenting as a painful finger: diagnosis by magnetic resonance imaging. *Ann Plast Surg* 1992;28:304–306.

301. DelSignore JL, Torre BA, Miller RJ. Extraskeletal chondroma of the hand. Case report and review of the literature. *Clin Orthop* 1990;254:147–152.

302. Stockley I, Norris SH. Trigger finger secondary to soft tissue chondroma. *J Hand Surg [Br]* 1990;15:468–469.

303. Hofmann AK, Wustner MC, Spier W. Compression neuropathy of the median nerve at the wrist joint caused by chondroma [German]. *Handchir Mikrochir Plast Chir* 1990;22:96–98.

304. Ando K, Goto Y, Hirabayashi N, et al. Cutaneous cartilaginous tumor. *Dermatol Surg* 1995;21:339–341.

305. Humphreys TR, Herzberg AJ, Elenitsas R, et al. Familial occurrence of multiple cutaneous chondromas. *Am J Dermatopathol* 1994;16:54–59.

306. Steiner GC, Meushar N, Norman A, et al. Intracapsular and paraarticular chondromas. *Clin Orthop* 1994;303:231–236.

307. Sowa DT, Moore JR, Weiland AJ. Extraskeletal osteochondromas of the wrist. *J Hand Surg [Am]* 1987;12:212–217.

308. Nather A, Chong PY. A rare case of carpal tunnel syndrome due to tenosynovial osteochondroma. *J Hand Surg [Br]* 1986;11:478–480.

309. Szendroi M, Deodhar A. Synovial neoformations and tumours. *Baillieres Best Pract Res Clin Rheumatol* 2000;14:363–383.

310. Yaffee HS. Peculiar nail dystrophy caused by an enchondroma. *Arch Dermatol* 1965;91:361.

311. Bansal M, Goldman AB, DiCarlo EF, et al. Soft tissue chondromas: diagnosis and differential diagnosis. *Skeletal Radiol* 1993;22:309–315.

312. Athanasou NA, Caughey M, Burge P, et al. Deposition of calcium pyrophosphate dihydrate crystals in a soft tissue chondroma. *Ann Rheum Dis* 1991;50:950–952.

313. del Rosario AD, Bui HX, Singh J, et al. Intracytoplasmic eosinophilic hyaline globules in cartilaginous neoplasms: a surgical, pathological, ultrastructural, and electron probe x-ray microanalyticstudy. *Hum Pathol* 1994;25:1283–1289.

314. Cates JM, Rosenberg AE, O'Connell JX, et al. Chondroblastoma-like chondroma of soft tissue: an underrecognized variant and its differential diagnosis. *Am J Surg Pathol* 2001;25:661–666.

315. Yamada T, Irisa T, Nakano S, et al. Extraskeletal chondroma with chondroblastic and granuloma-like elements. *Clin Orthop* 1995;315:257–261.

316. Thool AA, Raut WK, Lele VR, et al. Fine needle aspiration cytology of soft tissue chondroma. A case report. *Acta Cytol* 2001;45:86–88.

317. Anthouli-Anagnostopoulou FA, Papachristou G. Extraskeletal chondroma, a rare soft tissue tumor. Case report. *Acta Orthop Belg* 2000;66:402–404.

318. Heydemann J, Gillespie R, Mancer K. Soft tissue recurrence of chondromyxoid fibroma. *J Pediatr Orthop* 1985;5:725–727.

319. Ragsdale BD, Vihn TN, Sweet DE. *Radiology* as gross pathology in evaluating chondroid lesions. *Hum Pathol* 1989;20:930.

320. Nakamura R, Ehara S, Nishida J, et al. Diffuse mineralization of extraskeletal chondroma: a case report. *Radiat Med* 1997;15:51–53.

321. Chandramohan M, Thomas NB, Funk L, et al. MR appearance of mineralized extra skeletal chondroma: a case report and review of literature. *Clin Radiol* 2002;57:421–423.

322. Bianchi S, Zwass A, Abdelwahab IF, et al. Sonographic evaluation of soft tissue chondroma. *J Clin Ultrasound* 1996;24:148–150.

323. Dal Cin P, Qi H, Sciot R, et al. Involvement of chromosomes 6 and 11 in a soft tissue chondroma. *Cancer Genet Cytogenet* 1997;93:177–178.

324. Murphy BA, Kilpatrick SE, Panella MJ, et al. Extra-acral calcifying aponeurotic fibroma: a distinctive case with 23-year follow-up. *J Cutan Pathol* 1996;23:369–372.

325. Fetsch JF, Miettinen M. Calcifying aponeurotic fibroma: a clinicopathologic study of 22 cases arising in uncommon sites. *Hum Pathol* 1998;29:1504–1510.

326. Tai LH, Johnston JO, Klein HZ, et al. Calcifying aponeurotic fibroma features seen on fine-needle aspiration biopsy: case report and brief review of the literature. *Diagn Cytopathol* 2001;24:336–339.

327. Wick MR, Burgess JH, Manivel JC. A reassessment of "chordoid sarcoma." Ultrastructural and immunohistochemical comparison with chordoma and skeletal myxoid chondrosarcoma. *Mod Pathol* 1988;1:433–443.

328. Enzinger FM, Shiraki M. Extraskeletal myxoid chondrosarcoma. An analysis of 34 cases. *Hum Pathol* 1972;3:421–435.

329. Quagliuolo V, Azzarelli A, Cerasoli S, et al. Unusual types of chondrosarcoma: chondrosarcoma arising in soft tissue and nonskeletal cartilage. *Eur J Surg Oncol* 1988;14:691–695.

330. Dardick I, Lagace R, Carlier MT, et al. Chordoid sarcoma (extraskeletal myxoid chondrosarcoma). A light and electronmicroscopic study. *Virchows Arch [A]* 1983;399:61–78.

331. Hachitanda Y, Tsuneyoshi M, Daimaru Y, et al. Extraskeletal myxoid chondrosarcoma in young children. *Cancer* 1988;61:2521–2526.

332. Klijanienko J, Micheau C, Cote R, et al. Unusual extraskeletal myxoid chondrosarcoma in a child. *Histopathology* 1990;16:196–198.

333. Fletcher CDM, Powell G, McKee PH. Extraskeletal myxoid chondrosarcoma: a histochemical and immunohistochemical study. *Histopathology* 1986;10:489–499.

334. Mackenzie DH. The unsuspected soft tissue chondrosarcoma. *Histopathology* 1983;7:759–766.

335. Weiss S.W. Ultrastructure of the so-called "chordoid sarcoma." *Cancer* 1976;37:300–306.

336. DeBlois G, Wang S, Kay S. Microtubular aggregates within rough endoplasmic reticulum: an unusual ultrastructural feature of extraskeletal myxoid chondrosarcoma. *Hum Pathol* 1986;17:469–475.

337. Vuzevski VD, van der Heul RO. Comparative ultrastructure of soft tissue myxoid tumors. *Ultrastruct Pathol* 1988;12:87–105.

338. Kindbloom L-G and Angervall L. Myxoid chondrosarcoma of the synovial tissue. A clinicopathologic, histochemical and ultrastructural analysis. *Cancer* 1983;52:1886–1895.

339. Suzuki T, Kaneka H, Kojima K, et al. Extraskeletal myxoid chondrosarcoma characterized by microtubular aggregates in the rough endoplasmic reticulum and tubulin immunoreactivity. *J Pathol* 1988;156:51–57.

340. Fletcher CDM, McKee PH. Immunohistochemistry and histogenesis of extraskeletal myxoid chondrosarcoma [Letter]. *J Pathol* 1985;147:67–68.

341. Graadt van Roggen JF, Hogendoorn PC, Fletcher CD. Myxoid tumours of soft tissue. *Histopathology* 1999;35:291–312.

342. Michal M, Miettinen M. Myoepitheliomas of the skin and soft tissues. Report of 12 cases. *Virchows Arch* 1999;434:393–400.

343. Michal M, Sokol L. Benign polymorphous mesenchymal tumor (mesenchymal hamartoma) of soft parts. Report of two cases. *Am J Dermatopathol* 1997;19:271–215.

344. Turc-Carel C, Cin P, Rao U, et al. Recurrent breakpoints at 9q31 and 22g12.2 in extraskeletal myxoid chondrosarcoma. *Cancer Genet Cytogenet* 1988;30:145–150.

345. Aramburu-Gonzalez JA, Rodriguez-Justo M, Jimenez-Reyes J, et al. A case of soft tissue mesenchymal chondrosarcoma metastatic to skin, clinically mimicking keratoacanthoma. *Am J Dermatopathol* 1999;21:392–394.

346. Shapeero LG, Vanel D, Couanet D, et al. Extraskeletal mesenchymal chondrosarcoma. *Radiology* 1993;186:819–826.

347. Granter SR, Renshaw AA, Fletcher CD, et al. CD99 reactivity in mesenchymal chondrosarcoma. *Hum Pathol* 1996;27:1273–1276.

348. Hoang MP, Suarez PA, Donner LR, Y Ro J, Ordonez NG, Ayala AG, Czerniak B. Mesenchymal chondrosarcoma: a small cell neoplasm with polyphenotypic differentiation. *Int J Surg Pathol* 2000;8:291–301.

349. Naumann S, Krallman PA, Unni KK, et al. Translocation der(13;21)(q10;q10) in skeletal and extraskeletal mesenchymal chondrosarcoma. *Mod Pathol* 2002;15:572–576.

350. Leal-Khouri SM, Barnhill RL, Baden HP. An unusual cutaneous metastasis of a chondrosarcoma. *J Cutan Pathol* 1990;17:274–7.

351. Arce FP, Pinto J, Portero I, et al. Cutaneous metastases as initial manifestation of dedifferentiated chondrosarcoma of bone. An autopsy case with review of the literature. *J Cutan Pathol* 2000;27:262–267.

352. Patel NK, McKee PH, Smith NP, et al. Primary metaplastic carcinoma (carcinosarcoma) of the skin. A clinicopathologic study of four cases and review of the literature. *Am J Dermatopathol* 1997;19:363–372.

353. Sexton CW, White WL. Chondrosarcomatous cutaneous metastasis. A unique manifestation of sarcomatoid (metaplastic) breast carcinoma. *Am J Dermatopathol* 1996;18:538–42.

354. Sato N, Sato K, Matoba N, et al. Malignant mesenchymoma arising in an incisional scar of the abdominal wall. *Eur J Surg Oncol* 1998;24:449–450.

355. Banerjee SS, Coyne JD, Menasce LP, et al. Diagnostic lessons of mucosal melanoma with osteocartilaginous differentiation. *Histopathology* 1998;33:255–260.

356. Ackley CD, Prieto VG, Bentley RC, et al. Primary chondroid melanoma. *J Cutan Pathol* 2001;28:482–485.

357. Wilson PR, Strutton GM, Stewart MR. Atypical fibroxanthoma: two unusual variants. *J Cutan Pathol* 1989;16:93–98.

TUMORS OF NEURAL TISSUE

RICHARD J. REED
ZSOLT ARGENYI

GENERAL ANATOMIC RELATIONSHIPS: STRUCTURAL COMPONENTS

A *nerve*, an anatomic unit, is composed of nerve fibers, endoneurium, and perineurium. *Nerve fibers*, the functioning element, are aggregated to form axial bundles (parallel arrays of nerve fibers with longitudinal symmetry). Individually, each fiber consists of an axon, or axons, and related *Schwann cells* (1–3). *Axons* are cytoplasmic extensions from the peri-karyon of *neurons* in the central nervous system (CNS), or in sympathetic ganglia. The peripheral portion of an axon along its entire length from its origin to terminus is enclosed by enveloping Schwann cells. Along nonmyelinated nerve fibers, a single Schwann cell encloses segments of several axons in cytoplasmic invaginations. Along myelinated nerve fibers, a single Schwann cell encloses a segment of an axon in concentric layers of its cytoplasmic membrane; where neighboring Schwann cells abut, end-to-end, a node of Ranvier is formed. In sympathetic ganglia, neurons are rimmed by satellite cells; Schwann cells are substituted for satellite cells along axons. Ultrastructurally, microfilaments, specialized intermediate (neural) filaments, and microtubules are components of axons. Schwann cells have complex cytoplasmic processes, are surrounded by continuous basal lamina, and contain densely packed intermediate filaments.

The *perineurium*, a tubular fibrous sheath, delimits each nerve. It extends from the pia-arachnoid of the CNS to the terminus of each nerve, or to specialized sensory receptors. Slender, bipolar, or tripolar cells (*perineurial cells*) are isolated among the concentric fibrous lamellae of the perineurium. Ultrastructurally, discontinuous basal lamina, numerous pinocytotic vesicles, and tight intercellular junctions are characteristics of perineureal cells. The perineurium is a relatively impervious barrier.

The *endoneurium*, a delicate, mucinous matrix, is confined by the perineurium; it provides a cushion for the axial collection of nerve fibers. Components of the endoneurium include fibroblasts, mast cells, collagen, a myxoid matrix, and capillaries.

In proximal (axial) locations, several large nerves, in bundles, are encased in a dense fibrous matrix, the *epineurium*

(a fibrous sheath which, at the junction of the spinal nerves with the CNS, is continuous with the dura mater). Individual nerves, at some place along their course, leave the bundles to continue without an epineurium. Near the terminus of each nerve, nerve fibers extend beyond an open-ended perineurium into the mesenchyme; naked axons even extend into epithelium. Ensheathed receptors of the skin include mucocutaneous corpuscles, and the corpuscles of Vater–Pacini, Meissner, and Merkel. Meissner corpuscles are ovoid structures in which an axon is sinuously enclosed in stacks of distinctive cells. Pacinian corpuscles are spherical structures in soft tissue. In them, concentrically laminated, distinctive cells, and fibrous lamellae are arranged around a centrally located axon (Fig. 35-1). The ultrastructural features of the laminated cells of both Meissner and pacinian corpuscles are perineurial cell-like (4), with the exception of the innermost cells which ensheathe the central axon.

ONTOGENY AND REACTIONS TO INJURY AS RELATED TO THE INTERPRETATION OF PHENOTYPIC EXPRESSIONS OR PATTERNS IN NEOPLASIA

Neurosustentacular cells of peripheral nerves, related cells of the peripheral ganglia, melanocytes, and even cells of some cranial mesenchyme are all of neurocristic origin.

In reactions of peripheral nerves to injury, reserve cells of neural origin proliferate; they subsequently express either a schwannian, or perineurial phenotype. Expressions of phenotype are fortuitous: the environs, in which uncommitted reserve cells find themselves, influence the expressions. The available options probably include a capacity to function facultatively as endoneurial fibroblasts (5).

Histologic interpretations are based on images, both real and virtual; the virtual images are evoked from the pathologist's mental stores; the richness of the stores is a reflection of the experience of the pathologist. Virtual images, once recalled and compared with real images, form the basis for histologic interpretations. Various patterns, some relating to the

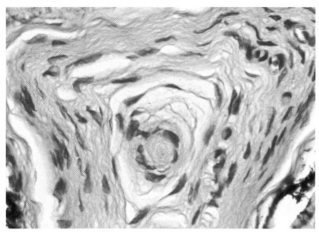

FIGURE 35-1. Pacinian corpuscle. This pacinian body has a distorted outline. At the periphery, there is a well-formed dense fibrous membrane. Elongated spindle cells are compressed among the compactly arranged collagen fibers. At the center, an acidophilic punctum is representative of a single axon. Cytoplasmic processes of sheath cells are clustered about the axon. There is an intermediate zone in which spindle cells are loosely spaced in a clear matrix. Regardless of the results of immunoreactions, the loosely spaced spindle cells have the morphologic features of perineurial cells. There is a morphologic continuum from periphery to, but not including, axon.

structural components of peripheral nerves, some to the embryologic development of their neurocristic precursors, and some to the reactions of normal nerves to injury, provide clues for the interpretation of the puzzling histologic patterns of nerve sheath tumors. In turn, the interpretations, often with an element of luck, can lead to the structuring of a proper histologic diagnosis. For example, the structure of

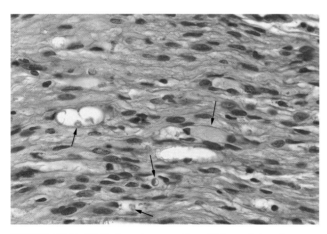

FIGURE 35-2. Wallerian degeneration. This peripheral nerve, bordering the site of an injury, shows poorly defined myelin sheaths; as a result, reticular fibers (basement membranes) of individual Schwann cells are more closely spaced. Scattered microcystic areas are representative of sites in which myelin sheaths have been disrupted. In some of the defects, there are globular deposits, some of which are concentrically laminated (*black arrows*); these "myelin figures" are collections of lipid membranes. Some of the Schwann cells are swollen and have pale, faintly granular cytoplasm (*green arrow*).

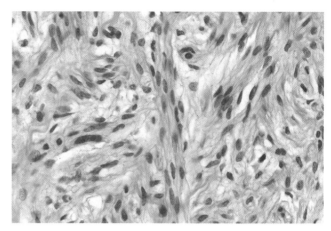

FIGURE 35-3. Extraneural neuroma. In this extraneural neuroma, Schwann cells cluster to form thin fascicles among collagen bundles of the preexisting soft tissue; the fascicles appear to be randomly distributed but their course has been directed by the distribution of proliferating axons, as the axons extend into the fibrous tissue in the process of repair.

Meissner corpuscles is recapitulated in the tactile corpuscle–like structures (tactoid bodies) of diffuse (extraneural) neurofibromas. Some of the features of wallerian degeneration (Fig. 35-2) are recapitulated in a most distorted manner in granular cell nerve sheath tumor. The intravaginal hyaline nodules of Renaut (3) may provide a model for the patterns manifested in nerve sheath myxomas.

When damaged, axons form multiple, sprout-like extensions. In the ensuing reparative process, newly formed Schwann cells accompany newly formed axons (Fig. 35-3). These patterns are incompletely recapitulated in spontaneous, intraneural neuromas. The distorted patterns that are manifested in intraneural neurofibromas, and even in some small schwannomas, may relate to a (temporary?) local excess of thin, nonmyelinated axons.

PHENOTYPES AND HISTOCHEMICAL AND IMMUNOHISTOCHEMICAL REACTIONS

Neurosustentacular cells, melanocytes, and even some mesenchymal cells are intermutable. In tumors of peripheral nerves, the structural qualities of either Schwann cells or perineurial cells are commonly expressed, but the expression of either histologic cell type may, in turn, be associated with immunohistochemical marker of a conflicting type. For example, the cells of tactile corpuscles mark with antibodies for S-100 protein (as do Schwann cells) but have the ultrastructural features of perineurial cells.

S-100 protein is a lightly acidic, calcium-binding protein of glial cells, but also is expressed in a variety of other cells, including melanocytes, lipocytes, chondrocytes, some sweat gland cells, and Schwann cells. *Neuron-specific enolase* (NSE) is a cytoplasmic product common to a variety of

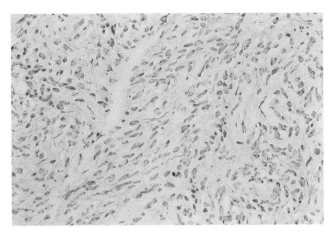

FIGURE 35-4. Extraneural neuroma (Bodian stain). The loosely spaced, delicate fibers are axons; axons are argyrophilic.

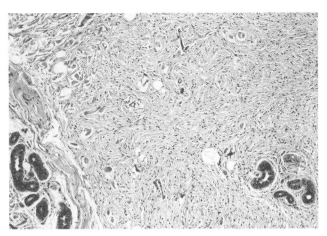

FIGURE 35-5. Extraneural sporadic cutaneous neurofibroma. A circumscribed, nonencapsulated tumor of the dermis is composed of loosely spaced spindle cells and wavy collagenous strands. Near the margin, collagen bundles of the dermis are entrapped in the lesion. A cluster of sweat glands also is present within the tumor.

cells including Schwann cells, and both neurons and their axons. An immunoreaction for the demonstration of neural filaments provides a pure demonstration of the reaction of axons. Silver impregnation techniques are the time-honored method of demonstrating axons (Fig. 35-4) but are less sensitive than immunohistochemical reactions; fewer axons are demonstrated. The luxol-fast blue stain, and antibodies for either myelin-basic protein (MBP) or CD57 (Leu-7) antigen demonstrate myelin products. An immunoreaction for glial fibrillary acidic protein (GFAP) is positive in glial cells; it is also positive in some of the cells in some tumors of salivary glands. In some large schwannomas of soft tissue, neoplastic Schwann cells are immunoreactive for GFAP. *Epithelial membrane antigen* (EMA) is a membrane-based glycoprotein commonly expressed in a variety of normal, and neoplastic tissue, including cells of the perineurium and sebaceous cells. Currently, peripherin is being promoted as a marker of neural crest derivatives.

Structural peculiarities take precedence over immunohistochemical findings; the commonness of a reaction for S-100 protein does not take precedence over the morphologic distinctions between schwannoma and neurofibroma. The commonness of a reaction for EMA should not be the basis for a grouping of morphologically dissimilar lesions in a category of " perineurioma," a currently popular practice.

NEUROFIBROMAS (HAMARTOMAS WITH PHENOTYPIC DIVERSITY)

Extraneural sporadic cutaneous neurofibromas (ESCNs) (the common sporadic neurofibromas) are soft, polypoid, and skin-colored, or slightly tan; they are small (rarely larger than a centimeter in diameter). They usually arise in adulthood. The identification of as many as four, small, cutaneous neurofibromas in a single patient, in the absence of

other confirmatory findings, would not qualify as stigmata of neurofibromatosis.

Histopathology. Under low magnification, most examples of ESCN are faintly eosinophilic; they are circumscribed but not encapsulated (Fig. 35-5); they are extraneural. Thin spindle cells with elongated, wavy nuclei are regularly spaced among thin, wavy collagenous strands (Fig. 35-6). The strands are either closely spaced (homogeneous pattern), or loosely spaced in a clear matrix (loose pattern) (1). The two patterns are often intermixed in a single lesion. Rarely, ESCNs are composed of widely spaced spindle, and stellate cells in a myxoid matrix. The regular spacing of adnexae is relatively preserved in cutaneous neurofibromas (Fig. 35-5). Small nerves entrapped in a cutaneous neurofibroma occasionally are enlarged and

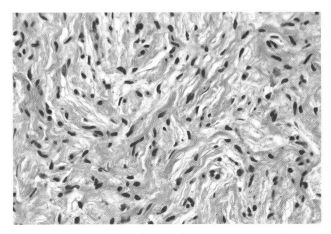

FIGURE 35-6. Extraneural sporadic cutaneous neurofibroma. Thin spindle cells are associated with thin, wavy collagen bundles. The cells and collagen bundles are loosely spaced in a clear or mucinous matrix.

hypercellular. Tactoid (tactile corpuscle-like) bodies, and pigmented, dendritic melanocytes are most uncommon.

Histogenesis. With silver impregnations (Bodian or Bielschowsky stain), only a few axons, mostly in small, entrapped nerves, are demonstrable. Immunohistochemically, axons are more uniformly, and generously represented. With monoclonal antibodies for NSE, an intense punctate, or fiber-like cytoplasmic reaction, in a background of diffuse cytoplasmic staining, identifies the axons of a cutaneous neurofibroma. A similar response, without diffuse cytoplasmic staining, characterizes the reaction for neural filaments. Both immunoreactions, and ultrastructural features have utility in the documentation of the schwannian (neurosustentacular) nature of the tumor cells in ESCN.

Differential Diagnosis. A schwannoma is intraneural (encapsulated); it usually does not contain axons as demonstrated by antibodies to neurofilaments.

In a neurotized nevus, nests and fascicles of nevocytic cells usually can be identified in scattered foci. Tactoid bodies are common in neurotized nevi, but rare in ESCN.

In the absence of an intraneural component, some cutaneous neurofibromas of neurofibromatosis are histologically indistinguishable from ESCN; cutaneous neurofibromas of neurofibromatosis that resemble, in histologic patterns, sporadic variants usually are larger than sporadic variants.

Some sporadic cutaneous neurofibromas, including subcutaneous variants, differ in patterns from ESCN. Confined by the perineurium of the nerve of origin, they are circumscribed and intraneural (1–3). Their internal patterns are indistinguishable from the patterns variously manifested in the intraneural components of plexiform neurofibromas.

On rare occasions, dermatofibromas, and subcutaneous, spindle cell lipomas may be mistaken for a nerve sheath tumor.

NEUROFIBROMATOSIS (PHENOTYPIC DIVERSITY EXPRESSED IN GENETICALLY DETERMINED HAMARTOMAS AND NEOPLASMS)

Multiple cutaneous neurofibromas are characteristic of most, but not all, examples of neurofibromatosis (von Recklinghausen's disease). Other important stigmata include plexiform (intraneural), and deep, diffuse (extraneural) neurofibromas, multiple peri-areolar neurofibromas, intraocular Lisch nodules, and macular, cutaneous hyperpigmentations (e.g., café-au-lait spots and bilateral axillary freckling) (6,7).

Neurofibromatosis type I (NF1) can arise as an autosomal dominant condition, but in nearly half of patients, it arises by spontaneous mutation (8). Cutaneous neurofibromas usually appear first in late childhood or in adolescence;

the disease progresses by showing gradual increases in the size and number of neurofibromas.

For NF1, the gene, which is huge, has been localized to the pericentromeric region of the long arm of chromosome 17. A high spontaneous mutation rate (9), an attribute of huge genes, would account for the high incidence of sporadic cases. The gene shows functional, and structural homology with guanosine triphosphatase–activating protein, which controls the ras oncogene. In turn, the role of the ras oncogene in growth, development, and differentiation may be aberrantly expressed in the NF1 phenotype (9). The protein product of the gene is called *neurofibromin* (10).

In NF1, superficial peripheral nerves, deep peripheral nerves, nerve roots, and the autonomic nerves of viscera and blood vessels may be affected. Large, pendulous plexiform neurofibromas have the flabby texture of a "bag of worms." Deep, diffuse neurofibromas are poorly defined at their limits with the adjacent soft tissue (3). Changes, that are associated with large neurofibromas of the skin and subcutaneous fat, provide an elephantiasic quality. Spinal nerve root tumors may cause compression of the spinal cord (8). Tumors of the CNS occur in 5% to 10% of patients (6). The pressure of an adjacent or intraosseous neurofibroma may result in erosive defects in bones. Nonspecific lesions, such as kyphoscoliosis, or an increase in the length of long bones, may occur. NF1, diffuse intestinal ganglioneuromatosis, and multiple endocrine neoplasia (MEN), type 2b, are unpredictably associated (11, 12). An association among juvenile xanthogranuloma, juvenile chronic myelogenous leukemia, and NF1 has been observed (13).

In localized or segmental neurofibromatosis, cutaneous neurofibromas are few in number, and the family history is negative (14–16).

In *neurofibromatosis type 2* (NF2, a genetically distinct variant), café-au-lait spots, neurofibromas, schwannomas, and a variety of intracranial tumors, including bilateral schwannomas of the acoustic nerves, are manifestations (10). The gene locus has been linked to chromosome 22q11-q13. The protein gene product, called *merlin*, is similar to a group of cytoskeleton-linked proteins (10).

The syndrome of *multiple schwannomas* (schwannomatosis or neurilemmomatosis) (17) is characterized by multiple schwannomas, and plexiform schwannomas. It has been characterized as a clinical entity, distinct from NF2 (18).

Café-au-lait spots occur in nearly all patients with neurofibromatosis. In the sequence in which clinical findings first appear, they usually precede cutaneous tumors (6). Although a few café-au-lait spots are occasionally seen in patients without neurofibromatosis, the presence of more than six spots, each exceeding 1.5 cm in diameter, is indicative of neurofibromatosis (6,8).

Histopathology. The histologic spectrum of neurofibromas in NF1 is broad. Cutaneous, extraneural variants (as manifested in ESCN); cutaneous or deep, circumscribed

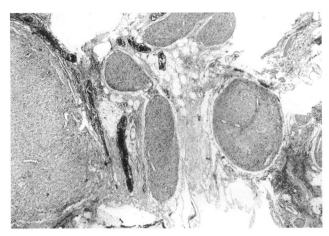

FIGURE 35-7. Components of a cutaneous, plexiform, intra-neural neurofibroma. For the most part, components of the plexus in this field are cut in cross-section. The tumor is intra-neural; it sits in fibrofat without an extraneural component. Each component is confined by a thickened perineurium.

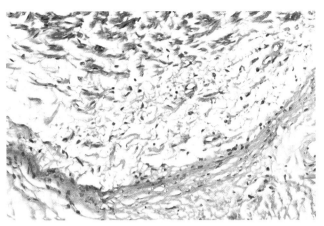

FIGURE 35-9. Intraneural neurofibroma; schwannian pattern of differentiation. A thickened perineurium forming a concave band near the bottom of the field, which defines the limits of the tumorous component at the interface with the adjacent soft tissue. At the top of the field, a distorted axial bundle (a rem-nant of the nerve of origin) is represented. The tumor is repre-sented in the space between the perineurium and the distorted axial bundle; thin, pale collagen bundles are loosely and ran-domly spaced in a stringy, myxoid matrix. Thin spindle cells with elongated, wavy nuclei are closely associated with some of the collagen bundles. The fibrous component of the lesion is asym-metrical in its relationships with both the long axis of the in-volved nerve and the central axial bundle.

(intraneural) variants; plexiform (intraneural) variants (Fig. 35-7); deep, diffuse (extraneural) variants; and various combinations of the above are manifested in an array of histologic patterns.

In many deep, circumscribed (intraneural) neurofi-bromas, and in most plexiform (intraneural) neurofibro-mas, axial bundles, which are composed of symmetrically arranged nerve fibers, are remnants of the axial bundle of the nerve of origin (3,19) (Figs. 35-8, 35-9, and 35-10). Their role in the histogenesis of NF is uncertain. The axial

bundle retains its symmetry in a field of distorted and asymmetrical patterns (Figs. 35-9 and 35-10). In some axial bundles, Schwann cells are hyperplastic, and tightly packed. In some areas, these remnants of the nerve of ori-gin focally evolve into micronodules composed of inter-lacing fascicles of Schwann cells; the micronodules qualify as *microscopic schwannomatosis* (3). Many of these cellular nidi (micronodules) may be independent of a true axial bundle, but all seem to function as growth centers (Fig. 35-11). From the periphery of these nidi (growth centers),

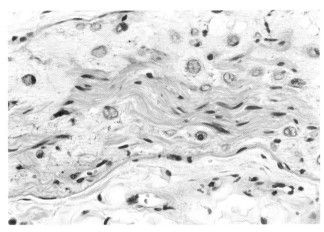

FIGURE 35-8. Plexiform intraneural neurofibroma; mucinous en-doneurial type. This small branch of a large, cutaneous, plexiform neurofibroma shows a well-defined, central bundle of Schwann cells (an axial bundle). In this central bundle, Schwann cell fasci-cles of the preexisting nerve are symmetrically arranged along the long axis of the nerve. The endoneurial space is widened and mucinous. In it, distinctive, rounded cells (endoneurial mucocytes) are loosely spaced. The expanding mucinous matrix has displaced some of the Schwann fascicles of the axial bundle away from their neighbors. The muciparous cells resemble the "cellules go-dronne" as seen in the "intravaginal hyaline system" of Renaut. The perineurium is delicate; it is a single layer of flattened cells.

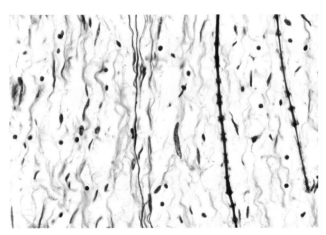

FIGURE 35-10. Intraneural neurofibroma; remnant of axial bundle (Bodian stain). Argyrophilic, myelinated and nonmyeli-nated axons are parallel, have axial symmetry, and are a rem-nant of the axial bundle. Wavy collagen bundles of the tumor are more asymmetrical in orientation.

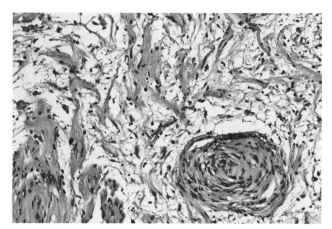

FIGURE 35-11. Intraneural neurofibroma; focal, microscopic schwannomatosis. Coarse collagen bundles are asymmetrically arranged in a loosely cellular, myxoid matrix. Near the right lower corner, collagen bundles and cells form a whorl. The whorl, as a nidus, is an example of microscopic schwannomatosis.

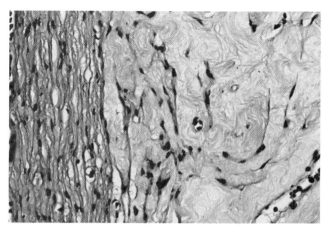

FIGURE 35-13. Intraneural neurofibroma, perineurial cell differentiation near the capsule of the tumor. The membrane to the *left* of the field is a thickened perineurium (capsule). In the fibrous matrix to the *right* of the perineurium, distinctive cells are loosely spaced; some blend with the inner surface of the perineurium. The loosely spaced cells have the morphologic features of perineurial cells.

cells and collagenous strands stream asymmetrically into the expanded endoneurial mucinous matrix; the expanded intraneural component becomes a tumor. In intraneural variants, similar patterns of streaming cells, and collagenous strands blend with (or arise from) the perineurium; the perineurium also appears to contribute to the tumor.

In the evolution of a neurofibroma, the contributions from each anatomic component of a peripheral nerve are variable. The cells of *perineurial variants* are bipolar or tripolar with rigid processes; they are loosely spaced in either a myxoid or fibrous matrix (Figs. 35-12 and 35-13). *Endoneurial (schwannian) variants* are characterized by a thickened perineurium, one or several axial bundles, and isolated cells in an expanded, mucinous endoneurial component (Figs. 35-9 through 35-15). In some examples, some of the

cells in an expanded, mucinous matrix resemble the "cellules godronné" of Renaut (round cells with mucinous matrix enclosed within the cytoplasm) (1,3) (Fig. 35-8). One or several axial bundles may be found among asymmetrical collagen bundles of the tumor. In the expanded endoneurial component of both perineurial and endoneurial (schwannian) variants, the matrix if it is rich in hyaluronic acid (3).

In a lesion in which the patterns of neurofibroma are otherwise preserved, and in the absence of mitotic activity, a spotty representation of scattered cells with enlarged, atypical nuclei is not a significant finding (Figs. 35-14 and 35-16); as a variable to be assessed in the absence of mitotic activity and necrosis, it is comparable to the ancient (atypi-

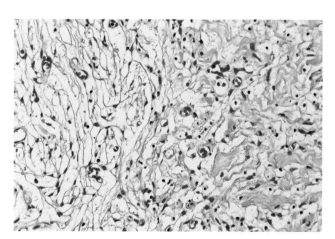

FIGURE 35-12. Intraneural neurofibroma; biphasic (perineurial and schwannian) patterns. To the *right*, wavy collagen bundles are loosely spaced; spindle cells are closely associated with the collagen bundles (schwannian pattern). To the *left*, distinctive, bipolar and tripolar cells are loosely spaced in a clear or myxoid matrix; these distinctive cells have perineurial qualities.

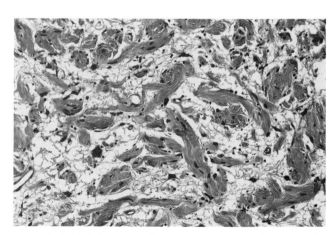

FIGURE 35-14. Intraneural neurofibroma; cytologic atypia. Coarse collagen bundles are loosely and randomly spaced in a myxoid matrix. Spindle cells are closely associated with the collagen bundles. Spindle and stellate cells are present among the collagen bundles in the myxoid matrix. Some of the cells in the myxoid matrix show nuclear atypism and variations in nuclear size and outline.

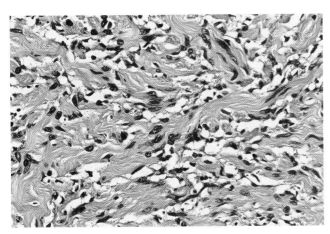

FIGURE 35-15. Intraneural neurofibroma; cellular pattern. Spindle cells are increased in number among the collagen bundles; focally, they are present within the collagen bundles. The cells have enlarged, wavy nuclei and scanty cytoplasm.

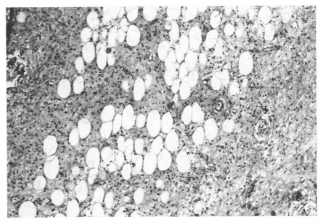

FIGURE 35-17. Extraneural (diffuse) neurofibroma. A delicately fibrous matrix is loosely cellular. The cells have scanty cytoplasm, and they appear as naked nuclei. Lipocytes are entrapped.

cal) change of schwannomas (3). Some neurofibromas are cellular (Fig. 35-15).

At the interface of *extraneural (diffuse) neurofibromas* with soft tissue, margins are poorly defined (Fig. 35-17), and lipocytes are often entrapped. The matrix of extraneural neurofibroma is either delicately fibrous, and faintly acidophilic, or more coarsely fibrous, and brightly acidophilic. In the absence of plexiform components, nerves within diffuse neurofibromas usually are small, internally symmetrical, and hypercellular; perineuria of such nerves often are hyperplastic. In cross-section, these nerves might be mistaken as evidence of Pacinian corpuscle–like differentiation (20). The patterns of both a plexiform (intraneural) neurofibroma, and a diffuse (extraneural) neurofibroma are combined (3) in *paraneurofibromas* (Fig. 35-18 and 35-19). Focal collections of structures resembling tactile corpuscles (tactoid bodies) (Fig. 35-20), and pigmented, dendritic melanocytes (a relatively common fea-

ture of deep, extraneural [diffuse] neurofibromas) (3), are rare in the intraneural components of plexiform, or circumscribed intraneural neurofibromas.

Ultrastructurally, the cells of neurofibromas (including those of tactoid bodies) mostly resemble perineurial cells (21), but cells with the characteristics of Schwann cells, as well as endoneurial fibroblasts, also have been identified: a morphologic continuum of neurosustentacular cells is manifested (3,22). Endoneurial fibroblasts, like common mesenchymal fibroblasts, do not have basal lamina. The average diameter of their collagen fibrils lies well below that of dermal collagen fibrils, which is about 100 nm (23).

Histogenesis. The immunohistochemical profile of neurofibroma is as follows: S-100 protein (positive), with variable expression of CD57 (Leu-7) antigen (positive), and myelin basic protein (positive). In extraneural cutaneous

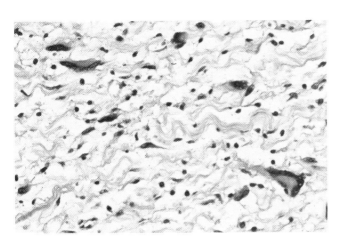

FIGURE 35-16. Intraneural neurofibroma; cellular atypia. Some of the cells among the collagen bundles are cytologically atypical, and some of the atypical cells are multinucleated.

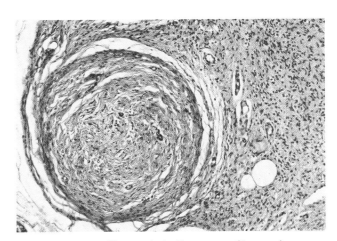

FIGURE 35-18. Diffuse and plexiform neurofibroma (paraneurofibroma). The round nodule to the left is a portion of an intraneural plexiform neurofibroma, it has been cut in cross-section. The delicate fibrous matrix to the right is a portion of a diffuse (extraneural) component.

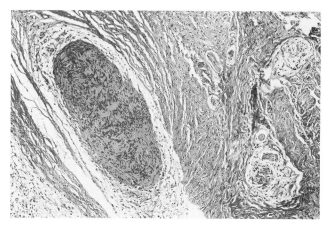

FIGURE 35-19. Diffuse and plexiform neurofibroma (paraneurofibroma) with focal microscopic schwannomatosis. The intraneural portions are pale, rounded, and faintly basophilic; in these components, wavy collagen bundles are loosely spaced. The extraneural component is a uniformly cellular fibrous matrix. Near the center of the field, a cellular nodule is confined within the intraneural matrix; in this cellular nodule, nuclei are arranged in palisades. The patterns of Verocay bodies are represented. The nodule is an example of microscopic schwannomatosis.

neurofibromas, axons, as demonstrated with NSE, or with antibodies to neurofilaments, are fairly uniform in distribution among collagen bundles. This finding is less consistent in deep, intraneural neurofibromas. CD34 expression has been interpreted as a reaction with endoneurial fibroblasts or monocytes (24).

The ultrastructural features of neurofibromas (a preponderance of cells that resemble perineurial cells [21], and the respective immunohistochemical findings (e.g., S-100 [positive] and EMA [negative]) are discordant qualities.

Schwann cells with enclosed axons, as demonstrated with monoclonal antibodies for either NSE or neural filaments, are present in cutaneous neurofibromas. They have

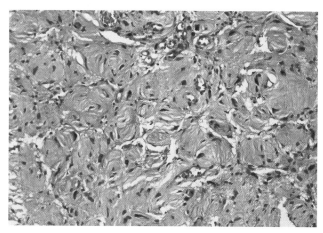

FIGURE 35-20. Extraneural neurofibroma; tactile corpuscle-like patterns. Spindle cells in stacked lamellae form tactile corpuscle-like structures as a regional variation in this extraneural neurofibroma.

been characterized as an integral part of neurofibromas, or simply as a consequence of the entrapment of uninvolved nerve fibers (21). Nonplexiform, but circumscribed neurofibromas, in von Recklinghausen disease contain abundant, peptide-rich nerves (25). Undoubtedly, similar associations exist in plexiform variants. The innervation of neurofibromas of NF1 apparently is much richer than has been appreciated in the past.

The extraneural distribution of the common dermal neurofibroma may be a manifestation of the extension of tumor through the open-ended terminal of perineurial sheaths, or through the thin perineurium of small dermal nerves (19). Deep, extraneural neurofibroma may represent a diffuse, neurocristic dysplasia that is expressed in mesenchymal patterns (3,26).

Differential Diagnosis. Plexiform (and pseudoplexiform) lesions of the skin and subcutaneous tissue include plexiform schwannoma (3), plexiform neuroma (27), the neuromas of the mucosal neuroma syndrome (28), nerve sheath myxoma (1,29), and plexiform fibrous histiocytoma (30). Even perineurioma, in all its current guises, has been proposed as having a plexiform variant, which apparently embraces some reported examples of nerve sheath myxoma (31).

Subcutaneous extraneural (diffuse) neurofibromas may be confused with the deep component of *dermatofibrosarcoma protuberans*. The confounding patterns account for the characterization of pigmented dermatofibrosarcoma protuberans as *pigmented storiform neurofibroma* (20,32).

In infancy, "plexiform" fibrous hamartoma also might be considered in the differential diagnosis of an extraneural neurofibroma.

The nodular myxoid components of a low-grade *malignant myxoid fibrous histiocytoma* might be misinterpreted as the pattern of a "plexiform" nerve sheath tumor.

In NF1, mucinous and proliferative endarteritis and aneurysms affect mainly muscular renal vessels, but similar changes may be manifested in other sites (3,33,34). Aneurysmal changes have been a prominent feature of muscular vessels in some examples of extraneural neurofibromas of the skin and soft tissue, particularly in the distribution of the trigeminal nerve (3). Such lesions may be mistaken for *hemangioma*.

TRUE NEOPLASMS OF SCHWANN CELLS

True neoplasms of Schwann cells are composed of ultrastructurally distinctive cells that are immunoreactive for S-100 protein. *Schwannomas (neurilemmomas; anaxonal, intraneural, Schwann cell tumors; "peripheral neurogliomas")* are benign, expansile neoplasms (1,21,35). The cells of schwannomas mostly have the characteristics of Schwann cells. Schwann cells are specialized sustentacular cells, normally distributed as a single layer about, and along, one or more axons. In a sense, they provide insulation that favors proper propagation of nerve impulses. In schwannomas, the population of Schwann cells exists independent of an axon plexus. As solitary, skin-colored tumors along the course of peripheral or cranial nerves, their usual size is between 2 and 4 cm; their usual location is the head or the flexor aspect of the extremities. Schwannomas are rare in the subcutaneous tissue; they are even less common in the dermis. In deep soft tissue, they may be large (36). Internal viscera (37) and bones may be involved. When small, most schwannomas are asymptomatic, but pain, localized to the tumor, or radiating along the nerve of origin, may be a complaint.

Histopathology. Schwannomas, with the exception of infiltrating, fascicular variants, are intraneural and symmetrically expansile; they are confined by the perineurium of the nerve of origin (Fig. 35-21). Most of the symmetrically bundled nerve fibers of the nerve of origin are displaced eccentrically. If identified in a histologic section, they usually are to be found between the tumor and the perineurium (3,35) (Fig. 35-21). Some of the nerve fibers may extend from the compressed, eccentric axial bundle into the tumor at the interface with the nerve of origin. The observations of Russell and Rubinstein (38) contradict the dictum that schwannomas are universally devoid of axons. Loosely and randomly spaced nonmyelinated axons have been observed in small peripheral schwannomas, and in small and medium-sized acoustic nerve schwannomas (38).

Two variant patterns, namely *Antoni A* and *Antoni B* types, have been described (39). In the Antoni type A tissue, uniform spindle cells are arranged back to back (Fig. 35-22); each cell is outlined by delicate, rigid, reticular fibers (basement membranes). The cells tend to cluster

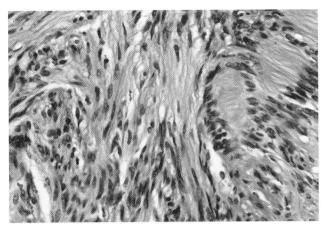

FIGURE 35-22. Schwannoma; Antoni A patterns. Pale spindle cells with elongated, wavy nuclei are arranged in fascicular patterns. To the right of the field, nuclear palisades are regularly spaced; two nuclear palisades and the enclosed cytoplasmic processes comprise a Verocay body. Cellular components of this type qualify as Antoni A tissue.

in stacks, and the respective nuclei often form palisades. Two neighboring palisades, the intervening cytoplasms of Schwann cells, and associated reticular fibers, all in combination, constitute a *Verocay body* (Fig. 35-22).

In Antoni type B tissue, files of elongated "Schwann" cells, arranged end-to-end, and individual "Schwann" cells are loosely spaced in a clear, watery, or myxoid matrix (1,40) (Figs. 35-23, 35-24, and 35-25); in some examples, the cells somewhat resemble glial cells; in other examples, they resemble perineurial cells.

Clusters of dilated, congested vessels showing fibrinoid necrosis, or with hyalinized walls; thrombi; and subendothelial collections of foam cells (40) (Fig. 35-26) are represented in both Antoni A and Antoni B tissue. Cystic

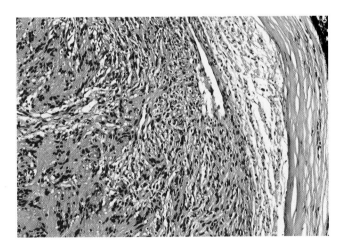

FIGURE 35-21. Schwannoma and nerve of origin. The schwannoma is uniformly cellular; focally, Schwann cells form nuclear palisades and Verocay bodies. To the *right*, a thickened perineurium defines the limits of the tumor with the neighboring soft tissue. The loosely cellular zone between the perineurium and the tumor is a compressed nerve of origin. The nerve maintains its identity at the periphery of the tumor; it is not enclosed within the substance of the tumor.

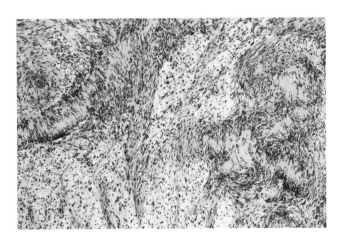

FIGURE 35-23. Schwannoma; mixed Antoni A and Antoni B patterns. The Antoni A component is cellular, and Verocay bodies are a prominent feature. The loosely cellular, pale zones are Antoni B patterns. In the Antoni B component, there is some variation in nuclear size and staining.

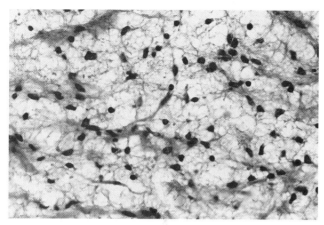

FIGURE 35-24. Schwannoma; Antoni B patterns. In this example, the cells of an Antoni B component are small with complex, delicate cytoplasmic processes. The cytologic features have a glial cell-like quality.

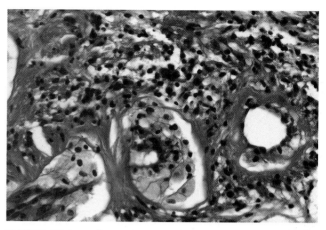

FIGURE 35-26. Schwannoma; Antoni B component, vascular changes. In this Antoni B component, several vessels are loosely clustered. They have thickened, hyalinized walls. There are prominent, subintimal collections of foam cells. Loose infiltrates of lymphoid cells are adjacent to the vessels, and among the foamy histiocytes. In part, the hyalin represents a stage in the organization of fibrinoid; fibrinoid degeneration and thrombosis are common vascular changes in some schwannomas.

changes (3,39) (Fig. 35-27), extravasated erythrocytes, and hemosiderin deposits are variable features.

Ultrastructurally, the tumor cells of a schwannoma manifest the features of Schwann cells (21). Axons usually are not a component. Long-spacing collagen may be represented (38).

The patterns in Antoni type B tissue are degenerative in nature; at the level of the light microscope, they have been characterized as "ancient change" (40). Ancient change also characterizes the nuclear atypia often seen in schwannomas. Ultrastructurally, tumor cells are widely separated by an electron-lucent, homogeneous matrix containing strands of fibrin, and detached segments of basement membrane. Autophagic lysosomes, some containing myelin figures, are seen in many cells. The cells show extensive loss of their basement membrane, disruption of their cell membrane, and degenerative changes in their nuclei (41).

Histogenesis. The immunohistochemical profile is S-100 protein (positive), collagen type IV and laminin (positive). In the capsule, cells are EMA (positive). A Bodian stain, and an immunoreaction for the demonstration of neural filaments reveal few or no axons, except in and near the peripherally displaced axial bundle.

Apoptosis is a deletion of selected cells in both physiologic, and pathologic processes (42,43). A modification of this process may be the operative phenomena promoting the expression of Antoni B patterns in a schwannoma.

Differential Diagnosis. For a nerve sheath tumor involving a significant sensory, or motor nerve, the distinctions between intraneural neurofibroma and schwannoma are important. The intact, but displaced symmetrical axial

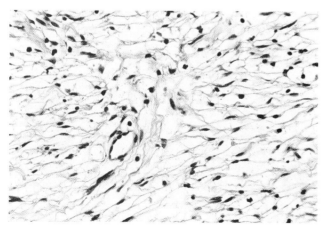

FIGURE 35-25. Schwannoma; Antoni B patterns. In this example, the cells of an Antoni B component are bi- or tri-polar, the cytoplasmic processes are elongated and straight, and the cells cytologically resemble perineurial cells.

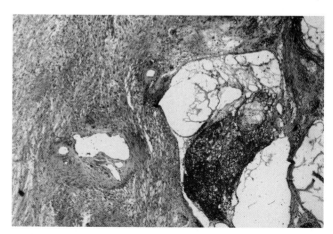

FIGURE 35-27. Schwannoma; microcystic and vascular changes. With this connective tissue stain, cells have a reddish tinge, and connective tissue is green. Vessels are dilated; their walls are fibrous and irregularly thickened. To the right, multiple, small cysts contain a loose meshwork of fibrin.

bundle (Fig. 35-21) of a schwannoma, if involving a functionally significant nerve, often can be preserved during surgical dissections. On the other hand, excision of an intraneural neurofibroma requires sacrifice of the nerve of origin (i.e., the centrally contained axial bundle must be sacrificed).

Palisaded and encapsulated neuroma (PEN) should be considered in the differential diagnosis of schwannoma. A demonstration of axons within the fascicles of tumor cells is sufficient to make the distinctions between PEN and schwannoma.

Variant Types of Schwannomas

Cellular Schwannoma

If other common features are preserved, scattered cells having large, hyperchromatic nuclei (Fig. 35-28) are of no significance. Cellular schwannoma (SC) has been promoted as a variant (1), but lesions, characterized as such in the literature, have shown a wide range of patterns. Increased cellularity per unit area, a preponderance of type A patterns, and a low mitotic rate (<10/10 HPF) are, in part, requisites for the diagnosis of "cellular schwannoma" (Fig. 35-29). Areas of atypia are acceptable in the definition. The criteria for the diagnosis of cellular schwannoma are of a type that generally would define borderline categories in other neoplastic systems.

The generic designation of cellular schwannoma, which embraces a variety of histologic patterns, has found, in several retrospective studies, a degree of legitimacy in the documentation of a favorable prognosis (1). Classes 1 and 2 (CS1 and CS2) are defined here.

In *CS1* (a restricted application of the designation in the manner of Harkin and Reed) (3), most examples are large

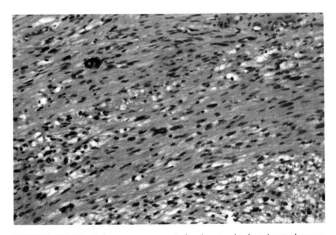

FIGURE 35-28. Schwannoma; cytologic atypia (ancient change of cytologic type). Spindle cells form interlacing fascicles. The cells show variations in nuclear size, staining, and outlines; in many of the nuclei, and chromatin is dense and smudgy. Mitoses are not a feature of "ancient change."

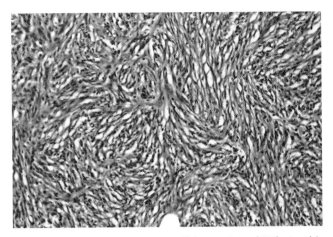

FIGURE 35-29. Schwannoma; cellular variant (CS1). In this schwannoma, patterns are uniformly cellular (Antoni A type). Uniform spindle cells are arranged in the pattern of interlacing fascicles. In this example, mitotic activity is not a significant feature.

tumors of the retroperitoneum and mediastinum (and may incidentally show immunoreactivity for glial fibrillary acidic protein [GFAP]) (44,45). The lesions of CS1 are mostly cellular with patternless areas in which cells form solid sheets alternating with areas in which intersecting fascicles of spindle cells (Fig. 35-29) produce storiform patterns (3). The basic patterns of a variant of schwannoma, such as a common schwannoma or an epithelioid schwannoma, are preserved, but in some examples most of the cells are cytologically atypical (Fig. 35-29). Cellular pleomorphism is acceptable. In some examples, nuclear atypia is uniform and extensive. By definition, mitoses are infrequent (<2/10 HPF). A background population of small lymphocytes also may contribute to the cellularity (3). Nuclear palisades, Verocay bodies, and Antoni type B components may be inconspicuous (3).

In *CS2*, (cellular schwannoma of Woodruff [46], and transformed schwannoma of Reed and Harkin [3]), some features are histologically worrisome. Increased cell density, storiform patterns, mitotic activity (even up to 20 or more mitoses per 10 HPF), zones of necrosis, and cytologic atypia might be cited as worrisome features (1,45–50). Some have argued that these lesions are unequivocally benign, but the prospective studies that would certify CS2 as something other than a low-grade, intraneural malignant schwannoma (transformed schwannoma of Reed and Harkin [3]) are not available. The patterns are of a type that, in other organ systems, would be consistent with a transition from benignancy to low-grade malignancy (Fig. 35-30). In practice, most of these lesions are amenable to local surgery. Confinement of such lesions by the perineurium of the nerve of origin may be prognostically, and therapeutically important in providing a distinction between these lesions and infiltrating low-grade malignant schwannomas (46).

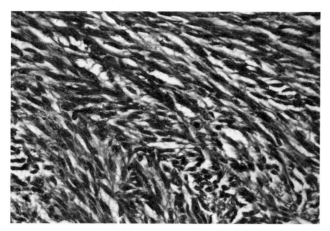

FIGURE 35-30. Schwannoma; cellular variant with mitotic activity (CS2). In this example of cellular schwannoma, the fascicles are hypercellular; nuclei are enlarged and show hyperchromatism. There are scattered mitotic figures.

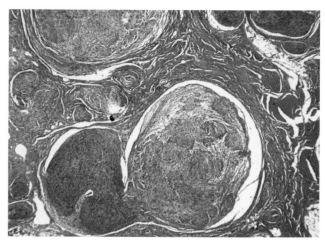

FIGURE 35-32. Plexiform schwannoma. Components of the plexus are mostly cut in cross-section, and are supported by a dense fibrous matrix. Within some of the components, both Antoni A and Antoni B patterns are represented.

Differential Diagnosis. The differential diagnosis of CS1 includes *leiomyoma*, low-grade *leiomyosarcoma*, and *gastrointestinal stromal tumor*. In the evaluation of a problematic lesion, an intense reaction for S-100 protein, and a negative reaction for smooth muscle antigen (SMA) and desmin would offer support for a diagnosis of schwannoma. Smooth muscle cells, in turn, react with antibodies to SMA and desmin. In gastrointestinal stromal tumors, divergent phenotypes may be expressed, but CD117 is the commonly expressed antigen. Variants of soft tissue sarcoma must be included in the differential diagnosis of CS1 and CS2.

Epithelioid Schwannoma

In the rare *epithelioid schwannoma* (with or without radial sclerosis) (3,51–53), spindle and round cells are clustered in epithelioid patterns and often have round nuclei (Fig. 35-31 and 35-32). Nuclear atypia and dense nuclear chromatin are common features. In some examples, the cells have acidophilic cytoplasm. In one variation, cells have round nuclei and scanty cytoplasm; some of the cells are radially arranged in palisades around distinctive zones of sclerosis (3,54–56). In the zones of sclerosis, fibrous lamellae are radially oriented; they interdigitate with cytoplasmic projections of the surrounding tumor cells (56). Such lesions have been characterized as epithelioid schwannoma with radial sclerosis (3), collagenous spherulosis in a schwannoma (56), and neuroblastoma-like epithelioid schwannoma (54,55). Neither the patterns nor the clinical behavior of these lesions justifies the last-mentioned characterization. Collagenous spherulosis, as originally defined for breast lesions, is distinct from the patterns of radial

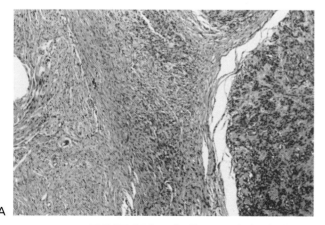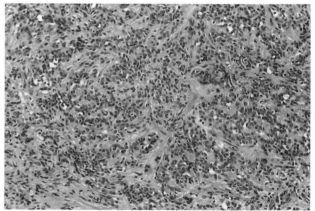

A   B

FIGURE 35-31. Plexiform epithelioid schwannoma, arising in extraneural neurofibroma. **A:** To the *right*, a portion of a plexiform lesion presents a sharp interface with an extraneural (diffuse) neurofibroma. Fascicles of uniform, epithelioid cells are loosely, and regularly spaced in the plexiform component. **B:** At higher magnification, the fascicles of uniform, small epithelioid cells are loosely spaced in a fibrous matrix.

sclerosis, as manifested in nerve sheath tumors. Some examples of epithelioid schwannoma have been characterized as cellular. Some epithelioid schwannomas are also plexiform (Figs. 35-31 and 35-32).

Glandular Schwannoma

Glands, having the features of sweat glands, are occasionally found within subcutaneous schwannomas (57–60). A demonstration of a component of myoepithelial cells has produced a proposal that the glands are nothing more than entrapped sweat glands (58,60). Yoshida and Toot (59) proposed *divergent differentiation* as an alternate explanation for the glandular inclusions. Glandular patterns of a different (entodermal?) type are a feature of some malignant schwannomas, they also have been observed in a benign neurofibroma (58). The "enteric" qualities include mucin-secreting goblet cells, and neuroendocrine markers, such as somatostatin.

Plexiform Schwannoma

These occur mostly in the subcutaneous tissue; they rarely are confined to the dermis (3,16,61–66). They may be a feature of the syndrome of *multiple schwannomas* (clinical schwannomatosis or neurilemmomatosis) (63,67), or they may be solitary (65). The NF2 gene and that of multiple schwannomas may be identical (68,69).

Histopathology. Plexiform schwannoma is intraneural. Spindle cells, often in solid Antoni A patterns, fill the expanded endoneurial space of a limited segment of a nerve plexus; each column and nodule of the tumor are surrounded by perineurium. The vascular changes and Antoni type B tissue of a common schwannoma are variable features. Cystic changes are uncommon. In some examples, fascicles of Schwann cells extend beyond the confines of the perineurium into the neighboring mesenchyme. The limited patterns in the adjacent soft tissue resemble those of a small, circumferential, extraneural neuroma (61). Some examples of plexiform schwannoma are "cellular," and some are epithelioid.

The category of plexiform schwannoma may be heterogeneous. Kao et al. (65) have documented a relationship between neurofibroma and plexiform schwannoma in one case. In our experience, plexiform schwannoma may be associated with a background of diffuse neurofibroma (Figs. 35-31 and 35-32). Examples of plexiform schwannoma that are focally rich in axons may be plexiform schwannoma ex plexiform neurofibroma or ex plexiform neuroma.

Schwannoma Arising in Neurofibroma (Emphasis on Relationships with Intraneural Microscopic Schwannomatosis)

Schwannomas in continuity with neurofibromas have been documented (70,71). *Intraneural microscopic schwannomato-* *sis* (3) (Figs. 35-11 and 35-19), a proliferative change affecting axial bundles of nerve fibers in intraneural neurofibromas, may, with progression, become a *schwannoma ex neurofibroma* (16). The phenomena of microscopic intraneural schwannomatosis may be operative in the evolution of some plexiform schwannomas. Rarely, remnants of an intraneural neurofibroma are found at the periphery of a cellular schwannoma (CS1).

Borderline Variants

Infiltrating (Extraneural) Fascicular Schwannoma of Infancy and Childhood

Infiltrating fascicular schwannoma (*IFS*) (plexiform malignant peripheral nerve sheath tumor of infancy and childhood [72]; fascicular schwannoma; congenital hamartoma of nerve [73]) is a rare Schwann cell neoplasm most often affecting an extremity. In contrast to all other variants of schwannoma, IFS is chiefly extraneural. True plexiform patterns (intraneural by definition) are not a prominent feature.

Histopathology. Uniform spindle cells form tortuous, interlacing fascicles that vary in size. In some of the thin fascicles, spindle cells tend to cluster in palisades with anuclear collections of cytoplasm separating neighboring palisades. IFS infiltrates skin and soft tissue and, in some examples, erodes bone. In one example, a richly cellular, and mitotically active intraneural component was identified (74); components of the original axial bundle were displaced peripherally.

In the only published collection (72), four of the six patients with follow-up had local recurrences. In addition, one patient, with an invasive lesion of the orbit, died.

The malignant nature of IFS has not been convincingly demonstrated. The histologic patterns overlap with those of both infiltrating and fascicular epithelioid malignant schwannoma (IFEMS) and neurotropic melanoma.

Histogenesis. The most characteristic feature of IFS is its extraneural invasion of soft tissue. The tumor cells of IFS are clearly identifiable, both immunohistochemically and ultrastructurally, as Schwann cells.

The nature of IFS is controversial. To assign IFS to the category of malignant nerve sheath tumor would only mask its undefined biologic nature. A malignant nerve sheath tumor unequivocally behaves in a malignant fashion, with a predictable capacity for local recurrence and metastasis. An assignment of IFS to the category of either cellular or plexiform schwannoma (74) would be an unwarranted extension of what is already too broadly defined. In the category of cellular schwannoma, as defined by Woodruff, some examples share the histologic features of malignant peripheral nerve sheath tumor but, in the available retrospective studies, all examples, *by definition*, have been biologically benign (examples with local recurrences excluded). IFS should be characterized as a borderline lesion of indeterminant malignant potential until its nature is better documented.

Psammomatous Melanotic Schwannoma

An uncommon tumor, psammomatous melanotic schwannoma (PMS), may be either sporadic, or a stigma of a complex (*Carney complex*) that includes some or all of the following: myxomas (including trichogenic and cardiac variants) (75), spotty pigmentation, pigmented adrenal cortical hyperplasia, large-cell calcifying Sertoli cell tumor (76), and endocrine overactivity (including Cushing syndrome) (77,78). Some examples of PMS have behaved in a malignant fashion.

Histologically, psammoma bodies, and pigmented, dendritic melanocytes are features. Most examples of PMS are quite distinct, but some show nuclear palisades and Verocay bodies (77,79).

Transformed (Borderline) Schwannoma (CS2)

This transformed (borderline) schwannoma (TBS) lesion of uncertain malignant potential (3), like its benign counterpart, is intraneural (confined by an expanded perineurium) (3). Its internal patterns, but not its setting, are reminiscent of patterns seen in minimal-deviation (low-grade) malignant schwannomas (MPNST) of neurofibromatosis (a lesion that is not confined by the perineurium of the nerve of origin). Some examples of TBS contain scattered globular deposits of melanotic pigment (3).

TBS, as defined by Reed and Harkin (3), shares many features with cellular schwannoma as defined by Woodruff et al. (46). The overlaps in patterns are given recognition here in the characterization of TBS as cellular schwannoma, class 2 (CS2).

Malignant transformation of benign schwannoma has been a rarely documented event (80–82). In one report (83), only histologically "high-grade" variants were represented. "High-grade," transformed malignant schwannomas, in contrast to TBS, show a greater degree of cellular atypia and pleomorphism, and a higher mitotic rate. They may show infiltrative growth beyond the confines of the perineurium (83), a quality that excludes TBS.

MALIGNANT SCHWANNOMA

Malignant peripheral nerve sheath tumor (neurofibrosarcoma, malignant schwannoma, MPNST, neurogenic sarcoma) is the characteristic malignancy arising in neurofibromatosis. Related malignancies may be *de novo*, or may

be transformations in other neurocristic neoplasms, such as schwannoma or ganglioneuroma. The criteria for the diagnosis of MPNST include some, or all, of the following: origin from, or continuity with, a major nerve or neurofibroma; association with classic stigmata of neurofibromatosis; identification of characteristic histologic patterns, and demonstration of immunohistochemical, or ultrastructural features of Schwann cells (and/or perineurial cells). It has been argued that, since most malignant schwannomas arise in association with neurofibromas of neurofibromatosis and since malignant schwannoma ex schwannoma is rare, the designation, malignant schwannoma, is inaccurate. The designation "malignant peripheral nerve sheath tumor," an alternative lacking discrimination, provides no distinctions between the common malignancy of neurofibromatosis and an uncommon lesion such as peripheral neuroepithelioma (primitive neuroectodermal tumor). It provides no distinctions between Schwann cell variants and perineurial variants. Epithelioid, and mesenchymal variants are not distinguished in the promotion of the designation, "malignant peripheral nerve sheath tumor."

MPNST (sheath or Schwann cell type) is the common malignant tumor of peripheral nerves (1,3,21,84–90). Its association with neurofibromatosis is established but, even in this setting, it is uncommon. In a series of 678 patients with neurofibromatosis, a MPNST was observed in only 21 (3.1%) of patients (89). In only 2 of the 678 patients did a MPNST primarily involve the skin and subcutis.

MPNST usually arise contiguous with either an extraneural, or intraneural component of a neurofibroma: in turn, they may be intraneural or extraneural. In the deep soft tissue, involvement of a large nerve trunk, such as a femoral, tibial, or intercostal nerve, is characteristic, but in some instances no such connections are apparent. MPNST may also arise as sporadic or *de novo* lesions (i.e., not associated with neurofibromatosis) (90). An origin in a benign schwannoma, as a documented phenomenon, rarely has been reported (83). For many examples of MPNST (sheath cell type), the patterns are expressive of the patterns of differentiation in embryonic mesenchyme (Fig. 35-33); fascicles of cells, often alternating light and dark (Fig. 35-34A and B), chondroid matrix, osteoid (Fig. 35-35), and rhabdomyoid cells (Fig. 35-36) are manifested. MPNST of perineurial type has been promoted as a variant, with the predictable proposal that such a lesion is a malignant perineurioma, but without evidence that there is a relationship between any of the benign "perineurioma" variants and MPNST of any type.

Histopathology. The variable patterns of differentiation in MPNST include (a) mesenchymal (fibrosarcomatous, osteosarcomatous and chondrosarcomatous [3], rhabdomyosarcomatous [1,88–92], and even liposarcomatous patterns); (b) glandular (entodermal) patterns (58); (c) epithelioid patterns in which individual spindle and round

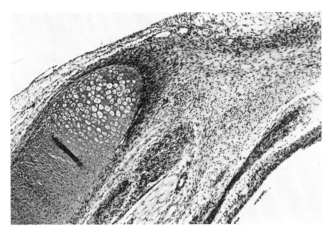

FIGURE 35-33. Fetal mesenchyme. Fetal mesenchyme shows varying patterns of differentiation. An island of immature cartilage is represented. In the neighboring mesenchyme, there are patterns of alternating light and dark fascicles. One fascicle of developing skeletal muscle fibers is represented in the myxoid matrix at the bottom of the field. These patterns are recapitulated in neoplastic patterns in many examples of malignant peripheral nerve sheath tumor.

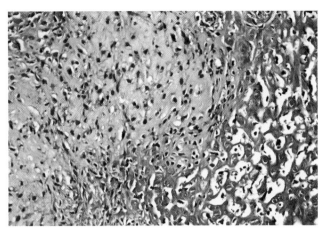

FIGURE 35-35. Malignant peripheral nerve sheath tumor; chondro-osseous differentiation. Chondroid differentiation is represented to the left of the center of the field; to the *right*, the patterns are those of neoplastic osteoid.

cells often have acidophilic cytoplasm (3,93,94), and are closely spaced in nests, fascicles, and sheets; and (d) neuroepithelioma-like patterns (95).

Histologically, *mesenchymal patterns* are preponderant in the setting of MPNST ex neurofibromatosis. Thin, spindle cells are arranged in interlacing fascicles in a fibromyxoid matrix. The fascicles are straight and can be traced across low-power fields; they are alternating light (pale) and dark (more intensely stained). Often the spindle cells are remarkably uniform (Fig. 35–34A and B). Neoplastic cells tend to be concentrically, or radially arranged about vessels, particularly near areas of necrosis. Having identified these basic features, an additional search for, and the identification of, specific expressions of mesenchymal differentiation

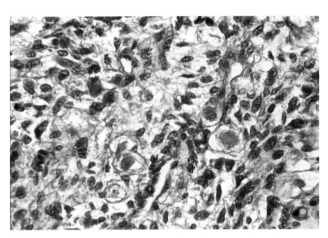

FIGURE 35-36. Malignant peripheral nerve sheath tumor; rhabdomyoblastic differentiation. In this field of undifferentiated small cells, there are scattered, rounded cells with plump, round nuclei. These round cells show concentrically arranged cytoplasmic myofibrils.

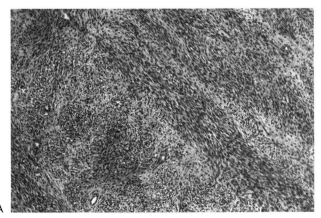

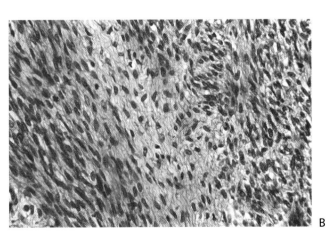

A   B

FIGURE 35-34. Malignant peripheral nerve sheath tumor; spindle cell variant. **A:** Atypical spindle cells form intersecting fascicles; the fascicles alternately are light and dark. **B:** At higher magnification, spindle cells are cytologically atypical but cytologic features are uniform.

provide strong support for a diagnosis of MPNST (Figs. 35-35 and 35–36). Patterns of specific mesenchymal differentiation, when found, usually are spotty in distribution. Having identified one specific pattern of mesenchymal differentiation, it is often possible for the observer to then find others. The mitotic rate provides a correlate for the diagnosis of MPNST. It is not a prime determinant of biologic potential. In the setting of neurofibromatosis, rates may be low (<10/10 HPF) or high (<50/10 HPF), and the outcome for either category may be poor, depending on other factors, such as the size and location of the lesions, and the age of the patient.

Epithelioid patterns are a variant expression of MPNST in the setting of neurofibromatosis. *De novo* malignant schwannomas (90) and "high-grade" MPNST arising in benign schwannomas (*malignant transformed schwannoma*) (83) tend to be intraneural in origin, and to be manifested in "epithelioid" patterns (93,94). The study of Hruban et al. (95) does not support this generalization but is compromised by including, as *de novo* variants, examples of both neuroepithelioma and MPNST arising in neurofibroma.

Histologically, in epithelioid variants, plump tumor cells in nests and sheets are closely spaced with scanty intercellular matrix (3,93,94) (Figs. 35-37 and 35-38). Nuclei are large and often rounded. In pleomorphic variants, tumor giant cells are common. Specific patterns of mesenchymal differentiation are variant features. In some examples, the cells form nests and cords in a sparsely cellular, myxoid or hyaline matrix. The "purely epithelioid" (epithelial) MPNST, a lesion with no "sarcomatous" component, is rare (3,96). In some "epithelial" examples, plump, acidophilic tumor cells manifest a striking cytoplasmic argyrophilia (3) (Fig. 35-39); they may represent large cell neuroendocrine carcinoma.

Malignant epithelioid peripheral nerve sheath tumors, some of which appear to have had their origin from, and

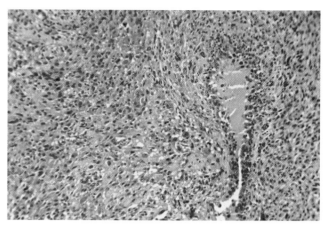

FIGURE 35-38. Epithelioid malignant peripheral nerve sheath tumor. Plump, rounded cells are arranged in patterns of ill-defined nests. Nuclei show variations in size and staining. A cleft to the right of the center of the field is outlined by palisades of tumor cells.

are in continuity with, a peripheral nerve, may manifest extraneural, infiltrating, and fascicular patterns (20,93) in the skin and subcutaneous tissue; they qualify as *infiltrating fascicular epithelioid malignant schwannomas* (IFEMSs). In the skin and subcutis, such a lesion, in recurrences, might be indistinguishable from so-called desmoplastic and neurotropic melanoma (Fig. 35-40).

The designation, MPNST, without additional qualifications, lacks discrimination; in the epithelioid category, the designation MPNST of epithelioid sheath cell type is more appropriate.

Zones of necrosis with peripheral palisades of tumor cells, a feature of both mesenchymal and epithelioid variants, are reminiscent of patterns in high-grade gliomas of the CNS.

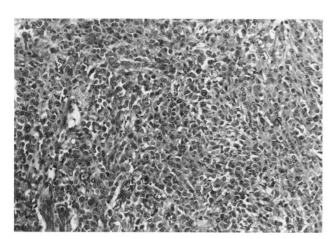

FIGURE 35-37. Epithelioid malignant peripheral nerve sheath tumor. Plump, atypical, spindle and epithelioid cells form solid sheets. Intercellular matrix is scanty.

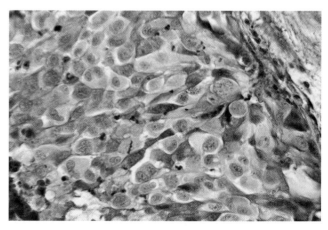

FIGURE 35-39. Neuroendocrine malignant peripheral nerve sheath tumor (Masson trichrome stain). Large atypical cells are closely clustered; they form distinct nests in a fibrous matrix. The preponderant cells have pale cytoplasm. Dark cells with dendritic processes are compressed among the pale cells. The dark cells are argyrophilic.

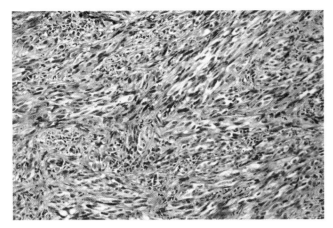

FIGURE 35-40. Fasciculated, malignant epithelioid peripheral nerve sheath tumor (neurotropic and melanoma-like). Broad fascicles of atypical spindle cells infiltrate a fibrous matrix; portions of this soft tissue lesion were intraneural.

Attempts to predict an association of MPNST with neurofibromatosis simply on the basis of histologic findings in the malignant component usually are defeated by common expressions of overlap in patterns of differentiation.

Ultrastructure. A light microscopic diagnosis of MPNST of sheath (Schwann) cell type is supported by a variety of features. Slender, overlapping cytoplasmic processes that envelop other processes, or cell bodies may be connected by intercellular junctions. Granular, flocculent material, preferably along and parallel to the plasma membrane may occasionally assume the linear form of basal lamina. Fine intracytoplasmic filaments should be absent or relative scanty (91).

Histogenesis. In this section, the figures reflect the whims of authors as they select, or reject, examples of "MPNST" for their studies. In 40% to 80% of cases of MPNST (20,96–97), the tumor cells are immunoreactive for S-100 protein. CD57 can be detected in 30% to 40% of the cases (97). Myelin basic protein is less commonly detected (10%) (98). Laminin and collagen type IV are found in about 25% to 30% of cases.

Of the many peripheral stigmata in neurofibromatosis, only neurofibromas are most predisposed to malignant transformations. Neurofibromas adjacent to MPNST often are cellular (Fig. 35-15).

Differential Diagnosis. In the absence of discernible stigmata of neurofibromatosis, differentiation of MPNST from fibrosarcoma is difficult. Patterns of interlacing fascicles, that are alternately light and dark, are characteristic of malignant schwannoma. In a mesenchymal variant of MPNST with patterns of specific differentiation but, with no history or stigmata of neurofibromatosis, a diagnosis of malignant mesenchymoma would be a consideration.

Monophasic synovial sarcoma should be considered in the differential diagnosis. Its genetic profile includes t(x; 18); for MPNST, the common changes are a loss of NF1 locus, and a loss of the band containing gene p53; the changes are

not specific. In 50% of monophasic synovial sarcomas, the cells are immunoreactive for cytokeratins and EMA.

For deep epithelioid variants of MPNST, malignant fibrous histiocytoma (99), rhabdomyosarcoma, leiomyosarcoma, and malignant melanoma are considerations.

If confronted with infiltrating and fascicular patterns in a tumor of the skin, a distinction between neurotropic melanoma (3,100) and cutaneous primary infiltrating and fascicular epithelioid MPNST may be impossible in the absence of melanocytic, lentiginous and junctional patterns in the overlying or adjacent epidermis. Fortunately, the distinction as to whether such a lesion is one or the other has no major therapeutic or prognostic implications: for both lesions the management would be similar. Patterns of radial sclerosis, as seen in rare epithelioid schwannomas, occasionally are a feature of dermal lesions in this overlap category of malignant fascicular epithelioid schwannoma and neurotropic melanoma.

Infiltrating fascicular schwannoma of infancy (IFS), in its histologic, but not its cytologic, patterns, shows overlaps with the patterns of both infiltrating fascicular epithelioid malignant schwannoma (IFEMS) and neurotropic melanoma (100).

Glandular, entoderm-like patterns (Fig. 35-41) may be more commonly associated with epithelioid than with mesenchymal variants of MPNST. If glandular patterns are represented in a problem lesion, then carcinosarcoma might be a consideration. Rarely, entoderm-like, glandular patterns, in the absence of sarcomatous components, are encountered in the soft tissue in the setting of neurofibromatosis; a lesion showing such patterns may represent a primary neuroendocrine carcinoma.

Ganglioneuroma of the deep soft tissue has been the rare site of origin for a MPNST (26,101–103).

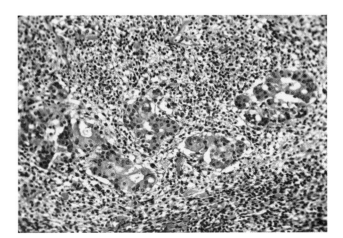

FIGURE 35-41. Small epithelioid cell malignant peripheral nerve sheath tumor; divergent glandular differentiation. Plump, columnar cells form solid nests and glandular patterns; the cells have small, round nuclei with uniform nuclear characteristics. The glandular spaces contain basophilic mucin. The glandular component is a random manifestation in an epithelioid, malignant peripheral nerve-sheath tumor.

Prognostication and Treatment. A moderate increase in cellularity, focal storiform patterns, mild nuclear atypia, and the presence of mitoses (<10/10 HPF) may be the only features that distinguish low-grade MPNST from neurofibroma (3,48,104,105). Such examples qualify as *minimal deviation variants of indeterminate malignant potential*; local surgery is an option in treatment.

In the setting of neurofibromatosis, MPNST, in its many guises, generally has a poor prognosis. High-grade tumors show high mitotic rates (as many as 50/10 HPF), dense cellularity, scanty stroma, marked nuclear atypia, pleomorphism, and palisaded zones of necrosis. For intraneural, high-grade MPNST ex schwannoma (confined by the perineurium of the nerve of origin), confinement favorably modifies the significance of the "high grade." In one series of epithelioid MPNST, superficial location (skin and subcutis) and small size were favorable prognostic parameters (93). In general, adverse prognostic factors include large tumor size, age 7 or more years, tumor necrosis 25% or more, and von Recklinghausen disease (106,107). A high mitotic rate and the need for resection by amputation have also been cited as factors related to a poor prognosis (95). Aggressive surgical treatment is required for high-grade tumors with extensive spread along the involved nerve (108).

TUMORS OF UNCERTAIN NATURE WITH NERVE SHEATH–LIKE FEATURES

Nerve sheath myxoma (NSM; neurothekeoma) was originally defined by Harkin and Reed (3) and was reintroduced by Gallager and Helwig (109) under the designation *neurothekeoma*. Additional designations include pacinian neurofibroma (110), bizarre cutaneous neurofibroma (111), cutaneous lobular neuromyxoma (112), perineurial myxoma (113), and myxoma of nerve sheath (114). In the accumulated studies, the patterns are divisible into a pure myxoid category, a pure "cellular" category, and an overlap category (115,116). Herein, in the fashion of Argenyi et al. (29), the category of nerve sheath myxoma will be divided into a small group, designated *mature nerve sheath myxoma (NSM1)* (a myxoid and loosely cellular lesion that mostly appears micronodular), and a larger group (*NSM2*) that includes both immature nerve sheath myxoma (cellular, or epithelioid and fascicular, neurothekeoma), and differentiating immature nerve sheath myxoma, in which immature (epithelioid) and mature (myxoid) patterns are mixed. Controversy as to the relationships between NSM1 and NSM2 continues. NSM1 certainly has a much clearer "immunohistochemical profile" (i.e., S-100 positive) than NSM2. Wang et al. (117) have reported a positive reaction for PGP 9.5 in NSM2, a finding offering support for the "neuroid" nature of NSM2. In all variations, NSM is a rare neoplasm of the dermis. To encounter somewhat similar lesions in the soft tissue is even more infrequent. NSM, in all its expressions, has been benign, although in cases of incomplete removal, rare examples, probably of the NSM2 type, have recurred. Axons are not a component of any of the variants. Neither neurofibromatosis nor multiple mucosal neuroma syndrome has been a documented association.

Mature Nerve Sheath Myxoma (Myxoid Neurothekeoma: NSM1)

Mature (micronodular) NSM ("classical" type of Argenyi et al. [29]) is most common in middle-aged adults (mean age 48 years) with a male–female ratio of approximately 1:2; characteristically, it is an asymptomatic, soft, skin-colored, or translucent papule or nodule ranging from 0.5 to 1.0 cm in diameter. It is typically located on the face and the upper extremities, but can occur anywhere on the body (118).

Histopathology. Symmetrically expansile, myxoid micronodules that vary in size are loosely clustered in a fibrous matrix in the reticular dermis. They form a multilobulated mass that is often poorly circumscribed, and not always symmetrical (Fig. 35-42). The myxoid matrix is rich in acid mucopolysaccharides (sulfated glycosaminoglycans). Bipolar and tripolar cells are widely and fairly regularly

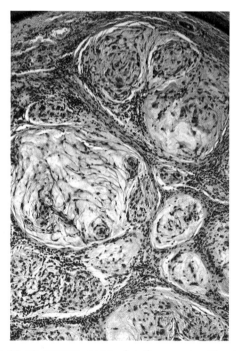

FIGURE 35-42. Mature nerve sheath myxoma. The lesion is plexiform; fascicles are represented in both longitudinal and cross-sections. Some of the fascicles are outlined by thin sheaths of condensed fibrous tissue. Tumor cells are loosely spaced in a prominent myxoid matrix. Some have thin polar extensions of cytoplasm; they morphologically resemble perineurial cells. Some are plump and epithelioid. Some of the thin cells form whorls about blood vessels of the fascicles. In this example, lymphoid infiltrates are prominent in the stroma.

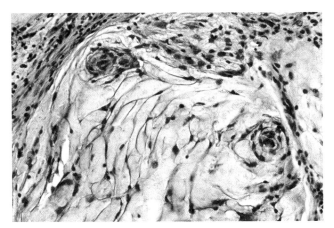

FIGURE 35-43. Mature nerve sheath myxoma. At higher magnification, many of the tumor cells have "perineurial cell-like" qualities. Some of the distinctive cells form whorls about vessels.

spaced (Fig. 35-43). Nuclei are elongated, and often angulated with inconspicuous nucleoli and uniformly distributed, dense chromatin. Cytoplasms are pale, and cell membranes are sharply defined. Centrally in the micronodules, cells tend to be arranged in loose whorls. Each micronodule is partially or completely outlined, in perineurium-like patterns, by a thin condensation of fibrous tissue. Continuity with adjacent nerves is rarely identified (3,109,113, 114,118).

Ultrastructurally in lesions of NSM1, a continuous basal lamina outlines most cells, but in some reports discontinuous basal lamina and pinocytotic vesicles have been features (118). Engulfment of collagen fibers in the manner of Schwann cells has been observed. Fibroblasts and mast cells are also represented (119).

Histogenesis. The immunohistochemical profile is S-100 protein (positive), collagen type IV (positive), and vimentin (positive) (29,120–123). A smaller number of cells are EMA (positive) (29,114,119).

Immature Nerve Sheath Myxoma (Cellular or Epithelioid and Fascicular Nerve Sheath Myxoma: NSM2)

The second and larger group (NSM2; *cellular neurothekeoma*) includes both immature (NSM2 A) and differentiating immature (NSM2 B) variants. In NSM2, the mean age is 24 years, but examples have been reported in children. Women are more commonly affected, and the upper body is the favored site (120). The lesions are firm, pink, red-brown papules or nodules measuring 0.5 to 3.0 cm, and some may produce symptoms (118).

Histopathology. In immature *NSM2 A*, fascicles of cells tend to be rather uniform in diameter, and their margins are poorly defined. They are arranged in infiltrating (dissecting) patterns among collagen bundles of the reticular dermis, or are supported by a fibrous matrix (Fig. 35-44A and B); they often extend into the subcutis. Exclusive of the fascicular component, individual tumor cells, and small, irregular clusters of tumor cells may infiltrate the reticular dermis; they may even extend into arrector muscles. In the fascicles, the cells are closely spaced; they tend to be polygonal, but in rare examples they are plump and spindle-shaped. Cytoplasm is conspicuous and tends to be acidophilic. Rigid cytoplasmic processes are prominent. The nuclei are plump, rounded or elongated, and somewhat irregular in outline. The chromatin is stippled, and nuclear membranes are heavy.

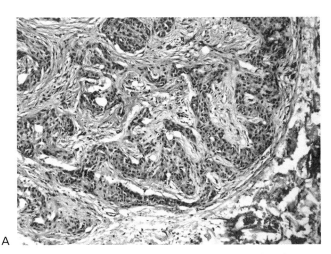
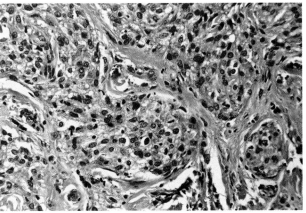

FIGURE 35-44. Immature nerve sheath myxoma. **A:** Pale, acidophilic epithelioid cells from tortuous, interconnected fascicles in a well-defined fibromyxoid matrix. The lesion is sharply circumscribed. In the fascicles, myxoid matrix is scanty. **B:** At higher magnification, the epithelioid cells of the fascicles are loosely attached to their neighbors. Defects among the tumor cells contain a mucinous matrix. The tumor cells show regular, round nuclei with well-defined nuclear membranes and stippled chromatin; nuclei are small.

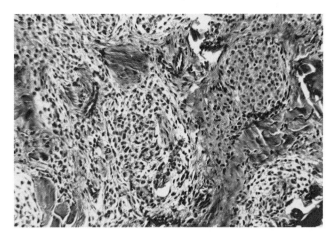

FIGURE 35-45. Nerve sheath myxoma; differentiating immature variant. In this example, cellular zones merge with myxoid zones, the lesion is fasciculated, and the fascicles extend among collagen bundles of the reticular dermis without inducing a tumor stroma.

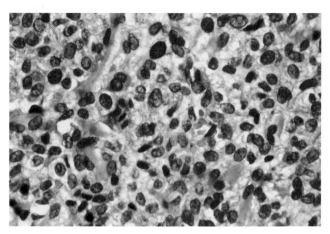

FIGURE 35-47. Atypical immature nerve sheath myxoma. Cells have scanty cytoplasm and enlarged, hyperchromatic nuclei. Nuclei vary in size and outline; some show prominent nucleoli.

In *NSM2 B*, some of the aggregates become locally expanded to form broad fascicles and nodules in which both immature (cellular), and mature (myxoid) patterns are represented (Fig. 35-45). In the myxoid zones, stellate cells are loosely spaced: their cytoplasmic processes are broader and more irregular in diameter than those of the cells of mature (NSM1) variants. The mature components tend to be focal, with a preference for the periphery of broad fascicles and nodules. Compact whorls of cells are focally prominent in all variations of NSM2. Spotty incomplete condensations of fibrous tissue are observed at the periphery of the broad fascicles and nodules.

In some examples of NSM2, the stroma consists of a sclerotic, fibrous matrix with no preservation of the interwoven fiber patterns of the reticular dermis (Fig. 35-44A).

Mitoses are not a prominent feature in most examples of both variants of NSM2. Atypical variants are characterized by nuclear atypia, and pleomorphism with scattered mitoses (Figs. 35-46 and 35-47), some of which may be atypical (113,123).

In some examples of NSM2, histiocytic, multinucleated giant cells are represented among the tumor cells. In lesions showing a component of such cells, the patterns overlap with those of plexiform fibrous histiocytoma (Fig. 35-48).

Rarely in lesions of NSM2, tumor cells extend within the perineurium, or in the endoneurial space of small nerves into the adjacent dermis.

Ultrastructurally, NSM2 A and B are composed preponderantly of undistinguished cells. Focal densities of the cell membranes that are suggestive of attachment plaques,

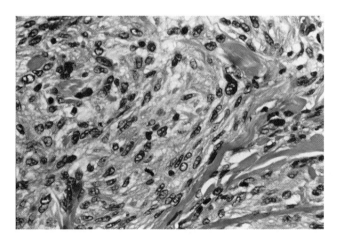

FIGURE 35-46. Atypical immature nerve sheath myxoma. Tumor cells of this atypical nerve sheath myxoma vary in size and outline; some are hyperchromatic. A mitotic figure is represented to the left and below the center of the field.

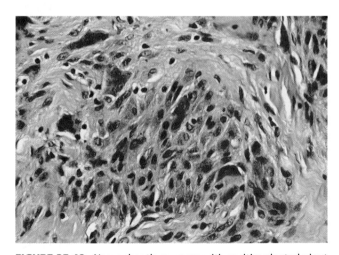

FIGURE 35-48. Nerve sheath myxoma with multinucleated giant cells. The basic pattern of this "plexiform" lesion suggested a variant of nerve sheath myxoma. Focally, as in this field, the patterns overlap with those of plexiform fibrous histiocytoma.

and focal, poorly formed, basal lamina–like material have been described. Some of the cells contain phagolysosome-like structures, irregularly arranged microfilaments, and rare microfilament-attached dense bodies (119). Mature fibroblasts are common. In a single case, perineurial cell–like features have been described (118).

Histogenesis. Immunohistochemically, the cells of NSM2 exhibit a variable and inconsistent phenotype. They are positive for vimentin and PGP 9.5, but do not stain convincingly for S-100 protein, or epithelial membrane antigen (120–122). Weak and variable expression of smooth muscle–specific actin, collagen type IV, NK1/C3, and CD57 have been reported (29,116–124). The immunohistochemical distinctions seem to contradict the position that NSM1 and NSM2 are related. They may provide evidence that the expressions of phenotype, and the respective histologic patterns are dependent on degree of differentiation.

Differential Diagnosis. Intraneural neurofibromas are rare in the dermis, and only slightly more common in the subcutis. Immunoreactive axons, a feature of intraneural neurofibroma, are not a feature of NSM1.

Cellular myxomas of the skin, including *angiomyxomas* (125) and *trichogenic myxomas* (75) are rare, and some are poorly documented. They are solid, uniform lesions: neither the micronodular qualities of NSM1 nor the fascicular and nodular qualities of NSM2 A and B are represented. In cellular myxomas, immunoreactions for S-100 protein are negative (29). Examples of cellular myxoma appear to have been included in some reports of NSM. Examples of "perineurioma" probably have been reported as NSM. Zelger et al. (31) suggest that some reported examples of NSM are perineuriomas.

Spindle cell nevus of the Spitz type, particularly dermal variants, might be confused with NSM2. A strong and uniform reaction for S-100 protein would favor a variant of Spitz nevus, or some other variant of nevus, such as a cellular blue nevus with prominent fascicular components. The pigmentation of deep penetrating nevus is not a feature of NSM2.

In rare examples, minimal deviation *neurotropic melanoma* would be a consideration. Most spindle cell melanomas are S-100 protein positive. Not all desmoplastic and neurotropic melanomas are immunoreactive for HMB45, but a positive reaction excludes NSM2. NSM2 A may be mistaken for a metastatic malignant melanoma (a lesion lacking a primary configuration). A positive reaction for S-100 protein and HMB45 would strongly favor a diagnosis of malignant melanoma.

Some examples of NSM2 B with involvement of the subcutis, and with numerous giant cells, would be difficult to distinguish from plexiform fibrous histiocytoma of children and young adults (30) (Fig. 35-48). In the nodular portions of plexiform fibrous histiocytoma, the cells are closely spaced, and often are admixed with multinucleated giant cells. Plexiform fibrous histiocytoma has a close as-

sociation with fascia. A myxoid matrix is not prominent, but focally may be a feature.

Sclerosing myofibroblastomas as well as rare myxoid, or epithelioid pilar leiomyomas of the skin should be considered in the differential diagnosis (126). In the cellular portions of myxoid leiomyomas, the cells clearly are smooth muscle in type. In some examples of NSM2 A, in which some of the cells are immunoreactive for smooth muscle actin, the tumor cells are consistently negative for desmin (29).

Epithelioid fibrous histiocytoma (*EFH*) (epithelioid cell histiocytoma, adventitial cellular myxofibroblastoma) (127, 128), a lesion favoring acral sites, tends to be polypoid, and is mostly confined to a widened papillary dermis. Some examples are mostly myxoid. Large vacuolated cells with muciparous qualities are occasionally a feature. Many of the dendritic histiocytes among tumor cells of EFH are reactive for factor XIIIa, and some are reactive for S-100 protein. Examples of EFH can be identified in some reports of NSM. It should be noted that PGP 9.5 has recently been found to be a ubiquitous marker and nonspecific as a marker in the practice of surgical pathology (129).

Biphasic nerve sheath tumor (large dendritic cells and small satellite cells nerve sheath tumor; dendritic cell neurofibroma with pseudorosettes) is a poorly defined, benign "plexiform" lesion of the skin (130,131). The tumorous components each are outlined by a sheath of cells that are immunoreactive for EMA; presumably, the cells forming the sheaths are representatives of the preexisting perineurium of the involved peripheral nerves; the lesions apparently are intraneural. Two cell types are represented: large dendritic cells and small, dark cells. The dark cells tend to cluster in patterns of satellitosis about the large dendritic cells. The tumor cells are immunoreactive for S-100 protein. The large cells are not neurons.

Granular Cell Tumors

Granular Cell Nerve Sheath Tumor

Granular cell nerve sheath tumors (GCNSTs) have been characterized as granular cell myoblastomas, granular cell schwannomas, and granular cell tumors. They usually are solitary but in about 10% of the cases are multiple; they may be multifocal. Forty percent of the cases involve the tongue (132), but the skin and the subcutaneous tissue also are a common site. Other reported sites include the esophagus, stomach, appendix, larynx, bronchus, pituitary gland, uvea, and skeletal muscle (133).

GCNSTs of the skin are well circumscribed, raised, firm, and nodular. Some examples are verrucoid at the surface. Generally, lesions range from 0.5 to 3.0 cm in diameter. The cut surface often is faintly yellow and homogeneous. Tenderness or pruritus has been an occasional complaint.

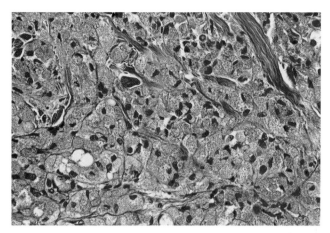

FIGURE 35-49. Granular nerve sheath tumor. In this example, the cells are plump and polygonal; fine granules, uniform in size, fill the cytoplasm of each cell. In this category, nuclear characteristics are variable from case to case; in this example, there is some variability in nuclear size and outline. An occasional nucleus contains an inclusion of cytoplasm. Nucleoli are variable in size.

Histopathology. Most GCNSTs are extraneural; rare examples have been intraneural, at least in part. Broad fascicles of tumor cells infiltrate the dermis among the collagen bundles (Fig. 35-49). Extension of tumor fascicles into the subcutis is common. The tumor cells are large and polygonal (Fig. 35-50); cell membranes are distinct. Faintly eosinophilic, uniform, small granules that are PAS (positive) and diastase-resistant fill the cytoplasms. Scattered, laminated, cytoplasmic globules with peripheral halos (residual bodies) (Fig. 35-50) are also represented. Nuclei usually are small, round to oval, and centrally located but, in some examples, are plump, irregular, and hyperchromatic with a central nucleolus. Mitoses are uncommon. Some clusters of tumor cells are surrounded by PAS (positive), diastase-resistant membranes, strands of collagen fibers, and occasional flattened, satellite

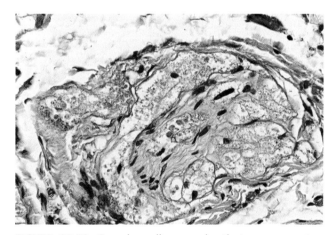

FIGURE 35-50. Granular cell nerve sheath tumor, neurotropism. Granular cells infiltrate the perineurium and the endoneurial space of this small nerve. In the cytoplasm of some of the cells, in addition to fine, uniform granules, there are larger, rounded, acidophilic bodies that are "residual body-like."

cells (132). Interstitial spindle cells have fibroblast-like qualities (20). Rarely, fascicles of tumor cells are entrapped in a dense fibrous matrix (sclerosing variant).

Neurotropic spread along peripheral nerves, both within, and at the advancing margins of the tumor, is often a feature (Fig. 35-50). Rarely, deep GCNSTs have an intraneural component that expands the involved nerve.

Some GCNSTs are associated with histologic signs of malignancy (134). Mitoses are an acceptable feature, and are not a marker for malignant transformation. GCNST infiltrates locally; it should be completely excised. Recurrences are common after incomplete excision.

Infiltration of skeletal muscle is a common feature of GCNST involving the squamous mucosae; in such areas, regenerating and degenerating muscle fibers are entrapped among fascicles of tumor cells. *Plexiform GCNST* is characterized by perineurial extensions of tumor along the neural plexus of the dermis in the absence of a discrete mass (135).

Ultrastructurally, tumor cells are outlined by basal lamina (136,137). The preponderant cytoplasmic granules are largely phagolysosomes. They appear as membrane-bound vacuoles measuring 200 to 900 nm in diameter. Some of the larger cytoplasmic bodies have the appearance of residual bodies, or myelin figures (133,137,138). The peripheral satellite cells of the fascicles are outlined by discontinuous lamina (139). Interstitial cells of the tumor contain angulate bodies (20).

Histogenesis. The granular cell category is heterogeneous. Not all examples mark as nerve sheath tumors; some of the divergent lesions are also atypical (139). The classic immunohistochemical profile is S-100 protein (positive), peripheral nerve myelin proteins, such as P2 protein and PO protein (positive) (140), PGP 9.5 (positive) (141), NSE (positive), and vimentin (positive).

Differential Diagnosis. A *xanthoma* is excluded by the identification of cytoplasmic granules (rather than vacuoles). A fascicular arrangement of cells favors GCNST.

Angulated, elongated columns of bland squamous cells occasionally extend from the epidermis into GCNST among the fascicles of tumor cells (*pseudoepitheliomatous hyperplasia*). On biopsy specimens from tumoral lesions of the tongue, genitalia, or the mucous membranes of the upper respiratory tract, esophagus, or anus, such patterns should be interpreted with caution. If confronted with such patterns, a careful search for a component of granular cells may avoid a mistaken diagnosis of carcinoma and, in turn, needless aggressive surgery.

Tumor cells with granular qualities are occasionally a feature of *lesions of diverse lineage*, such as basal cell carcinoma (142) and dermatofibroma (143). The granules of rare granular squamous cell carcinomas, in contrast to those of other benign and malignant granular cell tumors, are PAS (negative), and desmosomes are seen on electron microscopy (144). In the jawbones, a granular cell variant of ameloblastoma has been described. Granular cell change has been noted in smooth muscle tumors (145).

Granular Cell Epulis of Infancy

This is a polypoid tumor of the gingiva of the newborn, with a predilection for girls (146). It shares the basic histologic features of *GCNST* but is immunohistochemically distinctive. The immunohistochemical profile is NSE (positive), vimentin (positive), S-100 protein (negative), GFAP (negative), CD57 (negative), MBP (negative), lysozyme (negative), a1-ACT (negative), and laminin (negative). Interstitial cells are positive for S-100 protein; they do not contain angulate bodies (147).

Malignant Granular Cell Tumor

The malignant granular cell tumor (MGCT) is uncommon. Most of the reported cases have occurred on the skin or in the subcutaneous tissue. As in benign GCNST, a few cases have been reported from other areas, such as the sciatic nerve (148) and the viscera. A variety of malignant tumors may masquerade in granular cell patterns. In all instances, an acceptance of the diagnosis, MGCT, is predicated on circumspection.

In the skin and subcutaneous tissue, MGCT, a rapidly growing, poorly defined nodule or mass, may reach considerable size, and undergo ulceration (149). Extensive metastases to viscera, skin, and skeletal musculature occur, either with, or without regional lymph node metastases (150). Some lesions, even in the absence of demonstrable metastases, have been characterized as MGCT (151).

Histopathology. There are two types of MGCT (152). In one type, in spite of the clinically malignant course, the histologic appearance of the primary lesion, and even of the metastases, is that of a benign GCNST, except for occasional mitotic figures, and mild pleomorphism with nuclei that are slightly larger than those seen in most benign GCNSTs (150,152,153). In the general category of GCNST, these cytologic features are too common to provide a reliable identification of lesions with the potential for metastases. In evaluating the malignant potential of histologically benign, or indeterminant granular cell tumors, clinical data, such as large size of the tumor, rapid growth, ulceration, and invasion into adjacent tissue, are of greater diagnostic value than the histologic features (154). The average diameter of "histologically benign, clinically malignant," granular cell tumors has been found to be 9 cm, as compared with 1.85 cm for the benign variety (152,154).

In the second type of MGCT, both the primary lesion and the metastases are histologically malignant: they show transitions from typical granular cells through pleomorphic granular cells to pleomorphic, nongranular spindle and giant cells with numerous mitotic figures (155,156).

In benign GCNST, immunohistochemical tests for S-100 protein, NSE, and vimentin are regularly positive. In MGCT, the same tests often are negative.

Fibrolamellar Nerve Sheath Tumor

Fibrolamellar nerve sheath tumor (FNST) is a solitary tumor of the dermis.

Histopathology. FNST is nonencapsulated but sharply defined in the dermis. Coarse, rigid, brightly eosinophilic lamellae are arranged in parallel arrays in stacks of four or more. Neighboring stacks are random in orientation, one to the other, but in some areas the patterns that result from the abutment of neighboring stacks are storiform. Some examples are mostly myxoid; in them, the fibrous lamellae are more delicate, and widely spaced. Tumor cells, each with a small nucleus, scanty perikaryon, and rigid, thin, polar extensions of cytoplasm, resemble perineurial cells. They are isolated in clear, or mucinous matrix among the fibrous lamellae. Rarely, a few loosely clustered, pigmented dendritic melanocytes have been a feature.

FNST is histologically distinctive but may be simply an exaggeration of perineurial-like patterns that are occasionally manifested in cutaneous neurofibromas.

FNST shares features with *sclerosing fibroma*, as manifested either sporadically or in the setting of *Cowden* disease. An appreciation of subtle cytologic differences, and a demonstration of immunoreactivity by some of the tumor cells for S-100 protein strongly favor the diagnosis of FNST.

TUMORS OF PERINEURIAL CELLS ("PERINEURIOMAS")

Storiform Perineurial Cell Fibroma, Soft Tissue Type

Storiform perineurial cell fibroma, soft tissue type (SPCF; storiform perineurial fibroma; "soft tissue perineurioma") is a solitary, symmetrically expansile, and well-circumscribed tumor of the subcutis (3,157–159), but the deep soft tissue and even viscera may be involved. Clinical features are not well established. The lesion is a fibroma whose component cells express the phenotype of perineurial cells.

Histopathology. SPCF is circumscribed. At its periphery, the interface with soft tissue is defined by a thin capsule consisting of several, loosely spaced, delicate fibrous lamellae. Beneath the capsule, thin collagen fibers form a delicate fibrous matrix. Cells with plump, angulated nuclei, and rigid, polar cytoplasmic extensions are loosely spaced (Fig. 35-51). Fascicles in storiform patterns are variably represented. In most examples, small nerves are embedded in, or may be traced into, the tumor. The tumor cells tend to form thin concentric layers around entrapped small nerves, blood vessels, and collagen bundles. Small stacks of hyalinized fibrous lamellae occasionally are a focal variation in such lesions (Fig. 35-51).

Histogenesis. The cytologic features are similar to those of perineurial cells. In some examples, tumor cells are immunoreactive for vimentin and EMA (159), although the latter reaction may be weak or patchy, and best developed in

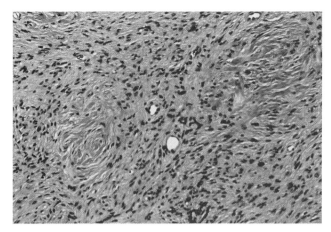

FIGURE 35-51. Storiform, perineurial cell nerve-sheath tumor (soft tissue "perineurioma"). Spindle cells are individually isolated in a delicate fibrous matrix. There are two collections of stacked, acidophilic fibrous lamellae.

cells in, or near the capsule. In other examples, scattered aggregates of tumor cells in more central locations are reactive for S-100 protein. Claudin-1, a tight junction–associated protein, recently has been reported as a common expression in membranous, granular patterns in perineuriomas (160). An abnormality of chromosome 22 has been reported (161).

Differential Diagnosis. Storiform patterns appear to be variations that are expressed in a variety of nerve sheath tumors, and perhaps variants of both schwannomas and neurofibromas may be included in this category. The evidence that SPCF is purely perineurial in character is unconvincing. For some problematic lesions, "cellular" schwannoma would be a diagnostic consideration.

Dermatofibrosarcoma protuberans, in its nodular, well-differentiated components, may be confused with SPCF. Fibrous histiocytoma of the subcutis, and dermatofibroma also are considerations in the differential diagnosis.

Dermatofibrosarcoma protuberans (DFSP) has been variously classified as a fibroblastic, fibrohistiocytic, or neurocristic tumor. The pigmented variant of DFSP (*Bednar tumor*) has been characterized as pigmented storiform neurofibroma. The nature of pigmented dermatofibrosarcoma is controversial but, in one study, perineurial cell–like qualities were observed (162). The cells of DFSP, like some cells of nerve sheath tumors, are immunoreactive for CD34 (163). DFSP is described in detail elsewhere (Chapter 33).

Pacinian Neurofibroma

The designation *pacinian neurofibroma* has been assigned to a variety of lesions. The list includes cellular blue nevus (164); a lesion of uncertain nature with perivascular, concentric lamellar fibrosis (165); diffuse neurofibroma with tactoid bodies (4); a giant pacinian corpuscle with an increased number of coarse fibrous lamellae (3); and nerve sheath myxoma (110).

Intraneural Symmetrically Concentric Perineurial Cell Tumor (Intraneural Perineurioma)

This tumor (PSCPCT; intraneural perineurioma, hypertrophic interstitial neuritis, hypertrophic mononeuropathy) (166–168) is an intraneural, solitary, segmental and cylindrical enlargement of a nerve. Sensorimotor defects are characteristic.

Histopathology. In the characterization of this lesion, distinctions are required between onion bulbs and pseudo-onion bulbs; pseudo-onion bulbs are composed of cells that are immunoreactive for EMA. If the cells of a concentrically arranged cluster are Schwann cells, the collection qualifies as an onion bulb pattern; if the concentrically arranged cells are mostly perineurial cells, the collection qualifies as a pseudo-onion bulb pattern. Cells with both the structural qualities and immunoreactivity of perineurial cells form concentric sheaths (pseudo-onion bulbs) around affected nerve fibers (Fig. 35-52), and even around small clusters of pseudo-onion bulbs (166). Collagen bundles and vessels may be similarly embraced. A specific and concentric orientation of cells about axons is a symmetric quality. Demyelination and degeneration of axons are associated phenomena; in the center of the clusters, axons may appear enlarged and irregular in outline.

Histogenesis. In PSCPCT, the concentrically arranged cells immunoreact with antibodies for EMA (166), and have the ultrastructural features of perineurial cells.

A defect in the integrity of the perineurial barrier has been proposed as the primary alteration. Delamination of the perineurium, and migration of perineurial cells into the endoneurium have been offered as an explanation for the origin of pseudo-onion bulbs (167).

PSCPCT is intraneural; the concentric ensheathing of nerve fibers is a symmetrical quality, and the ensheathing cells have perineurial cell-like qualities.

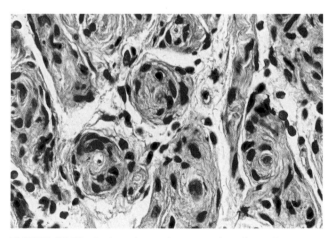

FIGURE 35-52. Perineurioma, intraneural variant. Axons are surrounded by concentric layers of spindle cells; the spindle cells are layered in onionskin patterns. The lesion is intraneural, and axial symmetry is preserved.

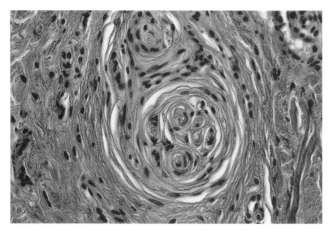

FIGURE 35-53. Hypertrophic neuropathy. In the center of the field, a small nerve is cut in cross-section. The perineurium is thickened. Spindle cells are arranged concentrically about nerve fibers (onionskin pattern). Some of the spindle cells blend with the thickened perineurium.

In common with descriptions of the clonal, chromosomal abnormalities in benign and malignant schwannomas, neurofibromas, meningiomas, and gliomas, deletion of 22q11,2-qter has been described in PSCPCT (166); it is cited as a finding favoring neoplasia (166).

Differential Diagnosis. The *hereditary degenerative neuropathies* are not localized and segmental (169). They are characterized by concentric hyperplasia of Schwann cells (onion bulbs) (Fig. 35-53).

Sclerosing Perineural Cell Fibroma, Acral Type (Sclerosing or Fibrous Perineurioma)

An uncommon, small, benign tumor found mainly on the hands has been characterized as either fibrous (dermal) perineurioma (170) or sclerosing (subcutaneous) perineurioma (171,172). It should be noted that most, if not all, the lesions in this category can be easily accommodated in the category of pacinian neurofibroma. The category of fibrous and sclerosing perineurioma expresses the penchant of some observers for new designations; it additionally expresses a currently popular penchant to group dissimilar lesions in the category of perineurioma.

These small tumors are basically fibrous lesions with focal areas of increased cellularity; they are fibromas whose component cells express the phenotype of perineurial cells. They are additionally distinguished by distribution; they mostly are acral in location. Some of the lesions have ill-defined margins; some are circumscribed, particularly along the deep margin. The cells are spindle shaped, or ovoid; they have round nuclei with uniformly distributed chromatin; they have pale or clear cytoplasm. Some of the cells appear to be outlined by a delicate membrane. In areas, the cells form thin, interconnected ribbons (retiform patterns). In other more cellular areas, the cells form whorls in patterns strongly suggestive of the arrangement of cells in a pacinian corpuscle. The cells are immunoreactive for EMA, and show ultrastructural features of perineurial cells. Some of the tumor cells are immunoreactive for muscle specific actin, and CD99.

The differential diagnosis includes glomus tumor. Obviously, lesions of this type might also be characterized as some type of pacinian neurofibroma.

An additional variant of "perineurioma," the retiform (reticular) perineurioma (173) is a soft tissue lesion sharing some of the features of the sclerosing, or fibrous variants. It should be obvious that the category of "perineurioma" has been compromised by this willingness to be extravagant in the application of the designation (Fig. 35-54A and B).

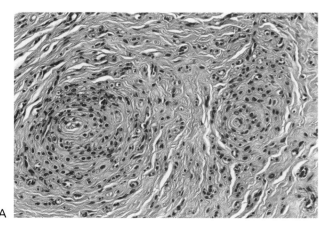

A

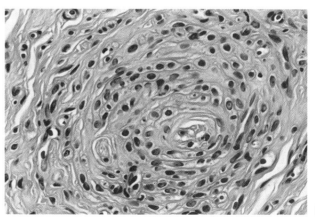

B

FIGURE 35-54. Sclerosing perineurial cell nerve sheath tumor (fibrous or sclerosing "perineurioma"). **A:** In two foci, bland, small cells with pale cytoplasm are arranged in whorls among delicate collagen fibers. The cells are round or slightly spindle shaped, and some appear to be isolated by basement membranes. The bland cytologic features are reminiscent of glomus cells. The concentric whorls are reminiscent of cellular arrangements in pacinian corpuscles. In the background, the lesion is sclerotic with small spindle cells among collagen bundles. **B:** At higher magnification, the cells form whorls about a central nidus. The cytologic features are more epithelioid than perineural.

NEUROMAS

Neuromas are hyperplasias of axons, and associated nerve sheath cells. In most, but not all, cutaneous neuromas, Schwann cells and axons are arranged in broad, interlacing (tortuous) fascicles; axons are easily demonstrated with silver impregnation techniques. Axons are also easily demonstrated with monoclonal antibodies, such as those for neurofilaments, but such reactions alone do not distinguish between the innervated fascicles of a neuroma and those of cutaneous neurofibroma.

Neuromas can be divided into four types: (a) extraneural (traumatic or acquired) neuromas; (b) intraneural (isolated and spontaneous, solitary or multiple) neuromas; (c) intraneural (multiple mucosal) neuromas, including those occurring in multiple endocrine neoplasia, type 2b; and (d) abnormalities of sensory receptors.

Extraneural Neuromas

Acquired (Traumatic) Neuroma

Traumatic neuromas are usually solitary, skin-colored or pink, firm papules or nodules at the sites of scars following local trauma. In mature neuromas, a lancinating type of pain may be elicited in response to local pressure.

Histopathology. Interlacing fascicles of regenerating nerve fibers extend from the proximal end of a damaged nerve; they extend through an acquired defect in the perineurium into the neighboring mesenchyme. They insinuate in asymmetrical patterns among collagen bundles (Fig. 35-55). With maturation, perineuria form around the extraneural fascicles. Tangled fascicles in a scar form the tumor. The distal end of a severed nerve does not contribute significantly to the neuroma. In pre-tumorous stages, nerve fibers

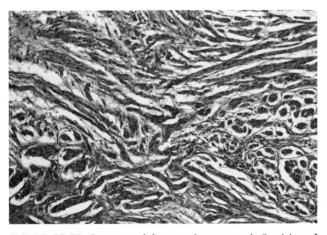

FIGURE 35-55. Extraneural (traumatic neuroma). Fascicles of Schwann cells are arranged haphazardly in a fibrous matrix. A thin perineurium has formed at the periphery of some of the fascicles; the thin perineuria are separated from the respective Schwann cell fascicles by a clear space.

of both the proximal, and distal segments of the disrupted nerve show wallerian degeneration (Fig 35-2).

Rudimentary Supernumerary Digits

These usually are asymptomatic, smooth or verrucous papules. Like intact supernumerary digits, they occur at the base of the ulnar side of the fifth finger. They are assumed to represent the residua of either autoamputation in utero, or postnatal destruction of a supernumerary digit (174).

Histopathology. Much of what comprises a rudimentary digit shows the histologic pattern of an acquired neuroma. Nerve fibers of the neuroma, that are located close to the epidermis, may terminate in closely spaced Meissner corpuscles (174).

Intraneural Neuromas

Palisaded and Encapsulated (Sporadic and Spontaneous) Neuroma

This neuroma (PEN) is uncommon. Solitary examples may arise in either early childhood, or adulthood (mean age, 45.5 years). Multiple neuromas arise in adulthood. Both solitary and multiple cutaneous intraneural neuromas usually are asymptomatic. In neither presentation are the lesions associated with the stigmata of *multiple endocrine neoplasia* (MEN).

PEN is a firm, rubbery, skin-colored, or pink papule or nodule (175–178); it commonly affects the "butterfly area" of the face. During biopsy, it often is enucleated from its dermal bed, and then submitted to the pathologist with little, if any, surrounding skin.

Histopathology. PEN is a bulbous expansion of a peripheral nerve, appearing as a well-circumscribed, ovoid, or rounded nodule in the dermis (Fig. 35-56). Intraneurally, Schwann cells form uniform, broad (often four or more cell layers), interlacing fascicles that are spaced in a clear, or mucinous matrix (Fig. 35-57). Nuclear palisades are ill-defined. Nuclear pleomorphism, and mitoses are not features. PEN is confined by a thin, expanded perineurial sheath. In many examples, the sheath is attenuated along the surface that approximates the epidermis. This variation is a consequence of the anatomy of a nerve: the perineurial sheath is open-ended in this site. At some site along the periphery, it is usually possible to identify, in continuity, extensions of tumor into the endoneurial space of small neighboring nerves.

The fascicles are rich in axons with silver stains (177) (Fig. 35-58) and with immunoreactions for neuron specific enolase (Fig. 35-59), and for neural filaments (178). A weak, sometimes discontinuous reaction for EMA is a feature in the capsule of PEN (178). The presence of axons sets PEN apart from schwannoma, including all the variants. In PEN, axon representation in the fascicles is variable from lesion to lesion (177). Axon density, as evaluated by an im-

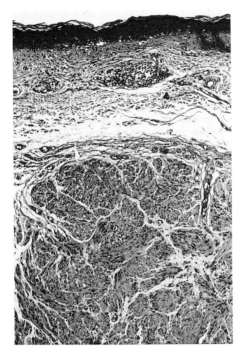

FIGURE 35-56. Palisaded and encapsulated (intraneural) neuroma. The lesion is encapsulated. Fascicles of Schwann cells are arranged in interlacing patterns; the fascicles are supported by a scanty clear or myxoid matrix. Focally, within some of the fascicles, the nuclei of the Schwann cells form ill-defined palisades.

munoreaction to peripherin may not be comparable to the relative density of axons with a Bodian stain (179).

Intraneural Plexiform Neuroma

Plexiform neuroma is an uncommon intraneural tumor of the dermis and subcutis. It has been characterized as a vari-

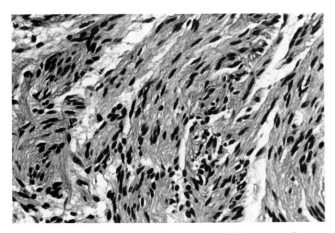

FIGURE 35-57. Palisaded and encapsulated (intraneural) neuroma. The Schwann cells form broad fascicles that are loosely spaced in a myxoid matrix. There are scattered nuclear palisades. In cross-section, some of the cells are vacuolated and have the features of nonmyelinated fibers. Myelinated fibers commonly are found in the fascicles.

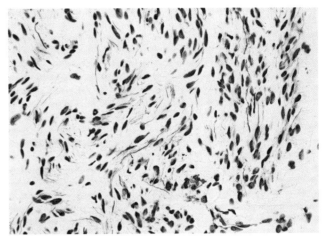

FIGURE 35-58. Palisaded and encapsulated (intraneural) neuroma (Bodian silver stain). The lesion is axon-rich.

ant of PEN (27), but some examples may represent incipient plexiform schwannoma.

Histopathology. Nodules and broad cords are circumscribed by the perineurium of the involved segment of nerve. The internal patterns of all the nodules, and broad cords are basically those of PEN.

Clustered, dilated vessels with sclerotic walls, and subendothelial collections of foam cells are features in common with schwannoma.

In contrast to fully developed plexiform schwannoma, plexiform neuroma, with both silver stains and immunoreactions for neural filaments, is rich in axons.

Mucosal Neuroma Syndrome

Multiple endocrine neoplasia (MEN), type 2b, first described in 1968 (28), is the only one of three types (i.e., types 1, 2,

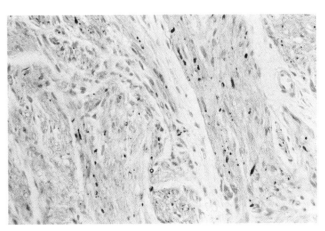

FIGURE 35-59. Palisaded and encapsulated (intraneural) neuroma (immunohistochemical reaction for neuron specific enolase). With a reaction for neuron specific enolase, axons are represented in large part as puncta.

and 2b) to show mucosal and cutaneous neuromas (*mucosal neuroma syndrome, MNS*). *Multiple* (*intraneural*) *neuromas*, many of which are periorificial, are often its earliest manifestation. First appearing in early childhood, they are seen as small nodules, often in large numbers, on the mucosa of the lips, tongue, oral cavity (180,181), and conjunctiva and sclera. Some patients show small, nodular neuromas, usually only in small numbers, on the skin of the face (181). Lesions occasionally are represented in large numbers on, and about, the nose, and on the eyelids. Quite frequently, the lips are thick, fleshy, and protruding (182). Marfanoid features, and skeletal abnormalities may be present (182).

MEN, type 2b; may be inherited as an autosomal dominant trait (180), *medullary thyroid carcinoma, bilateral pheochromocytoma* (181), and *diffuse alimentary tract ganglioneuromatosis* are associated disorders of variable frequency (183).

Histopathology. The neuromas of the MNS are intraneural, and plexiform. Characteristically, the involved nerves are slender. Many are uniform in diameter, but bulbous expansions also are a feature. Within the confines of the perineurium, fascicles, that are fairly uniform in diameter, and composed of two or more nerve fibers, are interlaced in asymmetrical patterns; they are closely spaced, back-to-back, in a clear, or mucinous (endoneurial) matrix. The fascicles of nerve fibers in the mucosal and cutaneous lesions are richly innervated.

Linear cutaneous neuroma (*dermatoneurie en stries*), a sporadic variant of an intraneural neuroma, is manifested clinically as a group of raised linearities (184,185). It differs from the mucosal neuroma syndrome in clinical presentation, and in the size of the altered nerves in the dermis.

Histologically, nerves of the dermis, and subcutis are slightly enlarged and hypercellular (Fig. 35-60A and B). Internally, Schwann cells are increased in number, and nerve fibers are tortuous; this combination of features results in loss of axial symmetry in the affected segments (Fig. 35-60B). It has been proposed that linear cutaneous neuromas are a manifestation of MEN, type 2b (184).

Multiple mucocutaneous neuromas may be encountered in the absence of other stigmata of MEN (186,187).

Ensheathed neuroma is a dermal microscopic lesion characterized by enlarged, hypercellular dermal nerves that are ensheathed by benign squamous epithelium (188).

Special Stains (*Applicable to All Neuromas*). With luxol-fast blue stain, some of the fibers in all forms of neuroma may be myelinated.

Electron Microscopy (*Applicable to All Neuromas*). Ultrastructurally, fascicles, which are composed of both myelinated, and nonmyelinated nerve fibers, are the chief feature of both extraneural (189) and intraneural neuromas; those of a mature, extraneural neuroma are ensheathed by multiple lamina of perineurial cells (189). Generally, perineurial cells do not outline the individual, asymmetrical fascicles of intraneural neuromas.

Histogenesis (*Applicable to All Neuromas*). The immunohistochemical profile is S-100 protein (positive), collagen type IV (positive), vimentin (positive), and NSE and neural filaments (positive).

In mature traumatic neuroma, the majority of the individual nerve fascicles are surrounded by cells that are immunoreactive for EMA, indicating perineurial differentiation (176). Collagens type I and III are deposited among the fascicles. The nerve fibers of the newly formed fascicles are supported by a matrix that is rich in acid mucopolysaccharides (176).

In spontaneous intraneural neuromas, such as PEN and those of the mucosal neuroma syndrome, the local proliferation of axons within the confines of the perineurium has not been adequately explained.

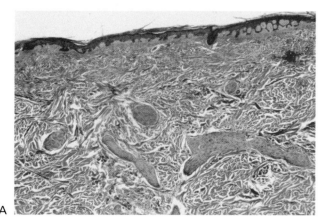

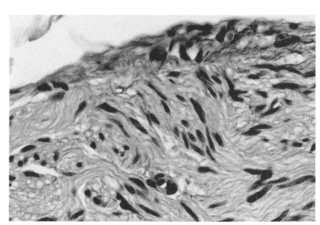

A   B

FIGURE 35-60. Linear (intraneural) neuroma. **A:** Nerves of the dermis are enlarged, showing Schwann cell hyperplasia. The cross-sectional diameter is increased. **B:** At higher magnification, interlacing fascicles of innervated Schwann cells form asymmetrical patterns; they are confined by a perineurium.

Pacinian Neuroma

Pacinian neuroma is found in the same anatomic sites as pacinian corpuscles (190); it is an occult, painful lesion.

Histopathology. Pacinian corpuscles form a localized cluster but are otherwise unremarkable. The corpuscles may vary in size.

If a cluster of corpuscles were continuous with an extraneural neuroma, it would be difficult to attribute the symptomatology to the cluster of corpuscles.

Patterns in which cells and fibers are concentrically layered are common in the setting of nerve sheath tumors. Some examples of nerve sheath tumors with such patterns have been characterized as "pacinian neurofibroma." Currently, some of these lesions are being characterized as "fibrous" or "sclerosing" perineurioma (170,171).

SMALL ROUND CELL TUMORS

This category includes primary, cutaneous, small-cell undifferentiated carcinoma (Merkel cell tumor); primitive neuroectodermal tumors (PNET), such as Ewing sarcoma and neuroepithelioma; neuroblastoma; primitive mesenchymal tumors, such as small cell osteosarcoma, and embryonal and alveolar rhabdomyosarcoma; rare melanomas of infancy that arise in the setting of giant congenital nevus (melanoblastoma of infancy) (191); and melanotic neuroectodermal tumor of infancy (192). In all of these lesions on hematoxylin-eosin–stained sections, cells with few distinguishing characteristics, other than scanty cytoplasm, and with closely spaced, "dark" nuclei, provide a challenge in differential diagnosis. In this category, some of the lesions that have been grouped as "primitive neuroectodermal tumors" share certain basic features, but mostly are to be distinguished by patterns of divergent differentiation, either morphologic or immunohistochemical (193). Small round cell tumors are more common in the soft tissue or bone (194,195). In the skin, cutaneous small (Merkel) cell undifferentiated carcinoma is most frequent.

Cutaneous Small (Merkel) Cell Undifferentiated Carcinoma

Cutaneous small cell undifferentiated carcinoma (CSCUC) (Merkel cell, neuroendocrine, or trabecular carcinoma) (196–203), an uncommon tumor, mostly occurs as a solitary nodule, usually on the head or on the extremities (202). Multiple lesions have been observed, either localized to one area or widely distributed. The tumors are usually few in number but occasionally are multitudinous. CSCUCs have a high rate of recurrence and metastasis (203).

The lesions of CSCUC are firm and red-pink. They usually are nonulcerated, and range in size from 0.8 to 4.0 cm in diameter.

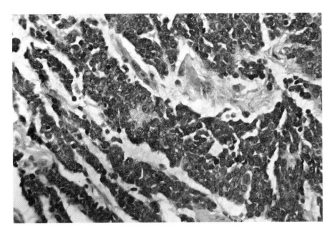

FIGURE 35-61. Merkel cell tumor. Atypical, but uniform, small blue cells form fascicles that vary in size. The cells have scanty cytoplasm; nuclei are crowded. Chromatin is delicate but uniformly distributed. Nucleoli are inconspicuous. There are scattered pyknotic nuclei. Each fascicle is outlined by a mucinous sheath that abuts on a fibrous matrix.

Histopathology. Tumor cells with scanty cytoplasm, and plump, round, or irregular nuclei are closely spaced in trabecular patterns and sheets (204a,204b) (Figs. 35-61 and 35-62). Less commonly, they are arranged in ribbons and festoons. Pseudorosettes are an occasional feature (205). Nuclear chromatin often is dense and uniformly distributed. In some examples, nuclei, focally or uniformly, show margination of chromatin. Nucleoli generally are inconspicuous. Nuclear molding may be a feature. Mitoses and nuclear fragments are regular features (196). In some CSCUC, the nests of cells are supported by scant, delicate, and paucicellular stroma. Lymphoid infiltrates are common at the margin and focally in the stroma. Contact with the epidermis is rare, but if a lesion invades the epidermis, the patterns may include intraepidermal collections of tumor cells (206,207). Patterns of keratinocytic

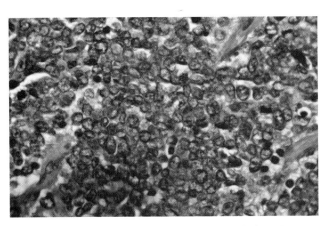

FIGURE 35-62. Merkel cell tumor. In this field, there is some central clearing of nuclei. The nuclei contain one or several nucleoli, and there are scattered mitotic figures.

dysplasia in the overlying epidermis, and even islands of squamous cell differentiation in the dermal nests are uncommon features (199,208,209). At the interface between the tumor and the epidermis, and at the margins of the tumor, dilated, thin-walled vessels commonly contain tumor cells.

The immunohistochemical profile is NSE (positive) (210), protein gene product (positive), chromogranins (positive), Ber-EP4 (positive) (210), and CD57 (positive) (211). A single punctate zone of cytoplasmic immunoreactivity for cytokeratins, especially CK20, or neurofilaments is most characteristic (212). EMA is expressed in 75% to 80% of CSCUC (213). A reaction for CK20 has been offered as a finding against the diagnosis of metastatic small-cell carcinoma of the lung (213). TTF-1, thyroid transcription factor-1, is specific for PSCUDC in situations in which the differential diagnosis includes PSCUD and CSCUC (214).

Ultrastructurally, cytoplasmic, membrane-bound, round, dense-core granules of neuroendocrine type measure 100 to 200 nm in diameter (198,205). Perinuclear bundles, or whorls of intermediate filaments that are 7 to 10 nm wide (215), and small desmosomes are regularly present. Tonofilaments attached to the desmosomes have been only found in a few cases (216).

Histogenesis. The origin of the CSCUC is controversial. Divergent differentiation is expressed in neuroendocrine, squamous, adnexal (213,217), and melanocytic phenotypes (218).

CSCUC shares genetic changes with tumors of neural crest origin, such as melanoma, pheochromocytoma, and neuroblastoma (219).

Differential Diagnosis. Cutaneous metastases from atypical carcinoids, or small-cell undifferentiated carcinoma (oat cell carcinoma) of the lung may be confused with primary CSCUC (220).

The nuclear characteristics of the cells of CSCUC differ from those of the cells of most lymphomas. Immunohistochemical studies are an aid in the differential diagnosis. If lymphoma remains a problem, even in the face of a negative reaction for leukocyte common antigen, reactions for the antigens L-26 and CD3 may provide more definitive information (221).

Primary small cell undifferentiated carcinomas have been observed in most organ systems. They are not peculiar to the skin, but those in the skin often have distinguishing characteristics. Small cell undifferentiated carcinomas of both the skin and lung are neuroendocrine carcinomas, but the former designation has a greater degree of specificity, and gives recognition to basic patterns that are expressed in distinctive primary neoplasms in a variety of organ systems. The nuclei of pulmonary small cell undifferentiated carcinomas (PSCUC) are irregular; they often have a pointed extremity. Patterns of squamous cell, and glandular differentiation are variable features of PSCUC. Clinicopathologic correlations are an aid in differential diagnosis.

The primary basaloid carcinomas and undifferentiated carcinomas of the skin appendages, including lymphoepithelial variants, also must be considered in differential diagnosis (222).

Tumors that are similar to CSCUC have been observed as isolated lesions in lymph nodes (223).

Peripheral Neuroblastoma

Neuroblastoma, as a primary soft tissue tumor, is a diagnosis of exclusion. The skin is a most unlikely site. In infancy, the differential diagnosis of undifferentiated, small-cell malignancies of the skin and soft tissue includes metastatic neuroblastoma. A thorough workup to rule out a metastasis from an occult site, such as the adrenal gland or paravertebral ganglia, is required. Metastatic neuroblastoma of infancy may present the picture of blueberry muffin baby (224) or as blanching subcutaneous nodules (225). Adult neuroblastomas have been documented (226,227).

Histopathology. Neuroblastomas are undifferentiated, small-cell malignancies. Solid sheets of undifferentiated cells often are the preponderant patterns, but septation, neuropil, differentiation, and Homer–Wright rosettes (often characterized as pseudorosettes), if identified, are an aid in diagnosis. Neuroblasts are distinguished by the formation of cell processes. The designation *neuropil* gives recognition to a matrix of cytoplasmic processes, including those of neurons, Schwann cells, and glial cells. It gives recognition to patterns of matrical differentiation in neuroectodermal tumors (Fig. 35-63). A sprinkling of larger, neuron-like cells with slightly eccentric, round nuclei, prominent central nucleoli, and marginated chromatin are features of neuroblastic differentiation (Fig. 35-64).

Depending on the degree of differentiation, the immunohistochemical profile is as follows: neural filaments

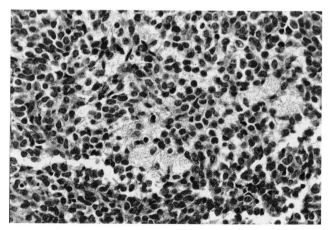

FIGURE 35-63. Differentiating neuroblastoma. Uniform, atypical, small blue cells form sheets. In areas, the diffuse patterns are interrupted by pale, rounded collections of delicate fibrils (neuropil).

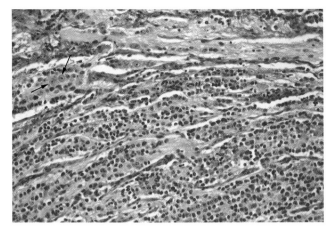

FIGURE 35-64. Differentiating neuroblastoma. The lesion is partitioned by delicate fibrous septa. Tumor cells are clustered among the septa; the hypocellular, fibrillated matrix among the cells is neuropil. Scattered cells have plump, round nuclei with a central nucleolus (*arrow*); these distinctive cells are differentiating ganglion cells.

(positive), NSE (positive), S-100 protein (positive), synaptophysin (positive), and even other neuroendocrine markers (228).

Metastatic neuroblastoma possesses an innate tendency for maturation (differentiation). As a consequence, metastases from a neuroblastoma may present as immature, or mature ganglioneuroma (229). The problems are complicated by the rare example in which a primary neuroblastoma of the adrenal gland with distant metastases undergoes complete regression in the primary site.

Ganglioneuroma

Ganglioneuroma is exceedingly uncommon in the skin (230–232). Rare examples appear to be in the nature of heterotopias (232). Some may represent divergent differentiation of phenotypically pluripotent neurocristic cells. Others may represent metastatic neuroblastoma that has matured into a ganglioneuroma.

Histopathology. The basic pattern of a ganglioneuroma is that of a neuroma in which characteristic ganglion cells are clustered and individually isolated (232). Small, primary ganglioneuromas of the skin may be characterized by numerous, mature ganglion cells, and an inconspicuous background of neurosustentacular cells (233). A desmoplastic variant has been reported (234).

Histogenesis. With immunoperoxidase stain for S-100 protein, Schwann cells are reactive (235). Like all neuromas, Schwann cell fascicles of a ganglioneuroma are innervated. Ganglion cells are reactive for NSE and chromogranins. Immaturity, as manifested by foci of small, dark cells, spongy neuropil, and lymphoid infiltrates, signals the need for additional studies to rule out a differentiating metastatic neuroblastoma. In immature gan-

glioneuroma, the neurons may not be associated with satellite cells.

PRIMITIVE NEUROECTODERMAL TUMORS

Ewing Sarcoma and Peripheral Neuroepithelioma

Originally, the designation *primitive neuroectodermal tumor* (PNET) served as a taxonomic convenience when confronted with the histologic pattern of a poorly differentiated, small round cell neoplasm showing some evidence of neuroectodermal differentiation. The designation has been attributed to A. P. Stout, but there is no mention of this designation in the commonly cited reference. Currently, the designation has supplanted that of neuroepithelioma, acquiring some degree of specificity.

Ewing sarcoma (EWS) and peripheral neuroepithelioma are PNETs; they are members of the category of small round cell tumors. EWS, including an atypical variant (236), is a rare malignant neoplasm of bone and soft tissue. *Peripheral neuroepithelioma* (PNE) (the "primitive neuroectodermal tumor") generally is a tumor of the deep soft tissue, with rare examples in bone. It has been reported in internal viscera. Askin's tumor is also cited as an example of primitive neuroectodermal tumor. Some examples of PNETs have had their origin in a peripheral nerve (237), or have been a component of malignant schwannoma (95).

Histopathology. PNETs are composed of small blue cells (238). In Ewing's category, the cells tend to be glycogen-rich. Nuclear characteristics are uniform; chromatin patterns tend to be open (238). In the neuroepithelioma category, the cells focally form pseudorosettes.

Histogenesis. Useful, but variably positive, reactions include NSE, CD57, and synaptophysin. In EWS and PNE, tumor cells are immunoreactive for CD99, MIC2 (239–242), the reaction is sensitive but not specific, and a positive reaction provides a distinction between PNET (positive) and neuroblastoma (negative).

Both EWS and PNE are characterized by the presence of chromosomal translocation t(11;22)(q24;q12), and the EWS gene has recently been identified at the breakpoint on chromosome 22 (243).

Differential Diagnosis. Neuroepithelioma-like patterns may be encountered as a regional variation in MPNST (95), and in the setting of cutaneous small-cell undifferentiated carcinoma (205).

Melanotic Neuroectodermal Tumor of Infancy

This tumor affects the tissues of the oral cavity, but also may be found in other sites (244–247). Polyphenotypic expressions of neural and epithelial markers, melanogenesis, and occasional glial and rhabdomyoblastic differentiation are variably represented. Its patterns have been compared to those of the retina at 5 weeks' gestation (247).

HETEROTOPIAS

Cephalic brain–like heterotopias (*CBHs*) (nasal gliomas) are found most commonly in the skin near the root of the nose (248–254), but they may be intranasal (40%) or extranasal (60%). Extranasal CBHs are smooth, firm, noncompressible, and skin-colored, ranging in size from 1 to 5 cm. They do not pulsate or transilluminate. On the external surface of the nose, they usually are not midline. Intranasally, CBHs present as a firm, smooth, red to purple protrusion, and usually measure 2 to 3 cm in diameter. They may resemble a hemangioma. Those that are both intranasal and extranasal are connected through a defect in the nasal bone (249). The other most commonly associated bony defects involve the fonticulus frontalis, the cribriform plate, and the space between nasal bone and cartilage (249). Some examples are connected by a fibrous cord to the dura. Other sites include the scalp, oropharynx, nasopharynx, tongue, and subcutaneous tissue overlying T-12 (250).

Histopathology. CBHs are not encapsulated. They are disorganized and commonly show admixtures of glial tissue (Fig. 35-65), randomly distributed, mature neurons, increased vascularity, focal calcification, and fibrous tissue (251). Strands of neural and fibrous tissue are interwoven (252). Fibrillary and gemistocytic astrocytes, activated oligodendrocytes, and giant astrocytes are variably represented. Astrocytes are the most conspicuous cellular component. In some examples, the astrocytic component may resemble a low-grade astrocytoma. Neurons usually are small. They may be absent (253). In some examples, they are focally prominent. Ependymal and retinal epithelium, and even choroid plexus–like components have been observed (254). Focal areas of oligodendroglial differentiation may be prominent; in such areas, the neuropil may be immunoreactive for both NSE and synaptophysin. The degree of differentiation in these heterotopias may reflect the age of the patient at the time of excision. Some examples are remarkable for the diversity of cell types, all representative of neuroectodermal differentiation. An oligodendroglioma arising in ectopic brain tissue of the nasopharynx has been reported.

Immunohistochemically, neurons react for NSE and neural filaments. Astrocytes and ependymal cells are, and oligodendroglial cells are not, immunoreactive for GFAP. The oligodendroglial cells share some immunoreactions with Schwann cells.

Differential Diagnosis. Encephaloceles (extracranial protrusions of brain-like tissue that are in continuity with the subarachnoid space) may show a high degree of organization (255). CBH and encephaloceles of the same anatomic sites have similar clinical features. A distinction between CBH and encephalocele is not always possible, but encephaloceles are connected to the subarachnoid space by a sinus tract, thus making an ordinary biopsy inadvisable. A rhinorrhea with leakage of spinal fluid, and septic encephalitis may ensue. Computerized tomography (255) and neurosurgical consultation should precede any operative intervention of either CBH or encephalocele (252).

CUTANEOUS MENINGIOMAS AND MENINGOTHELIAL HETEROTOPIAS

Beyond the confines of the CNS, cells with the features of meningothelial cells may be encountered in skin and soft tissue (256). They may be represented in patterns of a neoplasm (and properly characterized as *ectopic* meningioma). They may be represented in patterns similar to those manifested in the coverings of *meningoceles, meningomyeloceles,* and *meningoencephaloceles* (and properly characterized as heterotopia or dysplasia).

A definition of various pathways and phenomena provides an explanation for the presence of meningothelial cells in the skin and soft tissue.

Precursors of meningothelial cells may be displaced into the dermis, and subcutis during embryogenesis. Such remnants, located mainly in subcutaneous tissue of the scalp, forehead, and paravertebral regions of children and young adults (256–259), may develop into congenital meningeal heterotopias. They are relatively restricted in distribution along the lines of closure of the developing neural tube. Some of these lesions qualify as acelic meningeal heterotopias (rudimentary meningoceles) (259). For such examples, occult connections with the CNS may become apparent only at the time of surgery, as evidenced by the leakage of spinal fluid into the surgical defect. Histologic patterns include those of both the dura and the leptomeninges.

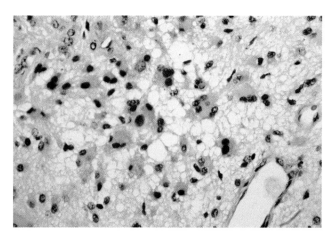

FIGURE 35-65. Parapharyngeal cephalic brain-like heterotopia. Astrocytes are supported by neuropil.

True ectopic meningomas, distributed along the course of cranial nerves of the sensory organs of the face and head, tend to occur in adults, and arise from extensions of arachnoidal lining cells along peripheral nerves (260). Some ectopic meningiomas arise in sites that are far from the axial skeleton. The histologic patterns of benign ectopic meningiomas recapitulate those of the meningiomas of the CNS.

Large intracranial meningiomas may extend in direct continuity through foramina (38) or old operative defects into the neighboring soft tissue; they qualify as *perforating* meningiomas. Their histology corresponds to that of the primary intracranial lesion and, once defined, is predictive of their behavior.

Anaplastic (*malignant*) *meningiomas*, including sarcomatous as well as papillary and hemangiopericytomatous variants, may aggressively invade bone, soft tissue, and scalp. They also may be associated with intracranial seeding, and with extracranial, mostly pulmonary metastases (38). Rarely, histologically benign meningiomas have seeded the brain surface or metastasized.

Histopathology. Heterotopias are not well circumscribed (260). The cells are cytologically bland, and loosely attached to their neighbors. They commonly outline thin, angulated clefts, a feature that may be mistaken as evidence of vascular differentiation (259,261) (Fig. 35-66). Whorls of cells and psammoma bodies, if identified, are an aid in diagnosis. The supporting matrix is fibrous and loosely fissured.

The histopathology and classification of true meningiomas, whether intracranial, ectopic, or metastatic, are complex. The basic features include sheets and nests of polygonal, or spindle cells, whorls of cells, psammoma bodies (Fig. 35-67), intranuclear inclusions of cytoplasm, immunoreactivity for EMA, and scanty, condensed stroma, or thin clefts at the interface between nests.

Anaplastic (malignant) meningiomas are characterized by dense cellularity, nuclear atypia, mitoses, necrosis, and

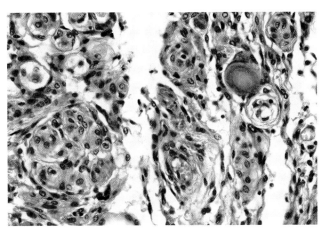

FIGURE 35-67. Cutaneous meningioma. Small, uniform spindle and epithelioid cells are arranged in nests and whorls; there are clefts among the nests. A psammoma body is represented.

invasion of the brain, and even soft tissue. The basic patterns of common meningiomas usually are preserved, but some examples are frankly sarcomatous.

Ultrastructurally, poorly formed basal lamina, rare desmosomes, abundant mitochondria, and elaborate interdigitating, cytoplasmic processes are all features of meningothelial cells.

Histogenesis. Like intracranial meningiomas, the cells of ectopic meningiomas, and meningeal heterotopias react immunohistochemically for vimentin and EMA (262–265). Depending on the histologic subtypes, the expression of certain antigens, especially cytokeratins and S-100 protein, is variable (259,265). The clonal nature of the antibody to S-100 protein may also influence test results.

Differential Diagnosis. Meningoceles, meningomyeloceles, and meningoencephaloceles, like meningeal heterotopias, present along the lines of closure of the neural tube. They consist of both dense and loosely laminated, vascularized fibrous tissue, some of which is arachnoidal in quality. If there is an associated encephalocele (or myelocele), then tissue of the CNS will also be represented.

Ependymal rests also may be found in the sacrococcygeal region. Some are organized in patterns that resemble microscopic myxopapillary ependymomas (266). They may provide an explanation for the origin of rare *ectopic ependymomas* in the sacrococcygeal region (267).

NEURAL TUMORS OF A DEGENERATIVE NATURE

In *impingement neurofasciitis* (*Morton or interdigital* "*neuroma*"), the compression of nerves, and soft tissue between bony or other hard surfaces may induce degenerative changes. The responses include demyelination and endoneurial fibrosis, mucinous and fibrinous degeneration of

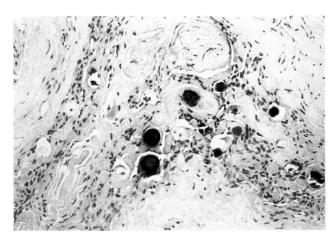

FIGURE 35-66. Meningeal heterotopia. Spindle cells with angulated, uniform nuclei form traceries among collagen bundles. There are clefts in some of the thin nests of spindle cells. The rounded, basophilic structures are psammoma bodies.

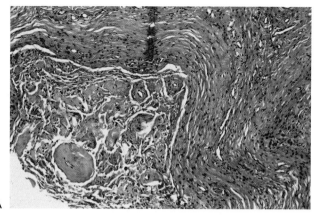
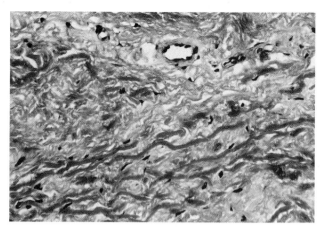

FIGURE 35-68. Impingement neuropathy (Morton's neuroma). **A:** To the left and extending to the bottom of the field, a nerve is cut in cross-section. The perineurium is thickened and fibrotic. Individual nerve fibers and small clusters of nerve fibers are loosely spaced in a myxoid matrix. There are scattered hyaline deposits in the endoneurial space. Vessels of the endoneurium, cut in cross-section, have thickened, hyalinized walls. **B:** The connective tissue adjacent to an affected nerve shows hyperelastosis; the elastic fibers are increased in diameter. Often in Morton's neuroma, the changes in the adjacent connective tissue are similar to those of elastofibroma dorsi.

soft tissue (fascia), deposition of pre-elastin over the surfaces of elastic fibers (in patterns resembling those seen in lesions of elastofibroma dorsi), and fibrinous bursitis (268) (Fig. 35-68). All of these phenomena, manifested in the interdigital area of so-called Morton neuromas, have nothing in common with the neuromas. In the altered nerves, localized oval zones of mucinous or fibrous matrix may focally displace the nerve fibers. Spindle and stellate cells are loosely arranged in whorls. Similar epiphenomena, characterized by Renaut as an "intravaginal hyaline system, often are encountered as incidental findings in "normal nerves."

The *ganglion cyst of nerve* is an uncommon tumor of a degenerative nature. In preferential sites, a superficial nerve impinges upon a bony protuberance.

Initially, the perineurium and endoneurium are mucinous, expanded, and paucicellular. In one or more sites, cystic changes ensue. The end result is a mucinous cyst that expands the endoneurial space, compresses the axial bundle, and distends the perineurial sheath. A condensation of fibrous tissue forms the wall of the cyst.

The ganglion cyst of nerve is distinguished from periarticular ganglion cyst by location.

NEUROTROPIC GROWTH (GENERAL COMMENTS)

Neurotropic growth of tumor is common in the skin. Generally, the identification of this phenomenon is sufficient to characterize any related primary neoplasm of the skin as aggressive (e.g., neurotropic melanoma [100], epidermoid carcinoma [269], and keratoacanthoma). Rarely, benign invasion of nerve sheaths by squamous epithelium has been

noted in re-excision specimens after a biopsy (270). The ensheathed neuroma is characterized by hyperplastic nerves that are ensheathed by benign squamous epithelium in the absence of a history of local trauma (271).

REFERENCES

1. Scheithauer BW, Woodruff JM, Earlandson RA. Tumors of the peripheral nervous system. In: Armed Forces Institute of Pathology, ed. *Atlas of tumor pathology*, 3rd series, fasc. 24. Washington, DC: Armed Forces Institute of Pathology, 1999.
2. Ortiz-Hidalgo C, Weller RO. Peripheral nervous system. In: Sternberg SS, ed. *Histology for pathologists*, 2nd ed. Philadelphia: Lippincott-Raven Press, 1997:285.
3. Reed RJ, Harkin JC. *Supplement: tumors of the peripheral nervous system*, 2nd series, fasc. 3. Washington, DC: Armed Forces Institute of Pathology, 1983.
4. Weiser G. An electron microscopic study of "pacinian neurofibroma." *Virchows Arch A* 1975;366:331.
5. Morris JH, Hudson AR, Weddell G. A study of degeneration and regeneration in the divided rat sciatic nerve based on electron microscopy. Part 1. *Z Zellforsch Mikrosk Anat* 1972;124:76.
6. Riccardi VM. Von Recklinghausen neurofibromatosis [Review]. *N Engl J Med* 1981;305:1617.
7. Crowe FW. Axillary freckling as a diagnostic aid in neurofibromatosis. *Ann Intern Med* 1964;61:1142.
8. Crowe FW, Schull WJ, Neel JV, eds. *Clinical, pathological, and genetic study of multiple neurofibromatosis*. Springfield, IL: Charles C. Thomas, 1956.
9. Goldberg NS, Collins FS. The hunt for the neurofibromatosis gene. *Arch Dermatol* 1991;127:1705.
10. Zvulunov A, Easterly NB. Neurocutaneous syndromes associated with pigmentary skin lesions. *J Am Acad Dermatol* 1995;32:915.
11. Shekitka KM, Sobin LH. Ganglioneuromas of the gastrointestinal tract: relation to von Recklinghausen disease and other multiple tumor syndromes. *Am J Surg Pathol* 1994;18:250.

12. DeLellis RA. Biology of disease: multiple endocrine neoplasia syndromes revisited: clinical, morphologic, and molecular features. *Lab Invest* 1995;72:494.
13. Zvulunov A, Barak Y, Metzker A. Juvenile xanthogranuloma, neurofibromatosis, and juvenile chronic myelogenous leukemia: world statistical analysis. *Arch Dermatol* 1995;131:904.
14. Jaakkola S, Muona P, James WD, et al. Segmental neurofibromatosis: immunocytochemical analysis of cutaneous lesions. *J Am Acad Dermatol* 1990;22:617.
15. Hager CM, Cohen PR, Tschen JA. Segmental neurofibromatosis: case reports and review. *J Am Acad Dermatol* 1997; 37:864.
16. Schultz ES, Kaufmann D, Tinschert S, et al. Segmental neurofibromatosis. *Dermatology* 2002;204:296.
17. Honda M, Arai E, Sawade S, et al. Neurofibromatosis 2 and neurilemmomatosis gene are identical. *J Invest Dermatol* 1995; 104:74.
18. Wolkenstein P, Benchikhi H, Zeller J, et al. Schwannomatosis; a clinical entity distinct from neurofibromatosis type 2. *Dermatology* 1997;195:228.
19. Masson P. *Human tumors: histology, diagnosis and technique*, 2nd ed. Detroit: Wayne State University Press, 1970.
20. Enzinger FM, Weiss SW. *Soft tissue tumors*, 3rd ed. St. Louis: Mosby-Year Book, 1995.
21. Erlandson RA, Woodruff JM. Peripheral nerve sheath tumors. *Cancer* 1982;49:273.
22. Friede RL. The organization of endoneurial collagen in peripheral nerves as revealed with the scanning electron microscope. *J Neurol Sci* 1978;38:83.
23. Lassmann H, Jurecka W, Lassmann G, et al. Different types of benign nerve sheath tumors. *Virchows Arch Pathol Anat* 1977; 375:197.
24. Khalifa MA, Montgomery EA, Ismid N, et al. What are the CD34+ cells in benign peripheral nerve sheath tumors: double immunostaining study of CD34 and S-100 protein. *Am J Clin Pathol* 2000:114:123.
25. Vaalasti A, Suomalainen H, Kuokkanen K, et al. Neuropeptides in cutaneous neurofibromas of von Recklinghausen's disease. *J Cutan Pathol* 1990;17:377.
26. Reed RJ. The neural crest, its migrants, and cutaneous malignant neoplasms related to neurocristic derivatives. In: Lynch HT, Fusaro RM, eds. *Cancer-associated genodermatoses*. New York: Van Nostrand Reinhold, 1982:177.
27. Argenyi ZB, Cooper PH, Santa Cruz D. Plexiform and other unusual variants of palisaded encapsulated neuroma. *J Cutan Pathol* 1993;20:34.
28. Gorlin RJ, Sedano HO, Vickers RA, et al. Multiple mucosal neuromas, pheochromocytoma and medullary carcinoma of the thyroid: a syndrome. *Cancer* 1968;22:293.
29. Argenyi ZB, LeBoit PE, Santa Cruz D, et al. Nerve sheath myxoma (neurothekeoma) of the skin: light microscopic and immunohistochemical reappraisal of the cellular variant. *J Cutan Pathol* 1993;20:294.
30. Enzinger F, Zhang R. Plexiform fibrohistiocytic tumor presenting in children and young adults: an analysis of 65 cases. *Am J Surg Pathol* 1988;12:818.
31. Zelger B, Weinlich G, Zelgre B. Perineurioma. A frequently unrecognized entity with emphasis on a plexiform variant. *Adv Clin Pathol* 2000;4:25–33.
32. Dupree WB, Langloss JM, Weiss SH. Pigmented dermatofibrosarcoma protuberans (Bednar tumor): a pathologic, ultrastructural, and immunohistochemical study. *Am J Surg Pathol* 1985;9:630.
33. Greene JF, Fitzwater JE, Burgess J. Arterial lesions associated with neurofibromatosis. *Am J Clin Pathol* 1974;62:481.
34. Salyer WR, Salyer DC. The vascular lesions of neurofibromatosis. *Angiology* 1974;25:510.
35. Masson P. Experimental and spontaneous schwannomas (peripheral gliomas). *Am J Pathol* 1932;8:367.
36. Ackerman LV, Taylor FH. Neurogenous tumors within the thorax: a clinicopathologic evaluation of forty-eight cases. *Cancer* 1951;4:669.
37. Stout AP. The peripheral manifestations of the specific nerve sheath tumor (neurilemmoma). *Am J Cancer* 1935;24:751.
38. Russell DS, Rubinstein LJ. *Pathology of tumours of the nervous system*, 5th ed. Baltimore: Williams & Wilkins, 1989.
39. Stout AP. *Tumors of the peripheral nervous system*, 1st series, fasc. 6. Washington, DC: Armed Forces Institute of Pathology, 1949.
40. Argenyi ZB, Balogh K, Abraham AA. Degenerative ("ancient") changes in benign cutaneous schwannoma: a light microscopic, histochemical, and immunohistochemical study. *J Cutan Pathol* 1993;20:148.
41. Sian CS, Ryan SF. The ultrastructure of neurilemmoma with emphasis on Antoni B tissue. *Hum Pathol* 1981;12:145.
42. Kerr JFR, Winterford CM, Harmon BV. Apoptosis: its significance in cancer and cancer therapy. *Cancer* 1994;73:2013.
43. Farber EM. Programmed cell death: necrosis versus apoptosis. *Mod Pathol* 1994;7:605.
44. Kawahara E, Oda Y, Ooi A, et al. Expression of glial fibrillary acidic protein (GFAP) in peripheral nerve sheath tumors. *Am J Surg Pathol* 1988;12:115.
45. Lodding P, Kindblom LG, Angerval L, et al. Cellular schwannoma: a clinicopathologic study of 29 cases. *Virchows Arch [A] Pathol Anat* 1990;416:237.
46. Woodruff JM, Godwin TA, Erlandson RA, et al. Cellular schwannoma: a variety of schwannoma sometimes mistaken for a malignant tumor. *Am J Surg Pathol* 1981;5:733.
47. Fletcher CDM, Davis SE, McKee PH. Cellular schwannoma: a distinct pseudosarcomatous entity. *Histopathology* 1987;11:21.
48. Hajdu SI. Schwannomas. *Mod Pathol* 1995;8:109.
49. Casadei GP, Scheithauer BW, Hirose T, et al. Cellular schwannoma. *Cancer* 1995;75:1109.
50. White W, Shiu MH, Rosenblum MK, et al. Cellular schwannoma: a clinicopathologic study of 57 patients and 58 tumors. *Cancer* 1990;66:1266.
51. Kindblom LG, Meis-Kindblom JM, Havel G, et al. Benign epithelioid schwannoma. *Am J Surg Pathol* 1998;22:762.
52. Smith K, Mezebish D, Williams JP, et al. Cutaneous epithelioid schwannomas: a rare variant of a benign peripheral nerve sheath tumor. *J Cutan Pathol* 1998;25:50.
53. Orosz Z. Cutaneous epithelioid schwannoma: an unusual benign neurogenic tumor. *J Cutan Pathol* 1999:26:213.
54. Fisher C, Chappell ME, Weiss SW. Neuroblastoma-like epithelioid schwannoma. *Histopathology* 1995;26:193.
55. Goldblum JR, Beals TF, Weiss SW. Neuroblastoma-like neurilemmoma. *Am J Surg Pathol* 1994;18:266.
56. Skelton HG, Smith KJ, Lupton GP. Collagenous spherulosis in a schwannoma. *Am J Dermatopathol* 1994;16:549.
57. Elston DM, Bergfeld WF, Biscotti CV, et al. Schwannoma with sweat duct differentiation. *J Cutan Pathol* 1993;20:254.
58. Woodruff JM, Christensen WN. Glandular peripheral nerve sheath tumors. *Cancer* 1993;72:3618.
59. Yoshida SO, Toot BV. Benign glandular schwannoma. *Am J Clin Pathol* 1993;100:167.
60. Kim YC, Park HJ, Cinn YW, et al. Benign glandular schwannoma. *Br J Dermatol* 2001;145:834.
61. Iwashita T, Enjoji M. Plexiform neurilemmoma: a clinicopathological and immunohistochemical analysis of 23 tumors from 20 patients. *Virchows Arch A Pathol Anat Histopathol* 1987;411:305.
62. Rongioletti F, Drago F, Rebora A. Multiple cutaneous plexiform schwannomas with tumors of the central nervous system. *Arch Dermatol* 1989;125:431.
63. Sasaki T, Nakajima H. Congenital neurilemmomatosis. *J Am Acad Dermatol* 1992;26:786.

64. Woodruff JM, Marshall MI, Godwin TA, et al. Plexiform (multinodular) schwannoma: a tumor simulating the plexiform neurofibroma. *Am J Surg Pathol* 1983;7:691.

65. Kao GF, Laskin WB, Olsen TG. Solitary cutaneous plexiform neurilemmoma (schwannoma): a clinicopathologic, immuno-histochemical, and ultrastructural study of 11 cases. *Mod Pathol* 1989;2:20.

66. Shishiba T, Niimura M, Ohtsuka F, et al. Multiple cutaneous neurilemmomas as a skin manifestation of neurilemmomatosis. *J Am Acad Dermatol* 1984;10:744.

67. Murata Y, Kumano K, Ugai K, et al. Neurilemmomatosis. *Br J Dermatol* 1991;125:466.

68. Rouleau GA, Merel P, Lutchman M, et al. Alteration in a new gene encoding a putative membrane-organizing protein causes neurofibromatosis type 2. *Nature* 1993;363:515.

69. Honda M, Arai E, Sawada S, et al. Neurofibromatosis 2 and neurilemmomatosis gene are identical. *J Invest Dermatol* 1995;104:74.

70. Feany MB, Anthony DC, Fletcher CD. Nerve sheath tunours with hybrid features of neurofibroma and schwannoma: a conceptual challenge. *Histopathology* 1998;32:405.

71. Zamecnik M. Hybrid neurofibroma/schwannoma versus schwannoma with Antoni B areas. *Histopathology* 2000;36:473.

72. Meis-Kindblom JM, Enzinger FM. Plexiform malignant peripheral nerve sheath tumor of infancy and childhood. *Am J Surg Pathol* 1994;18:479.

73. Argenyi ZB, Goodenberger ME, Strauss JS. Congenital neural hamartoma ("fascicular schwannoma"): a light microscopic, immunohistochemical, and ultrastructural study. *Am J Dermatopathol* 1990;12:283.

74. Woodruff JM, Erlandson RA, Scheithauer BW. Nerve sheath tumors: letter to editor. *Am J Surg Pathol* 1995;19:608.

75. Cohen C, Davis TS. Multiple trichogenic adnexal tumors. *Am J Dermatopathol* 1986;8:241.

76. Proppe KH, Scully RE. Large cell calcifying Sertoli cell tumor of the testis. *Am J Clin Pathol* 1980;74:607.

77. Carney JA. Psammomatous melanotic schwannoma: a distinctive, heritable tumor with special associations, including cardiac myxoma and the Cushing syndrome. *Am J Surg Pathol* 1990;14:206.

78. Carney JA, Hruska LS, Beauchamp GD, et al. Dominant inheritance of the complex of myxomas, spotty pigmentation, and endocrine overactivity. *Mayo Clin Proc* 1986;61:165.

79. Foad MS, Kleiner DE, Dugan EM. A case of psammomatous melanotic schwannoma in the setting of the Carney complex. *J Cutan Pathol*. 2000;27:556.

80. Carstens PHB, Schrodt GR. Malignant transformation of a benign encapsulated neurilemmoma. *Am J Clin Pathol* 1969;51:144.

81. McMenamin ME, Fletcher CD. Expanding the spectrum of malignant change in schwannomas: epithelioid malignant change, epithelioid malignant peripheral nerve sheath tumor, and epithelioid angiosarcoma: a study of 17 cases. *Am J Surg Pathol* 2001;25:13.

82. Nayler SJ, Leiman G, Omar T, et al. Malignant transformation in a schwannoma. *Histopathology* 1996;29:189.

83. Woodruff JM, Selig AM, Crowley K, et al. Schwannoma (neurilemmoma) with malignant transformation: a rare, distinctive peripheral nerve tumor. *Am J Surg Pathol* 1994;18:882.

84. Hirose T, Scheithauer BW, Sano T. Perineurial malignant peripheral nerve sheath tumor (MPNST): a clinicopathologic, immunohistochemical, and ultrastructural study of seven cases. *Am J Surg Pathol* 1998:22:1368.

85. Rosenberg AS, Langee CL, Stevens GL, et al. Malignant peripheral nerve sheath tumor with perineurial differentiation: "malignant perineurioma." *J Cutan Pathol* 2002;29:362.

86. Leroy K, Dumas V, Martin-Garcia, et al. Malignant peripheral nerve sheath tumors associated with neurofibromatosis type 1: a clinicopathologic and molecular study of 17 patients. *Arch Dermatol* 2001;137:908.

87. Takeuchi A, Ushigome S. Diverse differentiation in malignant peripheral nerve sheath tumours associated with neurofibromatosis-1: an immunohistochemical and ultrastructural study. *Histopathology* 2001;39:298.

88. Guccion JG, Enzinger FM. Malignant schwannoma associated with von Recklinghausen's neurofibromatosis. *Virchows Arch Anat Pathol* 1979;39:43.

89. D'Agostino AN, Soule EH, Miller RH. Sarcomas of the peripheral nerves and somatic soft tissues associated with multiple neurofibromatosis (von Recklinghausen's disease). *Cancer* 1963;16:1015.

90. D'Agostino AN, Soule EH, Miller RH. Primary malignant neoplasms of nerves (malignant neurilemmomas) in patients without manifestations of multiple neurofibromatosis (von Recklinghausen's disease). *Cancer* 1963;16:1003.

91. Taxy JB, Battifora H, Trujillo Y, et al. Electron microscopy in the diagnosis of malignant schwannoma. *Cancer* 1981;48:1381.

92. Woodruff JM, Perino G. Non–germ-cell or teratomatous malignant tumors showing additional rhabdomyoblastic differentiation, with emphasis on malignant triton tumor. *Semin Diagn Pathol* 1994;11:69.

93. Laskin WB, Weiss SW, Bratthauer GL. Epithelioid variant of malignant peripheral nerve sheath tumor (malignant epithelioid schwannoma). *Am J Surg Pathol* 1991;15:1136.

94. Lodding P, Kindblom L-G, Angervall L. Epithelioid malignant schwannoma: a study of 14 cases. *Virchows Arch A* 1986;409:437.

95. Hruban RH, Shiu MH, Senie RT, et al. Malignant peripheral nerve sheath tumors of the buttocks and lower extremity: a study of 43 cases. *Cancer* 1990;66:1253.

96. Dicarlo EF, Woodruff JM, Bansal M, et al. The purely epithelioid malignant peripheral nerve sheath tumor. *Am J Surg Pathol* 1986;10:478.

97. Wick MR, Swanson PE, Scheithauer BW, et al. Malignant peripheral nerve sheath tumor: an immunohistochemical study of 62 cases. *Am J Clin Pathol* 1987;87:425.

98. Daimaru Y, Hashimoto H, Enjoji M. Malignant peripheral nerve sheath tumors (malignant schwannomas): an immunohistochemical study of 29 cases. *Am J Surg Pathol* 1983;9:434.

99. Fletcher CDM. Pleomorphic malignant fibrous histiocytoma: fact or fiction? *Am J Surg Pathol* 1992;16:213.

100. Reed RJ, Leonard DD. Neurotropic melanoma: a variant of desmoplastic melanoma. *Am J Surg Pathol* 1979;3:301.

101. Reed RJ. Case 13. In: *Proceedings of the 49th Annual Anatomic Pathology Slide Seminar, American Society of Clinical Pathologists.* Chicago: American Society of Clinical Pathologists Press, 1983:97.

102. Ricci A, Parham DM, Woodruff JM, et al. Malignant peripheral nerve sheath tumor arising from ganglioneuroma. *Am J Surg Pathol* 1984;8:19.

103. Ghali VS, Gold JE, Vincent RA, et al. Malignant peripheral nerve sheath tumor arising spontaneously from retroperitoneal ganglioneuroma: a case report, review of the literature, and immunohistochemical study. *Hum Pathol* 1992;23:72.

104. Lin BT, Weiss LM, Medeiros LJ. Neurofibroma and cellular neurofibroma with atypia: a report of 14 tumors. *Am J Surg Pathol* 1997, 21:1443.

105. Liapis H, Dehner LP, Gutmann DH. Neurofibroma and cellular neurofibroma with atypia: a report of 14 tumors. *Am J Surg Pathol* 1999;23:1156.

106. Meis JM, Enzinger FM, Martz KL, et al. Malignant peripheral nerve sheath tumors (malignant schwannomas) in children. *Am J Surg Pathol* 1992;16:694.

107. Wanebo JE, Malik JM, Vandenberg SR, et al. Malignant peripheral nerve sheath tumors: a clinicopathologic study of 28 cases. *Cancer* 1993;71:1247.

108. Sordillo PP, Helson L, Hajdu SI, et al. Malignant schwannoma: clinical characteristics, survival, and response to therapy. *Cancer* 1981;47:2503.

109. Gallager RL, Helwig EB. Neurothekeoma: a benign cutaneous tumor of neural origin. *Am J Clin Pathol* 1980;74:759.

110. MacDonald DM, Wilson-Jones E. Pacinian neurofibroma. *Histopathology* 1977;1:247.

111. King DT, Barr RJ. Bizarre cutaneous neurofibromas. *J Cutan Pathol* 1980;7:21.

112. Holden CA, Wilson-Jones E, MacDonald DM. Cutaneous lobular neuromyoma. *Br J Dermatol* 1982;106:211.

113. Pulitzer DR, Reed RJ. Nerve-sheath myxoma (perineurial myxoma). *Am J Dermatopathol* 1985;7:409.

114. Goldstein J, Lifshitz T. Myxoma of the nerve sheath: report of three cases, observations by light and electron microscopy and histochemical analysis. *Am J Dermatopathol* 1985;7:423.

115. Rosati LA, Fratamico FCM, Eusebi V. Cellular neurothekeoma. *Appl Pathol* 1986;4:186.

116. Barnhill RL, Mihm MC. Cellular neurothekeoma: a distinctive variant of neurothekeoma mimicking nevomelanocytic tumors. *Am J Surg Pathol* 1990;14:113.

117. Wang AR, May D, Bourne P, et al. PGP9.5: a marker for cellular neurothekeoma. *Am J Surg Pathol* 1999;23:1401.

118. Barnhill RL, Dickerson GR, Nickeleit V, et al. Studies on cellular origin of neurothekeoma: clinical, light microscopic, immunohistochemical, and ultrastructural observations. *J Am Acad Dermatol* 1991;25:80.

119. Aronson PJ, Fretzin DF, Potter BS. Neurothekeoma of Gallager and Helwig: dermal nerve sheath myxoma variant. *J Cutan Pathol* 1985;12:506.

120. Laskin WB, Fetsch JF, Miettinen M. The "neurothekeoma:" immunohistochemical analysis distinguishes the true nerve sheath myxoma from its mimics. *Hum Pathol* 2000;31:1230.

121. Salami S, Chomeyko K. Neurothekeoma (N.T.), a clinicopathologic study of 13 new cases with emphasis on immunohistochemical and ultrastructural features. *J Cutan Pathol* 2000;27:571.

122. Strumia R, Lombardi AR, Cavazzini L. S-100 negative myxoid neurothekeoma. *Am J Dermatopathol* 2001;23:82–83.

123. Busam KJ, Mentzel T, Colpaert C, et al. Atypical or worrisome features in cellular neurothekeoma: a study of 10 cases. *Am J Surg Pathol* 1998;22:1067.

124. Argenyi ZB, Kutzner H, Seaba MM. Ultrastructural spectrum of cutaneous nerve sheath myxoma/cellular neurothekeoma. *J Cutan Pathol* 1995;22:137.

125. Allen PW, Dymock RB, MacCormac LB. Superficial angiomyxomas with and without epithelial components: report of 30 tumors in 28 patients. *Am J Surg Pathol* 1988;12:519.

126. Calonje E, Wilson-Jones E, Smith NP, et al. Cellular "neurothekeoma:" an epithelioid variant of pilar leiomyoma? Morphological and immunohistochemical analysis of a series. *Histopathology* 1992;20:397.

127. Wilson-Jones E, Cerio R, Smith NP. Epithelioid cell histiocytoma: a new entity. *Br J Dermatol* 1989;120:185.

128. Gomez CS, Calonje E, Fletcher CDM. Epithelioid benign fibrous histiocytoma of skin: clinicopathological analysis of 20 cases of a poorly known variant. *Histopathology* 1994;24:123.

129. Campbell LK, Thomas JR, Lamps LW, et al. Protein gene product 9.5 (PGP9.5) is not a specific marker of neural and nerve sheath tumors: an immunohistochemical study of 95 mesenchymal neoplasms. *Mod Pathol* 2003;16:963–969.

130. Michal M, Fanburg-Smith JC, Mentzel T, et al. dendritic cell neurofibroma with pseudorosettes: a report of 18 cases of a distinct and hitherto unrecognized neurofibroma variant. *Am J Surg Pathol* 2001;25:587.

131. Simpson RH, Seymour MJ. Dendritic cell neurofibroma with pseudorosettes: two tumors in a patient with evidence of neurofibromatosis. *Am J Surg Pathol* 2001;25:1458.

132. Aparicio SR, Lumsden CE. Light and electron microscopic studies on the granular cell myoblastoma of the tongue. *J Pathol* 1969;97:339.

133. Sobel HJ, Marquet E. Granular cells and granular cell lesions. *Pathol Annu* 1974;9:43.

134. Miracco C, Andreassi A, Laurini L, et al. Granular cell tumour with histological signs of malignancy: report of a case and comparison with 10 benign and 4 atypical cases. *Br J Dermatol* 1999;141:573.

135. Lee J, Bhawan J, Wax F, et al. Plexiform granular cell tumor: a report of two cases. *Am J Dermatopathol* 1994;16:537.

136. Ordonez NG. Granular cell tumor: a review and update. *Adv Anat Pathol* 1999;6:186.

137. Garancis JC, Komorowski RA, Kuzma JF. Granular cell myoblastoma. *Cancer* 1970;25:542.

138. Weiser G. Granularzelltumor (granulares neurom feyrter) und schwannsche Phagen: elektronenoptische untersuchung von 3 fallen. *Virchows Arch A* 1987;380:49 .

139. Lee MW, Chang SE, Song KY, et al. S-100 protein negative atypical granular cell tumor: report of a case. *Int J Dermatol* 2002;41:168.

140. Mukai M. Immunohistochemical localization of S-100 protein and peripheral nerve myelin (P2 protein, PO protein) in granular cell tumors. *Am J Pathol* 1983;112:139.

141. Mahalingam M, LaPiccolo D, Byers HR. Expression of PGP 9.5 in granular cell nerve sheath tumors: an immunohistochemical study of six cases. *J Cutan Pathol* 2001;28:282.

142. LeBoit PE, Barr RJ, Burall S, et al. Primitive polypoid granular-cell tumor and other cutaneous granular-cell neoplasms of apparent nonneural origin. *Am J Surg Pathol* 1991;15:48.

143. Cheng Sd, Usmani AS, DeYoung BR, et al. Dermatofibroma-like granular cell tumor. *J Cutan Pathol* 2001;28:49.

144. Gilliet F, MacGee W, Stoian M, et al. Zur histogenese granuliertzelliger tumoren. *Hautarzt* 1973;24:52.

145. Mentzel T, Wadden C, Fletcher CDM. Granular cell change in smooth muscle tumours of skin and soft tissue. *Histopathology* 1994;24:223.

146. Takahashi H, Fujita S, Satoh H, et al. Immunohistochemical study of congenital gingival granular cell tumor (congenital epulis). *J Oral Pathol Med* 1990;19:492.

147. Lack EE, Perez-Atayde AR, McGill TJ, et al. Gingival granular cell tumor of the newborn (congenital "epulis"): ultrastructural observations relating to histogenesis. *Hum Pathol* 1982;13:686.

148. Simsir A, Osborne BM, Greenebaum E. Malignant granular cell tumor: a case report and review of the recent literature. *Hum Pathol* 1996;27:853.

149. Shimamura K, Osamura RY. Malignant granular cell tumor of the right sciatic nerve: report of an autopsy case with electron microscopic, immunohistochemical, and enzyme histochemical studies. *Cancer* 1984;53:524.

150. Klima M, Peters J. Malignant granular cell tumor. *Arch Pathol* 1987;111:1070.

151. Gokasian ST, Terzakis JA, Santagada EA. Malignant granular cell tumor. *J Cutan Pathol* 1994;21:263.

152. Gamboa LG. Malignant granular-cell myoblastoma. *Arch Pathol* 1955;60:663.

153. Uzoaru I, Firfer B, Ray V, et al. Malignant granular cell tumor. *Arch Pathol Lab Med* 1992;116:206.

154. Strong EW, McDivitt RW, Brasfield RD. Granular cell myoblastoma. *Cancer* 1970;25:415.

155. Al-Sarraf M, Loud AV, Vaitkevicius VK. Malignant granular cell tumor: histochemical and electron microscopic study. *Arch Pathol* 1971;91:550.

156. Gartmann H. Malignant granular cell tumor. *Hautarzt* 1977;28:40.

157. Lazarus SS, Trombetta LD. Ultrastructural identification of a benign perineurial cell tumor. *Cancer* 1978;41:1823.

158. Tsang WYW, Chan JKC, Chow LTC, et al. Perineurioma: an uncommon soft tissue neoplasm distinct from localized hypertrophic neuropathy and neurofibroma. *Am J Surg Pathol* 1992; 16:756.

159. Mentzel T, Dei Tos AP, Fletcher CDM. Perineurioma (storiform perineurial fibroma): clinico-pathological analysis of four cases. *Histopathology* 1994;25:261.

160. Folpe AL, Billings SD, McKenney JK, et al. Expression of claudin-1, a recently described tight junction-associated protein, distinguishes soft tissue perineurioma from potential mimics. *Am J Surg Pathol* 2002;26:1620.

161. Giannini C, Scheithauer BW, Jenkins RB, et al. soft-tissue perineurioma: evidence for an abnormality of chromosome 22. Criteria for diagnosis, and review of literature. *Am J Surg Pathol* 1997;21:164.

162. Dupree WB, Langloss JM, Weiss SW. Pigmented dermatofibrosarcoma protuberans (Bednar tumor): a pathologic, ultrastructural, and immunohistochemical study. *Am J Surg Pathol* 1985;9:630.

163. Weiss SW, Nickoloff BJ. CD-34 is expressed by a distinctive cell population in peripheral nerve, nerve sheath tumors, and related lesions. *Am J Surg Pathol* 1993;17:1039.

164. Pritchard KW, Custer RP. Pacinian neurofibroma. *Cancer* 1952;5:297.

165. Prose PH, Gherardi GJ, Coblenz A. Pacinian neurofibroma. *Arch Dermatol* 1957;76:65.

166. Emory TS, Scheithauer BW, Hirose T, et al. Intraneural perineurioma: a clonal neoplasm associated with abnormalities of chromosome 22. *Am J Clin Pathol* 1995;103:696.

167. Stanton C, Perentes E, Phillips L, et al. The immunohistochemical demonstration of early perineurial change in the development of localized hypertrophic neuropathy: case studies. *Hum Pathol* 1988;19:1455.

168. Mitsumoto H, Wilbourn AJ, Goren H. Perineurioma as the cause of localized hypertrophic neuropathy. *Muscle Nerve* 1980; 3:403.

169. Anthony DC, Hevner RF. Advances in the genetics of hereditary peripheral neuropathies. *Adv Anat Pathol* 1995;2:283.

170. Skelton HG, Williams J, Smith KJ. The clinical and histologic spectrum of cutaneous fibrous perineurioma. *Am J Dermatopathol* 2001;23:190.

171. Fetsch JF, Miettinen M. Sclerosing perineurioma: a clinicopathologic study of 19 cases of a distinctive soft tissue lesion with a predilection for the fingers and palms of young adults. *Am J Surg Pathol* 1997;21:1433.

172. Burgues O, Monteagudo C, Noguera R, et al. Cutaneous sclerosing pacinian-like perineurioma. *Histopathology* 2001;39: 498.

173. van Roggen JFG, McMenamin ME, Belchis DA, et al. Reticular perineurioma: a distinctive variant of soft tissue perineurioma. *Am J Surg Pathol* 2001;485.

174. Shapiro L, Juhlin EA, Brownstein HM. Rudimentary polydactyly. *Arch Dermatol* 1973;108:223.

175. Fletcher CDM. Solitary circumscribed neuroma of the skin (so-called palisaded, encapsulated neuroma): a clinicopathologic and immunohistochemical study. *Am J Surg Pathol* 1989; 13:574.

176. Argenyi ZB, Santa-Cruz D, Bromley C. Comparative light-microscopic and immunohistochemical study of traumatic and palisaded and encapsulated neuromas of the skin. *Am J Dermatopathol* 1992;14:504.

177. Reed RJ, Fine RM, Meltzer HD. Palisaded, encapsulated neuromas of the skin. *Arch Dermatol* 1972;106:865.

178. Argenyi ZB. Immunohistochemical characterization of palisaded, encapsulated neuroma. *J Cutan Pathol* 1990;17:329.

179. Kossard S, Kumar A, Wilkinson B. Neural spectrum: palisaded encapsulated neuroma and Verocay body poor dermal schwannoma. *J Cutan Pathol* 1999;26:31.

180. Hurwitz S. Sipple syndrome. *Arch Dermatol* 1974;110:139.

181. Khairi MRA, Dexter RN, Burzynski NJ, et al. Mucosal neuroma, pheochromocytoma and medullary thyroid carcinoma: multiple endocrine neoplasia type 3 [Review]. *Medicine (Baltimore)* 1975;54:89.

182. Ayala F, Derosa G, Scippa L, et al. Multiple endocrine neoplasia, type IIb. *Dermatologica* 1981;162:292.

183. Carney JA, Go VLW, Sizemore GW, et al. Alimentary-tract ganglioneuromatosis: a major component of the syndrome of multiple endocrine neoplasia, type 2b. *N Engl J Med* 1976;295: 1287.

184. Guillet G, Gauthier Y, Tamisier JM, et al. Linear cutaneous neuromas (dermatoneurie en strie): a limited phakomatosis with striated pigmentation corresponding to cutaneous hyperrneury (featuring multiple endocrine neoplasia syndrome?). *J Cutan Pathol* 1987;14:43.

185. Mason GH, Pitt TE, Tay E. Cutaneous nerve hypertrophy. *Pathology* 1998;26:31.

186. Pujol RM, Matias-Guiu X, Miralles J, et al. Multiple idiopathic mucosal neuromas: a minor form of muptiple endocrine neoplasia type 2B or a new entity? *J Am Acad Dermatol* 1997;37: 349.

187. Truchot F, Grezard P, Wolf F, et al. Multiple idiopathic mucocutaneous neuromas: a new entity? *Br J Dermatol* 2001;145:826.

188. Requena L, Grosshans E, Kutzner H, et al. Epithelial sheath neuroma: a new entity. *Am J Surg Pathol* 2000;24:190–196.

189. Waggener JD. Ultrastructure of benign peripheral nerve sheath tumors. *Cancer* 1966;19:699.

190. Fletcher CDM, Theaker JM. Digital pacinian neuroma: a distinctive hyperplastic lesion. *Histopathology* 1989;15:249.

191. Reed RJ. Giant congenital nevi: a conceptualization of patterns. *J Invest Dermatol* 1993;100:300s.

192. Pettinato G, Manivel JC, d'Amore ESG, et al. Melanotic neuroectodermal tumor of infancy: a reexamination of a histogenetic problem based on immunohistochemical, flow cytometric, and ultrastructural study of 10 cases. *Am J Surg Pathol* 1991;15:233.

193. Pearson JM, Harris M, Eyden BP, et al. Divergent differentiation in small round-cell tumours of the soft tissues with neural features: an analysis of 10 cases. *Histopathology* 1993;23:1.

194. Navarro S, Cavazzana AO, Llombart-Bosch A, et al. Comparison of Ewing's sarcoma of bone and peripheral neuroepithelioma: an immunocytochemical and ultrastructural analysis of two primitive neuroectodermal neoplasms. *Arch Pathol Lab Med* 1994;118:608.

195. Kushner BH, Hajdu SI, Gulati SC, et al. Extracranial primitive neuroectodermal tumors: the Memorial Sloan-Kettering Cancer Center experience. *Cancer* 1991;67:1825.

196. Toker C. Trabecular carcinoma of the skin. *Arch Dermatol* 1972;105:107.

197. Tang CK, Toker C. Trabecular carcinoma of the skin. *Cancer* 1978;42:2311.

198. Ratner D, Nelson BR, Brown MD, et al. Merkel cell carcinoma. *J Am Acad Dermatol* 1993;29:143.

199. Akhtar S, Oza KK, Wright J. Merkel cell carcinoma: report of 10 cases and review of the literature. *J Am Acad Dermatol* 2000; 43:755.

200. Cerroni L, Kerl H. Primary cutaneous neuroendocrine (Merkel cell) carcinoma in association with squamous- and basal-cell carcinoma. *Am J Dermatopathol* 1997;19:610.

201. Gollard R, Weber R, Kosty MP, et al. Merkel cell carcinoma: review of 22 cases with surgical, pathologic, and therapeutic considerations. *Cancer* 2000;88:1842.

202. Raaf JH, Urmacher C, Knapper WK, et al. Trabecular (Merkel cell) carcinoma of the skin. *Cancer* 1986;57:178.

203. Skelton HG, Smith KJ, Hitchcock CL, et al. Merkel cell carcinoma: analysis of clinical, histologic, and immunohistochemical features of 132 cases with relation to survival. *J Am Acad Dermatol* 1997;37:734.

204a. Sibley RK, Dehner LP, Rosai J. Primary neurocrine (Merkel cell?) carcinoma of the skin. *Am J Surg Pathol* 1985;9:95.

204b. Sibley RK, Dahl D. Primary neuroendocrine (Merkel cell?) carcinoma of the skin: an immunocytochemical study of 21 cases. *Am J Surg Pathol* 1985;9:109.

205. Silva EG, MacKay B, Goepfert H, et al. Endocrine carcinoma of the skin: Merkel cell carcinoma. *Pathol Annu* 1984;19:1.

206. Smith KJ, Skelton HG III, Holland TT, et al. Neuroendocrine (Merkel cell) carcinoma with an intraepidermal component. *Am J Dermatopathol* 1993;15:528.

207. LeBoit PE, Crutcher WA, Shapiro PE. Pagetoid intraepidermal spread in Merkel cell (primary neuroendocrine) carcinoma of the skin. *Am J Surg Pathol* 1992;16:584.

208. Foschini MP, Eusebi V. Divergent differentiation in endocrine and non-endocrine tumors of the skin. *Semin Diagn Pathol* 2000;17:162.

209. Traest K, De Vos R, van den Oord JJ. Pagetoid Merkel cell carcinoma: speculations on its origin and the mechanism of epidermal spread. *J Cutan Pathol* 199;26:362.

210. Wick MR, Scheithauer BW, Kovacs K. Neuron-specific enolase in neuroendocrine tumors of the thymus, bronchus, and skin. *Am J Clin Pathol* 1983;79:703.

211. Michels S, Swanson PE, Robb JA, et al. Leu–7 in small cell neoplasms: an immunohistochemical study with ultrastructural correlations. *Cancer* 1987;60:2958.

212. Merot Y, Margolis RJ, Dahl D, et al. Coexpression of neurofilament and keratin proteins in cutaneous neuroendocrine carcinoma cells. *J Invest Dermatol* 1986;86:74.

213. Wick MR, Goellner JR, Scheithauer BW, et al. Primary neuroendocrine carcinomas of the skin: Merkel cell tumors. *Am J Clin Pathol* 1983;79:6.

214. Hanly AJ, Elgart GW, Jorda M, et al. Analysis of thyroid transcription factor-1 and cytokeratin 20 separates Merkel cell carcinoma from small cell carcinoma of lung. *J Cutan Pathol* 2000;27:118.

215. van Muijen GNP, Ruiter DJ, Warnaar SO. Intermediate filaments in Merkel cell tumors. *Hum Pathol* 1985;16:590.

216. Haneke E. Electron microscopy of Merkel cell carcinoma from formalin-fixed tissue. *J Am Acad Dermatol* 1985;12:487.

217. Gould E, Albores-Saavedra J, Dubner B, et al. Eccrine and squamous differentiation in Merkel cell carcinoma: an immunohistochemical study. *Am J Surg Pathol* 1988;12:768.

218. Isimbaldi G, Sironi M, Taccagni GL, et al. Tripartite differentiation (squamous, glandular, and melanocytic) of a primary cutaneous neurocrine carcinoma. *Am J Dermatopathol* 1993;15: 260. 216.

219. Vortmeyer AG, Merino MJ, Boni R, et al. Genetic changes associated with primary Merkel cell carcinoma. *Am J Clin Pathol* 1998;109:565.

220. Wick MR, Millns JL, Sibley RK. Secondary neuroendocrine carcinomas of the skin. *J Am Acad Dermatol* 1985;13:134.

221. Wick MR, Kaye VN, Sibley RK, et al. Primary neuroendocrine carcinoma and small-cell malignant lymphoma of the skin. *J Cutan Pathol* 1986;13:347.

222. Rios-Martin JJ, Solorzano-Amoreti A, Gonzalez-Campora R, et al. Neuroendocrine carcinoma of the skin with a lympho-epithelioma-like histological pattern. *Br J Dermatol* 2000;143: 460.

223. Eusebi V, Capella C, Cossu A, et al. Neuroendocrine carcinoma within lymph nodes in the absence of a primary tumor, with special reference to Merkel cell carcinoma. *Am J Surg Pathol* 1992;16:658.

224. Shown TE, Durfee ME. Blueberry muffin baby: neonatal neuroblastoma with subcutaneous metastases. *J Urol* 1970;104:193.

225. Hawthorne HC, Nelson JS, Witzleben CL, et al. Blanching subcutaneous nodules in neonatal neuroblastoma. *J Pediatr* 1970;77:297.

226. Aleshire SL, Glick AD, Cruz VE, et al. Neuroblastoma in adults: pathologic findings and clinical outcome. *Arch Pathol Lab Med* 1985;109:352.

227. Mackay B, Luna MA, Butler JJ. Adult neuroblastoma: electron microscopic observations in nine cases. *Cancer* 1976;37:1334.

228. Osborn M, Dirk T, Kaser H, et al. Immunohistochemical localization of neurofilaments and neuron-specific enolase in 29 cases of neuro-blastoma. *Am J Pathol* 1986;122:433.

229. Joshi VV, Silverman JF. Pathology of neuroblastic tumors. *Semin Diagn Pathol* 1994;11:107.

230. Gambini C, Rongioletti F. Primary congenital cutaneous ganglioneuroma. *J Am Acad Dermatol* 1996;35:353.

231. Hammond RR, Walton JC. Cutaneous ganglioneuromas: a case report and review of the literature. *Hum Pathol* 1996;27: 735.

232. Collins JP, Johnson WC, Burgoon LF Jr. Ganglioneuroma of the skin. *Arch Dermatol* 1972;105:256.

233. Rios JJ, Diaz-Cano SJ, Rivera-Hueto F, et al. Cutaneous ganglion cell choristoma. *J Cutan Pathol* 1991;18:469.

234. Franchi A, Massi D, Santucci M. Desmoplastic cutaneous ganglioneuroma. *Histopathology* 1999;34:82–84.

235. Lee JY, Martinez AJ, Abell E. Ganglioneuromatous tumor of the skin: a combined heterotopia of ganglion cells and hamartomatous neuroma. Report of a case. *J Cutan Pathol* 1988;15:58.

236. Hartman KR, Triche TJ, Kinsella TJ, et al. Prognostic value of histopathology in Ewing's sarcoma: long-term follow-up of distal extremity primary tumors. *Cancer* 1991;67:163.

237. Hashimoto H, Enjoji M, Nakajima T, et al. Malignant neuroepithelioma (peripheral neuroblastoma): a clinicopathologic study of 15 cases. *Am J Surg Pathol* 1983;7:309.

238. Banerjee SS, Agbamu DA, Eyden BP, et al. Clinicopathological characteristics of peripheral primitive neuroectodermal tumor of skin and subcutaneous tissue. *Histopathology* 1997;31:355.

239. Hasegawa Sl, Davison JM, Rutten A, et al. Primary cutaneous Ewing's sarcoma: immunophenotypic and molecular cytogenetic evaluation of five cases. *Am J Surg Pathol* 1998;22:310.

240. Sur M, Cooper K. PNET's everywhere. *Histopathology* 1999; 35:279–280.

241. Fellinger EJ, Garin-Chesa P, Glasser DB, et al. Comparison of cell surface antigen HBA71 (p30/32 mic2), neuron specific enolase, and vimentin in the immunohistochemical analysis of Ewing's sarcoma of bone. *Am J Surg Pathol* 1992;16:746.

242. Perlman EJ, Dickman PS, Askin FB, et al. Ewing's sarcoma—routine diagnostic utilization of MIC2 analysis: a pediatric oncology group/children's cancer group intergroup study. *Hum Pathol* 1994;25:304.

243. Ladanyi M, Garin-Chesa P, Rettig WJ, et al. EWS rearrangement in Ewing's sarcoma and peripheral neuroectodermal tumor: molecular detection and correlation with cytogenetic analysis and MIC2 expression. *Diag Mol Pathol* 1993;2:141.

244. Argenyi ZB, Schelper RL, Balogh K. Pigmented neuroectodermal tumor of infancy: a light microscopic and immunohistochemical study. *J Cutan Pathol* 1991;18:40.

245. Kapadia SB, Frisman DM, Hitchcock CL, et al. Melanotic neuroectodermal tumor of infancy: clinicopathological, immunohistochemical, and flow cytometric study. *Am J Surg Pathol* 1993;17:566.

246. Raju U, Zarbo RJ, Regezi JA, et al. Melanotic neuroectodermal tumors of infancy: intermediate filament-, neuroendocrine-, and melanoma-associated antigen profiles. *Appl Immunohistochem* 1993;1:69.

247. Pettinato G, Manivel JC, d'Amore ESG, et al. Melanotic neuroectodermal tumor of infancy: a reexamination of a histogenetic problem based on immunohistochemical, flow cytometric, and ultrastructural study of 10 cases. *Am J Surg Pathol* 1991;15:233.

248. Baran R, Kopf A, Schnitzler L. Le gliome nasal. *Ann Dermatol Syphiligr* 1973;100:395.

249. Christianson HB. Nasal glioma. *Arch Dermatol* 1966;93:68.

250. Skelton HG, Smith KJ. Glial heterotopia in the subcutaneous tissue overlying T-12. *J Cutan Pathol* 199;26:523–527.

251. Kopf AW, Bart RS. Nasal glioma. *J Dermatol Surg Oncol* 1978;4:128.

252. Fletcher CDM, Carpenter G, McKee PH. Nasal glioma: a rarity. *Am J Dermatopathol* 1986;8:341.

253. Yeoh GPS, Bale PM, de Silva M. Nasal cerebral heterotopia: the so-called nasal glioma or sequestered encephalocele and its variants. *Pediatr Pathol* 1989;9:531.

254. Mirra SS, Pearl GS, Hoffman JC, et al. Nasal "glioma" with prominent neuronal component. *Arch Pathol* 1981;105:540.

255. Berry AD, Patterson JW. Meningoceles, meningomyeloceles, and encephaloceles: a neuro-dermatopathologic study of 132 cases. *J Cutan Pathol* 1990;18:164.

256. Sibley DA, Cooper PH. Rudimentary meningocele: a variant of "primary cutaneous meningioma." *J Cutan Pathol* 1989;16:72.

257. Chan HH, Fung JW, Lam WM, et al. The clinical spectrum of rudimentary meningocele. *Pediatr Dermatol* 1998;15:388.

258. El Shabrawi-Caelen L, White WL, Soyer HP, et al. Rudimentary memingocele: remnant of a neural tube defect? *Arch Dermatol* 2001;137:45.

259. Lopez DA, Silvers DN, Helwig EB. Cutaneous meningioma: a clinicopathologic study. *Cancer* 1974;34:728.

260. Laymon CW, Becker FT. Massive metastasizing meningioma involving the scalp. *Arch Derm Syph* 1949;59:626.

261. Suster S, Rosai J. Hamartoma of the scalp with ectopic meningothelial elements: a distinctive benign soft tissue lesion that may simulate angiosarcoma. *Am J Surg Pathol* 1990;14:1.

262. Theaker JM, Fleming KA. Meningioma of the scalp: a case report with immunohistochemical features. *J Cutan Pathol* 1987;14:49.

263. Gelli MC, Pasquinelli G, Martinelli G, et al. Cutaneous meningiomas: histochemical, immunohistochemical, and ultrastructural investigation. *Histopathology* 1993;23:576.

264. Argenyi ZB, Theiberg MD, Hayes CM, et al. Primary cutaneous meningioma associated with von Recklinghausen's disease. *J Cutan Pathol* 1994;21:549.

265. Theaker JM, Gatter KC, Puddle J. Epithelial membrane antigen expression by the perineurium of peripheral nerve and in peripheral nerve tumors. *Histopathology* 1988;13:171.

266. Pultizer DR, Martin PC, Collins PC, et al. Subcutaneous sacrococcygeal ("myxopapillary") ependymal rests. *Am J Surg Pathol* 1988;12:672.

267. Anderson MS. Myxopapillary ependymomas presenting in the soft tissue over the sacrococcygeal region. *Cancer* 1966;19:585.

268. Reed RJ, Bliss BO. Morton's neuroma: regressive and productive intermetatarsal elastofibrositis. *Arch Pathol* 1973;95:123.

269. Lawrence N, Cottel WI. Squamous cell carcinoma of the skin with perineural invasion. *J Am Acad Dermatol* 1994;31:30.

270. Stern JB, Haupt HM. Reexcision perineural invasion: not a sign of malignancy. *Am J Dermatopathol* 1990;14:183.

271. Zelger BG, ZelgerB. Epithelial sheath neuroma: a benign neoplasm. *Am J Surg Pathol* 2001;25:696.

METASTATIC CARCINOMA OF THE SKIN: INCIDENCE AND DISSEMINATION

WAINE C. JOHNSON

Cutaneous metastases are of diagnostic importance because they may be the first manifestation of an undiscovered internal malignancy or the first indication of metastasis of a supposedly adequately treated malignancy. The site of the primary tumor, if unknown, may be suspected by the histopathology and appropriate immunoperoxidase studies. Cutaneous metastases are generally uncommon but have been reported more frequently in recent years. In a study of 7,316 patients with internal cancer, Lookingbill et al. (1) found 367 (5%) to have skin involvement. Of 4,020 patients with metastatic disease, Lookingbill et al. (2) reported that 420 (10%) had cutaneous metastases. Nine percent of 7,518 patients with internal cancer who were autopsied at Roswell Park Memorial Institute had skin metastases (3). The incidence of various tumors that are metastatic to the skin correlates well with the frequency of occurrence of the primary malignant tumor in each gender.

Review of 724 patients with cutaneous metastases in 1972 by Brownstein and Helwig (4) showed that, in women, commensurate with the greater frequency of carcinoma of the breast, 69% of all cutaneous metastases originated in the breast. Carcinoma of the large intestine accounted for 9% of cutaneous metastases, and carcinoma of the lungs and ovaries accounted for 4%. In recent years, the incidence of cutaneous metastasis from carcinoma of the lungs in women has significantly increased, and carcinoma of the lungs has become the most frequent cause of cancer deaths in women (as it is in men) (5,6). The study by Brownstein and Helwig (4) of cutaneous metastases in men revealed the following incidences of primary carcinoma: lungs, 24%; large intestine, 19%; oral cavity, 12%; and kidney and stomach, each 6%. Metastatic melanoma was found in 13% (discussed in Chapter 29).

Due to the relative rarity of carcinomas of the thyroid gland, pancreas, liver, gall bladder, urinary bladder, endometrium, prostate, testes, and neuroendocrine system, cutaneous metastases of these tumors are also relatively rare. A review by Schwartz (7) reported cutaneous metastatic disease as the first sign of internal cancer most commonly seen with cancer of the lung, kidney, and ovary.

Dissemination may take place through the lymphatics or the blood stream. In carcinomas of the breast and the oral cavity, metastases reach the skin largely through lymphatic channels and are often located in the overlying skin. In contrast, cutaneous metastatic lesions in other carcinomas are often the result of hematogenous dissemination and may appear in any area of the skin (8). Cutaneous metastases are more likely to be found in older individuals. Rare metastases found in the young are usually derived from a neuroblastoma or, less commonly, a rhabdomyosarcoma (9).

Cutaneous metastases usually appear as multiple, discrete, painless, and freely movable papules or nodules of sudden onset. Cutaneous metastases occur in about 10% of cases of metastases (2). The nodules are usually 1 to 3 cm in diameter, but much larger lesions have been reported (10). Metastases tend to occur on cutaneous surfaces near the site of the primary tumor, but exceptions to this include the scalp that may be as frequent as 5% of all cutaneous metastases. Metastasis to the umbilicus is relatively common and the underlying primary tumor is usually an adenocarcinoma of the stomach, ovaries, endometrium, or breast (11,12). A zosteriform pattern of skin metastasis has been reported to occur on the chest wall and abdominal wall, and the most frequent site of the primary was breast, ovary or lung, prostate, bladder, or stomach (13,14).

CARCINOMA OF THE BREAST

Cutaneous metastases that occur predominantly by lymphatic dissemination include inflammatory carcinoma, carcinoma en cuirasse, telangiectatic and nodular carcinoma, and carcinoma of the inframammary crease. Alopecia neoplastica and mammary carcinoma of the eyelid are probably caused by hematogenous spread (7).

Inflammatory breast carcinoma is characterized by an erythematous patch or plaque with an active spreading border that resembles erysipelas and usually affects the breast and nearby skin (7). Rarely, inflammatory metastatic carcinoma may arise from primary involvement of other organs. The inflammatory appearance and warmth are attributed to capillary congestion.

En cuirasse metastatic carcinoma is characterized by a diffuse morphea-like induration of the skin and rarely involves skin from other primary carcinomas. It usually begins as scattered papular lesions coalescing into a sclerodermoid plaque without inflammatory changes.

Telangiectatic metastatic breast carcinoma is characterized by violaceous papulovesicles resembling lymphangioma circumscriptum (7). A violaceous hue, which is often present, is caused by blood in dilated vascular channels.

The nodular form appears as multiple firm nodules that may show ulceration. An exophytic nodule may occur in the inframammary crease resembling a primary squamous cell or basal cell carcinoma and occurs more frequently in women with large breasts.

Alopecia neoplastica occurs as oval plaques or patches of the scalp and may be confused clinically with alopecia areata or a scarring alopecia. Metastatic mammary carcinoma in the eyelid clinically presents as a painless swelling with induration or as a discrete nodule (7).

Histopathology. In inflammatory carcinoma histologic examination of the skin reveals extensive invasion of the dermis and often the subcutaneous lymphatics by groups and cords of tumor cells. The tumor cells are similar to those in the primary growth and atypical in character with large, pleomorphic, hyperchromatic nuclei. There is marked capillary congestion, which is the reason for the clinical appearance of erythema and warmth (7). Often there is interstitial edema and a slight perivascular lymphoid infiltrate. The extensive lymphatic dissemination is caused by retrograde

lymphatic spread into the skin secondary to blockage of the deep lymphatics and lymph nodes (15). Fibrosis is not a significant feature. Some studies indicate only 1% to 4% of patients with metastatic breast carcinoma present with the inflammatory or erysipeloid type and that most of these patients have intraductal breast carcinoma (16).

In en cuirasse carcinoma, also referred to as *scirrhous carcinoma*, the indurated areas show fibrosis and may contain only a few tumor cells. The tumor cells may be confused with fibroblasts. The tumor cells have elongated nuclei similar to fibroblasts, but the nuclei are larger, more angular, and more deeply basophilic. The tumor cells often lie singly, but in some areas they may form small groups or single rows between fibrotic and thickened collagen bundles (Fig. 36-1). This latter feature of "Indian filing" is of particular diagnostic importance and may be seen in any histologic variety.

In telangiectatic carcinoma the tumor cells tend to be located more superficially in the dermis within dilated lymphatic vessels than those in inflammatory carcinoma. The blood vessels are congested with red blood cells, as in inflammatory carcinoma, but usually also contain aggregates of neoplastic cells (17). The presence of many dilated blood vessels immediately beneath the epidermis gives rise to the clinical appearance of hemorrhagic vesicles.

In nodular carcinoma there are variably sized groups of tumor cells in the dermis, and these nodular areas are surrounded by fibrosis. Depending on the tumor type, some cells may show a glandular arrangement, which may be quite ill defined (Fig. 36-2). Sometimes a nodule may be pigmented and clinically suggestive of a melanoma or pigmented basal cell carcinoma. The pigment results from melanin accumulation within the cytoplasm of neoplastic cells and in the stroma (18).

Carcinoma of the inframammary crease has been described as islands of epithelial cells with hyperchromatic

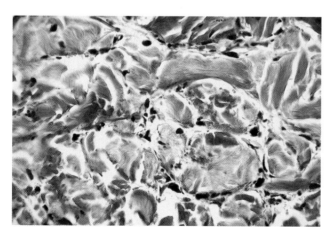

FIGURE 36-1. Metastatic breast carcinoma. Individual atypical tumor cells are seen between fibrotic collagen bundles, H&E × 400.

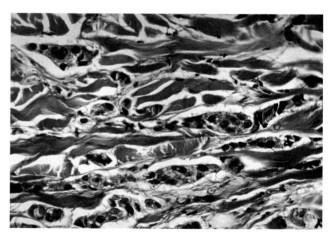

FIGURE 36-2. Metastatic breast carcinoma showing a glandular arrangement between collagen bundles, ×320.

nuclei extending contiguously with the epidermis from the dermis (19).

In hematogenous metastases the histologic picture varies with clinical presentation. In alopecia neoplastica, the features resemble those of en cuirasse type with single files of tumor cells between thickened collagen bundles (20). Metastatic mammary carcinoma involving the eyelid has been described in 13 patients (7), and in 8 of them the microscopic features had a prominent histiocytoid appearance (21).

Epidermotropic involvement from metastatic breast carcinoma may mimic malignant melanoma and/or Paget's disease (22).

The signet-ring cell histologic pattern of breast carcinoma (Fig. 36-3) may also be seen in carcinoma of the gastrointestinal tract and urinary bladder (23). This may be confused with a primary cutaneous signet-ring cell carcinoma that occurs most frequently in middle-aged men on the eyelid, and less frequently in the axilla (23). A primary mucinous carcinoma of the skin also may require distinction from metastatic lesions from the breast or colon (9). Rarely, a granular cell histologic pattern is seen (24).

Immunoperoxidase. Cutaneous metastases are positive with most cytokeratins, except for CK209 and often are positive with epithelial membrane antigen (EMA) and carcinoembryonic antigen (CEA). Reactivity with S-100 protein has been reported in as many as 24% of cases of primary and metastatic breast carcinoma (25). The presence of melanin granules and melanosomes within tumor cells that give a positive HMB-45 is rare and probably occurs secondarily to phagocytosis or melanocyte colonization of the tumor cells (18). In lesions in which there are cells positive with S-100 or HMB-45, reactivity with keratins, EMA, and/or CEA would rule out melanoma. A positive androgen receptor marker would be helpful in identifying metastatic breast cancer when estrogen receptors and progesterone receptors are negative (26). Primary

signet-ring carcinoma of the skin has been reported to be positive with CK7 and CK20, and this would aid in distinction from breast carcinoma, which is usually negative with CK20 (23).

Mucinous carcinoma of the skin, which is generally thought to derive from sweat glands, is positive with numerous cytokeratins, but is negative with cytokeratin 20. This would allow distinction from a metastatic mucinous adenocarcinoma of the colon, which would be positive with CK20 (27).

Expression of CK7 was found in the majority of cases of carcinoma, with the exception of those arising from the colon, prostate, kidney, thymus, carcinoid tumors of the lung and gastrointestinal tract, and Merkel cell tumors of the skin.

CARCINOMA OF THE LUNG

Metastasis to skin is more common in men, but the incidence of lung carcinoma in women is increasing (5,6). In 56 patients reported with skin metastasis from lung carcinoma, 7% had a skin nodule before the diagnosis of the primary tumor and 16% had a nodule at the same time (28). In 11 of 21 patients with cutaneous metastasis, the skin was the first extranodal site (1). Metastases may occur on any cutaneous surface, but the most common sites are the chest wall and posterior abdomen (7). Oat cell carcinoma shows predilection for the skin of the back (2). Most lesions present as a localized cluster of cutaneous papules or nodules or as a solitary nodule.

Histopathology. Cutaneous metastases were undifferentiated in approximately 40%, and adenocarcinoma and squamous cell carcinoma in approximately 30% each (4). The undifferentiated tumors were often of the small cell type with hyperchromatic nuclei and scant cytoplasm (4). Small cell carcinomas of the lung include oat cell carcinomas and carcinoid tumors. Carcinoid tumors of the lung are derived from the bronchus and consist of solid islands and nests of uniform cells (Fig. 36-4). Other sources of carcinoid tumors include stomach, small and large intestine, and primary in skin (29–31). The closely packed tumor cells may suggest a malignant lymphoma. Immunoperoxidase studies are extremely helpful in making this distinction. Larger cells require consideration of metastatic amelanotic melanoma and, again, immunoperoxidase studies may be required for distinction.

Squamous cell carcinomas metastatic to skin are usually poorly or moderately differentiated (4). They can usually be distinguished from primary squamous cell carcinoma by the absence of proliferation from the surface epidermis and seldom show an orderly pattern of differentiation from basaloid to prickle cells with centers of keratinization. They show occasional whorls of squamoid cells with imperfect keratinization and individually keratinized cells, and sometimes

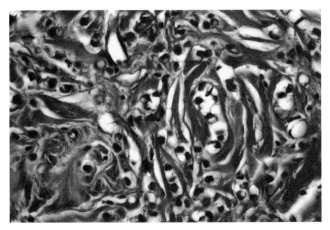

FIGURE 36-3. Metastatic breast carcinoma showing a signet-ring cell pattern, × 400.

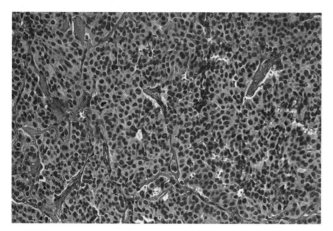

FIGURE 36-4. Metastatic small cell carcinoma from lung shows uniform pattern of carcinoid. H&E × 240.

have large, bizarre forms with frequent mitotic figures (4). In larger tumors, areas of central necrosis are often present. Most cutaneous metastatic squamous cell carcinomas arise in the lung, oral cavity, or esophagus. Tumors from the oral cavity tend to be more differentiated and nearly always appear on the head or neck. Squamous carcinoma metastatic from the esophagus shows essentially similar features to that from the lung (4).

Adenocarcinomas metastatic to skin from lung are often moderately differentiated, but some show well-formed, mucin-secreting, glandular structures. Individual tumor cells sometimes contain abundant cytoplasmic mucin, but usually lack large pools of mucin, which is more characteristically seen from gastrointestinal metastatic adenocarcinomas (4).

Immunoperoxidase. In addition to keratins that are positive in most metastatic carcinomas, most metastatic adenocarcinomas are positive with EMA and CEA. It has been stated that a positive reaction with CEA (seen in 50% of secondary neuroendocrine carcinomas) may be most helpful in differentiating between primary and secondary lesions (32). A rare exception to this consideration is the presence of duct-like structures in two instances of Merkel cell carcinoma, and these were CEA positive (33). This was assumed to be eccrine differentiation. Merkel cell carcinomas usually show a CK20 perinuclear dot, and/or diffuse activity, and this is rarely seen in metastatic neuroendocrine carcinomas (34). They may show reactivity to one or more of the following: protein gene product (PCP), chromogranin-A, CD56 antigen (Leu-7), and Synaptophysin (32). Negative reactions with lymphocyte common antigen (LCA) and other lymphoid markers are most helpful in ruling out malignant lymphomas (35). Thyroid transcription factor 1 (TTF-1) is positive in thyroid carcinoma and in small cell lung carcinoma and is negative in most cases of Merkel cell carcinoma (34,36).

GASTROINTESTINAL CARCINOMA

Carcinoma of the colon and rectum is the second most common type of primary cancer in men (7). Cutaneous lesions usually appear after the primary tumor has been

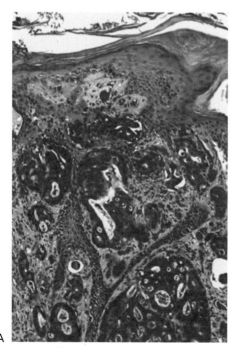
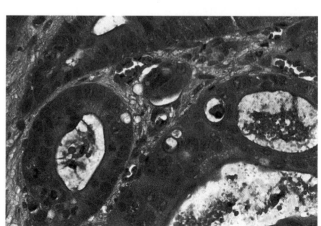

A   B

FIGURE 36-5. Metastatic carcinoma from colon shows secondary epidermal involvement. **A:** H&E × 40. **B:** H&E × 280.

recognized and occur more commonly on the abdomen or perineal areas, although the head and neck areas are sometimes involved. Metastases from gastric carcinoma may occur at any distant site, but the umbilical region is perhaps most common.

Histopathology. Most cutaneous metastases from the large intestine and all from the stomach as reported by Brownstein and Helwig (37) were adenocarcinomas (Fig. 36-5A, B). A mucinous carcinoma pattern with small groups of tumor cells that lie in large pools of mucin is common in lesions from the large intestine. Signet-ring cell differentiation is not usually seen in lesions from the large intestine but may be present in lesions from the stomach (4). The stomach metastases are usually anaplastic, infiltrating carcinomas with variable cellularity, a loose stroma, and varying proportions of signet-ring cells. The mucin present in metastatic carcinoma from the gastrointestinal tract as well as in mucinous carcinomas from the breast and lung is a nonsulfated, hyaluronidase-resistant, sialic acid–type of mucosubstance (38–40). Histochemical procedures show this mucin to be positive with colloidal iron, hyaluronidase resistant, Alcian blue positive at pH 2.5 and negative at pH 0.4, and aldehyde-fuchsin positive at pH 1.7 and negative at pH 1.0. It shows metachromasia with toluidine blue at pH 3.0, and is negative at pH 2.0, is PAS positive and diastase resistant, and is mucicarmine positive (41). In contrast, histochemical studies of adenoid squamous cell carcinoma show the mucin to be predominantly hyaluronic acid. Also, distinction from adenoid basal cell carcinoma and adenocystic carcinoma from lacrimal and salivary glands can be made based on the fact that these latter tumors contain a predominance of sulfated acid mucosaccharides (41). The differential diagnosis for metastatic carcinoma includes carcinomas of cutaneous adnexae such as sweat gland carcinomas.

Immunoperoxidase. A study by Chu et al. (42) showed CK20 positivity in almost all colorectal carcinomas (Fig. 36-6A and B) and Merkel cell tumors, pancreatic carcinomas (62%), gastric carcinomas (50%), cholangiocarcinomas (43%), and transitional cell carcinomas (29%). The same study showed that CK20 positivity was nearly absent in carcinomas from other organ systems and in malignant mesotheliomas (42).

ORAL CAVITY CARCINOMA

Most lesions metastasizing from carcinomas of the oral cavity are spread by lymphatic invasion and are located on the face or neck (4). They usually appear as multiple or solitary nodules and sometimes are ulcerated.

Histopathology. The lesions are almost always squamous cell in type and are usually moderately or well differentiated (4). They are located usually in the deeper dermis and subcutaneous tissue with sparing of the superficial cutis. In examples with ulceration and involvement of the upper corium, distinction from primary squamous cell carcinoma of skin may not be possible (4).

RENAL CELL CARCINOMA

The tumors are most commonly located in the head and neck area, although any site may be involved (7,43). They often present as solitary or a few nodules, and may be skin colored, reddish, or violaceous. They may occur as the first sign of internal cancer or as late as 10 years after diagnosis of the primary. They occur almost always in men.

Histopathology. The histologic features are usually those of a clear-cell adenocarcinoma. They are often localized intradermal nodules and may stretch the overlying epidermis (4) (Fig. 36-7A). The tumor cells show oval nuclei with abundant, clear cytoplasm and often are in a glandular configuration (Fig. 36-7B). The stroma is vascular, and extravasated red blood cells are frequent. Intracytoplasmic glycogen is uniformly present as demonstrated by staining with PAS stain and diastase-labile intracytoplasmic material. Frozen

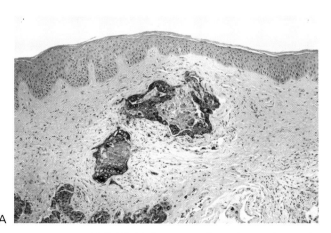
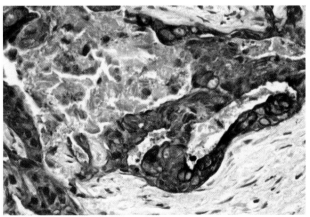

FIGURE 36-6. Metastatic carcinoma from colon, cytokeratin-20. **A:** × 40. **B:** × 320.

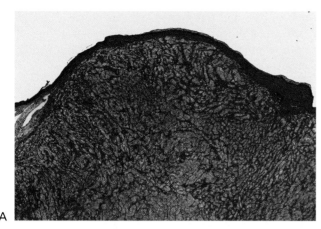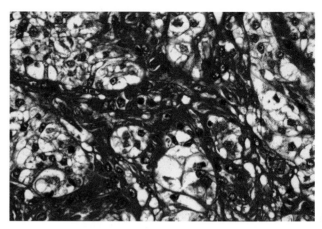

FIGURE 36-7. Metastatic carcinoma from kidney. **A:** Dermal infiltrate pressing on overlying epidermis, × 40. **B:** Shows clear cell pattern with stroma of dilated capillaries, × 320.

sections stained with oil red O show the presence of lipid droplets in many tumor cells (43). The histologic differential diagnosis includes adnexal tumors and especially eccrine acrospiroma. In contrast to the usual unilobular and hemorrhagic renal cell carcinoma, the eccrine acrospiroma tends to be multilobular and nonhemorrhagic, and often-distinct ductal structures are present. Sebaceous cell tumors also may be confused, but the markedly vascular stroma and hemorrhagic nature of the renal cell cancer is fairly distinctive.

Immunoperoxidase. In most cases, the tumor cells are reactive with pankeratin, AE1/AE3, CAM5.2, EMA, and CD10. They are usually negative with CK7 and CK20, and about 60% in one study were positive with vimentin (44,45).

CARCINOMA OF THE OVARY

The most frequent sites involved are the abdomen including the umbilicus, the vulva, or the back (7). Lesions of the

abdomen may be in the scar sites from surgery or diagnostic procedures (2).

Histopathology. The features are usually of a moderately or well-differentiated adenocarcinoma, often having a papillary configuration and containing psammoma bodies (4). Psammoma bodies in cutaneous metastases in 724 patients studied by these authors were found only in metastases from the ovary (but might also be seen in papillary carcinomas from other sites including, for example, the thyroid).

Immunoperoxidase. Papillary ovarian tumors were all CK7 positive and CK20 negative, mucinous ovarian carcinomas (Fig. 36-8) were CK7 positive and a few were CK20 negative (46).

CARCINOID AND NEUROENDOCRINE CARCINOMAS

These tumors are assumed to be derived from the neural crest tissues and have been classified as amine precursor uptake and decarboxylase (APUD) system (33). Lesions appear as solitary or multiple cutaneous papules or nodules and may occur at any site. Primary carcinoids giving rise to cutaneous metastases (Fig. 36-4) occur most frequently in the bronchi but have been reported in various sites, including the small intestines, sigmoid, colon, pancreas, stomach, thymus, and thyroid (31). In addition to carcinoid tumors, cutaneous metastases from neuroendocrine carcinomas of a variety of sites including the uterus, vulva, gall bladder, and fallopian tubes have been reported (7,47). Neuroblastoma, which is the most common cancer identified at birth, has been reported to metastasize to the subcutaneous tissue in 32% of patients with congenital neuroblastoma (7). Clinically, they have a fairly specific appearance, which has been described as like a "blueberry muffin." This term has also

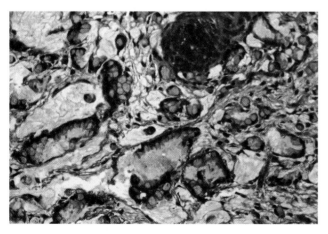

FIGURE 36-8. Metastatic mucinous ovarian carcinoma. H&E × 240.

been used to describe some cases of congenital leukemia. Cutaneous neuroblastoma is very rare in adults, and it is impossible to distinguish between primary and metastatic lesions except for finding an internal primary tumor (48).

Histopathology. Carcinoid metastases in the skin and subcutaneous tissue consist of solid islands, nests, and cords of tumor cells (Fig. 36-4). As a rule, the cells appear quite uniform in size and shape, have small, rounded nuclei, and abundant, clear, or eosinophilic cytoplasm occasionally containing numerous eosinophilic granules (49). However, in some instances the nuclei are hyperchromatic and there may be areas in which the nuclei show anaplasia by being irregularly shaped, large, and hyperchromatic. Carcinoids of the bronchus usually contain argyrophil granules in contrast to those of the small intestine, which usually contain argentaffin granules, which can be demonstrated by the Fontana–Masson stain (50). Cutaneous metastases of bronchial carcinoids may have either argyrophil or argentaffin granules (51). The histologic differential diagnosis may include sweat gland carcinoma or glomus tumor because of their arrangement in well-defined islands, as well as metastases from noncarcinoid neuroendocrine tumors, and primary Merkel cell carcinoma. The latter usually show more immature cells or greater cellular atypism, a greater number of mitotic figures, and a "trabecular" pattern. The presence of an intraepidermal component would also favor a primary Merkel cell carcinoma (33). Involvement of the deep dermis and multiple skin sites favor a metastatic lesion (47). Primary or metastatic neuroblastomas (peripheral neuroectodermal tumor) show identical features of undifferentiated, small, hyperchromatic cells with frequent rosettes of the Homer–Wright type and numerous mitoses (48). Some examples of undifferentiated lesions may not show rosettes. The histologic differential diagnosis includes other small cell carcinomas that sometimes show rosette-like structures, extraskeletal Ewing's sarcoma, lymphoma, and leukemia. Merkel cell carcinoma tends to display a trabecular arrangement, but this is not always specific.

Immunoperoxidase and Electron Microscopy. Immunoperoxidase studies are of great value in distinguishing a primary Merkel cell carcinoma of the skin from a metastatic neuroendocrine carcinoma. Merkel cell carcinomas are usually positive with CK20 (52) and are negative with TTF-1 and CK7 (34,36). If the lesion were positive for CEA in nonductal or nonglandular sites, this would strongly favor a metastatic lesion (32,33). The presence of a positive reaction with NSE and EMA is not necessarily helpful, since these can be reactive in primary or secondary neuroendocrine carcinomas as well as sweat gland carcinomas. Reactivity with CK20 favors a Merkel cell tumor. If the tumor is positive with S-100, this favors an eccrine sweat gland carcinoma, a metastatic breast carcinoma, or a malignant melanoma. If the tumor is positive with LCA, this identifies the lesion as a malignant lymphoma. A rare exception to this

rule was published by Nandedkar et al. (53). Calcitonin has been demonstrated in cutaneous metastasis of medullary carcinoma of the thyroid (54). Electron microscopic studies of carcinoid, neuroendocrine carcinomas, and primary Merkel cell carcinomas show "neurosecretory" membrane-bound, dense-core granules measuring 100 to 250 nm in diameter (31,47,51,55). These granules do not distinguish among members of this group. Immunoelectron microscopic studies confirm the presence of cytokeratin (AE1/AE3) arranged in paranuclear areas, while cytoplasmic synaptophysin and chromogranin positivity over dense-core granules tend to confirm light microscopic immunohistochemical studies (55). Neuroblastoma has been reported to be positive with NSE but often is negative with other commonly reactive antigens of neuroendocrine tumors such as EMA, chromogranin-A, and synaptophysin (48). Electron microscopy shows membrane-bound, dense-core granules concentrated in the cytoplasmic processes. Desmosomes and microtubules are usually seen in more differentiated tumors.

MISCELLANEOUS CARCINOMAS

In metastatic carcinoma from the liver the arrangement of malignant hepatocytes in irregular columns are fairly distinctive and, if there are acinar structures containing bile, the diagnosis is definite (56).

In choriocarcinoma the cutaneous metastases show the two types of cells that arise from the fetal trophoblast: cytotrophoblasts and syncytiotrophoblasts. The cytotrophoblasts usually grow in clusters, and the cells appear cuboidal with large, vesicular nuclei and a pale cytoplasm. The syncytiotrophoblasts, which have large and irregular nuclei and a basophilic cytoplasm, grow around the clusters of cytotrophoblasts in a plexiform pattern resembling chorionic villi (57). The syncytiotrophoblasts have been reported to be strongly positive for human chorionic gonadotropin (HCG) antigen (58).

Metastatic carcinoma of the prostate to skin is rare and usually occurs in the inguinal area, lower abdomen, or thighs, but distant sites of the scalp and face have been reported (7). Reactivity with prostate-specific antigen establishes the diagnosis (59).

Pancreatic cancer metastatic to skin is rare, and the most common site is the umbilical area (7,60). Histologically it usually represents an adenocarcinoma. Immunoperoxidase with a carbohydrate antigen (CA19–9) is found to be positive (60). This antigen is commonly present in adenocarcinoma of the pancreas but is not specific. It is usually negative in adenocarcinomas of the breast.

Cutaneous metastases from thyroid carcinoma tend to involve the abdominal skin or the head area (7). Medullary, follicular, and papillary thyroid carcinomas may retain their histologic patterns in the cutaneous metastases (Fig. 36-9).

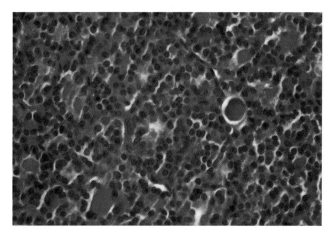

FIGURE 36-9. Metastatic carcinoma from thyroid. H&E × 220.

Immunoperoxidase studies often show a positive reaction to antithyroglobulin antibody 61 and to TTF-1 (34).

REFERENCES

1. Lookingbill DP, Spangler N, Sexton FM. Skin involvement as the presenting sign of internal carcinoma. *J Am Acad Dermatol* 1990;22:19.
2. Lookingbill DP, Spangler N, Helm KF. Cutaneous metastases in patients with metastatic carcinoma: a retrospective study of 4020 patients. *J Am Acad Dermatol* 1993;29:228.
3. Spencer PS, Helm TN. Skin metastases in cancer patients. *Cutis* 1987;39:119.
4. Brownstein MH, Helwig EB. Metastatic tumors of the skin. *Cancer* 1972;29:1298.
5. Fielding JE. Smoking and women. *N Engl J Med* 1987;317:1343.
6. Liu Y, Sturgis CD, Grzybicki DM, et al. Microtubule-associated protein-2: a new sensitive and specific marker for pulmonary carcinoid tumor and small cell carcinoma. *Mod Pathol* 2001;14:880–885.
7. Schwartz RA. Cutaneous metastatic disease. *J Am Acad Dermatol* 1995;33:161.
8. Brownstein MH, Helwig EB. Patterns of cutaneous metastasis. *Arch Dermatol* 1972;105:862.
9. Wesche WA, Khare VK, Chesney TM, et al. Non-hematopoietic cutaneous metastases in children and adolescents: thirty years experience at St. Jude Children's Research Hospital. *J Cutan Pathol* 2000;27:485–492.
10. Peris K, Fargnoli MC, Lunghi F, et al. Unusually large cutaneous metastases of renal cell carcinoma. *Acta Derm Venereol* 2001;81:77–78.
11. Steck WD, Helwig EB. Tumors of the umbilicus. *Cancer* 1965;18:907–915.
12. Powell FC, Cooper AJ, Massa MC, et al. Sister Mary Joseph's nodule: a clinical and histologic study. *J Am Acad Dermatol* 1984;10:610–615.
13. Kikuchi Y, Matsuyama A, Nomura K. Zosteriform metastatic skin cancer: report of three cases and review of the literature. *Dermatology* 2001;202:336–338.
14. Ahmed I, Holley KJ, Charles-Holmes R. Zosteriform metastasis of colon. *Dermatology* 2000;142:182–183.
15. Zala L, Jenni C. Das carcinoma erysipelatodes. *Dermatologica* 1980;160:80.
16. Cox SE, Cruz PD. A spectrum of inflammatory metastasis to skin via lymphatics: three cases of carcinoma erysipeloides. *J Am Acad Dermatol* 1994;30:304.
17. Ingram JT. Carcinoma erysipelatodes and carcinoma telangiectaticum. *Arch Dermatol* 1958;77:227.
18. Shamai-Lubovitz O, Rothem A, Ben-David E, et al. Cutaneous metastatic carcinoma of the breast mimicking malignant melanoma clinically and histologically. *J Am Acad Dermatol* 1994;31:1058.
19. Waisman M. Carcinoma of the inframammary crease. *Arch Dermatol* 1978;114:1520.
20. Carson HJ, Pellettiere EV, Lack E. Alopecia neoplastica simulating alopecia areata and antedating the detection of primary breast carcinoma. *J Cutan Pathol* 1994;21:67.
21. Hood CI, Font RL, Zimmerman LE. Metastatic mammary carcinoma in the eyelid with histiocytoid appearance. *Cancer* 1973;31:793.
22. Requena L, Sanchez Yus E, Nunez C, et al. Epidermotropically metastatic breast carcinomas. Rare histopathologic variants mimicking melanoma and Paget's disease. *Am J Dermatopathol* 1996;18:385–395.
23. Gonzales-Lois C, Rodriquez-Peralto JL, Serrano-Pardo R, et al. Cutaneous signet ring cell carcinoma. a report of a case and review of the literature. *Am J Dermatopathol* 2001;23:325–328.
24. Franzblau MJ, Manwaring M, Plumhof C, et al. Metastatic breast carcinoma mimicking granular cell tumor. *J Cutan Pathol* 1989 Aug.;16:218–221.
25. Stroup RM, Pinkus GS. S-100 immunoreactivity in primary and metastatic carcinoma of the breast: a potential source of error in immunodiagnosis. *Hum Pathol* 1988;19:949.
26. Bayer-Garner IB, Smoller B. Androgen receptors: a marker to increase sensitivity for identifying breast cancer in skin metastasis of unknown primary site. *Mod Pathol* 2000;13:119–22.
27. Ohnishi T, Takizawa H, Watanabe S. Immunohistochemical analysis of cytokeratin and human milk fat globulin expression in mucinous carcinoma of the skin. *J Cutan Pathol* 2002;29:38–43.
28. Brady LW, O'Neill EA, Farber SH. Unusual sites of metastases. *Semin Oncol* 1977;4:59.
29. McCracken GA, Washington CV, Templeton SF. Metastatic cutaneous carcinoid. *J Am Acad Dermatol* 1996;35:997–998.
30. Courville P, Joly P, Thomine E, et al. Primary cutaneous carcinoid tumour. *Histopathology* 2000;36:566–567.
31. Rodriquez G, Villamizar R. Carcinoid tumor with skin metastasis. *Am J Dermatopathol* 1992;14:263.
32. Wick MR, Swanson PE, Ritter JH, et al. The immunohistology of cutaneous neoplasia: a practical perspective. *J Cutan Pathol* 1993;20:481.
33. Smith KJ, Skelton HG III, Holland TT, et al. Neuroendocrine (Merkel cell) carcinoma with an intraepidermal component. *Am J Dermatopathol* 1993;15:528.
34. Byrd-Gloster AL, Khoor A, Glass LF, et al. Differential expression of thyroid transcription factor 1 in small cell lung carcinoma and Merkel cell tumor. *Hum Pathol* 2000;31:58–62.
35. Guinee DG Jr, Fishback NF, Koss MN, et al. The spectrum of immunohistochemical staining of small-cell lung carcinoma in specimens from transbronchial and open-lung biopsies. *Am J Clin Pathol* 1994;102:406.
36. Tot T. The value of cytokeratins 20 and 7 in discriminating metastatic adenocarcinomas from pleural mesotheliomas. *Cancer* 2001;92:2727–2732.
37. Brownstein MH, Helwig EB. Spread of tumors to the skin. *Arch Dermatol* 1973;107:80.
38. Johnson WC, Helwig EB. Histochemistry of primary and metastatic mucus-secreting tumors. *Ann N Y Acad Sci* 1963;106:794.

39. Johnson WC, Helwig EB. Histochemistry of the acid mucopoly-saccharides of skin in normal and in certain pathologic conditions. *Am J Clin Pathol* 1963;40:123.

40. Werner I. Studies on glycoproteins from mucous epithelium and epithelial secretions. *Acta Soc Med Ups* 1953;58:1.

41. Johnson WC. Histochemistry of the skin. In: Graham JH, Johnson WC, Helwig EB, eds. *Dermal pathology.* Hagerstown, MD: Harper & Row, 1972:75.

42. Chu P, Wu E, Weiss LM. Cytokeratin 7 and cytokeratin 20 expression in epithelial neoplasms: a survey of 435 cases. *Mod Pathol* 2000;13:962–972.

43. Connor DH, Taylor HB, Helwig EB. Cutaneous metastasis of renal cell carcinoma. *Arch Pathol* 1963;76:339.

44. Chu P, Arber DA. Paraffin-section detection of CD10 in 505 nonhematopoietic neoplasms. Frequent expression in renal cell carcinoma and endometrial stromal sarcoma. *Am J Clin Pathol* 2000;113:374–382.

45. Sim SJ, Ro JY, Ordonez NG, et al. Metastatic renal cell carcinoma to the bladder: a clinicopathologic and immunohistochemical study. *Mod Pathol* 1999;12:351–355.

46. Cathro HP, Stoler MH. Expression of cytokeratins 7 and 20 in ovarian neoplasia. *Am J Clin Pathol* 2002;117:944–951.

47. Fogaca MF, Fedorciw BJ, Tahan SR, et al. Cutaneous metastasis of neuroendocrine carcinoma of uterine origin. *J Cutan Pathol* 1993;20:455.

48. Van Nguyen A, Argenyi ZB. Cutaneous neuroblastoma. *Am J Dermatopathol* 1993;15:7.

49. Reingold IM, Escovitz WE. Metastatic cutaneous carcinoid. *Arch Dermatol* 1960;82:971.

50. Brody HJ, Stallings WP, Fine RM, et al. Carcinoid in an umbilical nodule. *Arch Dermatol* 1978;114:570.

51. Keane J, Fretzin DV, Wellington J, et al. Bronchial carcinoid metastatic to skin: light and electron microscopic findings. *J Cutan Pathol* 1980;7:43.

52. Scott MP, Helm KA. Cytokeratin 20: a marker for diagnosing Merkel cell carcinoma. *Am J Dermatopathol* 1999;21:16–20.

53. Nandedkar MA, Palazzo J, Abbondanzo SL, et al. CD45 (leukocyte common antigen) immunoreactivity in metastatic undifferentiated and neuroendocrine carcinoma: a potential diagnostic pitfall. *Mod Pathol* 1998;11:1204–1210.

54. Ordonez NG, Samaan NA. Medulary carcinoma of the thyroid metastatic to the skin: report of two cases. *J Cutan Pathol* 1987;14:251.

55. Mount SL, Taatjes DJ. Neuroendocrine carcinoma of the skin (Merkel cell carcinoma): an immunoelectron-microscopic case study. *Am J Dermatopathol* 1994;16:60.

56. Kahn JA, Sinhamohapatra SB, Schneider AF. Hepatoma presenting as a skin metastasis. *Arch Dermatol* 1971;104:299.

57. Cosnow I, Fretzin DF. Choriocarcinoma metastatic to skin. *Arch Dermatol* 1974;109:551.

58. Chhieng DC, Jennings TA, Slominski A, et al. Choriocarcinoma presenting as a cutaneous metastasis. *J Cutan Pathol* 1995;22:374.

59. Segal R, Penneys NS, Nahass G. Metastatic prostatic carcinoma histologically mimicking malignant melanoma. *J Cutan Pathol* 1994;21:280.

60. Taniguchi S, Hisa T, Hamada T. Cutaneous metastases of pancreatic carcinoma with unusual clinical features. *J Am Acad Dermatol* 1994;31:877.

61. Toyota N, Asaga H, Hirokawa M, et al. A case of skin metastasis from follicular thyroid carcinoma. *Dermatology* 1994;188:69.

APPENDIX

ELECTRON MICROGRAPHS

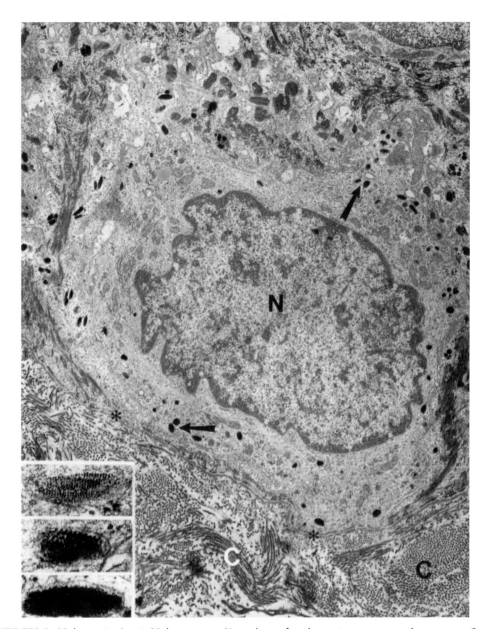

FIGURE EM-1. Melanocyte. **Inset:** Melanosomes. *N*, nucleus of melanocyte; *arrows*, melanosomes; *C*, colla-gen in the dermis; *asterisk*, basal lamina. **Insets:** Melanosomes in different stages of development: stage II (*upper*), stage III (*middle*), and stage IV (*lower*).

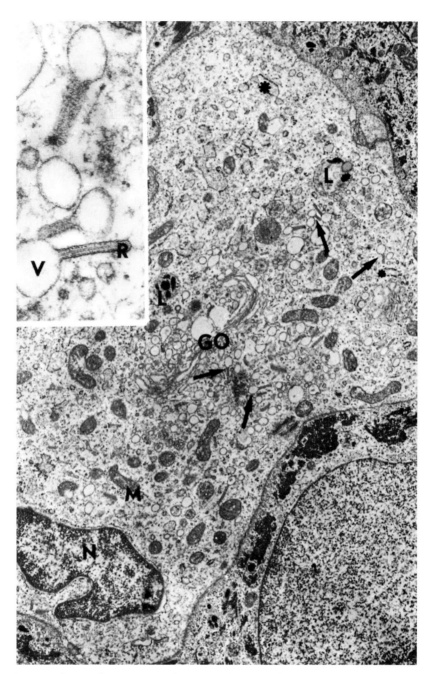

FIGURE EM-2. Langerhans cell. **Inset:** Langerhans granules. *N*, nucleus of Langerhans cell; *L*, lysosomes containing melanosomes; *GO*, Golgi complex; *M*, mitochondrium; *asterisk*, rough endoplasmic reticulum; *arrows*, Langerhans granules. **Inset:** Langerhans granules at higher magnification consisting of a vesicle (*V*) and a rod (*R*), both giving the appearance of a tennis racquet.

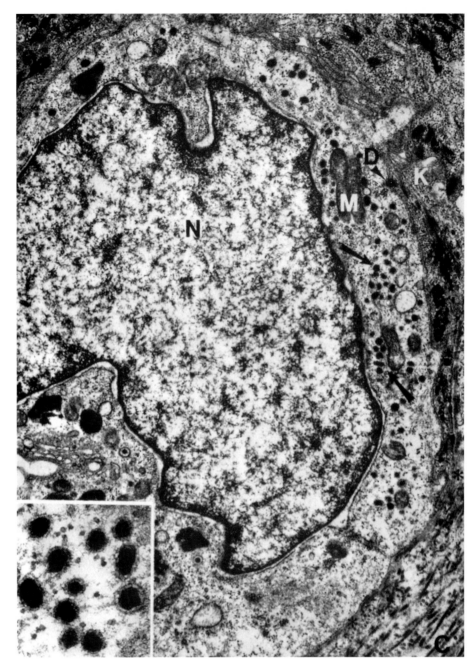

FIGURE EM-3. Merkel cell. **Inset:** Merkel granules. *N*, nucleus of Merkel cell; *asterisk*, on basal lamina; *M*, mitochondria; *arrows*, specific granules of the Merkel cell; *D with pointer*, desmosome between Merkel cell and keratinocyte (*K*); *C*, collagen with cross striation. **Inset:** Specific membrane-bound granules at higher magnification.

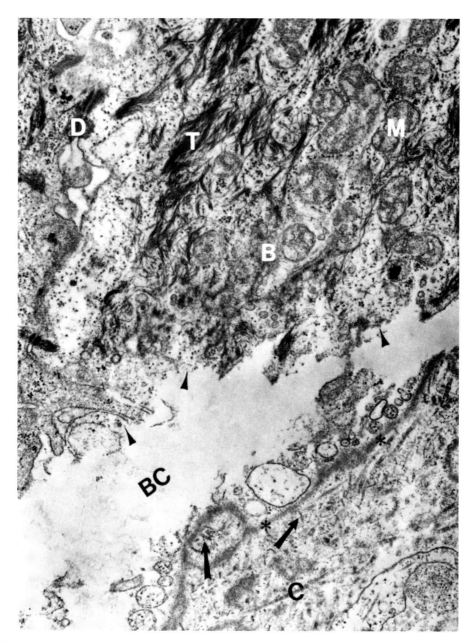

FIGURE EM-4. Epidermolysis bullosa simplex. The blister formed as the result of degenerative, cytolytic changes in the basal cells (*B*). The bulla cavity (*BC*) is situated above the basement membrane (*asterisk*). The basal cells are severely damaged, lacking a plasma membrane (*pointers*). *T*, tonofilaments; *M*, mitochondria; *D*, desmosome.

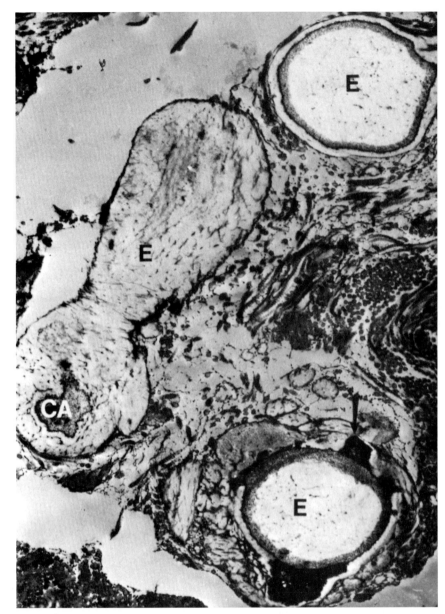

FIGURE EM-5. Pseudoxanthoma elasticum. The elastic fibers (*E*) are bizarrely shaped. Calcium (*CA*, *arrows*) is deposited on or around elastic fibers.

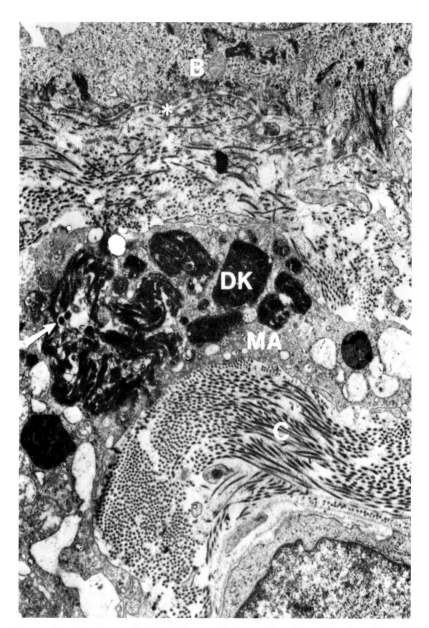

FIGURE EM-6. Incontinentia pigmenti. In this disease, dyskeratotic cells are found in the epidermis. Macrophages migrate into the epidermis, phagocytize these dyskeratotic cells as well as melanosomes, and subsequently return to the dermis. *MA*, macrophage containing dyskeratotic material (*DK*) and melanosomes (*arrow*); *B*, basal cell; *asterisk*, basal lamina; *C*, collagen.

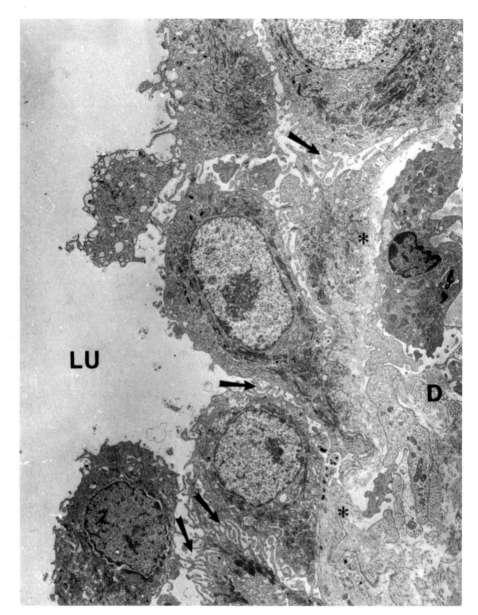

FIGURE EM-7. Pemphigus vulgaris, tombstone row. The dissolution of the intercellular cement led to the formation of a blister. At the base of the blister, one or two rows of keratinocytes are left. The cohesion of the basal cells with the dermis is well preserved. *LU*, blister lumen; *asterisks*, basement membrane; *arrows*, microvilli of keratinocytes; *D*, dermis.

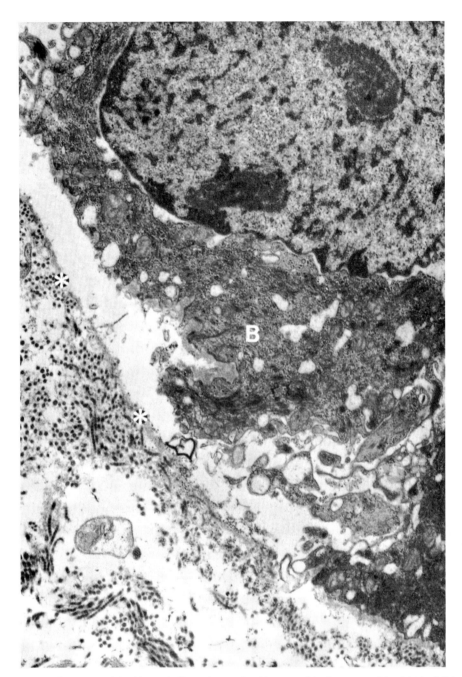

FIGURE EM-8. Bullous pemphigoid, noninflamed type. In this type of bullous pemphigoid, the blister forms between the basal cell (*B*) and the basement membrane (*asterisks*).

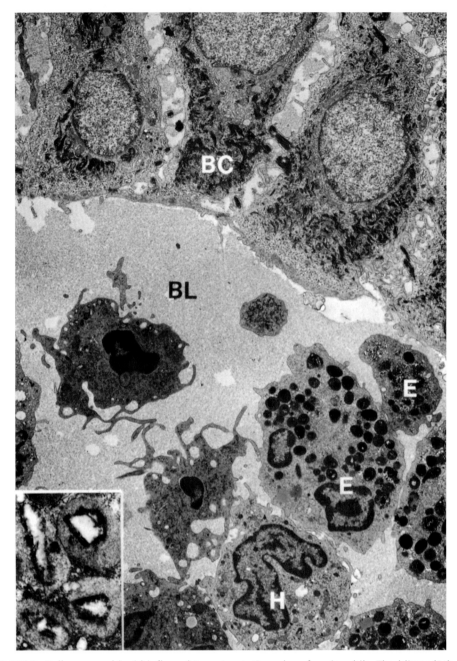

FIGURE EM-9. Bullous pemphigoid inflamed type. **Inset:** Granules of eosinophils. The blister (*BL*) contains several histiocytes (*H*) and eosinophils (*E*). The basement membrane has disappeared. The basal cells (*BC*) at the top of the blister are well preserved. **Inset:** Eosinophilic granules at higher magnification show a "crystal" at their center.

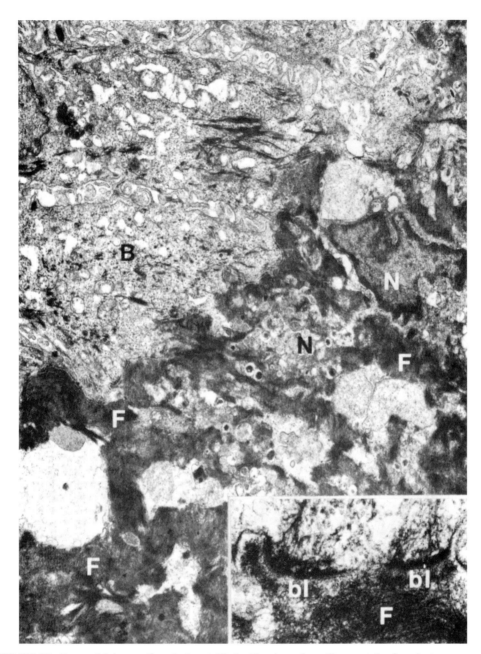

FIGURE EM-10. Dermatitis herpetiformis. **Inset:** Fibrin. The dermal papillae contain abundant amounts of fibrin (*F*). Between the meshes of fibrin, fragments of neutrophilic leukocytes (*N*) can be seen. *B*, basal cell. **Inset:** The fibrin (*F*) is attached to the dermal side of the basement membrane or basal lamina (*bl*). The basement membrane shows discontinuities.

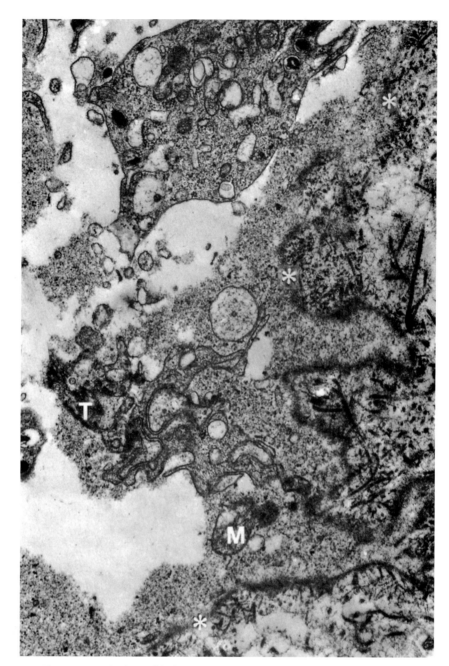

FIGURE EM-11. Herpes gestationis. In this disease, the blister forms either between basal cells and the basement membrane or, subsequent to dissolution of basal cells, between squamous cells and the basement membrane. A disintegrated basal cell containing tonofilaments (*T*) and mitochondria (*M*) and the basement membrane (*asterisks*) form the floor of the blister.

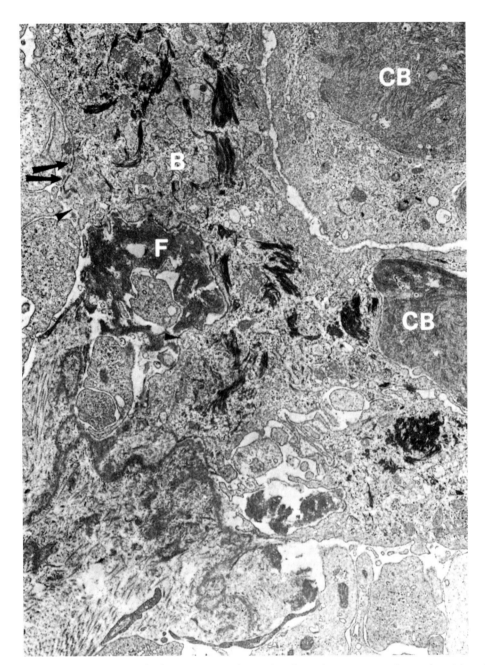

FIGURE EM-12. Lichen planus. The basement membrane is split up in some areas (*arrows*) and has disappeared in others (*pointers*). The lower epidermis contains colloid bodies (*CB*) consisting of numerous filaments and remnants of organelles. *F*, fibrin beneath the basal cell (*B*).

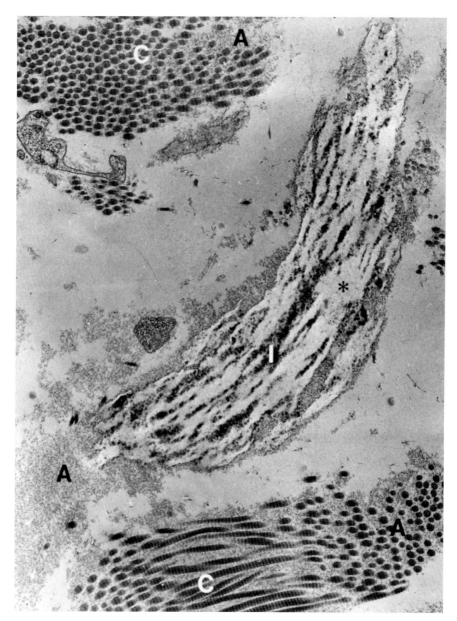

FIGURE EM-13. Solar degeneration. The elastic fiber contains in its amorphous matrix (*asterisk*) numerous electron-dense inclusions (*I*). Extensive amorphous material (*A*) can be seen around the elastotic fiber and among the collagen fibrils (*C*).

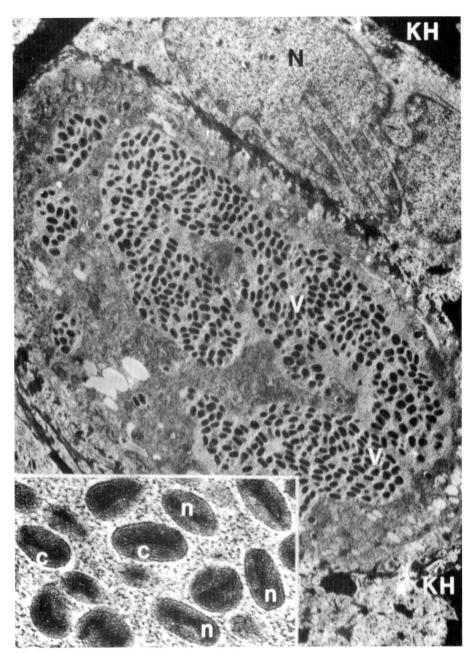

FIGURE EM-14. Molluscum contagiosum. **Inset:** High magnification of viruses. The granular cell contains an inclusion body consisting of numerous molluscum contagiosum viruses (*V*). The nucleus (*N*) of the cell has been displaced to the periphery of the cell. *KH*, keratohyaline granules. **Inset:** The virus consists of the dumb-bell-shaped nucleoid (*n*) surrounded by the capsid (*c*).

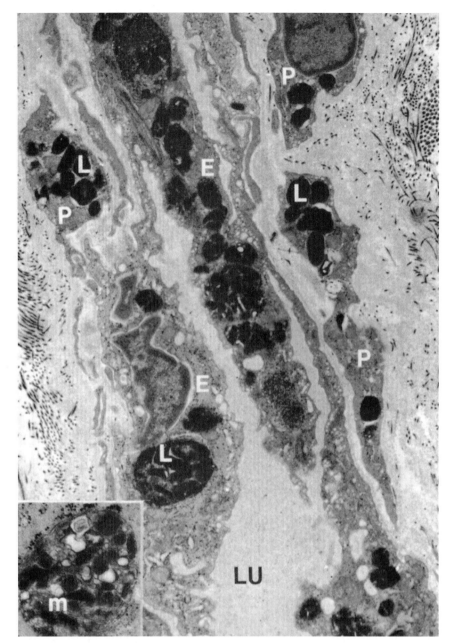

FIGURE EM-15. Angiokeratoma corporis diffusum (Fabry's disease). **Inset:** Lysosomal residual body. Endothelial cells (*E*) and pericytes (*P*) contain lipid deposits (*L*) within greatly enlarged lysosomes. *LU*, lumen of capillary. **Inset:** A large matured lysosome as a residual body shows laminated myelin figures (*m*).

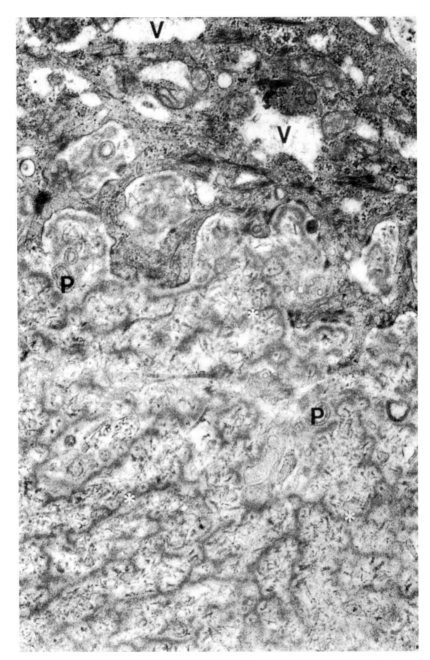

FIGURE EM-16. Discoid lupus erythematosus. The basal cell contains several vacuoles (*V*), which ultimately may cause disintegration of the cell. Many cross-sectioned projections (*P*) of the basal cell into the dermis can be seen, as can a greatly increased amount of basal lamina material (*asterisks*).

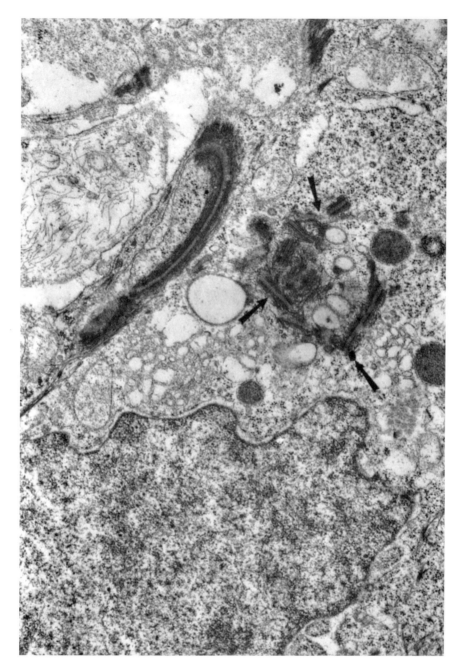

FIGURE EM-17. Squamous cell carcinoma. Desmosomes attached to tonofilaments (*arrows*) can be seen within the cytoplasm of the tumor cell.

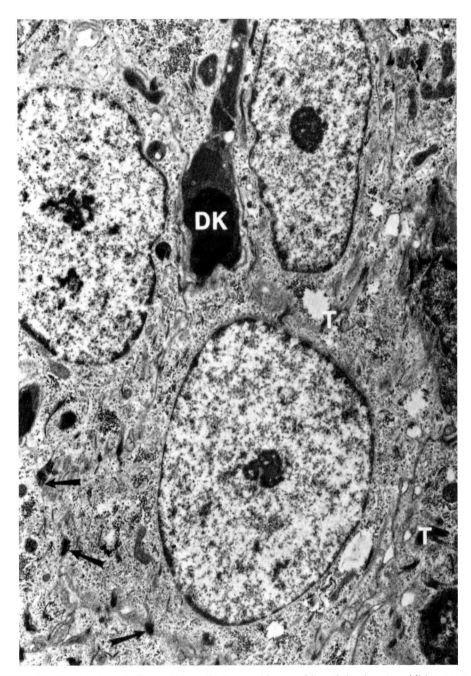

FIGURE EM-18. Basal cell epithelioma. The cells show evidence of keratinization. In addition to tonofilaments (*T*) and desmosomes (*arrows*), some dyskeratotic material (*DK*) is present.

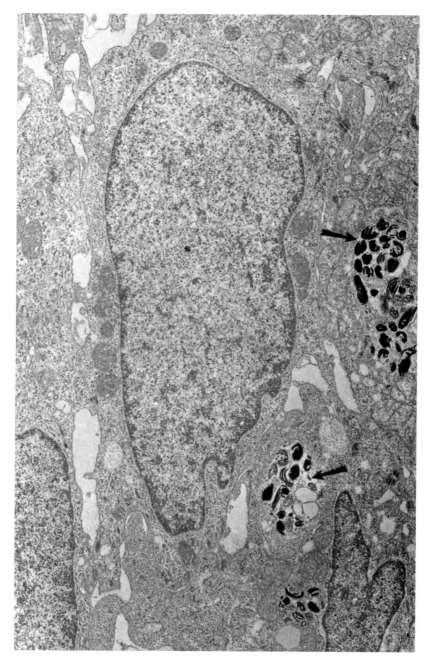

FIGURE EM-19. Pigmented basal cell carcinoma. Some of the tumor cells contain melanosome complexes located within lysosomes (*arrows*).

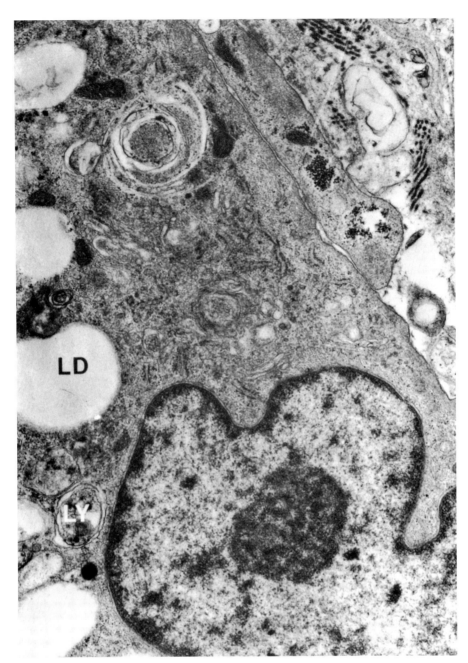

FIGURE EM-20. Dermatofibroma. The essential cells are fibroblasts, which, in addition to producing collagen, are engaged in phagocytosis and storage of lipid. *LY*, lysosome; *LD*, lipid droplets. (Courtesy of Dr. B. Mihatsch-Konz.)

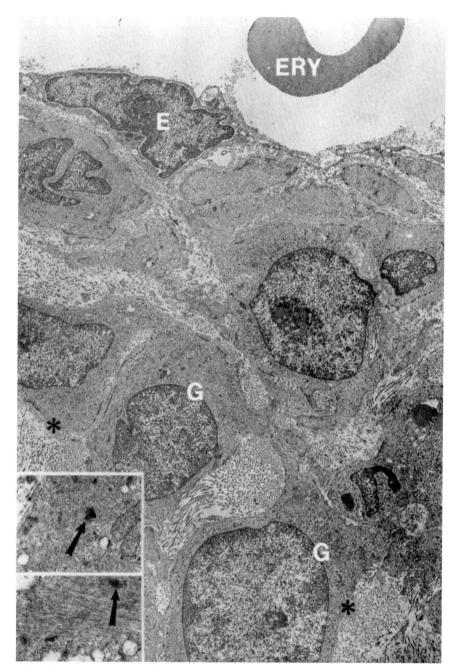

FIGURE EM-21. Glomus tumor. **Inset:** Myofilaments. The glomus cells are smooth muscle cells. Each glomus cell is surrounded by a basal lamina (*asterisk*). *E*, endothelial cell of capillary; *G*, glomus cell; *ERY*, erythrocyte within capillary lumen. **Insets:** The *upper* inset shows the myofilaments in cross-section, the *lower* inset in longitudinal section. *Arrows* point to so-called dense bodies.

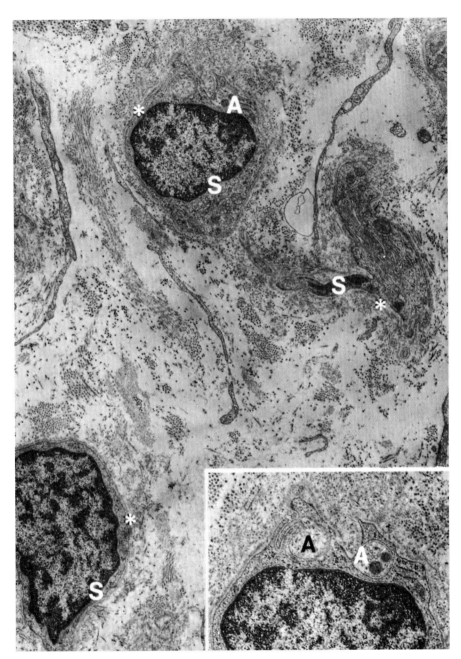

FIGURE EM-22. Neurofibroma. **Inset:** Axons in Schwann cell. The main cell type is the Schwann cell (*S*). Each cell is surrounded by a basal lamina (*asterisks*). Schwann cells contain axons (*A*) in their cytoplasm. **Inset:** Two axons (*A*) of the upper Schwann cell are shown at higher magnification.

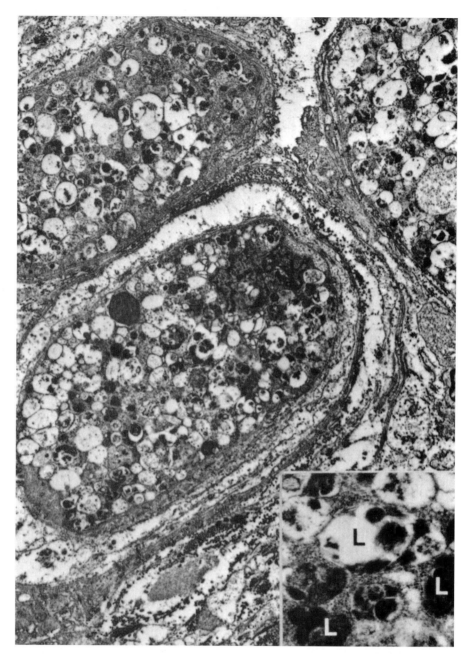

FIGURE EM-23. Granular cell tumor. **Inset:** Cytoplasmic granules. The cells contain numerous cytoplasmic granules, which are lysosomes. **Inset:** The lysosomes (*L*) are shown at higher magnification.

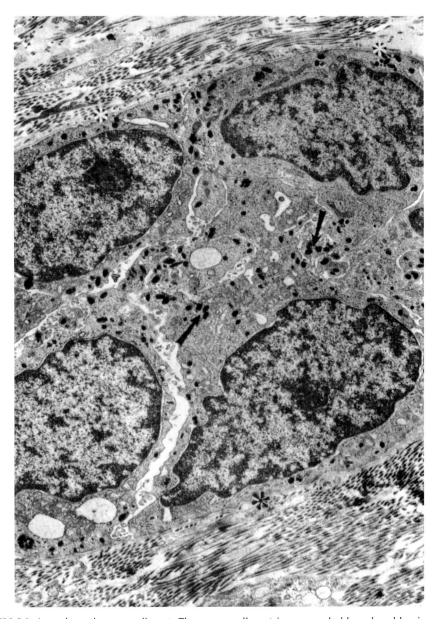

FIGURE EM-24. Intradermal nevus cell nest. The nevus cell nest is surrounded by a basal lamina (*asterisk*). There are no desmosomes between adjacent nevus cells. The nevus cells contain numerous melanosomes (*arrows*).

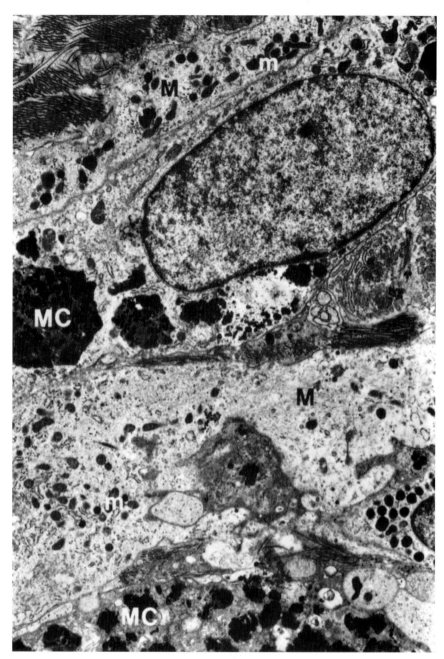

FIGURE EM-25. Malignant melanoma. In addition to malignant spindle-shaped melanocytes (*M*) containing an abundance of melanosomes (*m*), melanophages with melanosome complexes (*MC*) are found.

INDEX